High-Acuity Nursing

Seventh Edition

Kathleen Dorman Wagner, EdD, MSN, RN
Faculty Emerita, University of Kentucky College of Nursing
Lexington, Kentucky

Melanie G. Hardin-Pierce, DNP, RN, APRN, ACNP-BC
Associate Professor of Nursing, University of Kentucky College of Nursing
Lexington, Kentucky

Darlene Welsh, PhD, MSN, RN
Associate Professor of Nursing, University of Kentucky College of Nursing
Lexington, Kentucky

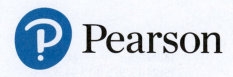

330 Hudson Street, NY, NY 10013

Vice President, Health Science and TED: *Julie Levin Alexander*
Director of Portfolio Management: *Katrin Beacom*
Executive Portfolio Manager: *Pamela Fuller*
Development Editor: *Pamela Lappies*
Portfolio Management Assistant: *Erin Sullivan*
Vice President, Content Production and Digital Studio: *Paul DeLuca*
Managing Producer, Health Science: *Melissa Bashe*
Content Producer: *Bianca Sepulveda*
Project Monitor: *Susan Watkins*
Operations Specialist: *Maura Zaldivar-Garcia*
Creative Director: *Blair Brown*
Creative Digital Lead: *Mary Siener*
Managing Producer, Digital Studio, Health Science: *Amy Peltier*

Digital Studio Producer, REVEL and eText 2.0: *Ellen Viganola*
Digital Content Team Lead: *Brian Prybella*
Digital Content Project Lead: *William Johnson*
Vice President, Product Marketing: *David Gesell*
Executive Product Marketing Manager: *Christopher Barry*
Sr. Field Marketing Manager: *Brittany Hammond*
Full-Service Project Management and Composition: *iEnergizer Aptara®, Ltd.*
Project Manager: *Sudip Sinha*
Inventory Manager: *Vatche Demirdjian*
Interior Design: *iEnergizer Aptara®, Ltd.*
Cover Design: *Studio Montage*
Cover Art: *Sabelskaya/Shutterstock*
Printer/Binder: *LSC Communications, Inc.*
Cover Printer: *Phoenix Color/Hagerstown*

Credits and acknowledgments borrowed from other sources and reproduced, with permission, in this textbook appear on the appropriate page within text.

Notice: Care has been taken to confirm the accuracy of information presented in this book. The authors, editors, and the publisher, however, cannot accept any responsibility for errors or omissions or for consequences from application of the information in this book and make no warranty, express or implied, with respect to its contents.

The authors and publisher have exerted every effort to ensure that drug selections and dosages set forth in this text are in accord with current recommendations and practice at time of publication. However, in view of ongoing research, changes in government regulations, and the constant flow of information relating to drug therapy and drug reactions, the reader is urged to check the package inserts of all drugs for any change in indications of dosage and for added warnings and precautions. This is particularly important when the recommended agent is a new and/or infrequently employed drug.

Library of Congress Cataloging-in-Publication Data
Names: Wagner, Kathleen Dorman, author. | Hardin-Pierce, Melanie G., author. | Welsh, Darlene, author.
Title: High-acuity nursing / Kathleen Dorman Wagner EdD, MSN, RN, Faculty Emerita, University of Kentucky College of Nursing, Lexington, Kentucky, Melanie G. Hardin-Pierce, DNP, RN, APRN, ACNP-BC, University of Kentucky College of Nursing, Lexington, Kentucky, Darlene Welsh, PhD, MSN, RN, University of Kentucky College of Nursing, Lexington, Kentucky.
Description: Seventh edition. | Boston : Pearson, [2018] | Revision of: High-acuity nursing / Kathleen Dorman Wagner, Melanie Hardin-Pierce, Darlene Welsh. | Includes bibliographical references and index.
Identifiers: LCCN 2017025338 | ISBN 9780134459295 | ISBN 0134459296
Subjects: LCSH: Intensive care nursing.
Classification: LCC RT120.I5 K53 2018 | DDC 616.02/8—dc23 LC record available at https://lccn.loc.gov/2017025338

1   17

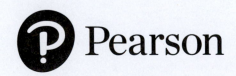

ISBN-10:   0-13-445929-6
ISBN-13: 978-0-13-445929-5

About the Authors

Kathleen Wagner, EdD, MSN, RN, is now faculty emerita, having recently retired from the University of Kentucky College of Nursing after many years of teaching pathophysiology, pathopharmacology, and high-acuity nursing to undergraduate nursing students. She was also the educational consultant for the Undergraduate Nursing Program at the University of Kentucky. She has a doctorate in instructional systems design and continues to work on a team developing Web-based clinical simulations for nursing students.

Melanie Hardin-Pierce, DNP, RN, APRN, ACNP-BC, is a tenured associate professor in the University of Kentucky College of Nursing, where she has over 30 years of experience as a critical care nurse and has taught high-acuity nursing to undergraduate and graduate nursing students. She currently teaches in the Doctor of Nursing Practice program and is the Coordinator of the Adult Geriatric Acute Care Nurse Practitioner DNP Option. In addition to teaching, she has been active in curriculum development in both baccalaureate and graduate nursing programs. She earned her Doctor of Nursing Practice degree at the University of Kentucky, having studied oral health in mechanically ventilated patients. She is a board-certified acute care nurse practitioner who practices as a critical care intensivist in the Veterans Health Administration Medical Center, Cooper Drive Division, Lexington. She is active in research of critically ill, mechanically ventilated patients; evidence-based practice; and interdisciplinary collaboration.

Darlene Welsh, PhD, MSN, RN, is Associate Professor, BSN Program Director, and Assistant Dean of Undergraduate Faculty Affairs at the University of Kentucky College of Nursing. Dr. Welsh earned a PhD in Educational Psychology and an MS in Nursing from the University of Kentucky. Her experiences in the care of critically ill patients include direct patient care, the conduct of research, and supervision of undergraduate and graduate students. Her research interests center on the provision of dietary instruction for patients with heart failure and interprofessional education for clinicians.

Thank You

We extend a heartfelt thanks to our contributors and reviewers, who gave their time, effort, and expertise to the development and writing of this new edition of our book.

Contributors

Jill Arzouman, DNP, RN, ACNS, BC, CMSRN
Director of Professional Practice
Banner University Medical Center
Tucson, Arizona
Chapter 1, High-Acuity Nursing
Chapter 2, Holistic Care of the Patient and Family

Susan K. Bohnenkamp, MS, RN, ACNS-BC, CCM
Clinical Nurse Specialist
Banner University Medical Center
Tucson, Arizona
Chapter 30, Alterations in White Blood Cell Function and Oncologic Emergencies

Pamela Branson, MSN, RN
Clinical Nurse Specialist
University of Kentucky
Lexington, Kentucky
Chapter 23, Alterations in Liver Function (with Melanie Hardin-Pierce)
Chapter 34, Determinants and Assessment of Oxygenation (with Melanie Hardin-Pierce)

Elizabeth Burckardt, DNP, ACNP
Department of Pulmonary and Critical Care Medicine
University of Louisville
Louisville, Kentucky
Chapter 38, Multiple Organ Dysfunction Syndrome (with Melanie Hardin-Pierce and Kathleen Dorman Wagner)

Heather L. Carlisle, PhD, DNP, RN-BC, FNP-BC, AGACNP-BC, CHPN
Clinical Assistant Professor
University of Arizona College of Nursing
Tucson, Arizona
Chapter 3: Palliative and End-of-life Care

Jennifer Cowley, MSN, RN
Senior Lecturer
University of Kentucky College of Nursing
Lexington, Kentucky
Chapter 25, Determinants and Assessment of Fluid and Electrolyte Balance
Chapter 26, Alterations in Fluid and Electrolyte Balance

Alexandra Dampier, DNP, APRN, NP-C, NRCME
Instructor
University of Kentucky College of Nursing
Lexington, Kentucky
Chapter 29, Alterations in Red Blood Cell Function and Hemostasis (with Angela Hensley)

Margaret M. Ecklund, MS, RN, CCRN-K, ACNP-BC
Clinical Nurse Specialist
Legacy Health
Portland, Oregon
Chapter 6, Nutrition Support
Chapter 7, Mechanical Ventilation

Nancy R. Eksterowicz, MSN, RNBC, APN2
Clinical Nurse, Pain Resource Nurse
University of Virginia Hospital
Charlottesville, Virginia
Chapter 5, Acute Pain Management

Julianne M. Evers, DNP, RN, CCRN
ICU Intensivist
Norton HealthCare
Louisville, Kentucky
Instructor
University of Kentucky College of Nursing
Lexington, Kentucky
Chapter 37, Shock States (with Melanie Hardin-Pierce)

Stephanie Fugate, MSN, ARNP, ACNP-BC
Instructor
University of Kentucky College of Nursing
Lexington, Kentucky
Chapter 27, Alterations in Kidney Function

Melanie Hardin-Pierce, DNP, RN, APRN, ACNP-BC
Associate Professor of Nursing
University of Kentucky College of Nursing
Lexington, Kentucky
*Chapter 17, Mentation and Sensory Motor Complications of
Acute Illness*
*Chapter 21, Determinants and Assessment of Gastrointestinal
Function*
Chapter 22, Alterations in Gastrointestinal Function
Chapter 23, Alterations in Liver Function (with Pamela
Branson)
Chapter 32, Metabolic Responses to Stress (with Samantha
Mancuso)
Chapter 34, Determinants and Assessment of Oxygenation
(with Pamela Branson)
Chapter 37, Shock States (with Julianne Evers)
Chapter 38, Multiple Organ Dysfunction Syndrome (with
Elizabeth Burckardt and Kathleen Dorman Wagner)

Angela B. Hensley, DNP, APRN, FNP-BC
Instructor
University of Kentucky College of Nursing
Lexington, Kentucky
*Chapter 29, Alterations in Red Blood Cell Function and
Hemostasis* (with Alexandria Dampier)

Dea J. Kent, DNP, RN, NP-C, CWOCN
Director, Nursing Home Oversight & Consulting
Community Healthcare Network
Fishers, Indiana
Chapter 10, Complex Wound Management
Chapter 36, Acute Burn Injury

Maureen E. Krenzer, MS, RN, ACNS-BC
Clinical Nurse Specialist
Chair, Pain Resource Nurse Committee
Rochester General Hospital
Rochester, New York
Chapter 24, Alterations in Pancreatic Function

Helen W. Lach, PhD, RN, CNL, FGSA, FAAN
Professor
Saint Louis University School of Nursing
St. Louis, Missouri
Chapter 4, The Older Adult High-Acuity Patient (with
Kristine L'Ecuyer)

Kristine M. L'Ecuyer, PhD, RN, CNL
Coordinator, Accelerated Master's of Science in Nursing
Saint Louis University School of Nursing
St. Louis, Missouri
Chapter 4, The Older Adult High-Acuity Patient (with Helen
W. Lach)

Sarah E. Lester, DNP, APRN, FNP-C, CNRN
Neurosciences Clinical Nurse Specialist
University of Kentucky
Lexington, Kentucky
Chapter 16, Determinants and Assessment of Cerebral Function
Chapter 19, Traumatic Brain Injury

Theresa Loan, APRN, PhD, FNP-BC
Professor
Department of Baccalaureate and Graduate Nursing
Eastern Kentucky University
Richmond, Kentucky
Chapter 13, Determinants and Assessment of Cardiac Function

**Samantha Mancuso, DNP, RN, APRN, AG-ACNP-BC,
CCRN**
University of Kentucky Medical Center
Lexington, Kentucky
*Chapter 31, Determinants and Assessment of Nutrition and
Metabolic Function*
Chapter 32, Metabolic Responses to Stress (with Melanie
Hardin-Pierce)

Angela C. Muzzy, RN, MSN, CCRN, CNS-BC
Clinical Nurse Specialist
Tucson Medical Center
Tucson, Arizona
Chapter 9, Basic Cardiac Rhythm Monitoring

Grace Nolde-Lopez, RN, MS, ANP-BC
Craig Hospital
Englewood, Colorado
Chapter 20, Acute Spinal Cord Injury

Gail L. Priestley, RN, MS, CCRN
Clinical Nurse Specialist
The University of Arizona Health Network
Tucson, Arizona
Chapter 12, Alterations in Pulmonary Function

Yvonne Rice, DNP, RN, APRN, AGACNP-BC, FNP-C
Instructor
Lead APP Trauma and Acute Care Surgery
University of Kentucky
Lexington, Kentucky
Chapter 35, Multiple Trauma

Kathleen Dorman Wagner, EdD, MSN, RN
Faculty Emerita
University of Kentucky College of Nursing
Lexington, Kentucky
Chapter 33, Diabetic Crises
Chapter 38, Multiple System Dysfunction (with Elizabeth
Burckardt and Melanie Hardin-Pierce)

Darlene Welsh, PhD, MSN, RN
Associate Professor of Nursing
University of Kentucky College of Nursing
Lexington, Kentucky
Chapter 8, Basic Hemodynamic Monitoring
Chapter 14, Alterations in Cardiac Function
Chapter 15, Alterations in Myocardial Tissue Perfusion
Chapter 18, Acute Stroke Injury
Chapter 28, Determinants and Assessment of Hematologic
Function
Chapter 39, Solid Organ and Hematopoietic Stem Cell
Transplantation

Maria D. Willey, DNP, APRN, NP-C, FNP-BC,
AGACNP-BC
Brooke Army Medical Center
San Antonio, Texas
Chapter 11, Determinants and Assessment of Pulmonary
Function

Accuracy Reviewer

Rachel Kinder, PhD, RN
Associate Professor
Western Kentucky University
Bowling Green, KY

Reviewers

Melissa A. Bathish, PhD, RN, CPNP-PC
Research Area Specialist/Lecturer/Student Resolutions
Officer
University of Michigan School of Nursing
Ann Arbor, Michigan

Maureen J. Dunn, RN, MSN
Nursing Instructor
Pennsylvania State University
Sharon, Pennsylvania

Antoinette France, MSNed, CCRN, RN
Salt Lake Community College
West Jordan, Utah

Sarah Gabua, DNP, RN, CNE
Full-time Faculty
Aspen University
Denver, Colorado

Deola Hardy, MSN, RN
RN Faculty
Baton Rouge General School of Nursing
Baton Rouge, Louisiana

Laura Logan, MSN, RN, CCRN
Nursing Faculty
Critical Care Clinical Instructor
Stephen F. Austin State University
Nacogdoches, Texas

Peter Miskin, DHSc, MScN, RN, PHN, CMSRN
Nursing Instructor
De Anza College
Cupertino, California
Adjunct Assistant Professor
Samuel Merritt University
Oakland, California

Diane Mulbrook, MA, BS
Assistant Professor of Nursing
Mount Mercy University
Cedar Rapids, Iowa

Bridget Nichols, RN, MSN, CCRN
Nurse Educator
The University of South Dakota
Sioux Falls, South Dakota
Avera Heart Hospital
Sioux Falls, South Dakota

Joan E. Niederriter, PhD, MSN, CMSRN, RN-BC
Associate Professor
Cleveland State University
Cleveland, Ohio

Jan Paauwe-Weust, DNP, RN
Assistant Professor in Nursing
Indiana State University School of Nursing
Terre Haute, Indiana

Joan Palladino, EdD, RN
Professor, Chair of the Department of Nursing
Western Connecticut State University
Danbury, Connecticut

Jill Price, PhD, MSN, RN
Dean, RNBSN Online Option
Chamberlain College of Nursing
Downers Grove, Illinois

Kristiann T. Williams, DNP, APRN, FNP-C
Associate Professor
Weber State University
Ogden, Utah

Maurita Wisniewski, MSN, RN, CCRN
Ohio Valley Hospital
McKees Rocks, Pennsylvania

Kerrie Young, RN, MSN, CCRN
Nursing Instructor
Amarillo College
Amarillo, Texas

Preface

When the first edition of *High-Acuity Nursing* was published in 1992, the term *high acuity* was largely confined to leveling patient acuity for determining hospital staffing needs rather than being applied to a type of nursing care or education. Since that time, the meaning of the term has been evolving to increasingly represent a distinct category of nursing that denotes care of complex patients outside of the critical care setting. For the purposes of this textbook, we continue to define *high acuity* in a way that is consistent with our original intent—that it represents a level of patient problems beyond uncomplicated acute illness on a health–illness continuum.

The high-acuity nurse cares for complex patients with unpredictable outcomes across care settings (to include critical care). Today, high-acuity patients are found in many healthcare settings, from high-skill, long-term-care facilities to critical care units. The patient population is older and faces an increased number of health issues upon entering the healthcare system. Hospitalized patients are being discharged earlier, often in a poorer state of health. In the home health setting, nurses provide care to patients with mechanical ventilators, central venous catheter lines, IV antibiotic therapy, and complicated injuries. Whereas critical care units are considered specialty areas within the hospital walls, much of the knowledge required to work within those specialties is generalist in nature. It is this generalist knowledge base that is needed by all nurses who work with patients experiencing complex care problems to ensure competent and safe nursing practice.

New to This Edition

The seventh edition of the book has been revised based on feedback from faculty and students.

- All chapters have been updated, and many have been reorganized and expanded.
- A new chapter focusing on palliative care and end-of-life issues has been added.
- New features that address Quality and Safety and Genetic Considerations have been added where appropriate.
- Posttest items have been revised to reflect changes in content and are written using NCLEX style.
- Emerging Evidence features have been updated.

Purpose of the Text

The *High-Acuity Nursing* text delivers critical information focusing on the adult patient, using learner-focused, active learning principles, with concise language and a user-friendly format. The book's design breaks down complex information into small, discrete chunks to assist learners in mastering the material. Self-testing is provided throughout the text, with short section quizzes and chapter posttests. All answers to the section review quizzes are provided to give learners immediate feedback on their command of section content before proceeding to the next chapter section.

The chapters in this book focus on the relationship between pathophysiology and the nursing process with the following goals in mind:

- To revisit and translate critical pathophysiological concepts pertaining to the high-acuity adult patient in a clinically applicable manner
- To examine the interrelationships among physiological concepts
- To enhance clinical decision-making skills
- To provide immediate feedback to the learner regarding assimilation of concepts and principles
- To provide self-paced learning

Ultimately, the goal is for the learner to be able to approach patient care conceptually, so that care is provided with a strong underlying understanding of its rationale.

This book is appropriate for use in multiple educational settings, including for undergraduate nursing students, novice nurses, novice critical care nurses, and home health nurses. It also serves as a review book for the experienced nurse wanting updated information about high-acuity nursing for continuing education purposes. Hospital staff development departments will find it useful as supplemental or required reading for nursing staff or for high-acuity or critical care classes.

Organization of the Text

The book is divided into ten parts: Introduction to High-Acuity Nursing, Therapeutic Support of the High-Acuity Patient, Pulmonary, Cardiovascular, Neurologic, Gastrointestinal, Fluid and Electrolytes, Hematologic, Nutrition and Metabolism, and Multisystem Dysfunction.

Part One: Introduction to High-Acuity Nursing is composed of four introductory chapters with topics that apply across high-acuity problems, including an introduction to high-acuity nursing and the care of high-acuity patients, and important considerations when caring for the high-acuity older adult. Part Two: Therapeutic Support of the High-Acuity Patient is composed of six chapters that focus on supportive interventions, including pain management, nutrition support, mechanical ventilation, hemodynamic monitoring, basic cardiac rhythm monitoring, and complex wound management. Parts Three through Ten cover topics that represent the more common complex health problems, assessments, and treatments associated with high-acuity adult patients.

All chapters contain Learning Outcomes, Section Review questions, and Chapter Review questions. Most chapters include Clinical Reasoning Checkpoint exercises. Each chapter is divided into small sections that cover one facet of the chapter's topic (e.g., pathophysiology or nursing management), and each section ends with a short self-assessment review quiz. Key words are bolded throughout the chapters to indicate glossary terms defined in the textbook's Glossary. Parts Three through Ten are composed of two different types of chapters: *Determinants and Assessment* chapters and *Alterations* chapters.

DETERMINANTS AND ASSESSMENT CHAPTERS Each part begins with an overview of normal concepts that provide a solid foundation for understanding the diseases being presented. Normal anatomy and physiology are reviewed, and relevant diagnostic tests and assessments are profiled. The therapeutic support and disease-focused (Alterations) chapters draw heavily on the normal concepts, diagnostic tests, and assessments covered in their corresponding *Determinants and Assessment* chapters.

ALTERATIONS CHAPTERS Following each *Determinants and Assessment* chapter is a series of organ- or concept-specific chapters that focus on a single topic area. The majority of *Alterations* chapters are based on body systems (e.g., Chapter 12, Alterations in Pulmonary Function) and include the pathophysiology, assessments, diagnostic testing, and collaborative management of disorders commonly seen in high-acuity adult patients. Several *Alterations* chapters focus on complications of high-acuity illness, such as multiple organ dysfunction syndrome and sensory motor complications of acute illness. The pathophysiologic basis of disease is emphasized in this textbook, based on the belief that strong foundational knowledge about the basis of disease improves learner understanding of the associated disease manifestations and rationales for treatment.

Summary

This text focuses on major problems and therapies frequently encountered in high-acuity patients. It is not designed as a comprehensive textbook of adult medical–surgical or critical care nursing. The book's format reduces the learner's sense of being overwhelmed by complex information. Learners are more apt to feel in command of the concepts, giving them the confidence to proceed to more complex concepts.

The seventh edition of *High-Acuity Nursing* has maintained the overall look and feel of the previous editions, with some valuable changes. Although the seventh edition has been updated and is offered in eText format as well as print, we have not compromised our interactive approach. The ultimate goal of this book continues to be to enhance the preparation of nurses for practice in today's healthcare settings.

Acknowledgments

With any publication, several years of sweat and tears go into its development. To our Executive Portfolio Manager, Pam Fuller, and our Development Editor, Pam Lappies, thank you so much for your patience, diligence, sense of humor, and work ethic—the book would have never made it to fruition without your hard work and guidance. It has been a true pleasure to work with you! To our Content Producer, Bianca Sepulveda, our Portfolio Management Assistant, Erin Sullivan, and our Project Manager at Aptara, Sudip Sinha, thank you all for your efforts and hard work. We would also like to warmly acknowledge the wonderful work of our Accuracy Reviewer, Dr. Rachel Kinder, PhD, RN, whose meticulous scrutiny of the information in the book chapters made our work much easier and significantly enhanced the quality and accuracy of the book. Warm thanks goes to Dr. Kathy Wagner for her mentorship and unwavering support in this "book business" and for inviting Darlene and Melanie to be part of *High-Acuity Nursing*.

Finally, our warm thanks also to our Chapter Review item writer, Pamela Fowler, who significantly added to the value of the tests.

In memory of a colleague, mentor, and friend, Pam Kidd, RN, PhD, ARNP, CEN, who died too soon and with Kathy coedited *High-Acuity Nursing* from its inception, we say her passion for teaching, warmth, and wit are deeply missed.

Kathleen Dorman Wagner
Melanie G. Hardin-Pierce
Darlene Welsh

Contents

Part Two Therapeutic Support of the High-Acuity Patient

14 Alterations in Cardiac Function   391

15 Alterations in Myocardial Tissue Perfusion   418

Part Five Neurologic

16 Determinants and Assessment of Cerebral Function   443

Part Six Gastrointestinal

27 Alterations in Kidney Function 692

Part Eight Hematologic

28 Determinants and Assessment of Hematologic Function 719

29 Alterations in Red Blood Cell Function and Hemostasis 743

30 Alterations in White Blood Cell Function and Oncologic Emergencies 767

Part Nine Nutrition and Metabolism

31 Determinants and Assessment of Nutrition and Metabolic Function 800

Chapter 1
High-Acuity Nursing

 Learning Outcomes

1.1 Describe the various healthcare environments in which high-acuity patients receive care.

1.2 Identify the need for resource allocation and staffing strategies for high-acuity patients.

1.3 Examine the use of technology in high-acuity environments.

1.4 Identify the components of a healthy practice environment.

1.5 Describe the importance of patient safety in the high-acuity environment.

This chapter provides an introduction to the environments in which adult high-acuity nursing care is provided. High-acuity care environments include any acute care areas in which complex patients with unpredictable outcomes are managed regardless of the exact environment. The patient may be in a critical care unit or in an intermediate care or general medical–surgical setting. This chapter also provides an overview of issues that nurses encounter when working in high-acuity care environments, particularly critical care. Emphasis is placed on the importance of developing a healthy practice environment in which patient safety is paramount.

Author's note: The American College of Critical Care Medicine (ACCM) and the American Association of Critical-Care Nurses (AACN) guidelines presented in this chapter remain current, although many of them were developed in the late 1990s to mid-2000s.

Section One: High-Acuity Environment

The creation of specialized units with specially trained personnel in which to care for patients has evolved over time and is now the accepted standard of care. This section provides an overview of how and why critical care units were initially developed, how patients are triaged according to the level of care required to best meet their needs, and a description of the different levels of care. The section ends with a profile of the high-acuity nurse.

Historical Perspective

Intensive care units (ICUs) were first developed in the early 1960s. There were multiple reasons for their development, including (1) the implementation of cardiopulmonary resuscitation (CPR) and the improved survival from sudden-death events; (2) better understanding of the treatment of hypovolemic shock related to recent war experiences; (3) the implementation of emergency medical services, resulting in improved transport systems; (4) the development of technologic inventions that required close observation for effective use (e.g., electrocardiographic monitoring); and (5) the initiation of renal transplant surgery. The first ICUs were recovery rooms. Patients admitted were still anesthetized. Problems resulted, however, when the volume of surgical procedures increased and recovery rooms quickly became full. The patient who required extra equipment and prolonged observation was placed in the newly created ICU.

Determining the Level of Care Needed

Although high-acuity patients are viewed historically as being in an acute care unit, because of the shortage of acute care beds this is no longer true. This shortage of beds combined with skyrocketing costs for healthcare requires practitioners to make decisions about where in the hospital high-acuity patients are placed so that they receive the

Table 1–1 Prioritization of Admission, Discharge, and Triage of Acutely Ill Patients in an ICU

Priority for ICU Placement	Description of Patient Characteristics
Priority 1	The patient is acutely ill, unstable, and requires intensive treatment and monitoring that cannot be provided outside of the ICU (e.g., mechanical ventilation, continuous vasoactive drug infusions). There are no limits on the extent of intended interventions. Examples may include patients requiring postoperative care or patients with acute respiratory failure necessitating mechanical ventilator support, shock or hemodynamic instability, or patients who require invasive monitoring and/or vasoactive drugs.
Priority 2	The patient requires intensive monitoring and may potentially need immediate intervention. There are no limits on the extent of intended interventions. Examples include patients with chronic comorbid conditions who develop an acute and severe medical or surgical illness.
Priority 3	The patient is critically ill and unstable, with a reduced likelihood of recovery because of underlying disease or the nature of the acute illness. The patient may receive intensive treatment to relieve acute illness; however, limits on therapeutic efforts may be set, such as no intubation or cardiopulmonary resuscitation. Examples include patients with metastatic malignancy complicated by infection, cardiac tamponade, or airway obstruction.
Priority 4	This patient is generally not appropriate for ICU admission. Determination of admission should be made on an individual basis, under unusual circumstances, and at the discretion of the ICU director. Examples include patients with peripheral vascular surgery, stable diabetic ketoacidosis, or conscious drug overdose, as well as patients with terminal and irreversible illness facing immediate death.

SOURCE: Data from American College of Critical Care Medicine (ACCM). (1999). Guidelines for Intensive Care Unit Admission, Discharge, and Triage. Critical Care Medicine.

most efficient and cost-effective care. This may mean the patient is placed in an ICU, an **intermediate care unit (IMC)**, also referred to as a **progressive care unit (PCU)**, or a medical–surgical acute care unit. These triage decisions require a systematic approach so that optimal outcomes and controlled costs are achieved.

The use of intermediate care or progressive care units may provide an efficient distribution of resources for the patient whose acute illness requires less monitoring equipment and staffing than is provided in an ICU. The intermediate care unit serves as a place for the monitoring and care of patients with moderate or potentially severe physiologic instability who require technical support but not necessarily artificial life support; it is reserved for those patients requiring less-than-standard intensive care but more-than-standard ward care. Guidelines for admission and discharge for adult intermediate care units were originally established by the American College of Critical Care Medicine (ACCM) (1998). The American Association of Colleges of Nursing (AACN) has supported these guidelines (Meyer, 2003).

The Society of Critical Care Medicine (SCCM) recommends using a prioritization model to help make decisions about appropriate admission, discharge, and triage of acutely ill patients in an ICU (ACCM, 1999). The model defines which patients may benefit most from receiving care in an ICU. This prioritization model is summarized in Table 1–1. Priority 1 includes the most critically ill, and Priority 4 includes those who are generally not appropriate candidates for ICU admission. While this model remains useful in today's practice environments, healthcare providers typically base ICU admission on individual patient need. For example, in some instances, patients with advanced cancer may be admitted into the ICU for the treatment of organ failure or for postoperative care. Some healthcare providers may consider this admission to be counter to the model guidelines (Kostakou, Rovina, Kyriakopoulou, Koulouris, & Koutsoukou, 2014).

Levels of Intensive Care Units

ICUs vary from hospital to hospital in terms of the services provided, the personnel, and their level of expertise. Large medical centers frequently have multiple ICUs defined by specialty area (e.g., neurosurgical ICU, trauma ICU). Small hospitals may have only one ICU designed to care for a variety of patients with medical or surgical disease processes. Although the types and varieties of ICUs may differ from one hospital to the next, all ICUs have the responsibility of providing services and personnel to ensure optimal care. The ACCM has identified three levels of ICUs as determined by resources available to the hospital (Haupt et al., 2003). These levels are summarized in Table 1–2.

Table 1–2 ACCM Definitions of ICU Levels of Care

ICU Level	Description of Services, Personnel
Level I	Hospitals with ICUs that provide comprehensive care for patients with a wide range of disorders. Sophisticated equipment is available. Units are staffed with specialized nurses and healthcare providers with critical care training. Comprehensive support services are available and include pharmacy, respiratory therapy, nutritional support, social services, and pastoral care. These units may be located within an academic teaching hospital or may be community based.
Level II	Hospitals with ICUs that have the capability of providing comprehensive care to most critically ill patients but not to specific patient populations (e.g., neurosurgical, cardiothoracic, trauma).
Level III	Hospitals with ICUs that have the ability to provide initial stabilization of critically ill patients but are limited in their ability to provide comprehensive care for all patients. These hospitals are able to care for ICU patients requiring routine care and monitoring.

SOURCE: Data from the American College of Critical Care Medicine (ACCM) as provided in Haupt et al. (2003).

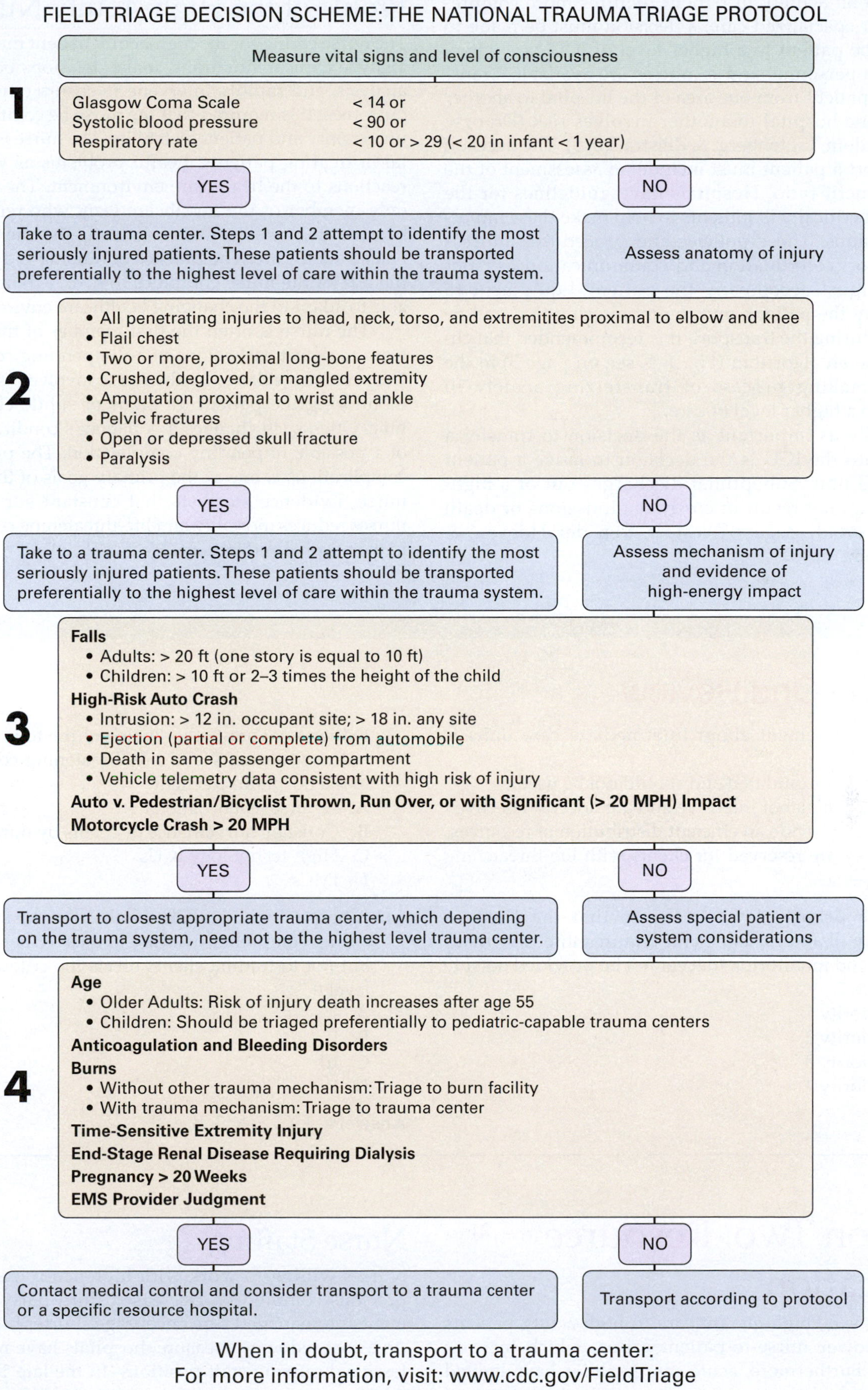

FIELD TRIAGE DECISION SCHEME: THE NATIONAL TRAUMA TRIAGE PROTOCOL

Measure vital signs and level of consciousness

1

Glasgow Coma Scale	< 14 or
Systolic blood pressure	< 90 or
Respiratory rate	< 10 or > 29 (< 20 in infant < 1 year)

YES — NO

Take to a trauma center. Steps 1 and 2 attempt to identify the most seriously injured patients. These patients should be transported preferentially to the highest level of care within the trauma system.

Assess anatomy of injury

2

- All penetrating injuries to head, neck, torso, and extremitites proximal to elbow and knee
- Flail chest
- Two or more, proximal long-bone features
- Crushed, degloved, or mangled extremity
- Amputation proximal to wrist and ankle
- Pelvic fractures
- Open or depressed skull fracture
- Paralysis

YES — NO

Take to a trauma center. Steps 1 and 2 attempt to identify the most seriously injured patients. These patients should be transported preferentially to the highest level of care within the trauma system.

Assess mechanism of injury and evidence of high-energy impact

3

Falls
- Adults: > 20 ft (one story is equal to 10 ft)
- Children: > 10 ft or 2–3 times the height of the child

High-Risk Auto Crash
- Intrusion: > 12 in. occupant site; > 18 in. any site
- Ejection (partial or complete) from automobile
- Death in same passenger compartment
- Vehicle telemetry data consistent with high risk of injury

Auto v. Pedestrian/Bicyclist Thrown, Run Over, or with Significant (> 20 MPH) Impact

Motorcycle Crash > 20 MPH

YES — NO

Transport to closest appropriate trauma center, which depending on the trauma system, need not be the highest level trauma center.

Assess special patient or system considerations

4

Age
- Older Adults: Risk of injury death increases after age 55
- Children: Should be triaged preferentially to pediatric-capable trauma centers

Anticoagulation and Bleeding Disorders

Burns
- Without other trauma mechanism: Triage to burn facility
- With trauma mechanism: Triage to trauma center

Time-Sensitive Extremity Injury

End-Stage Renal Disease Requiring Dialysis

Pregnancy > 20 Weeks

EMS Provider Judgment

YES — NO

Contact medical control and consider transport to a trauma center or a specific resource hospital.

Transport according to protocol

When in doubt, transport to a trauma center:
For more information, visit: www.cdc.gov/FieldTriage

Figure 1–1 Field Triage Decision Scheme: The National Trauma Triage Protocol
SOURCE: Centers for Disease Control (2012).

When an acutely ill patient requires more comprehensive or specialized care, a decision must be made to transfer the patient to a higher level of ICU care where additional personnel and resources are available. Transporting a patient from one area of the hospital to another or from one hospital to another involves risk (Droogh, Smit, Absalom, Ligtenberg, & Zijlstra, 2015). The decision to transport a patient must include an assessment of the risk-to-benefit ratio. Hospitals have guidelines for the transfer of critically ill patients to help make these important decisions. These policies and procedures address pretransport coordination and communication, personnel who must accompany the patient, equipment to accompany the patient, and the monitoring that will be required during the transport. It is recommended that clinicians use an algorithm (Fig. 1–1, see on page 3) in the decision-making process of transferring acutely ill patients to a higher level of care.

Equally as important as the decision to transfer a patient into the ICU is the decision to move a patient to an IMC unit. Suboptimal discharges out of a high-acuity unit may result in costly readmissions or death (Van Sluisveld, Zegers, Westert, Van der Hoeven, & Wollersheim, 2013).

Profile of the High-Acuity Nurse

The nurse caring for the high-acuity patient must be able to analyze clinical situations, make decisions based on this analysis, and rapidly intervene to ensure optimal patient outcomes. It is required that the nurse be comfortable with uncertainty and patient instability. The nurse is instrumental in treating patients' health problems as well as their reactions to the healthcare environment. The nurse is the only member of the healthcare team who remains at the bedside and, as a result, is frequently the one who coordinates patient care. The practice of nursing is dynamic, and the role of the nurse continues to evolve. Nurses must be able to adapt to the changing healthcare environment.

The nurse is often the first member of the healthcare team to detect early signs of an impending complication. Constant surveillance by the nurse involves assessing and monitoring the patient for signs of subtle changes over time. Often such changes in a patient's condition are clues of a possible impending complication. The prevention of complications is one of the primary goals of the acute care nurse. Evidence suggests that constant surveillance by nurses reduces mortality and life-threatening complications in the hospitalized patient (West et al., 2014).

Section One Review

1. Which statement about intermediate care units is correct?
   A. They are outdated and should not be used.
   B. They are labor intensive and are not cost effective.
   C. They provide an efficient distribution of resources.
   D. They are reserved for clients with life-threatening illnesses.

2. Which priority level indicates that the client is acutely ill and unstable and requires intensive treatment and monitoring that cannot be provided outside the ICU?
   A. Priority 1
   B. Priority 2
   C. Priority 3
   D. Priority 4

3. Evidence suggests that which of the following factors reduces mortality and life-threatening complications in the hospitalized client?
   A. A nurse–client ratio of 1:2
   B. Constant surveillance of clients by nurses
   C. High-technology ICUs
   D. IMCs

4. A hospital with an ICU that has the capability of providing comprehensive care to most critically ill clients but not to trauma clients meets the criteria for which level ICU?
   A. I
   B. II
   C. III
   D. IV

Answers: 1. C, 2. A, 3. B, 4. B

Section Two: Resource Allocation

Providing safe, high-quality care to high-acuity patients requires lower nurse-to-patient ratios, which increase expenses. Furthermore, acute care facilities have limited numbers of beds for patients who require high levels of care. Thus resource allocation is an important consideration.

Nurse Staffing

Nurses willing to work with high-acuity patients are a precious commodity. Decreased third-party reimbursement and managed care encourage shorter hospital stays. As a cost-reducing measure, hospitals have reduced professional nursing staff positions. In the late 1990s, hospital restructuring and reengineering forced bedside nurses to embrace what were considered new concepts at the time, such as role redesign, work transformation, and patient-centered care. Hospital employees, including nurses, were required to cross-train and "float" to care for patients outside their specialty areas. Unlicensed assistive personnel (UAP) were trained and supervised by nurses to complete patient care tasks. All these changes led to decreased job satisfaction and nurses leaving practice in high-acuity areas.

Other factors have contributed to the shortage of nurses. The most significant development was the passage of the Affordable Care Act in 2010, which increased access to care in the United States (U.S. Department of Health & Human Services, 2014). The influx of patients into the system resulted in shortages in nurses working in high-acuity areas. In addition, while the registered nurse (RN) workforce is rapidly aging, many older nurses are working longer and not retiring. This has caused a shift of nurses to less physically demanding settings in areas such as ambulatory care (Auerbach, Buerhaus, & Staiger, 2014). Nurse faculty members are also aging, and fewer young nurses are choosing academic nursing as a career. This results in a decreased ability to make education available to the next generation of nurses. Also, as the population continues to age, more patients will require high-acuity care.

Nursing-shortage issues are multifaceted and will continue to require comprehensive solutions. These may include federal funding for nursing education, changes in state regulations related to staffing standards, and increased public awareness. Legislation that advocates for minimum registered nurse-to-patient ratios in hospitals, promotes nursing advocacy for patients, and supports nurse training has been introduced at the national level of government (Rubin, 2015).

Nurse-to-Patient Ratios A decrease in the number of professional nurses has forced hospitals to increase nurse-to-patient ratios. The result: One nurse cares for more patients. What is the optimal nurse-to-patient ratio in high-acuity settings? The Academy of Medical-Surgical Nurses (AMSN) is not in favor of establishing predetermined ratios. Rather, the needs of the patient and the skill mix of the nursing staff must be considered when making decisions about staffing patterns (AMSN, 2011). Adequate resources must be available to evaluate the patient/family response to treatment, education, and pharmacological interventions (Dabney & Kalisch, 2015).

The position of the AACN is consistent with that of the AMSN. Staffing is both a process and an outcome. Optimal care is provided when the patient's needs are matched with the caregiver's competencies. The first principle of staffing should be to provide safe and effective patient care. The patient's acuity level and the intensity of the nursing care requirements should determine the nurse-to-patient ratio (AACN, 2005).

The reduction in professional nursing staff has encouraged an upgrade of nursing assistant skills. The American Nurses Association and the National Council of State Boards of Nursing support the use of UAP to enable the professional nurse to provide nursing care (American Nurses Association, 2005). When UAP provide direct patient care, they are accountable to, and work under, the direct supervision of the professional nurse. The RN must use leadership skills to safely and legally delegate tasks to the UAP.

Magnet Status: Recruiting and Retaining Nurses One potential solution to the nursing shortage has been the Magnet Recognition Program. This concept, originally developed in the 1980s by the American Nurses Credentialing Center, awards hospitals a **Magnet designation** if they are able to create working environments that are successful in recruiting and retaining professional nurses. In effect, these environments act like magnets to attract nurses. Hospitals that achieve "Magnet status" have practice models that promote professional nursing. Nurses who work at Magnet hospitals are more involved in decision making, report better relations with physicians, and have higher nurse-to-patient ratios. Hospitals with Magnet status report their patients have shorter ICU stays and shorter hospital stays. The Magnet hospital program has been successful over time, but it can be improved. Further studies are needed to evaluate the effects of Magnet hospital status on patient outcomes and to update and identify the essential components of Magnetism (Kramer et al., 2014).

Decreasing Resources, Increasing Care Needs

Decisions about allocation of resources must be made when there is a need to place patients in acute care areas (specifically in ICU or step-down units), but there are no beds available. Who is in need of the greatest healthcare resources when they are acutely ill?

Who Belongs in an ICU? The priority levels depicted in Table 1–1 were developed to assist clinicians in making these tough decisions about admission, discharge, and triage in high-acuity-care areas. Some could argue that ICU resources should be used for patients who have the greatest probability of benefiting or have a higher quality of life. If resource allocations were based on these principles, the actual precipitating event that created the need for resources would be irrelevant. Therefore, oncology patients, trauma patients, the young, and the old would be considered equally. Futility of treatment and informed refusal by the patient may be acceptable reasons for healthcare providers (HCPs) to limit treatment. Although these issues occur daily in the care of high-acuity patients, they also occur in a larger context of society that includes ethical, economic, and legal considerations (McHugh et al., 2015).

Oncology patients are often stereotyped as not being candidates for aggressive treatment. However, they frequently become acutely ill from therapeutic interventions. Should these patients be denied access to resources when their conditions are medically induced? During a patient's final hours, high-acuity care may be deemed appropriate because intensive efforts may be required to ensure suffering is minimized during and after removal from life support. The improvement of the quality of the dying and death experience is recognized as an important goal in modern medicine (Ñamendys-Silva, Plata-Menchaca, Rivero-Sigarroa, & Herrera-Gómez, 2015).

Age has been used to justify the withholding of resources from older adults. Extended care in the ICU has been questioned because of the high mortality rate among older adult patients. However, some studies of healthy older adult patients have shown that they often fare as well as younger patients (Mick & Ackerman, 2004). Older adult patients with minimal comorbidities appear to have similar health benefits following coronary artery bypass surgery when compared with younger patients. The severity of the illness, the admitting diagnosis, and the patient's previous health status contribute to patient outcomes. A high-acuity patient admitted to the hospital with a preexisting chronic medical condition may pose a greater risk of dying when compared to a patient who is not chronically ill.

It is difficult to predict who will benefit from care in high-acuity areas. Severity-of-injury scales and probability models were developed for this purpose. The Injury Severity Score, New Injury Severity Score, and Abbreviated Injury Scale are examples of severity-of-injury scales used in hospitals (Wong et al., 2016). However, the exclusive use of such indices has not been a completely accurate predictor of outcomes. Other factors must be taken into account.

For example, functional capacity, as well as age and treatment intensity, have been associated with patient outcomes (Baldwin, 2015; Peigne et al., 2016). Mortality is usually the outcome studied in high-acuity care. Outcomes may also include patient comfort, quality of life, functional status, and other variables in addition to living and dying. While the use of severity-of-injury scales is important to compare patient populations for research and resource allocation, patients and their families consider multiple outcomes when deciding whether to withdraw life support (Sim, Jung, Shin, Kim, & Park, 2015).

Families play an important role in resource utilization. Family involvement in these decisions about allocation of resources may ultimately decrease the use of technological resources and increase comfort measures during the last hours before death. Goals for care must be discussed with the patient and family, allowing ample time for meaningful discussion—and facilitating these decisions requires adequate training, excellent communication skills, and a collaborative effort by the interdisciplinary team. Palliative care bridges the gap between comfort and cure at the end of life and may be appropriate (Baker, Luce, & Bosslet, 2015). Patients who die in high-acuity areas consume significant resources. The constitution of end-of-life care is subjective, and cost alone cannot be used to justify the use of healthcare resources. Each patient situation is different (Oerlemans et al., 2015).

Emerging Evidence

- Investigators compared changes over time in surgical patient outcomes, nurse-reported quality, and nurse outcomes in a sample of 11 hospitals that attained Magnet status and 125 non-Magnet hospitals. Magnet hospitals demonstrated greater improvements in their work environments than other hospitals. On average, the changes in 30-day surgical mortality and failure-to-rescue rates over the study period were more pronounced in Magnet hospitals than in non-Magnet hospitals, by 2.4 fewer deaths per 1000 patients ($p < 0.01$) and 6.1 fewer deaths per 1000 patients ($p = 0.02$), respectively. Similar differences in the changes for Magnet hospitals and non-Magnet hospitals were observed in nurse-reported quality of care and nurse outcomes. Magnet recognition is associated with significant improvements over time in the quality of the work environment and in patient and nurse outcomes that exceed those of non-Magnet hospitals (*Kutney-Lee et al., 2015*).

- A total of 491 direct care registered nurses completed a survey measuring their professional quality of life (burnout, secondary traumatic stress, and compassion satisfaction). Significant predictors of burnout included a lack of meaningful recognition, more years of experience than other nurses, and being in the millennial generation (ages 21–33 years). Significant predictors of compassion satisfaction included receiving meaningful recognition, having higher job satisfaction than other nurses, being in the baby boomer generation (ages 50–65 years), and

having fewer years of experience than other nurses. No significant differences were noted across nurse specialties, units, or departments. Compassion fatigue in nurses has clear implications for nursing retention and the quality of life (*Kelly, Runge, & Spencer, 2015*).

- Thirty-six nurses were observed for 210 hours as they were exposed to 5070 mechanical alarms; 87.1% of pediatric ICU and 99.0% of non-ICU clinical alarms were nonactionable. Incremental increases in response time were noted as the number of nonactionable alarms in the preceding 120 minutes increased. Alarm fatigue could explain these findings. Future studies should evaluate the simultaneous influence of workload and other factors that can impact response time to clinical care alarms (*Bonafide et al., 2015*).

- Researchers evaluated the effectiveness of implementing quiet time in an ICU on levels of light, noise, and nurses' stress. Quiet time consisted of turning down unit lights for a designated period of time. An illumination light meter, a sound meter, and a visual analog stress scale were used for measurement 30 minutes before quiet time and 30 minutes, 1 hour, and 2 hours after quiet time. Light levels and nurses' stress levels were decreased after quiet time. Noise was decreased but not significantly. Quiet time is easily performed and promotes a healthy practice environment (*Riemer, Mates, Ryan, & Schleder, 2015*).

Section Two Review

1. Which statement is accurate concerning unlicensed assistive personnel (UAP)?
   A. UAP may not work in high-acuity environments.
   B. UAP may work independently as long as they notify the RN at the end of their shifts.
   C. UAP perform only those tasks delegated to them by a professional nurse.
   D. UAP are not governed by state boards of nursing.

2. What does the designation of Magnet status indicate?
   A. The hospital uses UAP to deliver most nursing care.
   B. The hospital uses practice models that promote professional nursing.
   C. The hospital has low nurse–client ratios.
   D. The hospital is not a desirable place for professional nurses to work.

3. According to some, ICU resources should be used for which clients?
   A. Those with cancer
   B. Those of advanced age
   C. Those with DNR orders
   D. Those who have the greatest possibility of benefiting

4. Which statement is correct regarding the improvement of the death and dying experience?
   A. It is a goal of modern medicine.
   B. It is the sole responsibility of the high-acuity nurse.
   C. It is not a standard of care in high-acuity units.
   D. It is the sole responsibility of the palliative care team.

Answers: 1. C, 2. B, 3. D, 4. A

Section Three: Use of Technology in High-Acuity Environments

In medical, business, academic, and many other work environments, technology influences how we communicate, document, evaluate, and conduct business—whether that business is making a product or taking care of patients. A major advantage of having technology available in the high-acuity environment is that the patient's status can be monitored continuously, using sensitive physiologic indicators of changing status. In the unstable patient, the ability to assess a possible problem before it becomes a full-blown complication may make the difference between life and death for that patient.

Technology is also a useful tool that can assist high-acuity nurses and other healthcare professionals in making critical decisions. Although decision making is viewed as somewhat artful and intuitive, computers use a scientific, programmed approach based on a massive database and algorithmic decision-making trees. Computer software programs are available to help diagnose patient conditions. Cellular smartphones and tablet technology also provide rapid access to a wide variety of medical-related applications that can assist with conversions and calculations, drug and disease information, diagnostics, and patient teaching.

While technology has provided the nurse with many advantages and improved patient outcomes, it has also given rise to some important issues. Nurses who care for acutely ill patients must be able to use technology in the caring process and still recognize its limits.

Patient Depersonalization

A major criticism of nurses who work with high-acuity patients is that they are too technologically oriented. The focus of nursing care in high-acuity patient care units is on monitoring patients for subtle physiologic changes. This monitoring requires the nurse to use multiple technologies. The patient interfaces with members of the healthcare team and medical equipment in the diagnosis and management of the patient's disease process. Difficulties arise when machines, rather than individual patient needs, become the focus of care of the high-acuity patient. Technology must be used to enhance care, not take the place of a nurse's personal knowledge, observation skills, and senses. A balance must be maintained between the use of technology and the humanistic aspect of nursing to promote efficient and high-quality care (Sabzevari, Mirzaei, Bagherian, & Iranpour, 2015).

Technical devices present mechanical impediments to touching the patient. Little surface area may be available for physical contact, and this may lead to a feeling of depersonalization. Technology may evoke fear in patients and contribute to their anxiety about their recovery process.

Overload and Overreliance Issues

Having responsibility for multiple pieces of equipment can increase the nurse's stress level. Because of the massive amount of patient data available, nurses may be reaching a saturation point in data processing. "Alarm fatigue" occurs when the number and frequency of alarms becomes overwhelming, resulting in delayed alarm responses and deliberate alarm deactivations, both of which adversely affect patient safety (Sendelbach, Wahl, Anthony, & Shotts, 2015).

Technology can be so intriguing that its primary purpose—to support the well-being of the patient—is lost. Technology may create demands where no demands existed before, such as what occurs with the fragmentation of patients into subpopulations (e.g., bone marrow transplant unit, cardiac surgery unit). Each subpopulation has its own special staff competing for hospital resources. The patient competes with machines for nursing surveillance. It is possible that nurses become so dependent on monitoring devices that they completely trust the equipment, even when the data conflict with their own clinical assessments.

Finding a Balance

The skilled nurse who practices in a high-acuity setting must be able to bridge the gap between complex technology and the art of caring. When new technologies are introduced at the bedside, it is commonplace for the nurse to focus initially on the technology because of the need to gain proficiency in the use of this technology to support patient care. To foster proficiency, it is important that the nurse be given the opportunity to become familiar with a technology before its actual use in patient care; thus, appropriate training in the use of high-tech equipment is crucial. A high degree of comfort with technology prevents it from becoming the focus of care. Nurses are at risk for becoming overly dependent on technology for clinical decision making, making it essential that the nurse validate the technologic data with nursing assessment data. The healthcare practitioner, not the technology, is ultimately responsible for clinical decisions. The element of human touch must never be removed from the bedside (Sabzevari et al., 2015).

Section Three Review

1. What are the hazards inherent in the use of technology? (Select all that apply.)
   A. Fragmenting clients into subpopulations
   B. Increasing the nurse's stress level
   C. Allowing more time for client contact
   D. Making the client overdependent on monitoring equipment
   E. Increasing nurse dependence on machines for decision making

2. Which statements are correct regarding the use of technical devices in high-acuity care? (Select all that apply.)
   A. They present mechanical impediments to touching.
   B. They are usually well accepted by clients.
   C. They may evoke fear in clients.
   D. They lead to a feeling of depersonalization.
   E. They may increase client anxiety.

3. What should be the focus of care of the high-acuity client?
   A. Bedside machines
   B. Individual client needs
   C. The alarms on the machines
   D. The nurse's needs

4. What should the nurse use to validate the technologic data?
   A. Nursing assessment data
   B. The healthcare provider
   C. Other technologic data
   D. Another nurse

Answers: 1. (A, B, E), 2. (A, C, D, E), 3. B, 4. A

Section Four: Healthy Practice Environment

Nurses work in demanding situations over long periods of time. The quest to provide high-quality patient care in a practice environment that has decreasing resources and increasing responsibilities creates conflict. This conflict creates feelings of personal and professional frustration and results in burnout and compassion fatigue (Hinderer et al., 2014). Practicing in a healthy environment increases job satisfaction and provides a buffer against stress and burnout. This section presents a discussion of a healthy high-acuity practice environment, nurse burnout, compassion fatigue, and coping with stress.

Healthy Practice Environment

In 2001, AACN made a commitment to promote healthy practice environments that support quality patient care and high levels of nurse satisfaction. Six standards were identified that are critical to create and sustain a **healthy practice environment** (AACN, 2005). These standards are listed in Table 1–3. AACN believes that the implementation of these standards will be an important step in meeting the commitment for a healthy practice environment. This will, in turn, lead to improved patient safety, enhanced recruitment and retention, and positive patient outcomes (AACN, 2005).

Table 1–3 AACN Standards for Healthy Practice Environments

Standard	Definition
Skilled communication	Nurses must be as proficient in communication skills as they are in clinical skills.
True collaboration	Nurses must be relentless in pursuing and fostering true collaboration.
Effective decision making	Nurses must be valued and committed partners in making policy, directing and evaluating clinical care, and leading organizational operations.
Appropriate staffing	Staffing must ensure the effective match between patient needs and nurse competencies.
Meaningful recognition	Nurses must be recognized and recognize others for the value each brings to the work of the organization.
Authentic leadership	Nurse leaders must fully embrace the imperative of a healthy practice environment, authentically live it, and engage others in its achievement.

SOURCE: Data from American Association of Critical-Care Nurses (ACCN). (2005).

Organizations can implement strategies to improve the practice environment, but it is the nurse who must validate their effectiveness. High-acuity nurses are the gatekeepers of patient safety. Structures, processes, and outcomes are required for quality care—that is, having the "right things in place" to do the "right things" so that the "right outcomes" will happen. A healthy and productive practice environment allows the nurse to give excellent care to patients while achieving job satisfaction (Kramer, Schmalenberg, & Maguire, 2010).

Stress, Burnout, and Compassion Fatigue

The term **burnout** has been used to describe feelings of personal and professional frustration, job dissatisfaction, job insecurity, and emotional and physical exertion. It is a syndrome of emotional exhaustion, depersonalization, and reduced personal accomplishments that occurs among individuals who work with people on a daily basis. When asked to describe burnout, healthcare professionals invariably talk about being overworked, feeling a lack of control, insufficient rewards, and conflicting values (Hinderer et al., 2014). Symptoms indicative of burnout are summarized in Box 1–1.

Patients' conditions change rapidly in high-acuity units, and this may be a source of burnout for nurses who work in these areas because it requires flexibility to manage rapidly changing circumstances. A patient with a poor prognosis may have a prolonged stay that involves the use of multiple technologies. Then, in the middle of a shift, a decision is made to cease these efforts. The patient may improve, requiring reevaluation and escalation of care. Conversely, a patient is declared dead by brain death criteria and immediately thereafter may become an organ donor. This requires the nurse to shift from caring for a patient to caring for organs for another patient. It is also quite common that within minutes after a patient's death, the nurse is told that a new patient is waiting to come into that very same bed. The nurse must mourn one patient's death and then minutes later invest energy in a new patient. A significant degree of uncertainty is confronted on a daily basis. A broad-based end-of-life-care curriculum may be instrumental in assisting the high-acuity nurse to cope with the daily stress of changing patient conditions.

Stress is a major component of burnout. A current reason for stress and subsequent burnout in nurses is decreased staffing, long working hours, and loss of concentration. Other sources of stress include manager unresponsiveness, lack of teamwork, and conflicts with other healthcare providers. Often this can lead to poor self-care, which can influence nurses' ability to appropriately care for patients (Boyle, 2015).

Secondary traumatic stress and compassion fatigue are also a threat to nurses who work in high-acuity environments. Experiencing the pain of others and constant exposure to tragedy over time takes a toll. **Compassion fatigue** results when the compassionate energy that has been expended by the nurse exceeds the ability to personally re-energize. Compassion fatigue is different from burnout in that it results from the stress nurses experience from the daily relationships with patients and families (Boyle, 2015).

Coping with Stress, Burnout, and Compassion Fatigue

The social environment of the nursing unit plays a role in nurses' perceived levels of stress. Stress can be either positive or negative. A positive social climate, characterized by strong managerial support and cohesiveness among the staff, serves as a buffer against the negative effects of stress. Environmental uncertainty, as measured by the number of admissions, discharges, and transfers in the high-acuity area, can result in emotional exhaustion. Nurses must enhance self-awareness of personal sources of tension. Once these sources are identified, strategies for alleviating stressors can be developed (Henderson, 2015).

Professional collegial relationships with healthcare providers, as well as delegation of appropriate patient care tasks to unlicensed personnel, can decrease stress and

---

BOX 1–1   Symptoms of Burnout

Behavioral
- Withdrawal
- Risk taking and impulsiveness
- Ambivalence
- Decreased productivity
- Contemplating career change
- Increased use of caffeine, alcohol, and nicotine

Physiologic
- Chronic fatigue
- Frequent minor ailments
- Sleep changes
- Appetite change
- Sexual difficulty

Psychologic
- Attempts to blame others
- Stereotyping patients
- Nightmares
- Depression
- Hostility and negativism
- Loss of tolerance

Cognitive
- Decreased ability to make decisions
- Poor judgment
- Lack of initiative
- Forgetfulness

burnout. The nurse assumes the central role at the bedside. While the physician or pharmacist may have a snapshot of the patient's condition, it is the high-acuity nurse who holds the video camera. Coordinating effective communication among multiple healthcare providers provides positive patient outcomes (Kramer et al., 2014).

Establishing critical incident stress debriefings (CISDs) may facilitate coping with specific situations. These are structured group discussions, usually occurring within several days following a crisis, designed to address symptoms of stress, assess the need for follow-up, and provide a sense of closure. These sessions are a formal way of managing stress before it becomes debilitating or

fosters burnout. The research is limited on the long-term benefits of CISDs; however, participants perceive such debriefings as important (Healy & Tyrrell, 2013). Another strategy for preventing burnout is to assist nurses during orientation in formulating clear ideas of their professional roles and responsibilities within the high-acuity environment. Offering new nurses the opportunity to meet in small groups provides a safe, confidential environment to share experiences. Promoting a sense of community can also enhance the ability to share stresses and joys, seek feedback for continuing performance improvement, and develop critical thinking skills (Maresca, Eggenberger, Moffa, & Newman, 2015).

Section Four Review

1. What are the components of a healthy work environment? (Select all that apply.)
   A. True collaboration
   B. Appropriate staffing
   C. Authentic leadership
   D. Individual priorities
   E. Skilled communication

2. Which factors can help buffer the negative effects of stress? (Select all that apply.)
   A. Environmental uncertainty
   B. Positive social climate
   C. Managerial support
   D. Cohesiveness among staff
   E. Ignoring stress as it develops

3. Critical incident stress debriefings (CISDs) can be used for which purposes? (Select all that apply.)
   A. Assess high-acuity clients
   B. Help families cope with stress
   C. Address staff symptoms of stress
   D. Provide staff with a sense of closure
   E. Assess the need for follow-up

4. The term *burnout* refers to which feelings? (Select all that apply.)
   A. Personal and professional frustration
   B. Loss of self-esteem
   C. Physical and emotional exertion
   D. Job dissatisfaction
   E. Job insecurity

Answers: 1. (A, B, C, E), 2. (B, C, D), 3. (C, D, E), 4. (A, C, D)

Section Five: Ensuring Patient Safety in High-Acuity Environments

Other than the operating room, there is no hospital environment in which the patient is more vulnerable than in high-acuity units, particularly critical care. For this reason, attendance to patient safety is of the upmost importance, as many patients cannot protect themselves and must rely fully on the competency of the nurse.

The Culture

Patient safety and healthy work environments are closely linked. For many years industry has examined work culture and its effect on job performance and outcomes; however, only recently has this been examined in healthcare. Reports from the Institute of Medicine (IOM) highlighted unsafe patient conditions and were instrumental in launching patient safety initiatives (IOM, Committee on Quality of

Health Care in America, 2001). Research has shown a correlation between working conditions, teamwork, and patient outcomes. High levels of teamwork result in decreased length of stay and decreased mortality (Pattison & Kline, 2015).

Healthcare errors have become recognized as a public health problem. Failure to disclose errors was part of the socialization process for many years. Now, errors are publicly reported in the media and on the internet. While some argue that healthcare professionals are human and apt to make mistakes, others feel that any medical mistake is unacceptable. For many years the fear of making mistakes was linked to a culture of blame. It was common for a nurse who reported an error to experience reprimands from unsupportive administrators and loss of respect from colleagues. The gradual shift to a culture of caring and support has been shown to increase error reporting and lead to systems improvement (Ulrich & Kear, 2014).

Patient Safety

The Joint Commission (TJC) is an accrediting organization committed to improving patient safety. Originally named

BOX 1–2 National Patient Safety Goals for Acute Care Hospitals 2015

- Improve the accuracy of patient identification.
- Improve the effectiveness of communication among caregivers.
- Improve the safety of using medications.
- Reduce harm associated with clinical alarm systems.
- Reduce the risk of healthcare-associated infections.
- Identify safety risks inherent in the patient population.
- Introduction of Universal Protocol for wrong site, wrong procedure, wrong person, wrong surgery.

SOURCE: Data from the Joint Commission. (2015).

the Joint Commission on Accreditation of Healthcare Organizations (JCAHO), the organization shortened the name in 2007. The Joint Commission's mission is to continuously improve the safety and quality of care provided to the public through the provision of healthcare accreditation that supports process improvement in healthcare organizations. The organization established "National Patient Safety Goals" for acute care hospitals in 2009. The goals for 2015 are summarized in Box 1–2. Each year these goals are reviewed and revised.

To improve the accuracy of patient identification, the nurse should use at least two patient identifiers when providing care, treatment, and services. For example, a nurse should check the patient's name band and ask the patient to state his or her name before drawing blood or giving a medication. Effectiveness of communication among caregivers should be improved. One way to accomplish this safety goal is to use a "read-back" process. For example, when reporting critical laboratory test results, the person giving the test result should verify the test result by having the person receiving the information record and read back the test results. The Situation, Background, Assessment, and Recommendation (SBAR) technique has been shown to be an effective tool for all hand-off communications (Whittingham & Oldroyd, 2014).

To improve the safety of using medications, The Joint Commission recommends that all medication labels be verified both verbally and visually by two people when the person preparing the medication may not be the person who will be administering it. Patient care areas have many alarms that add to the unit noise level, and information is displayed that desensitizes nurses to the very information to which they need to tend. While there is no single solution, hospitals must understand their systems and develop a coordinated approach to alarm management.

To reduce the risk of healthcare-associated infections, hospitals must implement evidence-based guidelines to prevent bloodstream infections associated with central lines. This includes annual education for healthcare workers who are involved with caring for patients with central lines. Education should include information about infections and the importance of prevention. Hospitals must identify and provide safe care for patients at risk for suicide. Patient safety is further enhanced when hospitals take a time-out before

every procedure to be certain that it is the right patient, appropriate procedure, and correct side of the body.

As another safety strategy, patients should be encouraged to actively participate in their own care. The patient and family should be educated on available reporting methods for concerns related to care, treatment, services, and patient safety issues. The Joint Commission requires hospitals to improve recognition and response to changes in patient condition. This means that hospitals must have a method that enables healthcare staff members to directly request additional assistance from a specially trained individual when the patient's condition appears to be worsening. Many hospitals have implemented rapid response teams (RRTs) to address this goal. While initial research is promising, further studies to determine effectiveness are warranted (White, Scott, Vaux, & Sullivan, 2015).

The Joint Commission requires adherence to a universal protocol. For example, a time-out process must be performed prior to starting a procedure, such as the bedside insertion of a percutaneous tracheostomy. The purpose of this time-out is to conduct a formal assessment that the correct patient, site, positioning, and procedure are identified; all relevant documents (such as a consent form) have been signed; and necessary equipment is available. The completed components must be clearly documented.

To receive The Joint Commission accreditation, the hospital must demonstrate and provide evidence that it is meeting these safety goals. High-acuity nurses must actively participate in ensuring these goals are met.

Technology and Patient Safety

Technology has been introduced to prevent errors. One example is the implementation of computerized provider order entry (CPOE) systems. These systems block incorrect medication orders; warn against drug interactions, allergies, and overdoses; provide current, accurate drug information; and alert to sound-alike drug names. While the initial cost is high, many hospitals have implemented computerized provider order entry and have benefited from cost savings and error reduction (Charles, Cannon, Hall, & Coustasse, 2014).

Manufactured devices may be a source of potential errors. Devices are carefully engineered to be fail-safe; however, adverse incidents do happen. The nurse must be competent in using the equipment. It is the responsibility of the nurse to report medical device failure when it occurs to the appropriate hospital department and to remove the item from service.

Barcode medication administration (BCMA) is another technology recently introduced to prevent errors. This system allows nurses to scan their badges, as well as patient wristbands, to access medication profiles. The nurse is then able to obtain the right medication, for the right patient, in the right dose, at the right time, and via the correct route (Seibert, Maddox, Flynn, & Williams, 2014).

Smartphones are commonplace and allow for text messaging, email retrieval, and application stores. The tablet personal computer allows for a wealth of clinical applications yet untapped (Furness, Bradford, & Paterson, 2013). While these systems have been effective in reducing errors, they are not infallible. The human component cannot be discounted.

Other Factors Contributing to Patient Safety

Patients trust their care to nurses who must cope with workforce shortages and ever-changing therapies and technologies. Since 2005, AACN's position is that the shortage of nurses working in high-acuity areas, overtime hours, and excessive documentation jeopardize patient safety. A strong educational foundation and solid orientation will allow for the high-acuity nurse to provide more efficient, safer care (AACN, 2005). Research has also shown that the educational level of the nurse is related to patient outcomes. Institutions with a higher percentage of nurses educated at the baccalaureate level or higher demonstrated lower mortality rates (Aiken, 2014).

The IOM has suggested performance standards for healthcare professionals that focus on patient safety. Furthermore, AACN (2005) believes that specialty certification addresses this need. Hospitals that create a culture of respect and professionalism are more likely to employ experienced, certified nurses in an environment where safety is valued. Research continues to indicate that adequate staffing, well-educated nurses, positive physician–nurse relationships, and responsible management are the keys to decreasing errors. Collegial relationships among all healthcare providers and trust will also contribute to patient safety (Pattison & Kline, 2015).

Section Five Review

1. What do the current client safety and healthy work environment cultures in the high-acuity environment promote?
   A. An increase in error reporting and systems improvement
   B. A decrease in error reporting
   C. A culture of blame
   D. The failure to publicly disclose medical errors

2. Which factors contribute to medical errors? (Select all that apply.)
   A. Staffing ratios
   B. Overtime
   C. Excessive documentation
   D. Specialty certification
   E. Responsible management

3. What must be done to ensure client safety before a percutaneous tracheostomy is placed at the bedside?
   A. One person should confirm the order.
   B. The correct client, site, and procedure should be identified during a time-out.
   C. Two people should confirm the order.
   D. Visitors should be asked to leave the room.

4. What is the proper procedure to ensure client safety when the nurse is preparing a medication that will be administered to the client by another person? (Select all that apply.)
   A. This should never be done.
   B. Confirm the order with the healthcare provider (HCP).
   C. Labels should be verbally verified by the two healthcare providers.
   D. Labels should be visually verified by the two healthcare providers.
   E. Document in the medication administration record prior to giving the medication.

Answers: 1. A, 2. (A, B, C), 3. B, 4. (C, D)

Clinical Reasoning Checkpoint

Case 1: RM is a 64-year-old with stage 4 metastatic colon cancer. She presents to the emergency department with shortness of breath. A chest x-ray reveals right lower lobe pneumonia. She is admitted to the hospital. She has advance directives that include no intubation or CPR.

1. Is RM a candidate for admission to the ICU? Why or why not?
2. Using the American College of Critical Care Medicine (ACCM) prioritization model, identify the patient's priority level for ICU placement.

Case 2: A patient with a history of new-onset seizures is admitted to a level III ICU. A diagnosis of brain tumor is made and surgery will be required. The healthcare provider (HCP) informs the patient that he needs to be transferred to another hospital that has a level I ICU.

3. After the HCP leaves the room, the patient says he doesn't understand why he needs to be transferred. As his nurse, explain the reason for the need for transfer.

Case 3: You would like to work in a high-acuity unit that has a healthy practice environment that supports quality patient care and high levels of nurse satisfaction. You are aware of the six standards identified by AACN that are critical to creating and sustaining a healthy work environment.

4. Provide at least one example of how you might see each of the six standards operationalized in the high-acuity unit.

Chapter 1 Review

1. The ICU nurse receives a call from the medical–surgical unit requesting transfer of a client to the ICU. The client is in acute respiratory failure and requires mechanical ventilation. He will require vasoactive drugs to help manage his profound hypotension. Based on the American College of Critical Care Medicine (ACCM) prioritization model, what is this client's priority for ICU placement?
   1. Priority 1
   2. Priority 2
   3. Priority 3
   4. Priority 4

2. A nurse is interviewing for a position in a community hospital. Hospital brochures describe a Level III ICU. Which statement describes the resources that the nurse would expect in this hospital?
   1. Those working in the ICU have specialty training and use specialized equipment to care for a wide variety of client illnesses and injuries.
   2. Staff and equipment in the unit are capable of providing comprehensive care for clients with a variety of illnesses and injuries.
   3. Staff in the unit can provide initial stabilization of clients for transfer to more advanced care.
   4. The hospital is a teaching facility with sophisticated equipment and provider expertise.

3. A hospital has been working to achieve Magnet status. Which statements by an ICU nurse reflect the benefits of Magnet status? (Select all that apply.)
   1. "I feel more ownership in the decisions being made to run the unit."
   2. "I don't have to supervise UAPs anymore."
   3. "It would be so much easier to work here if the physicians were friendlier."
   4. "Taking care of one less client each shift makes such a difference."
   5. "Our pay raise makes working here worth all the stress."

4. In the middle of a shift a nurse comes to the manager to discuss the acuity level and number of clients he has been assigned. Which statement would the manager interpret as indicating the nurse needs further education about nurse–client ratios?
   1. "I cannot provide the amount of care that all these clients need."
   2. "Our professional organizations would not approve of exceeding their recommended ratios."
   3. "Is there someone who can be called in to help me with this client load?"
   4. "I am worried I'm going to miss something with one of these clients."

5. New, fairly complex monitoring devices have been purchased to replace current monitors in the ICU. How should the nurse manager plan to introduce this equipment to the unit?
   1. Have one device placed in one room and rotate nurses through caring for clients on the monitor.
   2. Require that all nurses caring for clients on this monitor have extensive training on its use.
   3. Have all the old monitors replaced with the new devices so that nurses can learn by using the equipment.
   4. Tell the nurses to focus on how to use the monitor when caring for clients for the first few days.

6. What is the best advice that an experienced ICU nurse can offer to new nurses on how to remain focused on the client?
   1. "Learn about the equipment before caring for the client."
   2. "Don't come to work in the ICU until you are proficient in all the equipment we use."
   3. "Try to arrange equipment so that you have ample opportunity to use the power of your touch with the client."
   4. "Until you are comfortable with equipment, ask to be assigned with another nurse."

7. A coworker has become increasingly withdrawn from social activities on the unit. She is often late for work and is ambivalent about warnings from the nurse manager. She has become hostile and negative about proposed changes in the unit. The nurse should recognize that the coworker is exhibiting symptoms of which condition?
   1. Burnout
   2. Stress
   3. Job dissatisfaction
   4. Conflict

8. The nurse manager has made a commitment to improve the health of the ICU work environment. Which activities will help meet that goal? (Select all that apply.)
   1. Make every effort to assign clients so that their needs match the nurse's strengths.
   2. Set up a program in which a "nurse of the day" is chosen and honored each day.
   3. Engage the hospital nurse executive in efforts to improve the health of the entire environment.
   4. Role-model successful collaboration with healthcare providers.
   5. Communicate in a clear and effective manner.

9. The hospital is planning to implement a CPOE system. One of the nurses says, "I don't see how that is going to help." Which statement by another nurse is a good response to this concern?
   1. "You are right; these systems often contribute to medication errors."
   2. "I heard that these systems can cause drug–drug interactions."
   3. "Actually, hospitals that have used these systems generally see error reduction."
   4. "The systems may help prevent errors, but they are way too expensive for use in most hospitals."

10. The high-acuity unit's operations council is seeking suggestions concerning the use of technology to prevent errors on the unit. What statements by nurses are good responses to this request? (Select all that apply.)
    1. "Barcode medication administration has been shown to reduce medication errors."
    2. "We could completely eliminate errors if we had new tablet computers."
    3. "We need more of the newest infusion pumps. They are always accurate."
    4. "Don't purchase anything that isn't fail-safe."
    5. "If we had smartphones, we could look up so much information."

Answers to questions found inside your textbook are available on the faculty resources site. Please consult with your instructor.

References

Academy of Medical-Surgical Nurses (AMSN). (2011). Position statement: Staffing standards for patient care. Retrieved August 20, 2015, from http://www.amsn.org

Aiken, L. (2014). Baccalaureate nurses and hospital outcomes: More evidence. *Medical Care, 52*(10), 861–863. doi: 10.1097/MLR.0000000000000222

American Association of Critical-Care Nurses (AACN). (2005). AACN standards for establishing and sustaining healthy work environments: A journey to excellence. *American Journal of Critical Care, 14,* 187–197.

American College of Critical Care Medicine (ACCM). (1993). Guidelines for the transfer of critically ill patients. *Critical Care Medicine, 21,* 931–937.

American College of Critical Care Medicine (ACCM). (1998). Guidelines on admission and discharge for adult intermediate care units. *Critical Care Medicine, 26*(3), 608.

American College of Critical Care Medicine (ACCM). (1999). Guidelines for intensive care unit admission, discharge, and triage. *Critical Care Medicine, 27*(3), 633–638.

American Nurses Association (ANA). (2005). Delegation: Joint ANA and National Council of State Boards of Nursing Position Statement. Retrieved August 20, 2015, from http://nursingworld.org

Auerbach, D., Buerhaus, P., & Staiger, D. (2014). Registered nurses are delaying retirement, a shift that has contributed to recent growth in the nurse workforce. *Health Affairs, 33*(8), 1474–1480. doi: 10.1377/hlthaff.2014.0128

Baker, M., Luce, J., & Bosslet, G. (2015). Integration of palliative care services in the intensive care unit. *Clinics in Chest Medicine, 36*(3), 441–448. doi: 10.1016/j.ccm.2015.05.010

Baldwin, M. R. (2015). Measuring and predicting long-term outcomes in older survivors of critical illness. *Minerva Anestesiologica, 81*(6), 650–661.

Bonafide, C., Lin, R., Zander, M., Graham, C., Paine, C., Rock, W., ... Keren, R. (2015). Association between exposure to nonactionable physiologic monitor alarms and response time in a children's hospital. *Journal of Hospital Medicine, 10*(6), 345–351. doi: 10.1002/jhm.2331

Boyle, D. (2015). Compassion fatigue: The cost of caring. *Nursing, 45*(7), 48–51. doi: 10.1097/01.NURSE.000061857.48809.a1

Centers for Disease Control and Prevention. (2012). 2011 Guidelines for Field Triage of Injured Patients. Retrieved September 15, 2017, from https://stacks.cdc.gov/view/cdc/23038/Share

Charles, K., Cannon, M., Hall, R., & Coustasse, A. (2014, Fall). Can utilizing a computerized provider order entry (CPOE) system prevent hospital medical errors and adverse drug events? *Perspectives in Health Information Management,* 1–16.

Dabney, B., & Kalisch, B. (2015). Nurse staffing levels and patient-reported missed nursing care. *Journal of Nursing Care Quality, 30*(4), 306–312. doi: 10.1097/NCQ.0000000000000123

Droogh, J., Smit, M., Absalom, A., Ligtenberg, J., & Zijlstra, J. (2015). Transferring the critically ill patient: Are we there yet? *Critical Care, 19*(62). doi: 10.1186/s13054-015-0749-4

Furness, N., Bradford, O., & Paterson, M. (2013). Tablets in trauma: Using mobile computing platforms to improve patient understanding and experience. *Orthopedics, 36*(3), 205–208. doi: 10.3928/01477447-20130222-06

Haupt, M. T., Bekes, C. E., Carl, L. C., Gray, A. W., Jastremski, M. S., Naylor, D. F., ... Society of Critical Care Medicine. (2003). Guidelines on critical care services and personnel: Recommendations based on a system of categorization of three levels of care. *Critical Care Medicine, 31*(11), 2677–2683.

Healy, S., & Tyrrell, M. (2013). Importance of debriefing following critical incidents. *Emergency Nurse, 20*(10), 32–37.

Henderson, J. (2015). The effect of hardiness education on hardiness and burnout on registered nurses. *Nursing Economics, 33*(4), 204–209.

Hinderer, K., VonRueden, K., Friedmann, E., McQuillan, K., Gilmore, R., Kramer, B., & Murray, M. (2014). Burnout, compassion fatigue, compassion satisfaction, and secondary traumatic stress in trauma nurses. *Journal of Trauma Nursing, 21*(4), 160–169. doi: 10.1097/JTN.0000000000000055

Institute of Medicine (IOM), Committee on Quality of Health Care in America. (2001). Crossing the quality chasm: A new health system for the 21st century.

Retrieved November 24, 2016, from https://www.nap.edu/read/10027/chapter/1

Kelly, L., Runge, J., & Spencer, C. (2015). Predictors of compassion fatigue and compassion satisfaction in acute care nurses. *Journal of Nursing Scholarship*, 47(6), 522–528. doi: 10.1111/jnu.12162

Kostakou, E., Rovina, N., Kyriakopoulou, M., Koulouris, N. G., & Koutsoukou, A. (2014). Critically ill cancer patient in intensive care unit: Issues that arise. *Journal of Critical Care*, 29, 817–822.

Kramer, M., Brewer, B., Halfer, D., Hnatiuk, C., MacPhee, M., & Schmalenberg, C. (2014). The evolution and development of an instrument to measure essential professional nursing practices. *Journal of Nursing Administration*, 44(11), 569–576. doi: 10.1097/NNA.0000000000000128

Kramer, M., Schmalenberg, C., & Maguire, P. (2010). Nine structures and leadership practices essential for a magnetic (healthy) work environment. *Nursing Administration Quarterly*, 34(1), 4–17.

Kutney-Lee, A., Stimpfel, A., Sloane, D., Cimiotti J., Quinn, L., & Aiken, L. (2015). Changes in patient and nurse outcomes associated with magnet hospital recognition. *Medical Care*, 53(6), 550–557. doi: 10.1097/MLR.0000000000000355

Maresca, R., Eggenberger, T., Moffa, C., & Newman, D. (2015). Lessons learned: Accessing the voice of nurses to improve a novice nurse program. *Journal for Nurses in Professional Development*, 31(4), 218–224. doi: 10.1097/NND.0000000000000169

McHugh, N., Baker, R., Mason, H., Williamson, L., Van Exel, J., Deogaonkar, R., … Donaldson, C. (2015). Extending life for people with a terminal illness: A moral right and an expensive death? Exploring societal perspectives. *BMC Medical Ethics*, 16(14). doi: 10.1186/s12910-015-0008-x

Meyer, M. (2003). Avoid PCU bottlenecks with proper admission and discharge criteria. *Critical Care Nurse*, 23(3), 59–63.

Mick, D. J., & Ackerman, M. H. (2004). Critical care nursing for older adults: Pathophysiological and functional considerations. *Nursing Clinics of North America*, 39(3), 473–493.

Ñamendys-Silva, S., Plata-Menchaca, E., Rivero-Sigarroa, E., & Herrera-Gómez, A. (2015). Opening the doors of the intensive care unit to cancer patients: A current perspective. *World Journal of Critical Care Medicine*, 4(3), 159–162. doi: 10.5492/wjccm.v4.i3.159

Oerlemans, A., Van Sluisveld, N., Van Leeuwen, E., Wollersheim H., Dekkers, W., & Zegers, M. (2015). Ethical problems in intensive care unit admission and discharge decisions: A qualitative study among physicians and nurses in the Netherlands. *BMC Medical Ethics*, 16(9), 1–10. doi: 10.1186/s12910-015-0001-4

Pattison, J., & Kline, T. (2015). Facilitating a just and trusting culture. *International Journal of Health Care Quality Assurance*, 28(1), 11–26. doi: 10.1108/IJHCQA-05-2013-0055

Peigne, V., Somme, D., Guerot, E., Lenain, E., Chatellier, G., Fagon, J.-Y., & Saint-Jean, O. (2016). Treatment intensity, age and outcome in medical ICU patients: Results of a French administrative database. *Annals of Intensive Care*, 6(7), 1–8. doi: 10.1186/s13613-016-0107-y

Riemer, H., Mates, J., Ryan, L., & Schleder, B. (2015). Decreased stress levels in nurses: A benefit of quiet time. *American Journal of Critical Care*, 24(5), 396–402. doi: 10.4037/ajcc2015706

Rubin R. (2015). Bill takes aim at nationwide shortage of nurses. *Journal of the American Medical Association*, 313(18), 1787. doi:10.1001/jama.2015.3747

Sabzevari, S., Mirzaei, T., Bagherian, B., & Iranpour, M. (2015). Critical care nurses' attitudes about influences of technology on nursing care. *British Journal of Medicine & Medical Research*, 9(8), 1–10. doi: 10.9734/BJMMR/2015/18400

Seibert, H., Maddox, R., Flynn, E., & Williams, C. (2014). Effect of barcode technology with electronic medication administration record on medication accuracy rates. *American Journal of Health-System Pharmacy*, 71, 209–218.

Sendelbach, S., Wahl, S., Anthony, A., & Shotts, P. (2015). Stop the noise: A quality improvement project to decrease electrocardiographic nuisance alarms. *Critical Care Nurse*, 35(4), 15–23. doi: 10.4037/ccn2015858

Sim, Y., Jung, H., Shin, T., Kim, D., & Park, S. (2015). Mortality and outcomes in very elderly patients 90 years of age or older admitted to the ICU. *Respiratory Care*, 60(3), 347–355. doi: 10.4187/respcare.03155

The Joint Commission. (2015). National Patient Safety Goals Effective January 1, 2015. Retrieved November 21, 2016, from http://www.jointcommission.org/assets/1/6/2015_NPSG_HAP.pdf

Ulrich, B., & Kear, T. (2014). Patient safety and patient safety culture: Foundations of excellent health care delivery. *Nephrology Nursing Journal*, 41(5), 447–456, 505.

U.S. Department of Health & Human Services. (2014). Key features of the Affordable Care Act by year. Retrieved November 19, 2016, from http://www.hhs.gov/healthcare/facts/timeline/timeline-text.html

Van Sluisveld, N., Zegers, M., Westert, G., Van der Hoeven, J., & Wollersheim, H. (2013). A strategy to enhance the safety and efficiency of handovers of ICU patients: Study protocol of the pICUp study. *Implementation Science 2013*, 8(67). doi:10.1186/1748-5908-8-67

West, E., Barron, D., Harrison, D., Rafferty, A., Rowan, K., & Sanderson, C. (2014). Nurse staffing, medical staffing and mortality in intensive care: An observational study. *International Journal of Nursing Studies*, 51, 781–794. doi: 10.1016/j.ijnurstu.2014.02.007

White, K., Scott, I. A., Vaux, A., & Sullivan, C. M. (2015). Rapid response teams in adult hospitals: Time for another look? *Internal Medicine Journal*. doi: 10.1111/imj.12845

Whittingham, K., & Oldroyd, L. (2014). Using an SBAR—Keeping it real! Demonstrating how improving safe care delivery has been incorporated into a top-up degree programme. *Nurse Education Today*, 34(6), e47–e52.

Wong, T. H., Krishnaswamy, G., Nadkarni, N. V., Nguyen, H. V., Lim, G. H., Bautista, D. C. T., . . . Ong, M. E. H. (2016). Combining the New Injury Severity Score with an anatomical polytrauma injury variable predicts mortality better than the New Injury Severity Score and the Injury Severity Score: A retrospective cohort study. *Scandinavian Journal of Trauma, Resuscitation and Emergency Medicine*, 24(25), 1–11. doi: 10.1186/s13049-016-0215-6

Chapter 2
Holistic Care of the Patient and Family

 Learning Outcomes

2.1 Describe the impact of illness on the high-acuity patient and family.

2.2 Identify ways the nurse can help high-acuity patients cope with an illness and/or injury event.

2.3 Describe the principles of patient- and family-centered care in the high-acuity environment as it relates to educational needs of visitation and policies.

2.4 Explain the importance of awareness of cultural diversity when caring for high-acuity patients.

2.5 Identify environmental stressors, their impact on high-acuity patients, and strategies to alleviate those stressors.

This chapter focuses on the impact of hospitalization on patients who are admitted with a serious or critical illness and the role nurses play in providing holistic care to this vulnerable patient population. Admission to a high-acuity care environment is extremely stressful to both patient and family, and nurses are in a pivotal position to provide comfort and support that help buffer the patient and family from the environment. To reduce stress and increase comfort, complementary and alternative therapies may be provided when the patient indicates an interest. While these therapies may require some modifications based on the patient's condition and environmental factors, such therapies may still produce the desired effects. Holistic care suggests the need to consider the patient in the context of family as a unit; therefore, the needs and desires of the family should be taken into consideration when planning and implementing care. Nurses in high-acuity areas also face changing patient care goals that may shift from maintaining life to providing comfort and preparing the patient and family for death. High-acuity care environments are often noisy, brightly lit, and highly active areas that remain so 24 hours a day, every day. Such a fast-paced environment places on the patient additional sensory stresses that can negatively impact outcomes, and

therefore it requires thoughtful and creative solutions for reducing environmental stressors.

Section One: Impact of Acute Illness on Patient and Family

High-acuity illness results in psychosocial as well as physiological crises. The high-acuity patient and family often must face loss of health, loss of limb, disfigurement, or necessary changes in lifestyle, which in turn may alter the patient's self-image and self-esteem. This section provides a brief review of Kübler-Ross's stages of grief in the context of high-acuity illness. It then presents nursing considerations regarding the importance of incorporating the family into the plan of care and describes the concept of family meetings as one holistic approach.

Kübler-Ross's Stages of Grief

According to Kübler-Ross and Kessler (2005), patients may respond to losses in certain predictable phases. A summary of Kübler-Ross's stages of grief, manifestations, and nursing

Table 2–1 Kübler-Ross's Stages of Grief

Stage	Definition	Manifestations	Interventions
Denial	Diagnosis does not have an emotional meaning.	Patient may avoid talking about their illness.	Nurse provides accurate information when asked and clarifies statements but does not stress reality.
Anger	Patient rejects diagnosis.	Patient may act out, may be demanding and angry or quiet and withdrawn.	Nurse provides consistent nursing care and does not argue with the patient.
Bargaining	Patient attempts to regain control.	Patient may postpone reality by making a "deal"—for example, a deal with God.	Nurse is noncritical and engages in active listening.
Depression	Diagnosis is accepted.	Sadness and crying; patient attempts to improve relationships with family and friends.	Nurse assists patient with problem solving.
Acceptance	Patient's identity is changed.	Patient may openly participate in care.	Nurse promotes self-care and independence.

SOURCE: Data from Kübler-Ross & Kessler. (2005).

interventions appropriate for each stage is presented in Table 2–1.

Denial and Anger   The first stage of denial occurs because the diagnosis does not have an emotional meaning. The denial stage can have positive effects. It may protect the patient against the emotional impact of the illness and conserve energy by removing worry. The nurse should clarify questions and provide accurate information. The patient may become angry and uncooperative because he or she is projecting difficulties onto hospital procedures, equipment, and personnel. In the initial stages, a patient may worry more about the equipment being used than about the diagnosis because the diagnosis may be a threat to life. The patient may be demanding or exhibit signs of withdrawal. Both signs are indicative of anger toward self or others. The nurse should not argue with the patient. Consistent, dependable nursing care should be provided.

Bargaining, Depression, and Acceptance   These three stages are characterized by an attempt to regain control. Patients may express guilt about the illness or injury as a gesture of assuming responsibility for events over which they may or may not have actual control. In this stage a patient may make a bargain with God: "If You will make me well, then I will take better care of myself." The nurse should function as a noncritical listener. During the depression stage, the patient may verbalize fears about the future. New behaviors are initiated that reflect new limitations. The patient may feel sad and have frequent crying episodes. Relationships with family and friends may be reorganized. The nurse can assist by building communication to assist with problem solving. Acceptance, the final stage, involves identity change. The patient may begin to think of the illness as a growing experience. Limitations are accepted as consequences and not as defects. Promoting self-care and independence is an important nursing role during this stage.

Kübler-Ross's stages are not fixed but reflect a dynamic process of adjusting to an acute situation. The patient may regress to an earlier stage during periods of heightened anxiety. One aim in caring for the high-acuity patient is to foster a feeling of security. A patient may feel vulnerable because of physiological changes, such as paralysis. Changes in patient care routines can increase patient anxiety, even when these changes mean the patient is getting better. Examples include removing cardiac electrodes,

weaning from mechanical ventilation, reducing pain medication, and increasing mobility.

Nursing Considerations

As the nurse cares for the high-acuity patient in various stages of acute illness, the patient's family members must also be taken into consideration. The high-acuity patient cannot be considered in isolation. The patient alone defines the members of his or her family. The family may not always be the traditional mother, father, and children. Families may be composed of single parents, same-sex partners, or close friends. The family is defined as the patient perceives it to be.

Because the patient's support system is essential, the high-acuity nursing unit has evolved from a restrictive environment into a more inclusive environment for families. This change is the result of an increasing body of research that demonstrates positive outcomes when family members actively participate in the recovery process of their loved one. Because of this important role, the nurse must identify and meet family needs so that family members can fully participate in the care of the patient.

Families of high-acuity patients in ICUs frequently need information, comfort, support, assurance, and accessibility. ICU families have consistently ranked communication as their first priority. Increased communication is associated with higher levels of family satisfaction. Families want frequent communication about the patient's condition. They want to know why particular interventions are initiated. They experience high levels of emotional distress and need to be reassured frequently and honestly that the patient is receiving the best care possible. Communication must be open, honest, direct, frequent, and ongoing. Proactive communication in the form of a family meeting, beginning early in the patient's ICU stay, helps the nurse to develop a family-centered plan of care (Kodali et al., 2014).

An important aspect of the hospital stay is the family meeting, in which the patient's condition and prognosis are discussed, family concerns are addressed, and mutual decisions about treatment goals are made. Research has established the benefits of early and effective communication; however, despite the evidence, family meetings do not regularly occur in the high-acuity setting (Gay, Pronovost, Bassett, & Nelson, 2009). Barriers to and strategies for organizing family meetings are summarized in Box 2–1.

BOX 2–1 Organizing Family Meetings

Barriers

- Physician schedules
- Multiple specialists
- Inadequate training in communication skills
- Culture and language differences
- Clinician emotional stress
- Lack of designated meeting space
- Poorly defined goals for meetings

Strategies for Facilitation

- Identify convenient blocks of time for all participants.
- Use printed materials to supplement discussion.

- Educate physicians about reimbursement for time spent meeting with families.
- Incorporate daily goal sheets into the family meeting.
- Engage and empower nurses to take an active role in the meeting process.
- Involve other disciplines—social work, pastoral care, PT/OT, palliative care.
- Provide positive reinforcement to clinicians who routinely participate in family meetings.
- Support training in communication skills.
- Encourage family presence in the high-acuity nursing unit.

SOURCE: Data from Gay et al. (2009).

Section One Review

1. A client was involved in a motor vehicle crash and sustained multiple lower-extremity fractures. He will need additional surgery and prolonged physical therapy. The nurse finds the client drawing plans for remodeling his porch to accommodate a wheelchair. This behavior reflects which stage of illness?
   A. Denial
   B. Anger
   C. Depression
   D. Acceptance

2. When interacting with a client in denial, what is the nurse's best strategy?
   A. Reinforce reality
   B. Function as a noncritical listener
   C. Explain the current treatment plan
   D. Help the client recall the injury event

3. What is an appropriate nursing intervention for a client experiencing shock and disbelief about his or her diagnosis?
   A. Active listening
   B. Providing accurate information
   C. Exhibiting empathy
   D. Acknowledging loss

4. Which changes can induce anxiety in the high-acuity client? (Select all that apply.)
   A. Weaning from mechanical ventilation
   B. Increasing pain medication
   C. Increasing mobility
   D. Changing monitoring
   E. Promoting sleep

Answers: 1. D, 2. B, 3. B, 4. (A, C, D)

Section Two: Coping with Acute Illness

There is a growing body of research on the importance of the search for meaning in life-changing events. **Spirituality**, a sense of faith and transcendence, and a sorting out of old life views are frequently part of the experience of the patient and family during acute illness or injury. Questions such as *"Why me?"* and *"Why this?"* and *"Why now?"* become part of the patient's and family's quests for meaning. The nurse can provide a sounding board for such questions and can act as a nonjudgmental listener as patients and families sort out their answers.

Complementary and Alternative Therapies

Various strategies can be used to help patients cope with the psychological and physical stressors of an acute illness.

Complementary and alternative therapies (CAT), such as aromatherapy, therapeutic humor, massage therapy, therapeutic touch, and guided imagery, may be beneficial to the high-acuity patient as a way of reducing stress. CAT may be used in lieu of, or as a complement to, standard medical treatment. It is important to remember that all patients are in need of healing, even if they cannot be cured. The decision to use CAT must be an informed decision. Some patients, because of personal feelings or cultural differences, may not be comfortable with massage or touch therapy, in which case CAT will actually add stress and may inhibit relaxation.

Many patients who are using CAT do not tell their healthcare provider. As the number of patients using CAT increases, so does the risk for side effects. A patient may experience interactions from allopathic medications or adverse effects from overuse. The high-acuity nurse plays an important role in making sure the patient knows what to expect and in helping patients choose therapies that are safe and effective (Kramlich, 2014). The high-acuity nurse must be able to provide evidence-based practice to guide the patient to receive benefit from CAT. Assessing the patient's perceptions of CAT is important to avoid increasing the patient's stress level rather than decreasing it (Burhenn, Olausson, Villegas, & Kravits, 2014).

Aromatherapy **Aromatherapy** is the use of oils to reduce stress and anxiety. Aromatic plant oils such as lavender, jasmine, and others have been shown in small, limited studies to reduce stress and anxiety in acutely ill patients. In a study of 60 patients in a coronary ICU, lavender essential oil increased the quality of sleep and reduced anxiety in patients with coronary artery disease (Karadag, Samancioglu, Ozden, & Bakir, 2015). These oils may be inhaled or used as an enhancement to massage therapy. Aromatherapy is thought to work on physical, spiritual, and psychological levels, complementing medical treatment but not claiming to cure any condition. Aromatherapy is recognized by many state boards of nursing as a component of holistic nursing. Research on the therapeutic effects of essential oils is limited and must be expanded. Aromatherapy will continue to play an essential role in promoting comfort and relaxation in patients.

Therapeutic Humor Humor has been recognized for years as a way of relieving stress. Unlike aromatherapy, which is easy to apply, humor may be difficult for the high-acuity nurse to deliver. However, a skilled nurse may use humor as one complementary and alternative therapy. Humor may be effective in reducing pain, showing the human side of the healthcare team, and helping the patient and family cope. Some nurses may not be comfortable using humor because they feel it is unprofessional, but when used effectively, humor strengthens the bond between the patient, family, and nurse (Allen, 2014).

Massage Therapy and Therapeutic Touch Massage and therapeutic touch may help patients relax, reduce anxiety, and promote sleep. In addition, these therapies are designed to have a positive effect on the vascular, muscular, and nervous systems. The use of massage therapy to relieve pain is widespread as an acceptable intervention. Older adults with advanced cancer accompanied with persistent pain report better overall health when using massage therapy (Marchand, 2014). The high-acuity nurse may use massage

BOX 2–2 Contraindications to Massage Therapy

- Advanced osteoporosis
- Bone fractures
- Burns
- Deep vein thrombosis
- Eczema
- Phlebitis
- Skin infections

therapy to treat all components of pain, which include physical, spiritual, emotional, and social domains. Barriers such as noise, clinical procedures, and staff acceptance need to be addressed for this therapy to be effective (Martorella, Boitor, Michaud, & Gélinas, 2014). Contraindications to massage therapy, as summarized by Ernst, Pittler, and Wider (2006), are listed in Box 2–2.

Guided Imagery **Guided imagery** is a CAT that uses the patient's own positive experiences to promote a vision or fantasy that encourages relaxation. In imagery, the patient focuses on positive thoughts and experiences and blocks out negative ones. Nurses can guide patients through imagery by asking them to place themselves in environments where they remember feeling relaxed. Many people recall the beach or ocean as having a calming effect. An example of imagery is the thought of lying on a beach on a deserted island, listening to the rolling of the surf against the shore, watching the graceful sway of the palm trees, and feeling the cool breezes, while at the same time feeling the warmth of the sun on the skin. Imagery provides an opportunity for the patient to take a vacation or temporary mental escape from the day-to-day realities of the high-acuity environment. Imagery is a CAT that may be beneficial for patients experiencing extensive and painful dressing changes, anxiety, depression, mood disturbance, or pain. Relaxation and the ability to focus are essential for a successful imagery experience (Burhenn et al., 2014).

Box 2–3 provides a case example describing a complementary and alternative therapy (CAT) intervention.

BOX 2–3 Case Example 1: Using Imagery

Mrs. M, a 79-year-old woman, underwent an exploratory laparotomy for a perforated duodenal ulcer. She has a history of chronic airflow limitation and takes daily prednisolone. Her wound is healing by secondary intention, and she experiences significant pain during dressing changes.

The nurse prepares the environment by dimming lights and decreasing noise. He places a sign outside the patient's room indicating that an imagery session is in progress. The nurse promotes relaxation by encouraging the patient to imagine that each muscle is going limp, starting at the top of her head. He describes it as a heavy, good feeling. The nurse tells the patient to concentrate on each body section separately (neck, shoulders, and so on). The patient closes her eyes and concentrates on her body.

Nurse: As the old dressing is removed, your new tissue is getting fresh nutrients because dead skin and bacteria are being

removed along with the gauze. Imagine a tiny skin cell with hands that reach out to join another skin cell to make a firm chain. Although you are a little uncomfortable, you want the dressing to be removed because the new skin cells cannot grow underneath the debris from the old cells. As the new cells get nutrients, there is less drainage and less discomfort. Now, imagine that the skin is completely together just like it was before surgery. There is no need for more dressing changes. Each time your dressing is changed, concentrate on this image of the skin cells joining hands to make a firm chain that is completely joined together and healed. Imagine the cells getting fresh air and food that make them strong.

The goal of this imagery session is to describe positive aspects of the dressing change and replace the patient's fear with a positive image of healing.

Other CAT Modalities   In addition to the previously discussed therapies, the high-acuity patient may pursue other CAT modalities, such as meditation, yoga, t'ai chi, hypnosis, relaxation techniques, or music therapy. Manipulation of energy fields and acupuncture, diet, and dietary supplements also have gained popularity.

Section Two Review

1. How may complementary and alternative therapies be used? (Select all that apply.)
   A. In lieu of standard medical treatment
   B. As a complement to standard medical treatment
   C. Only with a physician's order
   D. In limited situations
   E. Only by a certified therapist

2. Which statement best describes the use of humor as therapy?
   A. Humor is not a way to relieve stress.
   B. Humor is a CAT that can be used with high-acuity clients.
   C. Humor is ineffective in reducing pain.
   D. Humor interferes with the bond between client and nurse.

3. Which conditions are contraindications to massage therapy? (Select all that apply.)
   A. Advanced osteoporosis
   B. Bone fractures
   C. Burns
   D. Deep vein thrombosis
   E. Chest pain

4. Guided imagery may be a useful strategy for clients with which conditions? (Select all that apply.)
   A. Anxiety
   B. Depression
   C. Pain
   D. Hypotension
   E. Delirium

Answers: 1. (A, B), 2. B, 3. (A, B, C, D), 4. (A, B, C)

Section Three: Patient- and Family-centered Care

Providing patient- and family-centered care in high-acuity environments is a continuing challenge as nurses and hospital administrators grapple with the pros and cons of actively involving the family in care of the patient. In addition, providing for the educational needs of the patients and their families is a nursing priority.

Educational Needs of Patients and Families

High-acuity patients have a right to know and understand what procedures are being done to and for them. Initially, when teaching high-acuity patients, the goal is to decrease stress and promote comfort rather than to increase knowledge. The patient and family may not recall what the nurse said 10 minutes later, but the patient's blood pressure may be decreased or the pain lessened. As adult learners, high-acuity patients focus on learning in order to solve problems. Thus, the nurse must assess what the patient considers to be problematic in order to make learning meaningful. Basic questions about what the patient and family want to know will assist the nurse in focusing content. It is also helpful to identify what the patient already knows. An interpersonal relationship allows for the patient to trust the abilities and knowledge of the nurse. For the high-acuity patient to learn, he or she must feel secure.

Several factors inhibit learning in high-acuity patients. Patients may be fatigued because of hypoxemia, anemia, or hypermetabolism. Barriers to communication, such as endotracheal tubes, many hourly interventions, and diagnostic tests, interfere with teaching and learning. Pain diminishes a person's ability to concentrate; drugs may depress the central nervous system and affect memory. The nurse should assess the patient for the presence of these factors. Physiologic needs take precedence over the need to know and the need to understand. Once the patient's condition has stabilized, however, the patient may be able to concentrate on learning. Educational needs of both patients and families must be taken into account to fulfill their needs and facilitate adaptation to critical illness (Polster, 2015). A summary of these educational needs, according to Palazzo (2001), are summarized in Table 2–2.

Engaging both patients and families in care improves outcomes. Governmental agencies such as the Agency for Healthcare Research and Quality (AHRQ) has developed guidelines for patient and family engagement (AHRQ, 2013).

Health Literacy   **Health literacy** is the degree to which patients and families have the ability to obtain, process, and understand basic health information to make informed decisions about their healthcare (Polster, 2015). In addition to English proficiency or the ability to read, health literacy encompasses numerical literacy, the ability to communicate with members of the healthcare team, filling out complex forms, and understanding concepts related to risk and probability. Patients most at risk for a low level of health literacy are those older than 65 years of age, members of minority groups, immigrants, those of a lower socioeconomic status, or those suffering from chronic illness. Some patients who normally take an active role in their healthcare may experience

Table 2–2 Educational Needs of Patients and Families

Educational Needs	Nursing Considerations
Current information about patient progress	Both families and patients need daily information on progress toward recovery. Trends in vital signs, results of laboratory tests, and wound healing are physiologic indicators that the nurse may discuss with the patient. In general, the high-acuity environment encourages a highly motivated learner.
Informed decision making	Most adults are self-directed and want to make informed decisions themselves, not have decisions made by someone else.
Acknowledgment of past	Adult learners have a lifetime of experiences that influence their values and opinions and shape their decisions.
Optimal learning environment	Using the right time and environment is conducive to the learning process. Transforming the high-acuity environment into a learning environment will enhance the learning process and improve retention. Presenting the information at the appropriate time is important.
Orientation to routines and care	Teaching patients and families procedures that will improve their daily life is productive. Teaching patients and families to perform complementary and alternative therapies to relieve pain, reduce stress, and induce sleep may be beneficial to all.
Motivation	Adults are motivated to learn something new when it will have a direct effect on their daily lives.

SOURCE: Data from Palazzo. (2001).

periods of low health literacy during times of depression, uncontrolled pain, or complex medical situations (Mattox, 2010). Patients with low health literacy are at risk for negative outcomes because they are unable to process basic health information that is crucial for their healthcare plan (Ingram & Kautz, 2012). Strategies for the high-acuity nurse to increase health literacy are listed in Box 2–4.

To ensure that patient and family goals for education are being met, the nurse should use return demonstration and teach-back techniques, supplementing the education with additional materials as appropriate.

Transfer Anxiety The transfer to a less acute unit may precipitate **transfer anxiety** in the patient or family. Transferring a medically stable patient out of the ICU is a routine procedure for healthcare providers, but patients and families may have mixed emotions about the event. Transfer anxiety has been defined as anxiety experienced by the individual who moves from a familiar, somewhat secure environment to an environment that is unfamiliar. Although discharge from the ICU is a positive step in terms of physical recovery, many patients experience high levels of anxiety with the transfer from the ICU to another high-acuity unit. In a systematic review of the effects of ICU transfer and discharge, patients and their families reported negative perceptions of care in medical–surgical units, such as less frequent monitoring and reduced nursing involvement (Cypress, 2013).

Several strategies can be used to decrease transfer anxiety. A structured transfer plan is often helpful. It should include strategies to encourage patient and family questions as well as their active involvement in the transfer plan. Optimally, it is best to transfer the patient during the daytime, although this is not always possible. The patient and family should receive information about unit routines and any new equipment and should be introduced to the receiving nurse before the transfer.

Box 2–5 provides a case example of transfer anxiety and how the nurse can deal with it.

Visitation Policies

There has been considerable debate about the effectiveness of open visitation policies in the ICU. Some feel that—although open visitation may be psychologically supportive—it comes with harmful physiologic consequences, interferes with time nurses need to spend caring for patients, and therefore leads

---

BOX 2–4 Strategies for Increasing Health Literacy

- Develop skills to determine low health literacy (observation of incomplete forms).
- Use available screening tests (Rapid Estimate of Adult Literacy in Medicine, or REALM).
- Provide more usable health information (non-print or multimedia resources).
- Incorporate validated tools to evaluate readability of existing health information.

SOURCE: Data from Mattox. (2010).

BOX 2–5 Case Example 2: Transfer Anxiety

Mrs. M, the 79-year-old patient who had an exploratory laparotomy (see Box 2–3), is improving. Her arterial blood gases (ABGs) have improved, and she is being weaned from mechanical ventilation. The nurse has been teaching her about wound care, explaining that there is a higher risk of a wound infection because she is also receiving corticosteroids. Up to this point, the patient has been eager to learn and has asked questions using a writing board; however, this morning she appears anxious.

Before teaching the patient, the nurse assesses the cause of her anxiety. Is it related to hypoxemia secondary to being weaned from mechanical ventilation? The nurse draws blood for an ABG, and the results are within normal limits. The patient's anxiety may be related to the fear of not being able to breathe without the ventilator. When questioned, the patient admits she is frightened about leaving the ICU and moving to another unit. The nurse explains to the patient that she will be assessed regularly to determine her ability to remain off the ventilator. Next, the nurse explains when Mrs. M will be transferred to a lower-acuity unit and the type of monitoring she will receive in the new unit.

to delays in care. Many ICUs in the United States continue to have restrictive visiting policies. However, the emphasis on family- and relationship-based care has changed restrictions on ICU visiting hours. Most patients and their family members prefer open visitation policies. Furthermore, patients who have family at the bedside seem to have less anxiety and hallucinations. The family can comfort the patient in ways not open to the staff and provide information to help the high-acuity nurse individualize the patient's plan of care (Hart, Hardin, Townsend, Ramsey, & Mahrle-Henson, 2013).

Finding a balance between patient, family, and staff needs is a priority. Observing patient–family interactions can provide information about the nature of the patient–family relationship and clues to family needs. The more acutely ill the patient, the more urgent it becomes for family members to be at the bedside to participate in decisions about the plan of care. The high-acuity nurse should perform a proactive assessment of the family's needs and incorporate this into the patient's plan of care (Hart et al., 2013).

Children are often restricted from visiting adult inpatient units because adults often believe they will be overwhelmed and unable to cope or understand. Hospital policies often prevent children from entering high-acuity units because of the risk of infection. Acute illness is a source of stress and disruption for the entire family, especially children. That said, visiting may reassure the child that the family member is alive and has not left them permanently. Negative behavioral and emotional responses have been shown to decrease after a child is allowed to visit a loved one in the ICU (Crider & Pate, 2011). In the instances where the high-acuity patient may not survive, the opportunity to "say goodbye" is very important. The nurse must use age-appropriate language when discussing illness with children. This allows for the planning of specific nursing interventions to best meet the needs of the child. The high-acuity nurse should collaborate with a certified child life specialist if one is available in the facility (Crider & Pate, 2011).

Historically, family members have been restricted from visiting during invasive procedures and cardiopulmonary resuscitation (CPR). Reasons for these restrictions have included fear that the family might lose control, the unpleasantness of what the families would see, insufficient room at the bedside, and increased risk of litigation. Many hospitals do not have written policies for family presence during CPR, yet it appears that many nurses believe families should be present. Advantages of having the family present, as summarized by Zavotsky et al. (2014), are listed in Box 2–6.

Families may need guidance regarding how to visit with the patient. The nurse may discuss the patient's appearance with the family prior to the visit. It is helpful for the family to know that they should speak to the patient in a normal tone of

---

BOX 2–6   Advantages of Family Presence During CPR

- The family is better equipped to make decisions regarding resuscitative efforts.
- The family is able to say goodbye.
- Witnessing the procedure provides a sense of control.
- The family has the ability to preserve the patient's dignity.
- The family who loses a loved one is provided a sense of closure.
- Families who witness CPR express fewer symptoms of posttraumatic stress disorder than those who do not.

SOURCE: Data from Zavotsky et al. (2014).

---

voice, to be comfortable simply being with the patient and not speaking at all, and to ask questions away from the bedside.

Flexible visitation can be established when nurses are consistent and communicate effectively with visitors. A contract between the nursing staff and family members may be effective. Staff must be prepared to set limits to visitation. Written hospital policies should include guidelines that define acceptable behavior and include a zero-tolerance policy that addresses unacceptable behavior, such as drug or alcohol usage, physical or verbal abuse, or the presence of weapons. Other resources can be helpful in meeting the needs of visitors, such as pastoral care, patient relations staff, social services, local support groups, physicians, and hospital administration.

The concept of patient- and family-centered care is being embraced by an increasing number of hospitals. In this care delivery model, family members are not kept away from the bedside of the acutely ill patient. Instead, they are welcomed and encouraged to be present and active in care. Although the nurse is instrumental in making family-centered care a core value in the high-acuity area, all members of the multidisciplinary team play a role in ensuring the family's needs are met. The essential components of patient- and family-centered care according to the Institute for Patient- and Family-Centered Care are listed in Box 2–7.

BOX 2–7   Core Concepts of Patient- and Family-Centered Care

- Dignity and Respect
- Information Sharing
- Participation
- Collaboration

SOURCE: Data from Institute for Patient- and Family-Centered Care.

Emerging Evidence

- Delirium is a common postoperative condition and can lead to increased cost and length of stay. The impact of preoperative education on postoperative delirium, anxiety, days of mechanical ventilation, and ICU length of stay was studied over an 18-month period. Patient education was effective in decreasing the number of mechanical ventilation days. There was no decrease in the level of anxiety, incidence of delirium, or number of ICU days. Further research is needed to determine interventions that will decrease delirium in high-acuity patients (*Chevillon, Hellyar, Madani, Kerr, & Kim, 2015*).

- A high percentage of alarms in high-acuity areas are false. These false alarms contribute to alarm fatigue and result in missed alarms and desensitization. Daily electrocardiogram electrode changes, proper skin preparation, education, and customization of alarm parameters decrease the number of false alarms (*Sendelbach & Funk, 2013*).
- To decrease stress related to family interactions in high-acuity areas, an evidence-based review of the literature produced

two recommendations. First, the interprofessional team should be kept abreast of treatment goals so that messages provided to the family are consistent. Second, a mechanism should be in place that allows for staff to request a debriefing, voice concerns with the treatment plan, decompress, or grieve (*Cypress, 2013*).

Section Three Review

1. When teaching high-acuity clients, what are the initial goals? (Select all that apply.)
   A. To reduce stress
   B. To promote comfort
   C. To increase knowledge
   D. To establish a trusting relationship
   E. To meet established education outcomes

2. Which strategy should the nurse use to reduce transfer anxiety?
   A. Introduce the client and family to the receiving nurse before the transfer occurs.
   B. Transfer the client during the night while he or she is sleeping.
   C. Do not include the family in the transfer until it's over.
   D. Inform the client that he or she will not receive as much nursing care in the lower-acuity unit.

3. What is the effect of unrestricted visiting hours on some clients?
   A. Fatigue
   B. Depression
   C. Fewer hallucinations
   D. Increased anxiety

4. Family presence during CPR contributes to which result?
   A. Ability of family to say goodbye
   B. Increased difficulty of family members moving through the grieving process
   C. Increased fear and anxiety
   D. Inability to promote a sense of closure

Answers: 1. (A, B), 2. A, 3. C, 4. A

Section Four: Cultural Diversity

Nurses work with patients and their families in the most intimate of situations—birth, illness, and often death. Working closely with patients and families during these times requires an appreciation of the diverse beliefs and attitudes that patients and their families bring with them into the hospital. It is a nursing obligation to provide culturally competent nursing care.

Cultural Competence

Cultural competence involves self-awareness—that is, being mindful of one's own beliefs and attitudes without letting them influence the care of patients with different backgrounds. With this self-awareness come knowledge, understanding, respect, and the ability to provide care within the cultural context of patients and their families (Hart & Mareno, 2013). The American Nurses Association (ANA) has recognized the need for nurses to provide culturally competent care. The ANA Code for Nurses (ANA, 2015) states that nurses should "practice with compassion and respect for the inherent dignity, worth and uniqueness of every individual" (p. 17). Nurses who are culturally competent are sensitive to the culture, race, gender, sexual orientation, social class, and economic status of their patients.

Cultural competence is more than just knowledge of another ethnic group. It is essential that the nurse provide culturally competent care to achieve equitable outcomes for all patients. Barriers to providing culturally competent care must be recognized and addressed by nurses in order for the profession to devise solutions (Hart & Mareno, 2013).

Cultural Assessment   The high-acuity environment is not always the most conducive environment for a thorough cultural assessment. However, the nurse cannot provide excellent care without knowledge of the patient's cultural background. Questions that may be asked or observed to better understand a patient's culture, as suggested by Lipson, Dibble, and Minarik (2001), are listed in Box 2–8.

Effective communication may be hindered by language differences. When family members serve as interpreters, the complete message may not be transmitted due to lack of medical vocabulary or family role conflicts. The family member may transmit the information with his or her own perceptions. Certain details may be eliminated due to embarrassment. When working with an interpreter, the high-acuity nurse must exhibit patience. Speaking in short units of speech and using simple language may convey the information more effectively. Observe the patient for nonverbal cues.

Other Sources of Diversity   In addition to assessing a patient's cultural background, other sources of diversity must be considered. Immigrants and refugees may have specific health beliefs and practices. It is important to determine

BOX 2–8   Cultural Assessment: Questions to Ask or Observe

1. Where was the patient born? Is the patient an immigrant? How long has the patient lived in this country?
2. What is the patient's ethnic affiliation?
3. Who makes up the patient's support system? Does the patient live in an ethnic community?
4. What is the primary (or secondary) language? What language does the patient or family prefer to speak or write?
5. How does the patient communicate nonverbally?
6. What is the patient's religious preference? Does it play an important role in the patient's life?
7. Does the patient have food preferences or prohibitions?
8. What is the patient's economic status?
9. Does the patient have specific health or illness practices or beliefs?
10. Does the patient or family have specific customs or beliefs related to illness, birth, or death?

SOURCE: Data from Lipson et al. (2001).

BOX 2–9   Using CRASH to Develop Cultural Competence

C	**C**onsider **C**ulture
R	show **R**espect
A	**A**ssess and **A**ffirm differences
S	**S**how **S**ensitivity and **S**elf-awareness
H	provide care with **H**umility

SOURCE: Data from Rust et al. (2006).

why these patients left their homeland and what drew them to the United States. Racial and ethnic considerations must be taken into account. **Race** refers to human biological variation, and **ethnicity** refers to a set of social, cultural, and political beliefs held by a group of individuals. Socioeconomic status (income, education, and occupation) may have a strong influence on healthcare beliefs and access to the healthcare system. Sexual orientation also should be taken into account. The nurse must collect these important data and communicate in a nonjudgmental manner.

Developing Cultural Competence

How, then, does a high-acuity nurse develop competence? One model proposed by Rust et al. (2006) suggests a core set of skills defined by the mnemonic CRASH (Box 2–9). In considering culture, the high-acuity nurse must assess individual patient characteristics such as national origin, faith, and education. Accounting for individual characteristics helps to prevent stereotyping. Conveying respect for the patient's unique health or illness beliefs is essential for developing cultural competence. Assessing and affirming differences is crucial as it relates to language preferences. Educational material must be presented in a language and at a level of understanding that meet the needs of the patient. Sensitivity is addressed during the initial assessment of health practices, health beliefs, dietary preferences, and home remedies. Providing culturally competent care requires looking at the patient's culture without judgment ("Culturally competent nursing care," 2015).

Section Four Review

1. Which statement best describes cultural diversity?
   A. Acute physical need makes attention to cultural diversity unimportant.
   B. Cultural diversity plays an important role in the care of the high-acuity client.
   C. There are four components in cultural diversity.
   D. Cultural diversity is composed of six components.

2. How can the nurse enhance communication with clients?
   A. Disregarding nonverbal cues
   B. Incorporating medical vocabulary
   C. Avoiding eye contact
   D. Speaking in small units of speech

3. Which term describes a set of social, cultural, and political beliefs held by a group of individuals?
   A. Race
   B. Socioeconomic status
   C. Ethnicity
   D. Sexual orientation

4. Which nursing skills demonstrate cultural competence? (Select all that apply.)
   A. Showing respect
   B. Assessing and affirming differences
   C. Showing sensitivity
   D. Providing care with humility
   E. Judging client actions

Answers: 1. B, 2. D, 3. C, 4. (A, B, C, D)

Section Five: Environmental Stressors

Sensory input involves all five senses: visual, auditory, olfactory, gustatory, and tactile. Individual perceptions of stimuli to the senses vary. People usually select stimuli that are most acceptable to them. However, during acute illness, the patient does not have control over the choice of the environment and its stimuli. Very young, very old, and postoperative or unresponsive patients are at greatest risk of experiencing **sensory perceptual alterations (SPAs)**. Acutely ill patients who develop SPAs may be at risk for the development of additional complications.

Sensory Perceptual Alterations

A combination of sensory overload and deprivation can exist in the high-acuity environment. The patient is deprived of normal sensory stimuli while being exposed to continuous strange stimuli. The nurse should assess what sounds are in the patient's normal environment and expose the patient to these sounds, if possible (through tape recordings). Visitors can be effective by discussing familiar topics with the patient. Unresponsive patients are particularly challenging because information about the patient's normal environment must be collected through a third person. It is difficult to assess whether unresponsive patients are experiencing sensory alterations because they cannot communicate.

Sensory Overload and Deprivation Sensory overload may occur when the patient is exposed to noise for continuous periods. The background environmental noise in a high-acuity unit includes annoying and frightening alarms, ringing telephones, pagers, staff conversations, loud overhead announcement systems, ventilators, cardiac monitors, the bubbling of chest tubes, and other strange and foreign sounds. However, patients report they are most disturbed by the staff's loud voices, especially at night when they interrupt sleep. The World Health Organization recommends sound levels of 35dB or less in patient rooms (Berglund, Lindvall, & Schwela, 1999). Noise in high-acuity areas often exceeds this level. Moreover, excessive noise has an adverse effect on both the physical and physiological state of the nurse resulting in stress for caregivers which may be detrimental to the quality of patient care (Riemer, Mates, Ryan, & Schleder, 2015).

Delirium Sensory perceptual alterations or other physical disruptions may cause **delirium** in the high-acuity patient. Although most clinicians would recognize delirium as an abnormal state, it is important for the nurse to ascertain the cause of the delirium. Features of delirium include an acute onset of fluctuating awareness, impaired ability to attend to environmental stimuli, and disorganized thinking (Andrews, Silva, Kaplan, & Zimbro, 2015). Delirium is often preceded by anxiety and restlessness that escalate to confusion and agitation. Hypoxemia, alcohol or barbiturate withdrawal, hyponatremia, drug adverse reactions, infections, and liver dysfunction can cause delirium. It is extremely important to rule out and treat any underlying causes of delirium rather than merely medicating the patient to control behavior.

Sleep Deprivation Alterations in the light or dark cycle, pain, environmental noise, caregiver interruptions, and stress can contribute to the inability of hospitalized patients to get adequate sleep and rest. Sedative hypnotics are often the preferred method for sleep disturbances, but this method has been linked to an increase in falls, delirium, and functional decline in patients, particularly in the elderly.

Interventions to Decrease Sensory Perceptual Alterations

Sensory perceptual alterations have a negative impact on the patient's physiological and psychological health, which can slow healing and may result in other complications. It is important for the nurse to implement a plan to minimize these alterations when possible.

Prevent Sleep Deprivation Interventions that contribute to the nonpharmacologic induction of sleep should be implemented. Planned rest periods that allow for 2 hours of uninterrupted sleep are essential to promoting rapid eye movement (REM) sleep (Ritmala-Castren, Virtanen, Leivo, Kaukonen, & Leino-Kilpi, 2015). REM sleep facilitates protein anabolism, restores the immune system, and promotes healing. Providing the patient with a few hours of REM sleep can be beneficial. Nurses should act as patient advocates to control the patient's environment and ensure adequate sleep and rest periods throughout the day and night. Closing the patient's door and posting a sign on it is often effective. Other nursing interventions include the following:

- Providing relaxing music of the patient's choice, or earplugs for those who prefer silence
- Controlling the patient's pain (essential to promoting REM sleep)
- Placing pagers on vibrate mode
- Turning down (or turning off) the volume of the overhead announcement system in patient care areas
- Decreasing the volume of alarms on equipment
- Adjusting light levels and offering eye masks to patients
- Encouraging ancillary services, such as physical therapy or respiratory therapy, to return after the patient has rested, if appropriate
- Limiting visitation during quiet time
- Helping the patient prepare mentally for quiet time through therapeutic touch or massage, guided imagery, or aromatherapy
- Planning a daily schedule for the patient that includes a quiet time every day so the patient can look forward to a time of relaxation and rest

Facilitate Communication Communicating with mechanically ventilated patients is very important to prevent SPA and promote a therapeutic nurse–patient relationship. The patient's inability to talk may cause high levels of stress, insecurity, and even panic. For many patients, the family's presence can promote a sense of security and relaxation. It is important for the high-acuity nurse to understand that family members are more likely than others to recognize when a patient is not behaving normally (Fink, Makic, Poteet, & Oman, 2015). However, patients and families can also become frustrated because they cannot understand lip reading. An experienced nurse is often helpful because he or she has more experience using lip-reading techniques with an intubated patient. Although many nurses use nonverbal communication with their patients, most of that communication is at a very concrete level—pertaining only to physical care and including short, task-oriented communication that does not provide emotional support. The behaviors that the nurse uses during these encounters can affect the quality of the interaction and patient outcomes, including satisfaction (Nilsen et al., 2014).

Patients use a variety of forms of nonverbal communication. Vital signs, such as an elevated heart rate or blood pressure, are one form of nonverbal communication. Facial expressions, such as smiling, grimacing, or even crying and laughing, can be valuable forms of communication. Hand gestures, such as grabbing the nurse's arm, holding hands, or even moving the legs around, are a method of communication. Some patients are able to write messages very clearly, whereas others attempt to write and simply become frustrated as they experience fine-motor difficulty or cannot see clearly. Large pen markers may be easier than thin pens or pencils for the patient to manipulate. Using computer keyboards or pointing to letters on alphabet boards requires gross motor skills. A coded eye-blink system may be used for patients who are unable to move anything else.

Section Five Review

1. Which noise do high-acuity clients report as being most annoying?
   A. Ambulance siren
   B. Staff's loud voices
   C. Television
   D. Equipment noise

2. The nurse is aware that REM sleep has which effects on the client? (Select all that apply.)
   A. Facilitates protein anabolism
   B. Lowers blood pressure and pulse
   C. Promotes healing
   D. Restores the immune system
   E. Reduces glycogen storage

3. Which nursing interventions would support the client's REM sleep? (Select all that apply.)
   A. Dimming lights during normal sleep time
   B. Putting up a wall clock in the client's room
   C. Reducing environmental noise
   D. Providing opioid analgesia at bedtime
   E. Limiting visitation during quiet time

4. What is a common characteristic of delirium? (Select all that apply.)
   A. Labile blood pressure
   B. Inability to attend to environmental stimuli
   C. Acute onset
   D. Disorganized thinking
   E. Agitation

Answers: 1. B, 2. (A, C, D), 3. (A, C, D, E), 4. (B, C, D, E)

Clinical Reasoning Checkpoint

This values clarification exercise is designed to help the learner explore personal values in relation to the profession of nursing and bioethical issues. By reflecting on personal values, we gain a better understanding of what factors may limit our ability to reason clearly and of when we may not be suitable for the role of patient advocate.

Values Clarification Exercise

Directions: To the left of each statement, place the number that best explains your position: 1 = mostly agree, 2 = somewhat agree, 3 = neutral, 4 = somewhat disagree, 5 = mostly disagree.

_____ 1. Infants with severe handicaps ought to be left to die.

_____ 2. Extraordinary medical treatment is always indicated.

_____ 3. My role as a nurse is to always resuscitate patients who could benefit from it, no matter what has been decided previously.

_____ 4. I must follow physician's orders.

_____ 5. Older patients should be allowed to die with dignity.

_____ 6. Medical technology has advanced the quality of life.

_____ 7. Children should not be involved in giving consent for treatments.

_____ 8. Families ought to make decisions about life or death situations without involving the patient.

_____ 9. Children should participate in human experimentation that is not harmful even if it is of no benefit to them.

_____ 10. Prisoners should participate in scientific experiments to repay society for their wrongdoings.

_____ 11. Women should seek medical care from female physicians to avoid potential discrimination.

_____ 12. Children whose parents refuse medical care for them should be removed from their families through court action.

_____ 13. Research using fetuses should be pursued vigorously.

_____ 14. Life-support systems should be discontinued after several days of flat electroencephalograms.

_____ 15. Health professionals are a scarce resource in many parts of the country.

_____ 16. Nursing is a subservient profession, especially to the medical profession.

_____ 17. As a nurse, I must relinquish my personal philosophy to support the philosophies of others.

_____ 18. All patients, regardless of differences, should be treated in a humanistic way.

_____ 19. I should give mouth-to-mouth resuscitation to a derelict if he needs it.

_____ 20. A child who is disabled has value.

_____ 21. All forms of human life have value.

_____ 22. I should be involved in decision making regarding ethical issues in practice.

_____ 23. Committees should decide who receives scarce resources, such as kidneys.

_____ 24. Patients' individual rights should be more important than the rights of society at large.

_____ 25. A person has the right to make a living will.

_____ 26. Underdeveloped countries should be given health and financial support by developed countries.

_____ 27. I should support all the positions on ethical issues taken by my professional association.

_____ 28. The care component of nursing practice is not as important as the cure component of medical practice.

_____ 29. The nurse's primary role in decision making on ethical issues is to implement the selected alternative.

_____ 30. I feel afraid when caring for a patient who is dying.

_____ 31. Children who have disabilities should be institutionalized.

_____ 32. Patients in mental health institutions and prisons should be given behavior modification therapy to make them conform to societal norms.

_____ 33. Personal possessions of patients should be removed to guarantee safekeeping during hospitalization.

_____ 34. Patients should have access to their own health information.

_____ 35. Withholding health information fosters the patient's recovery.

_____ 36. A patient with kidney failure is always able to get kidney dialysis when needed.

_____ 37. Society should bear the cost of extraordinary medical interventions.

_____ 38. Confidentiality is an important part of the nurse's role.

_____ 39. As a nurse, I should value responsibility.

_____ 40. Nurses have a right to withhold information to facilitate nursing research on human subjects.

_____ 41. The patient who refuses treatment should be dropped from the health supervision of an agency or professional.

_____ 42. Transplantations should be done whenever needed.

Personal Application

1. Add the number of 1s, 2s, 3s, 4s, and 5s that you have.

2. How many statements do you have clear ideas (1s and 5s) about?

3. Do these outweigh the number of ambivalent (neutral) statements you listed?

4. Look at the statements that you agree with (1s and 2s). Is there a relationship between the statements that influenced your responses (e.g., age of patient, patient acuity)?

5. Look at the statements that you disagree with (4s and 5s). Is there a relationship between these statements that influenced your responses?

6. Analyze the following cluster of statements. Is there any consistency in the way you rated these statements? What variables influenced your decision?

   Cluster 5, 8, 14, 25, 30: Relates to issues pertaining to death

   Cluster 3, 4, 16, 17, 22, 27, 28, 29, 38: Relates to the profession of nursing

   Cluster 2, 6, 14, 36, 37, 42: Relates to issues raised by advanced technology

   Cluster 1, 7, 9, 12, 20, 31: Relates to children

   Cluster 9, 10, 13, 40: Relates to human experimentation

   Cluster 3, 7, 8, 11, 12, 18, 19, 21, 24, 25, 33, 34, 35, 38, 41: Relates to patients' rights

   Cluster 9, 10, 24, 26, 32, 37: Relates to society's rights

   Cluster 15, 23, 36: Relates to allocation of resources

   Cluster 3, 4, 17, 18, 19, 22, 27, 29, 39: Relates to perceptions of obligations

SOURCE: Adapted from Steele & Harmon. (1983).

Chapter 2 Review

1. A client is crying about a below-knee amputation sustained as a pedestrian in a pedestrian–vehicle crash. She expresses fears about ambulating in physical therapy. The nurse interprets this situation as a sign that the client is in which stage of illness?

   1. Denial
   2. Bargaining
   3. Depression
   4. Acceptance

2. A client was recently admitted to the ICU after a myocardial infarction. The family wants to meet with the nurse. The nurse prepares for this meeting with the knowledge that at this stage of illness the family most needs which things? (Select all that apply.)

   1. Frequent updates on the client's condition
   2. Rationale for interventions being started
   3. Easy access to food
   4. A comfortable place to stay
   5. Social service information on insurance benefits

3. The nurse is considering use of a complementary and alternative therapy (CAT) to help a client cope with the pain associated with burn treatment. The nurse designs this plan with full consideration that which CAT is a risky strategy?
   1. Humor
   2. Aromatherapy
   3. Massage therapy
   4. Guided imagery

4. High-acuity clients have a right to know and understand what procedures are being done to and for them. The nurse sets which initial goals when teaching the client about these procedures? (Select all that apply.)
   1. To decrease the client's stress
   2. To promote client comfort
   3. To increase the client's knowledge
   4. To facilitate recall of events
   5. To decrease the client's fatigue

5. The nurse is conducting an admission assessment on a client who is an immigrant to the United States. How would the nurse demonstrate cultural competence when caring for this client?
   1. Consider that the client's culture may differ significantly from that of the nurse.
   2. Be respectful of the client and the family when providing care.
   3. When cultural differences are assessed, confirm their presence with the client or family.
   4. Use knowledge of typical members of the client's nationality to guide care.
   5. Be aware of the impact of cultural differences on the nurse.

6. A client has been an active participant in all aspects of hospitalization. This morning the client seems confused and has difficulty completing a form documenting consent to a procedure to be done tomorrow. What nursing actions are indicated? (Select all that apply.)
   1. Initiate a request for an order for sedating medication.
   2. Recommend that the planned procedure be delayed.
   3. Review the client's most recent laboratory results.
   4. Assess the client for other findings of depression.
   5. Have a family member complete the required form.

7. A 79-year-old client had a colon resection with colostomy two days ago for adenocarcinoma. She has had a patient-controlled analgesia pump for pain management. Since yesterday she has become increasingly anxious and agitated. Today she is suddenly yelling out for help, is combative, and has pulled out her nasogastric tube. The nurse should recognize that this client is exhibiting symptoms of which condition?
   1. Delirium
   2. Sleep deprivation
   3. Sensory overload
   4. Overdose of narcotics

8. The hospital supports open visitation throughout the facility. Family members visiting in the coronary care unit have been noisy and disruptive even after being asked to keep down the level of their voices. What nursing action is indicated?
   1. Ask the visitors to leave the unit.
   2. Tell the visitors they can stay if they are quiet.
   3. Ask the client if the visitors should leave.
   4. Call the client's physician for a "no visitors" order.

9. A client in the ICU speaks only broken English. The nurse has been unsuccessful in understanding information, and it is apparent the client does not understand the nurse. How should the nurse proceed?
   1. Have a family member stay in the room at all times.
   2. Ask a friend to interpret for the client.
   3. Write down all instructions and use a white board for the client.
   4. Call social services and request an interpreter.

10. A client has developed confusion while in the ICU. Medical reasons for the confusion have been ruled out and a diagnosis of sensory perceptual alterations made. What should the nurse tell visitors about this client?
    1. Only one person at a time should visit.
    2. Talk about familiar and calming things while in the room.
    3. The client cannot have visitors.
    4. Do not bring cell phones or other objects that make noise into the room.

Answers to questions found inside your textbook are available on the faculty resources site. Please consult with your instructor.

References

Agency for Healthcare Research and Quality (AHRQ). (2013). *Guide to patient and family engagement in hospital quality and safety.* Retrieved October 7, 2015, from http://www.ahrq.gov/professionals/systems/hospital/engagingfamilies/index.html

Allen, D. (2014). Laughter really can be the best medicine. *Nursing Standard, 28*(32), 24–25. doi:10.7748/ns2014.04.28.32.24.s28

American Nurses Association (ANA). (2015). *Code of ethics for nurses.* Retrieved January 11, 2017, from http://www .nursingworld.org/codeofethics

Andrews, L., Silva, S., Kaplan, S., & Zimbro, K. (2015). Delirium monitoring and patient outcomes in a general intensive care unit. *American Journal of Critical Care,* 24(1), 48–56. doi:10.4037/ajcc2015740

Berglund, B., Lindvall, T., & Schwela, D. H. (1999). *Guidelines for community noise.* Retrieved January 11, 2017, from http://apps.who.int/iris/handle/10665/66217

Burhenn, P., Olausson, J., Villegas, G., & Kravits, K. (2014). Guided imagery for pain control. *Clinical Journal of Oncology Nursing,* 18(5), 501–503. doi:10.1188/14. CJON.501-503

Chevillon, C., Hellyar, M., Madani, C., Kerr, K., & Kim, S. (2015). Preoperative education on postoperative delirium, anxiety, and knowledge in pulmonary thromboendarterectomy clients, *American Journal of Critical Care,* 24(2), 164–171. doi:10.4037/ajcc2015658

Crider, J., & Pate, M. (2011). Helping children say goodbye to loved ones in adult and pediatric intensive care units: Certified child life specialist–critical care nurse partnership. *AACN Advanced Critical Care,* 22(2), 109–112.

Culturally competent nursing care and promoting diversity in our nursing workforce. (2015). *Michigan Nurse,* 88(3), 7–11.

Cypress, B. (2013). Transfer out of intensive care: An evidence-based literature review. *Dimensions of Critical Care Nursing,* 32(5), 244–261. doi:10.1097/ DCC.0b013e3182a07646

Ernst, E., Pittler, M., & Wider, B. (Eds.). (2006). *The desktop guide to complementary and alternative medicine: An evidence-based approach* (2nd ed.). St. Louis, MO: Mosby/ Edinburgh, Scotland: Elsevier.

Fink, R., Makic, M., Poteet, A. W., & Oman, K. (2015). The ventilated patient's experience. *Dimensions of Critical Care Nursing,* 34(5), 301–308. doi:10.1097/ DCC.0000000000000128

Gay, E., Pronovost, P., Bassett, R., & Nelson, J. (2009). The intensive care unit family meetings: Making it happen. *Journal of Critical Care,* 24(4), 629.e1–629.e12.

Hart, A., Hardin, S., Townsend, A., Ramsey, S., & Mahrle-Henson, A. (2013). Critical care visitation: Nurse and family preference. *Dimensions of Critical Care Nursing,* 32(6), 289–299. doi:10.1097/01. DCC.0000434515.58265.7d

Hart, P., & Mareno, M. (2013). Cultural challenges and barriers through the voices of nurses. *Journal of Clinical Nursing,* 23, 2223–2233. doi:10.1111/jocn.12500

Ingram, R., & Kautz, D. (2012). When the patient and family just do not get it: Overcoming low health literacy in critical care. *Dimensions of Critical Care Nursing,* 3(1), 25–30. doi:10.1097/DCC.0b013e31823a5471

Institute for Patient- and Family-Centered Care. (n.d.). *Core concepts of patient- and family-centered care.* Retrieved November 28, 2016, from http://www.ipfcc .org/pdf/CoreConcepts.pdf

Karadag, E., Samancioglu, S., Ozden, D., & Bakir, E. (2015). Effects of aromatherapy on sleep quality and anxiety of clients. *Nursing in Critical Care,* 20(5), 1–8. doi:10.1111/nicc.12198

Kodali, S., Stametz, R., Bengier, A., Clarke, D., Layon, A., & Darer, J. (2014). Family experience with intensive care unit care: Association of self-reported family conferences and family satisfaction. *Journal of Critical Care,* 29(4), 641–644. doi:10.1016/j.jcrc.2014.03.012

Kramlich, D. (2014). Introduction to complementary, alternative and traditional therapies. *Critical Care Nurse,* 34(6), 50–56. doi:10.4037/ccn2014807

Kübler-Ross, E. K., & Kessler, D. (2005). *On grief and grieving: Finding the meaning of grief through the five stages of loss.* New York, NY: Scribner.

Lipson, J., Dibble, S., & Minarik, P. (Eds.). (2001). *Culture & nursing care: A pocket guide.* San Francisco, CA: UCSF Nursing Press.

Marchand, L. (2014). Integrative and complementary therapies for clients with advanced cancer. *Annals of Palliative Medicine,* 3(3), 160–171. doi:10.3978/j. issn.2224-5820.2014.07.01

Martorella, G., Boitor, M., Michaud, C., & Gélinas, C. (2014). Feasibility and acceptability of hand massage therapy for pain management of postoperative cardiac surgery clients in the intensive care unit. *Heart & Lung,* 43(5), 437–444. doi:10.1016/j.hrtlng.2014.06.047

Mattox, E. (2010). Identifying vulnerable patients at heightened risk for medical error. *Critical Care Nurse,* 30(2), 61–69.

Nilsen, M., Happ, M., Donovan, H., Barnato, A., Hoffman, L., & Sereika, S. (2014). Adaptation of a communication interaction behavior instrument for use in mechanically ventilated, nonvocal older adults. *Nursing Research,* 63(1), 3–13. doi:10.1097/NNR.0000000000000012

Palazzo, M. O. (2001). Teaching in crisis. Patient and family education in critical care. *Critical Care Clinics of North America,* 13, 83–92.

Polster, D. (2015). Information: Tools for success. *Nursing,* 45(5), 42–49. doi:10.1097/01.NURSE.0000463652.55908.75

Riemer, H., Mates, J., Ryan, L., & Schleder, B. (2015). Decreased stress levels in nurses: A benefit of quiet time. *American Journal of Critical Care,* 24(5), 396–402. doi:10.4037/ajcc2015706

Ritmala-Castren, M., Virtanen, I., Leivo, S., Kaukonen, K., & Leino-Kilpi, H. (2015). Sleep and nursing care activities in an intensive care unit. *Nursing and Health Sciences,* 17, 354–361. doi:10.1111/nhs.12195

Rust, G., Kondwani, K., Martinez, R., Dansie, R., Wong, W., Fry-Johnson, Y., . . . Strothers, H. (2006). A crash-course in cultural competence. *Ethnicity and Disease,* 16(2, suppl. 3), 29–36.

Sendelbach, S., & Funk, M. (2013). Alarm fatigue, a patient safety concern. *Advanced Critical Care,* 24(4), 378–386. doi:10.1097/NCI.0b013e3182a903f9

Steele, S., & Harmon, V. (1983). *Values clarification in nursing.* Norwalk, CT: Appleton-Century Crofts.

Zavotsky, K., McCoy, J., Bell, G., Haussman, K., Joiner, J., Marcoux, K., . . . & Tortajada, D. (2014). Resuscitation team perceptions of family presence during CPR. *Advanced Emergency Nursing Journal,* 36(4), 325–334. doi:10.1097/TME.0000000000000027

Chapter 3
Palliative and End-of-life Care

Learning Outcomes

3.1 Examine the role of palliative care for the high-acuity patient and family.

3.2 Identify ways the nurse can facilitate therapeutic communication for palliative care to help high-acuity patients and their families cope with an illness and/or injury event.

3.3 Describe the assessment and management of pain and other symptoms typically experienced by high-acuity patients.

3.4 Discuss nursing competencies to provide high-quality nursing care to patients and families at the end of life, including bereavement services.

3.5 Identify professional stressors, their impact on high-acuity nurses, and strategies to alleviate those stressors.

This chapter focuses on palliative and end-of-life care in the high-acuity setting, where a heavy emphasis is placed on technology and procedures as mainstays of healthcare. Technology provides vital information to help practitioners determine the severity of illness, treat underlying pathology, and assess the response to treatment. This also means there are more choices about when to use technology, more potential interventions for patients, and an increased need for education and advocacy in a treatment-focused environment. The low nurse-to-patient ratios in intensive care units promote close observation and rapid intervention when addressing the changing health status of patients and the psychosocial needs of families. In general, the ability of the nurse to provide dedicated attention to one or two patients at a time can aid in the provision of palliative care in the high-acuity environment.

In the past, being admitted to a critical care unit meant that the goals of care were directed toward maintaining the patient's life, and all interventions worked toward that goal. If the patient survived to be transferred, it was considered a "win," and if the patient died, it was considered a "defeat." Times have changed; now it is common for nurses to be required to switch care goals from maintaining life to providing palliative and possibly end-of-life care.

Section One: Palliative Care

Palliative care should be offered to patients early in the occurrence of a serious or life-threatening illness or when physical or emotional symptoms are interfering with treatment and/or quality of life. Unfortunately, palliative care is more likely to be suggested as patients move into the last stages of illness. Palliative care is a larger construct than just "end-of-life" care. Understanding the various trajectories of approaching death is important knowledge that enables clinicians to discern which clinical situations call for palliative care.

Historically, an acutely ill patient was once clearly distinguished from a terminally ill patient. Nurses and physicians focused their efforts on saving lives, not providing end-of-life care. Despite advances in technology, it is impossible to predict which patients will die in the acute care setting and which will live. There may not be a time when it is clear that care needs to shift from a cure-oriented to a comfort-oriented approach; consequently, distinctions between acute and terminal illnesses may be unclear. Therefore, it is incumbent on the high-acuity nurse to provide care that is comprehensive and includes attending to the comfort needs of patients and families. Patients attempting to prolong life as well as those who are at the end of life must have their pain controlled and receive ongoing communication regarding their prognosis. End-of-life care and high-acuity care must converge and not conflict. As a result, patients who do not die in the high-acuity setting should be referred to hospice when available.

What Is Palliative Care?

Palliative care is an interdisciplinary approach to relieve suffering and improve quality of life. The care is directed toward patients with life-threatening illness and their families. Nursing and medical treatments are combined with control of pain and symptoms. Common symptoms addressed by the team include shortness of breath, fatigue, constipation, nausea, loss of appetite, and difficulty sleeping. Less than a decade ago, intensive care and palliative care were thought to be mutually exclusive.

It is important for the high-acuity nurse to explain to patients and their families that palliative care may be provided at the same time that medical treatment is directed toward a cure (McAdam & Puntillo, 2015). Palliative care programs incorporate the services of medical and nursing specialists, social workers, and chaplains. Most insurance companies, including Medicare and Medicaid, often cover part or all of the costs for palliative care treatment. This may even include medical supplies and equipment (Center to Advance Palliative Care, n.d.).

National Consensus Project In 2001, in response to the poor state of end-of-life care in the United States, and due to the multidisciplinary nature of palliative care, six professional organizations joined forces to set guidelines to improve the delivery of palliative care services (Dahlin & Wittenberg, 2015). Dubbed the National Consensus Project for Quality Palliative Care (NCP), the consortium consists of members of the Hospice and Palliative Nurses Association (HPNA), the American Academy of Hospice and Palliative Medicine (AAHPM), the Center to Advance Palliative Care (CAPC), the National Association of Social Workers (NASW), the National Hospice and Palliative Care Organization (NHPCO), and the National Palliative Care Research Center (NPCRC) (National Consensus Project for Quality Palliative Care [NCP], n.d.). The NCP's Clinical Practice Guidelines for Quality Palliative Care is a document that promotes optimal palliative care by standardizing the care with the goal of improving palliative care throughout the United States (NCP, 2013). The NCP defines eight domains of palliative care, listed in Box 3–1.

Palliative Care in High-Acuity Settings

The delivery of palliative care can take place in a variety of settings on behalf of patients experiencing a wide array of medical diagnoses. Nurses, physicians, and other healthcare professionals must engage in complex planning with patients and their families to provide optimal care. Because of the multiple factors that can impact the quality of care, barriers must be addressed as interventions are planned and executed.

High-Acuity Patients and Palliative Care Cancer is the disease often associated with palliative care. However, other serious illnesses cause pain and symptoms that interfere with quality of life and lead to death. These may include

---

BOX 3–1 National Consensus Project Domains of Palliative Care

- Domain 1: Structure and processes of care
- Domain 2: Physical aspects of care
- Domain 3: Psychological and psychiatric aspects of care
- Domain 4: Social aspects of care
- Domain 5: Spiritual, religious, and existential aspects of care
- Domain 6: Cultural aspects of care
- Domain 7: Care of the patient at the end of life
- Domain 8: Ethical and legal aspects of care

SOURCE: Data from National Consensus Project for Quality Palliative Care. (n.d.).

---

cardiac disease (e.g., heart failure [HF]), chronic respiratory disorders (e.g., chronic obstructive pulmonary disease [COPD]), end-stage renal failure (ESRF), acquired immune deficiency syndrome (AIDS), and neurological diseases (e.g., Parkinson disease). Common advanced-illness experiences by patients in high-acuity settings include severe pneumonia, systemic inflammatory response syndrome (SIRS), sepsis, acute respiratory distress syndrome (ARDS), acute renal failure, multisystem organ dysfunction syndrome (MODS), bacterial endocarditis, viral infections (e.g., influenza), necrotizing fasciitis, meningitis/encephalitis, intra-abdominal pathogens (e.g., intra-abdominal abscesses, peritonitis, toxic megacolon), central line infection in an immunosuppressed patient, and urosepsis. Patients with multiple comorbidities may be at higher risk for mortality.

Palliative care in the hospital setting is needed for several reasons. Unmet needs of dying patients and concerns about the cost of high-acuity care and limited bed availability have fostered the growth of palliative care in hospital settings. The number of people who live with complex illnesses is growing. To meet the needs of these patients and their families, hospitals must find a way to deliver high-quality, cost-effective care. In the past, hospitals adopted a model that embraced treatment and quick discharge; however, not all patients fit this model. Palliative care, as a systematic approach to patient care in the ICU, provides an extra layer of support to critically ill patients and their families, as outlined in Box 3–2 (Center to Advance Palliative Care, 2013).

The goal of palliative care is to improve quality of life (Center to Advance Palliative Care, 2013). A nurse, physician, family member, patient, social worker, or case manager may initiate a referral to the palliative care team. Components of ICU palliative care in the ICU as identified by high-acuity care professionals are listed in Box 3–3.

Barriers to Providing Palliative Care The high-acuity nurse faces barriers to caring for patients who can benefit the most from palliative care. Patients, families, and, in some instances, members of the healthcare team may have inflated expectations of the outcome of medical therapies. They find it difficult to move from a process of curing to a process of caring, which delays attention to palliative needs. The high-acuity environment has been a place where healthcare professionals work in "silos." In general, barriers to the delivery of palliative care include misunderstandings, difficulties with initiating a discussion regarding

> **BOX 3–2**   Benefits of Palliative Care in the ICU
>
> - Decreased ICU length of stay
> - Decreased hospital length of stay
> - Increased family understanding
> - Increased consensus between families and providers
> - Increased consensus among provider groups
> - Decreased family anxiety and posttraumatic stress
> - Decreased use of ventilators
> - Decreased use of artificial hydration and nutrition
> - Increased number of family meetings
> - Increased percentage of patient status changes to do-not-resuscitate orders
>
> **SOURCE:** Adapted from Aslakson et al. (2014) and Baker et al. (2015).

> **BOX 3–3**   Components of Palliative Care in the ICU
>
> - Symptom management and comfort care
> - Communication among team members and with patients and families
> - Patient- and family-centered decision making
> - Emotional and practical support for patients and families
> - Spiritual support for patients and families
> - Continuity of care
> - Emotional and organizational support for ICU clinicians
>
> **SOURCE:** Adapted from Clarke et al. (2003).

palliative care, and cultural issues (Perrin & Kazanowsi, 2015). The high-acuity patient is often the recipient of fragmented care and ineffective, inconsistent communication.

To overcome these barriers, healthcare professionals must be educated and trained in all aspects of palliative care. Changing belief systems from denial of death and a culture of rescue in high-acuity areas may seem like an insurmountable endeavor. Education must focus on the limitations of critical care therapies, embracing treatment goals that are attainable, and the benefits of palliative interventions. Not only does the healthcare team need education, but the public at large must be included in the process. As availability of palliative care teams continues to increase, the evidence suggests that involvement of the team in patient care will result in positive outcomes for patients and families (Baker et al., 2015; Center to Advance Palliative Care, 2013; Huffines et al., 2013).

Section One Review

1. In which situations should palliative care be offered to a client? (Select all that apply.)
   A. When a life-threatening illness exists
   B. When emotional symptoms are interfering with quality of life
   C. When physical symptoms are interfering with quality of life
   D. Not until the client is in the last 6 months of life
   E. Only when physical symptoms interfere with treatment

2. What is true about insurance coverage for palliative care?
   A. Palliative care is covered by Medicare but not by Medicaid.
   B. Palliative care is covered by Medicaid but not by Medicare.
   C. Palliative care is typically covered, at least in part, by private insurance.
   D. Palliative care is not covered by most private or governmental insurances.

3. What are some benefits of palliative care in the intensive care unit (ICU)? (Select all that apply.)
   A. Increased use of ventilators
   B. Increased consensus among provider groups
   C. Greater emphasis on keeping the client hydrated
   D. Decreased need for do-not-resuscitate orders

4. What is the goal of palliative care in the ICU?
   A. To cure the underlying illness
   B. To improve quality of life for the client
   C. To reduce cost of hospitalization
   D. To delay death to the extent possible

Answers: 1. (A, B, C), 2. C, 3. B, 4. B

Section Two: Communication and Decision Making

Communication and continuous assessment of patient management goals are key components of end-of-life care in the critical care setting. Providers must be clear with each other, and with the patient and family, about the likely outcome of the illness. They must provide an anticipated timeline with goals and milestones in the care process. If it becomes necessary to change the goals of care from cure to palliation, that transition must be clearly explained and discussed with the patient and family.

Establishing Goals of Care

Palliative care includes the establishment of specific goals for patient treatment and family-centered care. Good communication skills are required along with patient and family inclusion as spirituality and other patient concerns are addressed.

A Multidisciplinary Approach When a patient has been referred to a palliative care team, the high-acuity nurse and other team members formulate a plan of care to meet the patient's psychological, social, cultural, and spiritual needs. Team meetings and family conferences are essential. During the family conference, goals are clarified, the decision-making process is supported, and communication is facilitated. The palliative care plan for the high-acuity patient is comprehensive and must address the multifaceted needs of the patient (Maani-Fogelman & Bakitas, 2015). Decisions and plans of care should be communicated to other healthcare providers, as well as the patient and family, and should be documented in the medical record in a timely manner. Box 3–4 outlines useful steps for caring for patients at risk of not surviving their ICU stay.

QSEN Highlight: Quality Improvement—Care and Communication Bundle Black et al. (2013) conducted a quality-improvement project to improve clinician–family communication in intensive care units with the use of communication bundles triggered at specific time frames after admission. They designed an intervention based on measures identified by the Institute of Health Improvement (IHI), consisting of two communication bundles to be completed by the end of the first 24 hours of ICU admission (day 1) and by the end of 72 hours (day 3). The day 1 bundle consisted of medical record documentation of the following elements: (1) surrogate decision maker identified, (2) code status addressed, (3) presence or absence of advance directives assessed, (4) pain assessment completed, (5) dyspnea assessment completed, and (6) ICU brochure provided. The day 3 communication bundle included documentation of the following elements: (1) completion of a multidisciplinary meeting (defined as at least one physician and one nurse) with patient and/or surrogate decision maker, (2) discussion of prognosis, (3) assessment of patient-specific goals, and (4) need for spiritual care assessed (i.e., offer of social work or pastoral care). After 21 months of implementation, significant increases ($p < 0.001$) were found in compliance for both day 1 activities (from 10.7% to 83.8%) and day 3 activities (from 1.6% to 28.8%).

Family-centered Care

Although the focus of care in high-acuity settings is on the critically ill patient, nurses and other clinicians realize that comprehensive patient care includes care of the patient's family (Steele & Davies, 2015). Family is whomever the patient identifies as such. In most cases, it is the people who provide the patient with emotional and practical support. It can refer to any significant other who participates in the care and well-being of the patient. A family-centered approach to care acknowledges the important relationship between the family and the critically ill patient. Therefore, no discussion of palliative care in the intensive care environment is complete without also discussing care of the patient's family. Proactive communication has been shown to increase satisfaction and decrease psychological burden in families of critically ill patients in the ICU (Black et al., 2013). However, family members' preferences for involvement in the decision-making process vary. Direct care nurses in intensive care settings tend to see their involvement in discussions of prognosis, goals of care, and palliative care as key elements of the delivery of quality patient care (Anderson et al., 2016).

Family members of critically ill patients are at high risk for developing long-term, significant morbidity from the hospital experience, with high rates of depression, anxiety, and posttraumatic stress disorder (PTSD) (Aslakson, Curtis, & Nelson, 2014). Providers in high-acuity settings should create supportive environments for the families of ICU patients and develop policies and routines that support the family. In addition to improving the physical environment (waiting and ICU rooms), hospital administrators can improve the physical environment for families, as well as create policies that provide families with access to consistent information about their loved ones' care (Kelley & Morrison, 2015). Specific tools can assist providers in communicating with patients and family members in an effort to improve the quality of care (Black et al., 2013; Singer et al., 2016). Three such tools are described in Box 3–5.

Spiritual Care Faith and/or religion play a critical role in helping patients and families cope with serious illness and end-of-life decision making, and most patients want their healthcare providers to be aware of the importance their spirituality holds for them (Chovan, Cluxton, & Rancour, 2015; Puchalski, 2014). Unfortunately, there is little specific, empiric information to guide high-acuity nurses in the spiritual assessment and support of patients and families. In-depth spiritual support may be optimized by engaging formally trained professionals such as chaplains and other spiritual care specialists in the patient's care. However, nurses can assess the need for further spiritual support by utilizing the FICA mnemonic for elaborating spiritual needs (Box 3–6).

End-of-life Decision Making

Nurses have a primary role in ensuring that the patient makes informed decisions regarding end-of-life care

---

BOX 3–4 Planning Palliative Care for ICU Patients

- Find out whether the patient has an advance directive, a durable power of attorney, and a documented preference about CPR.
- Hold a patient and family meeting to identify and communicate goals of care within the first 5 days of the ICU stay.
- Outline the steps to be taken to accomplish the goals of care, including criteria for how effectiveness will be evaluated.
- Communicate the care plan to staff and family, identifying the best persons to carry out each part of the plan.
- Use a multidisciplinary team approach to decision making regarding transition to end-of-life care and withdrawal of life support.
- If the patient lacks decision-making capacity or legal representation, a guardian should be assigned, or an ethics committee consulted, to protect the patient's interests.
- The goals in any palliative care plan are to provide optimal symptom management, psychosocial and spiritual support, patient- and family-centered care, coordination across settings, and staff support.

SOURCE: From McAdam & Puntillo. (2015).

BOX 3–5 Communication Tools for Family Meetings

Spikes

- **S**ETTING up the interview
- Assessing the patient's **P**ERCEPTION
- Obtaining the patient's **I**NVITATION
- Giving **K**NOWLEDGE and information
- Responding to **E**MOTION
- **S**UMMARIZING the discussion

Nurse

- **N**AMING
- **U**NDERSTANDING
- **R**ESPECTING
- **S**UPPORTING
- **E**XPLORING

The VALUE Checklist

- **V**ALUE family statements
- **A**CKNOWLEDGE and address family emotions
- **L**ISTEN and respond to family members
- **U**NDERSTAND the patient as a person
- **E**LICIT family questions

SOURCE: Adapted from Kelley & Morrison (2015); McAdam & Puntillo (2015); and Singer et al. (2016).

(American Association of Critical-Care Nurses [AACN], 2005). The nurse working with high-acuity patients serves as a patient advocate, intercedes for patients who cannot speak for themselves, and supports the decisions of the patient or the patient's designated surrogate. Understanding the impact of cultural, spiritual, and religious backgrounds on the patient's decision making is important. Nurses are also directed to uphold the choices and values of the patient even when these wishes conflict with those of healthcare providers and families (AACN).

Ethical and Legal Principles The Patient Self-Determination Act, passed as part of the Omnibus Budget Reconciliation Act of 1990, requires that all patients be given information about their right to formulate advance directives of two types: (1) advance directives (e.g., living wills) in which specific instructions from the patient may be made known, and (2) appointment directives (e.g., durable power of attorney for healthcare) in which a person is designated as having the patient's authority to make health decisions on the patient's behalf (American Cancer Society, 2014). Forms for these directives are available free of charge from the National Hospice and Palliative Care Organization. The use of healthcare directives has increased the role of the patient and family in making end-of-life decisions.

Advance Directives It is useful to have the patient's wishes for level of intervention defined before a medical crisis occurs. Only 26% of patients have executed an advance directive that defines the level of intervention the patient is willing to accept at the end of life (Rao, Anderson, Lin, & Laux, 2014). Advance directives may include directions to maximize therapies aimed at comfort and to limit use of life-sustaining therapies, such as cardiopulmonary resuscitation (CPR), feeding tubes, and artificial hydration. An example of an advance directive that uses layperson's terms is the Five Wishes document from the organization Aging with Dignity (http://www.agingwithdignity.org).

Living wills are not medical orders, but they can be used to guide such orders once the patient is admitted to the hospital. The presence of advance directives, when available, guides the hospital staff in identifying the patient's surrogate decision maker and assists in determining the level of care desired. If the patient has an advance directive, a copy should be provided in a prominent place in the patient's medical record. Directives can be placed in hospital charts and scanned into electronic records. Any changes in treatment preferences should be communicated and documented throughout the patient's hospital stay.

BOX 3–6 FICA Spiritual History Tool©

F – Faith and Belief

"Do you consider yourself spiritual or religious?" or "Is spirituality something important to you" or "Do you have spiritual beliefs that help you cope with stress/difficult times?" (Contextualize to reason for visit if it is not the routine history.)

If the patient responds "No," the healthcare provider might ask, "What gives your life meaning?" Sometimes patients respond with answers such as family, career, or nature.

(The question of meaning should also be asked even if people answer yes to spirituality.)

I – Importance

"What importance does your spirituality have in your life? Has your spirituality influenced how you take care of yourself, your health? Does your spirituality influence you in your healthcare decision making (e.g. advance directives, treatment etc.)?"

C – Community

"Are you part of a spiritual community?" Communities such as churches, temples, and mosques, or a group of like-minded friends, family, or yoga, can serve as strong support systems for some patients. Can explore further: "Is this of support to you and how? Is there a group of people you really love or who are important to you?"

A – Address in Care

"How would you like me, your healthcare provider, to address these issues in your healthcare?" (With the newer models including diagnosis of spiritual distress A also refers to the "Assessment and Plan" of patient spiritual distress or issues within a treatment or care plan.)

© C. Puchalski, 1996

SOURCE: Christina M. Puchalski, MD, FICA Spiritual History Tool, adapted from The FICA Spiritual History Tool #274, *Journal of Palliative Medicine*, Volume 17, Number 1, 2014, Puchalski, Christina.

Capacity In the high-acuity setting, it is important to establish whether the patient has decision-making capacity to consent to interventions and the ability to format a plan of care with providers. Often, the advanced stage of illness or injury and the severity of the underlying pathology impair the patient's decision-making capacity. The ability to make decisions about care depends on the patient's ability to understand the clinical facts of his or her health status and the consequences of treatment options. Elements of decision-making capacity include (1) ability to understand the information about options for care, (2) ability to reason and consider the options being offered, (3) ability to communicate a choice, and (4) ability to describe consequences of the decision (Berry & Griffie, 2015). Documentation of decision-making capacity should be included in the medical record and updated as the patient's condition changes. It is important to remember that the existence of a designated healthcare power of attorney does not mean that the patient is no longer in charge of decisions about his or her care. The power of attorney is empowered to make decisions only if and when the patient lacks capacity (Berry & Griffie, 2015).

Proxy Decision Making In the event that a patient is unable to make or communicate healthcare decisions and if no power of attorney for healthcare has been previously designated, it is imperative to identify a proxy decision maker. Input from the patient's family regarding goals of care and patient wishes should be sought. If patients have had discussions with their family members about what they would or would not want at the end of life, the emotional burden on the family may be lightened. Social service involvement can assist with the assessment of family dynamics and the identification of a surrogate decision maker. All family members should know the identity of the designated decision maker. This person is charged with making decisions that the patient would make if he or she were able to make them. The decisions should reflect the known wishes of the patient. If the patient's wishes are not known, then the decisions should reflect what would be in the best interest of the patient. The designated decision maker will have legal authority over the decision, but customarily other family members participate in the discussions (Hinderer, Friedmann, & Fins, 2015).

Code Status Conversations about code status can be challenging due to the public's misperception about high success rates of resuscitation as represented in the media. Rates of survival to hospital discharge are much lower for patients with end-stage conditions or who suffer from frailty or significant functional loss. Most hospitals have do-not-resuscitate forms that include check boxes for interventions such as intubation, chest compressions, and medications. Unfortunately, offering a menu of choices to uninformed patients and family members can lead to confusion and inconsistent choices.

Allow Natural Death Patients and families are often confused and frightened by terms such as *do not resuscitate* (DNR), *do not intubate* (DNI), and *comfort measures only* (CMO). Families interpret these to mean that nothing will be done for their loved one, and the nurse may not be equipped to provide adequate explanations. In 2000, the term *allow natural death* (AND) was introduced. Using this term implies that the patient is dying and that everything possible is being done to keep the patient comfortable and allow the dying process to occur naturally. The goal of AND is to prevent unnecessary suffering and allow nature to take its course. While AND is not different from DNR, the language is more acceptable to patients and families (Buscaino, Singh, Nissanov, & Wells, 2013).

Medical Orders Advance directive documents are not substitutes for medical orders. Some states utilize medical order forms that state patients' wishes regarding life-sustaining therapies. These portable medical order forms are intended to be used by patients with serious health problems. Two examples are Provider/Physician Orders for Life Sustaining Treatment or Medical Orders for Life-Sustaining Treatment (POLST or MOLST). The need for this type of form arose because advance directives did not give guidance to emergency medical services (EMS) personnel—for example, a request to limit CPR outside the hospital. Different from an advance directive, POLST forms are medical orders that are honored across all treatment settings. The POLST/MOLST forms specify the types of treatments that a patient would or would not receive at the end of life. These medical orders are signed by the patient's physician and do not expire. The orders can be revised by either voiding the form and completing a new form or making updates on the form. These orders are not recognized in every state, though the list of states that do accept them is growing. High-acuity nurses in states that recognize POLST or MOLST forms need to be aware of whether or not a regulatory mandate requires healthcare providers to honor the patient wishes documented on the form, or if the document is merely a guideline (Chovan et al., 2015; Mularski et al., 2013).

Section Two Review

1. What should occur during a family conference regarding goals of care for a terminally ill client? (Select all that apply.)
   A. Clarification of goals
   B. Support of the decision-making process
   C. Facilitation of communication
   D. Determination of method of payment
   E. Documentation of family understanding of unit regulations

2. Which options should be considered if a client is shown to lack decision-making capacity? (Select all that apply.)
   A. Legal representation should be established.
   B. The hospital should direct care.
   C. A guardian should be assigned.
   D. The attending physician should direct care.
   E. The hospital's ethics committee should be consulted.

3. What is the first step in using the SPIKE tool to facilitate communication during family meetings?
    A. Support the family decision-making process
    B. Summarize the client's condition to this point
    C. Suggest a treatment plan
    D. Set up the interview

4. Which statement is correct regarding the use of living wills?
    A. They are used to guide medical orders.
    B. They are a substitute for medical orders.
    C. They are the same as a durable power of attorney.
    D. They are not part of the medical record.

Answers: 1. (A, B, C), 2. (A, C, D), 3. D, 4. A

Section Three: Pain and Symptom Management

The most common physical and psychological symptoms among terminally ill patients are listed in Box 3–7. Symptoms rarely occur one at a time; rather they occur in clusters (Barsevick & Aktas, 2013; Stapleton, Holden, Epstein, & Wilkie, 2016). The two most frequently cited symptoms of dying patients are pain and fatigue (Oechsle, Goerth, Bokemeyer, & Mehnert, 2013). Effective symptom control may be one of the last interventions offered to dying patients and their families (Berry & Griffie, 2015). Adequate symptom management is most successful when undertaken in collaboration with patients, their caregivers, and a multidisciplinary team (Brant, 2014).

Pain Assessment and Management

Pain is noted in 36% to 90% of terminally ill patients (Chi & Demiris, 2016). More than 30% of patients in the ICU report "significant pain at rest," and more than 50% have significant pain when they are repositioned, suctioned, and provided with wound care (American Association of Critical Care Nurses [AACN], 2013). Some of the common causes of pain in critically ill patients are listed in Box 3–8.

Procedural Pain   Critically ill patients may undergo dozens of painful diagnostic and treatment procedures during the course of their hospitalization, including central and peripheral line placements, nasogastric tube placements, chest tube placement and removal, urinary catheter insertion and removal, wound debridement, dressing changes, and endotracheal suctioning. The seemingly innocuous procedure of turning a patient in the bed to prevent pressure ulcers can be immensely painful for a critically ill patient. The high-acuity nurse will become adept at anticipating these procedures and will pre-medicate patients for pain whenever possible. If a decision has been made to transition to comfort care or to end life support, the high-acuity nurse can evaluate the appropriateness of planned procedures and advocate for their discontinuation. The high-acuity nurse plays a key role in helping patients avoid iatrogenic suffering at the end of life (Brant, 2014; Paice, 2015).

BOX 3–8   Causes of Pain in High-Acuity Settings

- Pain from trauma or accidents
- Postsurgical pain
- Pre-existing chronic pain (back pain, arthritis)
- Procedures such as suctioning, turning, central-line cannula placement, chest tube placement/removal, and removal of wound drains
- Painful wounds or burns with dressing changes
- Intubation
- Cardiac conditions and infarction
- Acute abdominal pain
- Pancreatitis
- Sickle cell crisis
- HIV/AIDS
- Psychosocial and spiritual issues such as suffering

SOURCE: Based on End-of-Life Nursing Education Consortium (ELNEC) Workshop (2014).

BOX 3–7   Common Symptoms Experienced by Terminally Ill Patients

Physical
- Pain
- Fatigue and/or weakness
- Dyspnea
- Nausea and vomiting
- Insomnia
- Xerostomia (dry mouth)
- Anorexia
- Constipation
- Cough
- Peripheral edema
- Pruritus
- Diarrhea
- Dysphagia
- Dizziness
- Fecal and/or urinary incontinence
- Peripheral neuropathy

Psychological
- Anxiety
- Depression
- Hopelessness
- Meaninglessness
- Confusion
- Loss of libido
- Irritability
- Impaired concentration

SOURCE: Adapted from Barsevick & Aktas (2013) and Stapleton et al. (2016).

Pain Assessment Patient self-report is the gold standard for assessing pain, but self-report may be difficult due to the limited ability of the critically ill patient to communicate if intubated or unconscious (Brant, 2014; Fink, Gates, & Montgomery, 2015). If the patient is conscious and can answer yes or no questions by blinking or lifting fingers, the patient is capable of self-reporting pain.

Pain assessment tools for the unconscious patient include behavioral observations as well as assessing physiological parameters. Current behavioral assessment tools are equal in their usefulness. Experts recommend that the nurse consider the validity of the tool for the population receiving care and exercise consistency when using the tool. Pain assessment tools for the nonverbal patient include the Behavioral Pain Rating Scale, PAIN Algorithm, Behavioral Pain Scale (BPS), Nonverbal Pain Scale, Pain Behavior Assessment Tool, and the Critical Care Pain Observation Tool (CPOT) (AACN, 2013; Chow, 2014; Rose, Haslam, Dale, Knechtel, & McGillion, 2013). Other tools used in nonverbal older adults in other settings that may be used in the critical care setting include the Checklist of Nonverbal Pain Indicators (CNPI) tested in older adults with advanced dementia in acute and long-term care settings, and Pain Assessment in Advanced Dementia Scale (PAIN-AD), tested with chronic pain patients in long-term care (Fink et al., 2015; McAdam & Puntillo, 2015).

When the patient cannot self-report, or when the objective measures of pain assessment conflict, the high-acuity nurse should assume that pain may be present if the patient has a condition or procedure known to cause pain. In this case, an appropriate dose of pain medication, based on previously effective doses, may be administered as an analgesic trial. If the patient is receiving sedative agents that have little to no analgesic effect, the high-acuity nurse will ensure that pain medications are given first (Brant, 2014; McAdam & Puntillo, 2015; Reynolds, Drew, & Dunwoody, 2013).

Interventions When the ICU patient is approaching death, the most important aim of care should be to make the patient's dying as comfortable as possible. Early recognition and assessment of pain are more effective in controlling and managing pain than attempting to catch up after the patient experiences severe pain.

The various types of pain and their management are discussed in Chapter 4.

Barriers to Effective Pain Management There are many barriers to providing optimum pain management in the high-acuity setting; barriers related to patients, barriers related to nurses, and barriers related to hospital policies were reported in a qualitative study of 37 Jordanian critical care nurses (Batiha, 2013). One challenge for the high-acuity nurse is that patients may be on long-term opioids at home, which leads to the development of tolerance to pain medicines. Patients with high opioid tolerance typically require higher doses of pain medicine to achieve pain relief. Concerns about patients developing tolerance to or becoming dependent upon opioids are misplaced during end-of-life care. There is no ceiling effect from opioids. Doses can be increased until the desired effect is reached as long as intolerable side effects do not occur. It is desirable to use the least amount of medication necessary to achieve

the greatest comfort while maintaining the patient's awareness. Daily goals for pain control should be discussed, and high-dose analgesics, in conjunction with adjuvant therapies, may be required for some pain syndromes.

Patients on long-term high doses of opioids may become physically dependent on them, which may not be an issue with end-of-life care. If an opioid-dependent patient is receiving a continuous opioid infusion, and the family wishes to have the flow rate decreased to enable the patient to actively participate in end-of-life decision making, this must be done slowly and carefully to avoid precipitating painful opioid withdrawal symptoms. Titration of opioids is an important skill of the high-acuity nurse— one that has the potential to greatly impact the experience of critically ill patients and their families.

Principle of Double Effect In the high-acuity setting, nurses are sometimes concerned that the administration of analgesics in the amounts necessary to provide comfort could "cause" death and be considered euthanasia. Therefore, it is essential that high-acuity nurses understand the "double-effect" principle (Bakitas, Bishop, & Hahn, 2014). The double-effect principle states that an act may have two foreseen effects: one good and one potentially harmful. If the intention is the good effect, and the harmful effect was not intended, then the act is morally defensible. The double-effect principle provides support to nurses when their moral intent is directed primarily at alleviating suffering. It is commonly applied to the situation in which analgesics (particularly opioids) are administered to terminally ill patients in the amounts necessary to decrease pain and suffering. Because the administration of analgesic medication to a patient in pain is considered a beneficent act, even though unwanted side effects such as decreased blood pressure, slowed breathing, or altered mental status are possible, the act is ethically justified. The principle of double effect is supported by professional standards of care (Knight, Espinoza, & Freeman, 2015).

Management of Non-pain Symptoms

Effective symptom management is essential to high-quality end-of-life care. Nurses should assess, intervene, and report patient outcomes for interventions to control or alleviate symptoms. The treatment of symptoms is often cyclic, with new strategies identified and carried out when desired outcomes are not achieved.

Dyspnea Dyspnea is the subjective experience of feeling short of breath and is one of the most distressing symptoms that can be experienced by critically ill patients, often even more distressing than pain. Up to 75% of dying patients experience dyspnea (Mularski et al., 2013). Many pathologies cause dyspnea, ranging from cardiac, pulmonary, oncologic, traumatic, or metabolic origins, in addition to iatrogenic causes such as intubation. Specifically, dyspnea may be caused by parenchymal lung disease, infection, effusions, pulmonary emboli, pulmonary edema, asthma, or compressed airway. Anxiety and pain, commonly experienced by critically ill patients, can also exacerbate the sensation of breathlessness. While many of the causes may be treated, often the underlying cause cannot be reversed.

Assessment. As is the case for pain, the gold standard for assessing dyspnea is patient self-report. Simply ask the patient, "Do you feel short of breath?" A yes or no answer provides enough information, even without ascertaining the intensity and quality of dyspnea. However, in critical care settings, patients may be unable to report even the presence of dyspnea due to low level of consciousness. One model, the Respiratory Distress Observation Scale (RDOS), derives a composite dyspnea score by incorporating physiologic measures such as vital signs with behavioral observations, accessory muscle use, nasal flaring, and the patient's facial expressions of fear (Puntillo et al., 2013). This tool has eight items, each scored from zero to two, that measure the presence and intensity of respiratory distress.

Management. Attempts should be made to reverse the underlying causes of dyspnea if possible, as long as the intervention is not more unpleasant than the dyspnea (e.g., avoid repeated thoracenteses). Noninvasive positive pressure ventilation (NPPV) such as bilevel positive airway pressure (BiPAP) or nasal continuous positive airway pressure (CPAP) may be helpful. Medications to reverse pathology include beta agonists (e.g., albuterol), anticholinergics (e.g., ipratropium), steroids, antibiotics, and nitric oxide/oxygen blends. Most often the only feasible treatment is to treat the symptoms rather than their cause. Symptomatic relief of dyspnea is best achieved by close evaluation of the patient and the use of opioids, benzodiazepines, and nonpharmacologic interventions (e.g., oxygen, positioning, and increased ambient air flow). Morphine reduces muscle tension and increases pulmonary vasodilation but is not effective when inhaled. Benzodiazepines may be used in patients who are not able to tolerate opioids or for whom the respiratory benefits are minimal. Each medication should be titrated to effect, with the goal being the reduction of dyspnea as reported by the patient, rather than targeting a specific respiratory rate or oxygen saturation level (Dudgeon, 2015; Puntillo et al., 2013; Rocker et al., 2013). The nurse should reassure family and caregivers that dyspnea does not necessarily indicate suffocation or air hunger.

Delirium Delirium is a clinical diagnosis made at the bedside, requiring a careful history and physical exam. Unlike dementia, delirium is of sudden onset, characterized by fluctuating consciousness and inattention. It is not uncommon in the hours before death. Delirium may be caused by metabolic encephalopathy in renal or liver failure, hypoxemia, infection, hypercalcemia, malignancy, dehydration, constipation, urinary retention, and metastases to the brain. Delirium is also a common side effect of medications commonly used in the high-acuity setting, such as opioids, glucocorticoids, anticholinergics, antihistamines, antiemetics, and benzodiazepines (Heidrich & English, 2015). Early recognition of delirium is important to allow for final communication with loved ones while the patient remains lucid. If changes in mentation reverse themselves with time of day, this may be an indication of impending delirium.

Assessment. Numerous evidence-based assessment tools exist for identifying delirium in critically ill patients: the Cognitive Test for Delirium (CTD), Confusion Assessment Method-ICU (CAM-ICU), Intensive Care Delirium Screening Checklist, NEECHAM Scale, and the Delirium Detection Score, to name a few (Bush et al., 2014a; Grassi et al., 2015; Heidrich & English, 2015).

Management. Nonpharmacologic interventions include stopping all unnecessary medications that may have delirium as a side effect; providing a calendar, clock, newspaper, or other orienting objects; and gently correcting hallucinations or cognitive mistakes. Restraints should be avoided. Medications to manage end-of-life delirium include typical and atypical antipsychotics, including haloperidol, ziprasidone, and quetiapine (Bush et al., 2014b; Grassi et al., 2015; Heidrich & English, 2015). This is in contrast to alcohol-related delirium in which benzodiazepines are used. Reassure family and caregivers that delirium does not necessarily indicate physical pain.

Nausea and Vomiting Nausea may result from uremia, liver failure, hypercalcemia, bowel obstruction, severe constipation, infection, gastroesophageal reflux disease, vestibular disease, brain metastases, medications (cancer chemotherapy, antibiotics, nonsteroidal anti-inflammatory drugs, opioids, proton pump inhibitors), or radiation therapy (Chow, Cogan, & Mun, 2015). Up to 70% of patients with advanced cancer have nausea (Tipton, 2014). For cancer patients receiving chemotherapy and/or radiation, the side effects of nausea, vomiting, and retching are reported as among the most distressing (Chow et al., 2015). For noncancer patients, rates of nausea and vomiting are estimated at less than 50%, though this is likely underreported (Chow et al., 2015).

Assessment. A thorough history can provide clues as to the cause of the nausea. The high-acuity nurse should observe for triggers of nausea, which may include medications, meals, movement, smells, presence of epigastric pain, heartburn, constipation, thirst, or hiccups. Physical examination includes abdominal assessment, auscultating bowel sounds, inspecting the oral cavity for thrush, and assessing the rectum for impaction. Lab results should be monitored to rule out an electrolyte imbalance. Validated assessment tools include the Visual Analog Scale (VAS), Morrow Assessment of Nausea and Emesis (MANE), Rhodes Index of Nausea and Vomiting (INV-2), and the Functional Living Index Emesis (FLIE) (Chow et al., 2015).

Management. Prevention of nausea is the goal. If prevention is unsuccessful, antiemetics may be used to eliminate or decrease severity. If decreased bowel motility is suspected, metoclopramide is the drug of choice for nausea treatment. Nausea, as a result of chemotherapy, can generally be mitigated with glucocorticoids and serotonin receptor blockers such as ondansetron. Other causes of nausea may respond to antihistamines (meclizine) or anticholinergics (scopolamine). Anticipatory nausea (common with cancer patients) may be prevented with a benzodiazepine to reduce anxiety. If the cause of the nausea and vomiting is an intestinal obstruction, decompression with a nasogastric tube may be required. However, the discomfort of this treatment should be weighed against the benefit (Collis & Mather, 2015; McAdam & Puntillo, 2015).

Section Three Review

1. Which situations act as barriers to effective pain management in the high-acuity setting? (Select all that apply.)
   A. Knowledge deficits
   B. Cultural biases
   C. Lack of assessment tools
   D. Poor availability of effective medications
   E. Communication misunderstandings

2. Which statement is correct regarding the use of morphine to treat dyspnea?
   A. Morphine acts by increasing thoracic muscle tension.
   B. Morphine decreases pulmonary vasodilation.
   C. Morphine is no longer recommended for treatment of dyspnea.
   D. Morphine is not effective when inhaled.

3. What is true of delirium associated with end of life?
   A. It is of slow onset.
   B. It is common in the hours just before death.
   C. It is rarely metabolic in nature.
   D. It requires a brain scan for diagnosis.

4. What is the primary goal for management of nausea and vomiting in the terminally ill client?
   A. Prevention
   B. Early identification of cause
   C. Avoidance of drug therapy
   D. Restoring electrolyte balance

Answers: 1. (A, B, E), 2. D, 3. B, 4. A

Section Four: Withdrawal of Life-sustaining Treatment

Life-sustaining therapy (LST) is defined as any healthcare intervention that is focused on increasing the life span of the patient. Such therapies may include artificial nutrition, intravenous hydration, blood replacement products, mechanical ventilation, vasoactive and inotropic agents, cardiac devices, and renal replacement therapies. Decisions to withhold and/or withdraw life-sustaining therapies are commonly made in the high-acuity setting. Patients have the right to accept or refuse treatments, even if the treatments are considered lifesaving. Withdrawal or withholding of interventions may be initiated by the patient, family, or the critical care team. Withdrawal of life support is considered ethically acceptable if it reduces unnecessary patient suffering when the prognosis is considered hopeless and if it complies with the patient's previously stated preferences.

When decisions of withdrawal of life-sustaining treatments are contemplated, palliative care providers should be consulted. Quality-of-life decisions need to be discussed at family meetings attended by an interprofessional team of physicians, nurses, and/or social workers and chaplains to promote shared decision making among the patient, family, and healthcare providers. The team should assess what the patient and family understand about the patient's prognosis and then should gently confirm the medical facts.

It may be difficult for families to come to terms with the concept of medical futility. **Medical futility** is defined as a situation in which the continuation or initiation of medical treatment might have the expected medical effect, yet there is no benefit to the patient (Chow, 2014). Common reactions to bad prognoses include anger, fear, sadness, helplessness, and isolation. The high-acuity nurse acknowledges these emotions and assures patients and families of continued care regardless of the treatment decision.

Process of Withdrawal

As soon as a decision is made to withdraw life-sustaining treatment, the care team should evaluate all current therapies to assess whether these treatments make a positive contribution to the patient's comfort (McAdam & Puntillo, 2015). Documentation in the medical record should include the decisions and rationales for the plan of care. A do-not-resuscitate order must be placed in the chart as indicated by the plan of care agreement. Communication with families should describe how the withdrawal process will proceed and should provide assurances that symptoms will be carefully managed. The family should be given the option of being with the patient after withdrawal of life support, in which case they should be provided with information on what to expect when death occurs. A time to initiate withdrawal is usually agreed upon with the family.

If a series of therapies is to be discontinued, dialysis is usually stopped first. The withdrawal of dialysis may cause dyspnea from fluid volume overload, which may necessitate the use of opioids or benzodiazepines. Next, vasopressors, artificial feeding, intravenous fluids, invasive monitoring, and antibiotics are discontinued. The discontinuation of artificial feeding may elicit alarm from the family, because offering food has great social significations. Provide reassurance that the lack of nutrition at the end of life does not lead to suffering (Campbell & Gorman, 2015).

Withdrawal of mechanical ventilatory support requires adequate management of potential agitation, pain, and hypoxia. Opioid and benzodiazepine agents should be considered for administration before and after extubation to prevent agitation and pain. When the patient is dependent on ventilatory support or vasopressors and that support is removed, death typically occurs

BOX 3-9 Withdrawal of Life-sustaining Therapies

Preparation for withdrawal of technology includes:

- A preparatory clinical team meeting to review medications, concerns, and support for the process.
- Assessment of patient and family spiritual, religious, and cultural rituals and practices that need to be addressed and facilitated by the team. Arrangements for dressing the patient in religious garments and/or honoring rituals if possible.
- Removal of equipment such as transducer monitors, ventilators, and blood infusion devices from the bedside to allow the family access to the patient.
- Positioning of chairs and tissues in room, to promote comfort, before the family arrives. Placement of the bed in a low position with the side rails down to allow the family to be near the patient.

- Premedication of the patient as appropriate for pain, dyspnea, seizures, and agitation to facilitate comfort and alleviate symptoms that the family might find distressing.
- Clamping of arterial lines, central lines, and other invasive equipment. Discontinuation of unnecessary medications, intravenous lines, and nasogastric or oral gastric tubes to allow the patient to look as normal as possible.
- Covering the patient with a blanket, leaving arms out to provide the family with the opportunity to hold the patient's hand.
- Turning off of monitor screens in room to prevent distraction. This allows the family to concentrate on the patient, not the monitoring screen.
- Provision of basic hygiene, including cleansing and moisturizing the patient's mouth to promote respectful care of the body.

SOURCE: Data from B. R. Ferrell, N. Coyle, & J. Paice (Eds.), Oxford Textbook of Palliative Nursing (pp.463–474; 740–760). New York, NY: Oxford University Press. http://doi.org/10.1093/med/9780199332342.001.0001.

within minutes (Campbell & Gorman, 2015). Box 3–9 describes activities that the high-acuity nurse can undertake in preparation for the withdrawal of life-sustaining therapies.

Brain Death and Organ Donation

A key role of nurses in high-acuity settings is to support the patient's family during the stress of withdrawal of technological support for their loved one. Two situations that are particularly challenging include brain death and organ donation.

Brain Death In the United States, established criteria help clinicians recognize brain death as death. This may be difficult for families to acknowledge, because the patient appears to be physiologically functioning and can seem to still be alive. In brain death, however, the patient's higher brain functions are no longer viable. Brain death occurs when all functions of the brain cease. Brain death is defined as an irreversible cessation of all brain functions, including the functions of the brain stem (Arbour, 2013). Declaration of brain death requires two neurologic exams completed by qualified physicians (preferably one is a neurologist) no less than 6 hours apart. Hospitals have established brain death protocols to guide care in these situations.

If brain death is established, the family should be told that the patient has been declared brain dead and the family should be provided with explanations regarding continued autonomic functions that eventually cease (Arbour, 2013). Family members may confuse brain death with other conditions, such as a persistent vegetative state, in which there is still some limited brain activity. Care should be taken to ensure that family members understand that the brain-dead patient is dead. In order to communicate effectively and sensitively with families in this situation, it is important for high-acuity nurses to possess a thorough understanding of the medical implications of brain death, regardless of their personal conceptions about death. It is

better for nurses in this situation to avoid speaking to the patient who has been declared brain dead as one might speak to a comatose patient, as this may introduce ambiguity into the situation and confuse family members.

Organ Donation Brain death is linked to the organ donation and transplant process, as it allows for the retrieval of well-perfused organs from patients who have been certified as dead. How the conversations with families about death and brain death are held affects families' understanding and may positively or negatively affect organ donation.

In the ideal case, families faced with the death of a loved one, regardless of the manner of death, may find comfort in being able to help others through organ donation. It is critical, however, that the discussion of brain death be kept completely separate from the discussion about organ donation. Organ donation discussions must be conducted by an authorized Organ Procurement Organization (OPO) representative ("designated requestor"). Organ procurement criteria are ever changing, but in the high-acuity setting at the time of this writing, organs that may be donated include the heart, lungs, pancreas, liver, and bowel. Eyes, skin, bone, heart valves, and corneas may be donated postmortem. Some patient's cultural or religious beliefs require the body to remain intact, and families may perceive organ donation as a desecration of the body. In these cases, the involvement of the hospital ethics committee may be helpful.

After the Death

After the death of a patient, the family may wish to spend time at the bedside. The high-acuity nurse asks if they need assistance, supplies, or resources, and whether they wish to be alone or have someone remain with them. Families need adequate time to sit quietly, perhaps privately, without time constraints. The reality of critical care units is that the deceased patient's bed will soon be needed for another patient. In this case, the charge nurse and hospital staff make arrangements to ensure that the family has sufficient time at the bedside, even as another patient needs to be admitted to the unit (Berry & Griffie, 2015).

Bereavement

After the death of the patient, families are supported with bereavement services. In the immediate aftermath, families require logistical and emotional support, particularly information about the next steps in terms of the disposition of the body for funeral arrangements. High-acuity hospital units typically compile "death packets" in advance that contain the necessary information, which families find reassuring. Many hospices offer support services for any member of the community who has suffered the death of a loved one, free of charge, regardless of whether the loved one was enrolled in hospice. These services can be very helpful to patients in the short term (Brohard, 2014; Corless, 2015).

Often, feelings of grief among family members may linger a year or more after a loved one's death. In light of this fact, many critical care units organize bereavement follow-up programs. These programs typically involve regular follow-up with the surviving family members every month, as well as at the 1-year anniversary of their loved one's death. These programs serve the dual purpose of helping healthcare providers cope with the loss and ease compassion fatigue. Some hospitals also hold memorial services at regular intervals (typically annually or biannually) for family and friends of the patient to reconnect with the hospital staff and celebrate the lives of those whom they served (Berry & Griffie, 2015; Cook & Rocker, 2014).

Family Outcomes   As worthwhile as these activities are, the manner in which a family copes with death is highly variable. Family members of high-acuity patients often serve as surrogate decision makers. If the patient's course was a difficult one, during which life-and-death decisions needed to be made in the absence of clear direction from the patient, family members may be at high risk of developing long-term psychological problems. These may include depression, anxiety, and posttraumatic stress disorder (Adams et al., 2014).

Section Four Review

1. In a situation where multiple life-sustaining treatments will be withdrawn, which therapy is usually the first to be discontinued?
   A. Dialysis
   B. Artificial feeding
   C. Authentic leadership
   D. Invasive monitoring
   E. Mechanical ventilation

2. What is required to declare a client brain dead?
   A. Permission from the family
   B. Neurologic exams by two qualified physicians
   C. Lack of pulse for at least 10 minutes
   D. Cessation of respiratory effort

3. Which statement is true regarding organ donation discussions?
   A. They should be initiated by the attending physician.
   B. They should not occur until brain death has occurred.
   C. They must be conducted by a designated requestor.
   D. They should occur at the time of discussion of brain death.

4. Which statement is true regarding grief and bereavement?
   A. The majority of grief feelings should be resolved within 6 months of the death.
   B. Bereavement services are managed by social service workers, not nurses.
   C. Family members may continue to grieve for a year or more.
   D. Bereavement services begin at the time the client's body is released from the hospital.

Answers: 1. A, 2. B, 3. C, 4. C

Section Five: Professional Issues

End-of-life and palliative care is challenging for healthcare professionals who engage in patient care. Managing the stress associated with the caregiver role is an important skill for the high-acuity nurse. Techniques to effectively manage moral distress, conflict, and barriers to optimal care should be part of the professional nurse's skill set.

Moral Distress

Ethical dilemmas can lead to moral distress for nurses in high-acuity settings. Nurses feel that they know the right thing to do but are constrained by institutional policies in their practice settings (Browning, 2013). This disconnect between knowing what to do but not being able to do it, and then witnessing negative consequences from that disconnect, leads to moral distress. High-acuity nurses need to recognize that they can positively contribute to ethical dilemmas by identifying and addressing them. They need to know where they can turn for help when they experience moral distress. The AACN program "Four A's to Rise Above Moral Distress" provides important information about how nurses can be helped to identify, assess, and act when situations that can cause moral distress arise (AACN, n.d.; Browning, 2013).

Assessment of Sources of Conflict   The American Nurses Association (ANA) *Standards of Clinical Nursing Practice* state that essential components of professional nursing practice include care, cure, and coordination (ANA, 2001). The AACN position is that nurses who work with acutely ill patients should base their practice on individual professional accountability; thorough knowledge of the interrelatedness of body systems; recognition and appreciation of a person's wholeness, uniqueness, and significant social–environmental relationships; and appreciation of the collaborative role of all health team members (AACN, 2015). While working with patients in high-acuity areas, nurses are often faced with ethical dilemmas. Exposure to death and the saving of human lives calls for the nurse to frequently evaluate personal values. Personal values often influence decision making. It is important for the nurse to fully understand his or her personal values.

Evaluating one's personal philosophy can improve satisfaction when working with acutely ill patients. Clarifying one's values helps to anticipate problems that may be encountered in the practice setting and supports the development of positive coping strategies. This knowledge is carried with the professional nurse throughout his or her career, regardless of the practice setting or the age of the patient.

It is important that the nurse be careful not to impose his or her own values onto the values held by the patient. The healthcare team should honor any end-of-life cultural and religious preferences of the patient. There may be circumstances in which conflicts occur between the nurse's worldview and that of the patient, such as in decisions regarding withholding or withdrawing life-sustaining treatment. In these circumstances, the nurse should transfer care of the patient to another qualified high-acuity nurse (ANA, 2012).

Caring for the Caregiver

Nurses in high-acuity areas are challenged by having to prepare simultaneously for two opposing outcomes: survival and death. There is a delicate balance between providing both curative and palliative care while also being mindful that the care may not be successful. Performing well with the possibilities of two wildly different outcomes, while also managing the expectations of family members, creates a great deal of stress. Additional stress is incurred from role conflict, task overload, caring for brain-dead patients, communication challenges with other healthcare professionals, and communication issues with patients and family members (Harris, 2013).

In high-acuity settings, clinicians have reported such challenges in providing palliative care as misunderstanding and equating palliative care with end-of-life care, disagreement about the feasibility and desirability of providing palliative care in the ICU, and a lack of communication between primary care or other outpatient providers and ICU staff. Other barriers to the delivery of high-quality palliative care include the resuscitation of patients with a do-not-resuscitate order, conflicts about withholding life-prolonging treatment between the family and the patient as described in written advance directives, and inadequate staff training in pain management (End-of-Life Nursing Education Consortium [ELNEC], 2014). In addition, undesirable coping mechanisms of nurses and other providers may include depersonalizing or avoiding patients or families.

One way to help nurses and other clinicians cope with work-related stressors is to hold regular debriefings during the creation of plans of care, during patient care conferences, and especially after a patient dies. These debriefings are particularly helpful in processing one's thoughts about difficult or "bad" deaths and may take the form of case review, during which the factual information about the patient is discussed. This allows the circumstances of the case to be described in different ways by the respective staff in different roles. Providers are also given an opportunity to express emotional responses about the care of the patient and family that took place over the course of the patient's hospitalization. The debriefings provide an opportunity to acknowledge grief and loss, to review lessons learned, and to discuss strategies and additional professional resources to cope with grief in a mutually supportive atmosphere (Harris, 2013).

In addition to establishing a system of regular debriefings, clinicians in high-acuity environments should be encouraged to engage in self-care activities to help with coping and prevent burnout and compassion fatigue. Hospital administrators need to promote a work culture that encourages staff to take regular breaks. Clinicians should remind and support each other about the importance of basic health principles, such as adequate rest and sleep, good nutrition, physical exercise, meditation, humor, and music, to promote self-care and encourage use of earned time off (Malloy, Thrane, Winston, Virani, & Kelly, 2013).

Barriers to End-of-life Care in High-Acuity Settings

High-acuity nurses want to ensure patients at the end of life will die with dignity and peace Baker et al. (2015) identified barriers to providing end-of-life care in the high-acuity environment (Box 3–10).

BOX 3–10   Barriers to End-of-life Care

- Nursing time constraints
- Staffing patterns
- Communication challenges
- Treatment decisions based on physician, not patient, needs

SOURCE: Adapted from Attia et al. (2013); Baker et al. (2015); and Harris et al. (2014).

The Institute of Medicine (IOM) was one of the first organizations to recommend that end-of-life care be improved (IOM, 1997). While issues related to end-of-life care have been discussed in the media, the culture change in high-acuity environments has been slow. The healthcare team does not always know patients' preferences for resuscitation, and advance directives may have minimal impact on treatment decisions. Suggestions for improving end-of-life care in high-acuity environments, as summarized by McAdam and Puntillo (2015), are listed in Box 3–11.

Educational Focus   Educational programs must be developed for all members of the healthcare team to address end-of-life care. The education must be directed toward those individuals already in the workforce, as well as those who are completing their basic education requirements. The American Association of Colleges of Nursing (2002) developed the End-of-Life Nursing Education Consortium Curriculum Modules for this purpose.

The high-acuity nurse can make a positive impact on patients and their families at the end of life because of the constant presence at the bedside. The nurse, the critical

> **BOX 3–11**   Nursing Suggestions for Improving Care at the End of Life
>
> - Changing the environment to accommodate families (beds, showering facilities, music, and places for meditation and family gathering)
> - Improving management of pain and discomfort (in accordance with advance directives)
> - Knowing patient wishes for end-of-life care (advance directives that are legally binding)
> - Ceasing treatments earlier or not initiating aggressive treatments (when continued medical care seems futile)
>
> **SOURCE:** Adapted from Aslakson et al. (2014); and Wentlandt et al. (2016).

link to moderating discussion of difficult issues, can facilitate discussions about treatment preferences and management of signs and symptoms at the end of life. Nursing actions and interventions for end-of-life care, as identified by Wingate and Wiegand (2008) are summarized in Table 3–1.

Table 3–1 Summary of Nursing Actions and Interventions at the End of Life

Topic	Intervention
Treatment decisions	• Ensure that decisions are made by patients, families, and interprofessional team members • Make adjustments in the treatment plan on an on-going basis and ensure that they reflect the patient's values and interests
Capacity for end-of-life decisions	• Confirm that the patient is able to understand the information provided and communicate preferences for care; assist with determining capacity • Understand that a surrogate can make treatment decisions through a proxy directive created by the patient; assist with process • Support the patient's creation of a "living will" to identify treatment choices
Nursing care	• Understand and comply with resuscitation decisions • Deliver hydration and nutrition when anticipated results meet patient goals • Discontinue unnecessary equipment and alarms • Provide physical comfort interventions, including sedatives, analgesics, antiemetics, cooling or warming measures, oral care, and personal hygiene • Include desired family members, friends, and pets at the bedside • Honor cultural and religious practices for end-of-life care
Bereavement	• Access pastoral care for patient and family support • Participate in staff debriefing as needed to prevent burnout and compassion fatigue

SOURCE: Data partially from Delgado (2014); Mayer & Winters (2016).

Section Five Review

1. How can high-acuity nurses positively contribute to ethical dilemma management?
   A. By disconnecting from this issue
   B. By identifying these situations
   C. By avoiding moral distress
   D. By applying their own values to these conflicts

2. Which intervention is important for the nurse dealing with an ethical dilemma or other moral conflict?
   A. Explain personal values to the client
   B. Frequently evaluate personal values
   C. Revise personal philosophy to match the issue
   D. Refuse to provide care to those whose values conflict

3. Which actions can help the nurse cope with work-related stressors? (Select all that apply.)
   A. Participate in regular debriefing sessions.
   B. Get adequate sleep
   C. Exercise regularly
   D. Take regular vacations
   E. Focus on the technical aspects of client care

4. How can the nurse best facilitate end-of-life discussions? (Select all that apply.)
   A. Communicate solely with the client about these matters
   B. Build on previous discussions
   C. Establish goals of care
   D. Provide clear basic information about the client's condition
   E. Avoid talking about any poor prognosis

Answers: 1. B, 2. B, 3. (A, B, C, D), 4. (B, C, D)

Clinical Reasoning Checkpoint

Mr. S, a 78-year-old male, is admitted to a progressive care unit for the treatment of an acute exacerbation of systolic heart failure. His symptoms include complaints of severe shortness of breath and air, fatigue, and swelling in his lower legs and feet. Vital signs on admission are blood pressure 160/100, heart rate 110 beats per minute, and respiratory rate 32 breaths per minute. Physical exam reveals bilateral pulmonary crackles throughout all lung fields, 3+ ankle edema in both extremities, and S_1, S_2, S_3 heart sounds.

After 1 week of aggressive medical treatment, Mr. S receives little relief from his respiratory complaints and other symptoms. His blood pressure has decreased to 146/96, but other vital signs remain relatively unchanged. He develops pulmonary edema, and the need for mechanical ventilation is discussed. Mr. S tells his medical team and family that he is tired after years of medical treatment for heart failure and would like to "die peacefully" without further intervention. Palliative care is planned and implemented.

1. Describe appropriate treatment of the respiratory symptoms in this case.
2. Explain a factor that could motivate the medical team to consider mechanical ventilation under these circumstances.
3. What further documentation would assist the health care providers with delivering the care desired by the patient?
4. Describe appropriate treatment goals in this patient case.

Chapter 3 Review

1. Which statement, made by a newly licensed nurse, would the preceptor evaluate as a possible barrier to this nurse providing palliative care?
   1. "It is hard for me to give up on my clients."
   2. "My newly admitted client is suffering so much."
   3. "I don't think much more can be done for my client."
   4. "Even with all this equipment there is so much we don't know."

2. A client's spouse says, "I don't want palliative care for my husband. I want to keep trying to cure his disease." Which nursing response is best?
   1. "I know this is a hard decision."
   2. "Palliative care can only be given in the last six months of life."
   3. "We can provide palliative care as we continue to work toward a cure."
   4. "Let's schedule a conference with you, your husband, the physicians, and social workers."

3. The nurse would evaluate which of the following situations as indicating the client has decision-making capacity? (Select all that apply.)
   1. The client can verbalize options for care.
   2. The nonverbal client blinks to answer yes or no to questions about care.
   3. The client requires maximum sedation to control constant pain.
   4. The client says, "I refuse this treatment even though it might save my life."
   5. The client is confused and combative.

4. Paramedics bring a Medical Orders for Life-Sustaining Treatment (MOLST) form to the emergency department along with a client. The nurse would evaluate that this document is valid if which conditions exist? (Select all that apply.)
   1. The expiration date is for 9 months in the future.
   2. There is no physician signature on the document.

3. The client has updated the form in several areas and has initialed the updates.

4. The document lists "no mechanical ventilator" as a requirement of care.

5. The client is reported to have a terminal condition.

5. A client had been electively sedated and paralyzed to control intracranial pressure following a closed head injury. A painful, invasive procedure is scheduled today. What nursing action is indicated?

   1. Do not be concerned about pain since the client is nonresponsive.

   2. Ask the physician about whether ordered prn pain medication is indicated.

   3. Administer preprocedure pain medication.

   4. Request that sedating medication be withheld so a pain assessment can be completed.

6. A nurse manager is assigning the care of these ICU clients to staff nurses for this shift. Which clients would the manager consider assigning to a nurse with particularly astute palliative care skills? (Select all that apply.)

   1. A client whose shortness of breath was found to be secondary to advanced lung cancer.

   2. A client who was intubated for treatment of chronic obstructive lung disease.

   3. A client who just returned from surgery for a perforated appendix.

   4. A client who had a myocardial infarction and is scheduled for stent placement today.

   5. A client who is in renal failure secondary to a serious crushing injury to the legs.

7. A client has been declared brain dead and is being considered as an organ transplant donor candidate. Which statement should the nurse make when speaking to the client's family?

   1. "We will keep your loved one on life support until the decision about organ donation is made."

   2. "I am so sorry to hear of the death of your loved one."

   3. "Your loved one is in an area between life and death."

   4. "Machinery keeping your loved one's body alive will be discontinued after organs are harvested."

8. An older adult client has just died following a long, protracted illness. Which nursing statements would be helpful to the family of a client who has just died? (Select all that apply.)

   1. "I am so sorry that your loved one died."

   2. "Would you like for me to go with you to your loved one's room?"

   3. "We will need to know which funeral home you want us to call."

   4. "We will need for you to get your loved one's belongings out of the room as soon as possible."

   5. "There is a small room just off the waiting room where you can wait for the rest of your family to arrive."

9. A nurse's values conflict with those of the client's family regarding withdrawal of life-sustaining treatment. What action should the nurse take?

   1. Continue to care for the client as if the conflict did not exist.

   2. Try to help the family see the need to reverse their opinion.

   3. Ask for a reassignment.

   4. Discuss the need for a DNR with the client's health care provider.

10. Which occurrences in an ICU would alert the nurse manager that additional debriefing sessions may be needed for staff? (Select all that apply.)

    1. A newly credentialed physician has written palliative care order for two clients in the last week.

    2. A nurse who was unfamiliar with a client's DNR status initiated CPR after the client had a cardiac arrest.

    3. Family have argued openly about life-sustaining treatment for their loved one.

    4. Clients have reported "The nurses don't seem to care about me as a person."

    5. Over the last month the staff has provided care to three brain-dead clients while awaiting organ donation.

Answers to questions found inside your textbook are available on the faculty resources site. Please consult with your instructor.

References

Adams, J. A., Anderson, R. A., Docherty, S. L., Tulsky, J. A., Steinhauser, K. E., & Bailey, D. E., Jr. (2014). Nursing strategies to support family members of ICU patients at high risk of dying. *Heart & Lung: The Journal of Acute and Critical Care, 43*(5), 406–415. http://doi .org/10.1016/j.hrtlng.2014.02.001

American Association of Colleges of Nursing. (2002). *End-of-life competency statements for a peaceful death.* Washington, DC: Author.

American Association of Critical-Care Nurses (AACN). (2005). Acute and critical care choices: A guide to advance directives. Aliso Viejo, CA: The Association.

American Association of Critical-Care Nurses (AACN). (2013). *Assessing pain in the critically ill adult: AACN practice alert, 1–7.* Retrieved February 6, 2017, from https://www.aacn.org/clinical-resources /practice-alerts/assessing-pain-in-the-critically -ill-adult

American Association of Critical-Care Nurses. (2015). *AACN Scope and Standards for Acute and Critical Care Nursing Practice.* Retrieved August 30, 2016, from http://www.aacn.org/wd/practice/docs/scope-and-standards-acute-critical-care-2015.pdf

American Association of Critical-Care Nurses (AACN). (n.d.). *Four A's to rise above moral distress.* Retrieved March 24, 2016, from http://www.aacn.org/wd /practice/content/ethic-moral.pcms?menu=practice

American Cancer Society (ACS). (2014). *The Patient Self-Determination Act (PSDA).* Retrieved February 21, 2016, from http://www.cancer .org/treatment/findingandpayingfortreatment /understandingfinancialandlegalmatters /advancedirectives/advance-directives-patient-self-determination-act

American Nurses Association (ANA). (2001). *Standards of clinical nursing practice* (2nd ed.). Washington, DC: American Nurses Publishing.

American Nurses Association (ANA). (2012). *Nursing care and do-not-resuscitate (DNR) orders and allow natural death (AND) decisions.* Retrieved February 21, 2016 from http://www.nursingworld.org/MainMenuCategories /EthicsStandards/Ethics-Position-Statements /Nursing-Care-and-Do-Not-Resuscitate-DNR-and-Allow-Natural-Death-Decisions.pdf

Anderson, W. G., Puntillo, K., Boyle, D., Barbour, S., Turner, K., Cimino, J., . . . Pantilat, S. (2016). ICU bedside nurses' involvement in palliative care communication: A multicenter survey. *Journal of Pain and Symptom Management, 51*(3), 589–596.e2. http://doi .org/10.1016/j.jpainsymman.2015.11.003

Arbour, R. B. (2013). Brain death: Assessment, controversy, and confounding factors. *Critical Care Nurse, 33*(6), 27–46. http://doi.org/10.4037 /ccn2013215

Aslakson, R., Cheng, J., Vollenweider, D., Galusca, D., Smith, T. J., & Pronovost, P. J. (2014). Evidence-based palliative care in the intensive care unit: A systematic review of interventions. *Journal of Palliative Medicine, 17*(2), 219–235. http://doi.org/10.1089 /jpm.2013.0409

Aslakson, R. A., Curtis, J. R., & Nelson, J. E. (2014). The changing role of palliative care in the ICU. *Critical Care Medicine, 42*(11), 2418–2428. http://doi.org/10.1097 /CCM.0000000000000573

Attia, A. K., Abd-Elaziz, W. W., & Kandeel, N. A. (2013). Critical care nurses' perception of barriers and supportive behaviors in end-of-life care. *American Journal of Hospice and Palliative Care, 30*(3), 297–304. doi:10.1177/1049909112450067

Baker, M., Luce, J., & Bosslet, G. T. (2015). Integration of palliative care services in the intensive care unit. *Clinics in Chest Medicine, 36*(3), 441–448. http://doi .org/10.1016/j.ccm.2015.05.010

Bakitas, M., Bishop, M. F., & Hahn, M. E. (2014). Symptoms when death is imminent. In C. H. Yarbro, D. Wujcik, & B. H. Gobel (Eds.), *Cancer symptom management* (4th ed., pp. 699–721). Burlington, MA: Jones & Bartlett.

Barsevick, A. M., & Aktas, A. (2013). Cancer symptom cluster research. *Current Opinion in Supportive and Palliative Care, 7*(1), 36–37. http://doi.org/10.1097 /SPC.0b013e32835defac

Batiha, A.-M. (2013). Pain management barriers in critical care units: A qualitative study. *International Journal of Advanced Nursing Studies, 3*(1), 1–5. http://doi .org/10.14419/ijans.v3i1.1494

Berry, P. H., & Griffie, J. (2015). Planning for the actual death. In B. R. Ferrell, N. Coyle, & J. Paice (Eds.), *Oxford textbook of palliative nursing* (4th ed., pp. 515–530). New York, NY: Oxford University Press. http://doi .org/10.1093/med/9780199332342.001.0001

Black, M. D., Vigorito, M. C., Curtis, J. R., Phillips, G. S., Martin, E. W., McNicoll, L., . . . Levy, M. (2013). A multifaceted intervention to improve compliance with process measures for ICU clinician communication with ICU patients and families. *Critical Care Medicine, 41*(10), 2275–2283. http://doi.org/10.1097 /CCM.0b013e3182982671

Brant, J. M. (2014). Pain. In C. H. Yarbro, D. Wujcik, & B. H. Gobel (Eds.), *Cancer symptom management* (4th ed., pp. 69–90). Burlington, MA: Jones & Bartlett.

Brohard, C. (2014). Grief. In C. H. Yarbro, D. Wujcik, & B. H. Gobel (Eds.), *Cancer symptom management* (4th ed., pp. 673–681). Burlington, MA: Jones & Bartlett.

Browning, A. M. (2013). Moral distress and psychological empowerment in critical care nurses caring for adults at end of life. *American Journal of Critical Care, 22*(2), 143–151. http://doi.org/10.4037/ajcc2013437

Buscaino, K. S., Singh, U., Nissanov, J., & Wells, M. (2013). Do Not Resuscitate (DNR) versus Allow Natural Death (AND): A dichotomy in perception between provider and patient. *Journal of the American Medical Directors Association, 14*(3), B21. http://doi.org/10.1016/ j.jamda.2012.12.060

Bush, S. H., Bruera, E., Lawlor, P. G., Kanji, S., Davis, D. H. J., Agar, M., . . . Pereira, J. L. (2014a). Clinical practice guidelines for delirium management: Potential application in palliative care. *Journal of Pain and Symptom Management, 48*(2), 249–258. http://doi .org/10.1016/j.jpainsymman.2013.09.023

Bush, S. H., Leonard, M. M., Agar, M., Spiller, J. A., Hosie, A., Wright, D. K., . . . Lawlor, P. G. (2014b). End-of-life delirium: Issues regarding recognition, optimal management, and the role of sedation in the dying phase. *Journal of Pain and Symptom Management, 48*(2), 215–230. http://doi.org/10.1016/j .jpainsymman.2014.05.009

Campbell, M. L., & Gorman, L. M. (2015). Withdrawal of life-sustaining therapies: Mechanical ventilation, dialysis, and cardiac devices. In B. R. Ferrell, N. Coyle, & J. Paice (Eds.), *Oxford textbook of palliative nursing* (4th ed., pp. 463–474). New York, NY: Oxford University Press. http://doi.org/10.1093 /med/9780199332342.001.0001

Center to Advance Palliative Care. (2013). *Implementing ICU screening criteria for unmet palliative care needs* (pp. 1–13). Retrieved November 28, 2016, from https://media .capc.org/filer_public/80/be/80be3587-6ca1-4eb8-93f0-7fa0e30cd153/76_66_ipal-icu-implementing-icu-screening-criteria-for-unmet-palliative-care-needs.pdf

Center to Advance Palliative Care. (n.d.). *About palliative care.* Retrieved March 21, 2016, from https://www .capc.org/about/palliative-care

Chi, N. C., & Demiris, G. (2016). Family caregivers' pain management in end-of-life care: A systematic review. *American Journal of Hospice and Palliative Medicine*, 1–16. http://doi.org/10.1177/1049909116637359

Chovan, J. D., Cluxton, D., & Rancour, P. (2015). Principles of patient and family assessment. In B. R. Ferrell, N. Coyle, & J. Paice (Eds.), *Oxford textbook of palliative nursing* (4th ed., pp. 58–80). New York, NY: Oxford University Press. http://doi.org/10.1093 /med/9780199332342.001.0001

Chow, K. (2014). Ethical dilemmas in the intensive care unit. *Journal of Hospice & Palliative Nursing*, 16(5), 256–260. http://doi.org/10.1097/NJH.0000000000000069

Chow, K., Cogan, D., & Mun, S. (2015). Nausea and vomiting. In B. R. Ferrell, N. Coyle, & J. Paice (Eds.), *Oxford textbook of palliative nursing* (4th ed., pp. 175–190). New York, NY: Oxford University Press. http://doi .org/10.1093/med/9780199332342.001.0001

Clarke, E. B., Curtis, J. R., Luce, J. M., Levy, M., Danis, M., Nelson, J., & Solomon, M. Z. (2003). Quality indicators for end-of-life care in the intensive care unit. *Critical Care Medicine*, 31(9), 2255–2262. http://doi .org/10.1097/01.CCM.0000084849.96385.85

Collis, E., & Mather, H. (2015). Nausea and vomiting in palliative care. *British Medical Journal*, 351:h6249. http://doi.org/10.1136/bmj.h6249

Cook, D., & Rocker, G. (2014). Dying with dignity in the intensive care unit. *New England Journal of Medicine*, 370(26), 2506–2514. http://doi.org/10.1056/NEJMra1208795

Corless, I. B. (2015). Bereavement. In B. R. Ferrell, N. Coyle, & J. Paice (Eds.), *Oxford textbook of palliative nursing* (4th ed., pp. 487–499). New York, NY: Oxford University Press. http://doi.org/10.1093 /med/9780199332342.001.0001

Dahlin, C. M., & Wittenberg, E. (2015). Communication in palliative care: An essential competency for nurses. In B. R. Ferrell, N. Coyle, & J. Paice (Eds.), *Oxford textbook of palliative nursing* (4th ed., pp. 81–112). New York, NY: Oxford University Press. http://doi.org/10.1093 /med/9780199332342.001.0001

Delgado, S. (2014). Chapter 8: Ethical and legal considerations. In S. M. Burns (Ed.), *AACN: Essentials of critical care nursing* (pp. 215–229). New York, NY: McGraw-Hill Education.

Dudgeon, D. (2015). Dyspnea, terminal secretions, and cough. In B. R. Ferrell, N. Coyle, & J. Paice (Eds.), *Oxford textbook of palliative nursing* (4th ed., pp. 247–261). New York, NY: Oxford University Press. http://doi .org/10.1093/med/9780199332342.001.0001

End-of-Life Nursing Education Consortium (ELNEC). (2014). ELNEC Critical Care Curriculum. Presented at ELNEC Critical Care Workshop.

Fink, R. M., Gates, R. A., & Montgomery, R. K. (2015). Pain assessment. In B. R. Ferrell, N. Coyle, & J. Paice (Eds.), *Oxford textbook of palliative nursing* (4th ed., pp. 113–134). New York, NY: Oxford University Press. http://doi.org/10.1093/med/ 9780199332342.001.0001

Grassi, L., Caraceni, A., Mitchell, A. J., Nanni, M. G., Berardi, M. A., Caruso, R., & Riba, M. (2015). Management of delirium in palliative care: A review. *Current Psychiatry Reports*, 17(3), 1535–1645. http://doi .org/10.1007/s11920-015-0550-8

Harris, L. J. M. (2013). Caring and coping. *Journal of Hospice & Palliative Nursing*, 15(8), 446–454. http://doi .org/10.1097/NJH.0b013e3182a0de78

Harris, M., Gaudet, J., & O'Reardon, C. (2014). Nursing care for patients at end of life in the adult intensive care unit. *Journal of Nursing Education and Practice*, 4(6), 84–89. Retrieved November 30, 2016, from http:// www.sciedu.ca/journal/index.php/jnep/article /view/4190/2711

Heidrich, D. E., & English, N. K. (2015). Delirium, confusion, agitation, and restlessness. In B. R. Ferrell, N. Coyle, & J. Paice (Eds.), *Oxford textbook of palliative nursing* (4th ed., pp. 385–403). New York, NY: Oxford University Press. http://doi.org/10.1093 /med/9780199332342.001.0001

Hinderer, K. A., Friedmann, E., & Fins, J. J. (2015). Withdrawal of life-sustaining treatment. *Dimensions of Critical Care Nursing*, 34(2), 91–99. http://doi .org/10.1097/DCC.0000000000000097

Huffines, M., Johnson, K. L., Smitz Naranjo, L. L., Lissauer, M. E., Fishel, M. A. M., D'Angelo Howes, S. M., . . . Smith, R. (2013). Improving family satisfaction and participation in decision making in an intensive care unit. *Critical Care Nurse*, 33(5), 56–69. http://doi .org/10.4037/ccn2013354

Institute of Medicine (IOM). (1997). *Approaching death: Improving care at the end of life.* New York, NY: National Academy Press.

Kelley, A. S., & Morrison, R. S. (2015). Palliative care for the seriously ill. *New England Journal of Medicine*, 373(8), 747–755. http://doi.org/10.1056/ NEJMra1404684

Knight, P., Espinoza, L. A., & Freeman, B. (2015). Sedation for refractory symptoms. In B. R. Ferrell, N. Coyle, & J. Paice (Eds.), *Oxford textbook of palliative nursing* (4th ed., pp. 440–448). New York, NY: Oxford University Press. http://doi.org/10.1093 /med/9780199332342.001.0001

Maani-Fogelman, P., & Bakitas, M. A. (2015). Hospital-based palliative care. In B. R. Ferrell, N. Coyle, & J. Paice (Eds.), *Oxford textbook of palliative nursing* (4th ed., pp. 20–57). New York, NY: Oxford University Press. http://doi.org/10.1093/med/9780199332342. 001.0001

Malloy, P., Thrane, S., Winston, T., Virani, R., & Kelly, K. (2013). Do nurses who care for patients in palliative and end-of-life settings perform good self-care? *Journal of Hospice & Palliative Nursing*, 15(2), 99–106. http://doi.org/10.1097/NJH. 0b013e31826bef72

Mayer, D., & Winters, C. (2016). Palliative care I critical access hospitals. *Critical Care Nurse, 36*(1), 72–78.

McAdam, J., & Puntillo, K. (2015). The intensive care unit. In B. R. Ferrell, N. Coyle, & J. Paice (Eds.), *Oxford textbook of palliative nursing* (4th ed., pp. 740–760). New York, NY: Oxford University Press. doi:10.1093 /med/9780199332342.001.0001

Mularski, R. A., Reinke, L. F., Carrieri-Kohlman, V., Fischer, M. D., Campbell, M. L., Rocker, G., . . . White, D.B. (2013). An official American Thoracic Society workshop report: Assessment and palliative management of dyspnea crisis. *Annals of the American Thoracic Society, 10*(5), S98–S106. http://doi .org/10.1513/AnnalsATS.201306-169ST

National Consensus Project for Quality Palliative Care (NCP). (2013). In C. M. Dahlin (Ed.), *Clinical practice guidelines for quality palliative care* (3rd ed., pp. 1–74). Pittsburgh, PA: Author. Retrieved from www .nationalconsensusproject.org

National Consensus Project for Quality Palliative Care (NCP). (n.d.). *About us.* Retrieved March 20, 2016, from http://www.nationalconsensusproject.org /DisplayPage.aspx?Title=About%20Us

Oechsle, K., Goerth, K., Bokemeyer, C., & Mehnert, A. (2013). Symptom burden in palliative care patients: Perspectives of patients, their family caregivers, and their attending physicians. *Supportive Care in Cancer: Official Journal of the Multinational Association of Supportive Care in Cancer, 21*(7), 1955–1962. http://doi .org/10.1007/s00520-013-1747-1

Paice, J. A. (2015). Pain at the end of life. In B. R. Ferrell, N. Coyle, & J. Paice (Eds.), *Oxford Textbook of Palliative Nursing* (4th ed., pp. 135–153). New York, NY: Oxford University Press. http://doi.org/10.1093 /med/9780199332342.001.0001

Perrin, K. O., & Kazanowski, M. (2015). Overcoming barriers to palliative care consultation. *Critical Care Nurse, 35*(5), 44–52. http://doi.org/10.4037 /ccn2015357

Puchalski, C. M. (2014). The FICA spiritual history tool #274. *Journal of Palliative Medicine, 17*(1), 105–106. http://doi.org/10.1089/jpm.2013.9458

Puntillo, K., Nelson, J. E., Weissman, D., Curtis, R., Weiss, S., Frontera, J., . . . Campbell, M. (2013). Palliative care in the ICU: Relief of pain, dyspnea, and thirst—A report from the IPAL-ICU Advisory Board. *Intensive Care Medicine, 40*(2), 235–248. http://doi.org/10.1007 /s00134-013-3153-z

Rao, J. K., Anderson, L. A., Lin, F.-C., & Laux, J. P. (2014). Completion of advance directives among U.S. consumers. *American Journal of Preventive Medicine, 46*(1), 65–70. http://doi.org/10.1016 /j.amepre.2013.09.008

Reynolds, J., Drew, D., & Dunwoody, C. (2013). American Society for Pain Management nursing position statement: Pain management at the end of life. *Pain Management Nursing, 14*(3), 172–175. http://doi .org/10.1016/j.pmn.2013.07.002

Rocker, G. M., Simpson, A. C., Young, J., Horton, R., Sinuff, T., Demmons, J., . . . Marciniuk, D. (2013). Opioid therapy for refractory dyspnea in patients with advanced chronic obstructive pulmonary disease: Patients' experiences and outcomes. *Canadian Medical Association Open, 1*(1), E27–E36. http://doi .org/10.9778/cmajo.20120031

Rose, L., Haslam, L., Dale, C., Knechtel, L., & McGillion, M. (2013). Behavioral pain assessment tool for critically ill adults unable to self-report pain. *American Journal of Critical Care, 22*(3), 246–255. http://doi.org/10.4037 /ajcc2013200

Singer, A. E., Ash, T., Ochotorena, C., Lorenz, K. A., Chong, K., Shreve, S. T., & Ahluwalia, S. C. (2016). A systematic review of family meeting tools in palliative and intensive care settings. *American Journal of Hospice and Palliative Medicine, 33*(8), 797–806. http://doi.org/10.1177/1049909115594353

Stapleton, S. J., Holden, J., Epstein, J., & Wilkie, D. J. (2016). Symptom clusters in patients with cancer in the hospice/palliative care setting. *Supportive Care in Cancer: Official Journal of the Multinational Association of Supportive Care in Cancer, 1–9.* http://doi.org/10.1007 /s00520-016-3210-6

Steele, R., & Davies, B. (2015). Supporting families in palliative care. In B. R. Ferrell, N. Coyle, & J. Paice (Eds.), *Oxford Textbook of Palliative Nursing* (4th ed., pp. 500–514). New York, NY: Oxford University Press. http://doi.org/10.1093 /med/9780199332342.001.0001

Tipton, J. (2014). Nausea and vomiting. In C. H. Yarbro, D. Wujcik, and B. H. Gobel (Eds.), *Cancer symptom management* (4th ed., pp. 213–238). Burlington, MA: Jones & Bartlett.

Wentlandt, K., Seccareccia, D., Kevork, N., Workentin, K., Blacker, S., Grossman, D., & Zimmerman, C. (2016). Quality of care and satisfaction with care on palliative care units. *Journal of Pain and Symptom Management, 51*(2), 184–192.

Chapter 4
The Older Adult High-Acuity Patient

Learning Outcomes

4.1 Illustrate the characteristics of the aging population.

4.2 Analyze the age-related changes in neurologic and neurosensory function.

4.3 Analyze the age-related changes in cardiovascular and pulmonary function.

4.4 Analyze the age-related changes in integumentary and musculoskeletal function.

4.5 Analyze the age-related changes in gastrointestinal and genitourinary function.

4.6 Analyze the age-related changes in endocrine and immune function.

4.7 Compare dementia, delirium, and depression and evaluate their impact on older high-acuity patients and their families.

4.8 Analyze falls, pain, and pharmacology as factors that impact hospitalization in the older patient.

4.9 Evaluate the use of common geriatric assessment tools.

4.10 Analyze the nursing management of older patients with high-risk injuries and trauma.

4.11 Appraise special situations, including the culture of caring for older adults and end-of-life care.

An increasing percentage of hospital and high-acuity patients are older adults. They are a vulnerable population needing skilled care. A number of changes occur as a result of the normal aging process, and while these changes do not cause illness or disability, they do put the older adult at risk for complications and negative outcomes during hospitalization. The high-acuity nurse needs to be aware of these changes and risks in order to properly assess older patients and provide interventions to improve outcomes. This chapter reviews key aging changes and common problems nurses are likely to encounter in the older high-acuity patient and provides strategies for improving nursing management of these challenging patients.

Section One: Introduction to the Aging Patient

Aging affects the physical, psychological, social, spiritual, and economic aspects of a person's life experience. Lifestyle as well as genetic and environmental influences may impact the aging process. The changes from aging and chronic disease put older adults at risk for poorer outcomes during acute illness, especially high-acuity illness.

The Older Adult Patient

Nurses working in high-acuity areas should understand the age-related changes that make older patients vulnerable to complications and that may impact the outcome of their hospitalization. Physical characteristics are affected during the aging process and are marked by a gradual loss of efficiency in function of all organ systems. The challenge for nurses is to distinguish between changes associated with normal aging and those that occur due to a pathologic process. Physiologic changes as well as other comorbidities impact the ability to respond to a current illness and thus are important factors that determine the outcome and recovery.

Older adults may present with common problems in uncommon ways: Symptoms are less predictable; older patients may have multiple other comorbidities, may be taking multiple medications, and may experience adverse drug reactions; and they are at greater risk for disability and complications (Brummel et al., 2015; Manning, 2014). In addition, older adults have reduced physiological reserve of most body systems; they have reduced homeostatic mechanisms, which affect temperature control and fluid and electrolyte balance, decreased response to stress, and increased risk of infections (LeMone, Burke, Bauldoff, & Gubrud, 2015; Tabloski, 2014; Valiathan, Ashman, Asthana, 2016).

Older adult visits to the emergency department for severe acute illness are increasing (Pines, Mullins, Cooper, Feng, & Roth, 2013), and older patients have a higher risk of hospitalization, longer lengths of stay, and greater morbidity and mortality than younger age groups. Early identification of high-risk patients and greater vigilance are needed in the care of older adults. The implementation of early interventions and the application of protocols can improve care, promote optimal function, prevent complications, and provide for the best possible outcomes for hospitalized elderly patients.

Characteristics of the Older Adult Population

The older population is growing older, both in and out of the hospital setting (Figure 4–1). Because of advancements in sanitation, technology, and medicine over the past hundred years, people are living longer.

Demographics In the United States, the population aged 65 and over is expected to double in size within the next 15 years (Centers for Disease Control and Prevention [CDC], 2013). By 2030, almost one out of every five Americans, or more than 72 million people, will be 65 years or older. The fastest-growing group is people over the age of 85, who have the highest utilization of healthcare resources, and there are nearly 70,000 centenarians (Administration on Aging [AOA], 2014). This "age wave" will peak in 2030 when the baby boomers, who started turning 65 in 2011, will all be over the age of 85 (AOA, 2014). This has implications for all professionals in healthcare, including nurses in high-acuity settings, because older adults use a disproportionate amount of our healthcare resources, placing increased strain on available healthcare services.

General Health Older adults have a disproportionate amount of health problems; 85% have at least one chronic condition (Ward, Schiller, & Goodman, 2014), and 50% have at least two. The most common chronic diseases include hypertension, arthritis, cancer, diabetes, and heart diseases (AOA, 2014). All of these may be the cause of hospitalization or need to be considered when treating the older patient with acute illness. The high rates of chronic disease are related to high levels of disability, with nearly half of older adults having some difficulty with daily activities or

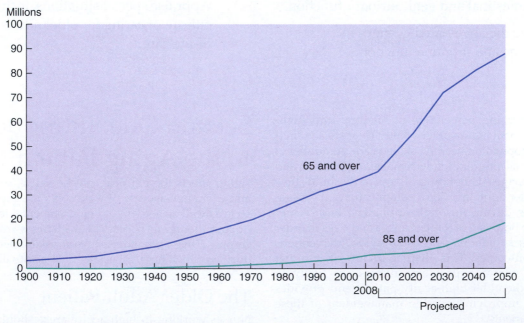

Figure 4–1 Population age 65 and over and age 85 and over, selected years 1900–2008 and projected 2010–2050.

SOURCE: Data from Population of Older Adults in the U.S., 1900–2008 and projected to 2050 from Federal Interagency Forum on Aging Related Statistics.

self-care (AOA, 2014), and these rates of disease and disability increase with age.

While older adults have more health problems than younger people, it is important to remember that as an age group they are very diverse in physical condition. The nurse should never assume the pre-illness health status of an older person without further investigation. While some older adults are frail with many health conditions, 14% of older adults have no chronic diseases (Ward et al., 2014), and nearly half of those over 65 report their health as very good or excellent (AOA, 2014). In 2013, only about 3.4% of older adults were living in institutional settings, with the highest rates among the oldest age groups (AOA, 2014). For this reason, the nurse should assess each older adult individually to determine baseline health and functional state prior to illness and strive to return the individual to this prior health state if possible.

Healthcare   Older adults make up a majority of patients in the general hospital setting: People over 65 have twice the rate of hospitalizations compared to younger adults (AOA, 2014). Older people make up about half of patients in the intensive care unit (Bell, 2014). Emergency department visits by older people are increasing, and these patients are more likely than younger people to be admitted to the hospital and have complications (Pines et al., 2013). Unfortunately, a high percentage of health resources are used in the last year of life, including critical care services, so the number of older adult high-acuity patients who are at the end of life is likely to increase.

Ethnic Diversity   Another change in the aging population in the United States is increasing racial and ethnic diversity. The minority population in adults older than 65 was about 17.5% in the year 2003 and is expected to rise to 28.5% by 2030 (AOA, 2014). Moreover, the Hispanic older adult population is expected to increase the most, from 7% in 2010 to nearly 20% in 2050 (CDC, 2013), while the African American population is expected to rise more modestly, from 8.3% to about 11% (an increase of 2.7%). With the growing immigrant and minority populations, nurses should strive to provide culturally competent care and meet the needs of an increasingly diverse population.

Section One Review

1. In the United States, what is the fastest-growing age group (by decade)?
   A. People over 55
   B. People over 65
   C. People over 75
   D. People over 85

2. About what percentage of older adults were living in institutional settings in 2013?
   A. 2.5%
   B. 3.4%
   C. 8%
   D. 10%

3. As a general statement, it would be correct to say that older adults have which characteristic?
   A. Pretty much alike
   B. Less likely to need to visit the ER
   C. Increasingly diverse
   D. Unlikely to have chronic diseases

4. Why are older adults more likely to present with a common problem in an uncommon way? (Select all that apply.)
   A. They take more medications.
   B. They have more comorbidities.
   C. They are less likely to care for themselves well.
   D. They are at greater risk for infection.
   E. They are less likely to follow care instructions correctly.

Answers: 1. D, 2. B, 3. C, 4. (A, B, D)

Section Two: Neurologic and Neurosensory Systems Changes

As a person ages, many changes occur in neurologic and neurosensory function. These changes make the older adult more prone to injury such as falls, and slower cognition may require adjustments in how the nurse conducts patient education. It is important to assess neurosensory alterations, as multiple senses such as hearing and sight can be significantly affected.

Neurologic System

The central nervous system (CNS) regulates the cognitive, behavioral, sensory, and homeostatic functions of the body. The rate of neurologic system changes associated with aging varies among individuals, organ systems, and among cell populations within organ systems (Tabloski, 2014). In the older adult, neurotransmitters are not synthesized at the same rate, which may lead to a decline in sympathetic and catecholamine response. This change may cause a decreased cardiac compensation in conditions such as fever, hypovolemia, or stress. In addition, declines in nervous system conduction may cause slower reflex responses. While

Table 4–1 Summary of Age-related Changes: Neurologic and Neurosensory Systems

Age-related Change	Physiologic Effect
CENTRAL NERVOUS SYSTEM	
Altered neurotransmitter synthesis	Altered sympathetic and catecholamine response Decreased cardiac compensation
Decreased nervous system conduction	Slower reflex response
Slower memory processes	Slower learning
More permeable blood–brain barrier	Increased risk of medication side effects or toxicity
Decreased brain volume and weight	Delayed onset of symptoms after intracranial bleeding Increased risk of medication side effects or toxicity
Formation of neurofibrillary tangles and senile plaque	Associated with development of Alzheimer disease
NEUROSENSORY	
Vision: decreased sensory receptors, corneal thickening and reshaping, cataracts, glaucoma	Decreased visual acuity and depth perception Pupils smaller with decreased response to light Cataracts: Increasingly cloudy vision as lens opacity increases Glaucoma: Loss of peripheral vision (blindness results if not treated)
Hearing: decreased sensitivity to sounds (particularly high-pitched sounds), increased cerumen impactions	Decrease in hearing and ability to hear high-pitched noises, especially in presence of background noise Increased processing and responding time to auditory stimuli
Touch: Decreased sensitivity in hands and feet	Decreased sensation in fingers, palms, and feet increases risk of injury (e.g., burns, trauma, undiscovered infection)
Proprioception, balance, and postural control: decreased	Decreased stability in walking, with increased risk of falls and traumatic injury

loss of memory is not normal, memory processes are slower and learning takes longer. The blood–brain barrier is more permeable, so medications may cross into the brain easily, increasing the risk of side effects or toxicity. In addition, dilation of the ventricles and a decrease in brain volume (probably due to loss of water) occur, which essentially increase the cranial dead space. Therefore, elderly persons may sustain a significant amount of hemorrhage after an injury-induced intracranial bleed before symptoms are apparent. Table 4–1 summarizes changes in the central nervous system in the older adult.

Nursing Implications of Central Nervous System Changes
In the high-acuity patient, age-related central nervous changes impact the neurologic exam. Nurses assess mental status, level of consciousness (LOC), delirium, and ability to communicate and follow commands, as well as short- and long-term memory (see discussion of geriatric assessment tests in Section Nine of this chapter). Comorbid conditions, hypoxia, electrolyte imbalances, and medications can potentially alter the patient's CNS assessment findings. Changes in fine and gross motor function, such as handgrip strength and reflexes, may be due to changes in CNS function. Nurses should be aware of the impact of CNS changes on the ability to perform self-care as well as the ability to follow or interpret instructions regarding self-care. In the high-acuity setting, age-related neurologic changes along with acute medical conditions and the environmental issues associated with high-acuity settings contribute to a risk for postoperative cognitive dysfunction, falls, restraint use, oversedation, and delirium. Changes in cognitive function through slower processing speed make learning new information take longer; however, patient teaching can still be effective. Table 4–2 provides a summary of the nursing implications of age-related changes to the neurological system.

Neurosensory Systems

As individuals age, there is a decline in all of the sensory receptors. Sensory impairments in older adults may occur as a result of normal changes of aging, the side effects of

Table 4–2 Nursing Implications: Neurologic and Sensory Changes

System	Implications
Neurologic	Assessment: Obtain baseline data (comorbid conditions, Glasgow Coma Scale [GCS], mental status, fall risk, muscle strength) Diagnosis and Planning: Risk for falls, hyperthermia, hypothermia, injury, confusion (acute or chronic), impaired memory, impaired bed mobility Implementation: Protect from hypothermia (minimize exposure to cool environment; keep covered during bathing; apply warmed blankets); allow more time for patient to answer questions and decrease background noise Evaluation: Evaluate mental status daily; re-evaluate fall risk with changes in patient status
Sensory	Assessment: Obtain baseline data (basic vision and hearing acuity; effectiveness and presence of sensory aids [glasses, hearing aids]; peripheral sensation; proprioception, balance, and postural control) Diagnosis and Planning: Impaired verbal communication, risk for injury, impaired walking Implementation: Provide patient with personal sensory aids (glasses, hearing aids) whenever feasible; explore alternative methods of communication based on existing sensory deficits (e.g., alphabet boards); provide walking aids as needed Evaluation: Evaluate effectiveness of meeting the patient's communication needs daily; prior to mobilizing the patient, re-evaluate proprioception, balance, and postural stability

medication, pathology of certain illnesses, and exposure to environmental insults and chemicals (Tabloski, 2014), although there is a great deal of diversity in the rate and severity of sensory decline. Visual acuity and depth perception decrease. Pupils are smaller, and pupillary response to light is decreased. The cornea becomes thicker, flatter, and more irregular in shape. The lens becomes more yellow and opaque; cataracts and glaucoma are common conditions, further complicating the accuracy of the eye exam.

Sensory changes affect the appetite and may contribute to nutritional status. Appetite and thirst dysregulation occurs, saliva production decreases, vision loss makes cooking more difficult, and diminished senses of taste and smell make food less appealing (Amarya, Singh, & Sabharwal, 2015). Auditory function declines, and there is decreased sensitivity to sound. An increase in cerumen impactions due to a decrease in function of the hair fibers of the ear canal causes blocking of sound and can affect hearing ability. In addition, older adults may have difficulty hearing high-pitched sounds and rushed speech, especially when there is background noise, and may require more time to process and respond to auditory stimuli. Touch sensitivity in the fingertips, palms, and lower extremities also deteriorates with aging. There is a decline in proprioception, balance, and postural control. Refer to Table 4–1 for a summary of the physiologic changes of aging associated with sensory function.

Nursing Implications of Neurosensory Changes   Sensory physiologic changes combine to alter the older adult's ability to interpret and adapt to the critical care environment in acute illness. In addition, these changes affect safety; increase vulnerability to confusion and depression, falls, and traumatic injuries; and negatively impact older adults' ability to interact in their environment. Changes in sensory function place the patient at increased risk for a variety of problems. Reduced pain sensation increases the risk of burns, traumatic injury, and infection, particularly in the lower extremities where decreased sensation may be most pronounced. The changes in sight and hearing associated with aging make the patient in a high-acuity environment vulnerable to sensory deprivation problems, which may increase the risk for development of confusion. When possible, the nurse should allow the patient to wear glasses and hearing aids to optimize communication. Refer to Table 4–2 for a summary of the nursing implications related to neurosensory changes associated with aging.

Section Two Review

1. The nurse understands that, in the older client, the diminished rate of neurotransmitter synthesis leads to which condition?
   A. Hypertension
   B. More rapid respiratory rate
   C. Increased cardiac response to stressors
   D. Decreased sympathetic nervous system response

2. The nurse understands that there is an increased risk of neurologic side effects or toxicity from drug therapies in the older client, related to which age-related change? (Select all that apply.)
   A. A smaller brain volume
   B. A more permeable blood–brain barrier
   C. Greater water content in the brain
   D. Atherosclerotic vascular changes
   E. Dilation of the ventricles

3. The nurse recognizes that older clients can have delayed manifestations of intracranial bleeding due to which age-related change?
   A. More dead space in the cranium
   B. Delays in reflex responses
   C. Decreased compensatory mechanisms
   D. Altered perceptions of pain

4. The nurse expects which age-related change when checking the pupils in the older client?
   A. Increased response to light
   B. Larger pupils
   C. Decreased response to light
   D. No pupil size change

Answers: 1. D, 2. (A, B, E), 3. A, 4. C

Section Three: Cardiovascular and Pulmonary Systems Changes

Coronary heart disease (CHD) is the leading cause of death in America; 82% of people who die of CHD are age 65 or older (AOA, 2014). With aging, pulmonary function decreases due to altered gas exchange, and chronic respiratory disorders are relatively common.

Cardiovascular System

Anatomic and physiologic cardiovascular changes alter the function of both the myocardium and the peripheral vasculature. Cardiovascular changes include decreased elasticity and increased stiffness of the arterial walls (arteriosclerosis), leading to higher blood pressure and increased left ventricular afterload. There is a loss of elastic and conductive tissue, as well as an increase in collagen, resulting in calcification, valve incompetence, conduction abnormalities, and arrhythmias. In addition, muscle cells of the myocardium increase in size, resulting in ventricular hypertrophy and decreased ventricular compliance (Tabloski, 2014). This change impacts the cardiac cycle by causing impaired diastolic filling and myocardial relaxation. Nurses monitor for changes in vital signs, extra heart sounds, murmurs, and electrocardiogram (ECG) changes. The peripheral vessels undergo a loss of elasticity and fat accumulation in the intima of the vessel wall (atherosclerosis), leading to peripheral vascular disease, the prevalence of which increases with age (Tabloski, 2014).

Neurohormonal changes including decreased vasomotor tone and baroreceptor response result in altered compensatory responses, hypertension, and decreased cardiac output. Paired with age-related changes in body composition, metabolic rate, and general state of fitness, age-associated physiologic changes combine to impact cardiovascular function and result in an increased prevalence of peripheral vascular disease and CHD in older adults.

Increases in prevalence of CHD occur in women and men but begin at a later age in women. The same risk factors associated with atherosclerosis in younger adults (lipid abnormalities, smoking, hypertension, diabetes) are predictive in older individuals as well. Modification of these risk factors can be effective in reducing the risk of atherosclerosis, even in older patients. Table 4–3 provides a summary of age-related changes in the cardiovascular system and their physiologic effects.

Nursing Implications of Cardiovascular Changes Normally, when myocardial demands increase, compensation occurs by an increased blood flow to the coronary arteries. If blood flow is limited due to pre-existing cardiovascular disease, a patient is more vulnerable to myocardial ischemia and infarction. Older adult patients with cardiac ischemia and acute myocardial infarction (AMI) may present with nonspecific or atypical symptoms. They may complain of shortness of breath or abdominal, throat, or back pain. In addition, they may have symptoms such as syncope, acute confusion, flu-like syndromes, stroke, and/or falls, which may delay or confuse their diagnosis and treatment.

Signs and symptoms may be more subtle or atypical in the older adult patient. Hypertension, acute coronary syndrome, and heart failure are prevalent in older adults in high-acuity settings. Age-related changes may impact differentiation of symptoms and interpretation of diagnostic tests. In addition, decline in kidney and liver function may influence laboratory findings such as cardio biomarkers (Davis, 2014).

Advances in cardiac surgery and in surgical techniques have improved morbidity and mortality statistics for older adults. Therapeutic treatments such as thrombolytic therapy, percutaneous transluminal coronary angioplasty (PTCA), coronary artery bypass graft (CABG), and valve replacements in the older adult will require vigilant clinical assessment and monitoring to prevent complications related to therapeutic interventions. Maintaining the patient's hemodynamic stability may be more challenging. Older adults require higher filling pressures to maintain adequate stroke volume and cardiac output. In

Table 4–3 Summary of Age-related Changes: Cardiovascular and Pulmonary Systems

Age-related Change	Physiologic Effect
CARDIOVASCULAR	
Heart muscle: hypertrophy or dilation, loss of elastic and conductive tissue, and increased fat and collagen content	Alterations in hemodynamics, reduced cardiac output, increased afterload, decreased compliance
Heart valves: calcification, fibrosis, or thickening	Valve stiffness or incompetence, alterations in hemodynamics, increased incidence of murmurs or extra heart sounds (S3 and S4)
Arterial and peripheral vessels: progressive thickening, loss of elasticity, increased lipid content, and increased stiffness	Increased incidence of atherosclerotic events, increased incidence of hypertension
Conduction system: decreased number of pacemaker cells, thickening of SA node, slower AV node conduction	Increased prevalence of arrhythmias or conduction abnormalities, alterations in heart rate, prolonged PR interval
Neurohormonal changes: Loss of vasomotor tone and baroreceptor response	Decreased compensatory abilities in response to stressors; increased susceptibility to orthostatic hypotension
PULMONARY	
Decreased elasticity of lung tissue and chest wall	Increased alveolar compliance, collapse of small airways, decreased PaO_2
Structural changes: calcification of thoracic wall, osteoporosis, or vertebral collapse	Decreased chest wall compliance, kyphosis, increased AP diameter
Decreased strength of respiratory muscles	Decreased maximal breathing capacity, decreased vital capacity
Reduced sensitivity of respiratory center	Blunted response to hypoxia or hypercapnia
Decreased cough reflex	Retention of secretions, increased susceptibility to aspiration, atelectasis, infection
Atrophy of cilia	Ineffective cough, inefficient cilia
Decreased alveolar surface area	Decreased PaO_2 (4 mmHg decrease per decade) Reduced ventilator efficiency

Table 4–4 Nursing Implications: Cardiovascular and Pulmonary Changes

System	Implications
Cardiovascular	Assessment: Obtain baseline data (comorbid cardiovascular conditions; arterial blood pressure; heart rate and sounds; peripheral pulses; ECG; cardiac biomarkers)
	Diagnosis and Planning: Alterations in cardiac output and tissue perfusion (myocardial and peripheral); circulatory fluid volume overload or deficit
	Implementation: Close monitoring for changes in cardiovascular status and complications of therapeutic interventions
	Evaluation: Signs of decreased tissue perfusion, increasing fluid imbalance, or decreased cardiac output; cardiac rhythm status; orthostatic hypotension
Pulmonary	Assessment: Obtain baseline data (comorbid pulmonary conditions; lung sounds; respiratory rate, depth, and regularity; coloring of skin and mucous membranes; arterial blood gases or pulse oximetry values)
	Diagnosis and Planning: Alterations in oxygenation, ventilation, and gas exchange; risk for prolonged mechanical ventilation (PMV)
	Implementation: Frequent pulmonary toilet (deep breathing and coughing exercises); progressive mobility/ambulation; high level of vigilance during periods of weaning from positive pressure ventilation; ventilator-associated pneumonia prevention
	Evaluation: Signs of respiratory muscle fatigue, hypoxia, or hypercapnia; changes in lung sounds

addition, volume assessment is imperative as older adults are sensitive to hypovolemia; at the same time, higher fluid volumes can increase the risk of pulmonary edema due to decreased ventricular compliance (Manning, 2014). Table 4–4 provides a summary of nursing implications related to cardiovascular changes in the older adult high-acuity patient.

Pulmonary System

Physiological changes in the respiratory system associated with aging may result from changes in the compliance of the chest wall and the lung tissue, as well as alterations in gas exchange. As the costal cartilage that connects the rib cage undergoes calcification, kyphosis may develop, which reduces chest wall compliance. Decreased chest wall compliance requires greater energy expenditure and leads to a decline in maximum inspiratory and expiratory force. There is also less oxygen carried by the blood due to aging, and therefore gas exchange occurs more slowly and less efficiently (Tabloski, 2014).

Other structural changes may include rib fractures from osteoporosis, as well as increased anteroposterior (AP) diameter. Loss of lung elasticity and elastic recoil leads to increased alveolar compliance and the collapse of small airways, which may cause a decrease in alveolar surface area, uneven alveolar ventilation ($\dot{V}/\dot{Q}$ mismatch), and decreased PaO_2 levels. Older adults have an altered ability to respond to hypoxemia and hypercapnia (Manning, 2014). Reduced respiratory reserve, decreased respiratory muscle strength, diminished cough reflex, and decreased function of cilia and epithelial cells result in increased susceptibility to pulmonary infections, acute lung injury, and sepsis. Refer to Table 4–3 for a summary of age-related pulmonary changes and their physiologic effects.

Nursing Implications of Pulmonary System Changes
Respiratory disorders are commonly encountered in patients in high-acuity areas. Potential nursing concerns are the risk for aspiration, atelectasis, and pneumonia. Older adults at risk for pulmonary complications include those who are recovering from surgery, suffering from rib fractures or chest injuries, or receiving narcotics; have artificial airways; have reflux; are deconditioned; and have altered nutritional or hydration status. Deep breathing and coughing exercises for older adults are an important nursing priority as respiratory muscles are weaker, the cough reflex is less effective, and the ciliary function is decreased. Nurses need to be able to accurately assess respiratory status to determine adequacy of gas exchange, ventilation, and perfusion, as well as to identify worsening respiratory function.

A number of issues relate to the increased complexity of care of the older adult patient on a mechanical ventilator. Changes in respiratory structure and function with aging should be considered when older patients are placed on a mechanical ventilator. The older patient may experience greater difficulty weaning from a ventilator due to poor respiratory muscle function, altered respiratory mechanics, or altered hemodynamics. Nurses monitor for signs of respiratory muscle fatigue (e.g., rapid shallow breathing, accessory muscle use, diaphoresis, and restlessness) with increased vigilance when attempting to wean an older patient from a ventilator in the high-acuity area. The patient is at increased risk of healthcare-associated pneumonia directly related to mechanical ventilation. Ventilator-associated pneumonia (VAP) is a bacterial pneumonia that often occurs in patients who are on a ventilator for more than 48 hours and is thought to be caused by the migration of oral pathogens into the lungs. VAP prevention guidelines are commonly implemented to avoid complications and associated increased morbidity and mortality (Manning, 2014). Nursing care of the mechanically ventilated patient to prevent VAP includes use of care bundles that include nursing interventions, such as optimal hand hygiene, keeping the head of the bed elevated greater than 30 degrees, providing frequent oral care, maintaining adequate endotracheal tube cuff pressure, use of polyurethane-cuffed tubes, consideration of suctioning intermittent subglottic secretions, assessing the need for ulcer prophylaxis, turning the patient frequently or using continuous lateral rotation therapy, deep vein thrombosis prophylaxis, and daily "sedation vacations" to assess for readiness to extubate and minimize the duration of ventilation (Manning, 2014).

Table 4–4 provides a summary of nursing implications related to pulmonary changes in the high-acuity older adult patient.

Section Three Review

1. The atypical presentation of some older clients experiencing acute myocardial ischemia/infarction may include which manifestations? (Select all that apply.)
   A. Hypothermia
   B. Falls
   C. Flu-like syndromes
   D. Higher than usual elevations of creatine kinase
   E. Acute confusion

2. Why is the risk of pulmonary infections higher in the older client?
   A. Increased lung elasticity
   B. Increased alveolar surface area
   C. Decreased chest anteroposterior (AP) diameter
   D. Loss of pulmonary epithelial cell function

3. When caring for the older client, which intervention should be a nursing priority for prevention of airway clearance and gas exchange complications?
   A. Deep breathing and coughing exercises
   B. High fluid intake
   C. Monitoring of respiratory rate and depth
   D. Assessing for adventitious breath sounds

4. In mechanically ventilated older clients, weaning is often more difficult for which major reason? (Select all that apply.)
   A. Weak respiratory muscle function
   B. Confused mental state
   C. Altered respiratory mechanics
   D. Changes in hemodynamics
   E. Reduced client coping skills

Answers: 1. (B, C, E), 2. D, 3. A, 4. (A, C, D)

Section Four: Integumentary and Musculoskeletal Systems Changes

Age-related changes in integumentary function make the skin more friable and vulnerable to injury. The musculoskeletal system loses mass and strength with aging; a weaker skeletal structure leads to stiffness and a higher risk of falls and fractures.

Integumentary System

The aging process is manifested in the changes in the appearance and function of the skin. Common integumentary changes such as wrinkling and sagging are due to a loss of elasticity of connective tissues as well as environmental influences. There is a loss of skin turgor resulting from decreased subcutaneous tissue, fragility of capillaries, flattening of the capillary bed, and frequent aspirin or blood thinner use. Older adults are prone to ecchymosis; skin becomes more transparent, and underlying veins are more visible. Because skin pigmentation declines, pallor is a less reliable sign of anemia or illness.

Lean body mass in muscle tissue is lost. The proportion of body fat increases as the proportion of body weight contributed by intracellular body water decreases (Tabloski, 2014). There is a loss of dermal and epidermal thickness; skin becomes thin and is more prone to breakdown and injury. Untreated skin problems can lead to pressure ulcers, discomfort, systemic infection, or functional impairments. The number and efficiency of sweat glands decreases with aging, predisposing the patient to hypothermia and hyperthermia as well as fluid and electrolyte imbalances (Tabloski, 2014). Table 4–5 provides a summary of the age-related changes in the integumentary system and their physiologic effects.

Nursing Implications of Integumentary Changes   Nurses should complete a thorough skin assessment to monitor for changes in skin integrity (Manning, 2014). It is important to identify potentially life-threatening skin infections and rashes due to medication hypersensitivity. Cellulitis may result from contamination of an open wound that affects the dermis layer of the skin. Bacteria may travel through the lymphatic system, where it can spread to deeper tissues or to the bloodstream. Skin assessment can also provide information regarding blood supply and venous drainage. Refer to Table 4–6 for a summary of nursing implications of integumentary changes.

Risk of Skin Breakdown.   Because the skin of an older adult is thin and fragile, the elderly are at risk for skin breakdown related to immobility and skin tears when they are moved. Compression of soft tissues under bony prominences, friction, and shearing can lead to tissue ischemia. Just a few hours on a backboard or on an operating room table may alter skin integrity in an older trauma patient. Although lying on the back with the head of the bed (HOB) elevated is a common and necessary position for an adult in the high-acuity setting, nurses should understand that it places increased weight on the coccyx. In addition, if the patient slides down in bed, repositioning is required, which often involves friction and shearing forces on the skin. The development of a pressure ulcer can cause significant delays in recovery, prolong hospitalization, and greatly impact quality of life. Risks may be higher in those with conditions that result in decreased oxygen and nutrient supply to the skin (Morehead & Blain, 2014). Priority nursing care to prevent pressure ulcers includes repositioning the patient frequently, optimizing nutritional status, and treating sacral skin with barrier moisturizers. Specialty beds with pressure-reducing surfaces may be warranted.

Thermoregulation Problems.   Because of age-related skin changes, older adults can have difficulty with

Table 4–5 Summary of Age-related Changes: Integumentary and Musculoskeletal Systems

Age-related Change	Physiologic Effect
INTEGUMENTARY	
Loss of elasticity of connective tissues; loss of dermal and epidermal thickness; decreased body water and increased body fat	Increased wrinkling and sagging, thinning of skin, susceptibility to breakdown and injury
Loss of lean body mass and subcutaneous tissue mass	Reduced insulation
Decreased skin pigmentation	Pallor
Atrophy of sweat glands	Decreased sweating, altered thermoregulation, fluid and electrolyte imbalances
Decreased exposure to sun	Vitamin D deficiency, osteoporosis, osteomalacia
MUSCULOSKELETAL	
Decreased muscle mass and strength	Alterations in mobility, muscle weakness, decreased exercise tolerance, and increased risk of falls
Deterioration of joint cartilage, increased joint stiffness, decreased joint mobility	Pain and decreased mobility of skeletal joints
Bone demineralization	Increased susceptibility to bone fractures and osteoporosis
Osteoporosis, degenerative spinal stenosis, thinning of vertebral cartilage	Spinal column compression, deformity, loss of height, compression of spinal nerves, pain

thermoregulation. Nursing care incorporates prevention of heat loss by monitoring room temperature, keeping the patient covered while bathing, and using warmed blankets when necessary.

Musculoskeletal System

Decreased muscle mass, bone demineralization, increased joint stiffness, and decreased joint mobility are common musculoskeletal issues in the older adult. In addition, decreased muscle strength is common with loss of selected muscle fibers, including respiratory muscles. Numerous age-related changes in other subsystems, such as reductions in neuronmuscular innervation, insulin activity, and levels of estrogen, testosterone, and growth hormone, as well as weight loss, protein deficiency, and physical inactivity, can contribute to loss of muscle mass and strength (Tabloski, 2014). Older adults are at high risk for development of weakness from lack of physical activity and prolonged immobility. In a study of healthy older men and women, after 10 days of bed rest

there was loss of lower-extremity strength, power, and aerobic exercise capacity with reduced physical activity, but there was no effect on physical performance (Kortebein, Symons, Ferrando, & Evans, 2008). Functional issues are typically not of immediate concern when the patient is severely ill. But the nurse needs to keep in mind that older adults lose strength and functional ability quickly from illness and immobility, leading older adults to experience what has long been called the "cascade to dependence" (Creditor, 1993).

Assessment of the musculoskeletal system must include data from the patient history, such as the prior functional level and the presence of osteoporosis, osteomalacia, or osteoarthritis. These conditions can contribute to potential complications such as pain, fractures, and falls and have implications for patient mobility. Osteoporosis is related to aging, particularly menopause in women, although men develop osteoporosis later in life. Osteoporosis can cause vertebral fracture, resulting in back pain and pronounced kyphosis, and increased risk of fracture with trauma impacting nursing care.

Table 4–6 Nursing Implications: Integumentary and Musculoskeletal Changes

System	Implications
Integumentary	Assessment: Obtain baseline data (comorbid integumentary conditions; skin integrity; Braden Scale for Predicting Pressure Sore Risk; rashes or cellulitis; nutritional status); monitor IV catheterization sites closely for infiltration Diagnosis and Planning: Increased risk for skin breakdown; imbalances in regulation of body temperature Implementation: Close monitoring for changes in skin integrity, particularly over bony prominences; measures to prevent pressure ulcers (routine turning and repositioning while avoiding friction and shearing forces); specialty bed use; application of barrier (e.g., transparent film or cream) to pressure area; protection against hypothermia (keep covered, warmed blankets); IV catheters secured with nonrestrictive dressings and paper tape to protect the skin Evaluation: Signs of changing skin integrity; changing Braden Scale for Predicting Pressure Sore Risk; signs of hypothermia (shivering, cold skin, drowsiness, confusion, depressed heart and respiratory rates); signs of IV catheter infiltration
Musculoskeletal	Assessment: Obtain baseline data (comorbid musculoskeletal conditions; mobility capabilities [muscle strength, balance, gait, pain]; ambulation aids [e.g., cane, walker]) Diagnosis and Planning: Increased risk for falls, prolonged immobility, decreased range of motion and muscle weakness Implementation: Early mobilization with high vigilance to maintain patient safety Evaluation: Functional ability for transfer and discharge planning

Osteoarthritis is the most common arthritic condition, affecting 12.1% of adults, with the rates highest in older adults (Centers for Disease Control and Prevention, 2015a). Joint involvement, particularly in weight-bearing joints, can result in pain and difficulty with mobility, especially after prolonged periods of bed rest. Patients with arthritis may be taking nonsteroidal anti-inflammatory medications (NSAIDs), which can impact kidney function and put them at risk for peptic ulcer disease.

Many conditions, such as degenerative spinal stenosis (narrowing of the spinal canal), thinning of the cartilage between the vertebrae, and development of bone spurs around the vertebrae, lead to compression of the spinal column or the spinal nerves and result in a variety of symptoms, including pain and deformity. Nurses assess musculoskeletal status, symptoms, and history that can influence nursing care. Refer to Table 4–5 for a summary of age-related musculoskeletal changes and their physiologic effects.

Nursing Implications of Musculoskeletal Changes The presence of degenerative arthritis and other musculoskeletal alterations has important implications for the care of patients in high-acuity settings. Posture, gait, balance, symmetry of body parts, and alignment of extremities may be altered. The threat to mobility is the most important challenge as patients suffer from weakness and joint-related pain, which may be chronic and impose limitations on comfort, recovery, and physical therapy. Fractures, particularly of the pelvis and femur, are more common with trauma and can be associated with significant blood loss. In the high-acuity setting, the nurse should provide early mobilization of patients (Lach, Lorenz, & L'Ecuyer, 2014). In a review of 19 studies evaluating disability outcomes in critically ill adults age 65 years and older, it was found that older adults are at great risk for disabilities following critical illnesses, and interventions that target immobility are associated with improved functional and cognitive outcomes (Brummel et al., 2015). Range of motion and early mobility are critical to help maintain muscle tone and strength throughout acute illness. In older adult patients, restraints should be avoided because their use can reduce mobility and function, leading to serious complications (American Academy of Nursing, 2015). Anticipatory planning for transfer and discharge should begin as soon as possible so that families can help older patients plan for next steps. Discharge-related factors include the patient's prehospital state, type of illness, potential for recovery, rehabilitation needs, and expected duration of acute illness. Most important, the nurse needs to share this information when the patient is transferred to a lower level of care. Continuity in care can reduce loss of functional ability and maximize recovery time. Refer to Table 4–6 for a summary of nursing implications relative to musculoskeletal changes.

Section Four Review

1. The older client is more susceptible to skin breakdown for which reasons? (Select all that apply.)
   A. Thinning of the skin
   B. Increased subcutaneous tissue
   C. Lower body fat content
   D. Thickening of capillary beds

2. When caring for the older client, which common nursing intervention is most likely to result in skin breakdown?
   A. Elevating head of bed 30 degrees
   B. Turning every 2 hours
   C. Using support surfaces
   D. Moisturizing sacral skin

3. When gathering a nursing history on an older client, what information from the client would indicate an increased risk for peptic ulcer disease?
   A. "I have been under intense stress lately."
   B. "I take nonsteroidal anti-inflammatory drugs daily."
   C. "I stopped taking my calcium supplement because it was difficult to swallow."
   D. "I drink about four cups of coffee each day."

4. Which musculoskeletal condition is most prevalent among older adults?
   A. Gout
   B. Rheumatoid arthritis
   C. Osteoarthritis
   D. Fractures

Answers: 1. A, 2. A, 3. B, 4. C

Section Five: Gastrointestinal and Genitourinary Systems Changes

Age-related changes in the gastrointestinal system can significantly alter the patient's nutritional status. Kidney function decreases with age, and older adults are at increased risk for urinary tract infection. This section provides a brief review of age-related alterations in the gastrointestinal and genitourinary systems and the nursing implications relative to those changes.

Gastrointestinal System

Physiologic changes in the gastrointestinal (GI) system include changes in the oral cavity, esophagus, stomach, small and large intestine, pancreas, and liver. Oral cavity changes that affect the teeth include wearing of tooth surfaces, thinning of enamel, cracking of teeth, tooth loss, and periodontal disease, all of which can affect appearance, swallowing, nutrition, and quality of life. Oral tissues become more fragile, and salivary production may be altered due to drug side effects, disease states, or altered nutrition. The sense of thirst may be diminished. Other possible conditions include osteoporosis or atrophy of the jawbone. Changes in the motility of the esophagus and esophageal sphincter function have not been found to be normal age-related changes, and therefore patients having difficulty swallowing or experiencing significant problems with reflux should be referred for further evaluation. Underlying vascular or neurological diseases in older people may contribute to altered esophageal motility and dysphagia, making safe administration of oral food and especially fluids difficult (Tabloski, 2014).

In the stomach, the secretion of digestive juices is diminished. Also, gastric acidity decreases, possibly due to chronic infection with *Helicobacter pylori*, which gradually destroys the secretory glands and parietal cells that produce gastric acids. The reduced acidity of the gastric pH increases the risk for growth of bacteria in the stomach, which in turn increases the risk of aspiration pneumonia in the older high-acuity patient. The absorptive capacity of cells of the small intestine is altered and impacts the absorption of vitamins and minerals. Changes in the large intestine include histological changes in the colon that contribute to muscle atrophy, slower transit rate, diminished sphincter tone, and diminished compliance of the rectum. The exocrine function of the pancreas is decreased, which

has important implications for the patient in the high-acuity setting. Blood flow to the liver is reduced, hepatocyte number is decreased, and hepatic regeneration is reduced. Although the liver has many functions, the most important age-related change in liver function is the decrease in the capacity to metabolize drugs. Table 4–7 provides a summary of age-related gastrointestinal changes and their physiologic effects.

Nursing Implications of Gastrointestinal System Changes

Because of age-related GI alterations, digestion may be affected, which has important consequences for the nutritional status of an older adult patient. Because jawbone changes and tooth loss affect chewing, nurses should assess this important foundation to healthy dietary intake. A thorough assessment includes a history of oral hygiene, diet, altered sensory perception, and elimination habits. Symptoms of concern that relate to the health of the GI system and that can impact nutritional status include abdominal pain, dysphagia, dyspepsia, nausea, vomiting, anorexia, weight loss, changes in stool characteristics, and gastrointestinal bleeding. Nurses should encourage adequate hydration, advocate for early enteral/parenteral nutrition, and monitor for delayed gastric emptying and signs of fecal impaction.

There is increased incidence of gastric ulcer development in older adults compared with younger adults. Medications that may affect the GI system include anticholinergics, laxatives, calcium channel blockers, aspirin and other NSAIDs, antacids, opioids, and antiemetics. The

Table 4–7 Summary of Age-related Changes: Gastrointestinal and Genitourinary Systems

Age-related Change	Physiologic Effect
GASTROINTESTINAL	
Tooth thinning, cracking, or loss; loss of dentition or tooth enamel; periodontal disease	Alterations in nutrition, appearance, swallowing, and quality of life
Alterations in oral tissues, atrophy of salivary glands and taste buds, diminished thirst	Alterations in nutrition
Delay in esophageal emptying, altered esophageal sphincter function	Increased susceptibility to indigestion, reflux, aspiration
Diminished digestive juices, decreased gastric acidity	Increased risk for bacterial overgrowth in stomach, increased risk of aspiration pneumonia
Decreased calcium absorption	Predisposition to constipation, altered bowel habits; increased risk of osteoporosis
Decreased GI muscle tone, altered stool transit time	Altered motility
Altered absorptive capacity of cells in small intestine	Alterations in absorption of vitamins and minerals
Muscle atrophy of colon, decreased sphincter tone	Slower GI transit rate, decreased rectal compliance
Decreased blood flow to liver, decreased number of liver cells.	Decreased ability to metabolize drugs
GENITOURINARY	
Atrophy of renal arterioles, glomerular sclerosis	Decreased renal blood flow; decreased glomeruli filtration rate; decreased creatinine clearance
Decreased number and function of nephrons	Decreased urine-concentrating ability; altered regulation of fluid and electrolyte balance
Decreased kidney efficiency	Increased risk of dehydration, fluid and electrolyte imbalances, medication toxicity
Weakening of bladder muscles and increased collagen content	Incomplete bladder emptying and limited distensibility; decreased bladder capacity and increased urine frequency
Decreased circulating estrogen and decreased tissue responsiveness to estrogen in women; prostatic hypertrophy in men	Changes in urethral sphincter and delayed bladder emptying; urinary incontinence

patient's history should be explored for surgical procedures, reflux problems, peptic ulcer disease, cancer, hepatitis, gallstones, and diabetes mellitus (DM). Nurses can advocate for stress ulcer prophylaxis and monitor for signs of bleeding.

Constipation is a significant concern in the older adult population and can lead to abdominal discomfort. Many factors contribute to constipation, including dehydration, side effects of medications, low fiber intake, cognitive impairments, and immobility (Tabloski, 2014). Other contributing factors to the development of constipation include physical illnesses such as metabolic and endocrine disorders (diabetes, hypothyroidism, and renal failure); neurologic disorders such as multiple sclerosis, Parkinson disease, or stroke; and psychologic status (somatization, anxiety, and depression; Tabloski, 2014). Nurses can ensure that steps are taken to prevent constipation and promote bowel function by understanding the risk factors associated with the development of constipation and the side effects of medications, ensuring adequate hydration and proper nutrition, and monitoring activity and bowel function. Table 4–8 summarizes nursing implications relative to GI system changes.

Genitourinary System

The kidney systematically loses function (i.e., glomerular filtration rate [GFR]) with age. Genitourinary (GU) changes are numerous and include fluid balance, decreased clearance of creatinine and some medications, renal failure, urinary tract infections (UTIs), and incontinence. Multiple factors contribute to increased vulnerability to fluid and electrolyte imbalances in the older adult, including decreased urine-concentrating ability; limitations in excretion of water, sodium, potassium, and hydrogen ions; and the GU system's declining ability to compensate. As an individual ages, renal blood flow decreases incrementally over time due to atrophy of the efferent and afferent arterioles, sclerotic glomeruli, and a decrease in the number and size of nephrons. These changes lead to a decline in glomerular filtration rate and a decrease in creatinine clearance. As renal tubular function declines, the function of the renin aldosterone system and the ability to concentrate urine are diminished, which affects the ability to regulate fluid and acid–base balance (Tabloski, 2014). Changes that affect the kidneys, ureters, urinary bladder, urethra, and prostate can impact the function of the genitourinary system. The ureters are vulnerable to reflux of the vesicoureteral junction, leading to reflux of urine and increased risk of infection.

While urinary incontinence is not normal with aging, age-related changes increase the risk of developing this condition. The bladder muscles weaken, which may lead to incomplete emptying, while collagen content increases, limiting distensibility and increasing the risk of urinary retention. Bladder capacity decreases and frequency of urination increases. Problems urinating may be due to altered sphincter muscles, neural controls, sensation, outlet size, muscle strength, or obstruction (Tabloski, 2014). In addition, the kidneys of older adults excrete more fluid and electrolytes at night, which results in greater nighttime urine volume and a potential for interrupted sleep patterns (Tabloski, 2014). Decreased estrogen in women can cause changes in the urethral sphincter and surrounding tissues, and men may experience prostatic hypertrophy. Refer to Table 4–7 for a summary of age-related changes in the GU system and their physiologic effects.

Nursing Implications of Genitourinary Changes Urinary tract infections are responsible for most cases of **bacteremia** (bacteria in the blood). In the hospital, UTIs are attributed to the presence of indwelling catheters, which should be removed as soon as possible. Initiatives to reduce catheter-associated urinary tract infections are recommended by the Centers for Disease Control and Prevention (2015b), along with guidelines and a toolkit to address these preventable infections.

Assessment for urinary tract infections is an important nursing task, as often symptoms are not apparent. The older adult patient may present with atypical manifestations of UTI, such as mental changes, confusion, nausea and vomiting, or abdominal pain, rather than the classic symptoms of fever, chills, frequency, urgency, dysuria, and suprapubic or flank pain. Other urinary symptoms may include nocturia, urgency, and incontinence.

Table 4–8 Nursing Implications: Gastrointestinal and Genitourinary Changes

System	Implications
Gastrointestinal	Assessment: Obtain baseline data (comorbid GI conditions; eating aids [e.g., dentures]; ability to chew; oral hygiene; diet; sensory perception; elimination habits; medication history [focus on drugs that alter GI motility])
	Diagnosis and Planning: Bowel incontinence, constipation, impaired dentition, diarrhea, dysfunctional gastrointestinal motility, imbalanced nutrition: less than body requirements
	Implementation: Close monitoring for changes in nutritional and GI status; promote hydration, proper nutrition, and bowel function
	Evaluation: Periodic evaluation of nutritional status; daily evaluation of bowel function and hydration status
Genitourinary	Assessment: Obtain baseline data (comorbid GU conditions; urinary patterns; medication history [focus on drugs that alter urinary function]; renal function)
	Diagnosis and Planning: Incontinence (continuous, functional, overflow, reflex, stress, or urge), self-care deficit: toileting; impaired urinary elimination, risk for infection: urinary tract
	Implementation: Close monitoring of intake and output balance and typical/atypical signs of urinary tract infection; facilitate normal toileting when feasible; avoid use of or minimize length of time for urinary catheterization; meticulous perineal care
	Evaluation: Daily evaluation of intake and output; periodic re-evaluation of renal function; daily reevaluation of need for continuance of urinary catheter when one is present

Atypical presentations can result in delay in diagnosis of urinary tract infection in older adults. Because of the many confounding comorbidities associated with alterations in GU function, renal disease may be overlooked.

Nurses should closely monitor hemoglobin, hematocrit, blood urea nitrogen (BUN), serum creatinine, electrolytes, urinalysis with culture, urine albumin, glucose, pH, microscopic examination of urinary sediment, and screening for bacteriuria. After high-acuity illness, bladder issues such as urinary incontinence should be evaluated and addressed. Refer to Table 4–8 for a summary of nursing implications relative to the GU system.

Section Five Review

1. The nurse is aware that in the older-adult high-acuity client, altered gastric pH increases the risk of which complication?
   A. Gastric ulcers
   B. Hepatitis
   C. Gastric cancer
   D. Pneumonia

2. Which age-related change in urinary system function should the nurse anticipate in the older adult?
   A. Decreased glomerular filtration rate
   B. Increased size of nephrons
   C. Decreased ureter lumen size
   D. Increased creatinine clearance

3. Dehydration and hyponatremia in the older adult are often associated with which physiologic alteration in the kidneys?
   A. Altered neural controls
   B. Changes in the urethral sphincter
   C. Declining renal tubule function
   D. Increased concentration of urine

4. The atypical presentation of urinary tract infection often seen in the older adult client includes which symptoms? (Select all that apply.)
   A. Abdominal pain
   B. Incontinence
   C. Nausea and vomiting
   D. High fever
   E. Confusion

Answers: 1. D, 2. A, 3. C, 4. (A, B, C, E)

Section Six: Endocrine and Immune System Changes

The endocrine system plays a crucial role in maintaining overall body homeostasis. As the functions of the various endocrine glands and organs diminish from aging, the reduced levels of hormones have profound effects on the body as a whole, resulting in an increasing risk of many chronic endocrine disorders. Age-related changes of the immune system make the older adult more vulnerable to infection and increase the risk for development of cancer. This section provides a brief review of age-related alterations in the endocrine and immune systems and the nursing implications relative to those changes.

Endocrine System

Age-related changes in the endocrine system result in menopause, as well as altered glucose metabolism and thyroid dysfunction. There is a decreased production of estrogen and progesterone, as well as testosterone, thyroid hormones, growth hormone, and insulin (Alvis & Hughes, 2015). The pancreas secretes less insulin, and insulin resistance increases, which results in a decreased ability to metabolize glucose. The prevalence of diabetes mellitus (DM) increases, with approximately 10.9 million Americans over the age of 65 (25.8%) with diagnosed or undiagnosed DM (Centers for Disease Control and Prevention,

2015c). As the aging body uses less thyroid hormone and the thyroid gland atrophies, the result is a decrease in T4 production and an increased risk for hypothyroidism. Basal metabolic rates decrease. Table 4–9 provides a summary of age-related endocrine changes and their physiologic effects.

Nursing Implications of Endocrine System Changes
Nurses should monitor blood glucose carefully in the older patient, with special attention to patients with diabetes. While control of blood glucose is important to prevent complications, with increasing age a less aggressive and more individualized approach to glucose control may be warranted, as hypoglycemia can have more significant effects on frail older patients (Mathur, Zammitt, & Frier, 2015). Illness, medications, and nutritional alterations influence glucose metabolism. Complications of diabetes, including retinopathy, neuropathy in the lower extremities, and vascular complications such as atherosclerosis, may affect treatment (Tabloski, 2014). Older adults with diabetes are particularly vulnerable to foot complications and foot ulcers; therefore, foot assessment and care require attention in the high-acuity area. A comprehensive approach to the care of the older adult with diabetes should involve the interdisciplinary team, including a diabetic educator, a pharmacist, and a dietician who can instruct patients about nutrition, glucose monitoring, and recognition and prevention of hypoglycemia.

Thyroid dysfunction may be related to a variety of symptoms in the older adult. Hypothyroidism is associated

Table 4–9 Summary of Age-related Changes: Endocrine and Immune Systems

Age-related Change	Physiologic Effect
ENDOCRINE	
Decreased production of estrogen, progesterone, testosterone, growth hormones	Vaginal atrophy, erectile dysfunction, loss of sexual drive
Decreased production of insulin and increased insulin resistance	Altered glucose metabolism, increased blood sugar levels, increased risk for diabetes mellitus (DM)
Thyroid atrophy and decreased production of thyroid hormones	Increased risk for hypothyroidism
Increased body fat and altered regulation of metabolism by hypothalamus	Decreased basal metabolic rate
IMMUNE SYSTEM	
Decreased T-cell function	Impaired cell-mediated immunity; delayed hypersensitivity reactions
Decreased B-cell function	Impaired humoral-mediated immunity; delayed antibody responses
Decreased production of lymphocytes	Increased susceptibility to infections
Appearance of autoantibodies	Increased prevalence of autoimmune disorders
Lower basal temperature	Decreased ability to muster a fever in response to inflammation and infection; loss of important indicator of infection

Table 4–10 Nursing Implications: Endocrine and Immune Changes

System	Implications
Endocrine	Assessment: Obtain baseline data (comorbid endocrine conditions [e.g., DM or hypothyroidism], blood glucose and HbA1C, triglycerides, cholesterol; thyroid function studies; skin integrity with focus on ankles and feet)
	Diagnosis and Planning: Risk for unstable blood glucose level, fatigue, risk for imbalanced fluid volume, risk for impaired skin integrity
	Implementation: *If diabetic,* routine evaluation of blood glucose; nutrition consult for appropriate nutrition planning; administer insulin or other glycemic agents as ordered. *If hypothyroid,* administer thyroid replacement therapy as ordered.
	Evaluation: Evaluate for therapeutic and nontherapeutic effects of drug therapies to treat diabetes or hypothyroidism. Evaluate skin integrity daily.
Immune	Assessment: Obtain baseline data (comorbid immune conditions; vaccination history; temperature; presence or recent use of invasive or indwelling lines; CBC with differential)
	Diagnosis and Planning: Risk for infection
	Implementation: Closely monitor for potential sources of infection; be aware of potential atypical presentation of infection in older adults; take preventive measures to avoid development of infection (e.g., good pulmonary hygiene, maintaining skin integrity, minimizing use of invasive and indwelling lines)
	Evaluation: Evaluate for signs of infection (typical and atypical presentations)

with reduced metabolic function, causing a slowing of both mental and physical function (Tabloski, 2014). Other symptoms can include intolerance to cold, weight gain, constipation, alterations in blood pressure, and anemia. Hyperthyroidism, although less common, may also occur and may be associated with cardiac issues (tachycardia and atrial fibrillation), congestive heart failure, weight loss, fatigue, and muscular weakness (Tabloski, 2014). Because these conditions often overlap with other clinical syndromes, thyroid conditions are often undiagnosed. Thyroid storm is a dangerous complication of hyperthyroidism and is related to an increased risk of death due to the associated cardiac complications. Table 4–10 provides a summary of the nursing implications relative to age-related endocrine changes.

Immune System

The immune system of an older person is more vulnerable than that of a younger person, and basic infection control measures should be adhered to carefully. Cell-mediated immunity declines with aging, and T-cell function decreases. Humoral-mediated immunity and antibody responses are impaired due to the aging of B cells (Alvis & Hughes, 2015). Numerous age-related physiologic changes also predispose an older adult to infection. Infection may present itself atypically in an older person. Because elderly patients have a lower basal temperature, fever (normally an

early sign of infection) may be absent. The nurse must assess infection by carefully examining sputum, urine, and wounds for color and texture changes. Nurses caring for older adults should be aware that changes in mental status, functional decline, hypothermia, unexplained hypo- or hyperglycemia, acidosis, tachycardia, and even falls could be related to an infectious process. Refer to Table 4–9 for a summary of age-related changes in the immune system and their physiologic effects.

Pneumonia and influenza remain among the top ten causes of death for older adults (Centers for Disease Control and Prevention, 2014). Because infection is difficult to treat in older adults and is associated with increased morbidity and mortality, it is important to prevent infection through administration of immunizations. Table 4–11 reviews guidelines for immunizations for older adults.

Nursing Implications of Immunologic Changes Nurses must identify and assess patients who are at high risk for infection. Nurses consider preexisting illnesses and recent history of diagnostic tests involving invasive or indwelling lines, and they implement careful monitoring of clinical signs. Because homeostasis is altered in an older adult during illness, the ability to generate a fever may be diminished. Breath sound assessment and monitoring of oxygen status are vital to identifying pneumonia early. A vaccination history is important to obtain, as influenza and pneumococcal vaccines decrease the risk for pneumonia. Box 4–1 lists the age-related changes that predispose the older adult patient to infection.

Table 4–11 Guidelines for Immunizations for Older Adults

Immunization	Older Adult Indications	Frequency
Influenza	Age 50 years and older Long-term-care residents Chronic medical diseases Healthcare workers	Annually
Pneumonia	Age 65 years and older Certain chronic health problems Altered immune function Residents of nursing homes Smokers	One dose each of pneumococcal vaccination (13-valent pneumococcal conjugate vaccine [PCV13] and 23-valent pneumococcal polysaccharide vaccine [PPSV23]), six months apart Give one dose if unvaccinated or if previous vaccination history is unknown, beginning with PCV13.
Tetanus, diphtheria, and pertussis booster	A one-time booster dose of Tdap (tetanus, diphtheria, and pertussis) vaccine should be administered to all adults who have completed a primary series, followed by Td (tetanus and diphtheria) boosters every 10 years.	One-time Tdap Td every 10 years
Zoster	Age 60 and older	One dose

SOURCE: Data from Centers for Disease Control and Prevention (2015a); Pilkinton & Talbot (2015).

BOX 4–1 Age-related Changes that Predispose to Infection

- Urinary retention
- Prostatic hypertrophy
- Decreased bladder tone
- Delayed gastric emptying
- Decreased cough strength
- Reduced ciliary action
- Flattened diaphragm
- Reduced muscle mass
- Stiffened thoracic cage
- Decreased skin elasticity
- Increased insulin resistance
- Decreased insulin secretion
- Decreased serum albumin (depending on nutritional state)

The presence of bacteremia increases vulnerability to the development of **sepsis**, a syndrome characterized by a systemic inflammatory response (SIRS) to infection, which can further deteriorate to severe sepsis and septic shock. The incidence of SIRS in older adults is significant, and mortality rates are high. Long-term mortality after severe sepsis of Veterans Affairs patients age 65 years and older was measured at 55% (Lemay, Anzueto, Restrepo, & Mortensen, 2014). Older adults are vulnerable to sepsis from bacteremia. Important risk factors include short- and long-term institutionalization, pressure ulcers, methicillin-resistant *Staphylococcus aureus* (MRSA), bacteremia hospitalization in the past 6 months, antimicrobial use in the past 3 months, indwelling catheters, mechanical ventilation, comorbidities, decline in functional status, dementia, diabetes with complications, and malnutrition (Tabloski, 2014; Lemay et al., 2014).

Because older patients do not exhibit the typical clinical manifestations of infection, the diagnosis may be delayed. Symptoms such as altered mental status (delirium, somnolence, and coma), tachypnea, anorexia, malaise, generalized weakness, falls, and urinary incontinence may be nonspecific expressions of infection in older adults. Clinical practice guidelines, protocols, or care bundles have been developed that outline the recommendations for treating patients with severe sepsis. Recent evidence from a retrospective study of adult patients in emergency departments indicates that age greater than 60 years and absence of fever were associated with a lack of recognition of sepsis (Stoneking et al., 2015). Older adults may respond well to treatment when symptoms are recognized and interventions are implemented in a timely manner.

Section Six Review

1. The nurse understands that age-related changes in the thyroid gland increase the risk for development of which thyroid-related problem in the older client?
   A. Hyperthyroidism
   B. Thyrotoxic storm
   C. Hypothyroidism
   D. Elevated basal metabolic rate

2. Which atypical signs of infection may be present in older clients? (Select all that apply.)
   A. Metabolic alkalosis
   B. Functional decline
   C. Altered mental status
   D. Recent history of falls
   E. Unexplained hypo- or hyperglycemia

3. The older client may not develop a fever as an early sign of infection due to which factor?
   A. Lower basal temperature
   B. Hyperthyroidism
   C. Elevated humoral immune function
   D. Increased circulating T-lymphocytes

4. What are some risk factors for the development of sepsis in older clients? (Select all that apply.)
   A. Institutionalization
   B. Pressure ulcers
   C. Altered mental status
   D. Indwelling urinary catheters
   E. Female gender

Answers: 1. C, 2. (B, C, D, E) 3. A, 4. (A, B, C, D)

Section Seven: Cognitive Conditions Impacting Hospitalization

The older adult is at high risk for three overlapping geriatric syndromes that can impact their hospital course: dementia, depression, and delirium. Often called the 3 Ds, these are common and often missed by health professionals or mistaken for one another as they can present with similar symptoms. Table 4–12 provides key features of each. An important consideration for the nurse is to recognize that loss of memory, confusion, and low mood are *not* a normal part of aging. The normal older adult retains memory and thinking abilities throughout life. So when the older patient exhibits these symptoms, a thorough evaluation and appropriate treatments are in order. Nurses should find out about the older patient's pre-illness cognitive status and mood to determine if changes are taking place during acute illness. The patient should be monitored for changes in orientation, thinking ability, or mood; any patient exhibiting these changes is at a very high risk for complications and safety problems in the hospital.

Dementia

Dementia is the term for the symptom of cognitive impairment seen in people with Alzheimer disease or other conditions that cause loss of memory and thinking ability. Alzheimer disease is responsible for the largest percentage of dementia in older adults, but Lewy body disease, vascular dementia, or small strokes are other causes. In a small percentage of people, dementia has a reversible cause such as hypothyroidism, vitamin B12 deficiency, depression, or delirium. Currently 5.2 million people over the age of 65 have Alzheimer disease. Due to the increase in the number of people over 65 in the United States, the annual number of new cases of both Alzheimer disease and other dementias is projected to double by the year 2050 (Alzheimer's Association, 2014).

Alzheimer disease is a degenerative disease causing gradual, progressive brain damage that increasingly impacts thinking and function. The disease is often not diagnosed until symptoms are significant, which means that patients with dementia may be admitted to the hospital without a diagnosis. The nurse may be the first to recognize the problem, so it is important to communicate findings to other health professionals. Red flags the nurse might notice include poor recall of information that the patient is expected to know, disorientation, failing to follow

Table 4–12 Differentiating Dementia, Depression, and Delirium

	Dementia	Depression	Delirium
Onset	Gradual, months to years	Weeks, may have past history	Sudden, hours to days with fluctuating course
Memory	Poor, worse for recent events	Poor, inability to concentrate	Poor, inattention
Thought	Disoriented, unable to understand complicated information	Apathy or lack of motivation, disoriented	Disoriented, unable to concentrate, may have hallucinations or delusions
Mood/speech	Repeats questions or stories, often socially appropriate until later stages	Low mood, quiet, or verbalizes negative thoughts	May be incoherent
Behavior	Usually appropriate until stress threshold is surpassed, then may exhibit agitation and increased confusion or combativeness	Usually appropriate but slow, less often agitation	Can be hyperactive and agitated, but some are hypoactive and less obvious; disturbed sleep
Nursing care approaches	Report memory problems and Mini-Cog score (see Section Nine in this chapter). Give frequent gentle reminders and reassurance. Avoid overstimulation. Provide opportunity for rest, sleep, and quiet time. Treat discomfort, which is often the cause of agitation.	Report low mood and score on the Geriatric Depression Scale (see Section Nine in this chapter). Provide support and encouragement. Encourage family involvement in care to extent possible.	Report changes in mental status on evaluation and Confusion Assessment Method score (see Section Nine in this chapter). Avoid overmedication (e.g., benzodiazepines). Use approaches similar to those for patients with dementia.

instructions, or difficulty finding the right words or completing sentences. Recognizing the problem in a hospitalized patient can help the nurse plan care to keep the patient safe and avoid problems such as agitation, falls, and other adverse events that result in a greater length of stay (Palmer et al., 2014). It is important to note that people with dementia are at high risk of developing delirium, an acute emergent condition.

Depression

Depression, another common illness in the older adult, is characterized by low mood. In the older adult, depression can be a lifelong problem, the result of chronic stress or losses common in this age group (retirement, widowhood, and social isolation), or related to illness. Depression is found in 9% to 19% of noninstitutionalized older adults (Federal Interagency Forum on Aging-Related Statistics, 2016). Rates are higher among those in institutional settings. Depression has a significant impact on the older adult's life and can be a life-threatening condition. The highest rate of suicide of any age group is among older men.

The patient with depression may have difficulty sleeping, poor appetite, or feelings of hopelessness. Other common symptoms are apathy, difficulty concentrating, and low self-esteem. Older adults also may present with physical symptoms such as aches and pains. Diagnosis is based on the presence of persistent symptoms that are not related to a recent loss and is very common in older people with conditions causing pain or disabling conditions.

While depression may not be addressed when the patient is in the high-acuity state, it is very treatable. The newer medications offer fewer side effects for older adults. The nurse should be aware of low mood or changes in mood and report concerns. For example, an exacerbation of depression may be triggered by withdrawal from treatment with hospitalization or acute illness. A depression can also be triggered by severe illness, such as stroke. Once the patient is stabilized, the depression can be addressed, as it may interfere with recovery. Long-term treatment should include a combination of pharmacotherapy and psychotherapy (Morgan, 2013).

Delirium

Delirium, sometimes called acute confusion, is the rapid onset of problems with cognition, characterized by fluctuating symptoms of inattention and confusion. Delirium is caused by an insult to the brain as a result of acute illness. It is a relatively common complication of critical illness that can develop across the lifespan. This section specifically addresses delirium in the older high-acuity patient.

In the healthy older adult, delirium may occur after a major injury or illness, but in the older adult who is frail or has underlying chronic illnesses or dementia, even a minor illness can precipitate delirium. Delirium often indicates a change in status and may be the first sign of a complication such as infection, bladder distention, or drug toxicity. Delirium increases the risk of long length of stay, readmission, nursing home placement, and even death, and it increases with complications of illness. In a retrospective study of 590 cardiac ICU patients ages 18 and older, those with delirium were older and had greater disease severity, longer ICU stays, and higher mortality (Pauley et al., 2015). Early identification of delirium is critical as it is usually reversible.

The older adult with delirium can have many symptoms, ranging from hypoactive behaviors (e.g., lethargy and inattentiveness) to hyperactive behaviors (e.g., agitation, restlessness, and even combativeness), making detection challenging. Nurses readily identify those patients with hyperactive symptoms because their behavior is noticeable. However, those with hypoactive delirium may not be noticed or considered either depressed or sedated. This "quiet" delirium is easy to miss but can be detected with routine assessment and monitoring to identify changes in cognitive level.

Section Seven Review

1. Which description of Alzheimer disease is most accurate?
   A. It is an acute problem with memory and thinking.
   B. It is the most common cause of progressive dementia.
   C. It is the result of brain inflammation.
   D. It is part of Lewy body disease.

2. Which statement is correct regarding hypoactive delirium in the older adult?
   A. It is sometimes misdiagnosed as depression.
   B. It is easy for the nurse to identify.
   C. It is usually associated with global hypoxia.
   D. It is generally irreversible even with early treatment.

3. Which assessment finding is the client with depression most likely to exhibit?
   A. Anxiety
   B. Confusion
   C. Low mood
   D. Inattention

4. What is the expected cognitive status of older adults?
   A. Loss of memory
   B. Confusion
   C. Low mood
   D. Memory retention

Answers: 1. B, 2. A, 3. C, 4. D

Section Eight: Factors Impacting Hospitalization

The many anatomic and physiologic age-related changes that occur in older adults must be taken into account during hospitalization to ensure safe, high-quality patient care. This section presents a discussion of three factors that should be considered when an older adult is admitted: falls, pain, and pharmacotherapy.

Falls

Falls are a common accident in acute care, resulting in injury and increasing length of stay in older patients. Medicare and Medicaid no longer pay for care resulting from hospital falls. Older patients are at higher risk of falls than younger people due to some of the aging-related changes discussed previously, such as musculoskeletal and sensory changes, combined with chronic conditions and acute illness. In a literature review of 23 studies to identify fall risk factors among older adults, factors associated with falls in older adult patients in acute care were identified (Zhao & Kim, 2015). Major factors, along with being in a geriatric unit, include advanced age, mental status deficits, cognitive problems, impaired mobility, stroke, hypertension, urinary incontinence, visual impairment, prolonged length of hospital stay, fall history, care dependency, and medications such as antidepressants, antipsychotics, and psychotropic drugs.

Fall prevention for older adults in acute care comprises several levels. The most basic level is a safe environment: use of appropriate beds and side rails, no clutter or tripping hazards, safe equipment such as bedside commodes, and safe basic care practices (call lights always in reach, safe footwear if ambulating). The second level is adequate surveillance to meet patient needs: frequent nursing rounds to address toileting needs, increased observation of delirious or confused patients, and routine ambulation or getting older patients up in the chair as able. These interventions address common fall risk factors (see assessment tools in Section Nine). Third-level fall prevention includes assessment of any additional fall risks, such as fall risk screening upon admission and planning interventions to address these risks. An example would be identifying the underlying causes of a patient's delirium to reduce confusion. This might prevent the patient from trying to climb over the side rails of the bed or interfering with tubes and lines. Evidence does not support use of restraints to prevent falls (Lach & Leach, 2014). Another important fall assessment includes identifying and addressing orthostatic hypotension.

Regarding staffing and care setting characteristics, an integrative review suggests that geriatric units had the highest fall rates, and the number of falls increases during change of shift, evening shifts, and night shifts (Zhao & Kim, 2015). Adequate RN staffing may be required to provide these assessments and plan appropriate care.

Pain

Pain is a common concern of older adults in acute care settings. Achieving adequate pain control for the older adult in the high-acuity setting can be challenging because of the types of pain, the causes of pain, and the physical manifestations of pain. Pain affects the older adult's ability to function, as well as quality of life. Pain can be due to an acute condition such as a fracture, postoperative pain, or a chronic disease such as osteoarthritis, back pain, and bone and joint disorders. A particular concern for the older adult is chronic pain. One in five persons over age 65 years is affected by chronic pain (Tabloski, 2014), which affects all aspects of life, health, and safety, as well as healthcare costs.

Pain Assessment   Age-related changes such as changes in cognition and sensory perception impact the ability of the patient to perceive and report pain. Barriers to pain assessment and management are numerous and include the individual's beliefs about pain and potential alterations in sensory and cognitive function that interfere with communication and the reporting of pain. A thorough nursing assessment is required. Many pain scales and assessment tools exist; however, assessment of nonverbal behavior, such as facial expressions, body language, and agitation, is equally important.

Pain Medications   Pain medication should be given routinely to manage severe pain. Although pain medications such as opiates control severe pain, they have side effects that may interfere with recovery from acute conditions. Undertreatment of acute as well as chronic pain has been commonly described among older adults and can lead to depression, social isolation, gait and mobility problems, nutrition and sleep disturbances, and physiologic responses such as hypertension and tachycardia (Tabloski, 2014). Other problems that result from poor pain control include agitation and delirium. Nonpharmacologic nursing interventions such as promoting sleep, maintaining a calm and peaceful environment, and promoting comfort help to create a healing environment and decrease the perception of pain.

Side effects of pain medications may present a challenge in the older patient. Nonsteroidal anti-inflammatory drugs (NSAIDs) can increase the risk of gastrointestinal bleeding and impaired renal function in frail older adults. Meperidine should be avoided because it commonly causes neurotoxicity and the risk of confusion or seizures in older patients (Tabloski, 2014). Frequent pain assessment and regular administration of pain medication at the lowest dose needed to treat pain may prevent or improve delirium. Nurses need to be vigilant in assessment, monitoring, and treatment of pain, as well as evaluation of the patient for any untoward reactions to treatments.

Pharmacotherapy

The administration of medications to the older adult is complicated, as these patients are at increased risk for drug toxicities and medication errors. The physiologic reasons for this increased risk involve changes in multiple body systems (Fig. 4–2). A multidisciplinary approach to pain management can be used to address the many components of pain (Kaye et al., 2014). Pain management programs are designed to avoid medication errors or adverse drug reactions (ADRs) by considering factors such as normal age-related physiologic changes that affect pharmacokinetics

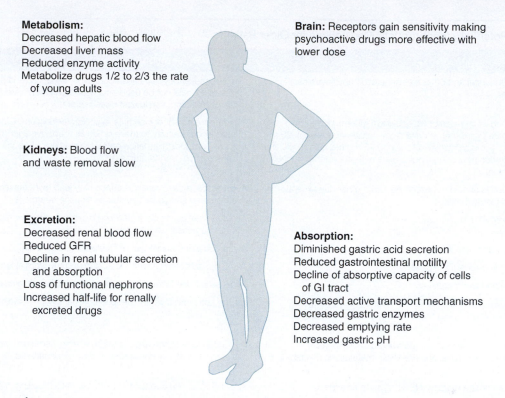

Metabolism:
Decreased hepatic blood flow
Decreased liver mass
Reduced enzyme activity
Metabolize drugs 1/2 to 2/3 the rate
   of young adults

Brain: Receptors gain sensitivity making
psychoactive drugs more effective with
lower dose

Kidneys: Blood flow
and waste removal slow

Excretion:
Decreased renal blood flow
Reduced GFR
Decline in renal tubular secretion
   and absorption
Loss of functional nephrons
Increased half-life for renally
   excreted drugs

Absorption:
Diminished gastric acid secretion
Reduced gastrointestinal motility
Decline of absorptive capacity of cells
   of GI tract
Decreased active transport mechanisms
Decreased gastric enzymes
Decreased emptying rate
Increased gastric pH

Figure 4–2 Aging body and drug use.

and pharmacodynamics, polypharmacy, self-medication, and poor medical compliance. Three major drug-related concerns are profiled here: physiologic changes, polypharmacy, and adverse drug reactions.

Physiologic Changes   When medications are administered to an older adult, changes in drug absorption, distribution, metabolism, and excretion should be considered due to the physiologic changes that occur in older adults. Factors that affect absorption include decreased surface area of the small intestine, decreased splanchnic blood flow, altered gastric pH, and decreased gastric motility. Distribution is affected by a decrease in lean body mass, increase in fat content, and decrease in total body water content. Altered liver and kidney function affect metabolism and excretion. Drugs metabolized by the liver or kidneys remain present and active for a longer period of time (Kaye et al., 2014), with an increased opportunity to produce side effects. Medications may be active in an older person's system longer and may be more potent. Therefore, drug dosage and frequency of administration may need to be altered or adjusted. The therapeutic window may be narrow, with one dose not being effective but a higher dose causing side effects. Typical signs of drug toxicity in older adults may involve CNS changes, orthostatic hypotension, falls, and incontinence rather than the more commonly seen nausea, vomiting, diarrhea, and rash.

Polypharmacy   The older adult may have several chronic illnesses that require management with numerous medications. These medications may counteract or interact with each other or cause side effects if withdrawn during hospitalization. Nurses should be aware of the physiologic changes of older adults and how these changes may impact the metabolism of specific drug groups (see Table 4–13). It is essential to

obtain a thorough medication history for older adult patients. Prescription medications, over-the-counter medications, vitamins and minerals, alcohol, caffeine, and tobacco as well as home remedies should be considered. Nursing care includes evaluating the effects of medications, monitoring drug levels, and anticipating side effects and interactions.

Adverse Drug Reactions   Experts in gerontology and pharmacology have identified medications that are potentially inappropriate for older patients because of increased risks for

Table 4–13 Physiologic Changes and Associated Drug Effects

Physiologic Changes	Effects
Heart dependent on endogenous catecholamines for effective pumping	Beta-blocking agents may precipitate heart failure.
Decrease in dopamine-making capacity of neurons	Phenothiazines further block dopamine uptake, precipitating Parkinson-like symptoms.
Dependence on prostacyclin-mediated renal vasodilation to maintain glomerular blood flow	Nonsteroidal anti-inflammatory agents (NSAIDs) that block prostacyclin may decrease renal blood flow and precipitate acute renal failure.
Dependence on elevated renin levels to maintain renal perfusion	Angiotensin-converting enzyme (ACE) inhibitors may decrease renal blood flow and precipitate acute renal failure.
Increased body fat	Effects of fat-soluble drugs (e.g., sedatives/hypnotics) are prolonged due to increased distribution volume in fat tissue.
Less body water	Blood levels of water-soluble drugs (e.g., alcohol) are higher due to decreased distribution volume.

Table 4–14 Potentially Inappropriate Medications for Older Patients

Drug	Recommendation and Concern
diphenhydramine (Benadryl) and other first-generation antihistamines (e.g., hydroxyzine)	Avoid because they can cause confusion, sedation, and anticholinergic effects. Should not be used as a hypnotic. When used to treat emergency allergic reaction, use lowest dose possible.
benzodiazepines: *long-acting*—chlordiazepoxide (Librium), diazepam (Valium), clorazepate (Tranxene); *short-acting*—lorazepam (Ativan), 60 mg oxazepam (Serax), 2 mg alprazolam (Xanax), 0.25 mg triazolam (Halcion). This category includes the nonbenzodiazepine receptor agonist hypnotics (zolpidem, zalepolon).	Avoid for treatment of insomnia, agitation, or delirium. Older adults have increased sensitivity to these drugs as they have a long half-life in older adults, producing sedation and increased risk of cognitive impairment, delirium, falls, and fractures.
digoxin (Lanoxin): Doses should not exceed 0.125 mg per day except when treating atrial arrhythmias.	Avoid as decreased renal clearance may lead to increased risk of toxic effects and should be avoided as first-line treatment.
meperidine (Demerol)	Avoid as may cause confusion and has many disadvantages compared to other narcotics; CNS toxicity.
ketorolac (Toradol), indomethacin	Avoid due to increased risk of GI bleeding, ulceration.
short-acting nifedipine (Procardia, Adalat)	Avoid due to potential for hypotension and myocardial ischemia.
clonidine (Catapres) and alpha agonists	Avoid as first-line therapy due to potential for CNS adverse effects, orthostasis.
tricyclic antidepressants: amitriptyline (Elavil), imipramine (Tofranil), chlordiazepoxide-amitriptyline (Limbitrol), perphenazine-amitriptyline (Triavil)	Strong anticholinergic and sedation properties, orthostasis.
muscle relaxants and antispasmodics: methocarbamol (Robaxin), carisoprodol (Soma), chlorzoxazone (Paraflex), metaxalone (Skelaxin), cyclobenzaprine (Flexeril)	Avoid due to anticholinergic adverse effects, sedation, weakness; may not be effective at low doses tolerated by older patients.
nonsteroidal anti-inflammatory drugs (NSAIDs), such as aspirin, ibuprofen	Avoid chronic use due to increased risk of GI bleeding and fluid retention.

SOURCE: Data from American Geriatrics Society. (2015).

side effects, decreased effectiveness, and possible existence of more effective treatments. The "Beers Criteria for Potentially Inappropriate Medication Use in Older Adults" (American Geriatrics Society, 2015) are widely used to safely prescribe medications for older patients. The criteria specify medications that should be avoided when possible, those that should be used only if no alternative is available, and those that should be used with caution, or, if used, may require frequent monitoring of the patient. Common side effects that often lead to drugs being added to this list include delirium or mental status effects, orthostatic hypotension leading to falls and fractures, and other anticholinergic effects. The updated criteria also address medications that are a problem in patients with impaired kidney function, putting them at increased risk for adverse drug events. Table 4–14 lists selected common medications that cause side effects in the elderly and are not recommended for use in this age group.

When an older adult is prescribed a new medication, the advice is to "start low and go slow." In other words,

use a low dose first and increase the dosage slowly as the patient's reaction is determined. Nurses should monitor patient reactions to any new medication and report any untoward changes, particularly in mental status. In addition, effective communication among healthcare providers and medication reconciliation are two crucial ways to reduce the risk of adverse effects related to polypharmacy issues.

Multiple sensory issues may be present that cause problems with patient management of a medication regimen. Short-term memory impairment may cause a person to take incorrect or multiple doses or skip doses. Impaired vision may affect accurate medication identification and dosage. Impaired agility in opening containers may lead to missed doses. Financial factors and transportation issues may keep the patient from filling prescriptions.

A summary of nursing care considerations specific to this patient population can be found in the special feature titled "Nursing Care: The Older Adult High-Acuity Patient."

Nursing Care
The Older Adult High-Acuity Patient

Expected Patient Outcomes and Related Interventions

Outcome 1: Preserve organ function

  Assess and compare to established norms, patient baselines, and trends.
   Assess for comorbidities that are present in addition to admitting diagnosis.

Monitor organ status
   Neurologic—Cognitive status, pupillary response, Glasgow Coma Scale (GCS)
   Cardiovascular—Blood pressure, heart rate, heart rhythm (cardiac monitoring), heart sounds
   Pulmonary—Respiratory rate and depth, lung sounds, pulse oximetry, arterial blood gases (ABG) as warranted

Gastrointestinal—Bowel sounds, bowel palpation, nutrition status, bowel movements, signs of occult or gross GI bleeding

Hepatic—Liver size by palpation, liver function tests (LFTs)

Renal—Intake and output, renal function tests (BUN, creatinine)

Interventions to support organ function

Maintain adequate mean arterial pressure (greater than 60 mmHg).

Measures to support blood pressure—careful use of fluids or vasopressors

Careful monitoring of:

Intake and output balance (avoid over- or underhydration)

Cardiac rhythm (monitor for cardiac dysrhythmias and treat as needed)

Maintain adequate oxygenation.

Administer oxygen therapy as ordered.

Turn every 2 hours.

Elevate head of bed 30 degrees.

Have patient do deep breathing exercises, incentive spirometry every 2–4 hours.

Decrease energy expenditure.

Alternate rest and active periods.

Maintain comfortable room temperature (prevent chilling).

Maintain normothermia (reduce fever, warm blankets if hypothermic).

Assist with physical activities as needed.

Encourage early ambulation as tolerated (reduce stasis problems and functional decline).

Avoid drug-induced organ injury (related to polypharmacy).

Carefully monitor drug dosage, interactions, and toxicities.

Adjust drug dosages as needed.

Monitor drug levels periodically.

Monitor closely for signs or symptoms of adverse drug reactions.

Avoid drug combinations with same-organ toxicities.

Monitor liver and kidney function.

Outcome 2: Minimize impact of delirium

Assess and compare to established norms, patient baselines, and trends.

Monitor for early signs of delirium or other cognitive changes.

Administer the CAM-ICU test to assess for delirium (described in Section Nine in this chapter).

Interventions to reduce impact of delirium

Treat pain, anxiety, and agitation to promote adequate rest.

Treat pain with lowest effective dose of analgesic.

Avoid drugs that are associated with delirium in older adults.

Decrease environmental stimuli.

Maintain nutrition and hydration.

Enlist significant others to help in maintaining patient orientation.

Investigate possible drug-induced causes of delirium.

Outcome 3: Prevent skin breakdown

Assess and compare to established norms, patient baselines, and trends.

Assess for comorbidities that increase the risk for problems of skin integrity (e.g., diabetes, chronic heart failure, dehydration, malnutrition, postoperative).

Monitor skin color, temperature, skin integrity, evidence of stasis ulcers.

Assess pressure points frequently (e.g., heels, spine, coccyx, elbows, back of head).

Monitor nutrition and hydration status.

Interventions to prevent skin breakdown

Reposition frequently, especially if head of bed is elevated.

Handle the patient gently, avoiding shearing forces.

Use pressure-reducing surfaces.

Use skin cleansers that are nondrying.

Use lotions to keep skin lubricated.

Consult with a skin specialist as needed.

Section Eight Review

1. Which measures are useful in fall prevention? (Select all that apply.)
   A. Use of restraints
   B. Rounds to address toileting needs
   C. Assessment of fall risk
   D. Identification of orthostatic hypotension
   E. Administration of prn pain medication

2. Why are medications not absorbed as well in the older adult? (Select all that apply.)
   A. Increased gastric motility
   B. Decreased splanchnic blood flow
   C. GERD
   D. Altered gastric pH
   E. Increased fat content

3. Age-related changes may affect which factors of pharmacodynamics? (Select all that apply.)
   A. Absorption
   B. Swallowing
   C. Metabolism
   D. Excretion
   E. Distribution

4. When an older adult requires pain medication, how should it be administered?
   A. Routinely
   B. Sparingly
   C. On an as-needed (prn) basis
   D. Liberally

Answers: 1. (B, C, D), 2. (B, D), 3. (A, C, D, E), 4. A

Section Nine: Geriatric Assessment Tools for the High-Acuity Nurse

Geriatric assessment tools are commonly used to screen for problems in older patients. This section describes the most important and most widely used tools for addressing dementia, delirium, and depression, as well as physical issues, in the high-acuity setting. These screening tools take only a few minutes to administer and have been widely used in clinical settings. The shortest versions of the tools are described here and are easy to use in practice.

Assessment of Mental Status

The nurse can easily assess mental status using several brief cognitive assessment tests to detect dementia in geriatric patients. The Mini-Cog test takes just 3 minutes to administer and tests the patient's memory, ability to concentrate, and ability to follow directions. To take this test, the patient must be able to talk and write. The test consists of a clock drawing task and an uncued recall of three unrelated words. The nurse first asks the patient to repeat and recall the three words, then draw the face of a clock showing a specific time like three o'clock, complete with numbers and hands, on a piece of paper. When the patient finishes drawing the clock, the patient is asked to repeat the three words. A simple scoring method makes it fast and easy to determine if the patient has normal cognition. Scoring is based on the three rules: 1) The patient who recalls none of the words is classified as demented; 2) the patient who recalls all three words is classified as nondemented; and 3) the patient with intermediate (one to two) word recall is classified based on the clock-drawing task where the patient is considered to be normal or nondemented if all numbers are present in the correct sequence and the hands display the correct time in a legible manner. The clock drawing is considered abnormal or demented if the drawing is not readable, the numbers are not in the correct sequence, or the hands do not display the correct time. This test has high sensitivity for predicting dementia, and diagnostic value is not limited by the patient's education or language (Borson, Scanlan, Brush, Vitallano, & Dokmak, 2000). If a patient has an abnormal score, the nurse should try to determine if there has been a problem with memory or function before and if the memory or function change has been gradual or sudden. When testing older adults, sit the patient up when possible, make sure glasses are in place and there is enough light to see during testing, and avoid excess background noise during testing.

The Mini-Mental State Examination (MMSE) is another widely used cognitive assessment test for dementia that only takes 7 minutes to complete. The MMSE tests orientation, recall, attention, calculation, language manipulation, and constructional praxis with a sensitivity of 87% and a specificity of 82% in inpatients. A limitation of this test is that it is not sensitive for mild dementia, and results may be influenced by age, education, and language, motor and visual impairments (Anthony, LeResche, Niaz, von Korff,& Folstein, 1982; Freidl, Schmidt, Stronegger, Irmler, Reinhart, & Koch, 1996). Another limitation of the MMSE is in assessing progressive cognitive decline in patients over time (Hensel, Angermeyer, & Riedel-Heller, 2007).

The Montreal Cognitive Assessment (MoCA) is yet another brief assessment test to detect cognitive impairment in older adults (Nasreddine et al., 2005). This test takes 10 minutes to complete. It is more sensitive (greater than or equal to 94%) than the MMSE for detecting mild cognitive impairment, but with less specificity (less than or equal to 60%) (Davis et al., 2015). The MoCA is accessible online and in multiple languages at www.mocatest.org.

Delirium Assessment   Delirium is diagnosed through identification of symptoms that are consistent with the diagnosis: acute onset, a fluctuating course, and inattention. Also, delirium is usually temporary and reversible. In addition, the patient must show some level of agitation or an altered level of wakefulness (anything other than "0" on the Richmond Agitation and Sedation Scale [RASS], which is "alert and calm") or disorganized thinking. The RASS is one instrument that can be used to measure level of agitation or sedation. A classic screening instrument that walks the nurse through the patient assessment of delirium is the Confusion Assessment Method (CAM) (Inouye et al., 1990). An ICU version of the CAM (Ely et al., 2001), the CAM-ICU, provides specific tasks the nurse can have the patient complete to help determine cognitive status. (See Chapter 17, Table 17–1.) A positive CAM-ICU score indicates a rescue situation and should be reported immediately to the physician.

Geriatric Depression Scale

The Geriatric Depression Scale (GDS) has been widely used to screen for depressive symptoms in older adults (Yesavage et al., 1983). It has short forms that have been validated, so that administration can be as efficient and easy as possible, including a five-item version that indicates depression when these items are answered negatively (see Box 4–2). To assess depression, the nurse asks the patient to respond yes or no to a series of questions about their mood over the past two weeks. The score is based on the number of depressed answers. When a score that suggests depression is obtained, the patient should be queried about suicidal ideation: Has the patient thought about or planned suicide? If a score suggests depression and the patient reports suicidal thoughts or comments, the nurse should report these findings to the physician or managing provider for follow-up.

Skin Assessment

Because of the previously described changes in the older adult's skin, the nurse must identify those at high risk for problems. Assessment of the risk for skin breakdown

BOX 4–2 Geriatric Depression Scale (GDS)

"I am going to ask you about your mood and how you have been feeling. Choose the best answer for how you have felt over the past week or so."

1.*	Are you basically satisfied with your life?.....	YES / NO
2.	Have you dropped many of your activities and interests?..	YES / NO
3.	Do you feel that your life is empty?	YES / NO
4.	Do you often get bored?.............................	YES / NO
5.*	Are you in good spirits most of the time?....	YES / NO
6.	Are you afraid that something bad is going to happen to you?	YES / NO
7.*	Do you feel happy most of the time?	YES / NO
8.	Do you often feel helpless?........................	YES / NO
9.	Do you prefer to stay at home, rather than going out and doing new things?................	YES / NO
10.	Do you feel you have more problems with memory than most?	YES / NO
11.*	Do you think it is wonderful to be alive now?..	YES / NO
12.	Do you feel pretty worthless the way you are now?...	YES / NO
13.*	Do you feel full of energy?..........................	YES / NO
14.	Do you feel that your situation is hopeless?...	YES / NO
15.	Do you think that most people are better off than you are?	YES / NO
	Number of underlined [circled] answers: _____	

Score ≥ 4 suggests depression for 15-item version.
Score ≥ 2 suggests depression for 5-item version; if positive, ask all 15 items to increase accuracy.

* This item is on the five-item version of the GDS.

SOURCE: Data from Hoyle et al. (1999); Sheikh & Yesavage. (1986); and Weeks et al. (2003).

---

begins at admission and continues with daily assessment and re-evaluation of skin integrity. The Braden Scale for Predicting Pressure Sore Risk is used in most acute care settings. The subscales of sensory, perception, moisture, mobility, nutrition, and friction and shear are scored based on descriptive criteria. A lower score on the assessment tool indicates a higher risk for pressure sore development (Bergstrom & Braden, 2002; Bergstrom, Braden, Laguzza, & Holman, 1987). When a patient is identified at risk, nursing interventions are initiated to prevent ulcers by reducing the risk factors. A toolkit has been developed to help hospital staff implement pressure ulcer prevention practices (Berlowitz et al., 2014.)

Falls and Mobility Assessment

Acute care settings require routine fall-risk assessment. The most common tools that have been tested and validated for use in the hospital setting are the Morse Fall Scale and Hendrich II Fall Risk Model. These tools help identify patients at risk for falling and should be administered on admission and at the very least after any procedure or change in condition. Many facilities require daily screening. Key risk factors from the Hendrich II Fall Risk Model include confusion or disorientation, depression, altered elimination, dizziness, male gender, antiepileptic drugs or benzodiazepines, and difficulty getting up and walking around (Hendrich, 2013). The Morse Fall Scale includes the following risk factors: history of falling, multiple conditions, mental status changes, need for a walking aid or walking problems, and presence of IV therapy (Morse, Morse, & Tylko, 1989). Morse (2008) recommends determining the best cutoff for high-risk patients for each unit, as units may differ widely. Some settings have developed their own fall-risk assessment tools, but unless they have been validated, these tools may not be any more helpful than the nurse's judgments about fall risk.

As discussed previously, the nurse needs to provide routine care to address common risk factors for falls (toileting issues, safe environment) and identify and address any specific risk factors patients may have, such as therapy to increase muscle strength or changing medications that increase the risk of falling. Even in the high-acuity setting, restraints do not prevent falls, and they increase the risk of injuries (Lach & Leach, 2014).

Pain Assessment

It is essential to assess pain in relation to its impact on the older adult's ability to function. In the high-acuity setting, it is also important to assess pain in relation to its impact on the older adult's ability to recover from the present health condition that has caused admission into the current setting. The most important consideration in the assessment of the presence and severity of pain is the patient's account of the pain. If cognitive or communication problems are suspected, the assessment of pain should be supplemented with information from family and caregivers who can report recent changes that might indicate pain (Tabloski, 2014). Once pain has been quantified, nurses work with patients to set goals for pain management.

Laboratory Data Assessment

The slow decline in organ function seen in the older adult patient results in alterations in laboratory findings and what constitutes an "acceptable" range. It is important for the high-acuity nurse to be aware of age-related alterations in laboratory trends. Table 4–15 lists common laboratory tests, their normal ranges, and expected age-related changes.

Table 4–15 Laboratory Values in the Older Adult

Lab Test	Normal Value	Changes with Age
URINALYSIS		
Protein	0–5 mg/100mL	Rises slightly • Normal change due to aging • Urinary tract infection • Renal pathology
Glucose	0–15 mg/100mL	Declines slightly • Glycosuria noted after high serum glucose levels
Specific gravity	1.005–1.030	Lower maximum in older adults • Declining renal function impairs ability to concentrate urine
HEMATOLOGY		
RBC count	Men: 4.5–6/mcL Women: 4–5/mcL	Men: 3.7–6 mcL Women: : 4–5 mcL

Erythrocyte sedimentation rate (ESR)	At age less than 50:
	Men: 0–15 mm/hr
	Women: 0–20 mm/hr
		Increases in age over 50 years:
		   Men: 0–20 mm/hr
		   Women: 0–30 mm/hr
		Mild elevations are age related.
		Changes are influenced by changes in hematocrit; therefore, increases are not specific.
		Results are helpful in identifying malignancy, infection, and connective tissue disorders.

Hemoglobin	Men: 13.5–18g/dL Women: 12–16g/dL	Men: 11–17 g/dL Women: 11.5–16 g/dL • Anemia is very common in older adults and is multifactorial.

Hematocrit	Men: 40–54%
	Women: 36–46%
		Slight decrease:
		   Men: 38–42%
		   Women: 38–41%
		Decline in hematopoiesis

Leukocytes	5000–10,000/mcL	Decreases:
		   Men: 4200–16,000 mcL
		   Women: 3100–10,000 mcL
		Decreases should not be immediately attributed to age.

Lymphocytes	25%–35%	Average: 30% (T cells and B cells decrease) Increases risks of infection Immunizations warranted
Platelets	150,000–400,000/mcL	No change
BLOOD CHEMISTRY		
Albumin	3.5–5/100mL	May decrease Related to a decrease in liver size and enzymes Protein energy malnutrition is common.
Total serum protein	6–8 g/dL	No change Decreases may be indicative of malnutrition, infection, or liver disease.
Blood urea nitrogen (BUN)	5–25 mg/dL	Increases (mild to moderate) May be attributed to decreased glomerular filtration rate or decreased cardiac output
Creatinine	0.5–1.5 mg/dL	Increases to high normal of 1.9 mg/dL Related to decrease in lean body mass
Creatinine clearance	85–135 mL/min	Slightly decreasing over time due to decreasing GFR with aging Guideline for dosages of medications excreted by kidney
Glucose (FBS)	70–110 mg/dL fasting	Upper normal limit increases slightly, 70–120 mg/dL. Increased prevalence of DM in older adults Medications may be the cause of glucose intolerance.
Triglycerides	40–49 Years: 30–160 mg/dL	Normal range alters at age older than 50: 40–190 mg/dL
Cholesterol	Less than 200 mg/dL	Total cholesterol increases between ages 60 and 90, especially in women, and decreases after age 90. Risks for coronary heart disease (CHD)
Thyroxine (T4)	4.5–11.5 mcg/dL	No age-related changes Changes may be due to thyroid disease, acute or chronic illnesses, or caloric deficiencies.
Triiodothyronine (T3)	80–200 ng/dL	Decrease of 25%
Thyroid-stimulating hormone (TSH)	0.35–5.5 mcg/mL	Slight increase Sensitive indication of thyroid disease
Alkaline phosphate (ALP)	20–130 u/L	Increase by 8–10 u/L Increase greater than 20% usually due to disease Elevations may be found with bone abnormalities, drugs (narcotics), and eating a fatty meal.

SOURCE: Based on Kee. (2014).

Section Nine Review

1. Which brief and easy test is used to evaluate a high-acuity older client for dementia?
   - A. Geriatric Depression Scale (GDS)
   - B. Richmond Agitation and Sedation Scale (RASS)
   - C. Mini-Cog Mental Status Test
   - D. Confusion Assessment Method (CAM)

2. What is the best tool for assessing delirium in the high-acuity older adult?
   - A. CAM-ICU
   - B. CAM
   - C. GDS
   - D. Mini-Cog

3. How often should the nurse conduct a skin assessment?
   - A. Daily
   - B. After changes in condition
   - C. At least weekly
   - D. Once per shift

4. Which consideration is most important when assessing for the presence and severity of pain?
   - A. The documentation of the previous shift
   - B. The report of the client's family members
   - C. The client's account of the pain
   - D. The physician's assessment of the pain

Answers: 1. C, 2. A, 3. C, 4. C

Section Ten: High-Risk Injuries and Complications of Trauma

Traumatic injuries are a leading cause of death in older adults. Unfortunately, trauma affects the older adult more severely than the younger adult. The prognosis in the older adult is related to a variety of factors, such as decreased physiologic reserves and decreased organ functioning. This section provides an overview of selected traumatic injuries, their effects on the older adult, and the associated nursing implications.

Traumatic Injury: An Overview

Several factors increase the vulnerability of an older adult to environmental hazards and increase the risk of falls and other traumatic injuries. These include altered sensory function; changes in motor strength, postural stability, balance, and coordination; exacerbations of medical conditions; and medication therapies. While falls are the most common cause of injury, motor vehicle crashes (MVCs) account for the most fatalities. In a recent meta-analysis of 24 studies, older adults experienced higher mortality rates after traumatic brain injury due to complications, consequences of biological aging such as decreased physiologic reserve, prevalence of chronic disease, conservative management techniques, and the consequences of biological aging (McIntyre, Mehta, Aubut, Dijkers, & Teasell, 2013).

Nursing Considerations   An in-depth history should be performed to obtain information about past medical and surgical history, immunization status, and chronic diseases such as renal failure, respiratory diseases, cirrhosis, diabetes, heart disease, and previous myocardial infarctions. Nursing care is aimed at stabilizing the injuries and preventing complications. Priorities for the care of the older adult patient in the high-acuity area include assessment of airway, breathing, and circulation. Oxygenation status is monitored via peripheral oxygen saturation, lactic acid levels, arterial blood gases, and mixed venous oxygen saturation. Early hemodynamic monitoring is important. Hemodynamic status is monitored noninvasively via urine output, level of consciousness (LOC), and pedal pulses with the aid of noninvasive hemodynamic monitors, or invasively with cardiac output measurements. Assessment of hypovolemic shock is more challenging. Tachycardia, normally an early sign of hypovolemia, is often obscured as the heart rate may not respond to blood loss. Volume overload is an additional concern, particularly in a patient with cardiac and renal disease. Thermoregulatory mechanisms may be impaired (Tabloski, 2014), and therefore, heat loss should be prevented by monitoring room temperature, using warm IV solutions, or warming blankets.

Syncopal Episodes

Older adults commonly require acute care management of syncope. Previous cardiovascular disease and treatment for hypertension may precipitate a syncopal episode from either decreased cardiac output or inadequate cerebral circulation. Syncopal episodes require an in-depth assessment (Box 4–3). Cardiac dysrhythmias may contribute to accidents and could be related to numerous factors, such as anemia or hormonal or electrolyte imbalances. Other risk factors for injury are diminished senses, such as vision or hearing, and diminished reflexes, agility, and coordination. If confusion or agitation is present, it is important to determine if this is new or due to some preexisting condition.

BOX 4–3   Assessment of Syncope in the Older Adult

Focus Area: Decreased Perfusion

1. History of palpitation, shortness of breath, diaphoresis, chest pain?
2. History of previous acute myocardial infarction (AMI), cerebrovascular accident (CVA)?
3. Dizziness or loss of balance upon arising or changing position?
4. History of vomiting, diarrhea, gastrointestinal (GI) bleeding?
5. Lack of food and/or fluid intake, underweight?

Focus Area: Neurologic

1. Any weakness, tingling, or numbness?
2. Prior trouble with walking or balance?
3. Trouble completing activities of daily living (ADLs)?
4. Any difficulty with speech or communication?
5. History of memory changes or acute changes in memory and thinking?

Focus Area: Illness

1. Any history of diabetes? If so, how treated? Last meal, activity, and medication?
2. Any history of cancer? If so, how treated? Last radiation, chemotherapy treatment, complete blood count (CBC), platelet count?
3. Any infection: fever, respiratory symptoms, change in urination and/or urine output?
4. Any history of cardiovascular disease? If so, how treated?

Focus Area: Medications

1. Use of alcohol or recreational drugs?
2. Use of antihypertensives?
3. Use of antihistamines?
4. Use of sedatives?
5. Use of pain medications?
6. Use of over-the-counter (OTC) medications such as NSAIDS?
7. Use of herbal or homeopathic remedies?

A thorough medication history may reveal medications that increase the risk of injury such as antihypertensives, oral hypoglycemic agents that may induce syncope, or diuretics without potassium supplements, which may precipitate dysrhythmias and hypotension. In addition, beta-blocking agents are known to decrease the sympathetic nervous system response to hypovolemia, and therefore they alter the usual compensatory responses to injury and shock.

Specific Types of Traumatic Injury

Injuries that are considered high-risk injuries due to an associated increase in morbidity and mortality in the older adult include brain, spine, chest, abdominal, and pelvic injuries; major orthopedic traumas; and burns.

Brain and Spine Injuries   Subdural hematomas occur more frequently in the older adult following a brain injury. The age-related loss of brain volume and increased intracranial space between the brain and the dura permit a large amount of bleeding before the appearance of symptoms of intracranial bleeding. In addition, the classic signs of headache and vomiting due to increased intracranial hypertension may be absent due to cerebral atrophy. Nurses caring for older adults after an injury should assess for subtle LOC changes and cranial nerve deficits. Symptoms may show up some time after a brain injury, such as from a fall.

Chest Injuries   Chest injuries are associated with fractured ribs in older adults because of osteoporosis. Pre-existing pulmonary disease and diminished pulmonary reserve increase the risk of respiratory failure and the necessity of intubation and mechanical ventilation. In addition, in cases where an older adult requires chest compressions during cardiac arrest, rib fractures often result because of the stiff and brittle nature of the ribcage.

Abdominal Injuries   Abdominal trauma in the elderly has a high mortality rate due to postoperative, pulmonary, and infectious complications. Older adults have diminished sensation and abdominal wall muscle tone, so the typical signs of peritoneal irritation, such as involuntary guarding and muscular rigidity, may be missing. Fragile ribs and a weakened abdominal wall increase the likelihood of abdominal injury with very little force.

Pelvic Injuries   Pelvic fractures are associated with severe hemorrhage related to the close proximity of the pelvic bones to the large pelvic blood vessels (e.g., aorta, femoral arteries, and veins). Because older adults have fewer compensatory responses to combat hypovolemia, early control of hemorrhage is essential to prevent shock. Embolization of major pelvic arteries may need to be performed as well as early stabilization with external fixation.

Orthopedic Trauma   Loss of bone mass and osteoporosis increase the susceptibility of the older adult to traumatic injuries, such as hip, femur, humerus, wrist, head, or spine injuries, which often result in significant fractures. Bone fractures result in acute pain and immobility. Early stabilization of fractures is important to prevent complications of prolonged immobility, such as pneumonia, pulmonary emboli, and deep vein thrombosis. Prolonged wound healing is an additional challenge and increases susceptibility to infection.

Burn Injury   Flame injuries associated with cooking, and scald injuries associated with bathing, are common. Older adults tend to have greater depth and breadth of burn due to their thinner skin, slower reaction times, reduced mobility, and diminished sensation. Prolonged healing is also a factor, particularly in the presence of malnutrition prior to injury. Older adults do not scar as much as younger patients, and therefore pressure garments are not essential.

Section Ten Review

1. Which factor increases the older adult's risk of traumatic injuries?
   A. Increasing age
   B. Sensory changes
   C. Decreased glomerular filtration
   D. Decreased cough reflex

2. Why is subdural hematoma a common complication of brain injury in the older client?
   A. Increase in intracranial space between the brain and dura
   B. Decreased reaction time
   C. Decreased sympathetic nervous system response to hypovolemia
   D. Decreased muscle tone

3. How do the effects of burn injury in an older adult compare to those in a young person?
   A. Greater depth and size of burn, prolonged healing, and decreased scarring
   B. Increased scarring that requires pressure garments for healing
   C. Smaller burn area due to the thicker skin of the older adult
   D. Smaller burn area, shorter healing time, and more scarring

4. Why are older adults prone to abdominal injury with very little force?
   A. Ribs are thickened and brittle.
   B. Abdominal wall is weakened.
   C. Abdominal skin is thicker.
   D. Reaction time is slowed.

Answers: 1. B, 2. A, 3. A, 4. B

Section Eleven: Special Considerations—A Culture of Caring and End-of-life Care

Older adults are more vulnerable to adverse outcomes and are at greater risk for functional decline or a loss of independence as a result of hospitalization. For this reason, special attention must be given to the needs of this patient population to improve outcomes.

A Culture of Caring for Older Adults

Delivering high-quality and safe patient care to the older adult requires an understanding of the special needs of this patient population. Box 4–4 provides a summary of key steps the nurse can follow to deliver optimal care for the older high-acuity patient. An exemplary program to help nurses address these issues is the Hartford Institute for Geriatric Nursing (HIGN) at New York University's (NYU) College of Nursing, funded by the John A. Hartford Foundation. The HIGN published a Global Vision Statement on Care of Older Adults (Mezey, 2011) that has been endorsed by over 40 national nursing organizations in recognition of their combined support of evidence-based practices for the

---

BOX 4–4   Steps to Optimize Care of the Older High-Acuity Patient

1. Find out what the patient was like prior to the current illness, particularly the functional and cognitive states. The patient could have been living alone, completely independent, or residing in a nursing home. This can have a major impact on how the nurse views the patient; during critical illness, the nurse may make incorrect assumptions about the patient's prehospitalization state.

2. Identify preadmission conditions and medications that may impact the patient's response to the current illness.

3. Expect the unexpected. Diseases in older adults often have an altered presentation, so any change in vital signs or cognitive state could indicate a new problem, such as infection, delirium, or complications. The nurse may need to use good nursing detective skills to determine what is really going on.

4. Pay special attention to basic nursing care. Pressure ulcers, falls, and incontinence are common geriatric syndromes and are preventable or manageable with good skin care, turning, and attention to voiding. Medicare does not pay for hospital

costs associated with preventable complications such as these, increasing hospital attention to these problems.

5. Prevent immobility and delirium, two of the most common and modifiable risk factors for functional and cognitive decline.

6. Maximize the patient's ability to communicate by having eyeglasses and hearing aids available and in place when possible. Speak slowly and loudly (avoiding shouting or using a high-pitched voice) and face the patient when speaking.

7. Learn key aging-related changes that may impact older patients in the high-acuity area.

8. Use appropriate and brief geriatric assessment tools (e.g., Mini-Cog Mental Status Test) to identify common problems, particularly dementia, delirium, and depression.

9. Work with other members of the interdisciplinary team to address problems. The complex problems of the older adult require complex interventions. Bring in social workers, geriatric physicians, physical or occupational therapists, dieticians, and psychologists or other professionals to assist in meeting the patient's needs.

care of older adults in all settings, which challenges nurses working in all settings to meet the physiological, functional, and psychological needs of older adults.

To address the needs of hospitalized older adults, the NYU HIGN coordinates the Nurses Improving Care for Healthsystem Elders (NICHE) program. This collaborative program originated in 1981 and currently operates within a network of 620 hospitals and healthcare facilities in 46 states, Canada, Bermuda, and Singapore. It is the leading nurse-driven program designed to help hospitals improve the care of older adults, with a vision for all patients 65 and older to be given sensitive and exemplary care (Nurses Improving Care for Healthsystem Elders, 2015). NICHE sponsors an annual conference and resources; information is available through its website. Programs such as "The Dementia Friendly Hospital Initiative" (Palmer et al., 2014) are also available to support staff who provide specialized care to patients with dementia.

End-of-life Care

In most acute care settings the focus of patient care is of a healing nature, and the needs of the older adult at the end of life may be neglected. However, as the population of older adults increases and technology continues to be used to improve and prolong life, nurses will need to be prepared to care for older adults at the end of life who no longer benefit from critical care technologies and treatments. Nurses are being taught to incorporate palliative care models aimed at the relief of symptoms and freedom from the stress of a life-threatening illness into acute care settings, including critical care units. Despite the challenges with medications and pain management in older patients, many options exist to ensure optimal pain relief (Kaye et al., 2014). Nurses are challenged with the task of blending high-tech and high-touch care in order to enhance the quality of life of older adults at the end of life. Many hospitals or systems offer specialists who consult on appropriate palliative care to increase comfort for patients and families and advise staff on appropriate therapies, such as pain medication.

Resuscitation   Initiating resuscitation assumes that the individual wishes to survive the current crisis, which may or may not be a valid assumption. Before initiating resuscitation, certain ethical and physiological issues should be taken into consideration.

Ethical Issues.   Numerous ethical issues surround resuscitation efforts in all patients, not just older adults. Issues for debate include benefits, likelihood of failure or adverse effects, futility, and decision making. A great deal of debate has surrounded the patient's wishes and the right to make one's own medical treatment decisions at the end of life. For example, in the later stages of dementia, intensive treatments may not be appropriate, and healthcare providers should help families make decisions about resuscitation and heroic measures for patients who may not benefit. In the absence of planning, families may be making decisions while coping with high-acuity illness. Even healthier older patients may reach the point where continued intensive treatments are not likely to benefit them. Nurses provide education and information about patient status and provide supportive care to families making difficult decisions. Nurses can ensure that patients and families are well educated on the issues of cardiopulmonary resuscitation (CPR), do not resuscitate (DNR) and allow natural death (AND) orders, and other advance directives.

Physiological Issues.   During resuscitation efforts on an older adult, a number of physiologic factors should be considered. An increase in heart rate is a normal compensatory response to low cardiac output states; however, the heart rate of an older adult has less ability to increase in response to stressors (a negative chronotropic response). Vasopressor or inotropic agents (drugs that increase blood pressure

Emerging Evidence

- Implementation of bundles of nursing care to prevent the effects of ICU-acquired delirium and weakness have shown promise in the area of ventilation, delirium prevention, and early mobility. In an evaluation of the effectiveness and safety of implementing the "Awakening and Breathing Coordination, Delirium Monitoring/Management, and Early Exercise/Mobility Bundle" into everyday practice, a study of 269 patients aged 19 and older spent 3 fewer days breathing without mechanical assistance, experienced less delirium, and were more likely to be mobilized during their ICU stay (Balas et al., 2014). Valid and reliable tools to assess sedation or agitation level and delirium status were a key component of this care bundle. The interventions used in this study may be applicable to other high-acuity settings (Balas et al., 2014).

- Long-term disability has been identified as a potential complication following critical illness. Brummel et al. (2015) analyzed 19 studies that evaluated disability outcomes in critically ill patients age 65 and older. Findings suggest that older adults who survive a critical illness have physical and cognitive declines resulting in disability at greater rates than hospitalized non–critically ill and community-dwelling older adults. Factors such as heavy sedation, physical restraints, and immobility contribute to poor outcomes. In addition, the authors recommend interventions that address modifiable risk factors, such as immobility, delirium, and minimizing ventilation (Brummel at al., 2015).

- Older adults who experience prolonged immobility during hospitalization are at risk for functional decline. Aging is associated with decreases in muscle mass, muscle strength, and joint mobility. In addition, other factors such as medical conditions, treatment devices and equipment, restraints, and staff priorities contribute to immobilization of older adults in high-acuity settings. Although potential barriers to mobility may exist in high-acuity settings, mobilization can be performed to some degree on every patient. Early and consistent mobilization is now recommended with the use of protocols, algorithms, care bundles, order sets, or checklists in order to prevent complications of immobility. Mobilization plans should be considered for all patients and should include careful patient assessment, clinician's judgment, and interprofessional consultation (Lach et al., 2014).

and heart rate) may be required when the cardiac output is low and the heart rate does not increase.

The lack of chronotropic response in the older adult has implications in fluid and electrolyte imbalance because compensatory tachycardia may not occur in response to hypovolemia. Nurses must rely on other indicators of hypovolemia, such as changes in hemodynamic values and decreased blood pressure. In addition, older adults are unable to increase their metabolic rates in proportion to the metabolic demands of increased heat production. Decreased muscle mass and decreased peripheral vasoconstriction prevent heat conservation in the elderly, and therefore nurses must monitor for hypothermia. A warm environment and warmed IV fluids may be warranted. Consideration of age should be incorporated into standard resuscitation protocols to ensure the best outcome for older patients.

Section Eleven Review

1. Nurses are challenged with the task of blending which types of care to enhance the quality of life of older adults at the end of life?
   A. High-tech and high-touch
   B. Resuscitation and pain management
   C. Palliative and resuscitation
   D. High-tech and palliative

2. What are the ethical concerns surrounding resuscitation? (Select all that apply.)
   A. Futility
   B. Likelihood of failure
   C. Paternalism
   D. Decision making
   E. Family absence

3. In caring for the older adult experiencing high levels of stress, the nurse would expect which heart rate response?

A. The heart rate decreases as the client's stress level increases.
B. The heart rate remains below what would be expected in a younger adult with an equal stress level.
C. Tachycardia is at a rate equal to what would develop in a younger adult with an equal stress level.
D. Tachycardia is at a rate higher than would be seen in a younger adult with an equal stress level.

4. Which changes of aging decrease the older adult's ability to conserve body heat? (Select all that apply.)
   A. Decreased muscle mass
   B. Decreased peripheral vasoconstriction
   C. Increased nervous system conduction
   D. Increased cardiovascular elasticity
   E. Increased compliance of the chest wall

Answers: 1. A, 2. (A, B, D), 3. B, 4. (A, B)

Clinical Reasoning Checkpoint

A thin 84-year-old female is admitted to the unit with pneumonia.

Patient History

The family tells the nurse that the patient has been living alone in an apartment and managing well, but she has been experiencing increased shortness of breath with a productive cough for the past week. Her daughters report that she has not been eating the food they prepare for her and that she has been experiencing periods of incontinence of both stool and urine for the past week. She has been having mild diarrhea for the past 3 days. She had a myocardial infarction 2 years ago and has a history of atrial fibrillation that is treated with digoxin and warfarin. She takes metoprolol (Lopressor) for her hypertension (last taken this morning). She takes ibuprofen for osteoarthritis of her back and knees.

1. On admission to the ICU, what initial nursing interventions would the nurse expect to perform related to the pneumonia?

2. What impact will the patient's beta-blocker use have on her compensatory responses to her injuries, illnesses, and/or hospitalization?

Admission Physical Examination

A brief neurologic exam reveals no gross focal or cognitive deficits; however, it is difficult to get the patient to follow commands, and she is oriented to person only. She is tachycardic (heart rate 120 bpm), and her blood pressure is 92/58. Her lung sounds are diminished in the bases bilaterally, and her respiratory rate is 24. The pulse oximeter reads an oxygen saturation of 86%. She has a temperature of 102.2°F (39°C). Her 12-lead ECG is negative for acute ischemic changes; however, she is in atrial fibrillation.

Orders Received

IV antibiotics are ordered, and orders are received for blood and sputum cultures, chest x-ray, complete metabolic panel, and CBC.

Clinical update: Later that day the patient becomes increasingly confused, with an HR increase to 145/minute, and her RR is now 32/minute with use of accessory muscles. Her blood pressure drops to 80/45 mmHg. She is transferred to the ICU for respiratory distress and pneumonia with possible sepsis. Her pulse oximeter reading is now 82%.

3. What is the likely etiology of the change in mental status for this patient, and what might be other etiologies of her change in mental and functional status?

4. What might be possible etiologies of her less-than-optimal oxygenation level and hypotension?

Current Laboratory Data

Significant lab results from the earlier blood draw include a creatinine of 1.8 and sodium of 125. The ICU nurse inserts an indwelling urinary catheter, and a small amount of dark urine is returned.

5. What would the nurse suspect related to kidney function in this patient, and what data would the nurse review?

6. What interventions would the nurse expect related to kidney function for this patient?

Clinical update: Routine fall precautions are in place for this patient.

7. Why are fall precautions important in the care of this patient? What musculoskeletal changes of aging predispose this woman to fractures and falls?

Chapter 4 Review

1. Because older clients are very diverse in their baseline health, history, and ethnicity, the nurse should use which strategies when developing a plan of care? (Select all that apply.)
   1. Obtain a good history from the client or the family.
   2. Use standardized plans of care.
   3. Monitor the client closely.
   4. Develop the plan based on the client's chronological age.
   5. Individualize the care provided.

2. An 83-year-old client fell at home this morning. The nurse continues to do frequent neurological status checks for several hours after the client is admitted. What is the primary rationale for this nursing decision?
   1. The stress of trauma tends to make older clients confused.
   2. Hospitalization causes delirium in many older clients.
   3. It takes longer for evidence of cerebral bleeds to appear in older clients.
   4. Older clients tend to underreport sensory changes.

3. A 72-year-old client has had cardiac valve dysfunction for several years. Upon being hospitalized with symptoms, the client says, "I guess it is time to have that valve replacement my doctor mentioned several years ago." How should the nurse respond?
   1. "Typically those surgeries are not done after age seventy."
   2. "Those surgeries are generally more successful in older adults."
   3. "I'm sure your physician will do a thorough diagnostic workup before that decision is made."
   4. "You should have had the surgery years ago when it was first discussed."

4. The daughter of an older adult who has been acutely ill talks to the nurse in the hall and says, "I don't see why you have to get her up in the chair. She has been so sick." How should the nurse reply to this concern?
   1. "It is so much easier to change her bed when she is in the chair."
   2. "Getting her up will help her remain mobile."
   3. "We don't want her to get lazy."
   4. "We have good reasons for all our interventions."

5. A hospitalized older adult has an indwelling urinary catheter that was placed 3 days ago. The nurse, aware of the potential for urinary tract infection, increases surveillance for which symptoms? (Select all that apply.)
   1. Confusion
   2. Abdominal pain
   3. Edema in the ankles
   4. Nausea
   5. Flank pain

6. The nurse assistant says, "I don't see how this client can have such a bad infection. He doesn't even have a fever." How should the nurse respond?
   1. "Check his temperature again in 15 minutes."
   2. "Older people's temperature may not rise to the fever range."
   3. "How did you measure his temperature?"
   4. "His core temperature is probably much higher than his oral temperature."

7. The nurse would be watchful for the development of depression in which clients? (Select all that apply.)
   1. A client who has chronic pain
   2. A newly widowed client
   3. A client just diagnosed with upper respiratory infection
   4. A client just diagnosed with diabetes mellitus
   5. A client who just had a below-the-knee amputation

8. Because of the changes in pharmacokinetics and pharmacodynamics brought about by aging, the nurse routinely monitors an older client for which effect?

   1. Lack of response to many pain medications
   2. Low blood levels of most medications
   3. Longer effects of some medications
   4. Increased rash response to many medications

9. The nurse would like to quickly test the mental status of a client who may be developing Alzheimer disease. Which tool would best evaluate this high-acuity older adult?

   1. GDS
   2. RASS
   3. CAM-ICU
   4. Mini-Cog

10. The nurse is caring for an older adult who was hospitalized following severe trauma in a motor vehicle crash. The nurse is mindful of which consideration when monitoring this client?

    1. Peripheral oxygen saturation will be helpful in determining oxygenation status.
    2. Hemodynamics must be monitored in a noninvasive manner.
    3. Level of consciousness will vary and is not a reliable indicator of status.
    4. Tachycardia will occur with hemorrhage.

Answers to questions found inside your textbook are available on the faculty resources site. Please consult with your instructor.

References

Administration on Aging (AOA). (2014). *A profile of older Americans: 2014.* Retrieved November 30, 2016, from http://www.aoa.acl.gov/Aging_Statistics /Profile/2014/docs/2014-Profile.pdf

Alvis, B. D., & Hughes, C. G. (2015). Physiology considerations in geriatric patients. *Anesthesiology Clinics, 33*(3), 447–456. doi:10.1016/j.anclin. 2015.05.003

Alzheimer's Association. (2014). *Alzheimer's Association Report: 2014 Alzheimer's disease facts and figures, 10*(2), e47–e92. Retrieved December 1, 2016, at https://www .alz.org/downloads/Facts_Figures_2014.pdf, http:// dx.doi.org/10.1016/j.jalz.2014.02.001

Amarya, S., Singh, K., & Sabharwal, M. (2015). Changes during aging and their association with malnutrition. *Journal of Clinical Gerontology and Geriatrics, 6*(3), 78–84. doi:10.1016/j.jcgg.2015.05.003

American Academy of Nursing. (2015). *Choosing wisely: Fifteen things nurses and patients should question.* Retrieved November 30, 2016, from http://www .aannet.org/initiatives/choosing-wisely

American Geriatrics Society. (2015). Updated Beers Criteria for potentially inappropriate medication use in older adults. *Journal of the American Geriatrics Society, 63*(11), 2227–2246.

Anthony, J. C., LeResche, L., Niaz, U., von Korff, M. R., & Folstein, M. F. (1982). Limits of the "Mini-Mental State" as a screening test for dementia and delirium among hospital patients. *Psychological Medicine, 12*(2); 397–408.

Balas, M. C., Vasilevskis, E. E., Olsen, K. M., Schmid, K. K., Shostrom, V., Cohen, M. Z., . . . Burke, W. J. (2014). Effectiveness and safety of the Awakening and Breathing Coordination, Delirium Monitoring/ Management, and Early Exercise/Mobility Bundle. *Critical Care Medicine, 42*(5), 1024–1036. doi:10.1097 /CCM.0000000000000129

Bell, L. (2014). The epidemiology of acute and critical illness in older adults. *Critical Care Nursing Clinics of North America, 26*(1), 1–5. doi:10.1016/j.ccell .2013.10.001

Bergstrom, N., & Braden, B. J. (2002). Predictive validity of the Braden Scale among black and white subjects. *Nursing Research, 51*(6), 398–403.

Bergstrom, N., Braden, B. J., Laguzza, A., & Holman, V. (1987). The Braden Scale for Predicting Pressure Sore Risk. *Nursing Research, 36*(4), 201–210.

Berlowitz, D., Lukas, C. V., Parker, V., Niederhauser, A., Silver, J., Logan, C., . . . Zulkowski, K. (2014). *Preventing pressure ulcers in hospitals: A toolkit for improving quality of care.* Retrieved December 1, 2016, from http:// www.ahrq.gov/professionals/systems/hospital /pressureulcertoolkit/index.html

Borson, S., Scanlan, J., Brush, M., Vitaliano, P., & Dokmak, A. (2000). The Mini-Cog: A cognitive "vital signs" measure for dementia screening in multi-lingual elderly. *International Journal of Geriatric Psychiatry, 15*(11), 1021–1027.

Brummel, N. E., Balas, M. C., Morandi, A., Ferrante, L. E., Gill, T. M., & Ely, W. (2015). Understanding and reducing disability in older adults following critical illness. *Critical Care Medicine, 43*(6), 1265–1275.

Centers for Disease Control and Prevention (CDC). (2013). *The state of aging and health in America 2013.* Retrieved November 30, 2016, from http://www.cdc.gov/aging /help/dph-aging/state-aging-health.html

Centers for Disease Control and Prevention (CDC). (2014). CDC national health report: Leading causes of morbidity and mortality and associated behavioral risk and protective factors—United States, 2005–2013. *Morbidity and Mortality Weekly Report, 63*(04), 3–27.

Centers for Disease Control and Prevention (CDC). (2015a). *National statistics; NHIS arthritis surveillance.* Retrieved November 30, 2016, from http://www.cdc.gov/arthritis/data_statistics/national-statistics.html

Centers for Disease Control and Prevention (CDC). (2015b). *Catheter-associated urinary tract infections (CAUTI).* Retrieved December 1, 2016, from http://www.cdc.gov/HAI/ca_uti/uti.html

Centers for Disease Control and Prevention (CDC). (2015c). *Diabetes report card 2014.* Retrieved December 1, 2016, from http://www.cdc.gov/diabetes/pdfs/library/diabetesreportcard2014.pdf

Centers for Disease Control and Prevention (CDC). (2016). *2016 recommended vaccinations for adults by age.* Retrieved February 6, 2017, from https://www.cdc.gov/vaccines/schedules/downloads/adult/adult-schedule-easy-read-bw.pdf

Creditor, M. C. (1993). Hazards of hospitalization of the elderly. *Annals of Internal Medicine, 118*(3), 219–223.

Davis, D. H., Creavin, S. T., Yip, J. L., Noel-Storr, A. H., Brayne, C., & Cullum, S. (2015). Montreal Cognitive Assessment for the diagnosis of Alzheimer's disease and other dementias. *Cochrane Database of Systemic Reviews.*

Davis, L. L. (2014). Cardiovascular issues in older adults. *Critical Care Nursing Clinics of North America, 26*(1), 61–89.

Ely, E. W., Inouye, S. K., Bernard, G. R., Gordon, S., Francis, J., Mey, L., . . . Dittus, R. (2001). Delirium in mechanically ventilated patients: Validity and reliability of the confusion assessment method for the intensive care unit (CAM-ICU). *Journal of the American Medical Association, 286*(21), 2701–2710.

Federal Interagency Forum on Aging-Related Statistics. (2016). *Older Americans 2016: Key indicators of well-being.* Retrieved February 6, 2017, from https://agingstats.gov/docs/LatestReport/OA2016.pdf

Freidl, W., Schmidt, R., Stronegger, W. J., Irmler, A., Reinhart, B., & Koch, M. (1996). Mini mental state examination: Influence of sociodemographic, environmental and behavioural factors and vascular risk factors. *Journal of Clinical Epidemiology, 49*(1):73.

Hendrich, A. (2013). *Fall risk assessment for older adults: The Hendrich II Fall Risk Model.* Retrieved December 1, 2016, from https://consultgeri.org/try-this/general-assessment/issue-8.pdf

Hensel, A., Angermeyer, M. C., & Riedel-Heller, S. G., (2007). Measuring cognitive change in older adults: Reliable change indices for the Mini-Mental State Examination. *Journal of Neurology, Neurosurgery, and Psychiatry, 78*(12): 1298. Epub 2007 Apr 18.

Hoyle, M. T., Alessi, C. A., Harker, J. O., Josephson, K. R., Pietruszka, F. M., Koelfgen, M., . . . Rubenstein, L. C. (1999). Development and testing of a five-item version of the Geriatric Depression Scale. *Journal of the American Geriatrics Society, 47*(7), 873–878.

Inouye, S. K., van Dyck, C. H., Alessi, C. A., Balkin, S., Siegal, A. P., & Horwitz, R. I. (1990). Clarifying confusion: The confusion assessment method. A new method for detection of delirium. *Annals of Internal Medicine, 113*(12), 941–948.

Kaye, A. D., Baluch, A. R., Kaye, R. J., Niaz, R. S., Kaye, A. J., Liu, H., & Fox, C. J. (2014). Geriatric pain management, pharmacological and nonpharmacological considerations. *Psychology & Neuroscience, 7*(1), 15–26. doi:10.3922/j.psns.2014.1.04

Kee, J. L. (2014). *Laboratory and diagnostic tests* (9th ed.). Upper Saddle River, NJ: Pearson.

Kortebein, P., Symons, T. B., Ferrando, A., & Evans, W. J. (2008). Functional impact of 10 days of bed rest in healthy older adults. *Journal of Gerontology, 63A*(10), M1076–M1081.

Lach, H. W., & Leach, K. (2014). Changing the practice of restraint use in acute care. *Evidence Based Practice Guideline Series.* Iowa City, Iowa: University of Iowa, The John A. Hartford Center of Geriatric Nursing Excellence.

Lach, H. W., Lorenz, R. A., & L'Ecuyer, K. M. (2014). Aging muscles and joints: Mobilization. *Critical Care Nursing Clinics of North America, 26*(1), 105–113. doi:10.1016/j.ccell.2013.10.005

Lemay, A. C., Anzueto, A., Restrepo, M. I., & Mortensen, E. M. (2014). Predictors of long-term mortality after severe sepsis in the elderly. *American Journal of the Medical Sciences, 347*(4), 282–288.

LeMone, P., Burke, K., Bauldoff, G., & Gubrud, P. (2015). *Medical-surgical nursing: Clinical reasoning in patient care* (6th ed.). Hoboken, NJ: Pearson Education Inc.

Manning, J. (2014). Acquainting critical care nurses with older patients' physiological changes. *Nursing Critical Care, 9*(6), 21–27. doi:10.1097/01

Mathur, S., Zammitt, N., & Frier, B. (2015). Optimal glycaemic control in elderly people with type 2 diabetes: What does the evidence say? *Drug Safety, 38*(1), 17–32. doi:10.1007/s40264-014-0247-7

McIntyre, A., Mehta, S., Aubut, J., Dijkers, M., & Teasell, R. (2013). Mortality among older adults after a traumatic brain injury: A meta-analysis. *Brain Injury, 27*(1), 31–40. doi:10.3109/02699052.2012.700086

Mezey, M. (2011). *Specialty nursing association global vision statement on care of older adults.* New York, NY: Hartford Institute for Geriatric Nursing, New York University College of Nursing. Retrieved February 6, 2017, from https://www.researchgate.net/publication/26768469_Specialty_Nursing_Association_Global_Vision_Statement_on_Care_of_Older_Adults

Morehead, D., & Blain, B. (2014). Driving hospital acquired pressure ulcers to zero. *Critical Care Clinics of North America, 26,* 559–567.

Morgan, J. H. (2013). Late-life depression and the counseling agenda: Exploring geriatric logotherapy as a treatment modality. *International Journal of Psychological Research, 6*(1), 94–101.

Morse, J. M. (2008). *Preventing patient falls* (2nd ed.). New York, NY: Springer.

Morse, J. M., Morse, R. M., & Tylko, S. J. (1989). Development of a scale to identify the fall-prone patient. *Canadian Journal on Aging, 8*(4), 366–367.

Nasreddine, Z. S., Phillips, N.A., Bedirian, V., Charbonneau, S., Whitehead, V., Collin, I., . . . Chertkow, H. (2005). The Montreal Cognitive Assessment, MoCA: A brief screening tool for mild cognitive impairment. *Journal of the American Geriatrics Society, 53*(4): 695.

Nurses Improving Care for Healthsystem Elders (NICHE). (2015). *The NICHE program.* Retrieved December 1, 2016, from http://www.nicheprogram.org

Palmer, J. L., Lach, H. W., McGillick, J., Murphy-White, M., Carroll, M. B., & Armstrong, J. L. (2014). The dementia friendly hospital initiative education program for acute care nurses and staff. *Journal of Continuing Education in Nursing, 45*(9), 416–424.

Pauley, E., Lishmanov, A., Schumann, S., Gala, G. J., van Diepen, S., & Katz, J. N. (2015). Delirium is a robust predictor of morbidity and mortality among critically ill patients treated in the cardiac intensive care unit. *American Heart Journal, 170*(1), 79–86. doi:10.1016/j.ahj.2015.04.013

Pilkinton, M. A., & Talbot, K. (2015). Update on vaccination guidelines for older adults. *Journal of American Geriatrics Society, 63*(3), 584–588.

Pines, J. M., Mullins, P. M., Cooper, J. K., Feng, L. B., & Roth, K. E. (2013). National trends in emergency department use, care patterns, and quality of care of older adults in the United States. *Journal of the American Geriatrics Society, 61,* 12–17.

Sheikh, V. I., & Yesavage, V. A. (1986). Geriatric Depression Scale: Recent evidence and development of a shorter version. In T. L. Brink (Ed.), *Clinical gerontology: A guide to assessment and intervention* (pp. 165–174). New York, NY: Haworth.

Stoneking, L. R., Winkler, J. P., DeLuca, L. A., Stolz, U., Stutz, A., Luman, J. C., . . . Denninghoff, K. R. (2015). Physician documentation of sepsis syndrome is associated with more aggressive treatment. *Western Journal of Emergency Medicine, 16*(3), 401–407. doi:10.5811/westjem.2015.3.25529

Tabloski, P. A. (2014). *Gerontological nursing* (3rd ed.). Upper Saddle River, NJ: Pearson.

Valiathan, R., Ashman, M., & Asthana, D. (2016). Effects of aging on the immune system: Infants to elderly. *Scandinavian Journal of Immunology, 83*(4), 255–266. doi:10.1111/sji.12413. e-pub ahead of print.

Ward, B. W., Schiller, J. S., & Goodman, R. A. (2014). Multiple chronic conditions among US adults: A 2012 update. *Preventing Chronic Disease, 11,* 130389. http://dx.doi.org/10.5888/pcd11.130389

Weeks, S. K., McGann, P. E., Michaels, T. K., & Penninx, B. W. (2003). Comparing various short-form Geriatric Depression Scales leads to the GDS-5/15. *Journal of Nursing Scholarship, 35*(2), 133–137.

Yesavage, J. A., Brink, T. L., Rose, T. L., Lum, O., Huang, V., Adey, M., & Leirer, V. O. (1983). Development and validation of a geriatric depression screening scale: A preliminary report. *Journal of Psychiatric Research, 17*(1), 37–49.

Zhao, Y. L., & Kim, H. (2015). Older adult inpatient falls in acute care hospitals: Intrinsic, extrinsic, and environmental factors. *Journal of Gerontologic Nursing, 41*(7), 29.

Chapter 5
Acute Pain Management

 ## Learning Outcomes

5.1 Examine the multidimensional nature of pain and the impact on treatment decisions.

5.2 Discuss issues related to the undertreatment of pain.

5.3 Identify potential sources and effects of pain.

5.4 Assess acute pain in the high-acuity adult patient.

5.5 Demonstrate effective management of pain for the high-acuity adult patient.

5.6 Perform focused assessments of the patient receiving opioid drug therapy to prevent opioid-induced respiratory depression.

5.7 Identify considerations associated with pain management in special populations.

5.8 Discuss the nursing management of patients undergoing procedural sedation.

High-acuity patients are at increased risk for acute pain related to their admitting diagnoses, immobility, required therapies, and diagnostic procedures. Unrelieved acute pain can increase morbidity and mortality and may lead to persistent pain. For these reasons, it is crucial that nurses who work with this patient population have a strong understanding of acute pain and its assessment and treatment options. This chapter focuses on the nature of pain and its potential sources in high-acuity patients. Systematic, thorough assessment of pain is a crucial part of providing high-quality and safe care to the patient. Nurses caring for high-acuity patients should utilize validated tools to assess pain, use around-the-clock dosing of prescribed analgesics for continuous pain, advocate for optimal treatment modalities, and understand the safety issues associated with potent analgesics. Management of pain requires careful consideration, particularly in special populations.

Section One: The Multifaceted Nature of Pain

To fully appreciate the complex multifaceted nature of pain, a basic understanding of the physiology of pain is needed. This section provides foundational information regarding pain, including definitions, a review of basic physiologic concepts, and a discussion of the multiple facets (aspects) of pain.

A Working Definition of Acute Pain

The International Association for the Study of Pain (IASP) defines pain as "An unpleasant sensory and emotional experience associated with actual or potential tissue damage, or described in terms of such damage" (International Association for the Study of Pain [IASP], 2014, para.1).

Differentiating Nociception and Pain While the terms *pain* and *nociception* are often used interchangeably, **nociception** refers only to the physiological response to tissue damage or injury. Acute nociceptive stimulation serves a major protective function by acting as an early warning system of impending or actual tissue injury and typically diminishes as the injury heals. **Pain**, however, involves psychosocial as well as physiological responses to injury. The psychosocial responses to pain are expressed through emotions (such as fear and anxiety) and are significantly influenced by learned behaviors, personal experience, and cultural influences. Therefore, every individual's response to pain will be different.

Pain intensity is subjective and cannot be objectively validated. Therefore, the nurse must accept the patient's self-report and use it as the foundation for the pain assessment. McCaffery's definition of pain is perhaps the most clinically relevant: "Pain is whatever the experiencing person says it is, existing whenever the experiencing person says it does" (McCaffery & Pasero, 1999, p. 17).

A Multifaceted Model of Pain

The multifaceted conceptualization of pain is based on the theoretical model by Loeser and Cousins (1990), which is conceptualized as four overlapping spheres: nociception, pain, suffering, and pain behaviors. Only the outermost facet, pain behaviors, can be observed by someone other than the person experiencing the pain. The relative contribution of each of the four facets to the pain experience is variable. Each facet is present to some degree in any pain experience. This multifaceted model of pain remains an effective framework for describing the pain experience. Acute pain responses are influenced by psychological variables such as cultural influences, level of anxiety, coping styles (anger versus passive response), locus of control (internal and/or external), response to diagnoses and adverse surgical outcomes, and personality traits.

Defining Acute Pain   The term *acute pain* is used to define the nociceptive reaction to an inflammatory (nociceptive) response following trauma, surgery, or a disease-related process resulting in cellular or tissue damage. The sensation of acute pain is continually changing and transient, noting a rapid onset and relatively brief duration (less than 6 months). Acute pain is accompanied by a high level of emotional and autonomic nervous system arousal.

The First Facet: Nociception   There are five types of sensory receptors, each with the ability to detect changes in a specific type of sensory input (see Table 5–1). Sensory receptors require a certain level of excitation (called the threshold) before they will transmit input. The term *nociception* refers to the activation of normally silent pain sensory receptors called **nociceptors**. Noxious (pain-causing) stimuli that are mechanical, thermal, or chemical activate nociceptors in the affected tissue. When nociceptors react to noxious stimuli, they act as a communication mechanism that facilitates the pain processes of transduction, transmission, modulation, and perception.

Transduction.   Pain transduction refers to the transformation of a noxious stimulus to a nociceptive impulse. A noxious stimulus strong enough to threaten tissue integrity transmits a message from the site of injury or tissue damage to the brain and results in pain. Tissue damage triggers the release of biochemical mediators (prostaglandins, bradykinin, and others). These mediators sensitize the nerves, producing cellular activity. When cells are stimulated by electrical energy, ion exchange occurs across the neuronal membrane, resulting in an action potential along the afferent fibers until the transmission ends in the dorsal horn at the presynaptic junction. Transduction of the messages from the nociceptors begins in the peripheral nervous system and initiates the exchange of sodium and potassium across the neuronal membranes, causing depolarization.

Transmission.   Pain transmission refers to conduction of the pain impulse through the nervous system once a noxious stimulus has been transformed into a nociceptive impulse. When the nerve fibers are stimulated, the impulse travels the length of the afferent or sensory nerve fibers, ending in the dorsal horn at the presynaptic junction. Two types of nerve fibers carry pain impulses— *A delta fibers* and *C fibers*. *A delta fibers* are small in diameter and are myelinated, conducting pain impulses rapidly along the myelin sheath, causing conduction of sharp, pinprick-like pain. *C fibers* are small in diameter but are usually unmyelinated, which results in a slow conduction rate and transmission of deep aching, throbbing sensations.

Role of the Central Nervous System in Transmission. Although the transmission of the impulse along the spinothalamic pathways appears relatively simple and straightforward, the process is complex. The noxious stimulus is transmitted from the periphery to the central nervous system (CNS) along the spinal cord to the brain. Three areas of the CNS are involved in pain transmission (in order of their location in the CNS): (1) the periventricular and periaqueductal gray (PAG) areas, located in the third ventricle, hypothalamus, and upper brainstem; (2) the raphe magnus nucleus, located in the brainstem; and (3) the pain inhibitory complex, located in the spinal cord dorsal horn. It is important to understand the role of the nervous system in order to identify how pain can be interrupted or modified.

Sensitization.   Once nociception transmission occurs, the surrounding nerve fibers become hypersensitive, causing the sensation of pain. This is the body's protective mechanism that is activated by inflammatory mediators at the site of the injury or trauma to prevent additional injury. However, if the pain intensity is maintained or noxious stimulation is persistent, cell damage occurs and additional chemical mediators are released. This results in expansion of the number of involved nociceptors, expanding the area of pain. This is known as **peripheral sensitization** and can decrease the patient's pain threshold, causing a repeated painful stimulus to be more intense and prolong the duration of pain. A classic example of peripheral sensitization can be noted following a small paper cut on a finger. Whenever the area is bumped, pain

Table 5–1 Sensory Receptors

Receptor	Function
Pain receptors (nociceptors)	Detection of tissue damage
Thermoreceptors	Detection of temperature changes
Electromagnetic receptors	Detection of light on eye retina
Chemoreceptors	Detection of smell, taste, concentration of arterial blood oxygen and carbon dioxide, and others
Mechanoreceptors	Detection of mechanical changes in cells adjacent to receptors (e.g., position and tactile senses)

is more intense and the pain is prolonged. **Central sensitization** is caused by the increased excitability of neurons in the CNS and is a complex abnormal response to a barrage of prolonged nociceptive activation. Central sensitization is thought to be responsible for the reorganization of both the peripheral nerves and the nerves in the CNS, producing abnormal sensation. With central sensitization, a sensation that is not normally painful, such as touch, will cause pain along the distribution of the injured nerve. This is referred to as **hyperalgesia**.

Modulation.   The body's attempt to alter pain transmission in response to specific physiologic events, such as pain and stress, is called **modulation**. Modulation is an adaptive process that releases endogenous (internal) neurotransmitters called endogenous opioid peptides. These influence pain impulses by producing analgesia at various stages of transmission. When these substances are released, they bind to special receptor sites along the ascending pain pathway and modify the pain transmission. Endogenous opioid peptides have been identified as being of three types: enkephalins, beta-endorphins, and dynorphins.

In addition to modulating pain, these neurotransmitters can stimulate euphoria, affect appetite, activate sex hormones, and enhance the immune system. Endorphins bind to the specific receptors in the dorsal horn to block the transmission of pain signals and act similarly to drugs such as morphine. Many factors, such as stress and pain, can decrease or increase the release of endogenous endorphins. It is now known that chronic administration of exogenous (external) opioids actually inhibits the production of endogenous (internal) endorphins (Sharma & Verma, 2015). This will be important when reviewing pharmacologic treatment for pain.

Perception.   Pain perception refers to the patient's subjective experience surrounding the pain. How a person perceives pain results from the other pain processes of transduction, transmission, and modulation. This process helps explain why behavior modification, relaxation, and other nonpharmacologic treatments can alter how pain is perceived.

The Second Facet: Pain   In order for perception of pain to occur, most nociceptor fibers enter the spinal cord through the dorsal route into the dorsal horn and terminate in the lamina. The afferent fibers terminate in the dorsal horn of the spinal cord, to the higher-order neuronal pathways to the brain (thalamus and cerebral cortex).

A major dual pathway consists of the neospinothalamic tract and paleospinothalamic tract. An example of this dual pathway is as follows: A delta pain fibers primarily transmit thermal and mechanical pain through the neospinothalamic tract. The theory underlying the A delta route of transmission is that pain impulses travel along *first-order* neurons to the dorsal horn of the spinal cord, terminating primarily in the lamina marginalis. Upon reaching the lamina marginalis in the dorsal horn, the impulse excites *second-order* neurons and immediately crosses to the opposite side of the spinal cord. The impulse then ascends

through the brainstem to the thalamus, where it is consciously acknowledged. From the thalamus it travels to the cerebral cortex, frontal lobe, and limbic system, where analysis of pain quality takes place.

Emotional reaction to pain occurs within the limbic system. A person can perceive pain only when transmission of the noxious stimulus terminates within the brain. It is unknown whether the patient's ability to perceive pain remains intact when cortical function is compromised or when cortical function has been chemically altered by sedative–hypnotics. It is clear that the negative physiologic outcomes related to the activation of the body's stress response occur regardless of whether or not the patient perceives pain at the cortical level. This explains why it is important to assume that high-acuity patients have pain during painful disease processes or procedures even if they are unable to communicate or lack the ability to respond with behavioral manifestations.

The Third Facet: Suffering   The multifaceted model describes the term *suffering* as a negative affective response that is generated in the higher nervous centers of the brain. It further states that suffering can be caused by pain or a variety of situations such as stress, anxiety, fear, loss of a loved one, and depression. The concept of suffering seems closely connected to the personal meaning of the pain. The clinician's objective assessment of suffering is restricted to observing for the presence or absence of pain behaviors. It is now commonly acknowledged that suffering is particularly associated with chronic pain. While suffering is an intensely personal experience, it is accompanied by a range of emotions. Suffering is not the same as pain, but pain often is closely associated and described as suffering. The sufferer will experience spiritual distress and feel voiceless. A loss of one's self through pain or illness can threaten a person's sense of wholeness. A growing area for nursing research includes the impact that approaches such as healing and spirituality have on pain. Nurses have a responsibility to recognize suffering in the high-acuity patient by carefully assessing physical, mental, and spiritual suffering and by treating pain while providing support through understanding and presence.

The Fourth Facet: Pain Behaviors   It is no coincidence that the outside circle of the multifaceted model of pain is pain behavior. **Pain behavior** refers to a person's physical reaction to the conscious perception of pain; it is what leads the observer to conclude that pain is being experienced. There are two types of pain behaviors: those that are intended to communicate pain (pain-*expressing* behaviors) and those that are intended to lessen or control the pain (pain-*controlling* behaviors). Common pain-expressing behaviors include crying, groaning, rubbing the painful part, or lying motionless. It is often difficult for the observer to differentiate pain-controlling from pain-expressing behaviors. For example, rubbing or massaging the painful part may be a means of moderating the sensory input (pain-controlling behavior) rather than a means of communicating (expressing) the pain to others.

Section One Review

1. Which description correctly applies to acute pain? (Select all that apply.)
   A. A short duration
   B. Continually changing
   C. Rapid onset
   D. Little emotional arousal
   E. May follow cellular or tissue damage

2. What is the term that refers to the activation of pain receptors and the pain pathway by a noxious stimulus strong enough to threaten tissue integrity?
   A. Acute pain
   B. Suffering
   C. Nociception
   D. Neuropathy

3. Tissue damage triggers the release of which biochemical mediators?
   A. A delta and C fibers
   B. Enkephalins, beta-endorphins, and dynorphins
   C. Prostaglandins and bradykinin
   D. Transduction, transmission, perception, and modulation

4. Loeser and Cousins's multifaceted model of pain includes which combination of facets?
   A. Nociception, perception, modulation, and remission
   B. Nociception, pain, suffering, and pain behaviors
   C. Transduction, transmission, modulation, and perception
   D. Perception, anxiety, remorse, and fear

Answers: 1. (A, B, C, E), 2. C, 3. C, 4. B

Section Two: Acute Pain in the High-Acuity Patient

Acute pain in the high-acuity patient is commonplace and expected in relation to the multiple potential sources of pain inherent in the types of illnesses and therapies associated with this patient population. This section presents a discussion of potential sources of acute pain in the high-acuity patient and how the combination of stress and pain negatively affects the patient's status.

Potential Sources of Pain

High-acuity patients are at risk for brief acute as well as persistent acute types of pain. The initial insult requiring admission to the hospital is often linked to acute pain (e.g., traumatic injury, organ ischemia, surgical manipulation). In addition, common in high-acuity patients are invasive lines and tubes (e.g., chest tubes, **intravenous** [into a vein] lines, endotracheal and tracheostomy tubes), all of which irritate delicate tissues and cause varying degrees of pain. In general, the greater the tissue injury, the greater the pain intensity. However, lack of widespread tissue injury does not preclude intense pain. The patient may also be required to undergo painful procedures, such as lumbar puncture, line insertions, or endoscopic examinations. Forced immobility results in myofascial or musculoskeletal pain. Pain in brain-injured patients is often overlooked because it is often assumed that brain tissue is not sensitive and clinicians are concerned that drugs such as opioids may mask the neurologic assessment and symptoms of neurologic deterioration. Nevertheless, in a mixed-methods study by Roulin and Ramelet (2015), 23 items specific to the assessment of pain in brain-injured patients were identified. The critical nature of an illness along with attachment to multiple tubes and potential chronic conditions such as back pain, neuropathy or arthritis may cause patients to experience a decreased pain threshold, and pain may be exacerbated.

Many of the conditions and treatments the high-acuity patient experiences activate the nociceptor or free nerve endings. Nociceptors are located in the afferent (sensory) peripheral nervous system in muscles and blood vessels. Persistent acute pain may be present due to the undertreatment of pain or to the continued or repeated stimulation of nociceptors (sensitivity). The pathophysiology of persistent acute pain may result in altered **neuroplasticity**, which refers to adaptive structural and functional nervous system changes. This adaptation may lead to chronic or persistent pain despite healing of the wound and trauma. While this chapter does not directly address chronic pain, clinicians caring for high-acuity patients need to be aware that the undertreatment of acute pain may have long-term consequences. Due to the changes in the nervous system that occur, the clinician needs to be vigilant about subtle changes in the quality of the pain.

Types of Acute Pain

Acute pain is divided into three types: somatic, visceral, and neuropathic.

Somatic Pain   **Somatic pain** occurs when nerves from skin, subcutaneous tissue, bones, muscle, and blood vessels are activated. Examples of somatic pain are incisional pain, tissue irritation, bone pain from fractures, joint pain from arthritis, and peripheral vascular disease–related pain. The patient will generally describe somatic pain as constant and achy. While musculoskeletal pain is generally considered somatic, special attention should be paid to clinical findings of refractory muscle spasms, excessive fatigue, or muscle disuse syndrome.

Visceral Pain   **Visceral pain** involves the internal organs or body cavity linings such as chest (lungs or heart) and abdomen, bladder or intestinal distention, or organ metastasis. The patient will likely describe visceral pain as cramping or splitting.

Neuropathic Pain A pain that occurs when there is a direct injury to a peripheral nerve, spinal cord, or the brain, is considered **neuropathic pain**. The patient generally describes the pain as shooting, burning, shock-like, or like lightning and will experience numbness and weakness. Resolution of pain from direct nerve injury is slow and depends largely on the level of injury to the nerve.

- Medical conditions such as diabetes, side effects from drugs, or chemotherapy can cause neuropathic pain that may be both acute and chronic.
- Entrapments and pinched nerves can occur along the spine or along the brachial plexus nerves that travel through the thoracic outlet. These conditions can result from positioning or ancillary muscles weakened from disuse and are rarely recognized in the long-term high-acuity patient.
- Completely severed nerves may continue to sprout with interruption in the transmission and will form abnormal and painful nerve growth known as *neuromas*. Neuromas can occur several weeks to months after nerve injury and are considered to be more chronic or persistent pain.

The Effects of Stress and Pain on the Body

In the high-acuity patient, pain can result from a variety of sources, such as tissue injury, ischemia, metabolic or chemical mediators, inflammation, or muscle spasm. Pain is also affected by stress. The stress response is crucial to self-preservation. It initiates events that increase the body's chances of survival by minimizing organ damage. When the sympathetic nervous system is activated, blood vessels decrease perfusion in order to limit blood loss while optimizing circulation to vital organs.

The initiation of the immune response to tissue injury when the body experiences a massive insult protects against infection and ischemia; however, the stress response, if not interrupted, can cause physiological changes to every organ system. A high-stress response increases vascular shunting, resulting in hypoperfusion of vital organs.

Stress increases serum levels of endogenous opioid peptides, which may result in counter-regulation of hormonal responses. Tissue injury is a strong stress response stimulus. The acute pain created by injured tissue initially increases both hormonal and sympathetic nervous system responses. The stress response will initially increase heart rate, blood pressure, cardiac workload, and oxygen demands. However, if the pain becomes prolonged, the sympathetic response to pain diminishes as a result of a parasympathetic rebound effect, which results in the normalization of vital signs. This is an important consideration when assessing pain in the high-acuity patient. Although the sympathetic response is important to assess, reliance on it as the sole indicator of acute pain may significantly misrepresent the intensity of pain.

Patients experiencing moderate to high levels of pain are often at increased risk for developing stasis-related complications because of immobility. Initially, pain is naturally associated with limiting activity, which encourages a person to rest and, therefore, aids in the healing process. This decrease in activity, however, is also associated with negative outcomes, such as pulmonary complications and deep vein thrombosis (DVT) because of venous stasis and decreased perfusion to the extremities. Pulmonary complications, such as atelectasis and stasis pneumonia, result from splinting that decreases spontaneous ventilatory movement and oxygenation. For example, pulmonary complications are frequently noted in patients who have had thoracic surgery, abdominal surgery, or trauma, and prolonged bed rest is a significant risk factor in the development of DVT. With decreased levels of pain, patients may become more active earlier in their recovery period, thus significantly decreasing the risk of developing stasis complications.

Section Two Review

1. Which statement reflects the relationship between pain and stress?
   A. Increased levels of stress worsen pain.
   B. Increased levels of stress worsen pain, only if anxiety is also present.
   C. Increased levels of stress worsen chronic pain but not acute pain.
   D. There is no significant relationship between pain and stress.

2. Which is the best description of the stress response?
   A. An avoidable reaction
   B. A maladaptive response to crises
   C. A crucial part of self-preservation
   D. An unpredictable reaction to pain

3. When the stress response becomes too great, it is associated with which physiologic changes? (Select all that apply.)
   A. Organ hypoperfusion
   B. Enhanced hormone function
   C. Increased vascular shunting
   D. Elevated endogenous opioid peptide levels
   E. Decreased oxygen demand

4. If acute pain is sustained for a prolonged period of time, how does it affect the nervous system?
   A. Sympathetic response diminishes.
   B. Parasympathetic response diminishes.
   C. Sympathetic response increases.
   D. There is no effect.

Answers: 1. A, 2. C, 3. (A, C, D), 4. A

Section Three: Pain Assessment

The American Association of Critical-Care Nurses (AACN) and other professional organizations are in agreement that pain is one of the most common symptoms in the high-acuity setting and must be assessed routinely using appropriate assessment tools (AACN, 2013). Assessing and reassessing pain in the high-acuity patient requires the nurse to utilize reliable and valid assessment tools that are easy to use, allow for easy documentation of findings, are easily understood by the communicative patient, and include standardized behavioral indicators in patients who are incapable of self-reporting or whose reports are unreliable (Stites, 2015). The use of objective pain assessment tools may supplement the subjectivity of pain assessment (Ware et al., 2015).

Pain level or intensity may vary in each individual primarily because of the neuro-biopsychological nature of pain. To manage pain effectively, it is essential to use self-report pain assessment tools whenever possible. These assessment tools help clinicians establish baseline criteria for evaluating pain and facilitate the development of appropriate comfort interventions. The ongoing challenge for caregivers and researchers is to find an effective alternative means of assessment for unconscious patients and other patients who cannot self-report their levels of pain (e.g., incoherence). While pain intensity is a key measure for pain, and every attempt should be made to solicit an intensity score from the patient, it is only one component of the assessment process and cannot always be obtained.

Pain History

The patient's pain history provides valuable information regarding preexisting pain experiences, treatment modalities, and medication history. In addition, pain history may also provide information regarding the patient's usual pain behaviors and pain relief methods used at home. Knowledge of an individual's usual pain behaviors would be of particular value if the patient should lose the ability to communicate during hospitalization. Box 5–1 lists important information that can be obtained through a pain history.

Unidimensional and Multidimensional Pain Assessment

Tools for measuring single or multiple dimensions of the pain experience are available for clinical use. The specific needs of the patient influence the type of pain assessment conducted by the nurse. Communication limitations, the capacity to understand instructions, the degree of urgency for pain relief measures, and other patient factors should be considered when selecting an assessment tool.

Unidimensional Pain Assessment   Unidimensional pain assessment tools provide the patient with a means to rate a single pain dimension, such as pain intensity, affective distress, or the subjective meaning of the pain. Intensity

---

BOX 5–1   Pain History

- Drug allergies
- Prior acute pain experiences
- Chronic pain problems—Location? Description of pain? How often? For how long?
- Activity level maintained during pain?
- Any recent changes in usual pain or discomfort pattern?
- How does the patient express pain at home (e.g., paces, lies motionless, cries, distraction)?
- How does the pain make the person feel (e.g., sad, angry, frustrated)?
- Usual relief measures:
  - Drug therapy (including over-the-counter and herbal substances)—Which drug(s)? How much? How often? Level of relief?
  - Nonpharmacologic—What type (e.g., hot water bottle, ice, heating pad)? Level of relief?

---

measurements should never be used as a complete assessment, nor should numeric scales be tied to medication doses. When the specific cause of pain is apparent (e.g., postsurgical incision pain), a unidimensional pain assessment tool is often considered sufficient to measure changes after an initial assessment occurs. Unidimensional tools are especially useful in evaluating the effectiveness of interventions used to decrease the pain. Unidimensional tools are also used as part of a multidimensional pain assessment. Examples of unidimensional pain assessment tools include the Visual Analog Scale, the Numeric Rating Scale, and verbal descriptor scales such as the Adjective Rating Scale. These tools are simple to use and take little time to administer.

Visual Analog Scale (VAS).   The VAS (Figure 5–1a) has been shown to be an effective measurement of pain intensity. There are several variations of the VAS. The most common is a horizontal or vertical line with one end labeled "no pain" and the opposite end labeled "worst pain imaginable." The patient self-reports the level of the pain along this line. The line is usually 10 centimeters in length. Once the patient has indicated the point on the scale that best represents the current level of pain, a centimeter ruler is placed on the scale and a numeric rating of 0 to 10 is given. On some VAS variations, a numeric scale is present on the reverse side, with a slide-rule type of device for converting the VAS to a numeric score.

Numeric Rating Scale (NRS).   The NRS (Figure 5–1b) is a variation of the VAS. It uses a sequence of numbers from which the patient chooses the level of pain. The most common use of the NRS is measurement of pain intensity based on a continuum of pain, with 0 being "no pain" and the higher numbers (5 through 10) indicating increasing pain up to the "worst pain imaginable." The most common and clinically supported NRS is the 0 to 10 scale. The NRS has also been used to rate numerically other dimensions of pain. An advantage of using the NRS is that the directions for using it have been translated into a variety of languages (Pasero & McCaffery, 2011).

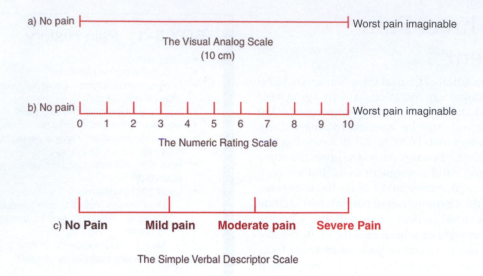

Figure 5–1 Examples of unidimensional pain assessments.

Verbal Descriptor Scales. As a unidimensional assessment tool, a verbal descriptor scale, such as the Adjective Rating Scale (ARS), may be used to measure any of the pain dimensions. For example, as a sensory dimension measure, the scale might include a list of adjectives, such as *sharp*, *cutting*, and *lacerating*. Using this list of words, the patient is asked to choose the adjective that best describes his or her current pain. The words should reflect different levels of the dimension being measured. Using this type of tool has several potential disadvantages. Careful choice of descriptor words is necessary if this type of scale is to be a useful pain assessment tool. The Verbal Descriptor Scale (VDS) is a useful scale for use with older adults who are unable to rate their pain using the numeric rating scales (Figure 5–1c).

FACES Pain Scale Revised. The FACES Pain Scale Revised (FPS-R) is useful for all older adults, including those with mild to moderate cognitive impairment. Some older adults will find this tool easy to use and may prefer it to the Numerical Rating Scale. This scale requires that patients have either verbal ability or the ability to point to the image on the scale that most closely represents their pain (International Association for the Study of Pain [ISAP], 2001).

Adapting the Unidimensional Pain Assessment Tool for the Severely Ill Patient A patient who is extremely ill or weak may be able to use unidimensional tools with the nurse's assistance. For example, the nurse can run a pencil along a VAS and have the patient nod or indicate in some way where the "point" of pain is on the scale. Sometimes, the patient may be able to point to the number on an NRS or to the location on the line of a VAS that best indicates the intensity of pain. As an alternative, the patient may be able to raise the number of fingers that indicate the level of pain, with no fingers raised being "no pain" and 5 or 10 fingers raised being the "worst pain imaginable."

Nurses frequently assume that extreme illness, weakness, or mild confusion prevents the patient from being able to self-report pain. This is not necessarily true. Self-report methods should be attempted in this patient group even though it may require patience and flexibility on the part of the nurse. If pain assessment is to be accurate using these methods, the nurse must give brief but clear directions to the patient and repeat these directions as needed during the assessment procedure.

Multidimensional Pain Assessment Multidimensional pain assessment tools provide the patient with a means to express the affective and evaluative aspects of the pain experience in addition to the sensory aspect. These tools work best for patients with more complex pain, such as pain of unknown origin or chronic pain. Examples of multidimensional tools include the McGill Pain Questionnaire (MPQ), the short-form MPQ (SF-MPQ), the Multidimensional Affect and Pain Survey (MAPS), and the Brief Pain Inventory. The most frequently used measurement of sensory and affective pain is the MPQ. This questionnaire measures four aspects of the pain experience: sensory, affective, evaluative, and miscellaneous. Each pain category is measured using a cluster of descriptive words. The patient's choice of words assists the clinician in determining the category from which the pain is originating and aids the clinician in choosing a therapeutic pain regimen that is individualized to the patient's needs. While easy to implement, it is rarely practical in the high-acuity patient. Both unidimensional and multidimensional tools have strengths and limitations associated with their use (Table 5–2).

The clinician should be aware that discrepancies may exist between the patient's self-reported level of pain and nurse-observed pain behaviors. For example, a patient may describe pain intensity as a 7 out of 10 while watching television or talking on the phone. This individual may be using coping skills that subjectively do not reflect high-pain scores. A patient's use of distraction and relaxation techniques can be misinterpreted as stoicism or exaggeration of self-reported pain levels.

Table 5–2 Advantages and Disadvantages of Pain Assessment Tools

UNIDIMENSIONAL TOOLS	
Advantages	**Disadvantages**
Provides baseline data	Measures only one dimension of the pain experience
Provides a means of comparing pre- and post-intervention pain intensity	Unable to measure degree of anxiety or stress accompanying the pain
Provides a standardized method for assessment of pain intensity	Requires relatively high cognitive level
Can be clearly documented and reported	Requires some means of communication
Adaptable for patients who cannot verbalize	
Easy to perform	
Short assessment time	
MULTIDIMENSIONAL TOOLS	
Advantages	**Disadvantages**
Provides baseline data	Valid only if patient understands vocabulary
Provides a standardized method for assessment of pain	Long length of completion time (McGill Pain Questionnaire)
Can be clearly documented and reported	Requires a high cognitive level
Assesses multiple aspects of the pain experience	
Provides data for choosing nonpharmacologic interventions	
Adaptable for patients who cannot verbalize	

Assessment of Pain in the Adult with Altered Communication Status

While the gold standard is patient self-report, the most common challenge for high-acuity nursing is pain assessment for the noncommunicative, sedated, or intubated patient. Patients who cannot communicate their pain—such as those who are ventilated and sedated, are immobilized, or have a cognitive status that precludes a report of pain—are at risk for undertreatment and rely on the nurse to advocate and intervene for pain control. Many high-acuity patients have altered communication abilities for a variety of reasons, such as altered levels of consciousness and extreme weakness. Figures 5–2 and 5–3 provide an example of an integrated pain assessment form developed by nurses for use with patients. The form includes a 10-point behavioral pain scale, which is used for vulnerable patients, such as those in critical care settings. Nurses may rate observed pain behaviors in any adult who is unable to self-report pain level by using the behavioral pain scale. Higher scores on this scale suggest greater levels of pain.

Despite a patient's inability to interpret the meaning of a painful event or communicate the level of pain being experienced, the physiologic stress response to pain still occurs, resulting in negative outcomes. With careful assessment of the high-acuity patient, the clinician can observe the environment and the individual's experience. If the situation or treatment is likely to inflict or exacerbate pain, and the patient can neither communicate the intensity nor exhibit pain behaviors, the clinician must assume that pain is present ("assume pain present" can be charted as **APP**) and then attempt an analgesic trial, carefully monitoring for side effects or subtle changes in

behaviors. The clinician should also encourage family members or caregivers who are familiar with the patient to provide input.

The American College of Critical Care Medicine/Society of Critical Care Medicine (ACCM/SCCM) 2013 clinical practice guidelines for the management of pain, agitation, and delirium in adult patients recommend the use of behavioral observation tools such as the Behavioral Pain Scale (BPS) or the Critical Care Pain Observation Tool (CPOT) (Davidson, Winkelman, Gélinas, & Dermenchyan, 2015). The CPOT is a valid and reliably tested tool when used in nonverbal high-acuity adults. It can be used to assess the presence of pain in unconscious or conscious patients who are either intubated or extubated. This scale measures four of five indicators of pain, including facial expression, body movements, muscle tension, ventilator compliance, or vocalization in extubated patients (Gélinas, Puntillo, Joffe, & Barr, 2013). It is important for the nurse to recognize that behavioral scales such as CPOT do not measure intensity. Higher numbers only indicate that pain is present. Caution should be used when choosing doses to alleviate pain and should never be determined by the number obtained through observation. In general, the nurse assumes pain is present based on a positive score and treats the pain while monitoring side effects until the score is zero.

Pain and Vital Sign Changes

During acute pain the nervous system responds and can cause variations in vital signs that may not be seen in nonpainful procedures. This is often observed in high-acuity patients during suctioning, turning, and other painful procedures. Arbour, Choinière, Topolovec-Vranic, Loiselle,

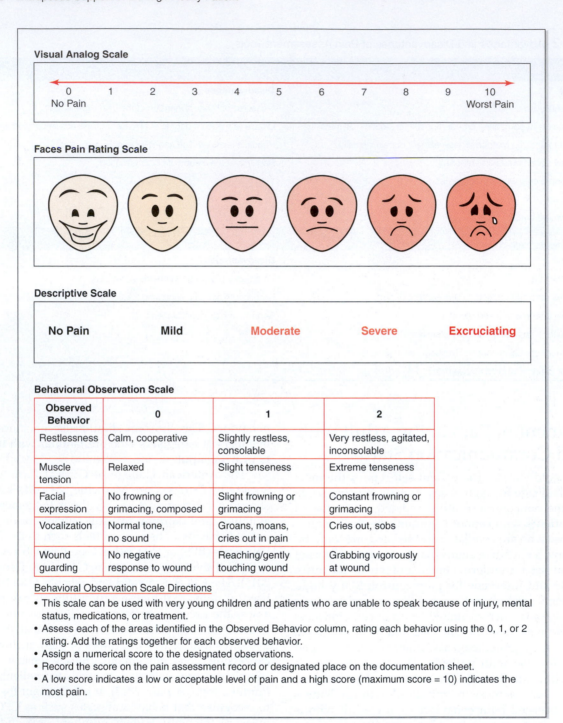

Visual Analog Scale

| 0 | 1 | 2 | 3 | 4 | 5 | 6 | 7 | 8 | 9 | 10 |
| No Pain | | | | | | | | | | Worst Pain |

Faces Pain Rating Scale

Descriptive Scale

| No Pain | Mild | Moderate | Severe | Excruciating |

Behavioral Observation Scale

Observed Behavior	0	1	2
Restlessness	Calm, cooperative	Slightly restless, consolable	Very restless, agitated, inconsolable
Muscle tension	Relaxed	Slight tenseness	Extreme tenseness
Facial expression	No frowning or grimacing, composed	Slight frowning or grimacing	Constant frowning or grimacing
Vocalization	Normal tone, no sound	Groans, moans, cries out in pain	Cries out, sobs
Wound guarding	No negative response to wound	Reaching/gently touching wound	Grabbing vigorously at wound

Behavioral Observation Scale Directions
- This scale can be used with very young children and patients who are unable to speak because of injury, mental status, medications, or treatment.
- Assess each of the areas identified in the Observed Behavior column, rating each behavior using the 0, 1, or 2 rating. Add the ratings together for each observed behavior.
- Assign a numerical score to the designated observations.
- Record the score on the pain assessment record or designated place on the documentation sheet.
- A low score indicates a low or acceptable level of pain and a high score (maximum score = 10) indicates the most pain.

Figure 5–2 Pain assessment tools (Part 1).

SOURCE: Based on "Pain assessment tools," developed by Pain Committee (2003). University Hospital, University of Kentucky.

and Gélinas (2014) concluded that while respiratory rate increase could be a potential indicator of pain in the nonverbal patient, vital signs are not specific for the detection of pain. The nervous system quickly returns to homeostasis despite pain. Absence of physiologic indicators (e.g., change in heart rate or blood pressure) does not preclude pain. Fear and anxiety along with physiologic conditions in the high-acuity patient can lead to variations in vital signs. Currently, there is no evidence that changes in vital signs

can predict pain. In addition, patients with persistent pain, for example, adapt to the stress response and do not demonstrate the same physiologic changes.

In summary, many techniques are available to nurses to assess the presence and dimensions of pain in high-acuity patients. Individualized care can be provided by considering the patient's specific needs for pain control. A hierarchy of pain assessment techniques is suggested in Table 5–3.

University of Kentucky Hospital
Chandler Medical Center
Lexington, Kentucky

PAIN ASSESSMENT/MANAGEMENT FLOW SHEET

Date _____ Use the following codes to document assessments of patients with c/o pain AND REASSESS these patients within a reasonable time frame following interventions.

Pain Rating Scales: 0/10   FACES   FLACC   Behavioral Other _____   Pain Management Goal: _____

Time	*Body Site (s)	*Description	*Pain Level before INTV	*Intervention(s)	*Pain Level after INTV	*Level of Arousal (S-4)	*Behavior Patterns	*SE from INTV	*Tx for SE	Comments: See Nsg Notes (Place check mark)	Nurse Initials
2400–0100											
0100–0200											
0200–0300											
0300–0400											
0400–0500											
0500–0600											
0600–0700											
0700–0800											
0800–0900											
0900–1000											
1000–1100											
1100–1200											
1200–1300											
1300–1400											
1400–1500											
1500–1600											
1600–1700											
1700–1800											
1800–1900											
1900–2000											
2000–2100											
2100–2200											
2200–2300											
2300–2400											

Codes

Body Sites

A = Abdomen	A = Arm (R or L)
C = Chest	L = Leg (R or L)
F = Face	T = Throat
H = Head	UB = Upper Back
J = Jaw	LB = Lower Back
N = Neck	Other: _____

Description

A = Ache	*Pediatrics:*
B = Burning	O = "Owie" or "boo = boo"
D = Dull	H = "Hurt"
P = Pressure	Other: _____
S = Sharp	
St = Stabbing	
T = Throbbing	

Level of Arousal

S = Sleeping, Easily Aroused
1 = Awake & Alert
2 = Occasionally Drowsy
3 = Freq. Drowsy, Drifts off to Sleep Easily
4 = Somnolent, Minimal or No Response to Stimuli

Interventions (INTV)

D = Distraction	*Pediatrics:*
GI = Guided Imagery	C = Cuddling or holding
H = Heat	Mu = Music
M = Massage	NP = Nonpharmacologic (i.e.,
Med = Medication (see MAR	bubbles, pinwheel, etc.)
of PCA sheet)	P = Play
R = Reposition	
Rel = Relaxation	
T = Teaching (i.e., PCA use)	

Behavior Patterns

A = Anxious	I = Inconsolable
G = Grimacing	U = Unnoticeable
P = Peaceful, Calm, Restful	APP = Assumed Pain Present
R = Restless, Thrashing	Other: _____

Side Effects (SE) / **Treatment of SE**

Side Effects (SE)	Treatment of SE
C = Confusion	A = Med Adjustment
I = Itching	C = In & Out Catheter
N = Nausea	F = Foley Catheter
R = Resp. Depression	Med = Medication
U = Urinary Retention	S = Safety Measures
V = Vomiting	Other: _____

Signature	Initials	Signature	Initials	Signature	Initials
Signature	Initials	Signature	Initials	Signature	Initials

8/02

Figure 5–3 Pain assessment and management flow sheet (Part 2).

SOURCE: Based on "Pain assessment & management flow sheet," developed by Pain Committee (2003). University Hospital, University of Kentucky.

Table 5–3 Hierarchy of Pain Assessment Techniques

Action	Considerations
Self-report	Consider scales such as the Verbal Numeric Scale or the Verbal Descriptor Scale, or the use of signals such as nodding, blinking, or hand signals for the ventilated patient.
Search for potential causes of pain	Pathologic conditions may create pain without triggering a behavioral or physiologic response.
Observation of patient behaviors	A valid approach, but behaviors are not indicative of pain intensity and may reflect other sources of distress.
If surrogate reporting	May not always be accurate and should be combined with other evidence when possible.
Attempt an analgesic trial	Provide a cautious analgesic trial. Pain behaviors may improve.

SOURCE: Data from Herr et al. (2011).

Section Three Review

1. The Numeric Rating Scale is most commonly used to measure what part of the pain experience?
   A. Affective
   B. Evaluative
   C. Intensity
   D. Coping

2. If a client is mildly confused, the nurse should initially try to assess pain using which method?
   A. Vital signs
   B. Self-report
   C. Facial expression
   D. Body posturing

3. What is a major weakness of multidimensional tools?
   A. The client must comprehend the vocabulary.
   B. They measure only pain intensity.
   C. The nurse performs the assessment.
   D. They are unable to measure degree of anxiety.

4. Which is a disadvantage of the Critical Care Pain Observation (CPOT) tool?
   A. Its validity has not been established.
   B. Its reliability has not been established.
   C. It cannot be used with nonverbal clients.
   D. It does not measure intensity.

Answers: 1. C, 2. B, 3. A, 4. D

Section Four: Management of Acute Pain

Effective pain management is facilitated by use of an organized, systematic approach. The World Health Organization (WHO) Analgesic Ladder provides an example of such an approach. The ladder suggests general pain management choices based on the level of pain (i.e., mild, mild-to-moderate, or moderate-to-severe). In addition, it provides a step-by-step approach to adjusting the pharmacologic choices if the patient's pain is persistent or increases. It is a model for treating acute pain and can be effectively applied in the high-acuity setting.

The high-acuity patient is particularly at risk for moderate to severe pain; thus, discussion will focus on management at this level of the ladder. The drugs of choice for acute pain management at this level are generally a combination of opioids and nonopioids. The addition of nonopioid and adjuvant therapies to further enhance the effects of opioid therapy reduces side effects by decreasing the amount of opioids needed to achieve analgesia. This is known as **pharmacologic multimodal analgesia**.

Pharmacologic Pain Management

The pharmacologic management of pain involves modulation of pain transmission at different levels of the nervous system. While opioids continue to be the mainstay of analgesic therapy, a combination of analgesics, each with a different mechanism, can improve pain control outcomes, although data reflecting improved outcomes in high-acuity patients are limited (Pandharipande & McGrane, 2015).

Multimodal Therapy Using multiple agents to interrupt the transmission of pain via different pathways is known as **multimodal analgesia**. The effectiveness of an intervention before the onset of intense pain and the continuation of the intervention throughout the duration of the pain by attacking or blocking the pain through various physiologic pathways have been well documented. While opioid therapy remains the cornerstone of acute pain management, a multimodal approach to pain management takes advantage of the additive or synergistic effects of different classes of analgesics and techniques. Multimodal regimens may include a combination of local anesthetics (e.g., epidurals, regional or peripheral nerve blocks, wound infiltration, intravenous lidocaine infusions), N-methyl-D-aspartate receptor antagonists

(NMDA antagonists) such as **ketamine** (provides analgesia by blocking specific receptors within the neurons), nonsteroidals, acetaminophen, anticonvulsants (gabapentinoids), and alpha2 agonists (e.g., clonidine [Catapres]) with or without opioids.

Opioid Analgesics Opium refers to a mixture of alkaloids from the poppy seed. **Opiates** are naturally occurring alkaloids such as morphine or codeine. The term **opioids** broadly describes all compounds that work at the opioid receptor sites. The term *narcotic* originally was used to describe medications for sleep, then was used to describe opioids, but now is largely used as a legal term for a broader category of stimulants and is associated with drugs that are likely to be abused.

The peripheral nervous system, the spinal cord, and the CNS have areas where modulation can occur due to the presence of opioid receptors. Most action occurs within the spinal cord at the dorsal horn, where sensory information from the peripheral nervous system triggers a response from the **endogenous** (internal to the body) system to modify the excitability of nerves and trigger changes within the CNS. By administering systemic (**exogenous**, external to the body) opioids, the analgesic system is activated. Exogenous opioids are involved in mood control, immune response, and other processes. Opioids function as neurotransmitters and play a role in hormonal secretion as well as cardiovascular control. Opioid receptors located on the presynaptic terminals on the A delta and C fibers will block the release of pain neurotransmitters from the nociceptor fibers, resulting in pain relief.

Therapeutic use of opioids begins with the selection of a specific opioid drug and route of administration. After the choice of drug and route are determined, decisions are made regarding the suitable initial dose, frequency of administration, optimal doses of nonopioid analgesics, and incidence and severity of side effects. The importance of careful adjustment of these medications for therapeutic effects cannot be overemphasized because dosing needs and analgesic responses vary greatly among individual patients. All clinicians need to have a complete understanding of equianalgesics between different opioids, as well as conversions to and from the oral and intravenous formulations.

Local anesthetics block nerve conduction near the site of infiltration by inhibiting sodium channels at the nerve endings. The nerve excitability is blocked. Both processes reduce pain and inflammation before the nociceptors are activated at the CNS.

Nonopioid Analgesics Effective pain management can be enhanced by a combination of opioid and nonopioid therapy. A better level of analgesia is often achieved in combination than when either is administered alone. Nonopioids include such drugs as acetaminophen, aspirin, and nonsteroidal anti-inflammatory drugs (NSAIDs).

Nonselective NSAIDs block cyclooxygenase (COX-1 and COX-2) enzymes by inhibiting the formation of prostaglandins, proteolytic enzymes, and bradykinin, thus decreasing the inflammatory process. The use of NSAIDS in high-acuity patients is uncommon because of specific contraindications in patients with renal dysfunction, gastrointestinal (GI) bleeding, platelet abnormalities, congestive heart failure, cirrhosis, asthma, or recent cardiac surgery (Pandharipande & McGrane, 2015). Careful use of NSAIDs in the high-acuity patient can be beneficial in select burn patients.

Acetaminophen is an effective analgesic and antipyretic agent and can decrease the total amount of opioids when treating moderate to severe pain. With the addition of the intravenous formulation now available in the United States, patients who cannot take oral medication can benefit from therapeutic dosing. Caution should be used in patients with mild hepatic or renal insufficiency, malnutrition, or dehydration. Acetaminophen is contraindicated in patients with chronic alcoholism or severe liver disease.

Additional Analgesics Additional analgesics include drugs that can assist in reducing certain types of pain. Their assistance may be indirect (by decreasing other symptoms associated with the underlying condition) or direct, as a coanalgesic. Traditionally, these drugs are generally used in addition to opioid and nonopioid analgesics for patients experiencing chronic pain. However, drugs such as NMDA antagonists (ketamine), alpha2 adrenergic agonists (dexmedetomidine), anticonvulsants (gabapentin and pregabalin), corticosteroids, and acetylcholine esterase inhibitors are widely used to treat postoperative pain and can reduce the need for high doses of opioids.

Neuropathic pain is present in some high-acuity patients. The clinician and the patient may become frustrated when the patient's pain either fails to respond to NSAIDs and opioid therapy or the patient can obtain only minimal relief. The patient may describe the pain as burning, electric, tingling, or shooting. Examples of neuropathic pain may be peripheral neuropathy, nerve injury, postherpetic neuralgia, trigeminal neuralgia, and phantom pain. Several specific examples of adjuvant drugs include corticosteroids, which are often used in treating cancer-related pain. Corticosteroids can shrink tumors that are impinging on nerves or decrease neurogenic inflammation. Tricyclic antidepressants (TCAs such as amitriptyline) and anticonvulsants have been used effectively for many years for the treatment of neuropathic pain. The exact mechanism of the TCAs is not completely understood, but it is generally believed that the inhibition of reuptake of serotonin and norepinephrine within the dorsal horn, along with alpha-adrenergic blockade, sodium channel effects, and perhaps N-methyl-D-aspartate (NMDA) receptor antagonism, plays a major role in altering the neurotransmitters. The anticonvulsants appear to stabilize the nerve membrane and depress the excitatory pathways in the CNS.

Low-dose systemic intravenous lidocaine and ketamine have become important adjuvants in the high-acuity patient who exhibits signs of hyperalgesia or neuropathic pain. Intravenous lidocaine suppresses inflammatory cells by inhibiting impulses from injured nerves. Ketamine is an NMDA blocker and is an effective adjuvant treatment that is opioid sparing with fewer adverse effects (Angst & Clark, 2010).

A well-thought-out pain management plan utilizes a multimodal approach targeting specific types or mechanisms of pain and may reduce opioid-related adverse effects by decreasing the amount of opioids needed as noted in a review of the literature related to the care of postsurgical patients (Golembiewski & Dasta, 2015).

Routes of Administration Many routes are available for administration of analgesia. The oral, subcutaneous, intramuscular, transdermal, and IV routes can be accessed by the nurse; however, most other routes require initial access by an anesthesiologist. Whenever local anesthetics are administered, it is important for the healthcare provider to monitor the patient for systemic anesthetic toxicity. Signs and symptoms of this complication include a 25% drop in baseline heart rate, tinnitus, slurred speech or thick tongue, and mental confusion. Table 5–4 provides a comparison of pharmacologic pain interventions.

Oral. The oral route is most commonly used for opioids. This route is also the most inexpensive and convenient. For the high-acuity patient, however, the oral route may not be available because of a nothing-by-mouth status or intubation. Although these patients are not able to take medications orally, they may have feeding tubes that act as an alternate medication route. When oral or enteral routes are used in the high-acuity patient, the clinician should monitor gastric function to ensure absorption. Patients may vomit medications before the analgesic has time to absorb. Patients with diarrhea or rapid gastric emptying or dumping syndrome may not absorb pills effectively.

Intravenous. The IV route can be used by the nurse or self-administered by the patient using IV patient-controlled analgesia (PCA). The most common method of PCA allows the patient to self-dose intravenously by pushing a button that is attached via a cord to an infusion device. The infusion device can be programmed for the patient to self-administer doses of opioid without becoming overly sedated. Other forms of PCA are administered through the subcutaneous and the epidural routes.

When IV access is not possible, the rectal or sublingual routes should be considered in preference to the traditional use of subcutaneous (subcu) and intramuscular (IM) routes because these two routes can cause tissue trauma and pain. In addition, the absorption of medications using subcu and IM routes is affected by individual patient factors such as heat, fever, and vasoconstriction that can either delay effectiveness or pose additional safety risks because peak effectiveness will be altered.

Intraspinal. Intraspinal opioids can be administered in a variety of ways:

- Single-dose epidural or intrathecal
- Intermittent scheduled-dose epidural or intrathecal
- Intermittent patient-controlled epidural anesthesia (PCEA) or intrathecal

- Continuous infusion of opioid alone or in combination with local anesthetic epidural or intrathecal
- Continuous infusion plus patient-controlled opioid alone or in combination with local anesthetic

Epidural. The goal of epidural analgesia is to instill analgesics into the epidural space to minimize discomfort and optimize the patient's recovery while minimizing side effects. The epidural route requires insertion of a small catheter into the area located just before the dura mater. The analgesia is then available to cross the dura mater into cerebral spinal fluid. An opioid, or a combination of opioid and local anesthetic, is delivered by injection or by using an infusion device.

The opioids diffuse across the dura mater and bind at opioid receptors. The local anesthetic selectively blocks sensory nerve fibers that make up the spinal nerve roots, acting as a neural blockade. The spinal nerve roots pass through the epidural space to the spinal cord, thus creating a convenient space to infuse drugs. Combinations of opioid and local anesthetic agents are used to modulate the transmission of pain through different pathways. This route requires low doses of analgesic, whether administered alone or in combination.

Side effects are minimized because lower concentrations are delivered directly to the site of action and little drug is available for systemic absorption. Opioids are more potent via the epidural than via IV because there is less protein binding (than in plasma); thus, more opioids are available at the receptors, resulting in less vascular uptake.

Neural blockade provides analgesia without the CNS effects of sedation, drowsiness, and respiratory depression that can occur when analgesics are given systemically (PO, IV, or IM). The benefits include longer-acting analgesia, avoidance of peaks and valleys in pain control, lower doses, and earlier ambulation by postoperative patients.

Intrathecal. The **intrathecal** route for analgesia requires the passage of a small needle or catheter directly into the cerebrospinal fluid (CSF) space. Opioid flows through the CSF and rapidly binds to opioid receptors in the spinal cord. Even smaller amounts of an intrathecally administered drug are required to achieve the same effects as epidural administration. The injection of preservative-free morphine into the CSF has been a postoperative technique since the late 1970s. Traditionally, nurse monitoring is recommended to ensure adequate ventilation and appropriate level of consciousness. Given that morphine is considered hydrophilic (not readily dissolvable in fat), it will remain available in high concentrations for 12 to 48 hours (Mugabure, 2013). This method places the spinal cord at some degree of risk, however, because of the potential for mechanical or chemical irritation or damage. Because there is no added protection from the dura mater to prevent bacterial flow, there is a higher risk of infection through a direct and continuous intrathecal infusion. Many methods are available to deliver intrathecal medications, including percutaneous catheters, implanted ports, and implanted pumps. Use of the epidural or intrathecal routes requires

Table 5–4 Pharmacologic Interventions

Type/Route of Analgesia	Advantages	Limitations
NONSTEROIDAL ANTI-INFLAMMATORY DRUGS (NSAIDS)		
Oral (alone)	Effective for mild to moderate pain.	Relatively contraindicated in patients with renal disease, risk of or actual coagulopathy, and risk of or active GI irritation or bleeding. May mask fever.
Oral (as an adjunct to opioid)	Potentiating effect results in opioid sparing.	Cautions as above.
Parenteral (ketorolac)	Effective for moderate to severe pain. Useful where opioids are contraindicated, especially to avoid respiratory depression and sedation. May advance to opioid.	Cautions as above.
OPIOIDS		
Oral (PO)	As effective as parenteral in appropriate doses. Route of choice. Noninvasive, inexpensive. Use as soon as oral medication tolerated.	Oral route may not be available for high-acuity patients. Slower onset of action.
Intramuscular	Avoid when other routes are available.	Injections are painful and absorption unreliable. May cause tissue trauma.
Subcutaneous	Less painful and preferable to IM, especially when slow infusion technique (1–3 mL/hr) is utilized. A butterfly needle can be placed for continuous infusions.	Bolus injections are painful and absorption unreliable.
Transdermal fentanyl patch	Useful when oral route is unavailable. Noninvasive.	Difficult to titrate due to delay of effective blood fentanyl concentrations. Contraindicated in opioid naïve patients.
Rectal	Does not require functional IV. May be appropriate in the patient unable to tolerate oral medications.	Absorption may be unpredictable, affected by defecation. May not be acceptable to all patients. Contraindicated in patients with painful anal conditions or those at risk for infection (neutropenia).
Intravenous (IV)	Parenteral route of choice after major surgery or when oral route is unavailable. Suitable for titrated bolus or continuous infusion.	Requires intravenous access. Significant risk of respiratory depression with inappropriate dosing; requires monitoring.
Patient-controlled analgesia (PCA)	Can be used with intravenous, subcutaneous, or epidural routes. Provides steady level of analgesia. Provides patient control. Avoids peaks and troughs.	Requires special locked infusion pumps and staff education. Requires monitoring, significant risk of respiratory depression with inappropriate dosing. Requires patient (only) to participate in the administration.
Epidural and intrathecal	Provides good analgesia. May be utilized for postoperative pain or for cancer pain in specific circumstances. May be used as a one-time injection (bolus) or as a continuous infusion.	Requires special infusion pumps and staff education. Requires daily follow-up by an experienced physician or pain team. Risk of respiratory depression higher with bolus dose than with continuous infusion; requires monitoring.
LOCAL ANESTHETICS	Available via multiple routes. Anti-inflammatory properties.	Require daily follow-up by experienced physician or pain team. Screen for allergies.
Epidural and intrathecal	Effective regional analgesia. Opioid sparing. Opioid and local anesthetic combination improves analgesia while reducing requirement. Continuous or patient controlled.	Requires careful monitoring, special pumps, and staff education. Follow-up by anesthesiologist or pain team. Risk of hypotension, weakness, and numbness. Increased risk for infection, hematoma.
Peripheral nerve block	Effective regional analgesia. Used postoperatively or for trauma pain. Opioid sparing. May be one-time injection or continuous infusion.	Requires careful monitoring, special pumps, and staff education.
Lidocaine IV	Potentiates opiates. Decreases peripheral and central sensitization.	Requires nursing monitoring. Contraindicated if patient has heart block.
Ketamine	Decreases risk for opioid-induced respiratory depression. Decreases withdrawal potential. Decreases hyperanalgesia.	Check with state board of nursing for RN restrictions. Hallucinations at high dosing.

SOURCE: Data partially from Dillon & Gibbs. (2016), Ducharme. (2016), and Weaver. (2016).

close communication between anesthesiology and nursing staff and careful monitoring of the patient. Generally, this route is contraindicated in high-acuity patients who are septic or anticoagulated.

Peripheral Nerve Block. A **peripheral nerve block (PNB)** is used to directly block pain transmission by bathing the nerve or surrounding area with local anesthetics. Peripheral nerve blocks are used for moderate to severe pain and can be administered either through a single injection or a continuous infusion. The peripheral nerve path that is transmitting the pain is located largely by ultrasound or occasionally by a nerve stimulator. The sites most frequently used for peripheral nerve blocks are the intercostal nerves medial to the insertion site of chest tubes, brachial plexus for rotator cuff repair, axillary for hand trauma or surgery, and lower extremities such as the femoral nerve prior to total knee arthroplasty. The duration of the analgesia depends on the half-life of the local anesthetic that has been injected. A low concentration of local anesthetics can also be infused continuously.

Pleural Infusion. The **pleural infusion** route primarily is used when multiple rib fractures are present. A small catheter is placed into the pleural space (between the visceral and parietal pleura) and a local anesthetic is injected or infused. Infusions can be administered via a continuous infusion pump or via an elastomeric pump (ON-Q pain relief system) that automatically and continuously delivers a regulated flow of local anesthetic to a patient's surgical site, fractured ribs, or in close proximity to nerves. By administering a local anesthetic via this route, multiple intercostal nerves can be blocked at one time without repeated needle sticks to the skin.

IV Lidocaine (Local Anesthetic) Bolus or Infusion Local anesthetics are an important part of multimodal therapy because they effectively block pain at the site of tissue damage by interrupting the nociceptive impulses that transmit the pain signals and act as an anti-inflammatory agent. The perioperative use of IV lidocaine in low concentrations decreased postoperative pain and minimized the use of opioids in adults undergoing complex spinal surgery (Farag et al., 2013). Intravenous lidocaine should be avoided in patients with second- or third-degree heart block, severe sinoatrial block (without a pacemaker), liver or kidney disease, or a history of adverse reaction to local anesthetics. During intravenous lidocaine administration, the high-acuity nurse should monitor the patient closely for rare but serious signs and symptoms of lidocaine toxicity. The signs and symptoms of toxicity follow a predictable progression from mild symptoms, such as numbness of the tongue, lightheadedness, and/or visual disturbances, progressing to moderate to severe, such as muscle twitching, unconsciousness, and seizures, followed by coma, respiratory arrest, and vascular depression. Because lidocaine has such a short half-life and is lipophilic, turning off the infusion with the onset of mild symptoms decreases the systemic levels within 30 to 60 minutes. Severe symptoms require that the high-acuity nurse immediately respond by stopping the infusion, initiating

CPR as necessary, administering oxygen, and maintaining an open airway while the emergency response team is activated. Severe toxicity can be completely reversed with the administration of lipid emulsion therapy at an infusion of 1.5 mL/kg over 1 minute. A continuous infusion of lipids of 0.25 mL/kg/min and repeated boluses should be administered for persistent cardiovascular collapse.

IV Ketamine Administration As noted, ketamine provides analgesia by blocking specific receptors within the neurons. These receptors are known as N-methyl-D-aspartate (NMDA) receptors. By blocking NMDA receptors, glutamate is released and binds to very specific opioid receptors (sigma receptors). Ketamine is a powerful dissociative anesthetic that produces a cataleptic-like state. Its primary action occurs on the cortex and limbic system in the brain. When low subanesthetic doses are used, analgesia is produced by changing or modulating central sensitization and opioid tolerance.

Dexmedetomidine **Dexmedetomidine** is a sedative agent typically used to provide moderate sedation in the mechanically ventilated patient, especially when performing a procedure. However, as a selective alpha2 agonist it has analgesic properties. Its potency is increased when given with opioids.

Propofol **Propofol**, primarily used as an anesthetic, is also used to decrease level of consciousness and to produce amnesia during procedures. Intravenous injection induces hypnosis, with minimal excitation, and works within 40 seconds from injection. It is thought to produce sedation and anesthesia by inhibiting the neurotransmitter GABA.

Nonpharmacologic Interventions

The National Institutes of Health (NIH) National Center for Complementary and Alternative Medicine defines complementary therapies or CAM as "a large and diverse group of interventions, practices, and disciplines that are based on physical procedures or techniques administered or taught to others by a trained practitioner" (NIH, 2015, para. 1). In general, these therapies are used to improve and maintain health through the mind and body connection and to treat symptoms of illness. Evidence suggests that meditation can enhance quality of life, reduce stress, and improve mental health. Mindfulness meditation and other meditation practices can engage neurobiological mechanisms involved in cognition and emotions with positive effects (NIH, 2015).

Complementary therapies are often used concurrently with medications to manage pain. The role of the clinician is to assist the patient in identifying the safety and effectiveness of therapies or interventions. When appropriate, the clinician identifies the risks and potential benefits of complementary therapies. All clinicians involved in the patient's care have a role in providing the necessary support for utilization of these therapies as outlined in the care plan. Guidelines for choice of nonpharmacologic interventions include pain problem identification, effectiveness for a specific patient, and the skill of the clinician. Table 5–5 provides some simple guidelines for promoting relaxation and possibly reducing pain levels in high-acuity patients.

Table 5–5 Simple Guidelines Promoting Relaxation in High-Acuity Patients

Technique	Description
Guided imagery	Ask the patient to imagine a safe and peaceful scene that is restful and happy. Instruct the patient to imagine the sounds and smells or the sensations, such as warmth or coolness. Initially the patient may want to describe the scene. If the patient is unable to communicate, you may want to guide him or her with suggestions. Allow your voice to become rhythmic as you guide the patient through a special image. Watch the patient's eyelids for fluttering as this may be an indication that the patient is imagining the scene.
Focused breathing	Instruct the patient to breathe normally. Do not require him or her to take deep breaths. Coach the patient to breathe in through the nose and out the mouth. Repeat "INHALE SLOWLY–EXHALE SLOWLY," prolonging the exhale. When the patient begins to maintain the rhythm, instruct the patient to think about the air as it fills the nose, sensing the air as it moves through the throat and down into the lungs. Picture the lungs opening to receive the fresh air. Instruct the patient to think only of the air, exhaling all other thoughts away with each breath. Ask the patient to close the eyes and visualize the air softly moving throughout the body. As the air passes through the body, it caresses and calms, flowing and ebbing. Allow the patient to continue practicing the breathing for several minutes.
Progressive muscle tension/ relaxation	Instruct the patient to slowly tense and then relax each muscle group. Help the patient to focus on the difference between muscle tension and relaxation, encouraging more awareness of physical sensations. Instruct the patient to start by tensing and relaxing the muscles in the toes and progressively working up to the neck and head. Have the patient tense muscles for at least 5 seconds and then relax for 30 seconds, and repeat.
General tips	Unless your patient requests specific cognitive therapies, normalize nonpharmacologic therapies. Some patients may have preconceived ideas about therapies, such as hypnosis and relaxation therapies. Always speak in a clear, slow, calm, and concise voice. If the person has difficulty hearing, get close and speak loudly and clearly, but do not yell. Provide a quiet environment using soft music or rhythmic background sounds. Use these techniques for short periods and return frequently as the person requires practice.

In general, especially with acute pain, complementary interventions are useful in combination with analgesia and do not take the place of analgesics. Complementary therapies can be initiated when pain is under reasonable control. Assessment of the patient's past experience with complementary therapies is beneficial, as patients may have experience with therapies that are compatible with their coping style and have been helpful in the past. The provision of adequate support materials (written or audio) will increase the benefit of such interventions. A patient who is fatigued, frightened, or in considerable pain will not be able to concentrate well enough to follow instructions or to perform time-consuming or complicated interventions.

Emerging Evidence

- Mindfulness meditation has long been shown to reliably reduce pain or pain awareness. It is believed that meditation works by engaging mechanisms supporting cognitive control. It has previously been postulated that this stimulates our own (endogenous) opioid activation system. A new study in healthy human volunteers suggests that mindfulness meditation decreases pain independently from the endogenous opioid. This finding supports the use of nonpharmacological therapies for the treatment of chronic or persistent pain (*Zeidan et al., 2016*).
- Researchers examined the relationship between anxiety and pain in a sample of 123 ICU patients who were not delirious or comatose.

Psychiatrists used the Hamilton Anxiety Rating Scale and the Faces Anxiety Scale to measure anxiety levels and the Numeric Rating Scale for Pain instrument to measure pain. The use of opioids and anxiolytics was also examined. Significant positive correlations were noted for anxiety and pain ratings on a daily basis. Levels of anxiety and pain positively impacted the use of anxiolytics but not opioids in this sample of patients. The treatment of anxiety along with pain should be considered for critically ill patients (*Oh et al., 2015*).

Section Four Review

1. The World Health Organization (WHO) Analgesic Ladder provides the clinician with what information?
   A. General pain management choices based on level of pain
   B. Nonpharmacologic interventions based on level of pain
   C. Specific pain management choices based on severity of pain
   D. Pharmacologic and nonpharmacologic pain-management choices

2. Which statement regarding nonopioid therapy is correct?
   A. Nonopioids have more severe side effects than opioids.
   B. Nonopioids are harder to access than opioids.
   C. Nonopioids can manage pain as effectively as opioids.
   D. Combining opioids and nonopioids enhances analgesia effectiveness.

3. What is the most common route used for PCA?
   A. Intramuscular
   B. Intravenous
   C. Subcutaneous
   D. Epidural

4. The guidelines for choosing appropriate nonpharmacologic interventions include which of the following? (Select all that apply.)
   A. Skill of clinician
   B. Effectiveness for client
   C. Pain problem identification
   D. Type of opioid being used
   E. Type of nonopioid being used

Answers: 1. A, 2. D, 3. B, 4. (A, B, C)

Section Five: Issues in Inadequate Treatment of Acute Pain

The American College of Critical Care Medicine reports that patients routinely experience pain, both at rest and with routine care, and that procedural pain is common among adults in critical care settings (Barr et al., 2013). The undertreatment of pain is multifactorial and involves complex social and system issues including inadequate attention to education regarding pain management in pharmacy, medicine, and nursing professional programs. The challenge for the high-acuity nurse is distinguishing the social and economic effects of misuse and abuse of opioids within the community from a pain management plan in the high-acuity setting including strong opioids. This section provides a brief overview of some of the major pain-related misconceptions that often lead to undertreatment. Knowing the terminology provides some distinctions between pain behaviors and the disease of addiction.

Definitions

It is important to differentiate among *tolerance*, *dependence*, and *addiction*, terms that are misused and have potentially negative connotations. These are the definitions:

- **Tolerance**. A decrease in effectiveness or diminishing side effects for the same dose that had previously been effective or caused the side effects.

- **Physical dependence**. When a drug is abruptly reduced or stopped, or an antagonist is given, symptoms of withdrawal occur. Generally, the person will experience increased pain, nausea, malaise, chills, sweating, and confusion (American Society of Addiction Medicine [ASAM], 2001).

- **Addiction**. A chronic neurologic and biologic disease. It is characterized by behaviors that include one or more of the following: impaired control of drug use, compulsive use despite harm to self or others, craving, and use of drug for purposes other than pain relief.

- **Opioid pseudoaddiction**. A term applied to patients who develop behaviors that mimic those associated with addiction. The individual may be labeled as drug craving or drug seeking. Pseudoaddiction, however, results from inadequate pain management, not

psychological dependence. A variety of responses are noted in patients who experience unrelieved pain, from acceptable drug seeking to pathologic behaviors. Unfortunately, it is often extremely difficult for nurses and physicians to discriminate between these two types of behaviors, particularly in situations in which patient's contact with the physician or nurse is limited, such as in the emergency department. Behaviors that suggest undertreatment of pain but are frequently misread as drug seeking rather than pain relief seeking include escalating demands for different or more pain medications, clock watching, preoccupation with obtaining pain medications, and anger. Pseudoaddiction results in a patient's distrust and suspicion of staff and avoidance of the patient by staff. Pseudoaddiction is distinguishable from actual addiction by resolution of aberrant behaviors when pain is relieved.

Reasons for Opioid Undertreatment of Pain

The practice of undertreating pain with minimal drug use is known as **oligoanalgesia**. Physicians underprescribe opioids by two methods: prescribing subtherapeutic doses and prescribing time intervals for drug doses that are longer than the pharmacologic duration of action. Nurses undertreat pain by administering less than the prescribed dose for the patient and administering opioids at longer intervals than prescribed. Patients often contribute to their own undertreatment of pain by not requesting as needed (prn) pain medications, taking medication at longer-than-ordered intervals, taking less than the amount prescribed, or refusing to take the drug at all (Pasero, Quinn, Portenoy, McCaffery, & Rizos, 2011).

Inadequate treatment of pain is a complex problem based on misconceptions widely held by physicians, nurses, and patients. There are four common misconceptions regarding opioid use that contribute to inadequate treatment: fear of addiction, physical dependence, tolerance, and respiratory depression.

Fear of Addiction (Psychological Dependence) Fear of addiction is probably the major cause of undertreatment of pain. The term **opiophobia** has been used to describe the irrational fear of prescribing (or consuming) adequate amounts of opiates for therapeutic results. In fact, very few hospitalized patients who receive opioids become addicted; as the pain subsides, so does the use of the opioids. The term *addiction* should be used with extreme caution. The indiscriminate labeling of a person who uses drugs as being an addict carries a strong social stigma that may negatively label an individual.

Fear of Physical Dependence   Some of the fear associated with physical dependence is generated from the belief that opioid withdrawal is life threatening, the symptoms associated with physical dependence are difficult to control, and the presence of symptoms of physical dependence prevent decreases in opioid doses as the pain decreases. In addition, many people believe that addiction is the natural progression of physical dependence. It is true that any patient who receives repeated doses of opioids is at risk for some degree of withdrawal symptoms if the opioid is suddenly stopped. These symptoms, however, can be effectively managed by gradual reduction in opioid dosage as the patient's pain subsides.

Fear of Tolerance   Fear of tolerance is usually seen in patients with long-term pain associated with either a disease process or painful treatments (e.g., patients with burns, cancer, or life-threatening illnesses). Patients, physicians, and nurses have expressed fear that opioids lose their effectiveness over time and may not work when really needed. A part of this fear is the belief in an imaginary dose ceiling, beyond which the drugs cannot be taken. In fact, this feared dose ceiling does not seem to exist. As tolerance to an opioid develops, so does the patient's tolerance to the side effects of sedation and respiratory depression. Tolerance is treated by decreasing the dose interval or increasing the dose. Nursing management should focus on patient education about the concept of tolerance and on monitoring for the therapeutic and nontherapeutic effects of the adjusted dosage.

Fear of Respiratory Depression   Physicians and nurses are particularly sensitive to the fear of respiratory depression. All opioids have the capability of causing respiratory depression, yet it need not be a life-threatening problem and should not prevent therapeutic opioid use. Nursing assessment should focus on close observation of the patient's response to opioids. **Sedation**, a calm, relaxed state due to the administration of a sedating drug, almost always develops before respiratory depression; therefore, the nurse should observe and document whether the patient becomes oversedated following the administration of opioids. Respiratory depression is dose related, and low doses are generally considered safe in the absence of obstructive sleep apnea. Monitoring for oversedation is the only way to determine what dose of an opioid will cause respiratory depression in any given patient. It is important to watch the individual's response, especially to the first dose.

Use of a standard assessment for opioid oversedation is considered best practice. In the high-acuity patient, the most commonly used scales to assess and document sedation are the Pasero Opioid-Induced Sedation Scale (POSS), the Richmond Agitation and Sedation Scale (RASS), and the Aldret (a scale commonly used to assess readiness for discharge from the postoperative care unit). The POSS is a simple scale comprised of five descriptive criteria, including S (sleep, easy to arouse), 1 (awake and alert), 2 (slightly drowsy, easily aroused), 3 (frequently drowsy, arousable, drifts off to sleep during conversation), and 4 (somnolent, minimal or no response to verbal and physical stimulation). Criteria 3 and 4 are considered an unacceptable level of opioid sedation (Nisbet & Mooney-Cotter, 2009). Nurses who use the POSS in the postanesthesia care unit have reported an increased confidence in administering opioids, knowing that they can administer them safely (Kobelt, Burke, & Renker, 2014).

Nursing Approach in Acute Pain Management

The way in which an analgesic is administered is probably more important than which drug is administered. In the acute care setting, the nurse maintains significant control over how analgesics are administered. Nursing activities that have an impact on therapeutic pain management include the following:

- Selecting an appropriate opioid or nonopioid from the analgesics ordered
- Evaluating when to administer the analgesic
- Evaluating how much analgesic to administer
- Obtaining a change in prescription when required

Effective pain management requires objective assessment skills and specific knowledge of opioids and nonopioids. In addition, the nurse must individualize the care plan to best meet the patient's individual comfort needs.

There are two major approaches to effective pain management: preventive and titration.

Preventive Approach   Using the preventive approach, analgesics are administered before the patient complains of pain. For example, when pain is occurring consistently over a 24-hour period, administering analgesics on a regular around-the-clock (ATC) schedule is more effective than administering them prn. This method helps to maintain a consistent therapeutic level of analgesic in the bloodstream and diminishes the likelihood of undertreatment of pain. Administering pain medication on a prn basis can cause prolonged delays in treating the patient's pain. If prn analgesia is to be used, it is important for the clinician to know the half-life and effectiveness of the medication being administered in order to predict when the patient is likely to need another dose. Maintaining awareness of pain by offering pain medication on a routine basis is more effective for pain control than requiring the patient to ask for medication prn. The patient may wait for the pain to become severe before requesting analgesia, or the clinician may be delayed in getting the drug to the patient. Either situation makes adequate pain relief more difficult to obtain.

At times prn administration is an acceptable option— for example, changing to prn late in the postoperative course to help decrease side effects, or when the pain is incidental, intermittent, or unpredictable. In addition, prn analgesics may be used as supplemental doses to regularly scheduled analgesics, primarily when a certain known activity causes pain (e.g., ambulation, sitting up in a chair, coughing, and deep breathing).

It is recommended that the nurse, as a patient advocate, be alert to the patient's comfort status and be proactive in consulting with the physician regarding changing the prn order to ATC if a more effective analgesia schedule is required. The nurse also has an important role in educating the patient and family regarding effective analgesia scheduling.

Titration Approach The titration approach calls for adjusting and individualizing therapy based on the effects the drug is having on the patient rather than the milligrams being administered. The goal is to gain the desired level of pain relief with minimum side effects. When using this approach, the clinician should consider the following:

- **Dose.** Analgesic potency helps provide a rational basis for choosing the appropriate starting dose.
- **Interval between doses.** Assess the patient regarding the amount of time it takes for the pain to increase. For example, if the nurse is administering an analgesic every 4 hours and the patient notices that the pain increases quickly after 3 hours, the interval should be changed to 3 hours.
- **Route of administration.** Use a conversion chart for equal analgesic dosing when switching from one route to another (see Table 5–6). In general, the oral dose is the preferred route unless oral administration is no longer possible, making it necessary to switch to the IV route. The most common reason for switching from IV to oral is that the pain is subsiding.

Equianalgesic conversion should be done without loss of pain control.

- **Choice of drug.** In general, effective analgesia with opioids is dose related and rarely requires a switch to another opioid. Unrelieved pain is not considered a reason for switching from one opioid to another. The most common reason for switching from one class of opioids to another is for the management of side effects. When switching from one opioid to another, it is important to monitor the patient for a heightened risk of incomplete tolerance. The patient who is already tolerant to the original opioid may not be tolerant to the new opioid. In such cases, it is recommended to reduce the starting doses by 25% to 50%. Opioids are classified as full (pure) opioid agonists, partial agonists, or mixed agonist–antagonists. Full agonists are more potent than partial agonists. Agonist–antagonists activate one type of opioid receptor and at the same time block another type. Withdrawal-like symptoms can occur when switching a patient from a pure agonist to an agonist–antagonist.

Regardless of the approach chosen to treat pain, undertreatment can still occur. Improved education for all healthcare professionals about pain and its treatment is a crucial first step in reversing this problem. In addition, when there is perceived undertreatment of pain, the high-acuity nurse must act as the patient's advocate through open communication with interprofessional team members.

Table 5–6 Equianalgesic Doses of Selected Opioids

This chart only reflects short-acting or instant-release formulation. All conversions are approximate.

Drug	Route	Equianalgesic Dose	Onset (Minutes)	Peak (Minutes)	Duration (Hours)
Morphine	IV	10 mg	2–5	10–20	2–4
	PO	30 mg	15–30	30–60	3–6
Hydromorphone	IV	1.5 mg	2–5	10–20	4–5
	PO	7.5 mg	15–30	30–60	
Fentanyl	IV	100 mcg	1–2	10–15	0.5–1
Oxycodone	PO	20 mg	10–15	30–60	4–5
Hydrocodone	PO	10 mg	30–60	30–60	3–6
Oxymorphone	PO	10 mg	30–60	30–60	3–4

SOURCE: Based on information obtained from Wilson et al. (2014).

Section Five Review

1. A common physiologic consequence of chronic opioid use that results in a person's requiring an increasing dose of opioids to maintain the same level of analgesia defines which term?
   A. Pseudoaddiction
   B. Tolerance
   C. Psychological dependence
   D. Physical dependence

2. Which statement is correct regarding opioid use and respiratory depression?
   A. Respiratory depression precedes the onset of sedation.
   B. Respiratory depression worsens as tolerance develops.
   C. Sedation occurs before respiratory depression.
   D. Respiratory depression is a common problem in hospitalized clients.

3. The use of prn analgesics is appropriate in which situations? (Select all that apply.)
   A. When pain is intermittent
   B. When pain is consistent
   C. When pain is unpredictable
   D. When used as a supplement to scheduled doses
   E. When the client fears addiction

4. When the titration approach to pain management is used, the emphasis is on what?
   A. The client's analgesic response
   B. Total milligrams per day
   C. Physical dependence
   D. Psychological dependence

Answers: 1. B, 2. C, 3. (A, C, D), 4. A

Section Six: Monitoring for Opioid-induced Respiratory Depression

Respiratory depression is a feared but essentially preventable complication of opioid analgesia. The relationship between an opioid analgesic dose and the effects on analgesia and respiratory depression varies based upon genetics, gender, age, comorbidities, concurrent sedating medications, and route of administration. Pharmacologic interventions using an opioid antagonist such as naloxone (Narcan) reverse opioid effects; however, rapid reversal is not without risks. Therefore, it is to the patient's advantage for the nurse to anticipate and prevent respiratory depression, thereby best assuring that rapid opioid reversal is not necessary.

Assessment

A variety of factors (variables) increase the likelihood of respiratory depression in patients receiving opioids. These factors can be divided into patient and iatrogenic variables (see Box 5–2).

Clinically significant respiratory depression is defined by more than respiratory rate. It encompasses rate and quality of respirations. Respirations should be assessed for 60 seconds and compared to the patient's baseline, allowing time for the nurse to evaluate trends in ventilation. The duration of the assessment provides an opportunity to evaluate quality of respirations, which includes depth,

regularity, and snoring that may be associated with airway obstruction. Assessment during sleep is best accomplished before waking or stimulating the patient because arousal stimulates respiration and prevents an accurate evaluation of the patient's respiratory status during sleep. It should be noted again that the night shift is a more frequent time for unanticipated respiratory depression.

Sedation Assessment Sedation occurs prior to opioid-induced respiratory depression. Opioid analgesia depresses both respiratory effort and rate, relaxes pharyngeal tone, and depresses the response to hypoxia and hypercarbia. Sedative effects of opioids generally precede respiratory depression. The use of a valid and reliable tool in sedation assessment is key to monitoring sedation. Two tools that have been tested in the arena of opioid analgesia are the POSS (Box 5–3) and the RASS, both of which are valid and reliable. The advantage of the POSS is that it includes recommended nursing actions for each level of sedation, providing direction for intervention for oversedation.

Use of Technology in Assessment Technological monitoring adds complexity and time to the nursing assessment; however, this is offset by early recognition of ventilatory changes. Continuous monitoring of oxygen saturation by pulse oximetry (SpO_2) and end tidal carbon dioxide ($EtCO_2$) levels allows trending of critical parameters for earlier recognition of impending respiratory depression.

Pulse Oximetry. Pulse oximetry measures oxygen saturation in arterial blood and pulse rate. Continuous monitoring of oxygen saturation has been recommended when

---

BOX 5–2 Patient- and Therapy-related Variables for Opioid-induced Respiratory Depression

Patient Variables

Age

Pulmonary disease or compromise

History of obstructive sleep apnea (OSA; history of snoring or witnessed apnea during sleep)

Body mass index (BMI) greater than 30 kg/m²

Neck circumference greater than 17.5 inches

Impaired renal or hepatic function

Neurologic disorder resulting in muscle weakness

Iatrogenic (Therapy) Variables

Level of Risk:
- Lowest Risk: Continuous epidural infusion
- Moderate to High Risk: Basal or continuous intravenous infusion
- Highest Risk: First 24 hours postoperatively

Hospital Environment Variables

- Night shift
- Patients admitted to units where nurses are unfamiliar with their care
- Poor environment of care, such as poor nursing–management or nursing–physician communication
- Poor staffing and less education of nursing staff providing care

SOURCE: Data from Needleman et al. (2011); Ramachandran et al. (2011).

BOX 5–3 Pasero Opioid-induced Sedation Scale (POSS)

S = Sleep, easy to arouse
   Acceptable: No action necessary; supplemental opioid may be given if needed.

1 = Awake and alert
   Acceptable: No action necessary; supplemental opioid may be given if needed.

2 = Slightly drowsy, easily aroused
   Acceptable: No action necessary; supplemental opioid may be given if needed.

3 = Frequently drowsy, arousable, drifts off to sleep during conversation
   Unacceptable: Decrease opioid dose by 25% to 50%. Administer acetaminophen or an NSAID, if not contraindicated, to control pain; monitor sedation and respiratory status closely until sedation level is less than 3.

4 = Somnolent, minimal or no response to physical stimulation
   Unacceptable: Stop opioid. Notify anesthesia provider; very slowly administer dilute IV naloxone (0.4 mg naloxone in 10 mL saline; 0.5 mL over 2-minute period); administer acetaminophen or an NSAID, if not contraindicated, to control pain; monitor sedation and respiratory status closely until sedation level is less than 3.

SOURCE: Pasero Opioid-Induced Sedation Scale (POSS) by Chris Pasero from Pain Assessment in the Patient Unable to Self-Report: Position Statement with Clinical Practice Recommendations (Herr et al., 2011). Reproduced by permission of Chris Pasero.

---

initiating opioid analgesia for patients at high risk for opioid-induced respiratory depression in order to facilitate the identification of trends. One study found that pulse oximetry monitoring, along with nursing notification of violation of alarm limits via wireless pager, led to a decrease in intensive care transfers and decreased rescue events among hospitalized patients (Taenzer, Pyke, McGrath, & Blike, 2010).

Capnography. Opioids suppress ventilation; therefore, monitoring of $EtCO_2$, respiratory rate, and oxygenation is appropriate. Normal $EtCO_2$ levels are 35–45 mmHg. Decreased respiratory rate (hypoventilation) increases $EtCO_2$ levels, and patients with pulmonary disease may have elevations in baseline $EtCO_2$ levels due to chronic ventilation problems. Assessment and documentation of the patient's baseline $EtCO_2$ as a comparison to current levels allows for trending of ventilatory status. The nurse should report an upward trend of $EtCO_2$ levels from normal or from the patient's baseline.

In summary, pulse oximetry only measures oxygenation, and $EtCO_2$ only measures ventilation; therefore, to adequately reflect patient status, monitoring of both is necessary. The combination of technological monitoring, careful monitoring of respiratory rate and quality, and monitoring of the patient's sedation level with a valid and reliable tool provides a more comprehensive overview of the patient status.

Nursing Interventions

Assessment of the patient's risk factors (individual and iatrogenic) must be documented in a manner that allows the information to be accessible across the continuum of care to all providers. The plan of care for patients at a higher risk for respiratory depression should include a greater frequency and intensity of monitoring (e.g., the use of continuous technological monitoring during opioid analgesia). Continuation of a higher level of monitoring should be based upon the patient's response to opioid therapy as evidenced by level of sedation, respiratory rate and quality, oxygenation saturation, and $EtCO_2$ levels. The patient's risk and the plan of care should be communicated at care transitions during handoff communication.

Once oversedation and a downward trend in respiratory rate and quality have been identified, monitoring frequency and intensity must be increased. Rapid opioid dose reductions may be considered when pain levels allow. Opioid-sparing therapies, such as the use of nonsedating analgesics (e.g., NSAIDs or acetaminophen) may decrease this downward trend. Working collaboratively with the prescribing healthcare provider to consider the omission of or dosage decrease of other sedating agents may also be effective in reducing the risk of advancing sedation and respiratory depression. For example, a nonsedating antiemetic such as ondansetron (Zofran) can replace a sedating agent such as promethazine (Phenergan). Stimulation of the patient may be adequate to prevent hypoventilation until the analgesic effect decreases. This approach requires individual nursing attention or transfer to a higher level of care.

Opioid Reversal Agent Naloxone (Narcan) may be required if the patient develops severe respiratory depression (respiratory rate below eight breaths per minute or increasing sedation with minimal patient response to physical stimulation, an oxygen saturation below 90%, and/or ongoing upward trend of $EtCO_2$). The half-life of naloxone is 30–81 minutes, which can result in an extended time during which the patient may be in extreme pain. Use of naloxone can also result in opioid withdrawal symptoms and other potentially major complications (see Box 5–4).

The naloxone dose should be administered slowly to avoid the sudden onset of pain or opioid withdrawal, in order to avoid precipitation of a sympathetic crisis. The exact PCA opioid reversal protocol will be specified by the prescribing healthcare provider or agency policy. Increased frequency and intensity of monitoring should continue until the analgesic dose has been metabolized because naloxone has a relatively short duration of action, allowing symptoms to return.

BOX 5–4 Potential Negative Effects of Rapid Reversal of Opioids

- Rapid onset of opioid withdrawal symptoms
- Severe pain
- Sympathetic nervous system crisis (tachycardia, tachypnea, hypertension)
- Myocardial ischemia, myocardial infarction, pulmonary edema
- Reduced effectiveness of opioid therapy if resumed following reversal

Additional information on naloxone is provided in the feature "Related Pharmacotherapy: Opiate Reversal Agent." Note that pain experts recommend a dilute solution of naloxone to avoid the creation of complications related to unrelieved pain and to prevent creation of a stress response. One ampoule of naloxone, 0.4 mg, can be diluted in 10 mL of saline and can be administered at 0.5 mL by IV push every 2 to 3 minutes until the patient is responsive. Titration of naloxone is discontinued as soon as the patient becomes responsive and respirations become normal.

Sedatives and analgesics in large doses are frequently administered in the ICU and contribute to delirium, which is subsequently associated with a longer hospital stay and decreased quality of life after discharge from the ICU. Delirium is also associated with increased mortality. Skrobik et al. (2010) measured outcomes after implementing a protocol to manage analgesia, sedation, and delirium for 604 patients. The education protocol included nonpharmacologic management of symptoms and individualized titration of sedation, analgesia, and delirium therapies. The use of coanalgesics such as acetaminophen and NSAIDs was encouraged. The protocol was associated with better outcomes in terms of superior analgesia, lower mean doses of opioids, shorter duration of mechanical ventilation, and shorter ICU and hospital length of stay. Decreasing the mean doses of opioids and sedative use was accomplished by individualizing the care of each patient.

Related Pharmacotherapy
Opiate Reversal Agent*

Opioid Antagonist

Naloxone hydrochloride (Narcan)

Actions and Uses

Short-acting narcotic antagonist. Used for rapid reversal of narcotic overdose. Rapidly reverses sedation, respiratory depression, and hypotension associated with overdose. Naloxone replaces the opioid at the Mu receptor sites; therefore, once reversal occurs, the opioid analgesic effects will rapidly cease.

Dosages (Adults)

Bolus administration:

Opiate overdose: 0.4–2 mg IV and repeat every 2–3 min up to 10 mg if needed; administer over 10–15 seconds minimally

Postoperative opiate depression: 0.1–0.2 mg IV and repeat every 2–3 min up to 3 doses if needed; administer over 10–15 seconds minimally

IV infusion administration:

Dilution required (2 mg in 500 mL NS or D_5W) to make concentration of 4 mcg/mL

Major Side Effects and Adverse Effects

- Rapid loss of analgesia
- Rapid opiate withdrawal (if dependence exists)
- Nausea and vomiting
- Hyperventilation
- Tremors

Nursing Implications

- Cautious use when used with suspected or known narcotic dependence
- For administering undiluted bolus—minimum delivery rate = over 10–15 seconds
- Monitor closely for manifestations of opioid withdrawal

*Nurses who work with patients receiving PCA therapy need to be knowledgeable about the agency's opioid reversal protocol.

SOURCE: Data from Wilson et al. (2014).

Section Six Review

1. What statement about opioid-induced respiratory depression is accurate?
   A. It is not of concern, since it can be immediately reversed with an opioid antagonist such as naloxone.
   B. It prevents tachypnea in the anxious client with pain.
   C. Prevention is best for the client in order to decrease risk and side effects or complications of reversal.
   D. It occurs more frequently during the first 24 hours postoperatively.

2. What is the safest modality for opioid analgesia?
   A. Client-controlled analgesia
   B. IV bolus
   C. Oral
   D. Epidural

3. Use of continuous SpO_2 and $EtCO_2$ monitoring for early recognition of impending respiratory depression has which major advantage?
   A. They monitor oxygenation status.
   B. They monitor oxygenation and ventilation status.
   C. They monitor ventilation status.
   D. They monitor sedation and ventilation status.

4. What statements about evaluating client risk for opioid-induced respiratory depression are accurate?
   A. It is not necessary until pain becomes severe.
   B. It only is important in opioid-naïve clients.
   C. It is the responsibility of the physician.
   D. It provides essential information to communicate at transitions in care.

Answers: 1. C, 2. D, 3. B, 4. D

Section Seven: Pain Management in Special Patient Populations

Several important patient-focused factors influence acute pain management. These factors include age, concurrent medical disorders, and history of substance abuse. A basic understanding of these factors helps to facilitate effective pain management.

Pharmacology and Aging

Elderly patients are more sensitive to analgesic agents and often require less medication to provide effective analgesia. In addition, the effects of the analgesic agents may last longer. The use of naloxone to reverse opioid-induced respiratory depression is rare but more prevalent in older patients, who are receiving CNS depressants or who have developed other conditions such as pneumonia and renal failure.

Therefore, all drugs should be administered with caution. Chronologic age does not have a direct relationship with deterioration of organ function; thus, aging individuals vary greatly in their capacity to absorb, metabolize, and excrete drugs. It can be stated, however, that older adults as a group are at higher risk for drug toxicity than younger adults for a variety of reasons. Drug reactions may be dose related or the result of the drug's interaction at the cellular level. Older adults tend to take more drugs, including analgesics, on a long-term basis often related to the presence of chronic illnesses that require drug therapy. These medications may interact with analgesics, producing symptoms. Older adults tend to have less body water and increased body fat. Less body water causes high blood levels of water-soluble drugs because of decreased distribution volume. Increased body fat causes prolonged effects of fat-soluble drugs because of increased distribution volume in fat tissue. Other complicating factors that increase the risk of adverse reactions or subtherapeutic dosing include the possibility of short-term memory impairment, which may cause a person to take incorrect dosages, miss doses, or take multiple doses. Impaired vision may lead to under- or overdosage. Impaired agility in opening containers may encourage a patient to miss a dose. Financial factors, as well as limited transportation, may keep the patient from filling prescriptions. Often these complicating factors are missed when taking a pain history.

Opioid use in the older adult has a wider distribution in the body with little difference in pharmacokinetics. This increases the risk for respiratory depression and increased cognitive impairment; thus, opioids should be initiated with caution until sensitivity is determined. Studies have shown that opioids are underutilized in older patients who could significantly benefit from their use; however, there is no reason for underutilization if opioids are administered according to an appropriate pain management plan (Katzung, 2009).

In obtaining a medication history, the nurse should reconcile the patient's prescription and over-the-counter (OTC) preparations; OTC supplements; alcohol, caffeine, and tobacco use; and home remedies. The nurse should be aware that certain drugs often prescribed for older adults, such as diuretics, anticholinergics, and sedatives, have a great number of undesirable side effects in this patient population. In assessing the older adult, symptoms suggesting drug toxicity may include incontinence, rather than the more commonly seen nausea, vomiting, diarrhea, and rash. Because of multiple age-related illnesses and chronic conditions, this population tends to require more prescription medications than younger patients prior to hospital admission, as well as during hospitalized care. Of particular concern is **polypharmacy**, or the use of multiple medications, increasing the potential for drug interactions, metabolic changes, and cognitive changes that could lead to the misinterpretation of new disease onset and the prescribing of additional medications to treat what is believed to be a "new" condition (Rochon, 2016).

Patients with Concurrent Medical Disorders

While opioids remain first-line therapy, high-acuity patients frequently have more than one organ with decreased function at any single time. Impaired function of the liver and kidneys has serious implications for analgesic therapy. Analgesics are primarily metabolized in the liver, with a small percentage excreted unchanged. The kidneys have the major responsibility for opioid excretion. When either of these organs has decreased functioning, serum drug levels increase, placing the patient at increasing risk for the development of adverse effects.

Certain opioids (e.g., morphine) are converted into polar glucuronidated metabolites (M6-glucuronide) in the liver and then excreted through the kidneys. The glucuronidated metabolites maintain analgesic capabilities that may be stronger than the actual opioid. If kidney function is significantly impaired, these metabolites may accumulate in the blood, resulting in prolonged and deeper analgesia. This can compromise the patient by precipitating severe respiratory depression, deep sedation, or intractable nausea.

Meperidine is a synthetic opioid that is poorly absorbed through the oral route. With repeated use of meperidine, normeperidine (a toxic metabolite of meperidine) can accumulate in the presence of renal insufficiency or high drug doses, resulting in CNS stimulation, which can precipitate tachycardia and seizure activity. When kidney or liver impairment is present, doses of most opioids must be reduced and the patient monitored closely for the development of unwanted effects. Many healthcare facilities have removed meperidine from their drug formularies as a choice for pain treatment due to the risk of CNS toxicity with repeated dosing, and because other, more acceptable alternatives are now available.

Management of the Tolerant Patient with Superimposed Acute Pain

Patients who have been receiving relatively high-dose, long-term opioid therapy for chronic or cancer pain, or those who regularly misuse or abuse opioids, pose a challenge in the high-acuity setting. These patients may have developed tolerance. Tolerance, a diminished patient response to a drug secondary to adaptation, can occur after repeated opioid administrations. Under these circumstances, dosages may need to be increased to achieve the desired effect. Hyperalgesia is a heightened sensitivity to pain, which decreases the pain threshold. In such cases, the opioid dose requirements may be significantly higher than what is usually recommended to reach a satisfactory level of analgesia. A thorough pain history provides valuable information regarding the potentially altered dose requirements of this patient population.

It is recommended that the patient's routine opioid dose at home be maintained or slightly increased and multimodal therapy added. This will avoid opioid withdrawal and limit hyperalgesia. When the patient is able to take oral medications, this can easily be accomplished by continuation of the patient's home opioid dose in a long-acting oral form and titration of either a short-acting oral opioid or PCA for acute pain coverage. As healing occurs and pain diminishes, short-acting opioids should be weaned accordingly.

A patient restricted to IV therapy requires conversion from the home oral opioid dose to an hourly IV dose. PCA can then be delivered, starting with a conservative continuous PCA dose with additional opioid delivered in the patient-controlled incremental format. The continuous dose and the incremental dose can be slowly titrated upward to control pain while monitoring for oversedation or respiratory depression. Interpatient variability requires individual dose titration. Chronic opioid use can complicate the treatment of a patient in severe acute pain.

Hyperalgesia

Both the use of high-dose opioids over a prolonged time and the effects of chronic pain on the CNS can produce **hyperalgesia**. Hyperalgesia is not the same as tolerance. Unlike tolerance, exposure to a drug induces changes that cause decreased response to the drug's effects over time; hyperalgesia is characterized by increasing pain despite repeated upward titration of opioids. In general, the pain will be reported as diffuse and extend beyond the original area of the pain. Increasing opioids only makes the pain worse (Davis, Shaiova, & Angst, 2007). Hyperalgesia should be suspected when the opioid becomes less effective in the absence of disease progression, especially in conjunction with unexplained pain reports. Treatment for hyperalgesia requires careful, gradual withdrawal of the offending opioid when appropriate. Use of nonopiates such as NSAIDs, lidocaine IV infusion, heat and/or ice, the addition of muscle relaxants, the use of anticonvulsants such as gabapentin (Neurontin) or pregabalin (Lyrica), SSRIs (e.g., venlafaxine [Effexor] or duloxetine [Cymbalta]), and tricyclic antidepressants can help decrease sensitization of the CNS. The use of acupuncture or transcutaneous electrical nerve stimulation (TENS) units along with relaxation therapy has been demonstrated to decrease hyperalgesia (Heinl, Drdla-Schutting, Xanthos, & Sandkëhler, 2011). Furthermore, switching from morphine or hydromorphone to methadone or buprenorphine is considered an effective treatment but requires experienced clinicians to transition the patient's therapy.

The Known Active or Recovering Substance Abuser as Patient

Nurses caring for high-acuity patients are likely to encounter a patient with active substance abuse prior to admission. High-risk behavior coincides with traumatic injuries involving alcohol and drug use. Patients with chemical dependencies have increased morbidity. Pain management of the high-acuity patient who is either an active or recovering substance abuser has important nursing implications. Recognizing the distinction between drug abuse or misuse and chemical dependency is important when considering analgesic therapy. The nurse caring for patients with chemical dependency must recognize the importance of treating pain despite the challenges. This discussion presents a brief overview of some of the issues and nursing implications related to controlling pain when caring for the patient with substance abuse.

An Ethical Code The American Society of Pain Management Nurses views addiction as a treatable disease that is chronic and relapsing (Oliver et al., 2012). It is characterized by uncontrolled, compulsive use and overconsumption of substances despite known harmful effects. Treating pain in this population poses a dilemma that is largely attributable to the medical maxim "Do no harm." Can and should pain in addicted patients be treated using substances that are in themselves addicting, thereby potentially contributing to the addiction? Experts in the fields of pain and addiction answer yes to this question. All people, regardless of whether they are substance abusers or not, have the right to have their pain relieved; thus, relief of pain temporarily overrides the problem of addiction (Oliver et al., 2012).

Assessing Opioid Misuse or Abuse It can be extremely difficult to evaluate whether a person's behavior stems from drug seeking related to addiction or from relief seeking related to undertreated pain. This is true particularly in healthcare settings, where there is often limited assessment and evaluation time involved. However, persons with or without active substance abuse can exhibit relief-seeking behaviors when pain is not adequately controlled.

Healthcare providers should be aware of behaviors and evidence that suggest active addiction. Box 5–5 lists some of the more common behaviors and evidence of active substance abuse. The problem of differentiating pseudoaddiction and addiction-driven behaviors may become even more difficult if the person has previously experienced inadequate pain relief. Previous negative relief-seeking experiences tend to foster maladaptive behaviors that can be misconstrued by the healthcare team as drug seeking and perpetuate suspicion and distrust, which encourage the practice of oligoanalgesia. One way to identify addictive behaviors is to initiate treatment and observe the behaviors: Pseudoaddiction behaviors cease when pain relief is achieved, whereas addiction behaviors continue when the primary motivation is something other than pain relief. It is crucial to closely observe and document changes in behavior prior to and during pain relief interventions.

The probability of opioid abuse has been linked to certain risk factors. This has led to the development of

---

BOX 5–5 Evidence Suspicious of Active Substance Abuse

Behavioral Evidence

- Frequent occurrences of significant impairment in communication or physical abilities
- Swings in mood and changes in personality
- Drug hoarding
- Withdrawal or alienation from family or friends
- Heavy alcohol use in social settings
- Obtaining drugs from others
- Use of multiple pharmacies
- Forging prescriptions
- Change in appetite, unexplained weight change
- Changes in speech pattern (e.g., slurred, rapid)
- Fatigue or drowsiness (depressants); restlessness, irritability (stimulants)
- Impaired memory
- Altered appearance and hygiene

Physical Evidence

- Inappropriately dilated or constricted pupils
- Red or watery eyes
- Hand tremors, stumbling gait
- Altered sleep patterns
- Persistent inflammation of nostrils, runny nose
- Deteriorating health
- Altered vital signs (elevated [stimulants]; decreased [depressants])
- Evidence of substance abuse (e.g., needle marks)

---

screening tools to help determine which patients may be at the highest risk for opioid abuse in order to determine the appropriate level of monitoring necessary during pain control interventions. Two such tools are the Opioid Risk Tool (ORT) and the Screener and Opioid Assessment for Patients with Pain (SOAPP) (Moore, Jones, Browder, Daffron, & Passik, 2009; Webster & Webster, 2005). The authors of both tools emphasize that all patients deserve treatment for pain despite the level of risk or the presence of aberrant behaviors. These tools are proposed to be used solely to determine the level of monitoring required (Webster & Webster, 2005).

Major Considerations in Pain Management

Clinicians often confuse physical dependence with addiction when managing pain in the active or recovering addict. The use of opioids may renew physical dependence, but that does not predict whether the person will relapse into addiction. Undertreatment of acute pain is more likely to reactivate the behaviors associated with addiction. Stress is also known to increase substance craving, and inadequate pain relief often increases stress, which may result in an escalation of substance use in the acute abuser or relapse in the recovering abuser. Although managing pain in this population may be difficult, it is not impossible. Employing recommendations of experts, such as those developed by the American Society of Pain Management Nurses

(ASPMN, 2008), can be useful in guiding medical and nursing pain interventions in this population.

Clinical Management Considerations The National Cancer Institute (NCI, 2011) offers the following guidelines that can be applied to pain treatment of the high-acuity patient with a history of substance abuse:

- **Involve a multidisciplinary team.** Substance abuse is complex and requires interdisciplinary care, such as pain expert physicians, nurses, social workers, and, if available, an addiction medicine expert.
- **Set realistic goals for therapy.** The risk of relapse increases with the heightened stress associated with life-threatening disease. Prevention of relapse may be impossible, requiring altered goal setting for management to include structured therapy, support, and limit setting.
- **Evaluate and treat comorbid psychiatric disorders.** The substance abuser is at extreme risk for anxiety, personality disorders, and depression. Presence of these disorders may require treatment during acute disease states.
- **Prevent or minimize withdrawal symptoms.** Obtain a complete drug history, keeping in mind that many patients abuse multiple drugs. Laboratory drug screening tests can provide a baseline of currently abused substances. Healthcare professionals should be familiar with the manifestations of commonly abused substances (see Table 5–7).
- **Consider the impact of tolerance.** Patients with a known history of recent opioid abuse may require 1.5 times or more opioids to provide analgesia to achieve pain relief.
- **Apply appropriate pharmacologic principles to treat chronic pain.** Analgesic dose individualization is an important principle; focusing on dose size rather than achievement of pain relief may result in pain undertreatment and subsequent development of pseudoaddiction behaviors.
- **Use a multimodal approach to treatment when benefits outweigh risks.** Recognize specific drug abuse behaviors (see Table 5–7).
- **Use nondrug approaches concurrently with analgesics as appropriate.** These may include further patient education, relaxation and coping techniques, and complementary pain-relieving interventions.

Other clinical pain management suggestions include the following:

- Avoid (if possible) analgesics that have the same pharmacologic basis as the abused drug.
- Choose extended-release and long-acting analgesics (e.g., fentanyl and methadone) rather than short-acting ones, and restrict short-acting opiates for breakthrough pain.
- Avoid naloxone (Narcan) unless life-threatening toxic effects are present because use of naloxone will precipitate immediate opiate withdrawal.
- Administer analgesics orally rather than intravenously when possible.

Table 5–7 Commonly Abused Substances and Withdrawal Manifestations

Substance	Common Examples	Common Street Names	Withdrawal Onset and Manifestations
Opiates (CNS depressants)	Codeine, hydromorphone (Dilaudid), morphine, oxycodone (Percodan with aspirin), others Heroin, opium	Morphine: morph, M Dilaudid: little D, dillies, lords Percodan: percs Heroin: horse, smack, H Opium: hop, tar	**Onset:** 4–6 hours following last dose **Manifestations:** Mild initially and becoming more severe; dilated pupils, runny nose, diarrhea, abdominal pain, chills, gooseflesh, insomnia, aching joints and muscles, nausea and vomiting, muscle twitching and tremors (may become severe), mental depression
Alcohol (CNS depressant)	Beer, wine, whiskey, many others	Liquor, beer, booze, wine	**Onset:** 12–48 hours **Manifestations:** Headache, anxiety, depression, nervousness, shakiness, irritability, fatigue, clouded thinking, emotionally lability; GI: nausea, vomiting, anorexia; CV: heart palpitations; EENT: enlarged, dilated pupils; skin: clammy, pale, sweaty palms; musculoskeletal: tremors, abnormal movements **Severe (complicated) withdrawal:** Rapid muscle tremors, seizures, tachycardia, cardiac dysrhythmias, profuse sweating, hallucinations, others
Barbiturates (CNS depressants)	Phenobarbital, pentobarbital	Barbs, red devils, goof balls, yellow jackets, downers	**Onset:** 12–20 hours following last dose **Manifestations:** Similar to alcohol withdrawal in the absence of alcohol; other mental changes: blank facial expression, slurred speech, flat affect; severe withdrawal can result in respiratory and heart failure, seizures, and death
Cocaine (CNS stimulant)	—	Coke, blow, snow, nose candy	**Onset:** 4–8 hours **Manifestations:** Few physical withdrawal symptoms; strong psychological symptoms, including rapid onset of depression, fatigue or sleepiness, strong craving for more cocaine, loss of pleasure; may also experience paranoia, agitation
Amphetamines (CNS stimulants)	Methylphenidate (Ritalin), pemoline (Cylert)	Speed, uppers, dexies, crank, meth, ice, crystal	**Onset:** 4–8 hours **Manifestations:** Depression, severe craving, mental confusion, insomnia, restlessness, paranoia, possible psychosis
Ecstasy (3,4-methyl-enedioxymethamphetamine [MDMA])	None	XTC, Adam, roll, E	**Onset:** Rapid **Manifestations:** Depression, anxiety, panic attacks, sleeplessness, depersonalization, paranoid delusions, drug craving
Anabolic-androgenic steroids	Depo-Testosterone, clomiphene citrate (Clomid), stanozolol (Winstrol)	Roids, juice, Arnolds, stackers, gym candy	**Onset:** Not fully documented **Manifestations:** Mood swings, fatigue, restlessness, anorexia, insomnia, reduced sex drive, desire for more steroids

Section Seven Review

1. Older adults tend to have increased body fat. What is the primary clinical significance of this statement?
   A. Larger doses of opioids are required to achieve pain relief.
   B. Fat-soluble drugs may have prolonged effects.
   C. There is reduced distribution volume, so drug concentration is lower.
   D. Pain relief using opioids should be avoided.

2. Accumulation of morphine metabolites in the blood because of renal dysfunction can cause what condition?
   A. Severe respiratory depression
   B. Seizures
   C. Tachycardia
   D. CNS stimulation

3. Accumulation of the metabolite of meperidine (normeperidine) in the blood can result in what condition?
   A. Severe sedation
   B. Bradycardia
   C. Severe respiratory depression
   D. Seizures

4. Which statement is accurate about the known substance abuser who is hospitalized?
   A. The client should receive no opioids.
   B. The client may require higher-than-usual opioid dose ranges.
   C. The client should receive only one type of opioid.
   D. The client may require lower-than-usual opioid dose ranges.

Answers: 1. B, 2. A, 3. D, 4. B

Section Eight: Procedural Sedation or Analgesia

It is important that the high-acuity nurse have a clear understanding of the four different stages of pharmacological sedation in order to effectively communicate with members of the healthcare team. A clarification of terms leads to increased patient safety. This section focuses on the fourth level of sedation, which encompasses general anesthesia. Level four is within the scope of nursing practice of the certified registered nurse anesthetist (CRNA) only. The American Association of Nurse Anesthetists (AANA, 2016) supports the use of practice guidelines established by the American Society of Anesthesiologists (ASA), which designate four primary levels of sedation: minimal, moderate, deep, and anesthesia (Table 5–8). Levels one through three are within the scope of practice for the high-acuity RN. The fourth level, anesthesia, can be managed by the CRNA.

Most often, minimal to moderate sedation is used to induce relaxation with insignificant variation in vital signs when patient cooperation is needed for a procedure. The goal for procedural sedation is to produce an altered mental status by administering pharmacological agents, primarily through the intravenous route. The patient should have an altered level of consciousness yet be able to maintain a patent airway and respond to verbal and environmental stimuli throughout the procedure. The Ramsay Sedation Scale (see Table 5–8) was developed in 1974 to assess sedation in the ICU. This scale correlates with sedation definitions that have been outlined by The Joint Commission (TJC). A comparison of these definitions is summarized in Table 5–8.

Purpose of Moderate Sedation or Analgesia

A high-acuity patient who is moderately sedated can tolerate uncomfortable procedures such as diagnostic colonoscopy, endoscopic retrograde cholangiopancreatography (ERCP), upper endoscopy, or electrical cardioversion. The patient is able to respond purposefully to verbal commands, breathe spontaneously and maintain his or her airway, cough and swallow, and cardiovascular function is not affected. The number and types of procedures performed outside of the operating room are increasing, and nurses often provide the sedation.

Nursing Management of the Patient Undergoing Procedural Sedation

Nurses must be properly trained and able to demonstrate a baseline knowledge of the pharmacology, be able

---

Table 5–8 Ramsay Sedation Scale Modified to Correlate with TJC Definitions of Minimal Sedation, Moderate Sedation, Deep Sedation, and General Anesthesia

Score	Modified Ramsay Sedation Scale Score Definition	TJC Sedation Definition
1	Awake and alert, minimal or no cognitive impairment	*Minimal sedation (anxiolysis)* is a drug-induced state during which patients respond normally to verbal commands. Although cognitive function and coordination may be impaired, ventilatory and cardiovascular functions are unaffected.
2	Awake but tranquil, purposeful responses to verbal commands at conversational level	*Moderate sedation/analgesia* is a drug-induced depression of consciousness during which patients respond purposefully to verbal commands, either alone or accompanied by light tactile stimulation. No interventions are required to maintain a patent airway, and spontaneous ventilation is adequate. Cardiovascular function is usually maintained.
3	Appears asleep, purposeful responses to verbal commands at conversational level	
4	Appears asleep, purposeful responses to commands but at a louder-than-usual conversational level, requiring light glabellar tap, or both	
5	Asleep, sluggish purposeful responses only to loud verbal commands, strong glabellar tap, or both	*Deep sedation/analgesia* is a drug-induced depression of consciousness during which patients cannot be easily aroused but respond purposefully following repeated or painful stimulation. The ability to independently maintain ventilatory function may be impaired. Patients may require assistance in maintaining a patent airway, and spontaneous ventilation may be inadequate. Cardiovascular function is usually maintained.
6	Asleep, sluggish purposeful responses only to painful stimuli	
7	Asleep, sluggish withdrawal to painful stimuli only (no purposeful responses)	
8	Unresponsive to external stimuli, including pain	*General anesthesia* is a drug-induced loss of consciousness during which patients are not arousable, even by painful stimulation. The ability to independently maintain ventilatory function is often impaired. Patients often require assistance in maintaining a patent airway, and positive pressure ventilation may be required because of depressed spontaneous ventilation or drug-induced depression of neuromuscular function. Cardiovascular function may be impaired.

SOURCE: From Mace et al. (2006). *Pain Management and Sedation: Emergency Department Management.* Reproduced by permission of The McGraw-Hill Companies.

to recognize cardiac arrhythmias, and be equipped and prepared to respond to any complication prior to administering procedural sedation and analgesia. In order to demonstrate competency, the high-acuity nurse is required to complete advanced cardiac life support (ACLS) training and should be aware of hospital policies related to the administration of procedural sedation. The nurse may administer moderate sedation only in the presence of a licensed independent practitioner. Rules regarding the specific drugs that fall within the RN scope of practice vary from state to state, and all nurses should be familiar with their specific state board of nursing restrictions or requirements.

Institutions that provide sedation are required to abide by strict policies, clinical guidelines, and protocols. The policies must contain age-appropriate considerations and should include descriptions of the necessary equipment and supplies, mandatory education requirements, processes for validating competency, required interface with risk management and quality improvement, and mandatory documentation. If a patient is undergoing a procedure with moderate sedation and progresses to a state of deep sedation, the high-acuity nurse must be prepared to manage the compromised airway and ensure oxygenation and ventilation. If the patient progresses to a state of general anesthesia, the nurse must be competent to manage oxygenation and ventilation as well as an unstable cardiovascular system.

Before the Procedure   Prior to beginning any procedure that requires procedural sedation, the nurse should ensure that the proper equipment is available and ready for use (AANA, 2016). The essential equipment for procedural sedation is listed in Box 5–6. The next step is to verify that the physician has explained the procedure to the patient or family, if indicated, and that the patient or family has given informed consent. This includes, but is not limited to, the medications to be administered, risks, benefits, possible adverse reactions, and alternative treatments.

Patient safety is always a priority. Whenever a procedure requiring written consent or an invasive procedure is about to be performed, The Joint Commission requires that a time-out be performed by the team. It is essential that the nurse managing the care of the patient undergoing moderate sedation has no additional responsibilities during administration that might result in leaving the patient unattended or might compromise continuous monitoring (AACN, 2010).

During the Procedure   Careful assessment of respiratory rate and quality should be monitored at least every 5 minutes. Oxygenation is best monitored with a combination of continuous oxygen saturation measurement using pulse oximetry (SpO_2) and capnography to measure end tidal carbon dioxide ($EtCO_2$). Capnography is recommended for moderate sedation. Capnography is a more sensitive indicator of early respiratory depression than is pulse oximetry or clinical assessment. The high-acuity nurse is continually monitoring cardiac status through variations in rate and rhythm using continuous cardiac rhythm monitoring. A broad knowledge of cardiac arrhythmias and their treatments is essential. Other physiologic measurements that must be monitored during the sedation and recovery period include respiratory rate, blood pressure, heart rate and rhythm, and level of consciousness (sedation). In addition, careful attention to skin condition and pressure areas is important as the sedated patient may not be aware of pain associated with immobility. Any significant changes must be reported to the physician or other advanced practice provider and immediately addressed.

Postprocedure   The high-acuity nurse must monitor the patient's sedation level, and the nurse should continue to monitor vital signs until the patient is fully awakened from the sedation. Depending upon the procedure performed, the nurse should also assess for pain, wound drainage, nausea and vomiting, intake and output, and neurovascular status. Following the procedure or sedation, the patient may report a brief period of amnesia. Other side effects may include headache, hangover, or unpleasant memories of the diagnostic procedure. No patient should be sent to an unsupervised area such as radiology or other diagnostic testing areas until fully awakened from sedation. In the event the patient does need to leave the primary patient care area to have another procedure before fully recovered, a nurse must accompany him or her.

Drugs Used for Moderate Sedation

A wide variety of drugs are used to attain a state of moderate sedation. These may include but are not limited to etomidate, propofol, ketamine, fentanyl, and midazolam. Drugs used for moderate sedation are summarized in the feature "Related Pharmacotherapy: Short-acting Intravenous Anesthetics Used for Moderate Sedation." Not all sedating medications have analgesic properties, and a combination of analgesics and sedatives is selected to achieve analgesia and sedation while maintaining a patent airway. Even though higher doses of opioids can cause sedation, they should never be used as a primary sedating agent due to the risks associated with respiratory compromise. To achieve the best results, these IV medications should be administered through separate IV lines. The patient's level of pain should be assessed using a behavioral pain rating scale, and analgesics should be administered as indicated by the patient's condition.

BOX 5–6   Equipment Needed for Moderate Sedation

- Intravenous access
- Pulse oximeter
- Capnography equipment
- Blood pressure monitor
- Cardiac monitor
- Emergency medications
- Emergency cart with defibrillator
- Suction equipment
- Positive pressure breathing device (Ambu bag)
- Supplemental oxygen
- Appropriate artificial airways (e.g., oral airways, endotracheal tubes)

Related Pharmacotherapy
Short-acting Intravenous Anesthetics Used for Moderate Sedation

Hypnotics or Sedative Hypnotics

Propofol (Diprivan)

Actions and Uses

Short-acting hypnotic/sedative hypnotic that induces and maintains anesthesia. If concurrent analgesia is desired, it may be given with a short-acting opioid, such as fentanyl.

Dosage (Adult)

Moderate sedation: 5 mcg/kg/min for minimum of 5 minutes; increase dose by 5–10 mcg/kg/min every 5–10 minutes until desired sedation level is achieved.

Major Side Effects and Adverse Effects

- Cardiovascular and respiratory depression
- Nausea and vomiting
- Overdose: Severe cardiopulmonary depression (hypotension, apnea, cardiopulmonary arrest)

Nursing Implications

- Cautious use with hypovolemic states, and in elderly and patients with poor cardiac function.
- Increased infection risk: Vials carry high risk for infection due to composition of the solution, which makes it an excellent bacterial growth medium. Discard open vial within 6 hours. Store unopened vials at 22°C (71.6°F).

Opioids

Fentanyl (Sublimaze)

Actions and Uses

Opioid analgesic that causes CNS depression. Useful for short-term analgesia needed for painful procedures or treatments. Often used in conjunction with short-term anesthesia agents.

Dosage (Adult)

Moderate to severe pain: 50–100 mcg
Premedication to anesthesia: 25–100 mcg, administered 30–60 minutes prior to procedure

Major Side Effects and Adverse Effects

- Cardiovascular and respiratory depression
- Overdose: apnea, cardiovascular collapse, cardiopulmonary arrest, others

Nursing Implications

- Monitor patient for opioid toxicity (severe respiratory depression, pinpoint pupils, and coma).
- Cautious use in older adults as it may result in severe respiratory depression.

Benzodiazepines

Midazolam (Versed)

Actions and Uses

Short-acting benzodiazepines are CNS depressants that can produce an unconscious state and amnesia. They are useful for inducing anesthesia and for moderate sedation. For the purpose of moderate sedation, they are often used in combination with a short-acting opioid analgesic, such as fentanyl.

Dosage (Adult)

Moderate sedation: 1–2.5 mg; repeat in 2 minutes as needed

Major Side Effects and Adverse Effects

- Cardiac and respiratory depression (hypotension, cardiac dysrhythmias, airway obstruction, apnea, respiratory arrest, and others)
- Nausea and vomiting, hiccups
- Overdose: deep sedation, unstable vital signs

Nursing Implications

- For sedation purposes: Drug should be delivered slowly (over at least 2 minutes) to minimize adverse cardiac and respiratory complications.
- Contraindicated in patient with glaucoma or if patient has vital signs that are abnormally low

Dissociative Anesthetic

Ketamine (Ketalar)

Actions and Uses

Ketamine places the patient in a dreamlike state that is dissociated from his or her environment (dissociative anesthesia). Other actions include analgesia, amnesia, sedation, and immobility. It is most useful for pediatric use during minor procedures or diagnostic tests.

Dosage (Adult)

Induction: 1 mg/kg to 4.5 mg/kg IV initial dosing

Major Side Effects and Adverse Effects

- Cardiovascular and respiratory stimulation
- Sensory and neuro: nystagmus and diplopia, increased muscle tone (may develop seizure-like activity)
- Nausea and vomiting
- Adverse psychological reactions: may develop hallucinations, confusion, excited state, and delirium lasting for approximately 1 hour

Nursing Implications

- 100 mg/mL concentration requires dilution for IV use
- Adverse psychological reactions: most common in 15–65 age range. To minimize, maintain patient in a quiet, low-stimulus environment. Premedicating patient with a benzodiazepine prior to ketamine induction reduces risk of this reaction.
- Use is contraindicated in patients with severe hypertension or known hypersensitivity.
- Do not mix ketamine and barbiturates or diazepam; mix and deliver separately.

Sedation should never be defined by the drug(s) used but by the goal of therapy. The use of single large-bolus doses of any medication carries more risk for respiratory and cardiovascular depression than titrated intravenous administration to a defined end point. Drugs that can be titrated have rapid onset and offset and allow for adjustments in dose and dose interval.

Possible Complications of Moderate Sedation

Undergoing moderate sedation is not without risks for complications, so a high state of nursing vigilance is required during the recovery phase.

Unintentional Deep Sedation   Sedation is a continuum, and it is not always possible to predict how a patient will respond to the medication. Therefore, the nurse who is administering moderate sedation must be prepared to rescue a patient who progresses to a state of deep analgesia

(sedation). The Joint Commission recommends that healthcare personnel administering moderate sedation be qualified to rescue a patient from unintentional deep sedation. This includes the ability to manage a compromised airway and provide ventilation if necessary. If the patient progresses to a deeper state of sedation than required for the procedure, all efforts must be focused on returning the patient to the original level of sedation. It is not acceptable to continue the procedure if the patient is oversedated.

Other Possible Complications   Adverse events may include cardiopulmonary arrest, airway compromise, hypoxemia, aspiration, significant hypotension, significant bradycardia or tachycardia, prolonged sedation, or death. If necessary, the nurse should be prepared to initiate resuscitative measures, including CPR, cardioversion, or defibrillation if indicated (ASPMN, 2008). Untoward events must be documented and reported according to established protocols. Reporting of adverse events through the proper channels allows for follow-up and continuous quality improvement.

Section Eight Review

1. When a client is sedated at level two (moderate sedation), the nurse would expect to assess which client level of response?
   A. Fully conscious but pain free
   B. Altered level of consciousness but able to respond to verbal stimuli
   C. Not responsive to verbal stimuli but able to maintain a patent airway
   D. Does not respond to verbal or environmental stimuli

2. When propofol (Diprivan) is used, what can the nurse expect will be required with an unused vial?
   A. Special handling with gloves
   B. Protection from the sunlight
   C. Disposal after 6 hours
   D. Placement in a freezer after 2 hours

3. A client receives ketamine (Ketalar) as anesthesia. The nurse is aware that to minimize the chance of adverse psychological reactions, what should occur?
   A. A sedative may be required.
   B. Frequent stimulation is required.
   C. A reversal drug will be administered.
   D. A quiet, low-stimulation environment must be maintained.

4. What is a major complication of conscious sedation for which monitoring is needed?
   A. Unintentional deep sedation
   B. Anaphylactic reaction
   C. Status epilepticus
   D. Hypertensive crisis

Answers: 1. B, 2. C, 3. D, 4. A

Clinical Reasoning Checkpoint

Twenty-four hours ago, 38-year-old Mr. Heung received multiple trauma injuries in a motor vehicle crash. He sustained fractures of his left femur and left humerus, both of which required open reduction; he also required repair of a liver laceration. In addition, he had rib fractures and a left pneumothorax, resulting in placement of a chest tube. Mr. Heung is intubated and breathing with the assistance of a positive pressure mechanical ventilator. His medical history is noncontributory, and his family history is negative for diabetes, cancer, or heart disease. Mr. Heung is drowsy and oriented only to his name. He cannot speak

due to the endotracheal tube. A central venous IV line is present in his right subclavian vein. He also has a nasogastric tube in place to intermittent suction and a Foley catheter.

The following questions relate to this case.

1. The importance of assessing a patient for potential sources of pain, particularly when the patient is unable to self-report pain, was discussed in this chapter. List the potential sources of pain for Mr. Heung based on the facts of the case.

2. James, a new ICU nurse, is preparing to assess Mr. Heung's pain but is uncertain which type of assessment would be the most appropriate to use in his patient's situation. He asks his coworker, Donna, a more experienced ICU nurse, what would be the best approach for assessing Mr. Heung's pain. Based on what you have learned about pain assessment in the high-acuity patient, what should Donna tell him?

3. Mr. Heung's wife expresses concern that her husband is receiving IV opiates for his pain and tells the nurse that she is afraid he will become addicted. How should you, the nurse, respond to Mrs. Heung to reduce her fears?

4. The nurse notes that a new order has been written for meperidine (Demerol) for Mr. Heung. The nurse is aware that this analgesic agent is no longer recommended.

   A. Briefly explain the reason meperidine is no longer recommended.

   B. What is the appropriate action for the nurse to take?

Chapter 5 Review

1. A client who was severely injured in a motor vehicle crash is comatose. The family asks if the client is in pain from the injuries sustained. How should the nurse respond to this concern?

   1. "Since he is in a coma, he isn't feeling any pain."

   2. "We are giving him sedatives to prevent him from feeling the pain."

   3. "When clients sustain this much injury, the pain response is blunted."

   4. "We are not certain, so he is receiving pain-controlling medications."

2. A client who had cardiac surgery yesterday says, "I don't want to take any more pain medication than I absolutely have to." The nurse encourages use of pain medications to help prevent which responses to unrelieved pain and stress? (Select all that apply.)

   1. Counterregulation of normal hormone responses

   2. Decrease in vascular shunting

   3. Hypoperfusion of the extremities

   4. Initial elevation of blood endorphin levels

   5. Blood stasis

3. A client must have multiple painful treatments for a burn injury. Why would the nurse encourage this client to take pain medications before these treatments?

   1. Multiple episodes of acute, unrelieved pain may result in chronic, persistent pain even after the wound has healed.

   2. Offering pain medication is standard in all such procedures.

   3. The client may have cardiac complications from the acute pain.

   4. There is really no reason to encourage this client to take pain medications, and the nurse should rely on the client's judgment.

4. A client sustained multiple fractures requiring operative intervention. Two days after surgery, the client is agitated and repeatedly hitting his left foot on the bedrail. What should be the nurse's initial intervention?

   1. Administer the ordered analgesic

   2. Contact the client's physician

   3. Have the client indicate pain level on a visual analog scale

   4. Document these new behaviors

5. A client who has severe injuries does not speak or understand English well. The nurse providing care for this client observes that she is agitated and restless. The nurse assigns this client a pain intensity score of 8/10 (8 out of a possible 10). What is true of this method of assigning a score?

   1. It is probably an accurate representation of the client's pain.

   2. It is an acceptable alternative pain-assessment tool.

   3. It is acceptable only under special circumstances such as these.

   4. It is an inappropriate use of a unidimensional tool.

6. A client has the following pain-management orders: morphine 10 mg (IM) every 4 hours prn; ibuprofen 400 mg (PO) every 6 hours. What is the primary purpose of ordering this combination of medication?

   1. The level of analgesia is enhanced.

   2. Sedation is increased if both medications are used.

   3. The respiratory depressive effects are reduced.

   4. The opioid dose can be significantly reduced.

7. A client is afraid to take morphine, stating, "I might stop breathing. That happened to my niece." How should the nurse respond to this fear? (Select all that apply.)

   1. "Using morphine does put you at high risk for respiratory problems."

   2. "We would see you getting overly sedated before your respirations are affected."

   3. "Respiratory depression is related to how much you are getting in a dose, and your dose is very low."

   4. "We will be closely monitoring your level of sedation and your respirations."

   5. "Your niece's nurse must have made a dosage error."

8. A client was admitted for treatment of burns over 65% of the body. History reveals that the client takes opioids at home to control chronic back pain. What would the nurse expect regarding the client's opioid dosage while hospitalized?

   1. It should be lower since the client is not opioid naïve.
   2. It will be approximately the same, with some prn doses for breakthrough pain.
   3. There may be a slight increase in the amount of opioids required.
   4. The dosage required for pain control may be significantly higher.

9. A client received moderate sedation for a procedure and is still very drowsy. It is necessary to move the client to another area of the hospital in order to admit a critically ill client. How should the nurse proceed?

   1. Call transport and request the transfer, advising that someone will need to stay with the client at all times.
   2. Assign a UAP to transport the client to the new area to be met by the nurse assuming care.
   3. Ask the unit clerk of the new area to come and get the client.
   4. Personally transport the client, remaining in attendance until sedation has cleared.

10. A client is to have moderate sedation for a procedure. The nurse has started the client's IV and is waiting for the physician doing the procedure to finish talking with the family in the next room. Which nursing actions are indicated? (Select all that apply.)

    1. Monitor the client's current respiratory rate.
    2. Initiate a cardiac monitor.
    3. Begin titrating the ordered sedation medication.
    4. Prepare the client for endotracheal intubation and mechanical ventilation.
    5. Be certain a signed informed consent is present on the chart.

Answers to questions found inside your textbook are available on the faculty resources site. Please consult with your instructor.

References

American Association of Critical-Care Nurses (AACN). (2010). Sedation guideline. Retrieved June 23, 2016, from www.aacn.org/WD/Practice/Docs/Sedation.doc

American Association of Critical-Care Nurses (AACN). (2013). Assessing pain in the critically ill adult. Retrieved December 5, 2016, from http://www.aacn.org/wd/practice/content/practicealerts/assessing-pain-critically-ill-adult.pcms?menu=practice

American Association of Nurse Anesthetists (AANA). (2016). Non-anesthesia provider procedural sedation and analgesia. Retrieved December 6, 2016, from http://www.aana.com/resources2/professionalpractice/Pages/Non-anesthesia-Provider-Procedural-Sedation-and-Analgesia.aspx

American Society of Addiction Medicine (ASAM). (2001). Definitions related to the use of opioids for the treatment of pain: Consensus statement of the American Academy of Pain Medicine, the American Pain Society, and the American Society of Addiction Medicine. Retrieved December 6, 2016, from http://www.asam.org/docs/publicy-policy-statements/1opioid-definitions-consensus-2-011.pdf

American Society of Pain Management Nurses (ASPMN). (2008). Procedural sedation consensus statement. Retrieved December 6, 2016, from http://www.aspmn.org/Documents/PS_-2-11-08.pdf

Angst, M., & Clark, J. D. (2010). Ketamine for managing perioperative pain in opioid-dependent patients with chronic pain: A unique indication? *Anesthesiology, 113*(3), 514–515.

Arbour, C., Choinière, M., Topolovec-Vranic, J., Loiselle, C. G., & Gélinas, C. (2014). Can fluctuations in vital signs be used for pain assessment in critically ill patients with brain injury? *Pain Research and Treatment,* Volume 2014. http://dx.doi.org/10.1155/2014/175794

Barr, J., Fraser, G. L., Puntillo, K., Ely, E. W., Gélinas, C., Dasta, J., . . . Jaeschke, R. (2013). Clinical practice guidelines for the management of pain, agitation, and delirium in adult patients in the intensive care unit. *Critical Care Medicine, 41*(1), 263–306.

Davidson, J. E., Winkelman, C., Gélinas, C., & Dermenchyan, A. (2015). Pain, agitation, and delirium guidelines: Nurses' involvement in development and implementation. *Critical Care Nurse, 35*(3), 17–31. doi:10.4037/ccn2015824

Davis, M. P., Shaiova, L. A., & Angst, M. S. (2007). When opioids cause pain. *Journal of Clinical Oncology, 25*(28), 4497–4498.

Dillon, D. C., & Gibbs, M. A. (2016). Chapter 36: Local and regional anesthesia. In J. E. Tintinalli, J. S. Stapczynski, J. Ma, D. M. Yealy, G. D. Meckler, & D. M. Cline (Eds.), *Tintinalli's emergency medicine: A comprehensive study guide* (8th ed.). Retrieved December 6, 2016, from http://accessmedicine.mhmedical.com/content.aspx?bookid=1658&sectionid=109427979

Ducharme, J. (2016). Chapter 35: Acute pain management. In J. E. Tintinalli, J. S. Stapczynski, J. Ma, D. M. Yealy, G. D. Meckler, & D. M. Cline (Eds.), *Tintinalli's emergency medicine: A comprehensive study guide* (8th ed.). Retrieved December 6, 2016, from http://accessmedicine.mhmedical.com/content.aspx?bookid=1658&sectionid=109405019

Farag, E., Ghobrial, M., Sessler, D. I., Dalton, J. E., Liu, J., Lee, J. H., . . . Kurz, A. (2013). Effect of perioperative intravenous lidocaine administration on pain, opioid consumption, and quality of life after complex spine surgery. *Anesthesiology, 119*(4), 932–940. doi:10.1097/ALN.0b013e318297d4a5

Gélinas, C., Puntillo, K. A., Joffe, A. M., & Barr, J. (2013). A validated approach to evaluating psychometric properties of pain assessment tools for use in nonverbal critically ill adults. *Seminars in Respiratory and Critical Care Medicine, 34*(2), 153–168. doi:10.1055/s-0033- 1342970

Golembiewski, J., & Dasta, J. (2015). Evolving role of local anesthetics in managing postsurgical analgesia. *Clinical Therapeutics, 37*(6), 1354–1371.

Heinl, C., Drdla-Schutting, R., Xanthos, D. N., & Sandkëhler, J. (2011). Distinct mechanisms underlying pronociceptive effects of opioids. *Journal of Neuroscience, 31*(46), 16748–16756.

Herr, K., Coyne, P. J., Manworren, R., McCaffery, M., & Merkel, S. (2011). Pain assessment in the nonverbal patient: Position statement with clinical practice recommendations. *Pain Management Nursing, 12*(4), 230–250.

International Association for the Study of Pain (ISAP). (2001). Faces Pain Scale–Revised home. Retrieved December 5, 2016, from http://www.iasp-pain.org/Education/Content.aspx?ItemNumber=1519

International Association for the Study of Pain (ISAP). (2014). IASP taxonomy. Retrieved December 5, 2016, from http://www.iasp-pain.org/Taxonomy%20#Pain

Katzung, B. G., (2009). Special aspects of geriatric pharmacology. In B. G. Katzung, S. Masters, & A. Trevor (Eds.), *Basic & clinical pharmacology* (11th ed., pp. 1051–1060). New York, NY: McGraw-Hill Medical.

Kobelt, P., Burke, K., & Renker, P. (2014). Evaluation of a standardized sedation assessment for opioid administration in the post anesthesia care unit. *Pain Management Nursing, 15*(3), 672–681.

Loeser, J. D., & Cousins, M. J. (1990). Contemporary pain management. *The Medical Journal of Australia, 153,* 208–212, 216.

Mace, S. E., Ducharme, J., & Murphy, M. F. (2006). *Pain management and sedation: Emergency department management.* New York, NY: McGraw-Hill.

McCaffery, M., & Pasero, C. (1999). *Pain: Clinical manual for nursing practice* (2nd ed.). St. Louis: C.V. Mosby.

Moore, T. M., Jones, T., Browder, J. H., Daffron, S., & Passik, S. D. (2009). A comparison of common screening methods for predicting aberrant drug-related behavior among patients receiving opioids for chronic pain management. *Pain Medicine, 10*(8), 1426–1433. doi:10.1111/j.1526-4637.2009.00743.x

Mugabure, B. B. (2013). Recommendations for spinal opioids clinical practice in the management of postoperative pain. *Journal of Anesthesiology and Clinical Science, 2*(28), 1–9. doi:10.7243/2049-9752-2-28

National Cancer Institute (NCI). (2011). Substance abuse issues in cancer (PDQ®): Supportive care–Health professional information (NCI). Retrieved December 6, 2016, from http://www.uofmhealth.org/health-library/ncicdr0000062835#ncicdr0000062835-overview

National Institutes of Health (NIH), National Center for Complementary and Integrative Health, U.S. Dept. of Health and Human Services. (2015). Advance research on mind and body interventions, practices, and disciplines. Retrieved December 6, 2016, from https://nccih.nih.gov/about/plans/2011/objective1.htm

Needleman, J., Buerhaus, P., Pandratz, V. S., Leibson, C. L., Stevens, S. R., & Harris, M. (2011). Nurse staffing and inpatient hospital mortality. *New England Journal of Medicine, 364*(11), 1037–1045.

Nisbet, A. T., & Mooney-Cotter, F. (2009). Comparison of selected sedation scales for reporting opioid-induced sedation assessment. *Pain Management Nursing, 10*(3), 154–164.

Oh, J., Sohn, J.-H., Shin, C. S., Na, S. H., Yoon, H.-J., Kim, J.-J., . . . Park, J. Y. (2015). Mutual relationship between anxiety and pain in the intensive care unit and its effect on medications. *Journal of Critical Care, 30*(5), 1043–1048. http://dx.doi.org/10.1016/j.jcrc.2015.05.025

Oliver, J., Coggins, C., Compton, P., Hagan, S., Matteliano, D., Stanton, M., . . . Turner, H. (2012). American Society for Pain Management Nursing position statement: Pain management in patients with substance use disorder. *Pain Management Nursing, 13*(3), 169–183.

Pandharipande, P., & McGrane, S. (2015). Pain control in the critically ill adult patient. *UpToDate.com.* Retrieved December 6, 2016, from http://www.uptodate.com/contents/pain-control-in-the-critically-ill-adult-patient#references

Pasero, C., & McCaffery, M. (2011). *Pain assessment and pharmacologic management.* St. Louis, MO: Elsevier/Mosby.

Pasero, C., Quinn, T. E., Portenoy, R. K., McCaffery, M., & Rizos, A. (2011). Section IV: Opioid analgesics. In C. Pasero & M. McCaffery (Eds.), *Pain assessment and pharmacologic management* (pp. 277–622). St. Louis, MO: Elsevier/Mosby.

Ramachandran, S. K., Haider, N., Saran, K. A., Mathis, M., Morris, M., & O'Reilly, M. (2011). Life-threatening critical respiratory events: A retrospective study of postoperative patients found unresponsive during analgesic therapy. *Journal of Clinical Anesthesia, 23*(3), 207–213.

Rochon, P. A. (2016). Drug prescribing for older adults. *UpToDate.com.* Retrieved December 6, 2016, from http://www.uptodate.com/contents/drug-prescribing-for-older-adults

Roulin, M., & Ramelet, A. (2015). Generating and selecting pain indicators for brain-injured critical care patients. *Pain Management Nursing, 37*(3), 221–232.

Sharma, A., & Verma, D. (2015). Endorphins: Endogenous opioid in human cells. *World Journal of Pharmacy & Pharmaceutical Sciences, 4*(1), 357–374.

Skrobik, Y., Ahern, S., Leblanc, M., Marquis, F., Awissi, D. K., & Kavanagh, B. P. (2010). Protocolized intensive care unit management of analgesia, sedation, and delirium improves analgesia and subsyndromal delirium rates. *Anesthesia & Analgesia, 111*(2), 451–463.

Stites, M. (2015). Pain, agitation, and delirium guidelines: Nurses' involvement in development and implementation, *Critical Care Nurse, 35,* 17–31.

Taenzer, A. H., Pyke, J. B., McGrath, S. P., & Blike, G. T. (2010). Impact of pulse oximetry surveillance on rescue events and intensive care unit transfers. *Anesthesiology*, *112*(2), 282–287.

Ware, L. J., Herr, K. A., Booker, S. S., Dotson, K., Key, J., Poindexter, N., . . . Packard, A. (2015). Psychometric evaluation of the revised Iowa Pain Thermometer (IPT-R) in a sample of diverse cognitively intact and impaired older adults: A pilot study. *Pain Management Nursing*, *16*(4), 475–482.

Weaver, C. (2016). Chapter 37: Procedural sedation. In J. E. Tintinalli, J. S. Stapczynski, J. Ma, D. M. Yealy, G. D. Meckler, & D. M. Cline (Eds.), *Tintinalli's emergency medicine: A comprehensive study guide* (8th ed.). Retrieved December 6, 2016, from http://accessmedicine .mhmedical.com/content.aspx?bookid=1658&sectio nid=109428134

Webster, L. R., & Webster, R. M. (2005). Predicting aberrant behaviors in opioid-treated patients: Preliminary validation of the Opioid Risk Tool. *Pain Medication*, *6*(6), 432–442.

Wilson, B. A., Shannon, M. T., & Shields, K. M. (2014). *Pearson Nurse's drug guide 2015.* New York, NY: Prentice Hall.

World Health Organization. (1996). *Cancer pain relief with a guide to opioid availability* (2nd ed.). Geneva, Switzerland: World Health Organization.

Zeidan, F., Adler-Neal, A. L., Wells, R. E., Stagnaro, E., May, L. M., Eisencach, J. C., . . . Coghill, R. C. (2016). Mindfulness-meditation-based pain relief is not mediated by endogenous opioids. *Journal of Neuroscience, 36* (11), 3391–3397.

Chapter 6
Nutrition Support

Learning Outcomes

6.1 Explain nutritional alterations associated with selected disease states.

6.2 Discuss enteral nutrition, including benefits, potential complications, gastric versus postpyloric feeding, and barriers to providing enteral nutrition.

6.3 Discuss the parenteral methods used to provide nutrition for the high-acuity patient, including potential complications.

6.4 Describe refeeding syndrome and prevention strategies.

The high-acuity patient is at high risk for development of significant nutritional deficits related to the level of physiologic stress placed on the body during the crisis. Nutritional deficits, in turn, complicate illness and negatively impact patient outcomes. Clinical studies indicate that severely malnourished patients have a greater risk of developing complications and increased mortality (Eman et al., 2010; Lim et al., 2012; Rubinson, Diette, Song, Brower, & Krishnan, 2004). This chapter focuses on nutritional alterations that occur during high-acuity illness and the ways in which patients are supported nutritionally. Baseline nutritional status is an important determinant for deciding when and what type of nutritional support to initiate. Normal nutrition and metabolism concepts, including assessments, are presented in Chapter 31: Determinants and Assessment of Nutrition and Metabolic Function.

Section One: Nutritional Alterations in Specific Disease States

The dysfunction of any organ results in a relative loss of its ability to maintain metabolic processes and perform its functions. This section provides an overview of some of the major nutritional alterations associated with major organ disorders and their nutritional implications.

Hepatic Failure

The liver plays a vital role in nutrition and metabolism. Major metabolic functions of the liver include synthesis and excretion of plasma proteins, synthesis of bile acids, conversion of ammonia to urea, storage of fat-soluble vitamins, maintenance of adequate coagulation, and metabolism of carbohydrates, proteins, and lipids.

The liver plays a key role in the metabolism of carbohydrates, the body's preferred energy source. The liver converts complex carbohydrates to simple sugars (glucose) that can be used for immediate energy needs. Excess glucose is converted to glycogen and stored in the liver as energy reserves for later use. During times of physiologic stress, when energy needs rapidly accelerate, the liver converts stored glycogen back to glucose. When glycogen stores are depleted, the liver converts protein and stored fat (triglycerides) to glucose as an energy source.

All plasma proteins, except gamma globulins and immunoglobulins, are produced in the liver. Most of the circulating plasma proteins are also secreted by the liver, including albumin, prealbumin, and transferrin. Decreased serum albumin is a major indicator of severe liver dysfunction; however, with its half-life of 14 to 21 days, the deficit is not immediately evident.

The liver is the primary site for lipid synthesis and degradation. Because of the limited storage space for glucose as glycogen, excess glucose is converted to triglycerides by the liver. Triglycerides are then stored in adipose tissue deposits as a reserve energy source. Cholesterol, phospholipids, and lipoproteins, which are also produced by the liver, are necessary for cell wall integrity and transmission of nerve impulses.

Hepatic failure may result as a consequence of liver disease, including but not limited to cirrhosis, hepatitis, and drug toxicity (e.g., acetaminophen toxicity). Metabolic alterations associated with hepatic failure include disorders of synthesis and storage functions, and disorders of metabolic and excretory functions (Grossman & Porth, 2014; Holecek, 2015). Table 6–1 lists the disorders associated with the loss of these metabolic functions.

Reduced nutrient intake as a result of general malaise, nausea, vomiting, and/or diarrhea can result in hypercatabolism. Coagulopathy and gastrointestinal and esophageal varices often complicate feeding tube placement because of the increased potential for bleeding. Progressive malnutrition leads to increased breakdown of skeletal muscle with release of branched-chain amino acids (BCAAs) and aromatic amino acids (AAAs). Excessive uptake of AAAs by the central nervous system may contribute to hepatic encephalopathy, a characteristic of late hepatic failure, because the liver is unable to convert aromatic amino acids and ammonia (a by-product of protein and amino acid metabolism) to urea for excretion in the urine (Holecek, 2015).

Energy expenditure is typically increased in high-acuity patients with hepatic failure; therefore, they require high carbohydrate intake, normal-to-moderate protein intake, but low fat intake. Excessive fat intake contributes to progressive liver dysfunction with accumulation of fatty deposits in the liver cells. Because of the numerous metabolic alterations associated with hepatic failure, overfeeding is just as detrimental as underfeeding.

The patient with liver failure particularly benefits from having energy expenditure measured by indirect calorimetry. Severe protein restrictions that were once routinely used to reduce hepatic encephalopathy are no longer considered appropriate because this practice was found to exacerbate protein depletion; however, the appropriate amount and type of protein intake remain controversial. There is no evidence to support that BCAA-enriched formulas improve patient outcomes (McClave et al., 2016).

Table 6–1 Nutrition-Metabolic Alterations in Hepatic Failure

Liver Functions	Associated Disorders
Synthesis and storage	Hypoglycemia
	Hypoalbuminemia
	Decreased cholesterol production
	Impaired fat absorption
Metabolic and excretory	Impaired conversion of ammonia to urea
	Elevated serum ammonia levels
	Increased levels of circulating steroid hormones
	Decreased drug metabolism
	Hyperbilirubinemia

SOURCE: Data from Grossman & Porth (2014), Holecek (2015).

Table 6–2 Liver Disease: Summary of Major Nutritional Derangements and Recommendations

Major Derangements	Recommendations
Protein-calorie malnutrition Micronutrient deficiencies (especially zinc and vitamins A, D, E, and K) Altered amino acid metabolism (decreased circulating branched-chain amino acids [BCAAs] and increased circulating aromatic amino acids [AAAs]) Preferred source of calories is fat, not carbohydrates Marked insulin resistance (especially in cirrhosis)	Perform thorough nutritional assessment, using dry weight or usual weight Use indirect calorimetry rather than Harris-Benedict equation to estimate caloric needs Monitor: zinc, vitamins A, D, E, and prothrombin time (PT) Administer 1.2–2 g/kg per day of standard protein Small, frequent meals (four to six per day), including late evening meal (especially in cirrhosis) For alcohol-induced disease: Consider nitrogen-balance-maintaining diet (includes standard amino acids and replacement of potassium, phosphate, magnesium, and thiamine)

SOURCE: Data from Grossman & Porth (2014) and McClave et al. (2016).

Fluid and electrolyte imbalance and infection contribute to hepatic encephalopathy and should be corrected before initiating feeding with significant amounts of branched-chain amino acids (Abdelsayed, 2015; Grossman & Porth, 2014). Table 6–2 provides a summary of the major nutritional derangements associated with liver disease and nutrition-related recommendations.

Lung Failure

Respiratory failure is the inability of the lungs to maintain adequate pulmonary gas exchange, as evidenced by abnormalities in the respiratory components of arterial blood gases (PaO_2, SaO_2, pH, and $PaCO_2$). Malnutrition (undernutrition) is a common problem associated with many chronic pulmonary diseases, such as chronic obstructive pulmonary disease (COPD). When present, malnutrition adversely affects pulmonary structures and functions, which increases the work of breathing and can precipitate respiratory failure.

In the absence of adequate calorie and protein intake, the respiratory muscles are catabolized to meet acute energy requirements. As respiratory muscle is consumed, the patient's ability to properly ventilate becomes impaired, ultimately leading to hypoventilation and respiratory ventilation failure. Furthermore, as protein deficiency progresses, decreased intravascular colloid osmotic pressure may lead to pulmonary edema and adversely impact ventilation and perfusion.

Hypoventilation results in the retention of CO_2 and, if allowed to progress, can lead to respiratory acidosis. Carbon dioxide is produced by the body as an end-product of metabolism. The greatest quantity of CO_2, however, comes from the ingestion of carbohydrates. Therefore, in patients who have problems with CO_2 retention, excessive carbohydrate and overall calorie intake may contribute to increased CO_2 levels and ventilation failure. Elevations in CO_2 may clinically present as an increased respiratory rate, bounding pulse, ruddy face, and lethargy. Hospitalized patients receiving only intravenous glucose have a significant increase in their **respiratory quotient (RQ)**. The RQ is a ratio of the amount of CO_2 that is produced to the amount of oxygen that is consumed. An RQ greater than 1.0 suggests that the patient is receiving too much carbohydrate.

Phosphorus levels should be closely monitored in patients with impaired gas exchange. Phosphorus is a component of 2,3-diphosphoglycerate (2,3-DPG), which facilitates oxygen transport. Low levels of 2,3-DPG diminish hemoglobin's ability to release oxygen to the tissues. Elevated levels of 2,3-DPG lower hemoglobin's affinity for oxygen, thereby contributing to impaired gas exchange. In addition, low phosphorus may further exacerbate respiratory muscle function at the cellular level. Subsequently, mechanical ventilator weaning should not be attempted until phosphorus stores are replenished (McClave et al., 2016).

Dietary Clinical Implications Balanced nutrient intake is important for all patients, particularly for patients with potential or actual alterations of oxygenation and ventilation. The nutritional needs of patients with respiratory failure are similar to those of other hypermetabolic, hypercatabolic patients. For example, increased work of breathing increases energy expenditure. However, food intake may decline because of cough, dyspnea, fatigue, anorexia, and/or early satiety. Although nitrogen balance, blood urea nitrogen, and creatinine should be monitored frequently to individualize protein dosing, protein intake of 1.2–2 g/kg/day for patients with stable COPD is recommended to prevent loss of lean muscle mass (Schols et al., 2014). A fluid-restricted, energy-dense formula (1.5–2 kcal/mL) may be the optimal choice (McClave et al., 2016). Sodium and fluid restriction may be indicated for patients with pulmonary edema. Best practice guidelines include a balanced diet as the patient emerges from the critical phase of illness (Snider et al., 2015).

Table 6–3 summarizes the major nutritional derangements in pulmonary disease and the nutritional recommendations for patients with severe pulmonary disease.

Kidney Failure

The main function of the kidneys is to maintain homeostatic balance of fluids, electrolytes, and organic solutes (waste products of normal metabolism). The majority of solute load consists of nitrogenous wastes that are derived primarily from protein breakdown. Elevation of these waste products is called **azotemia** and results in complex metabolic disturbances. Kidney failure is classified as acute or chronic on the basis of presenting symptoms and underlying causes.

Acute Kidney Injury Acute kidney injury (AKI) is characterized by a sudden inability to excrete metabolic wastes and is often characterized by **oliguria** (diminished urinary output of less than 500 mL of urine in 24 hours), a sudden increase in serum blood urea nitrogen (BUN) and creatinine levels, and electrolyte abnormalities such as an elevated potassium level. Causes of AKI include decreased perfusion to the kidneys, a disease process within the kidneys, and obstruction to the outflow of urine.

Metabolic alterations of AKI include hypercatabolism, hypermetabolism, volume overload, and electrolyte imbalances. Inadequate nutritional intake, underlying comorbid conditions, and loss of nutrients in the dialysate in patients receiving hemodialysis can contribute to hypermetabolic and hypercatabolic responses. Serum levels of potassium, phosphorus, and magnesium are usually elevated as a result of catabolism of lean body mass and decreased electrolyte excretion by the kidneys. Fluid volume overload is a major concern during the oliguric phase of AKI. Replacement of kidney function during AKI can be accomplished through hemodialysis, peritoneal dialysis, or other forms of continuous hemofiltration to correct metabolic acidosis, volume overload, uremia, and electrolyte imbalances.

Energy and protein needs are determined by hypermetabolic needs, the underlying cause of AKI, and other comorbidities. In patients with mild acute kidney injury, 25–30 kcal/kg/day is usually sufficient to meet nutritional requirements (Bellizzi et al., 2015; McClave et al., 2016). Energy needs can be measured by indirect calorimetry. If unavailable, use of predictive formulas may be beneficial to avoid excessive caloric intake. Increased protein intake may necessitate more frequent dialysis. In the absence of dialysis, protein intake should be restricted

Table 6–3 Pulmonary Disease: Summary of Major Nutritional Derangements and Recommendations

Major Derangements	Recommendations
Weight loss related to increased REE Decreased body mass (fat and nonfat) Decreased ventilatory drive Decreased micronutrients, hypophosphatemia in particular	Perform thorough nutritional assessment. Supplemental nutritional support may be of benefit in patients with COPD, pulmonary failure, and acute respiratory distress syndrome (ARDS). Avoid overfeeding with carbohydrates (causes elevated CO_2 levels). Indirect calorimetry may assist in establishing caloric needs. Achieving a balanced diet is a realistic goal. Limited carbohydrate intake may be of benefit in reducing CO_2 load. Replace phosphate when hypophosphatemia is present. In patients with acute respiratory distress syndrome (ARDS), use fluid-restricted formulations if restriction is needed.

SOURCE: Data from McClave et al. (2016) and Reeves et al. (2014).

to approximately 1.2–2 g/kg/day. (For patients receiving continual renal replacement therapy [CRRT], or frequent hemodialysis, amino acid losses are increased [Umber, Wolley, Golper, Shaver, & Marshall, 2014].) Therefore, increased protein up to 2.5 g/kg/day is indicated for nutrition support (McClave et al., 2016). Many patients can be maintained on regular enteral formulas. For those patients who have electrolyte imbalances and elevated BUN and creatinine levels, specialty renal formulas are available that contain little or no electrolytes and are low in protein. Patients require close monitoring of their fluid and electrolyte status. Nutritional goals fluctuate relative to changes in the patient's underlying clinical condition and/or need for dialysis. It is important not to overly restrict protein in patients with AKF, as this can lengthen healing time.

Chronic Kidney Failure

Chronic kidney failure (CKF) is characterized by a progressive worsening of the kidneys' ability to excrete waste products, maintain fluid and electrolyte balance, and produce hormones. Uremia often develops and is the result of increased circulating solute waste in the bloodstream that the kidneys cannot eliminate. Clinically, uremia presents as malaise, weakness, muscle cramping, itching, nausea, delayed gastric emptying, vomiting, and complaints of a metallic taste in the mouth, which may promote anorexia. Anorexia may also be related to unappetizing and/or restricted renal-specific diets.

Energy supply must be adequate to meet the nutritional needs of the high-acuity patient who is hypermetabolic. Individuals receiving dialysis require protein supplementation to adjust for protein losses. The exact nutritional supplementation must be individualized based on multiple factors, such as the patient's general condition and nutritional status, stage of renal failure, type and frequency of dialysis, metabolic state, and comorbidities. Table 6–4 provides a summary of major nutritional derangements and nutritional recommendations for the patient with kidney disease.

Heart Failure

Many patients with moderate to severe heart failure develop a state of malnutrition known as cardiac **cachexia**. Unlike the adipose tissue loss in starvation, cardiac cachexia is characterized by a loss of lean body mass greater than 10%. Although it was once believed that the heart was spared from the muscle-wasting effects of malnutrition, it is now known that cardiac muscle is also affected. Loss of muscle mass in a cachectic heart results in less effective cardiac pumping and persistent circulatory failure. As cardiac failure continues and cardiac output decreases, tissues become increasingly deprived of oxygen. This is a form of tissue injury, and unless the underlying condition is corrected, the effects of hypermetabolism further the loss of lean muscle mass.

The nutritional needs of high-acuity patients with cardiac disease should be closely monitored, as the fluid volume associated with nutritional intake can have a negative effect on hemodynamics. Oxygen consumption increases with food intake. For patients who are able to take food orally, the postprandial elevation of oxygen consumption can be significant enough to cause hemodynamic instability.

The presence of food in the gastrointestinal tract results in greater blood flow through the splanchnic circulation. This increased blood volume occurs when blood is shunted from other vital organs, such as the heart, kidneys, and/or brain; therefore, intake for patients with cardiac disease should be limited to frequent, small amounts of food. For patients who require enteral or parenteral nutrition support, continuous infusion of the formula may be beneficial to regulate the effects of the nutrients. Nutrition delivery is dictated by individualized tolerance and route of administration.

The energy needs of patients with heart failure are based on current weight, activity restrictions, and the severity of cardiac disease. Low-density caloric formulas may be beneficial in helping obese patients reach a healthier weight, which places less stress on the heart. For undernourished patients with severe heart failure, energy needs may increase by as much as double their resting energy

Table 6–4 Renal Disease: Summary of Major Nutritional Derangements and Recommendations

Major Derangements	Recommendations

Protein-calorie malnutrition
Hypermetabolism
Accelerated protein breakdown
Impaired protein synthesis
Altered glucose utilization
Impaired lipid metabolism
Hypercalemia
Hypercalcemia
	Perform thorough nutritional assessment.
	Monitor serum electrolytes.
	Acute renal failure and receiving nutritional support:
	• Provide balanced mix of essential and nonessential amino acids.
	• If severely malnourished or hypercatabolic, provide protein intake of 1.2–2 g/kg per day.
	Not on dialysis, may benefit from:
	• Low protein diet (0.6–0.8 g/kg per day), limited volume; low potassium intake.
	• Essential amino acid supplementation.
	On dialysis, may benefit from:
	• Maintenance hemodialysis—protein intake up to 2.5 g/kg per day.
	• CRRT up to 2.5 g/kg/day
	• Supplement: water-soluble vitamins
	   ○ Phosphate binders per electrolyte monitoring.
	   ○ Timing of enteral feeding and PO intake with HD treatments important to coordinate.

SOURCE: Data from Bellizzi et al. (2015) and McClave et al. (2016).

expenditure (REE). Anorexia is also frequently observed in patients with cardiac failure; dyspnea, fatigue, and unappetizing, restricted diets may contribute to lack of appetite.

Sodium restriction varies as to the level of clinical stability. Sodium is restricted to not less than 2 g/day (Reilly et al., 2015). Diuretics commonly used to manage heart failure tend to reduce body stores of potassium, magnesium, and thiamine. Thiamine deficiency leads to vasodilation of the peripheral blood vessels, which can potentially produce high-output heart failure (Awtry & Colucci, 2015). These deficiencies should be monitored, replenished, or supplemented on a regular basis as they may impair cardiac contractility and are reversible.

Obesity

It is important to recognize the needs of the high-acuity bariatric patient. Malnutrition is less evident in the patient with a BMI greater than 25. Obese patients are more likely to have fuel utilization issues compared to lean patients but will have impaired wound healing if malnourished. Actual and ideal weight and waist circumference are important measures, not the adjusted body weight. Biomarkers for metabolic syndrome, including cholesterol, triglyceride, and serum glucose, help plan for nutrition needs. Comorbidities are included for a comprehensive evaluation of need. High-protein, hypocaloric formula is the recommendation, with caloric density for volume limitation. If a patient has a history of bariatric surgery, supplemental thiamine is indicated and evaluation and replacement of micronutrient deficiencies such as vitamin B_{12}, folate, trace minerals, and fat-soluble vitamins (McClave et al., 2016).

Burns

Burn patients are among those with the highest expected energy, protein, and fluid needs. The extent of the hypermetabolic response is related to the severity of the burn. In severe burn injury, caloric intake is increased to 100% above normal levels (Czapran et al., 2015; LeMone, Burke, Bauldoff & Gubrud, 2015). Indirect calorimetry is often standard practice for evaluating actual energy expenditure to optimize feeding. The energy demands of the burn patient are not self-limiting, and the hypermetabolic state and increased energy expenditure continue through the recovery and rehabilitative phase. Early nutrition support is recommended within 4–6 hours of injury, with protein replacement in the range of 1.5–2 g/kg/day (McClave et al., 2016).

Increased energy expenditure may persist longer in the burn patient than in patients with other types of tissue injuries. Individualized nutritional and energy requirements are crucial for successful wound healing and skin grafting. As with any extensive wounds, vitamin supplementation is essential for healing and the maintenance of overall immune function. Vitamins A, B complex, and C, along with zinc, support wound healing. Standardized protocols for vitamin supplementation are followed to enhance skin grafting success and prevent nutritional deficiencies.

Patients with burn injuries over more than 40% of total body surface area experience massive fluid shifts due to increased circulating histamines, prostaglandins, and cytokines. These substances increase capillary permeability, leading to loss of protein and subsequent fluid shift from the intravascular space to the interstitial space. Fluid resuscitation in the burn patient uses various formulas, such as the Parkland Formula and the Consensus Formula. Fluid resuscitation is initiated at the time of burn injury and generally continues for about 48 hours, until capillary seal is re-established, fluid shifts stabilize, and the patient regains hemodynamic stability. Table 6–5 provides a summary of major nutritional derangements and nutritional recommendations in acute burn injury.

Traumatic Brain Injury

Although the brain consumes 20% of the body's oxygen supply and receives 15% of the resting cardiac output, it cannot store glucose (Curtis & Epstein, 2014). Patients with traumatic brain injury (TBI) are severely hypermetabolic and catabolic due to the massive release of catecholamines (norepinephrine and epinephrine) and cortisol. The increased circulation of these hormones is responsible for the conversion of glycogen to glucose for energy.

Glucagon acts on the liver to convert amino acids into glucose; stored fat is also converted into glucose. Decreased insulin release from the pancreas, combined with rapid conversion of stored nutrients into glucose, results in

Table 6–5 Acute Severe Burn Injury: Summary of Major Nutritional Derangements and Recommendations

Major Derangements	Recommendations
Severe hypermetabolism and hypercatabolism Weight loss Decreased lean body mass Massive protein and calorie demands Energy expenditure: estimated at 20% to 30% above measured level to meet demands Gastric ileus is common.	Perform thorough nutritional assessment: • Emphasis: protein and energy needs • Ongoing assessment Indirect calorimetry may be of use (if feasible). Take an aggressive nutrition approach: • Enteral route: Initiate within 4–6 hours of postburn, locate tube postpyloric if possible. • High-calorie, high-protein supplementation. • Research does not support routine use of anabolic agents or specific nutrients.

SOURCE: Data from Czapran et al. (2015) and McClave et al. (2016).

hyperglycemia, which has been identified as a significant predictor of outcome from brain injury (Terzioglu, Ekinci, & Berkman, 2015). Patients with fever, seizure activity, and decerebrate or decorticate muscle posturing have an even higher rate of energy expenditure, and oxygen demand often exceeds supply.

To meet the high energy needs of the brain, cardiac output is increased along with the amount of oxygen that the brain extracts from the blood. However, if oxygen demand continues to exceed supply, hypoxemia occurs. The brain tries to compensate for the hypoxemia via vasodilation of the blood vessels to increase blood flow and oxygen delivery to the brain; however, this compensatory response contributes to the increased intracranial pressure that is the hallmark of brain injury. Hypoxemia leads to anaerobic metabolism in the brain tissue. Anaerobic metabolism cannot adequately supply the brain's energy needs and causes lactic acidosis (Bistrian & Driscoll, 2015; Curtis & Epstein, 2014).

Predictive energy requirement formulas, such as the Harris–Benedict equation, have been known to underestimate energy needs in this patient population. To prevent the deleterious effects of underfeeding, use of indirect calorimetry may be beneficial. Accelerated catabolic rate and increased nitrogen losses associated with traumatic brain injury are particularly notable in the first few days to weeks following the initial injury. The exact mechanism of significant urinary nitrogen losses is unclear. Immobility, decreased nitrogen efficiency, steroid administration, and decreased nutrient intake have all been suggested as causative factors.

Providing adequate energy and protein for a positive nitrogen balance is paramount to successful treatment, and aggressive nutrition support is recommended for patients with TBI. Patients with a decreased level of consciousness or a poor cough or gag reflex are also at increased risk for pulmonary aspiration. Also, because TBI patients are often unable to safely and/or adequately consume oral nutrition, alternative methods such as enteral nutrition should be employed, with consideration of an early gastrostomy tube for stable access.

Even though gastrointestinal motility is greatly diminished, absorption of nutrients by the small bowel is usually maintained. Therefore, placement of a postpyloric small-bore feeding tube may be preferred. Endoscopic feeding tube placement may be necessary. Enteral feeding during drug-induced coma is efficacious and well tolerated by many patients, thus limiting the need for parenteral nutrition. If postpyloric feeding placement may be delayed, initiating feeding with a gastric-placed tube is recommended so as not to delay nutritional intake, monitoring for response (McClave et al., 2016).

Section One Review

1. A high-acuity client with hepatic failure may typically experience which condition? (Select all that apply.)
   A. Breakdown of skeletal muscle protein
   B. Increased energy expenditure
   C. Conversion of glycogen back to glucose
   D. Hyperglycemia
   E. Impaired fat absorption

2. Which nutritional goals would be set for the client experiencing pulmonary failure?
   A. Higher sodium content
   B. Very low protein content
   C. Lower carbohydrate content
   D. Higher fat content

3. A high-acuity client with acute kidney failure may typically experience abnormalities in which areas? (Select all that apply.)
   A. Protein catabolism
   B. Fluid levels
   C. Metabolic rate
   D. Glucose levels
   E. Electrolyte levels

4. Nutritional intake is supplemented with vitamins A, B complex, and C, as well as zinc, for which reason?
   A. To promote red blood cell count
   B. To promote wound healing
   C. To lower BUN level
   D. To lower cholesterol

Answers: 1. (A, B, C, E), 2. C, 3. (A, B, C, E), 4. B

Section Two: Enteral Nutrition

For the high-acuity patient who is highly catabolic (nitrogen loss greater than 15–20 g/day), nutritional support should be initiated as soon as possible. The goal is to minimize further breakdown of the skeletal muscle and visceral protein stores. Nutrition support should be provided via the enteral route in critically ill patients with a functional GI tract (McClave et al., 2016). Unless there is known traumatic disruption or chronic malabsorptive disease, it is generally assumed that the GI tract is capable of absorbing nutrients, fluids, and electrolytes. Patients with a high-acuity illness or injury who are unable to safely consume oral nutrition require a small-bore feeding tube (Harvey et al., 2014).

Criteria for Selection of Enteral Nutrition

Selection of the specific type of enteral feeding is based on three criteria: GI integrity and function, baseline nutritional status, and severity and duration of illness. When assessing GI function, it is important to first determine when the patient is expected to be able to receive oral nutrition.

Gastrointestinal Integrity and Function Enteral nutrition should be considered when the patient (a) cannot or should not take in food orally *or* (b) oral intake is insufficient or unreliable; *and* (c) if the patient has a functional GI tract and access can be safely achieved. Feeding tube placement is recommended within 24 to 48 hours of admission. The specific type of feeding tube placed is related to the anticipated time of recovery, the patient's level of consciousness, the patient's comfort, and cost effectiveness (McClave et al., 2016).

Illness Severity and Possible Duration Energy expenditure and calorie and protein requirements increase with the severity of illness. The hypermetabolism of the metabolic stress response can persist for extended periods in the presence of physiologic complications such as extensive wounds or sepsis. Advances in the understanding of the metabolic stress response and the immunologic functions of the intestines have led to a greater appreciation for the need to provide nutrition support to the high-acuity patient early during the course of illness or injury (Casaer & Ziegler, 2015; Dwyer, 2015).

Timing of Nutrition Support Providing nutrition early in the course of illness or injury is a treatment priority. Enteral nutrition (EN) feedings should be initiated within 24 to 48 hours of admission and the volume increased over a 48- to 72-hour time frame to the goal volume (McClave et al., 2016). Sepsis guidelines recommend early, limited enteral nutrition (Elke, Kott, & Weiler, 2015). Early delivery of protein and calories supported favorable outcomes (Elke, Wang, Weiler, Day, & Heyland, 2014). Feeding protocols that target volume versus rate promote the nurse's critical thinking and flexibility to deliver the prescribed amount in a 24-hour period (McClave et al., 2016).

Readiness for enteral feeding should not be determined by the presence of bowel sounds alone. Active bowel sounds have been used as criteria to initiate feeding, but there is no scientific evidence to support this practice. Bowel sounds are a poor indicator of small bowel motility and nutrient absorption, as they are the result of air passing through the intestinal tract. Many interventions prevent the normal passage of air through the GI tract, such as nasogastric suctioning, sedation, and nothing-by-mouth (NPO) status. Therefore, waiting for bowel sounds places the patient at undue risk for malnutrition (McClave et al., 2016).

Benefits of Enteral Nutrition

A major benefit of enteral nutrition is that it helps maintain GI barrier function. Reductions in GI barrier function are associated with increased bacterial translocation, systemic inflammatory response syndrome (SIRS), and multiple organ dysfunction syndrome (MODS). In animal models, fasting is associated with increased translocation of bacteria from the GI tract into mesenteric lymph nodes, portal circulation, and the peritoneal cavity (Dwyer, 2015). The major benefits and contraindications of enteral nutrition are summarized in Box 6–1.

Although invasive, feeding tube insertion has less inherent risk of mechanical and infectious complications than central venous line insertion for total parenteral nutrition (TPN) administration. The cost of enteral formulas is significantly lower than the daily cost of TPN. Even the most expensive specialty enteral formulas do not equal the cost of providing TPN.

Common Contraindications for Enteral Nutrition

Many patients who were once thought to require TPN are now often successfully fed via the enteral route; contraindications to enteral nutrition have diminished as its safety and efficacy have been demonstrated in many types of high-acuity patients. Enteral nutrition can be provided to patients with GI fistulas if the tube can be positioned distal to the site of the fistula. Mechanical obstruction is the only absolute contraindication to enteral feedings.

BOX 6–1 Major Benefits and Contraindications for Enteral Nutrition

Major Benefits
- Maintenance of GI barrier function
- Maintenance of GI immunologic function
- More physiologic than parenteral nutrition
- Possible decrease in severity of metabolic stress response
- More cost-effective than parenteral nutrition
- Decreased risk of infectious complications
- Enhanced wound healing

Contraindications
- Absolute contraindication
  - Mechanical obstruction of GI tract
- Relative contraindications
  - Severe hemorrhagic pancreatitis
  - Necrotizing enterocolitis
  - Prolonged ileus
  - Severe, intractable diarrhea
  - Protracted vomiting
  - Enteric high-output fistulas
  - Intestinal dysmotility
  - Intestinal ischemia
- Nasal septal defect
- Esophageal varices
- Written advance directive declining a feeding tube

Types of Enteral Feedings

Numerous enteral formulas are available. Commonly used formulas are lactose free and nutritionally complete and contain a mixture of carbohydrates, proteins, fats, vitamins, trace elements, and water. Choosing the appropriate formula for the high-acuity patient is based on the patient's energy and protein requirements, the underlying disease state or organ function, intestinal absorptive and digestive function, and fluid requirements. In addition, the location of the feeding tube tip, cost, and feeding duration must all be considered. Differences between formulas lie in how the nutrients are structured, their varying osmolality, and their range in caloric density, typically 1 to 2 kcal/mL. Interdisciplinary collaboration for planning care ensures the data for the best formula and strategy. Table 6–6 summarizes selected enteral feeding formulas and the patients they are most appropriate for.

Free Water   Free water—that is, water containing no additives—may be ordered for the patient receiving enteral feedings for a variety of reasons, including hydration, flushing to maintain tube patency, diluting medications, and reconstitution of the enteral nutrition formula (Dwyer, 2015). Free water can come from a variety of sources, such as tap water, sterile water, or purified water. The normal daily fluid requirement is about 30 mL of water/kg of body mass plus replacement of fluids that are lost from the body (e.g., sweating, diarrhea, and wound output) (Bistrian & Driscoll, 2015). The fluid content of enteral feedings often is not sufficient to meet the patient's daily hydration requirements; therefore, additional free water may be ordered to ensure adequate hydration.

In high-acuity patients, particularly those with a compromised immune system, care must be taken to provide a safe (uncontaminated) water source to prevent possible infection. For this reason, in the high-acuity setting, sterile water is recommended (McClave et al., 2016).

Table 6–6 Summary of Selected Enteral Feeding Formulas

Type of Formula	Comments	Formula Contents	Brand Name Examples
Complete formulas	Suitable for most patients requiring enteral feedings	• 1 kcal/mL • Protein: approximately 14% total kcal • Fat: approximately 30% total kcal • Carbohydrates: approximately 60% total kcal • Recommended daily intake of all minerals and vitamins is 1,500 mL/day.	Compleat Ensure Isocal Nutren Isolan Sustacal Resource
High-calorie complete	Appropriate for patients on fluid restriction	• As above; provides 1.5–2 kcal/mL	Ensure Plus Sustacal HC Comply Nutren 1.5 Resource Plus Isocal HCN Magnacal TwoCal HN
Complete lactose free, high residue	Appropriate to prevent or treat diarrhea, constipation	• Same as complete formulas and also provides fiber	Jevity Profiber Nutren 1.0 with fiber Fiberlan Sustacal with fiber Ultracal Ensure with fiber FiberSource Accupep HPF
Disease-specific formulas	Available for kidney failure, respiratory failure, liver failure with hepatic encephalopathy, diabetes	• Contain essential amino acids, fat greater than 50% total kcal, high amounts of branched-chain amino acids	Amin-Aid Travasorb Renal Aminess Pulmocare NutriVent Hepatic-Acid II Travasorb Hepatic Glucerna
Formulas for immunocompromised, systemic inflammatory response syndrome (SIRS), or physiological stress states	Appropriate for patients with AIDS, burns, trauma, sepsis, SIRS, ARDS	• Immunomodulating formulas contain enhanced arginine, omega-3 fatty acids nucleotides, beta carotene, 1–1.3 kcal/mL. • Formulas for physiologic stress contain increased branched-chain amino acids, high protein, or both, 1–1.2 kcal/mL.	Impact Immun-Aid Perative Oxepa Physiologic stress formulas include: TraumaCal Impact Replete

SOURCE: Data from Bistrian & Driscoll (2015) and LeMone et al. (2015).

Nursing Care
The Patient Receiving Supplemental Enteral Nutrition

Expected Patient Outcomes and Related Interventions

Outcome 1: The patient will achieve adequate nutritional status.

Assess and compare the patient's nutritional status to established norms, patient baselines, and trends.

Type and severity of malnutrition
Perform assessment of nutritional status or other nutrition-specific assessment. Weight and height.
Consult a dietician.
Evaluate nitrogen balance status: obtain urine urea nitrogen (UUN) and 24-hour protein intake.
Assess vitamin and mineral status (e.g., zinc, iron, magnesium, phosphate, folic acid, vitamins A, D, and E).
Determine the number and type of calories needed to meet nutritional requirements.
Indirect calorimetry
Respiratory quotient (RQ)
Fick method
Harris–Benedict equation with stress factors included
Monitor intake and output closely, including all losses from the GI tract.
Monitor the patient's response to treatment.
Daily weights
Baseline and periodic reassessment of anthropometric measurements
Periodic re-evaluation of vitamin and mineral status (e.g., zinc, iron, magnesium, phosphate, folic acid, vitamins A, D, and E), and white blood cell (WBC) count
Do not place feedings on hold for repositioning.
Do not hold feeding for residual volumes less than 500 mL.
Periodic interdisciplinary team review of plan of care

Institute measures to initiate and maintain enteral feedings using an evidence-based protocol.

Insert or assist with insertion of enteral feeding tube. Gastric placement is best option to get feeding initiated.
If postpyloric route is chosen, consider prokinetic agent(s) as ordered to facilitate passage through pyloric sphincter. Fluoroscopic guidance may be necessary.
Ensure that feeding tube tip is properly located with radiograph before initiating feedings.
Secure device with commercial tube holder or commercial bridle to deter self-removal.
Administer enteral nutrition as prescribed.
Frequently assess for intolerance.

Patients are at risk for:
Diarrhea
Fluid and electrolyte imbalance

Under-nutrition
Infection

Outcome 2: The patient will experience no aspiration.

Assess and compare the patient's pulmonary status to established norms, patient baselines, and trends.

Risks for aspiration
Altered level of consciousness
GI intolerance
High gastric residual volume
Gastric or abdominal distension
Gastric or abdominal discomfort
Improperly positioned feeding tube

Institute measures to prevent aspiration.

Position head of bed at 30- to 45-degree elevation when delivering enteral tube feeding. Use pump to deliver a set hourly tube-monitored feeding rate.
Perform routine oral care with subglottic suctioning of oral secretions.
Verify tube placement before initiating enteral feedings; secure feeding tubes with bridle device to prevent tube displacement.

Patients are at risk for:
Aspiration

Outcome 3: The patient will maintain adequate fluid volume.

Assess and compare the patient's fluid volume status to established norms, patient baselines, and trends.

Indications of dehydration (e.g., hypotension, tachycardia, decreased urinary output, and thirst)

Institute measures to maintain adequate fluid volume.

Identify factors that may cause diarrhea (e.g., bacterial contamination of feeding formula, sorbitol-containing medications, and prokinetic agents).
Decrease rate of bolus feeding or change to continuous rate to prevent rapid fluid shifts and/or diarrhea.
Provide fiber supplement to bulk up stools and prevent diarrhea.
Consider probiotic administration.
Check infusion rates for enteral feeding administration.
Provide free water as prescribed to offset the high osmolarity of tube feedings.

Patients are at risk for:
Incontinence
Diarrhea
Disturbed body image
Hypovolemia
Infection

SOURCE: Data from DiLibero et al. (2015); McClave et al. (2016); and Parks et al. (2013).

Feeding Tube Placement

A number of weighted or nonweighted small-bore (8 to 12 Fr) feeding tubes made of Silastic or polyurethane are available. Enteral feeding access can be achieved by a variety of methods that include blind or radiologic-assisted placement of a small-bore feeding tube, percutaneous placement of a gastrostomy and/or jejunostomy tube, and surgical placement of a gastrostomy or jejunostomy tube. The expected duration of need for enteral feedings helps determine the type of placement. For example, if a patient is expected to require prolonged or permanent enteral feedings, percutaneous or surgical placement may be the best approach. The small-bore feeding tube is the least invasive and most economical device. This polyurethane weighted or nonweighted tube can be used for gastric or transpyloric feeding.

Successful postpyloric placement of the feeding tube via the nasal or oral cavity often requires advanced clinician skill, special patient positioning and tube design, and the use of prokinetic medications to help assist with tube positioning and advancement. Passage of the feeding tube from the stomach into the small bowel is associated with upper GI motility. Motor function of the upper GI tract is frequently altered in critically ill patients; those on mechanical ventilation; and those with chronic conditions, such as diabetes mellitus, vagotomy, and intestinal pseudo-obstruction (Bryant, Phang, & Abrams, 2015). Repeated attempts to position the feeding tube postpyloric can cause patient discomfort and delay initiation of feeding. Repeated abdominal x-rays to verify tube position and clinician time contribute to increased cost. Electromagnetic devices are available at the bedside to follow the tip for placement. While helpful, this image may not replace the verification by radiograph as tubes may be malpositioned and the accuracy of electromagnetic devices has not been established (Bryant et al., 2015).

Gastric Versus Postpyloric Feeding

One of the ongoing controversies of nutrition support is whether high-acuity patients should be fed by means of intragastric or postpyloric feeding. In some patients, when repeated blind attempts to place the feeding tube postpyloric delays onset of feeding, it may be beneficial to initiate gastric feeding with a more concentrated formula at a low hourly rate. Delayed gastric emptying (gastroparesis) associated with critical illness is a primary reason for preference of feeding into the small bowel instead of the stomach. Some clinicians believe that transpyloric feeding decreases the risk of aspiration, but that belief is not supported by the literature (McClave et al., 2016).

Medications such as histamine H2-receptor antagonists (H2-blockers) (e.g., cimetidine [Tagamet]) and proton pump inhibitors (e.g., omeprazole [Prilosec]) increase intragastric pH, thereby reducing the protection normally provided by more acidic gastric pH against bacterial colonization. Aspiration of colonized bacteria is the major mechanism for the entry of bacteria into the lungs and contributes to the development of healthcare-associated pneumonia, particularly in mechanically ventilated patients. Other medications that cause relaxation of the lower esophageal sphincter, such as theophylline, dopamine, anticholinergics, calcium channel blockers, and meperidine, also increase the risk of aspiration. Aspiration of colonized oral secretions is most associated with the cause of healthcare-associated pneumonia, supporting routine oral care and elevation of the head of the bed (McClave et al., 2016).

Complications of Enteral Nutrition

Complications of enteral feedings are classified into five categories: gastrointestinal, nutritional, mechanical, metabolic, and infectious. Table 6–7 lists potential enteral complications, possible causes, and suggested treatment.

Clinicians may halt feedings inappropriately based on a single high gastric residual volume (GRV) of 400 to 500 mL of enteral feeding formula. Although a single high GRV should raise the suspicion of intolerance, one high value does not necessarily indicate feeding failure. Such practices promote malnutrition. The current recommendation for patients is the elimination of routine GRV evaluation (McClave et al., 2016). Steps to reduce aspiration risk and improve tolerance of gastric feedings include prokinetic agents, continuous infusion of enteral feed, comprehensive oral care, and head of bed elevation.

If the patient demonstrates overt signs of regurgitation, vomiting, or aspiration, enteral feedings should be held, and the patient should be assessed and re-evaluated for alternative strategies to meet nutritional goals. Promotility agents may be useful if high GRVs persist.

Supportive Drug Therapy

Malnourished patients generally require supplemental vitamins and minerals to restore essential micronutrients. A multivitamin and mineral supplement may be given, or therapy may be tailored to correct specific deficiencies. See the "Related Pharmacotherapy: Nursing Implications of Vitamin and Mineral Supplement Administration" feature for nursing implications of vitamin and mineral supplements.

Table 6–7 Complications Associated with Enteral Nutrition

Complication	Possible Cause	Suggested Treatment
GASTROINTESTINAL		
Nausea/vomiting	Hyperosmolar feeding	Start isotonic feeding.
	Rapid infusion rate	Start feedings slowly and advance as tolerated.
	Obstruction	Reassess GI function.
	Delayed gastric emptying	Start prokinetic agent (metoclopramide, erythromycin) to increase gastric emptying: feed distal to pylorus.
	Contaminated solution or infusion set	Hang canned formula for no longer than manufacturer's recommendation; change container and infusion set every 24 hours; use good hand-hygiene technique before handling formulas.
	Medication side effect	Consider alternative medication. Consider antiemetic.
Diarrhea	Antibiotics may alter intestinal flora, causing bacteria overgrowth: *Clostridium difficile* infection and pseudomembranous colitis.	Send stool specimens for culture and sensitivity, WBC count, ova, parasites, and *C. difficile* cytotoxin. Flexible sigmoidoscopy provides faster and more reliable diagnosis than stool studies; treatment of choice for *C. difficile* toxin is IV/PO metronidazole (Flagyl) or PO vancomycin (Vancocin); hold any antidiarrheal agents until infectious source is ruled out.
	Liquid medications containing sorbitol or other concentrated sugar base have a laxative effect (common cause of diarrhea in patients receiving liquid medications).	Use non-sorbitol medication products; if crushing medications, use a crusher to avoid tube obstruction.
	Iatrogenic without other cause	Consider fiber supplement in divided doses over a 24-hour period.
NUTRITIONAL		
Malnutrition	Underfeeding (delivering less than prescribed amount of EN) can result in malnutrition; existing malnutrition is associated with loss of microvilli, villous brush border enzymes, and subsequent reduction in intestinal absorptive surface area.	Minimize interruptions to enteral tube feeding delivery; holding enteral feedings for frequent procedures or instillation of medications may prevent patient from receiving needed energy and protein. Minimize high gastric residuals with high-calorie, low-volume enteral formula and prokinetic agents.
Hypoalbuminemia	While not a complication of EN therapy, an existing low serum albumin complicates effectiveness and tolerance of EN; a low intravascular osmotic pressure prevents nutrients from being absorbed from the GI tract.	Poor tolerance is evident in patients with serum albumin less than 2.5 mg/dL; benefits of albumin administration should outweigh cost and potential complications.
MECHANICAL		
Feeding tube occlusion	Medications, from failure to flush tubing properly; viscous formulas	***Prevention* is key.** Irrigate feeding tube with 30–50 mL warm water every 4 hours, before and after medication administration.
		Alternate positive/negative pressure with syringe to dislodge clot.
		Warm water may dissolve clots. There is no evidence to use colas or juice to open occlusion.
		Do not attempt to dislodge clots with stylet; may cause esophageal or gastric mucosal perforations.
METABOLIC		
Hypoglycemia	Sudden cessation of feeding	Provide supplemental glucose.
Hyperglycemia	Stress response, diabetic or glucose intolerance	Usually resolves as stress is alleviated; initiate feedings slowly; monitor blood glucose every 6 hours.
Electrolyte imbalance	Dehydration or fluid overload	Monitor fluid status; monitor electrolytes and replace as needed.
	Excess losses (diarrhea, fistula, nasogastric drainage, ascites)	Replace fluid and electrolytes as needed.
		Provide appropriate organ failure formula.
INFECTIOUS		
Aspiration pneumonia	High-risk patients include those who are comatose, weak, debilitated, or intubated or have tracheostomies or neuromuscular disorders.	Elevate head of bed at least 30 degrees; feed into small bowel distal to pylorus. Provide comprehensive oral care with subglottic suctioning, toothbrush and chlorhexidine mouth rinse to reduce oral colonization. Dye should not be added to enteral feeding to identify aspiration of gastric contents, as dye lacks the required sensitivity and has been associated with several adverse events.

SOURCE: Data from Bistrian & Driscoll (2015) and McClave et al. (2016).

Related Pharmacotherapy
Nursing Implications of Vitamin and Mineral Supplement Administration

Fat-soluble Vitamins

Vitamins A, D, E, K

Action and Uses

The fat-soluble vitamins are absorbed in the GI tract. Vitamins A and D are stored in the liver. Toxicity may develop if these vitamins are taken in excessive amounts.

Major Adverse Effects

Usually well tolerated. Hypersensitivity during parenteral administration is rare but potentially life threatening.

Nursing Implications

Monitor carefully for hypersensitivity reactions during parenteral administration. Have emergency equipment available.

Administer vitamin A with food.

Avoid administering vitamin K intravenously.

Teach patient the importance of eating a well-balanced diet.

If indicated, provide a list of foods high in specific vitamins.

Caution that excessive intake of these vitamins may lead to vitamin toxicity.

Water-soluble Vitamins

Vitamin C (ascorbic acid)

Vitamin B complex: thiamine (B_1), riboflavin (B_2), niacin (nicotinic acid), pyridoxine hydrochloride (B_6), pantothenic acid, and biotin

Action and Uses

These vitamins are used to prevent or treat deficiency problems. If the diet is deficient in one vitamin, it is usually deficient in other vitamins as well; therefore, multivitamin preparations are often administered. Most of these vitamins are well absorbed from the GI tract.

Major Adverse Effects

Usually well tolerated; hypersensitivity reactions are rare but can be life threatening.

Nursing Implications

Monitor for responses to replacement therapy.

Monitor sensitivity reactions from parenteral administration.

Have emergency equipment available.

Do not exceed recommended daily allowances.

Minerals

Sodium, potassium, magnesium, calcium, copper, fluoride, iodine, zinc, manganese, chromium, selenium

Action and Uses

Minerals are inorganic chemicals that are vital to a variety of physiologic functions. Also called trace elements, minerals are part of a balanced diet. Recommended daily intake has not been established for all mineral substances. The dosage of prescribed minerals depends on the specific deficiency, route of administration, and patient's general health.

Major Adverse Effects

Hypersensitivity reactions are rare but can be life threatening.

Nursing Implications

All mineral preparations should be diluted prior to administration.

Prior to administration of iodine, assess for history of hypersensitivity to iodine or seafood; if hypersensitive, notify the physician, pharmacist, or nurse practitioner.

Except for fluoride and zinc, administer with or after meals.

SOURCE: Data from Dwyer (2015).

Section Two Review

1. A client has a relatively well-functioning gastrointestinal tract but is unable to take adequate nutrients by mouth. What is the best method for administering nutritional support to this client?
   A. Nasoenteric feedings
   B. Oral diet
   C. Withholding nutrition
   D. TPN

2. What are some advantages of enteral nutrition over TPN? (Select all that apply.)
   A. Lower risk of bacterial translocation
   B. Providing central venous access
   C. Maintaining GI morphology and function
   D. Lower cost
   E. Decreased risk of infection

3. Nasoenteric feeding is best imitated by placement into which organ?
   A. Esophagus
   B. Stomach
   C. Small bowel
   D. Large bowel

4. Bacterial overgrowth (*C. difficile* infection and pseudomembranous colitis) may cause diarrhea in patients receiving enteral nutrition. What are the suggested diagnostic and treatment interventions? (Select all that apply.)
   A. Sending stool specimens for testing
   B. Performing flexible sigmoidoscopy
   C. Administering antidiarrheal agents
   D. Administering metronidazole (Flagyl) or vancomycin (Vancocin)
   E. Assessing white blood cell count (WBC)

Answers: 1. A, 2. (A, C, D, E), 3. B, 4. (A, B, D, E)

Section Three: Total Parenteral Nutrition

Total parenteral nutrition (TPN) is a nutritionally complete, intravenously delivered solution composed of macronutrients (carbohydrates, proteins, lipids), micronutrients (electrolytes, vitamins, trace minerals) and water. Its use is indicated when oral or enteral nutrition is not possible or when absorption or function of the gastrointestinal tract is not sufficient (or unreliable) to meet the nutritional needs of the patient. TPN is contraindicated in patients with a functioning, usable GI tract capable of absorbing adequate nutrients; when sole dependence is anticipated to last fewer than 7 days; when aggressive support is not warranted; and when the risks of TPN outweigh the potential benefits. TPN is recommended as soon as possible after ICU admission if high nutritional risk and enteral nutrition is not feasible. With the exception of severe hemorrhagic pancreatitis, necrotizing enterocolitis, prolonged ileus, and distal bowel obstruction, some enteral nutrition is recommended in addition to TPN to maintain GI integrity (McClave et al., 2016). For more information, see the "Nursing Care: The Patient Receiving Parenteral Nutrition" feature.

Nursing Care
The Patient Receiving Parenteral Nutrition

Expected Patient Outcomes and Related Interventions

Outcome 1: The patient will achieve adequate nutritional status.

Assess and compare the patient's nutritional status to established norms, patient baselines, and trends.
  [Refer to Outcome 1 in "Nursing Care: The Patient Receiving Supplemental Enteral Nutrition"]

Institute measures to initiate and maintain parenteral nutrition.
  Assist with insertion of central line for TPN (or peripheral line for peripheral parenteral nutrition [PPN]), using bundle approach.
  Hand hygiene
  Sterile barrier precaution
  Chlorhexidine skin antisepsis
  Optimal site selection
  During line insertion, monitor for signs and symptoms of:
    Pneumothorax
    Catheter fracture
    Subclavian or carotid artery puncture
    Air embolism
    Cardiac dysrhythmias
  Administer parenteral nutrition as prescribed.
  Frequently assess for intolerance and/or infectious, metabolic, or mechanical complications.
  Monitor for hyperglycemia, abnormal liver, and renal function.
  Monitor intake and output closely, including all losses from the GI tract.
  Monitor the patient's response to treatment.
  Daily interdisciplinary team monitoring for line need and prompt removal.

Related conditions
  Increased risk for hypovolemia
  Increased risk for electrolyte imbalance
  Increased risk for malnutrition (under-nutrition)
  Increased risk for infectious complications

Outcome 2: The patient will maintain normal fluid and electrolyte balance.

Assess and compare the patient's fluid and electrolyte balance to established norms, patient baselines, and trends.
  Monitor the patient closely for signs of dehydration and electrolyte imbalance.

Institute measures to maintain fluid and electrolyte balance.
  Maintain strict intake and output monitoring, including all emesis and tube drainage.
  Maintain IV access and administer IV fluids as ordered.
  Report abnormal electrolytes to provider and replace electrolytes as ordered.

Related conditions.
  Increased risk for hypovolemia
  Increased risk for malnutrition

Outcome 3: The patient will experience no central line–associated infection

Assess and compare the patient's central line status to established norms, patient baselines, and trends.
  Signs and symptoms of central line–associated sepsis:
    Sudden onset of fever, rigors, or chills that coincide with parenteral infusion
    Erythema, swelling, tenderness, or purulent drainage from catheter site
    Sudden temperature elevation that resolves on catheter removal
    Leukocytosis

Sudden onset of glucose intolerance that may develop up to 12 hours before temperature elevation

Bacteremia/septicemia/septic shock

Institute measures to prevent central line–associated infection.

Catheter insertion

For central venous catheter (CVC) line: insert in subclavian vein; avoid lower extremity insertions.

Meticulous hand hygiene and aseptic technique

Central line insertion: maximal sterile barrier precautions (cap, mask, sterile gown, sterile gloves, sterile drape)

PICC insertion: recommend same as central line placement

Skin antisepsis: aqueous chlorhexidine gluconate

SOURCE: Data from Bistrian & Driscoll (2015), Marschall et al. (2014), and Tapia et al. (2015).

Catheter site dressings: either gauze dressings or transparent dressings (transparent dressing can be left in place for duration of catheter insertion)

In-line filters may decrease phlebitis but no clear support for prevention of infection

Consider use of antimicrobial- or antiseptic-impregnated catheter

Catheter replacement:

Central catheters, including PICCs: Timing of replacement is controversial for reducing infection—advocacy for no routine replacement and removal when there is no longer a need for central access.

Related conditions

Increased risk for infectious complications

Delivery of Parenteral Nutrition

Total parenteral nutrition (TPN) with greater than 10% glucose is delivered through a central line (Figure 6–1) to allow higher blood volumes in the larger central veins to rapidly dilute and disperse the solution, which decreases the vessel irritation associated with the increased osmolarity of the solution. Multilumen central venous catheters are commonly used. These catheters allow for one central venous access, with multiple ports for hemodynamic monitoring (e.g., central venous pressure [CVP]) and fluid and medication delivery without risk of drug incompatibility. If TPN is expected to be needed for more than a few weeks, a more permanent device, such as a subcutaneously tunneled central catheter or implanted vascular access device, should be placed.

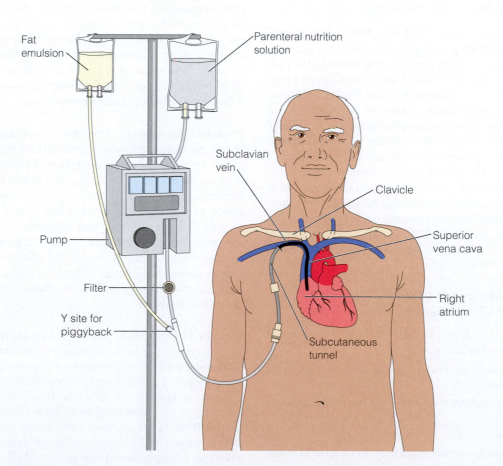

Figure 6–1 Total parenteral nutrition through a catheter in the right subclavian vein.

SOURCE: From LeMone, Burke, Bauldoff, & Gubrud (2015). Reproduced by permission of Pearson Education, Inc.

A peripherally inserted central catheter (PICC) also allows central venous access for TPN administration. A PICC line is inserted peripherally, usually into the basilic vein, and advanced so that the tip of the catheter rests in the superior vena cava. A PICC line is often inserted and managed by a vascular access team of nurses.

TPN has sometimes been referred to as *hyperalimentation* or *hyperal*. These terms are not preferred because they incorrectly imply that the patient is receiving more calories, protein, and other nutrients than may be required. TPN solutions are designed to meet the individual energy and protein needs of a patient based on the clinical condition, underlying disease states, and organ function.

Glucose concentrations of 10% or less can be delivered as peripheral parenteral nutrition (PPN). PPN is infused into smaller, peripheral veins (e.g., the basilic vein) and is often used for short-term nutrition support (7 to 10 days) or as a supplement during transitional phases to enteral or oral nutrition routes (McClave et al., 2016).

Complications of Total Parenteral Nutrition

TPN therapy is not without risks. Complications range from mild to severe, and they may increase hospital length of stay or precipitate a potentially life-threatening crisis. The three major categories of TPN therapy complications are infectious, metabolic, and mechanical.

Infectious Complications Both the TPN solution and the indwelling catheter are prime sites for infection, because of the high glucose content; any break in the system is a potential site for localized infection that can progress to a systemic infection if left unchecked. **Central line–associated bloodstream infection (CLABSI)** has a significant mortality rate, and hospital stays are reportedly longer and more expensive as a result of complications and treatment associated with central lines (Bistrian & Driscoll, 2015). Some of the more common reasons for CLABSI include lack of sterility during placement of central lines and inadequate precautions taken during maintenance of the central line and insertion site (e.g., changing tubing, dressings, bags). CLABSI events are preventable, and bundled care practices have improved outcomes (Marschall et al., 2014).

Clinical Manifestations of CLABSI. The clinical signs and symptoms of CLABSI include:

- Sudden onset of fever, rigors, or chills that coincide with parenteral infusion
- Erythema, swelling, tenderness, or purulent drainage from the catheter site
- Sudden temperature elevation that resolves on catheter removal
- Leukocytosis
- Sudden glucose intolerance that may occur up to 12 hours before temperature elevation
- Bacteremia/septicemia/septic shock

Prevention and Treatment of CLABSI. To minimize the risk of central line infections, one port of multilumen catheters should be dedicated to TPN administration. The catheter insertion site and access port require meticulous care. Although transparent dressings allow for easier observation of the catheter entrance site, they have a tendency to trap moisture and, hence, lead to a higher incidence of infection than traditional, sterile gauze dressings (Bistrian & Driscoll, 2015).

The insertion site should be monitored for signs of leakage, erythema, edema, and inflammation. Chlorhexidine solution, a local antiseptic, should be used for insertion site care. In addition, the use of catheters impregnated with either chlorhexidine/silver sulfadiazine or minocycline/rifampin combinations may also reduce the incidence of central line–associated infection. Treatment often includes topical and systemic antibiotics and catheter removal (Bistrian & Driscoll, 2015).

Metabolic Complications Metabolic complications of TPN are similar to those of enteral nutrition. (Refer to Section Two for complications, possible causes, and suggested treatment.) Other possible metabolic derangements caused by TPN are hyperglycemia, prerenal azotemia, and hepatic dysfunction.

Hyperglycemia. Hyperglycemia, or elevated blood glucose over 180 mg/dL, commonly occurs in parenteral and enteral nutrition. Elevated glucose levels have been shown to reduce neutrophil chemotaxis and phagocytosis and may be an independent risk factor for infection. Glycemic control can be achieved by increasing insulin in the TPN solution, maintaining a continuous insulin drip during TPN administration, or administering sliding-scale insulin subcutaneously at regular intervals.

Prerenal Azotemia. Prerenal azotemia is caused by overaggressive protein administration and is aggravated by underlying dehydration. Presenting signs and symptoms include an elevated serum BUN, elevated serum sodium, and clinical signs of dehydration. If the cause of prerenal azotemia is not found and corrected within 24 hours, the patient may develop kidney damage, with progressive deterioration in level of consciousness as the azotemia worsens and can ultimately lead to coma. Close monitoring of body weight, fluid balance, and adequate protein intake is important in preventing this complication.

Hepatic Dysfunction. Hepatic dysfunction can develop secondary to the macronutrient concentrations in TPN solutions, particularly excessive glucose concentrations. Steatohepatitis (fatty liver), intrahepatic and extrahepatic cholestasis (suppression of bile flow), and cholelithiasis (formation of gallstones) may be reflected in elevated-serum liver function tests (including aspartate aminotransferase [AST], amino alanine transferase [ALT], alkaline phosphatase [Alk phos; ALP], and bilirubin) during the course of TPN and usually return to normal spontaneously when the infusion is stopped.

Mechanical Complications   Mechanical complications related to central venous catheter insertion include pneumothorax, catheter fracture, subclavian or carotid artery puncture, air embolism, and dysrhythmias.

Pneumothorax.   Pneumothorax, the most common mechanical complication, is caused by the puncture or laceration of the pleura on insertion of the needle or catheter for central line placement. Air enters the pleural space, with partial or complete collapse of the lung. Most pneumothoraces produce symptoms, although some are totally asymptomatic. In general, the larger the collapse, the more pronounced the symptoms. Commonly seen are shortness of breath, restlessness, hypoxia, decreased or absent lung sounds on the side of the collapse, and chest pain radiating to the back. Treatment depends on the severity of the collapse and respiratory compromise. Moderate-to-large collapse requires a chest tube to restore negative pressure within the chest cavity.

Catheter Fracture and Occlusion.   Over time the catheter can become less pliable, resulting in fractures or breakage. Occlusion can occur if the catheter tip lodges against the vessel wall or is "pinched" between the clavicle and first rib. Other occlusions can result from fibrin buildup, blood or lipid deposition, and drug precipitates. Another type of occlusion, "withdrawal occlusion," allows infusion of a solution but prevents blood withdrawal.

Artery Puncture.   Inadvertent puncture or laceration of the subclavian or carotid arteries is indicated by a flashback of arterial blood in the syringe, pulsatile blood flow, bleeding from the catheter site or development of a large hematoma, and hypotension. Treatment involves withdrawing the syringe or catheter and applying direct pressure to the site until bleeding ceases.

Air Embolism.   Air embolism may occur whenever the central venous system is open to air. Signs and symptoms vary with the amount of air pulled into the venous system but may include respiratory distress, tachycardia, hypotension, sudden cardiovascular collapse, neurologic deficits, or cardiac arrest. Immediate action is required. Occlude the catheter nearest to the entry site in the skin. Place the patient on the left side and in the Trendelenburg position. This allows an air embolus to float into the right ventricle of the heart, away from the pulmonary artery. Prevention is the key. Always use Luer-Lok or other secure connectors and air-eliminating filters on central line tubing.

Cardiac Dysrhythmias.   Dysrhythmias during central venous catheter insertions are the result of the catheter or guide wire placement within the myocardium causing cardiac irritation. Persistent dysrhythmias may indicate malpositioning of the catheter. The result may be atrial, junctional, or ventricular dysrhythmias, which may cause decreased cardiac output, decreased blood pressure, or loss of consciousness. The appropriate intervention is to partially withdraw the catheter or guide wire and repeat a chest x-ray to verify catheter placement. If the placement is good and the dysrhythmia continues, an antiarrhythmic may be required.

Section Three Review

1. When is TPN indicated?
   A. Adequate amounts of nutrients can be delivered through the GI tract.
   B. Adequate amounts of nutrients cannot be delivered through the GI tract.
   C. A functioning, usable gastrointestinal tract is capable of absorbing adequate nutrients.
   D. Aggressive nutritional support is not warranted.

2. How should TPN with more than 10% glucose be administered?
   A. Through a nasoenteric feeding tube
   B. Through a peripheral vein
   C. Through a surgically placed jejunal feeding tube
   D. Through a central vein

3. What is the primary cause of CLABSI, a potentially lethal complication of TPN?

   A. A malpositioned catheter or guide wire during the central line insertion
   B. Lack of sterility during central line placement and inadequate line maintenance
   C. Inadvertent puncture or laceration of the subclavian or carotid artery
   D. Puncture or laceration of the vein on insertion of the needle or catheter

4. Hyperglycemia is a potential metabolic complication of TPN and increases the risk for the development of which problem?
   A. Prerenal azotemia
   B. Hepatic dysfunction
   C. Infection
   D. Cardiac dysrhythmias

Answers: 1. A, 2. D, 3. B, 4. A

Section Four: Refeeding Considerations

Refeeding syndrome (RFS) is a complication associated with reinitiating nutritional support in a person who is significantly malnourished, particularly with protein-energy malnutrition such as marasmus or kwashiorkor. No universal definition for RFS exists, but it is considered life threatening because it presents with low levels of serum phosphorus, magnesium, and potassium.

During periods of starvation, stored fat and protein become the body's primary fuel source; however, once refeeding is initiated the pancreas is stimulated to release more insulin. The increased insulin causes an increased uptake of glucose and other electrolytes, such as phosphorus, potassium, and magnesium, into the cells. This causes rapid depletion of serum electrolyte levels, causing hypophosphatemia, hypokalemia, and hypomagnesemia, which, if severe, has the potential to cause life-threatening respiratory and cardiac muscle dysfunction and failure and neurologic symptoms. Figure 6–2 shows the RFS trajectory. Table 6–8 lists clinical consequences of RFS.

Identifying individuals at risk for refeeding syndrome prior to initiating nutrition therapy is an important initial step in prevention. Patients at particular risk for developing RFS include older adults and those with cancer, cachexia, HIV/AIDS, chronic alcoholism, severe obesity state with subsequent rapid weight loss, and anorexia nervosa (Crook, 2014). Box 6–2 lists common conditions associated with RFS. In patients with the potential to develop refeeding syndrome, both initial and frequent evaluation of serum phosphorus, potassium, and magnesium is recommended (Parli et al., 2014).

The key to management of RFS is prevention. As the recognition of RFS improves, management guidelines have evolved. It is recommended that nutritional support be initiated at 25% of goal and advanced slowly and cautiously, only after serum electrolytes have been stabilized (Parli et al., 2014). If symptoms of RFS occur, nutritional intake should be reduced or halted until symptoms are corrected and resolved.

Table 6–8 Clinical Consequences of Refeeding Syndrome

System Derangements	Symptoms
Electrolyte imbalances	• Hypokalemia • Hypophosphatemia • Hypomagnesemia
Glucose intolerance	• Hyperglycemia
Cardiac	• Dysrhythmia • Heart failure
Respiratory	• Diaphragmatic fatigue • Respiratory failure • Failure to wean from mechanical ventilation
Hematologic	• Hemolysis • Anemia
Immunologic	• Immunosuppression • Infection/septicemia
Neurologic	• Encephalopathy • Delirium
Musculoskeletal	• Weakness • Rhabdomyolysis

SOURCE: Data from Parli, Ruf, & Magnuson (2014).

If nutritional therapy is halted because of the onset of RFS symptoms, it can be resumed following resolution of the symptoms at 25% or less of the previous rate. Fluid and electrolyte abnormalities can be corrected while continuing nutrition therapy (Parli et al., 2014). Potassium, phosphorus, and magnesium replacements are accomplished with weight-based strategies per serum laboratory values. Advancement of nutrition therapy should occur over a period of 3 to 7 days, with caloric intake increasing by 10% to 25% per day or 200 to 250 kcal/day after electrolytes have stabilized. Caution should be exercised with patients receiving parenteral nutrition as full caloric replacement can be accomplished more easily, which increases the risk of RFS. Additional interventions that should be considered when initiating nutrition therapy in a patient who is at risk for developing RFS include multivitamin and thiamine supplements, as well as frequent monitoring of all serum electrolyte levels, heart rate, and ECG rhythms (Parli et al., 2014).

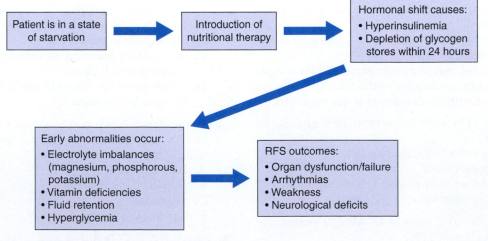

Figure 6–2 Refeeding syndrome trajectory.
SOURCE: Data from Byrnes & Stangenes (2011).

BOX 6–2   Common Conditions Associated with Refeeding Syndrome

- Weight loss (less than 85% of ideal body weight)
- Cachexia
- Eating disorders (anorexia or bulimia)
- Dysphagia or chewing disorders
- Malabsorption (short bowel syndrome, cystic fibrosis, pancreatitis; inflammatory bowel disease)
- Poorly controlled diabetes
- Inadequate or absent nutrition for more than 7 days
- Severe malnourishment (marasmus or kwashiorkor)
- Post–bariatric surgery
- HIV/AIDS

- Chronic liver disease
- Neurological deficits
- Alcoholism
- Radiation therapy
- Cancer
- Neglect or failure to thrive
- Poor social circumstances (homelessness, starvation)
- Postoperative
- Lives at skilled nursing or assisted living facility
- Older adult

SOURCE: Data from Parli et al. (2014).

Emerging Evidence

- Researchers conducted a retrospective cohort study of 88 adults with abdominal trauma to determine the feasibility and benefit of early enteral feeding. Patients receiving early feeding (within 72 hours of surgical ICU [SICU] admission) were compared with a matched sample of patients receiving delayed enteral feeding. There were no differences between the groups' feeding intolerances or mortality at 28 days. The early feeding group had fewer infectious complications ($p = 0.04$) and shorter ICU and hospital lengths of stay ($p < 0.01$) when compared to the delayed feeding group. Early enteral feeding within 72 hours of ICU admittance was associated with improved outcomes without risk of increasing feeding intolerances in patients with abdominal trauma *(Yin et al., 2015)*.
- Researchers evaluated the impact of a prescribed protein delivery on mortality and time to discharge using data from the International Nutrition Survey (2013). Percentages of prescribed protein and energy intake compared between patients admitted to the ICU for more than 4 days ($n = 2828$) and those who were patients for more than 12 days ($n = 1584$). Achieving more than 80% of prescribed protein intake was associated with reduced mortality, but more than 80% of prescribed energy intake was not. Time to discharge alive was shorter in patients in the 12-day group and longer with the greater than 80% prescribed energy in the 4-day group. The conclusion was that at least 80% of prescribed protein intake may be important to survival and shorter ICU and hospital length of stay in ICU patients *(Nicolo, Heyland, Chittams, Sammarco, & Compher, 2016)*.
- Hooper et al. (2016) assessed the diagnostic accuracy of urinary measures to screen for water-loss dehydration (insufficient fluid intake) in adults older than 65 years who were participants in either of two large clinical trials of older adults who reside in long-term care facilities ($n = 162$) or who live in community settings ($n = 151$). Neither urine specific gravity, urine color, or osmolality were diagnostic for water-loss dehydration *(Hooper et al., 2016)*.

Section Four Review

1. Which statement is accurate regarding refeeding syndrome?
   - A. It only affects clients with diabetes.
   - B. It occurs in the absence of marasmus or kwashiorkor.
   - C. It occurs when feeding is stopped suddenly.
   - D. It occurs upon reinitiation of feeding in a patient in a starved state.

2. The risk of developing RFS is increased by which conditions? (Select all that apply.)
   - A. Acute kidney failure
   - B. Acute respiratory failure
   - C. Blood transfusion
   - D. Alcoholism
   - E. Severe weight loss

3. Refeeding syndrome is related to release of which hormone?
   - A. Estrogen
   - B. Insulin
   - C. Testosterone
   - D. Growth

4. Which client is at highest risk for refeeding syndrome?
   - A. A client who has been NPO and is now being started on clear liquids.
   - B. A client who has been unable to swallow who is now being started on thickened liquids.
   - C. A client who will be started on enteral feedings via a gastric tube.
   - D. A client who will be started on parenteral feedings.

Answers: 1. D, 2. (D, E), 3. B, 4. D

Clinical Reasoning Checkpoint

Mr. X is a 49-year-old African American male admitted to a telemetry unit with acute hypoxic respiratory failure secondary to pneumonia. On arrival, he is orally intubated and mechanically ventilated.

Vital signs: BP 112/62, HR 124, RR 18, temp 39.2°C (102.6°F)

Ventilator settings: TV 700 mL, AC mode at rate of 18/min, FiO_2 80%, PEEP of 8 cm H_2O.

History of present illness: Mr. X has been experiencing increased shortness of breath with a productive cough for the past 3 days. He has not eaten much for the past 4 to 5 days due to nausea and vomiting. He smokes one pack of cigarettes per day and has a history of alcohol abuse. His breath smells strongly of alcohol on admission.

1. Can nutrition support improve Mr. X's outcomes? If yes, how?
2. What are the consequences of malnutrition in this patient?
3. Mr. X's nitrogen requirement is 0.8–1 gram of protein/day based on an estimated 25 kcal/kg/day caloric requirement. What modes of delivery are preferred for his nutrition? Why?
4. A small-bore feeding tube is placed. Enteral nutrition is ordered. Are there contraindications to enteral nutrition?

Chapter 6 Review

1. A client who developed acute kidney failure while hospitalized has been started on hemodialysis. Which change in nutritional therapy would the nurse anticipate?
   1. Water-soluble vitamins will be restricted.
   2. Protein intake will be liberalized up to 2.5 g/kg/day.
   3. Fluid intake will be encouraged.
   4. High phosphorus foods will be increased.

2. A client required hospitalization to treat pulmonary edema. The client's respiratory quotient has slowly increased and is now in excess of 1.0. Which dietary adjustment would the nurse consider?
   1. Increasing the amount of free water offered
   2. Decreasing the amount of dietary carbohydrate
   3. Holding the client NPO with glucose intravenous fluid supplementation
   4. Decreasing the amount of dietary protein

3. A client has been hospitalized after sustaining 60% body surface burns. The nurse anticipates which approach regarding this client's nutrition?
   1. The client will be held NPO for the first 1-2 days of hospitalization.
   2. TPN will be started within the first 2 hours following admission.
   3. Postpyloric enteral feeding will begin with 4 to 6 hours of admission.
   4. Small amounts of oral fluids will be offered starting at admission.

4. The nurse is advocating for early nutritional support for a patient via an enteral tube. Which statement indicates an understanding of enteral feeding initiation?
   1. "Once the client has been NPO for 2 days, enteral feeding can begin."
   2. "We can't start the enteral feedings until the client bowel sounds return."
   3. "Enteral feeding is less risky for the client than parenteral feeding."
   4. "Because this client has an intestinal obstruction, enteral feeding is our only option."

5. A client is scheduled to begin postpyloric enteral feeding today. How would the nurse explain the benefits of this procedure?
   1. "You won't have to have a feeding tube in your nose."
   2. "This will reduce the risk of getting formula in your lungs."
   3. "This will help you get more nutrition, as your stomach isn't working correctly yet."
   4. "We can give your feedings all at one time rather than hooking you to a feeding machine all the time."

6. A client who has been receiving TPN for 3 days suddenly develops glucose intolerance. The nurse should assess for which other findings? (Select all that apply.)
   1. Fever
   2. Tenderness at the catheter site
   3. Decreased heart rate
   4. Decreased serum sodium
   5. Shortness of breath

7. During a dressing change, the client, who is receiving TPN via a central venous catheter, develops dyspnea and tachycardia. What should the nurse do?

1. Sit the client up in high Fowler's position.

2. Place the client on the left side.

3. Pinch the TPN tubing to occlude flow.

4. Tap the in-line filter to remove air bubbles.

8. A central venous catheter has been placed to initiate a client's TPN. Post procedure x-ray reveals a possible small pneumothorax. The nurse would increase surveillance for which finding suggesting this pneumothorax is extending. (Select all that apply.)

1. Restlessness

2. Chest pain that radiates to the back

3. High fever

4. Dyspnea

5. Tachypnea

9. A severely malnourished client is brought to the emergency department. Total parenteral nutrition will be initiated. The health care team should implement which plan for this client's nutritional support?

1. Rapid administration of TPN to reverse the malnutrition as quickly as possible

2. Restriction of sodium and potassium in the feeding

3. Addition of a second TPN site of normal saline to correct dehydration

4. Gradual advancement of nutritional support

10. When providing care for a client at risk for refeeding syndrome, which interventions would the nurse implement? (Select all that apply.)

1. Place the client on a cardiac monitor.

2. Monitor electrolytes frequently.

3. Keep the client on strict bed rest.

4. Administer thiamine supplements as ordered.

5. Administer multivitamins as ordered.

Answers to questions found inside your textbook are available on the faculty resources site. Please consult with your instructor.

References

Abdelsayed, G. G. (2015). Diets in encephalopathy. *Clinics in Liver Disease 19*(3), 497–505.

Awtry, E. H., & Colucci, W. S. (2015). Cardiac manifestations of systemic disease. In D. L. Longo, A. S. Fauci, D. L. Kasper, S. L. Hauser, J. L. Jameson, & J. Loscalzo (Eds.), *Harrison's principles of internal medicine* (18th ed.). Retrieved December 7, 2016, from http://www.accessmedicine.com/content.aspx?aID=9109738

Bellizzi, V., Chiodini, P., Cupisti, A., Viola, B. F., Pezzotta, M., De Nicola, L., . . . Di Iorio, B. (2015). Very low-protein diet plus ketoacids in chronic kidney disease and risk of death during end-stage renal disease: A historical cohort controlled study. *Nephrology Dialysis Transplantation, 30*(1), 71–77.

Bistrian, B. R., & Driscoll, D. F. (2015). Enteral and parenteral nutrition therapy. In D. L. Longo, A. S. Fauci, D. L. Kasper, S. L. Hauser, J. L. Jameson, & J. Loscalzo (Eds.), *Harrison's principles of internal medicine* (18th ed.). Retrieved December 7, 2016, from http://www.accessmedicine.com/content.aspx?aID=9100156

Bryant, V., Phang, J., & Abrams, K. (2015). Verifying placement of small-bore feeding tubes: Electromagnetic device images versus abdominal radiographs. *American Journal of Critical Care, 24*(6), 525–531.

Byrnes, M. C., & Stangenes, J. (2011). Refeeding in the ICU: An adult and pediatric problem. *Current Opinion in Clinical Nutrition and Metabolic Care, 14*(2), 186–192.

Casaer, M. P., & Ziegler, T. R. (2015). Endocrine and metabolic considerations in critically ill patients 2: Nutritional support in critical illness and recovery. *Lancet Diabetes Endocrinology, 3*(9), 734–745. http://dx.doi.org/10.1016

Crook, M. A. (2014). Refeeding syndrome: Problems with definition and management. *Nutrition, 30*(11–12), 1448–1455.

Curtis, L., & Epstein, P. (2014). Nutritional treatment for acute and chronic traumatic brain injury patients. *Journal of Neurosurgical Sciences, 58*(3), 151–160.

Czapran, A., Headdon, W., Deane, A. M., Lange, K., Chapman, M. J., & Heyland, D. K. (2015). International observational study of nutritional support in mechanically ventilated patients following burn injury. *Burns, 41*(3), 510–518.

DiLibero, J., Lavieri, M., O'Donoghue, S., & DeSanto-Madeya, S. (2015). Withholding or continuing enteral feedings during repositioning and the incidence of aspiration. *American Journal of Critical Care, 24*(3), 258–261.

Dwyer, J. (2015). Nutritional requirements and dietary assessment. In D. L. Longo, A. S. Fauci, D. L. Kasper, S. L. Hauser, J. L. Jameson, & J. Loscalzo (Eds.), *Harrison's principles of internal medicine* (18th ed.). Retrieved December 7, 2016, from http://accessmedicine.mhmedical.com/content.aspx?bookid=331&sectionid=40726807

Elke, G., Kott, M., & Weiler, N. (2015). When and how should sepsis patients be fed? *Current Opinion in Clinical Nutrition & Metabolic Care, 18*(2), 169–178.

Elke, G., Wang, M., Weiler, N., Day, A. G., & Heyland, D. K. (2014). Close to recommended caloric and protein intake by enteral nutrition is associated with better clinical outcome of critically ill septic patients: Secondary analysis of a large international nutrition database. *Critical Care, 18*(1), R29. doi:10.1186/cc13720

Eman, S. M., Shahin, B., Meijers, J. M., Schols, J. M., Tannen, A., Halfens, R. J., & Dassen, T. (2010). The relationship between malnutrition parameters and pressure ulcers in hospitals and nursing homes. *Nutrition, 26*(9), 886–889.

Grossman, S., & Porth, C. M. (2014). Disorders of hepatic and biliary function. In C. M. Porth & G. Matfin (Eds.), *Pathophysiology: Concepts of altered health states* (9th ed., pp. 949–981). Philadelphia, PA: Lippincott Williams & Wilkins.

Harvey, S., Parrott, F., Harrison, D. A., Bear, D. E., Segaran, E., Beale, R., . . . Rowan, K. M. (2014). Trial of the route of early nutritional support in critically ill adults. *New England Journal of Medicine, 371*(18), 1673–1684.

Holecek, M. (2015). Ammonia and amino acid profiles in liver cirrhosis: Effects of variables leading to hepatic encephalopathy. *Nutrition 31*(1), 14–20.

Hooper, L., Bunn, D., Abdelhamid, A., Gillings, R., Jennings, A., Maas, K., . . . Fairweather-Tait, S. (2016). Water loss (intracellular) dehydration assessed using urinary tests: How well do they work? Diagnostic accuracy in older people. *American Journal of Clinical Nutrition, 104*(1), 121–131.

International Nutrition Survey. (2013). Retrieved February 9, 2017, from http://criticalcarenutrition.com/docs/INS%202013/INS_REDCap_23April2013.pdf

LeMone, P., Burke, K., Bauldoff, G., & Gubrud, P. (2015). *Medical surgical nursing: Clinical reasoning in patient care.* Hoboken, NJ: Pearson.

Lim, S. L., Ong, K. C. B., Chan, Y. H., Loke, W. C., Ferguson, M., & Daniels, L. (2012). Malnutrition and its impact on cost of hospitalization, length of stay, readmission and 3-year mortality. *Clinical Nutrition, 31*(3), 345–350.

Marschall, J., Mermel, L. A., Fakih, M., Hadaway, L., Kallen, A., O'Grady, N. P., . . . Yokoe, D. S. (2014). Strategies to prevent central line–associated bloodstream infections in acute care hospitals: 2014 update. *Infection Control and Hospital Epidemiology, 35*(S2), 89–107.

McClave, S. A., Taylor, B. E., Martindale, R. G., Warren, M. M., Johnson, D. R., Braunschweig, C., . . . American Society for Parenteral and Enteral Nutrition. (2016). Guidelines for the provision and assessment of nutrition support therapy in the adult critically ill patient: Society of Critical Care Medicine (SCCM) and American Society for Parenteral and Enteral Nutrition (A.S.P.E.N.). *Journal of Parenteral and Enteral Nutrition, 40*(2), 159–211. doi:10.1177/0148607115621863 Retrieved December 7, 2016, from http://pen.sagepub.com/content/40/2/159?etoc

Nicolo, M., Heyland, D., Chittams, J., Sammarco, T., & Compher, T. (2016). Clinical outcomes related to protein delivery in a critically ill population: A multicenter, multinational observation study. *Journal of Parenteral and Enteral Nutrition, 40*(1), 45–51.

Parks, J., Klaus, S., Staggs, V., & Pena, M. (2013). Outcomes of nasal bridling to secure enteral tubes in burn patients. *American Journal of Critical Care, 22*(2), 136–142.

Parli, S. E., Ruf, K. M., & Magnuson, B. (2014). Pathophysiology, treatment, and prevention of fluid and electrolyte abnormalities during refeeding syndrome. *Journal of Infusion Nursing, 37*(3), 197–202.

Reeves, A., White, H., Sosnowski, K., Tran, K., Jones, M., & Palmer, M. (2014). Energy and protein intakes of hospitalised patients with acute respiratory failure receiving non-invasive ventilation. *Clinical Nutrition, 33*(6), 1068–1073.

Reilly, C. M., Anderson, K. M., Baas, L., Johnson, E., Lennie, T. A., Lewis, C. M., & Prasun, M. A. (2015). American Association of Heart Failure Nurses Best Practices paper: Literature synthesis and guideline review for dietary sodium restriction. *Heart & Lung, 44*(4), 289–298.

Rubinson, L., Diette, G. B., Song, X., Brower, R. G., & Krishnan, J. A. (2004). Low caloric intake is associated with nosocomial bloodstream infections in patients in the medical intensive care unit. *Critical Care Medicine, 32*(2), 350–357.

Schols, A. M., Ferreira, I. M., Franssen, F. M., Gosker, H. R., Janssens, W., Muscaritoli, M., . . . Singh, S. J. (2014). Nutritional assessment and therapy in COPD: A European Respiratory Society statement. *European Respiratory Journal, 44*(6), 1504–1520.

Snider, J. T., Jena, A. B., Linthicum, M. T., Hegazi, R. A., Partridge, J. S., LaVallee, C., . . . Wischmeyer, P. E. (2015). Effect of hospital use of oral nutritional supplementation on length of stay, hospital cost, and 30-day readmissions among Medicare patients with COPD. *Chest, 147*(6), 1477–1484.

Tapia, M. J., Ocón, J., Cabrejas-Gómez, C., Ballesteros-Pomar, M. D., Vidal-Casariego, A., Arraiza-Irigoyen, C., . . . Olveira, G. (2015). Nutrition-related risk indexes and long-term mortality in noncritically ill inpatients who receive total parenteral nutrition (prospective multicenter study). *Clinical Nutrition, 34*(5), 962–967.

Terzioglu, B., Ekinci, O., & Berkman, Z. (2015). Hyperglycemia is a predictor of prognosis in traumatic brain injury: Tertiary intensive care unit study. *Journal of Research in the Medical Sciences, 20*(12), 1166–1171.

Umber, A., Wolley, M. J., Golper, T. A., Shaver, M. J., & Marshall, M. R. (2014). Amino acid losses during sustained low efficiency dialysis in critically ill patients with acute kidney injury. *Clinical nephrology, 81*(2), 93–99.

Yin, J., Wang, J., Shang, S., Yao, D., Mao, Q., Kong, W., . . . Li, J. (2015). Early versus delayed enteral feeding in patients with abdominal trauma: A retrospective cohort study. *European Journal of Trauma Surgery, 41*(1), 99–105.

Chapter 7
Mechanical Ventilation

 ## Learning Outcomes

7.1 Identify criteria used to determine the need for mechanical ventilator support.

7.2 Select the equipment necessary to initiate mechanical ventilation.

7.3 Describe the modes of mechanical ventilation.

7.4 Explain the commonly monitored ventilator settings.

7.5 Cite indications for noninvasive ventilatory support.

7.6 Discuss the major complications of mechanical ventilation with intubation.

7.7 Describe artificial airways and implications for practice.

7.8 Describe the nursing care of the patient requiring ventilatory support.

7.9 Describe options of weaning a patient from mechanical ventilation and the nurse's role in this process.

This chapter provides an overview of mechanical ventilator support for the high-acuity adult patient. Nurses caring for an individual on ventilator support collaborate closely with the interdisciplinary team to organize delivery of care during the initiation, ongoing care, and weaning from support. Content includes ventilation both with an artificial airway and noninvasive support, including benefits and complications. Knowledge of the most recent research findings on artificial airways and types of tracheostomy tubes supports the delivery of evidence-based care.

This chapter builds on content covered in two other chapters: Chapter 11: Determinants and Assessment of Pulmonary Function and Chapter 12: Alterations in Pulmonary Function. It is recommended that the reader become familiar with the material in those two chapters before beginning this one.

Section One: Determining the Need for Ventilatory Support

Mechanical ventilators are life-support machines that augment and support the **ventilation** portion of the respiratory process. The invasiveness of the artificial airway and the physiologic alterations associated with mechanical ventilation place the patient at substantial risk for development of major complications; therefore, the relative benefits and risks of using mechanical ventilation are weighed. Mechanical ventilation is a supportive intervention only. It is meant to support the patient's oxygenation and ventilation status while interventions are initiated to correct the underlying problem. Ventilator support is best initiated as a semi-elective procedure before the patient's condition becomes severely compromised by hemodynamic instability. Early support may improve the patient's outcome.

How then is the decision made to place a patient on a mechanical ventilator? Evidence supports criteria to aid the healthcare team in rapidly determining which patients may require ventilatory support. These criteria generally are not based on specific medical diagnoses but rather on ventilation and oxygenation status (see Table 7–1).

Acute respiratory failure (*ARF*) is a commonly used and broad term for labeling failure of ventilation, failure of oxygenation, or a combination of both. It is clinically defined as a $PaCO_2$ greater than 50 mmHg with a pH less than 7.30 and/or PaO_2 less than 60 mmHg. Patients requiring mechanical ventilation generally develop one type of ARF as their initial primary pulmonary dysfunction. Therefore, for the purposes of this chapter, ARF is divided into its two component parts (acute ventilatory failure and oxygenation

Table 7-1 Criteria for Ventilatory Support

Criteria	Critical Values
Acute ventilatory failure	PaCO$_2$ greater than 50 mmHg, pH less than 7.30
Acute oxygenation failure (hypoxemia)	PaO$_2$ less than 60 mmHg
Pulmonary mechanics:	
Respiratory rate (f)	f greater than 35 breaths/min and increased work of breathing
Vital capacity (VC)	VC less than 10 to 15 mL/kg (normal: 65 to 75 mL)
Maximum inspiratory pressure (MIP) Chest retractions Asymmetrical chest motions	Less than –25 to 0 cm H$_2$O (normal: –100 to –50 cm H$_2$O)

SOURCE: Data from Bristle et al. (2014); Tobin (2013).

failure) because the presence of either is an independent criterion for mechanical ventilation.

Acute Ventilatory Failure

Acute ventilatory failure (AVF) is the most common indication for ventilator support. AVF is the inability of the lungs to maintain adequate alveolar ventilation. It is diagnosed on the basis of the acid–base imbalance it creates—acute respiratory acidosis, which is expressed as PaCO$_2$ greater than 50 mmHg and pH less than 7.30. A variety of problems can cause AVF, such as brain trauma, apnea neuromuscular dysfunction, pneumonia, sepsis, acute respiratory distress syndrome (ARDS), heart failure, ineffective airway clearance, and drug-induced central nervous system (CNS) depression. Essentially, any problem that decreases movement of air to and from the alveoli (alveolar hypoventilation) can precipitate AVF.

Generally speaking, AVF is a direct indication for rapid intubation and mechanical ventilatory support. Other criteria may be used, such as level of consciousness or a particular degree of respiratory acidosis, in making the decision to initiate mechanical support. Patients with severe chronic obstructive pulmonary disease (COPD) or other nonreversible conditions may have firm opinions as to whether they want life-support devices such as mechanical ventilators; they should have the opportunity for informed consent that includes an explanation by the provider of risks and benefits of being intubated and placed on a mechanical ventilator. Advance directives assist the interdisciplinary team partner and the patient's family or proxy to understand the patient's wishes for intubation and ventilation when the patient is unable to make an informed decision. Conversations and review of documentation prior to a crisis situation promote an understanding of the goals of care.

Hypoxemic Respiratory Failure

The second major indication for mechanical ventilatory support is hypoxemia, which is frequently quantified as a PaO$_2$ of less than 60 mmHg (the clinical definition of oxygenation

failure). A low ventilation–perfusion ($\dot{V}/\dot{Q}$) ratio is the most common cause of hypoxemia. A low $\dot{V}/\dot{Q}$ refers to a state in which there is an excess of perfusion in relation to ventilation. The cause of a low $\dot{V}/\dot{Q}$ may be an obstructing mucous plug in the distal airway, causing a reduction in alveolar ventilation. Examples of conditions that are associated with a low $\dot{V}/\dot{Q}$ include asthma, pneumonia, COPD, and atelectasis.

Low ($\dot{V}/\dot{Q}$) is associated with a phenomenon called shunting. **Shunting** refers to the state in which pulmonary capillary perfusion is normal but alveolar ventilation is lacking. Pulmonary capillary blood that circulates through a nonfunctioning alveolar unit cannot pick up oxygen from that alveolus. Although some shunting is normal, if many alveolar units become nonfunctioning, a significant decrease in oxygen saturation (SaO$_2$) will occur, causing hypoxemia. Severe shunting is associated with respiratory distress syndromes of both the infant and adult and severe pneumonia. Pulmonary embolism and acute lung injury events can manifest with hypoxemic respiratory failure (Kress & Hall, 2015; Tobin, 2013).

Pulmonary Mechanics

Pulmonary function (pulmonary mechanics) testing may be used to decide if mechanical ventilatory support is needed. Such testing provides the clinician with crucial information about respiratory muscle strength and airflow. When evaluating the need for mechanical ventilation, pulmonary function tests can provide data used in identifying hypoventilation. Several of the more common tests used as criteria are vital capacity, negative inspiratory force, and respiratory rate (f). **Vital capacity (VC)** is the maximum amount of air that is expired after a maximal inspiration, indicating a person's greatest breathing capacity. VC decreases in the presence of restrictive pulmonary diseases such as atelectasis, pneumonia, and other disorders that reduce lung compliance. Negative inspiratory force (NIF) measures the amount of negative pressure that a person is able to generate from a maximal inspiratory effort. It reflects the strength of the respiratory muscles. Abnormally low NIF levels develop with respiratory muscle fatigue or neuromuscular diseases. A sustained respiratory rate of over 35 breaths per minute significantly increases the work of breathing, leading to respiratory muscle fatigue. Pulmonary mechanics also play a crucial role in determining readiness for removal from mechanical ventilation.

Special Considerations

Older adults are at risk for respiratory failure due to pulmonary and nonpulmonary reasons. Age-related changes in pulmonary physiology place the older adult at risk for respiratory failure. These changes include decreased chest wall compliance, which increases the work of breathing; decreased oxygenation because of structural lung changes; and decreased lung volume and strength, which reduce cough effectiveness and increase the risk for infection. A reduced sensitivity to hypoxemia and high CO$_2$ level (hypercapnia) plus changes in drug metabolism may increase the respiratory depressive effects of narcotics and sedatives. Many pulmonary diseases, such as COPD, become more evident with age. Age-related changes in other organs as well as comorbid conditions alter respiratory function. For example, heart disease has multiple effects, including potential low ejection fraction with heart failure, which can precipitate pulmonary edema and hypoxemia; and renal disease can alter buffer and fluid volume, precipitating acid–base imbalances and pulmonary congestion. Poor nutrition and decreased muscle strength can be additional risk factors due to overall functional deconditioning (LeMone, Burke, Bauldoff, & Gubrud, 2015; Weatherspoon & Weatherspoon, 2012).

Section One Review

1. The term *acute ventilatory failure* refers to the inability of the lungs to do what?
   A. Expand
   B. Diffuse gases
   C. Exchange oxygen and carbon dioxide
   D. Maintain adequate alveolar ventilation

2. Acute respiratory acidosis is defined clinically as:
   A. $PaCO_2$ greater than 50 mmHg and pH less than 7.30
   B. PaO_2 less than 60 mmHg
   C. $PaCO_2$ greater than 45 mmHg and pH less than 7.35
   D. PaO_2 less than 80 mmHg

3. A low $\dot{V}/\dot{Q}$ exists when what occurs?
   A. Ventilation is in excess of perfusion.
   B. Perfusion is in excess of ventilation.
   C. Blood is shunted away from the alveoli.
   D. There is an obstruction in the pulmonary capillaries.

4. The term *pulmonary shunt* refers to what condition?
   A. Movement of air directly from one alveolus to another
   B. Normal pulmonary capillary perfusion, reduced alveolar ventilation
   C. An opening between the pulmonary artery and the heart
   D. Normal alveolar ventilation, reduced pulmonary capillary perfusion

Answers: 1. D, 2. A, 3. B, 4. B

Section Two: Required Equipment for Mechanical Ventilation

Mechanical ventilation with intubation is a complex intervention that requires a plan of care and the necessary equipment. Adequate preparation will facilitate smooth implementation.

Initial Equipment Necessary for Establishment of a Patent Airway

Mechanical ventilation requires the use of artificial airways. Artificial airways can be divided into two groups: endotracheal tubes and tracheostomy tubes.

Endotracheal Tubes The endotracheal (ET) tube is a specially designed semirigid and radiopaque tube. Its slightly curved shaft is designed for ease of passage through the curved upper airway. In adults, the tubes require a cuff if positive pressure ventilation is to be initiated. The cuff is a balloon that is attached around the circumference of the tube toward the distal end of the ET tube (Figure 7–1).

When it is inflated, the tube seals the space between the tube and the trachea so air is directed through the tube into the lower airway, ensuring a predictable tidal volume or pressure (Figure 7–2).

Neonatal and small pediatrics ET tubes do not have cuffs, because in children younger than 5 years of age, the cricoid cartilage offers a sufficient seal once the tube is inserted. ET tubes are also available with an evacuation lumen exiting above the cuff to suction out subglottic secretions that accumulate at the back of the throat on top of the inflated cuff (Figure 7–3). These secretions can harbor bacteria and contribute to the risk of ventilator-associated pneumonia (VAP).

Choice of Endotracheal Tube Size and Route. The size of the ET tube to be inserted will depend primarily on the age and size of the person to be intubated. ET tube sizes range from 2 to 11 mm, which reflects the diameter of the inside lumen. In the adult, the route of entry also determines ET tube size. A smaller-size tube is required if it is to be inserted nasally because the nasal airway passage is significantly smaller than the oral airway passage. A staff member credentialed in endotracheal intubation is designated to perform the intubation.

Current guidelines recommend the use of the orotracheal as opposed to the nasotracheal route. Although the nasotracheal tube may be more comfortable for the patient,

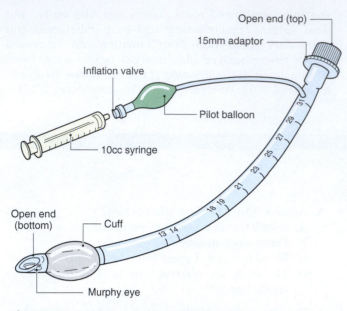

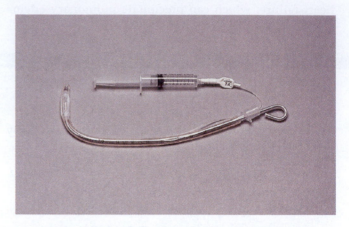

Figure 7–1 Features of an endotracheal tube. The photo image on the right shows an endotracheal tube with a stylet (metal guide wire) in place.

SOURCE: Nathan Eldridge/Pearson Education, Inc.

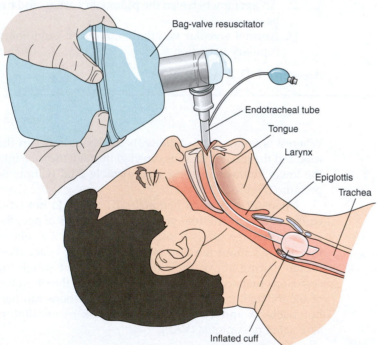

Figure 7–2 Endotracheal tube with cuff inflated.

Figure 7–3 Endotracheal tube with evacuation (suction) lumen.

it carries greater risk of sinusitis and other infections. Other problems associated with the smaller tube needed to intubate nasally include increased airway resistance, increased chance of tube kinking, and more difficulty suctioning effectively. Nasotracheal intubation should be reserved for situations where facial trauma or other considerations make oral intubation impossible.

Intubation Equipment. Before beginning intubation, the nurse ensures that the following items are at hand (Vollman & Sole, 2011):

- Soft-cuffed ET tubes (in a variety of sizes)
- Stylet—to guide the tube in place by keeping it stiff (orotracheal route only)

- Topical anesthetic—to promote comfort and local anesthesia
- Laryngoscope handle with blade attached and functional light source—to open and visualize the airway
- Magill forceps—to assist with removal of foreign bodies from the airway/pharynx and guiding the tube past the pharyngeal area
- Suction machine or set up to wall-mounted suction head
- Suction catheter kit with sterile gloves
- Yankauer (oral) suction catheter—to clear the airway of secretions
- Syringe for cuff inflation
- Water-soluble lubricant—to apply to the ET tube to facilitate insertion
- Commercial endotracheal tube-holding device (or adhesive tape if device not available)—to secure the ET tube following insertion
- Personal protective equipment
- Sedative medication (under guidance of credentialed provider) and intravenous access—for patient comfort and safety and facilitating insertion process
- Stethoscope—to auscultate bilateral lung sounds after insertion
- CO_2 detector—to aid in identification of tube location

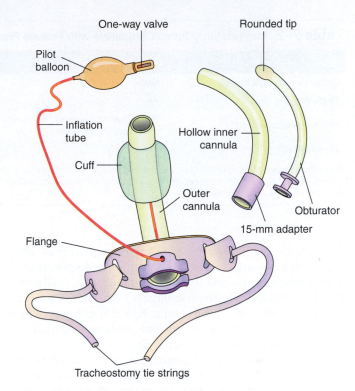

Figure 7–4 Single cannula air-cuff tracheostomy tube with obturator.

Tracheostomy Tubes Generally, when mechanical ventilation is initiated, a tracheostomy is not the initial access to the airway because it is more invasive and takes longer to perform. An emergency tracheostomy might be performed for upper airway obstruction secondary to head or neck surgery, severe edema (such as inhalation burns), or a tumor obstruction. Tracheostomy is more commonly performed on the patient who requires prolonged intubation because of failure to wean from the ventilator. Tracheostomy tubes are used for secretion management if the individual is weaned from the ventilator support. Prolonged use of an ET or nasotracheal tube is associated with complications, including laryngeal damage, ventilator-associated pneumonia, and pressure sores at the lips (or nares) and in the oral cavity. The appropriate timing of tracheostomy varies and remains a subject of controversy despite multiple retrospective and prospective studies performed to evaluate this clinical question. These studies suggest that early tracheostomy (within 7–10 days of intubation), especially among patients with traumatic brain injury, is associated with significant improvements in duration of mechanical ventilation, intensive care unit and hospital length of stay, reduced ventilator-associated pneumonia, reduced hospital costs, and improved patient survival (Hyde et al., 2015; Wang et al., 2011; Young, Harrison, Cuthbertson, & Rowan, 2013).

Benefits of transition to tracheostomy tubes are the potential for less sedation, early mobility, oral intake, communication, and the move to a less intensive level of care. Unless there are clear indications for ongoing need, a tracheostomy tube may be best timed at 7 to 10 days of intubation with an inability to wean (Cheung & Napolitano, 2014).

Tracheostomy tubes may be placed by percutaneous approach using dilators at the bedside with sedation. They are also placed via open surgical approach in the operating room using anesthesia and cutting away of tracheal ring. Each facility has preferences for the type of tracheostomy tube procedure performed and type of tube that is initially placed (Akulian, Yarmus, & Feller-Kopman, 2015).

Tracheostomy tubes vary in type and size, including diameter and length (see Figure 7–4).

Initial tubes are likely made of plastic material and have a cuff, similar to the ET tube, around the circumference of the tube near the distal end. The inflated air cuff helps ensure tidal volume delivery from the ventilator by creating a seal (Skillings & Curtis, 2011). Size and length of tubes vary per patient size and need. Commonly used sizes have an outer diameter of 6 to 8 mm and are 70 to 80 mm in length. Tubes may have a single cannula or disposable or reusable inner cannulas. Tube material may also range from Teflon to metal. Cuffs are commonly filled with air, but variations can be sterile water-filled cuffs or foam cuffs. Refer to Table 7–2 for a comparison of tracheostomy tubes that are compatible with positive pressure mechanical ventilators.

Table 7–2 Tracheostomy Tubes Compatible with Positive Pressure Mechanical Ventilators

Type	Cuff Inflated with	Fenestrated*	Comments
Single cannula, tight to shaft	Water	No	Promotes air flow when cuff is deflated
Single cannula, air cuff	Air	No	Standard trach tube
Single cannula, foam cuff	No air instilled, passively inflates with atmospheric pressure	No	Not used with speaking valves
Dual cannula	Air/Cuffless	Yes/No	(* See fenestration comments below)

*Fenestrated tubes have an opening on the posterior wall of the outer cannula above the cuff. The fenestrated inner cannula allows air flow to facilitate speech and passage of air flow with weaning. Inner cannulas can either be removed and cleaned or disposed. Fenestration can lead to granuloma formation in the airway or become malpositioned.

Securing the Artificial Airway   Any type of artificial airway must be secured in place to prevent tube displacement and to minimize trauma to mucous membranes (Vollman & Sole, 2011). Initially, in an emergency situation, the tube can be secured with adhesive tape; however, commercially available ET tube stabilizers are the preferred method of securing the ET tube (see Figure 7–5).

Tracheostomy tubes commonly are secured with twill tape or a commercially available tracheostomy holder with Velcro fasteners. The tracheostomy tube also may be initially sutured in place to prevent accidental dislodgment. The tract created by the tube in place matures over time, but caution is still required for timely replacement or exchange of the tube with decannulation (Dawson, 2014).

Supportive Equipment   In addition to the artificial airway and mechanical ventilator, other supplies and equipment must be readily available for the care of the patient, including the following:

- Two oxygen sources, one for the ventilator and one for a manual resuscitation bag to provide 100% oxygen. The manual resuscitation bag should have a mask attachment available for manual hyperinflation for accidental extubation or decannulation.
- Suction equipment and at least one suction source.
- Closed system suction set up, or disposable sterile suction kits, gloves, containers, sterile water.
- Oral pharyngeal airway or a bite block if the oral route is used (to prevent closure of the airway if the patient should bite down on the tube)—also facilitates access to the oropharynx for suctioning. Used if the commercial tube holder does not have a bite block in place.
- Cuff manometer to check the ET or tracheostomy tube cuff pressure on a regular basis.
- A manual resuscitation bag to provide adequate backup in case of ventilator failure and for open system suctioning.
- If positive end-expiratory pressure (PEEP) is to be used on the ventilator, a manual resuscitation bag with a PEEP attachment is recommended if a closed suctioning system is not to be used.
- Secure intravenous access for medication administration.
- Appropriate sedation and muscle relaxant agents available as needed.

Postintubation Assessment   Immediately following intubation, the position of the endotracheal tube is assessed for proper placement in the trachea. While the patient is receiving breaths via a manual resuscitation bag, both lung fields are auscultated for equal breath sounds. Air sounds or gurgling noises over the epigastric area indicate that the endotracheal tube is malpositioned in the esophagus. Once the airway is secured, a chest x-ray should be performed to confirm correct placement (2–3 cm above the carina).

An immediate method to ensure proper tube placement is to measure carbon dioxide in exhaled air using capnography or a disposable CO_2 detector (Goodrich, 2011). However, carbon dioxide monitors may produce false negatives if the cardiac output is too low to generate the return of CO_2 from the blood to the lungs and false positives if the patient has ingested a carbonated beverage prior to intubation.

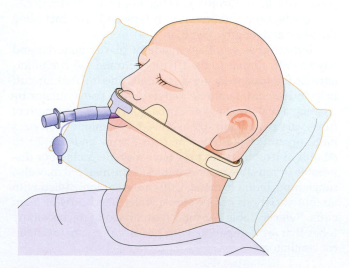

Figure 7–5 Securing the endotracheal tube.

Section Two Review

1. In the adult, an inflated ET tube cuff is necessary for positive pressure mechanical ventilation primarily because it does what?
   A. Prevents stomach contents from getting into the lungs
   B. Seals off the nasopharynx from the oropharynx
   C. Prevents air from getting into the stomach
   D. Seals off the lower airway from the upper airway

2. In an emergency situation, what is the most common entry route for airway access?
   A. Oral intubation
   B. Nasal intubation
   C. Tracheostomy
   D. Oropharyngeal airway

3. Which statement is true about securing the artificial airway?
   A. The inflated cuff provides sufficient securing.
   B. The airway is generally sutured in place.
   C. A nasotracheal tube does not require securing.
   D. Artificial airways are optimally secured using a commercial tube holder.

4. Supportive equipment when a person has an artificial airway in place includes which of the following? (Select all that apply.)
   A. At least one oxygen source
   B. Suctioning equipment
   C. Manual resuscitation bag and mask
   D. A backup ventilator in the room
   E. Oral pharyngeal airway or bite block

Answers: 1. D, 2. A, 3. D, 4. (B, C, E)

Section Three: Types of Mechanical Ventilators

Ventilators are classified according to their mechanism of force, which is either negative or positive pressure.

Negative Pressure Ventilators

Negative pressure ventilators were the first type of ventilator to be developed, as early as the middle 1800s. Negative pressure ventilation uses negatively applied pressure to the thorax by external means. To use a negative pressure ventilator, the patient's entire body (e.g., an iron lung) or thoracic region (e.g., a cuirass) is encased in an airtight unit. At regular intervals, the air pressure in the sealed unit is reduced to below atmospheric pressure. The resulting negative pressure is transmitted through the thorax, which results in a pressure gradient that causes air to move into the lungs. The amount of negative pressure used is based on the desired tidal volume (V_T) —the higher the desired V_T, the higher the negative pressure required.

Positive Pressure Ventilators

Positive pressure ventilation is the mainstay of ventilatory support in acute care settings (Figure 7–6). Positive pressure ventilators most commonly require an artificial airway to deliver ventilatory support but may be done with a face or nasal mask (noninvasive ventilation). Gases are delivered into the lungs through the ventilator's circuitry, which is attached to an artificial airway (ET or tracheostomy tube). There are multiple models of positive pressure ventilators available, and several different models may be used within one institution (see Figure 7–5 for an example).

Positive pressure ventilators are commonly described on the basis of their cycling mechanism. The term *cycle* refers to the mechanism by which the inspiratory phase is stopped and the expiratory phase is started. There are four major cycling mechanisms: pressure cycled, volume cycled, time cycled, and flow cycled.

Because the cycling mechanisms actually limit the length of inspiration, the term *cycle* is often replaced by the term *limit* (e.g., pressure-limited mechanism). Many ventilators provide more than one cycling mechanism; however, only one cycling mechanism can be used at a time. With this increased flexibility, the healthcare team can alter the type of cycling based on the changing needs of the patient without switching ventilators. The remainder of this section briefly describes ventilators based on the cycling mechanism used.

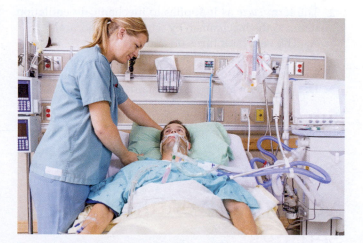

Figure 7–6 Intubated male patient with positive pressure mechanical ventilator at the patient's left.
SOURCE: Tyler Olson/Shutterstock

Pressure-cycled Ventilation   Pressure-cycled ventilation delivers a preset pressure of gas to the lungs. The pressure delivered (expressed in cm H_2O) is constant while the volume of air it delivers varies with the lung's compliance and airway resistance. This presents potentially serious support problems because stiffening lungs, a leak in the system, or a partially obstructed airway can significantly alter the volume of gas delivered with each breath. Maintaining an adequate tidal volume (V_T or TV) is crucial for normal lung functioning. Pressure-cycled ventilation is increasingly used as a method to protect the injured lung from further damage from high inspiratory pressures and is an option on most ventilators.

Airway pressure release ventilation (APRV) is an inverse-ratio, pressure-controlled, intermittent mandatory ventilation. It allows spontaneous breathing with prolonged application of high mean airway pressure. The increased airway pressure helps to recruit (open up) collapsed airless alveoli to improve alveolar ventilation and gas exchange (Facchin & Fan, 2015). Delivery of breaths is coordinated by pressure high and low, and time high and low. Evidence supports improved organ perfusion, but the increased work of breathing with spontaneous effort is a concern (Ferdowsali & Modock, 2013).

Volume-cycled Ventilation   Volume-cycled ventilation delivers a preset volume of gas (measured in mL or L) to the lungs, making volume the constant and pressure the variable. Within a certain preset safety range (pressure limits), the ventilator will deliver the established volume of gas regardless of the amount of pressure it requires. This has the advantage of being able to overcome changes in lung compliance and airway resistance. As lung compliance decreases or airway resistance increases, the pressure at which the gas is delivered to the lungs will increase sufficiently to deliver the desired volume of gas to the lungs. Volume-cycled ventilation has the potential to generate high pressures, especially in less compliant lungs, in order to deliver the set volume. Therefore, the risk of barotrauma is greater. **Barotrauma** is injury to pulmonary tissue, particularly the alveoli, as a result of excessive pressure.

Time-cycled Ventilation   When time-cycled ventilation is used, the length of time allowed for inspiration is controlled. These ventilators hold time constant, but volume and pressure may vary. Time-cycled ventilators frequently are referred to as time-cycled–pressure-limited ventilators because they also limit the maximum amount of pressure that can be delivered. The microprocessor ventilators can use time cycling and also have the advantage of being able to limit volume and pressure.

Flow-cycled Ventilation   Pressure support ventilation (PSV) is an example of flow-cycled ventilation. A preset pressure augments the patient's inspiratory effort and continues as long as the patient continues to inhale at a certain flow rate. As the patient reaches the end of inspiration, flow decreases. At a predetermined level of flow (e.g., 25% of peak inspiratory flow) inspiration ends. Tidal volume, rate, and time are variable (Lamb, 2015).

Section Three Review

1. Negative pressure ventilators adjust the tidal volume by doing what?
   A. Adjusting the amount of negative airflow
   B. Adjusting the amount of positive airflow
   C. Altering the amount of negative pressure applied
   D. Altering the amount of positive pressure applied

2. The term *cycle* as it applies to mechanical ventilation refers to the mechanism by which what occurs?
   A. The ventilator turns on and off.
   B. Inspiration ceases and expiration starts.
   C. The concentration of oxygen is controlled.
   D. The rate of airflow is maintained.

3. Volume-cycled ventilation differs from pressure-cycled ventilation because it does what?
   A. Adjusts volume as pulmonary pressure changes
   B. Increases airflow as compliance increases
   C. Decreases airflow as airway resistance decreases
   D. Can adjust pressure to changes in lung compliance

4. Pressure-cycled ventilation uses which of the following as a constant?
   A. Pressure
   B. Time
   C. Volume
   D. Flow rate

Answers: 1. C, 2. B, 3. D, 4. A

Section Four: Commonly Monitored Ventilator Settings

Positive pressure ventilators offer many variables that can be manipulated to precisely meet the individual pulmonary needs of the patient. Certain settings and values related to each variable must be monitored by anyone taking care of a mechanically ventilated patient whether in a critical care unit, on a general floor, or in the home. Although positive pressure ventilators deliver ventilator support in varying ways (different modes), the principles of nursing care to monitor mechanically ventilated patients are similar. The most commonly monitored settings include tidal volume (V_T), fraction of inspired oxygen (FiO_2), ventilation mode, respiratory rate (f), positive end-expiratory

increases. Although alveolar pressure is not measured directly, it can be approximated through measurement of the plateau pressure. Plateau pressure relates to the pressure being exerted on the alveoli when inspiration is complete at the end of a positive pressure ventilation and is easily measured at the end of inspiration. The plateau pressure is a reflection of lung compliance. Lung compliance is the measure of the lungs' ability to stretch and expand during ventilation. Low compliance means the lung is stiff, requiring higher pressure to inflate the alveoli, as with fibrosis or ARDS. High compliance is when the lung has less ability to recoil, as with emphysema or COPD.

Barotrauma. Recall that excessive pressure can cause barotrauma. A tidal volume of more than 10 mL/kg may overdistend the alveoli, increasing pressure, which may result in injury or rupture of the alveolar membrane. A rupture would allow air to enter the pleural space (pneumothorax) or air in the tissues (subcutaneous emphysema).

Volutrauma. The overdistension of the alveoli can cause more subtle alveolar injury than is seen with barotrauma. When volutrauma occurs, overstretching the alveolar cells triggers release of inflammatory mediators and stimulation of the inflammatory response. Volutrauma increases the permeability of the lungs' microvasculature, which may result in pulmonary edema (Celli, 2015; LeMone et al., 2015; Tobin, 2013).

Normal-volume Settings The selection of tidal volume may range from 4 to 10 mL/kg of ideal body weight (adult) based on the patient's lung status. Patients with normal lungs can be ventilated in the higher ranges, whereas those with restrictive or obstructive disease should be managed with lower tidal volumes. The goal is to adequately ventilate the lungs while maintaining a plateau pressure of less than 30 cm H_2O. Some patients with pulmonary diseases cannot be adequately ventilated (i.e., normal partial pressure of alveolar carbon dioxide in the alveoli [$PaCO_2$]) at these lower pressures and volumes. A technique called permissive hypercapnia may be considered for use in this patient population. This technique deliberately allows hypoventilation by using low tidal volumes, and the healthcare team must determine goals for the $PaCO_2$ and pH (Celli, 2015; LeMone et al., 2015; Marino, 2014).

Fraction of Inspired Oxygen (FiO₂)

FiO_2 is the **fraction of inspired oxygen**. It is expressed as a decimal, although clinicians often discuss it in percentages, in terms of oxygen concentrations. At sea level, the room air that is inhaled into the alveoli is composed of oxygen that is 0.21 of the total concentration of gases in the alveoli. A mechanical ventilator is able to deliver a wide range of FiO_2, from 0.21 to 1 (an oxygen concentration of 21% to 100%).

Initially, in an acute decompensation event, FiO_2 is commonly set at 0.5 to 1 to deliver 50% to 100% oxygen to the patient. The setting is then increased or decreased based on the patient's PaO_2 and clinical picture. The goal is

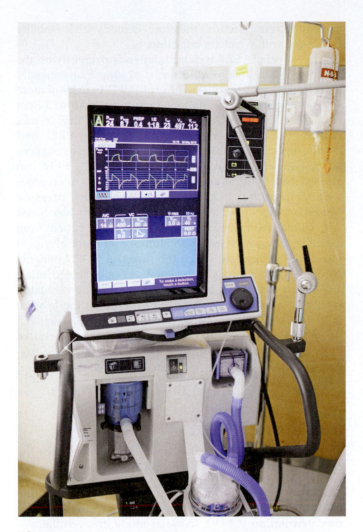

Figure 7–7 Positive pressure mechanical ventilator and control panel.
SOURCE: Happy Together/Shutterstock

pressure (PEEP), continuous positive airway pressure (CPAP), pressure support (PS), peak inspiratory pressure (PIP), plateau pressures, and alarms. The appearance of the control panel varies widely with different types of ventilators. Figure 7–7 shows an example of a control panel.

Tidal Volume

Tidal volume (V_T or TV) is the amount of air that moves in and out of the lungs in one normal breath. Normal spontaneous V_T ranges from 7 to 9 mL/kg (or 500–800 mL in an adult). If volume-cycled ventilation is to be used, the desired V_T is set by the provider when mechanical ventilation is initiated, determined by patient need. Current trends in ventilator management are to use smaller tidal volumes (6–10 mL/kg) and prevent high peak airway pressures and possible barotrauma. The goal V_T is the maximum volume allowed to keep the peak airway pressure less than 30 mmHg while maintaining adequate ventilation (Celli, 2015; LeMone et al., 2015; Tobin, 2013).

Adverse Effects of High Tidal Volumes The risk of lung injury increases as tidal volume or peak alveolar pressure

to maintain the PaO_2 within an acceptable range for the individual, using the lowest level of FiO_2. Prolonged use of FiO_2 greater than 0.60 may cause complications associated with oxygen toxicity.

When maintenance of some degree of patient-initiated breathing is desirable, care must be taken to set the FiO_2 at the lowest level that will deliver an acceptable PaO_2. The use of high concentrations of oxygen on individuals who are CO_2 retainers (COPD) may increase the PaO_2 excessively and obliterate the hypoxic drive to breathe. Patients who are CO_2 retainers have a hypoxic drive to breath; otherwise, the normal stimulus to breathe is a high $PaCO_2$. This means that CO_2 retainers' respiratory rate is determined by their PaO_2 level. In these patients a high PaO_2 will cause them to have a decreased drive to breathe. Although oxygen remains an important life-saving therapy in critical care, accumulating evidence has demonstrated the role of hyperoxia in the pathogenesis of several life-threatening conditions. The toxic effects of supraphysiological oxygen concentrations are driven by cell damage, cell death, and inflammation. Given that critically ill patients are prone to inflammation, cardiovascular instability, and depleted antioxidant mechanisms, the most rational practice may be to supply oxygen conservatively and titrate the therapy carefully to the patient's needs. At this time, our understanding of oxygen toxicity is limited in humans, and conflicting research findings hamper the development of compelling guidelines. Drugs such as amiodarone can increase the risk of hyperoxia-mediated lung injuries because a serious adverse event of amiodarone is pulmonary toxicity (Helmerhorst, Schultz, van der Voort, de Jonge, & van Westerloo, 2015; Marino, 2014; Tobin, 2013).

Respiratory Rate

Properly setting the respiratory (breathing) rate (f) on the ventilator is important in establishing adequate *minute ventilation* ($\dot{V}_E$), the amount of air that moves in and out of the lungs in 1 minute. Normal V_E is 5 to 7 L/min. V_T (tidal volume) and f (rate) are the two variables that make up V_E. It can be calculated using the following equation:

$$V_E = V_T \times f$$

These variables are significant because if either one is manipulated, it will affect V_E. If V_E becomes too low, hypoventilation will occur, possibly precipitating acute respiratory acidosis. In the carbon dioxide–retaining COPD patient, hypoventilation that results in increased CO_2 levels can complicate liberation from mechanical ventilation. In addition, the respiratory alkalosis produced by hyperventilation will shift the oxyhemoglobin dissociation curve to the left, impairing the release of oxygen at the tissue level (Celli, 2015; Marino, 2014; Tobin, 2013).

Positive End-expiratory Pressure

Positive end-expiratory pressure (PEEP) is set to provide pressure at the end of expiration, to prevent alveolar collapse. PEEP supports oxygenation, and levels of 5 cm H_2O provide support. As PEEP levels increase, cardiac output may decrease because of the increase in intrathoracic pressure and

decreasing venous return; therefore, hemodynamic stability is assessed with ventilator adjustments.

The level of PEEP required depends primarily on the severity of lung injury. Mild forms of lung injury usually require between 5 and 10 cm H_2O of PEEP. In cases of more severe lung injury, the patient may require 10 to 20 cm H_2O. There is lack of consensus of the best PEEP to use, with a recommendation for judicious use of PEEP and monitoring clinical indicators of tolerance such as oxygenation levels and airway pressures (Tobin, 2013). PEEP can also be used to offset **auto-PEEP**, which refers to an unintentional buildup of positive end-expiratory pressure caused by alveolar air trapping. It is particularly associated with COPD. Air trapping prevents the COPD patient from exhaling fully, which leaves a volume of air in the alveoli at the end of expiration. When the lungs of COPD patients become hyperinflated, the patient may not be able to inhale sufficiently to trigger a breath on the mechanical ventilator. Applying a small amount of PEEP to match the level of auto-PEEP can offset the effects of the auto-PEEP such that the patient can trigger the ventilator to cycle properly. An assessment of pleural pressure monitoring has been suggested as an option to measure the effectiveness and required level of PEEP (Lamb, 2015).

Ventilation Modes

The ventilation mode refers to that which initiates the cycling of the ventilator to initiate inspiration.

Assist-control Mode Most ventilators have an **assist-control (AC) mode** also referred to as **controlled mandatory ventilation (CMV)**. In assist mode, the ventilator is sensitive to the inspiratory effort of the patient. When the patient begins to inhale, the assist mode triggers the ventilator to deliver a breath at the prescribed settings (called a *ventilator* or *mechanical breath*). The assist part of the mode is sensitive to spontaneous inspiratory effort of the patient, allowing the patient to maintain some control over the rate of breathing. At the same time, the control part of the mode acts as a backup should the patient decrease the breathing effort below the preset rate. When AC mode is used, every breath is a ventilator breath at the preset tidal volume. AC mode commonly is used initially as a resting mode, particularly in patients with acute respiratory failure or respiratory muscle fatigue because it takes over the work of breathing, thereby resting the respiratory muscles and reducing oxygen consumption. The major disadvantage of AC mode is the potential development of respiratory muscle atrophy, or ventilator-induced diaphragm dysfunction, from the ventilator performing the work of breathing. Prolonged use of this mode can make weaning more difficult due to respiratory muscle weakness. Furthermore, the patient may be at risk for respiratory alkalosis secondary to breathing above the set respiratory rate (sometimes referred to as overbreathing) (Celli, 2015; Marino, 2014).

Synchronous Intermittent Mandatory Ventilation Mode Using the **synchronous intermittent mandatory ventilation (SIMV)** mode, the patient spontaneously breathes through the ventilator circuit, maintaining much of the work of breathing. Interspersed at regular intervals, the ventilator provides a preset ventilator breath. The intervals are based on the SIMV rate set by the operator. For example, if the SIMV is set at 12, the ventilator will deliver a breath approximately every 5 seconds to make 12 breaths per minute. Between mandatory breaths, the patient's breathing will vary in V_T and rate because it is composed of spontaneous breaths, not ventilator breaths. SIMV synchronizes a mandatory breath to follow the patient's exhalation to prevent stacking of breaths (adding a ventilator breath on top of the patient's own inhalation). SIMV has certain advantages over the other modes. It decreases the risk of hyperventilation and provides a better ventilation-perfusion distribution, and it may reduce sedation needs as there is more synchrony with ventilation for the patient. This mode can cause respiratory muscle fatigue while an individual is in the weaning process, however, if there are inadequate rest periods (Celli, 2015; Marino, 2014; Tobin, 2013).

Pressure Support Ventilation Mode

Pressure support ventilation (PSV), introduced into the United States during the mid-1980s, is defined as an adjunct weaning mode that enhances spontaneous inspiratory effort by application of positive pressure. It is triggered by the patient's spontaneous breathing effort and may decrease the effort (work) required to achieve a tidal volume. PSV applies and maintains the preset pressure throughout the entire inspiration phase.

One use for PSV is to decrease the work of breathing by overcoming increased airway resistance (R_{aw}) imposed by an artificial airway and ventilator circuitry. In this application, pressure support ventilation may be used as an aid to ventilator weaning. Patients on SIMV and continuous positive airway pressure (CPAP) weaning mode are at increased risk for respiratory muscle fatigue and ventilatory failure because they must breathe harder to maintain adequate tidal volumes. In these patients, PSV decreases the work of breathing by supporting the tidal volume during spontaneous breaths. It can also be used as a primary ventilatory mode to assist patients who are breathing spontaneously, including patients receiving CPAP. This application requires a stable lung condition as well as reliable respiratory control. Apnea parameters are set for safety depending on the basic mode the ventilator is functioning in to ensure patient safety.

Three major factors determine the patient's tidal volume: the preset pressure support level, the degree of patient effort, and the level of airway resistance and lung compliance. When using desired tidal volume as the basis for manipulating the level of PSV, the PSV level is increased until the desired tidal volume is reached. When the level of PSV is used to offset the resistance imposed by the artificial airway, the PSV level commonly is adjusted to provide just enough support to overcome estimated resistance, increasing patient comfort. Pressure support ventilation frequently is adjusted in increments of 5 cm H_2O, with levels commonly ranging from 5 to 15 cm H_2O (Celli, 2015; Marino, 2014; Tobin, 2013).

Pressure-regulated Volume-controlled Mode

Pressure-regulated volume-controlled (PRVC) ventilation is a dual-control mode of ventilation. This mode resembles AC mode in that rate and tidal volume are preset and breaths can be initiated by the patient (assisted breath) or the ventilator (controlled breath). Like pressure support ventilation, pressure is constant throughout inspiration; however, the pressure readjusts on a breath-to-breath basis to achieve the set tidal volume. As the patient's pulmonary condition changes, the pressure required to deliver the tidal volume adjusts automatically. Oxygenation is improved through a decelerating inspiratory flow pattern (Bristle et al., 2014).

High-frequency Oscillating Ventilation

High-frequency oscillating ventilation (HFOV) combines high respiratory rates, greater than four times normal, and tidal volumes smaller than anatomical dead space (1–4 mL/kg). An oscillatory pump within the ventilator delivers the high frequency (3–15 Hz) of gas. The airway pressure oscillates around a constant mean airway pressure. The mean airway pressure is set by adjusting the inspiratory flow rate and expiratory back pressure valve. The principle of the constant mean airway pressure is to maintain alveolar recruitment, which is opening up alveoli, while avoiding high peak airway pressures, therefore preventing overdistention and improving oxygenation. A potential consequence of this mode is the requirement of sedation and neuromuscular blockade (Bristle et al., 2014; Facchin & Fan, 2015).

High-frequency Percussive Ventilator

High-frequency percussive ventilator (HFPV) is a mode utilized for patients with severe respiratory failure to improve oxygenation with lower peak pressures, thereby reducing the risk of lung injury. The ventilator that is used for this mode of ventilation is pneumatically powered, pressure limited, and time cycled with a high-frequency flow interrupter. Tidal volumes are small with 300 to 700 oscillations per minute. The delivery of gas flow promotes secretion mobilization, supporting improved oxygenation (Kunugiyama & Schulman, 2012; Marino, 2014).

Airway Pressure Release Ventilation

Airway pressure release ventilation (APRV) is a pressure control mode utilized in critical care since the 1980s. It uses a combination of CPAP with intermittent, time-cycled pressure release toward a lower value. The movement from P_{high} to P_{low} aids in carbon dioxide elimination. Alveolar recruitment is increased with this mode, with support of spontaneous breathing. The timing is set at $Time_{high}$ and $Time_{low}$ for the delivery to coordinate with the pressure (Ferdowsali & Modock, 2013). APRV is indicated for ARDS but contraindicated for severe COPD as the hyperinflation may induce barotrauma (Bristle et al., 2014; Marino, 2014).

Extracorporeal Membrane Oxygenation

Extracorporeal membrane oxygenation (ECMO) is an invasive procedure utilized by credentialed teams in specialty centers. Large-bore catheters are inserted to provide blood flow to achieve gas exchange for severe lung injury using a lung protective strategy. Transfer of oxygen across the membrane is saturation dependent, and carbon dioxide transfer is partial-pressure dependent (Bristle et al., 2014).

Peak Inspiratory Pressure or Peak Airway Pressure

When using volume-cycled ventilation, the tidal volume is preset to deliver a certain number of milliliters or liters of air. The pressure it takes to deliver that amount of volume varies, depending primarily on airway resistance and lung compliance. The highest level of pressure applied to the lungs during inspiration is called the *peak inspiratory pressure* (PIP) or *peak airway pressure* (PAP or P_{Peak}). PIP is measured with all modes of ventilation. In pressure-cycled ventilation, the PIP is set and the tidal volume is variable, depending on lung compliance. The PIP is measured in centimeters of water pressure (cm H_2O) and may be visualized on an airway pressure manometer or on a data screen. In the adult, PIP volumes of less than 40 cm H_2O are considered desirable. It is known that high PIPs greatly increase the risk of barotrauma and have negative effects on other body systems.

An increasing PIP trend signifies that increasing amounts of pressure are necessary to deliver the preset tidal volume, or, in the case of pressure cycled mode, an increasing PIP means that increased pressures are required to ventilate the lung. It is most commonly indicative of increasing airway resistance or decreasing lung compliance, suggesting a worsening of the patient's pulmonary status. A decreasing PIP signifies that less pressure is needed to deliver the tidal volume. It may indicate an improvement in airway resistance or lung compliance, suggesting possible improvement of the patient's pulmonary status (Marino, 2014) or can occur if there is a disconnection in the ventilator circuitry.

Alarms

The patient's life depends on correct functioning of the ventilator and maintenance of a patent airway. To protect the patient, ventilators are equipped with a system of alarms to alert the caregiver to problems. In any alarm, the nurse should always check the patient before the ventilator. In addition, the nurse should collaborate with the respiratory therapist to troubleshoot ventilator operation. In the event of ventilator or power failure, the nurse manually ventilates the patient using a manual resuscitation bag (see Figure 7–2) attached to an oxygen source that is kept at the bedside.

Alarms are set according to patient condition and need. Agency and unit standards, with interdisciplinary input, establish parameters for safe monitoring and responsibility for patient support in response to alarms. The high-acuity nurse receives special training and competency testing during orientation to ensure safe practice and patient safety related to ventilator alarms and alarm troubleshooting (The Joint Commission, 2014).

Low Exhaled Volume Alarm The low exhaled volume alarm indicates that there is a loss of tidal volume or a leak in the system. When this alarm goes off, the nurse should focus rapidly on checking to see whether the ventilator tubing has become disconnected or whether the artificial airway cuff is inadequately filled with air or has a leak. The cuff can be checked by feeling for air leaking out of the nose and mouth. The pilot balloon attached to the artificial airway indicates the status of cuff inflation. The nurse may also hear gurgling sounds from the mouth or note that the patient can suddenly vocalize, which also indicates a leak or insufficiently inflated cuff. A leaking cuff may be checked by orally suctioning above-cuff secretions, followed by cuff deflation and reinflation to observe its ability to attain and then maintain a tracheal seal. If the cuff is ruptured, the nurse must notify the medical team immediately and prepare for reintubation. If a cuff must be deflated for any reason, deep oral suctioning should precede deflation to prevent flooding the lower airway with contaminated secretions from the upper airway.

High-pressure Alarm

The high-pressure alarm is triggered by increased airway resistance. Examples of clinical conditions that cause a high-pressure alarm include coughing, biting on the tube, secretions in the airway, or water in the tubing. After clearing the tubing of moisture and ensuring patency, the nurse should assess the patient for coughing, visible secretions, distress, or oxygen desaturation. If any of these conditions are present, the nurse will need to suction the patient to clear the airway. After interventions, the nurse resets the alarm and reassesses the patient to determine if the problem was solved.

Alarms should never be ignored or turned off. Some alarms can be muted temporarily, for example, during suctioning. Box 7–1 presents the rules regarding the proper response to an alarm.

Initial Ventilator Settings

Standard settings may be used as a guideline when mechanical ventilation is initiated. These initial settings may be determined by the provider or the respiratory therapist. Initial settings will vary based on the patient's clinical situation and underlying lung disease. In emergent situations, the FiO_2 is often initially set at 1 and can

---

BOX 7–1 Troubleshooting Ventilator Alarms

- Check the patient first. If the patient appears to be in no distress, then check connections and the machine. Do not bypass or turn off ventilator alarms. The intubated patient is unable to communicate or call for assistance. Deep sedation or neuromuscular blockade renders the patient unable to protect airway or have effective spontaneous breathing.
- If the cause of an alarm is not immediately found or cannot be immediately corrected, the patient should be removed from the ventilator and manually ventilated using a resuscitation bag and oxygen until the problem is corrected. A respiratory therapist should be called to the bedside.
- The nurse should collaborate with the respiratory therapist and provider regarding patient distress and interventions for assessing the patient or tending to ventilator adjustment.

SOURCE: Data from LeMone et al. (2015).

be titrated by pulse oximetry to maintain adequate oxygen saturation. Arterial blood gases (ABGs) are checked after the initiation of mechanical ventilation and adjustments in ventilator settings are made based on the ABG results. FiO_2 is adjusted to attain and maintain SaO_2 greater than 90% and PaO_2 greater than 60 mmHg. Tidal volume and rate may be altered to correct pH and $PaCO_2$ abnormalities. If hemodynamic stability allows, PEEP may be used to support oxygenation. Pressure support can augment volume-regulated (SIMV, AC mode) and spontaneous modes of ventilation by increasing airway pressures and relieving "air hunger" in patients with COPD and emphysema. Modes of ventilation may be selected based on empirical evidence, the performance of each device available to clinicians, and the clinical outcome and response to therapy. The goal of mechanical ventilation is to provide gas exchange safely, avoiding ventilator-induced lung injury and monitoring alarms. Mechanical ventilation is a means to support ventilation while the patient's underlying critical illness is resolved (Celli, 2015; Marino, 2014; Mireles-Cabodevila, Hatipoglu, & Chatburn, 2013).

Section Four Review

1. Barotrauma is associated with which ventilator setting?
   A. Assist control mode
   B. High tidal volumes
   C. Low FiO_2
   D. Rapid respiratory rates

2. What can a low minute ventilation ($\dot{V}_E$) cause?
   A. Acute metabolic alkalosis
   B. Acute respiratory alkalosis
   C. Acute metabolic acidosis
   D. Acute respiratory acidosis

3. PEEP affects the alveoli by doing what?
   A. Increasing alveolar fluid
   B. Decreasing their relative size
   C. Sealing off nonfunctioning units
   D. Maintaining them open at end expiration

4. What does an increasing PIP most commonly indicate?
   A. Increasing airway resistance and/or decreasing lung compliance
   B. Decreasing airway resistance and/or decreasing lung compliance
   C. Increasing airway resistance and increasing lung compliance
   D. Decreasing airway resistance and decreasing lung compliance

Answers: 1. B, 2. D, 3. D, 4. A

Section Five: Noninvasive Alternatives to Mechanical Ventilation

The combination of positive pressure ventilation and artificial airways places the patient at risk for multiple complications and significantly increases patient morbidity and mortality. In an effort to reduce risks of upper-airway disturbance, glottis function, and infections, several alternative noninvasive methods have been developed for delivery of positive airway pressure without requiring the insertion of artificial airways.

Noninvasive ventilatory methods can be effective alternatives to traditional invasive techniques for acute respiratory failure secondary to COPD, acute cardiogenic pulmonary edema, immunocompromised patients, and weaning facilitation. It is less likely to be effective with pneumonia or ARDS. Agitated patients with large volumes of secretions are challenging to manage with NPPV (Gregoretti, Pisani, Cortegiani, & Ranieri, 2015; Tobin, 2013). Advantages of noninvasive modes are avoidance of the risks associated with oral or nasal intubation, such as dental, laryngeal injury, sinusitis, ventilator-associated pneumonia, oversedation, and inability to verbalize.

Two noninvasive alternatives are noninvasive intermittent positive pressure ventilation (NIPPV) and continuous positive airway pressure (CPAP) (Gregoretti et al., 2015).

Noninvasive Intermittent Positive Pressure Ventilation

One alternative to conventional mechanical ventilator support that does not require intubation is **noninvasive intermittent positive pressure ventilation (NIPPV)**. This type of ventilator emits pressurized air, or "breaths," at prescribed intervals. A positive pressure ventilator machine and an interface device are required.

Masks and Interfaces   NIPPV is applied using a variety of *interfaces*, often a mask, in place of the invasive endotracheal or tracheostomy tube. In the acute care setting, the two most commonly used interfaces are oronasal and nasal masks. The oronasal mask covers both the mouth and the nose, and the nasal mask covers only the nose (see Figure 7–8). Choice of interface device depends primarily on patient comfort and effectiveness of ventilation. For example, a patient may find the oronasal mask to be claustrophobic and prefer the nasal mask. A distressed patient breathing through the mouth may get

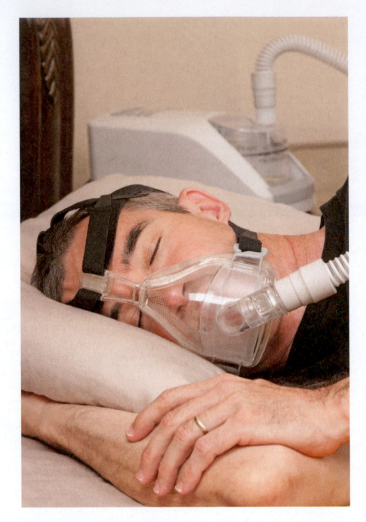

Figure 7–8 A patient using an oronasal mask with CPAP to treat sleep apnea.

SOURCE: Brian Chase/Shutterstock

more benefit from the oronasal mask. Other interface options include nasal pillows (which fit into the nares), full-face masks, helmets, and a large, cannula-type device (Schallom et al., 2015).

By collaborating with the respiratory therapist and provider, the team can provide the best choice of interface device and plan of care for use of NPPV and NIPPV. Attention to skin integrity, especially at the bridge of the nose and cheeks, helps prevent skin breakdown. A full-face mask along with proactive placement of a hydrocolloid may deter the development of a pressure injury. Planning for NPPV and NIPPV interface removal with oxygen support for meals and oral care requires coordination between the nursing team, respiratory therapist, and patient. For individuals too dyspneic or dependent on support, a small-bore feeding tube may be an option to ensure nutrition. Aspiration risks are high with any form of intake, especially with full-face masks, and the nurse should proceed with caution and maintain head-of-the-bed elevation. Eyedrops to lubricate the corneas may be a comfort and help to avoid eye irritation if there is air flow escape from the interface device.

Types of Noninvasive Intermittent Ventilation　Any positive pressure mechanical ventilator can be used for NPPV and NIPPV, including standard ICU ventilators, smaller portable home ventilators, and bilevel devices.

Standard ICU and Acute Care Ventilators.　Acute and critical care ventilators offer the advantages of volume or pressure-cycled ventilation modes, increased monitoring, alarms, and accurate titration of oxygen and tidal volumes. Rebreathing CO_2 is a lesser risk than with a single limb circuit because the ventilator circuit consists of two tubes (inspiratory and expiratory limbs). Gas from the ventilator is delivered to the patient via the inspiratory limb or tubing. Exhaled air, including CO_2, is removed by a separate expiratory limb or tubing so the patient does not rebreathe exhaled gas.

Portable Ventilators.　Smaller ventilators are primarily used in the home setting for patients with chronic respiratory failure. They can be used in either volume-cycled or pressure-cycled modes, depending on the ventilator model. The smaller size makes these ventilators a convenient option for long-term use. They have fewer alarms and monitoring capabilities than acute care ventilators.

Bilevel Devices.　Clinicians sometimes exchange the term *bilevel* with *bipap*, which actually refers to the trade name, *BiPAP*, one of the first bilevel machines produced by Respironics. Bilevel devices were specifically developed for noninvasive ventilation and were designed to compensate for the required NIPPV air leak. These devices maintain a minimal PEEP level (usually about 4 cm H_2O) to continually flush CO_2 from the system. Smaller and less complex than standard ventilators, bilevel devices provide positive pressure support to the patient throughout the breathing cycle. They have a single limb or hose that carries inspired air (Figure 7–9).

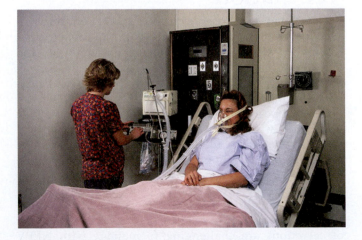

Figure 7–9 Patient receiving BiPAP via face mask. Machine is capable of CPAP and BiPAP.

SOURCE: Ron May/Pearson Education, Inc.

Gas from the bilevel device is delivered through the single limb or hose, and the patient's exhaled air goes out through the same tube and the air exhaust port on the interface device and tubing, making hypercapnia from rebreathing CO_2 a potential problem. To prevent hypercapnia, bilevel devices have continuous positive air flow to help expel exhaled CO_2 from the mask. Bilevel devices are also designed to compensate for leaks. A backup breathing rate can be set in the case of apnea, but setting FiO_2 is usually less precise, and the devices have fewer alarms and monitoring capabilities than a standard mechanical ventilator. Various models have more sophisticated monitoring and oxygen titration features. Some autotitrate-type models are able to respond to patient demand and adjust pressures based on need within set parameters. Recording cards (smart cards) can be used within the machine to record volumes and times of use.

Settings for bilevel devices use a different terminology than standard ventilators. The inspiratory positive airway pressure (IPAP) equates with the peak inspiratory pressure (PIP), and the expiratory positive airway pressure (EPAP) equates with positive end-expiratory pressure (PEEP). The patient's level of support for tidal volume is the difference between the IPAP and EPAP. Backup rates may be set in the spontaneous-timed (S/T) mode for concerns of apnea. Flow delivery is set with volume and ramp, to accommodate needs and comfort (Gregoretti et al., 2015).

Average Volume-assured Pressure Support (AVAPS)

Average volume-assured pressure support (AVAPS) is a mode with bilevel positive airway pressure with pressure-spontaneous/timed function with a fixed tidal volume that automatically adjusts to a patient's needs. AVAPS has been used for COPD and hypercapneic encephalopathy, with evidence supporting its benefit for rapid recovery of consciousness when compared to traditional BiPAP alone (Claudett et al., 2015).

Indications and Contraindications for Use

At home, NIPPV is used primarily for patients who cannot fully support their own ventilatory efforts for prolonged periods (e.g., patients with neuromuscular disease). In the ICU setting, NIPPV is used for patients in acute respiratory distress as a treatment option to avoid intubation. NIPPV has been used successfully for patients with hypercapnic failure, such as those with COPD or congestive heart failure, and with postoperative patients. It has also been used for immunocompromised patients who are at increased risk of bleeding and infection with intubation and for patients who do not wish to be intubated. NIPPV can support oxygenation and gas exchange for individuals with hypoventilation secondary to restrictive lung disease, such as that caused by severe obesity. NIPPV has been used for selected patients with hypoxemic respiratory failure (such as ARDS and pneumonia) with results based on patient acuity and response to treatment of the underlying disease. Use of NIPPV in the critically ill patient requires intense monitoring so that intubation is not delayed if the patient's condition deteriorates further. It is not indicated as an alternative to imminent decline and intubation. Use of NIPPV may be useful in supporting patients whose respiratory status has deteriorated after withdrawal from conventional mechanical ventilation to avoid reintubation. It is a less invasive option for patients with irreversible disease who desire less aggressive therapy, and it carries less risk of complications, such as ventilator-associated pneumonia (Tobin, 2013).

Contraindications for using NIPPV include an unstable hemodynamic status, cardiac dysrhythmias or myocardial ischemia, apnea, the inability to clear one's own secretions or maintain airway patency, nausea with emesis, and the inability to achieve a proper mask fit (Tobin, 2013).

As with intubation and mechanical ventilation, a review of advance directives and goals of care is important to determine the best plan of care. For the patient who does not desire intubation, NIPPV may be a suitable option, but the duration of therapy may be a challenge if the underlying disease is progressive and the individual becomes dependent on the NIPPV (Gregoretti et al., 2015).

Continuous Positive Airway Pressure

Continuous positive airway pressure (CPAP) is a mode of mechanical assistance that provides a continuous level of positive airway pressure for a spontaneously breathing person. The level of pressure remains the same throughout the breathing cycle; hence, CPAP does not provide assisted ventilation on inspiration as does NIPPV. Like PEEP, CPAP improves oxygenation by opening alveoli and is used in pressures ranging from 5 to 20 cm H_2O. CPAP does not require a mechanical ventilator; instead, it is delivered by a special flow generator (i.e., a blower) via an interface device. The same type of interface device used with NIPPV can be used with CPAP.

CPAP most commonly is used to treat obstructive sleep apnea, a disorder in which the tissues of the oropharynx collapse, periodically obstructing the airway. The constant pressure of CPAP acts like a splint to hold the airway open. When employed as a treatment for obstructive sleep apnea, the desirable level of CPAP is determined through a sleep study in a laboratory setting. In establishing the correct level of CPAP, the goal is to set the CPAP level at the point at which the patient stops having the apnea episodes or when the frequency and duration of episodes is at an acceptable level.

The CPAP level can be determined at home rather than in a sleep laboratory setting. In the home setting, special equipment adjusts the level of positive pressure and monitors apneic events, pressures, and oxygen saturation. Some of the newer CPAP units adjust airway pressure automatically, responding to snoring, apnea or hypopnea, or airflow limitation. Supplemental oxygen may be added to the circuit, dependent on patient need (Donovan, Boeder, Malhotra, & Patel, 2015).

Complications of NIPPV

Many of the potential complications of NIPPV are the same as those of positive pressure mechanical ventilation, although the severity and frequency of the complications are significantly reduced with NIPPV compared to the potential complications of mechanical ventilation. Complications specific to delivery of positive pressure through an interface device include conjunctivitis, gastric distention, nasal dryness, skin irritation, and aspiration. In addition, hypoventilation is a common complication associated with mechanical problems.

Conjunctivitis is caused by air leaking from the mask around the bridge of the nose and blowing on the eyes. This problem may be easily corrected by adjusting the interface device to eliminate the leak or fitting of a new mask. Lubricating eyedrops may be helpful. Gastric distention is caused by air swallowing. Inspiratory pressures used for NIPPV are usually less than 20 cm H_2O, which reduces air entry into the esophagus. Simethicone may be helpful in reducing gastric distention. Fortunately, with long-term use, gastric distention often becomes less of a problem. Nasal-related complaints include dryness, bleeding, and congestion. These problems may be relieved by use of heated humidification or nasal sprays. Skin irritation and pressure ulcers may develop under the straps and mask. To minimize or prevent this problem, masks must be fitted carefully and not strapped tightly to the face. A protective skin covering, such as a hydrocolloid, can be used over the bridge of the nose. Alternating interfaces—for example, using nasal pillows—may also reduce skin irritation. Aspiration is a rare, but serious, problem. It can be avoided by limiting NIPPV therapy to patients who can clear their own airways and who are not fed anything by mouth until stable. Anxiety and claustrophobia may be limiting factors to compliance and success (Piesiak, Brzecka, Kosacka, & Jankowska, 2015).

Hypoventilation is the major mechanical problem associated with NIPPV therapy. Hypoventilation can occur through two mechanisms: (1) when there is an inadequate seal to attain the preset pressure or (2) when there is inadequate airflow. Improving the seal or adjusting the flow (when possible) may relieve this problem. If patients continue to hypoventilate despite NIPPV, setting adjustments or consideration of intubation may be necessary (Tobin, 2013).

Nursing Considerations

To best ensure a patient's success in using NIPPV, a combination of explanations, patience, and coaching is required. The therapy should be explained and demonstrated at each step, giving the patient an opportunity to ask questions and adapt to the sensations of the masks and air pressures. The following list provides a suggested set of steps that should be included in the initiation of NIPPV:

1. Select the interface device and size.
2. Position head of bed at 45° angle.
3. Allow the patient to feel the airflow.
4. Allow the patient to hold the device to the face without straps.
5. Apply dressings to the nasal bridge and other pressure points.
6. Provide oral care and lip moisture.
7. Let the patient breathe through the mask briefly.
8. Connect the tubing to the mask (set IPAP low at 8 or less) to help the patient adjust to the feeling of positive airflow.
9. Continue to hold the mask in place.
10. As the patient becomes more comfortable, attach the head straps securely, avoiding a fit that is too tight.
11. As the patient becomes more comfortable, gradually increase the pressure to the level desired.

Patients are monitored for device synchrony, air leaks, and clinical response with pulse oximetry. Positive patient outcomes include a decreasing toward normal respiratory rate, improved oxygenation, and decreased use of accessory muscles. The nurse is positioned to coordinate the team effort, including the respiratory therapist, provider, physical therapist, dietitian, social worker, and family to ensure the following:

- Understanding of and compliance with the NIPPV or CPAP therapy
- Adequate nutritional intake and oral care
- Intact skin integrity
- Optimal mobility
- Reduced anxiety and pain management and optimal sleep pattern
- Home care planning if device is needed

Home ventilatory support therapy requires planning to ensure that data are collected to provide insurance coverage. When patient qualification has been verified, the nurse can establish a partnership with the home care vendor and planner to coordinate instructions to the patient or the primary caregiver. Teaching needs include the following:

- Signs and symptoms of complications
- Circumstances under which to call the physician
- Proper use and maintenance of equipment
- Application and removal of interface device and securing straps
- Troubleshooting problems

Follow-up visits by a home health nurse or a respiratory therapist are usually ordered as a means of monitoring both the equipment and the patient.

Section Five Review

1. Which of the following statements describes NIPPV?
   A. It requires a flow generator (blower).
   B. It combines negative and positive pressure principles.
   C. It uses a positive pressure device.
   D. It independently manipulates inspiratory and expiratory pressures.

2. NIPPV is most useful for a client who
   A. Requires only support of tidal volume.
   B. Cannot fully support his or her own expiratory effort.
   C. Requires only support for nocturnal hypercapnia and hypoxemia.
   D. Cannot fully support his or her own ventilatory effort over long periods of time.

3. Which statement best reflects nasal CPAP?
   A. It is used as a treatment of obstructive sleep apnea.
   B. It requires a positive pressure mechanical ventilator.
   C. The pressure level cannot be adjusted once it has been set.
   D. It allows manipulation of inspiratory and expiratory pressures.

4. Common complications of noninvasive methods of ventilatory support include what conditions? (Select all that apply.)
   A. Conjunctivitis
   B. Nasal congestion
   C. Hypoventilation
   D. Otitis media
   E. Aspiration

Answers: 1. C, 2. D, 3. A, 4. (A, B, C, E)

Section Six: Major Complications of Mechanical Ventilation

Positive pressure ventilation (PPV) affects virtually all body systems. These effects can lead to multiple system complications. Table 7–3 summarizes the multisystem effects of positive pressure ventilation.

Cardiovascular Complications

During normal spontaneous inhalation, air is drawn into the lungs because of a drop in intrathoracic pressure. At the same time, the decreased intrathoracic pressure increases venous return to the heart by drawing blood into the heart and the major thoracic vessels. As blood is moved into the right heart, the right heart chamber enlarges and stretches, enhancing right ventricular preload and stroke volume. During normal exhalation, there is an increase in

Table 7–3 Multisystem Effects of Positive Pressure Ventilation

System	Effects of PPV	Associated Clinical Manifestations
Cardiovascular	Decreased cardiac output Decreased preload Decreased stroke volume Increased afterload	Decreased blood pressure (particularly in presence of hypovolemia & heart failure); if compensation is present, normal blood pressure, increased heart rate, increased systemic vascular resistance
Pulmonary	Increased gas flow to nondependent lung and to central lung tissue Increased blood flow to peripheral lung tissues Alveolar distension with risk for barotrauma and volutrauma Lower airway contamination causing ventilator-associated pneumonia (VAP) Risk for oxygen toxicity	Decreased PaO_2 Barotrauma or volutrauma manifestations: increased agitation and coughing with frequent high-pressure alarm, diminished or absent breath sounds, subcutaneous emphysema on palpation, deteriorating BP and ABG VAP manifestations: increased adventitious breath sounds, changes in sputum color and quantity; fevers, leukocytosis; positive chest x-ray, and increased oxygen requirement Oxygen toxicity manifestations: ARDS-like presentation
Neurovascular	Decreased venous return from the head Decreased blood flow to head if cardiac output is decreased	Possible increased intracranial pressure; possible altered level of consciousness
Renal	Redistribution of blood flow through kidneys Decreased blood flow to the kidneys associated with decreased cardiac output	Decreased urine output; increased serum sodium and creatinine levels; water retention
Gastrointestinal	Decreased blood flow into the intestinal viscera Increased risk of gastric stress ulcer formation, gastrointestinal bleed, hepatic dysfunction (increased bilirubin)	Epigastric pain or burning; occult or gross blood in stool; decreasing hemoglobin and hematocrit; increasing bilirubin

SOURCE: Tobin (2013).

the flow of blood from the pulmonary circulation to the left heart, increasing left ventricular preload and stroke volume. At the end of spontaneous exhalation, the output of blood decreases in both the right and left heart.

Positive pressure ventilation reduces cardiac output by decreasing venous return to the heart in three major ways. First, the presence of positive intrathoracic pressure increases external pressure on the inferior vena cava and blood flowing into the right atrium, decreasing cardiac output. Second, cardiac output is reduced through the increase of right ventricular afterload secondary to increased lung volume. Third, the amount of pressure being exerted on the alveoli can increase pulmonary vascular resistance and right ventricular afterload. As the level of pressure is increased, venous return to the heart decreases. The more the heart and pulmonary capillaries are squeezed by the presence of positive pressure, the lower the cardiac output, and hypotension may result with low cardiac output, particularly if the patient is not well hydrated when PEEP is initiated. This helps explain why high levels of PEEP can dramatically reduce cardiac output. Other factors that influence the effects of PPV on the cardiovascular system include lung and thoracic compliance, airway resistance, and the patient's volemic state (Tobin, 2013).

Pulmonary Complications

Normally during spontaneous breathing the relationship between ventilation and perfusion $\dot{V}/\dot{Q}$ is relatively balanced, with most inhaled gases flowing toward the diaphragm. The distribution of gases to the alveoli normally favors the peripheral and dependent lung areas. Likewise, pulmonary perfusion normally is the greatest in dependent areas, thus matching the lung zones with the most ventilation with the lung zones with the most perfusion.

Altered Ventilation and Perfusion PPV alters the relationship of ventilation to perfusion in the lungs. Gases flow through the path of least resistance, which during PPV increases ventilation to the nondependent lung areas and large airways. This is largely due to the decreased functioning and stiffening of the diaphragm associated with passive PPV. PPV gas flow increases ventilation to the healthy lung areas, while flow decreases to the diseased areas because it meets increased resistance in diseased lung tissue.

When PPV is used, the positive pressure is transmitted to the pulmonary vessels, pushing the blood to the peripheral lung and to dependent areas. Because perfusion is now the greatest in the periphery and in the dependent lung areas and ventilation is greatest in the nondependent and larger airways, the relationship of ventilation to perfusion is altered to some degree. In areas with the most perfusion, there is decreased ventilation, and in areas with adequate ventilation, perfusion is reduced. This can create problems with oxygenation because of increased shunting, which can be reflected in deteriorating PaO_2 levels. Under certain circumstances, shunt and $\dot{V}/\dot{Q}$ matching can significantly improve during PPV. This is typically seen when PEEP is applied to treat refractory hypoxemia associated with increased shunt and decreased functional residual capacity (e.g., ARDS). When nonfunctional alveoli are recruited and become functional (reopen and take part in gas exchange), shunt is reduced, $\dot{V}/\dot{Q}$ matching is improved, and PaO_2 levels may significantly improve.

Barotrauma and Volutrauma There is increasing evidence that the pulmonary injury associated with PPV results from alveolar distention created by a combination of excessive alveolar pressure (barotrauma) and volume (volutrauma) (Celli, 2015). The higher the positive pressure or volume applied, the greater the risk of trauma. Patients who are at the highest risk for development of barotrauma and volutrauma are those requiring high levels of PEEP and high peak airway pressures (PAP, PIP) or high tidal volumes. Barotrauma or volutrauma can manifest itself as pneumothorax, subcutaneous emphysema, or pneumomediastinum (air within the mediastinum). Clinically, it should be suspected if (1) the patient has a sudden onset of agitation and cough associated with a frequent high-pressure alarm, (2) the blood pressure and ABG rapidly deteriorate, (3) breath sounds suddenly are diminished or absent, or (4) subcutaneous emphysema can be palpated on the anterior neck or chest. If a pneumothorax or pneumomediastinum is diagnosed by chest x-ray, insertion of a chest tube should be anticipated.

Oxygen Toxicity Oxygen toxicity is associated with the use of an oxygen concentration of 60% or greater (FiO_2 of 0.6 or greater) for more than 48 hours. The use of 100% oxygen concentration (FiO_2 of 1) can cause pulmonary changes within 6 hours. Oxygen toxicity damages the endothelial lining of the lungs and decreases alveolar macrophage activity. It also decreases mucus and surfactant production. If it is allowed to continue for more than 72 hours, the patient may develop a pattern of symptoms similar to ARDS. The early signs and symptoms of oxygen toxicity are nonspecific (malaise, fatigue, and substernal discomfort). Because early symptoms are difficult to assess, the nurse should be aware of who is at risk for developing oxygen toxicity on the basis of the length of time that the patient has received an O_2 concentration of 60% or higher. Unfortunately, the signs and symptoms of oxygen toxicity are similar to changes that may be due to the underlying disease process or ventilator-induced lung injury (VILI). Although every effort should be made to decrease oxygen concentrations to nontoxic levels, the need to maintain adequate oxygenation and safe ventilatory pressures is paramount (Tobin, 2013).

Ventilator-associated Pneumonia (VAP) Healthcare-associated pulmonary infection is a common major complication of mechanical ventilation that develops in patients intubated for more than 48 hours. Criteria for VAP include radiographic finding of new or progressive infiltrate, fever, leukocytosis or leukopenia, worsening gas exchange, purulent secretions, cough, and dyspnea (Nair & Niederman, 2015).

The passing of an ET or tracheostomy tube from the upper airway into the lower airway introduces upper airway contaminants into the lower airway. The presence of an artificial airway bypasses the normal upper airway defense mechanisms, reduces cough effectiveness, stimulates mucus production, and decreases the mucociliary motion that helps to remove bacteria from the lower airway. Upper-airway secretions pool above the ET tube cuff, forming a biofilm that provides an environment in which bacteria can multiply. The biofilm can become dislodged and disseminated into the lungs by ventilator-induced breaths. *Ventilator-associated event* (VAE) has been a term used for surveillance by the Centers for Disease Control and Prevention, with a low sensitivity and specificity for diagnosing VAP, and may be less useful for the intensive care unit population (Nair & Niederman, 2015).

Multiple factors contribute to the development of VAP. These risk factors can be divided into three categories: device related, host related, and personnel related.

- Device-related risk factors include nasogastric and orogastric tubes, either of which can interrupt the gastroesophageal sphincter, leading to increased gastroesophageal reflux—and provide a route for bacteria to translocate from the stomach to the upper airway. Enteral feedings increase gastric pH and gastric volume, increasing the risk of aspiration. Medications that prevent stress ulcer formation create an alkaline pH in which bacteria multiply. The endotracheal tube itself is a risk factor for VAP. Secretions pool above the ET tube cuff and can be aspirated into the lungs.

- Host-related risk factors include underlying medical conditions such as COPD and immunosuppression. The patient's mental status and inability to cough and clear secretions are important in the risk of VAP. Upright positioning of the patient decreases the risk of lower airway contamination from bacteria harbored on dental plaque and oropharyngeal secretions.

- Personnel-related risk factors include improper hand hygiene while working with mechanically ventilated patients. Use of closed suctioning systems may reduce the risk of contamination of the airway by personnel.

Signs and symptoms of a pulmonary infection include development of adventitious breath sounds and changes in sputum color or quantity. Systemically, infection may be evidenced by fever and increased white blood cell (WBC) count. Positive chest x-ray and sputum culture findings are important diagnostic tools. Reduction of oral bacteria and secretions is crucial to prevention of VAP; thus, effective oral hygiene should include brushing of teeth, rinsing the mouth, and frequent removal of oral secretions. Many institutions have developed VAP bundled orders, based on evidence, that include elevating head of the bed, routine oral care procedures with subglottic suctioning, and other interventions (American Association of Critical-Care Nurses [AACN], 2008; AACN, 2010).

Systemic antibiotics are used for the treatment for VAP bacterial-related infections. Inhaled antibiotics are suggested as an adjunctive therapy to systemic therapy for VAP to reduce the emergence of new resistance (Palmer, 2015).

Neurovascular Complications

PPV can cause a change in neurovascular status through two major mechanisms: increased intracranial pressure (ICP) and decreased cerebral perfusion pressure (CPP). Patients who have existing intracranial or neurovascular problems are at particular risk when moderate-to-high ventilation pressures are required. The increased intrathoracic pressure associated with PPV decreases venous return from the head. The higher the pressure required to ventilate the patient, the greater the effects on the ICP.

Blood flow to the head (cerebral perfusion pressure) may be reduced. If cardiac output drops sufficiently to reduce systolic blood pressure, cerebral perfusion may become compromised. CPP is influenced by two factors: ICP and mean arterial pressure (MAP). This relationship is expressed as follows:

$$CPP = MAP - ICP$$

MAP is determined by the systolic and diastolic blood pressures. Therefore, as systolic blood pressure decreases, so will MAP, causing a reduction in CPP. If CPP drops too low, cerebral hypoxia can result.

Renal Complications

PPV is associated with decreased urinary output. The mechanisms for this decrease are multiple, and some are unclear; however, three major mechanisms that may contribute to decreased renal function include decreased cardiac output, redistribution of renal blood flow, and hormonal alterations.

Decreased Cardiac Output Recall that positive pressure ventilation reduces CO, which then reduces perfusion to the kidneys. As kidney perfusion drops, glomerular filtration rate falls, resulting in decreased urine output. In most mechanically ventilated patients, CO can be managed through natural compensatory mechanisms and hydration therapy, which maintain adequate arterial blood pressure and renal blood flow.

Redistribution of Renal Blood Flow Positive pressure ventilation increases internal pressures not only in the thorax, but also in the abdomen, creating a redistribution of intrarenal blood flow. Renal perfusion may be altered by decreased blood flow to the outer renal cortex and increased flow to the inner cortex and outer medullary tissue, where the juxtamedullary nephrons are located. The blood flow redistribution can result in a significant decrease in urinary output, and less sodium and creatinine are excreted. When sodium is resorbed, water also is resorbed to maintain homeostasis, thus reducing urine output.

Hormonal Alterations The cardiovascular changes induced by positive pressure may stimulate the release of antidiuretic hormone (ADH), renin, aldosterone, atrial natriuretic factor, and catecholamines. These hormones may affect renal blood flow and renal function, but observed effects vary with a patient's clinical status, hydration, and underlying disease.

Gastrointestinal Complications

Gastrointestinal bleeding occurs through development of stress ulcers. Stress ulcers develop as a result of either gastric hyperacidity or, more commonly, from a transient visceral hypoxic episode. In the mechanically ventilated patient, the tissue hypoxia may be related to acute respiratory failure or may result from increased resistance to blood flow in the viscera. Stress ulcers, which usually are shallow erosions in the mucosal lining, often cause slow, insidious bleeds and, therefore, may not be diagnosed early in their development. For this reason, it is important to check stools for occult blood (guaiac). In addition,

some patients with no history of liver disease develop hepatic dysfunction.

Clinically, the patient who develops a stress ulcer exhibits a decreasing hematocrit and guaiac positive stools. If bleeding becomes significant, the stools may be black or dark red. If the ulcer is in the stomach, nasogastric aspirate will be guaiac positive, and the aspirate will appear bright red to dark red. Because mechanical ventilation for longer than 48 hours increases the risk for development of stress ulcers, preventive interventions are recommended. These include the use of antacids, histamine (H_2) antagonists, or proton pump inhibitors. Alternatively, sucralfate provides mucosal protection without pH alteration and may have advantages in reducing bacterial overgrowth in the stomach.

Acalculous cholecystitis has been associated with mechanical ventilation that exceeds 72 hours with an unclear etiology, although associated with other critical illness risk factors. Increased pressure on the liver can decrease perfusion and create hepatic dysfunction (Tobin, 2013).

Section Six Review

1. PPV affects the cardiovascular system by doing what?
   A. Increasing cardiac output
   B. Decreasing venous return to the heart
   C. Increasing arterial blood pressure
   D. Increasing venous return to the heart

2. Changes in cardiac output resulting from positive pressure ventilation are associated with which manifestation?
   A. Increased arterial blood pressure
   B. Increased urinary output
   C. Decreased arterial blood pressure
   D. Decreased pulse rate

3. Positive pressure ventilation (PPV) alters the relationship of ventilation to perfusion in what way?
   A. Ventilation increases in nondependent lung areas.
   B. Ventilation increases in the small airways.
   C. Perfusion increases in the nondependent lung areas.
   D. Perfusion increases near the large airways.

4. Which assessment finding in a client receiving PPV should make the nurse suspect pulmonary barotrauma or volutrauma?
   A. Onset of increased lethargy
   B. Increase in arterial blood pressure
   C. Increase in breath sounds over a lung field
   D. Increased cough with high-pressure alarm triggering

Answers: 1. B, 2. C, 3. A, 4. D

Section Seven: Artificial Airway Complications

Artificial airways have their own set of complications that are primarily related to airway trauma, local tissue ischemia, and bypassing the normal upper airway defenses that warm and humidify the air.

Nasal or Oral Damage

Placing an artificial airway through the nasal passage can traumatize nasal mucous membranes during the passing of the tube. After the nasotracheal tube is in place, ischemia and possibly necrosis of the nares may develop as a result of the pressure the tube exerts on the internal nasal wall.

For this reason, choosing the proper size tube is crucial in minimizing the risk of damage. Anchoring the tube to the cheeks rather than to the top of the nose also helps prevent pressure damage. Furthermore, a nasotracheal tube can occlude the eustachian tubes, which increases the risk of development of ear pressure problems or inner ear infection. The oral intubation approach can also cause damage. Pressure from the oral ET tube may cause ulcerations and possible necrosis of the inner cheek or lip. Oral endotracheal tubes should be repositioned on a regular interval, no less than every 24 hours, to prevent pressure damage to the lips and mouth. Dental trauma or tongue pressure sores can develop from the presence of an ET tube. Commercial tube holders offer an option of pressure relief on the skin and a clip for the tube that allows movement of the tube without retaping (Vollman & Sole, 2011).

Cuff Trauma

Although the use of ET and tracheal cuffs is necessary to mechanically ventilate the patient properly, cuffs can cause potentially severe tracheal and laryngeal injuries. The use of excessive cuff pressures is the major contributing factor in these injuries. Arterial capillary blood flow pressure through the trachea is low (less than 30 mmHg). A high-pressure force, such as is delivered by an overinflated cuff, exerts a pressure that is higher than tracheal capillary pressure, causing circulation in the cuffed area to be compromised. Decreased or obliterated blood flow to an area of tissue causes ischemia, which, if allowed to continue for an extended period, can produce necrosis. Necrosis of the trachea, larynx, or both can result in development of fistulas, fibrosis, and ulceration. Moreover, although rare, increased pressure can lead to erosion of nearby vessels such as the innominate artery, creating hemorrhage risk.

Proper monitoring and control of cuff pressures decrease the risk of complications significantly. Cuff pressures must be monitored at least once every shift via a cuff manometer (Figure 7–10).

Safe cuff pressures range from 20 to 25 mmHg (27 to 34 cm H_2O). A minimum occluding pressure technique may also be used to reduce the risk of pressure-related cuff damage. Using this technique, the cuff is inflated only to the point at which it seals the airway during the mechanical ventilation. Cuff pressure should be regularly checked using the minimum occluding pressure technique and should not exceed 30 mmHg (Richard & Mercat, 2014).

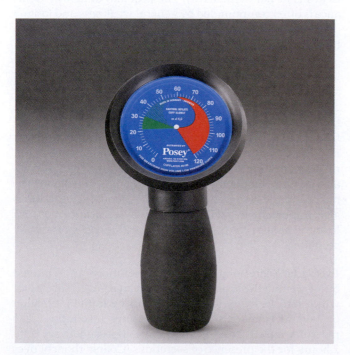

Figure 7–10 Example of a cuff manometer.

SOURCE: Images provided Courtesy Posey Company, Arcadia, California

Artificial airways can damage one or both vocal cords as a result of the traumatic introduction of the tube, or damage can be caused by the pressure of the tube against the cords. Fistula formation is also a major concern. Should tracheal injury from a cuff cause a fistula to form between the trachea and esophagus, gastric secretions can be aspirated into the lungs. Tracheoesophageal (TE) fistulas should be suspected if food or tube-fed food is aspirated during tracheal suctioning. This infrequent, but serious, complication is diagnosed with computed tomography (CT) scan and contrast studies. Use of low-pressure cuffs with proper cuff inflation technique and use of correct tube size can minimize cuff-related complications (Goodrich, 2011).

Tracheostomy Tubes

Tracheostomy tubes, considered longer-term artificial airways, have a separate set of complications.

Tracheomalacia, the weakening or erosion of the tracheal cartilage, is a rare complication that can arise when tracheal wall tissue becomes damaged from the presence of the tube, cuff, or suctioning over a prolonged time. Overinflation of the cuff is considered the major risk factor. The trachea becomes more compliant and may stretch, causing difficulty in maintaining a cuff seal. It may develop in malnourished patients with tracheostomy tubes left in for longer times. Proper cuff inflation that is routinely monitored can help prevent development of tracheomalacia. Use of a tube of a different length or diameter may help solve the cuff leak issue and ensure a seal. Moving the inflation point of the cuff allows time for the area to heal. For intractable cases of tracheomalacia, tracheal stents may be placed to keep the airway diameter open.

Granulation tissue can develop at any point in the trachea as a consequence of the tube rubbing on the tracheal wall or from suction trauma. Formation of granulation tissue can cause obstruction to airflow. Laryngoscopy can identify the degree of the problem, and solutions may include changing the tracheostomy tube to a different length, a steroid trial, or surgical removal.

Tracheal stoma erosion can develop as the stoma size is enlarged in patients with tracheostomies. This can present as excess secretions from the stoma opening with redness and skin excoriation. Packing material such as an alginate may help wick secretions away from the skin. Protective barrier ointments may help to avoid skin breakdown. The first line of prevention for skin-related complications is a skin cleaning and protection plan beginning at the insertion time. Care for skin under the phalange of sutured tracheostomies helps avoid maceration and pressure injury (Plowright, 2014).

Accidental decannulation is an emergency situation. A spare tube of the same or smaller size to reinsert immediately in the stoma may maintain the airway patency and ability to ventilate. The newer stoma (less than 7 days) may close and not allow recannulation. This may require oral intubation to support ventilation in a critically compromised patient (Cheung & Napolitano, 2014).

Section Seven Review

1. The presence of a nasotracheal tube can affect the ears because it can do what?
   A. Occlude the eustachian tubes
   B. Exert direct pressure on the inner ears
   C. Cause inner ear ischemia
   D. Directly damage the eustachian tubes

2. Endotracheal tube cuff pressures can damage the trachea when cuff pressure is:
   A. Increased during coughing.
   B. Reduced due to a leak.
   C. Lower than surrounding capillary pressure.
   D. Higher than surrounding capillary pressure.

3. What is the upper limit of safe tracheal cuff pressure?
   A. 15 mmHg
   B. 20 mmHg
   C. 25 mmHg
   D. 30 mmHg

4. Clients with tracheostomy tubes with overinflation of the cuff are at risk to develop what condition?
   A. High blood pressure
   B. Gastrointestinal bleeding
   C. Tracheomalacia
   D. Ventilator-associated pneumonia

Answers: 1. A, 2. D, 3. D, 4. C

Section Eight: Care of the Patient Requiring Mechanical Ventilation

The general goals and outcome criteria appropriate to the management of a patient receiving mechanical ventilation may be divided into two major categories: support of physiologic needs and support of psychosocial needs. Support of the patient's physiologic needs is accomplished through interventions that promote optimal oxygenation, treat impaired gas exchange, provide adequate ventilation, protect the airway, support tissue perfusion, ensure functional mobility, and provide adequate nutrition. Support of the patient's psychosocial needs centers around interventions to (1) reduce anxiety and pain, (2) provide a balance of sleep and activity, (3) promote communication, and (4) support spiritual needs. Support of family and patient includes ensuring understanding of the goals of mechanical ventilation and the plan of care.

Nursing Management of Physiologic Needs

The patient's nursing management is planned around interventions to attain the patient care goals. The first three goals—promote optimal oxygenation, provide adequate ventilation, and protect the patient's airway—are all addressed through implementation of the three pulmonary-related nursing diagnoses. An additional goal in which the nurse takes a pivotal role is to prevent complications associated with mechanical ventilation (and critical illness), particularly ventilator-associated pneumonia (VAP), stress-induced mucosal injury (SIMI), and complications of immobility such as venous thromboembolism

(VTE). See the "Nursing Care: Prevention of Common Complications in the Patient on Mechanical Ventilation" feature for a summary of some of the major assessments, interventions, and nursing diagnoses specifically focusing on these potential complications.

Ineffective Airway Clearance   The patient who requires conventional positive pressure ventilation will have an endotracheal or tracheostomy tube inserted to access and limit airflow external to the tube from the lower airway. The length and relatively small internal diameter of ET tubes make it difficult, if not impossible, for the patient to clear his or her own airway. The problem of airway clearance is often compounded by general weakness and fatigue or diminished level of responsiveness, any of which also hinders airway clearance.

Airway clearance is a top-priority interdisciplinary-team goal in management of the patient with an artificial airway. The primary reason that airway patency becomes compromised is airway obstruction caused by excessive, thick, or pooled secretions. If airway patency is not maintained and airflow becomes compromised, the patient's respiratory status will deteriorate, potentially resulting in respiratory failure. Frequent assessment of the patient's airway with suctioning as needed is a crucial role for the nurse and the respiratory therapist. Adequate hydration is also important in facilitating airway clearance because level of patient hydration alters the thickness of airway secretions.

Excessive Secretions.   Excessive secretions are removed by suctioning the artificial airway on an as-necessary basis, which may be every few minutes during initial intubation or several times a shift with ongoing intubation. The patient's breath sounds should be assessed every 1 to 2 hours for the presence of secretions. Coarse rhonchi over the trachea is the most sensitive indicator of the need for endotracheal suctioning (Sole, Bennett, & Ashworth, 2015).

Nursing Care

Prevention of Common Complications in the Patient on Mechanical Ventilation

Expected Patient Outcomes and Related Interventions

Outcome: The patient experiences no complications of mechanical ventilation

Assess and compare to established norms, patient baseline, and trends

Monitor for signs of pneumonia

Fever, increased WBC, increased adventitious sounds

Change in color and consistency of secretions

Positive chest x-ray with evidence of pulmonary infiltrates

Worsening ABG trends

Confusion in the older adult

Monitor for signs of stress-induced mucosal injury (SIMI)

Occult or gross blood in GI secretions or stool

Decreasing hemoglobin, hematocrit, and RBC counts

Interventions to prevent common complications of mechanical ventilation

Institute ventilator bundle orders

Elevate head of bed 30 degrees or higher unless contra-indicated (AACN, 2008; Burns, 2014).

Use ET tube with continuous suction above cuff if patient is to be intubated more than 48 hours; no routine changing of ventilator circuits (Burns, 2014).

Perform oral hygiene two or more times per day (AACN, 2010).

Use soft toothbrush to brush teeth, gums, and tongue; moisturize oral mucosa and lips q 2–4 hours.

During perioperative period in adults undergoing cardiac surgery, use chlorhexidine gluconate (0.12%) oral rinse twice per day.

Early progressive mobility has been shown to reduce complications and promote functional recovery. Coordinating the effort of mobilizing a ventilator-dependent patient is part of interdisciplinary planning (Reames, Price, King, & Dickinson, 2016).

Identify risk factors for unplanned extubations and plan for patient agitation, physical and surveillance needs, and monitor response to therapy to ensure safety (Kiekkas, Aretha, Panteli, Baltopoulos, & Filos, 2013).

Administer related drug therapy and monitor for therapeutic and nontherapeutic effects

Antisecretory therapy, either histamine 2 receptor agonist (H_2RA) or proton pump inhibitor (PPI)

Mucosal protectant therapy, sucralfate

Coughing, whether it sets off the ventilator's high-pressure alarm or not, may indicate a need for suctioning. The nurse often may hear the secretions without the use of a stethoscope, particularly during coughing. Coughing, however, can occur as a result of tracheal irritation or bronchospasm or because the tip of the airway is touching the carina. The last two situations can precipitate severe coughing spasms. Because coughing may occur without the presence of secretions in the large airways, the nurse should assess the situation first. Unnecessary suctioning causes needless trauma to the delicate mucous membranes in the trachea and also depletes oxygen levels. Interventions to facilitate airway clearance include the following:

- Assess before suctioning, and suction if needed.
- Perform preoxygenation of the patient and lung hyperinflation using a manual resuscitation bag or mechanical ventilator prior to suctioning.
- Follow approved protocols for suctioning.
- Monitor the patient closely for adverse effects of suctioning, such as dysrhythmias and hypoxemia (usually by observing SpO_2 levels).

In most circumstances, the nurse will maintain oxygenation during suctioning if the following common protocol is maintained:

Step 1: **Hyperoxygenate or hyperventilate.** Deliver 100% oxygen accompanied by one of two methods:
- *Manual method:* Manually ventilate the patient with a manual resuscitation (Ambu) bag for four to five breaths (two-handed ventilating will deliver significantly larger breaths than one-handed ventilating), or
- *Machine method:* Most mechanical ventilators have a 100% button that will deliver oxygen at 100% for 2 minutes (particularly important if closed suction systems are being used).

Step 2: **Suction.** Use moderate, not high, suction pressure, ranging from 100 mmHg to 120 mmHg. Advance the suction catheter only so far as to recover secretions. Apply suction only on withdrawal, rotating the catheter while using intermittent suction and withdrawing the catheter within 10 seconds. Repeat steps 1 and 2 until the airway is cleared.

Step 3: **Return the patient to the ventilator.** If an in-line closed system suction unit is used, flush the catheter and tubing with saline bolus, and relock the access valve.

Routine saline instillation is not recommended prior to suctioning. This practice does not facilitate secretion removal, increases the risk of bacterial contamination of the lower airways, and may precipitate hypoxemia (Chulay & Seckel, 2011).

Suction catheters can be divided into two major groups: open and closed systems. Both systems are used for suctioning artificial airways, but only open systems are used without an artificial airway in place. Each type of system has its own suctioning protocol. Closed system catheters are self-contained within a sheath attached directly to the artificial airway (see Figure 7–11).

A closed-catheter system remains in the artificial airway system between suctioning, allowing it to be used multiple times, with rinsing with saline after the suctioning event. Open systems generally are single-use catheters that require sterile gloves for entry into the airway.

Thick Secretions. Thick secretions are a common challenge to maintaining effective airway clearance. Gas delivered directly into the lower airway bypasses the warming and humidification that the upper airway normally provides, altering airway secretions. Properly hydrating the patient is an important means of thinning secretions because secretions are composed primarily of water. Mechanically ventilated patients receive warmed, humidified gases that facilitate liquefying secretions. Spontaneously breathing patients on a tracheostomy collar need humidified oxygen or air delivered to promote hydration. Follow lab values of BUN, creatinine, sodium, and serum osmolality to ensure adequate systemic hydration and collaborate to ensure adequate water intake.

Pooled Secretions. Pooled secretions can cause obstruction of major airways or can plug the tip of the artificial airway. Methods to improve cough effectiveness, such as the assisted cough technique, are used for specific populations (e.g., spinal cord injury patients).

Oral secretions also pool above the cuff of the endotracheal tube, presenting a risk of VAP. Frequent oral care and subglotttic suctioning are important to reduce the volume of these secretions. Special endotracheal tubes are available that permit continuous removal of subglottic secretions via

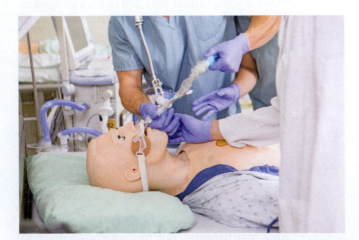

Figure 7–11 Healthcare team adjusting endotracheal tube on simulated patient in hospital.
SOURCE: Tyler Olson/123RF.com

an additional suction port located just above the cuff (Chulay & Seckel, 2011).

Impaired Gas Exchange

Impaired gas exchange is a major reason for placing a patient on a mechanical ventilator. It can involve problems of oxygenation, problems of CO_2 elimination, or often both. Oxygenation problems most often result from imbalances in the relationship between ventilation and perfusion ($\dot{V}/\dot{Q}$). Mechanical ventilators are effective in improving oxygenation but do not directly manipulate it. The ventilator facilitates oxygenation in the following ways: (1) The positive airflow of the ventilator delivers oxygen to the alveoli where diffusion takes place; (2) the FiO_2 setting is adjusted as required to attain and maintain desired PaO_2, SaO_2 and SpO_2 levels; and (3) PEEP is added as needed to optimize gas exchange through manipulation of the alveoli.

Other nursing measures to improve oxygenation include turning the patient on a regular basis and maintaining a patent airway (refer to "Ineffective Airway Clearance"), closely attending to the patient's comfort needs to improve breathing patterns, and ensuring progressive mobility.

Ineffective Breathing Pattern

Ventilators can manipulate CO_2 levels directly by causing alveolar hyperventilation or hypoventilation. This fact increases the risk of the patient developing an acid–base imbalance.

Alveolar Hyperventilation Hyperventilation is associated with decreasing CO_2 levels and respiratory alkalosis. It can be patient induced if the patient is on the AC or CMV mode and is hyperventilating for any reason (e.g., anxiety, pain, brain injury) because the patient can exhale too much CO_2. This occurs because every breath that the patient takes in on these modes is a ventilator breath with a preset tidal volume. Alveolar hyperventilation also can be induced mechanically by setting the rate or tidal volume too high on the ventilator. Sometimes, as in patients with increased intracranial pressure, mild respiratory alkalosis is induced intentionally to facilitate cerebral vasoconstriction through reduced CO_2 levels since CO_2 acts as a natural vasodilator (Tobin, 2013).

Alveolar Hypoventilation Hypoventilation is associated with increasing CO_2 levels and respiratory acidosis. Hypoventilation may be patient induced—for example, in the patient on SIMV mode (or other spontaneous breathing mode) whose breathing is too shallow. It also can be induced mechanically by setting the rate or tidal volume too low on the ventilator.

Nursing Considerations A changing ABG trend may indicate destabilization of the patient's respiratory or metabolic status, and the underlying cause should be investigated. It is the nurse's responsibility to monitor the ABG trends, observe the patient's condition, notify the provider of increasing abnormalities, collaborate with respiratory therapists, and monitor the ventilator settings at established intervals. The nurse also can facilitate gas exchange by taking actions to maintain airway clearance and effective breathing patterns.

Patients may be placed on the mechanical ventilator because of ineffective breathing patterns, which consist of any significant changes in the breathing rate, rhythm, or depth from the patient's baseline normal values (e.g., tachypnea, bradypnea, apnea, hypoventilation, hyperventilation). Changes in breathing patterns can affect ventilation, oxygenation, and acid–base status, as previously described.

After the patient is placed on the ventilator, breathing patterns that remain too rapid must be controlled to prevent hyperventilation problems. The nurse should assess for possible causes of the rapid pattern and take steps to relieve the problem when possible. Rapid breathing patterns may stem from fear, anxiety, pain, or such physiologic problems as acid–base imbalance or head injury.

Protection of the Airway Protecting the airway is a major goal in caring for the mechanically ventilated patient. Any artificial airway can be dislodged fairly easily and either partially or completely. Steps must be taken to minimize the possibility of dislodgment, which could precipitate respiratory compromise. During bedside care, the highest risk of dislodgment occurs while moving the patient from side to side in bed, when transferring the patient into or out of bed, and during transport out of the unit. Ensuring proper fit and placement of the commercial tube holder prior to movement provides safety. Furthermore, it is advisable to have the ICU nurse accompany the patient when being transported off the unit for procedures and to ensure adequate securing of device before transport.

If the patient is not fully oriented or is uncooperative, he or she may pull out the airway. Interventions to reorient and remind the patient are indicated, as are measures to relieve pain and anxiety. Ensuring adequate supervision and meeting physical and emotional needs support best practice. When less restrictive measures are not sufficient, soft wrist restraints may be necessary, which requires a healthcare provider's order. When restraints are in use, neurovascular checks are routinely performed distal to the restraints and protocols are followed to ensure that care needs are met, including turning, positioning, and skin care. The purpose of the restraints must be explained and reinforced to both the patient and family, emphasizing that the restraints are in place for protection of the airway (Kiekkas et al., 2013).

Alteration in Cardiac Output

The general goal of supporting tissue perfusion can be addressed by increasing cardiac output. Positive pressure ventilation profoundly affects the normal hemodynamics of the body by increasing intrathoracic pressures and decreasing venous return to the heart, which decreases cardiac output. The use of PEEP further compromises cardiac output by further decreasing venous return. While on the mechanical ventilator, the patient may have a flow-directed catheter inserted in the pulmonary artery

to closely monitor hemodynamic status, particularly if there is a history of cardiovascular problems.

If the patient does not have a pulmonary artery catheter inserted, the nurse can assess for the clinical manifestations of decreased cardiac output, such as confusion, restlessness, decreased urine output, flattened neck veins, and clammy, cool skin. Management of abnormal hemodynamics depends on the underlying cause of the instability; however, attaining and maintaining optimal hydration is a major factor in achieving hemodynamic stability.

Alteration in Nutrition Many patients who require mechanical ventilation have preexisting malnutrition associated with their chronic illness or inadequate nutritional support during hospitalization or a combination of both. This patient population is at high risk for imbalanced nutrition that does not meet the body's requirements. During the acute phase of illness, the patient will receive nothing orally. The presence of an ET tube, even with a properly inflated cuff, places the patient at high risk for aspiration of microparticles that can leak around the endotracheal cuff and contaminate the lower airway. This leakage can precipitate complications associated with aspiration.

A malnourished state with a negative nitrogen balance significantly decreases the patient's chances of successfully weaning from the mechanical ventilator due to respiratory muscle atrophy and weakness. Regaining nutritional integrity is a crucial aspect of care management because it has a direct impact on the patient's ability to improve his or her condition.

Collaboration with the dietitian and provider allows for nutritional assessment and formula delivery to meet each individual's needs. A small-bore feeding tube is placed with a functional gastrointestinal system and verified for enteral feeds and hydration. Total parenteral nutrition via a central catheter may be an alternative option for gastrointestinal dysfunction. Constipation with abdominal distention can develop during mechanical ventilation due to immobility, illness, and narcotics used for comfort. Simethicone may be used for individuals with abdominal distention secondary to gas accumulation in the bowel.

Nursing Management of Psychosocial Needs

The following is a brief discussion of psychosocial needs specific to the patient requiring mechanical ventilation.

Anxiety and Pain High-acuity patients, in general, are at high risk for experiencing pain and anxiety related to their underlying illness, procedures, immobility, routine care, and the critical care environment itself. The high-acuity patient who is also being mechanically ventilated has additional potential sources of pain and anxiety. Pain is commonly associated with the insertion and continuing presence of the ET tube and frequent suctioning. A high level of anxiety is often associated with having to breathe through an ET tube that is attached to a ventilator, and the inability to communicate orally. Anxiety is a common complaint of patients who have chronic respiratory problems.

Many chronic pulmonary diseases are progressive in nature; thus, a pattern of increasing disability is experienced. As many chronic pulmonary diseases progress, patients experience an increasing pattern of hospital admissions for complications of their diseases.

When patients are experiencing acute respiratory distress, their anxiety may intensify. Severe dyspnea is frequently associated with fear of suffocation or dying. All energy is focused toward breathing when acute distress exists. Being placed on a mechanical ventilator may be received by the patient either with relief or with an increased state of anxiety.

Management of the patient's anxiety and pain while on the mechanical ventilator requires collaborative and independent nursing interventions. Sedation commonly is ordered to decrease anxiety levels, which, in turn, helps the patient breathe with the ventilator. When oxygen consumption is significantly elevated, a neuromuscular blocking agent may be used to paralyze the respiratory muscles, producing rapid apnea and total skeletal muscle paralysis. Neuromuscular blocking agents do not alter the responsiveness level of the patient. Therefore, while in the paralyzed state, this group of patients should receive intermittent IV sedation and analgesia at regular intervals to reduce anxiety, relieve pain, and enhance mental rest. Goals of minimal sedation and progressive mobility lead to fewer critical care complications.

Sleep Pattern Disturbance   While on the ventilator, the patient experiences interruptions throughout the 24-hour day. Airway clearance and other maintenance nursing interventions frequently require disturbing a resting or sleeping high-acuity patient. Clustering interventions, especially during sleep periods, promotes better rest. Dimmed lights, noise reduction, and a coordinated routine—while ensuring safety with alarms and monitoring—help provide an atmosphere for rest. Observing the mode of ventilation and adjusting per need may help ensure better sleep patterns (LeMone et al., 2015; Tobin, 2013).

Communication and Sensation   The presence of an artificial airway prevents the patient from communicating verbally. The patient who is fully responsive may become very frustrated when he or she cannot talk. Patient and family teaching should include that the loss of audible speech is temporary while the cuffed tube is in place, due to airflow alteration by the vocal cords. Alternative communication methods are available. To evaluate appropriate types of communication alternatives, the nurse must evaluate the patient's visual status and collaborate with the speech or language therapist to determine whether the patient wears eyeglasses, which may improve interaction.

Simple needs often can be expressed through lip reading or hand signals. Determining the best strategy and ensuring that all team members utilize it will promote the most effective results. Communication boards, dry-erase boards, and computers may be useful options. Technology-savvy individuals may find success with texting or using social media.

Speaking valves are one-way valves, bias closed on exhalation, that can be added to the ventilator circuit for tracheostomy patients after assessment and collaboration to facilitate voice with cuff deflation. If the valve is an option, a plan of care is developed for its use and monitoring safety (Morris, Bedon, McIntosh, & Whitmer, 2015).

Family Support   The psychosocial needs of the patient's family are important while the patient's physical needs are being managed on the ventilator. How families perceive the use of a ventilator varies. The family may express relief that the patient's breathing status is now protected. This is particularly true of families of patients who have had several past intubations. The patient's family initially may find the presence of the artificial airway and mechanical ventilator a frightening experience. The frequent alarms and the patient's inability to communicate verbally are the basis for many questions asked of the nurse.

Section Eight Review

1. What is the primary reason that airway patency becomes compromised in the mechanically ventilated client?
   A. Ineffective cough to clear mucus
   B. Oversedation
   C. Presence of thin watery secretions
   D. Dehydration

2. Which manifestation is an indication for suctioning?
   A. Low airway pressure alarm
   B. Low respiratory rate
   C. Course crackles over the trachea
   D. Normal oxygenation

3. A mechanically ventilated client who is malnourished is at high risk for failure to wean for what reason?
   A. Impaired gas exchange
   B. Decreased cardiac output
   C. Increased airway resistance
   D. Respiratory muscle weakness

4. A client who is mechanically ventilated is not sleeping well. What nursing action would address this problem?
   A. Cluster activities
   B. Administer sedatives
   C. Administer neuromuscular blocking agents
   D. Space activities evenly throughout the 24-hour day

Answers: 1. A, 2. C, 3. D, 4. A

Section Nine: Weaning the Patient from the Mechanical Ventilator

The term *mechanical ventilator weaning* includes all the activities involved in freeing a patient from mechanical ventilator support and attaining total independence from the ventilator. Withdrawing this support is an interdisciplinary effort that requires coordination among the provider, respiratory therapist, nurse, and patient. Ventilator weaning may be a relatively simple and rapid withdrawal process, or it may be complex and extremely slow. The majority of patients requiring mechanical ventilator support are weaned rapidly with little difficulty. The remaining few are those who require prolonged weaning or are unable to wean. This small but significant group consists primarily of patients who have a history of chronic pulmonary disease or who have required prolonged mechanical ventilation due to critical illness. The key to successful weaning is the correction of the underlying disorder that caused the ventilator dependence.

Patients who are being evaluated for ventilator weaning fall into three categories:

- Patients whose liberation from the ventilator is rapid when the reason for mechanical ventilation is resolved
- Patients who wean from mechanical ventilation slowly and gradually and whose condition requires more deliberate planning than the usual routine weaning activities
- Patients who are considered ventilator dependent and may require long-term ventilatory support

Readiness for Weaning

Just as criteria are used in making the decision to place a patient on a mechanical ventilator, criteria are used when determining readiness for withdrawal from ventilator support. Successful weaning involves using a systematic approach, including determination of readiness to wean, weaning, and postextubation (removal of the artificial airway) follow-up. Weaning predictor tests have limited usefulness with no clear definitive path beyond clinical decisions of the team (Blackwood, Burns, Cardwell, & O'Halloran, 2014; Tobin, 2013).

Traditional Methods to Determine Readiness to Wean Successful weaning depends on the physiologic and psychologic readiness of the patient. The traditional criteria for determining readiness to wean are similar to the criteria used in deciding to place the patient on the mechanical ventilator. These criteria can be divided into initial and comprehensive patient screenings.

Initial Patient Screening. Consideration for readiness for weaning begins when the cause of respiratory failure is resolved or significantly improved. Other necessary criteria include adequate oxygenation (while receiving FiO_2 less than 0.50 and PEEP less than 8), hemodynamic stability, and spontaneous ventilatory effort. Predictors of weaning success are open to physician and team interpretation. The interpretation of a test result depends on the clinician's belief and pretest probability of disease (Tobin, 2013). A comprehensive, interdisciplinary, protocol-driven approach is best for successful liberation from mechanical ventilation (Blackwood et al., 2014).

Alternative Indications of Readiness to Wean   Table 7–4 provides a summary of the bedside weaning parameters.

The Weaning Process: Duration

Weaning the patient from mechanical ventilator support requires careful planning; therefore, interdisciplinary planning and reassessment are key for successful outcomes. The strategies used will vary based on individual

Table 7–4 Bedside Weaning Parameters

Parameter	Target Range	Comments
Rapid Shallow Breathing Index (RSBI, f/V_T)	Fewer than 105 breaths/min/L (spontaneous breathing)	Consists of the patient's respiratory rate divided by the tidal volume Obtain at least 1 minute after disconnection while receiving O_2 therapy More useful for study protocol than in weaning protocols
Vital Capacity (VC)	Greater than 10 mL/kg (ideal body weight [IBW]	Requires patient cooperation; is not a consistent predictor of readiness to wean
Breathing Rate (f)	Fewer than 35 spontaneous breaths/min	Breathing more than 35/min = negative indicator for weaning success
Spontaneous Tidal Volume (V_T)	Greater than 4 to 6 mL/kg (IBW)	
Maximum Inspiratory Pressure (MIP, P_{Imax}) (or Negative Inspiratory Force [NIF])	Less than −20 to −30 cm H_2O	Measured after 20 sec of airway occlusion Cease if desaturation or cardiac dysrhythmias develop
Minute Ventilation ($\dot{V}_E$)	Less than 10 L/min	
Airway Occlusion Pressure ($P_{0.1}$)	Less than −6 cm H_2O	Upper airway pressure is measured after airway occluded for 100 msec during inspiratory phase. Requires special valve systems

Emerging Evidence

- According to a Cochrane Database systematic review of 11 trials, there exists some evidence of a reduction in duration of mechanical ventilation, weaning duration, and ICU length of stay (ICU-LOS) with use of standardized protocols (*Blackwood et al., 2014*).

- In a study that compared nasal-oral mask with full-face mask in a convenience sample of critically ill patients (100 in each group), the full-face mask caused fewer pressure ulcers on the bridge of the nose and was more comfortable. Preventive application of hydrocolloid dressing, frequent reassessment, and use of full-face mask interfaces may reduce risk (*Schallom et al., 2015*).

- The results of a descriptive study of 42 adult patients on mechanical ventilators, to assess for cues for suctioning after closed-system suctioning, demonstrated that patients on mechanical ventilators should be routinely assessed for coarse rhonchi over the trachea area to determine the need for suctioning. Lung sound assessment is a less sensitive indicator (*Sole et al., 2015*).

- Lai et al. (2016) investigated the outcomes of 1821 patients requiring prolonged mechanical ventilation (defined as more than 21 days) and identified risk factors associated with its mortality rate after admission to a respiratory care center between January 2006 and December 2014. The mean age of the sample was 69.8 ± 14.2 years, and 521 patients (28.6%) were aged > 80 years. Upon admission, the APACHE II scores were 16.5 ± 6.3, and 1311 (72%) patients had at least one comorbidity. Pulmonary infection was the most common diagnosis (n = 770, 42.3%). A total of 320 patients died with an in-hospital mortality rate of 17.6%. A multivariate stepwise logistic regression analysis indicated that patients were more likely to die if they were > 80 years of age, had lower albumin levels (< 2 g/dL) and higher APACHE II scores (≥15), required hemodialysis, or had a comorbidity. In conclusion, the in-hospital mortality for patients requiring PMV in our study was 17%, and mortality was associated with disease severity, hypoalbuminemia, hemodialysis, and an older age (*Lai et al., 2016*).

patient needs and time on ventilator support. Based on a time trajectory, there are two ways to wean a patient: rapid weaning and slow weaning.

Rapid Weaning (Short Term) A patient with no significant lung disease (e.g., recovering from surgery or a drug overdose) requires short-term mechanical ventilation. Once the underlying problem is corrected (e.g., reversal of anesthesia effects), the patient is evaluated for weaning. If weaning criteria are met, the patient is placed on spontaneous breathing mode (CPAP, PSV, or T-piece) and provided with humidified oxygen with T-piece for 30 to 120 minutes. During the trial period, the patient is monitored for comfort, cardiac rhythm status, and ABG status. If these criteria remain within acceptable limits (PaO$_2$ greater than 60 mmHg on FiO$_2$ of less than 40%, and pH above 7.30), the patient is extubated. Rapid weaning may also be accomplished using low levels of PSV or CPAP. The patient is given a brief trial period and then extubated. In a randomized study of 160 adults on mechanical ventilation for more than 24 hours, no difference was found when comparing proportional assist ventilation plus (PAV+), T-tube, and PSV regarding extubation failure, duration of mechanical ventilation, or ICU or hospital stay (Teixeira et al., 2015). Figure 7–12 illustrates a typical T-piece (blow-by) configuration

Slow Weaning (Long Term) Slow weaning is performed on patients who are unable to wean rapidly for a variety of reasons. A patient with underlying chronic lung disease (e.g., emphysema or pulmonary fibrosis) complicated by some acute problem (e.g., sepsis, pneumonia), or a patient who has had a prolonged illness frequently cannot be weaned as rapidly as a patient with normal lungs. Difficult-to-wean patients often are in a poorer state of general health than the fast-weaning group. Their ability to make the transition back to spontaneous negative pressure breathing from long-term positive pressure breathing is

slow and requires retraining and strengthening of the respiratory muscles. Problems associated with difficult weaning include excessive respiratory muscle work of breathing, respiratory muscle fatigue, anemia, malnutrition, excessive secretions, infection, unstable hemodynamic state, fear, and anxiety.

Slow weaning is a complex process. Over time, multiple weaning strategies may need to be employed in response to changes in the patient's clinical status. Long-term weaning requires close monitoring of the patient's multisystem functions, as well as psychosocial status, as progressive mobility is introduced. Management of problems as they arise significantly improves the chances for successful weaning.

The Weaning Process: Methods

Weaning the patient from the ventilator can be done manually or by using the mechanical ventilator.

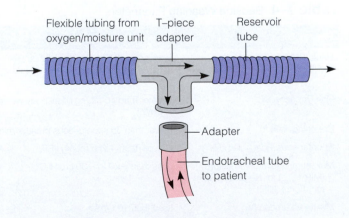

Figure 7–12 T–piece (blow-by) configuration.

Manual Weaning (Spontaneous Breathing Trials) The original method of withdrawing a patient from a ventilator was manual weaning, and it is still used today. Manual weaning is accomplished by following a schedule of disconnecting the patient from the mechanical ventilator for increasingly longer periods of time. When this method is used, the patient is disconnected from the ventilator and a humidified oxygen source is attached to the artificial airway using a T-piece. The nurse and respiratory therapist are responsible for closely monitoring the patient for signs of weaning intolerance.

Manual weaning requires close patient contact throughout the weaning period, with the nurse playing a crucial role in patient monitoring, pulmonary hygiene, and coaching breathing during the trial period. The nurse's calm reassurance is instrumental in assisting the patient past the period of anxiety often associated with removal from the mechanical ventilator. Manual weaning is performed on an increasing schedule, either throughout a 24-hour period or only during day and evening hours, maintaining the patient on mechanical ventilation throughout the night for rest. The amount of time the patient is kept off the ventilator may start at 5 minutes and increase to the entire day, except at night, before full independence. Manual weaning must be individually designed, based on the patient's changing status from day to day, with consideration of the overall plan of a weaning protocol (Blackwood et al., 2014).

Manual weaning is a strengthening exercise for the respiratory muscles. Complete removal from the ventilator forces the respiratory muscles to take over the complete work of breathing, without any assistance from the ventilator for increasing blocks of time. Conditioning is increased through use of the weaning procedure and good nutrition and hydration. Inspiratory muscle training for selected patients in the ICU may show benefits to overall outcomes (Elkins & Dentice, 2015).

Manual weaning has several disadvantages. First, it may be a frightening experience for the patient who is more accustomed to positive pressure breathing. Abrupt removal from the ventilator may precipitate high anxiety, which can hinder the weaning process. Second, manual weaning is time-consuming for the nurse. During the period that the patient is off the ventilator, particularly in the early stages of weaning, the nurse's bedside presence to coach and monitor tolerance, and to provide encouragement, may be a challenge to fulfill.

Ventilator Weaning Spontaneous breathing trials can also be done using the ventilator. Rather than placing the patient on a T-piece, the patient is placed on CPAP with or without low levels of pressure support. The length of time of spontaneous breathing is increased as tolerated, similar to T-piece weaning. Using the ventilator for spontaneous trials offers the advantages of maintaining CPAP, which may be important for some patients, and ventilator monitoring for safety.

Ventilator weaning is generally thought to be less traumatic for the patient because it does not involve intermittent removal from the ventilator. A variety of alternative modes are used for ventilator weaning. The choice of weaning mode is based on the clinician's preferences, the type of equipment available, and the patient's needs and clinical status. There is no significant difference in weaning failure with manual versus ventilator weaning (Teixeira et al., 2015).

Table 7–5 provides a summary of the common manual and ventilator weaning modes.

Weaning may not be a smooth undertaking. In patients with underlying disease, a changing condition

Table 7–5 Common Weaning Modes

Weaning Mode	Description	Advantages	Disadvantages
T-Piece (spontaneous breathing trials)	Patient is provided supplementary oxygen and humidity. Time off the ventilator is gradually increased.	Strengthening exercise for respiratory muscles All breaths are spontaneous.	Potential for apnea Requires close monitoring, can cause patient anxiety
SIMV	Frequency of mandatory ventilator breaths is slowly decreased, which requires the patient to gradually take over own work of breathing.	Maintains respiratory muscle strength and reduces atrophy Maintains more normal gas distribution Reduces cardiovascular side effects Maintains some of the work of breathing	May increase the work of breathing as a result of demand valve system Rate must be manually manipulated.
PSV	Provides positive pressure during the inspiration phase to support tidal volumes and decrease work of breathing	Decreased work of breathing, as it attempts to overcome tube resistance Increased patient comfort Minimal cardiovascular side effects	All breaths are spontaneous. Flow pattern may not be adequate. Inspiratory flow rate may be too high or too low.
Mandatory minute ventilation (MMV)	Guarantees an ongoing stable level of minute ventilation ($\dot{V}_E$) As the patient increases or decreases ventilatory effort, the ventilator adjusts itself automatically to continue to provide the same level of $\dot{V}_E$.	Good control of $PaCO_2$ Protection from hypoventilation during weaning Facilitates transition from ventilator to spontaneous breathing	May not respond quickly enough to an apneic episode Potential for development of hypercapnia in presence of a rapid shallow breathing pattern

SOURCE: Data from Teixeira et al. (2015); Tobin (2013).

can require temporary cessation of weaning. This is particularly true if the patient should develop pneumonia. Such a status change may first manifest itself in a sudden intolerance to weaning.

Whatever the method used, it requires a comprehensive approach to weaning, coordinated by a team leader. Success using structured, interdisciplinary protocols helps guide the weaning process and ongoing patient assessments. Continuing efforts are made to optimize all aspects of care. During weaning, the respiratory therapist is generally in charge of making setting changes to the mechanical ventilator while the nurse and respiratory therapist closely monitor the patient for signs of failure to wean. If failure-to-wean signs develop, the patient should be returned to the preweaning ventilator settings and the plan reviewed for amendments.

Special Considerations for Older Adults

Older adults can have outcomes from mechanical ventilation similar to those of younger patients. However, common complications of critical illness, such as delirium, side effects of sedative agents, and deconditioning, can adversely prolong ventilation and length of stay for older adults. Higher mortality rates and poorer functional outcomes occur in patients with multiple organ failure or prolonged intubation. The best mode for weaning older adult patients has not been identified.

Older adults, without significant comorbid illness, become frail in the high-acuity setting and vulnerable to complications. To avoid fatigue, nursing care and procedures should be spaced at intervals allowing time for rest. Sleep can be enhanced by obtaining information on and trying to maintain the patient's usual schedule, promoting a day–night schedule, reducing noise, and following nonpharmacologic approaches.

Priorities for care include cautious use of sedative–hypnotic agents that can cause confusion because older adult patients are at increased risk for developing delirium. Delirium protocols provide guidance for care planning. All medications should be evaluated for potential adverse drug interactions. Efforts can be made to enhance quality stimulation and communication. Hearing aids and eyeglasses should be used if needed by the patient. Malnutrition may be present on admission or develop while the patient is in the hospital and can contribute to muscle weakness. Early progressive mobility is needed to limit muscle atrophy from prolonged bed rest. These approaches are not limited to the care of older adults but represent important care for any high-acuity patient. In older adult patients, however, the approaches assume a greater imperative given their vulnerability and reduced capacity to recover from severe insults (Reames et al., 2016).

Postextubation Follow-up

Extubation is carried out as soon as it is determined that patients can sustain spontaneous breathing, usually indicated by maintaining their own airways and coughing adequately to mobilize secretions. An air leak test is helpful to evaluate the potential for airway obstruction postextubation. To conduct an air leak test, the oropharynx is suctioned, the ET cuff is deflated, and the patient is evaluated for the ability to breathe around the tube. When these criteria are met, rapid tube removal is recommended. Quick tube removal is important because the ET tube increases the work of breathing.

Following extubation, particular attention must be given to excellent pulmonary hygiene, including a routine of mobilizing secretions with optimal positioning. Various aerosol therapies, percussion, and postural drainage may be ordered to prevent or treat complications, if indicated. Noninvasive ventilation may be helpful for patients at high risk for fatigue and reintubation.

Glottic edema is a potential postextubation complication resulting in stridor, which can be mild or severe. When severe, it can cause total obstruction of the airway and require reintubation. Patients are also at risk postextubation for aspiration as a result of swallowing dysfunction. There is a high incidence of aspiration (up to 50%) in patients who have been intubated for more than 48 hours. Many of these patients develop silent aspiration (aspirating without coughing). Aspiration may contribute to postextubation respiratory failure. Patients must be monitored carefully when oral intake is resumed, and a formal swallow evaluation may be appropriate for high-risk patients (AACN, 2010).

Patients with tracheostomy tubes may be considered for decannulation when they no longer need ventilator support. With spontaneous breathing, assessment for secretion clearance, tolerance to cuff deflation, and oxygen need suggest success with possible decannulation. An interim step is exchanging a tracheostomy tube with either a cuffless tube or a tight-to-shaft tube that may be capped. This promotes airflow around the perimeter of the tube, vocalization, and secretion clearance. If this tube is tolerated without setback, decannulation may be considered. When the tube is removed, the stoma is covered with petrolatum gauze to provide a seal that allows for effective coughing and phonation. The time required for a stoma to close varies among individuals (Cheung & Napolitano, 2014).

Terminal Weaning

Terminal weaning is the intentional removal of the mechanical ventilator when the patient is expected to die without it. Many institutions have a policy and specific protocols for terminal weaning. Medications are generally ordered to be administered as needed to maintain patient comfort by minimizing pain, respiratory distress, agitation, and anxiety. Withdrawal from the ventilator can be accomplished with a slow weaning process or rapid withdrawal. The nurse closely monitors the patient's status and provides medications as needed (prn). Furthermore, the nurse plays an important role in supporting the patient's family through this end-of-life process (Currow, Higginson, & Johnson, 2013).

Section Nine Review

1. In what manner are the vast majority of clients requiring mechanical ventilation weaned?
   A. Rapidly, with difficulty
   B. Rapidly, without difficulty
   C. Slowly, with difficulty
   D. Slowly, without difficulty

2. The majority of difficult-to-wean clients have which condition?
   A. Pneumonia
   B. Congestive heart failure
   C. Acute respiratory distress syndrome
   D. Chronic pulmonary disease

3. Which question would be asked during the initial client screening criteria for weaning eligibility?
   A. Is the urinary output greater than 620 mL/24 hr?
   B. Is the prealbumin 10 mg/dL or greater?
   C. Is the client's clinical condition improving?
   D. Have drugs been discontinued that decrease the respiratory drive?

4. Which term refers to weaning by intermittently removing the client from the ventilator for increasing periods of time.
   A. Manual
   B. Ventilator
   C. SIMV
   D. Pressure support ventilation

Answers: 1. B, 2. D, 3. C, 4. A

Clinical Reasoning Checkpoint

Deborah M, a 44-year-old morbidly obese female, has just been transferred to the surgical ICU from the postop recovery room following bariatric surgery. Her medical history is positive for hypertension and type 2 diabetes; she also has a history of sleep apnea. Her social history is positive for smoking half a pack of cigarettes every day for 25 years. She is a divorced mother with three children. The recovery room nurse informs you that Ms. M self-extubated and the decision was made to allow her to remain extubated. She is awake but drowsy and is currently receiving 4 liters of oxygen by nasal cannula. She is attached to a cardiac monitor and pulse oximetry.

1. What risk factors does Ms. M have for developing pulmonary problems while in the ICU?

2. By 6 hours postop, you are becoming concerned that Ms. M's pulmonary status is deteriorating. What priority assessment data do you want to obtain at this time?

Clinical Update You now have access to your initial assessment data:

Parameter	Previous	Current
Vital Signs		
• Respiratory Rate: • Blood Pressure: • Heart Rate:	• 22–24 breaths/min • 142–146 (SBP) and 84–88 (DBP) • 74–86 beats/min, regular	• 32–36 breaths/min, shallow • 156/92 • 94–102 beats/min, regular
• SpO$_2$:	• 99%	• 90%
• ABG	On admission to SICU: • pH: 7.40 • PaCO$_2$, 42 mmHg • PaO$_2$, 99 mmHg • HCO$_3$ 28 mEq/L	• pH: 7.30 • PaCO$_2$, 52 mmHg • PaO$_2$, 85 mmHg • HCO$_3$ 28 mEq/L

3. Examine the data that you just collected on Ms. M (see clinical update).
   • In looking at her trends, what is your analysis of her current status?
   • Does she qualify for initial consideration for mechanical ventilation?
   • Briefly explain your answer.

Clinical Update Bedside pulmonary function tests (PFTs) are ordered, and the results are as follows:

Vital capacity (VC): 14 mL/kg
Minute ventilation ($\dot{V}_E$): 13 L/min
Negative inspiratory force (NIF): −18 cm H$_2$O

4. Examine Ms. M's pulmonary function test results. Explain the significance of these results.

5. You are assigned to prepare for Ms. M's reintubation. List the necessary pieces of equipment.

6. Ms. M is placed on a positive pressure ventilator, with volume cycling, assist-control mode, with 5 cm H$_2$O of PEEP. Briefly explain each of these terms:
   • Positive pressure ventilator
   • Volume cycling
   • Assist-control mode
   • PEEP of 5 cm H$_2$O
   • FiO$_2$ of 0.30

Chapter 7 Review

1. A client is admitted to the hospital with a diagnosis of acute respiratory failure and may require mechanical ventilation. The client has a low ventilation-perfusion ratio as a result of pulmonary shunting. Which ABG result would the nurse anticipate in this client?
   1. PaO_2 55 mmHG
   2. pH 7.30
   3. $PaCO_2$ 30 mmHG
   4. PaO_2 100 mmHG

2. A client admitted in respiratory failure becomes increasingly tachypneic and hypoxic and requires emergent intubation. The nurse can expect which artificial airway to be inserted?
   1. Oral endotracheal tube
   2. Nasotracheal tube
   3. Tracheostomy tube
   4. Oral pharyngeal airway

3. A client is placed on volume-cycled ventilation. The nurse plans care for this client based on which characteristic of this method of ventilation?
   1. A set volume will be delivered, which will help overcome the client's airway resistance changes.
   2. There is no need for placement of an artificial airway.
   3. The volume delivered by the ventilator will vary depending upon pressure changes.
   4. This type of ventilator is able to deliver higher oxygen levels than other types.

4. A client's ventilatory setting is at 10 cm H_2O of PEEP. Which assessment findings would the nurse evaluate as indicating a possible negative consequence to this ventilator setting? (Select all that apply.)
   1. Pneumothorax
   2. Increased sedation
   3. Decrease in blood pressure
   4. Lower respiratory rate
   5. Temperature elevation

5. Before being placed on noninvasive positive pressure ventilation (NIPPV), a client has these ABGs: pH 7.25, $PaCO_2$ 66 mmHg, PaO_2 90 mmHg, HCO_3 23 mmHg. One hour after being placed on NIPPV the client's ABGs are pH 7.32, $PaCO_2$ 46 mmHg, PaO_2 92 mmHg, HCO_3 24 mmHg. What should the nurse do? (Select all that apply.)
   1. Increase the oxygen
   2. Plan for immediate intubation
   3. Increase the expiratory pressure
   4. Check the mask for an air leak
   5. Continue monitoring

6. A client on mechanical ventilation has decreasing hemoglobin and hematocrit with dark stools. The nurse should prepare for which intervention?
   1. Administer an enema
   2. Administer an iron supplement
   3. Discontinue the proton pump inhibitor
   4. Test stools for blood

7. A client has an oral endotracheal tube and has been on mechanical ventilation for 3 days. Why is it important for the nurse to monitor and maintain cuff pressure at no more than 30 mmHg?
   1. So that secretions from the upper airway can enter the lower airway
   2. To prevent necrosis of the trachea
   3. To allow for air movement around the cuff
   4. To increase circulation in the lungs

8. A nurse is having difficulty clearing secretions from a client's endotracheal tube. What actions should the nurse take? (Select all that apply.)
   1. Increase the frequency of suctioning
   2. Increase the client's fluid intake
   3. Instill saline into the endotracheal tube before suctioning
   4. Check to see that adequate humidification is delivered via the ventilator
   5. Increase suction pressure

9. A client is successfully weaned off mechanical ventilation using spontaneous breathing (T-piece) trials. The nurse explains to the student nurse that using the T-piece supports weaning in which manner?
   1. It requires the client to gradually take over the work of breathing.
   2. It supports the client's tidal volume during inspiration.
   3. It ensures that the client maintains a stable minute volume.
   4. It supports the client by maintaining open alveoli at the end of expiration.

10. A client is placed on a mechanical ventilator at these settings: tidal volume 450 mL, rate 8 breaths per minute, FiO_2 50%. The client's $PaCO_2$ has increased from 45 mmHg to 55 mmHg. What ventilator setting does the nurse expect to be altered to decrease the $PaCO_2$?
    1. Decrease rate to 6 breaths per minute
    2. Increase FiO_2 to 60 percent
    3. Decrease tidal volume to 400 mL
    4. Increase rate to 12 breaths per minute

*Answers to questions found inside your textbook are available on
the faculty resources site. Please consult with your instructor.*

References

Akulian, J. A., Yarmus, L., & Feller-Kopman, D. (2015). The role of cricothyrotomy, tracheostomy, and percutaneous tracheostomy in airway management. *Anesthesiology Clinics, 33*(2), 357–367.

American Association of Critical-Care Nurses (AACN). (2008). AACN practice alert: Ventilator associated pneumonia (VAP). Retrieved December 12, 2016, from http://www.aacn.org/wd/practice/docs/practicealerts/vap.pdf

American Association of Critical-Care Nurses (AACN). (2010). AACN practice alert: Oral care for patients at risk for ventilator-associated pneumonia. Retrieved December 12, 2016, from http://www.aacn.org/wd/practice/docs/practicealerts/oral-care-patients-at-risk-vap.pdf?menu=aboutus

Blackwood, B., Burns, K., Cardwell, C., & O'Halloran, P. (2014). Protocolized versus non-protocolized weaning for reducing the duration of mechanical ventilation in critically ill adult patients. *Cochrane Database of Systematic Reviews, 11*. doi:10.1002/14651858.CD006904.pub3

Bristle, T. J., Collins, S., Hewer, I., & Hollifield, K. (2014). Anesthesia and critical care ventilator modes: Past, present, and future. *AANA Journal, 82*(5), 387–400.

Burns, S. (2014). *AACN essentials of critical care nursing* (3rd ed.). New York, NY: McGraw-Hill Companies.

Celli, B. (2015). Chapter 323: Mechanical ventilator support. In D. L. Kasper, A. S. Fauci, D. L. Longo, S. L. Hauser, J. L. Jameson, & J. Loscalzo (Eds.), *Harrison's principles of internal medicine* (19th ed., pp. 1740–1744). New York, NY: McGraw-Hill.

Claudett, K. H., Claudett, M. B., Wong, M. C., Martinez, A. N., Soto Espinoza, R. S., Montalvo, M., . . . Andrade, M. G. (2013). Noninvasive mechanical ventilation with average volume assured pressure support (AVAPS) in patients with chronic obstructive pulmonary disease and hypercapnic encephalopathy. *BMC Pulmonary Medicine, 13*(12). doi:10.1186/1471-2466-13-12

Cheung, N. H., & Napolitano, L. M. (2014). Tracheostomy: Epidemiology, indications, timing, technique, and outcomes. *Respiratory Care, 59*(6), 895–919.

Chulay, M., & Seckel, M. (2011). Suctioning: Endotracheal or tracheostomy tube. In D. J. Lynn-McHale Wiegand (Ed.), *AACN procedure manual for critical care* (6th ed., pp. 79–87). Aliso Viejo, CA: American Association of Critical-Care Nurses.

Currow, D. C., Higginson, I. J., & Johnson, M. J. (2013). Breathlessness—current and emerging mechanisms, measurement and management: A discussion from an European Association of Palliative Care workshop. *Palliative Medicine, 27*(10), 932–938. doi:10.1177/0269216313493819

Dawson, D. (2014). Essential principles: Tracheostomy care in the adult patient. *Nursing in Critical Care, 19*(2), 63–72. doi:10.1111/nicc.12076

Donovan, L. M., Boeder, S., Malhotra, A., & Patel, S. R. (2015). New developments in the use of positive airway pressure for obstructive sleep apnea. *Journal of Thoracic Disease, 7*(8), 1323–1342. doi:10.3978/j.issn.2072-1439.2015.07.30

Elkins, M., & Dentice, R. (2015). Inspiratory muscle training facilitates weaning from mechanical ventilation among patients in the intensive care unit: A systematic review. *Journal of Physiotherapy, 61*, 125–134.

Facchin, F., & Fan, E. (2015). Airway pressure release ventilation and high-frequency oscillatory ventilation: Potential strategies to treat severe hypoxemia and prevent ventilator-induced lung injury. *Respiratory Care, 60*(10), 1509–1521. doi:10.4187/respcare.04255

Ferdowsali, K., & Modock, J. (2013). Airway pressure release ventilation: Improving oxygenation. *Dimensions of Critical Care Nursing, 32*(5), 222–228.

Goodrich, C. A. (2011). Endotracheal intubation (perform). In D. L. Wiegand (Ed.), *AACN procedure manual for critical care* (6th ed., pp. 9–21). Aliso Viejo, CA: American Association of Critical-Care Nurses.

Gregoretti, C., Pisani, L., Cortegiani, A., & Ranieri, V. M. (2015). Noninvasive ventilation in critically ill patients. *Critical Care Clinics, 31*, 435–457. http://dx.doi.org/10.1016/j.ccc.2015.03.002

Helmerhorst, H., Schultz, M., van der Voort, P., de Jonge, E., & van Westerloo, D. (2015). Bench-to-bedside review: The effects of hyperoxia during critical illness. *Critical Care, 19*(1), 284.

Hyde, G. A., Savage, S. A., Zarzaur, B. L., Hart-Hyde, J. E., Schaefer, C. B., Croce, M. A., & Fabian, T. C. (2015). Early tracheostomy in trauma patients saves time and money. *Inquiry, 46*(1), 110–114.

Joint Commission, The. (2014). National patient safety goal on alarm management. Retrieved December 12, 2016, from http://www.jointcommission.org/assets/1/18/jcp0713_announce_new_nspg.pdf

Kiekkas, P., Aretha, D., Panteli, E., Baltopoulos, G. I., & Filos, K. S. (2013). Unplanned extubation in critically ill adults: Clinical review. *Nursing in Critical Care, 18*(3), 123–134. doi:10.1111/j.1478-5153.2012.00542

Kress, J., & Hall, J. (2015). Chapter 321: Approach to the patient with critical illness. In D. Kasper, A. Fauci, D. Longo, S. Hauser, J. Jameson, & J. Loscalzo (Eds.), *Harrison's principles of internal medicine* (19th ed., pp. 1729–1740). New York, NY: McGraw-Hill Education.

Kunugiyama, S. K., & Schulman, C. S. (2012). High-frequency percussive ventilation using the VDR-4 ventilator: An effective strategy for patients with refractory hypoxemia. *AACN Advanced Critical Care, 23*(4), 370–380. doi:10.1097/NCI.0b013e31826e9031

Lai, C., Shieh, J., Chiang, S., Chiang, K., Weng, S., Ho, C., . . . Cheng, K. (2016). The outcomes and prognostic factors of patients requiring prolonged mechanical ventilation. *Scientific Reports, 6*, 28034. doi:10.1038/srep28034

Lamb, K. D. (2015). Year in review 2014: Mechanical ventilation. *Respiratory Care, 60*(4), 606–608.

LeMone, P., Burke, K., Bauldoff, G., & Gubrud, P. (2015). *Medical-surgical nursing: Clinical reasoning in patient care* (6th ed.). Hoboken, NJ: Pearson Education.

Marino, P. (2014). *The ICU book* (4th ed.). Philadelphia, PA: Lippincott Williams & Wilkins.

Mireles-Cabodevila, E., Hatipoglu, U., & Chatburn, R. (2013). A rational framework for selecting modes of ventilation. *Respiratory Care, 58*(2), 348–366.

Morris, L. L., Bedon, A. M., McIntosh, E., & Whitmer, A. (2015). Restoring speech to tracheostomy patients. *Critical Care Nurse, 35*(6), 13–28. doi:10.4037/ccn2015401

Nair, G. B., & Niederman, M. S. (2015). Ventilator-associated pneumonia: Present understanding and ongoing debates. *Intensive Care Medicine, 41,* 34–48. doi:10.1007/s00134-014-3564-5

Palmer, L. B. (2015). Ventilator-associated infection: The role for inhaled antibiotics. *Current Opinion in Pulmonary Medicine, 21,* 239–249. doi:10.1097/MCP.0000000000000160

Plowright, C. (2014). Safe care of patients with tracheostomies. *Nursing Times, 110*(31), 12–14.

Piesiak, P., Brzecka, A., Kosacka, M., & Jankowska, R. (2015). Efficacy of noninvasive volume targeted ventilation in patients with chronic respiratory failure due to kyphoscoliosis. *Advances in Experimental Medicine and Biology, 838,* 53–58. doi:10.1007/5584_2014_68

Reames, C. D., Price, D. M., King, E. A., & Dickinson, S. (2016). Mobilizing patients along the continuum of critical care. *Dimensions of Critical Care Nursing, 35*(1), 10–15. doi:10.1097/DCC.0000000000000151

Richard, J. M., & Mercat, A. (2014). Tracheal cuff management as part of a lung-protective strategy. *Respiratory Care, 59*(11), 1810–1811. doi:10.4187/respcare.03745

Schallom, M., Cracchiolo, L., Falker, A., Foster, J., Hager, J., Morehouse, T., . . . Kollef, M. (2015). Pressure ulcer incidence in patients wearing nasal-oral versus full-face noninvasive ventilation masks. *American Journal of Critical Care, 24*(4), 349–357. doi:10.4037/ajcc2015386

Skillings, K. N., & Curtis, B. L. (2011). Tracheostomy tube care. In D. L. Wiegand (Ed.), *AACN procedure manual for critical care* (6th ed., pp. 96–104). Aliso Viejo, CA: American Association of Critical-Care Nurses.

Sole, M. L., Bennett, M., & Ashworth, S. (2015). Clinical indicators for endotracheal suctioning in adult patients receiving mechanical ventilation. *American Journal of Critical Care, 24*(4), 318–325. doi:10.4037/ajcc2015794

Teixeira, S. N., Osaku, E. F., de Macedo Costa, C. L., Fernandes Toccolini, B., Lamberti Costa, N., Cândia, M. F., . . . Duarte, P. A. (2015). Comparison of proportional assist ventilation plus, T-tube ventilation, and pressure support ventilation as spontaneous breathing trials for extubation: A randomized study. *Respiratory Care, 60*(11), 1527–1535. doi:10.4187/respcare.03915

Tobin, M. J. (2013). *Principles and practice of mechanical ventilation.* New York, NY: McGraw-Hill Medical.

Vollman, K. M., & Sole, M. L. (2011). Endotracheal tube and oral care. In D. J. Lynn-McHale Wiegand (Ed.), *AACN procedure manual for critical care* (6th ed., pp. 31–38). Aliso Viejo, CA: American Association of Critical-Care Nurses.

Wang, F., Wu, Y., Bo, L., Lou, J., Zhu, J., & Chen, F. (2011). The timing of tracheotomy in critically ill patients undergoing mechanical ventilation: A systematic review and meta-analysis of randomized clinical trials. *CHEST, 140*(6), 1456–1465.

Weatherspoon, D. L., & Weatherspoon, C. A. (2012). Pulmonary problems. In J. W. Foster & S. A. Prevost (Eds.), *Advanced practice nursing of adults in acute care* (pp. 398–443). Philadelphia, PA: F.A. Davis.

Young, D., Harrison, D. A., Cuthbertson, B. H., & Rowan, K. (2013). Effect of early vs late tracheotomy placement on survival in patients receiving mechanical ventilation: The TracMan randomized trial. *Journal of the American Medical Association, 309*(20), 2121–2129.

Chapter 8
Basic Hemodynamic Monitoring

Learning Outcomes

8.1 Describe the major parameters of interest when monitoring a patient's hemodynamic status.

8.2 Describe noninvasive and minimally invasive hemodynamic monitoring technologies, including impedance cardiography, Doppler ultrasound, central venous pressure, direct arterial blood pressure measurement, and arterial pulse contour analysis technology.

8.3 Explain pulmonary artery (PA) catheters, including their purpose, required competencies, interpretation of data, functional components, and care of the catheter.

8.4 Apply knowledge of catheter insertion, management, and process for obtaining measurements using the PA catheter.

8.5 Describe right atrial and right ventricular pressures, including the purposes, measurement, waveform analysis, clinical findings, and treatment of abnormal pressures.

8.6 Explain pulmonary artery and pulmonary artery wedge pressures (a measure of left ventricular end diastolic pressure [LVEDP]), including the purposes, measurement, waveform analysis, clinical findings, and related interventions for treating abnormal pressures.

8.7 Describe vascular resistance (systemic and pulmonary) and its measurements, including treatments for abnormal levels.

This chapter focuses on basic concepts of hemodynamics and hemodynamic monitoring technologies and requires a working knowledge of the determinants of cardiac output: preload, afterload, and contractility. This chapter provides an overview of current hemodynamic monitoring technologies and common hemodynamic parameters that can be measured either directly or indirectly. It is organized by degree of invasiveness of the various technologies, beginning with noninvasive and ending with the most invasive technology, the pulmonary artery catheter.

Section One: Introduction to Hemodynamic Parameters

Monitoring cardiovascular blood flow, pressures, and volumes to evaluate tissue perfusion and oxygenation has become an essential part of providing high-quality care to high-acuity patients in multiple settings, such as surgery, diagnostic procedure departments (e.g., cardiac cath lab, ultrasound), and critical care areas. This section introduces the concept of hemodynamics and provides an overview of the determinants of cardiac output, the major parameter of interest to hemodynamic monitoring. Each hemodynamic parameter is presented individually and in detail in later sections.

Table 8–1 provides the hemodynamic parameters presented in this chapter, their formulae, and normal ranges.

Hemodynamics

Hemodynamics is a physiologic term that refers to the forces involved in the flow of blood as it circulates through the cardiovascular system. As the word implies, these forces are constantly changing (i.e., they are dynamic) to meet constantly altering tissue oxygen needs. Hemodynamic monitoring is the evaluation of cardiovascular function as the heart and blood vessels respond to physiologic or pathophysiologic alterations and involves the measurement of pressure, volume, and flow of blood. Hemodynamic monitoring technologies are often organized in terms of their level of invasiveness to the patient: noninvasive, minimally (or less) invasive, and invasive. Each device typically has some capacity to assess preload, afterload, contractility, and cardiac output. Hemodynamic monitoring is a rapidly evolving area in high-acuity care; therefore, as new technologies become available, it is important to evaluate the evidence for each in terms of both accuracy and patient outcome.

At the most basic level, hemodynamics can be measured by obtaining the blood pressure (using a blood pressure cuff and sphygmomanometer), heart rate (by auscultating or palpating), and urine output, all basic assessments that are easily acquired. In potentially unstable situations, however, basic hemodynamic assessments are often inadequate to accurately reflect the rapidly changing hemodynamic status—for example, during major surgery or critical illness. In such situations, more advanced hemodynamic monitoring methods are needed to accurately measure rapid changes in pressure, volume, or flow of blood to facilitate prompt diagnosis and initiate an effective treatment strategy.

Cardiac Output and Cardiac Index

Having a basic understanding of cardiac output and its determinants is key to understanding hemodynamic monitoring. **Cardiac output (CO)** is the amount of blood pumped by the heart each minute. The formula used to derive CO is simple: CO is the product of the heart rate (HR) multiplied by the stroke volume (SV) [CO = HR × SV]. Any change in HR or SV will alter CO. The normal range of CO is 4 to 8 L/min.

Cardiac Index   While measuring CO provides important information, it is not sensitive to the size of the person; yet, a person's body size significantly impacts what constitutes adequate cardiac output. Thus, in addition to CO, **cardiac index (CI)** is measured as a more accurate hemodynamic indicator of CO because it relates the CO to the patient's body size. The CI is far more meaningful than the CO for bedside clinical decision making. The formula for calculating CI is [CI = CO/BSA], with a normal range of 2.4 to 4 L/min/m². Most hemodynamic monitors calculate body surface area (BSA) if the patient's height and weight are entered into the monitor's computer system.

A clinical example illustrates the significance of body size in evaluating the adequacy of cardiac output. Consider the CO required by two different-size individuals: a large, muscular, male football player and a petite woman (examine their assessment data below). Both individuals

Table 8–1 Hemodynamic Parameters, Formulae, and Normal Ranges

Parameter	Formula	Normal Values
Cardiac index (CI)	CO/BSA	2.4 to 4.0 L/min/m²
Cardiac output (CO)	HR × SV (Heart rate × Stroke volume)	4 to 8 L/min
Left ventricular stroke work index (LVSWI)	(MAP − PAWP) × (SVI) × (0.0136)	50 to 62 g/m²/beat
Mean arterial pressure (MAP)	[(SBP) + 2 (DBP)]/3	70 to 90 mmHg
Mean pulmonary artery pressure (Mean PAP)	[(systolic) + 2 (diastolic)]/3	12 to 20 mmHg
Pulmonary artery diastolic (PAD) pressure	None	8 to 15 mmHg (2 to 5 mmHg higher than PAWP)
Pulmonary artery systolic (PAS) pressure	None	20 to 30 mmHg
Pulmonary artery wedge pressure (PAWP)	None	4 to 12 mmHg
Pulmonary vascular resistance (PVR)	[(Mean PAP) − (PAWP) × 80]/CO	50 to 250 dynes [a unit of force] · sec · cm⁻⁵
Pulmonary vascular resistance index (PVRI)	[(Mean PAP) − (PAWP) × 80]/CI	255 to 315 dynes · sec · cm⁻⁵/m²
Right atrial pressure (RAP)	None	2 to 6 mmHg
Right ventricular (RV) pressure	RV systolic/RV diastolic	20 to 30 mmHg/2 to 8 mmHg
Right ventricular stroke work index (RVSWI)	(Mean PAP − RAP) × (SVI) × (0.0136)	7.9 to 9.7 g/m²/beat
Stroke volume (SV)	CO/HR	50 to 100 mL/beat
Stroke volume index (SVI)	CI/HR	25 to 45 mL/beat/m²
Systemic vascular resistance (SVR)	[(MAP) − (RAP) × 80]/CO	800 to 1200 dynes · sec · cm⁻⁵
Systemic vascular resistance index (SVRI)	[(MAP) − (RAP) × 80]/CI	1970 to 2390 dynes · sec · cm⁻⁵/m²

have the same CO, 4 L/min, which technically falls within the normal range of 4 to 8 L/min. A quick bedside physical assessment of these individuals would yield significantly different clinical pictures. The CO of 4 L/min provides an adequate CI and serves the oxygen transport needs of the petite woman (CI = 2.65 liters/min/m²); however, the low CI of the football player is inadequate to meet his oxygen transport needs (CI = 1.64 L/min/m²); he is likely to have signs and symptoms of low cardiac output or shock.

Parameter	Football Player	Petite Woman
Cardiac output (L/min)	4	4
Weight (kg)	113	52
Height (cm)	194	158
BSA (m²)	2.44	1.51
Cardiac index (L/min/m²)	1.64	2.65
Hemodynamic status	Shocky	Adequate

Heart Rate

Heart rate is the first determinant of cardiac output and is an easily measured parameter. The heart rate is dictated by the heart's pacemaker sites, with influence from the sympathetic and parasympathetic nervous systems. It rapidly compensates for changes in CO by speeding up or slowing down. Anything that decreases HR, such as certain drugs (e.g., beta adrenergic or calcium channel blockers) or heart dysrhythmias (e.g., heart block), can rapidly decrease CO. Severe tachycardia can also reduce CO by shortening ventricular filling time during diastole, preventing sufficient blood volume from entering the ventricles before systole and causing a decrease in SV.

Stroke Volume Stroke volume (SV) is the second determinant of CO. It is defined as the amount of blood ejected by each heartbeat. Three factors significantly influence SV: preload, afterload, and contractility. These factors interact to determine the CO by their effects on SV (Figure 8–1). An adequate cardiac output is required to deliver oxygen to the tissues and organs; therefore, measures that directly and indirectly reflect CO and its determinants are the primary measures of interest for hemodynamic monitoring.

Preload. Preload is the pressure or stretch exerted on the walls of the ventricle by the volume of blood filling the ventricle at the end of diastole (ventricular filling). It is typically used as an indication of the volume status of the patient. Too little preload (volume) will not adequately stretch the ventricular muscle to produce the best contraction (i.e., the best SV). Too much preload overstretches the ventricular muscle, which results in poor contractility, a reduced SV, and a drop in CO. According to Starling's law, preload, then, has to be "just right" to get the best ventricular contraction and, therefore, the optimal CO. Although clinical emphasis is often placed on left ventricular preload, both ventricles have the property of preload.

Causes of low preload are typically fluid volume deficits. There are two types of fluid deficit: absolute and relative. An absolute volume deficit results from loss of volume from the vascular system, as in hemorrhage or dehydration. A relative hypovolemia results from drugs or conditions that cause severe vasodilation, generalized edema, or third spacing, any of which reduces venous return to the right heart. With vasodilation, more fluid stays in the peripheral vascular system, and less returns to the right atrium without any loss of volume from the intravascular space.

Causes of elevated preload are typically associated with the failing heart or volume overload. Inadequate CO from the left ventricle (LV) results in "backward failure." As the left heart fails and blood backs up into the pulmonary veins and lungs, the volume in the pulmonary circulation increases, as does pulmonary vascular resistance (PVR). Increased PVR ultimately results in inadequate emptying of the right ventricle (RV) with right ventricular hypertrophy as blood being pumped into the pulmonary artery meets resistance. As a result, right preload increases and CO decreases.

Afterload. Afterload is the resistance to ventricular contraction. Simply stated, afterload is the pressure the ventricle must overcome to open the aortic or pulmonic valve and eject blood out of the ventricle into the systemic or pulmonary circulation, respectively. Afterload can be viewed as the pressure in the aorta pushing against the valve to hold it in the closed position. However, fixed lesions, such as aortic stenosis, and heart anomalies, such as coarctation of the aorta, also represent afterload the ventricle must overcome before it can eject the stroke volume. As afterload increases, the heart works harder, requiring more oxygen. When afterload is high, the ventricle does not fully empty, which translates into a reduced SV and low CO.

Afterload can also be too low, as seen with peripheral vasodilation. When the pressure or resistance in the aorta is low, the left ventricle needs to generate very little pressure to open the aortic valve and eject blood into the circulation. It therefore will not contract as vigorously. The net effect is a weak contraction, resulting in a reduced CO and a low systolic blood pressure. Like preload, afterload must be "just right" for the best CO.

Contractility. Contractility is a property of myocardial muscle fibers that allows them to shorten. It is one of three determinants of stroke volume and is therefore an important factor in determining CO. A vigorous contraction improves CO by increasing the SV; a weak contraction, such as develops with heart failure or hypovolemia, decreases CO by decreasing SV. Measurements of contractility are discussed in Section Seven.

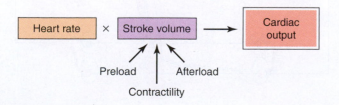

Figure 8–1 The determinants of cardiac output.

Section One Review

1. Which basic measures can be used to evaluate hemodynamic status? (Select all that apply.)
   A. Urine output
   B. Temperature
   C. Heart rate
   D. Blood pressure
   E. Respiratory rate

2. How is cardiac index (CI) best defined?
   A. The amount of blood pumped through the body every hour
   B. The amount of blood pumped through the body every minute
   C. The amount of blood pumped by the heart each minute corrected for body weight
   D. The amount of blood pumped by the heart each minute corrected for body size

3. Stroke volume is heavily influenced by which hemodynamic factors? (Select all that apply.)
   A. Contractility
   B. Afterload
   C. Preload
   D. Elasticity
   E. Oxygen status

4. Which term best represents afterload?
   A. Resistance
   B. Contraction
   C. Force
   D. Flow

Answers: 1. (A, C, D), 2. D, 3. (A, B, C), 4. A

Section Two: Noninvasive and Minimally Invasive Hemodynamic Technologies

There is great interest in finding an acceptable device to measure cardiac output that can be used in place of the highly invasive pulmonary artery (PA) catheter. The ideal hemodynamic monitor should be noninvasive, valid, reliable under various hemodynamic situations, easy to use, continuous, and cost effective. To date, there is no single hemodynamic monitoring technology that meets all these criteria. Less-invasive devices have three potential advantages: They are associated with fewer complications, they provide continuous or near continuous hemodynamic data, and the data accuracy is at an acceptable level and sensitive to rapid changes in the patient's hemodynamic status (Johnson & Mohajer-Esfahani, 2014; Lorne et al., 2014). This section presents an overview of major trends in noninvasive and minimally invasive technologies.

Noninvasive Technologies

Two major noninvasive hemodynamic monitoring technologies available at this time are impedance cardiography and Doppler ultrasound.

Impedance Cardiography Impedance cardiography (ICG) is used to assess cardiac function by measuring resistance to the flow of a high-frequency, low-amplitude current. It is based on the principle that electricity seeks the path of least resistance (the blood-filled aorta) and travels with less effort through fluid than through bone, tissue, or air. Impedance cardiography measures beat-by-beat changes in impedance in the aorta to determine CO. Electrodes are placed bilaterally (usually paired) at the base of the neck and on the lateral chest at the level of the diaphragm (Figure 8–2). A small high-frequency electrical current is transmitted through the outer electrodes, following the path of least resistance (the blood in the aorta), and is sensed by the inner electrodes.

Impedance cardiography has many applications in outpatient and inpatient settings. It can be used to measure a variety of hemodynamic parameters, including flow (SV/SVI and CO/CI), resistance (SVR/SVRI), and contractility

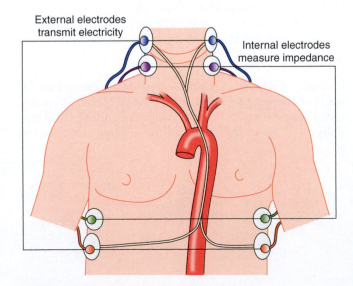

Figure 8–2 Impedance cardiography.

(LV [left ventricle] ejection time, velocity index, and other parameters). Impedance cardiography has been used to measure cardiac output trends in patients undergoing general surgery, with ICG being a reliable method for monitoring (Lorne et al., 2014). A study of the use of ICG in hypertension management revealed that blood pressure management improved when hemodynamics were monitored with ICG technology (Khraim & Pike, 2014). Although ICG can be used to measure cardiac output, stroke volume and other hemodynamic parameters, interference from motion, large body mass, dysrhythmias, and other patient variables make accurate use in critical care environments challenging (Johnson & Mohajer-Esfahani, 2014). Refer to Table 8–2 for additional information about impedance cardiography.

Doppler Ultrasound Doppler ultrasound (US), or Doppler echocardiography, a noninvasive or minimally invasive technology first used in the 1940s, continues to be used widely in clinical practice today. Fluid replacement goals during elective surgery can be met with treatments based on CO and intravascular fluid volume measurements using Doppler ultrasound (Waldron et al., 2014). The prediction of arterial pressure response to fluid administration along with successful volume expansion was achieved through the use of Doppler US in a study of mechanically ventilated patients with acute circulatory failure (Garcia et al., 2014).

Doppler US measures blood flow velocity in the vessel and, when applied to hemodynamic monitoring, helps determine CO, preload, afterload, and contractility status. Technologies using Doppler US have specific algorithms, based on the patient's height and weight, that determine the cross-sectional area of the vessel or valve. When the Doppler probe is placed over a specific area, the blood flow velocity and heart rate are measured.

For hemodynamic monitoring, the probe is either inserted into the esophagus (esophageal Doppler US), a minimally invasive technique, or placed externally at the sternal notch (transcutaneous Doppler US), a noninvasive technique (Johnson & Mohajer-Esfahani, 2014).

The patient's SV and CO may be calculated once blood flow velocity and cross-sectional area of the vessel or valve are known. Each specific device may have proprietary names for the parameters obtained, but generally the devices measure the peak velocity for each particular stroke beat, which then can be used to determine the time it takes for that column of blood to travel. This velocity time can be used with the cross-sectional area of the pulmonic or aortic valve (based on a height–weight nomogram) to determine the SV. Doppler US can calculate beat-to-beat rates to obtain the heart rate. CO is calculated using the formula CO = HR × SV.

Using Doppler US, preload is measured as the corrected flow time (FTc), which is the duration of blood flow during systole corrected for heart rate. Typically the FTc in adults is 330 to 360 milliseconds. The measurement of preload is based on the principle that the heart takes a given amount of time to eject a volume of blood for a given **inotropic** (contractile) force and a given end diastolic volume. High inotropic activity results in a higher SV and flow time; poor inotropic activity results in a low SV and flow time. A low end diastolic volume results in a low SV and a short flow time, whereas a high end diastolic volume leads to a high SV and a long flow time. Afterload can impact the FTc as well: High resistance to the ejection of blood results in a shortened FTc, whereas low afterload (such as in the case of vasodilators) causes a rise in the FTc. Suffice it to say that a short FTc is indicative that preload may be low, and a high FTc is a sign that preload may be high.

Minimally Invasive Hemodynamic Technologies

Minimally invasive (sometimes referred to as less invasive) hemodynamic technologies are defined here as devices that either require entry into a large vessel, but not the heart and pulmonary artery, or that enter the body in any orifice. There are two major types of central access lines used to measure hemodynamic parameters: central venous pressure IV lines and arterial access lines. An example of a minimally invasive device that requires placement of a sensor in the body is the transesophageal Doppler technology already described.

Central Venous Access and Measurement The central venous pressure (CVP) is an indicator of central blood volume and is influenced by a variety of factors, including cardiac output, systemic venous return to the heart,

Table 8–2 Noninvasive Technologies for Hemodynamic Monitoring

Technology	Description of Device
Impedance cardiography	Uses high-frequency, low-amplitude current to measure the resistance to electrical current flow Requires 4 to 6 external skin electrodes Measures: • Directly: volume of electrically participating tissue • Indirectly: stroke volume, cardiac output, contractility indicators
Doppler ultrasound	Measures blood flow velocity in the vessel using a Doppler signal Calculates aortic flow time and peak velocity of blood flow (a contractility measurement) The flow time is corrected for heart rate and is a preload value. *Esophageal probe* (may be considered minimally invasive): • The esophagus lies in close proximity to the ascending aorta. • An esophageal probe (the size of an 18-gauge nasogastric tube [NGT]) is inserted into the esophagus orally. *Transcutaneous probe* (noninvasive): • Doppler probe is placed on sternal notch to obtain waveforms. • Aorta and pulmonary artery outflow tracts are used to determine flow time and peak velocity. • Continuous cardiac output is monitored via an artery. • Each technology uses a proprietary algorithm (mathematical) to determine the hemodynamic indicators.

and total blood volume. The CVP can be used to measure central blood volume, right ventricular filling pressure, and central venous oxygenation saturation (Pinsky, 2015; Walley, 2015). Measuring CVP requires only that a central venous catheter (CVC) line be inserted with the distal tip located in the superior vena cava near the entrance to the right atrium. For temporary use, the right subclavian or internal jugular vein is commonly selected as the insertion site; however, other more peripheral vascular entry points can also be used as long as the catheter tip is located appropriately.

The CVP central line can be used to deliver fluids and medications, take blood samples, or obtain CVP hemodynamic measurements. If the CVC line has multiple lumens, the CVP is obtained through the distal port and measures the pressure in the vena cava and right atrium (right heart preload; right atrial pressure [RAP]), reflecting venous return to the heart. It provides valuable information about the patient's fluid status trends (normovolemia vs. fluid deficit vs. fluid excess); however, it does not provide information regarding left heart and arterial side fluid status. A normal CVP ranges from 2 to 6 mmHg and is a mean pressure. While measuring CVP can provide information about right heart function, research reveals mixed results for using CVP to estimate fluid volume replacement needs (Leatherman & Marini, 2015).

There are two major methods of measuring CVP: the transducer- or computer-based method and the visual method. While the CVP is often measured using a transducer- or computer-based monitoring system, it does not require that level of technology. When the patient has no central line available, CVP can be estimated by observing internal jugular venous pulsation. To perform this quick check of CVP, the head of the bed is elevated to 45 degrees and the patient's head is supported by a small pillow. A centimeter ruler is placed vertically at the sternal angle, and the level of internal jugular pulsation is observed and measured. Elevated CVP is present if the pulsations are higher than 3 to 4 cm above the sternal angle (Berman, Synder, & Frandsen, 2016).

While complications associated with CVC lines are rare, they are important to monitor for pneumothorax or hemothorax (particularly with subclavian vein access), hematoma, arterial puncture (particularly with internal jugular vein access), and infection.

Mechanical complications related to central venous catheter insertion include pneumothorax, catheter fracture, subclavian or carotid artery puncture, air embolism, and dysrhythmias.

Pneumothorax. Pneumothorax, the most common mechanical complication, is caused by the puncture or laceration of the pleura on insertion of the needle or catheter for central line placement. Air enters the pleural space, with partial or complete collapse of the lung. Most pneumothoraces produce symptoms, although some are totally asymptomatic. In general, the larger the collapse, the more pronounced the symptoms. Commonly seen are shortness of breath, restlessness, hypoxia, decreased or absent lung sounds on the side of the collapse, and chest pain radiating to the back. Treatment depends on the severity of the collapse and respiratory compromise. Moderate-to-large collapse requires a chest tube to restore negative pressure within the chest cavity.

Catheter Fracture and Occlusion. Over time the catheter can become less pliable, resulting in fractures or breakage. Occlusion can occur if the catheter tip lodges against the vessel wall or is "pinched" between the clavicle and first rib. Other occlusions can result from fibrin buildup, blood or lipid deposition, and drug precipitates. Another type of occlusion, withdrawal occlusion, allows infusion of a solution but prevents blood withdrawal.

Artery Puncture. Inadvertent puncture or laceration of the subclavian or carotid arteries is indicated by a flashback of arterial blood in the syringe, pulsatile blood flow, bleeding from the catheter site or development of a large hematoma, and hypotension. Treatment involves withdrawing the syringe or catheter and applying direct pressure to the site until bleeding ceases.

Air Embolism. Air embolism may occur whenever the central venous system is open to air. Signs and symptoms vary with the amount of air pulled into the venous system, but they may include respiratory distress, tachycardia, hypotension, sudden cardiovascular collapse, neurologic deficits, or cardiac arrest. Immediate action is required. Occlude the catheter nearest to the entry site in the skin. Place the patient on the left side and in the Trendelenburg position. This allows an air embolus to float into the right ventricle of the heart, away from the pulmonary artery. Prevention is the key. Always use Luer-Lok or other secure connectors and air-eliminating filters on central line tubing.

Cardiac Dysrhythmias. Dysrhythmias (rhythm irregularities) during central venous insertions are the result of a malpositioned catheter or guide wire. The result may be atrial, junctional, or ventricular dysrhythmias, which may cause decreased cardiac output, decreased blood pressure, or loss of consciousness. The appropriate intervention is to partially withdraw the catheter or guide wire. If the dysrhythmia continues, an antiarrhythmic may be required.

Arterial Access and Measurements Blood pressure is a function of blood flow (CO) and the elasticity of the blood vessels; therefore, it can be used as an indirect measure of CO. The basic physiology of systemic blood pressure is presented in Chapter 13.

Arterial Access Line. When a hemodynamically unstable patient requires frequent monitoring of systemic blood pressure and mean arterial pressure (MAP) or frequent arterial blood gases (ABGs) need to be drawn, an arterial access line ("art" line) may be inserted. Arterial pressure monitoring is common in high-acuity settings, especially in critical care units. It facilitates continuous and accurate monitoring of blood pressure, which allows the nurse to monitor the patient's response to interventions and vasoactive medications without disturbing the patient to take a manual blood pressure reading.

Advantages of direct (invasive) blood pressure monitoring in the high-acuity patient include the following:

- Information about minute-to-minute changes in blood pressure
- Increased accuracy of measurement in the hypotensive patient
- More precise titration of medications and fluids
- Capacity to obtain ABGs and blood samples without pain and discomfort to the patient
- Ability to analyze arterial pulse contours

A disadvantage of peripheral artery (e.g., radial or femoral) blood pressure (BP) monitoring is that the peripheral BP may not accurately reflect the central BP status (within the aorta); therefore, therapies based on a peripheral BP reading may not meet the actual needs of the patient (Alarcon & Fink, 2014).

Insertion of the Arterial Access Line.   The nurse typically is responsible for setting up the equipment for catheter insertion, calibrating the equipment to ensure accurate readings, and assisting the healthcare provider (HCP) with the procedure. The equipment needed to monitor systemic arterial blood pressures is the same as that used to monitor pulmonary artery (PA) pressures, except that a small catheter is used and inserted into a peripheral artery (usually the radial, although the ulnar artery can also be used).

Once the arterial catheter is in place, the nurse is responsible for patient safety and comfort and the maintenance of the system. Securing the pressure tubing to prevent dislodgement and possible exsanguination is an important nursing responsibility. Safety measures to prevent exsanguination include covering all caps along the monitoring system, securing all connections, and ensuring that all monitor alarms are on.

Monitoring circulation distal to the insertion site is another important nursing function. Skin color and temperature and all pulses distal to the insertion site are regularly assessed and documented. Any alteration in circulation is promptly brought to the attention of the appropriate HCP. The site is observed frequently for signs of infection: redness, warmth, edema, and drainage. Unit-specific protocols and responsibilities related to arterial monitoring are typically described in hospital policy and procedure manuals.

Arterial Waveform.   The arterial waveform has a characteristic morphology that is related to the cardiac cycle (Figure 8–3). When the aortic valve opens, blood is ejected into the aorta. This forms a steep upstroke on the arterial waveform, called the anacrotic limb. The top of this limb represents the peak, or highest systolic

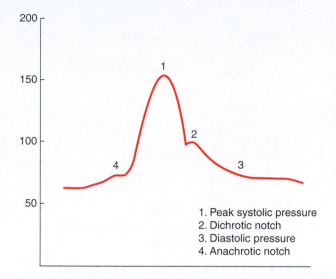

Figure 8–3 Components of the systemic arterial pressure waveform.

SOURCE: Reprinted with permission. Copyright © 2000 Edwards Lifesciences. Swan-Ganz® is a trademark of Edwards Lifesciences Corporation, registered in the U.S. Patent and Trademark Office.

pressure, which appears digitally on the monitor as the systolic pressure. After this peak pressure, the waveform descends. This descent forms the dicrotic limb and represents systolic ejection of blood that is continuing at a reduced force. The descending, or dicrotic, limb is disrupted by the dicrotic notch, which is an important point on the waveform. The dicrotic notch represents closure of the aortic valve and the beginning of ventricular diastole. The lowest portion of the waveform (baseline) represents the diastolic pressure and is reflected digitally on the monitor.

Arterial Pulse Contour Analysis.   There is increasing interest in analyzing arterial pulsatile waveforms to continuously measure CO as an alternative to inserting the more invasive PA catheter. Pulse waveforms are generated by many monitors, including pulse oximeters, arterial lines, and PA catheters. The use of the pulse contour analysis is based on the principle that the SV may be measured by assessing the beat-to-beat changes in the amplitude of the pulse pressure as displayed on the waveform. SV affects systolic blood pressure such that, with a reduction in SV, a change is seen in the beat-to-beat pulse amplitude (or variation in stroke volume). Moreover, the systemic vascular resistance (SVR) can be calculated when the CVP is simultaneously measured with standard methodologies. Figure 8–4 shows an example of an arterial pulse contour waveform.

A variety of technologies can be used to measure cardiac output in real time by arterial-pressure waveform analysis. Devices such as the VolumeView/EV 1000 by Edwards Lifesciences calibrate the arterial pressure waveform analysis with an independent invasive cardiac output measurement (Monnet & Teboul, 2015). Other devices (FloTrac by Edwards Lifesciences, LiDCORapid by LiDCO)

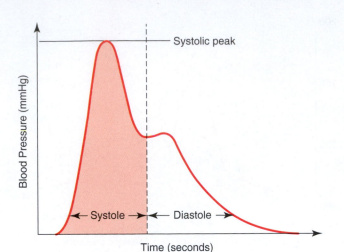

Figure 8–4 LiDCOrapid Cardiac Sensor System (Covidien).

use a standard arterial catheter without calibration. The FloTrac device automatically adjusts for changing vascular conditions (e.g., vasodilation and hyperdynamic conditions) and can be attached to any arterial catheter, providing continuous hemodynamic readings through a special FloTrac sensor.

While these devices provide continuous cardiac output measurements, there are some disadvantages to their use. Calibrated devices provide accurate estimates of cardiac output; however, using them can be time consuming due to the frequent need for recalibration (Monnet & Teboul, 2015). In addition, the reliability of uncalibrated devices can be low when the patient's vascular resistance dramatically changes (Monnet & Teboul, 2015).

Box 8–1 provides additional information on arterial pulse contour analysis.

> **BOX 8–1** Summary of Arterial Pulse Contour Analysis Devices
>
> - They require arterial access using a regular arterial line.
> - They require placement of a special arterial thermodilution catheter in the femoral, axillary, or brachial artery.
> - They require initial calibration and recalibration using transpulmonary thermodilution.
> - They do not require a thermodilution CO for calibration.
> - They measure continuous CO by analyzing the arterial pulse contour.
> - They measure arterial pulse contour using a special blood flow sensor.

Mean Arterial Pressure. The mean arterial pressure (MAP) is an approximation of the average pressure in the systemic circulation throughout the cardiac cycle. The normal range is 70 to 90 mmHg. The MAP is provided as a digital readout when an arterial line (or automatic blood pressure equipment) is in use. The MAP obtained from an arterial line is the most accurate because the mean is actually measured rather than calculated. When direct arterial monitoring is not available, the MAP must be calculated. Keep in mind that MAPs calculated from cuff pressures (automatic or manual) have a potential for error because of extraneous factors such as incorrect cuff size, differences in hearing, sensitivity of the instrument, and patient movement.

The formula for MAP reflects the components of the cardiac cycle. In normal heart rates, systole accounts for one-third of the cycle and diastole for two-thirds. The formula is MAP = [(SBP) + 2(DBP)]/3, where SBP is systolic BP, and DBP is diastolic BP.

Section Two Review

1. What do Doppler ultrasound hemodynamic monitors measure?
   A. Pulmonary artery wedge pressure
   B. Blood flow velocity
   C. Pulse pressure variation
   D. Systolic blood pressure

2. Using pulse contour analysis hemodynamic monitors, how is stroke volume measured?
   A. Cardiac output
   B. Beat-to-beat changes in pulse amplitude
   C. Heart rate
   D. Central venous pressure

3. What is the normal range for mean arterial pressure (MAP)?
   A. 60–70 mmHg
   B. 140/80 mmHg
   C. 70–90 mmHg
   D. 100–120 mmHg

4. Where should the tip of the central venous pressure (CVP) line be positioned?
   A. Right atrium near the opening to the tricuspid valve
   B. Pulmonary artery
   C. Vena cava near the entrance to the right atrium
   D. Subclavian vein

Answers: 1. B, 2. B, 3. C, 4. C

Emerging Evidence

- In a small study of 10 healthy males, heart rate, blood pressure, stroke volume, cardiac output, systemic vascular resistance, and other hemodynamic parameters were measured in three trunk postures with impedance cardiography. Stroke volume was higher when the upper trunk alone was elevated when compared to elevating the entire trunk in a 60-degree Fowler's position *(Kubota, Endo, Kubota, Ishizuka, & Furudate, 2015)*.
- FloTrac or Vigileo device assessments of cardiac output in various patient positions were significantly higher than cardiac output readings obtained with thermodilution techniques via pulmonary artery catheterization in a sample of eight morbidly obese patients *(Tejedor et al., 2015)*.
- The use of less invasive hemodynamic monitoring techniques such as esophageal Doppler monitoring, arterial pressure contour analysis, and FloTrac, in lieu of pulmonary artery catheterization, was not associated with an increase in patient mortality over a 5-year period in intensive care settings *(Kirton, Calabrese, & Staff, 2015)*.

Section Three: Introduction to Pulmonary Artery Catheters

The remainder of this chapter provides an overview of pulmonary artery catheters and hemodynamic parameters that can be obtained using them. Various terms are used by healthcare professionals to refer to a pulmonary artery catheter, including right heart catheter, Swan or Swan–Ganz catheter, and flow-directed thermodilution catheter. This chapter uses the term pulmonary artery (PA) catheter.

The PA catheter is a balloon-tipped catheter that is inserted through a central vein and floated into position in the pulmonary artery (Figure 8–5). The catheter was first used in clinical practice in the late 1960s and was the first bedside device capable of providing a comprehensive hemodynamic profile. It was the only device used for bedside hemodynamic monitoring for several decades. In the late 1990s a series of papers was published that stirred debate concerning the clinical use of the PA catheter. While its use has declined as newer, less invasive technologies have become available, it remains an important bedside monitoring option, particularly when comprehensive hemodynamic monitoring is needed, as in severe heart failure and shock states.

Purpose of PA Catheters

The pulmonary artery (PA) catheter is an invasive diagnostic tool that can be used at the bedside for the following purposes:

- To determine the direct pressures or volumes within the right heart and PA, and for the indirect measurement of left heart pressures
- To determine cardiac output (CO)
- To sample pulmonary artery mixed venous blood (SvO_2)
- To provide various therapies (e.g., IV fluids, medications, or temporary cardiac pacing)

Required Provider Competencies

Hemodynamic data are used to make major clinical management decisions for high-acuity patients. As with all diagnostic tests, the validity of the test results is only as good as the accuracy of the data collected. Therefore, hemodynamic monitoring in the high-acuity patient population requires competency in both technical and physiological aspects. Nurses who are expected to work with hemodynamic monitors require specialized training in the correct use of the equipment and analysis of the data. The nurse must follow three steps in hemodynamic assessment with the PA catheter:

1. **Obtain accurate data.** Correct procedures for calibrating and using the equipment for hemodynamic

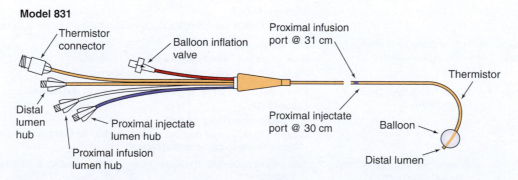

Figure 8–5 Five-lumen pulmonary artery catheter.

monitoring are necessary for measurement accuracy (Miller, 2014). Procedures include appropriate leveling and zeroing, use of minimal transducer tubing, maintenance of system patency free from air bubbles, square wave testing, and patient positioning.

2. **Correctly analyze waveforms.** Waveforms are best assessed when they are printed and correlated with the electrocardiogram (ECG) and respiratory cycles (Miller, 2014). Certain modes of mechanical ventilation and rapid, spontaneous respirations make locating end expiration difficult. Capnography is sometimes used to identify physiological end expiration.

3. **Integrate the data with the patient assessment.** Integration is accomplished by looking at all the data in the hemodynamic profile collectively. These data are discussed in detail in this chapter; however, it should be recognized that they must be correlated with findings in the physical assessment of CO. It is also important to recognize that ongoing education is required to ensure patient safety and positive clinical outcomes.

Interpretation of Data

Data collection is not the end point of hemodynamic monitoring. Abnormal pressures and changes in trends must be recognized, correlated with the patient's condition, and acted on. Careful clinical assessment, integrated with the data collected from a PA catheter, provides a basis for nursing interventions and the titration of potent vasoactive medications and the administration of fluids.

Several guidelines must be followed when interpreting readings:

- Always assess patient trends rather than an isolated reading.
- Question abnormal readings. Recheck the reading after zeroing and calibrating the equipment. Assess the patient for additional data to support the reading.

- Compare the readings with the patient's normal values and *not* with the normal values listed in a textbook.
- Do not be fooled by normal readings. The patient may have normal readings temporarily because of compensatory mechanisms. Continue to assess the patient.
- Assess the interrelationships among the readings. The goal is to obtain a picture of the patient's hemodynamic status, not simply a number.

Standard PA Catheter Construction and Components

The PA catheter is constructed of a radiopaque polyvinyl-chloride. Several sizes and various options are available. Many have a heparin coating to reduce the risk of thrombus formation. All PA catheters have color-coded extrusions, or ports, on the proximal end that provide access to the various catheter lumens. The catheter is marked at 10-cm intervals to facilitate correct placement. A standard PA catheter has five lumens, as shown in Figure 8–5.

The PA catheter is a complex, multilumen device that can be somewhat intimidating at first sight. It becomes much easier to understand when considering its component parts. The following describes each of the separate sections of the standard (basic) PA catheter. When indicated, special nursing considerations are included. Table 8–3 provides a summary of the component parts of a five-lumen standard thermodilution PA catheter.

Proximal Injectate Lumen and Hub   The proximal lumen terminates in the most proximal chamber of the heart, the right atrium (RA). Most catheter manufacturers imprint the word *proximal* on either the hub or the tubing close to the hub. On most catheters, the proximal port tubing is blue for rapid visual identification. One way to remember this is to link the blue tubing to the "blue" desaturated blood found in the right atrium.

Table 8–3 Summary of Component Parts of a Five-lumen Standard Thermodilution PA Catheter

Component	Typical Descriptors	Uses
Proximal injectate lumen and hub	Hub or tubing label: Proximal Color: Blue	Measures RA pressure (RAP) For bolus thermodilution CO: injectate pushed through this port Infusion of IV fluids Caution: DO NOT run vasoactive drugs via port if using it for bolus CO injectate.
Proximal infusion lumen and hub (optional)	Hub or tubing label: Infusion Color: White or clear	IV infusions Provides backup injectate port for bolus CO measurement Caution: Same as proximal injectate lumen and hub
Distal lumen and hub	Hub or tubing label: Distal Color: Yellow	Connected to transducer for continuous PA pressure and waveform Obtain PAWP Sampling of mixed blood for SvO_2 Caution: DO NOT infuse medications or IV solution through this port unless specifically ordered to do so by prescribing provider.
Thermistor	Proximal hub attaches to cable for CO measurement	Temperature sensing for (1) obtaining core body temperature, and (2) thermodilution CO measurement
Balloon inflation lumen and valve	Proximal hub contains gate valve device and syringe	Inflating for flow-directed catheter insertion or readvancing catheter, and for wedging the catheter tip to obtain PAWP measurement Caution: Keep valve locked at all times; ensure that balloon is deflated when not performing PAWP; follow agency policy for withdrawing catheter tip if spontaneous wedge occurs.

When connected to a transducer, the proximal port allows for monitoring of the right atrial pressure (RAP). When bolus thermodilution cardiac output (CO) is used, a bolus of IV fluid (called injectate) is pushed through this lumen to determine CO. To avoid inadvertently creating a bolus of potent medications, vasoactive drugs should not be infused through the proximal lumen when it is being used for thermodilution CO measurements. Intravenous fluids and intermittent medications can also be infused through this port.

Proximal Infusion Lumen and Hub (Optional) When present, the proximal infusion lumen terminates in the right atrium and is labeled *infusion* on the hub or the tubing near the hub. On most catheters, the tubing of this port is white or clear for rapid visual identification. This port is used primarily as the main line for IV fluid infusions and is especially helpful in patients with poor peripheral venous access. This optional port can be used to obtain CO determinations if the proximal injectate lumen becomes occluded. However, the individual values obtained from this port may not be as reproducible as those obtained from the proximal injectate port. To avoid inadvertent bolus of potent medications, do not infuse vasoactive medications through the lumen selected for bolus thermodilution CO determination.

Distal Lumen and Hub The distal lumen terminates at the distal tip of the PA catheter, opening in the pulmonary artery. Most catheter manufacturers imprint the word *distal* on either the hub or the tubing close to the hub. On most catheters, the tubing of this port is yellow for rapid visual identification. The distal port is connected to a transducer for continuous monitoring of the pulmonary artery pressure (PAP) and waveform. The pulmonary artery wedge pressure (PAWP) is obtained through this port by careful balloon inflation. In addition, mixed venous blood oxygen saturation (SvO_2) can be continuously monitored or intermittently sampled from this port. This port terminates in the pulmonary artery; therefore, the venous blood returning from all parts of the body has been well mixed in the right atrium and ventricle before it is pumped into the pulmonary artery. Medications and IV solutions are not infused through this port, except under certain conditions when indicated by an HCP.

Thermistor The thermistor detects changes in the temperature of the blood, which is an essential part of cardiac output determination. The wire terminates near the tip of the catheter and is exposed to the blood flowing through the pulmonary artery. It allows for continuous monitoring of core body temperature. The proximal end attaches to a cable linking it with the device used to measure CO. This device is either a CO module compatible with the bedside monitoring system or a freestanding CO computer. The continuous CO model of the PA catheter has a copper metal filament surrounding part of the PA catheter. When connected to the monitor, thermal energy is emitted by the thermal filament to calculate CO based on thermodilution principles.

Balloon Inflation Lumen and Valve This lumen is contiguous with the small balloon at the distal end of the catheter. A gate-valve mechanism on the hub locks this port in an open or closed position. The valve should be kept locked at all times except when doing the balloon inflation to obtain a pulmonary artery wedge pressure (PAWP). The balloon is slowly inflated with a syringe that withdraws to only 1.5 mL while the PA waveform is continuously monitored. Inflation is stopped as soon as the waveform changes to a PA wedge waveform. The maximum recommended inflation volume specified in the catheter instructions should not be exceeded. Deflation of the balloon is always passive because manual deflation may damage balloon integrity. It is crucial that the balloon never be left in the inflated position because it obstructs circulation distal to the balloon. Directly after PAWP values are obtained, it is best to expel all air from the syringe and reconnect with the syringe fully deflated to prevent accidental reinflation of the balloon.

Hemodynamic Monitoring Equipment

A typical hemodynamic monitoring system is shown in Figure 8–6. Except for the catheter, the system components are the same as for pulmonary arterial pressure monitoring or systemic arterial pressure monitoring.

Transducer Pressures within the heart and pulmonary artery are measured using a transducer. A transducer is a translator: It translates mechanical energy sensed by the catheter into electrical energy, displayed on the monitor screen as a waveform. It is the nurse's responsibility to ensure that the transducer is translating correctly. To that end, the nurse must zero and level the catheter according to unit or hospital policies and procedures.

Leveling the Transducer. Leveling the transducer corrects for hydrostatic pressure changes in vessels above and below the heart. The transducer is referenced (or leveled) and zeroed at the phlebostatic axis. The **phlebostatic axis** approximates the level of the right atrium and represents the level of the catheter tip. In the supine position, the external landmark for the right atrium is the fourth intercostal space, one half the anterior and posterior diameter of the chest (Miller, 2014). Improper positioning of the transducer leads to inaccurate readings; every time the patient's position changes, the transducer must be re-referenced to ensure that the readings are taken in the same place each time.

Zeroing the transducer corrects for any drift or deviation from baseline that may occur. Current transducers have minimal zero drift, so routine rezeroing is unnecessary.

Pressure Bag To overcome the pressure within the pulmonary artery and prevent blood from backing up into the pressure tubing, a pressure bag is placed around the flush solution bag and inflated to 300 mmHg. Depending on hospital policy, the flush solution may or may not contain heparin.

Special Pulmonary Artery Catheters

Several types of PA catheters have the standard design properties of all PA catheters plus additional properties that meet special therapeutic or measurement needs. These specialty catheters include the following:

- Pacing port: temporary cardiac pacing (atrial, ventricular, or atrioventricular [AV] sequential)

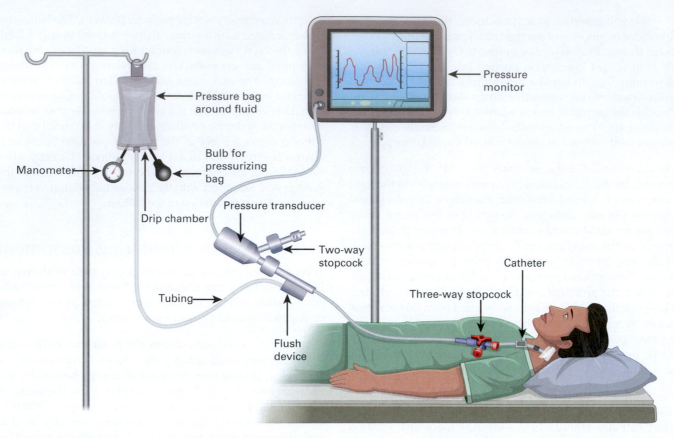

Figure 8–6 Hemodynamic monitoring equipment.

- Continuous cardiac output (CCO): automatic continuous CO measurement via thermal filament method of thermodilution
- Oximetry: continuous measurement of mixed venous oxygen saturation (SvO_2)
- Volumetrics: continuous measurement of CO, right ventricular end diastolic volume (RVEDV) and right ventricular ejection fraction (RVEF).

Care of Central Venous Catheters

Historically, with the increasing use of central venous catheters (CVCs; e.g., central lines and PA catheters) in the acute care setting, particularly in critical care units, there was an increase in healthcare-associated CVC infections. Moreover, central line–associated bloodstream infections (CLABSIs) are potentially life threatening with over 30,000 cases reported each year in U.S. acute care facilities

(Centers for Disease Control and Prevention [CDC], 2016). The CDC *Guidelines for the Prevention of Intravascular Catheter-Related Infections* were developed in 2002 and updated in 2011 (CDC, 2011) to address this potentially fatal complication. With the adoption of rigorous guidelines for central line insertion and care, a 46% decrease in CLABSIs was documented from 2008 to 2013 (CDC, 2015). The CDC care recommendations emphasize the need for meticulous care of any CVC line, following the agency policy and procedures based on best available evidence. The updated CDC guidelines are listed in Box 8–2.

Development of a healthcare-associated CVC infection is considered a nursing-sensitive indicator and sentinel (or "never") event by The Joint Commission (TJC) and is the focus of a safe-practice guideline of the National Quality Forum/Agency for Healthcare Research and Quality (NQF/AHRQ). An online toolkit from The Joint Commission provides information on the various aspects of CVC care, including CLABSI prevention (TJC, 2015).

BOX 8–2 Guidelines for the Prevention of Intravascular Catheter-related Bloodstream Infections

Catheter Site Dressing Regimens

- Use a chlorhexidine-impregnated sponge dressing for temporary short-term catheters in patients older than 2 months if the CLABSI rate has not been substantially reduced despite adherence to basic preventive measures, including education and training, use of chlorhexidine for skin antisepsis, and maximal sterile barrier (MSB).

- Replace gauze dressings used on short-term CVC sites every 2 days. (Category II)
- Replace transparent dressings used on short-term CVC sites at least every 7 days, except in pediatric patients in whom the risk of dislodging the catheter may outweigh the benefit of changing the dressing.

Needleless Intravascular Catheter Systems

- When needleless systems are used, a split septum valve may be preferred over a mechanical valve due to the increased risk of infection with some mechanical valves.
- Minimize contamination risk by scrubbing the access port with an appropriate antiseptic (chlorhexidine, povidone-iodine, an iodophor, or 70% alcohol) and accessing the port only with sterile devices.

Recommendations for Central Venous Catheters

- Avoid using the femoral vein for central venous access in adult patients. (Category IA)
- Use a subclavian rather than a jugular site in adult patients to minimize infection risk for nontunneled CVC placement.

Skin Preparation

- Prepare clean skin with a > 0.5% chlorhexidine-based preparation before central venous catheter insertion and during dressing changes. If there is a contraindication to chlorhexidine, alternatives include tincture of iodine, an iodophor, or 70% alcohol.

SOURCE: Adapted from CDC (2011).

Maximal Sterile Barrier Precautions

- Use maximal sterile barrier (MSB) precautions, including the use of a cap, mask, sterile gown, sterile gloves, and a sterile full-body drape for insertion of CVCs, PICCs, or guide wire exchange.

Replacing Administration Sets

- In patients not receiving blood, blood products, or lipid fat emulsions, replace administration sets that are continuously used, including secondary sets and add-on devices, no more frequently than at 96-hour intervals, but at least every 7 days. (Category IA)
- The frequency for replacing intermittently used administration sets is an unresolved issue. The frequency for replacing needles to access implantable ports is also an unresolved issue.

Replacement of Peripheral and Midline Catheters

- Replace peripheral catheters no more frequently than every 72 to 96 hours to reduce risk of infection and phlebitis in adults.

Catheter Securement Devices

- Use a sutureless securement device to reduce the risk of infection for intravascular catheters.

Section Three Review

1. Which port of the PA catheter is used to obtain RAP?
   A. Proximal
   B. Distal
   C. Thermistor wire
   D. Balloon inflation

2. Why should vasoactive drugs never be infused through the port used for thermodilution CO determinations?
   A. The lumen is too small.
   B. A bolus injection of a potent drug will occur every time CO is obtained.
   C. CO readings will be less accurate.
   D. Some vasoactive drugs are not compatible with the catheter material.

3. What is the best way to deflate the balloon on the PA catheter?
   A. Slowly pull back on the syringe plunger.
   B. Quickly pull back on the plunger to limit deflation time.
   C. Allow the balloon to deflate passively.
   D. Remove the syringe from the hub directly after inflation.

4. When leveling the transducer, the phlebostatic axis approximates which level?
   A. Superior vena cava
   B. Right atrium
   C. Right ventricle
   D. Heart apex

Answers: 1. A, 2. B, 3. C, 4. B

Section Four: Pulmonary Artery Catheter Insertion and Measurements

While the use of the PA catheter has steadily declined because of questionable cost versus benefits results, it has a place in providing a comprehensive hemodynamic profile in patients who experience profound hypo- or hypertension, sepsis, heart failure, severe fluid imbalances, and other remarkable complications (Magder, 2015). This section presents an overview of the activities involved in the insertion, management, and general measurements of the PA catheter.

Catheter Insertion and Management

Insertion of a PA catheter is performed only by healthcare professionals who have undergone specific training. The bedside nurse is often needed to assist with the insertion; therefore, a basic understanding of the procedure and related nursing roles is necessary.

Preprocedure Patient and Family Education   The patient may be awake when the catheter is inserted, and it can be a frightening experience if he or she does not know what to expect. Patient and family education should include the following information about the procedure:

- The purpose of the catheter is to assess heart function and fluid status, allowing more precise management of the patient's condition.

- The site will be scrubbed with an antiseptic solution, and a pinch, sting, or burning sensation may be felt when the local anesthetic is injected.

- A temporary sensation of pressure should be expected when a large IV catheter (the sheath introducer) is inserted into the subclavian, jugular, or femoral vein.

- The long, thin, balloon-tipped catheter will not be felt as it is threaded through the sheath introducer, floated through the right heart, and positioned in the pulmonary artery.

- After the procedure, the patient should expect to be attached to multiple IV lines that will restrict some freedom of movement. In addition, the family should be prepared to see additional equipment during their next visit with the patient.

- During the procedure, most patients find it helpful and reassuring to receive general information on how things are going and an estimated time to completion.

Insertion of the PA Catheter   The insertion of a PA catheter is performed in critical care units, cardiac catheterization laboratories, and operating rooms. The complication rate related to this procedure is low; however, it is not without potential risks, such as pneumothorax, damage to the blood vessels or heart, dysrhythmias, infection or bleeding, bleeding at the insertion site, and death. Except in rare emergency situations, informed consent should be obtained prior to catheter insertion. In addition, prior to insertion, several steps are taken that help ensure that insertion is completed safely and with ease and that accurate data are produced (Box 8–3).

The insertion of a PA catheter is always a sterile procedure involving maximal barrier precautions. All persons in the room should perform hand hygiene prior to

the procedure and wear a cap and mask. The nurse ensures that the person inserting the PA catheter is wearing a sterile gown and gloves and that the patient has a full-body drape. The patient's skin is prepared with a 2% chlorhexidine gluconate solution. Along with the healthcare provider, the nurse is responsible for careful observation and monitoring of the patient during the insertion process.

Once positioned, the percutaneous sheath introducer (a short central line) is typically secured in place and the PA catheter is threaded through the introducer lumen into the right heart. The balloon is inflated once the catheter tip enters the right atrium, and the catheter is "floated" into the pulmonary artery following the natural direction of blood flow. During the procedure, the monitor is closely observed for the distinct wave patterns that should develop as the catheter tip moves through the right heart chambers and into the pulmonary artery. The balloon should be deflated after the catheter is positioned in the pulmonary artery and during times of catheter repositioning during the insertion process.

Postprocedure Management   After the catheter has been inserted, the nurse assumes responsibility for patient safety and comfort and system maintenance. The nurse is also responsible for maintaining the catheter site, documenting pressures in the heart and PA, and obtaining accurate cardiac output measurements.

A chest x-ray is obtained immediately to confirm catheter position and to assess for a pneumothorax due to the percutaneous introducer insertion. Until proper placement of the catheter has been confirmed, the catheter is not used to infuse medications or fluids. It is the nurse's responsibility to recognize abnormal waveforms and trends and intervene promptly, including notifying the HCP when indicated. The nurse must know and follow unit-specific policies and procedures related to hemodynamic monitoring.

Obtaining Accurate Hemodynamic Measurements   To best ensure that hemodynamic measurements are accurate, the American Association of Critical-Care Nurses (AACN; Miller, 2014) has made recommendations regarding patient repositioning and waveform measurement.

BOX 8–3   Steps in Preparation for PA Catheter Insertion

1. **Provide patient and family teaching.**
   Explain the catheter, its purpose, and related equipment.
2. **Gather all supplies.**
   See agency policy and procedure (will include PA catheter, introducer, pressure cables and modules, transducer system, leveling device, sterile garb, IV normal saline and pressure bag, and other items).
3. **Prime the pressure monitoring system to remove all air.**
   - Be sure to prime through all stopcocks and to remove all air from the IV bag of fluid before priming the system.

- Perform an additional flush with 10 mL of IV fluid by attaching the syringe to the stopcock at the transducer and quickly flushing the tubing with the syringe. This will help flush out any remaining air bubbles.
4. **Inspect the tubing.**
   - Be sure that all air bubbles have been removed. Repeat fast flush with syringe if needed.
5. **Place the IV bag in the pressure bag and inflate to 300 mmHg.**
6. **Connect to the bedside monitor and zero balance and level the transducer.**

SOURCE: Data from Butterworth et at. (2013), Edwards Lifesciences (2015), Miller (2014).

Repositioning the Patient.   Repositioning the patient is an important consideration in continuous hemodynamic monitoring.

- The following are acceptable positions for PA catheter measurements:
  - Preferred position: supine, with head of bed (HOB) elevated from 0 to 60 degrees
  - Not preferred: lateral position after referencing and zeroing the system
- Obtain readings in a position of comfort; flat positioning contraindicated in patients with spontaneous respirations and dyspnea
- The transducer should be leveled and referenced to the phlebostatic axis using a laser or a carpenter's level with each position change. Specific referencing recommendations are available for placing the patient in a lateral position.

Measuring Waveforms.   Changes in intrathoracic pressure during the respiratory cycle (inspiration and expiration) significantly alter hemodynamic pressures. Obtaining accurate measurements requires reading pressure waveforms at end expiration when pleural pressure is at its lowest level. Furthermore, measurement of waveforms should be done from an analog tracing that includes a simultaneous ECG tracing.

PA Catheter Measurements

The measurements that can be read using the PA catheter depend on the exact type of catheter; however, all catheters are able to measure cardiac output, preload, and afterload.

Measuring Cardiac Output   The PA catheter uses a thermodilution method to calculate CO. Temperature changes are detected by an injectate temperature probe in the blood flowing from a proximal point on the catheter to the thermistor near the distal tip. When measuring CO, data is relayed to the computer through a special cable attached to the thermistor connector at the proximal end of the PA catheter. The thermistor monitors changes in the temperature of the blood and the duration of the changes, then relays the data to the CO computer where it is analyzed and a time–temperature CO "curve" is formed (Figure 8–7). The area under the curve represents the CO, which is calculated and displayed by the computer in liters per minute (L/min). The thermistor also allows for constant monitoring of core body temperature.

There are two thermodilution methods: intermittent CO fluid bolus method and continuous CO thermal filament method.

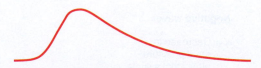

Figure 8–7 A normal cardiac output curve.

Intermittent Fluid Bolus Thermodilution Method.   The traditional method of thermodilution CO requires the use of **injectate**, a 10-mL bolus of IV normal saline that is injected through the proximal injectate port of the PA catheter into the right atrium. The temperature of this fluid is cooler than blood temperature and may be iced or room temperature. The injectate temperature is sensed by an in-line temperature probe and relayed to the CO computer. The CO computer has two temperatures stored in it: the temperature of the blood and the temperature of the fluid bolus. The presence of the cooler fluid injectate bolus that mixes with pulmonary artery blood results in a transient drop in the temperature of the blood flowing through the pulmonary artery. As blood continues to be pumped into the pulmonary artery, the blood temperature rapidly rewarms to the prebolus level.

Continuous CO Thermal Filament Thermodilution Method. A major breakthrough in the CO thermodilution method was the invention of new PA catheter technology that can automatically and continuously measure CO. The new technology uses a thermal (heating) filament about 11 cm in length that is part of the PA catheter wall. When correctly placed, the thermal filament lies within the heart, between the right atrium and right ventricle. An intermittent signal is sent to the filament every 30 to 60 seconds to warm the blood flowing by the filament (Edwards Lifesciences, 2015). The heating element is located proximal to the thermistor. Heat is applied to the blood at the heating element, and the temperature change is read downstream at the thermistor.

Measuring Preload   Preload is reflected in two PA catheter measurements, the right atrial pressure (RAP) and the **pulmonary artery wedge pressure (PAWP)**. The RAP directly measures right ventricular preload, and the PAWP measures left ventricular preload. The PAWP is an indirect measure of pressure in the left ventricle at the end of diastole (or left ventricular end diastolic pressure [LVEDP]). LVEDP provides an estimate of the volume status of the patient. Right heart preload is obtained by measuring the mean RAP. When the tricuspid valve is open, the RAP is used as a proxy for right ventricular end diastolic pressure (RVEDP). Like the LVEDP (measured by the PAWP), the RVEDP is an estimate of the patient's volume status.

RAP and PAWP are presented in detail in Sections Five and Six, respectively.

Measuring Afterload   Afterload, or resistance, is a calculated variable that can be obtained using PA catheter measurements. The left-sided afterload is known as the **systemic vascular resistance (SVR)**; the right-sided afterload is known as the **pulmonary vascular resistance (PVR)**. Both measures and their formulae are discussed in depth in Section Seven.

Measuring Contractility   Cardiac contractility is not directly measured at the bedside. Several hemodynamic parameters can be used, however, to give some indication of contractility, including SV (and SVI) and **ventricular stroke work index (VSWI)**. The VSWI is the amount of work involved in moving blood in the ventricle with each heartbeat, which is described in Section Seven.

Section Four Review

1. The thermodilution method of CO determination is based on which factor?
   A. A change in blood temperature over time
   B. The length of time it takes for dye to be circulated
   C. The temperature of the injectate
   D. The volume of the injectate

2. The client requires insertion of a PA catheter. Which nursing action is indicated?
   A. Use strict sterile technique while inserting the catheter.
   B. Prepare to assist with the insertion of the catheter.
   C. Ask that the client be placed on the surgery schedule for insertion.
   D. Prep the inside of the client's left elbow for the insertion.

3. Which action is priority following insertion of a PA catheter?
   A. Obtain a chest x-ray
   B. Infuse heparin through the port
   C. Infuse an antibiotic through the port
   D. Place the client in High-Fowler position

4. Which statement is correct regarding continuous CO measurements?
   A. They are less accurate than bolus thermodilution CO measurements.
   B. They provide two updates on CO readings every hour.
   C. They depend on user technique for accuracy.
   D. They depend on the blood being warmed.

Answers: 1. A, 2. B, 3. A, 4. D

Section Five: Right Atrial and Ventricular Pressures

The right side of the heart is a relatively low-pressure system that receives venous return from the body. Pressures and volumes can be measured in the right-heart chambers, but although right atrial pressure is routinely measured, right ventricular pressure is measured only during PA catheter insertion.

Right Atrial Pressure

Right atrial pressure (RAP) is an estimate of right ventricular preload (i.e., the volume status of the right heart). Recall that preload is the stretch exerted on the walls of the ventricle by the volume of blood filling the ventricle at the end of diastole. The RAP is used as an estimate of right ventricular end diastolic pressure (RVEDP) because the tricuspid valve remains open until the end of right ventricular diastole, allowing right ventricular pressure to be transmitted to the right atrium.

Obtaining Measurements The RAP is obtained from the proximal port of the PA catheter, which opens into the right atrium. It is always read as a mean pressure, and the normal range is 2 to 6 mmHg. The RAP waveform is monitored by attaching a transducer to the proximal (blue) port of the PA catheter. The right atrial waveform has a characteristic undulating pattern consisting of three positive and two negative excursions. These undulations are a result of mechanical events in the cardiac cycle. The positive excursions consist of a, c, and v waves. The rise in atrial pressure during atrial systole forms the a wave. Closure of the tricuspid valve early in systole produces the c wave (not always well visualized). The v wave is produced by an increase in pressure from passive atrial filling that occurs against a slightly bulging atrioventricular valve during ventricular systole. The negative excursions consist of the x and y deflections. The x descent follows both the a and c waves and results from the drop in atrial pressure after atrial systole. The y descent is a result of passive right atrial emptying into the right ventricle when the tricuspid valve opens just prior to atrial systole. The RAP can also be obtained using a device to measure central venous pressure (CVP); CVP is an equivalent measurement of RAP. Figure 8–8 illustrates a labeled atrial waveform.

Waveform Analysis Assessment of the waveform begins with obtaining a graphic readout from either the bedside or a central monitoring system. This printout should include both the ECG and RAP tracings in order

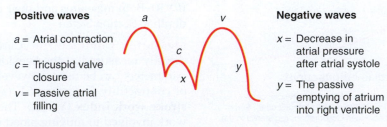

Positive waves

a = Atrial contraction

c = Tricuspid valve closure

v = Passive atrial filling

Negative waves

x = Decrease in atrial pressure after atrial systole

y = The passive emptying of atrium into right ventricle

Figure 8–8 A labeled right atrial waveform.

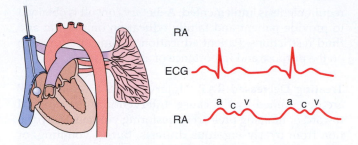

Figure 8–9 Right atrial waveform with the *a* and *v* wave components identified.

SOURCE: "Right atrial waveform with the a and v wave components identified" from Edwards Lifesciences. Reprinted with permission. Copyright © 2000 Edwards Lifesciences. Swan-Ganz® is a trademark of Edwards Lifesciences Corporation, registered in the U.S. Patent and Trademark Office.

to correlate the mechanical events of the heart (RAP tracing) with the electrical events (ECG tracing) (Figure 8–9). The *a* wave is a ventricular diastolic event, and the *v* wave is a systolic event. The *c* wave marks the end of diastole. The RVEDP is marked in the RAP tracing by the *c* wave when visible. The *c* wave marks end diastole and may be located on the monitor strip (simultaneous printout of the ECG and RAP tracings) by drawing a line straight down from the *QRS* (Q, R, S waves) complex. If the *c* wave is not visible, the *a* wave may be used. The *a* wave represents atrial systole and, therefore, follows the *P* wave on the ECG tracing.

Any pressure in the thoracic cavity is transmitted to the great vessels and the cardiac chambers. Thus, measurement of the RAP is obtained at end expiration to eliminate intrathoracic pressures. Spontaneously breathing patients generate a negative-pressure breath on inspiration. This is reflected in the RAP waveform as a downward deflection. Patients on a ventilator with mandatory positive pressure breaths show a rise in their RAP waveform on inspiration. An addition of positive end expiratory pressure greater than 10 cm H_2O may result in elevation of

the entire waveform above the baseline pressure. Interpretation of the RAP is based on trends in data and not the absolute number. Find the end expiration phase of the RAP waveform in the mechanically ventilated patient in Figure 8–10.

Conditions Leading to Alterations in RAP Normally, pressure and volume are proportional: An increase in volume generates an increase in pressure, and a decrease in volume generates a decrease in pressure. This is the basis for using pressures as proxies for volume status. Keeping this in mind, increases in RAP are often associated with fluid excess problems, and decreases in RAP are often associated with fluid deficit problems; however, other factors can also alter RAP, as described here.

Causes of Increased RAP and Associated Clinical Findings. The RAP increases with fluid volume excess problems (e.g., heart failure or excessive fluid intake), and any pathologic condition that increases the pressures or vascular volumes in the lungs can increase pulmonary resistance, which in turn increases the work of the right ventricle. These circumstances can lead to the inability of the ventricle to empty itself during systole. However, there are certain abnormal circumstances in which the RAP increases without increasing volume. Consider a balloon that is inflated with a given volume of water, and imagine squeezing the balloon: The pressure inside the balloon increases, but the volume does not change. Clinically, this is seen in pathologic conditions such as cardiac tamponade or tension pneumothorax.

Clinical findings associated with an increased RAP vary according to the cause and duration but are generally those of fluid volume excess. When elevated RAP is a result of left-heart failure, signs and symptoms of left ventricular failure will also be found.

Causes of Decreased RAP and Associated Clinical Findings. A decreased RAP indicates low right-heart preload. This results from either absolute or relative

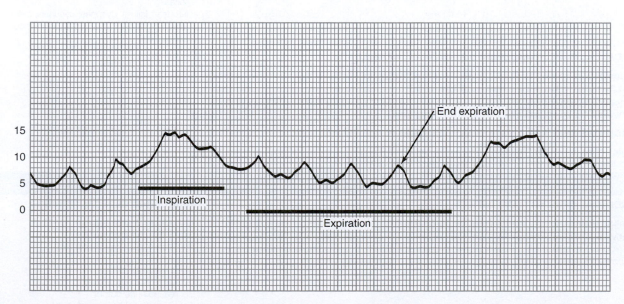

Figure 8–10 End expiration phase on RAP waveform in a patient receiving mechanical ventilation.

hypovolemia. Poor venous return to the heart for any reason results in a reduction in RAP. In high-acuity patients, examples of causes of absolute deficit include hemorrhage or excessive diuresis, and examples of causes of relative deficit are drug-induced vasodilation or third-spacing of fluid.

Clinical findings accompanying decreased RAP depend on the severity of the condition. Typical findings are those of fluid volume deficit. Should the deficit be sufficient to compromise CO, the patient will develop signs of shock.

Table 8–4 lists common causes and associated clinical findings of increased and decreased RAP.

Interventions for Treating Abnormal RAP Interventions for treating abnormal levels of RAP are determined by the cause; therefore, determining the cause of abnormal pressures should be a major early goal.

Treating Increased RAP. In general, care is directed toward optimizing preload by reducing volume—for example, by adding diuretic therapy. Overall goals are to decrease venous return to the right heart, increase contractility, and decrease the workload of the heart. Preload is reduced by restricting fluid and sodium and administering diuretics or vasodilating medications. Nursing care includes careful and frequent assessment of the patient's response to interventions. This includes keeping meticulous intake and output records and obtaining daily weights. A care plan designed to decrease patient energy requirements is implemented. A dietary consult is obtained to provide patient and family education on sodium and fluid restrictions. Patient education includes information on the purpose and importance of all medications.

Treating Decreased RAP. Interventions for a low RAP are determined by the cause. Interventions are directed toward optimizing preload by restoring volume. Dehydration from overly vigorous diuresis, burns, vomiting, or diarrhea is corrected by oral replacement when possible or by careful intravenous hydration. Hemorrhage may need surgical correction. Crystalloid IV fluids and blood products replace volume lost by hemorrhage. The hypovolemia or low-preload state related to sepsis is treated with replacement fluids, the administration of appropriate antibiotics to treat the sepsis, and careful adjustment of vasoconstricting medications, such as dopamine and norepinephrine.

Vasodilating medications are also a potential cause of low preload because pooling of blood in a dilated vascular system reduces venous return to the heart. Intravenous nitrates and nitroprusside (Nipride) are typically titrated by the nurse, based on orders from the HCP. Oral medications with vasodilating properties should be identified and discussed with the HCP prior to administration. The nurse performs careful and frequent assessment of the patient's response to these interventions. Intake and output are monitored and evaluated, and changes in the patient's weight provide important information.

Table 8–4 Conditions That Alter Right Atrial Pressure and Associated Clinical Findings

Increased RAP	
CONDITIONS CAUSING FLUID EXCESS	**ASSOCIATED CLINICAL FINDINGS**
Chronic or severe left heart failure: Increased volume in pulmonary circulation causing increased pressure against which the right ventricle must pump, reducing right ventricular emptying **Excessive fluid intake:** Excessive IV fluids or too rapid IV infusion; excessive oral fluid intake	Jugular venous distention (JVD) Tachycardia Right ventricular gallop (S3, S4, or both) Liver enlargement and tenderness Edema (dependent or generalized) Ascites If left heart failure: dyspnea, cyanosis, pulmonary crackles, shortness of breath, increased fatigability
CONDITIONS CAUSING INCREASED PULMONARY AFTERLOAD	
Pulmonic valve stenosis: Reduced valve opening preventing full ejection of right ventricular volume into pulmonary artery; fluid buildup in right ventricle **Pulmonary hypertension:** High pressure in lungs increasing afterload against which the right ventricle must pump, reducing right ventricular emptying	
CONDITIONS THAT APPLY EXTERNAL PRESSURE ON THE HEART	
Cardiac tamponade and tension pneumothorax: Rapid fluid buildup in the pericardial space resulting in pressure against the heart, increasing to right ventricular filling	
Decreased RAP	
CONDITIONS CAUSING FLUID DEFICIT	**ASSOCIATED CLINICAL FINDINGS**
Absolute deficit: Hemorrhage, diuresis, dehydration (e.g., vomiting or diarrhea), extensive burns **Relative fluid deficit:** Vasodilation (e.g., drug induced), certain shock states (e.g., anaphylactic, neurogenic, systemic inflammatory response syndrome [SIRS]), third-spacing of fluids, severe hypoalbuminemia	Tachycardia, hypotension Diminished pulse amplitude Flat neck veins in supine position Reduced CO Thirst and poor skin turgor Dry mucous membranes Decreased urine output If severe: clinical findings of shock

Right Ventricular Pressure

The **right ventricular (RV) pressure (or RVP)** is not continuously monitored with a traditional PA catheter but is observed and documented during insertion of the catheter. It is the responsibility of the nurse to recognize an RV waveform. The RV pressure is measured as a systolic and diastolic pressure. The systolic pressure represents the pressure necessary to exceed the pressure in the pulmonary artery (RV afterload), open the pulmonary valve, and eject blood into the pulmonary circulation. The right end diastolic pressure directly reflects the preload status of the right ventricle and should approximate the RAP. The normal RV pressure ranges are RV systolic, 20 to 30 mmHg, and RV diastolic, 2 to 8 mmHg.

Waveform Recognition The RV waveform has a characteristic pattern. It consists of a steep upstroke and a sharp downstroke (Figure 8–11). Compare this waveform to the right atrial waveform in Figure 8–9. Although there is a marked increase in systolic pressure, the RV diastolic pressure remains essentially the same as the RAP. That is important information in identifying the waveform of a catheter that has slipped back into the right ventricle.

Clinical Implications The RV waveform should be seen only during PA catheter insertion, as the catheter is floated through the RV. Observation of this waveform at any time other than insertion indicates that the PA catheter tip has retreated from its proper position in the PA. A dislodged PA catheter tip has two important implications from a technical perspective and from a patient safety perspective. First, all parameters obtained from a dislocated catheter, including the CO, are incorrect. Second, and most important, the patient is at risk for cardiac dysrhythmias. The displaced catheter tip can irritate the right ventricular endothelium, triggering potentially life-threatening abnormal cardiac rhythms (e.g., premature ventricular contractions or ventricular tachycardia). In addition, the

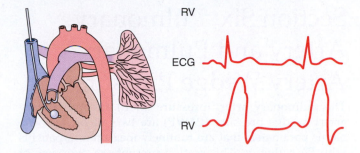

Figure 8–11 Right ventricular (RV) waveform.

SOURCE: "Right ventricular (RV) waveform" from Edwards Lifesciences. Reprinted with permission. Copyright © 2000 Edwards Lifesciences. Swan-Ganz® is a trademark of Edwards Lifesciences Corporation, registered in the U.S. Patent and Trademark Office.

right bundle branch portion of the cardiac conduction system lies close to the surface of the right ventricular septum; consequently, irritation can cause cardiac conduction disturbances such as heart block and bundle branch blocks. Therefore, it is important that the nurse quickly recognize the abnormal presence of the RV waveform and its corresponding pressures and report this complication immediately to the appropriate HCP to expedite repositioning of the catheter.

Some hospitals or units have specific nursing protocols to follow when a PA catheter retreats into the RV, such as pulling the catheter back into the right atrium or inflating the balloon to foster flotation of the catheter tip back into the PA. It is the responsibility of the nurse to be aware of unit policy and state licensure guidelines related to repositioning a PA catheter to a different location.

Once the catheter has been inserted, the exposed portion of the catheter is considered contaminated and should not be advanced unless a sterile contamination sheath is placed over the catheter before insertion. The use of these sheaths allows repositioning of the catheter without increasing the risk of infection.

Section Five Review

1. The RAP is measured through which port of the PA catheter?
   - **A.** Proximal
   - **B.** Distal
   - **C.** Medial
   - **D.** Thermistor

2. The RAP is a reflection of which factor?
   - **A.** PAWP
   - **B.** Right-heart afterload
   - **C.** Left-heart function
   - **D.** Right-heart preload

3. What is the correct value range for the normal mean RAP?
   - **A.** Less than 4 mmHg
   - **B.** 2 to 6 mmHg
   - **C.** 6 to 12 mmHg
   - **D.** 14 to 20 mmHg

4. What is the most accurate description of the RV waveform?
   - **A.** Almost flat
   - **B.** A soft undulating pattern
   - **C.** Sharply notched with a slow downstroke
   - **D.** A steep upstroke followed by a sharp downstroke

Answers: 1. A, 2. D, 3. B, 4. D

Section Six: Pulmonary Artery and Pulmonary Artery Wedge Pressures

The pulmonary artery pressure (PAP) and pulmonary artery wedge pressure (PAWP) are two major hemodynamic parameters that are routinely measured in patients with PA catheters. This section presents an overview of both parameters.

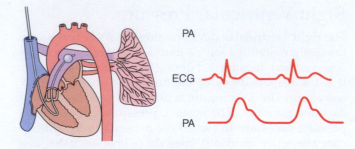

Figure 8–12 PA waveform.

SOURCE: "PA waveform" from Edwards Life sciences. Reprinted with permission. Copyright © 2000 Edwards Lifesciences. Swan-Ganz® is a trademark of Edwards Lifesciences Corporation, registered in the U.S. Patent and Trademark Office.

Pulmonary Artery Pressure

Pulmonary artery pressure (PAP) normally reflects both right and left heart pressures and is read as a systolic and diastolic pressure. The **pulmonary artery systolic (PAS) pressure** reflects the highest pressure generated by the RV during systole, with a normal range of 20 to 30 mmHg. The **pulmonary artery diastolic (PAD) pressure** reflects the lowest pressure within the pulmonary artery and has a normal range of 8 to 15 mmHg.

The PAD pressure is an important measurement because it is normally 2 to 5 mmHg higher than the pulmonary artery wedge pressure (PAWP). After the PAD pressure has been demonstrated to correlate with the PAWP, it is used to monitor left ventricular preload status. Certain cardiovascular disorders (e.g., mitral stenosis, heart rate greater than 125/min) and pulmonary disorders (e.g., chronic obstructive pulmonary disease, pulmonary embolism) alter the relationship of PAD to PAWP, and in such cases PAD cannot be used to monitor PAWP.

Waveform Analysis   The PAP is obtained from the distal port of the PA catheter. The PA waveform is monitored continuously by a transducer attached to the distal port of the catheter. The PA waveform has a characteristic pattern (Figure 8–12). It consists of a steep upstroke and a downstroke that is distinguished by a dicrotic notch formed by the closure of the pulmonic valve.

On entry of the catheter into the PA from the right ventricle, the top of the waveform stays essentially the same height, but the bottom or diastolic portion of the waveform elevates. If the catheter tip retreats into the right ventricle, the diastolic pressure drops and the dicrotic notch is lost. Familiarity with these waveform properties allows the nurse to identify catheter position correctly. This is important because catheter retreat into the right ventricle could result in dysrhythmias.

The PA pressure waveform represents arterial pressure on the right side of the heart. The systolic upstroke of the PA pressure tracing represents right ventricular ejection and is preceded by ventricular electrical depolarization. The PA pressure may be obtained clinically by printing out both the ECG and PA pressure tracings. The PA systolic pressure will follow the *QRS* wave of the ECG. Correlate the ECG with the PA pressure tracing in Figure 8–12.

Elevated Pulmonary Artery Pressure   Pulmonary artery pressure is heavily influenced by alterations in heart function or changes in pulmonary pressures. When PAP becomes abnormally elevated, the associated clinical findings will reflect the underlying cause of the abnormality.

Elevated PAS.   The PA pressure is generated by the right ventricle; therefore, any condition that acutely or chronically increases the afterload of the right ventricle (i.e., increases the pulmonary vascular resistance) results in an elevated PAS pressure. Examples include pulmonary hypertension from any cause, including chronic lung disease, pulmonary embolism, and hypoxemia.

The clinical findings of elevated PAS pressure vary according to the cause, severity, and duration of the elevated pressure. Assessment of the patient with pulmonary hypertension may reveal signs of right-heart failure, including distended neck veins, peripheral edema, a tender liver, and ascites. Palpation of the chest may reveal a right ventricular lift, and auscultation may reveal S3 and S4 heart sounds. The patient with a pulmonary embolus may present as a medical emergency with dyspnea, chest pain, hemoptysis, and hemodynamic instability.

Elevated PAD.   Conditions that affect the left heart, such as angina or myocardial infarction, fluid overload, mitral stenosis, and left-to-right intracardiac shunts, are associated with a high PAD pressure.

Clinical findings associated with left-heart failure may result in some or all of the following signs and symptoms: dyspnea, tachycardia, S3 or S4 heart sounds, and bilateral crackles in the lungs. CO is reduced, and PAWP is elevated.

Treatment of Elevated PAP   Interventions for an elevated PAS or PAD pressure are determined by the cause. In general, care is directed toward reducing preload by administering diuretics and restricting fluid and sodium intake. In addition, some novel therapies aimed at pulmonary vascular vasodilation have been developed to treat pulmonary hypertension. Cardiac contractility is improved by the use of positive inotropic medications, such as digoxin

(Lanoxin), dobutamine (Dobutrex), dopamine, and amrinone (Inocor). Nursing care includes careful administration of potent medications, intake and output measurements, and daily weights. Care is focused on reducing the workload of the heart by planning physical activities that are followed by rest periods.

Low Pulmonary Artery Diastolic Pressure A low PAD pressure typically indicates a low preload state related to inadequate venous return to the left heart. Clinical findings associated with low preload states include tachycardia, flat neck veins, clear lungs, dry oral mucosa, poor skin turgor, hypotension, and decreased urine output. If severe, the signs and symptoms of advanced shock, such as cool and clammy skin, also may be seen.

Interventions are directed toward improving left ventricle (LV) preload through volume replacement. Nursing care includes managing fluid replacement through an ongoing assessment of the patient's hydration status and hemodynamic parameters. It is important to assess changes in patient weight and intake and output data.

Pulmonary Artery Wedge Pressure

Pulmonary artery wedge pressure (PAWP) is also known as pulmonary artery occlusion pressure (PAOP) and pulmonary capillary wedge pressure (PCWP). For the purposes of this chapter, it is referred to as PAWP. The PAWP reflects left ventricular end diastolic pressure (LVEDP), which is a measure of preload in the left ventricle. The concept of preload applies to both the right and left ventricles, but emphasis is placed on the left ventricle because it functions as a systemic pump that determines patient outcomes.

Left ventricular preload is measured directly only during a cardiac catheterization or following open heart surgery when a left ventricular line is placed. It is indirectly measured with a PA catheter through measurement of the PAWP.

Obtaining Measurements The PAWP is obtained through the distal port of the PA catheter. To obtain a PAWP, the catheter balloon is inflated slowly, allowing the catheter to float and "wedge" in a small branch of the pulmonary artery. Inflation (usually around 0.9 mL) is stopped as soon as the characteristic PAWP pattern is observed. The inflated balloon stops the forward flow of blood through that vessel. Because there are no valves in the pulmonary circulation, the catheter wedged in the pulmonary artery "sees" forward, through the pulmonary capillaries, pulmonary veins, left atrium, and into the left ventricle. Because the mitral valve remains open until the end of ventricular diastole, the left atrium and ventricle essentially function as one open chamber until the mitral valve closes. This is why the PAWP reflects the pressure in the left ventricle at end diastole.

PAWP Waveform Analysis The normal PAWP range is 4 to 12 mmHg. Like the RAP, when the c wave is not visible (as is the usual case with the PAWP tracing), the

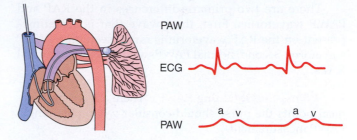

Figure 8–13 Pulmonary artery wedge pressure waveform.

SOURCE: "Pulmonary artery wedge pressure waveform" from Edwards Lifesciences. Reprinted with permission. Copyright © 2000 Edwards Lifesciences. Swan-Ganz® is a trademark of Edwards Lifesciences Corporation, registered in the U.S. Patent and Trademark Office.

PAWP is read as the mean of the a wave. The PAWP waveform (Figure 8–13) is similar in appearance to the right atrial waveform shown in Figure 8–9. In the absence of mitral valve disease, the PAWP is considered an accurate estimate of left ventricular preload. It provides information about the volume status of the left ventricle and aids in the evaluation of left ventricular compliance. An elevated PAWP suggests a stiff, noncompliant left ventricle that contracts poorly. A low PAWP indicates that preload is low.

The first positive wave is the a wave, produced by the rise in atrial pressure caused by left atrial contraction. The second positive wave is the v wave, formed as the left atrium fills during ventricular systole. The c wave, not typically seen on the PAWP waveform, is produced by closure of the mitral valve at the initiation of ventricular systole.

As shown in Figure 8–14, the two negative PAWP waveforms are the x and y descents. The first negative descent is the x wave, which reflects decreased volume in the left atrium after atrial systole. The y descent results from the pressure drop in the left atrium when the mitral valve opens just prior to atrial contraction, permitting passive emptying of the left atrium.

The PAWP is read and interpreted in the same manner as is the RAP (i.e., a dual-channel strip in which the RAP and ECG waveforms are printed out simultaneously). The a wave is near the end of the QRS complex of the ECG (Leatherman & Marini, 2015). The mean of the a wave is documented. Find the correlation between the a wave of the PAWP tracing and the ECG in Figure 8–13.

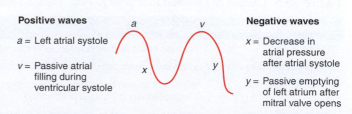

Positive waves

a = Left atrial systole

v = Passive atrial filling during ventricular systole

Negative waves

x = Decrease in atrial pressure after atrial systole

y = Passive emptying of left atrium after mitral valve opens

Figure 8–14 A labeled PAWP waveform.

There are two primary differences in the RAP and PAWP waveforms. First, the *c* wave that is sometimes present on the RAP waveform is rarely seen on a PAWP waveform. Second, normal PAWPs are higher than normal RAPs.

Key Points for Obtaining PAWP   There are several technical points the nurse should consider when obtaining a PAWP measurement.

- Observe the waveform constantly during inflation, and stop inflation as soon as the PAWP is identified.

- Use the smallest inflation volume possible, and do not exceed the maximum recommended volume (typically less than 1.25 mL). This reduces the risk of balloon rupture.

- Maintain inflation only long enough to obtain a stable reading.

- Obtain the PAWP at end expiration, when intrathoracic pressure is most stable and less affected by respiratory variation.

- Because active air withdrawal can damage the balloon, allow it to deflate passively.

- If resistance is felt during balloon inflation, stop! *Do not continue!* The balloon tip may be lodged in a very small vessel or stuck against a structure. Continuing to inflate may cause vessel damage or rupture. Allow the balloon to passively deflate, and call the HCP.

- If no resistance is felt during balloon inflation with the appropriate volume of air and a PAWP waveform does not appear, the balloon may have ruptured. Using the appropriate stopcock, turn the balloon lumen port off to the patient. Label the lumen "Do Not Use," and notify the HCP.

Pulmonary infarction can result from leaving the PA balloon inflated for too long or when a deflated tip becomes lodged in the PA branch. A PAWP waveform will appear on the monitor. The patient should be turned or made to cough to relieve a lodged balloon. Open the stopcock on the port and remove the syringe to allow passive deflation of the balloon.

Elevated PAWP   Any condition that increases the left ventricular end diastolic blood volume results in an elevated PAWP. Table 8–5 lists conditions that are associated with elevated PAWP.

Clinical Findings.   Clinical findings related to an elevated PAWP vary according to the degree of elevation but typically include tachycardia, exertional dyspnea, orthopnea, paroxysmal nocturnal dyspnea (PND), crackles in the lung fields, an S3 or S4 gallop at the heart apex, and neck vein distension.

Interventions.   Interventions are directed toward optimizing preload by administering diuretics and vasodilators and restricting sodium and fluid. Intravenous and oral nitrates dilate the venous bed and displace fluid, which lower preload by reducing the venous return to the heart. Control of dysrhythmias helps the heart to pump more effectively. Afterload is reduced by administration of arteriole vasodilators, such as nitroprusside (Nipride), and ACE inhibitors, such as captopril (Capoten). By dilating the peripheral arterioles, these drugs reduce afterload, promote emptying of the ventricle, and effectively reduce cardiac work and myocardial oxygen requirements. Contractility is enhanced by careful titration of inotropic medications, such as digoxin, dobutamine (Dobutrex), and amrinone (Inocor). If these interventions fail to improve PAWP and CO, an intraaortic balloon pump may be required.

The nurse is responsible for careful titration of potent vasoactive medications to improve hemodynamics. Manipulation of medications and treatments is based on astute physical assessments correlated with current hemodynamic parameters obtained from the PA catheter. Critical thinking at the bedside is crucial to improved patient outcomes. Frequent nursing assessments, accurate intake and output records, and daily weights are crucial to follow the response to treatment.

Low PAWP   A low PAWP typically is related to inadequate circulating blood volume. Clinical findings are those of fluid deficit, including flat neck veins, clear lungs, low pulse pressure, decreased urine output, hypotension, tachycardia, and likely complaints of thirst. Interventions include careful replacement of fluid or blood products by correlating the PAWP with an ongoing assessment of the patient's response to treatment. Hourly urine output, careful intake and output records, and daily weights are indicated.

Table 8–5 Causes of Elevated Pulmonary Artery Wedge Pressure

Associated Condition	Description
Fluid overload	From excessive fluid replacement or kidney failure
Left ventricular failure	Inadequate ventricular emptying from poor contractility
Myocardial ischemia	Insufficient oxygen to cardiac muscle decreases available ATP for energy, resulting in decreased cardiac muscle compliance and impaired contractility
Mitral stenosis	High left atrial pressure transmitted back into the pulmonary vasculature, elevating pulmonary pressures
Cardiac tamponade	Increases the resistance to ventricular filling due to external pressure being applied against the cardiac wall; RAP, PAD, and PAWP elevate and become similar (called diastolic equalization, a hallmark of cardiac tamponade)

Section Six Review

1. The normal range for PAD pressure is which set of values?
   A. 2 to 8 mmHg
   B. 4 to 10 mmHg
   C. 6 to 12 mmHg
   D. 8 to 15 mmHg

2. A PAD is 2 mmHg. The nurse should anticipate performing which intervention?
   A. Administering diuretics and implementing fluid restrictions
   B. Volume replacement
   C. Administering a positive inotropic agent
   D. No intervention needed

3. What is the normal range of the PAWP?
   A. 2 to 10 mmHg
   B. 4 to 12 mmHg
   C. 8 to 16 mmHg
   D. 10 to 18 mmHg

4. In heart failure, what is the expected PAWP?
   A. Well within the normal range
   B. Low-normal or below-normal range
   C. High-normal or above-normal range
   D. High or low

Answers: 1. D, 2. B, 3. B, 4. C

Section Seven: Vascular Resistance and Stroke Work

Throughout the chapter, afterload and contractility have been addressed in a variety of contexts. Alterations in afterload or contractility significantly impact the patient's hemodynamic status; therefore, evaluating and normalizing afterload or contractility problems are an important part of the overall treatment strategy in hemodynamically unstable patients. Measurements of systemic and pulmonary vascular resistance are the major means of evaluating afterload; stroke volume and ventricular stroke work index are indirect measures of contractility.

Systemic Vascular Resistance

Systemic vascular resistance (SVR) is an estimate of left ventricular afterload. It represents an average of the resistance of all the vascular beds. Recall that afterload is the resistance (opposing force) the left ventricle must overcome to open the aortic valve and eject the stroke volume into the systemic circulation. Afterload is one of the primary determinants of myocardial oxygen demand. The harder the heart works to pump blood out of the ventricle, the higher the myocardial oxygen requirement. A high SVR can reduce SV and CO. This is an important aspect to consider during regulation of potent vasoactive medications. These medications may improve MAP and afterload but may also decrease SV.

Most monitors calculate the SVR; however, it is helpful to understand the components that make up the formula. Left ventricular afterload is the product of a change in pressure (MAP − RAP) times a conversion factor (80) divided by flow (CO). To individualize SVR to the patient, the CI is substituted for the CO in the formula. Table 8–1 lists the equations and normal ranges for SVR and SVRI. The indices of CI and SVRI are far better indicators of the patient's hemodynamic status than the CO and SVR alone because the indices are referenced to body size.

Elevated SVR or SVRI   A high SVR or SVRI may be the result of multiple problems. In hypothermia, peripheral vasoconstriction occurs as a compensatory mechanism to keep the core body temperature warm. In this circumstance, warming the patient may be the only intervention necessary to dilate the constricted peripheral vasculature, normalize SVR, and improve CO.

Hypovolemia can produce an elevated SVR due to the compensatory mechanisms that are activated. Inadequate circulating blood volume induces vasoconstriction. This mechanism results in the shunting of as much peripheral blood volume as possible back to the vital organs (heart, lungs, and brain). Careful fluid replacement normalizes the SVR.

In cardiac failure, hypotension initiates similar compensatory mechanisms. The peripheral vascular beds constrict in an attempt to increase the blood return to the heart, thereby increasing the blood pressure. However, in this situation, returning more blood (more preload) to an already failing heart does not help. The vasoconstriction itself results in an increased afterload, which means the already struggling heart must now overcome more pressure to open the aortic valve and eject the stroke volume.

Collaborative Management.   The patient with increased SVR needs help in reducing both preload and afterload. Preload is reduced using diuretic and nitrate (vasodilator) therapies. Afterload reduction is done cautiously in a patient with low blood pressure. A vasodilator, such as nitroprusside (Nipride), or an ACE inhibitor, such as captopril (Capoten), may be administered. Milrinone (Primacor) is a positive inotropic agent that improves myocardial contractility and causes vasodilation to reduce both afterload and preload. Reducing afterload makes it easier for the heart to eject SV, lessens cardiac work and myocardial oxygen demand, and improves CO.

Low SVR or SVRI   Widespread vasodilation is the major cause of low SVR. It can result from drug-induced vasodilation (e.g., nitrate drugs, ACE inhibitors) or as a physiologic response to certain shock states, such as sepsis, neurogenic shock, and anaphylaxis. As vasodilation increases, CO drops and the patient becomes hypotensive.

If the low SVR is drug induced, either the drug dosage is adjusted or the drug is withdrawn. In the treatment of shock, SVR is improved with the careful titration of vasoconstricting medications such as dopamine, phenylephrine, or norepinephrine. Careful fluid resuscitation can also be initiated to "fill up the vascular tank" to treat the relative fluid deficit caused by widespread vasodilation.

Pulmonary Vascular Resistance

Pulmonary vascular resistance (PVR) is an estimate of right ventricular afterload. It represents an average of the resistance of pulmonary vascular beds. Most hemodynamic monitors calculate PVR. However, it is helpful to understand the components that make up the formula. Right ventricular afterload is the product of change in pressure (mean PAP − PAWP) multiplied by 80 (a conversion factor) and divided by flow (CO). Table 8–1 lists the equation and normal ranges for PVR and PVRI.

High PVR or PVRI   PVR or PVRI is elevated with hypoxemia (causes pulmonary vasoconstriction), acute lung injury, acute respiratory distress syndrome, pulmonary hypertension, and pulmonary congestion. A high PVR reduces right ventricular SV and CO, increasing the work and oxygen demands of the right ventricle. Treatment for high PVR includes the administration of pulmonary vasodilators, and, if warranted, correction of anemia, acidosis, or hypoxemia (Douglas, 2015).

Stroke Volume

Recall that SV is one of the two determinants of cardiac output and that it is influenced by preload, afterload, and contractility. Therefore, determining the SV (or SVI) can provide valuable information about contractility, particularly if the status of preload and afterload is already known. Stroke volume cannot be directly measured at the bedside and requires calculating its various components. Table 8–1 lists the formulae and normal values for SV and SVI.

Anything that alters preload, afterload, or contractility will alter SV; therefore, when abnormal values are obtained, it is important to place these data in the broader context of the patient's other clinical findings.

Ventricular Stroke Work

Measuring ventricular stroke work (VSW) or ventricular stroke work index (VSWI) can provide important information about ventricular function through measuring the work involved in one ventricular contraction.

Left Ventricular Stroke Work Index   A great deal of information goes into calculating the left ventricular stroke work index (LVSWI) because it represents work that is influenced by two factors: (1) the pressure the heart beats against (afterload) and (2) the volume the ventricle must pump forward. Variables in the calculation of LVSWI are first collected. These include SVI, MAP, and PAWP. Table 8–1 provides the formula and normal values for LVSWI.

In some situations it helps to compare the LVSWI with the PAWP. PAWP reflects volume and LVSWI represents pressure. When the left ventricle becomes stiff (decreased compliance), the PAWP does not accurately reflect the workload of the left ventricle because the relationship between volume and pressure is not direct. In this case it is best to calculate LVSWI rather than PAWP.

Once the LVSWI is obtained, it is plotted on the y axis of a ventricular function curve (Figure 8–15). PAWP is plotted on the x axis. This provides a picture of how the left ventricle is performing in light of the pressure and volume conditions. As noted in the diagram, an LVSWI between 40 and 60 g/m²/beat and a PAWP between 8 and 20 mmHg is best for left ventricular ejection. Low LVSWI may be an indication that the patient is hypovolemic or has cardiac failure. If both the LVSWI and the PAWP are low, more volume may be needed to improve contractility. High LVSWI may be an indication of hypervolemia. If both the LVSWI and the PAWP are high, diuretics and vasodilators may be needed.

Contractility is optimized when preload and afterload are optimized. If the CO remains low after both preload and afterload have been optimized, inotropic agents to improve CO may be considered, because increasing the contractile force of a weak ventricle improves SV and CO.

Right Ventricular Stroke Work Index   Right ventricular stroke work index (RVSWI) is the amount of work involved in moving blood in the right ventricle with each beat. The formula represents the pressure generated (mean PAP) multiplied by the volume pumped (SVI). Like LVSWI, the RVSWI increases or decreases with changes in either pressure (mean PAP) or volume pumped (SVI). As shown in Table 8–1, the normal values for RVSWI are significantly lower than those for LVSWI, because the right heart works within a low-pressure environment. Increased and decreased values are treated much the same as for LVSWI.

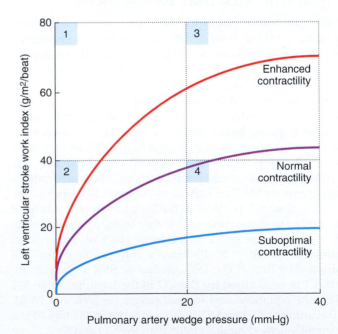

Quadrant 1: Optimal function; Quadrant 2: Hypovolemia;
Quadrant 3: Hypervolemia; Quadrant 4: Cardiac failure

Figure 8–15 Ventricular function curve.

Section Seven Review

1. Afterload to the left ventricle is estimated by determining which hemodynamic value?
   A. Systemic vascular resistance (SVR)
   B. Pulmonary vascular resistance (PVR)
   C. Right atrial pressure (RAP)
   D. Pulmonary artery wedge pressure (PAWP)

2. Using the following hemodynamic parameters, calculate SVR: MAP = 90 mmHg, RAP = 6 mmHg, CO = 6.2 L/min, BSA = 1.8 m^2.
   A. 622 dynes · sec · cm^{-5}/m^2
   B. 1083 dynes · sec · cm^{-5}/m^2
   C. 1274 dynes · sec · cm^{-5}/m^2
   D. 1832 dynes · sec · cm^{-5}/m^2

3. Afterload to the right ventricle can be estimated using which hemodynamic measurement?
   A. Systemic vascular resistance (SVR)
   B. Pulmonary artery wedge pressure (PAWP)
   C. Pulmonary vascular resistance (PVR)
   D. Right atrial pressure (RAP)

4. When assessing left ventricular function, the LVSWI should be used instead of the PAWP in the presence of which condition?
   A. Hypovolemia
   B. Heart failure
   C. Decreased compliance
   D. Hypervolemia

Answers: 1. A, 2. B, 3. C, 4. C

Clinical Reasoning Checkpoint

You are the nurse caring for a patient in the ICU. The healthcare team has just placed a pulmonary artery catheter into this patient.

1. Indicate which hub or lumen you would use to perform the following:
   A. Monitor RAP
   B. Connect the transducer for continuous monitoring of PA pressures
   C. Monitor PAWP
   D. Administer IV fluid boluses
   E. Obtain a sample for mixed venous oxygen saturation
   F. Measure core body temperature

2. Match the hemodynamic measurements with their corresponding component of CO:
   1. _____PAWP   A. Preload RV
   2. _____CVP   B. Afterload LV
   3. _____SVR   C. Ventricular stroke work index
   4. _____PVR   D. Preload LV
   5. _____Contractility   E. Afterload RV

3. Calculate the derived hemodynamic parameters:
   A. Your patient has a BP of 60/40 mmHg. Calculate the MAP. What is your interpretation of this MAP? What physical assessment findings would you expect in a patient with this MAP? What interventions would you anticipate for a patient with this MAP?
   B. Your patient has the following: MAP 47 mmHg, RAP 12 mmHg, and CO 3.4 L/min. Calculate the SVR. What is your interpretation of this SVR?
   C. Your patient has the following: mean PAP 40 mmHg, PAWP 18 mmHg, and CO 3.4 L/min. Calculate the PVR. What is your interpretation of this PVR?

Chapter 8 Review

1. The client with cirrhosis of the liver has significant ascites. The client is cold, clammy, and confused. The nurse interprets these findings as indicating which physiological condition?
   1. Increased preload from increased venous return to the heart
   2. Decreased afterload from peripheral vasodilation
   3. Decreased preload from a relative volume depletion
   4. Increased afterload from ankle edema

2. A client has had an arterial line inserted into the radial artery. Which nursing interventions should the nurse add to this client's plan of care? (Select all that apply.)
   1. Regularly assess the color of the client's hand.
   2. Measure pulses distal to the insertion site.
   3. Remove the caps along the monitoring system.
   4. Secure all line connections.
   5. Observe insertion site for redness, warmth, or edema.

3. A client has a PA catheter inserted. Which port should the nurse use for infusion of IV fluids?
   1. Proximal
   2. Distal
   3. Yellow port
   4. Balloon port

4. The nurse has obtained a pulmonary wedge pressure (PAWP) from a PA catheter. What interventions are necessary? (Select all that apply.)
   1. Manually deflate the balloon to ensure all air is removed.
   2. Tape the syringe used for inflation to the head of the client's bed.
   3. Leave the balloon inflated.
   4. Expel all air from the syringe and reattach to the catheter.
   5. Leave the balloon deflated.

5. The nurse is preparing a client for insertion of a pulmonary artery (PA) catheter. Which information should the nurse provide?
   1. "You will be taken to the operating room and given general anesthesia for this procedure."
   2. "You will not feel the catheter as it is inserted."
   3. "You will have no discomfort with this procedure."
   4. "Once this procedure is completed, you will be free of IV lines."

6. A client has just been assisted with hygienic care, including a bed bath and linen change. It is time to obtain hemodynamic measurements. Which intervention should the nurse perform?
   1. Position the client with the head of the bed at 90 degrees.
   2. Allow the client to rest in a position of comfort.
   3. Place the transducer on a level with the client's clavicles.
   4. Expose the client's shoulders by pulling down the gown.

7. A nurse notices an RV waveform on the bedside monitor during routine hemodynamic monitoring. Which action is a nursing priority?
   1. No action is necessary for this normal finding.
   2. Assess the client for altered cardiac output.
   3. Auscultate the lungs for crackles.
   4. Notify the appropriate healthcare provider immediately.

8. The nurse assesses that the dicrotic notch of a PA waveform has disappeared. What action should the nurse take?
   1. Remove the catheter.
   2. Notify the appropriate healthcare provider.
   3. Nothing, as this is normal in systole.
   4. Gently pull on the catheter until the notch reappears.

9. Hemodynamic monitoring of a client reveals an elevation of the pulmonary artery systolic (PAS) pressure. The nurse would assess for which findings? (Select all that apply.)
   1. Left ventricular lift on palpation
   2. Tenderness over the right costal margin
   3. S3 and S4 heart sounds
   4. Flat neck veins
   5. Peripheral edema

10. A client in septic shock has low systemic vascular resistance (SVR). The nurse would anticipate participating in which interventions? (Select all that apply.)
    1. Administering vasoconstricting medications
    2. Keeping the head of the client's bed elevated at 30 degrees
    3. Fluid resuscitation
    4. Diuretic therapy
    5. Restricting oral fluids

Answers to questions found inside your textbook are available on the faculty resources site. Please consult with your instructor.

References

Alarcon, L. H., & Fink, M.P. (2014). Physiologic monitoring of the surgical patient. In F. Brunicardi, D. K. Andersen, T. R. Billiar, D. L. Dunn, J. G. Hunter, J. B. Matthews, & R. E. Pollock (Eds.), *Schwartz's principles of surgery* (10th ed.). Retrieved July 16, 2015 from http://accessmedicine.mhmedical.com.ezproxy.uky.edu/content.aspx?bookid=980&Sectionid=59610854

Berman, A., Synder, S. J., & Frandsen, G. (2016). Assessing health. In A. Berman, S. J. Synder, & G. Frandsen (Eds.), *Kozier & Erb's fundamentals of nursing practice: Concepts, process, and practice* (10th ed., pp. 513–596).

Retrieved December 15, 2016, from http://instructors.coursesmart.com/9780133974546/firstsection#X2ludGVybmFsX0J2ZGVwRmxhc2hSZWFkZXI/eG1saWQ9OTc4MDEzMzk3NDU0Ni81MTM=

Butterworth, J. F., IV, Mackey, D. C., Wasnick, J. D. (2013). Chapter 5: Cardiovascular monitoring. In J. F. Butterworth, IV, D. C. Mackey, & J. D. Wasnick (Eds.), *Morgan & Mikhail's clinical anesthesiology* (5th ed.). Retrieved December 16, 2016, from http://accessmedicine.mhmedical.com.ezproxy.uky.edu/content.aspx?bookid=564&Sectionid=42800535

Centers for Disease Control and Prevention (CDC). (2011). Guidelines for the prevention of intravascular catheter-related infections. Retrieved December 16, 2016, from http://www.cdc.gov/hicpac/pdf/guidelines/bsi-guidelines-2011.pdf

Centers for Disease Control and Prevention (CDC). (2015). Bloodstream infection event (central line-associated bloodstream infection and non-central line-associated bloodstream infection). Retrieved December 16, 2016, from http://www.cdc.gov/nhsn/PDFs/pscManual/4PSC_CLABScurrent.pdf

Centers for Disease Control and Prevention (CDC). (2016). Healthcare-associated infections (HAI) progress report. Retrieved December 16, 2016, from http://www.cdc.gov/hai/progress-report/index.html

Douglas, I. S. (2015). Acute right heart syndromes. In J. B. Hall, G. A. Schmidt, & J. P. Kress (Eds.), *Principles of critical care* (4th ed.). Retrieved July 22, 2015, from http://accessmedicine.mhmedical.com.ezproxy.uky.edu/content.aspx?bookid=1340&Sectionid=80031364

Edwards Lifesciences. (2015). *Quick guide to cardiopulmonary care.* Retrieved February 12, 2017, from http://www.edwards.com/eu/Specialties/CriticalCareMedicine/Pages/QuickGuide.aspx

Garcia, M. I. M., Romero, M. G., Cano, A. G., Aya, H. D., Rhodes, A., Grounds, R. M., & Cecconi, M. (2014). Dynamic arterial elastance as a predictor of arterial pressure response to fluid administration: A validation study. *Critical Care, 18*, 626–637.

Johnson, A. & Mohajer-Esfahani, M. (2014). Exploring hemodynamics: A review of current and emerging noninvasive monitoring techniques. *Critical Care Nursing Clinics of North America, 26*, 357–375.

Khraim, F., & Pike, R. (2014). Impedance cardiography-guided treatment of hypertension: A review of the literature. *Canadian Journal of Cardiovascular Nursing, 24*(4), 7–12.

Kirton, O. C., Calabrese, R. C., & Staff, I. (2015). Increasing use of less-invasive hemodynamic monitoring in 3 specialty surgical intensive care units: A 5-year experience at a tertiary medical center. *Journal of Intensive Care Medicine, 1*, 30–36.

Kubota, S., Endo, Y., Kubota, M., Ishizuka, Y., & Furudate, T. (2015). Effects of trunk posture in Fowler's position on hemodynamics. *Autonomic Neuroscience: Basic and Clinical, 189*, 56–59.

Leatherman, J. W., & Marini, J. (2015). Chapter 28: Interpretation of hemodynamic waveforms. In J. B. Hall, G. A. Schmidt, & J. P. Kress (Eds.), *Principles of*

critical care (4th ed.). Retrieved December 15, 2016, from http://accessanesthesiology.mhmedical.com/content.aspx?sectionid=80030289&bookid=1340&jumpsectionID=80030295&Resultclick=2

Lorne, E., Mahjoub, Y., Diouf, M., Sleghem, J., Buchalet, C., Guinot, P. G., . . . Dupont, H. (2014). Accuracy of impedance cardiography for evaluating trends in cardiac output: A comparison with oesophageal Doppler. *British Journal of Anaesthesia.* Retrieved December 15, 2016, from http://bja.oxfordjournals.org/content/early/2014/05/28/bja.aeu136.full.pdf. doi:10.1093/bja/aeu136

Magder, S. (2015). Invasive hemodynamic monitoring. *Critical Care Clinics, 31*, 67–87.

Miller, L. R. (2014). Hemodynamic monitoring. In S. M. Burns (Ed.), *AACN essentials of critical care nursing* (pp. 69–118). New York, NY: McGraw-Hill.

Monnet, X., & Teboul, J. L. (2015). Minimally invasive monitoring. *Critical Care Clinics, 31*, 25–42.

Pinsky, M. R. (2015). Chapter 32: Assessing the circulation: Oximetry, indicator dilution, and pulse contour analysis. In J. B. Hall, G. A. Schmidt, & J. P. Kress (Eds.), *Principles of critical care* (4th ed.). Retrieved December 16, 2016, from http://accessanesthesiology.mhmedical.com/content.aspx?sectionid=80030766&bookid=1340

Tejedor, A., Rivas, E., Ríos, J., Arismendi, E., Martinez-Palli, G., Delgado, S., & Balust, J. (2015). Accuracy of Vigileo/Flotrac monitoring system in morbidly obese patients. *Journal of Critical Care, 30*(3), 562–566.

The Joint Commission (TJC). (2015). *CLABSI toolkit - Chapter 3:* CLABSI prevention strategies, techniques, and technologies. Retrieved December 16, 2016, from http://www.jointcommission.org/topics/clabsi_toolkit__chapter_3.aspx

Waldron, N. H., Miller, T. E., Thacker, J. K., Manchester, A. K., White, W. D., Nardiello, J., . . . Gan, T. J. (2014). A prospective comparison of a noninvasive cardiac output monitor versus esophageal Doppler monitor for goal-directed fluid therapy in colorectal surgery patients. *Society for Technology in Anesthesia, 118*(5), 966–975.

Walley, K. R. (2015). Chapter 35: Ventricular dysfunction in critical illness. In J. B. Hall, G. A. Schmidt, & J. P. Kress (Eds.), *Principles of critical care* (4th ed.). Retrieved December 16, 2016, from http://accessmedicine.mhmedical.com/content.aspx?bookid=1340&sectionid=80030978

Chapter 9
Basic Cardiac Rhythm Monitoring

 Learning Outcomes

9.1 Explain membrane permeability changes that occur in cardiac cells and the relationship between membrane permeability and serum electrolyte levels.

9.2 Describe the cardiac conduction system, the normal electrocardiogram (ECG) complex, and nursing responsibilities for the patient who requires cardiac monitoring.

9.3 Interpret ECG patterns using a systematic approach.

9.4 Identify factors that place a person at risk for developing dysrhythmias.

9.5 Differentiate among common dysrhythmias arising from the sinoatrial (SA) node and their treatments.

9.6 Compare and contrast basic atrial dysrhythmias and their treatments.

9.7 Distinguish among common junctional dysrhythmias and their treatments.

9.8 Differentiate among common ventricular dysrhythmias and their treatments.

9.9 Distinguish among the four conduction abnormalities, known as heart blocks, and their treatments.

9.10 Discuss pharmacologic and countershock interventions for specific dysrhythmias and their nursing implications.

9.11 Identify indications for pacemaker and implantable cardioversion or defibrillation therapy, types of devices, and nursing implications for the patient receiving these therapies.

This chapter is written at an introductory knowledge level for individuals who provide nursing care for high-acuity patients requiring electrocardiogram (ECG) monitoring. An essential review of the cardiac cycle is included in order to promote understanding of cardiac dysrhythmias, including guidelines for ECG interpretation. The chapter also provides a systematic approach to understanding automaticity and conduction that can then be applied to practical situations. While the chapter profiles basic cardiac dysrhythmias of atrial, junctional, and ventricular origin, it is not intended as a comprehensive lesson on every potential dysrhythmia a nurse may encounter in the clinical setting.

Section One: Cellular Membrane Permeability

This section provides a review of membrane permeability changes in cardiac cells and the relationship between membrane permeability and serum electrolyte levels.

Resting Cardiac Cell

Electrolytes, particularly sodium and potassium (and calcium to a lesser degree), affect cardiac function. Under resting conditions, intracellular potassium (K^+) concentration is

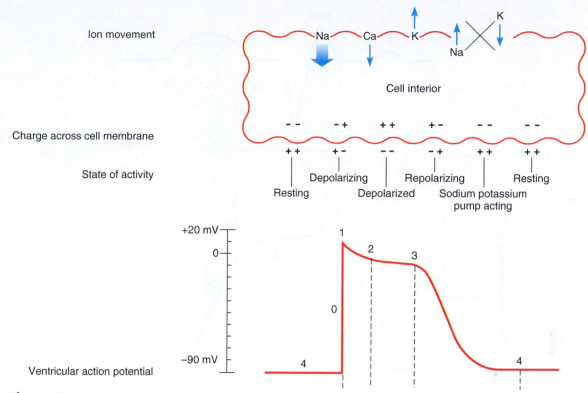

Figure 9–1 Action potential of a cardiac cell. In the resting state (phase 4), the cell membrane is polarized: the cell's interior has a negative charge compared to that of extracellular fluid. On depolarization (phase 0), sodium ions diffuse rapidly across the cell membrane into the cell, and calcium channels open. In the fully depolarized state (phase 1), the cell's interior has a net positive charge compared to its exterior. During the plateau period (phase 2), calcium moves into the cell and potassium diffusion slows, prolonging the action potential. In phase 3, calcium channels close, the sodium-potassium pump removes sodium from the cell, and the cell membrane again becomes polarized with a net negative charge.

greater inside the cell than outside, while sodium (Na^+) and calcium (Ca^{++}) concentrations are greater outside the cell. As a result, during the resting state, the inside of the cell is more electrically negative relative to the outside of the cell due to the differences in ion concentrations. This negatively charged resting state is referred to as the **polarized** state.

Active Cardiac Cell—Action Potential

When activated, the resting (polarized) cell undergoes a change in polarity that is produced by an action potential. It is caused by stimulation of cardiac cells that extends across the myocardium to produce heart contraction or relaxation.

Depolarization and Repolarization   When the cardiac cell receives an electrical stimulus, sodium and calcium shift into the cell and potassium shifts out, causing the cell to become more positively charged. This alteration in ion charge is called **depolarization**, which normally results in myocardial contraction. **Repolarization** refers to recovery of the cell to its resting state. During repolarization, K^+, Na^+, and Ca^{++} ions shift back to their original

places relative to the cell membrane, and the cardiac cell returns to a negative charge. Repolarization normally results in myocardial relaxation. Figure 9–1 illustrates the action potential of a cardiac cell.

Action Potential Phases   The **action potential** is a five-phase cycle that produces changes in the cell membrane's electrical charge (Figure 9–1): depolarization (phase 0), early repolarization (phase 1), **plateau phase** (phase 2), repolarization (phase 3), and **resting membrane potential** (phase 4).

Depolarization (Phase 0).   During depolarization, the cell is almost impermeable to sodium unless a stimulus occurs. This stimulus may be electrical in origin, such as the firing of the sinoatrial (SA) node (an internal stimulus) or emergency **defibrillation** (an external stimulus). Chemical changes may also precipitate depolarization. For example, hypoxemia, respiratory acidosis, and pharmaceutical agents (e.g., sodium bicarbonate) may serve as chemical stimuli. In depolarization, more sodium moves into the cell through the fast sodium channels and creates a fast response action potential. The inside of the cell becomes positively charged.

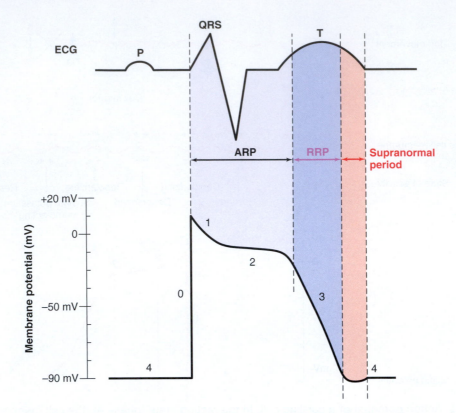

Figure 9–2 Refractory periods: Absolute, relative, and supernormal.

Repolarization (Phases 1–3). The process of repolarization takes place over phases 1, 2, and 3. In early repolarization (phase 1), sodium channels close; during the plateau phase (phase 2), calcium channels open. The calcium channels open and close slowly compared to the fast sodium channels. The influx of calcium maintains the positive charge (depolarization) a little longer. Chemical blockage of these channels (i.e., sodium and calcium channel blockers) is used to treat a variety of cardiac abnormalities. In phase 3, potassium shifts back into the cell to create the original electrochemical gradient.

Resting Membrane Potential (Phase 4). During the resting membrane potential phase, repolarization is completed, the original electrochemical gradient is in place, and the cell is ready to be depolarized again.

Refractory and Supranormal Periods During specific periods of the action potential, the cardiac cells are completely or relatively resistant to accepting a new impulse. Beginning in phase 0 and ending at the midpoint of phase 3, the cell cannot respond to another stimulus regardless of the strength of the stimulus. This is called the **absolute refractory period** because the cell absolutely cannot respond to any new electrical impulse; it is completely resistant to stimuli because the Na^+ channel is still inactivated by the previous stimulation (Figure 9–2).

Eventually (beginning at the midpoint of phase 3 and lasting until the beginning of phase 4), the cell recovers

sufficiently to allow a stronger than normal electrical stimulus to trigger depolarization. This period is called the **relative refractory period** because the cell is relatively (but not completely) unresponsive. Phase 4 represents a time in which a weaker than normal stimulus can produce depolarization. This is called the **supranormal period**. Examples of serious abnormal cardiac rhythms that can result from depolarization during the relative refractory and supranormal periods are supraventricular and ventricular tachycardia. Table 9–1 summarizes the phases of the action potential.

Table 9–1 Phases of an Action Potential

Phase 0	Depolarization	Movement of sodium into cell (fast channels open)
Phase 1	Early repolarization	Closure of fast sodium channels
Phase 2	Plateau	Calcium moves into cell (slow channels open)
Phase 3	Repolarization	Potassium moves into cell
Phase 4	Resting membrane potential	Electrochemical gradient returned to normal potential Sarcolemma (the fine transparent tubular sheath that envelops the fibers of skeletal muscles) almost impermeable to sodium

Section One Review

1. Which set of electrolytes has the greatest effect on normal cardiac function?
   A. Potassium and magnesium
   B. Potassium and calcium
   C. Sodium and calcium
   D. Sodium and potassium

2. Match the phase of the action potential with the electrical event.
   __Phase 0   **a.** Repolarization
   __Phase 1   **b.** Plateau
   __Phase 2   **c.** Depolarization
   __Phase 3   **d.** Resting membrane potential
   __Phase 4   **e.** Early repolarization

3. During the plateau phase, which channel is open?
   A. Potassium
   B. Sodium
   C. Calcium
   D. Chloride

4. During which period can a stronger than normal stimulus produce depolarization?
   A. Resting membrane potential
   B. Absolute refractory period
   C. Relative refractory period
   D. Supranormal period

Answers: 1. D, 2. Phase 0 (c. Depolarization), Phase 1 (e. Early repolarization), Phase 2 (b. Plateau), Phase 3 (a. Repolarization), Phase 4 (d. Resting membrane potential), 3. C, 4. C

Section Two: Cardiac Conduction and the Electrocardiogram

The cardiac cycle is perpetuated by an intrinsic electrical circuit in the heart. Specialized areas of myocardial cells influence this electrical pathway. While the ECG demonstrates the electrical activity of the heart, it does not demonstrate actual mechanical activity—as it is possible to have a normal ECG with compromised muscle contraction of the heart. This could be caused by such diagnoses as acute coronary syndrome, heart failure, or severe acidosis. (Examples will be discussed later in this chapter.) A thorough understanding of the electrical conduction system remains an essential component of learning and understanding ECG interpretation.

Electrical Conduction of the Heart

Certain cardiac cells have a unique characteristic called **automaticity**, which is the ability to spontaneously depolarize (i.e., they can create a repetitive impulse without requiring external stimulation). Such cells are known as **pacemaker cells**. Physiologically, they differ from regular cardiac cells in that they have a constant sodium influx; thus, they slowly depolarize at a steady rate until the threshold is reached and an action potential created. Furthermore, through the characteristic of **conductivity**, the ability of a system to transmit energy, impulses generated by pacemaker cells are then transmitted to the surrounding myocardium.

There are three potential pacemakers of the heart: a primary pacemaker in addition to two other backup or lower-rate pacemakers. Essentially, this hierarchy of potential pacemakers provides a three-level system should one or two of the pacemakers ever fail. The three potential pacemakers include the following:

- Sinus (or SA) node, which generates an impulse at 60 to 100 beats per minute (bpm) and is located in the upper right atrium near where the superior vena cava comes into the heart.

- Atrioventricular (AV) junction, which generates an impulse at 40 to 60 bpm and is located in the base of the right atrium near the tricuspid valve. The AV node is available if the SA node pacemaker fails.

- Ventricular Purkinje fibers, which generate an impulse at 20 to 40 bpm and are located in the ventricular walls as a network. These fibers are available if the SA node and AV junction pacemakers fail.

The primary pacemaker of the heart is the SA node because its impulse generation is normally the fastest.

The Normal Conduction Pathway   The impulses are transmitted from the atria to the ventricles along a cardiac conduction pathway (Figure 9–3).

Normally, the impulse originates in the SA node and travels through special conductive (internodal) pathways to the AV node. The impulse is delayed at the AV node for about 0.1 second to allow the atria to depolarize and contract. The impulse then continues down the conduction pathway to the bundle of His. From the bundle of His, the impulse rapidly travels through the right and left bundle branches located in the septum and into a network of special conductive fibers called **Purkinje fibers**, which carry electrical impulses directly to ventricular muscle cells.

The Electrocardiogram

The **electrocardiogram (ECG)** is a graphic representation of the electrical, not mechanical, activity of the heart. The ECG has a relatively predictable pattern composed of positive and negative deflections (waves) that deviate from a flat base line. This is known as the *isoelectric* line. Deflections that rise above the isoelectric line are positive waves, and

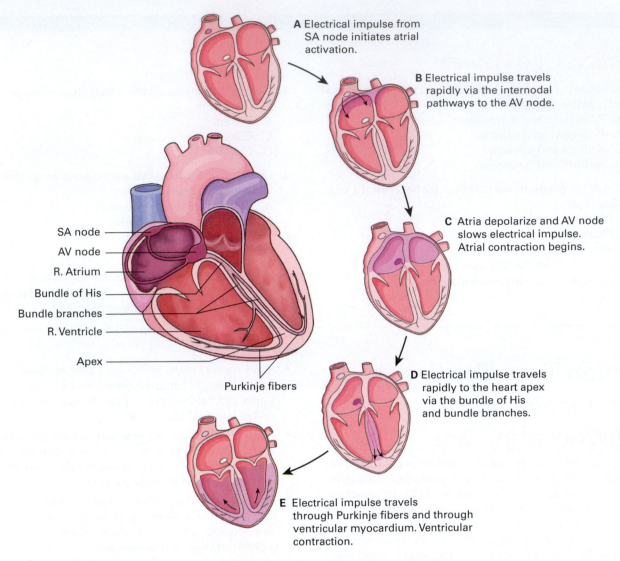

A Electrical impulse from SA node initiates atrial activation.

B Electrical impulse travels rapidly via the internodal pathways to the AV node.

C Atria depolarize and AV node slows electrical impulse. Atrial contraction begins.

SA node
AV node
R. Atrium
Bundle of His
Bundle branches
R. Ventricle
Apex
Purkinje fibers

D Electrical impulse travels rapidly to the heart apex via the bundle of His and bundle branches.

E Electrical impulse travels through Purkinje fibers and through ventricular myocardium. Ventricular contraction.

Figure 9–3 Electrical conduction system in the heart.

those that fall below the line are negative. The isoelectric line represents the absence of electrical activity and is an important reference point for measuring the various waves of the ECG complex.

The Normal ECG Pattern   The normal ECG pattern consists of multiple components, including the *P* wave and *PR* interval; *QRS* complex; *ST* segment; and *QT* interval (Figure 9–4).

The exact appearance of the various ECG pattern components changes based on which specific view (the lead) is being used. A 12-lead ECG provides 12 different views of the electrical output of the heart, and each view represents a different portion of the heart (e.g., anterior wall vs. inferior wall). Therefore, each ECG lead will have its own unique morphology. The techniques for assessing a cardiac rhythm strip are the same for each lead and are presented in this section. The 12-lead ECG is primarily used for diagnostic purposes and requires additional training for accuracy in interpretation. Generally, the high-acuity nurse continuously monitors one or two leads on a cardiac or hemodynamic monitoring system, which allows the nurse

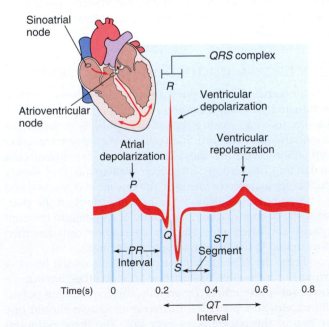

Figure 9–4 Normal ECG waveform and intervals.

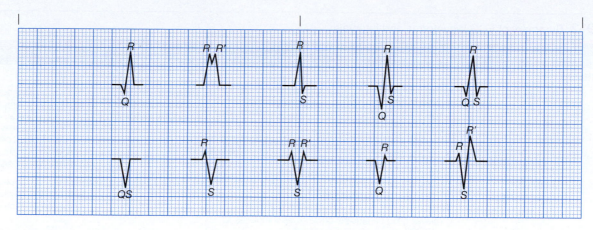

Figure 9–5 Examples of *QRS* complex variations.

to quickly gain expertise in differentiating normal from abnormal rhythms.

P Wave and PR Interval. The *P* wave indicates atrial depolarization, stimulated by the firing of the SA node. The *PR* interval depicts conduction of the impulse from the SA node through the internodal pathway to the AV node and downward to the ventricles.

QRS Complex. The *QRS* complex reflects ventricular depolarization. Atrial repolarization is also occurring during this period; however, it is hidden by the *QRS* complex because ventricular depolarization has greater amplitude than atrial depolarization. The normal *QRS* complex is spiked in appearance, and its shape varies between individuals and may consist of one to three waves (Figure 9–5).

The waves that comprise the complex are as follows:

- **Q wave**—A negative deflection that precedes a positive deflection. It begins at the end of the *PR* interval. There can be only one with each *QRS* complex; however, it may not be present.

- **R wave**—One or more positive deflections. If there is more than one, they are labeled as *R* and *R′* (R prime).

- **S wave**—A negative deflection that follows the *R* wave. If there is no *R* wave in the complex, it is labeled as a *QS* wave.

ST Segment and T Wave. The *ST* segment is a line that begins directly after the *QRS* complex and ends at the beginning of the *T* wave (Figure 9–4). It is normally located at the isoelectric line. The *ST* segment represents the completion of ventricular depolarization and the beginning of ventricular repolarization.

The *T* wave directly follows the *ST* segment and appears as a rounded, slightly asymmetrical, positive deflection when the *QRS* complex is positive. It represents repolarization of the ventricles. The *T* wave is often referred to as the resting phase of the cardiac cycle. The upstroke of the *T* wave occurs during the absolute refractory period; however, the downstroke represents a relative refractory period, during which time a sufficiently strong electrical stimulus can trigger depolarization. The heart is vulnerable

during the relative refractory period. An abnormal impulse (dysrhythmia) of sufficient electrical strength that triggers prematurely, on the downstroke of the *T* wave, can result in development of a potentially life-threatening dysrhythmia (e.g., ventricular tachycardia or ventricular fibrillation)—sometimes called the **R on T phenomenon**.

A variety of factors can alter the appearance of the *T* wave and *ST* segment because of altered ventricular repolarization. For example, the *T* wave becomes flattened or inverted in the presence of myocardial ischemia. Specific electrolyte abnormalities also alter the *T* wave appearance. For example, a patient with elevated serum potassium level (hyperkalemia) develops a tall, peaked *T* wave. The *ST* segment can become depressed with myocardial ischemia and elevated with myocardial injury.

QT Interval. The *QT* interval represents ventricular depolarization and repolarization. It is measured from the beginning of the *QRS* complex to the end of the *T* wave.

Table 9–2 summarizes the ECG waveforms and intervals.

Cardiac Monitoring Systems

Cardiac monitoring is used whenever a patient's heart rate and rhythm must be continuously monitored. Although there are many types of monitoring systems, all systems use four basic components: an oscilloscope display system (ECG machine or cardiac monitor), a monitor cable, lead wires, and electrodes (Figure 9–6). Electrical impulses sent out from the heart are detectable on the skin throughout the body. **Electrodes**, which are small adhesive patches with conducting gel placed on the skin, pick up (sense) the electrical impulses and send them through attached lead wires to a cable on the ECG machine or cardiac monitor, where the ECG rhythm can be viewed or printed out on special paper. The ends of the lead wires are typically color coded (white, black, brown, green, and red) in order to help identify each lead for correct placement.

All cardiac monitors use lead cable systems to record cardiac electrical activity. Leads are electrographic pictures of the various surfaces of the heart (i.e., anterior, lateral, or other walls of the heart). Lead II tends to be the favored

Table 9–2 Summary of ECG Waveforms and Intervals

	Description	Evaluation	Normal Parameters	Significance
WAVEFORMS				
P wave	Atrial depolarization	Appearance: Do all P waves look alike? Relationship to QRS complex: Does one P wave precede every QRS complex?	All P waves look alike. One P wave precedes every QRS complex.	If not identical, all or some may be of atrial or junctional, not SA node, origin. If more than one P wave precedes a QRS complex, a conduction problem (heart block) may be present.
QRS complex	Ventricular depolarization	Measure: From beginning of Q wave to end of S wave, where it returns to baseline. Appearance: Varies with individual—not all three waves need be present; however, all complexes should look alike in the same lead.	Less than 0.12 sec	Widening QRS complex suggests bundle branch block or other conduction delay.
INTERVALS				
R–R Interval	Represents rate of ventricular depolarization (therefore heart rate)	Regularity: Distance from one R wave to next R wave—is distance regular or irregular?		If R–R interval is constant, it is a *regular* rhythm. If R–R intervals vary, it is an *irregular* rhythm.
PR interval	Impulse travel time from the atrium to the ventricles	Measure: From beginning of P wave to beginning of QRS complex. Regularity: Is interval the same from one to the next?	0.12–0.20 sec	If greater than 0.20 sec, a conduction delay, called an AV heart block, is present.
QT interval	Length of time it takes the ventricles to depolarize *and* repolarize	Measure: From beginning of Q wave to end of T wave. Length: Varies with heart rate (HR). At HR of 60 to 100 bpm, length should be less than 1/2 of HR.	Less than half of the R–R interval	Length greater than 0.50 sec is considered dangerously prolonged.

lead among clinicians—as all of the waveforms are generally upright and more easily distinguishable and measurable. However, it is important to note that lead II does not look at the whole picture of the heart's electrical conduction system, and ECG changes could be missed if other leads are never evaluated. A basic lead system is composed of three electrodes: one positive, one negative, and one ground. Each lead system looks at cardiac depolarization from a different location, producing P waves, QRS complexes, and T waves of varying configurations. Although a

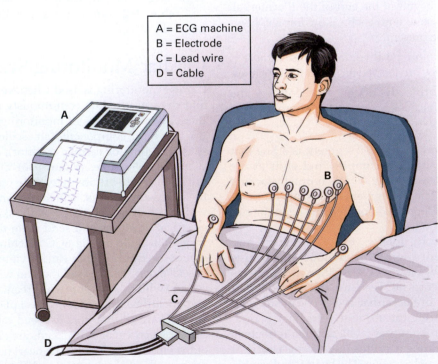

A = ECG machine
B = Electrode
C = Lead wire
D = Cable

Figure 9–6 Components of ECG monitoring system.

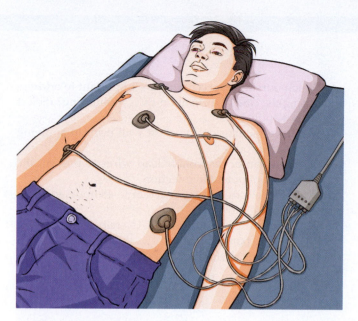

Figure 9–7 Placement of electrodes.

minimum of three electrodes is required, often five electrodes are used, either to monitor two leads simultaneously or to allow selection of different leads. The lead wires are either attached directly to a bedside monitor or to a remote receiver (telemetry). The ECG can also be sent to a central terminal in the high-acuity unit where the rhythms are observed. Some units have designated telemetry technicians who monitor patients' ECG rhythms continuously and can notify the nurse should any changes occur. Regardless of the type of system used, proper lead placement is essential for accurate cardiac monitoring, and lead placement is verified by the nurse at the beginning of each shift. Figure 9–7 shows placement of a five-electrode lead system.

Nursing Care of a Patient Who Requires Cardiac Monitoring

Several routine nursing actions are required when caring for a patient requiring continuous cardiac monitoring.

Electrode Management   To prevent the potential transmission of infection from one patient to another, appropriately cleaned or disposable lead wires should be applied to each new patient. The patient's skin must be prepared before attaching the ECG electrodes. Electrode site preparation includes clipping excessive hair and cleansing the skin with soap and water or with alcohol. This will help ensure optimal skin contact. Sites may be rotated on a routine basis to prevent skin irritation or breakdown. It is important to clean gel residue from previous sites and document skin condition under the pads.

Monitor Alarms   While alarms are a critical component to the safety of patients, it is important to review and adjust alarm settings to specific patient condition and diagnosis. With more than 90% of clinical alarms being false, reducing alarm fatigue and improving patient safety surrounding alarms has become a priority for The Joint Commission and healthcare organizations. Excessive alarms in the clinical setting result in desensitization, ignoring alarms, and silencing them before fully evaluating, which in turn can lead to serious patient harm. "Nuisance" alarms should be addressed promptly by individualizing alarms to decrease the burden of alarm fatigue. The alarms are left on and audible to the interdisciplinary team at all times unless the patient's condition indicates otherwise.

ECG Strip Analysis   An ECG rhythm strip is recorded and placed in the patient record on a regular basis per unit protocol, when the cardiac rhythm changes, or with any change in patient condition. Each strip is analyzed using a systematic process such as outlined in Section Three.

Patient Electrical Safety   Ensuring patient safety during ECG monitoring is imperative. Frayed wires and/or electrical outlet damage can cause electricity to go directly to the patient. Always check for frayed wires or components before performing ECG monitoring.

Patient and Family Education   Patients need to know why they require ECG monitoring. They need reassurance that they are protected from electric shocks from the equipment. Patients and families should also be informed that the alarms can sound as a result of patient movement and other factors, in addition to cardiac abnormalities.

Emerging Evidence

- To reduce the number of false ECG alarms in a 16-bed adult medical cardiovascular care unit, a quality improvement bundle project consisted of adjusting default settings, changing ECG electrodes daily, standardizing skin preparation, and using disposable leads. The mean number of alarm signals per day was reduced from 28.5 to 3.28, an 88.5% reduction (Sendelbach, Wahl, Anthony, & Shotts, 2015).
- Atrial fibrillation is quite common in the critically ill and accounts for up to 60% of dysrhythmias. In a retrospective 2-year cohort study conducted by *Gupta, Tiruvoipati, and Green (2015)*, 412 patients with atrial fibrillation were compared with patients who did not have atrial fibrillation for mortality, their duration of mechanical ventilation, and their length of stay while hospitalized. While atrial fibrillation was not independently associated with a higher risk for death, patients with atrial fibrillation were noted to have higher mortality rates, prolonged mechanical ventilation, and longer lengths of stay. *(Gupta, Tiruvoipati, & Green, 2015).*

- With advances in technology and the desire for less invasive diagnostics, the research and development of portable wireless ECG monitoring systems has been increasing. In preliminary uses and trials, these systems have been shown to produce high-resolution, real-time, excellent quality tracings and an improved patient satisfaction related to having to wear less hardware (Prats-Boluda et al., 2015; Wang, Doleschel, Wunderlich, & Heinen, 2014).
- While rare (but significant), patients with mesial temporal lobe epilepsy are at risk for sudden unexpected death. The pathophysiology is unclear. Typically, during a seizure, these patients experience tachycardia. However, there are those who also develop bradycardia and even asystole. The benefit of incorporating continuous ECG monitoring with these patients may help to quickly identify potentially lethal dysrhythmias so that lifesaving interventions can be implemented (Dawson, Gupta, Madden, Pacheco, & Olson, 2015).

Section Two Review

1. What information about a *PR* interval greater than 0.20 second is correct?
   A. It is normal.
   B. It indicates a pacemaker other than the SA node is firing.
   C. It indicates a delay in conduction.
   D. It is too fast to maintain adequate cardiac output.

2. Ventricular depolarization is reflected in which component?
   A. *P* wave
   B. *PR* interval
   C. *T* wave
   D. *QRS* complex

3. What component wave of the ECG may show changes associated with the presence of cardiac ischemia?
   A. *P* wave
   B. *PR* interval
   C. *QRS* complex
   D. *T* wave

4. Which nursing interventions are important to address during the care of a client on ECG monitoring? (Select all that apply.)
   A. Shave the hair on the chest wall prior to applying the electrodes.
   B. Use clean or disposable lead wires to prevent the spread of potential infection.
   C. Rotate electrode sites every 24 to 48 hours to avoid skin breakdown.
   D. Record and analyze an ECG strip if the cardiac rhythm changes.
   E. Set alarms to standard parameters.

Answers: 1. C, 2. D, 3. D, 4. (B, C, D)

Section Three: Basic Interpretation Guidelines

Learning the normal ECG waves and intervals and a systematic way to interpret an ECG rhythm strip is an important first step in being able to monitor high-acuity patients and accurately interpret abnormal patterns. This section focuses on normal waves and intervals while Sections Five through Nine focus on abnormal rhythm patterns.

ECG Graph Paper

The ECG is printed on graph paper with small and large blocks. The horizontal axis of the graph paper represents time, and the vertical axis represents voltage. Therefore, on the horizontal axis each small block of the graph paper is equal to 1 mm, or 0.04 sec, and each small block on the vertical axis is equivalent to 1 mm, or 0.1 mV. Vertically, each large box is 5 mm (0.5 mV). For the purposes of basic ECG interpretation, time is the most important factor to consider; and for this reason, voltage will not be discussed further. Horizontally, because each small block equals 0.04 sec, a large block, composed of five small blocks, equals 0.20 sec; and five large blocks represent 1 second (Figure 9–8).

Eight Steps of ECG Interpretation

Following are the eight steps to follow when interpreting an ECG:

1. Measure the heart rate.
2. Examine the *R–R* interval.

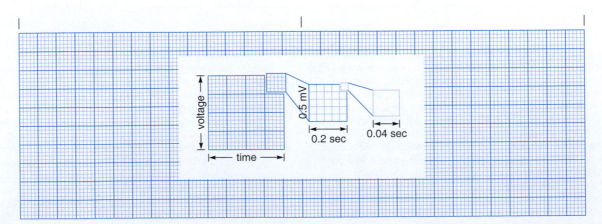

Figure 9–8 ECG paper is a graph divided into millimeter-size squares. Time is measured on the horizontal axis. With a paper speed of 25 mm/sec, each small (1-mm) box equals 0.04 seconds, and each larger (5-mm) box equals 0.2 seconds. The amplitude of any wave is measured on the vertical axis in millimeters.

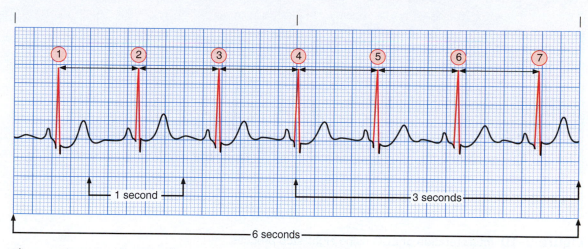

Figure 9–9 Calculation of heart rate.

3. Examine the *P* wave.
4. Measure the *PR* interval.
5. Determine if each *P* wave is followed by a *QRS* complex.
6. Examine and measure the *QRS* complex.
7. Examine and measure the *QT* interval.
8. Diagnose the rhythm.

Once the rhythm is diagnosed, the nurse needs to determine the rhythm's clinical significance and initiate any appropriate follow-up actions.

Measure the Heart Rate   Two methods are commonly used to determine heart rate by visual examination of an ECG strip: block counting and 6-second strip methods. There are two ways to measure rate using the block (box) counting method. To use the first method, divide 300 by the number of 0.20-sec boxes between two *R* waves. To use the second method, divide 1500 by the number of 0.04-sec blocks between two *R* waves. During this process, it is helpful to remember that 300 large boxes or 1500 small boxes represent 60 sec in time. The block counting method has certain advantages over the 6-sec rhythm strip method. It can determine an accurate heart rate when the rate is regular; it can be used to determine the rate of the underlying rhythm when frequent ectopic beats are present; and when an irregular rhythm is present, it can be used to determine the slowest and fastest rates. Its primary disadvantage is that it takes additional time to count the blocks and then calculate.

The second method of measuring heart rate is based on a 6-sec rhythm strip. This method can be used with either a regular or irregular rhythm. ECG paper is marked at the top or bottom margin in 3-second intervals (called hash marks). *QRS* complexes in a 6-sec strip (30 large blocks) are multiplied by 10 to obtain the heart rate per minute (6 × 10 = 60 sec). The primary advantage of this method is that the heart rate can rapidly be estimated; the major disadvantages are that it is less accurate and provides less information about the beat-to-beat rhythm pattern within the 6-sec strip than would be obtained using

the block-counting method. Figure 9–9 demonstrates this method of rate calculation.

Examine the R–R Intervals   The regularity of the *R* waves is examined. If the *R* waves appear in regular intervals (are constant), the rhythm is a regular rhythm. If the *R* waves do not occur at constant intervals, it is an irregular rhythm. The closer the *R* waves are to each other, the faster the heart rate; the farther apart the *R* waves are, the slower the heart rate.

Examine the P Waves   The *P* wave is a smooth, rounded, upward deflection. Under normal circumstances, when the SA node is serving as the primary pacemaker, all *P* waves will look the same. However, if another cardiac cell is acting as the primary pacemaker in place of the SA node (e.g., premature atrial contractions or junctional rhythm), the *P* waves will have an altered shape or can be absent.

Measure the PR Interval   Measure the *PR* interval, which reflects the amount of time it takes an impulse to travel from the atria to the ventricles. The interval is measured from the beginning of the *P* wave to the beginning of the *QRS* complex. The normal *PR* interval is 0.12 to 0.20 sec. A longer *PR* interval (greater than 0.20 sec) suggests a conduction delay, usually in the area of the AV node (e.g., first-degree AV block).

P Waves Precede Each QRS   Determine if each *P* wave is followed by a *QRS* complex. Normally, there should be a stable one-to-one relationship between the two waves. If *P* waves are present but are not followed consistently by a *QRS* complex, a second- or third-degree heart block (Section Nine) is present.

Examine and Measure the QRS Complex   Examination of the *QRS* complexes begins with identifying the complex components. The normal *QRS* complex is less than 0.12 sec (usually between 0.6 and 0.10 sec). Recall that the actual configuration of the *QRS* complex varies with the individual (Figure 9–5); however, regardless of its configuration, all *QRS* complexes should look identical for that individual.

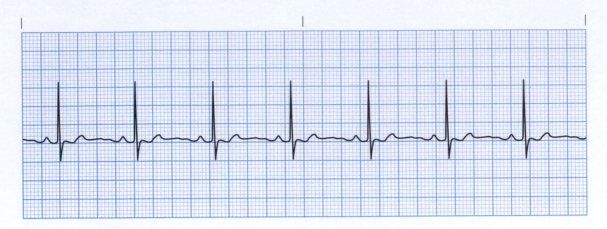

Figure 9–10 Interpretation of ECG using eight-step process.

1. **Measure the rate.** There are 7 complexes in 6 seconds: $7 \times 10 =$ Heart rate of 70. **Or** R–R interval = 21 small boxes. Divide 1500 by the number of small boxes in a minute. $1500 \div 21 = 71$ bpm.
2. **Examine the R–R interval.** The interval is regular; therefore, the rhythm is regular.
3. **Examine the P wave.** The P waves are the same configuration.
4. **Measure the PR interval.** The interval is constant and measures 4 small boxes (0.4) or 0.16 seconds.
5. **Check to see whether the P waves are followed by a QRS complex.** P waves are followed by QRS complex.
6. **Examine and measure the QRS complex.** The complexes are the same configuration and measure 2 small boxes (0.04) or 0.08 seconds.
7. **Measure the QT interval.** The interval measures at 8 small boxes or 0.32 seconds.
8. **Diagnose the rhythm.** Normal sinus rhythm.

An abnormally wide *QRS* complex suggests delayed conduction through the bundle branches (known as a bundle branch block or intraventricular conduction delay), abnormal conduction within the ventricles, or early activation of the ventricles through a bypass route.

Measure the QT Interval   Recall that the *QT* interval is measured from the beginning of the *Q* wave to the end of the *T* wave. It normally is less than half the *R–R* interval (the distance between two *R* waves in two consecutive *QRS* complexes). The interval is usually less than 0.40 sec in length, depending on the heart rate. As heart rate increases, the *QT* interval shortens; and as heart rate decreases, the *QT* interval lengthens. For higher risk patients (as described below), the *QT* interval should be corrected for heart rate (*QTc*) by using the formula:

$$QTc = QT / \text{square root of the } R - R \text{ interval}$$

A *QTc* greater than 0.50 sec is considered to be dangerously prolonged because it increases the risk of dysrhythmias caused by the *R* on *T* phenomenon.

Monitoring the *QT* interval is becoming standard practice in many high-acuity environments. Particular attention to it should be given to patients with low serum potassium or magnesium levels, those with a new onset of bradycardia, or those who overdose on prodysrhythmic drugs or are taking medications known to prolong *QT* intervals (such as haloperidol, quinidine, or procainamide).

Diagnose the Rhythm   Various rhythms and/or ectopic heartbeats may be present in high-acuity patients. These rhythms are discussed in greater detail in Sections Five through Nine. Some rhythms have deleterious hemodynamic consequences while others are benign. Knowledge of basic ECG rhythm interpretation allows the nurse to quickly identify any potential life-threatening cardiac conduction abnormalities and take appropriate action.

Figure 9–10 illustrates the application of the principles discussed in this section. This should provide a consistent and comprehensive approach to ECG interpretation. If the heart rate is 60–100 bpm, *R–R* intervals are regular, *P* waves look alike, *PR* interval is 0.12–0.20 sec, every *P* wave is followed by a *QRS* complex, *QRS* complex is less than 0.12 sec, and *QT* interval is less than half the *R–R* interval, then the rhythm is interpreted as normal sinus rhythm.

Clinical Significance

Nurses working in high-acuity areas receive special training in interpreting cardiac rhythm strips; however, correct interpretation of a cardiac rhythm alone is not sufficient to protect the patient. The nurse must also understand the clinical significance of any abnormal rhythm. When a dysrhythmia is diagnosed, the nurse must know whether it requires follow-up interventions and their order of priorities and the degree of urgency, because time may be a critical factor with potentially life-threatening dysrhythmias.

ECG Interpretation Exercise 1: Basic Strip Interpretation

1. Identify the *P* wave, *QRS* complex, and *T* wave in the ECG strip.

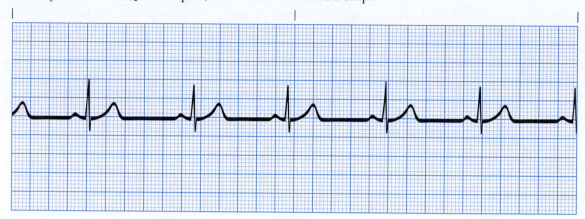

2. Measure the *PR* interval, *QRS* complex and *QT* interval in the ECG strip.

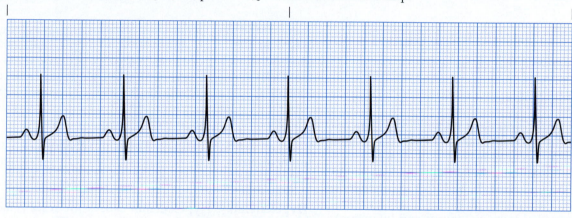

PR interval: _____   *QRS* complex: _____   *QT* interval: _____

3. Measure the *PR* interval, *QRS* complex, and *QT* interval in the ECG strip.

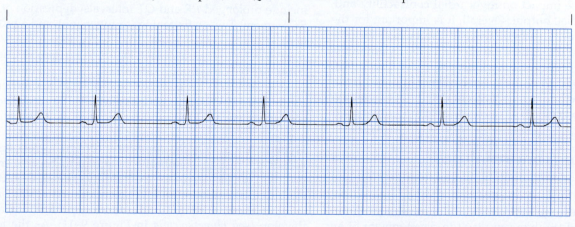

PR interval: _____   *QRS* complex: _____   *QT* interval: _____

4. Calculate the heart rate using the small block (0.04 second) calculation method strip in item 3 of this exercise.

Heart rate: _____ bpm

Section Three Review

1. The cardiac rhythm strip reveals 5 large blocks between *R* waves. What is the client's heart rate?
   A. 45 bpm
   B. 60 bpm
   C. 90 bpm
   D. 110 bpm

2. The *R–R* interval on a client's cardiac rhythm strip is constant. What does the nurse know about the client's heart rate and rhythm?
   A. The rate is slow.
   B. The rate is rapid.
   C. The rhythm is irregular.
   D. The rhythm is regular.

3. The *PR* interval is the time between the:
   A. beginning of the *P* wave and the beginning of the *QRS* complex.
   B. beginning of the *P* wave and the end of the *T* wave.
   C. end of the *P* wave and end of the *QRS* complex.
   D. end of the *R* wave and end of the *P* wave.

4. A client's *QRS* complex measures 0.16 second. This interval is:
   A. normal
   B. short
   C. long
   D. half the length of the *PR* interval

Answers: 1. B, 2. D, 3. A, 4. C

Section Four: Risk Factors for Development of Dysrhythmias

Dysrhythmias are abnormal heart rhythms, and there are many possible causes. Dysrhythmias are not necessarily pathologic, and they occur in healthy as well as diseased hearts. Frequent causes of dysrhythmias in the high-acuity patient include degenerative changes in the conduction system, fluid and electrolyte imbalances, acute coronary syndromes (myocardial ischemia, injury, and infarction), heart failure, and the effects of drug ingestion.

The major complication associated with dysrhythmias is their negative impact on myocardial contractility and, ultimately, cardiac output. Overall, it is important for the nurse to recognize dysrhythmias early and assess for possible causes and the patient's response to the dysrhythmia (e.g., change in level of consciousness, chest discomfort, changes in blood pressure). Timely reporting and treatment of dysrhythmias may prevent deleterious hemodynamic consequences.

Electrolyte Abnormalities

Recall from Section One that the cardiac cell action potential requires shifts of electrolytes, notably potassium, sodium, and calcium. Moreover, development of an abnormality in one electrolyte can result in development of an abnormality in other electrolytes. For this reason, if a person develops an electrolyte abnormality, it may result in an alteration in the cardiac impulse production or conduction. High-acuity patients frequently develop electrolyte abnormalities related to their disease processes or therapies. This increases their risk of developing cardiac dysrhythmias. It is important for the high-acuity nurse to be familiar with the critical or panic values of the various electrolytes. Extreme values are often referred to as critical or panic

values. Mild to moderate electrolyte abnormalities are generally benign, requiring relatively simple replacement therapy. However, extremes in serum electrolyte levels are not well tolerated by the body (particularly the heart) and can precipitate potentially life-threatening events. Hospital laboratory departments provide institution-level normal and abnormal ranges as well as the critical values.

Potassium Abnormalities   Potassium abnormalities are a particular risk factor for development of dysrhythmias, especially in extreme ranges.

Hypokalemia.   Hypokalemia causes the resting membrane potential to become more negative. This means that it takes a greater stimulus to reach threshold for excitation and open the sodium channels. ECG pattern changes include prolonged *PR* and *QT* intervals, depression of the *ST* segment, *T* wave flattening (or inversion), and a prominent *U* wave, which is an extra wave that follows the *T* wave (refer to *Hypokalemia* in Figure 9–11) (Jang & Cheng, 2014). Bradydysrhythmias (abnormally slow rhythms) and conduction blocks are common, and premature ventricular contractions (PVCs) can occur as a result. The critical value for hypokalemia is less than 2.5 mEq/L (Kee, 2014).

Hyperkalemia.   On the opposite spectrum, hyperkalemia causes the resting membrane potential to become more positive, which decreases excitability. The ECG pattern evolves as the potassium level increases. At a potassium level of about 6 mEq/L, tall, narrow, peaked *T* waves develop (see *Hyperkalemia* in Figure 9–11). As the level increases, the *PR* interval becomes prolonged and the *P* wave may disappear (Jang & Cheng, 2014). At a potassium level of 8 mEq/L or higher, the peaked *T* waves disappear and *QRS* complex widens (see Severe hyperkalemia in Figure 9–11), which is considered an ominous sign of impending cardiac arrest (Jang & Cheng, 2014). Eventually the cell becomes too positive to respond and depolarize, and **asystole** (no heartbeat) occurs. The critical value of hyperkalemia is greater than 7.0 mEq/L (Kee, 2014).

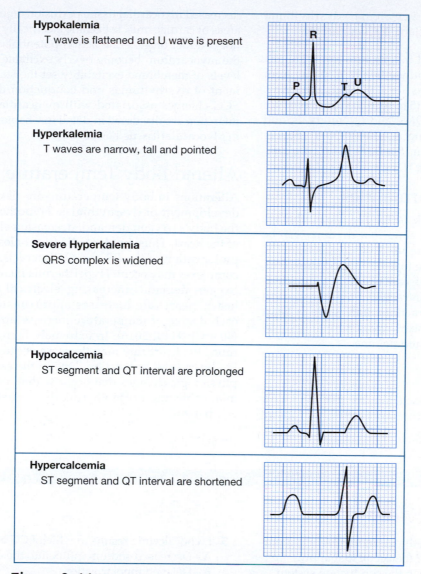

Hypokalemia
T wave is flattened and U wave is present

Hyperkalemia
T waves are narrow, tall and pointed

Severe Hyperkalemia
QRS complex is widened

Hypocalcemia
ST segment and QT interval are prolonged

Hypercalcemia
ST segment and QT interval are shortened

Figure 9–11 Effects of potassium and calcium disturbances on ECG pattern.

Calcium Abnormalities Calcium is important in nerve impulse transmission and skeletal and myocardial muscle contractions.

Hypocalcemia. A low calcium level is a common abnormality in high-acuity patients, often resulting from multiple factors such as chronic kidney failure, hypoparathyroidism, severe vitamin D deficiency, sepsis, or other electrolyte abnormalities (e.g., hypomagnesemia and hyperphosphatemia), or it can be drug induced (Jang & Cheng, 2014). Hypocalcemia may prolong the *QT* interval (see *Hypocalcemia* in Figure 9–11), decreases myocardial function, and increases the risk for development of abnormal rhythms resulting from increased cardiac cell excitability (Kee, 2014).

Hypercalcemia. Hypercalcemia is rarely seen in high-acuity patients and is primarily found in patients with hyperparathyroidism or malignancies (Jang & Cheng, 2014). The cardiac effects of hypercalcemia include strengthened contractility and shortened ventricular

repolarization, which shortens the *QT* interval; it can also cause atrioventricular heart blocks in severe hypercalcemia (Jang & Cheng, 2014).

Magnesium Abnormalities Magnesium is primarily located in bone and within cells with very little normally being found in the serum. It plays an important role in neuromuscular function.

Hypomagnesemia. Decreased levels of magnesium most commonly result from gastrointestinal losses (e.g., diarrhea) or renal losses (e.g., non–potassium-sparing diuretics). It is often seen in the presence of hypokalemia and hypocalcemia; therefore, if either of these abnormalities exists, a magnesium level should be obtained. Furthermore, it enhances digitalis toxicity in patients who are receiving diuretics, just as hypokalemia does. Hypomagnesemia increases the irritability of the nervous system and can produce dysrhythmias. Prolongation of the *PR* and *QT* intervals and widening of the *QRS* complex can be seen in hypomagnesemia and in severe cases can trigger a potentially life-threatening ventricular dysrhythmia known as torsades de pointes (Jang & Cheng, 2014).

Hypermagnesemia. Elevated magnesium levels are primarily seen in patients with kidney failure resulting from the inability to excrete excess ions through the urine. Increased levels of magnesium (5 to 10 mEq/L) can produce bradycardia; prolonged *PR*, *QRS*, and *QT* intervals; and widened *QRS* complexes (Jang & Cheng, 2014). Severe hypermagnesemia (greater than 15 mEq/L) can cause complete AV heart block or asystole (Jang & Cheng, 2014).

Fluid Volume Abnormalities

Fluid volume status is a risk factor for dysrhythmias. Tachydysrhythmias, or rapid abnormal rhythms, can be noted in patients with a severe fluid volume deficit. The heart rate increases in response to a diminished stroke volume. Fluid volume overload can result in ventricular enlargement and decreased contractility. In patients with a diminished myocardial contractility state such as heart failure, premature beats and heart rate abnormalities may appear in response to excess fluid volume.

Hypoxemia

Hypoxemia and myocardial ischemia are risk factors for the development of dysrhythmias. During periods of decreased myocardial tissue perfusion, injured or infarcted areas of cardiac muscle become electrically inactive and do not conduct or generate action potentials. Other areas of the myocardium become overly excitable. These varying levels of membrane excitability set the stage for development of dysrhythmias and conduction defects. Specific ECG changes associated with myocardial ischemia and infarction are discussed in detail in Chapter 15: Alterations in Myocardial Tissue Perfusion.

Altered Body Temperature

Alterations in body temperature are risk factors for the development of dysrhythmias. Hypothermia decreases the body's oxygen demand, decreasing electrical activity of the heart. Thus, **bradycardia** (rate of less than 60 bpm), prolongation of the *PR* and *QT* intervals, and wide *QRS* complexes may occur. Hyperthermia increases the body's oxygen demand, increasing electrical activity of the heart. Heart rate increases approximately 10 bpm for each degree of temperature increase up to about 105°F (40.5°C) (Hall, 2016). In extremely high body temperatures, the heart rate may decrease because of deteriorating heart muscle function. Due to the cardiac and other physiologic changes that occur with hyper- or hypothermia, achieving normothermia is a nursing priority for any patient.

Section Four Review

1. Frequent causes of dysrhythmias in high-acuity clients include which conditions? (Select all that apply.)
   A. Degenerative changes in the conduction system
   B. Fluid and electrolyte imbalances
   C. Neuromuscular illnesses
   D. Drug ingestion
   E. Myocardial ischemia

2. Hypokalemia results in which ECG abnormality?
   A. Delayed conduction
   B. Increased automaticity
   C. Tall, peaked *T* waves
   D. Inverted *P* waves

3. Hypocalcemia results in which ECG abnormality?
   A. Decreased sodium influx into the cell
   B. Delayed repolarization
   C. Prolonged *QT* interval
   D. Spontaneous conduction

4. Injured and infarcted areas of myocardium have what effect on action potentials and electrical activity? (Select all that apply.)
   A. Do not generate action potentials
   B. Do not conduct action potentials
   C. Do not interfere with the conduction of action potentials
   D. Are electrically inactive
   E. Are overactive electrically

Answers: 1. (A, B, D, E), 2. A, 3. C, 4 (A, B, D)

Section Five: Sinus Dysrhythmias

Sinus dysrhythmias are abnormal electrical impulse patterns that originate at the SA node and include sinus bradycardia and sinus tachycardia.

Sinus Bradycardia

Sinus bradycardia is defined as a heart rate less than 60 bpm. It originates from the SA node, as evidenced by a regular *P* wave preceding each *QRS* complex. The only abnormality noted in this rhythm is the rate. Sinus bradycardia can be present in athletes because they have strong

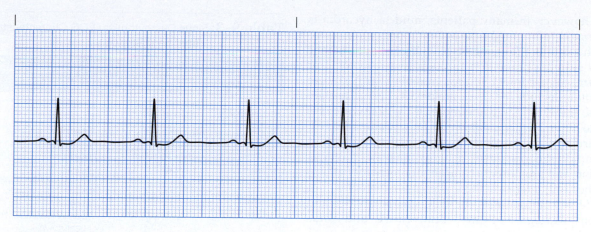

Figure 9–12 Sinus bradycardia.

1. Rate: 60
2. *R–R* interval: regular
3. *P* wave: regular, upright, matching
4. *PR* interval: 0.18

5. *P* wave precedes *QRS*: yes
6. *QRS* complex: 0.08
7. *QT* interval: 0.40

cardiac muscle contractions; therefore, a slower heart rate can still maintain an efficient cardiac output (CO). Sinus bradycardia commonly results from stimulation of the parasympathetic nervous system or as a side effect of some cardiovascular drugs, such as digitalis, beta adrenergic agonists, and calcium blocking agents.

Sinus bradycardia is not treated unless the person experiences symptoms of decreased CO such as syncope, hypotension, or angina. If the rate drops too low, the risk of ectopic (abnormal) pacemakers firing increases, and lethal ventricular dysrhythmias can result. Symptomatic sinus bradycardia is treated by administering atropine because it blocks the parasympathetic innervation to the SA node, allowing normal sympathetic innervation to gain control and increase SA node firing. A pacemaker may be required if the bradycardia is prolonged and the patient remains symptomatic. Sinus bradycardia is illustrated in Figure 9–12.

Sinus **tachycardia** is an abnormally rapid heart rate that ranges from 100 to 150 bpm and originates in the SA node. There are no other abnormal characteristics associated with this rhythm (Figure 9–13). The rapid rate results from sympathetic nervous system stimulation that can be in response to fear, increased physical activity, hypermetabolic states (such as fever), or pain. It can also be a compensatory response if the patient is experiencing decreased cardiac output as seen, for example, with hypovolemia or heart failure. Sinus tachycardia can produce angina if the cardiac output decreases to the point of reducing coronary circulation or if myocardial oxygen demand is increased without an increase in coronary circulation.

When sinus tachycardia develops, the nurse assesses the patient for signs of decreased cardiac output, such as decreasing level of consciousness, hypotension, and

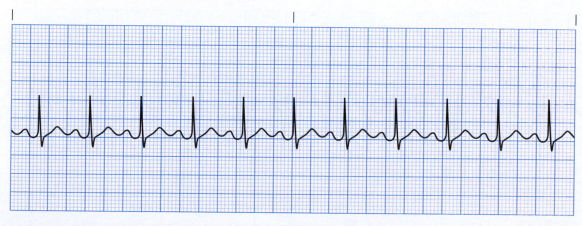

Figure 9–13 Sinus tachycardia.

1. Rate: 110
2. *R–R* interval: regular
3. *P* wave: Regular, upright, matching
4. *PR* interval: 0.20

5. *P* wave precedes *QRS*: yes
6. *QRS* complex: 0.08
7. *QT* interval: 0.32

angina; however, in many patients, mild tachycardia is well tolerated. It is treated if the patient becomes symptomatic, with treatment focusing on relieving the sympathetic nervous system stimulation through pharmacologic or nonpharmacologic interventions. Possible pharmacologic interventions include sedatives, antianxiety agents, analgesics, and antipyretics. Furthermore, if the tachycardia is related to hypovolemia, a fluid bolus may be administered. Nonpharmacologic nursing measures that may decrease the sympathetic response include imagery, massage, distraction, and promoting a calm environment for patients who indicate an interest in these alternative therapies.

Table 9–3 summarizes the ECG characteristics and treatment strategies of sinus bradycardia and sinus tachycardia.

Table 9–3 Sinus Dysrhythmias: ECG Characteristics and Treatment Strategies

Rhythm	Characteristic	Symptomatic Treatment Strategies
Sinus bradycardia	Rate less than 60 bpm	Atropine/pacemaker
Sinus tachycardia	Rate greater than 100 bpm and less than 150 bpm	Antianxiety measures Pain relief measures Antipyretics Oxygen Calcium channel blockers Beta-blocking agents Fluids Vagal nerve stimulus (cough or bear down) Carotid artery massage

ECG Interpretation Exercise 2: Sinus Dysrhythmias

1.

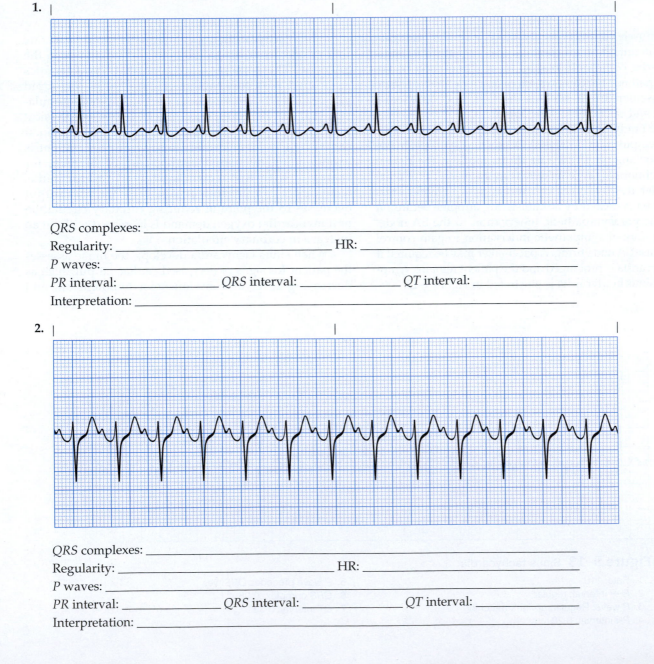

QRS complexes: _____

Regularity: _____ HR: _____

P waves: _____

PR interval: _____ QRS interval: _____ QT interval: _____

Interpretation: _____

2.

QRS complexes: _____

Regularity: _____ HR: _____

P waves: _____

PR interval: _____ QRS interval: _____ QT interval: _____

Interpretation: _____

3.

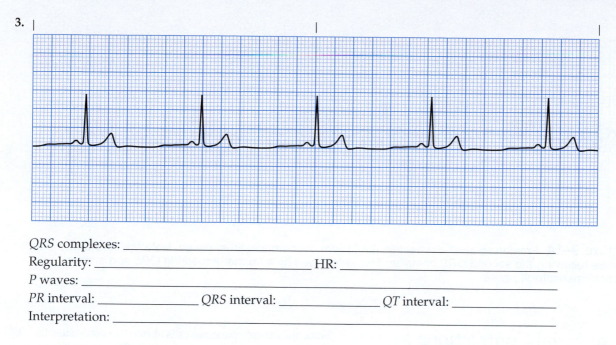

QRS complexes: _____

Regularity: _____ HR: _____

P waves: _____

PR interval: _____ QRS interval: _____ QT interval: _____

Interpretation: _____

Section Five Review

1. Sinus bradycardia originates from which area of the heart?
   A. Intranodal pathways
   B. Atrioventricular (AV) junction
   C. Purkinje fibers
   D. Sinoatrial node

2. Atropine can be used to treat sinus bradycardia because it has what effect on the heart?
   A. Inhibits the AV node
   B. Stimulates the sympathetic nervous system
   C. Blocks the parasympathetic nervous system
   D. Enhances ventricular conduction

3. Sinus tachycardia may result from what factors? (Select all that apply.)
   A. Parasympathetic stimulation
   B. Anxiety
   C. Pain
   D. Fever
   E. Beta-adrenergic blocking agents

4. Decreasing level of consciousness associated with sinus dysrhythmias indicates what occurrence?
   A. Increased ventricular contractility
   B. Decreased cardiac output
   C. Increased atrial filling
   D. Decreased AV conduction

Answers: 1. D, 2. C, 3. (B, C, D), 4. B

Section Six: Atrial Dysrhythmias

Atrial dysrhythmias originate from ectopic impulses within the atria. They may develop when the SA node is not firing properly or when an irritable focus (or multiple foci) develops in the atria. Common atrial dysrhythmias include premature atrial contractions (PACs), supraventricular tachycardia (SVT), atrial fibrillation (AFib), and atrial flutter (AFL). Each of these dysrhythmias is characterized by a rapid atrial rate; and, if associated with a rapid ventricular response, the patient can become symptomatic. The term **ventricular response** refers to impulses that pass through the AV node, triggering ventricular depolarization and contraction. Symptoms are caused by decreased CO secondary to tachycardia, which decreases ventricular filling time and stroke volume (SV), and may include a fluttering sensation in the chest, dyspnea, lightheadedness, or angina. In patients experiencing rapid AFib, CO is also decreased by loss of the atrial kick, which is the additional CO that results from a normal atrial contraction.

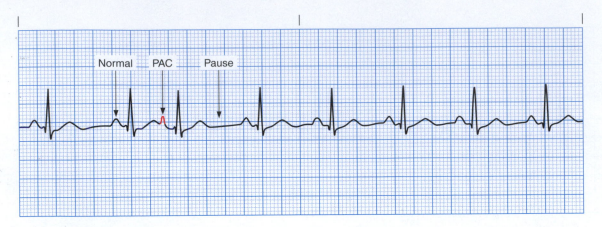

Figure 9–14 Premature atrial contraction (PAC) with noncompensatory pause. Note the PAC that occurs following the second *QRS* complex. This is followed by a normal-appearing *QRS* and a short (noncompensatory) pause.

Premature Atrial Contractions

Premature heartbeats can originate from any excitable focus outside of the normal SA node pacemaker; therefore, they are referred to as ectopic pacemakers. Premature beats are a relatively common phenomenon, and in healthy people they are benign. In the presence of cardiovascular disease, however, ectopic pacemakers can trigger potentially life-threatening cardiac dysrhythmias. Premature heartbeats are usually caused by enhanced automaticity of cardiac cells resulting from a stimulus such as caffeine, nicotine, alcohol, or stress. In patients with cardiovascular disease, the most dangerous cause is cardiac ischemia.

Premature atrial contractions (PACs) are a common type of premature beat that originates from one (**unifocal**) or more (**multifocal**) ectopic pacemakers located in the atria. A *P* wave is visible, unless it is hidden in the preceding *T* wave. The premature *P* wave often looks different from the normal SA node *P* wave—its appearance depending on the exact location of the originating impulse. The underlying rhythm is usually regular with the PAC causing a brief irregularity. There is a characteristic short pause following a PAC called a *noncompensatory pause* (i.e., the *R–R* interval from the *R* wave preceding the PAC to the *R* wave following the PAC is less than two regular *R–R* intervals measured on the underlying regular rhythm). PACs are generally benign and do not require intervention; however, they may serve as an early warning for the development of more serious atrial dysrhythmias and warrant continued close observation of the patient if cardiac disease is known or suspected. Figure 9–14 shows an example of a PAC.

Supraventricular Tachycardia

Supraventricular tachycardia (SVT) refers to a tachycardia that originates anywhere above the ventricles and usually has a rate between 150 and 250 bpm. The rhythm is regular, but *P* waves are not distinguishable because they are buried in the preceding *T* wave due to the rapid rate (Figure 9–15).

Since the ectopic pacemaker is above the ventricles, the *QRS* complex appears normal (narrow). The causes of SVT are similar to those of sinus tachycardia and premature atrial contractions.

The heart rates associated with SVT are extremely rapid, and the patient usually becomes symptomatic, showing signs of decreased cardiac output, as with other tachycardias. Treatment may include Valsalva's maneuver (forceful exhalation against a closed airway) or antidysrhythmic agents such as adenosine, calcium channel blocking agents, beta adrenergic blocking agents, or digoxin. In cases where the patient is experiencing distress, such as hypotension, altered mental status, or signs of shock, or is unresponsive to drug therapy, a synchronized cardioversion is used to rapidly correct the dysrhythmia. Antidysrhythmic agents and cardioversion are presented in Section Ten.

Atrial Flutter

Atrial flutter (AFL) has a faster atrial rate than supraventricular tachycardia, generally between 250 and 350 bpm. The atria are firing so rapidly that the AV node is unable to respond to every impulse; therefore, the ventricular rate depends on the number of impulses that pass through the AV node, resulting in a ventricular response. The ventricular response is often regular but can be irregular, depending on the regularity of impulse conduction through the AV node. Regardless of the regularity of the ventricular response (measured as *R–R* intervals), the atrial firing rate is regular. There are no *P* waves present; however, there are atrial oscillations that appear as flutter waves (sometimes referred to as *F* waves). These *F* waves often have a distinct sawtooth appearance in one or more leads that makes the dysrhythmia easily recognizable. Atrial flutter is described by the number of atrial oscillations (*F* waves) between each *QRS* complex (e.g., "5:1 flutter" as shown in Figure 9–16).

The severity of symptoms displayed by the patient depends largely on the ventricular rate; a fast ventricular rate decreases stroke volume because there is less time for

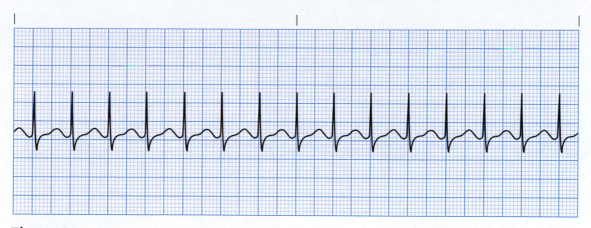

Figure 9–15 Supraventricular tachycardia.

1. Rate: 150
2. *R–R* interval: irregular
3. *P* wave: unable to definitively distinguish; may be the tall peaked spike following *QRS*
4. *PR* interval: cannot calculate
5. *P* wave precedes each *QRS*: cannot identify
6. *QRS* complex: 0.08
7. *QT* interval: unable to definitively measure

diastole. Therefore, the goal is to control the ventricular rate and restore the patient to sinus rhythm. Calcium channel blockers and beta-blocking agents are used to slow down the ventricular rate (see Section Ten). With a high success rate, synchronized cardioversion is the preferred method of treating this dysrhythmia. By synchronizing the countershock to the patient's ECG pattern, the patient's abnormal rhythm resets without the risk of causing the *R* on *T* phenomenon. (Synchronized cardioversion is presented later in this chapter.) Due to the risk of clot formation in the "fluttering" atria, anticoagulation should be considered in this patient population, especially if

cardioversion is considered. If persistent, radiofrequency ablation, an elective procedure to destroy cells that produce dysrhythmias, may also help to resolve this rhythm disturbance (Rosenthal, 2015).

Atrial Fibrillation

Atrial fibrillation (AFib) is a condition in which the atria are contracting so fast—greater than 350 bpm—that they are unable to have adequate filling or contraction. Rather than one ectopic pacemaker generating impulses, multiple foci are all firing in a disorganized fashion throughout

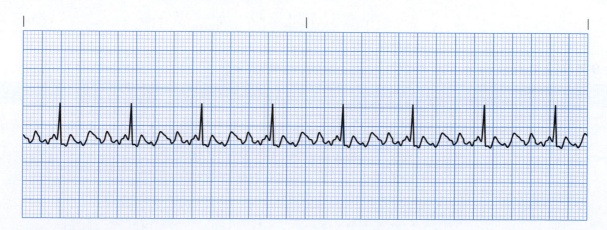

Figure 9–16 Atrial flutter.

1. Rate: ventricular = 80; atrial = about 320
2. *R–R* interval: regular
3. *P* wave: cannot distinguish, flutter (sawtooth) waves present
4. *PR* interval: cannot calculate
5. *P* wave precedes *QRS*: cannot identify
6. *QRS* complex: 0.10
7. *QT* interval: cannot be determined

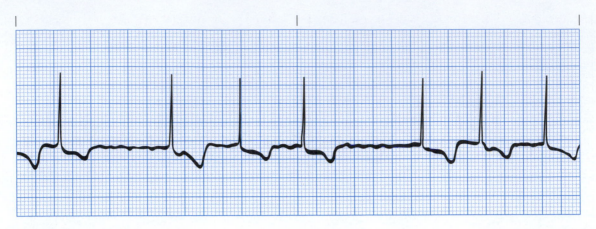

Figure 9–17 Atrial fibrillation.

1. Rate: atrial = unable to calculate; ventricular = about 70 in 6-sec strip
2. *R–R* interval: regular
3. *P* wave: undistinguishable
4. *PR* interval: cannot calculate
5. *P* wave precedes each *QRS*: cannot identify
6. *QRS* complex: 0.04–0.06
7. *QT* interval: cannot be determined

the atria. This chaotic electrical activity causes the atria to quiver rather than contract in an organized fashion, resulting in loss of the normal atrial kick contribution to cardiac output. Therefore, the ventricles are inadequately filled, and stroke volume is diminished by approximately 20% to 25%. Due to inadequate emptying, blood that remains in the atria is prone to forming clots, which increases the risk of thrombotic stroke or pulmonary embolism. The greatest risk of this occurring is when the rhythm returns to a sinus rhythm—due to the atria now fully contracting (active "atrial kick") and expelling the clot(s) into the ventricles and then to either the brain or the lungs.

Atrial fibrillation is the most common chronic dysrhythmia seen in the older adult population and can often be associated with heart failure. It should be immediately considered when a patient presents with a highly irregular heart rhythm. Its three major characteristics include (1) an absence of *P* waves, (2) a normal *QRS* configuration with highly irregular *R–R* intervals (an "irregularly irregular" rhythm), and (3) the presence of fibrillatory waves (*F* waves) (Figure 9–17).

This highly irregular heart rhythm results from unpredictable conduction of impulses through the AV node with the heart rate ranging between 140 and 200 bpm. When assessing a pulse with atrial fibrillation, the nurse can feel a

Table 9–4 Atrial Dysrhythmias: ECG Characteristics and Treatment Strategies

Rhythm	Characteristic	Treatment Strategies
Premature atrial contractions	*PR* interval may be shortened, normal, or prolonged *QRS* complex normal Noncompensatory pause	May not be treated if asymptomatic Reduce stress, caffeine, alcohol intake, smoking Beta-blocking agents
Supraventricular tachycardia	*P* waves not distinguishable (buried) *R–R* interval regular Atrial rate 150–250 bpm	Adenosine Vagal maneuvers (e.g., carotid massage) Beta-blocking agents Calcium channel blocking agents Synchronized cardioversion
Atrial flutter	*R–R* interval may be regular or irregular Atrial rate may be up to 350 bpm Sawtoothed or flutter waves	Beta-blocking agents Calcium channel blocking agents Synchronized cardioversion
Atrial fibrillation	*R–R* interval irregularly irregular Atrial rate greater than 350 bpm	Digitalis Amiodarone Beta-blocking agents Calcium channel blocking agents Synchronized cardioversion

*Note: If atrial fibrillation duration is greater than 48 hours, anticoagulation must be considered before rhythm conversion is attempted to avoid clot dislodgement from the atria.

pulse deficit; there is a difference between the apical heart rate and the peripheral pulse rate because the stroke volume is not adequate enough with some beats to produce a palpable pulse.

Conversion of atrial fibrillation back to a normal sinus rhythm is desirable if the dysrhythmia is new; however, in some cases it is resistant to conversion. If conversion is not possible, it is important to control the heart rate because doing so improves hemodynamics. If the patient does not respond to or does not tolerate pharmacologic treatments (e.g., hypotension) or becomes unstable, synchronized cardioversion is considered. Long-standing, asymptomatic atrial fibrillation may not require treatment. However, patients generally require anticoagulation, such as warfarin therapy, to prevent the formation of blood clots in the atria to reduce the risk of stroke and pulmonary embolism. Drugs that are particularly effective in controlling the ventricular rate are digoxin (Lanoxin), amiodarone (Cordarone), beta adrenergic blocking agents, and calcium channel blocking agents.

Table 9–4 summarizes the ECG characteristics and treatment strategies for the atrial dysrhythmias.

ECG Interpretation Exercise 3: Atrial Dysrhythmias

1.

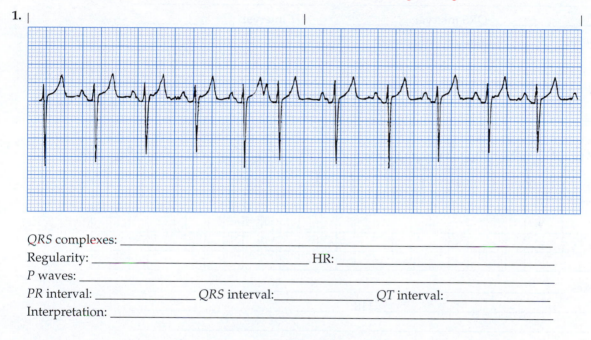

QRS complexes: _____

Regularity: _____ HR: _____

_P_ waves: _____

_PR_ interval: _____ _QRS_ interval: _____ _QT_ interval: _____

Interpretation: _____

2.

QRS complexes: _____

Regularity: _____ HR: _____

_P_ waves: _____

_PR_ interval: _____ _QRS_ interval: _____ _QT_ interval: _____

Interpretation: _____

3.

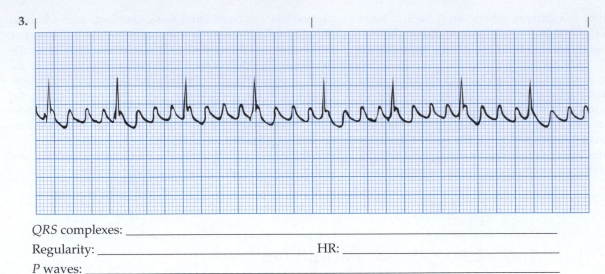

QRS complexes: _____

Regularity: _____ HR: _____

P waves: _____

PR interval: _____ QRS interval: _____ QT interval: _____

Interpretation: _____

4.

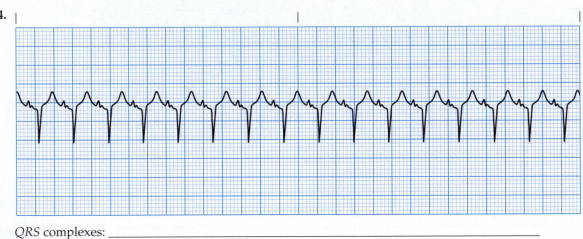

QRS complexes: _____

Regularity: _____ HR: _____

P waves: _____

PR interval: _____ QRS interval: _____ QT interval: _____

Interpretation: _____

Section Six Review

1. Atrial dysrhythmias produce symptoms of lighthead-edness or angina for which reason?
 A. Cardiac output is decreased.
 B. Ventricular conduction is delayed.
 C. SA node is competing for pacemaker status.
 D. Coronary vasodilation occurs.

2. Which are characteristic of premature atrial contractions (PACs)? (Select all that apply.)
 A. There is no ventricular contraction.
 B. There is a premature *P* wave.
 C. The underlying rhythm is usually regular.
 D. There is a noncompensatory pause.
 E. The *QRS* configuration is abnormal.

3. Which are ECG characteristics of atrial fibrillation? (Select all that apply.)
 A. Absent *P* waves
 B. Irregular *R–R* interval
 C. Atrial rate greater than 160 bpm
 D. *PR* interval is greater than 0.20 second
 E. *F* waves are present

4. Atrial flutter typically has what atrial rate?
 A. Between 150 and 250 bpm
 B. Less than 60 bpm
 C. Between 250 and 350 bpm
 D. Greater than 400 bpm

Answers: 1. A, 2. (B, C, D), 3. (A, B, E), 4. C

Section Seven: Junctional Dysrhythmias

Junctional dysrhythmias refer to ectopic rhythms that originate in the atrioventricular (AV) junction. Recall that the AV junction can act as a backup pacemaker when the SA node fails to fire. Pacemaker cells in this area have an intrinsic rate of 40 to 60 bpm. After these pacemaker cells discharge, the energy spreads upward to depolarize the atria and downward to depolarize the ventricles. Because the ventricles usually are depolarized in a downward fashion, the *QRS* complex appears normal. The atria are depolarized in an abnormal manner so the *P* wave can be inverted or absent, depending on which lead is being viewed. For example, in lead II it is inverted. The timing of the *P* wave is abnormal, and its location in relation to the *QRS* complex varies in one of three ways:

- It may precede the *QRS* complex—impulse originates high in AV junction; occurs when atria depolarize first; *PR* interval is shorter than 0.12 sec.
- It may be buried in the *QRS* complex and be hidden—impulse originates in mid-AV junction; occurs when atria and ventricles depolarize simultaneously; therefore it is not visible.
- It can follow the *QRS* complex—impulse originates low in AV junction; occurs when ventricles depolarize first.

Considered a protective mechanism or a backup mode, junctional rhythms produce varying heart rates. A *junctional rhythm* (sometimes called a *junctional escape rhythm*) is characterized by a rate of 40 to 60 bpm (Figure 9–18). If the rate of the rhythm is between 60 and 100 bpm, it is called an *accelerated junctional rhythm* (Figure 9–19). *Junctional tachycardia* refers to

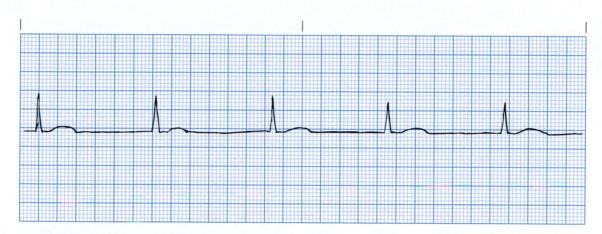

Figure 9–18 Junctional rhythm.

1. Rate: atrial = NA; ventricular = 50
2. *R–R* interval: regular
3. *P* wave: not present
4. *PR* interval: NA
5. *P* wave precedes each *QRS*: NA
6. *QRS* complex: 0.06
7. *QT* interval: 0.44

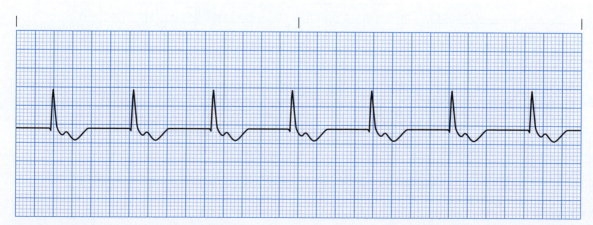

Figure 9–19 Accelerated junctional rhythm.

1. Rate: 70
2. *R–R* interval: regular
3. *P* wave: regular, follows *QRS*
4. *PR* interval: not measured; *P* wave follows *QRS*
5. *P* wave precedes each *QRS*: no; *P* wave follows *QRS*
6. *QRS* complex: 0.08
7. *QT* interval: 0.40

a junctional rhythm with a rate greater than 100 bpm. Digitalis toxicity can precipitate junctional rhythms because it decreases the automaticity of the AV node and slows conduction between the SA and AV nodes.

Usually, the patient can tolerate junctional rhythms; however, if the patient experiences symptoms of decreased cardiac output because the rate is too slow, atropine is administered. Often, the dysrhythmia is treated by withholding the medication that has caused it. A pacemaker may be inserted as a protective measure in case the junction fails or if the patient is symptomatic.

Table 9–5 compares the ECG characteristics and treatment strategies for junctional dysrhythmias.

Table 9–5 Junctional Dysrhythmias: ECG Characteristics and Treatment Strategies

Rhythm	Characteristic	Treatment Strategies
Junctional rhythm	Rate 40–60 bpm Inverted or absent P waves	May not be treated if patient is asymptomatic Atropine Pacemaker insertion
Junctional tachycardia (accelerated junctional rhythm)	Rate greater than 100 bpm Inverted or absent P waves	May not be treated if patient is asymptomatic Pacemaker insertion Withhold digitalis if associated with digitalis toxicity

ECG Interpretation Exercise 4: Junctional Dysrhythmias

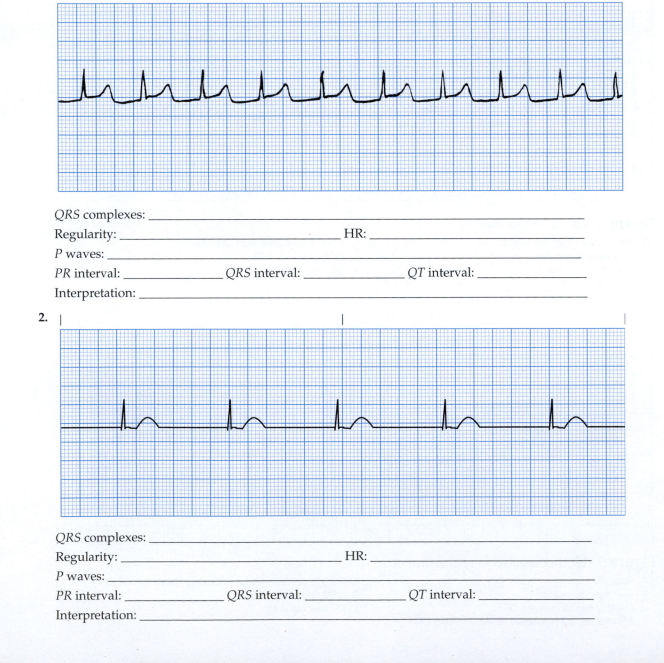

1.

QRS complexes: _____

Regularity: _____ HR: _____

P waves: _____

PR interval: _____ QRS interval: _____ QT interval: _____

Interpretation: _____

2.

QRS complexes: _____

Regularity: _____ HR: _____

P waves: _____

PR interval: _____ QRS interval: _____ QT interval: _____

Interpretation: _____

3.

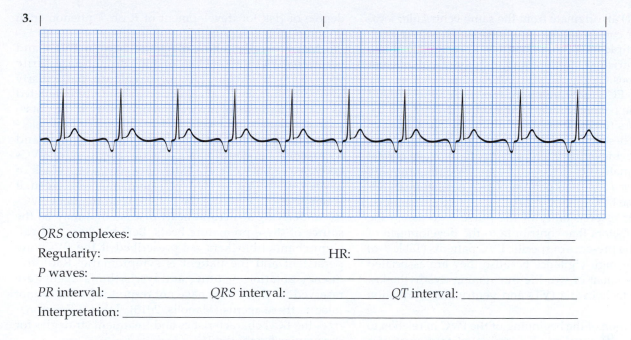

QRS complexes: _____

Regularity: _____ HR: _____

P waves: _____

PR interval: _____ QRS interval: _____ QT interval: _____

Interpretation: _____

Section Seven Review

1. Junctional tachycardia is classified as a junctional rhythm with what rate?
   A. Greater than 40 bpm
   B. Greater than 60 bpm
   C. Greater than 100 bpm
   D. Between 60 and 100 bpm

2. Which statement correctly describes the *P* wave in a junctional rhythm?
   A. It is bizarre in configuration.
   B. It is always absent.
   C. It can appear anywhere in relation to the *QRS* complex.
   D. It is flat.

3. What is the rate of an accelerated junctional rhythm?
   A. Less than 60 bpm
   B. 60 to 100 bpm
   C. 100 to 120 bpm
   D. Greater than 150 bpm

4. What interventions for junctional rhythms may be performed? (Select all that apply.)
   A. Administration of digitalis
   B. Administration of atropine
   C. Implantation of a pacemaker
   D. Cardioversion
   E. Defibrillation

Answers: 1. C, 2. C, 3. B, 4. (B, C)

Section Eight: Ventricular Dysrhythmias

Ventricular dysrhythmias are ectopic impulses that originate in the ventricle and can be life-threatening. When an impulse originates in the ventricles, it cannot use the normal conduction pathway, which results in a slow depolarization of the ventricles and a large and wide *QRS* complex. The ventricular impulse does not depolarize the atria; however, if independent atrial depolarization occurs, the resulting *P* wave is usually hidden in the widened *QRS* complex. Ectopic impulses of ventricular origin alter hemodynamics. This results in a decrease in cardiac output from loss of the atrial kick from backward depolarization and from pushing ventricular blood against closed valves. Three common ventricular dysrhythmias are premature ventricular contractions, ventricular tachycardia, and ventricular fibrillation.

Premature Ventricular Contractions

Premature ventricular contractions (PVCs) are ectopic impulses that originate in the ventricle and discharge before the next normal sinus beat is due. Hemodynamically, ventricular diastole that precedes a premature ventricular contraction is too brief, and therefore cannot contribute significantly to CO. Since the electrical stimulus originates outside of the atria, there is no *P* wave preceding the PVC, and the configuration of the *QRS* complex is usually large (higher voltage on an ECG monitor and wider than 0.12 sec). The waveform is also bizarre in appearance and is generally in the opposite direction of the person's usual *QRS* complex. There is a characteristic full *compensatory pause* (i.e., the *R–R* interval from the *R* wave preceding the PVC to the *R* wave following the PVC is equal to two regular *R–R* intervals of the underlying ECG pattern) (Figure 9–20). Unifocal (single focus) PVCs

(Figure 9–21) all originate from the same ventricular location so their configurations look identical; however, multifocal (multiple foci) PVCs (Figure 9–22) originate at two or more ventricular locations and therefore have different configurations.

During ECG interpretation, the nurse assesses and describes the patient's underlying cardiac rhythm and the type of PVCs (unifocal versus multifocal). The timing of the PVCs is described if they occur in a repeatable pattern. For example, **bigeminy** is a repeated pattern of one normal SA node–initiated beat followed by one PVC (Figure 9–23). **Trigeminy** is a repeated pattern of two normal beats followed by one PVC (Figure 9–24).

A major responsibility of the nurse is to assess the patient for factors that contribute to the development of PVCs and the presence of specific PVC patterns (Table 9–6) that warrant high vigilance because they are associated with development of two life-threatening dysrhythmias: ventricular tachycardia (VT) and ventricular fibrillation (VFib).

The location of the beginning of the PVC in relation to the preceding T wave is also evaluated to monitor for degree of risk for development of R on T phenomenon (Figure 9–25).

Many people who experience benign PVCs and occasional PVCs (less than 6/min) do not necessarily require any treatment. Electrolyte balance, particularly low potassium and/or magnesium, should be evaluated as potential causes of myocardial irritability. If the potassium or magnesium levels are low, the appropriate electrolyte supplementation is provided. Stress and hypoxemia can contribute to the development of PVCs because cardiac cells are extremely sensitive to lack of oxygen, which is corrected with supplemental oxygen. It is important to evaluate the patient with frequent PVCs for underlying structural heart disease that may be the source of these premature beats. Beta blockers and calcium channel blockers are prescribed if the PVCs are persistent and the patient is symptomatic. Radiofrequency ablation or other antidysrhythmia agents are reserved for those who have not responded to or cannot tolerate these agents (Manolis, 2016). Table 9–7 summarizes the ECG characteristics and treatment strategies for ventricular dysrhythmias.

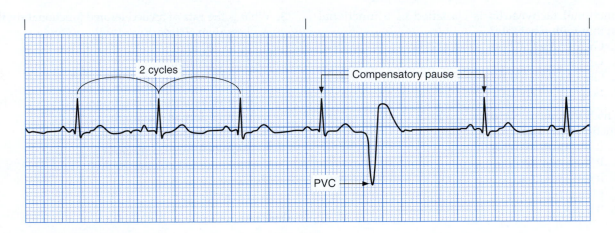

Figure 9–20 PVC with complete compensatory pause.

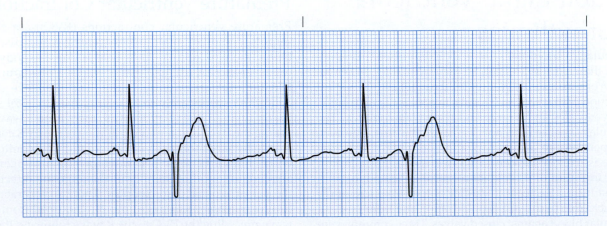

Figure 9–21 Unifocal PVCs. Note that the two PVCs are bizarre in appearance and the waveforms are in opposite directions of the underlying QRS complexes.

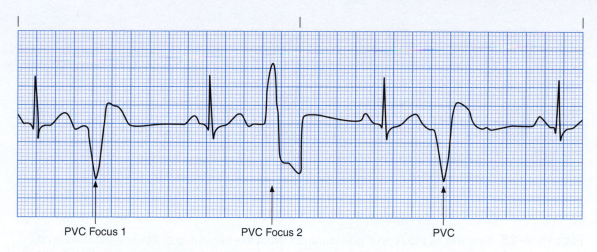

Figure 9–22 Multifocal PVCs. Note the differences in PVC configurations.

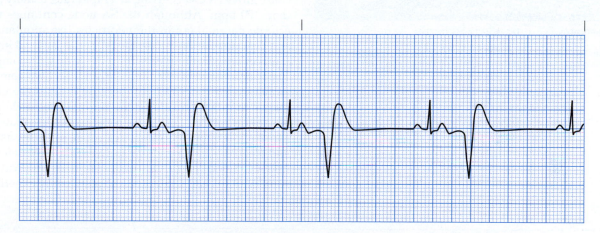

Figure 9–23 Ventricular bigeminy. Note that the heart rate is actually 40 bpm since PVCs do not contribute to the cardiac output.

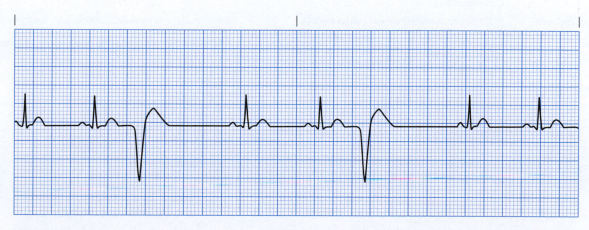

Figure 9–24 Ventricular trigeminy. Note that the PVCs are from the same focus (unifocal).

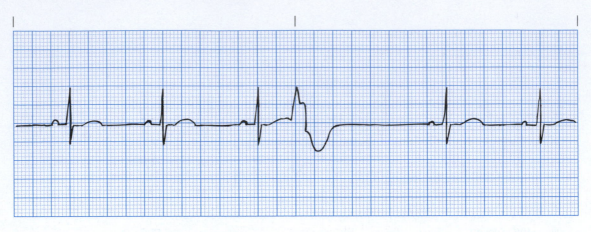

Figure 9–25 Example of the R on T phenomenon. Note the beginning of the ectopic beat on the downstroke of the T wave.

Table 9–6 Circumstances That Warrant Close Observation of Premature Ventricular Contractions

Type of Problem	Criteria for Concern
Ectopic frequency	More than 6 per minute
ECG pattern or number of ectopic beats	Two PVCs occurring together (couplets) A run of ventricular tachycardia (more than 3 PVCs in a row) Multifocal PVCs (from more than 1 ectopic focus)
Wave relationships	R on T phenomenon (PVC that occurs on the downstroke of the T wave preceding the PVC. The downstroke of the T wave is a relative refractory or vulnerable period wherein a stimulus that is strong enough can excite the heart and trigger VT or VFib.)

Ventricular Tachycardia

Ventricular tachycardia (VT) is classified as three or more consecutive PVCs occurring at a rapid rate, usually greater than 100 bpm. Although the SA node continues to fire, ectopic pacemakers in the ventricles fire spontaneously and bear no relationship to the SA node–initiated impulse. P waves are often hidden within the wide QRS complexes. The R–R interval is often regular, and the QRS complex is wide (greater than 0.12 sec) because it takes the impulse longer to move outside of the normal conduction pathway. Short runs of ventricular tachycardia (less than 30 sec) can be tolerated by some but must be fully assessed and treated—as ventricular tachycardia may deteriorate into sustained VT or ventricular fibrillation. With short runs, patients can sometimes be alert while experiencing

Table 9–7 Ventricular Dysrhythmias: ECG Characteristics and Treatment Strategies

Rhythm	Characteristic	Treatment Strategies*
Premature ventricular contractions	PR interval absent in premature beat QRS > 0.12 sec QRS configuration large and bizarre in appearance QRS configuration often in opposite direction of underlying normal QRS Compensatory pause	May not be treated if asymptomatic Reduce caffeine intake, reduce stress Correct low electrolyte levels Beta blockers Calcium channel blockers
Ventricular tachycardia	R–R interval usually regular, but can be irregular Absent P waves or P waves not associated with QRS complex Wide QRS but somewhat uniform Rate greater than 100 bpm May or may not have a pulse	With pulse: synchronized cardioversion, amiodarone, procainamide No pulse: Same treatment strategy as ventricular fibrillation
Ventricular fibrillation	R–R interval undeterminable Absent P wave and QRS Rate undeterminable Chaotic waveform No pulse present	CPR Defibrillation Epinephrine Vasopressin Amiodarone Search for and treat possible causes
Asystole	Complete absence of electrical impulses	Verify lead placement CPR Epinephrine Vasopressin Search for and treat possible causes

*Lists are not all-inclusive. Follow ACLS guidelines.

ventricular tachycardia, and a carotid pulse can be present; however, as cardiac output diminishes, and oxygen delivery to the body's tissues becomes compromised, a loss of consciousness will occur, and American Heart Association Advanced Cardiac Life Support (ACLS) measures will become necessary (Link et al., 2015).

Synchronized cardioversion may be used to convert VT; however, when pulseless VT is present, cardiopulmonary resuscitation (CPR) and defibrillation are required. Ventricular tachycardia requires the implementation of ACLS by trained interdisciplinary team members such as nurses, respiratory therapists, pharmacists, and physicians. Pharmacological treatment of ventricular tachycardia may include epinephrine, vasopressin, amiodarone, lidocaine, or magnesium. Figure 9–26 is an example of ventricular tachycardia. *Important:* It is critical for the

interdisciplinary team to be aware of the patient's and/or family's wishes regarding cardiopulmonary resuscitation. The patient's advance directives should be documented in the medical record and communicated during patient handoff reports.

Ventricular Fibrillation

Ventricular fibrillation, a fatal rhythm, is the most common cause of sudden cardiac arrest. Myocardial infarction and ventricular tachycardia can precede the development of ventricular fibrillation. The ECG pattern is chaotic due to weak, disorganized ectopic impulses from multiple locations in the ventricles. It is impossible to identify any *PQRST* waves, and the rhythm is grossly irregular (Figure 9–27). There are no contractions in the

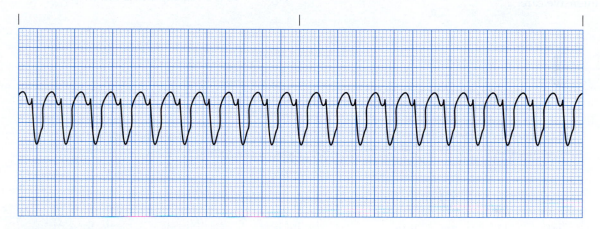

Figure 9–26 Ventricular tachycardia.

1. Rate: atrial = unable to calculate; ventricular = 180–190
2. *R–R* interval: regular
3. *P* wave: undistinguishable
4. *PR* interval: none
5. *P* wave precedes each *QRS*: no
6. *QRS* complex: 0.16
7. *QT* interval: unmeasurable

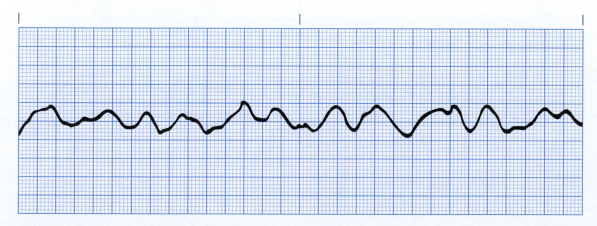

Figure 9–27 Ventricular fibrillation.

1. Rate: atrial = none; ventricular = none
2. *R–R* interval: undeterminable
3. *P* wave: none
4. *PR* interval: none
5. *P* wave precedes each *QRS*: no
6. *QRS* complex: none
7. *QT* interval: none

atria or ventricles; therefore, there is no cardiac output and the patient is unresponsive and pulseless, requiring immediate ACLS treatment.

Defibrillation is the treatment of choice for ventricular fibrillation. In public settings (e.g., airports, malls), an automated external defibrillator (AED) may be available to treat an individual experiencing sudden cardiac arrest. Pharmacotherapy includes a bolus of epinephrine, vasopressin, amiodarone, lidocaine, and magnesium. If the patient remains pulseless, CPR and attempts at defibrillation continue per ACLS guidelines. Once the patient has converted from ventricular fibrillation and has a pulse, a continuous infusion of the last drug used to convert the rhythm is initiated and post–cardiac arrest care is initiated. This may include, but is not limited to, establishing an advanced airway, mechanical ventilation, treating hypotension, and inducing hypothermia. These patients will require intensive care.

Asystole

Asystole represents complete cessation of electrical impulses. The patient is unconscious and pulseless. It is imperative that the nurse check that the rhythm is verified in two separate leads as fine ventricular fibrillation can mimic asystole and requires different interventions. Once confirmed, chest compressions are initiated immediately and continued with minimal interruptions. In addition to CPR, other treatments for asystole include epinephrine or vasopressin. During resuscitation, clinicians must consider and treat the various causes of asystole. Possible contributing factors of asystole include hypovolemia, hypoxemia, electrolyte imbalances (acidosis, potassium), hypothermia, various toxins, cardiac tamponade, tension pneumothorax, and pulmonary or coronary thrombosis (Pozner, 2015). Often, despite rigorous efforts, asystole is a terminal rhythm. Figure 9–28 is an example of asystole.

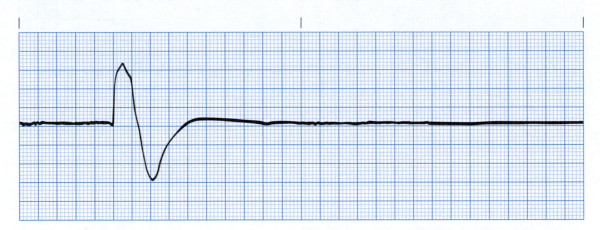

Figure 9–28 Asystole.

ECG Interpretation Exercise 5: Ventricular Dysrhythmias

1.
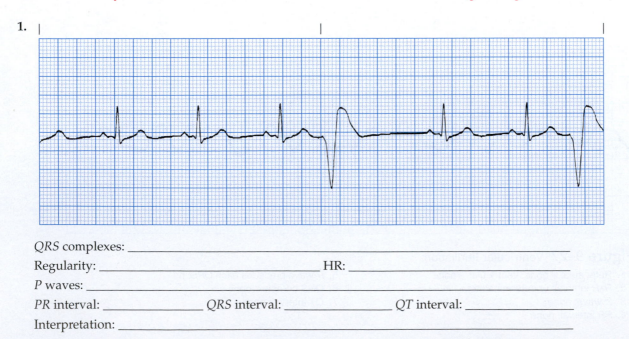

QRS complexes: _____

Regularity: _____ HR: _____

P waves: _____

PR interval: _____ QRS interval: _____ QT interval: _____

Interpretation: _____

2.

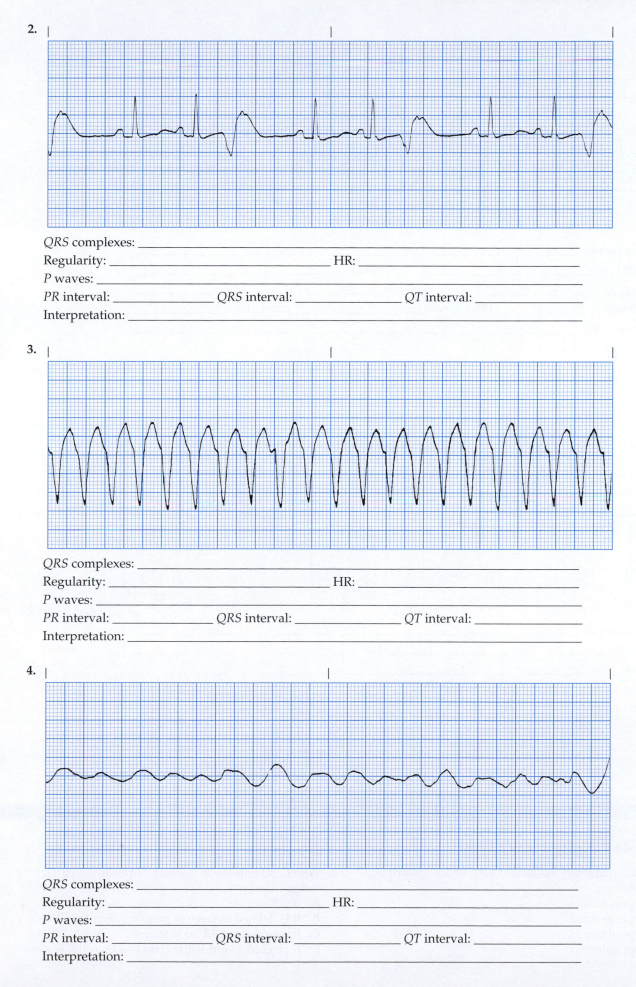

QRS complexes: _____

Regularity: _____ HR: _____

P waves: _____

PR interval: _____ *QRS* interval: _____ *QT* interval: _____

Interpretation: _____

3.

QRS complexes: _____

Regularity: _____ HR: _____

P waves: _____

PR interval: _____ *QRS* interval: _____ *QT* interval: _____

Interpretation: _____

4.

QRS complexes: _____

Regularity: _____ HR: _____

P waves: _____

PR interval: _____ *QRS* interval: _____ *QT* interval: _____

Interpretation: _____

5.

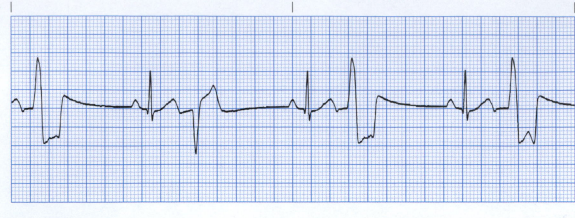

QRS complexes: _____

Regularity: _____ HR: _____

P waves: _____

PR interval: _____ QRS interval: _____ QT interval: _____

Interpretation: _____

6.

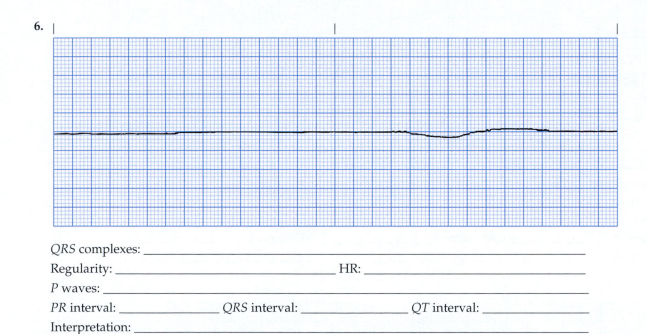

QRS complexes: _____

Regularity: _____ HR: _____

P waves: _____

PR interval: _____ QRS interval: _____ QT interval: _____

Interpretation: _____

Section Eight Review

1. PVCs are frequently associated with which underlying problem?
   A. Hyponatremia
   B. Hypocalcemia
   C. Hypoglycemia
   D. Hypokalemia

2. Which statement is correct regarding ventricular tachycardia?
   A. It is harmless.
   B. It is defined as three or more consecutive PVCs.
   C. It results from SA node fatigue.
   D. It produces ventricular rates less than 100 bpm.

3. Which of the following is considered a "short run" of ventricular tachycardia?
  A. 1 minute
  B. 45 seconds to 1 minute
  C. Less than 30 seconds
  D. Two PVCs

4. After the client has converted from ventricular fibrillation and has a pulse, which intervention should be initiated?
  A. Check electrolytes
  B. A bolus of vasopressin
  C. A bolus of epinephrine
  D. A continuous infusion of the last drug used to convert the rhythm

Answers: 1. D, 2. B, 3. C, 4. D

Section Nine: Conduction Abnormalities

Cardiac impulse conduction can be inhibited anywhere along the conduction pathway. A variety of factors can slow conduction, such as cardiac ischemia, digitalis, antiarrhythmic agents, and increased parasympathetic activity. When the delay occurs at the atrioventricular (AV) junction, it is called an AV block. Acute AV blocks are associated with myocardial infarction, whereas chronic AV blocks may develop from coronary artery disease. AV blocks are classified as partial (first degree and second degree) or complete (third degree), based on the relationship of the *P* wave to the *QRS* complex.

First-degree Atrioventricular Block

A first-degree AV block is a partial type of block that is denoted by a prolonged *PR* interval (more than 0.20 sec). There is a delay in conduction through the AV node; however, the *P* wave and *QRS* complex maintain a 1:1 relationship such that every *P* wave is followed by a *QRS* complex regardless of the *PR* interval length. The rest of the ECG is normal. The patient is usually asymptomatic, and no treatment is necessary. While first-degree AV block is usually benign, in the presence of acute myocardial infarction or coronary artery disease, the conduction delay can increase, leading to second- or third-degree AV block, both of which require treatment. Figure 9–29 is an example of first-degree AV block.

Second-degree Atrioventricular Block

Second-degree AV block has a more serious degree of blockage than first degree but is still classified as a partial heart block. There are two patterns of second-degree AV block: Mobitz I and Mobitz II.

Mobitz Type I (Wenckebach) In Mobitz type I, with successive beats, the *PR* interval lengthens progressively

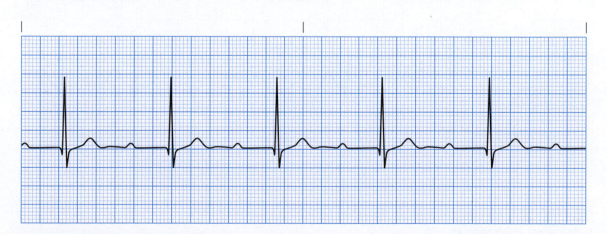

Figure 9–29 First-degree AV block.
  1. Rate: 50
  2. *R–R* interval: regular
  3. *P* wave: upright, regular, matching, precedes every *QRS*
  4. *PR* interval: 0.44
  5. *P* wave precedes *QRS*: yes, on 1:1 basis
  6. *QRS* complex: 0.10
  7. *QT* interval: 0.40

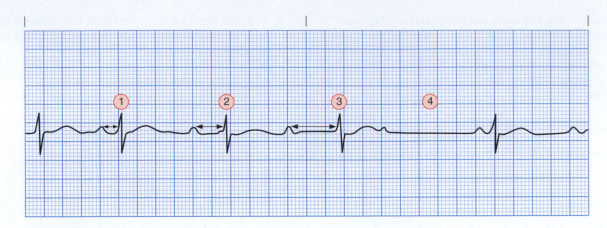

Figure 9–30 Mobitz type I (Wenckebach) second-degree block.

1. Rate: 0.50
2. *R–R* interval: irregular
3. *P* wave: regular, upright, matching; one per *QRS* except for 5th *QRS*, which has two *P* waves preceding *QRS*
4. *PR* interval: variable; progressively prolongs until *QRS* is lost for one beat
5. *P* wave precedes *QRS*: yes
6. *QRS* complex: 0.10
7. *QT* interval: 0.44

before the dropping of the *QRS* complex. The SA node fires regularly; however, the AV junction increasingly blocks the impulse for a longer time until there is an ultimate failure of the AV junction to conduct the impulse, hence the dropped *QRS* (Figure 9–30). After a drop in the *QRS* complex, the pattern repeats itself. In most cases, Mobitz type I is considered a benign rhythm.

Mobitz Type II In Mobitz type II second-degree AV block, the *PR* intervals are of constant duration before

dropping the *QRS* complex (Figure 9–31). *QRS* complexes are wide because the block is usually lower in the conduction system (bundle of His). This type of AV block is less common but is considered more serious because it is associated with progression to third-degree AV block and asystole.

Management of Second-degree AV Block The nurse determines the ventricular rate (number of *QRS* complexes) of the rhythm and the frequency of dropped beats.

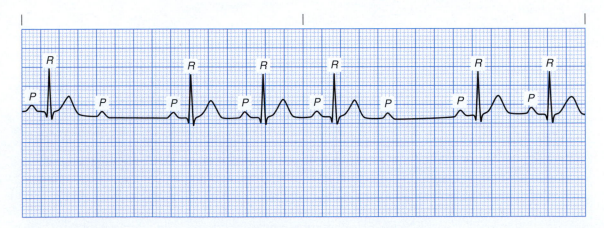

Figure 9–31 Mobitz type II second-degree AV block (3:1 conduction).

1. Rate: atrial = 80, ventricular = 60
2. *R–R* interval: regular
3. *P* wave: upright, matching, regular
4. *PR* interval: 0.20
5. *P* wave precedes *QRS*: yes, some *QRS* complexes have more than 1 *P* wave
6. *QRS* complex: 0.06–0.08
7. *QT* interval: 0.44

Angina, light-headedness, and dyspnea can occur because of decreased cardiac output. In the case of type I second-degree AV block, if the rate is below 60 bpm and the patient is asymptomatic, no treatment is initiated, but the patient is closely monitored. A patient with type II second-degree AV block, whether symptomatic or asymptomatic, will likely receive a pacemaker.

Regardless of the type of second-degree block, if the patient experiences symptoms, atropine is administered to temporarily increase the heart rate and relieve symptoms until more definitive therapies can be initiated as necessary. Dopamine or epinephrine may be given in severe symptomatic bradycardia to increase the arterial blood pressure and heart rate. A temporary (transvenous or transcutaneous) pacemaker may be initiated for symptomatic or severe second-degree AV block. Transcutaneous and transvenous pacing are extremely effective temporary measures to reestablish an adequate heart rate until either the patient's own rhythm recovers or a permanent pacemaker is placed.

Third-degree (Complete) Atrioventricular Block

With third-degree (complete) AV block, no impulses are conducted through the AV node, causing the atria and ventricles to contract independent of one another. There is no relationship between the *P* wave and the *QRS* complex because the atria and the ventricles are paced by separate pacemakers. The atria and ventricles fire at their inherent rates (atria = 60–100 bpm; ventricles = 25–40 bpm), but they do not function as a single unit. The *P–P* wave interval is regular, as is the *R–R* wave

interval, but there is no relationship between the *P* wave and the *QRS* complex; therefore, when assessing a rhythm strip showing complete AV block, it is noticeable that the *PR* interval varies from beat to beat. The *QRS* complex is usually wide because of the ventricular origin of its stimulus.

Complete heart block is usually associated with myocardial infarction and requires emergency treatment. The lack of coordination between the heart chambers results in greatly diminished cardiac output because of inadequate filling of the ventricles. In rare cases, the ventricular rate is fast enough to maintain cardiac output, and symptoms are less severe. Usually, however, the patient experiences an alteration in mental status and syncope. Complete heart block can progress to ventricular fibrillation. Treatment is the same as that for type II second-degree heart block. If symptomatic, the patient is administered atropine, dopamine, or epinephrine. External pacing and transvenous pacing may also be used. Figure 9–32 is an example of complete heart block.

Bundle Branch Block

A bundle branch block (BBB) results from an impairment in conduction through the bundle of His branches. Once the impulse enters the ventricles, its conduction through the right and left bundle branches can be impaired—also known as an intraventricular conduction delay. Instead of moving rapidly, the impulse travels slowly down the blocked side; thus, one ventricle depolarizes faster than the other. On the ECG, the *QRS* complex is prolonged (greater than 0.12 sec) and its appearance varies, depending on the affected side (right or left bundle branches). A 12-lead ECG

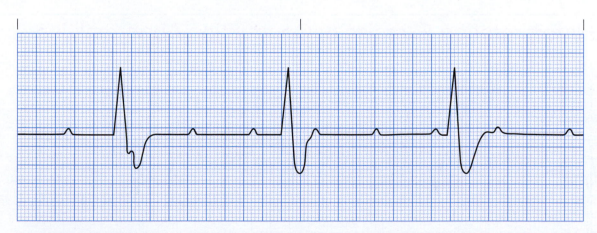

Figure 9–32 Third-degree (complete) heart block.

1. Rate: atrial = 90; ventricular = 30
2. *R–R* interval: regular
3. *P* wave: regular, upright, matching
4. *PR* interval: variable
5. *P* wave precedes each *QRS*: yes, multiple; no relationship with *QRS*
6. *QRS* complex: 0.10
7. *QT* interval: 0.40

Table 9–8 Conduction Abnormalities: ECG Characteristics and Treatment Strategies

Block	Characteristics	Treatment Strategies
First degree	PR interval greater than 0.20 sec R–R interval regular	Usually not treated unless patient is symptomatic Possibly medication related (e.g., digitalis)
Second degree, Mobitz type I	Atrial rate greater than ventricular rate R–R interval irregular PR interval gradually lengthens until a P wave is blocked (no QRS follows the P wave)	Withhold digitalis if associated with digitalis toxicity Atropine Dopamine Epinephrine Temporary pacemaker (transcutaneous, then transvenous, as indicated) Permanent pacemaker insertion
Second degree, Mobitz type II	Atrial rate greater than ventricular rate No consistent pattern to blocking of the P wave When present, PR interval consistent R–R interval usually irregular	Atropine Dopamine Epinephrine Temporary pacemaker (transcutaneous then transvenous as indicated) Permanent pacemaker insertion
Third degree, complete	No association of P waves and R waves R–R interval regular P-P interval regular QRS may be widened	Atropine Dopamine Epinephrine Temporary pacemaker (transcutaneous then transvenous as indicated) Permanent pacemaker insertion
Bundle branch block	QRS widened (greater than 0.12 sec) Appearance varies based on which branch is blocking (right or left)	No treatment required for the block itself

is necessary to determine from which side the block is occurring. Bundle branch blocks do not cause symptoms, and treatment is unnecessary except in the case of a new-onset left BBB in which the patient may be experiencing a myocardial infarction. Clinically, it is important to note that ECG changes associated with left BBB can mask acute myocardial infarction ECG changes. Therefore, a patient who presents with a new left BBB and symptoms of an acute coronary syndrome should be treated as a medical emergency (Davies & Scott, 2015).

Table 9–8 summarizes the ECG characteristics and treatment strategies of conduction abnormalities.

ECG Interpretation Exercise 6: Conduction Abnormalities

1.

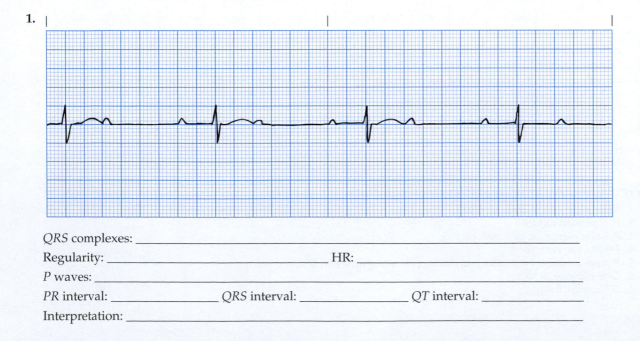

QRS complexes: _____

Regularity: _____ HR: _____

P waves: _____

PR interval: _____ QRS interval: _____ QT interval: _____

Interpretation: _____

2.

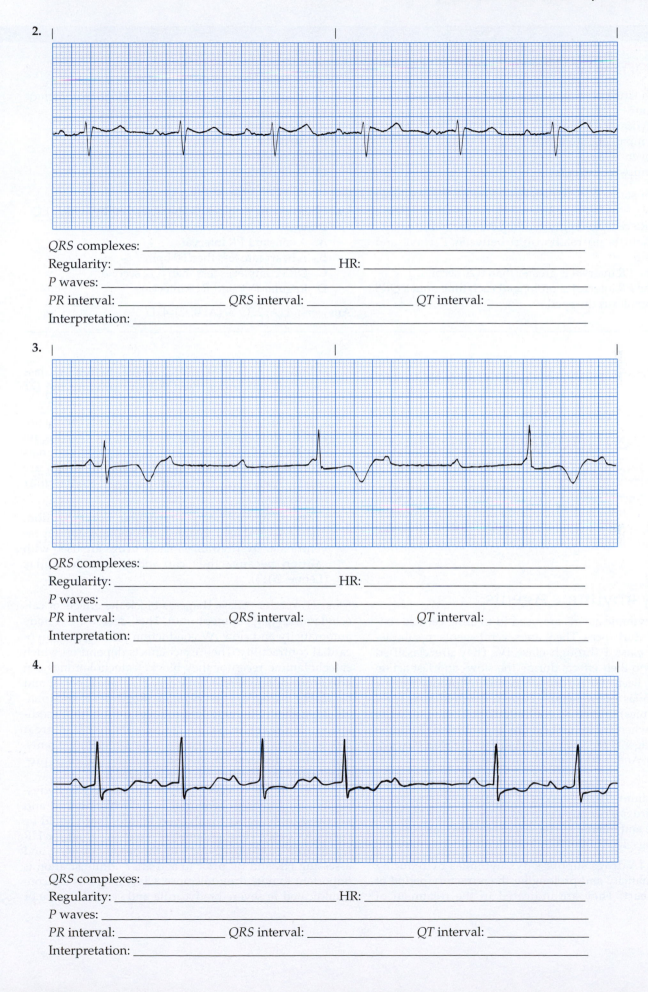

QRS complexes: _____

Regularity: _____ HR: _____

P waves: _____

PR interval: _____ QRS interval: _____ QT interval: _____

Interpretation: _____

3.

QRS complexes: _____

Regularity: _____ HR: _____

P waves: _____

PR interval: _____ QRS interval: _____ QT interval: _____

Interpretation: _____

4.

QRS complexes: _____

Regularity: _____ HR: _____

P waves: _____

PR interval: _____ QRS interval: _____ QT interval: _____

Interpretation: _____

Section Nine Review

1. Which situation may produce blocks in impulse conduction?
   A. Myocardial ischemia
   B. Sympathetic stimulation
   C. Fever
   D. Antipyretic agents

2. Which statement characterizes first-degree AV heart block?
   A. QRS complex is greater than 0.20 second.
   B. There is no relationship between P wave and QRS.
   C. The PR interval is greater than 0.20 second.
   D. The PR interval is prolonged each time until a QRS complex is dropped.

3. Treatment for second-degree heart block may include which treatments? (Select all that apply.)
   A. Pacemaker
   B. Atropine
   C. Epinephrine
   D. Defibrillation
   E. Beta-blocking agents

4. Complete heart block is characterized by which ECG change?
   A. A constant PR interval
   B. A heart rate less than 50 bpm
   C. QRS complexes less than 0.12 second
   D. Regular P–P and R–R intervals

Answers: 1. A, 2. C, 3. (A, B, C), 4. D

Section Ten: Pharmacologic and Countershock Interventions and Nursing Implications

Major treatments of cardiac dysrhythmias include a wide variety of antidysrhythmic agents and electric countershock. This section provides an overview of the four classes of antidysrhythmic agents and two types of electric countershock.

Antidysrhythmic Agents

Antidysrhythmic agents are used in treating cardiac conduction disturbances. There are several agents in subcategories of class I through class IV. They are classified according to their effects during the slow- and fast-action potentials. Each of these drugs is capable of producing new dysrhythmias or worsening current dysrhythmias (prodysrhythmics); therefore, continuous ECG monitoring is required when these medications are initiated. Antidysrhythmic agents are summarized in the "Related Pharmacotherapy: Antidysrhythmic Agents" feature.

Class I Agents   Class I antidysrhythmia drugs are known as fast sodium channel blockers. By blocking these channels, the drugs slow impulse conduction through the atria, ventricles, and bundle of His. There are three categories of class I drugs: IA, IB, and IC.

- Class IA drugs suppress dysrhythmias by reducing automaticity and prolonging the refractory period of the heart. They are indicated in the treatment of supraventricular and ventricular dysrhythmias. Class IA drugs can widen the QRS and prolong the QT intervals.

- Class IB drugs decrease refractory periods but do not affect automaticity to a great extent, thus having no significant ECG effects. In fact, repolarization is accelerated with these agents. Class IB drugs are used chiefly in the treatment of ventricular dysrhythmias.

- Class IC agents delay ventricular repolarization. They are used as a maintenance therapy for supraventricular dysrhythmias. These drugs are used with caution because they can induce dysrhythmias (Lehne, 2013).

Class II Agents   Class II agents block the effects of catecholamines (e.g., epinephrine). They decrease SA node automaticity and slow AV conduction velocity and myocardial contractility. Their exact effects depend on which catecholamine receptor they block. Catecholamines can affect four different receptors: alpha1, alpha2, beta1, and beta2. For example, phentolamine (Regitine) is an alpha-blocking agent; therefore, it produces peripheral vasodilation. However, most of the agents used to treat dysrhythmias in this category are beta-blocking agents. Thus, they decrease cardiac stimulation and may produce vasodilation and bronchoconstriction.

Drugs in this category are used in treating tachydysrhythmias. Although beneficial in reducing preload and afterload in the patient with heart failure, they should be used cautiously. Hold parameters (such as "Hold for HR less than 60") are established with the healthcare team, and assessing HR and BP prior to and after administration is important to note drug tolerance. Class II agents are contraindicated in severe bradycardia and second-degree or

Related Pharmacotherapy
Antidysrhythmic Agents

Class IA Sodium Channel Blockers

Procainamide (Procanbid), quinidine (Apo-Quinidine), disopyramide (Norpace, NAPAmide)

Action and Uses

Slow conduction and impulses in the atria, ventricles, and bundle of His

Dosages (Adult)

Procainamide: Arrhythmias—25–50 mg/min IV until arrhythmia is controlled (max. dose 1 gram). Maintenance—2–6 mg/min.

Major Side Effects

May widen QRS complex, prolong QT interval, and induce heart block

Nursing Implications

Monitor cardiac rhythm and immediately report the following: widening of QRS complex, changes in QT interval, disappearance of P waves, sudden onset of or increase in ectopic ventricular beats. Monitor blood pressure closely for hypotension.

Class IB Sodium Channel Blockers

Lidocaine (Xylocaine), mexiletine (Mexitil), phenytoin (Dilantin), tocainide (Tonocard)

Action and Uses

Suppresses automaticity in bundle of His, Purkinje fibers, and elevated electrical stimulation thresholds of ventricles during diastole

Dosages (Adult)

Lidocaine: Ventricular arrhythmias—50–100 mg IV bolus at 20–50 mg/min. Repeat in 5 minutes if needed. Max dose 300 mg/hr. Maintenance dose 1–4 mg/min.

Major Side Effects

Difficulty breathing or swallowing, convulsions, respiratory depression, neurotoxicity (drowsiness, dizziness, confusion), cardiovascular collapse

Nursing Implications

Stop infusion if ECG indicates excessive cardiac depression (prolongation of PR interval or QRS complex) and the appearance of dysrhythmias.
Monitor blood pressure and ECG continuously.
Assess respiratory and neurologic status.
Monitor serum blood levels.

Class IC Sodium Channel Blockers

Flecainide (Tambocor), propafenone (Rhymol)

Action and Uses

Slows conduction velocity throughout myocardial conduction system; increases ventricular refractoriness

Dosages (Adult)

Flecainide: Life-threatening ventricular arrhythmias—100 mg PO q 12 hrs (if needed can increase dose by 50 mg increments q 4 days); max. dose of 400 mg/day.
Propafenone: Atrial fibrillation—Extended release 225 mg PO q 12 hrs; max dose 425 mg/12 hrs.

Major Side Effects

Dizziness, nausea, dysrhythmias, chest pain; may increase digoxin levels

Nursing Implications

Correct serum potassium levels prior to administration.
Monitor serum blood levels.

Class II: Beta Blockers

Metoprolol (Toprol), atenolol (Tenormin), propranolol (Inderal), esmolol (Brevibloc), acebutolol (Sectral, Monitan)

Action and Uses

Reduces automaticity in the SA node and slows conduction in the AV node. Blocks sympathetically mediated increases in heart rate and blood pressure as the drug binds to beta1 receptors in cardiac muscle. Uses include treatment of hypertension, angina, and heart failure.

Dosages (Adult)

Metoprolol: Hypertension—50–100 mg PO/day. Also available in IV form for acute coronary syndrome treatment.

Major Side Effects

Anaphylactic reactions, severe hypotension, laryngospasm, bronchoconstriction, bradycardia

Nursing Implications

Monitor vital signs before and after administration.
Monitor for hypotension during initial titration phase and when increasing dosage.

Class III: Potassium Channel Blockers

Amiodarone (Cordarone, Pacerone), bretylium, sotalol (Betapace), ibutilide (Corvert), dofetilide (Tikosyn)

Action and Uses

Acts on cardiac tissue to prolong duration of action potential refractory period without altering the resting membrane potential. Used for treatment of life-threatening ventricular dysrhythmias, supraventricular dysrhythmias, atrial fibrillation.

Dosages (Adult)

Amiodarone: Arrhythmias—Loading dose—150 mg over 10-minute period; followed by 360 mg over next 6 hours. Maintenance dose—540 mg (0.5 mg/min) for 18 hours. After initial 24 hours may continue drug dose at 0.5 mg/min. Then convert IV to PO dosing for maintenance.

Major Side Effects

Dizziness, hypotension, bradycardia, sinus arrest, pulmonary toxicity

Nursing Implications

Correct serum potassium and magnesium levels prior to initiation of drug.
Monitor for hypotension during initial titration phase and when increasing dosage. Slow infusion if significant bradycardia or hypotension occurs.
Sustained monitoring is essential due to long half-life.

Class IV: Calcium Channels Blockers

Diltiazem (Cardizem), verapamil (Calan)

Action and Uses

Inhibits calcium transport into myocardial cells. Slows automaticity of the SA node and delays conduction in the AV node; depresses myocardial contractility. Uses include treatment of atrial dysrhythmias and hypertension.

Dosages (Adult)

Diltiazem: Atrial fibrillation or flutter—20 mg IV over 2–5 minutes; after 15 minutes, may repeat bolus. Continuous infusion: No greater than 15 mg/hr for up to 24 hr.

SOURCE: Dosages from Adams et al. (2014) and Wilson, Shannon, & Shields (2016).

Major Side Effects

Hypotension, bradycardia. Abrupt withdrawal may can precipitate angina.

Nursing Implications

Monitor for hypotension during initial titration phase and when increasing dosage.

Can elevate digoxin levels in the blood.

---

higher heart blocks. Because Class II drugs decrease the heart rate by blocking the sympathetic nervous system, the heart rate may not be able to adequately respond to situations requiring an increase in cardiac output, such as exercise, stress, or a crisis. In cases of cardiac arrest, the heart may be less sensitive to sympathomimetic drugs (e.g., epinephrine) because of the beta-blocking effect.

Class III Agents Class III agents block potassium channels, thereby delaying repolarization and prolonging the refractory period. A prolonged *QT* interval may develop and therefore should be measured routinely. Class III agents increase the fibrillation threshold, which makes the cells more resistant to ectopic stimuli. They are indicated in the treatment of atrial and ventricular dysrhythmias. Sotalol (Betapace) is an agent in this category. Amiodarone, another class III agent, is a first-line medication for ventricular tachycardia and ventricular fibrillation that is resistant to defibrillation.

Class IV Agents Class IV agents are calcium channel blockers. These drugs block the entry of calcium through the cell membranes, thereby decreasing depolarization. Automaticity in the SA node is reduced, AV node conduction is slowed, and an overall decrease in myocardial contractility is produced with Class IV agents. Verapamil and diltiazem are examples of calcium channel blockers commonly used for treating supraventricular tachydysrhythmias.

Other Agents Adenosine and digoxin do not fit within the four major classes. Both of these drugs reduce AV node automaticity and slow AV conduction. Digoxin is classified as a cardiac glycoside and inotropic agent. It can be used to treat supraventricular tachycardia, atrial fibrillation, and atrial flutter. Adenosine is classified as an antiarrhythmic and is first-line therapy to convert supraventricular tachycardia to normal sinus rhythm. It is administered rapidly, over 1 to 2 sec, as an IV bolus (Wilson, Shannon, & Shields, 2016). Adenosine has a very short half-life (approximately 10 sec) and is used to temporarily inhibit AV node conduction and block reentry of impulses from the ventricles. Consequently, the heart rate decreases significantly as the conduction of impulses through the AV node slows. An expected brief period of

asystole (up to 15 sec) is common after rapid administration. The goal is to reset the normal conduction of the heart. Side effects include facial flushing, dyspnea, and chest pressure. With adenosine use, it is important to have ACLS-trained providers present along with emergency response equipment.

Nursing Management of Patients Receiving Antidysrhythmic Agents Prior to administration of any antidysrhythmic agent, the nurse obtains the following baseline data: vital signs, ECG interpretation using the eight-step process, and a physical assessment of the cardiac, respiratory, and neurologic systems. These data are monitored during drug administration—especially in the initial phases. An infusion pump is used when the drugs are administered by the intravenous route. The patient should be instructed to report dizziness, palpitations, skin rashes, or wheezing. It must be noted that while the goal of these drugs is to suppress or convert dysrhythmias, virtually all antidysrhythmic drugs also have prodysrhythmic effects. Essentially, the drugs can worsen existing dysrhythmias and precipitate new ones.

Countershock

Countershock is the use of electric current that is delivered to the heart to reset a dysrhythmia. There are two major forms of countershock: elective cardioversion and emergency defibrillation.

Elective Cardioversion Cardioversion is a form of countershock that delivers an electrical current that is synchronized with the patient's heart rhythm. It is used to treat supraventricular tachycardia (SVT) that is resistant to medication, atrial fibrillation or atrial flutter, and ventricular tachycardia in an unstable patient. The unstable patient may have hypotension, dyspnea, or complaints of chest pain. The patient may also have symptoms suggestive of heart failure, myocardial ischemia, or infarction.

Once the patient is attached to the ECG monitor on the defibrillator, a sync button located on the defibrillator machine is pushed prior to each cardioversion attempt. This provides synchronization with, or a tracking of, the *R* wave (a dot appears above the *R* wave on the screen). This allows the machine to discharge after the *R* wave and before the downstroke of the *T* wave (during the absolute

Nursing Care
The Patient Undergoing Elective Cardioversion

Expected Patient Outcomes and Related Interventions

Outcome 1: Need for elective cardioversion confirmed

Assess and compare to established norms, patient baseline, and trends

Monitor vital signs and both mental and respiratory status to ascertain whether the patient is stable or unstable with rhythm. (Note: If patient does become unstable and time is of essence, certain steps listed below may be omitted as appropriate.)

Interventions to confirm dysrhythmia

Obtain a 12-lead ECG for further diagnosis of the rhythm.

Obtain expert consultation (if available) to confirm the rhythm and determine appropriate treatment.

Outcome 2: Optimal patient preparation for the procedure

Assess and compare to established norms, patient baseline, and trends

Assess the patient and family's knowledge of the situation and explain the dysrhythmia and need for cardioversion in understandable terms.

Interventions to confirm dysrhythmia

Fully explain the risks and benefits of the procedure to the patient and family.

Obtain informed consent as per institution policy. There is always risk of the cardioversion resulting in a more lethal rhythm, such as ventricular tachycardia or fibrillation.

Place patient on NPO status until the procedure is over to decrease the risk of aspiration.

Establish IV access—this will be used to premedicate with the administration of IV sedatives as ordered to allow for conscious sedation.

Have IV fluids readily available.

Ensure that the patient's chest is free of excess hair (clip if necessary) and any medication patches or moisture to allow for optimal conduction of the electricity while maintaining safety.

Place the patient in a supine (flat if possible) position for best access to the chest.

Have emergency equipment standing by, including oxygen (bag-valve-mask [BVM] device or 100% non-rebreather mask), suction, emergency medications, and the code cart.

Connect the patient to the ECG monitor on the defibrillator. When available, a multidisciplinary team is always the best approach for this procedure. Personnel may include nurses, physicians, anesthesiologists, and respiratory therapists.

Outcome 3: Successful cardioversion to sinus rhythm*

Assess and compare to established norms, patient baseline, and trends

Immediately preprocedure: Confirm presence of dysrhythmia or consult for expert opinion.

Following procedure: Confirm presence of corrected rhythm; take vital signs and assess neurological and respiratory status.

Interventions to perform elective cardioversion

Press the sync button on the defibrillator with *each* cardioversion attempt. This mechanism tracks and delivers the charge on the *R* wave of the *QRS*, thereby avoiding the relative refractory period.

After appropriate sedation, airway management, and applying the hands-free pads or paddles to the chest wall or thorax (Figure 9–33 for one example), the appropriate energy (joules) is selected on the defibrillator.

Just prior to the cardioversion shock delivery, the person in charge of pressing the shock button will state "All clear!" and ensure that no one is in contact with the patient or the bed to prevent accidentally shocking others.

The defibrillator will record the patient's rhythm before, during, and after the cardioversion. Document the ECG strips, amount of joules, number of attempts, and rhythm after the procedure.

If unsuccessful, repeated attempts may be made to cardiovert the rhythm.

Outcome 4: Maintains postprocedure stability

Due to the sedation, reorient the patient as needed and maintain fall precautions until sedation is metabolized.

Monitor and document the patient's pulmonary and cardiovascular status and vital signs frequently to ensure hemodynamic stability.

Continue to monitor ECG for dysrhythmias. Notify healthcare provider immediately if dysrhythmias return.

Assess the chest wall for any potential burns from the cardioversion and treat as appropriate.

Inform the patient and family of the outcome and future plan of care.

*For complete steps involved in a cardioversion, follow the guidelines for advanced cardiac life support (ACLS) and those of the defibrillator manufacturer and the institution.

---

refractory period). Synchronization is important because delivering energy during the relative refractory period may precipitate ventricular fibrillation. Generally, low voltages are delivered (less than 200 joules), depending on the dysrhythmia, patient's size, and heart's response to treatment. Cardioversion is repeated using higher voltages if it is unsuccessful at lower voltages.

Nursing Considerations. In preparation for the procedure, the nurse obtains informed consent and educates the patient as to the purpose of the cardioversion and what to expect during the procedure and afterward. Respiratory therapy may be asked to stand by should the patient require airway or breathing assistance. An ECG strip is obtained prior to and after the procedure and can be printed from the defibrillator unit. The patient may have a transesophageal echocardiogram performed prior to cardioversion to assess for clots in the atrium. IV access is also confirmed before the procedure. If hemodynamically stable, the patient is given a light sedative, or is placed under conscious (moderate) sedation, prior to treatment to minimize discomfort. Any serum electrolyte abnormalities (especially calcium, magnesium, and potassium) are reported to the provider. All metallic objects are removed from the patient. Conductive pads are placed on the chest below the right clavicle to the right of the sternum, and in the midaxillary line on the left. Pads may also be placed on the anterior and posterior chest walls.

Additional information regarding patient assessment and management can be found in the "Nursing Care: The Patient Undergoing Elective Cardioversion" feature.

After the procedure, the nurse assesses for potential complications, including an embolic event (especially cerebral), respiratory depression, skin burns, and dysrhythmias. An ECG strip should be obtained after the procedure and placed in the medical record, along with documentation of the specific joules used and treatments administered.

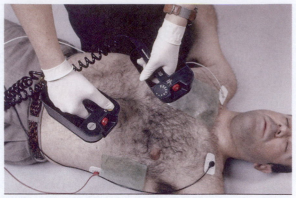

Figure 9–33 Placement of paddles for defibrillation.

Defibrillation

Defibrillation is an emergency procedure used to treat ventricular tachycardia in a pulseless patient or in ventricular fibrillation. Defibrillation is an unsynchronized electric shock that usually administers a larger number of joules (up to 360) than used in cardioversion. With defibrillation, conductive paste or gel pads are applied on the chest wall at the apex and base of the heart (Figure 9–33). Many defibrillators are also equipped with a hands-free cable and pads option. A continuous ECG recording is obtained during the procedure. The person delivering the current announces "All clear!" prior to dispensing the electrical current to ensure that no one is touching the patient or the bed. High-quality CPR and ACLS are immediately

resumed after the shock. When an IV line is available, pharmacological interventions take place. After 2 minutes or approximately five cycles of CPR, the pulse and rhythm are checked. If indicated, electric shock and pharmacological therapy are continued per guidelines.

In addition to traditional medical defibrillator devices, an automatic external defibrillator (AED) may also be used by medical and nursing service personnel, as well as laypersons, to treat ventricular tachycardia and ventricular fibrillation. Today, AED use is taught to the general public and devices can be found in many public places (airports, malls) and even purchased for personal use. The ECG pattern is detected through large patches placed on the patient's chest. If a lethal dysrhythmia is detected, the AED discharges to defibrillate the patient. Once turned on, the AED will instruct the user on its proper operation.

ECG Interpretation Exercise 7: Countershock

1.

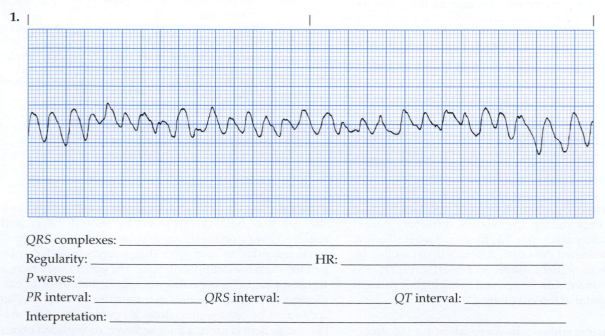

QRS complexes: _____

Regularity: _____   HR: _____

P waves: _____

PR interval: _____   QRS interval: _____   QT interval: _____

Interpretation: _____

2. What treatments, including medications, would the nurse anticipate with the above rhythm?

3.

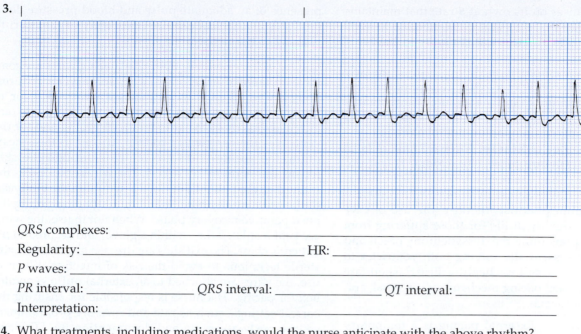

QRS complexes: _____

Regularity: _____ HR: _____

P waves: _____

PR interval: _____ QRS interval: _____ QT interval: _____

Interpretation: _____

4. What treatments, including medications, would the nurse anticipate with the above rhythm?

Section Ten Review

1. Beta blockers (class II agents) may produce which of the following side effects?
   A. Weight gain
   B. Hypokalemia
   C. Wheezing
   D. Hives

2. Which statement regarding the difference between cardioversion and defibrillation is correct?
   A. Defibrillation uses a lower amount of joules.
   B. Cardioversion is synchronized.
   C. Defibrillation cannot be repeated.
   D. Cardioversion is used only to treat atrial dysrhythmias.

3. Nursing responsibilities in administering antidysrhythmic agents include which activities? (Select all that apply.)
   A. Administering all continuous IV drips with an infusion pump
   B. Administering the drugs in 30–50 mL of IV fluid
   C. Obtaining vital signs before, during, and after administration
   D. Obtaining an ECG strip before, during, and after administration
   E. Monitoring cardiac, respiratory, and neurologic systems during administration

4. Nursing responsibilities surrounding cardioversion include which actions? (Select all that apply.)
   A. Ensuring the "sync" button is pushed prior to cardioversion
   B. Informing the client of what to expect during the procedure
   C. Obtaining an ECG recording before and after
   D. Reviewing electrolyte levels
   E. Place the client in High-Fowler position

Answers: 1. C, 2. B, 3. (A, C, D, E), 4. (A, B, C, D)

Section Eleven: Electrical Therapy

Patients with conduction disturbances may require temporary or permanent electrical therapy to maintain cardiac function through applying electrical stimulation that either acts as an artificial pacemaker or supplies intermittent corrective electrical shock to prevent sudden cardiac death.

Pacemakers

A pacemaker is a pulse generator used to provide an electrical stimulus to the heart when the heart fails to conduct or generate impulses on its own at a rate that maintains cardiac output. The pulse generator is connected to leads (wires) that provide an electrical stimulus to the heart when necessary.

Pacemakers are used in addition to drug therapy when one of three conditions exists: failure of the conduction system, failure to initiate an impulse spontaneously, or failure to maintain primary pacing control (spontaneous impulses may occur, but they are not synchronized). Another indication for pacemakers is in treatment of heart failure. Since 2001, cardiac resynchronization therapy (CRT) has been a treatment for patients suffering from left ventricular dysfunction. In combination with optimum pharmacotherapy, the use of CRT can improve the quality of life for those suffering from heart failure by preventing the dyssynchrony of left and right ventricles—essentially forcing both ventricles to beat simultaneously as in a healthy heart. There are three commonly used pacing mechanisms: external, epicardial, and endocardial.

External Pacemakers External pacing is a temporary measure. It delivers electric impulses to the myocardium transcutaneously through two electrode pads placed anteriorly, or anteriorly and posteriorly on the chest (Figure 9–34). It is important to note that during periods of hypoxia and acidosis, the myocardium is less responsive to external pacing. Because this type of pacing sends electricity through the skin and body tissue prior to affecting the myocardium, it may be a painful experience for the patient, who should be medicated accordingly. When caring for a patient receiving external pacing, the nurse notes the date and time external pacing is initiated, as well as the pacing rate, mode, and amount of current, known as milliamperes (mA), that are necessary to obtain full capture at the desired heart rate. An ECG strip is obtained and analyzed before and continuously monitored throughout this therapy. The presence of an adequate pulse and blood pressure demonstrates mechanical capture (the ability of the heart to respond to the electrical impulse).

Epicardial Pacemakers Epicardial pacing wires are commonly placed during open heart surgery procedures. They are temporary wires that are removed prior to patient discharge from the hospital. The wires are attached directly to the atria for atrial pacing and/or the ventricles for ventricular pacing. Affixed to the epicardium, the pacing wires are brought through the skin (below the sternum) for access. The wires are used in the event that the patient develops a symptomatic bradycardia or other dysrhythmia that requires pacing during the postoperative recovery phase. When not in use, the wires are kept insulated (i.e., within a glove) and secured to the patient's chest. The exit sites are dressed and treated with sterile technique to avoid the risk of infection. When in use, the wires are attached to an external pulse generator box for pacing. The nurse is responsible for ensuring the correct settings, such as rate and mA, are programmed, continuously assessing and documenting the ECG and patient response to the pacing, and changing the battery per manufacturer recommendations. Gloves should always be worn when handling epicardial pacing wires to avoid accidental microshocks to the patient (Hardin & Kaplow, 2016).

Transvenous Pacemakers Temporary transvenous pacing is achieved through electrical stimulation of the right ventricular or right atrial endocardium by an electrode-tipped catheter. Two approaches are available for placing a pacing wire: direct insertion of the pacing wire or insertion of a special pulmonary artery catheter that has an embedded pacing port. Both approaches use a central vein, often the subclavian or internal jugular, for insertion. The insertion process may be performed in an operating room, in a cardiac catheterization laboratory, or at the bedside, and it

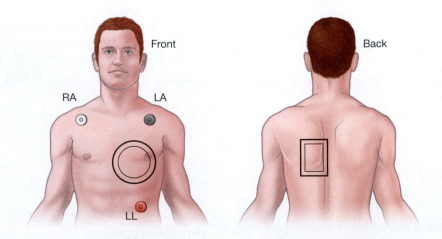

Figure 9–34 External (transcutaneous) conductor pad placement.

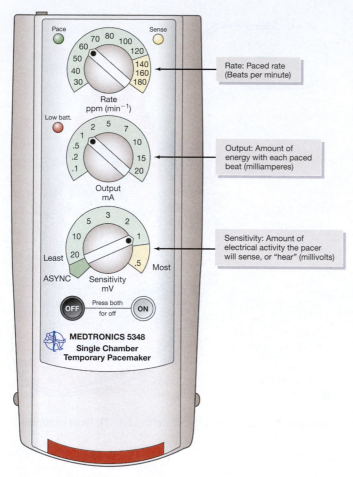

Figure 9–35 Temporary pacemaker generator.

is used as a temporary measure until the patient can, if necessary, have a permanent pacemaker placed. The insertion process is done under sterile conditions with full barrier precautions as this mimics a central venous line placement. Bedside fluoroscopy may be needed to aid in correct placement. Once placed, the lead wires are attached to an external pulse generator box (as described in epicardial pacing in the previous section) and pacing is begun (Figure 9–35). The nurse obtains an ECG rhythm strip prior to and after insertion.

When the procedure is complete, a chest x-ray is required to ensure proper placement of the lead wire in addition to ensuring that the patient did not experience complications from the central line placement (e.g., pneumothorax). Care of the transvenous pacing wire and site is performed using sterile technique as this line poses risks for bloodstream infection. As with epicardial pacing wires, gloves should be worn at all times when handling pacemaker wires to prevent microshock.

Permanent Implanted Pacemakers   Permanent pacemakers use an internal pulse generator. Placement is a planned procedure performed in the operating room or in a cardiac catheterization laboratory. This generator is typically located in a subcutaneous tissue pocket (above the muscles and ribs, below the clavicle) in the chest wall. The leads are passed transvenously into the heart and rest within the endocardium, as shown in Figure 9–36.

Endocardial pacers are usually inserted through the subclavian or jugular vein into the atria and/or ventricle(s), where they are lodged. The generator is a small, thin, sealed device that contains a battery and is programmed according to the needs of the patient (Figure 9–37).

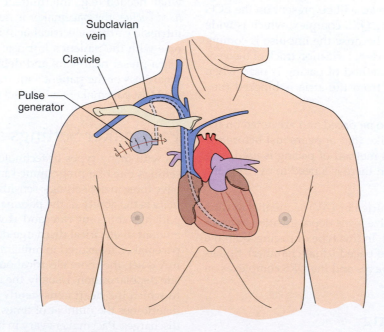

Figure 9–36 Location of permanent pacemaker.

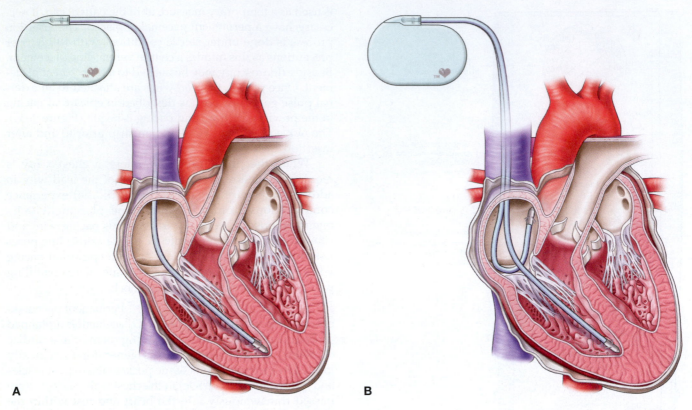

A   **B**

Figure 9–37 Permanent pacemakers, showing pulse generator and pacing catheter: **A,** Single chamber. **B,** Dual chamber.

Chambers Paced   Pacemakers have the ability to pace the atrium, the ventricle, or both (dual or AV sequential) chambers. (Refer to Figure 9–37 A and B.)

Ventricle.   Most pacemakers are designed to pace the ventricles. In this case, a spike will be present on the ECG rhythm strip just before the *QRS* complex, which is wide and bizarre in appearance because the impulse is coming from outside of the normal depolarization track of the ventricle (Figure 9–38). This method of pacing is used when transmission of impulses from the atria is blocked (i.e., complete heart block).

Atrium.   The atria can also be paced and are noted on the ECG rhythm strip as a spike that appears just before the *P* wave (Figure 9–39). This method of pacing is used with sinus node disease or when there is a need to override the intrinsic sinus rate.

Dual Chamber.   Atrioventricular (AV) sequential or dual pacing is used to synchronize heart depolarization in order to maintain cardiac output. In this type of pacing, both the atria and the ventricles are paced (dual chamber). Spikes appear before both the *P* waves and the *QRS* complexes on the ECG (Figure 9–40).

Pacemaker Sensing

Pacemakers have the capability of sensing intrinsic (heart-generated) electrical activity and may be either set on demand or fixed pacing. In *demand pacing*, the pacemaker is

able to sense intrinsic heart activity and will not generate a pacemaker impulse unless it fails to sense an intrinsic impulse within a set time interval. In this setting, the pacemaker acts as a backup system that only triggers beats when needed (e.g., intermittent bradycardia problems). In *fixed pacing*, the pacemaker is not sensitive to the patient's intrinsic cardiac electrical activity and does not synchronize with the patient's intrinsic impulses. The pacemaker has a preset heart rate and delivers impulses at that rate regardless of the patient's intrinsic cardiac electrical activity. Most pacemakers will be set on demand pacing.

Pacemaker Settings and Modes

As with many types of technology-based devices, desired settings must be programmed into the device. Pacemakers have three major settings: sensitivity, output, and rate. *Sensitivity* is the ability of the pacemaker sensor to recognize the patient's inherent rate and rhythm. *Output* is the small amount of electrical discharge delivered to the heart by the pacemaker, measured in milliamperes (mA). The higher the mA is set, the more electrical output is delivered to stimulate depolarization. Usually, the mA is set at the lowest level to which the heart consistently responds. The *rate* setting determines the number of times per minute the pacemaker discharges. Pacemakers vary in how they respond to electrical events in the heart. There are three major modes in which pacemakers are described: chamber(s) paced, chamber(s) sensed, and the response to sensing.

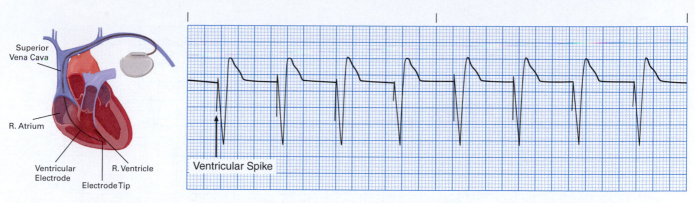

Figure 9–38 Ventricular pacemaker spikes occur before the *QRS*.

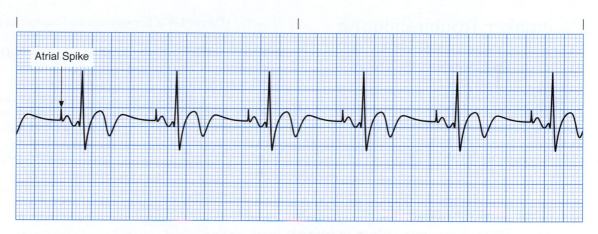

Figure 9–39 Atrial pacemaker spikes occur before the *P* wave.

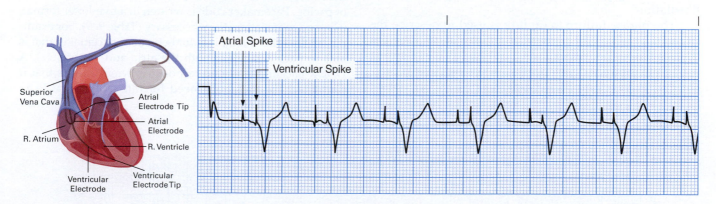

Figure 9–40 AV sequential pacing: Both atria and ventricles are paced.

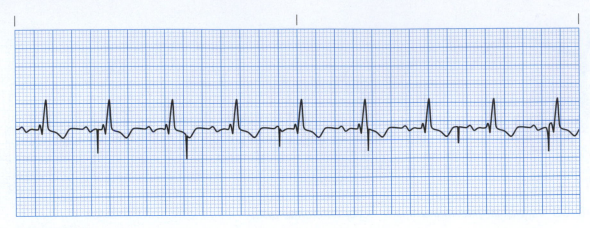

Figure 9–41 Failure to sense.

Pacemaker Troubleshooting

The number of times the pacemaker fires is determined by the sensitivity setting of the pacemaker. If the sensitivity is too low, the pacemaker may not sense the patient's own cardiac electrical activity and will pace more frequently. At a higher sensitivity level, the pacemaker is better able to sense the patient's own cardiac electrical activity and is inhibited from firing, thus avoiding competing with the patient's own intrinsic rate. Most pacemakers are set on demand, with a high-sensitivity setting.

If the pacemaker does compete with or does not recognize the patient's own impulse generation (i.e., his own heart rhythm), the term **failure to sense** is used (Figure 9–41). This is a potentially dangerous situation because the pacemaker can discharge an impulse during the relative refractory or supranormal periods of ventricular repolarization, precipitating ventricular fibrillation.

The phrase **failure to capture** is used to describe the situation in which the pacemaker initiates an impulse but the heart does not respond or the stimulus is not strong enough to produce depolarization. A pacing spike is present, but P waves or QRS complexes or both are absent (Figure 9–42). For sensing and capturing to occur, the pulse generator must have adequate battery function, the leads must be firmly attached to the pacemaker and the endocardium, and the lead wires must be intact with a high enough mA output.

Failure to fire occurs when a pacemaker fails to send out an electrical impulse at the appointed time. Common causes are a loose pacemaker wire connection and a dead pacemaker battery. The lack of a visible pacemaker spike followed by a pause will be noted on the cardiac monitor. Failure to fire can be intermittent or sustained; and if sustained, the ECG will show a reversion to the patient's underlying rhythm.

Pacemaker Classification

Pacemakers are classified according to a uniform system that is universally used to describe how the device functions according to where the pacing leads are and the mode of pacing. Pacemaker code is written in a five-letter format, using no more letters than necessary (Table 9–9). For example, a DDD pacemaker is a dual-chamber pacemaker that is able to pace and sense both the atria and ventricle(s). A DDDR pacemaker is rate responsive, which means that it can detect the metabolic need for rate adjustment (e.g.,

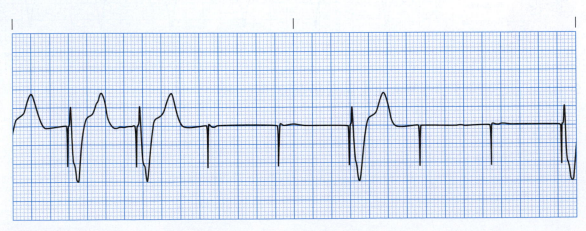

Figure 9–42 Failure to capture.

Table 9–9 Generic Pacemaker Code

Chamber Paced (First Letter)	Chamber Sensed (Second Letter)	Pacemaker Response (Third Letter)	Programmable Functions (Fourth Letter)	Antitachycardia Functions (Fifth Letter)
A = Atrium	Atrium	Triggered	Programmable/multiprogrammable	Pacing
V = Ventricle	Ventricle	Inhibited	Rate responsive	Shock
D = Dual	Dual	Dual	Communication	Dual
O = None	None	None	None	None

SOURCE: Adapted from Bernstein et al., 2002.

during exercise) and adjust accordingly if the native pacemaker fails to achieve this rate.

Implantable Cardioverter-defibrillator

An implantable cardioverter-defibrillator (ICD), sometimes called an automated implantable cardioverter-defibrillator (AICD), is placed in patients who have had prior aborted sudden cardiac death or proven sustained ventricular tachycardia. It also may be placed prophylactically in high-risk groups, such as those with various forms of cardiomyopathy. The device is a fully implantable, battery-operated system designed to recognize and terminate ventricular tachyarrhythmias that can cause sudden death. Pacemaker capabilities may also be included in the ICD.

ICDs are capable of distinguishing ventricular tachycardia (VT) from ventricular fibrillation (VFib) (thus delivering defibrillation shocks only when absolutely necessary); antitachycardia pacing (to treat VT without resorting to cardioversion shocks unless necessary); providing backup bradycardia pacing (eliminating the need for a standard pacemaker); and storing cardiac events so that they can be retrieved for analyzing the patient's response to treatment. Generator longevity depends on how often the device's features are used but typically lasts 5 to 10 years.

Implantation of the ICD is accomplished percutaneously through the subclavian or cephalic vein. The lead is positioned in the heart transvenously, and the generator is implanted subcutaneously in the upper chest. Once in place the device is programmed and tested using electrophysiologic studies. In essence, VFib is intentionally induced in a controlled environment. The ICD is set to deliver shocks at the joules and rate necessary to convert the VFib to a sinus rhythm.

If the ICD malfunctions, it may be necessary to deactivate the device by applying a special magnet over the ICD. The nurse must be familiar with the correct procedure for deactivating the device. If the ICD malfunctions, or if the heart does not respond to shocks delivered, life-support measures are initiated. During cardiopulmonary resuscitation (CPR), the rescuer may feel a mild shock (similar to a static electricity shock) if the device fires. External defibrillation is performed as described in Section Ten. However, one should avoid placing the paddles over the actual ICD device. Patients who need an ICD require extensive training and must understand the difference between heart attack and cardiac arrest. The ICD does not prevent a myocardial infarction, but it does attempt to prevent cardiac arrest.

Patient Education   The patient is taught that the ICD can "reorganize" the heart rhythm as well as stimulate the heart (if the pacemaker action is available). Patients should be prepared for what to experience with an internal shock and how to react when the ICD is preparing to shock (e.g., pull over if driving, sit down). Patients are encouraged to keep a diary of shocks received, activities before and after treatment, symptoms, and response after shock. They should contact their cardiologist when they receive a shock.

Patients with ICDs must understand and adhere to certain restrictions and limitations. For example, individuals may be restricted from driving in some states. Patients should avoid strong electromagnetic fields and are advised to consult their provider prior to having an MRI. The ICD may be temporarily reprogrammed for the MRI procedure to avoid inappropriate sensing. Arc welders and large industrial motors should be avoided. Some cellular phones can interfere with the operation of defibrillators if held closer than 6 inches from the pulse generator; therefore, patients are encouraged to use cell phones on the ear opposite their ICD.

Electrical Therapy Nursing Considerations

Caring for a patient with a pacemaker or ICD requires specialized nursing care, including preparing the patient for insertion of an endocardial pacemaker or applying and using an external pacing device correctly. In hospital units where pacing is more common (e.g. cardiac care units), nursing competencies will likely include pacemaker training. During pacemaker therapy, the patient's ECG pattern is monitored to determine if the pacemaker is pacing at the correct rate (demand versus fixed), capturing with each impulse, and sensing the patient's own rhythm. In addition, the nurse assesses the threshold (minimal amount of output required to initiate depolarization) of the pacemaker. The learner is referred to the literature associated with each pacing and defibrillation device to determine the correct method of checking the threshold for that device. It is helpful if patients with histories of dysrhythmias carry copies of their most recent ECGs. Patients are encouraged to carry the device information card in their wallet or wear a medical alert bracelet to identify themselves as having pacemakers or ICDs. The type of device, manufacturer, and model number should be readily available to healthcare providers.

ECG Interpretation Exercise 8: Pacemakers

Directions: In the ECG rhythm strips below, identify the pacemaker malfunction, if any.

1.

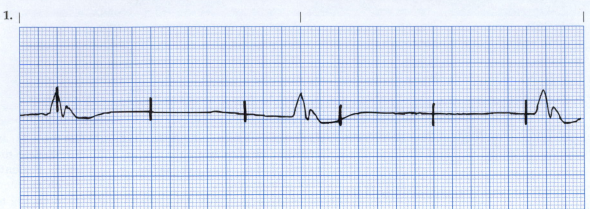

This client has a _____ pacemaker set at a rate of _____ bpm.

Interpretation: _____

2.

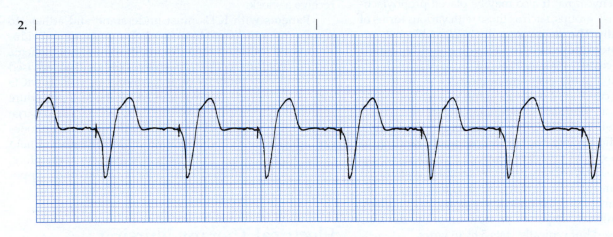

This client has a _____ pacemaker set at a rate of _____ bpm.

Interpretation: _____

3.

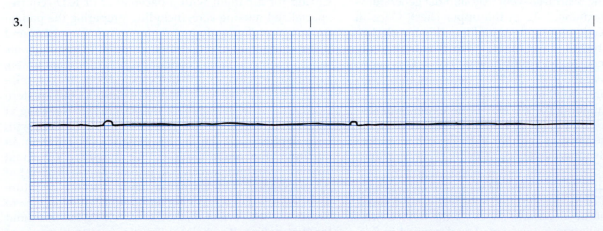

This client has a _____ pacemaker set at a rate of _____ bpm.

Interpretation: _____

Section Eleven Review

1. Which statement correctly describes an epicardial pacing device?
   A. It is placed through the subclavian vein.
   B. It is applied to the chest wall.
   C. It is inserted in open heart surgery.
   D. It is used exclusively for AV sequential pacing.

2. *Failure to sense* means which situation exists?
   A. The pacing device is turned off.
   B. Depolarization is not occurring.
   C. The client is tachycardic.
   D. The pacing device is competing with the client's own rhythm.

3. The phrase *failure to capture* refers to which situation?
   A. Depolarization does not occur after a pacer-generated impulse.
   B. Atria and ventricles are not contracting in a synchronous manner.
   C. The pacing device needs to be replaced.
   D. The client will require cardioversion.

4. When should clients with an ICD device contact their healthcare provider?
   A. When they get the flu
   B. When they have a fever
   C. When they go out of the country
   D. When they receive a shock

Answers: 1. C, 2. D, 3. D, 4. D

Clinical Reasoning Checkpoint

A 72-year-old male patient develops an irregular heart rhythm accompanied by dizziness and nausea and tells his wife that his heart is "just not working right." His skin is unusually cool and pale. His wife assists him to their vehicle and drives him to the local ED. On admission, the nurse obtains the rhythm strip below.

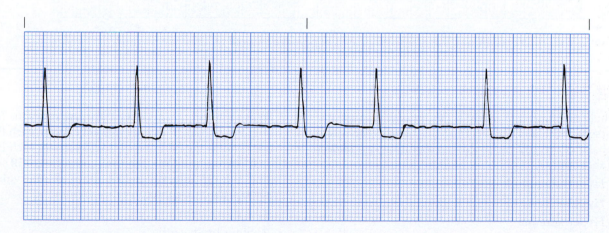

1. What is this rhythm?
2. How does this rhythm affect the patient's cardiac output and vital signs?
3. What interventions and medications would you anticipate being ordered for this dysrhythmia?

Clinical Update: The patient is admitted to the coronary care unit. Three hours later, the monitor alarm indicates the following rhythm.

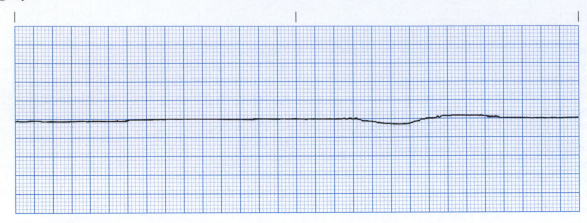

4. Identify this rhythm.

5. What interventions and medications would you anticipate being ordered for this dysrhythmia?

Clinical Update: The patient is successfully resuscitated, and a pacemaker is inserted. A few hours later the following rhythm was noted.

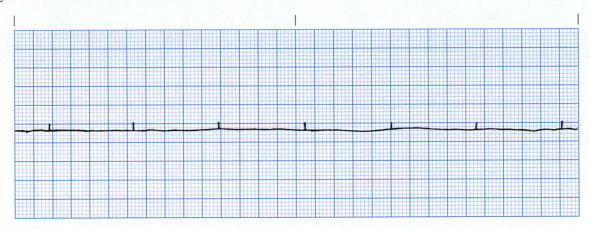

6. What is your interpretation of this strip? What are the possible causes?

Chapter 9 Review

1. When evaluating a client's laboratory results, the nurse is particularly concerned that which electrolyte imbalances would cause rhythm disturbances? (Select all that apply.)

   1. Hyperkalemia
   2. Hypokalemia
   3. Hypernatremia
   4. Hyponatremia
   5. Hypermagnesemia

2. The nurse should intervene if which finding is observed on the cardiac monitor? (Select all that apply.)

   1. *R–R* intervals are regular.
   2. *PR* interval is 0.30 second.
   3. *P* waves precede *QRS* complexes.
   4. *QRS* interval is 0.20 second.
   5. The *ST* segment is on the isoelectric line.

3. When interpreting an ECG, the nurse notes the following: HR 75 bpm, *R–R* intervals are regular, each *P* wave looks alike, the *PR* interval is 0.15 second, each *P* wave is followed by a *QRS*, the *QRS* complex is 0.10 second, and the *QT* interval is half the *R–R* interval. How should the nurse interpret this rhythm?

   1. A dysrhythmia
   2. Sinus bradycardia
   3. Normal sinus rhythm
   4. Heart block

4. A clients's morning potassium is 2 mEq/L. As a result, the nurse increases surveillance for which situation?

   1. Decreased fluid volume
   2. Malnutrition
   3. A decrease in cardiac output
   4. Decreased urine output

5. A client has sinus bradycardia. The nurse would intervene if the client developed which findings related to this diagnosis? (Select all that apply.)
   1. Dizziness
   2. Hypotension
   3. Angina
   4. Fever
   5. A heart rate of 60

6. A client in the emergency department has been diagnosed with atrial fibrillation. His vital signs are stable, but he reports that he has felt these "palpitations" in his chest for over two weeks. The nurse would discuss which topics with the client before he is discharged home? (Select all that apply.)
   1. The purposes and use of anticoagulation
   2. Discussion of need for immediate cardioversion
   3. Possible side effects of beta-blocking agents
   4. Signs and symptoms of stroke and pulmonary embolism
   5. Dietary restrictions when taking potassium supplements

7. A client develops a dysrhythmia. The rate is 50 bpm and the P waves are inverted. The PR interval is 0.10 second. QRS complex is normal. What nursing measure is essential for this client?
   1. Assess for symptoms of decreased cardiac output.
   2. Call the code team.
   3. Prepare the client for cardioversion.
   4. Ask the client to cough or bear down.

8. A client is having frequent episodes of a dysrhythmia. There are three PVC in a row with a rate of 110. There are no identifiable P waves, the R–R interval is regular, and the QRS complex is 0.20 second. How would the nurse interpret this rhythm?
   1. Bigeminy
   2. Trigeminy
   3. Ventricular tachycardia
   4. Ventricular fibrillation

9. The client's ECG strip reveals a rate of 80 bpm, P waves preceding every QRS, a QRS following each P wave, a PR interval of 0.28 second, and a QRS of 0.08 second. How should the nurse interpret this rhythm?
   1. Normal sinus rhythm
   2. First-degree AV block
   3. Type I second-degree block
   4. Left bundle branch block

10. A client has an ICD inserted. Which information is most important for the nurse to provide to this client?
   1. There are no driving restrictions.
   2. Magnetic fields will not interfere with the device.
   3. Cellular phones will not interfere with the device's operation.
   4. The client should wear a medical alert bracelet.

Answers to questions found inside your textbook are available on the faculty resources site. Please consult with your instructor.

References

Adams, M. P., Holland, L. N., & Urban, C. Q. (2014). *Pharmacology for nurses: A pathophysiologic approach* (4th ed.). Upper Saddle River, NJ: Prentice Hall.

Beasley, B. M. (2014). *Understanding EKGs: A practical approach* (4th ed.). Upper Saddle River, NJ: Pearson Brady.

Bernstein, A. D., Daubert, J. C., Fletcher, R. D., Hayes, D. L., Lüderitz, B., Reynolds, D. W., . . . Sutton, R. (2002). The revised NASPE/BPEG generic code for antibradycardia, adaptive-rate, and multisite pacing. North American Society of Pacing and Electrophysiology/British Pacing and Electrophysiology Group. *Pacing & Clinical Electrophysiology, 25*(2), 260–264.

Davies, A., & Scott, A. (2015). Conduction blocks and cardiac pacing. In A. Davies & A. Scott (Eds.), *Starting to read ECGs: A comprehensive guide to theory and practice* (pp. 81–105). London, UK: Springer.

Dawson, E. A., Gupta, P. K., Madden, D. J., Pacheco, J., & Olson, D. M. (2015). Arrhythmias in the epilepsy monitoring unit: Watching for sudden unexpected death in epilepsy. *Journal of Neuroscience Nursing, 47*(3), 131–134.

Gupta, S., Tiruvoipati, R., & Green, C. (2015). Atrial fibrillation and mortality in critically ill patients: A retrospective study. *American Journal of Critical Care, 24*(4), 336–341.

Hall, J. E. (2016). Cardiac arrhythmias and their electrocardiographic interpretation. In A. C. Guyton & J. E. Hall (Eds.), *Textbook of medical physiology* (13th ed., pp. 155–166). Philadelphia, PA: Elsevier Saunders.

Hardin, S. R., & Kaplow, R. (2016). *Cardiac surgery essentials for critical care nursing* (2nd ed.) Sudbury, MA: Jones & Bartlett Publishers.

Jang, J. L., & Cheng, S. (2014). Fluid and electrolyte management. In A. Hirbe, A. Rosenstock, H. Otepka, H. Godara, & M. Nassif (Eds.), *The Washington manual of medical therapeutics* (34th ed., pp. 400–441). Philadelphia, PA: Wolters Kluwer Health | Lippincott Williams & Wilkins.

Kee, J. L. (2014). *Laboratory and diagnostic tests with nursing implications* (9th ed.). Upper Saddle River, NJ: Pearson.

Lehne, R. A. (2013). *Pharmacology for nursing care* (8th ed.). St. Louis, MO: Elsevier Saunders.

Link, M. S., Berkow, L. C., Kudenchuk, P. J., Halperin, H. R., Hess, E. P., Moitra, V. K., . . . Donnino, M. W. (2015). Part 7: Adult advanced cardiovascular life support: 2015 American Heart Association guidelines update for cardiopulmonary resuscitation and emergency cardiovascular care. *Circulation*, *132*(18 suppl 2), S444–S464.

Manolis, A. (2016, February 15). *Ventricular premature beats.* Retrieved December 19, 2016, from http://www.uptodate.com/contents/ventricular-premature-beats

Osborn, K. S., Wraa, C. E., Watson, A. B., & Holleran, R. S. (2014). *Medical-surgical nursing preparation for practice* (2nd ed.). Upper Saddle River, NJ: Pearson.

Pozner, C. N. (2015, June). *Advanced cardiac life support (ACLS) in adults.* Retrieved December 19, 2016, from http://www.uptodate.com/contents/advanced-cardiac-life-support-acls-in-adults

Prats-Boluda, G., Ye-Lin, Y., Bueno Barrachina, J. M., Senent, E., Rodriguez de Sanabria, R., & Garcia-Casado, J. (2015). Development of a portable wireless system for bipolar concentric ECG recording. *Measurement Science and Technology*, *26*. doi:10.1088/0957-0233/26/7/075102

Rosenthal, L. (2015, December 30). *Atrial flutter treatment and management.* Retrieved December 19, 2016, from http://emedicine.medscape.com/article/151210-treatment

Sendelbach, S., Wahl, S., Anthony, A., & Shotts, P. (2015). Stop the noise: A quality improvement project to decrease electrocardiographic nuisance alarms. *Critical Care Nurse*, *35*(4), 15–23.

Wang, Y., Doleschel, S., Wunderlich, R., & Heinen, S. (2014). A wearable wireless ECG monitoring system with dynamic transmission power control for long-term homecare. *Journal of Medical Systems*, *39*(35). doi:10.1007/s10916-015-0223-5

Wilson, B. A., Shannon, M. T., & Shields, K. M. (2016). *Pearson nurse's drug guide 2016.* Hoboken, NJ: Pearson Education, Inc.

Chapter 10
Complex Wound Management

Learning Outcomes

10.1 Describe the anatomic structures and functions of the skin and the effects of wounds on skin integrity.

10.2 Explain wound physiology, including the physiologic events that occur in each phase of wound repair and the methods of wound closure.

10.3 Discuss physiologic and environmental factors that affect wound healing.

10.4 Identify the common clinical assessments used to evaluate wound healing.

10.5 Discuss treatment modalities used in wound management and their rationale.

10.6 Explain wound infections, including conditions that predispose a patient to developing an infection, diagnostic criteria, and treatment interventions.

10.7 Describe necrotizing soft-tissue infections, including pathophysiology, signs and symptoms, risk factors, and treatment strategies for necrotizing fasciitis and Fournier gangrene.

10.8 Discuss enterocutaneous fistula, including pathophysiology, risk factors, clinical presentation, and collaborative management.

10.9 Review pressure ulcers, including etiology, risk factors, assessment tools, and collaborative management.

The high-acuity patient is at increased risk for developing interruptions of skin integrity for multiple reasons, such as prolonged immobility, malnutrition, decreased immune system functioning, multiple organ failure, and increased susceptibility to infection. This chapter focuses on severe insults to the integumentary system and complex wound management. Acute burn injury is presented as a stand-alone topic in Chapter 36.

Section One: Anatomy and Physiology of the Skin and Effects of Wounds

The skin (or integument) is a tough membrane covering the entire body surface and is the largest organ of the body. It provides vital protection from the external environment and helps maintain homeostasis within the internal environment (Kent & Wraa, 2013). Wounds to the skin disrupt skin integrity, thereby interfering with protective and homeostatic functions. This section presents a brief review of the anatomy and physiology of the skin and an introduction to wounds.

Normal Skin Anatomy

Skin is composed of two layers of tissue: the epidermis and the dermis (Figure 10–1). Commonly, the subcutaneous tissue is named as the third layer of the skin. The skin is a complex organ, and its importance is often overlooked. In the high-acuity patient, however, the skin, maintenance of its integrity, and preservation of its function are imperative.

The **epidermis**, the avascular outermost layer, is composed of stratified squamous epithelial cells and is divided into five sublayers, called stratum. Each stratum contains specific structures that synergistically work together to maintain the skin integrity and preserve its function.

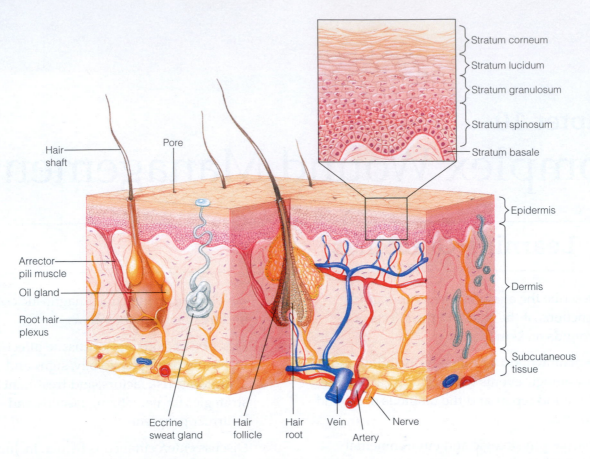

Figure 10–1 Anatomy of the skin. The skin is composed of two layers of tissue: the epidermis and dermis. Subcutaneous tissue is located at the base of the dermis (hypodermis).

Important cells in these layers include the melanocyte (pigmentation of skin) and the Langerhans cells (skin immune system). The epidermal epithelium is constantly being shed or worn away (epidermal renewal), with turnover time ranging from 26 to 42 days. Complete epidermal renewal takes about 2 months (Wysocki, 2016).

The innermost layer of skin is the **dermis**, the thickest tissue layer of the skin. It provides support to the epidermis and is made up of two major proteins (elastin and collagen) that provide elasticity and strength to the skin. Fibroblasts are the primary cells in the dermis; however, it also contains mast cells, macrophages, and lymphocytes. The dermis contains the dermal appendages of the skin—hair follicles and the sebaceous and sweat glands. It is vascularized and innervated, projecting capillaries into the epidermis to deliver nutrients and oxygen to the epidermal layer (Wysocki, 2016).

The dermal vasculature provides nutritional support, immune surveillance, wound healing, thermal regulation, hemostasis, and the inflammatory response. Dermal nerve endings respond to cold, heat, touch, pain, and pressure, serving an important protective and sensing function (Wysocki, 2016).

The epidermis and dermis are two distinct layers that share the basement membrane zone (BMZ), which is the interface between the two layers. The BMZ allows communication between different cell types and contains collagen. It is the area affected with blister formation, mechanical trauma, and full-thickness wounds (Wysocki, 2016).

The **hypodermis** is a subcutaneous layer below the dermis that consists of adipose tissue and blood vessels. It is not physiologically a true skin layer but is called the *cutis* or *subcutaneous tissue*. The hypodermis attaches the dermis to underlying structures and provides the body with structure and support, energy, cushioning, insulation, and skin mobility (James, Berger, & Elston, 2016; Wysocki, 2016). Some structures, such as the hair follicles and sweat glands, extend into this layer (Wysocki, 2016).

Skin functions differently across the lifespan. Infants, especially premature infants, have the most permeable skin, which increases their risk for hypothermia and toxicity from some topical agents. Adults with normal skin have less permeable skin, while older adults have increasing permeability and friability of their skin, which places them at greater risk for skin injuries and complications as a result of deteriorating functionality in their integument (Wysocki, 2016).

Wounds: A Disruption of Skin Functions

A wound creates an alteration and disruption of the anatomic and physiologic functions of the skin. A wound can be created intentionally, as with a surgeon's knife; by accidental trauma, such as occurs in a motor vehicle crash; or by mechanical forces, as with pressure ulcer formation or in friction and shear wounds. It is important for the nurse to know the normal structures of the skin as this knowledge aids in determining the extent of tissue involvement in an open wound. The extent of tissue involvement in most wounds is typically classified as partial thickness or full thickness. An exception to this simple classification system is the more complex staging system used specifically to describe pressure ulcer injury.

A **partial-thickness wound** involves only partial loss of the skin layers; it is confined to the epidermal and part of the dermal layers. Partial-thickness wounds are shallow, approximately 0.2 cm in depth (Doughty & Sparks, 2016).

They are painful as a result of nerve-ending exposure. A stage II pressure ulcer is an example of a partial-thickness wound.

A **full-thickness wound** involves total loss of both the epidermis and the dermis and often of deeper tissue layers such as subcutaneous tissue, muscle, or bone. These wounds extend to at least the subcutaneous tissue. A stage III or IV pressure ulcer is an example of a full-thickness wound. The time frame for repair and the repair process itself vary greatly for partial-thickness and full-thickness wounds (Doughty & Sparks, 2016).

Section One Review

1. The components of the dermis include which structures? (Select all that apply.)
   A. Epithelial cells, subcutaneous tissue
   B. Adipose tissue, subcutaneous tissue
   C. Sweat and sebaceous glands
   D. Fibroblasts and blood vessels
   E. Mast cells and hair follicles

2. What are the functions of the hypodermis? (Select all that apply.)
   A. Providing energy
   B. Providing cushioning
   C. Providing insulation
   D. Storing water
   E. Allowing for skin mobility

3. A stage II pressure ulcer is an example of which type of wound?
   A. Superficial
   B. Partial thickness
   C. Full thickness
   D. Superficial full thickness

4. Full-thickness wounds extend to at least which layer of skin?
   A. Epidermis
   B. Dermis
   C. Subcutaneous
   D. Muscle

Answers: 1. (**C**, D, E), 2. (A, B, C, E), 3. B, 4. C

Section Two: Wound Physiology

Acute wounds occur suddenly and progress rapidly through a predictable series of repair events that result in wound closure. Acute wounds are usually a consequence of a traumatic injury or surgery. In contrast, chronic wounds fail to proceed through an orderly and timely repair process, resulting in lengthy closure or failure to close. Chronic wounds are complex and may be characterized by vascular compromise, prolonged or chronic inflammation, cells that have ceased to properly function, or repetitive injury to an existing wound or ulcer (Doughty & Sparks, 2016; Holloway, Harding, Stechmiller, & Schultz, 2016). The ability to repair tissue damage is important to survival. When injured, the body immediately begins the process of restoring the integrity and physiologic functions of the tissue. A basic understanding of the wound repair process and wound closure helps the nurse to assess, diagnose, plan, and evaluate nursing interventions for the patient with altered skin integrity.

Phases of Wound Repair

From the moment of injury, overlapping physiologic processes work to restore a protective barrier. Wound repair occurs by one of two mechanisms: regeneration or scar formation. Partial-thickness wounds heal by regeneration, or replacement of the damaged tissue with healthy tissue. Epidermal cells from the epidermal appendages are the source of new epithelium. Full-thickness wounds heal by scar formation, or replacement of lost tissue with connective tissue that lacks some of the properties of the original tissue.

There are three phases of wound repair (also called the wound-healing cascade): inflammation, proliferation or repair, and remodeling or maturation. Normal repair is complex and depends on the cells involved in one phase to produce the chemical stimuli and substances important in progressing to the next phase (Doughty & Sparks, 2016; Holloway et al., 2016).

Inflammation Phase   The inflammatory phase occurs immediately after injury and lasts about 3 days. This is a critical phase because the wound environment is being prepared for subsequent tissue development. The major events that occur in this phase are **hemostasis** (i.e., control of bleeding) and the removal of cellular debris and bacteria (Holloway et al., 2016).

Immediately upon injury, vascular and cellular events are initiated. Thromboplastin is released from injured cells that activate the clotting cascade. Platelets aggregate at the injury site to form a plug and seal the break in the vessel wall. The platelets also liberate growth factors that are

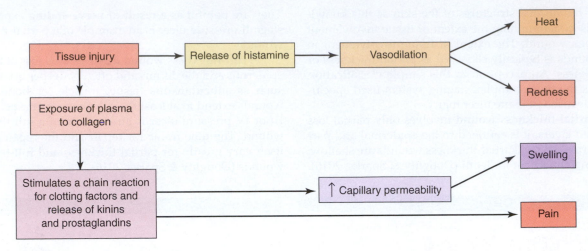

Figure 10–2 Basic inflammatory response. There are four cardinal signs of inflammation: heat, redness, swelling, and pain.

essential in tissue development during the subsequent phase of healing (e.g., platelet-derived growth factor, epidermal growth factor). A great deal of interest currently revolves around the activities of these factors and immune-regulatory and pro-inflammatory cytokines that influence tissue-level cellular response in the healing process.

Once hemostasis is achieved, the blood vessels dilate to bring needed nutrients, chemicals, and white blood cells (WBCs) to the injured area. WBCs quickly adhere to the endothelium (layer of tissue lining the blood vessels) and begin to control any bacterial contamination of the wound. Macrophages appear and engulf bacteria and remove dead tissue (Holloway et al., 2016). The chemical and vascular events during this phase of wound repair produce the four cardinal signs of inflammation: heat, redness, swelling, and pain (Holloway et al., 2016) (Figure 10–2). An example of a wound in the inflammatory phase of wound repair is shown in Figure 10–3.

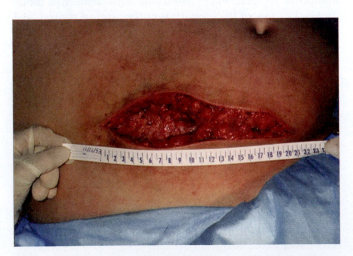

Figure 10–3 A new full-thickness surgical wound left open for secondary intention in the normal inflammatory phase of healing.

SOURCE: Kathy Cisney

The inflammatory phase is essential to the wound healing process. The absence of an inflammatory response to injury, as may happen in the immunosuppressed patient, impairs wound healing. Prolonged inflammation due to wound infection also impairs wound healing. In both cases the usual wound processes from the inflammatory phase to the proliferation phase of wound repair are altered or halted.

Proliferation or Repair Phase The **proliferative phase** begins about 3 days after injury and continues for several weeks. The major processes that occur during this phase are focused on building new tissue to fill the wound space and restoring a functional barrier. The key cell during this phase is the fibroblast. Fibroblasts arrive at day 3 postinjury and peak around the 7th day (Holloway et al., 2016). Fibroblasts produce glycosaminoglycans (hyaluronic acid), proteoglycans, and collagen, the main extracellular substances in granulation tissue (Holloway et al., 2016). The major events during this phase are angiogenesis, epithelialization, collagen formation, granulation tissue formation, and contraction.

Angiogenesis. **Angiogenesis** is the formation of new blood vessels to reestablish perfusion to the wound bed. The process is driven by growth factors, cytokines, and the hypoxic gradient from within healthy tissue near the wound to the center of the wound. The new vessels actually originate as capillaries and form a matrix in the wound bed. These vessels grow until they meet another capillary, and then they begin a connection process that allows blood to circulate and new cells to grow (Holloway et al., 2016).

Epithelialization. **Epithelialization** involves the migration of epithelial cells across a wound's surface. The cells rapidly undergo mitotic divisions and migrate along fibrin strands to reestablish layers of epithelium to cover the defect. A moist environment enhances epithelialization. Debris or bacteria on the surface inhibit both the spread of epithelial cells and the healing process. Epithelialization serves to provide a barrier against the external environment and further bacterial invasion.

Collagen Formation. The proliferative phase provides strength to the healing wound. Fibroblasts produce **collagen**, the major component of new connective tissue. Fluid collections, hematomas, dead tissue, and foreign materials act as physical barriers that prevent fibroblast penetration. Therefore, one of the primary goals of wound management is the removal of these materials. The wound space fills with fiber bundles, which enlarge and form a dense collagenous structure that binds the tissues firmly together.

As the population of fibroblasts decreases, collagen fibers become dominant in the wound. Collagen cross-linking provides tensile strength to the wound. The synthesis of collagen requires several nutrients and minerals. Thus, the nutritional status of the patient becomes very important during wound healing. This is discussed in greater detail in Section Three.

Granulation Tissue Formation. Early **granulation tissue** arises from the previously described provisional matrix characterized by unstructured collagen and high amounts of fibronectin. The vascular endothelium proliferates, and a great deal of capillary budding appears. These buds give the new granulation tissue its characteristic pink–red color. Granulation tissue formation is affected by perfusion, oxygen, nutrition, and glucose levels (Doughty & Sparks, 2016).

Contraction. As new granulation tissue is formed, the wound margins begin to contract or pull together toward the center of the wound, and the surface area of the wound decreases. This process is known as **contraction**. Specialized fibroblasts (myofibroblasts) exert tractional forces on the matrix, reducing wound size (Doughty & Sparks, 2016).

Remodeling or Maturation Phase Usually by the third week after a disruption in skin integrity, the remodeling or maturation phase begins. The **remodeling phase** or **maturation phase** is the final repair process, and it continues beyond 1 year (Doughty & Sparks, 2016). Major events of this final phase include increased collagen reorganization and increased tensile strength. The final product of all the events that occur during full-thickness wound healing is the scar, which has covered the defect and restored the protective barrier against the external environment. Factors affecting the final appearance of the scar include wound tension, body location, and wound closure technique. Around day 21, the wound only demonstrates 20% of the tensile strength of any intact dermis. Even when the wound is completely healed, only about 70% to 80% of the tensile strength of normal skin is regained at 18 months post wounding, and the patient is at risk for recurrent breakdown (Doughty & Sparks, 2016; Holloway et al., 2016).

Classifications of Wound Closure

Wound closure is classified as primary, secondary, or tertiary intention (Figure 10–4). The rate of wound healing depends on the method used to close the wound, which in turn depends on the amount of tissue damage or loss and the potential for wound infection. Successful wound healing requires a cascade of events and a series of physiologic

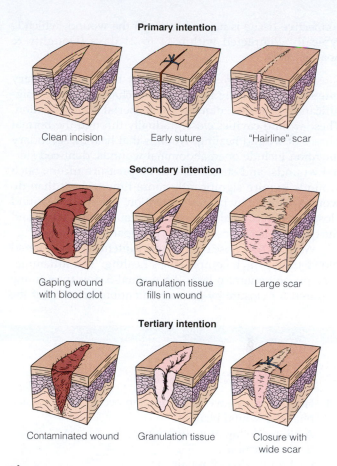

Primary intention

Clean incision   Early suture   "Hairline" scar

Secondary intention

Gaping wound   Granulation tissue   Large scar
with blood clot   fills in wound

Tertiary intention

Contaminated wound   Granulation tissue   Closure with
                                                         wide scar

Figure 10–4 Wound healing by primary, secondary, and tertiary intention.

responses before resulting in durable repair. A full-thickness wound heals differently, depending on the classification of repair (primary versus secondary intention), but proceeds through the same phases of healing.

Primary Intention **Primary intention** refers to closing the wound by mechanical means. This method is used when there is minimal tissue loss and skin edges are well approximated. Clean lacerations and most surgical incisions are closed using primary intention.

Mechanical means used to close wounds include tape, sutures, staples, and glue. Adhesive skin closure with microporous tape is best used in areas that are not over hairy surfaces or joints; when exposed to water, these tapes eventually fall off. Absorbable sutures are used to close dermal and subcutaneous layers, and nonabsorbable sutures are used for external closure. Staples allow for rapid closure and are frequently used on the extremities, torso, and scalp. Tissue glue is applied topically along the wound as a form of closure. These methods may be used singly or in combination.

Wounds that repair by primary intention are rather small, decreasing the distance new blood vessels and epithelial cells must migrate. Hemostasis resulting in the formation of a clot plays a major role in wounds healing by primary intention. Proliferation, consisting mainly of epithelialization, begins within hours after injury and is usually complete within 24 to 48 hours. A limited amount of connective tissue is needed to mend the wound, which is typically completed within 14 to 21 days (Doughty & Sparks, 2016).

Secondary Intention Wounds that heal by **secondary intention** are usually large wounds characterized by significant tissue loss, damage, or bacterial contamination. These wound cavities close gradually through the normal phases of wound healing. Wounds that heal by secondary intention include open abdominal wounds, dehisced sternal wounds, and stages III and IV pressure ulcers. Such wounds require significantly more time to heal than do wounds healing by primary intention. The time to wound closure is determined by the rate of wound contraction and the depth of tissue loss (Doughty & Sparks, 2016).

Wounds that close by secondary intention have altered blood flow, which compromises healing. The inflammatory phase generally lasts the normal 3-day time frame required for closure by primary intention; however, if the wound has heavy bacterial loads or large amounts of devitalized tissue, this phase can last significantly longer. The proliferation phase is prolonged, beginning with granulation tissue formation, followed by contraction, and ending with epithelialization. The maturation or remodeling phase mirrors that of wounds healing by primary intention. Newly closed or healed wounds lack tensile strength and require protection from stress for the first 2 to 3 months (Doughty & Sparks, 2016).

Tertiary Intention **Tertiary intention** is a method of delayed wound closure that uses a combination of primary and secondary intention. The wound is left open until the risk of infection has resolved and the wound is free of debris. Topical wound therapies and dressing type are tailored to meet specific wound needs. The wound is later closed by primary intention. Abdominal incisions complicated by significant infection often require this approach (Doughty & Sparks, 2016).

Section Two Review

1. Heat, redness, swelling, and pain occur during which phase of wound healing?
   A. Remodeling or maturation
   B. Contraction
   C. Proliferative or repair
   D. Inflammatory

2. Which statement accurately describes epithelialization?
   A. It is enhanced by a moist environment.
   B. It is enhanced by a dry, sterile environment.
   C. It removes debris.
   D. It spreads on surfaces laden with debris.

3. In the proliferation phase, what is the action of fluid collections, hematomas, and dead tissue?
   A. Serve as scaffolds for fibroblast proliferation
   B. Form barriers against fibroblast penetration
   C. Serve as protective covers for new epithelial cells
   D. Provide a moist environment to enhance epithelialization

4. How would an incision for a cholecystectomy usually be allowed to heal?
   A. Tertiary intention
   B. Secondary intention
   C. Primary intention
   D. Delayed secondary intention

Answers: 1. D, 2. A, 3. B, 4. **C**

Section Three: Factors That Affect Wound Healing

Acutely ill patients experience many risk factors that increase the likelihood of impaired wound healing. These include impaired oxygenation, compromised nutritional status, age, preexisting disease, medications, and obesity. These factors increase the risk of delayed wound healing, wound infection, and wound dehiscence. Nursing is challenged to provide the optimal environment that supports the wound-healing process.

Oxygenation and Tissue Perfusion

Many drugs and treatments to accelerate healing have been investigated. However, perfusion of injured tissue with well-oxygenated blood may be most important. Adequate oxygen supply to wounds is required by immune and inflammatory cells to produce proteins, reestablish vascular structure and epithelium, and provide resistance to bacterial invasion. Adequate oxygenation promotes neovascularization and optimizes collagen deposition, which increases the tensile strength of wound beds. Adequate levels of oxygen in the wound bed are also a major determinant of susceptibility to infection. The more hypoxic the wound is, the more anaerobic activity can be accelerated (Howard, Asmis, Evans, & Mustoe, 2013).

The availability of oxygen to tissue and wound beds depends on vascular supply, vasomotor tone, arterial oxygen tension, and the diffusion distance for oxygen to cross the capillary membrane. Edema and necrotic debris increase the diffusion distance for oxygen to reach cells in the wound. For optimal wound perfusion and oxygenation, patients must be warm, have adequate intravascular volume, and have adequate control of pain and anxiety. Stress associated with cold, pain, and fear cause peripheral vasoconstriction and can decrease oxygen delivery to wounds. The nurse should ensure a warm environment for the patient with a wound, not only in his or her room but also during invasive procedures and during transport.

Many conditions interfere with the delivery of oxygen to the wound: thrombosis, radiation, obesity, diabetes, cardiovascular disease, cigarette smoking, hypotension, hypothermia, hypovolemia, and the administration of vasoactive drugs. Significant blood loss, which frequently occurs in traumatically injured patients, results in hypovolemia, hypotension, and decreased tissue perfusion. Poor glycemic control with levels greater than 200 mcg/dL impairs wound healing, altering neutrophil function and epithelial migration, and may increase risk for wound dehiscence (Endara et al., 2013). Smoking and tobacco use adversely affect wound healing. By-products such as nicotine, carbon monoxide, and hydrogen cyanide reduce oxygenation, impair the immune response, reduce fibroblast activity, and increase platelet adhesion and thrombus formation. Smoking is associated with significantly higher infection rates (Doughty & Sparks, 2016).

Nursing care for the patient with an acute (e.g., surgical or traumatic) wound must include supportive measures to enhance tissue perfusion and prevent infection. Implementation of interventions to prevent hypothermia and hypovolemia, reduce pain and anxiety, reduce any risks for complications that are modifiable, and manage edema is standard (Graybill, Stojadinovic, Crumbley, & Elster, 2016; Whitney, 2016). Hyperbaric oxygen therapy may be used as an adjunct therapy in hypoxic conditions, such as gas gangrene, necrotizing fasciitis, and traumatic crush injuries (Graybill et al., 2016).

Nutrition

Wound healing is an anabolic metabolic process—that is, it requires energy to build new tissue. Therefore, adequate nutrition is a critical factor in wound repair. Inadequate nutrition predisposes the acutely ill patient to altered immune function and poor wound healing. It is essential that patients with wounds receive optimal nutritional support. Metabolic processes involved in wound healing rely heavily on adequate nutritional substrates. Physiologic and psychological stress, traumatic injury, and fever further increase the basal metabolic rate, depleting nutritional reserves. Because of these demands, malnutrition in the acutely ill patient is common.

Carbohydrates, proteins, fat, minerals, vitamins, and normovolemia are fundamental to normal cellular integrity and tissue repair and regeneration. The body's first priority is adequate energy (kilocalories). About 50% to 60% of caloric needs are met through carbohydrates, 20% to 25% through protein, and the rest through fat.

Protein Proteins are especially important, as they are the building blocks of collagen, a cellular matrix that forms the basis of tissue granulation. A patient with a wound may lose 100 grams of protein a day through wound drainage or exudate. Postinjury demands for protein are increased (Stotts, 2016a). Protein is required for collagen synthesis, immune responses, formation of granulation tissue, and

fibroblast proliferation. Therefore, it is desirable for patients to maintain a positive nitrogen (protein) balance to enhance wound healing. A protein deficiency prolongs the inflammatory phase of wound healing and impairs fibroblast proliferation, collagen and protein matrix synthesis, angiogenesis, and wound remodeling (Gould et al., 2015). Amino acid supplementation with arginine or glutamine is often prescribed to enhance the functioning of growth factors and immune cells and to support collagen deposition.

Fats Fats serve as building blocks for prostaglandins, which regulate cell metabolism, inflammation, and circulation. Fats are a rich energy source and play a crucial role in protecting protein from being tapped as a major source of energy.

Vitamins and Minerals Vitamins are needed to build new tissues and aid in normal immune function. Micronutrients such as fat-soluble vitamins (A, D, E, and K) participate in the wound healing process; and vitamins A, C, and B complex and the mineral zinc play especially important roles in wound healing, as listed in Table 10–1.

Fluids An adequate fluid volume status (normovolemia) is a factor that affects perfusion and oxygen delivery to healing tissues. Hypoperfusion to the subcutaneous capillary bed can result from vasoconstriction from systemic causes (low volume states or heart failure) or local causes (arterial insufficiency, vasoconstriction, or edema). The degree of hypoperfusion of the subcutaneous capillary bed is responsive to fluid status, temperature, and postoperative pain. Measures to maintain normovolemia, normothermia, and pain management can positively influence wound healing outcomes and infection rates. Mild to moderate normovolemic anemia does not appear to adversely affect wound oxygen tension and collagen synthesis, unless the hematocrit falls below 15% (Barbul, Efron, & Kavalukas, 2015).

Maintaining adequate nutrition and hydration in the high-acuity patient remains a challenge, demanding the expertise of a variety of professionals of the healthcare team. A multidisciplinary approach is imperative in wound healing and in accomplishing overall positive patient outcomes. The diet must provide the essential nutrients for optimal wound healing.

Age

Aging affects almost every stage of wound healing; the wound-healing process is markedly slower as patients age. Patients of advanced age have reduced collagen and fibroblast synthesis, impaired wound contraction, and slower reepithelialization of open wounds (Gould et al., 2015). In addition to the physiologic effects, patients are more likely to have nutritional deficiencies and pulmonary or cardiovascular diseases that further diminish local oxygenation to wounds and immunologic resistance. Nursing and collaborative-care healthcare teams aim to correct reversible comorbidities, optimize nutritional status, and provide evidence-based wound care (Doughty & Sparks, 2016).

Table 10–1 Essential Nutrients in Wound Healing

Vitamin A	Collagen synthesis Promotes tissue formation Facilitates epithelialization Inflammatory response Reverses inhibitory effects of long-term corticosteroid therapy
Vitamin B complex	Co-factor in enzymes Aids in WBC function, antibody formation, resistance to infection Facilitates fibroblast function and collagen synthesis Deficiency leads to decreased epithelialization
Vitamin C	Capillary wall integrity Collagen synthesis Activates WBCs and macrophages in wound; enhances their migration Fibroblast function Immune function
Vitamin K	Essential for blood clotting Deficiency can lengthen inflammatory phase
Copper	Co-factor for connective tissue and collagen production
Arginine	Amino acid involved in nitric oxide production, which is essential for collagen formation and angiogenesis Enhances immunity
Zinc	Essential for protein synthesis and collagen formation Supports immunity
Glutamine	Amino acid that plays role in preserving nitrogen balance, protein synthesis, cellular structure, and cellular metabolism and respiration

Diabetes Mellitus

Wound healing in the patient with diabetes is compromised as a result of macrovascular and microvascular changes, poor glycemic control, and loss of sensation. Diabetes is associated with abnormal and prolonged inflammation, reduced collagen synthesis, decreased tensile strength, impaired epithelial migration, and compromised vasculature. Hyperglycemia is associated with compromised neutrophil function and impaired epithelial migration. Glucose levels have direct effects on several phases of wound healing, and the importance of glycemic control cannot be overstated. The nurse caring for the acutely ill diabetic patient with a wound can promote a significant, positive impact on wound healing through scrupulous attention to glucose monitoring and maximizing glycemic control (less than 200 mcg/dL). Obesity, insulin resistance, hyperglycemia, and diabetic renal failure contribute significantly and independently to the impaired wound healing observed in diabetics. Careful correction of blood sugar levels improves the outcome of wounds in diabetic patients (Barbul et al., 2015).

Medications

Steroid therapy, used to block the inflammatory component of many diseases, has a well-known inhibitory effect on wound healing. Corticosteroids suppress inflammation and reduce proliferation of keratinocytes and fibroblasts, impairing both granulation and epithelial resurfacing. Patients taking greater than 30 to 40 mg/day experience the greatest effect (Doughty & Sparks, 2016). Chronic corticosteroid use may also result in a deficiency of zinc, which is necessary for wound healing.

There is controversy as to whether nonsteroidal anti-inflammatory drugs (NSAIDs) impact wound healing, but a side effect of these medications is platelet inhibition, which influences the wound healing cascade mechanism (Hopf, Shapshak, Junkins, & O'Neill, 2016). Other medications that interfere with wound healing include chemotherapeutic agents and immunosuppressant drugs. Chemotherapeutic agents impair the production of WBCs and fibroblasts, disrupting both the inflammatory and proliferation phases of repair and increasing the risk of infection. Immunosuppressant drugs increase susceptibility to infection and alter the body's ability to exhibit signs of infection (Doughty & Sparks, 2016).

Obesity

The obese patient (body mass index of 30 or greater) experiences an increased incidence of dehiscence, herniation, and infection (Gallagher, 2016). Adipose tissue is poorly vascularized, which increases the risk of ischemia. Adipose tissue is difficult to suture, which makes the obese patient at risk to develop a wound dehiscence. A binder or splint (pillow) to the incision provides support during straining or coughing and takes excess tension off the incision.

Topical Therapy

Implement best-practice dressing strategies to eliminate necrotic tissue and heavy bacterial loads. Use topical therapies that keep the wound surface clean and moist. A dry wound environment leads to cell death and desiccation. Antiseptic agents (hydrogen peroxide, povidone-iodine, acetic acid) are cytotoxic to fibroblasts and should be generally avoided as wound dressings. The only exception to this is a limited use of a diluted hypochlorite solution (Dakin's solution) (Ramundo, 2016) or povidone-iodine use on dead avascular eschar (Raetz & Wick, 2015). Silver-impregnated dressings have become a popular and safe choice for an antimicrobial topical approach to wounds, and cadexomer iodine dressings are safe as well (Ramundo, 2016).

Section Three Review

1. Small-vessel changes that impair tissue perfusion and oxygenation occur with which condition?
   A. Malnutrition
   B. Elevated sodium levels
   C. Diabetes
   D. Steroid therapy

2. What is the most important nutritional substance for wound healing?
   A. Glucose
   B. Fat
   C. Vitamins
   D. Protein

3. What is the most important factor supporting wound healing?
   A. Preventing infection
   B. Total parenteral nutrition
   C. Perfusion with well-oxygenated blood
   D. Potassium replacement

4. A dry wound environment has which effect?
   A. It enhances epithelialization.
   B. It leads to cell desiccation.
   C. It reduces bacterial load.
   D. It prevents necrosis.

Answers: 1. C, 2. D, 3. C, 4. B

Section Four: Clinical Assessment of Wound Healing

In assessing wound healing, it is important to assess the patient's preexisting health problems, focusing on conditions that alter tissue perfusion and oxygenation and impair the body's resistance to infection. It is also important to collect data on the medication and treatment history that may impair the healing process. The physical assessment should include evaluation of the wound by inspection and palpation as well as the collection and evaluation of objective data to assess the patient's tissue perfusion and oxygenation, immunologic, and nutritional status. Systematic assessment and comprehensive evaluation of both patient and wound provide a consistent method for assessing wound healing.

Wound Assessment

Assessment entails the inspection and collection of data that lead to a comprehensive individualized plan of care. Physical assessment parameters address wound etiology, wound duration, and intrinsic and extrinsic factors impairing wound healing. The first wound assessment is considered the baseline assessment to which all subsequent assessments are compared. Wound assessment includes documentation of the following wound characteristics: anatomic location, extent of tissue involvement (classification as a partial-thickness or full-thickness wound, or according to another appropriate classification system: e.g., pressure ulcers, skin tears, vascular ulcers, diabetic foot ulcers), the type of tissue present in the wound base (viable or nonviable), tissue color, measurements of wound size, appearance and amount of wound exudate, characteristics of the wound edge, periwound skin condition, and bacterial burden. The frequency of reassessment varies depending on the patient's overall condition, wound severity, type of dressing used, and goals of therapy (Nix, 2016).

Inspection

Wound tissue assessment occurs after dressing removal and wound cleansing. Wounds, incision lines, casts, pins, and surrounding skin integrity are inspected for signs of infection and skin alterations. The healing process and the effectiveness of wound care are evaluated.

Wound Measurement   Changes in wound dimensions may indicate improvement or decline in wound status. The nurse should measure and record the length, width, and depth of the wound, measuring the wound from the widest width perpendicular to its length (Figure 10–5). Depth

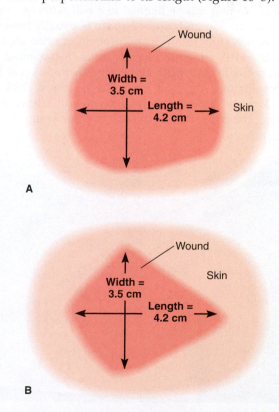

Figure 10–5 Measurement of wound size.

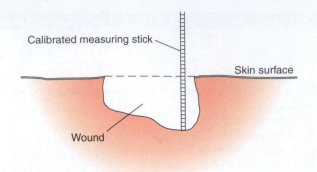

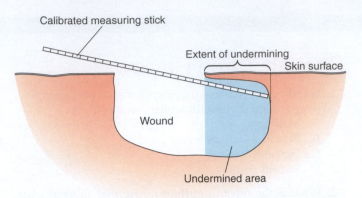

Undermining = 1.2 cm

Figure 10–6 Wound depth is measured at the deepest level of the wound.

Figure 10–8 Cross-sectional schematic of a wound with tunneling. Documentation must include the tunnel's depth, width, and position within the wound bed, commonly using clock terms (e.g., "Wound tunnels at 3 o'clock position").

can be determined by inserting a sterile, cotton-tipped applicator into the deepest part of the wound and grasping the applicator (or a calibrated measuring tool) where it meets the wound's edge (Figure 10–6). Irregular wound beds are difficult to measure accurately, so it is important to take measurements of depth and length from the same point each time. Unfortunately, linear measurement is not exact but does provide a way to detect a trend.

The entire full-thickness wound bed should be probed for the presence of tunneling. **Tunneling** is a narrow passageway or sinus tract in which there is unhealed, detached tissue under the skin created by the separation of, or destruction to, fascial planes. It is measured by inserting a sterile probe (or sterile cotton-tipped swab) into the passageway until resistance is met, as shown in Figure 10–7. These areas may become infected and develop into an abscess.

Undermining can be likened to a cliff without tissue underneath it. The undermined space is usually broader than a tunnel. Undermining and tunneling, often seen in stages III and IV pressure ulcers, can be documented by measuring depth and width and noting the location of the tunneling or undermining using the face of a clock as a model, with 12 o'clock being the patient's head and 6:00 being the patient's feet (Nix, 2016). For example, if a

wound on the anterior aspect of the left leg has tunneling on the medial side, the measurement would be x centimeters at the 9 o'clock position (Figure 10–8). For a wound with tunneling on the lateral side, the measurement would be x centimeters at the 3 o'clock position.

Wound tracings made with a clean wound tracing sheet and permanent marker can also be used to measure wound size. Many organizations require that all wounds be documented with a photograph. It should be noted that there are guidelines for wound photography in place through several organizations such as the Wound Ostomy Continence Nurses Society (WOCN), the National Pressure Ulcer Advisory Panel (NPUAP), and the American Professional Wound Care Association (APWCA).

Presence of Exudate or Drainage   The fluid produced by wounds is called **exudate**. Exudate must be assessed for volume (none, light, moderate, or heavy), type (clear, serosanguineous, sanguineous, purulent), and odor (absent, faint, moderate, or strong). The amount of exudate generally varies with the type of wound. An unexpected increase in wound exudate may be indicative of a clinical condition such as infection (Nix, 2016). Exudate normally bathes the wound continuously, keeping it moist, supplying nutrients, and providing the best conditions for migration and mitosis of epithelial cells and control of bacteria at the wound surface. Highly odorous, purulent wound exudate is abnormal and should be brought to the attention of the attending healthcare provider. In some cases, unusual, excessive, or copious wound drainage can be measured more accurately if a pouching system (commercial wound manager or custom appliance) is used to contain the drainage after collection with a bag (gravity drain) or canister (suction).

Appearance of Wound Tissue   Wound tissue characteristics are an indication of the state of healing. Normal progression from the inflammatory phase to proliferation in a full-thickness wound results in a vascular granulating wound surface. Healthy granulation tissue presents as a red, vascular, granular tissue with a berrylike appearance. In Figure 10–9, the wound has progressed to the proliferation phase, with the beginning of granulating tissue buds.

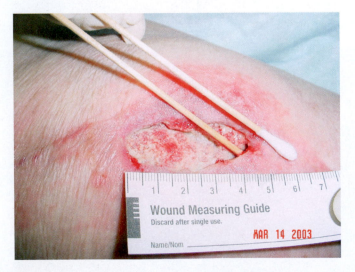

Figure 10–7 Tunneling wound.

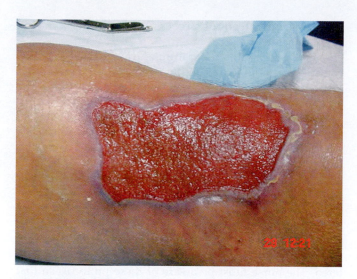

Figure 10–9 Healthy wound bed granulation and epithelialization tissue.

Just as a 100% granulating wound base is an indication of normal wound healing, nonviable tissue provides information about wound status. Nonviable tissue may be associated with impaired tissue oxygenation, wound desiccation, or increased bioburden. **Bioburden** refers to the degree of foreign material and debris resulting from bacteria and tissue injury that cause a delay in the wound healing process. **Eschar**, a type of nonviable tissue, is a black, gray, or yellow-tan necrotic tissue, thick and leathery, that appears even with the skin margin but extends more deeply. The extent or depth of tissue involvement is unknown until the tissue is removed or debrided. **Slough**, another type of nonviable tissue, is a moist, slimy, gray, tan, or yellow necrotic tissue attached to the wound base. The ideal local wound environment is free from slough and eschar. Pale and dusky granulation tissue suggests poor blood supply.

Wounds with nonviable tissue or tissue necrosis remain in the inflammatory phase, delaying and impairing healing. Necrotic tissue also provides an environment for organism growth, predisposing the wound to infection. Wounds may have a combination of nonviable (eschar or slough) and viable tissue. Documentation should reflect the extent to which each exists in the wound bed (e.g., 20% slough and 80% granulation). One easy method to utilize to document the tissue is the red-yellow-black (RYB) system, where red is the granulation tissue, yellow is slough, and black is eschar. This is also documented as a percentage (e.g., 20% red, 50% yellow, and 30% black tissue).

Inspection of Wound Edges   The wound edges should be attached (approximated) to each other without undermining. Edges should be moist and flush with the wound base, allowing epithelial cells to migrate from the edges across the surface once granulation and wound contraction are complete. Prematurely closed and/or rolled wound edges impair the epithelialization needed to close the wound. Premature closure is not uncommon in chronic wounds; in such cases, surgical intervention is required to open the edges to allow for epithelial migration and wound closure (Nix, 2016). In full-thickness wounds, epithelial cells migrate up to 3 cm from the wound edge, requiring split-thickness grafting or myocutaneous flaps for closure, as these wounds are too large and do not contract enough to allow for complete epithelial coverage and scar closure.

Inspection of Periwound Skin   Periwound assessment provides information about the effectiveness of the treatment plan and topical therapy (Nix, 2016). Impaired periwound skin integrity compromises and complicates wound healing. The periwound skin should be described by color (erythema, pale, white, or blue), texture (moist, dry, indurated, boggy, macerated, or rash), temperature (hot, warm, or cool), and integrity (denuded, erosion, or pustules) (Nix, 2016). Periwound skin should not be erythematous or tender; the wound margins should not be macerated. Maceration is evident when the periwound skin is white or pale, developing when drainage from the wound is in prolonged contact with healthy skin tissue around the wound. If not corrected, maceration leads to altered skin integrity and further wound compromise.

Periwound skin integrity can also be altered by frequent tape removal. Simple measures to protect the periwound area include the use of skin barriers before application of tape or other adhesives or the use of other protectant agents prior to covering the wound.

Palpation of Periwound Area   Palpation of the wound and surrounding areas assists in recognizing changes in size, consistency, moisture, and texture. The periwound area may be reddened around the wound base due to inflammation, which may indicate deeper tissue injury or infection. A boggy or soft periwound area occurs with maceration. If the area is hardened or indurated, then edema, infection, deep tissue injury, or necrosis is suspected (Stotts, 2016a). Visible or palpable bone increases the risk for osteomyelitis, which is a serious complication that should be reported to the attending healthcare provider.

Assessment of Tissue Perfusion and Oxygenation Status

Adequate tissue perfusion and oxygenation is the most important factor to assess in wound healing. Tissue oxygen levels depend on adequate cardiac output, hemoglobin, and the perfusion and oxygen content of the blood. Local and systemic factors that alter tissue perfusion and oxygenation include necrosis, debris, and foreign materials in the wound; pain and stress; hypothermia; tobacco use; and obesity (Whitney, 2016).

Microcirculation (in the capillary beds that feed the wound area) and vascular perfusion status may be assessed using transcutaneous oxygen measurement (TCOM). TCOM can measure the oxygen tension of the wound tissue with a heated electrode that vasodilates the wound capillary bed. TCOM values of less than 40 mmHg indicate hypoxia and impaired wound healing (Doughty, 2016).

To assess circulation into and from a wound, assess the proximal and distal pulses by palpation or by Doppler ultrasound. Proximal pulses demonstrate adequate circulation to the area. Measure capillary refill time in seconds. Compare the skin temperature bilaterally. Sensorimotor assessment distal to the wound may be done by testing for discrimination between sharp and dull pressures.

Assessment of Immunologic Status

An intact immunologic response to injury, regardless of the cause of injury, is a key factor in proper wound healing. The patient is assessed for the three predisposing elements for wound infection: susceptible host, compromised wound, and infectious organism. Factors that cause local and systemic resistance to infection are assessed. Compromised wounds containing devitalized tissue, hematomas, and debris are debrided to prevent an environment conducive to bacterial proliferation. The patient is assessed for sources of pathogenic organisms.

Assessment of immunologic status includes WBC, fibrinogen, body temperature, wound cultures, and serum antimicrobial levels. The inflammatory phase of wound healing releases WBCs. It is not uncommon for patients with wounds to have elevated WBC counts during the initial phase of wound healing. Elevated WBCs in later phases are more indicative of an infectious process.

Neutrophils are the primary cells involved in phagocytosis. Elevated neutrophil counts are indicative of an acute infection as mature and immature neutrophils are released in response to an increased need for phagocytosis. Neutrophils are essential in the presence of infection if wound healing is to occur. Adequate amounts of fibrinogen are needed to convert to fibrin. This aids in localizing the infectious process by providing a matrix for phagocytosis.

Increased body temperature is triggered by microorganisms, bacterial toxins and antigens, and the inflammatory process. Because fever is a manifestation of both the inflammatory and the infectious process, it is important to assess the patient's overall clinical picture for etiologic factors of the fever. Patients in a hypothermic state experience decreased tissue perfusion and oxygenation and decreased leukocyte activity.

Antimicrobial medications should be appropriate for organisms validated by culture and sensitivity testing. Monitoring concentrations of antimicrobial agents in the blood confirms therapeutic drug levels and determines toxicity. The best assessment can be made by drawing serum peak and trough samples, depending on the antimicrobial administered. The nurse must be aware of these protocols so that accurate therapeutic concentrations and toxicity can be assessed.

Assessment of Nutritional Status

A complete and thorough nutritional assessment for all patients with altered skin and tissue integrity is imperative. The assessment must include baseline height and weight, serial weight monitoring, and regular assessment of intake and output. Laboratory serum protein values, such as albumin and prealbumin, are commonly used as measures of malnutrition. However, there is no single laboratory test to confirm or diagnose the scope of malnutrition or nutritional issues (Stotts, 2016b). Clinical observations and laboratory data should be included in the entire discussion of nutritional status for patients (Stotts, 2016b).

Section Four Review

1. Assessment of a wound bed reveals yellow-colored tissue that is slimy and attached to the wound base. How would the nurse document this assessment?
   A. Infection
   B. Eschar
   C. Slough
   D. Macerated tissue

2. Which findings are associated with maceration of periwound skin? (Select all that apply.)
   A. The area is "boggy."
   B. The skin is indurated.
   C. The skin is pale.
   D. The area is reddened.
   E. The area is warm to touch.

3. Which techniques can be used to assess wound size? (Select all that apply.)
   A. Measuring widest width perpendicular to length
   B. Marking on clean wound tracing sheet
   C. Drawing on plastic wrap
   D. Relating wound to a common object (e.g., "size of a quarter")
   E. Measure depth with a disposable ruler

4. In assessing a wound, the nurse notes that it contains granulation tissue that is pale and dusky. What is the cause?
   A. Drainage in the wound
   B. Maceration
   C. Infection
   D. Poor blood supply

Answers: 1. C, 2. (A, C, E), 3. (A, B), 4. D

Section Five: Principles of Wound Management

The process of wound healing is affected by many patient factors, as presented in Section Three. Wound management decisions are based on these factors and are designed to construct a physiologically positive local wound environment. There are three important principles of wound management: controlling or eliminating the etiology or causative factors, providing systemic support to reduce existing and potential co-factors, and maintaining an optimal physiologic local wound environment (Bryant & Nix, 2016). To accomplish closure, a variety of interventions may be required within each principle. For example, maintaining an optimal physiologic wound environment depends on an adequate moisture level, temperature control, pH regulation, and control of organism bioburden (Bryant & Nix, 2016).

Nurses have the opportunity to favorably manipulate certain environmental factors that promote wound healing. Local wound care includes cleansing, debridement, and selection of appropriate wound dressing materials. Wound care (cleansing and debridement) requires an order from a physician or other qualified provider.

Wound Cleansing

Wound cleansing involves removing debris, microorganisms, contaminants, exudate, and devitalized tissue, usually by flushing the surface of the wound with a nontoxic irrigating solution such as normal saline. The fluid should be warmed to body temperature if possible, as cool fluid inhibits phagocytic and cellular growth in the wound. The size and condition of the wound determine the method of cleansing. The effective and safe pressure range for wound cleansing is 4 to 15 pounds per square inch (psi) to avoid trauma to the wound bed. A large wound with a significant amount of necrosis requires high-pressure (8 to 15 psi) irrigation with enough solution to adequately remove the debris.

Several devices can be used to perform high-pressure irrigation, and numerous irrigation kits are commercially available; however, basic hospital equipment can also be used for normal pressure irrigations. For example, a 35 mL syringe used with a 19-gauge angiocath delivers a pressure of about 8 psi to the wound.

The goal of cleansing proliferative, granulating wounds is to remove inorganic debris from the wound using a gentle flushing technique. The use of pressures higher than 15 psi may force bacteria deeper into the tissue. Wounds are not scrubbed, as this can cause trauma to healthy tissue, but they should be cleansed with gauze material mechanically to assist in removing surface debris (mechanical debridement) (Bryant & Nix, 2016; Ramundo, 2016).

Debridement

Debridement, the removal of nonviable tissue, foreign matter, and debris from the wound bed, is a naturally occurring event in the wound repair process. However, a buildup of nonviable necrotic tissue stresses this natural process and overwhelms the phagocytic demand on the wound, retarding wound healing. Wound healing cannot take place until nonviable tissue is removed. Debridement reduces the local bioburden, controls and potentially prevents wound infections, and facilitates visualization of the wound (Ramundo, 2016).

The five methods of debridement are sharp, mechanical, chemical, autolytic, and biosurgical. They may be used alone or in combination during the wound repair process (Ramundo, 2016).

- **Sharp debridement** is the preferred method for removal of necrotic tissue using a scalpel or scissors. Sharp debridement selectively removes devitalized tissue, foreign material, and debris. Sharp debridement may be done in a sterile fashion at the bedside or in surgery, and often results in bleeding from the wound. **Conservative sharp debridement** is the removal of necrotic tissue with a clean method and does not generally result in blood loss. Both types of sharp debridement are generally performed by a physician or another healthcare provider with a demonstrated skill set to perform such procedures.

- **Mechanical debridement** is accomplished with wet-to-dry gauze dressings, irrigation, hydrotherapy, or low-frequency ultrasound. The most common method of mechanical debridement is wiping the wound with gauze or a similar material.

- **Chemical debridement** involves the removal of necrotic tissue using enzymes or sodium hypochlorite. The topical application of enzymes is a selective form of debridement. Collagenase is a pharmaceutical enzyme that digests collagen in necrotic tissue. Dakin's solution is a dilution of sodium hypochlorite (bleach) and sterile water. As a debriding agent, it denatures protein, loosening slough and making it easier to remove it from the wound.

- **Autolytic debridement** is a selective, painless form of debridement whereby usual body processes effectively remove nonviable necrotic tissue. Autolysis is stimulated by a moist environment and adequate leukocyte function and neutrophil count. Moisture-retentive dressings include semiocclusive (transparent films) and occlusive (hydrocolloid wafers) dressings. These dressings are contraindicated in patients with impaired immunity, actively infected wounds, or extensive tissue necrosis. Moisture-retentive dressings allow endogenous enzymes in the wound to selectively liquefy necrotic tissue. In addition, the growth factors and inflammatory cells in the wound fluid hasten the inflammatory and proliferative phases of wound healing (Ramundo, 2016). It is vital that clinicians do not mistake the wound fluid for an infectious process. It is normal to have a fluid collection under the dressing. After removal of the dressing, the nurse should irrigate the wound with normal saline prior to assessing the wound.

Moisture-retentive dressings are changed daily to weekly, depending on the type of wound, amount of exudate, and class of dressing used. Patients who are immunocompromised and those with diabetes may not respond favorably or as expected with autolytic debridement, secondary to their limited ability to mount an inflammatory response.

- **Biosurgical (maggot) debridement** was first used to remove necrotic tissue while leaving healthy tissue alone in the wounds of soldiers on the battlefield. Today there is renewed interest in this method of debridement in clinical centers. This form of debridement uses sterile larvae that are introduced into the wound bed. It is generally considered a last-resort option when other methods of debridement have been ineffective or if the patient is a nonsurgical candidate.

Dressings

Dressings are placed over wounds for multiple purposes: debridement, protection from the external environment, provision of a physiological environment conducive to wound healing, and provision of immobilization, support, and comfort. Dressings assist in the assessment of quality and quantity of drainage, pressure reduction, and absorption. They prevent infection, control wound drainage, and minimize scarring.

The condition of the wound bed determines the type of dressing used. As a wound changes, dressing care is modified. It is essential for the nurse to continue assessing the wound throughout the healing process with valid scales such as the Pressure Ulcer Scale for Healing (PUSH) to evaluate the effectiveness of the wound management plan. The PUSH scale categorizes the ulcer with respect to surface area, exudate, and type of wound tissue. Subscales for each of these ulcer characteristics are assigned, then added to obtain the total score. A comparison of total scores measured over time provides an indication of the improvement or deterioration in ulcer healing.

Wounds healing by primary intention require dressings that absorb exudate and protect the wound from trauma and contamination; therefore, a dry dressing is applied. The length of time a dressing is required for primary intention wounds is usually 1 to 3 days. Wounds healing by secondary or tertiary intention require dressing materials that provide a warm, moist local environment conducive to healing; debride necrotic tissue; absorb exudate; and protect the wound from further trauma and contamination. Specific types of dressings and their care are summarized in Table 10–2. As noted in the table, a variety of dressings can be used, including alginates, hydrocolloids, and traditional moist gauze dressings.

Negative Pressure Wound Therapy

Negative pressure wound therapy (NPWT) is the application of subatmospheric pressure to the wound bed using suction to enhance granulation and contraction and collect wound fluid. Multiple commercial systems are available, such as Vacuum-Assisted Closure (VAC) (Kinetic Concepts Inc.), RENASYS (Smith & Nephew), and others. NPWT is not recommended in inadequately debrided, necrotic, or malignant wounds; where vital organs are exposed; in wounds with no exudate; or in individuals with untreated coagulopathy, osteomyelitis, or local or systemic clinical infection. Cautious use by an experienced healthcare professional is recommended for individuals on anticoagulant therapy, in actively bleeding wounds, or where the wound is in close proximity to major blood vessels (National Pressure Ulcer Advisory Panel et al., 2014).

In NPWT, a wound filler dressing and suction tubing are sealed to the skin with transparent film dressing and connected to a suction device and collection container. Wound filler dressings may consist of open-cell foam, silicone tubing wrapped with gauze (plain or antimicrobial), nonadherent matrix, or nonwoven polymer (Figure 10–10). NPWT provides subatmospheric pressure to the wound bed ranging from −40 to −200 mmHg, depending on the patient, the wound, and the goal of therapy. The majority of NPWT systems allow for continuous and intermittent suction settings. Continuous therapy is generally used at −125 mmHg. Intermittent suction may be used if wound healing has stalled. NPWT improves local wound perfusion by decreasing edema and bacterial contamination and improves neovascularization, granulation, and wound contraction (Netsch, Nix, & Haugen, 2016).

NPWT can be used in a variety of complex wounds, such as deep wounds, stage III and IV pressure ulcers, leg ulcers, and diabetic foot ulcers (Anghel & Kim, 2016; Armstrong & Lavery, 2005; Blume, Walters, Payne, Avata, & Lantis, 2008; Kim et al., 2014; Sajid et al., 2015; Tuncel, Erkorkmaz, & Turan, 2013; Vaidhya, Panchal, & Anchalia, 2015). Prior to application of NPWT, the wound must be debrided of necrotic tissue and the wound must be well vascularized. The wound filler dressing may be changed

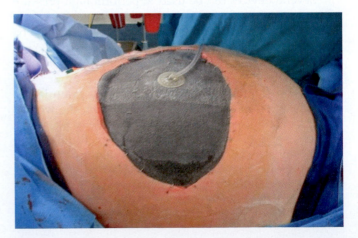

Figure 10–10 Negative pressure wound therapy.

SOURCE: Trish Martin

Table 10–2 Wound Dressings

Type	Indications	Considerations
Gauze: plain or hypertonic saline	Use with full-thickness wounds healing by secondary intention Nonviable wound base with or without infection Deep wounds with tunneling	Cleanse wound, apply gauze, cover with secondary dressing No solution should be visibly dripping from the dressing as it is placed into the wound; solution will retard wound closure, increase bacteria, and macerate periwound skin None of the dressing should touch intact skin
Antimicrobial: antiseptics, cadexomer iodine, honey, Hydrofera Blue, mupirocin, silver dressings	Partial- or full-thickness wounds Critical colonization, infection, or biofilms Wounds with foul odor	Cleanse wound Avoid saline with silver, use sterile water instead Apply appropriate secondary dressing
Transparent film: Tegaderm (3M) Opsite (Smith & Nephew) Suresite (Medline)	Shallow partial-thickness wounds Dry to minimally exudative wounds Not recommended for infected wounds Use with caution in immunosuppressed patients or diabetics with uncontrolled glucose	Cleanse wound, dry periwound skin Allow 1- to 2-inch border around wound Typical change time is every 3 days and prn due to leakage or displacement Use skin barrier on periwound skin prior to dressing application May be used as a primary or secondary dressing
Hydrocolloid: DuoDerm (ConvaTec) Replicare (Smith & Nephew)	Partial- or full-thickness wounds without depth Minimal to moderate exudate Not recommended for infected wounds Use with caution in immunosuppressed patients or diabetics with uncontrolled glucose	Like transparent film, except change every 3 to 5 days; prn due to leakage or displacement Remove carefully to avoid mechanical injury or skin tear
Calcium alginate: Kaltostat (ConvaTec) Restore CalciCare (Hollister)	Partial- or full-thickness wounds with or without depth Moderate to heavily exudative Do not pack into a tunnel, because fibers can be left behind	Cleanse wound, dry Change every 1 to 3 days Irrigate wound to evacuate alginate Wound fluid may have a green color as a by-product of the dressing
Hydrogel: *Sheet:* Vigilon (Bard) Elast-Gel (Southwest Technologies) *Amorphous:* PolyMem (Ferris Mfg Corp) Mepilex (Mölnlycke Health Care)	Partial- or full-thickness wound Dry to minimally exudative Change daily to every 3 days Partial- or full-thickness wounds with (filler) or without (sheets) depth Minimal to heavy exudate, depending on brand or type Primary or secondary dressing	Cleanse wound, dry Change every 1 to 3 days Water in gel form is comfortable and will not adhere Some foams have adherent border, provide thermal insulation, and absorb light to heavy amounts of exudate Change every 1 to 3 days, depending on amount of exudate Comfortable; does not adhere to wound; appropriate for use on fragile skin
Fiber gel: Aquacel (ConvaTec)	Partial- or full-thickness wounds Moderate exudate	Cleanse wound, dry; change every 1 to 3 days prn exudate
Collagen: Puracol (Medline) Promogran (Systagenix Wound Management)	Full-thickness wounds with or without depth Uninfected wounds, minimal to moderate exudate Chronic wounds without necrosis Contraindicated in bovine sensitivity	Dressing change frequency depends on brand, amount of exudate, and manufacturer's recommendations
Contact layer: Restore TRIACT technology (Hollister) Mepitel (Mölnlycke)	Partial- or full-thickness wounds with or without depth Can use in infected wounds, donor sites, split-thickness skin grafts (STSGs)	Cleanse wound, dry; line wound bed, apply secondary dressing Not intended to be changed with each dressing change

every 12 hours for infected wounds or every 72 hours in the absence of infection. Patients may experience pain from the interaction of the wound filler with the wound bed, the amount of pressure, and the suction technique. Pain etiology should be assessed and interventions employed to alleviate the pain. These include changing the type of dressing, adding a nonadherent contact layer prior to the wound filler dressing, using lower pressure (75–80 mmHg), switching from intermittent to constant suction, instilling normal saline to moisten the dressing prior to removal, instilling with topical lidocaine (Xylocaine) without epinephrine, and changing the type of NPWT system (Netsch, Nix, & Haugen, 2016).

Additional information about wound management can be found in the "Nursing Care: The Patient with an Acute or Chronic Wound" feature.

Nursing Care
The Patient with an Acute or Chronic Wound

Expected Patient Outcomes and Related Interventions

Assess and compare to established norms, patient baselines, and trends.

Patient history
Comorbidities, current medications, social history, habits (e.g., smoking), allergies
Assessments
Immune status (e.g., WBC with differential count, proteins [e.g., albumin, prealbumin, total proteins])
Blood glucose levels
Hydration status (e.g., intake and output balance, edema or third-spacing, fluid loss from wound[s], skin turgor)
Nutrition status (e.g., nutritional assessment, daily dietary intake, plasma proteins and total proteins, serum electrolytes)
Oxygenation status (e.g., SpO_2, ABG [PaO_2 and SaO_2], hemoglobin, lung sounds, respiratory rate and depth)
Perfusion status (e.g., BP, HR, MAP, peripheral pulses, capillary refill, peripheral limb color and temperature)
Wound(s)
Length, width, and depth; etiology; age of wound(s); treatments
Pressure points (e.g., heels, spine, coccyx, trochanters, elbows, back of head)

Interventions to promote wound healing and prevent complications

Monitor wound for changes in size, shape, and appearance
Principles of wound management:
- Debridement—sends signals that trigger platelet aggregation, leukocytosis, phagocytosis to clean up debris, and growth factors to heal with new collagen synthesis
- Dressings—provide moisture for epithelial migration in a dry wound, or moisture retention and absorption to prevent maceration and further collagen damage in a wet wound
- Offloading devices—alleviate pressure and restore circulation for healing (e.g. special shoes, splints, wheelchair cushions, special bed surfaces)
- Nutrition—dietary consultation to determine caloric, protein, and nutrient requirements
- Vascular status should be optimized for healing
- Bioburden and infection must be controlled with antimicrobial agents, specialized dressings, and debridement
- Perineal care of the incontinent patient to prevent skin breakdown and/or wound contamination
- Keep periwound skin dry and protected from moisture and fecal or urine contaminants—use moisture barrier ointments
- Avoid soap on skin as high pH and residue are irritating; instead use skin cleansers containing nonionic surfactants that do not strip natural body oil; can use products that are antibacterial, cleansing, moisturizing, and protecting
- Use emollients and moisturizers to prevent moisture loss and add moisture to the skin
- Consult a wound or skin care expert to assist in developing or re-evaluating the plan of care

Nutrition interventions
Offer high-calorie, high-protein diet with supplements
Monitor daily weights, intake and output
Consult dietician within 24 hours of admission
Monitor prealbumin levels weekly to assess response to nutritional therapies

Pain management
Assess pain level and report any increase in pain
Assess effectiveness of pharmacologic interventions

Section Five Review

1. What size syringe would the nurse select to irrigate a wound?
   A. 35 mL
   B. 50 mL
   C. 60 mL
   D. 100 mL

2. What type of dressing would be indicated to cover a wound healing by primary intention?
   A. Dry
   B. Hydrocolloid
   C. Antimicrobial
   D. Polyurethane

3. Which equipment is part of a negative pressure wound therapy system? (Select all that apply.)
   A. Wound expander dressing
   B. Suction tubing
   C. Transparent film dressing
   D. Collection container
   E. Hydrocolloid dressing

4. Which agent is used to assist in chemical wound debridement?
   A. Acetic acid
   B. Collagenase
   C. Betadine (povidone-iodine)
   D. Half-strength hydrogen peroxide

Answers: 1. A, 2. A, 3. (B, C, E), 4. B

Section Six: Wound Infections: Etiology, Diagnosis, and Treatment

Intact skin provides a barrier to microorganism invasion and infection. Once epidermal integrity is disrupted, the wound quickly becomes contaminated by body fluids and normal skin flora (*Acinetobacter*, *Streptococcus*, and *Staphylococcus*). The effect of the microorganism burden, or bioburden, on the wound is vast and complicated. All wounds have some level of microorganism burden; most do not become infected.

The evolution of bioburden consists of five microbial states: contamination, colonization, critical colonization, biofilm, and infection. The presence of nonreplicating microbes is called **contamination**. Wound **colonization** occurs if the microflora replicate but do not adversely affect wound healing. Contamination and colonization are normal. **Critical colonization** describes a level of microorganism burden that affects skin cell proliferation and tissue repair, altering wound healing but not invading the wound tissue. As microorganisms adhere to the wound, they develop a biofilm. A **biofilm** is a group of mixed microorganisms embedded in a matrix that is attached to the wound, making it difficult to kill the microorganisms. About 6% of acute wounds develop biofilms, and about 60% of chronic wounds have a biofilm presence (Percival, McCarty, & Lipsky, 2015). **Wound infection** occurs when the microorganisms multiply and invade wound tissues. According to laboratory tests, a wound is considered infected when tissue contains greater than 10^5 colony-forming units (CFUs) as the gold standard. However, wounds can also be considered infected with less than 10^5 CFUs because of interaction that takes place when multiple microbes are present. More than 90% of chronic wounds have polymicrobes, often containing up to 4 species (Stotts, 2016a). However, the mere presence of certain types of bacteria can interfere with wound healing. Beta-hemolytic *Streptococcus* is a virulent strain of bacteria that can cause infections even at very low concentrations. The adverse effects of microbes in wounds are summarized in Box 10–1.

The classic clinical signs of a wound infection include increased exudate, erythema, induration, local warmth, edema, increased pain, and at times fever. The diagnosis of a wound infection relies heavily on the understanding that immunocompromised or immunosuppressed patients may not manifest an inflammatory response or the classic symptoms. Wound cultures are obtained to determine the appropriate antibiotic selection and therapy (Stotts, 2016a).

Predisposing Factors for Wound Infection

Three elements predispose the patient to developing a wound infection: a susceptible host, a compromised wound, and an infectious organism.

Susceptible Host   One of the major determinants of a subsequent infection after surgery or trauma is the patient's own defense mechanisms. The patient who is a **susceptible host** has some degree of local or systemic impairment of resistance to bacterial invasion. Local impairment may be the result of dead, foreign material or hematomas directly in the wound or some interference in blood supply to the area as a result of vascular disease. The causes of systemic impairment may include diabetes, immune deficiency, acute or chronic use of steroids, kidney disease, malnutrition, cardiovascular disease, pulmonary disease, extremes of age, obesity, cancer, and the use of immunosuppressive therapies. Health habits such as tobacco and drug use or abuse are predisposing factors (Percival et al., 2015; Stotts, 2016a). These patients usually have an impaired and acute inflammatory response.

Compromised Wound   A **compromised wound** is one that contains devitalized tissue, which is tissue that has been separated from the circulation and the body's antimicrobial defenses. Bacteria proliferate on wounds that contain dead tissue, hematomas, or foreign material. Debridement of these materials is essential to prevent an environment conducive to bacterial growth.

Infectious Organism   Many different organisms are capable of initiating a wound infection. Organisms come from endogenous or exogenous sources. Endogenous sources arise within the patient. A variety of microorganisms exist on and in the human body—on normal skin and in gastrointestinal flora. Microorganisms in these areas are not pathogenic until they are released from the sites they normally inhabit and are allowed to proliferate in a sterile area of the body. Exogenous organisms enter the body from the external environment when the skin barrier has been broken. The external environment may be the accident scene (for trauma patients) or the healthcare setting.

Diagnosis and Treatment of Wound Infection

In diagnosing wound infection it is important to consider the patient's physical assessment and individual risk factors for wound infection along with the clinical presentation of the wound. The nurse may note a change in the characteristic amount and odor of drainage, from serosanguineous to purulent and malodorous. Fever and elevated WBCs indicate a more invasive infection. Table 10–3 outlines laboratory and diagnostic tests used to monitor patients for wound healing and infection. If clinical symptoms of infection appear, or when a clean wound fails

---

BOX 10–1   Adverse Effects of Microbes on Wound Healing

- Microbes compete with host cells for nutrients and oxygen.
- Bacteria release exotoxins that are cytotoxic.
- Bacteria endotoxins within their cell walls activate host inflammatory response.
- Wound infections delay wound healing.

Table 10–3 Laboratory Tests Related to Wound Healing

Test and Normal Values	Expected Abnormality	Treatment
White blood cells (WBC): 4500–11,000/mm^3	Increased with inflammation and acute infection Decreased with thrombocytopenia, cancers, anemias, or liver disease	Diagnose and track infection. WBC alone does not tell healthcare providers anything without differential.
Platelets: 150,000–400,000/mm^3	Increased with inflammation and infection Indication of concealed bleeding (e.g., gastrointestinal [GI])	Basic element of coagulation. Decreased count can drive treatment.
Red blood cells (RBC): Female: 4–5.5 million/mm^3 Male: 4.5–6.2 million/mm^3	May be decreased due to bleeding from the wound Menses in women Renal disease Decrease might indicate depleted blood volume Chronic infections	Monitor for need for medications or blood administration to increase value.
Hemoglobin (Hgb): Female: 12–15 g/dL Male: 14–16.5 g/dL	May be decreased due to bleeding from the wound, hypoxia, anemias, or overhydration Some prescription medications can decrease count	Monitor with hematocrit for need for medications or blood administration to increase value.
Hematocrit (HCT): Female: 35–47% Male: 42–52%	May be decreased due to bleeding from the wound	Monitor for need for medications or blood administration to increase value.
Total proteins: 6.3–8.3 g/dL	May be decreased with malnutrition Decrease indicates immunosuppression	Monitor need for nutritional supplements.
Serum albumin: 3.5–5.5 g/dL	May be decreased with malnutrition injury because albumin catabolism increases as a result of injury	Monitor need for nutritional supplements. Half-life is 21 days; it is easily influenced by medications and fluid status.
Serum prealbumin: 16–40 mg/dL	Reflects immune and inflammatory status	Current protein status.
Wound culture and sensitivity: Negative	Will be positive if there is contamination, colonization, or infection	Assess for wound infection and which antibiotic will be effective in treating it.

SOURCE: Osborn et al. (2014). *Medical-Surgical Nursing: Preparations for Practice* (2nd ed.). Upper Saddle River, NJ: Pearson. Reproduced by Permission of Pearson Education.

to progress to the proliferation phase within 2 weeks of appropriate topical wound therapy, wound cultures are obtained. The aim of wound culturing is the identification of the specific aerobic or anaerobic microorganisms, or both, causing the infection and their susceptibility to antibiotics. The culture technique is critical in isolating the infectious microorganism. The wound culture should be collected from clean, healthy, viable wound tissue. The infectious agent of concern inhabits healthy tissue rather than purulent exudate, necrotic tissue, eschar, or slough. Obtaining a specimen for gram stain is also recommended (Stotts, 2016a). The results guide the appropriate administration of systemic antibiotics.

Local wound management for infection refers back to the three principles of wound management discussed in the prior section. Topical therapy decisions are directed at decreasing local bioburden, cleansing, debridement, and moist wound healing. The use of commercially safe and clinically effective topical antimicrobials assists in controlling the wound bioburden, potentially reducing the need for antibiotics and halting the development of resistant microorganisms (Stotts, 2016a).

Systemic signs of wound infection require treatment with systemic antibiotics that are sensitive to the causative microorganism. Until wound culture results are known, broad-spectrum antibiotics are prescribed. Antibiotic-resistant microorganisms such as methicillin-resistant *Staphylococcus aureus* (MRSA), vancomycin-resistant *Enterococci* (VRE), and *Acinetobacter* may be involved in acute-care wound infections. Fungal wound infections have become a recent concern.

Wound assessment, diligent management of wound bioburden, provision of individual patient system support, administration of antibiotics, and monitoring of therapeutic drug levels when indicated are important in supporting wound healing and avoiding sepsis in this population.

Prevention of Wound Infections

One of the greatest priorities in wound care is the prevention of infection. Prevention begins with recognizing the three elements that predispose the patient to a wound infection, as previously described: susceptible host, compromised wound, and infectious organism.

For elective surgical procedures, prevention begins preoperatively with skin preparation, mechanical and antibiotic bowel preparations, timely prophylactic administration of antibiotics, and sterile draping of the operative site. Intraoperatively, careful surgical technique minimizes injury, and aseptic technique prevents endogenous and exogenous bacterial contamination.

For patients with traumatic injury, resuscitation and lifesaving measures often take priority over the immediate treatment of wounds. After the resuscitative phase is completed, prompt and proper management of the wounds reduces the likelihood of subsequent infection. It is not uncommon for traumatically incurred wounds to be contaminated with dirt, grass, glass, twigs, leaves, stool, shrapnel, or bullet or knife fragments. Management of these wounds begins with cleansing via high-pressure irrigation and debridement to remove bacteria and foreign debris.

The importance of hand hygiene to prevent the transmission of infectious organisms was determined more than a century ago. Hand hygiene is still considered one of the most important methods of preventing wound infections. This is especially true in high-acuity settings, where susceptible hosts, compromised wounds, and infectious organisms are in close proximity to each other.

Section Six Review

1. Local impairment of resistance to bacterial invasion may be the result of which factor?
   A. Foreign material
   B. Malnutrition
   C. Cancer
   D. Immunosuppressive drugs

2. What is an example of an endogenous source of organisms?
   A. Debris in the wound
   B. The accident scene
   C. The gastrointestinal tract
   D. The hospital setting

3. Which conditions are criteria for a diagnosis of wound infection? (Select all that apply.)
   A. Purulent drainage from a wound
   B. Negative wound culture
   C. Signs of inflammation
   D. Elevated systemic temperature
   E. Increased odor from the wound

4. Which elements predispose the client to a wound infection? (Select all that apply.)
   A. Immunocompetency
   B. Susceptible host
   C. Devitalized wound tissue
   D. Infectious organism
   E. Total protein of 7.4 g/dL

Answers: 1. A, 2. C, 3. (A, C, D, E), 4. (B, C, D)

Section Seven: Necrotizing Soft-tissue Infections

Necrotic tissue is dead, devitalized tissue. It is an impediment to wound healing and provides an environment for microorganism growth and infection (Baranoski, Ayello, & Langemo, 2016). Infection of the skin and soft tissue becomes complicated when the inflammatory process affects deep tissue layers or when management requires surgical intervention (Singhai, 2016). Necrotizing soft-tissue infections (NSTIs) are rare but potentially fatal infections involving the skin, subcutaneous tissue, fascia, and/or muscle (Van Driessche & Kirsner, 2016). Two types of life-threatening NSTIs may occur in high-acuity patients: necrotizing fasciitis and Fournier gangrene.

Necrotizing Fasciitis

Necrotizing fasciitis (NF) is a severe, deep, soft-tissue infection that leads to necrosis of the subcutaneous tissue and fascia without involvement of the underlying muscle. It can progress rapidly along the fascial plane, causing extensive local tissue destruction, necrosis, and systemic toxicity if not promptly diagnosed and treated. Necrotizing fasciitis is classified as type I, II, III, or IV based on the causative microorganisms. The etiology of NF appears to be multifactorial. In many cases there is prior skin injury or trauma to the area (surgery, burn, muscle injury, insect bite, needlestick). It tends to develop in a susceptible host with preexisting risk factors, as summarized in Box 10–2.

Mortality rate in the past has been reported as 70%, but incidence of NF in adults is reported at 0.4 cases per 100,000. Mortality increases with years of age (Van Driessche & Kirsner, 2016).

Signs and Symptoms NF can affect any part of the body but most commonly involves the extremities, perineum, or abdomen. The extent of involvement in these tissues can range from simple contamination to an unpredictable clinical course and finally to septic shock, multisystem organ failure, and death.

BOX 10–2 Predisposing Risk Factors for Necrotizing Fasciitis

- Chronic disease
  - Heart disease
  - Diabetes mellitus
  - Renal failure
  - Alcoholism
  - Underlying malignancy
  - Peripheral vascular disease
  - Chronic liver disease
- Drugs
  - Steroids
  - Intravenous drug abuse
- Immunosuppression
  - Steroids
  - Cancer chemotherapy
- Malnutrition
- Advancing age
- Obesity

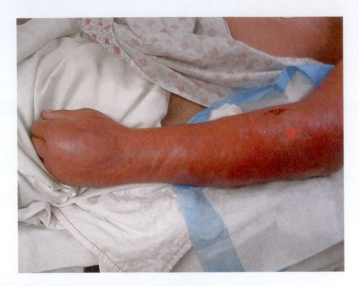

Figure 10–11 Appearance of inflammation in necrotizing fasciitis. Note erythema, edema, and taut appearance of the skin.

SOURCE: Trish Martin

NF is difficult to diagnose in the beginning stage because symptoms mimic nonsevere soft-tissue infections. Early signs include those associated with the inflammatory process: erythema, edema, and pain in the affected area (Figure 10–11). In the early stages it is not easily recognizable because the underlying necrosis is far more extensive than that noted on the skin (Figures 10–12(A) and 10–12(B)). In a study of 138 clinical and laboratory features of 29 NF patients compared with 59 age- and gender-matched patients with severe cellulitis, one important manifestation in NF is severe

pain at onset that is out of proportion to the physical clinical presentation of erythema or edema, and that characteristic of severe pain seems to be the main differential of this condition, as compared to cellulitis (Borschitz, Schlicht, Siegel, Hanke, & von Stebut, 2015). As the infection continues, the skin may change color from red-purple to dusky blue before progressing to necrosis and the formation of hemorrhagic bullae. The development of bullae, or blisters, is important in the differential diagnosis of NF because they are rarely associated with other skin infections such as cellulitis or phlebitis; however, they are considered a late sign in the pathological process (Hakkarainen, Kopari, Pham, & Evans, 2014) (Figure 10–13). In later stages, crepitus may be palpated in the affected area or may be seen radiographically. Crepitus results from gas-forming organisms and anaerobic infection.

The underlying disease process is common to all types of NF, but the speed of development and associated clinical features differ greatly depending on the causative microorganism(s). Some types of NF progress more slowly, evolving over days, while others, initially more insidious, progress rapidly. Tissue necrosis can extend 3 cm of tissues per hour (Davis & Stöppler, 2016), with lots of variability of spread reported in the literature in case-related scenarios.

NF is often compared to cellulitis as a general point of differentiation. Laboratory findings in NF patients as compared to those who had cellulitis have some significant differences. For example, C-reactive protein (CRP) is a serum marker that can indicate acute inflammation. The median CRP for cellulitis patients was 49 mg/dL, while the median CRP in NF patients was 254 mg/dL. In addition, blood creatinine levels were elevated in NF patients. NF patients showed an increase in activated partial thromboplastin time (aPTT), as well as the international normalized ratio

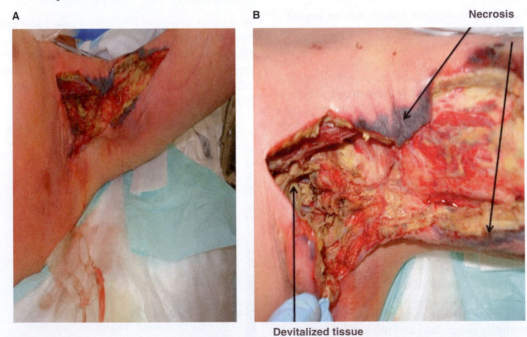

Figure 10–12 Note how necrosis of the subcutaneous tissue and fascia is far more extensive than that of the skin, A. Note the dusky blue discoloration of the skin around the wound, B. When the wound is further opened and debrided, note the devitalized tissue and necrosis. Also note the absence of frank purulence.

SOURCE: Trish Martin

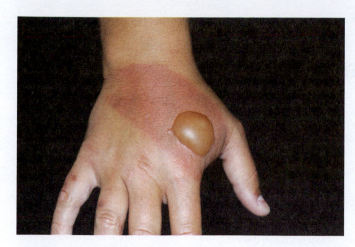

Figure 10–13 Bullae. Bullae are filled with serous and hemorrhagic fluid.

SOURCE: Trish Martin

(INR). However, the NF patient tended to have a decreased erythrocyte and hemoglobin count compared to the patient with cellulitis (Borschitz et al., 2015; Weng et al., 2014).

To diagnose NSTI more rapidly and reliably, and to distinguish it from severe cellulitis or abscess, a clinical scoring system has been developed. The laboratory risk indicator for necrotizing fasciitis (LRINEC) model, developed by Wong and colleagues after observation of 89 patients with NF and 225 control patients, is based on lab measurements of C-reactive protein, WBC count, hemoglobin, sodium, creatinine, and glucose (Wong, Khin, Heng, Tan, & Low, 2004). The total possible score is 13; a score greater than or equal to 6 is highly indicative of NF, with a 92% positive predictability and a 96% negative predictability. Although the LRINEC scoring model is widely used, it has never been validated in prospective trials, and its use is limited when competing inflammatory states are present. Clinical presentation in combination with the LRINEC model should complement each other (Hakkarainen et al., 2014). Wound cultures may reveal a mixture of aerobic and anaerobic organisms, although the most common causative organism is *Streptococcus*. There has been a great deal of attention in the media about "flesh-eating bacteria," which is a strain of *Streptococcus*, group A beta-hemolytic *streptococci* (GAS). Approximately 9000 to 11,500 cases of invasive GAS disease occur each year in the United States (3.2 to 3.9/100,000 population), resulting in 1000 to 1800 deaths annually. NF is responsible for an average of about 6% to 7% of these invasive cases (Centers for Disease Control & Prevention, 2014).

Depending on the causative organism, NF is categorized as type I, II, III, or IV:

- Type I is caused by two or more pathogens (polymicrobial) and is the most common type of NF, accounting for 70% to 90% of cases (Misiakos et al., 2014). In fact, in type I NF, an average of 4.4 pathogens are identifiable (Misiakos et al., 2014). This type of NF is associated with multiple comorbid conditions, including diabetes mellitus, and often occurs in the trunk and perineum areas of the body (Misiakos et al., 2014).

- Type II is a monomicrobial infection caused by GAS, either alone or with *Staphylococcus aureus*. The incidence of community-acquired methicillin-resistant *S. aureus* (MRSA) soft-tissue infection accounts for 10% to 30% of all patients with this type of NF and seems to have a strong incidence after small incisions and the use of NSAID medication (Misiakos et al., 2014). Type II infections tend to occur in otherwise healthy, young, immunocompetent hosts. This type of NF typically appears on the limbs of the patient (Misiakos et al., 2014).

- Type III is caused by marine organisms, mainly *Vibrio*. These infections are associated with seafood ingestion (raw oysters) and wound contamination with seawater (Misiakos et al., 2014). In addition, the *Clostridium* species appears as type III NF, and it typically manifests in traumatic crush-type injuries or in intestinal or obstetric surgical wounds. This *Clostridium* species seems to be prevalent with drug addicts. Common sites of infection are the limbs, trunk, and perineum (Misiakos et al., 2014).

- Type IV is a fungal infection related to *Candida* and is rare, mainly affecting immunocompromised patients, and is very aggressive clinically (Misiakos et al., 2014).

Pathogenesis of NF   The pathogens causing NF invade the subcutaneous tissue and proliferate rapidly. They then invade and block blood vessels and the lymphatic system, causing vasoconstriction and thrombosis. Hypoxic conditions in the subcutaneous tissue impair neutrophil actions. Decreased blood flow to the area impairs the delivery of oxygen, nutrients, and antibiotics and results in necrosis of the skin and fascia. This tissue ischemia promotes rapid bacterial spread (Misiakos et al., 2014).

Treatment   Treatment of NF includes intravenous administration of broad-spectrum antibiotics that cover the commonly suspected organisms, aggressive surgical debridement, wound management, and dressing changes. There is no clear optimal approach for medication interventions for the treatment of NF. However, it is agreed that the medication approach should treat multiple organisms in combination (Stevens & Baddour, 2014). Antibiotic regimens vary widely but typically consist of intravenous administration of penicillin or piperacillin-tazobactam for gram-positive cocci; aminoglycoside, cephalosporins, or carbapenems for gram-negative aerobes; and clindamycin for anaerobes. If the patient has a severe penicillin hypersensitivity, clindamycin or metronidazole with an aminoglycoside or fluoroquinolone may be used. Empiric MRSA coverage with vancomycin or linezolid may be appropriate in areas with high rates of community- and hospital-acquired MRSA. Antimicrobial therapy should have special consideration for group A *Streptococcus* (GAS) and *Clostridium* species as these are very common (Stevens & Baddour, 2014). Antibiotics alone may suppress the systemic sequelae of the infection, but they do not address the underlying source, leading to the demise of the patient; however, aggressive surgery often may limit the postoperative amount of antibiotics required (Misiakos et al., 2014). Mortality approaches 100% without surgical intervention (Stevens & Baddour, 2014), and aggressive surgical

Related Pharmacotherapy
Combination Antimicrobials for NSTIs

Penicillin G

Megacillin

Action and Uses

Beta-lactam antibiotic. Acts by interfering with synthesis of muco-peptides essential to formation and integrity of bacterial cell wall. Highly active against gram-positive cocci and gram-negative cocci.

Dosages (Adult)

Moderate to severe infections: 1.2–24 million units; given in divided doses every 4 hours (intermittent infusion); or continuous infusion (dividing total dose over 24-hr. period)

Major Side Effects

Systemic anaphylaxis
Urinary, delayed skin reactions

Nursing Implications

Treatment may be started before wound cultures are known.
Administer intravenous solutions over at least an hour to avoid electrolyte imbalance from potassium or sodium content.

Aminoglycosides

Gentamicin

Action and Uses

Active against a wide variety of aerobic gram-negative bacteria and certain gram-positive organisms such as MRSA

Dosages (Adult)

Moderate to severe infection: 1–2 mg/kg (loading dose); 3–5 mg/kg per day, divided into three doses (maintenance dose)

Major Side Effects

Nephrotoxicity
Decreased creatinine clearance

Nursing Implications

Monitor renal function, particularly in patients with impaired renal function, advancing age, or therapy beyond 10 days.
Draw blood specimens for peak concentrations 30 to 60 minutes after completion of IV administration. Draw blood specimens for trough concentrations just before administration of IV dose. Use nonheparinized tubes to collect blood samples.

Antitrichomonal

Metronidazole (Flagyl)

Action and Uses

Synthetic compound that has trichomonacidal and amebicidal activity as well as antibacterial activity against anaerobic bacteria and some gram-negative bacteria

Dosages (Adult)

Anaerobic infections: 15 mg/kg (loading dose); 7.5 mg/kg every 6 hrs (maintenance dose); maximum dose = 4 g/24 hrs

Major Side Effects

Overgrowth of *Candida*
Nausea

Nursing Implications

Administer IV slowly over an hour.
Assess for signs of central nervous system toxicity.
Commonly used treatment regimens include MRSA prophylactic treatment.
Choices include vancomycin, linezolid, daptomycin.

---

intervention is always necessary for NF treatment. Additional information regarding antibiotic therapy for necrotizing soft-tissue infections can be found in the "Related Pharmacotherapy: Combination Antimicrobials for NSTIs" feature.

All nonviable tissues, including fascia, must be surgically debrided. The patient may require debridement in the operating room every couple of days (Figure 10–14(A)). Negative pressure wound therapy (NPWT) may be used (Figure 10–14(B)). More aggressive surgery, such as amputation of an extremity, may be required if the patient does not heal or develops septic shock. Given the high rate of systemic toxicity, these patients often require intensive monitoring, hemodynamic resuscitation, and nutritional support, all of which have been shown to decrease mortality. Patients with NF are at high risk for developing multisystem organ dysfunction. Judicious control of glucose and other therapeutic approaches for septic shock are used to optimize the host response to infection. Hyperbaric oxygen therapy (HBOT) and intravenous immunoglobulin (IVIG) are possible adjunct therapies. Use of HBOT in the treatment of NF is not well established. IVIG is a reasonable option to neutralize streptococcal toxins in severe cases, having been demonstrated as effective in similar toxic shock syndrome cases (Stevens & Baddour, 2014).

Once systemic manifestations of an infectious process disappear, wound exudate decreases in volume and granulation tissue develops and begins to fill in the wound defect. Wound closure may be assisted by delayed primary closure (Figure 10–15) or surgical skin grafts or flaps. Skin grafting with a split-thickness skin graft (STSG) is most commonly needed in large wounds to achieve rapid, safe wound closure. Skin is taken from a donor site and placed on healthy granulation tissue to cover the defect (Figure 10–16). Revascularization of the grafted skin occurs, closing the wound over time.

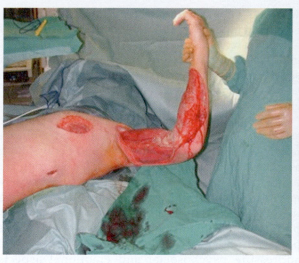
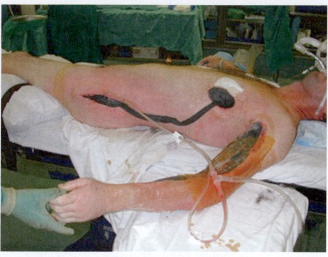

A   **B**

Figure 10–14 After wide surgical debridement of NF of the arm A, a NPWT system is placed B.

SOURCE: Trish Martin

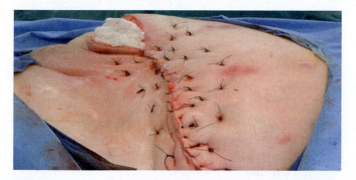

Figure 10–15 Delayed primary closure of the abdomen after NF has been resolved.

SOURCE: Trish Martin

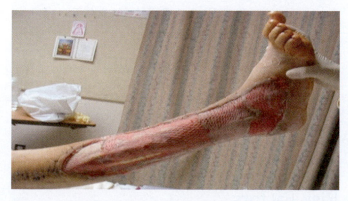

Figure 10–16 Split-thickness skin graft.

SOURCE: Trish Martin

Fournier Gangrene

Fournier gangrene (FG) is a form of type I necrotizing fasciitis that develops in the perineal, genital, and perianal regions but can spread to the abdominal wall, causing soft-tissue necrosis and sepsis (Sroczynski, Sebastian, Rudnicki,

Sebastian, & Agrawal, 2013). It is ten times more common in males than females (Pais, 2016). FG can arise spontaneously or from a perineal abscess, an infection of a Bartholin's gland or the scrotum, or a genitourinary procedure, but in at least 60% of the cases, diabetes is present (Pais, 2016). Skin color changes, and crepitus, similar to those in NF, can occur (Figure 10–17). As with NF, a surgical approach is always warranted, and these patients present with unique needs, given the anatomical location of FG. Sometimes diverting colostomies or fecal management systems are warranted due to location, which can be challenging for care (Pais, 2016).

Treatment of FG is similar to that for patients with other types of NF: administration of broad-spectrum antibiotics

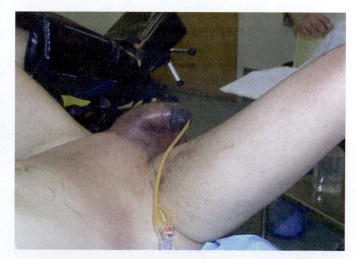

Figure 10–17 Fournier gangrene. Note the dusky-blue discoloration moving from the penis and extending proximally along the abdomen. Soft-tissue necrosis extends from the penis through the muscle planes of the abdomen.

SOURCE: Trish Martin

for polymicrobial infections, aggressive surgical debridement, and wound management. Wound management may include dressing changes with moist saline gauze, advanced topical therapies with or without an antimicrobial, or NPWT. Adequate pain management is essential prior to and during dressing changes. A temporary diverting colostomy or urinary diversion may be required to lessen wound contamination and promote healing. In a study of 86 patients with FG, patients who experience FG face persistent medical and mental health problems, including secondary complications, impaired sexual function, impaired physical function, and often years of treatment with multiple specialists (Czymek et al., 2013).

Nursing Care

Patients with NSTIs require comprehensive management involving nursing and other health-professional best practices. Knowledge about NSTIs can assist nurses in advocating for differential diagnosis, immediate treatment, and a plan of care. Many patients require intensive nursing care, assessment, and monitoring for sepsis and multisystem organ dysfunction. Administering antibiotics as scheduled is imperative, as is performing therapeutic lab draws for specific antibiotics to monitor dosing level effectiveness.

Nursing wound management is often complicated and time consuming, demanding knowledge of dressing techniques along with wound base and periwound tissue assessment. The nurse is responsible for ensuring that the patient receives nutrition and hydration as ordered to maximize healing potential. Pain impairs wound healing; therefore, nursing assessment and pain management prior to and during dressing changes are vital to positive patient outcomes. Nursing care is comprehensive, addressing psychosocial and emotional aspects for patients with a life-threatening, disfiguring, rapid disease process.

Section Seven Review

1. What are some predisposing risk factors for NF? (Select all that apply.)
   A. Heart disease
   B. Immunosuppression
   C. Diabetes mellitus
   D. Obesity
   E. Young adulthood

2. Which assessment is associated with NF?
   A. Pain out of proportion to apparent injury
   B. Enlarged lymph nodes
   C. Frank purulence
   D. Pitting edema

3. *Flesh-eating bacteria* is a lay term for which organism?
   A. *Staphylococcus aureus*
   B. Group A beta-hemolytic *streptococci*
   C. Marine vibrios
   D. *Streptococcus aureus*

4. Which antibiotics are likely to be prescribed for the treatment of NF? (Select all that apply.)
   A. Penicillin
   B. Aminoglycoside
   C. Clindamycin
   D. Erythromycin
   E. Carbapenem

Answers: 1. (A, B, C, D), 2. A, 3. B, 4. (A, B, C, E)

Section Eight: Enterocutaneous Fistulas

A **fistula** is a tubelike passage that forms a connection between different sites (e.g., a cavity and a tube, or a cavity and a free surface). An **enterocutaneous fistula (ECF)** is a passageway that develops between a segment of the GI tract and the skin or wound bed. A simple fistula is a short, direct track connecting bowel and skin. Complex fistulae are associated with an abscess or multiple organ involvement (type 1) or appear as an opening into a wound (type 2) (Bryant & Best, 2016). The vast majority of ECFs occur as a complication of abdominal surgery (85%), usually involving a bowel anastomosis, repair of an enterotomy, or unrecognized bowel injury. ECFs may be iatrogenic or due to underlying disease processes such as Crohn disease, ulcerative colitis, or diverticular disease. Of course any of these comorbid conditions in addition to abdominal surgery increases the risk of ECF occurrence (Stein, 2015). Management of ECFs is complex and challenging and often requires a multidisciplinary team of surgeons, wound ostomy nurses, nutritionists, physical therapists, and occupational therapists. Patients with ECFs have fluid and electrolyte imbalances, malnutrition, and altered skin integrity requiring complex wound management.

Risk Factors

Certain risk factors, as summarized in Box 10–3, are known to increase the chances of developing an ECF. In malnourished states, tissue repair and regeneration are compromised and bowel anastomoses are more likely to fail, which allows GI contents to leak into the peritoneum. Patients who have been on long-term and/or high-dose steroids are at risk for developing an ECF as a result of poor wound healing. Chemotherapy and radiation therapy to the abdomen cause decreased tissue integrity and interfere with

BOX 10–3 Conditions That Increase the Risk of Enterocutaneous Fistulas

- Malnutrition at the time of surgery
- History of steroid use
- History of chemotherapy or radiation therapy to the abdomen
- Inflammatory bowel disease
- Trauma to the abdomen, abdominal compartment syndrome

wound healing after abdominal surgery. ECFs can occur in patients who had abdominal surgery for trauma, especially if a bowel injury is missed at the initial operation or if the patient developed abdominal compartment syndrome and required damage control surgery in which the abdomen was left open to heal by secondary intention. An exposed bowel can develop secondary bowel injury during the process of dressing changes. It is important for the nurse to prevent these problems by protecting the bowel with a nonadherent contact layer dressing until sufficient granulation has covered the exposed bowel.

Clinical Presentation

The first sign of an ECF appears as a local wound infection if the abdominal incision is healing by primary intention. The skin around the sutures or staples may become erythematous, and the skin becomes shiny and tight. Within a couple of days, the appearance and odor of GI contents may be noted. A small amount of drainage may seep out of the sutures and appear on the patient's gown or bed linens.

For patients with open abdomens healing by secondary intention, the drainage may not be visible in the wound bed but may only be apparent on the dressings as they are removed from the wound (Figure 10–18). Drainage on the dressings may change from serosanguineous to green or brown and may have a fecal odor. In these situations, it is imperative that the nurse notify the healthcare provider immediately. Early recognition is crucial to prevent life-threatening metabolic, septic, and nutritional complications (Badrasawi, Shahar, & Sagap, 2014). In addition, it is very important to protect the skin in the area surrounding the fistula.

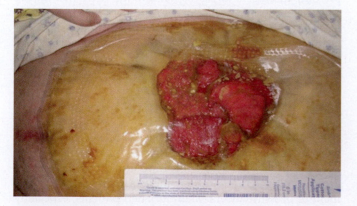

Figure 10–18 Enterocutaneous fistula. Note the green stool drainage in the wound bed.

SOURCE: Trish Martin

An upper GI contrast study or CT scan may be ordered to determine the exact anatomic location of the ECF. A fistulagram may be performed by a radiologist who introduces dye into the fistula, followed by radiologic examination to visualize the scope of the fistula. Location is an important prognostic factor. ECFs that form in the proximal GI tract (small bowel) are associated with worse patient outcomes (Gyorki et al., 2010; Martinez, Luque-de-Leon, Mier, Blanco-Benavides, & Robledo, 2008). These ECFs have a higher output of GI drainage, which results in severe fluid and electrolyte imbalances and malnutrition because nutrients and water are not absorbed. High-output drainage is generally defined as ECF drainage greater than 500 mL/day (Bryant & Best, 2016). ECFs that form in the distal GI tract (colon) do not have as much drainage, and the stool from the ECF has a thicker consistency. Small-bowel ECFs tend to take longer to heal and require longer courses of treatment and hospitalization than ECFs that develop in the colon.

Collaborative Management

Management of patients with ECFs includes correction of fluid and electrolyte imbalances, nutritional support, and complex wound management. With high-output ECFs, the nurse should monitor the patient for signs of hypovolemia. Serum electrolytes should be monitored for the development of hypokalemia, hypochloremia, and acidosis, depending on the location of the ECF in the GI tract. The nurse should ensure accurate measurement of ECF drainage so that fluids and electrolytes can be replaced accordingly.

Evidenced-based nutritional support may include enteral or parenteral nutrition or fistuloclysis; however, the literature is scarce as to which route is optimal (Badrasawi, Shahar, & Sagap, 2014). There is increasing evidence that enteral nutrition is associated with maintenance of GI mucosal integrity and improved immunologic host response, as well as fewer complications for the patient (Badrasawi, Shahar, & Sagap, 2014). Enteral nutrition has been found to be useless in patients with an ECF and high-output drainage. Parenteral nutrition may be required in conjunction with enteral nutrition to allow administration of full nutritional requirements (Badrasawi, Shahar, & Sagap, 2014). Fistuloclysis is a feeding technique in which the fistula itself serves as the entry portal for nutrition. This method has been found to be nutritionally sound, cost efficient, and effective. It has been used in the small bowel when enteral nutrition could not be absorbed or when parenteral nutrition is not indicated (Badrasawi, Shahar, & Sagap, 2014; Coetzee, Rahm, Boutall, & Goldberg, 2014). Nutritional support decisions are individualized based on the location of the ECF, the output from the ECF, and the patient's overall metabolic and nutritional requirements.

Management of skin integrity in patients with an ECF is extremely complex and challenging for the high-acuity nurse. If available, a wound ostomy nurse should be consulted to help manage these complex wounds. Skin protection, drainage quantification, and drainage containment must be considered when developing the plan of care for these patients. The enzyme content of the ECF drainage, coupled with the prolonged exposure of the perifistular skin to effluent, leads to alteration in skin integrity. Skin care may include application of ostomy appliances to help protect the skin and contain drainage. As noted, peri-wound barrier products can be used to protect the skin from ECF drainage (Bryant & Best, 2016).

Decreasing ECF output is important in reducing fluid and electrolyte imbalances and promoting wound healing. Reduction of ECF drainage may be accomplished by reducing GI secretions via administration of H_2 receptor antago-nists or proton pump inhibitors. Bowel transit may be slowed with antimotility agents. The use of antisecretory agents, such as somatostatin and octreotide, is controversial. These agents reduce secretion of GI hormones (gastrin and cholecystokinin), in turn decreasing gastric and pancreatic secretions. These agents may reduce fistula drainage and decrease time to closure of ECFs; however, it is not known whether they increase the overall likelihood of spontaneous closure of ECFs.

Section Eight Review

1. What are risk factors for the development of an ECF after abdominal surgery? (Select all that apply.)
   A. Hypoalbuminemia
   B. Long-term use of steroids
   C. Radiation therapy to the abdomen
   D. Abdominal compartment syndrome
   E. Immunosuppression

2. Which rate of ECF drainage is defined as high output?
   A. 100 mL/hour
   B. 200 mL/day
   C. 500 mL/hour
   D. 500 mL/day

3. The client with a high-output ECF is at risk for developing which abnormalities? (Select all that apply.)
   A. Alkalosis
   B. Hypokalemia
   C. Hypochloremia
   D. Hypomagnesemia
   E. Hypovolemia

4. Which products can be used to achieve skin protection, drainage quantification, and drainage containment of an ECF?
   A. Wet-to-dry dressings
   B. Ostomy appliances
   C. Hydrocolloid wafers
   D. Skin-barrier protection products

Answers: 1. (A, B, C, D), 2. D, 3. (B, C, E), 4. B

Section Nine: Pressure Ulcers

A pressure ulcer is a localized injury to the skin and/or underlying tissue, usually over a bony prominence, that occurs when blood circulation to an area is decreased due to compression of the skin between the bone and another surface. The resulting tissue ischemia leads to necrosis and ulcer formation. Heels, the sacral area, ischial areas and trochanters, and the lower back are the most common sites for pressure ulcers. Less common sites include the elbows, occiput of the head, spine, nose, and ears. Patient position can also be a factor for where the ulcer develops; common sites for this type of pressure ulcer are listed in Table 10–4.

Table 10–4 Common Sites for Pressure Ulcers by Patient Position

Patient Position	Pressure Ulcer Sites
Supine	Scapula, occiput, sacrum, heels
Lateral	Ear, shoulder, trochanter, medial knee, malleolus, foot edge
Prone	Nose, forehead, chest, iliac crests, foot edges, toes

Etiology of Pressure Ulcers

Intrinsic factors that contribute to the development of pressure ulcers are those internal conditions that relate to the patient's physical or mental health, such as nutritional status, mobility, incontinence, age, and skin condition. Extrinsic factors are those that derive from the immediate environment—such as skin hygiene, medications, shear, and friction—and place the patient at increased risk. A pressure ulcer is simply a response to the stress that the tissues are under. Basically, pressure ulcers are the internal response to the external mechanical load on the skin. The factors mentioned also stress the skin, but the key is the tolerance of the duration of the pressure present on the bony prominence (Ayello, Baranoski, Cuddigan, & Harris, 2016).

Risk Factors for Pressure Ulcer Development

Patients whose activity is restricted—such as those with strokes, spinal cord injury resulting in tetraplegia or paraplegia, and fractures—are at increased risk for development of pressure ulcers. Malnourished patients, especially those with protein-calorie malnutrition or those who are very thin, have skin that is prone to ulceration. Also, patients who are incontinent or whose skin is exposed to moisture—such as excessive perspiration, wound drainage, and urinary or fecal incontinence—are at increased risk for skin breakdown. Critically ill patients who receive vasopressor medications for hypotension and patients with comorbid conditions—such as diabetes mellitus, hypertension, and respiratory and/or vascular disease—are also at increased risk (Ayello et al., 2016).

Predicting Risk for Pressure Ulcers

A widely used, clinically validated tool that allows nurses to score a high-acuity patient's risk for development of pressure ulcers is the Braden Scale for Predicting Pressure Ulcer Risk (Table 10–5). Scores range from 6 to 23; lower scores indicate a higher risk. A score of 18 or lower places the patient at risk for a pressure ulcer and should prompt the nurse to implement strategies to reduce risk to the patient. It is incumbent upon the nurse to be familiar with the institution's policies and procedures for the prevention and management of pressure ulcers.

In addition to the total score of the Braden Scale, each score on the subsets must be assessed individually. The nursing intervention for the patient can be found clearly by identifying the low score for each subscale (Ayello et al., 2016). In addition, those patients who are over 65 years of age should be considered to be at a higher level of risk than scored (Qaseem, Mir, Starkey, & Denberg, 2015).

Table 10–5 Braden Scale for Predicting Pressure Ulcer Risk

Note: Bed- and chairbound individuals or those with impaired ability to reposition should be assessed upon admission for their risk of developing pressure ulcers. Patients with established pressure ulcers should be reassessed periodically.

Patient Name:_____ Room Number:_____ Date:_____

Sensory Perception	1. Completely Limited	2. Very Limited	3. Slightly Limited	4. No Impairment	Indicate Appropriate Numbers Below
Ability to respond meaningfully to pressure-related discomfort	Unresponsive (does not moan, flinch or grasp) to painful stimuli, due to diminished level of . consciousness or sedation. OR limited ability to feel pain over most of body surface.	Responds only to painful stimuli. Cannot communicate discomfort except by moaning or restlessness. OR has a sensory impairment which limits the ability to feel pain or discomfort over 1/2 of body.	Responds to verbal commands, but cannot always communicate discomfort or need to be turned. OR has some sensory impairment which limits ability to feel pain or discomfort in 1 or 2 extremities.	Responds to verbal commands. Has no sensory deficit which would limit ability to feel or voice pain or discomfort.	
Moisture	**1. Constantly Moist**	**2. Very Moist**	**3. Occasionally Moist**	**4. Rarely Moist**	
Degree to which skin is exposed to moisture	Skin is kept moist almost constantly by perspiration, urine. Dampness is detected every time patient is moved or turned.	Skin is often, but not always, moist. Linen must be changed at least once a shift.	Skin is occasionally moist, requiring an extra linen change approximately once a day.	Skin is usually dry. Linen only requires changing at routine intervals.	
Activity	**1. Bedfast**	**2. Chairfast**	**3. Walks Occasionally**	**4. Walks Frequently**	
Degree of physical activity	Confined to bed.	Ability to walk severely limited or nonexistent. Cannot bear own weight and/or must be assisted into chair or wheelchair.	Walks occasionally during day, but for very short distances, with or without assistance. Spends majority of each shift in bed or chair.	Walks outside the room at least twice a day and inside room at least once every 2 hours during waking hours.	
Mobility	**1. Completely Immobile**	**2. Very Limited**	**3. Slightly Limited**	**4. No Limitations**	
Ability to change and control body position	Does not make even slight changes in body or extremity position without assistance.	Makes occasional slight changes in body or extremity position but unable to make frequent or significant changes independently.	Makes frequent though slight changes in body or extremity position independently.	Makes major and frequent changes in position without assistance.	
Nutrition	**1. Very Poor**	**2. Probably Inadequate**	**3. Adequate**	**4. Excellent**	
Usual food intake pattern	Never eats a complete meal. Rarely eats more than 1/3 of any food offered. Eats 2 servings or less of protein (meat or dairy products) per day. Takes fluids poorly. Does not take a liquid dietary supplement. OR is NPO and/or maintained on clear liquids or IVs for more than 5 days.	Rarely eats a complete meal and generally eats only about 1/2 of any food offered. Protein intake includes only 3 servings of meat or dairy products per day. Occasionally will take a dietary supplement. OR receives less than optimum amount of liquid diet or tube feeding.	Eats more than 1/2 of most meals. Eats a total of 4 servings of protein (meat, dairy products) each day. Occasionally will refuse a meal, but will usually take a supplement if offered. OR is on a tube feeding or TPN regimen which probably meets most of nutritional needs.	Eats most of every meal. Never refuses a meal. Usually eats a total of 4 or more servings of meat and dairy products. Occasionally eats between meals. Does not require supplementation.	

(continued)

Table 10–5 Continued

Friction and Shear	1. Problem	2. Potential Problem	3. No Apparent Problem
	Requires moderate to maximum assistance in moving. Complete lifting without sliding against sheets is impossible. Frequently slides down in bed or chair, requiring frequent repositioning with maximum assistance. Spasticity, contractures, or agitation lead to almost constant friction.	Moves feebly or requires minimum assistance. During a move, skin probably slides to some extent against sheets, chair restraints, or other devices. Maintains relatively good position in chair or bed most of the time, but occasionally slides down.	Moves in bed and in chair independently and has sufficient muscle strength to lift up completely during move. Maintains good position in bed or chair at all times.

Note: Patients with a total score of 16 or less are considered to be at risk of developing pressure ulcers. (15 or 16 = low risk; 13 or 14 = moderate risk; 12 or less = high risk

Total Score:_____

Generally, an agency will have a policy regarding pressure ulcer risk assessment; however, the Braden Scale is often used upon admission and then daily to trend risk over time.

Pressure Ulcer Staging

Pressure ulcers are staged according to the depth of injury using a staging classification system developed to ensure consistency in the assessment and documentation of these wounds. A caveat to this is that if the wound is necrotic and covered with eschar, it cannot be staged because the depth cannot be measured—debridement of the wound would be necessary. In 2007 and 2014 the National Pressure Ulcer Advisory Panel (NPUAP) updated its guidelines for pressure ulcer staging to describe six stages of pressure

ulcer development (Table 10–6). Table 10–7 shows four stages of pressure ulcers using the NPUAP guidelines.

Collaborative Management of Pressure Ulcers

Preventive measures are the best strategy to avoid or reduce the development of pressure ulcers. Once a pressure ulcer develops, the goals of treatment are to maintain or improve oxygenation to the area, prevent infection, and promote healing. Products to treat these wounds range from those that absorb exudate, thereby keeping the wound dry, to those that protect and insulate the wound. Treatment decisions are guided by the ulcer characteristics. Stage I ulcers require frequent turning and removal of

Table 10–6 National Guidelines for Pressure Ulcer Staging from the National Pressure Ulcer Advisory Panel (NPUAP)

Stage of Wound	Guideline
Suspected Deep-tissue injury (sDTI)	sDTI is characterized by purple or maroon tissue over bony prominence areas from pressure or shear with intact skin. It often feels boggy (soft) or indurated (hard) or warmer or cooler than adjacent tissue. It should be classified as an sDTI, and close monitoring for further deterioration should be performed.
Stage I	Intact skin with nonblanchable area of redness. A keynote for other clues, especially for those with darker skin tones, is any change in color, warmth, edema, or pain over a bony prominence area of pressure.
Stage II	Partial-thickness avulsion of skin into dermis layer and may present as a shallow open ulcer without slough (dead cells). It also can present as either an intact serum-filled blister or a serum-filled blister that has ruptured.
Stage III	Involves full-thickness loss in which the hypodermis or subcutaneous fat layer may be exposed. Slough may be present, and structures such as tendon or bone are not visible. When located on the nose, ear, back of head, or ankle, the ulcer may be shallow due to decreased fat tissue in these areas. Tunneling and undermining may be present.
Stage IV	Full-thickness wound with exposed tendon, muscle, and/or bone. Most often has slough or eschar (dead tissue). The same information regarding anatomical location and depth of wound from stage III is applicable at this stage.
Unstageable	Eschar and/or slough that cover the wound area cannot be staged because the underlying tissue cannot be assessed. It is therefore classified as unstageable until the slough/eschar is removed, and then the wound should be documented related to its defining characteristics.

Table 10–7   Pressure Ulcer Appearance by Stage

Appearance by Stage		Description
Stage I	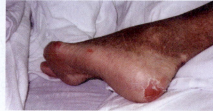 SOURCE: Kathy Cisney	A sign of risk. Intact skin with nonblanchable redness of a localized area, usually over a bony prominence. The area may be painful, firm, soft, warmer, or cooler than adjacent tissue. May be difficult to detect in people with dark skin.
Stage II	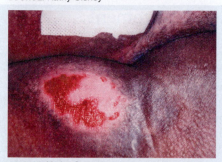 SOURCE: Kathy Cisney	Partial-thickness loss of dermis presenting as a shallow open ulcer with a red or pink wound bed. May also present as an intact or open blister. The ulcer may be shiny or dry, without bruising or slough (loss of tissue).
Stage III	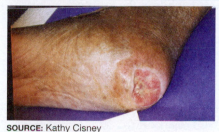 SOURCE: Kathy Cisney	Full-thickness tissue loss. Subcutaneous fat may be visible but bone, tendon, or muscle are *not* exposed. Slough may be present but does not obscure the depth of tissue loss. *May* include undermining and tunneling.
Stage IV	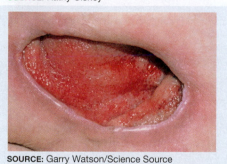 SOURCE: Garry Watson/Science Source	Full-thickness skin loss with exposed bone, tendon, or muscle. Slough or eschar (dead tissue such as a scab) may be present on some parts of the wound bed. Often includes undermining and tunneling.

SOURCE: Based on National Pressure Ulcer Advisory Panel, European Pressure Ulcer Advisory Panel and Pan Pacific Pressure Injury Alliance. Prevention and Treatment of Pressure Ulcers: Quick Reference Guide (2014). Emily Haausler (Ed.). Cambridge Media: Osborne Park, Western Australia.

pressure (called off-loading), which often can prevent progression of the ulcer. Stage II and III ulcers need a moist healing environment. Stage IV wounds require packing to fill dead space and/or absorb exudate.

Multiple facets influence the nursing and medical care of the patient who has a pressure ulcer. Such patients may need a special pressure-reducing support surface, because one pressure ulcer being present escalates the patient to the highest risk level. Off-loading bony prominences prophylactically cannot be overstated, and the more critically ill the patient is, the more likely a hypoxic event will occur. If a hypoxic event occurs, the patient's risk for development of a suspected deep-tissue injury (sDTI) increases, because of the overall deterioration of the patient. Hypoxia in the high-acuity patient can translate into ischemic skin (Honaker, Forston, Davis, Wiesner, & Morgan, 2013).

Local wound care must be based on the wound characteristics, such as location, depth of tissue loss, amount of exudate, presence of cellulitis, condition of wound edges and periwound skin, and wound tissue characteristics. For example, a dry wound may need a treatment regimen that donates moisture; a wet wound needs a treatment to dry it a bit; a shallow wound requires a covering, while a deep wound requires packing (Ayello et al., 2016).

Collaboration with an interdisciplinary team (consisting of dieticians, case managers, social workers, and consultative healthcare providers such as cardiovascular and infectious disease specialists, physical therapists, and surgeons) is warranted when treating the patient who has a significant pressure ulcer (multiple stage II or a single stage III or IV). Nutritional consultation with a dietician to ensure that the high-acuity patient has caloric, fluid, and protein requirements being met is important. The dietician may have strong recommendations for lab work and remedies for nutritional supplementation to aid in wound healing. Consultation with a certified wound nurse is imperative as this nurse has the expertise to recommend advanced dressings that can potentially streamline the wound care and make it more cost efficient and time efficient. The surgeons may need to provide surgical or local sharp debridement for the patient, and the infectious disease provider can handle the complex antibiotic needs that can occur should a wound become infected. Discharge to home will be more complex if the patient has a wound. In addition, the wound is an extra stressor for the high-acuity patient, and this may take a physiological toll on him or her.

Adjunct therapies such as hyperbaric oxygen, application of growth factor, biosynthetic agents, and negative pressure therapy may be used. These therapies require the nurse to consult the wound care team consisting of dieticians, case managers, social workers, and consultative healthcare providers (cardiovascular and infectious disease specialists, physical therapists, and surgeons). In addition, the patient may need a pressure-reducing mattress and/or chair cushion if a wound is present on the sitting or lying surface as well as for prevention, given the fragility of a high-acuity patient.

A collaborative and comprehensive approach to wound care is essential. The plan must focus on alleviating pressure, treating the ulcer with specialized wound care, education, nutrition, rehydration, mobility, and specialized beds.

Nursing Management

Once a pressure ulcer develops, the nurse is responsible for assessing the wound at periodic intervals for improvement and response to treatment. The nurse should be familiar with the institution's policies and procedures for accurate documentation. A pressure ulcer must be coded as community acquired or healthcare facility acquired because the Centers for Medicare & Medicaid Services (CMS) do not reimburse for care of pressure ulcers acquired in healthcare facilities or for those pressure ulcers identified on admission that worsen while in the facility.

Emerging Evidence

- In a review of the records of 230 hospitalized patients who developed pressure ulcers compared to a matched control group, Braden Scale scores performed upon admission to an acute care facility were predictive of a healthcare-associated pressure ulcer (HAPU) at some point during the hospital stay. However, the nutrition subscale is important, as a low body weight index was predictive of sacral pressure ulcer development. Further, Braden Scale scores on hospital day 7 were predictive of a HAPU during week 2 of the stay *(Miller, Frankenfield, Lehman, Maguire, & Schirm, 2016)*.
- A study of 230 nurses in six critical care units examined the effectiveness of a unit-based education on implementation of a sustainable bowel management program in a critical care setting. The study findings showed a statistically significant ($p < .001$) improvement in knowledge scores and in self-efficacy scores *(Pittman, Beeson, Carter, & Collin, 2015)*.
- A study of 552 intensive care unit patients with and without pressure ulcers compared key variables sorted into the following categories: (1) disease status, (2) physical conditions, and (3) conditions of hospitalization. The variables of peripheral arterial diseases ($p = .002$), mechanical ventilation greater than 72 hours ($p < .001$), respiratory failure ($p < .001$), liver failure ($p = .04$), and severe sepsis or septic shock ($p = .02$) were statistically significant and independent predictors of acute skin failure in ICU patients *(Delmore, Cox, Rolnitzky, Chu, & Stolfi, 2015)*.
- The International Skin Tear Advisory Panel conducted a systematic literature review and 3-phase Delphi consensus with a panel of international reviewers to provide the best available evidence for product selection related to the treatment of skin tears, and these recommendations are reported *(LeBlanc et al., 2016)*.
- Support surfaces are an integral component of pressure ulcer prevention and treatment, but there is insufficient evidence to guide clinical decision making in this area. This article is the report for the first evidence- and consensus-based algorithm for support surface selection that has undergone content validation *(McNichol, Watts, Mackey, Beitz, & Gray, 2015)*.

Section Nine Review

1. A client who continually moves back to the supine position after turning is at risk for pressure ulcers at which sites? (Select all that apply.)
   A. Scapula
   B. Toes
   C. Medial knee
   D. Sacrum
   E. Heel

2. A client is assessed to have a Braden score of 18. Based on this score, what should the nurse do?
   A. Do nothing, but repeat the assessment in 72 hours.
   B. Institute measures to reduce the risk of pressure ulcers.
   C. Consult respiratory therapy to administer inhaled bronchodilator treatment.
   D. Allow the client to remain in a supine position for more than 2 hours.

3. Pressure ulcers are staged according to which finding?
   A. Depth
   B. Location
   C. Size measured laterally
   D. Presence or absence of eschar

4. A client with a stage 1 pressure ulcer would most benefit from which treatment modality?
   A. A moist healing environment
   B. Off-loading
   C. Packing
   D. An absorbent dressing

Answers: 1. (A, D, E), 2. B, 3. A, 4. B

Clinical Reasoning Checkpoint

Mr. A, a 54-year-old male, had a cyst on his right lower extremity (RLE) that got progressively worse and looked infected, so he went to his local emergency department. The cyst was incised and drained. The patient was placed on oral antibiotics and sent home with dressing changes. One week later he returned to the emergency department complaining of severe leg pain. He has a medical history of hypertension, type 2 diabetes mellitus, and IV drug abuse. His vital signs were BP 180/65 mmHg, HR 90/min, temperature 100.9°F, and RR 16 bpm. His RLE is shown in Figure CRC10–1.

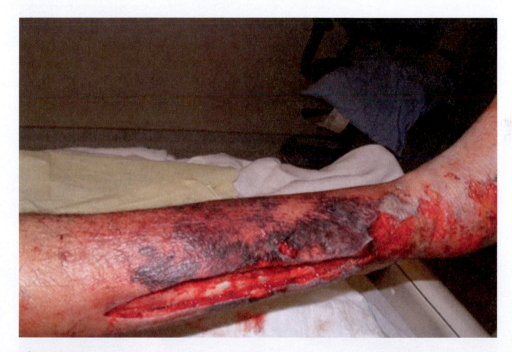

Figure CRC10–1

SOURCE: Trish Martin

1. What is your assessment of Mr. A's RLE?

2. Serum labs are drawn including WBC, sodium, hemoglobin, creatinine, and glucose. If Mr. A has necrotizing fasciitis (NF), what results would you anticipate?

3. Wound cultures are taken. Results reveal the presence of *Streptococcus A* and *Staphylococcus aureus.* What antibiotics would you anticipate administering, and what organisms would they cover?

4. Figure CRC10–2 shows the nurse practitioner assisting the surgeon in the operating room in the debridement of Mr. A's wound. What are they doing, and why?

5. Figure CRC10–3 is a picture of Mr. A's leg after debridement. Assess the wound bed.

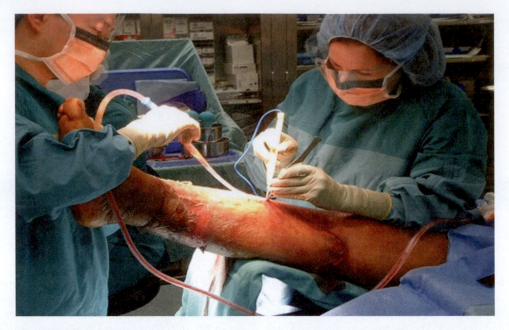

Figure CRC10–2

SOURCE: Trish Martin

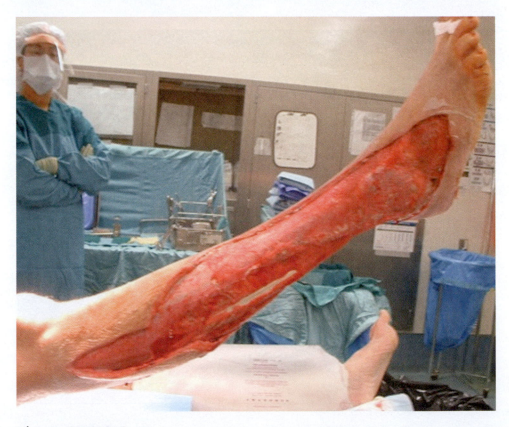

Figure CRC10–3

SOURCE: Trish Martin

6. Mr. A returns to the high-acuity unit postoperatively with a NPWT system (Figure CRC10–4). What is the purpose of this type of dressing?

7. You are discharging a patient with an open abdominal wound. You have taught his wife how to do the dressing changes. The patient smoked two to three packs of cigarettes per day prior to his admission. The patient is anxious to go home to resume smoking. What information is important for you to provide to this patient about the effects of smoking on his wound healing?

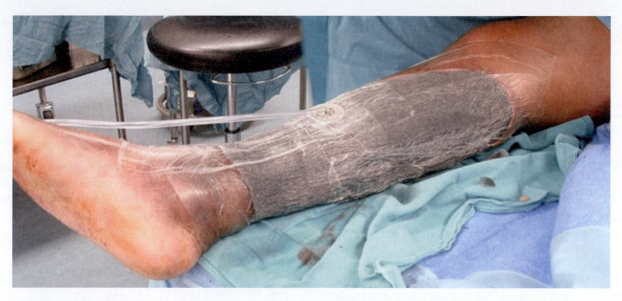

Figure CRC10–4

SOURCE: Trish Martin

Chapter 10 Review

1. A client is admitted from home care with a pressure ulcer that extends into the subcutaneous tissue. How would the nurse describe this wound?

   1. Stage II pressure ulcer
   2. Partial thickness wound
   3. Stage III pressure ulcer
   4. Full thickness wound

2. A client is having surgery for a ruptured appendix today, and the incision is expected to be closed by tertiary intention. What education about the wound will the nurse provide? (Select all that apply.)

   1. "When you see your incision, you will notice it is closed with adhesive strips."
   2. "Your incision will be open to allow for drainage."
   3. "Your incision will be allowed to heal on its own."
   4. "You will require another procedure to close the incision."
   5. "You will need to return in five to seven days to have your sutures removed."

3. The nurse is providing care to clients with abdominal surgical wounds. The nurse would prioritize use of a pillow to splint the wound during coughing and strain with which client?

   1. A 60-year-old client after elective hysterectomy
   2. A 34-year-old client with central obesity
   3. A 40-year-old client who drinks a glass of wine twice a week
   4. A 50-year-old client who takes zinc supplements

4. Palpation of periwound skin reveals induration. The nurse would conduct further assessment for which complications? (Select all that apply.)

   1. Infection
   2. Deep-tissue necrosis
   3. Maceration
   4. Edema
   5. Deep-tissue injury

5. A client is receiving autolytic debridement with a hydrocolloid wafer dressing. The nurse notes a collection of yellow fluid under the dressing on the day before the dressing is scheduled to be changed. What nursing action is indicated?

   1. Remove the dressing to culture the wound.
   2. Irrigate the wound with normal saline.
   3. Leave the dressing intact.
   4. Call the healthcare provider.

6. A client is receiving negative pressure wound therapy (NPWT). Upon removal of the sponge, the nurse notes that granulation tissue has grown into the sponge. The client complains of pain. What actions should the nurse take? (Select all that apply.)

   1. Stop the procedure immediately and collaborate with the healthcare provider.
   2. Wet the sponge with normal saline.
   3. Discuss changing the sponge more frequently with the healthcare provider.
   4. Wet the sponge with hydrogen peroxide.
   5. Tell the client this is an expected event that indicates healing is occurring.

7. A client is brought to the emergency department after being injured in a tornado. The client was found in a muddy ditch and has multiple cuts and abrasions from debris. What nursing measures are indicated to prevent infections in these wounds? (Select all that apply.)

   1. Cleanse the wounds as soon as possible.
   2. Require hand hygiene for all persons who come in contact with the client.
   3. Assist with debridement as indicated.
   4. Place the client in strict isolation.
   5. Administer antibiotics as directed.

8. A client presents to the emergency department with a minor abrasion on the leg that occurred while he was mowing the lawn. The client states, "This is such a small scratch, but it hurts a lot." Assessment reveals slight redness and edema at the site, which feels slightly warm to touch. Which assessment findings are of most concern to the nurse? (Select all that apply.)

   1. The injury is on the client's leg.
   2. The pain from the scratch is out of proportion to its size.
   3. There is slight redness at the site.
   4. There is slight edema at the site.
   5. The site is warm to the touch.

9. The skin around a client's abdominal sutures is reddened. Which finding would most increase the nurse's concern that an enterocutaneous fistula (ECF) has developed?

   1. Abdominal skin is flaccid
   2. There is drainage on the client's gown.
   3. There is the odor of feces in the room.
   4. The client reports having no appetite.

10. A client will be admitted following extensive surgery for Fournier gangrene. The nurse who will provide care for this client should prepare for which postoperative interventions? (Select all that apply.)

   1. Strict isolation from all other clients
   2. Antibiotic therapy
   3. Special fecal management care
   4. Pain management
   5. Special respiratory therapy interventions

Answers to questions found inside your textbook are available on the faculty resources site. Please consult with your instructor.

References

Anghel, E. L., & Kim, P. J. (2016). Negative-pressure wound therapy: A comprehensive review of the evidence. *Plastic Reconstructive Surgery, 138*(3 Suppl), 129S–137S.

Armstrong, D. G., & Lavery, L. A. (2005). Diabetic Foot Study Consortium. Negative pressure wound therapy after partial diabetic foot amputation: A multicentre, randomised controlled trial. *Lancet, 366*, 1704–1710.

Ayello, E. A., Baranoski, S., Cuddigan, J. E., & Harris, W. S. (2016). Pressure ulcers. In S. Baranoski & E. A. Ayello (Eds.), *Wound care essentials: Practice principles* (4th ed., pp. 309–339). Philadelphia, PA: Wolters Kluwer.

Badrasawi, M., Shahar, S., & Sagap, I. (2014). Nutritional management in enterocutaneous fistula. What is the evidence? *The Malaysian Journal of Medical Sciences, 22*(4), 6–16. PMCID: PMC4683844

Baranoski, S., Ayello, E. A., & Langemo, D. (2016). Wound assessment. In S. Baranoski & E. A. Ayello (Eds.), *Wound care essentials: Practice principles* (4th ed., pp. 99–120). Philadelphia, PA: Wolters Kluwer.

Barbul, A., Efron, D. T., & Kavalukas, S. L. (2015). Wound healing. In F. Brunicardi, D. K. Andersen, T. R. Billiar, D. L. Dunn, J. G. Hunter, J. B. Matthews, & R. E. Pollock, (Eds.), *Schwartz's principles of surgery* (10th ed., Chapter 9). Retrieved February 17, 2017, from http://accessmedicine.mhmedical.com.ezproxy.uky.edu/content.aspx?bookid=980&sectionid=59610850

Blume, P. A., Walters, J., Payne, W., Avata, J., & Lantis, J. (2008). Comparison of negative pressure wound therapy using vacuum-assisted closure with advanced moist wound therapy in the treatment of diabetic foot ulcers: A multicenter randomized controlled trial. *Diabetes Care, 31*, 631–636.

Borschitz, T., Schlicht, S., Siegel, E., Hanke, E., & von Stebut, E. (2015). Improvement of a clinical score for necrotizing fasciitis: "Pain out of proportion" and high CRP levels aid the diagnosis. *PLoS ONE, 10*(7), e0132775. doi:10.1371/journal.pone.0132775

Bryant, R. A., & Best, M. (2016). Management of draining wounds and fistulas. In R. Bryant & D. Nix (Eds.), *Acute and chronic wounds: Current management concepts* (5th ed., pp. 509–529). St. Louis, MO: Elsevier.

Bryant, R., & Nix, D. (2016). Principles of wound healing and topical management. In R. Bryant & D. Nix (Eds.), *Acute and chronic wounds: Current management concepts* (5th ed., pp. 287–302). St. Louis, MO: Elsevier.

Centers for Disease Control & Prevention (2014). *Group A streptococcal (GAS) disease.* Retrieved December 22, 2016, from http://www.cdc.gov/groupAstrep/about/faqs.html

Coetzee, E., Rahm, Z., Boutall, A., & Goldberg, P. (2014). Refeeding enteroclysis as an alternative to parenteral nutrition for enteric fistula. *Colorectal Diseases, 16*(10), 823–830.

Czymek, R., Kujath, P., Bruch, H. P., Pfeiffer, D., Nebrig, M., Seehofer, D., & Guckelberger, O. (2013). Treatment, outcome and quality of life after Fournier's gangrene: A multicentre study. *Colorectal Disease, 15*(12), 1529–1536. doi:10.1111/codi.12396

Davis, C. P., & Stöppler, M. C. (2016). *Necrotizing fasciitis: Flesh eating disease.* Retrieved December 22, 2016, from http://www.medicinenet.com/necrotizing_fasciitis/article.htm

Delmore, B., Cox, J., Rolnitzky, L., Chu, A., & Stolfi, A. (2015). Differentiating a pressure ulcer from acute skin failure in the adult critical care patient. *Advances in Skin & Wound Care, 28*(11), 514–524.

Doughty, D. (2016). Arterial ulcers. In R. Bryant & D. Nix (Eds.), *Acute and chronic wounds: Current management concepts* (5th ed., pp. 174–189). St. Louis, MO: Elsevier.

Doughty, D. B., & Sparks, B. (2016). Wound-healing physiology and factors that affect the repair process. In R. Bryant & D. Nix (Eds.), *Acute and chronic wounds: Current management concepts* (5th ed., pp. 62–79). St. Louis, MO: Elsevier.

Endara, M., Masden, D., Goldstein, J., Gondek, S., Steinberg, J., & Attinger, C. (2013). The role of chronic and perioperative glucose management in high-risk surgical closures: A case for tighter glycemic control. *Plastic and Reconstructive Surgery, 132*(4), 996–1004.

Gallagher, S. (2016). Skin care needs of the obese patient. In R. Bryant & D. Nix (Eds.), *Acute and chronic wounds: Current management concepts* (5th ed., pp. 477–486). St. Louis, MO: Elsevier.

Gould, L., Abadir, P., Brem, H., Carter, M., Conner-Kerr, T., Davidson, J., . . . Schmader, K. (2015). *Wound Repair & Regeneration, 23*(1), 1–13. doi:10.1111/wrr.12245

Graybill, J., Stojadinovic, A., Crumbley, D., Elster, E. (2016). Traumatic wounds: Bullets, blasts, and vehicle crashes. In R. Bryant & D. Nix (Eds.), *Acute and chronic wounds: Current management concepts* (5th ed., pp. 433–446). St. Louis, MO: Elsevier.

Gyorki, D. E., Brooks, C. E., Gett, R., Woods, R. J., Johnston, M., Keck, J. O., . . . Keck, A. G. (2010). Enterocutaneous fistula: A single-centre experience. *ANZ Journal of Surgery, 80*(3), 178–181. doi:10.1111/j.1445-2197.2009.05086.x

Hakkarainen, T. W., Kopari, N. M., Pham, T. N., & Evans, H. E. (2014). Necrotizing soft tissue infections: Review and current concepts in treatment, systems of care, and outcomes. *Current Problems in Surgery, 51*(8), 344–362. doi:10.1067/j.cpsurg.2014.06.001.NIH

Holloway, S., Harding, R., Stechmiller, J. K., & Schultz, G. (2016). Acute and chronic wound healing. In S. Baranoski & E. A. Ayello (Eds.), *Wound care essentials* (4th ed., pp. 82–98). Philadelphia, PA: Wolters Kluwer.

Honaker, J. S., Forston, M. R., Davis, E. A., Wiesner, M. M., & Morgan, J. A. (2013). Effects of non contact low-frequency ultrasound on healing of suspected deep tissue injury: A retrospective analysis. *International Wound Journal, 10*(1), 65–72. DOI:10.1111/j.1742-481X.2012.00944.x.

Hopf, H. W., Shapshak, D., Junkins, S., & O'Neill, D. K. (2016). Managing wound pain. In R. Bryant & D. Nix (Eds.), *Acute and chronic wounds: Current management concepts* (5th ed., pp. 371–382). St. Louis, MO: Elsevier.

Howard, M. A., Asmis, R., Evans, K. K., & Mustoe, T. A. (2013). Oxygen and wound care: A review of current therapeutic modalities and future direction. *Wound Repair & Regeneration, 21*(4), 503–511.

James, W. D., Berger, T., & Elston, D. (2016). Skin: Basic structure and function. In W. D. James, T. Berger, & D. Elston (Eds.), *Andrews' diseases of the skin: Clinical dermatology* (12th ed., pp. 1–10). Philadelphia, PA: Elsevier.

Kent, D., & Wraa, C. (2013). Nursing assessment of the patient with integumentary disorders. In K. S. Osborn, C. E. Wraa, A. B. Watson, & R. Holleran (Eds.), *Medical-surgical nursing: Preparation for practice* (2nd ed., pp. 1830–1841). Upper Saddle River, NJ: Pearson.

Kim, P. J., Attinger, C. E., Steinberg, J. S., Evans, K. K., Powers, K. A., Hung, R.W., . . . Lavery, L. (2014). The impact of negative-pressure wound therapy with instillation compared with standard negative-pressure wound therapy: A retrospective, historical, cohort, controlled study. *Plastic and Reconstructive Surgery, 133*, 709–716.

LeBlanc, K., Baranoski, S., Christensen, D., Langemo, D., Edwards, K., Holloway, S., . . . Woo, K. (2016). The art of dressing selection: A consensus statement on skin tears and best practice. *Advances in Skin & Wound Care, 29*(1), 32–46. PMID: 26650095

Martinez, J. L., Luque-de-Leon, E., Mier, J., Blanco-Benavides, R., & Robledo, F. (2008). Systematic management of postoperative enterocutaneous fistulas: Factors related to outcomes. *World Journal of Surgery, 32*(3), 436–443.

McNichol, L., Watts, C., Mackey, D., Beitz, J., & Gray, M. (2015). Identifying the right surface for the right patient at the right time: Generation and content validation of an algorithm for support surface selection. *Journal of Wound Ostomy & Continence Nursing, 42*(1), 19–37. doi:10.1097/WON.0000000000000103

Miller, N., Frankenfield, D., Lehman, E., Maguire, M., & Schirm, V. (2016). Predicting pressure ulcer development in clinical practice: Evaluation of Braden Scale scores and nutrition parameters. *Journal of Wound Ostomy & Continence Nursing, 43*(2), 133–139. doi:10.1097.WON.0000000000000184

Misiakos, E. P., Bagias, G., Patapis, P., Sotiropoulos, D., Kanavidis, P., & Machairas, A. (2014). Current concepts in the management of necrotizing fasciitis. *Frontiers in Surgery, 1*(36), 1–10. doi:10.3389/fsurg.2014.00036

National Pressure Ulcer Advisory Panel, European Pressure Ulcer Advisory Panel, and Pan Pacific Pressure Injury Alliance. (2014). In E. Haesler (Ed.), *Prevention and treatment of pressure ulcers: QUICK reference guide.* Osborne Park, Western Australia: Cambridge Media. Retrieved December 21, 2016, from http://www.npuap.org/wp-content/uploads/2014/08/Quick-Reference-Guide-DIGITAL-NPUAP-EPUAP-PPPIA-Jan2016.pdf

Netsch, D. S., Nix, D. P., & Haugen, V. (2016). Negative pressure wound therapy. In R. Bryant & D. Nix (Eds.), *Acute and chronic wounds: Current management concepts* (5th ed., pp. 325–335). St. Louis, MO: Elsevier.

Nix, D. P. (2016). Skin and wound inspection and assessment. In R. Bryant & D. Nix (Eds.), *Acute and chronic wounds: Current management concepts* (5th ed., pp. 103–118). St. Louis, MO: Elsevier.

Osborn, K., Wraa, C. Watson, A., & Holleran, R. (2014). *Medical-surgical nursing: Preparation for practice* (2nd ed.). Upper Saddle River, NJ: Pearson.

Pais, V. M. (2016). Fournier gangrene. *Medscape*. Retrieved December 22, 2016, from http://emedicine.medscape .com/article/2028899-overview#a3

Percival, S., McCarty, S., & Lipsky, B. (2015, July 1). Biofilms and wounds: An overview of the evidence. *Advanced Wound Care* (New Rochelle), 4(7), 373–381.

Pittman, J., Beeson, T., Carter, B., & Collin, T. (2015). Implementation of a bowel management program in critical care. *Journal of Wound Ostomy & Continence Nursing*, 42(4), 389–394. doi:10.1097. WON.0000000000000146

Qaseem, A., Mir, T. P., Starkey, M., & Denberg, T. S. (2015). Risk assessment and prevention of pressure ulcers: A clinical practice guideline from the American College of Physicians. *Annals of Internal Medicine*, 162(5), 359–369.

Raetz, J. G., & Wick, K. H. (2015). Common questions about pressure ulcers. *America Family Physician*, 92(10), 888–894.

Ramundo, J. M. (2016). Wound debridement. In R. Bryant & D. Nix (Eds.), *Acute and chronic wounds: Current management concepts* (5th ed., pp. 277–287). St. Louis, MO: Elsevier.

Sajid, M. T., Mustafa, Q., Shaheen, N., Hussain, S. M., Shukr, L., & Ahmed, M. (2015). Comparison of negative pressure wound therapy using vacuum-assisted closure with advanced moist wound therapy in the treatment of diabetic foot ulcers. *Journal of College of Physicians and Surgeons Pakistan*, 25, 789–793.

Singhai, H. (2016). Skin and soft tissue infections—Incision, drainage, and debridement. *Medscape*. Retrieved December 22, 2016, from http://emedicine .medscape.com/article/1830144-overview

Sroczynski, M., Sebastian, M., Rudnicki, J., Sebastian, A., & Agrawal, A. K. (2013). A complex approach to the treatment of Fournier's gangrene. *Advances in Clinical and Experimental Medicine*, 22(1), 131–135.

Stein, S. L. (2015). Overview of enteric fistulas. *UpToDate*. Retrieved December 22, 2016, from http://www. uptodate.com/contents/overview-of-enteric-fistulas?s ource=machineLearning&search=enterocutaneous+fist ula&selectedTitle=1%7E24&anchor=H322535&sectionR ank=1#H322535

Stevens, D. L., & Baddour, L. M. (2014). Necrotizing soft tissue infections. *UpToDate Online*. Retrieved December 22, 2016, from http://www.uptodate.com /contents/necrotizing-soft-tissue-infections

Stotts, N. (2016a). Wound infection: Diagnosis and management. In R. Bryant & D. Nix (Eds.), *Acute and chronic wounds: Current management concepts* (5th ed., pp. 266–277). St. Louis, MO: Elsevier.

Stotts, N. (2016b). Nutritional assessment and support. In R. Bryant & D. Nix (Eds.), *Acute and chronic wounds: Current management concepts* (5th ed., pp. 382–393). St. Louis, MO: Elsevier.

Tuncel, U., Erkorkmaz, Ü., & Turan, A. (2013). Clinical evaluation of gauze-based negative pressure wound therapy in challenging wounds. *International Wound Journal*, 10, 152–158.

Vaidhya, N., Panchal, A., & Anchalia, M. M. (2015). A new cost-effective method of NPWT in diabetic foot wound. *Indian Journal of Surgery*, 77(Suppl 2), 525–529.

Weng, C. L., Wang, C. H., Chen, I. C., Hsiao, K. Y., Chang, K. P., Wu, S. Y., & Hong-Mo, S. (2014). Red cell distribution width is an independent predictor of mortality in necrotizing fasciitis. *American Journal of Emergency Medicine*, 32(10), 1259–1262. doi:10.1016/j. ajem.2014.08.001

Whitney, J. D. (2016). Perfusion and oxygenation. In R. Bryant & D. Nix (Eds.), *Acute and chronic wounds: Current management concepts* (5th ed., pp. 393–401). St. Louis, MO: Elsevier.

Wong, C. H., Khin, L. W., Heng, K. S., Tan, K. C., & Low, C. O. (2004). The LRINEC (Laboratory Risk Indicator for Necrotizing Fasciitis) score: A tool for distinguishing necrotizing fasciitis from other soft tissue infections. *Critical Care Medicine*, 32(7), 1535–1541.

Wysocki, A. B. (2016). Anatomy and physiology of skin and soft tissue. In R. Bryant & D. Nix (Eds.), *Acute and chronic wounds: Current management concepts* (5th ed., pp. 45–62). St. Louis, MO: Elsevier.

Chapter 11
Determinants and Assessment of Pulmonary Function

Learning Outcomes

11.1 Explain the conducting airways and the concept of ventilation.

11.2 Discuss external respiration and pulmonary gas diffusion.

11.3 Describe pulmonary perfusion and its components.

11.4 Differentiate between respiratory and metabolic acid–base imbalances and levels of compensation.

11.5 Interpret arterial blood gases, including compensatory status.

11.6 Conduct a focused respiratory nursing history and assessment.

11.7 Describe tests used to evaluate pulmonary function.

11.8 Discuss noninvasive and invasive methods of monitoring gas exchange and applications.

This chapter provides foundational knowledge of pulmonary physiology and assessment of pulmonary function to provide the learner with a deeper understanding of pulmonary disease.

Section One: Mechanics of Breathing—Ventilation

The respiratory process has three vital components: ventilation, diffusion, and perfusion. This section provides an overview of ventilation.

The Conducting Airways

The respiratory tract can be divided into the conducting and respiratory airways. The conducting airways consist of the nasal passages, mouth, pharynx, larynx, trachea, bronchi, and bronchioles. These airways serve as an air conduit to move air to and from the atmosphere and the alveoli. They also provide important protective functions by humidifying, filtering, and warming the air passing through them. In addition, much of the conducting airway contains a mucociliary system that removes pathogens and foreign materials by capturing them on the mucus layer and transporting them through ciliary movement toward the pharynx, where they are swallowed and destroyed in the stomach.

In high-acuity patients who require an artificial airway (e.g., tracheostomy or endotracheal tube), the initial conducting airway is bypassed, which significantly reduces the protective functions and increases the risk of aspiration and ventilator-associated pneumonia (VAP). In such cases, the protective functions are artificially replaced using special equipment that provides humidity, warmth, and, in some cases, filtering services.

The tracheobronchial tree consists of the trachea, which branches into the right and left bronchi. It may be helpful to think of the trachea as the base of the tree and the alveoli as the tiny terminal fruit clusters. At the junction of the Y formed by the two primary bronchial branches is the **carina**. This structure is heavily enervated and extremely sensitive to stimulation. The carina becomes clinically significant when touched by a suction catheter or endotracheal tube, which can trigger bronchospasm or severe coughing. The right bronchus is shorter and larger in diameter than the left bronchus and is at almost a straight angle with the trachea. The left bronchus is longer, smaller in diameter, and at a more acute angle than the right bronchus. The bronchial anatomic structure has clinical significance because the size and positioning of the right bronchus make it more vulnerable to the introduction of pathogens and foreign particles as well as for the misplacement of an endotracheal tube. The trachea and bronchial walls contain a C-shaped cartilage structure, which is present down to the bronchiole level. The cartilage gives structure and protection to the larger airways.

Toward the terminal end of the bronchial tree are the bronchioles, which are surrounded by smooth muscle but lack cartilage. Bronchioles regulate resistance to air flow by constricting or dilating (bronchoconstriction and bronchodilation). Figure 11–1 is an illustration of the anatomy of the respiratory system.

Ventilation

Ventilation is the first of the three components of the respiratory process and is defined as the mechanical movement of air flow to and from the atmosphere and the alveoli. Ventilation involves the actual work of breathing and requires nervous system control and adequate functioning of the lungs and conducting airways, thorax, and respiratory muscles. Decreased functioning of any one of these factors will affect the body's ability to ventilate properly.

Ventilation is accomplished through a bellows-like action. Air moves in and out of the lungs as a result of the changing size of the thorax caused by contraction of the diaphragm and intercostal muscles. When the thorax enlarges, the intrapulmonary pressure drops to below atmospheric pressure. Air then moves from the area of higher pressure to the area of lower pressure, resulting in air flowing into the lungs (inspiration), until the pressure

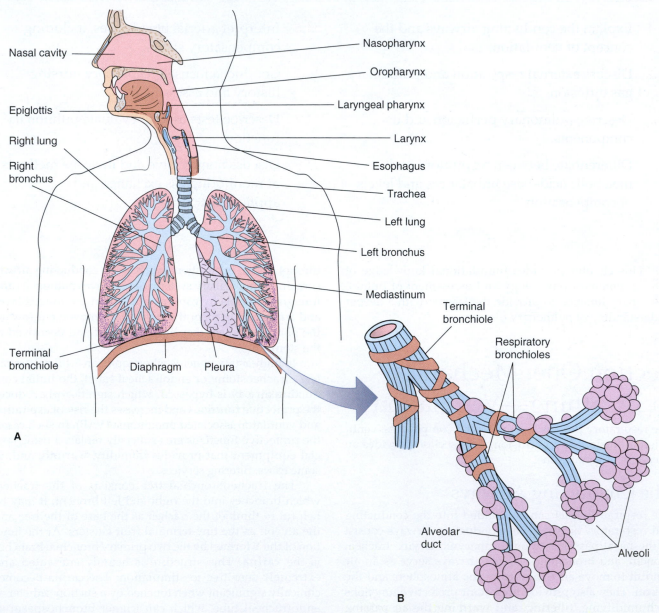

Figure 11–1 Anatomy of the respiratory system. A, Major anatomic features. B, Terminal airways.

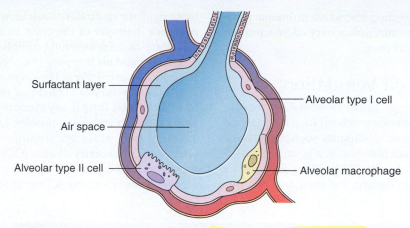

Figure 11–2 The surfactant layer. Type II cells secrete surfactant, a lipoprotein that lines the inner wall of the alveoli, reducing surface tension to prevent alveolar collapse.

in the lungs becomes slightly higher than atmospheric pressure. At this point, the diaphragm and intercostal muscles relax, and air flows back out of the lungs (expiration) until once again pressures are equalized.

Lung tissue has a constant tendency to collapse because of several important properties. First, the fluid lining of the alveoli has a naturally high surface tension, creating a tendency for the alveolar walls to collapse. To prevent this, special cells (type II cells) in the alveoli secrete a lipoprotein called **surfactant**. Surfactant has a detergent-like action that reduces the surface tension of the fluid lining the alveolar sacs (Figure 11–2), thereby reducing the tendency toward collapse. Second, the lungs are composed of elastic fibers. The elastic force of these fibers constantly seeks to return to a resting state (i.e., collapsed lungs). To maintain the lungs in an inflated state, the elastic forces must constantly be overcome by opposing forces.

The thorax is the primary opposing force that maintains the lungs in an expanded state. The thoracic bony structure provides a cage-like framework that maintains the lungs in a baseline inflated state even at rest because of the attraction that exists between the visceral and parietal pleurae. The pleurae are slick-surfaced, moist membranes. The **parietal pleura** adheres to the thoracic walls, diaphragm, and mediastinum; the **visceral pleura** adheres to the lung parenchyma. To understand the pleural attraction, it may help to think of placing two moistened sheets of smooth glass together. Although it would be relatively easy to glide one sheet over the other in a parallel fashion, it would be very difficult to pull them directly apart at a 180-degree angle. The glass sheets represent the two pleurae. Under normal circumstances, the parietal and visceral pleurae act as one membrane. Therefore, as the thorax increases and decreases in size, the lungs increase and decrease in volume.

Lung Compliance   The ease with which the lungs are able to expand is measured in terms of lung compliance. For example, it is much more difficult to blow up a small balloon than a large balloon. To inflate the small balloon, you would need to blow harder (exert more pressure force) to obtain the same volume you would obtain with less

force in the large balloon. The small balloon is less compliant than the large balloon. **Compliance (C_L)** is defined in terms of lung volume (mL) and pressure (cm H_2O) as

$$C_L = \Delta V / \Delta P$$

where C_L is lung compliance, ΔV is change in volume (mL), and ΔP is change in pressure (cm H_2O).

Like a bag of assorted-size balloons, alveoli also come in many sizes. Each size of alveolus has a certain filling capacity beyond which it can become overexpanded and even burst. As the alveoli approach their filling capacity, they become less compliant—that is, it takes more force to completely expand the alveoli and even greater force to hyperexpand them. A clinical example of alveoli becoming less compliant is acute respiratory distress syndrome (ARDS). Patients with ARDS experience decreased alveolar compliance and often require higher levels of positive end–expiratory pressure (PEEP) to open and expand alveoli that have become significantly noncompliant because of the disease process. Use of PEEP ideally increases lung compliance. However, if too much PEEP (measured in cm H_2O pressure) is applied, alveoli become so hyperexpanded that compliance further decreases, the alveoli are at risk of rupture, and ventilation is compromised. PEEP is explained in detail in the Chapter 7: Mechanical Ventilation.

Many pulmonary and extrapulmonary problems influence compliance. Compliance is very sensitive to any condition that affects the lung's tissues, particularly if the disorder causes a reduction in pulmonary surfactant, which is crucial to maintenance of functional alveoli. When there is a deficiency of surfactant, compliance is decreased. Decreased compliance is sometimes referred to as *stiff lungs*, meaning that it takes more force (pressure) to increase lung volume. For example, whereas a person with normal lungs can inhale 50 to 100 mL of air for every 1 cm H_2O of pressure exerted, a person with decreased compliance might be able to inhale 30 to 40 mL/cm H_2O of pressure. Decreased compliance causes tidal volume to decrease and, therefore, increases the work of breathing. The breathing rate also increases to compensate for the decreased tidal volume. Pulmonary problems causing decreased compliance are called restrictive pulmonary disorders and include pneumonia, pulmonary edema, pulmonary fibrosis, and pneumothorax.

Effects of Aging on Ventilation

As a person ages, the lungs undergo many progressive changes from a combination of age-related lung changes and a lifetime of exposure to air pollutants such as cigarette smoke, chemicals, and urban pollution (Calhoun et al., 2015; Cefalu, 2011; Vaz Fragoso & Gill, 2012). Many changes are predictable: The diaphragm flattens, the chest wall becomes more rigid, the respiratory muscles weaken, and the anterior–posterior diameter of the chest increases. All these factors contribute to decreased lung compliance, altered pulmonary mechanics, and **air trapping** (the abnormal retention of air in the lungs on exhalation). However, a person who has never smoked and who has maintained normal lungs throughout life may exhibit little if any clinically significant changes in ventilation. In contrast, in older adults with a history of smoking and other environmental exposures, chronic obstructive pulmonary disease (COPD) is considered a leading cause for hospitalization as well as a leading cause of morbidity and mortality (Criner et al., 2015).

Section One Review

1. The conducting airways serve which major functions? (Select all that apply.)
   A. Gas exchange
   B. Filtering
   C. Immune protection
   D. Humidifying
   E. Warming

2. During expiration, the intrapulmonary pressure causes air to flow out of the lungs for which reason?
   A. Because the intrapulmonary pressure is higher than atmospheric pressure
   B. Because the intrapulmonary pressure is equal to perfusion pressure
   C. Because the intrapulmonary pressure is lower than atmospheric pressure
   D. Because the intrapulmonary pressure is equal to alveolar pressure

3. What is the purpose of surfactant?
   A. To decrease lung compliance
   B. To increase alveolar surface tension
   C. To cleanse the alveoli
   D. To decrease alveolar surface tension

4. What is the primary function of type II alveolar cells?
   A. Filtration
   B. Gas exchange
   C. Immune protection
   D. Surfactant production

Answers: 1. (B, D, E), 2. A, 3. D, 4. D

Section Two: Pulmonary Gas Exchange—Respiration and Diffusion

Respiration is the process by which the body's cells are supplied with oxygen and carbon dioxide is eliminated from the body. Respiration can be further divided into internal and external respiration. **Internal respiration** refers to the movement of gases across systemic capillary–cell membranes in the tissues. **External respiration** refers to the movement of gases across the alveolar–capillary membrane (i.e., pulmonary gas exchange) and is the focus of this chapter. Both external and internal respiration use diffusion as their means of exchanging gases. Figure 11–3 illustrates external and internal respiration and the cardiopulmonary circuit.

Diffusion

Diffusion is the second of the three components of the respiratory process. Oxygenation of tissues is dependent on the process of diffusion as the vital mechanism for both external and internal respiration. **Diffusion** is the movement of gases down a pressure gradient from an area of high pressure to an area of low pressure. The alveolar–capillary membrane is extremely thin, offering little resistance to diffusion in normal circumstances. The membrane can thicken when pulmonary pathologic processes exist, reducing diffusion (e.g., pulmonary edema, acute respiratory distress syndrome). When diffusion is reduced, the carbon dioxide tension may remain at normal levels initially because carbon dioxide diffuses 20 times faster than oxygen; however, the oxygen tension decreases rapidly.

Five factors affect diffusion through the alveolar–capillary membrane: partial pressures, gas gradient, lung surface area, alveolar–capillary membrane thickness, and length of gas exposure in the lungs. In addition, the oxyhemoglobin dissociation curve plays an important role in determining the affinity of oxygen to hemoglobin, which directly affects diffusion.

Partial Pressures of Gases   Atmospheric air is composed of molecules of nitrogen, oxygen, carbon dioxide, and water vapor. The combination of all these gases exerts

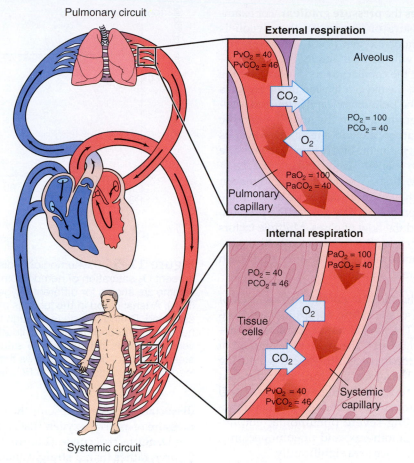

Pulmonary circuit

External respiration

PvO$_2$ = 40
PvCO$_2$ = 46

Alveolus

CO$_2$

PO$_2$ = 100
PCO$_2$ = 40

O$_2$

PaO$_2$ = 100
PaCO$_2$ = 40

Pulmonary
capillary

Internal respiration

PaO$_2$ = 100
PaCO$_2$ = 40

PO$_2$ = 40
PCO$_2$ = 46

Tissue
cells

O$_2$

CO$_2$

PvO$_2$ = 40
PvCO$_2$ = 46

Systemic
capillary

Systemic circuit

Figure 11–3 External and internal respiration and the cardiopulmonary circuit.

about 760 mmHg of pressure at sea level. The respiratory process, however, does not actively involve the use of the water vapor or nitrogen but, rather, the exchange of oxygen and carbon dioxide.

Oxygen and carbon dioxide both exert a certain percentage of the total air pressure. Oxygen in the alveoli exerts an average of 100 mmHg pressure. This **partial pressure** of oxygen is called PO$_2$, or oxygen tension. When the PO$_2$ refers to oxygen in the arterial blood, it is abbreviated as PaO$_2$ ("a" for arterial), and when it refers to venous blood, it is specified as PvO$_2$ ("v" for venous). Carbon dioxide (CO$_2$) in the alveoli exerts an average of 40 mmHg pressure, and this partial pressure is called PCO$_2$. The abbreviations "a" and "v" used to describe PO$_2$ also apply to PCO$_2$.

Venous blood returning to the lungs from the tissues is oxygen poor because the blood has delivered its load of oxygen to the tissues for use. Venous blood is rich in carbon dioxide (measured as PvCO$_2$) because CO$_2$ is the major waste product of cellular metabolism and is transported through the blood for removal by the lungs. Table 11–1 compares the average partial pressures of oxygen and carbon dioxide in arterial and venous blood.

Pressure Gradient The difference between the partial pressures of gases in the alveoli and the pulmonary capillary blood dictates which direction each gas flows based on the law of diffusion (i.e., gases move from an area of higher pressure to an area of lower pressure) (Figure 11–4). This

Table 11–1 Comparison of Average Partial Pressures in Arterial and Venous Blood

	Arterial Blood (PaO$_2$) (mmHg)	Venous Blood (PvO$_2$) (mmHg)
Oxygen	100	40
Carbon dioxide	40	46

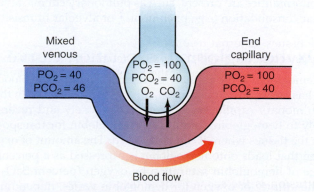

Mixed
venous

PO$_2$ = 40
PCO$_2$ = 46

PO$_2$ = 100
PCO$_2$ = 40
O$_2$ CO$_2$

End
capillary

PO$_2$ = 100
PCO$_2$ = 40

Blood flow

Figure 11–4 Gas distribution and pressure gradients.

difference is referred to as the **pressure gradient**. For example, if the partial pressure of oxygen in the alveoli is 100 mmHg and the venous oxygen (PvO_2) is 40 mmHg, oxygen in the alveoli will diffuse across the alveolar–capillary membrane into the capillary blood to equalize the partial pressures. Because the oxygen tension in the alveolus is much higher than in the pulmonary capillary blood, oxygen diffuses down the gradient from the alveolus into the blood passing by. The carbon dioxide tension, however, is lower in the alveolus than it is in the blood, causing a pressure gradient that diffuses CO_2 out of the blood and into the alveolus for elimination by the lungs. The rate at which diffusion occurs depends on the actual pressure difference between the two areas where diffusion occurs. The greater the pressure difference, the more rapid the flow of gases. Multiple factors increase the gradient. For example, exercise and positive pressure mechanical ventilation increase the pressure gradient in the lungs, increasing the rate of diffusion.

Lung Surface Area   The total functional surface area of normal lungs is immense, providing an optimal environment for gas exchange. The greater the available alveolar–capillary membrane surface area, the greater the amount of oxygen and carbon dioxide that can diffuse across it during a specific time period. Therefore, any lung disorder that significantly decreases functional lung surface area will decrease diffusion and impair gas exchange. Many pulmonary conditions, including severe pneumonia, emphysema, lung tumors, pneumothorax, and pneumonectomy, can reduce functioning surface area significantly.

Alveolar–Capillary Membrane Thickness   The thickness of the alveolar–capillary membrane is of major importance. The thinner the membrane, the more rapid the rate of diffusion of gases. Several conditions can increase membrane thickness, thereby decreasing the rate of diffusion, such as fluid in the alveoli or interstitial spaces or both (e.g., pulmonary edema), an inflammatory process involving the alveoli (e.g., pneumonia), and lung conditions that cause fibrosis (e.g., ARDS or pneumoconiosis).

Length of Gas Exposure   During periods of high cardiac output, such as occurs with heavy exercise or stress, blood flow is faster through the alveolar–capillary system than it is at rest. Under these circumstances, diffusion takes place during a shortened exposure time. In healthy lungs, oxygen exchange is usually not impaired with high cardiac output states; however, hypoxemia may result if diffusion abnormalities are present, such as pulmonary edema, alveolar consolidation (e.g., pneumonia), or alveolar fibrosis.

Oxyhemoglobin Dissociation Curve

Hemoglobin is the primary carrier of oxygen in the blood. It has an affinity, or attraction, for oxygen molecules. In the pulmonary capillaries, oxygen binds loosely and reversibly to hemoglobin, forming oxyhemoglobin for transport to the tissues where it can be released. The amount of oxygen that loads onto hemoglobin is expressed as a percentage of hemoglobin saturation by oxygen (percent SaO_2). The affinity of oxygen for hemoglobin varies, depending on certain physiologic factors. The **oxyhemoglobin**

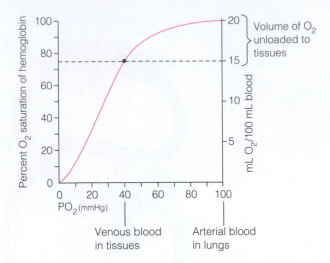

Figure 11–5   Oxyhemoglobin dissociation curve. The percent O_2 saturation of hemoglobin and total blood oxygen volume are shown for different oxygen partial pressures (PO_2). Arterial blood in the lungs is almost completely saturated. During one pass through the body, about 25% of hemoglobin-bound oxygen is unloaded to the tissues. Thus, venous blood is still about 75% saturated with oxygen. The steep portion of the curve shows that hemoglobin readily offloads and on-loads oxygen at PO_2 levels below 50 mmHg.

dissociation curve represents the relationship of the partial pressure of arterial oxygen (PaO_2) and hemoglobin saturation (SaO_2). The curve (Figure 11–5) is depicted as an S-curve rather than a straight line, showing that the SaO_2 does not maintain a direct relationship with the PaO_2.

The top portion of the curve (PaO_2 greater than 60 mmHg) is flattened into a horizontal position. In this portion, a large alteration in PaO_2 produces only small alterations in the percentage of hemoglobin saturation. For example, note that a 10 mmHg decrease of PaO_2 from 80 mmHg to 70 mmHg would produce very little change in SaO_2 (see Figure 11–5). Clinically, this means that although administering supplemental oxygen may significantly increase the patient's PaO_2, the resulting SaO_2 increase will be small in proportion. The patient's oxygenation status is better protected at the top of the curve.

The bottom portion of the curve (PaO_2 less than 60 mmHg) is steep. In this portion, any alteration in PaO_2 yields a large change in percentage of hemoglobin saturation (SaO_2). For example, a 10 mmHg decrease in PaO_2 from 60 mmHg to 50 mmHg decreases the SaO_2 from about 85% to about 75% (a decrease of approximately 10%). Clinically, this means that administration of supplemental oxygen sufficient to increase the PaO_2 should yield large increases in SaO_2. However, any abnormalities in the ventilation–perfusion relationship would interfere with reoxygenation.

Low PaO_2 at the tissue level stimulates oxygen release from hemoglobin to the tissues. High PaO_2 at the pulmonary capillary level stimulates hemoglobin to bind with more oxygen. Other factors can change the curve, shifting it to the right or the left (Figure 11–6). A shift to the right prevents hemoglobin from binding as readily with oxygen in the lungs, although oxygen can be released at the tissue level more readily. A shift to the left causes hemoglobin to bind more readily with oxygen in the lungs but inhibits

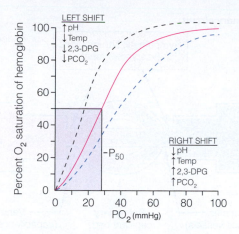

Figure 11–6 Oxyhemoglobin dissociation curve right and left shifts. Normally, when hemoglobin is 50% saturated with oxygen (P_{50}) the PaO_2 will be 27 mmHg. The P_{50} changes when physiologic factors are altered, shifting the curve. A shift to the left increases the affinity of oxygen to hemoglobin, inhibiting its release to tissues. A shift to the right decreases the affinity of oxygen to hemoglobin, making it release to tissues more readily.

release at the tissue level. Factors that shift the curve to the right and left are listed in Table 11–2. Slight shifts are adaptive. For example, an increased body temperature increases oxygen demand, causing a slight right shift, which increases release of oxygen to the tissues to meet

Table 11–2 Factors Affecting the Oxyhemoglobin Dissociation Curve

Left Shift	Right Shift
Alkalosis	Acidosis
Hypothermia	Hyperthermia
Hypocapnia	Hypercapnia
Decreased 2,3-DPG*	Increased 2,3-DPG

*2,3-DPG = 2,3-diphosphoglycerate.

increasing tissue oxygen demand. Severe or rapid shifts, however, can produce life-threatening tissue hypoxia.

The Effects of Aging on Diffusion

Due to aging processes, total lung surface area decreases, the alveolar–capillary membrane thickness increases, and alveoli are destroyed. These changes result in decreased diffusion across the alveolar–capillary membrane, altering the ventilation–perfusion relationship. Overall, gas exchange becomes less efficient, placing the older high-acuity patient at risk for hypoxemia and/or hypercapnia. In addition, over time, the airways become larger, which increases dead space ventilation, and terminal airways lose supportive structures, which can result in air trapping. These are physiologic changes that can lead to carbon dioxide retention.

Section Two Review

1. Pressure gradient affects the diffusion of gases in which way?
   A. The more rapid the ventilatory rate, the greater the gradient
   B. The greater the difference, the more rapid the gas flow
   C. The less rapid the ventilatory rate, the greater the gradient
   D. The smaller the difference, the more rapid the gas flow

2. Which disease process would increase the thickness of the alveolar–capillary membrane?
   A. Pneumothorax
   B. Pneumonia
   C. Lung tumor
   D. Pneumonectomy

3. Which statement is correct regarding the normal relationship between oxygen and hemoglobin?
   A. Oxygen binds loosely and reversibly to hemoglobin.
   B. Hemoglobin is attracted to oxygen molecules.
   C. The affinity of hemoglobin to oxygen is constant.
   D. The relationship is expressed in mmHg (pressure).

4. On the oxyhemoglobin dissociation curve, at a PaO_2 less than 60 mmHg, any change in PaO_2 yields how much of a change in SaO_2?
   A. No change
   B. A small change
   C. A large change
   D. An unpredictable change

Answers: 1. B, 2. B, 3. A, 4. C

Section Three: Pulmonary Gas Exchange—Perfusion

Perfusion is the third and final component of the respiratory process. For our purposes, **perfusion** refers to the pumping or flow of blood to tissues and organs.

Perfusion can be divided into two circulatory systems: systemic and pulmonary (refer to Figure 11–3). The *systemic system* is vast, running from the aorta through the right side of the heart. The *pulmonary system* is much smaller, beginning with the pulmonary artery in the right ventricle, then continuing through the lungs and back into the left ventricle.

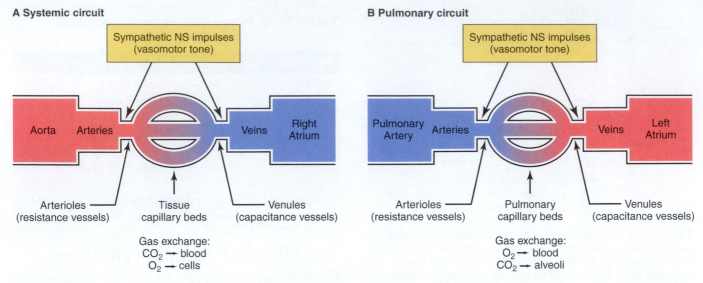

A Systemic circuit

B Pulmonary circuit

Figure 11–7 Two perfusion systems. A, Systemic and B, Pulmonary.

The pulmonary system is dependent on adequate perfusion in the systemic system, and adequate perfusion in both systems is required for oxygenation of the tissues in the entire body. Both perfusion systems are composed of a complex network of blood vessels of varying sizes and functions (Figure 11–7). Pulmonary perfusion is altered by multiple factors: cardiac output (CO), gravity, ventilation-to-perfusion relationship, shunt, and pulmonary vascular resistance (PVR).

Cardiac Output

Cardiac output (CO) is a determined by stroke volume (SV) and heart rate (HR), where CO = SV × HR. Normal cardiac output is between 4 and 8 liters per minute. Stroke volume is a function of ventricular preload, afterload, and contractility. A common measurement that is used clinically to reflect adequacy of perfusion is the **mean arterial pressure (MAP)**. This can be approximated using the equation MAP = $(2[P_{dias}] + P_{sys})/3$, where P_{dias} is diastolic blood pressure and P_{sys} is systolic blood pressure. Ideally, the MAP is maintained between 70 and 100 mmHg in adults (Kitamura, Katz, & Ruoff, 2014). A MAP of less than 60 mmHg is inadequate for perfusing major organs, such as the brain, heart, and kidneys. Typically, the clinical goal is to maintain the MAP at 70 or above to prevent organ hypoperfusion, which can result in organ ischemia and **multiple organ dysfunction syndrome (MODS)**.

Gravity

The effects of gravity on blood are an important consideration in pulmonary gas exchange. Since blood has weight, it is gravity dependent; thus it naturally accumulates the most in the dependent areas of the body. In the lungs, blood accumulates in the dependent areas of the lung fields. Gravity has a significant influence on the relationship between ventilation and pulmonary perfusion.

Ventilation–perfusion Relationship

The normal diffusion of gases requires a certain balance of alveolar ventilation (movement of gas into the alveoli) and pulmonary perfusion (blood flow through the pulmonary capillaries). Normal gas exchange cannot take place in affected areas if a significant imbalance in this relationship develops. For this reason, it is important to gain a basic understanding of the relationship of ventilation (V or V̇) to perfusion (Q or Q̇). This relationship is expressed as a ratio of alveolar ventilation to pulmonary capillary perfusion **V̇/Q̇ ratio**. For ideal gas exchange to occur, we might expect that for every liter of fresh air coming into the alveoli, 1 liter of blood would flow past it, creating a 1:1 ratio of ventilation to perfusion. In reality, for approximately every 4 liters of air flowing into the alveoli, about 5 liters of blood flow past (an average ratio of 4:5, or 0.8) (Figure 11–8).

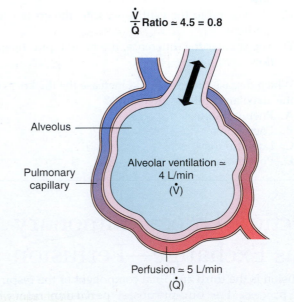

$$\frac{\dot{V}}{\dot{Q}} \text{ Ratio} \simeq 4.5 = 0.8$$

Alveolus

Pulmonary capillary

Alveolar ventilation ≈ 4 L/min (V̇)

Perfusion ≈ 5 L/min (Q̇)

Figure 11–8 The relationship of ventilation to perfusion.

The balance of ventilation to perfusion is greatly affected by the PaO_2 and $PaCO_2$. This balance depends on the adequate diffusion of oxygen and carbon dioxide across the alveolar–capillary membrane, as well as on the movement of oxygen into and carbon dioxide out of the alveoli.

Although normal values are given for PaO_2 (100 mmHg) and $PaCO_2$ (40 mmHg), these numbers only express an average. The actual partial pressures of oxygen and carbon dioxide vary throughout the lungs because ventilation is not distributed evenly due to gravity-dependent factors. In an upright person, alveolar ventilation is moderate in the lungs because of increased negative pleural pressures in relation to the lung bases. This makes the alveoli in the lung apices more resistant to air flow during inspiration. When breathing spontaneously, air flow naturally moves toward the diaphragm, which results in more air movement into the bases and peripheral lung during inspiration (air flow follows the path of least resistance). Pulmonary capillary perfusion is largely gravity dependent, making perfusion greatest in the dependent areas of the lungs (the bases in an upright person). Consequently, because ventilation and perfusion are both greatest in the bases of the lungs, the greatest amount of gas exchange occurs in this portion of the lung fields.

In the upper lungs, there is moderate alveolar ventilation and significantly reduced perfusion, making an excess of ventilation to available perfusion. This results in a "high" $\dot{V}/\dot{Q}$ ratio—that is, a $\dot{V}/\dot{Q}$ ratio that is higher than the average of 0.8. In the lower lungs, there is a moderate increase in ventilation with a significant increase in perfusion. This results in a "low" $\dot{V}/\dot{Q}$ ratio (lower than the average of 0.8).

The clinical significance of ventilation–perfusion balance becomes apparent when considering its implications in high-acuity patients. This patient population often requires prolonged bed rest, usually in a relatively horizontal position. Because blood is relatively gravity dependent, it will shift from the lung bases to whichever lung area is in the dependent position; however, air continues to be drawn toward the diaphragm (Figure 11–9).

Keeping the principles of $\dot{V}/\dot{Q}$ ratio in mind, what could happen if a patient is positioned on the right side when there is significant pneumonia in the right lung fields? Because the patient is lying on the right side, maximum pulmonary capillary perfusion will be on the right. Pneumonia is associated with secretions and other factors that cause obstruction of air flow into the affected lung alveoli. Therefore, because air flow follows the path of least resistance, it will avoid the diseased right lung area. This combination of a significant decrease in ventilation in the presence of normal-to-increased perfusion causes a mismatching of ventilation to perfusion, creating a low $\dot{V}/\dot{Q}$ ratio. If sufficient mismatching occurs, PaO_2 and oxygen saturation levels can decrease significantly. Positioning this

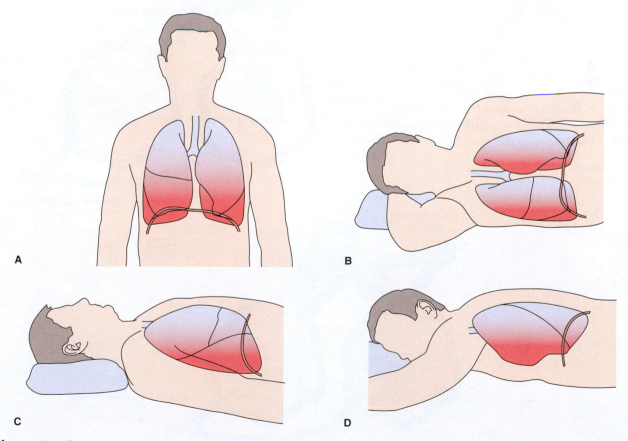

Figure 11–9 Positioning and ventilation-to-perfusion relationship. A, Upright position—Air moves toward diaphragm and blood gravitates to bases. B, Side-lying position—Air moves toward diaphragm while blood gravitates to lateral dependent lung fields. C, Supine position—Air moves toward diaphragm while blood gravitates to posterior dependent lung fields. D, Prone position—Air moves toward diaphragm while blood gravitates to the anterior dependent lung fields.

Table 11–3 Comparison of High and Low
V̇/Q̇ Ratios

High V̇/Q̇ Ratio	Low V̇/Q̇ Ratio
Normal to increased alveolar ventilation associated with decreased perfusion	Decreased alveolar ventilation associated with normal to increased perfusion
Alveolar gas effect: Increased cardiac output Decreased alveolar CO_2 Normally exists in upper lung fields	**Alveolar gas effect:** Decreased oxygen in alveoli Increased CO_2 in alveoli Normally exists in lower lung fields
Abnormally present with: Decreased cardiac output Pulmonary emboli Pneumothorax Destruction of pulmonary capillaries	**Abnormally present with:** Hypoventilation Obstructive lung diseases Restrictive lung diseases
Arterial blood gas effects: Increased PaO_2 Decreased $PaCO_2$ Increased pH	**Arterial blood gas effects:** Decreased PaO_2 Increased $PaCO_2$ Decreased pH

patient on the left side may be better tolerated because V̇/Q̇ matching would be improved. This, then, is one reason why some high-acuity patients tolerate being turned on one side more than another.

For patients in acute respiratory distress syndrome (ARDS), prone positioning may improve oxygenation. When supine, blood gravitates to the posterior lung fields, causing alveoli to fill with fluid and collapse. Placing patients in the prone position may reverse the effect of gravity and recruit lung tissue to improve oxygenation. Table 11–3 compares high and low V̇/Q̇ ratios.

Pulmonary Shunt

The term **pulmonary shunt (true shunt or physiologic shunt)** refers to the percentage of cardiac output that flows from the right heart into the left heart without undergoing pulmonary gas exchange (Sethi & McCool, 2016). Pulmonary shunting is a major cause of hypoxemia in high-acuity patients. It also helps explain how problems in ventilation and perfusion originate. There are two types of true shunts—anatomic shunt and capillary shunt (Figure 11–10).

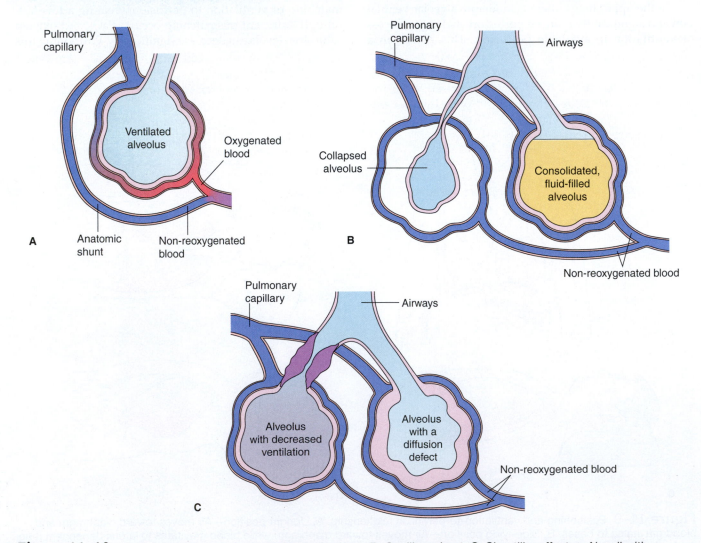

Figure 11–10 Types of pulmonary shunt. A, Anatomic shunt. B, Capillary shunt. C, Shuntlike effects—Alveoli with decreased ventilation may respond well to oxygen therapy.

Anatomic Shunt Not all blood that flows through the lungs participates in gas exchange. The term **anatomic shunt** refers to blood that moves from the right heart into the left heart without coming into contact with alveoli. Normally, this is approximately 2% to 5% of blood flow. Normal anatomic shunting occurs as a result of the emptying of the bronchial and several other veins into the venous system of the lungs.

Abnormal anatomic shunting can occur with certain heart or lung problems. For example, a ventricular septal defect (a hole in the heart wall dividing the right and left ventricles) shunts unoxygenated venous blood from the right heart directly into the oxygenated blood in the left heart by way of the defect. Traumatic injury to pulmonary blood vessels and tissues and certain types of lung tumors can also cause abnormal anatomic shunting.

Capillary Shunt **Capillary shunt** is the normal flow of blood past completely unventilated alveoli. This means that the blood flowing by the affected alveoli does not take part in diffusion. Capillary shunt results from such conditions as consolidation, atelectasis, or fluid in the alveoli. It is this type of shunt that most commonly develops in high-acuity adult patients.

Absolute Shunt The combined amount of anatomic shunt and capillary shunt is called **absolute shunt**. The total percentage of cardiac output involved in absolute shunt has important clinical implications. Lung tissue that is affected by absolute shunt is refractory to oxygen therapy because it involves nonfunctioning alveoli. No matter how much oxygen is administered, diffusion cannot take place if alveoli are completely bypassed or nonfunctioning. Shunting of more than 15% of cardiac output can result in severe respiratory failure. In fact, patients with acute respiratory distress syndrome (ARDS) generally have an absolute shunt of more than 20% of their cardiac output. The hallmark of ARDS is **refractory hypoxemia** (hypoxemia that is not significantly affected by administration of increasing levels of oxygen), which is consistent with the clinical picture of absolute shunt. Estimates of the amount of shunt can be made using several formulas.

Shuntlike Effect **Shuntlike effect** is not a true shunt because the shunting is not complete. Shuntlike effect occurs when there is an excess of perfusion in relation to alveolar ventilation—in other words, when alveolar ventilation is reduced but not totally absent. Common causes include bronchospasm, hypoventilation, or pooling of secretions. Because the alveoli are still functioning to some extent, hypoxemia secondary to shuntlike effect is very responsive to oxygen therapy.

Venous Admixture **Venous admixture** refers to the effect that pulmonary shunt has on the contents of the blood as it drains into the left heart and out into the system as arterial blood. Beyond the shunted areas, the fully reoxygenated blood (from normal alveolar units) mixes with the completely or relatively unoxygenated blood (from true shunt or shuntlike-effect alveolar units). The oxygen concentrations remix in the combined blood to establish a new balance, resulting in a PaO_2 that is higher than PaO_2 in blood affected by the shunt but lower than what it would be if the alveoli were normal (Figure 11–11).

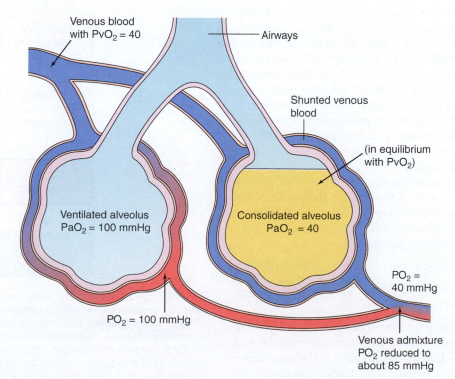

Figure 11–11 Venous admixture. Occurs when reoxygenated blood mixes with non-reoxygenated blood distal to the alveoli.

Table 11–4 P/F (PaO$_2$/FiO$_2$) Ratio

Equation*	$\dfrac{\text{PaO}_2}{\text{FiO}_2}$
Components	PaO$_2$ = partial pressure of arterial oxygen (mmHg) FiO$_2$ = fraction of inspired oxygen (O$_2$ concentration; decimal)
Normal values	350–450 Minimum clinically acceptable level = 286 Inverse relationship: The lower the ratio value drops below normal, the more intrapulmonary shunt worsens.
Example	A patient has a PaO$_2$ of 92 mmHg on an FiO$_2$ of 60%: $$\dfrac{92}{0.60} = 153$$ This is below the minimum acceptable level.

*This formula is best used when PaCO$_2$ is stable.

SOURCE: Based on Cairo (2016).

Estimating Intrapulmonary Shunt   Several formulas for calculation of estimations of intrapulmonary shunt can provide significant information when assessing the oxygenation status of the high-acuity patient. Increasingly, nurses who take care of this patient population are expected to have a basic understanding of these calculations and their significance. Calculating the P/F (PaO$_2$/FiO$_2$) ratio is the simplest way to estimate intrapulmonary shunt. It is best used when the patient's PaCO$_2$ is stable because it is not sensitive to changes in that value. Table 11–4 shows how to calculate a P/F ratio.

Pulmonary Vascular Resistance

Pulmonary vascular resistance (PVR) measures the resistance to blood flow in the pulmonary vascular system, which is a low-resistance system. In effect, it represents right ventricular afterload in much the same way that systemic vascular resistance (SVR) represents left ventricular afterload (a high-resistance system). Recall that the right ventricle pumps oxygen-poor blood into the pulmonary capillaries by way of the pulmonary artery. The amount of right ventricular force required to pump the blood into the lungs depends on the resistance to flow present in the pulmonary vascular system. This resistance to flow is called pulmonary vascular resistance.

Three main factors determine the amount of pulmonary resistance: the length of the vessels, the radius of the vessels, and the viscosity (thickness) of the blood. Of these factors, the major determinant is vessel radius (caliber), which is altered by the following:

- The volume of blood in the pulmonary vascular system
- The amount of pulmonary vasoconstriction
- The degree of lung inflation

Factors related to the volume of blood in the pulmonary vascular system include capillary recruitment and distention. Of these factors, recruitment is the most influential. The small pulmonary capillaries open up (are recruited) in response to an increase in blood flow. Under circumstances in which pulmonary blood flow is low

(e.g., shock), the smaller capillaries may receive so little blood that they collapse. Pulmonary vasoconstriction occurs in response to hypoxia, hypercapnia, and acidosis and is a major cause of increased PVR in the high-acuity patient. When an area of the lung becomes hypoxic, such as is seen in shunt, vasoconstriction is triggered to divert blood flow to more functional areas of the lungs and reduces the impact of shunt. In cases involving a generalized pulmonary disease process (e.g., late-stage emphysema), pulmonary vasoconstriction becomes global and PVR increases significantly. The degree of lung inflation also influences the diameter of the pulmonary capillaries. As the lung inflates, capillaries become stretched. In states

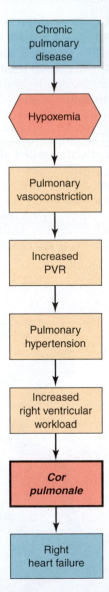

Figure 11–12 Cor pulmonale. Severe chronic pulmonary diseases are associated with a pattern of increasing hypoxemia that causes the lungs to vasoconstrict. The pulmonary vascular vasoconstriction increases PVR, which results in pulmonary hypertension. The right heart is required to work harder to pump blood into the pulmonary vascular system, and, over time, the right ventricle dilates and hypertrophies in response to the increased PVR. The adaptation of the right ventricle is called cor pulmonale.

of high lung inflation, capillaries become compressed, which decreases their diameter and increases PVR.

Calculating pulmonary vascular resistance requires the presence of a flow-directed pulmonary artery catheter, where, $PVR = (\overline{PAP} - PCWP) \times \frac{80}{CO}$. The calculation measures resistance, which is a function of pressure and flow. Pressure is determined by the mean pulmonary artery pressure and the pulmonary capillary wedge pressure. Flow is measured as the cardiac output. Table 11–5 summarizes the calculation of pulmonary vascular resistance.

Cor Pulmonale **Cor pulmonale** refers to right ventricular hypertrophy and dilation secondary to pulmonary disease and is a complication of increased PVR. Cor pulmonale can cause right-heart failure and is a major cause of death in the patient with end-stage chronic obstructive pulmonary disease (COPD). It is the result of a sequence of events precipitated by pulmonary hypertension. As PVR increases, pressure in the pulmonary artery is increased, making it more difficult for the right ventricle to push blood into the lungs during systole. The right heart becomes congested because less blood is moved out with each contraction. Over time, this congestion causes the right-heart chambers to dilate. The right-heart muscle hypertrophies to compensate for the increased work of contraction. Figure 11–12 shows how the heart is affected by pulmonary hypertension.

Table 11–5 Pulmonary Vascular Resistance (PVR)

Equation	$PVR = (\overline{PAP} - PCWP) \times \frac{80}{CO}$
Components	$\overline{PAP}$ = mean pulmonary artery pressure PCWP = pulmonary capillary wedge pressure CO = cardiac output 80 = conversion factor
Normal values	50–150 dynes·sec·cm^{-5}
Example	A patient has a $\overline{PAP}$ of 22 mmHg, a PCWP of 9 mmHg, and a CO of 4.5 L/min $PVR = (22-9) \times \frac{80}{4.5}$ $PVR = 13 \times 17.78$ $PVR = 231.14$
Factors associated with increased PVR	Alveolar hypoxia, decreased pH, alveolar hypercapnia; positive pressure ventilation; histamine, prostaglandin, angiotensin, catecholamines; sympathetic nervous system stimulation

SOURCE: Data from Levitzky (2013).

Section Three Review

1. Which statement is true regarding the relationship of ventilation to perfusion in an upright person?
   A. It varies throughout the lung.
   B. Ventilation is best in the apices.
   C. Perfusion is best in peripheral lung areas.
   D. It maintains a 1:1 relationship.

2. A client has developed left lower lobe pneumonia; however, the remaining lung fields are clear. It is time to reposition the client in bed. Of the following positions, which is most likely to optimize the ventilation–perfusion relationship?
   A. Lying on the right side
   B. Supine
   C. Lying on the left side
   D. Horizontal in the bed

3. Normal blood flow past completely unventilated alveoli is the definition of which term?
   A. Physiologic shunt
   B. Anatomic shunt
   C. Capillary shunt
   D. Venous admixture

4. Oxygen therapy is most effective in treating which condition?
   A. Shuntlike effect
   B. Anatomic shunt
   C. Capillary shunt
   D. Absolute shunt

Answers: 1. A, 2. A, 3. C, 4. A

Section Four: Acid–base Physiology and Disturbances

The acid–base status is another type of determinant of gas exchange because the lungs play a critical role in maintaining acid–base homeostasis. The lungs are also the source of severe acid–base imbalances in the presence of certain pulmonary disease states.

Acid–base Physiology

The body contains many acid and base substances. **Acids** are substances that dissociate or lose ions. **Bases** are substances capable of accepting ions. A **buffer** is a substance that reacts with acids and bases to maintain a neutral environment of stable pH. The **pH** represents the free hydrogen ion (H^+) concentration. An increase in H^+ concentration lowers pH and increases acidity. A decrease in H^+ concentration increases pH and increases alkalinity. Acid–base balance is crucial to the effective functioning of body systems. Severe imbalances can be lethal.

The body's acids include volatile and nonvolatile acids. **Volatile acids** can convert to a gas form for excretion (carbonic acid). Carbonic acid rapidly converts to carbon dioxide for excretion from the lungs. The lungs excrete a very large amount of acid each day in this manner. **Nonvolatile (metabolic) acids** cannot be converted to gas and must be excreted through the kidneys. Examples of nonvolatile acids include lactic acid and ketones. Unlike the lungs, the kidneys are capable of excreting only a small amount of acid each day and respond slowly to changes. Hydrogen ions are excreted in the proximal and distal tubules of the kidneys in exchange for sodium.

Maintaining Acid–base Balance: Buffer Systems and Compensation

Normal cellular function is dependent on maintaining acid–base balance; the body is intolerant of abnormal acid–base states. The body has three mechanisms to maintain acid–base balance: the buffering mechanism, the respiratory compensation mechanism, and the metabolic (renal) compensation mechanism.

Buffer Mechanism The body is intolerant of wide changes in pH and works constantly to maintain the pH range between 7.35 and 7.45 (Figure 11–13). A normal pH is maintained if the ratio of bicarbonate (HCO_3) to carbon dioxide (CO_2) remains approximately 20:1 (HCO_3/CO_2).

Respiratory Compensation Mechanism Compensation is the process whereby an abnormal pH is returned to within normal limits through counterbalancing acid–base activities. Compensation occurs over time; thus, it is referred to in terms of the degree (or level) to which the body has achieved compensation. There are four levels of compensation: uncompensated (acute), partially

compensated, compensated (chronic), or corrected. An uncompensated (acute) acid–base state is one in which the pH is abnormal because other buffer and regulatory mechanisms have not begun to correct the imbalance. A partially compensated acid–base state is one in which the pH is abnormal; however, the body buffers and regulatory mechanisms have begun to respond to the imbalance. A compensated acid–base state is one in which the pH has returned to within normal limits, with the acid–base imbalance being neutralized but not corrected. Finally, a corrected acid–base state is one in which all acid–base parameters have returned to normal ranges following a state of acid–base imbalance. Table 11–6 summarizes the characteristics and provides examples of the levels of compensation.

Buffering mechanisms represent chemical reactions between acids and bases that maintain a neutral environment. Bases react with excess hydrogen ions (H^+) and acids react with excess HCO_3 to prevent shifts in pH. Buffering mechanisms are triggered quickly in response to any change in pH.

Metabolic (Renal) Compensation Mechanism The bicarbonate buffer system is the major buffering system in the body. Its components are regulated by the lungs (CO_2) and kidneys (HCO_3). The following reversible reaction (carbonic acid equation) represents the shifts that occur as carbonic acid (H_2CO_3) is shifted depending on body needs (left shift makes pH more acid, and right shift makes pH more alkaline):

$$H^+ + HCO_3 \leftrightarrow H_2CO_3 \leftrightarrow CO_2 + H_2O$$
$$\text{More Acid} \longleftarrow \longrightarrow \text{More Alkaline}$$

Additional nonbicarbonate buffers include hemoglobin, serum proteins, and the phosphate system, the latter of which is mainly a function of the kidneys. The bicarbonate system is relatively slow to respond, taking hours to days to respond to acid–base disturbances.

The metabolic compensation mechanism controls the rate of elimination or resorption of hydrogen and bicarbonate ions in the kidney. In situations of increased acid loads (acidosis), H^+ elimination and bicarbonate resorption are increased. In alkalosis, H^+ is resorbed and HCO_3^- is excreted. Metabolic compensation is slow. It begins in hours but takes days to reach maximum compensation. This delayed compensatory mechanism helps explain why so many respiratory problems initially cause acute (uncompensated) acid–base disturbances.

Respiratory (Pulmonary) Compensation Mechanism The respiratory buffer system is the rapid-response compensatory mechanism for metabolic acid–base derangements. It responds within minutes of development of a disturbance. The lungs have two ways of compensating: (1) alveolar hypoventilation in response to metabolic alkalosis and (2) alveolar hyperventilation in response to metabolic acidosis. Hypoventilation (slow and/or shallow breathing) retains CO_2, which is then available to shift the carbonic acid equation toward the left (see the preceding discussion), shifting the pH toward acid. Hyperventilation (rapid and/or deep breathing) blows off CO_2, which then

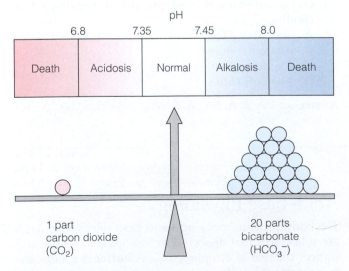

Figure 11–13 Acid–base balance. The normal ratio of bicarbonate to carbon dioxide is 20:1. As long as this ratio is maintained, the pH remains within the normal range of 7.35 to 7.45.

Table 11–6 Levels of Compensation

Level of Compensation	Characteristics	Example
Uncompensated (acute)	Abnormal pH with one abnormal value and one normal value	pH 7.20, $PaCO_2$ 60 mmHg, HCO_3 24 mEq/L *Interpretation:* The pH and $PaCO_2$ match (acid). HCO_3 is normal. No compensation is occurring. An uncompensated (acute) acidosis state exists.
Partially compensated	Abnormal pH with two abnormal values ($PaCO_2$ and HCO_3 are moving in opposite directions)	pH 7.30, $PaCO_2$ 60 mmHg, HCO_3 30 mEq/L *Interpretation:* The pH and $PaCO_2$ match (acid). HCO_3 is alkaline or moving in the opposite direction from the $PaCO_2$. The pH is still abnormal. A partially compensated acidosis state exists.
Compensated (chronic)	Normal pH plus two abnormal values ($PaCO_2$ and HCO_3 are moving in opposite directions)	pH 7.38, $PaCO_2$ 50 mmHg, HCO_3 30 mEq/L *Interpretation:* The pH (acid side of normal range) and $PaCO_2$ (acid) match. HCO_3 is alkaline (opposite of $PaCO_2$). A (chronic) compensated acidosis state exists.
Corrected	Normal pH and two normal values. No acid–base disturbance currently exists.	pH 7.36, $PaCO_2$ 43 mmHg, HCO_3 26 mEq/L *Interpretation:* A normal acid–base state in a person who, until recently, had an acid–base disturbance.

shifts the carbonic acid equation back toward the right, driving the pH up, toward alkaline (Barrett, Barman, Boitano, & Brooks, 2016).

Respiratory Acid–base Disturbances

Primary respiratory disturbances are reflected by changes in the $PaCO_2$, either above normal as in respiratory acidosis or below normal as in respiratory alkalosis.

Respiratory Acidosis Respiratory acidosis occurs when the pH drops below 7.35 and the $PaCO_2$ rises above 45 mmHg. **Hypercapnia**, elevated carbon dioxide (CO_2), indicates alveolar hypoventilation. The lungs are not blowing off enough carbon dioxide, causing an excess of carbonic acid. Carbon dioxide is considered an acid because it combines with water to form carbonic acid. It is essential to determine the cause of hypoventilation and then to correct it when possible. Box 11–1 lists some of the major causes of acute respiratory acidosis.

Table 11–7 Comparison of Acute and Chronic Respiratory Acidosis

Parameter	Uncompensated	Compensated	
	Acute	Partial	Chronic
pH	↓	↓	Normal
$PaCO_2$	↑	↑	↑
HCO_3	Normal	↑	↑

A "chronic" abnormal acid–base state implies a state of compensation. Chronic respiratory acidosis is usually associated with one of the two main types of chronic obstructive pulmonary disease: chronic bronchitis or emphysema. The elevation of carbon dioxide occurs gradually over many years; therefore, the body is able to compensate to maintain a normal pH by elevating the bicarbonate. Because individuals with COPD have little respiratory reserve, additional stressors can cause decompensation, which produces respiratory failure. Table 11–7 compares the effects of acute and chronic acidosis on ABG levels.

Respiratory Alkalosis Respiratory alkalosis occurs when the pH is greater than 7.45 and the $PaCO_2$ falls below 35 mmHg. The decreased carbon dioxide indicates alveolar hyperventilation. The lungs are eliminating too much carbon dioxide, creating a carbonic acid deficit. In the presence of respiratory alkalosis, there is insufficient carbon dioxide available to combine with water to form carbonic acid (H_2CO_3). The key to effective treatment of respiratory alkalosis is to determine the cause of the hyperventilation and provide the intervention necessary to correct the problem. Common causes of acute respiratory alkalosis are listed in Box 11–2.

Chronic respiratory alkalosis is uncommon. The same factors causing acute respiratory alkalosis could cause a chronic state if the problem remained uncorrected. Table 11–8 compares the effects of acute and chronic respiratory alkalosis on ABG levels.

BOX 11–1 Common Causes of Acute Respiratory Acidosis

Alveolar hypoventilation, caused by:

- Respiratory depression
  - Oversedation
  - Overdose
  - Brain injury
- Decreased ventilation
  - Respiratory muscle fatigue
  - Neuromuscular diseases
  - Mechanical ventilation (underventilation)
- Altered diffusion or ventilation–perfusion mismatch
  - Pulmonary edema
  - Severe atelectasis
  - Pneumonia
  - Severe bronchospasm

<table>
<tr><td></td></tr>
</table>

BOX 11–2 Common Causes of Acute Respiratory Alkalosis

Alveolar hyperventilation, caused by:

- Hypoxia
- Brain injury
- Fever
- Mechanical ventilation (overventilation)
- Pain
- Anxiety, fear

Table 11–8 Comparison of Acute and Chronic Respiratory Alkalosis

Parameter	Uncompensated	Compensated	
	Acute	Partial	Chronic
pH	↑	↑	Normal
PaCO$_2$	↓	↓	↓
HCO$_3$	Normal	↓	↓

Metabolic Acid–base Disturbances

While the focus of this chapter is the pulmonary system, a discussion of acid–base imbalances would not be complete without considering metabolic imbalances. Primary metabolic disturbances are reflected by abnormal base excess (BE) levels and changes in bicarbonate (HCO$_3$) levels.

Base Excess or Deficit Base excess (BE) or **base deficit (BD)** is a measure of the amount of buffer required to return the blood to a normal pH state. The normal range is ±2 mEq/L (Kee, 2014). Base excess or deficit is a purely nonrespiratory measurement because it is not affected by carbonic acid concentrations; therefore, abnormal levels are specific to a metabolic acid–base disturbance. A base *excess* is present if the value is greater than +2 mEq/L, reflecting either an excess of base or a deficit of fixed acids. It signals the presence of a metabolic alkalosis state. A base *deficit* is present if the value is less than −2 mEq/L, reflecting an excess of fixed acids or a deficit of base in the blood. It signals the presence of a metabolic acidosis state.

Keep in mind that a patient may simultaneously experience a metabolic and respiratory acid–based disturbance. For this reason, the nurse must examine the entire arterial blood gas and the patient's clinical status to determine the exact nature of an acid–base disturbance.

Metabolic Acidosis Metabolic acidosis can be defined clinically as pH less than 7.35 and HCO$_3$ less than 22 mEq/L, with a base deficit (less than −2 mEq/L). Metabolic acidosis can be caused by an increase in metabolic acids or excessive loss of base. Examples of conditions that can cause an increase in hydrogen ion (H$^+$) concentration include the following:

- Diabetic acidosis as a result of elevated ketones
- Uremia associated with increased levels of phosphates and sulfates

- Ingestion of acidic drugs, such as aspirin (salicylate) overdose
- Lactic acidosis caused by increased lactic acid production

Examples of conditions that precipitate a decrease in bicarbonate (HCO$_3$) levels include the following:

- Diarrhea, which causes loss of alkaline substances
- Gastrointestinal fistulas, leading to loss of alkaline substances
- Loss of body fluids from drains below the umbilicus (except urinary catheter), causing loss of alkaline fluids
- Drugs causing loss of alkali, such as laxative overuse
- Hyperaldosteronism, which causes increased renal loss

Lactic Acidosis. Acid metabolites, such as lactic acid (lactate), result from cellular breakdown and anaerobic metabolism. The normal range for an arterial serum lactate is 0.5 to 2 mmol/L and 0.5 to 1.5 mmol/L for a venous blood sample (Kee, 2014). High-acuity patients are at particular risk for developing elevated levels of lactate because lactic acidosis is closely associated with shock and other severe physiologic insults. During a shock episode, cellular hypoxia rapidly drives up serum lactate levels, usually higher than 5 mEq/L. This rise often precedes decompensatory signs, such as decreased urine output and decreased blood pressure, and thus may be an indicator of impending shock. Other conditions that can cause lactic acidosis include severe dehydration, severe infection, severe trauma, diabetic ketoacidosis, and hepatic failure (Kee, 2014).

Table 11–9 compares the effects of acute and chronic metabolic acidosis on arterial blood gases.

Metabolic Alkalosis Metabolic alkalosis can be defined clinically as pH greater than 7.45 and bicarbonate (HCO$_3$) level greater than 26 mEq/L, with a base excess (greater than +2). Metabolic alkalosis occurs when the amount of alkali (base) increases or excessive loss of acid occurs.

A common cause of increased alkali is ingestion of alkaline drugs associated with the overuse of antacids or overadministration of sodium bicarbonate during a cardiac arrest emergency. Examples of conditions that result in a decrease in acid include the following:

- Loss of gastric fluids from vomiting or nasogastric suction
- Treatment with steroids, especially those with mineralocorticoid effects

---

Table 11–9 Comparison of Acute and Chronic Metabolic Acidosis

Parameter	Uncompensated	Compensated	
	Acute	Partial	Chronic
pH	↓	↓	Normal
PaCO$_2$	Normal	↓	↓
HCO$_3$	↓	↓	↓

Table 11–10 Comparison of Acute and Chronic Metabolic Alkalosis

| Parameter | Uncompensated | Compensated | |
	Acute	Partial	Chronic
pH	↑	↑	Normal
$PaCO_2$	Normal	↑	↑
HCO_3	↑	↑	↑

- Diuretic therapy with certain drugs, such as furosemide (Lasix), causing loss of potassium
- Binge–purge syndrome

Table 11–10 compares the effects of acute and chronic metabolic alkalosis on arterial blood gases.

Section Four Review

1. Respiratory compensation involves the excretion or retention of which gas or substance?
   A. CO_2
   B. HCO_3
   C. H_2O
   D. K^+

2. Metabolic compensation involves changes in the renal excretion or resorption of which combination of gases or substances?
   A. H^+, CO_2
   B. HCO_3, H^+
   C. Glucose, HCO_3
   D. CO_2, HCO_3

3. Client situations associated with respiratory alkalosis include which condition?
   A. Sedation
   B. Neuromuscular blockade
   C. Pulmonary edema
   D. Anxiety

4. Which condition may cause metabolic acidosis because of a decrease in bicarbonate levels?
   A. Diarrhea
   B. Uremia
   C. Aspirin ingestion
   D. Diabetic ketoacidosis

Answers: 1. A, 2. B, 3. D, 4. A

Section Five: Arterial Blood Gases

The interpretation of arterial blood gases provides valuable information on the patient's acid–base and oxygenation status. In Section Four, determinants of acid–base status (pH, $PaCO_2$ and bicarbonate [HCO_3]) were presented. This section focuses on the determinants of oxygenation status and interpretation of the entire arterial blood gas.

Determinants of Oxygenation Status

There are three major determinants of oxygenation status: PaO_2, SaO_2 (or SpO_2), and hemoglobin.

PaO₂ PaO_2 represents the partial pressure of the oxygen dissolved in arterial blood (3% of total oxygen), not the total amount of oxygen available. The normal range is 80 to 100 mmHg (Pagana, 2015). Although it accounts for only a small percentage of total oxygen in the blood, it is an important indicator of oxygenation because PaO_2 and oxygen saturation (SaO_2) maintain a relationship. This relationship is reflected in the oxyhemoglobin dissociation curve, which was discussed in Section Two.

SaO₂ and SpO₂ Oxygen saturation (SO_2) refers to the percentage of oxygen that is bound to hemoglobin (called oxyhemoglobin) in the blood. SO_2 can be measured in arterial blood (SaO_2 or SpO_2) or venous blood (SvO_2); however, the ABG only measures SaO_2. The degree of saturation is important in determining the amount of oxygen available for delivery to the tissues. The normal value of SaO_2 and SpO_2 is greater than 95% (Kee, 2014). The **SaO₂** may be obtained as one aspect of the arterial blood gas values ("a" for arterial). It is a direct measure of arterial blood oxygen saturation. **SpO₂** specifically refers to the saturation of oxygen when measured using pulse oximetry ("p" for pulse). Pulse oximetry is a noninvasive means of intermittently or continuously monitoring oxygen saturation using light waves. It is an indirect measurement of oxygen saturation. The SaO_2 and SpO_2 values should be essentially the same.

When SpO_2 is to be used as the primary device for monitoring oxygen saturation, it is recommended that an arterial blood gas be obtained to compare the SaO_2 with the SpO_2 values to evaluate them for any disparities. Further, when there is any doubt of the validity of SpO_2 readings, an ABG should be drawn and evaluated. Additional information on pulse oximetry is available in Section Eight.

Hemoglobin Hemoglobin (Hgb or Hb) is the major component of red blood cells. The normal range is 12 to 15 g/dL in women and 13.5 to 18 g/dL in men (Kee, 2014). Hemoglobin is composed of protein and heme, which contains iron. Oxygen binds to the iron atoms located on the four heme groups of each hemoglobin molecule. Hemoglobin is the major carrier of oxygen in the blood and is, therefore, an important factor in tissue oxygenation.

Arterial Blood Gas

Arterial blood gas (ABG) values are typically reported as normal at sea level (760 mmHg) partial pressures, room air (21% oxygen), and a blood temperature of 37°C (98.6°F). Significant alterations in any of these factors must be considered during interpretation.

Age affects some of the normal ABG values. Acid–base–related values (pH, $PaCO_2$, and HCO_3) may remain unchanged throughout adult life (Pagana, 2015). However, oxygenation-related values diminish. For example, the older adult has a 25% to 30% decrease in PaO_2 between the ages of 30 and 80 years (Pagana, 2015). Normal ABG values are ranges that have been established for normal, healthy adults. However, in high-acuity patients, it is important to establish a baseline for the individual because abnormal values may become the acceptable baseline for some individuals. For example, a patient with chronic lung disease may have a PaO_2 of 60 mmHg and a $PaCO_2$ of 50 mmHg as a normal baseline. Attempts to return this individual's ABG values to those of a normal, healthy person would have serious consequences.

Table 11–11 provides a summary of normal ABG values.

Table 11–11 Normal Arterial Blood Gas Values

Component	Range
ACID–BASE	
pH	7.35–7.45
$PaCO_2$	35–45 mmHg
HCO_3	24–28 mEq/L
BE	±2 mEq/L
OXYGENATION STATUS	
PaO_2	80–100 mmHg
SaO_2	Greater than 95%
Hgb	13.5–18 g/dL (males)
	12–15 g/dL (females)

SOURCE: Data sources for PaO_2 normal range are from Pagana (2015); all other laboratory ranges are from Kee (2014).

Arterial Blood Gas Interpretation A single ABG measurement represents only a single point in time. Arterial blood gases are most valuable when trends are evaluated over time, correlated with other values, and incorporated into the overall clinical picture. Interpretation of ABGs includes determination of acid–base state, level of compensation, and oxygenation status. Determination of the acid–base state

Table 11–12 Steps in Determining Acid–Base and Oxygenation Status

Step	Normal Values	Questions
ACID–BASE INTERPRETATION		
Step 1: Evaluate pH	pH = 7.35 to 7.45; midpoint = 7.40 If less than 7.40 = acid If greater than 7.40 = alkaline	Ask: • Is the pH within normal range? • Is pH on acid or alkaline side of 7.40?
Step 2: Evaluate $PaCO_2$	$PaCO_2$ = 35 to 45 mmHg If less than 35 mmHg = alkaline If greater than 45 mmHg = acid	Ask: • Is $PaCO_2$ within normal range? • If not, does it deviate to acid or alkaline side?
Step 3: Evaluate HCO_3	HCO_3 = 22 to 26 mEq/L If less than 22 mEq/L = acid If greater than 26 mEq/L = alkaline	Ask: • Is HCO_3 within normal range? • If not, does it deviate to alkaline or acid side?
Step 4: Determine Acid–Base Status	The acid–base status has now been determined for the individual components of $PaCO_2$ and HCO_3.	Ask: • Which individual component matches the pH acid–base state? • The match determines the *primary* acid–base disturbance.
OXYGENATION STATUS INTERPRETATION		
Step 5: Evaluate PaO_2	PaO_2 = 80 to 100 mmHg	Ask: • Is it within normal range? • What is this person's baseline? • Is it within acceptable range for this person? • If not, is it too low or too high?
Step 6: Evaluate SaO_2	SaO_2 = greater than 95%	Ask: • Is it within acceptable range?
Step 7: Evaluate Hgb	Hgb = 12 to 15 g/dL (females) Hgb = 13.5 to 17 g/dL (males)	Ask: • Are there enough oxygen carriers?
Step 8: Evaluate patient	Although ABG interpretation is an important adjunct to assessing a patient's status, it cannot take the place of direct evaluation of the patient.	Ask: • Does patient's clinical picture match the acid–base and oxygen interpretation? • Does the patient have a chronic disorder that is associated with long-term alterations in ABGs? • Are there any acute processes occurring that need to be taken into consideration? • Does the patient have a fever?

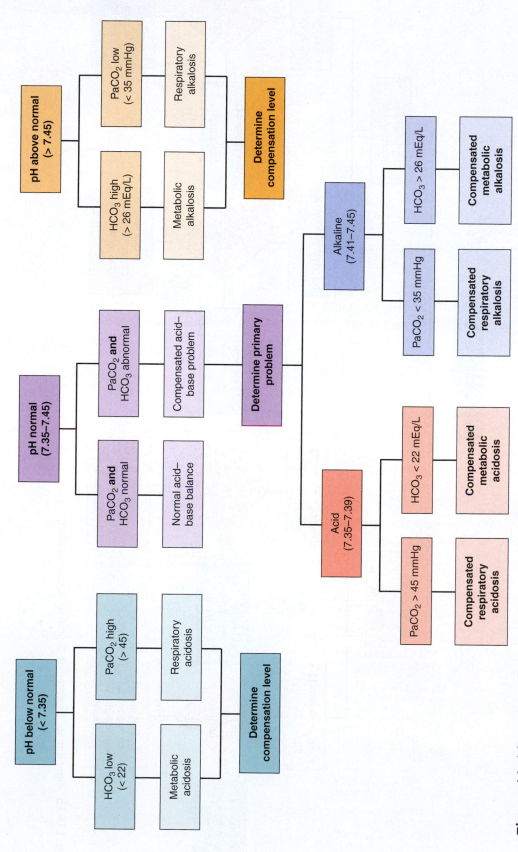

Figure 11–14 Algorithm for interpreting primary acid–base disturbances.

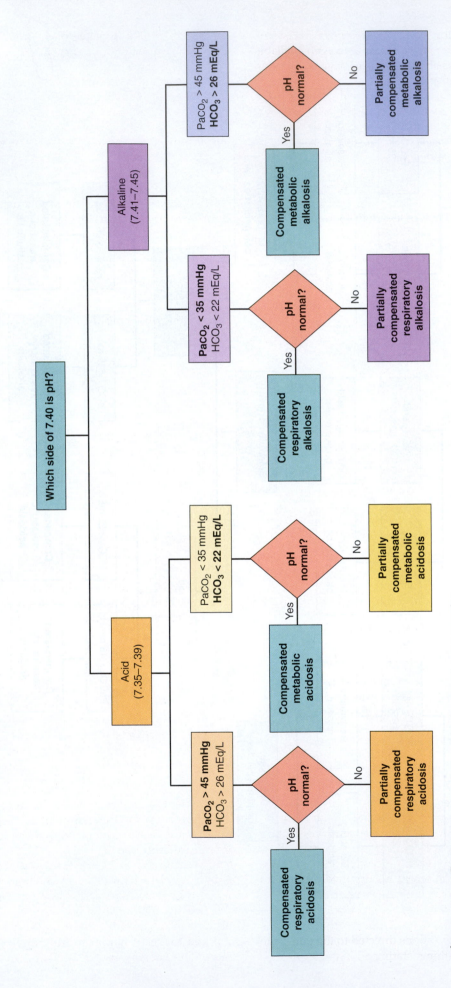

Figure 11–15 Algorithm for interpreting degree of compensation.

was discussed in Section Four. The oxygenation status reflects alveolar ventilation, the amount of oxygen available in arterial blood for possible tissue use, oxygen-carrying capacity, and oxygen transport.

The severity of hypoxemia is frequently referred to as mild, moderate, or severe. However, the exact associated PaO_2 levels are somewhat arbitrary and vary among experts. For the purposes of this chapter, the levels of hypoxemia are defined as follows:

- Mild hypoxemia: PaO_2 60 to 75 mmHg
- Moderate hypoxemia: PaO_2 45 to 59 mmHg
- Severe hypoxemia: PaO_2 of less than 45 mmHg

A step-by-step process for ABG interpretation evaluates each component to determine acid–base balance and oxygenation status, as presented in Table 11–12. Although acid–base balance determination is presented first, oxygenation status is often analyzed first, based on the needs of the patient and the preference of the person performing the analysis. Figures 11–14 and 11–15 provide algorithms for interpreting primary acid–base disturbances and level of compensation.

Supplemental ABG exercises are provided at the end of this chapter. Take the time to practice determining acid–base states and oxygenation status using the steps and algorithms provided in this section.

Section Five Review

1. Normal values for arterial blood gases include which value?
   A. pH 7.5
   B. $PaCO_2$ 20 mmHg
   C. HCO_3 26 mmHg
   D. SaO_2 75 mmHg

2. An increase in bicarbonate would have which effect on the pH?
   A. More acidic
   B. More alkaline
   C. More neutral
   D. No change

3. A client who typically has normal ABG values is found to have a PaO_2 of 73 mmHg. Which classification of hypoxia exists?
   A. Mild
   B. No hypoxia is present
   C. Moderate
   D. Severe

4. What factor must always be evaluated to place ABGs in the proper context?
   A. Laboratory values
   B. Supplemental oxygen therapy
   C. Mode of ventilation
   D. Client status

Answers: 1. C, 2. B, 3. A, 4. D

Section Six: Focused Respiratory Nursing History and Assessment

Many high-acuity patients are at increased risk for being admitted with pulmonary diseases or developing respiratory complications. This section provides a review of the focused respiratory system assessment as it applies to the high-acuity adult patient.

Nursing History

When a patient is admitted to the hospital in acute distress, the nurse initially assesses airway, breathing, and circulation (ABCs) and immediately takes appropriate action based on those assessments. As soon as is feasible, information regarding the immediate events leading to admission should be obtained. A recent history gives important clues to the etiology and chain of events related to the current problem. The presence of severe respiratory distress limits the amount of health history information a patient is able to relate. Minimize questions directed to the patient to reduce the stress on breathing, stating all inquiries in such

a way that they require very brief answers. Historical data that is particularly important to assess in the patient with acute pulmonary problems include the following factors.

Social History   Assess tobacco and alcohol use. Tobacco use is associated with many pulmonary diseases, and current use may further aggravate acute pulmonary problems. The number of cigarettes smoked per day and the number of years a patient has smoked should be assessed. Alcohol use in association with prescribed drug therapy may adversely affect the patient's respiratory condition. Problems with alcohol withdrawal can complicate the cardiopulmonary status should delirium tremens develop.

Nutritional History   The nutritional state of a pulmonary patient is crucial to assess because malnutrition is contributory to the development of respiratory failure. Furthermore, many patients with chronic pulmonary disorders are admitted to the hospital in a malnourished state, which negatively impacts outcomes. There are several ways in which this can happen. First, a protein–calorie deficit weakens muscles, including the respiratory muscles. Second, malnutrition is associated with a weakened immune system, which increases susceptibility to infection and makes it harder to fight against existing infections. The increased stress associated with an acute infection can precipitate acute respiratory failure. Third, a high-carbohydrate diet increases the overall carbon dioxide load in the body. This may lead to ventilatory complications in certain patients. If there is concern that malnutrition is present, a nutritional assessment, laboratory testing of proteins, and a nutrition consult may be considered.

Cardiopulmonary History

Because the lungs, heart, and blood vessels comprise a common circuit, factors that alter any part of the circuit can cause a subsequent alteration in other parts. It is often difficult to differentiate between problems of pulmonary and cardiovascular etiology. Because of this, obtaining sufficient data regarding the cardiovascular system is invaluable in planning the management of the patient. Of particular importance are data concerning preexisting cardiovascular conditions such as a history of hypertension, coronary artery disease, or previous myocardial infarction. Preexisting pulmonary problems such as asthma or emphysema, as well as prehospital activity tolerance, can also help to differentiate pulmonary and cardiac problems.

Sleep–Rest History

Pulmonary problems frequently interfere with sleep and rest for a variety of reasons. If the respiratory problem is severe enough to cause hypoxia, the patient often exhibits restlessness associated with inadequate oxygenation of the brain. Pulmonary disorders often increase the work of breathing, which can interfere with rest and sleep. Patients in respiratory distress may sleep poorly because they fear that they will cease to breathe when they are unaware. Others cannot sleep because of their level of general discomfort. Dyspnea and air hunger are anxiety-producing and threatening experiences for pulmonary patients.

Common Complaints Associated with Pulmonary Disorders

If a respiratory problem is suspected, the nurse should focus on obtaining information concerning the most common respiratory complaints: dyspnea, chest pain, cough, sputum, and hemoptysis. This can be accomplished by interviewing the patient and/or family (subjective data) and by performing a nursing assessment (objective data). Regular assessment of the common respiratory symptoms is also important in monitoring the patient for acute changes in respiratory status.

Dyspnea

Dyspnea is a subjective (patient-based) symptom. The two major subcategories of dyspnea are orthopnea and paroxysmal nocturnal dyspnea. The nurse may also observe certain signs and symptoms during clinical assessments that suggest the presence of dyspnea.

Subjective Data. Dyspnea is the feeling of difficulty breathing or shortness of breath. Physiologically, dyspnea is associated with increased work of breathing—a supply-and-demand imbalance. Increased work of breathing occurs when ventilatory demands go beyond the body's ability to respond. Progressive dyspnea is noted commonly in both restrictive and obstructive pulmonary disorders.

Orthopnea is a type of dyspnea closely associated with cardiac problems or severe pulmonary disease. It refers to a state in which the patient assumes a head-up position to relieve dyspnea. Orthopnea may be mild (the patient may need several pillows to sleep comfortably in bed), or it may be severe (the patient may need to sit upright in a chair or in bed). When taking the patient's history, it is important to ask how many pillows are required for breathing comfortably while at rest. Requiring additional pillows to breathe comfortably while lying down is sometimes referred to as pillow orthopnea. For example, a patient who states that three pillows are required for sleep would have three-pillow orthopnea.

One type of dyspnea is of particular interest in differentiating cardiac from pulmonary disorders. **Paroxysmal nocturnal dyspnea (PND)** is associated with left-heart failure. The typical patient report is that of waking during the night, after being asleep for several hours, with a sudden onset of severe orthopnea. On sitting up or getting out of bed, the dyspnea is relieved, and the patient is able to resume sleep. Paroxysmal nocturnal dyspnea is a form of transient mild pulmonary edema. It is believed that fluids that have been congested in the lower extremities during the day because of gravity drainage shift to the heart and lungs, causing a fluid volume overload when the person is horizontal (as in sleep) for several hours.

Objective Data. Objectively, the nurse may note tachypnea; nasal flaring; use of **accessory muscles** in the neck, chest, or abdomen; or abnormal arterial blood gases. The patient may voluntarily assume a high-Fowler sitting position secondary to orthopnea. Severe tachypnea—a respiratory rate of more than 30 breaths per minute—significantly increases the work of breathing. If tachypnea continues for a prolonged period, respiratory muscle fatigue can occur, which may ultimately cause acute respiratory failure.

Chest Pain

When a patient is admitted with reports of chest pain, it is critical to differentiate pain caused by pulmonary disease from pain caused by cardiac disease.

Subjective Data. When assessing chest pain, it is important to note how long the pain has been present, if it radiates, and what the triggering and alleviating factors are. The type of chest pain the patient describes can be helpful in differentiating cardiogenic (originating from the heart) from pleuritic (originating from the pleura) pain. Cardiogenic pain generally is described as dull, pressure-like discomfort often radiating to the jaw, back, or left arm. If asked to point to the painful area, the patient often uses the palm of the hand, indicating a somewhat general area. Cardiogenic pain is unaffected by breathing. In contrast, pleuritic pain frequently is described as sharp and knifelike, and the patient is able to point to the focal area with one finger. When the patient is between breaths or the breath is held, pain decreases or ceases. The pain increases with deep breathing but does not radiate. A pleural friction rub may sometimes be auscultated at the focal pain point.

Most pulmonary disorders affecting only the lung parenchyma (lung tissue) are not associated with chest pain as an early symptom because the parenchyma is insensitive to pain. For example, lung cancer frequently goes undetected until a routine chest x-ray is taken and read or the tumor impinges on innervated thoracic structures, causing deep pain. Like lung tissue, the attached visceral pleura is insensitive. The parietal pleura, however, is well innervated, and when inflammation (called **pleurisy** or **pleuritis**) occurs, it can trigger the sharp pain, as previously described.

Objective Data. Objective data the nurse may note include splinting, shallow respirations, tachypnea, facial changes associated with pain, and increased blood pressure and pulse.

Cough Coughing is an important reflex activity that assists the mucociliary escalator in removing secretions and foreign particles from the lower airway. It is triggered by irritation, the presence of foreign particles, or obstruction of the airway.

Subjective Data. The patient should be asked to provide the following information about cough: frequency, character (dry, productive, congested), duration, triggers, pattern of occurrence, and alleviating factors.

Objective Data. The nurse can observe the strength, character, and frequency of the cough.

Sputum The characteristics of sputum or changes in the characteristics provide important information about a pulmonary disease.

Subjective Data. It is important to obtain a description of sputum production in a pulmonary patient. If a disease is associated with chronic production of sputum, the patient should be asked to describe the usual quantity, characteristics, and color as well as any changes associated with the current pulmonary problem.

Objective Data. Sputum may consist of a variety of substances, such as mucus, pus, bacteria, or blood. Sputum should be monitored on a regular basis for quantity, characteristics (thin, thick, tenacious), color, and odor. Sputum changes should be noted and documented because they may reflect a change in the patient's pulmonary status.

Hemoptysis Hemoptysis is the expectoration of bloody secretions. It is important to determine the source of the bleeding, which may be the upper airway (e.g., the oral cavity or nose) or the lower airway (e.g., the lungs).

Subjective Data. In patients who are experiencing respiratory problems, the presence of hemoptysis can be a significant finding and may be of cardiovascular or pulmonary origin.

Common causes of cardiovascular-related hemoptysis include pulmonary embolism and cardiogenic pulmonary edema secondary to left-heart failure. The most common source of hemoptysis, however, is lung disease, particularly as a result of infection and neoplasms. Lung diseases associated with hemoptysis include bronchitis, bronchiectasis, pneumonia, tuberculosis, fungal and parasitic infections, and lung tumors.

Objective Data. When hemoptysis is noted, it should be assessed for color, consistency, and quantity. The frequency and duration also should be noted and documented.

Focused Respiratory Assessment

The focused respiratory assessment is an important part of evaluating the patient for status changes throughout the shift. The onset of acute respiratory distress can be rapid and severe. The nurse should be alert to changes from previously assessed baseline data and data trends. When such changes are noted, a rapid and focused respiratory assessment should be immediately conducted, focusing on key data that strongly suggest an acute alteration in respiratory function. Box 11–3 lists key abnormal data.

Inspection Skin coloring should be inspected closely for cyanosis. Observe the lips, earlobes, and beneath the tongue for central cyanosis, which may indicate prolonged hypoxia. In patients with dark skin tones, cyanosis can be observed on the lips and tongue, which will appear ashen-gray. Cyanosis is not a reliable indicator of hypoxia because it is dependent on the amount of reduced hemoglobin present. Its value, therefore, is as supportive data rather than diagnostic data. When present, cyanosis is a late sign of respiratory distress.

Inspect the shape of the chest and observe chest movement for symmetry of expansion and the rate, depth, and pattern of breathing. Note use of accessory muscles to assist in breathing. If the patient has sustained chest trauma or has chest tubes in place, the chest should be observed for changes in appearance and palpated for subcutaneous emphysema and areas of tenderness. The chest may also be palpated for tactile fremitus and chest expansion. Chest percussion is useful for detecting the presence of air, fluid, or consolidation under the area being percussed.

Auscultation Auscultation is one of the most important pulmonary assessment tools. The diaphragm of the

---

BOX 11–3 Key Abnormal Data Suggesting Altered Respiratory Function

- Suddenly increased restlessness and agitation (hypoxia)
- Suddenly decreased level of responsiveness, increased lethargy (hypercapnia)
- Significant change in pattern of breathing:
  - Respiratory rate less than 10/min or greater than 30/min
  - Shallow or erratic breathing
- Increased cyanosis or duskiness
- Increased use of accessory muscles
- Increased dyspnea or orthopnea
- Increase in adventitious breath sounds or development of abnormal breath sounds
- Changing trends in vital signs (blood pressure, pulse, respirations):
  - Increasing trends indicate that compensation is occurring
  - Decreasing trends indicate that decompensation activities may be occurring
- Presence of pain

Table 11–13 Normal Breath Sounds

Breath Sound	Inspiratory or Expiratory Pattern	Normal Location	Description
Vesicular	/\	Peripheral lung fields	Whispering, rustling quality; quiet and low pitched; inspiratory phase is longer than expiratory phase; no distinct pause between inspiration and expiration
Bronchial (tubular)	/\	Over the trachea and larynx	High-pitched, loud sound; pause heard between inspiratory and expiratory phases; expiration phase is longer than inspiration (abnormal if heard in peripheral lung; may indicate a consolidation, such as pneumonia)
Bronchovesicular	/\	In all lobes near major airways	Sound is between vesicular and bronchial

stethoscope is best for hearing most breath sounds, auscultating in a pattern that allows comparison of one lung to the other.

Normal Breath Sounds. The three types of normal breath sounds are vesicular, bronchial (tubular), and bronchovesicular. Table 11–13 differentiates the various normal sounds.

Abnormal Breath Sounds. The chest should be auscultated routinely for diminished or absent sounds in any field. The presence of abnormal breath sounds is associated with a change in lung status, such as partial or complete obstruction of a part of the airway by secretions or fluid, or loss of elasticity in the lung fields. Adventitious breath sounds are heard on top of other breath sounds. They are never considered normal. Adventitious sounds may be caused by fluid or secretions in the airways or alveoli, by alveoli opening or collapsing, or by bronchoconstriction. When abnormal breath sounds are present, the nurse should assess and document the location and when in the respiratory cycle they are heard. Adventitious sounds are classified as crackles, rhonchi, wheeze, stridor, pleural rub, and diminished or absent lung sounds.

Crackles are associated with either fluid or secretions in the small airways or alveoli, or with the opening of alveoli from a collapsed state. Crackles are heard most commonly during inspiration as relatively discrete, delicate popping sounds of short duration. They may be described as fine or coarse. Fine crackles are delicate, high pitched, and of short duration. The classic description of fine crackles is that they sound similar to the noise made by rubbing hair between the fingers next to the ear. Conditions such as atelectasis and pneumonia are associated with fine crackles. Coarse or loud crackles are louder, lower-pitched sounds of longer duration than fine crackles, similar to the sound of Velcro separating. They are heard in conditions such as bronchitis and pulmonary edema.

Rhonchi are heard as coarse, bubbly sounds. They are most commonly present during expiration and are auscultated over the larger airways. Rhonchi are associated with an accumulation of fluid or secretions in the larger airways, such as in pneumonia.

A **wheeze** is caused by air passing through constricted airways. The constriction may be caused by bronchospasm, fluid, secretions, edema obstructing the airway, or an obstructing tumor or foreign body. A wheeze has a musical quality that may be high pitched or low pitched. It may be heard on inspiration or expiration and is of long duration.

Stridor is a type of wheeze caused by upper-airway obstruction from inflamed tissue or a foreign body. It is described as a high-pitched inspiratory wheeze heard louder over the neck than the chest wall. In high-acuity adult patients, it may develop from airway edema resulting from such problems as thermal burn inhalation injury or airway trauma during extubation.

Pleural rub is caused by an inflammation of the pleural linings (membranes). When inflammation occurs, the linings become resistant to free movement. The characteristic sound is heard during breathing and ceases between breaths or with breath holding. Also referred to as pleural friction rub, it has been described as sounding like leather rubbing together or creaking.

Diminished or absent breath sounds are caused by diminished or absent air flow to an area of the lungs. A loss or decrease of sounds in discrete lung areas often results from problems such as lung consolidation, as seen with pneumonia, tumors, or pneumothorax. When assessed, the nurse should document the location. In patients with lung hyperinflation disorders, such as chronic obstructive pulmonary disease (COPD) and acute asthma, generalized loss of breath sounds may indicate a potentially life-threatening hypoventilation situation.

Vital Signs and Hemodynamic Values Vital signs and hemodynamic values provide crucial baseline data and are important indicators of changing patient status when trended over time. In addition to vital signs, a pulse oximeter reading should be obtained. If a central venous or pulmonary artery catheter is in place, important hemodynamic monitoring assessments include central venous pressure (CVP), pulmonary artery pressure (PAP), pulmonary artery wedge pressure (PAWP), mean arterial pressure

(MAP), and cardiac output (CO). Hemodynamic monitoring generally is initiated when severe cardiac involvement is suspected or fluid status is questioned. If the patient's condition is purely pulmonary in nature, data collected from hemodynamic monitoring may be of insufficient value to warrant such an invasive procedure. The presence of pulmonary hypertension can alter hemodynamic measurements

Section Six Review

1. When a client is admitted in acute respiratory distress, the initial history should focus on which priority?
   A. Smoking history
   B. Events leading to current admission
   C. Nutritional history
   D. Events leading to previous admissions

2. What are the most common complaints associated with pulmonary disease? (Select all that apply.)
   A. Cough
   B. Sputum
   C. Cyanosis
   D. Dyspnea
   E. Chest pain

3. How is the chest pain typical of pleuritic pain best characterized?
   A. Sharp
   B. Pressurelike
   C. Radiating
   D. Dull

4. What is the cause of crackles?
   A. Secretions in the large airways
   B. Inflammation of the pleural linings
   C. Air passing through constricted airways
   D. Fluid or secretions in the small airways or alveoli

Answers: 1. B, 2. (A, B, D, E), 3. A, 4 D

Section Seven: Pulmonary Function Evaluation

The provider or medical team generally initiates orders for pulmonary function testing to assist in diagnosing a pulmonary problem or updating or evaluating a patient's pulmonary status. Actual implementation and interpretation of the tests often become an interdisciplinary undertaking.

Pulmonary Function Tests

Ventilation is measured in a variety of ways using pulmonary function tests (PFTs). These tests provide baseline data and also provide a means to monitor the progress of functional impairments associated with pulmonary diseases. They help differentiate a restrictive pulmonary problem from an obstructive one. In addition, PFTs are useful for monitoring the effectiveness of therapeutic interventions (Figure 11–16). Diagnostic pulmonary function

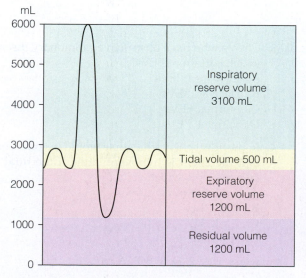
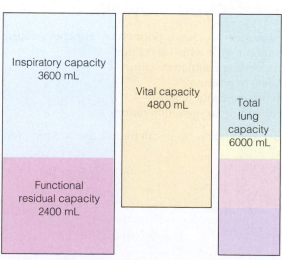

Figure 11–16 Pulmonary function tests. The relationship of lung volumes and capacities. Volumes (mL) shown are for an average adult male.

testing is usually conducted in a pulmonary laboratory using special computerized equipment that accurately measures pulmonary volumes, capacities, and air flow. Simpler measures of pulmonary function, however, can be measured at the bedside using a spirometer.

Bedside Pulmonary Function Measurements

High-acuity patients with or without direct pulmonary involvement are at risk of developing pulmonary complications associated with immobility and respiratory muscle fatigue. Pulmonary function may be monitored in patients who are at particular risk for ventilatory decompensation. Performing bedside PFTs requires the patient's cooperation; patients who are admitted in severe respiratory distress (e.g., COPD exacerbation) may be too dyspneic to tolerate bedside PFTs during their acute distress period (Cydulka & Bates, 2016).

The bedside PFTs of particular interest are tidal volume, vital capacity, and minute ventilation. Both tidal volume and vital capacity help monitor respiratory muscle strength. As the patient experiences respiratory muscle fatigue, these values decrease. Bedside PFTs can be measured using a respiratory spirometer and are frequently used as part of weaning criteria during mechanical ventilation. Normal values vary with height, weight, gender, and age.

Tidal volume (VT or TV) is the amount of air that moves in and out of the lungs with each normal breath. When VT drops below 4 mL/kg, a state of alveolar hypoventilation develops, and the patient rebreathes dead-space air in the conducting airways rather than exchanging gases with the atmosphere. Acute respiratory failure results when hypoventilation becomes severe and results in hypercapnia and acidosis.

Vital capacity (VC) is the maximum amount of air expired after a maximal inspiration. Normal vital capacity differs with a person's gender, height, weight, and age. It decreases with age and in the presence of acute or chronic restrictive pulmonary diseases.

Minute ventilation ($\dot{V}_E$ or $M_{\dot{V}}$) is the total volume of air expired in 1 minute during exhalation. It is a rapid method of measuring total lung ventilation changes, but it is not considered an accurate measure of alveolar ventilation. Minute ventilation is not a direct measurement but a simple calculation,

$$\dot{V}_E = VT \times f$$

where f = frequency of breaths per minute. Normal minute ventilation is 5 to 10 L/min. When it increases to greater than 10 L/min, the work of breathing is significantly increased. Minute ventilation less than 5 L/min indicates that the patient is at risk for problems associated with hypoventilation.

Forced Expiratory Volumes

Forced expiratory volumes (FEVs) are an important diagnostic measurement that helps differentiate restrictive pulmonary problems from obstructive problems and measures airway resistance. They are also important in determining the severity of obstructive diseases. FEVs measure how rapidly a person can forcefully exhale air after a maximal inhalation, measuring volume (in liters) over time (in seconds). Patients who have a restrictive airway problem are able to push air forcefully out of their lungs at a normal rate, whereas persons who have an obstructive disorder have a delayed emptying rate (a reduced rate of expiratory air flow). Generally, FEV testing is not conducted routinely as a bedside trending parameter.

Section Seven Review

1. In the acutely ill client, pulmonary function testing helps monitor for which condition?
   A. Impending ventilatory failure
   B. Acute hypoxemia
   C. Acute metabolic acidosis
   D. Impending oxygenation failure

2. Minute ventilation $\dot{V}_E$ is calculated using which formula?
   A. $\dot{V}_E = \dot{V}C \times f$
   B. $\dot{V}_E = VT/f$
   C. $\dot{V}_E = \dot{V}C \times VT$
   D. $\dot{V}_E = VT \times f$

3. Clients who have obstructive pulmonary disease have which pattern of FEVs?
   A. Increased FEVs
   B. Delayed FEVs
   C. Normal FEVs
   D. Variable FEVs

4. In the adult client, the nurse would become concerned that the client is hypoventilating if the tidal volume falls to below which value?
   A. 4 mL/kg
   B. 5 mL/kg
   C. 7 mL/kg
   D. 9 mL/kg

Answers: 1. A, 2. D, 3. B, 4. A

Section Eight: Noninvasive and Invasive Monitoring of Gas Exchange

High-acuity patients frequently require monitoring of their oxygenation or ventilation status. When possible, noninvasive technologies such as pulse oximetry and capnography are used. However, when hemodynamic monitoring is also needed, an invasive arterial line is inserted because it can continuously monitor blood pressure, measure arterial oxygen saturation, and provide ready access to arterial blood for ABG sampling.

Pulse Oximetry

Pulse oximetry is a noninvasive technique for monitoring arterial capillary hemoglobin saturation (SpO_2) and pulse rate. It uses infrared light absorption to determine oxyhemoglobin saturation (Kress & Hall, 2015; Shoemaker, Belzberg, & Wo, 1998; Taenzer, Pyke, McGrath, & Blike, 2010). It also detects pulsatile flow to differentiate between venous and arterial blood. A sensor is placed on the forehead, finger, nose, or ear, and an oximeter provides a constant assessment of arterial oxygen saturation (Figure 11–17). Fingers are most commonly used for sensor placement; however, the adequacy of peripheral circulation must be taken into consideration when choosing the best sensor location.

Pulse oximetry is best used as an adjunct to a variety of assessment modalities in providing continuous information for evaluation of oxygenation status. Ideally, the continuous arterial oxygen saturation readings reflect the patient's oxygenation status and alert the clinician to subtle or sudden changes. In some patients, use of oximetry may reduce the frequency of invasive ABG measurements if acid–base and ventilation are not problems.

Causes of Inaccurate Readings   Many factors can affect the accuracy of pulse oximetry in high-acuity patients. In general, these factors can be divided into problems of technical (mechanical) origin and those of physiologic origin. Technical problems include motion artifact, external light sources, and improper sensor placement. Motion artifact refers to patient movement that the sensor misinterprets as being a pulse. New technologies are being developed that are more tolerant of motion. Bright lights within the patient's immediate environment can compete with the pulse oximeter's light source. When this is a problem, the sensor should be covered up to protect it from the external lighting. Nail polish or artificial nails can also compete with the oximeter's light source, thus requiring removal. An improperly placed sensor may not be able to register arterial pulsations because of lack of sufficient arterial flow.

Physiologic factors that alter the accuracy of SpO_2 to predict blood oxygen content (and ultimately delivery of oxygen to the tissues) include hemoglobin level, acid–base imbalance, vasoconstriction (e.g., peripheral vascular disease, hypothermia, shock, hypovolemia, and vasopressors in high doses), and some cardiac dysrhythmias (Glass, 2016). The level of hemoglobin greatly affects the oxygen content of the blood. When a patient is severely anemic, the SpO_2 may remain high, indicating sufficient oxygen saturation of available hemoglobin. The actual oxygen content of the blood, however, may be inadequate to meet tissue oxygenation needs, thus increasing the risk of tissue hypoxia. Hemoglobin levels should be monitored and taken into consideration when analyzing SpO_2 measurements.

When an acid–base imbalance exists, acidosis may cause a lower saturation reading and alkalosis may cause a higher reading because of shifts in the oxyhemoglobin dissociation curve. Severe peripheral vasoconstriction creates a low-flow arterial state in which the pulsatile force is too weak to be accurately read by pulse oximetry. When severe vasoconstriction is present, the sensor may read more accurately if it is removed from distal sites (fingers, toes) and attached to a more central location, such as the bridge of the nose or the earlobe. The hypothermic patient generally requires warming to normothermic levels before pulse oximetry can be used. In addition, patients who have abnormal levels of carboxyhemoglobin (carbon dioxide and carbon monoxide) may have a high SpO_2 even though the oxyhemoglobin level is very low. This false reading occurs because pulse oximetry cannot differentiate carboxyhemoglobin from oxyhemoglobin.

Capnography

Capnometry provides the numeric measurement of carbon dioxide (CO_2). **Capnography**, also referred to as end tidal CO_2 monitoring, is the noninvasive monitoring on a graphic display of CO_2 concentration that is exhaled by the patient during breathing (Glass, 2016). Capnography results in a single-value capnometric measurement called the $EtCO_2$ (end tidal CO_2). Continuous bedside monitoring of CO_2 is accomplished using infrared light absorption or mass spectrometry. Infrared analyzers measure carbon dioxide based on its strong absorption band at a distinctive wavelength. A **capnogram** displays the capnography measurements as a continuous waveform that can be read, breath by breath, throughout the breathing cycle. CO_2 can

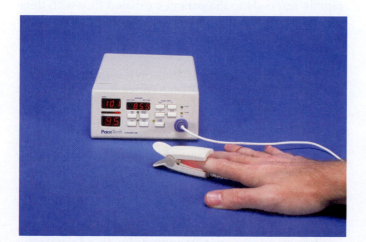

Figure 11–17 Pulse oximetry sensor.

SOURCE: Richard Logan/Pearson Education, Inc.

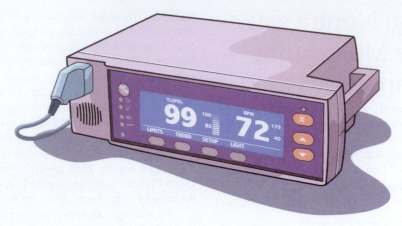

Figure 11–18 Example of a capnograph monitor. Measures and displays end tidal carbon dioxide, SpO_2, and respiratory and pulse rates.

be sampled using either sidestream or mainstream techniques. Figure 11–18 shows an example of a capnograph monitor.

Capnography Applications   Capnography is commonly used to monitor the adequacy of ventilation in surgical and procedural anesthesia, postoperative recovery, critical care units, and emergency departments (EDs). Current ACLS guidelines for CPR and emergency care call for the use of capnography to confirm endotracheal tube placement and monitor the adequacy of ventilation (Callaway et al., 2015). Other applications include the detection of inadvertent enteric feeding tube placement and assessment of the adequacy of ventilation.

End tidal carbon dioxide monitoring may be used to assess ventilatory status and provide an early warning of changes in ventilation. An abnormally low $EtCO_2$ (less than 30 mmHg) is most commonly associated with hyperventilation, hypothermia, pulmonary embolism, or decreased cardiac output (Glass, 2016). Increased $EtCO_2$ (greater than 44 mmHg) is associated with increased production of carbon dioxide (e.g., fever or increased cardiac output) or hypoventilation (e.g., respiratory center depression or neuromuscular diseases).

The usefulness of bedside capnography is not without limitations. In patients with morbid obesity, severe pulmonary edema, or ventilation–perfusion abnormalities, the $EtCO_2$ may not accurately reflect $PaCO_2$ (Vissers & Danzl, 2016). However, it may still be helpful if a correlation between $PaCO_2$ and $EtCO_2$ can be established and used for trending. Unfortunately, many high-acuity patients develop ventilation–perfusion abnormalities, which may limit the usefulness of $EtCO_2$ monitoring.

Types of Capnography CO_2 is sampled for capnography in three ways. Infrared analyzers are applied either sidestream or mainstream, and colorimetric capnography uses pH-sensitive paper to estimate $EtCO_2$ ranges.

Sidestream.   When a sidestream analyzer is used, a small volume of exhaled gas is diverted from the main airway circuit through a small tube and is analyzed in a special chamber apart from the airway circuit. The major disadvantage to using sidestream gas samples is that the values are indirect estimated measurements. The major advantage is that it can be used with patients who are not intubated.

Mainstream.   Mainstream infrared analyzers are placed in-line as part of the airway circuit and continuously measure the $EtCO_2$ directly, in real time (Glass, 2016). The major disadvantage to the mainstream technique is that it requires the patient to be intubated.

Colorimetric Capnography.   Colorimetric capnography uses pH-sensitive paper that changes color based on the patient's exhaled pH to represent a range of $EtCO_2$. It is most commonly used in emergency departments to assess for proper endotracheal (ET) tube placement (Vissers & Danzl, 2016); however, it is also used in the field by emergency squads and in ICU settings. A CO_2 detector device is attached to the ET tube following tube insertion, the patient is given six breaths, and the device is read at full-end expiration (Nellcor, 2011) (Figure 11–19). The device rapidly responds to the patient's exhaled CO_2 with three color ranges. For example, with a Nellcor EASYCAP II, the detector device has a color range of purple to yellow with interpretation as follows:

- Color range A (purple): 0.03% to less than 0.5% $EtCO_2$ (less than 4 mmHg CO_2); interpretation: ET tube is not in the trachea.

- Color range B (brown): 0.5% to less than 2% $EtCO_2$ (4 to less than 15 mmHg CO_2); interpretation: ET tube may be in the esophagus, or patient may have hypocarbia or low pulmonary blood flow.

- Color range C (yellow): 2% to 5% $EtCO_2$ (15 to 38 mmHg CO_2); interpretation: ET tube is properly located in the trachea (Nellcor, 2011).

While colorimetric capnography is adequate for assessing proper ET tube placement, it does not provide precise $EtCO_2$ data and therefore has limited applications (Vissers & Danzl, 2016).

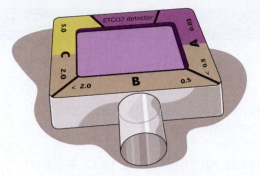

Figure 11–19 Disposable EtCO$_2$ detector device.

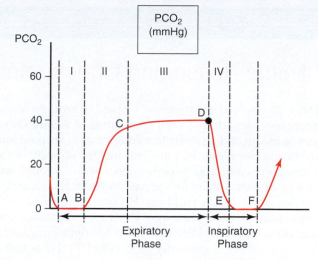

Figure 11–20 Normal capnogram pattern divided into phases. Phase I, initial exhalation phase representing anatomical dead space; Phase II, rapid increase in CO$_2$ representing mixture of dead space and alveolar CO$_2$; Phase III, alveolar plateau representing alveolar CO$_2$; Phase IV, inspiratory phase.

The Capnogram   The capnogram is the waveform that is visible on the capnography screen. A normal capnogram shows an EtCO$_2$ within several mmHg of arterial PaCO$_2$ at the end of the plateau phase (the end tidal CO$_2$). In a normal capnogram, the carbon dioxide concentration is 0 at the beginning of expiration, gradually rising until it reaches a plateau (Figure 11–20). The end tidal carbon dioxide is the highest concentration at the end of exhalation. EtCO$_2$ monitoring is used in the clinical setting as a noninvasive indirect method of measuring PaCO$_2$. In a normal person, EtCO$_2$ is 30 to 43 mmHg, typically 4 to 6 mmHg below PaCO$_2$ (Marino, 2014).

Invasive Blood Gas Monitoring

The arterial catheter (commonly called an arterial line or art line) is an invasive means of monitoring a patient's hemodynamic status (e.g., blood pressure, mean arterial pressure, heart rate), as well as pulmonary gas exchange status. Arterial catheters are most commonly inserted into a radial artery but can also be inserted into a femoral or other artery. A major advantage of drawing blood, including arterial blood gases, from an indwelling arterial line is that frequent samples can be obtained without causing additional trauma and pain to the patient from repeated needlesticks.

Section Eight Review

1. What is pulse oximetry used to measure?
   A. Mixed venous saturation
   B. Transcutaneous oxygen saturation
   C. Venous oxygen capillary hemoglobin saturation
   D. Arterial oxygen capillary hemoglobin saturation

2. Which conditions impair the accuracy of pulse oximetry? (Select all that apply.)
   A. Pulmonary embolism
   B. Excessive movement
   C. Vasodilation
   D. Hypothermia
   E. Improper sensor placement

3. EtCO$_2$ is an indicator of which alveolar factor?
   A. Acid–base state
   B. Compensation
   C. Oxygenation
   D. Ventilation

4. Colorimetric capnography uses what measure to estimate EtCO$_2$?
   A. pH
   B. PaCO$_2$
   C. Inhaled CO$_2$
   D. HCO$_3$

Answers: 1. D, 2. (B, D, E), 3. D, 4. A

Clinical Reasoning Checkpoint

RM, a 45-year-old construction worker, is brought to the emergency department with complaints of severe shortness of breath and a productive cough that is keeping him up during the night. His medical history is positive for chronic bronchitis and hypertension. He has smoked one pack of cigarettes a day for the past 35 years. He is married and has three adult children. He was diagnosed with emphysema several years ago. During auscultation, you hear rhonchi, particularly evident in his right lung fields. His temperature is currently 38°C (100.4°F). He is tentatively diagnosed with bacterial pneumonia.

1. RM's emphysema disease state alters the surface area of his lungs in which way?

2. RM has developed consolidations in his alveoli from pneumonia. (a) Describe the type of pulmonary shunt this creates; and (b) explain how this will affect his receiving oxygen therapy.

Clinical Update: RM has an arterial blood gas drawn on room air. The results are pH 7.28, $PaCO_2$ 53, PaO_2 56 mmHg, HCO_3 36 mEq/L, and SaO_2 92. He has just had a portable chest x-ray done. The results show cor pulmonale.

3. Interpret his ABG, including degree of compensation.

4. What is his P/F ratio at this time, and what is its significance?

5. RM asks you to explain what cor pulmonale is. What will you tell him?

Supplemental ABG Exercises

For the following, interpret the acid–base status as normal, metabolic or respiratory, alkalosis or acidosis. Indicate the state of compensation as uncompensated (acute state), partially compensated, or compensated (chronic state). Indicate the oxygenation status as adequate or inadequate, when indicated.

1. pH 7.58, $PaCO_2$ 38 mmHg, HCO_3 30 mEq/L
   Interpretation:
   Compensation:

2. pH 7.20, $PaCO_2$ 60 mmHg, HCO_3 26 mEq/L
   Interpretation:
   Compensation:

3. pH 7.39, $PaCO_2$ 43 mmHg, HCO_3 24 mEq/L
   Interpretation:
   Compensation:

4. pH 7.32, $PaCO_2$ 60 mmHg, HCO_3 30 mEq/L
   Interpretation:
   Compensation:

5. pH 7.5, $PaCO_2$ 50 mmHg, HCO_3 38 mEq/L
   Interpretation:
   Compensation:

6. pH 7.45, $PaCO_2$ 30 mmHg, HCO_3 20 mEq/L
   Interpretation:
   Compensation:

7. pH 7.40, $PaCO_2$ 40 mmHg, HCO_3 24 mEq/L
   Interpretation:
   Compensation:

8. pH 7.37, $PaCO_2$ 48 mmHg, HCO_3 29 mEq/L, PaO_2 80 mmHg, SaO_2 95%
   Acid–base state:
   Oxygenation status:

9. pH 7.48, $PaCO_2$ 30 mmHg, HCO_3 24 mEq/L, PaO_2 90 mmHg, SaO_2 98%
   Acid–base state:
   Oxygenation status:

10. pH 7.48, $PaCO_2$ 33 mmHg, HCO_3 25 mEq/L, PaO_2 68 mmHg, SaO_2 98%
    Acid–base state:
    Oxygenation status:

11. pH 7.38, $PaCO_2$ 38 mmHg, HCO_3 24 mEq/L, PaO_2 269 mmHg, SaO_2 100%
    Acid–base state:
    Oxygenation status:

12. pH 7.17, $PaCO_2$ 18 mmHg, HCO_3 7 mEq/L, PaO_2 100 mmHg, SaO_2 99%
    Acid–base state:
    Oxygenation status:

Chapter 11 Review

1. A client has developed a pulmonary problem that has resulted in decreased lung compliance. How will this affect the client's respiratory system?
   1. It will increase the client's tidal volume.
   2. It will increase the client's work of breathing.
   3. It will decrease the client's overall oxygen consumption.
   4. It will decrease the client's carbon dioxide level.

2. A client who has developed right middle-lobe pneumonia will experience decreased ventilation in the affected lung areas for which reasons? (Select all that apply.)
   1. The pressure gradient is abnormal.
   2. Gas moves from an area of low pressure to an area of high pressure.
   3. Decreased perfusion causes decreased ventilation.
   4. Gas follows the path of least resistance.
   5. The consolidation in the tissues will increase the pressure.

3. A client with pneumonia develops what is believed to be an absolute pulmonary shunt. Oxygen therapy has been initiated per venti-mask. The nurse would expect which effect on the client's hypoxemia?
   1. It will be unchanged.
   2. It will worsen.
   3. It will be relieved.
   4. It will initially improve, then worsen again.

4. A client is diagnosed with DKA after being admitted to the hospital with a serum glucose of 650 mg/dL and positive serum ketones. Blood gases are: pH 7.25, $PaCO_2$ 36 mmHg, HCO_3 14 mEq/L. This pH is most likely a result of which acid–base disturbance?
   1. Metabolic acidosis
   2. Respiratory acidosis
   3. Respiratory alkalosis
   4. Metabolic alkalosis

5. A client has the following ABG results: pH 7.50, $PaCO_2$ 30 mmHg, HCO_3 20 mEq/L, PaO_2 88 mmHg, SaO_2 98%. How would the nurse interpret these results?
   1. Compensated metabolic acidosis
   2. Partially compensated metabolic acidosis
   3. Partially compensated respiratory alkalosis
   4. Compensated respiratory acidosis

6. A client is admitted to the hospital with complaints of severe chest pain and dyspnea. The client has an oral temperature of 38.3°C (101°F). Why is it important for the nurse to obtain a nutritional history from this client? (Select all that apply.)
   1. Hypoglycemia weakens respiratory muscles.
   2. High-carbohydrate diets increase carbon dioxide levels.

3. High-carbohydrate intake weakens respiratory muscles.
4. Poor nutritional status increases susceptibility to infection.
5. Vitamin C intake above the recommended daily amount causes oxidative changes in lung tissue.

7. Pulmonary function tests are performed on a client diagnosed with right middle-lobe pneumonia. The client's tidal volume and vital capacity are both below normal. The nurse would plan care based on which interpretation of these results?
   1. The client has respiratory muscle fatigue.
   2. The client has increasing atelectasis.
   3. The client has loss of pulmonary surfactant.
   4. The client is hyperventilating.

8. A client has been in the ICU and intubated for 1 week. $EtCO_2$ is attached to the client's mechanical ventilator circuit to assess for which development?
   1. Early tissue metabolic changes
   2. Oxygenation failure
   3. Early changes in ventilation
   4. Ventilatory dependency

9. A client comes to the emergency department complaining of shortness of breath and chest pain. The ABG results are: pH 7.45, $PaCO_2$ 35 mmHg, PaO_2 60 mmHg, HCO_3 24 mEq/L. What should be the nurse's first intervention?
   1. Set up for intubation.
   2. No intervention is necessary.
   3. Place the client on oxygen.
   4. Administer sodium bicarbonate.

10. A client is admitted to the emergency department with complaints of shortness of breath, cough, and fever. Which clinical manifestations would the nurse interpret as indicating early respiratory distress? (Select all that apply.)
    1. Increased respiratory rate
    2. Tachycardia
    3. Agitation
    4. Cyanosis
    5. Confusion

Answers to questions found inside your textbook are available on the faculty resources site. Please consult with your instructor.

References

Barrett, K. E., Barman, S. M., Boitano, S., & Brooks, H. L. (2016). Chapter 35: Gas transport and pH. In K. E. Barrett, S. M. Barman, S. Boitano, & H. L. Brooks (Eds.), *Ganong's review of medical physiology* (25th ed.). Retrieved December 26, 2016, from http://

accessmedicine.mhmedical.com/content.aspx?bookid=1587&sectionid=97166353&jumpsectionID=97166374

Cairo, J. M. (2016). *Pilbeam's mechanical ventilation: Physiological and clinical applications* (6th ed.). St. Louis, MO: Elsevier.

Calhoun, C., Shivshankar, P., Saker, M., Sloane, L., Livi, C., Sharp, Z., . . . LeSaux, C. (2015). Senescent cells contribute to the physiological remodeling of aged lungs. *The Journals of Gerontology, Series A, Biological Sciences and Medical Sciences, 71*(2),153–160. doi:10.1093/Gerona/glu241

Callaway, C. W., Soar, J., Aibiki, M., Böttiger, B. W., Brooks, S. C., Deakin, C. D., . . . Zimmerman, J. (2015). 2015 international consensus on cardiopulmonary resuscitation and emergency cardiovascular care science with treatment recommendations. *Circulation, 132* (Suppl. 1), S84–S145.

Cefalu, C. A. (2011). Theories and mechanisms of aging. *Clinics in Geriatric Medicine, 27*(4), 491–506.

Criner, G. J., Bourbeau, J., Diekemper, R. L., Ouellette, D. R., Goodridge, D., Hernandez, P., . . . Stickland, M. K. (2015). Prevention of acute exacerbations of COPD: American College of Chest Physicians and Canadian Thoracic Society Guideline. *Chest, 147*(4), 894–942.

Cydulka, R. K., & Bates, C. G. (2016). Chapter 70: Chronic obstructive pulmonary disease. In J. E. Tintinalli, J. Stapczynski, O. Ma, D. M. Yealy, G. D. Meckler, & D. M. Cline (Eds.), *Tintinalli's emergency medicine: A comprehensive study guide* (8th ed.). Retrieved December 26, 2016, from http://accessmedicine.mhmedical.com/Content.aspx?bookId=1658&sectionId=109429760

Glass, C. (2016). Chapter 16: Blood gases. In J. E. Tintinalli, J. Stapczynski, O. Ma, D. M. Yealy, G. D. Meckler, & D. M. Cline (Eds.), *Tintinalli's emergency medicine: A comprehensive study guide* (8th ed.). Retrieved December 26, 2016, from http://accessmedicine.mhmedical.com/content.aspx?sectionid=109385181&bookid=1658&Resultclick=2

Kee, J. L. (2014). *Laboratory and diagnostic tests with nursing implications* (9th ed.). Upper Saddle River, NJ: Pearson.

Kitamura, B. C., Katz, E. D., & Ruoff, B. E. (2014). Commonly used formulas and calculations. In J. R. Roberts & J. R. Hedges (Eds.), *Clinical procedures in emergency medicine* (pp. 1477–1488). Philadelphia, PA: Elsevier Saunders.

Kress, J. P., & Hall, J. B. (2015). 321: Approach to the patient with critical illness. In D. Kasper, A. Fauci, S. Hauser, D. Longo, J. Jameson, & J. Loscalzo (Eds.), *Harrison's principles of internal medicine* (19th ed.). Retrieved December 26, 2016, from http://accessmedicine.mhmedical.com/Content.aspx?bookId=1130&sectionId=79745589

Levitzky, M. G. (2013). Chapter 4: Blood flow to the lung. In M. G. Levitzky (Ed.), *Pulmonary physiology* (8th ed., pp. 97–103). New York, NY: McGraw Hill. Retrieved December 26, 2016, from http://accessmedicine.mhmedical.com/content.aspx?bookid=575&sectionid=42512982

Marino, P. L. (2014). *The ICU book* (4th ed.). Philadelphia, PA: Wolters Kluwer Health/Lippincott Williams & Wilkins.

Nellcor. (2011). *Adult colorimetric CO_2 detector.* Retrieved December 26, 2016, from http://www.covidien.com/imageServer.aspx/doc253945.pdf?contentID=34084&contenttype=application/pdf

Pagana, K. D. (2015). *Mosby's diagnostic and laboratory test reference* (12th ed.). St. Louis, MO: Elsevier Mosby.

Sethi, J., & McCool, F. D. (2016). Evaluating lung structure and function. In I. J. Benjamin, R. C. Griggs, E. J. Wing, & J. G. Fitz (Eds.), *Andreoli and Carpenter's Cecil essentials of medicine* (9th ed., pp. 190–206). Philadelphia, PA: Elsevier Saunders.

Shoemaker, W. C., Belzberg, H., & Wo, C. C. J. (1998). Multicenter study of noninvasive monitoring systems as alternatives to invasive monitoring of acutely ill emergency patients. *Chest, 114*(6), 1643–1652. PubMed: 9872201

Taenzer, A. H., Pyke, J. B., McGrath, S. P., & Blike, G. T. (2010). Impact of pulse oximetry surveillance on rescue events and intensive care unit transfers: A before-and-after concurrence study. *Anesthesiology, 112*(2), 282–287. PubMed: 20098128

Vaz Fragoso, C. A., & Gill, T. M. (2012). Respiratory impairment and the aging lung: A novel paradigm for assessing pulmonary function. *Journal of Gerontology: Series A, Biological Sciences and Medical Sciences, 67A*(3), 264–275. doi:10.1093/Gerona/glr198

Vissers, R. J., & Danzl, D. (2016). Chapter 29: Intubation and mechanical ventilation. In J. E. Tintinalli, J. Stapczynski, O. Ma, D. M. Yealy, G. D. Meckler, & D. M. Cline (Eds.), *Tintinalli's emergency medicine: A comprehensive study guide* (8th ed.). Retrieved December 26, 2016, from http://accessmedicine.mhmedical.com/content.aspx?sectionid=109427490&bookid=1658&Resultclick=2

Chapter 12
Alterations in Pulmonary Function

Learning Outcomes

12.1 Explain the basic differences between restrictive and obstructive pulmonary diseases.

12.2 Discuss the pathophysiologic basis of respiratory failure.

12.3 Describe acute respiratory distress syndrome (ARDS).

12.4 Explain the types, pathophysiology, and management of acute pulmonary embolism.

12.5 Discuss the types, pathophysiology, and management of acute bacterial and viral pneumonias.

12.6 Describe the principles and management of patients undergoing thoracic surgery and chest drainage.

12.7 Implement a general plan of care for a patient with an acute alteration in respiratory function.

High-acuity patients may be admitted in acute pulmonary distress, or severe pulmonary disorders may develop after admission. It is critical that nurses working in high-acuity environments be able to rapidly recognize acute pulmonary diseases and complications and their treatments. It is suggested that Chapter 11: Determinants and Assessment of Pulmonary Function be read prior to this chapter for important foundational information that will enhance the reader's understanding of the material in this chapter.

Section One: Review of Restrictive and Obstructive Pulmonary Disorders

Pulmonary diseases may be divided into acute and chronic problems. Acute problems have a rapid onset, are episodic, and frequently are confined to the lungs. In contrast, chronic problems usually have a slow, often insidious onset, and the pulmonary impairment either does not change or slowly worsens over an extended period. Chronic pulmonary problems generally involve other organs as part of the disease process. Patients with chronic pulmonary problems, such as emphysema, may develop an acute problem (e.g., pneumonia) that may further stress their pulmonary status.

Pulmonary diseases may be divided further into problems of inflow of air (restrictive) and outflow of air (obstructive). By being able to differentiate between obstructive and restrictive pulmonary diseases, the nurse can apply appropriate nursing diagnoses regardless of the medical diagnosis of the specific pulmonary disease process.

Restrictive Pulmonary Disorders

Restrictive disorders are associated with decreased lung compliance (CL), decreased lung expansion, and reduced lung volumes because of parenchymal disease or because of a disease of the pleura, chest wall, or neuromuscular system. Unlike obstructive lung diseases, including asthma and COPD, which show a normal or increased total lung

Table 12–1 Common Restrictive Pulmonary Disorders

External Problems	Internal (Parenchymal) Problems
Obesity	Pneumonia
Neuromuscular diseases:	Atelectasis
Myasthenia gravis	Heart failure
Muscular dystrophy	Pulmonary edema
Guillain-Barré syndrome	Pulmonary fibrosis
Spinal cord trauma	Pulmonary tumors
Chest wall disorders:	Pneumothorax
Extensive chest burns	Asbestosis
Scoliosis	
Flail chest	

BOX 12–1 Clinical Manifestations of Restrictive Pulmonary Disorders

- Increased respiratory rate
- Decreased tidal volume (VT)
- Normal to decreased PaO_2
- Shortness of breath
- Cough
- Chest pain or discomfort
- Fatigue
- History of weight loss

capacity (TLC), restrictive disease are associated with a decreased TLC. Restrictive lung diseases may be caused by internal problems, such as a decrease in the number of functioning alveoli (e.g., atelectasis or pneumonia), a loss of lung tissue (e.g., pneumonectomy or lung tumors), or by external problems (e.g., chest burns or morbid obesity). Table 12–1 provides a more complete listing of restrictive disorders.

Restrictive disorders are problems of volume (the amount of air, measured in mL or L, which flows in and out of the lungs) rather than air flow (the rate or speed at which air moves into or out of the lungs). In other words, the volume of air that is inhaled can be exhaled at a normal rate of flow. The patient with a restrictive disorder will have a reduced tidal volume (VT) and total lung capacity (TLC). Air cannot move into the alveoli as readily as it should because of limited expansion (decreased lung compliance), which can lead to alveolar hypoventilation. Hypoxemia will result if alveolar oxygen diffuses into the blood at a faster rate than it is replaced by ventilation. When this occurs, the PaO_2 falls at approximately the same rate as the $PaCO_2$ rises, assuming that diffusion is normal. The causes of restrictive lung diseases are sometimes represented by the mnemonic PAINT, for pleural, alveolar, interstitial, neuromuscular, and thoracic cage abnormalities.

Restrictive pulmonary problems often disturb the relationship of ventilation to perfusion ($\dot{V}/\dot{Q}$ ratio). In mild to moderate restrictive disease, the $\dot{V}/\dot{Q}$ ratio may stay normal because both ventilation and perfusion may be fairly equally disturbed. In many acute restrictive diseases, perfusion becomes diminished because of edema that results from an inflammatory process. Perfusion can also become reduced by compression or blockage of the pulmonary vasculature. In severe disease, a low $\dot{V}/\dot{Q}$ ratio may develop because ventilation is greatly diminished, whereas perfusion may be fairly normal or moderately disturbed. A low $\dot{V}/\dot{Q}$ ratio is associated with hypoxemia with a decreasing pH and increasing $PaCO_2$. Box 12–1 lists the typical signs and symptoms associated with restrictive pulmonary disorders.

Obstructive Pulmonary Disorders

Chronic obstructive pulmonary disease (COPD) is the term commonly applied in the clinical setting to pulmonary disorders that hinder expiratory air flow. The more accurate and preferred term for these disorders, however, is *chronic air flow limitation*. Currently, these two terms are often used interchangeably. Some of the major obstructive disorders include the following:

- Emphysema
- Chronic bronchitis
- Asthma
- Cystic fibrosis

In obstructive pulmonary disorders, air can flow into the lungs but then becomes trapped. The inability to exhale rapidly causes a prolongation of expiratory time. If expiratory time becomes significantly prolonged, the alveoli are unable to empty before the person inhales again, trapping CO_2 within them. Expiratory times are measured using **forced expiratory volume (FEV)** testing, which is a measure of dynamic lung function. FEV testing determines how rapidly a person can forcefully exhale air after a maximal inhalation.

Obstructive problems may be caused by airway narrowing, such as bronchospasm, bronchoconstriction, and edema by airway obstruction, as seen with increased secretions and mucus plugging. Obstructive disorders are associated with increased lung compliance (hyperinflated lungs) accompanied by a loss of elastic recoil. The $\dot{V}/\dot{Q}$ ratio may be disturbed with this group of disorders. In disease processes that do not destroy alveoli, such as chronic bronchitis, the $\dot{V}/\dot{Q}$ ratio may be low (i.e., ventilation is reduced, whereas perfusion remains normal). If lung tissue is actually destroyed, such as occurs with emphysema, the $\dot{V}/\dot{Q}$ ratio may remain normal because both ventilation and perfusion are equally impaired. A normal $\dot{V}/\dot{Q}$ ratio does not necessarily indicate healthy lungs. It indicates only that a balance exists between ventilation and blood flow. Box 12–2 lists the typical clinical manifestations associated with obstructive pulmonary disorders.

Restrictive and obstructive diseases differ in their effect on lung volume, air flow, pathophysiology, blood gas disturbances, and physical assessment. Table 12–2 compares these two disease processes.

BOX 12–2 Clinical Manifestations of Obstructive Pulmonary Disorders

- Mucus hypersecretion (except with pure emphysema)
- Wheezes, rhonchi
- Dyspnea (episodic or progressive)
- Diminished breath and heart sounds
- Barrel chest (increased anteroposterior [AP] diameter)
- Progressive hypercapnia and respiratory acidosis
- Progressive or episodic hypoxemia (particularly in later stages)
- Cor pulmonale
- Accessory muscle use
- Increased expiratory time (expiration time longer than inspiration time)
- Pulmonary function tests (PFTs): Normal to increased TLC, increased functional residual capacity (FRC), decreased forced expiratory volume (FEV), decreased vital capacity (VC)

Table 12–2 Comparison of Pulmonary System Alterations in Restrictive and Obstructive Pulmonary Diseases

Restrictive Disorders	Obstructive Disorders
Characteristics	
Decreased lung expansion	Increased lung expansion
Decreased lung compliance	Increased lung compliance
Normal air flow	Decreased expiratory air flow; prolonged expiratory time
Pulmonary Function Testing	
Decreased total lung capacity (TLC)	Decreased forced expiratory
Decreased tidal volume (VT)	volumes (FEVs)
Pathologic Disturbances	
Internal Problems	
Decreased functioning alveoli	Bronchoconstriction
Loss of pulmonary tissue	Bronchospasm
Loss of respiratory muscle strength	Airway edema
	Airway obstruction
	Airway collapse
	Pooling of copious secretions
External Problems	
Disorders that decrease lung compliance external to the lungs	
Associated Blood Gas Disturbances	
Decreased PaO$_2$	
Normal to low V̇/Q̇ ratio	Increased PaCO$_2$
Increased intrapulmonary shunt	Decreased pH (if not
Increased PaCO$_2$ and decreased pH if	compensated)
ventilatory pump failure is present	Normal to decreased PaO$_2$
	(may stay stable until severe disease state)
Associated Lung Sounds	
Rhonchi, if secretions build up in large airways	Wheezes (most common)
	Rhonchi, if secretions build up in large airways
	Diminished breath sounds (severe bronchospasm)

Status Asthmaticus Asthma differs from the other obstructive pulmonary diseases in that the air flow obstruction is episodic rather than continuous. For many years, asthma was considered a reversible disease in that lung function and gas exchange were thought to return to normal with treatment. Today, however, experts know that the process is not always completely reversible with some patients (particularly those with frequent exacerbations) eventually developing permanent remodeling of the airways (Nakawah, Hawkins, & Barbandi, 2013). Physiologic changes that characterize acute asthma exacerbations include inflammation, which causes airway edema with narrowing of airway passages, and hyperresponsiveness of airways to irritants, which results in bronchospasm and mucus plugging.

The classic triad of asthma symptoms includes paroxysmal episodes of dyspnea, wheeze, and cough triggered by a stimulus. Some of the more common triggering stimuli include allergens, exercise, stress, and infections. Commonly, asthma is managed with combinations of inhaled corticosteroids and bronchodilators.

Status asthmaticus, also referred to as acute severe asthma, is a severe exacerbation of asthma signs and symptoms that does not respond to the usual drug therapy. If it persists, status asthmaticus can become a life-threatening emergency from airway obstruction. Death from status asthmaticus is rare but is usually due to hypoxia, cardiopulmonary arrest, or complications that arise from mechanical ventilation such as worsening of air trapping (Leatherman, 2015). The ability to rapidly recognize a life-threatening episode of status asthmaticus is crucial for healthcare professionals who work in emergency settings (Schivo, Phan, Louie, & Harper, 2013). A particularly ominous clinical finding is a sudden decrease in wheezing or loss of breath sounds, which may indicate complete airway obstruction from mucus plugs and impending cardiopulmonary arrest. Box 12–3 lists some of the major features of life-threatening status asthmaticus.

Recommendations for treatment of status asthmaticus include oxygen, intravenous corticosteroids, possibly inhalation of heliox (a combination of helium and oxygen) to improve air flow, and repeated doses of a short-acting sympathomimetic inhalation agent such as albuterol (Leatherman, 2015). Corticosteroids are the mainstay of treatment of this inflammatory disease and must be given early, as they take several hours to become

BOX 12–3 Major Features of Life-threatening Status Asthmaticus

- Pulsus paradoxus of 25 mmHg or greater
- Use of accessory muscles
- Significant lung hyperinflation
- Arterial blood gas (ABG) showing hypoxemia with or without hypercapnia
- Reduced peak expiratory flow rate or FEV$_1$ (30% or less of predicted value)
- Sudden onset of decreased wheezing or reduced (or no) breath sounds
- Coma or confusion
- Inability to speak or only one-word phrases
- Fatigue

Related Pharmacotherapy
Agents Used for Treatment of Pulmonary Diseases

Beta Agonists

Short-acting: albuterol (Proventil, Ventolin, ProAir), pirbuterol (Maxair), levalbuterol (Xopenex), racemic epinephrine (Vaponefrin)
Long-acting: salmeterol (Serevent), formoterol (Foradil)

Action and Uses

Stimulate beta 2 adrenergic (epinephrine) receptors in the lung
Relax bronchial smooth muscle and cause bronchodilation
Used for obstructive diseases (asthma, exercise-induced asthma, COPD)
Short-acting drugs used as rescue medications for asthma
May be used hourly or as continuous nebulizer for acute exacerbations
Long-acting drugs used routinely for control and nighttime symptoms

Dosages (Adult)

Albuterol: 2–4 mg (PO) 3 to 4 x/day or sustained release 4–8 mg 2 x/day. Inhalation: 1–2 inhalations every 4–6 hrs
Salmeterol: 1 powder diskus (50 mcg) inhaled 2 x/day (12 hrs apart)

Major Adverse Effects

Tachycardia, hypertension, tremors
Potential paradoxical response of increased bronchospasm
Hypokalemia (primarily in higher doses)

Nursing Implications

Document heart rate and blood pressure, therapeutic response (improved air flow, wheezing), side effects
Patient education: correct use of inhalers, spacers, nebulizers
Patient education: long-acting inhalers not to be used as rescue medications, risk of toxicity
Drugs available as metered-dosed inhaler, dry powder inhaler, and small volume nebulizer

Anticholinergic Bronchodilators

Short-acting: ipratropium bromide (Atrovent)
Long-acting: tiotropium (Spiriva)
Combination ipratropium bromide and albuterol (Combivent)

Action and Uses

Bronchodilation; blockade of cholinergic-induced bronchoconstriction
Maintenance therapy primarily for COPD

Dosages (Adult)

COPD: two inhalations of meter-dose inhalers (MDI) 4 x/day (at no less than 4 hr intervals). Nebulizer: 500 mcg every 6–8 hrs

Major Adverse Effects

Poor absorption via inhalation limits systemic side effects (anxiety, dizziness, headache, nervousness)
Cough, dry mouth (more common)

Nursing Implications

Avoid eye exposure during nebulizer treatments (pupil dilation)
Caution: older MDI contained soy base (soy and peanut allergy)

Assess history for soy or peanut allergy: ensure formulation does not contain soy
Caution in patients with narrow-angle glaucoma, prostatic hypertrophy
Document heart rate and blood pressure, therapeutic response, side effects
Patient education: correct use of inhalers, nebulizers
Drugs available as MDI, dry powder inhaler, and small volume nebulizer

Corticosteroids

IV: methylprednisolone (Solu-Medrol), hydrocortisone (Solu-Cortef)
Oral: prednisone
Inhaled: beclomethasone dipropionate (QVAR)
    flunisolide (AeroBid)
    fluticasone (Flovent)
    budesonide (Pulmicort)
    combinations of steroid and beta agonists (Advair)

Action and Uses

Anti-inflammatory agents, reduce airway edema (reduces airway obstruction) associated with asthma, COPD
Used as a controller for asthma and COPD to reduce airway inflammation
Additional higher doses given IV for acute exacerbations

Dosages (Adult)

Status asthmaticus: 2 mg/kg (IV) initially, then 1–5 mg/kg every hour

Major Adverse Effects

Fewer side effects with inhaled steroids
Systemic (IV and oral formulations): insomnia, mood changes (euphoria or delirium possible), hypertension, hyperglycemia, hypokalemia, fluid retention, adrenal suppression, poor wound healing, GI bleeding, immune suppression or infection especially fungal, acute adrenal insufficiency with sudden withdrawal after long-term use
Local: oral or pharyngeal fungal infections, cough, hoarse voice, bronchospasm

Nursing Implications

High-acuity formulation is primarily intravenous; oral and inhaled used for stable patients
Onset of effect is hours; used as a controller for asthma and COPD, not rapid response for bronchospasm
Use with spacer or reservoir device for inhaled steroids to prevent oral thrush; brush teeth, rinse mouth after dosing
Patient education: oral hygiene, use of spacer, inhaler technique to reduce oral infections and hoarseness
Drugs available primarily as MDI and dry powder inhaler
Avoid stopping systemic corticosteroids abruptly and monitor for acute adrenal insufficiency (e.g., hypotension, shock)

Methylxanthines

Theophylline (Theo-Dur), aminophylline

Action and Uses

Bronchodilation by blocking phosphodiesterase
Potential anti-inflammatory effects
Stimulates ventilation
Used as a third-line bronchodilator for chronic obstructive disease, occasionally used in acute care settings

Dosages (Adult)

Theophylline: Loading dose of 5 mg/kg (PO or IV). Maintenance dose of 0.4 mg/kg/hr (nonsmoker); 0.6 mg/kg/hr (smoker); 0.2 mg/kg/hr with heart failure (HF) or cirrhosis.
Aminophylline: Loading dose of 6 mg/kg (IV) over 30 min. Maintenance dose of 0.6 mg/kg/h (nonsmoker); 0.8 mg/kg/h (smoker); 0.1–0.2 mg/kg/hr (HF or cirrhosis).

Major Adverse Effects

Multiple: tachycardia, dysrhythmias, anxiety, insomnia, seizures, tremors, nausea, vomiting, anorexia
Severe adverse effects have limited use in recent years

Nursing Implications

Monitor serum theophylline levels (goal = 5–15 mcg/mL), toxicity common if level greater than 20 mcg/mL
Monitor I & O (diuretic effect), heart rate, blood pressure, cardiac rhythm
Assess for therapeutic effect, side effects
Administer IV loading dose by infusion, slowly over 20–30 minutes. Maximum 20–25 mg/minute or continuous infusion.

Mucolytics

Acetylcysteine (Mucomyst)
Dornase alfa (Pulmozyme), also called DNase

Action and Uses

Decrease viscosity of respiratory secretions
Acetylcysteine: used acutely to improve airway clearance in diseases with thick mucus production (bronchitis, bronchiectasis) and during bronchoscopy to clear mucous plugs
Dornase: synthetic pancreatic enzyme, breaks down DNA material from neutrophils (DNase)
Used chronically in some diseases (cystic fibrosis)

Dosages (Adult)

1–10 mL of 20% solution (inhalation) every 4–6 hrs; 2–20 mL of 10% solution every 4–6 hrs. Direct instillation: 1–2 mL of 10%–20% solution every 1–4 hrs.

SOURCE: Dosages are from Wilson et al. (2017).

Major Adverse Effects

Acetylcysteine: bronchospasm (do not use for asthma), bad odor and taste, nausea
Dornase alfa: pharyngitis, chest pain

Nursing Implications

Assess for effectiveness on cough, clearance of secretions, possible bronchospasm, and side effects
Administer bronchodilator prior to acetylcysteine

Pulmonary Vasodilators

Inhaled: nitric oxide (iNO) off-label use in acute respiratory distress syndrome (ARDS) for adults, iloprost (pulmonary hypertension)
Intravenous: epoprostenol (Flolan), treprostinil (Remodulin)
Subcutaneous: treprostinil (Remodulin)
Oral: bosentan, sildenafil

Action and Uses

Specialized treatment (rescue therapy for life-threatening hypoxemia) and pulmonary hypertension
Selectively vasodilate pulmonary vasculature
Reduce pulmonary hypertension
Improve oxygenation: V̇/Q̇ matching improves due to improved perfusion to ventilated alveoli

Dosages (Adult)

Epoprostenol: For primary pulmonary hypertension, initial dose 2 ng/kg/min (IV), increase by 2 ng/kg/min every 15 min until dose-limiting effects develop.
Sildenafil: For pulmonary arterial hypertension, 20 mg (PO) 3 x/day (4–6 hrs apart); 10 mg (IV) 3 x/day.

Major Adverse Effects

Multiple, depending on agent
Nitric oxide: hypotension, methemoglobinemia
Treprostinil: hypotension, headache, flushing, jaw pain

Nursing Implications

Monitor heart rate, blood pressure, therapeutic effects and side effects
iNO: Observe for rebound pulmonary hypertension and hypoxemia as dose is tapered
Treprostinil (prostaglandin) therapy for pulmonary hypertension is specialized and complex: Refer to specialized literature

---

effective. Development of ventilatory failure (hypercapnia) is unusual but can result from fatigue due to the increased work of breathing. Fatigue and decreasing level of consciousness may signal the need for mechanical ventilation (Albertson, Sutter, & Chan, 2015; Chung et al., 2014). Mechanical ventilation in acute asthma presents particular risks during intubation and challenges in ventilator management due to the bronchospasm and air trapping. Ventilator management goals are to achieve adequate gas exchange and avoid complications. Ventilator strategies include lower tidal volumes and slower respiratory rates to avoid high inspiratory pressures, minimize air trapping, and allow for extended expiratory time. Complications of mechanical ventilation in status asthmaticus include barotrauma and hypotension, both induced by pulmonary hyperinflation (Leatherman, 2015). A summary of some of the major drugs used to treat disorders such as asthma can be found in the "Related Pharmacotherapy: Agents Used for Treatment of Pulmonary Diseases" feature.

Section One Review

1. Restrictive pulmonary diseases are associated with which condition?
   A. Increased lung expansion
   B. Increased lung compliance
   C. Decreased lung expansion
   D. Decreased airflow into lungs

2. Which pulmonary disorder is considered a restrictive disease?
   A. Pneumonia
   B. Asthma
   C. Emphysema
   D. Chronic bronchitis

3. Obstructive pulmonary diseases are associated with which condition?
   A. Decreased lung expansion
   B. Decreased lung compliance
   C. Decreased airflow into lungs
   D. Decreased expiratory airflow

4. Beta agonist agents such as albuterol are given to relieve which acute airway problem?
   A. Airway edema
   B. Bronchoconstriction
   C. Airway inflammation
   D. Pulmonary hypertension

Answers: 1. C, 2. A, 3. D, 4. B

Section Two: Acute Respiratory Failure

In Chapter 11, perfusion was described in terms of two circuits: pulmonary and systemic. For the purposes of this chapter, it is helpful to reconsider these circuits in a slightly different manner—that is, to view the heart and lungs as a complex integrated cardiopulmonary system that shares volume and pressure with the rest of the systemic circulation—whatever affects one part of the system potentially affects the whole.

The cardiopulmonary system is very sensitive to pressure changes within it, requiring compensatory adjustments to maintain homeostasis. Primary problems of cardiac origin can create secondary pulmonary problems. For example, left-heart failure can cause cardiogenic pulmonary edema. The opposite is also true—pulmonary problems can affect cardiac status, as in cor pulmonale (right-heart failure of pulmonary origin). If a pulmonary disorder decreases the ability of the lungs to maintain adequate acid–base balance and oxygenation, the heart must work harder to make more blood available for diffusion, causing a compensatory increase in vital signs (increased blood pressure and pulse). The patient's lungs work harder by increasing the respiratory rate (tachypnea) and depth (hyperventilation).

Respiratory Insufficiency and Failure

Respiratory disorders vary greatly in the way they affect lung function. The amount of diffusion surface area that becomes impaired is a major factor in altering gas exchange. The extent of impairment coupled with the rate of disease onset contributes greatly to the ability of the body to cope adequately through compensatory mechanisms. The terms *chronic* (compensated) *respiratory insufficiency* and *acute respiratory failure* are used to differentiate the level of compensation.

Chronic Respiratory Insufficiency   **Respiratory insufficiency** is a state in which an acceptable level of gas exchange is maintained only through cardiopulmonary compensatory mechanisms. Chronic pulmonary problems have a slow onset and often are progressive in nature. The body has time to compensate for growing pulmonary gas exchange deficits, thereby maintaining an adequate level of oxygenation and acid–base balance until late-stage disease. A person can lead a relatively normal life in a state of chronic respiratory insufficiency. Arterial blood gases typically noted include a normal pH, an elevated $PaCO_2$ accompanied by an elevated HCO_3 (compensated respiratory acidosis), and a normal to low PaO_2. Respiratory insufficiency, with its compensated arterial blood gas status, is not a normal state and should be considered impending respiratory failure, particularly in unstable patients.

High-acuity patients often walk a fine line between respiratory insufficiency and respiratory failure, and their ability to compensate is reduced. Decompensation results from any stressor (such as acute infection) that is severe enough to push patients beyond their ability to meet the added demands—that is, they develop a supply-and-demand imbalance, respiratory muscle fatigue, and impending respiratory failure. Without rapid recognition and timely interventions to relieve the underlying problem, the patient's condition often deteriorates rapidly into acute respiratory failure.

The nurse plays a crucial role in early recognition of impending respiratory failure. Clinical signs of impending failure include tachypnea, tachycardia, increased use of accessory respiratory muscles (e.g., trapezius, sternocleidomastoid, or abdominals), nasal flaring, abnormal chest wall movements, labored breathing, and a decreasing SpO_2. The patient may also be diaphoretic or orthopneic, complain of air hunger, and appear anxious. When clinical signs suggest increased respiratory muscle fatigue or impending respiratory failure, an ABG is usually ordered. Patient outcomes may be improved with early recognition of impending respiratory failure in conjunction with

Table 12–3 Acute Respiratory Failure and Its Components

Type of Failure	Clinical Definition	Clinical Manifestations
Acute respiratory failure	$PaCO_2$ greater than 50 mmHg with a pH less than 7.30 and/or PaO_2 less than 60 mmHg	See below
Oxygenation failure	PaO_2 less than 60 mmHg	Pulmonary: dyspnea, tachypnea, increased pulmonary vascular resistance Cardiovascular: increased blood pressure, heart rate, cardiac dysrhythmias, cyanosis; weak, thready pulse Central nervous system: altered level of responsiveness; restlessness, confusion
Ventilation failure	$PaCO_2$ greater than 50 mmHg with a pH less than 7.30 (acute respiratory acidosis)	Pulmonary: tachypnea Vascular: headache; flushed, wet skin Cardiovascular: bounding pulse, increased blood pressure and heart rate Central nervous system: anesthetic effects of carbon dioxide: lethargy, drowsiness, coma (CO_2 narcosis)

aggressive interventions to treat the underlying cause, decrease oxygen demands, and increase oxygen supply.

Acute Respiratory Failure Acute respiratory failure **(ARF)** is a life-threatening state that can result from many pulmonary diseases. It is caused by an imbalance in supply and demand and develops when the cardiopulmonary system is unable to maintain adequate gas exchange. Normally, the cardiopulmonary system is able to meet the demands of the body by increasing its work to supply adequate oxygen and rid the body of carbon dioxide. If the body's demands become higher than the cardiopulmonary system can meet, the system will fail, precipitating acute respiratory failure.

Components of Acute Respiratory Failure. The term *acute respiratory failure* is a general one that pertains to both gas exchange gases: oxygen and carbon dioxide. To better understand the complexity of respiratory failure, it is helpful to break it down into its two component parts: failure of oxygenation and failure of ventilation. Sometimes both failure components are present initially; however, more commonly a failure of one or the other system occurs initially. For this reason, it is important to be able to differentiate the two failure components.

Failure of Oxygenation. In a state of **oxygenation failure**, the primary problem is one of hypoxemia. Carbon dioxide (CO_2) diffuses across the alveolar–capillary membrane approximately 20 times more rapidly than does oxygen. For this reason, CO_2 levels may remain normal when diffusion is impaired, even though the patient is showing signs of moderate to severe hypoxemia. Conditions that can cause oxygenation failure are frequently restrictive pulmonary disorders, such as **acute respiratory distress syndrome (ARDS)** and pneumonia. Should these conditions worsen or should the patient develop respiratory muscle fatigue, CO_2 levels will rise due to hypoventilation, which may result in ventilatory failure.

Hypoxemia is accompanied by multiple compensatory mechanisms that work to regain an adequate oxygenation state. Clinically, it is important to maintain the PaO_2 at 60 mmHg or higher because of oxygen's decreased affinity to hemoglobin at a lower PaO_2. At this crucial point, any further decrease in PaO_2 will result in a large decrease in hemoglobin saturation (SaO_2). The clinical manifestations and clinical definition of oxygenation failure are presented in Table 12–3.

Failure of Ventilation. Ventilatory failure (acute respiratory acidosis) is caused by alveolar hypoventilation—that is, the inability to move air into the alveoli, which decreases gas exchange, leading to a buildup of carbon dioxide. It can be caused by any problem that interferes with adequate movement of air flow (e.g., neuromuscular disorders, respiratory muscle fatigue, and COPD).

Clinical manifestations of ventilatory failure reflect hypercapnia (elevated carbon dioxide). Most of the symptoms associated with hypercapnia are the result of the strong vasodilator effect of carbon dioxide. The term **CO_2 narcosis** is sometimes used to describe ventilatory failure, based on its effects on level of consciousness. The clinical manifestations and clinical definition of ventilatory failure are presented in Table 12–3.

Complications of Respiratory Failure. Acute respiratory failure can affect virtually all body systems by causing organ hypoxia. If the respiratory failure is coupled with decreased cardiac output, the patient is at particular risk for hypoperfusion or hypoxic organ shock complications, such as those seen with multiple organ dysfunction syndrome (MODS), including ARDS. The presence of hypercapnia, with its accompanying respiratory acidosis and vasodilation states, adds another pathophysiologic burden on the body because cellular function rapidly becomes impaired in acidotic states. In addition, the generalized vasodilatory effects can increase intracranial pressure and decrease cardiac output and systemic vascular resistance.

As a general rule, ventilation failure is considered a more serious problem than oxygenation failure. Acute respiratory acidosis can quickly deteriorate to systemic acidosis, which is poorly tolerated by the body. Oxygenation failure, however, is associated with better compensatory mechanisms and, therefore, is better tolerated.

Pathogenesis of Respiratory Failure. The sequence of events that leads to the development of respiratory failure is a complicated one. It is initiated by the presence of a disease process that either directly (e.g., pneumonia) or indirectly (e.g., Guillain-Barré syndrome) interferes with normal lung function. As pulmonary function deteriorates, the patient develops $\dot{V}/\dot{Q}$ ratio abnormalities and decreasing PaO_2. The body recognizes increased oxygen demand and responds by increasing the rate and depth of respirations to move more air into and out of the alveoli (compensation). This compensatory mechanism decreases $PaCO_2$ to regain an adequate level of ventilation and acid–base balance. Compensatory mechanisms (including increased work of breathing) require more energy; thus, the body's metabolic rate increases. More oxygen is consumed by the tissues and more carbon dioxide is produced as an end-product of metabolism. The overall effect of the sequence is a progressive increase in arterial carbon dioxide and a decrease in arterial oxygen. A state of acute respiratory failure exists when the patient meets these clinical criteria: $PaCO_2$ greater than 50 mmHg with a pH of less than 7.30 and/or a PaO_2 of less than 60 mmHg when the patient is breathing room air.

Should the sequence of events that precipitated the acute respiratory failure not be corrected adequately, the level of respiratory failure worsens, causing a further increase in the work of breathing. The patient develops respiratory muscle fatigue, which can eventually lead to respiratory muscle failure and decompensation with worsening of both ventilation and oxygenation. If this sequence of events is allowed to continue, arterial blood gas concentrations steadily deteriorate, leading to the death of the patient.

Management of the Patient with Acute Respiratory Failure

Management goals for the patient in acute respiratory failure include the following:

- Treat the underlying cause.
- Support the patient.
- Prevent or treat complications.

Detailed information on the management of patients with specific pulmonary disorders are found in the remaining sections of this chapter.

Section Two Review

1. Which arterial blood gas pH results would the nurse most commonly note with chronic respiratory insufficiency?
   A. pH within normal limits
   B. pH above normal range
   C. pH below normal range
   D. Variable pH

2. *Failure to oxygenate* refers to which primary problem?
   A. Ventilation
   B. Hypoxemia
   C. Arterial pH
   D. Carbon dioxide

3. The primary problem associated with failure to ventilate is which condition?
   A. Alveolar hypoventilation
   B. Capillary hypoperfusion
   C. Alveolar hyperventilation
   D. Capillary hyperperfusion

4. What is the result of increased metabolic demand?
   A. Decreased oxygen consumption
   B. Decreased carbon dioxide production
   C. Increased oxygen consumption
   D. Increased carbon dioxide consumption

Answers: 1. A, 2. B, 3. A, 4. C

Section Three: Acute Respiratory Distress Syndrome

Adult respiratory distress syndrome (ARDS) was first described in 1967 as a respiratory failure syndrome characterized by bilateral pulmonary filtrates (Ashbaugh, Bigelow, Petty, & Levine, 1967). In those early years, it was referred to as "adult" RDS to differentiate it from infant hyaline membrane disease. As the disorder became better understood, the word *adult* was replaced by *acute* to acknowledge the similarities between the adult and child versions of the disorder.

In 1994, the American-European Consensus Conference convened to standardize the definition of ARDS (Bernard et al., 1994). Acute respiratory distress syndrome (ARDS) was conceptualized as the most severe expression of **acute lung injury (ALI)**. ALI was described as a continuum of severity from mild, subclinical injury at one end of the continuum to severe injury (ARDS) at the opposite end. The new "Berlin definition" of ARDS was published in 2012 as an attempt to simplify diagnosis and improve the predictive ability of the criteria. The new criteria define three levels of ARDS severity, dropping the concept of ALI in favor of calling it mild ARDS. This definition also removes the heart failure exclusion criteria (pulmonary artery wedge pressure [PAWP] over 18 and/or left atrial hypertension) to allow patients with heart failure to meet the ARDS criteria. Table 12–4 shows a comparison of the 1992 and 2011 ARDS definitions (ARDS Definition Task Force, 2012).

Etiologic Factors

Acute respiratory distress syndrome is a syndrome of inflammation and increased permeability that occurs within one week of a known clinical insult or new or

Table 12–4 ARDS 1992 and 2011 Consensus Definitions

1992 American-European Consensus Conference (AECC) Definition	2011 Berlin Definition
Acute onset	Acute onset within 1 week of known insult or worsening of respiratory status
Bilateral infiltrates on chest radiograph (frontal view)	Bilateral opacities by chest imaging (not explained by other pulmonary disorders)
Pulmonary artery wedge pressure (PAWP) 18 mmHg or less and/or no left atrial hypertension (HF)	Pulmonary edema: not explained by heart failure or fluid overload
Oxygenation status measured as P/F ratio (regardless of positive end–expiratory pressure [PEEP] level): ALI = 300 mmHg or less ARDS = 200 mmHg or less	Oxygenation status measured as P/F ratio (on PEEP of 5 cm H_2O or higher): Mild: 200–300 Moderate: 100–200 Severe: 100 or less

SOURCE: Data from ARDS Definition Task Force (2011) and Bernard et al. (1994).

worsening respiratory symptoms associated with bilateral opacities on chest imaging, and acute hypoxic respiratory failure that cannot be explained by, but may coexist with, left atrial or pulmonary capillary hypertension. The hypoxic respiratory failure can be mild (PaO_2/FiO_2 200–300 mmHg on > 5 cm H_2O PEEP), moderate (PaO_2/FiO_2 100–200 mmHg on > 5 cm H_2O), or severe (PaO_2/FiO_2 < 100 mmHg on > 5 cm H_2O) (Fanelli et al., 2013). ARDS results from predisposing medical insults, either direct (aspiration) or indirect (sepsis, trauma). Predisposing factors have one thing in common: All are known to trigger a systemic inflammatory response that, if sufficiently strong, may involve the lungs, leading to diffuse lung injury (Villar, Sulemanji, & Kacmarek, 2014). Currently, there is not a complete explanation as to why, in similar pathologic conditions, a few people develop ARDS but most do not. It has been suggested that the answer depends to some extent on the characteristics and severity of the primary injury and the presence of coexisting predisposing factors (Mikkelsen, Lanken, & Christie, 2015). Table 12–5 lists some of the more common predisposing factors.

Table 12–5 Common Predisposing Disorders of ARDS

Direct	Indirect
Pneumonia[a]	Sepsis[a]
Gastric aspiration[b]	Severe traumatic injury with shock requiring massive blood transfusions[b] (each factor alone [traumatic injury, shock, massive blood transfusions] can lead to ARDS; the combination increases the risk significantly)
Near drowning	Acute pancreatitis
Direct severe chest contusion	Drug overdose
Inhalation injury	

[a] Most common predisposing disorders
[b] Common predisposing disorders
SOURCE: Data from Monahan (2013).

The risk of ARDS appears to be additive when multiple risk factors are present. Further, genetic factors that produce a more extreme inflammatory response may also play a role in the severity of this syndrome (Mikkelsen et al., 2015).

Diagnosis

Defining ARDS and differentiating it from other acute pulmonary disorders has been a difficult task since it was first described. The ARDS Definition Task Force defined ARDS on the basis of clinical criteria. Using these criteria, the severity of ARDS can be diagnosed based on the ratio of PaO_2 to FiO_2 (P/F ratio) (Table 12–4). Differentiating ARDS from other pulmonary disorders can be difficult, but it is important to make this differentiation because therapy differs among the various disease states. Several criteria assist in making a differential diagnosis:

1. **Bronchoalveolar lavage (BAL) fluid.** Bronchoalveolar fluid is obtained during a bronchoscopic examination into a lung lobe. Fluid obtained from the BAL may contain cells that help distinguish among ARDS, infections, and other inflammatory diseases (Mikkelsen et al., 2015).

2. **Brain natriuretic peptide (BNP).** This marker of heart strain is suggested as a helpful test to distinguish ALI/ARDS from HF if the BNP level is less than 100 pg/mL. Low BNP levels imply that HF is not present (Hansen-Flaschen & Siegel, 2015).

3. **Chest radiography.** Heart enlargement is typically noted in HF but not in ARDS. Pulmonary infiltrates noted in heart failure are usually greatest in the dependent lung fields; pulmonary infiltrates noted in ARDS are more diffuse (throughout the lung fields) (Reilly & Christie, 2015).

There is also investigational interest in finding serum and BAL molecular markers that measure acute lung injury similar to measuring serum troponin for myocardial cell injury. Biomarkers have been investigated, including pro-inflammatory cytokines such as interleukin 6, surfactant protein D, angiopoietin-2, and tumor-necrosis factor alpha (TNFα) as well as elements of coagulation and fibrinolysis (protein C, plasminogen) that are also activated in the inflammatory process. To date, none of these biomarkers have been supported for use in clinical practice (Chesnutt & Matthay, 2015).

Pathogenesis

ARDS is not a disease but a pattern of pathophysiologic lung changes resulting in a corresponding pattern of clinical manifestations (i.e., a syndrome). It is a distinct type of acute lung injury resulting in severe respiratory failure. ARDS is caused by diffuse inflammatory injury to the alveolar–capillary membrane, resulting in disruption of both the pulmonary capillary endothelium and the alveolar epithelium. Invasion of lung tissue by polymorphonuclear neutrophils (PMNs), which activate a variety of inflammatory by-products, is believed to be central to the

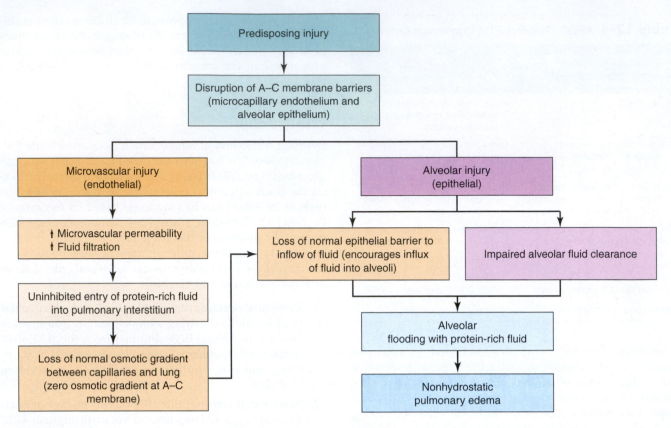

Figure 12–1 Pathogenesis of nonhydrostatic pulmonary edema.

SOURCE: Data from Siegel (2015a).

inflammatory injury. Disruption of the pulmonary capillary endothelium allows plasma proteins and fluid to escape into the pulmonary interstitial spaces. Injury to the alveolar epithelial lining permits fluid and plasma proteins to flood into the alveoli, resulting in nonhydrostatic pulmonary edema (Siegel, 2015a). Figure 12–1 provides a graphic map of one possible explanation of the pathogenesis of this form of pulmonary edema.

The hydrostatic pulmonary edema of HF has a different pathogenesis. Normally, hydrostatic pressure in the alveoli is greater than in the pulmonary interstitium, which protects the alveoli from abnormal inflow of interstitial fluid. In situations where left-heart pressures create an elevated backup pressure into the pulmonary veins (as seen in HF), the resulting elevated hydrostatic capillary pressure causes increased flow out of the capillaries into the interstitium because fluid passes through a semipermeable membrane (alveolar–capillary membrane) from greater pressure to lower pressure. Eventually, if interstitial pressures become sufficiently elevated, the alveoli begin to take in fluid as well (the mechanism for this form of alveolar flooding is not fully understood). Although the pathophysiology of lung edema in ARDS is due to increased permeability, the edema of ARDS can be worsened by increased hydrostatic pressures resulting from fluid overload (Krüger & Ludman, 2014).

ARDS can be triggered by either a local (pulmonary) inflammatory problem or a distant systemic problem (particularly sepsis or systemic inflammatory response syndrome [SIRS]). ARDS is the lungs' expression of this widespread inflammatory event. No matter what initial direct or indirect insult triggers the onset of ARDS, the subsequent sequence of events remains relatively predictable. Figure 12–2 illustrates a theoretical pathogenesis pathway of ARDS.

ARDS can be described as having two phases: the exudative phase and the fibroproliferative phase (Reilly & Christie, 2015). These phases reflect the early phase of acute injury followed by a phase of lung repair and are summarized in Table 12–6.

Clinical Presentation

Because ARDS is the result of another underlying illness or injury, the patient's clinical presentation will reflect both processes. Respiratory symptoms due to ARDS typically develop within 48 to 72 hours of the precipitating event (e.g., sepsis) and progress rapidly (Weinberger et al., 2014). The respiratory rate increases, accompanied by hypoxemia and dyspnea. The increased ventilation, a compensation for hypoxemia, results in respiratory alkalosis in arterial blood gases. Early chest radiography may demonstrate only mild bilateral infiltrates.

As ARDS progresses, cyanosis and accessory muscle use may be noted. A cough develops, frequently producing sputum that is typical of pulmonary edema. The heart rate increases and diffuse crackles may be auscultated. Arterial blood gas findings show a pattern of increasing hypoxemia

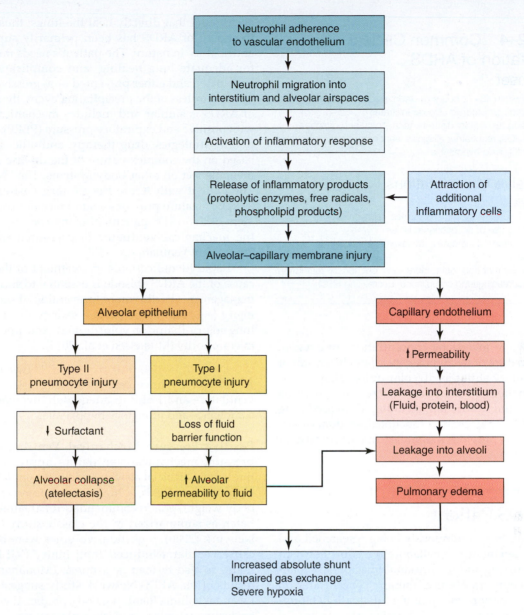

Figure 12–2 Theory of pathogenesis of ARDS.

SOURCE: Data from Chesnutt & Matthay (2015) and Weinberger et al. (2014).

Table 12–6 Phases of ARDS

Phase	Characteristics	Pathology
Exudative phase (1 to 3 days)	Diffuse microvascular injury and alveolar damage Invasion of inflammatory cells into interstitium Development of hyaline membranes[a] in alveolar spaces	Destruction of type I pneumocytes resulting in diffuse alveolar damage (DAD) Damage to type II epithelial cells with decreased surfactant production
Fibroproliferative phase (3 to 7 days)	Lung repair period Degree of recovery is dependent on: • Severity of primary lung injury • Influence of secondary forms of injury (e.g., barotrauma, healthcare-associated infection, oxygen toxicity)	Hyperplasia of type II pneumocytes Resolution of inflammatory process with clearing of fluid and cellular debris Proliferation of fibroblasts in basement membrane of alveoli Development of intra-alveolar and interstitial fibrosis[b] Lung remodeling Degree of lung repair = variable Full repair of lung architecture: return to normal compliance and gas exchange over 6- to 12-month period Permanent damage to lung architecture: if basement membrane becomes disrupted, cannot repair correctly

[a] Hyaline membranes consist of plasma proteins and cellular debris.

[b] Severity of pulmonary disability in survivors of ARDS depends on extent of fibrosis.

SOURCE: Data from Weinberger et al. (2014) and Monahan (2013).

that is refractory to increasing concentrations of oxygen. The refractory nature of the hypoxemia is largely a result of increasing capillary shunt as alveolar units collapse and become dysfunctional. Pulmonary function tests will be consistent with lung restriction, including decreased lung compliance (CL) and decreased functional residual capacity (FRC). Box 12–4 provides a summary of the typical clinical presentation of ARDS.

Collaborative Management of the ARDS Patient

Treatment of ARDS is continuously being researched and improved. Management is a collaborative effort between medicine and nursing and requires multidisciplinary planning and interventions. Medical therapy concentrates on promoting oxygenation, maintaining adequate hemodynamics, and promoting healing. Nursing plays a crucial role, focusing on implementing supportive measures to maintain the patient until the alveolar–capillary membrane regains its integrity and the syndrome resolves; monitoring the patient's status, the therapeutic and nontherapeutic effects of medical therapy; and monitoring for possible multisystem complications. No specific therapies have

been found that directly heal the lungs; thus, historically, treatment of ARDS has been primarily supportive and anticipatory in nature. The patient's needs must all be met for adequate lung healing, and complications must be anticipated and either prevented or aggressively treated.

Regardless of the precipitating event, the management of ARDS is similar and includes mechanical ventilation with positive end expiratory pressure (PEEP), patient positioning strategies, drug therapy, and other interventions based on the complex nature of the disease and its detrimental effect on other body systems. The "Nursing Care: The Patient with Acute Respiratory Distress Syndrome (ARDS)" feature provides a summary of nursing management of the ARDS patient. Nursing care that is specific to the mechanical ventilator is presented in Chapter 7: Mechanical Ventilation.

Rapid identification and treatment of the underlying cause of the ARDS episode is essential to successful ARDS management. Furthermore, prevention of secondary lung injury (e.g., aspiration, oxygen toxicity, ventilator-induced lung injury [baro- or volutrauma], and pneumonia) is a major priority (Mikkelsen et al., 2015).

Mechanical Ventilation Strategies   Two mainstays of ARDS therapy have been positive pressure mechanical ventilators and PEEP to adequately overcome low lung compliance and refractory hypoxemia.

Positive Pressure Mechanical Ventilation.   Positive pressure mechanical ventilators apply positive force through an artificial airway to deliver ventilatory support. Until the late 1990s, a high tidal volume (10–15 mL/kg body weight) was recommended for treatment of ARDS. Later, as summarized in the classic study by the ARDS Network (2000), high tidal volumes were discovered to cause ventilator-induced lung injury (VILI). This lung injury is also termed *volutrauma* (Monahan, 2013). The results of the ARDS Network study suggest that using a low tidal volume (6 mL/kg body predicted weight), called protective ventilation, with a plateau pressure of 30 cm H_2O or less significantly reduces mortality as well as ventilator days in ARDS patients regardless of the precipitating cause. More recently, the lower tidal volume approach has been recommended for most at-risk patients to prevent lung injury and development of ARDS (Fuller, Mohr, Drewry, & Carpenter, 2013).

Nursing Care
The Patient with Acute Respiratory Distress Syndrome (ARDS)

Expected Patient Outcomes and Related Interventions

Outcome 1: Support of pulmonary gas exchange

Assess and compare to established norms, patient baseline, and trends

Vital signs, lung sounds, chest x-ray, P/F ratio, peak airway pressure, SpO_2, ABG, CBC, intake and output, daily weights, hemodynamic parameters, ET tube position, secretions (amount and consistency)

Interventions to decrease lung fluid

Conservative fluid therapy, as ordered

(Goal: prevent fluid overload while maintaining adequate CO)

Diuretic therapy, as ordered

Interventions to increase pulmonary gas exchange

Mechanical ventilation

Optimal PEEP therapy, as ordered (Goal: maintain PaO_2 of 60 mmHg at FiO_2 of 0.6 or less)

Monitor for desired and adverse effects

Protective ventilation (VT of 6 mL/kg or less ideal body weight [IBW]; Goal: prevent ventilator-induced lung injury [VILI])

Reposition every 2 hours (if other alternative position therapy not being used; Goal: improve $\dot{V}/\dot{Q}$ relationship)

Prone positioning or continuous lateral rotation therapy (CLRT) therapy, as ordered

Prevent accidental dislodgement of endotracheal (ET) tube

Monitor for development of pressure ulcers

Monitor closely for adverse effects

Interventions to maintain airway patency and protect airway

Secure ET tube with tape or other stabilizing device

Suction ET tube and mouth as needed

Maintain ET tube cuff pressure

Administer related drug therapy and monitor for therapeutic and nontherapeutic effects

Diuretic agents (e.g., furosemide [Lasix])

Corticosteroids (e.g., methylprednisolone)

Nitric oxide (iNO) therapy

Beta adrenergic agonist therapy (e.g., IV albuterol; IV use is not yet available in the United States)

Outcome 2: Optimize oxygen delivery to body systems

Assess and compare to established norms, patient baseline, and trends

Arterial blood pressure, heart rate, temperature, mean arterial pressure (MAP), complete blood count (CBC), hemodynamic parameters, pain, and anxiety

Interventions to maintain adequate oxygen delivery (DO_2) to body systems

Maintain MAP greater than 70 mmHg, BP greater than 90 mmHg systolic

Maintain adequate urine output

Correct lactic acidosis

Maintain adequate levels of hemoglobin

Interventions to reduce metabolic demands

Maintain afebrile state

Control pain and anxiety

Reduce extraneous body movements

Administer related drug therapy and monitor for therapeutic and nontherapeutic effects

Vasopressor agents (e.g., dopamine, dobutamine)

Sedation agents (e.g., midazolam [Versed], lorazepam [Ativan], propofol [Diprivan])

Analgesic agents (e.g., morphine [MScontin], fentanyl [Actiq])

Neuromuscular blockade (e.g., cisatracurium [Nimbex])

Outcome 3: Maintain nutritional balance

Assess and compare to established norms, patient baseline, and trends

Daily weights, temperature, serum electrolytes, CBC, serum albumin, prealbumin, renal function tests (BUN, creatinine), nitrogen balance (e.g., metabolic cart study), edema, bowel sounds, bowel movements

Interventions to maintain nutritional balance

Provide nutritional support: enteral nutrition (Goal: initiate within 24 hours of intubation)

Monitor tube tip placement

SOURCE: Data partially from Siegel (2015c).

Elevate head of bed 30 degrees or greater

Frequent oral care: oral airway cleaning and suctioning

Administer related drug therapy and monitor for therapeutic and nontherapeutic effects

Agents to reduce metabolic demand (see Outcome 2)

Intravenous fluids, as ordered

Bowel regimen agents: stool softeners, bulking agents, laxatives

Oral hygiene agents (e.g., chlorhexidine [Peridex])

Related nursing diagnoses

Impaired nutrition: less than body requirements

Risk for aspiration

Diarrhea or constipation

Risk for electrolyte imbalance

Outcome 4: Minimize pain, anxiety, and delirium; promote sleep

Assess and compare to established norms, patient baseline, and trends

Patient self-assessment of pain, anxiety, lack of sufficient rest; when patient cannot communicate, evaluate for signs of pain or anxiety (e.g., facial grimacing, restlessness); assess for presence of pain-producing invasive tubes or lines or altered skin integrity

Interventions to reduce anxiety and delirium and promote rest

Cluster activities to provide periods of undisturbed rest

Maintain a restful environment (e.g., turn down lights between procedures; reduce environmental noise levels)

Explain all procedures and treatments

Keep call light within patient reach, as appropriate

Support meaningful sensory stimulation: glasses, hearing aids as appropriate

Minimize use of delirium-producing drugs as possible (e.g., benzodiazepines [diazepam, lorazepam, etc.])

Daily reduction of sedatives and analgesia combined with evaluation of spontaneous breathing

Administer related drug therapy and monitor for therapeutic and nontherapeutic effects

Sedation agents (e.g., midazolam, lorazepam, or propofol)

Analgesic agents (e.g., morphine, fentanyl)

Outcome 5: Promote communication and provide family support

Assess and compare to established norms, patient baseline, and trends

Glasgow Coma Scale, mental status, delirium assessment, ability to communicate through alternative means

Interventions to promote communication and provide family support

Frequent reminders that patient is unable to talk at present time

Frequent reorientation of family members to ventilator equipment

Ask yes/no questions

Use alternative communication boards (e.g., alphabet or picture boards, writing boards)

Provide patient and family with updates on patient status

Positive End Expiratory Pressure (PEEP).

A major complicating factor in ARDS is the massive collapse of alveoli, which causes a significant shunt, decreased lung compliance, and severe hypoxemia. This explains the refractory nature of ARDS to conventional oxygen therapy. Recall that atelectasis is a type of capillary shunt, which is absolute in nature. Regardless of the oxygen concentration delivered, the gas never enters the affected alveoli for gas exchange. Until PEEP became available, there was no way to force alveoli open once they had collapsed.

PEEP applies positive pressure into the patient's airway at the end of expiration and prevents the alveoli from closing. PEEP maintains the alveoli in an open state throughout the breathing cycle, which increases gas diffusion time, thereby increasing gas exchange. PEEP also reduces shunt by recruiting collapsed alveoli (popping them open). Once open, PEEP may prevent another type of damage to alveoli from the stress of opening and closing with each ventilator cycle, termed *atelectrauma* (Monahan, 2013). The goal in using PEEP is to achieve an adequate PaO_2 (usually at least 60 mmHg) while reducing the inspired oxygen concentration (FiO_2) to less than 0.6 (60%) because high concentrations of oxygen eventually cause oxygen toxicity.

The level of desired PEEP is individually evaluated. Current recommendations are to optimize the amount of PEEP to achieve oxygenation goals and avoid toxic oxygen levels (Reilly & Christie, 2015). Although PEEP has been invaluable for treatment of ARDS, it is not without hazards, including decreased cardiac output, overdistention of alveoli, and **pneumothorax** (abnormal presence of air in the intrapleural space), among others.

The use of smaller tidal volumes, while reducing the risk of alveolar injury from overdistention, creates another concern for microatelectasis despite the use of PEEP. This microatelectasis is also termed "derecruitment" (Mikkelsen et al., 2015). Alveolar collapse can occur when the ventilator is disconnected or during suctioning. Recruitment maneuvers—strategies to reopen these closed alveoli by momentarily using higher pressures or volumes—are under investigation. They can improve oxygenation but to date have not changed outcomes in ARDS (Reilly & Christie, 2015).

According to the ARMA trial (ARDS Network, 2000), **low tidal volume ventilation (LTVV)** reduces the damaging effects (volutrauma) of excessive stretching of lung tissue and alveoli that occurs with higher tidal volumes, and is the standard of care for people with ARDS requiring mechanical ventilation.

Although the ARMA trial, the largest clinical trial supporting this paradigm, was criticized both for its design and for ethical concerns, its results (ARDS Network, 2000), followed by two flawed but concordant meta-analyses (Petrucci & Lacovelli, 2004; Putensen, Theuerkauf, Zinserling, Wrigge, & Pelosi, 2009) including ten randomized trials total, have supported the standard that the use of low tidal volumes improves survival in ARDS. The research evidence suggests that a strategy of low tidal volume ventilation (6–8 mL/kg ideal body weight) reduces absolute mortality by about 7% to 9%, as compared to using 10 mL/kg or more tidal volumes (~ 42% mortality in control groups vs. ~ 34% in the LTVV groups). This translates to a number needed to treat of between 11 and 15 people with ARDS to prevent one death by using LTVV.

In addition to using lower tidal volumes to ventilate patients with ARDS, alternative mechanical ventilation options may be initiated when conventional therapy has not been effective in attaining adequate gas exchange. Some of the more common alternatives include pressure control ventilation, reverse inspiratory-to-expiratory (I:E) ratio ventilation, airway pressure release ventilation, high-frequency ventilation, and bilevel ventilation. It is important to note,

Table 12–7 Protective Mechanical Ventilation Settings to Reduce Ventilator-induced Lung Injury

Parameter	Setting
Tidal volume (V_T)	6 mL/kg (IBW) or less
PEEP (optimal PEEP)	Minimum level that achieves SaO_2 90% or greater at FiO_2 of 0.6 (60%) or less
Permissive hypercapnia[a]	No specific settings. Develops as tidal volume is reduced and ventilator rate is increased. Goal: Maintain pH within ordered range, using HCO_3 infusion prn.
Plateau pressure	30 cm H_2O or less

[a] Permissive hypercapnia—V_T, f, $\dot{V}_E$, and other settings can be manipulated to allow $PaCO_2$ to elevate, keeping the pH within specified acidotic parameters (such as 7.25–7.30) to reduce PAP to within desired range; contraindicated in patients with unstable intracranial pressure or hemodynamic status.

SOURCE: Data from Mikkelsen et al. (2015).

however, that while some of these alternative options have the advantage of reducing problems of barotrauma and volutrauma, none of them stand out as superior to the use of low tidal volume ventilation for use in ARDS in the adult population (Reilly & Christie, 2015).

Table 12–7 summarizes mechanical ventilation settings that support oxygen exchange while protecting the lungs.

Patient Positioning Strategies There has been increasing interest in the effects of various types of patient positioning in improving patient outcomes. Two major types of therapy, continuous lateral rotation therapy and prone positioning, are briefly described here.

Continuous Lateral Rotation Therapy (CLRT). Beds that provide CLRT (also called Kinetic Therapy™ or oscillation therapy) continuously rotate the patient's body from side to side (with brief pauses), thus shifting pressure and fluid. Manual turning is a traditional nursing intervention to prevent pressure ulcers, improve pulmonary function and cardiovascular tone, prevent circulatory stasis, and improve muscle and mental function (Makic, Rauen, Watson, & Poteet, 2014). Manual turning is inconsistently practiced in many ICUs according to Kalisch and Xie (2014). CLRT is commonly employed in high-acuity units as an alternative to manual turning for the purpose of reducing stasis of fluid and gas-related complications.

Research evaluating CLRT concluded that this therapy decreases pulmonary complications such as atelectasis but does not reduce mortality (Hanneman et al., 2015). A recent study of 15 ventilated general ICU patients (not specifically ARDS), comparing manual turning with CLRT, concluded that automated turning may reduce pulmonary complications; however, they found no statistically significant differences between groups in turning-related adverse events, duration of mechanical ventilation, ICU length of stay, or ICU mortality (Hanneman et al., 2015). Figure 12–3 shows an example of a CLRT bed.

Prone Position Therapy. Prone positioning (proning) is the periodic placement of a patient in a face-down (prone) position for the purpose of increasing oxygenation while potentially reducing therapeutic oxygen concentration

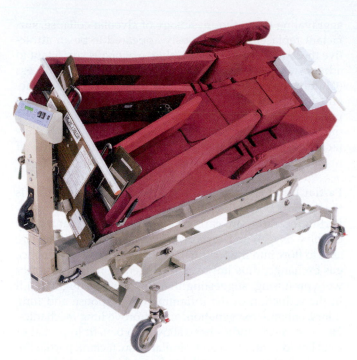

Figure 12–3 RotoRest bed. A form of CLRT therapy.
SOURCE: Courtesy of KCI Licensing, Inc. 2008.

(Hudack, 2013). Prone positioning can be achieved in a variety of ways, such as manually, using special pillows or proning devices, and mechanically, using automated proning beds.

While the exact mechanism for improved oxygenation is not completely known, understanding the effects of the supine position on the injured lung helps explain why the prone position might be therapeutic. The supine position results in atelectasis in the lower, posterior (dependent) areas of the lung. Factors that may contribute to this loss of lung volume include more air flow or ventilation to the anterior portion of the lung and posterior lung compression by the heart and abdominal organs (Schwartz, Atul Malhotra, & Kacmarek, 2015). At the same time, gravitational forces maintain blood flow to the now-atelectatic dependent lung regions, resulting in increased shunt.

Physiology of Prone Positioning. The prone position may improve oxygenation by recruiting alveoli (increasing functional residual capacity [FRC]), redistribution of perfusion and improved removal of secretions (Mikkelsen et al., 2015). More air now enters the posterior lung units, with the weight of the heart and abdominal organs shifted off that lung tissue while blood flow remains increased to the posterior lung fields, reducing shunt (Schwartz et al., 2015). A major advantage of prone positioning is that improved oxygenation can be achieved using a noninvasive, relatively simple procedure. Evidence suggests that there is a window of opportunity in which prone positioning is therapeutic in ARDS patients, namely the early phase of the disease (Chiumello, Algieri, Brioni, & Babini, 2015). Research for years has demonstrated that proning improves

oxygenation in ARDS but does not improve survival. In 2013, The Proning Severe ARDS Patients (PROSEVA) study comparing the prone position and the supine position in 466 adults who met the American–European consensus criteria for ARDS from 26 ICUs suggested improved survival in patients with severe ARDS. In this study, prone position was conducted for longer periods as well, at least 16 hours per day (Guérin et al., 2013). In patients with severe ARDS, early application of prolonged prone-positioning sessions significantly decreased 28-day and 90-day mortality (Guérin et al., 2013)

Appropriate Application of Prone Positioning. Given the results of studies to date and the potential for complications, the prone position should be reserved for patients with severe hypoxemia, with careful assessment of clinical response (Schwartz et al., 2015). It is highly recommended that the patient be thoroughly assessed prior to the decision to use this technique (Chiumello et al., 2015). Not all patients can tolerate being placed in the prone position and may develop worsening oxygenation or hemodynamic instability. Uncontrolled intracranial pressure has been identified as a contraindication. Prone positioning of morbidly obese patients is safe and feasible (De Jong et al., 2013). Prone positioning of patients with spinal fracture is contraindicated.

Careful preparation prior to the turn is essential to minimize positioning-related complications such as accidental ET tube dislodgement, pressure ulcers, loss of venous access, intolerance of enteral feeding, or eye injury (Chiumello et al., 2015). Increased pressure ulcers of the face and thorax reported in the PROSEVA study were attributed to the longer duration of prone position (Girard et al., 2014). Nursing care should anticipate and address these risks to prevent complications with a well-coordinated multidisciplinary plan of care.

Fluid Management Although the lung edema of ARDS is due primarily to increased alveolar-capillary permeability, it can be aggravated by increased hydrostatic pressure from high intravascular volume. However, fluid resuscitation is vital to maintaining organ perfusion. How to balance these competing issues of fluid balance has been a concern in the management of ARDS patients. The largest study to date on this topic supports conservative fluid management in hemodynamically stable patients following initial resuscitation, because avoiding fluid gain in stable patients improves oxygenation and results in less time on mechanical ventilation (National Heart, Lung, and Blood Institute Acute Respiratory Distress Syndrome Clinical Trials Network, 2006). Another fluid management strategy, using albumin and furosemide to alter fluid balance, also demonstrated improved oxygenation but no change in survival rates (Mikkelsen et al., 2015; Wiedemann et al., 2006).

Pharmacologic Therapy Pharmacologic treatment has failed to significantly improve ARDS patient outcomes (Koh, 2014). Currently, several therapies warrant description.

Corticosteroids. The use of corticosteroids as a treatment for ARDS remains controversial and is based on the inflammatory nature of the disease pathology. Inflammation and lung injury from the by-products of inflammation are a major source of lung destruction in ARDS pathogenesis. Some patients recover within the first week of ARDS, but in others the inflammation does not resolve and progresses to a fibrotic phase of the disease (Chudow, Carter, & Rumbak, 2015).

High-dose steroids have not been shown to be effective and may be harmful (Mikkelsen et al., 2015). A large, randomized, controlled trial conducted by the ARDS Clinical Trials Network found improvement in oxygenation but no improvement in mortality. Of note, late steroid use (after 14 days) was associated with increased mortality and greater neuromuscular weakness and is not recommended (Siegel, 2015b).

In this review of eight controlled trials using different doses and timing of steroids, Meduri et al. (2009) found that early, prolonged low to moderate dose steroid administration improved survival rates. These investigators also found frequent infections without fever in the patients receiving steroids and stressed the importance of obtaining active surveillance cultures (BAL fluid sampling at 5-7 day intervals). Meduri, Annane, Chrousos, Marik, and Sinclair (2009) recommend avoidance of neuromuscular blocking agents to minimize weakness and a slow tapering of the steroids after the respiratory failure has resolved to reduce the risk of rebound inflammation. These studies, while conflicting, add to the body of information regarding the place of anti-inflammatory agents in the treatment of ARDS and highlight serious complications of infection and muscle weakness.

Inhaled Vasodilators. Nitric oxide (iNO) and prostacyclins are potent vasodilators. Nitric oxide should not be confused with nitrous oxide (N_2O, "laughing gas"), which is used for mild anesthesia. Nitric oxide is normally produced by the body and plays an important role in pulmonary blood flow regulation. The pathology of ARDS includes acute pulmonary hypertension as a result of pulmonary vasoconstriction in early ARDS, as well as impairment of hypoxic pulmonary vasoconstriction (Chudow et al., 2015). Inhalation of vasodilators increases PaO_2 by selectively redistributing pulmonary blood flow to working alveoli, thereby reducing shunt (Reilly & Christie, 2015). Inhaled vasodilator therapy has been shown to improve oxygenation in the first days of use, but not to improve survival from ARDS. Inhaled nitric oxide therapy may also carry an increased risk of acute kidney failure (Perner et al., 2015). Despite a lack of effect on survival, inhaled vasodilators may have a role for patients with the most severe, life-threatening hypoxemia when other strategies have failed (Chudow et al., 2015). For additional information on iNO as a pulmonary vasodilating agent, refer to the "Related Pharmacotherapy: Agents Used for Treatment of Pulmonary Diseases" feature.

Surfactant Replacement Therapy. Surfactant therapy, used in treating infant distress syndrome, is a well-known, highly successful therapy. Because ARDS in adults results in decreased surfactant production and inactivation,

aggravating the pathophysiology of alveolar collapse, surfactant replacement previously appeared to be an attractive therapy; however, trials using exogenous surfactant in adults with ARDS have not met with the same success (Chudow et al., 2015). Several features of current surfactant therapy have been identified that pose challenges, particularly the composition of the formula and the method of delivery (aerosol versus direct instillation). Surfactant is not currently available for adults outside of research protocols (Mikkelsen et al., 2015).

Partial Liquid Ventilation. Partial liquid ventilation is the introduction of perfluorocarbon liquid into the lungs. Perfluorocarbons are carbon-based molecules that readily dissolve oxygen and carbon dioxide. Perfluorocarbons are able to flow into the terminal airways, where they enhance gas exchange, thus improving oxygenation. Early studies were promising, suggesting that this therapy might result in the reduction of the inflammatory response and lung injury, enhance oxygenation, and improve lung mechanics. However, later studies have shown no benefit to partial or total liquid ventilation and, similar to surfactant, partial liquid ventilation is not available for routine use (Mikkelsen et al., 2015).

Neuromuscular Blocking Agents. Once a common adjunct to mechanical ventilation in severe ARDS, neuromuscular blockade has been used less frequently in the past decades due to concerns of prolonged muscle weakness and other complications including deep vein thrombosis (DVT), corneal abrasions, and patient awareness during paralysis (Greenberg & Vender, 2013). Papazian et al. (2010) reported improved oxygenation (the PaO_2–FiO_2 ratio was higher, and the $PaCO_2$ value lower) and outcomes using cisatracurium (a neuromuscular blocking agent) early for 48 hours in 177 patients with severe ARDS compared to 162 who received a placebo. Neuromuscular blockade may improve patient–ventilator synchrony and improve oxygenation by several mechanisms, including reduction of ventilator-associated lung injury (Slutsky & Ranieri, 2013). Authors caution that this therapy carries the risk of profound muscle weakness and requires frequent reassessment of patient needs and peripheral nerve stimulation (train-of-four monitoring) (Greenberg & Vender, 2013).

Nutrition. In addition to the role of nutrition as an important supportive measure in acute illness, enteral formulas with omega-3 fatty acids and antioxidant supplements that could potentially reduce inflammation in ARDS have been studied (Chudow et al., 2015). Once again, studies have yielded conflicting results (Desai, McClave, & Rice, 2014). General guidelines for nutritional support in ARDS include early enteral feeding and avoidance of excessive calories to avoid excess CO_2 production (Hanson, Rutten, Rollins, & Dobak, 2015). Enteral nutrition can safely be provided to patients in the prone position (Linn, Beckett, & Foellinger, 2015).

Other Emerging Drug Therapy. There remains high interest in finding new therapies that can effectively reduce mortality in patients with ARDS. Possibilities for the future include stem cells, nebulized heparin, keratinocyte growth factor, angiotensin-converting enzyme 2 (Curley & Laffey, 2015) and aerosolized albuterol (Chudow et al., 2015).

Extracorporeal membrane oxygenation (ECMO) is an advanced therapy offered at specialized hospitals that has expanded the options available to patients with the most severe ARDS. ECMO therapy oxygenates the patient's blood and removes carbon dioxide by circulating the blood through an external circuit (similar to dialysis). ECMO is not a new therapy but had not shown improvements in survival in ARDS until recently. Renewed interest developed when ECMO was used as a rescue therapy during an H1N1 influenza epidemic and the results of a study showing improved survival in ARDS (Mikkelsen et al., 2015).

Prognosis

The mortality rate associated with ARDS varies widely, depending on its etiology and comorbidity factors, and ranges from about 30% to 40% (Reilly & Christie, 2015). The underlying cause of ARDS appears to affect prognosis, with the highest mortality seen with sepsis and the lowest with ARDS due to trauma. A number of patient risk factors, such as age and comorbid diseases and number of organs involved (e.g., liver disease, renal and liver disease), may also affect mortality (Mikkelsen et al., 2015). Three interventions, however, have reduced mortality rates: PEEP, mechanical ventilation using low (protective) tidal volumes, and conservative fluid management following initial resuscitation (Burnham, Janssen, Riches, Moss, & Downey, 2014). Mortality in patients with ARDS is more often the result of multiple organ failure than from the hypoxemia of ARDS (Carlucci, Graf, Simmons, & Corbridge, 2014).

There is research interest in finding methods to more accurately predict the prognosis in a patient with ARDS.

More accurate prediction could assist teams in counseling families (Perner et al., 2015), in designing research studies, and in identifying patients likely to need more aggressive therapies (Villar et al., 2015). Work is under way to validate a number of biological markers (Terpstra, Aman, van Nieuw Amerongen, & Groeneveld, 2014), as well as lung injury scoring (Kangelaris et al., 2014). Finally, earlier identification of patients at high risk of developing ARDS may allow early treatment or prevention strategies (Mikkelsen et al., 2015).

Quality of life for ARDS survivors is an issue receiving a great deal of attention. For those who survive, lung repair occurs slowly and terminates by about 6 months following onset. A small number of patients will develop fibrosis from impaired healing, leading to persistent symptoms and decreased quality of life. Burnham et al. (2014) describe the processes involved in the development of fibrosis and conclude that identifying markers of fibrosis early could identify patients who would benefit from targeted therapies.

In the long term, most survivors of ARDS do not have severe pulmonary dysfunction. They do report serious impairment in physical, psychological, and emotional function related to persistent muscle weakness, pain, depression, anxiety, and cognitive changes such as memory loss (Jones, 2013). This sequelae of critical illness has been termed *post-intensive care syndrome* or *PICS* (Davidson, Harvey, Bemis-Dougherty, Smith, & Hopkins, 2013).

These post-ICU impairments have profound implications for patients' quality of life, needs for rehabilitation, family support, and healthcare costs. Caregivers also experience stress with prolonged responsibilities (Perner et al., 2015). Interventions such as daily interruption of sedatives and early rehabilitation show promise in improving outcomes by minimizing muscle weakness and delirium (Jones, 2013). Nursing plays a pivotal role in these prevention strategies.

Section Three Review

1. Which condition is the most common indirect predisposing disorder of ARDS?
   A. Gastric aspiration
   B. Severe trauma
   C. Sepsis
   D. Pneumonia

2. The pulmonary edema associated with ARDS is caused by which condition?
   A. Capillary microembolism
   B. Left ventricular failure
   C. Loss of surfactant
   D. Injured alveolar–capillary membrane

3. *Permissive hypercapnia* is contraindicated in which client population?
   A. Those with unstable intracranial pressure
   B. Those requiring mechanical ventilation
   C. Those whose ARDS is related to traumatic injury
   D. Those who are over age 45 years

4. Which statement correctly describes the primary purpose of CLRT?
   A. It prevents pneumonia.
   B. It saves manual turning time.
   C. It prevents decubitus ulcers.
   D. It prevents reduced stasis of fluid and gas.

Answers: 1. D, 2. D, 3. A, 4. D

Section Four: Pulmonary Embolism

Pulmonary embolism (PE) is responsible for approximately 100,000 deaths each year (Thompson & Hales, 2015) and is the leading cause of preventable in-hospital deaths (Flanders & Zwerneman, 2014). The incidence of PE appears to have increased in recent years, but that increase correlates with improvements in diagnostic techniques with advanced computed tomography (CT) scans (Meyer & Schmidt, 2015). Although many pulmonary emboli are asymptomatic, others lead to rapid death, with as many as 25% of patients dying before being admitted to the hospital (Meyer & Schmidt, 2015). This section provides an overview of the types, causes, signs and symptoms, and treatment of pulmonary emboli, but the focus is on thromboembolism.

Pulmonary embolism is the blockage of a pulmonary blood vessel caused by a thromboembolism or other bloodborne material that has passed through the venous system, into the right side of the heart, and into the pulmonary artery. Emboli become lodged in the lungs because of the natural blood flow of the venous system. As blood flows into the lungs for gas exchange, it moves through a pulmonary vascular system of decreasing size that begins at the pulmonary artery trunk and ends in the microvasculature of the pulmonary capillary system. This system makes the lungs act as a filtering organ, stopping any material that is too large to squeeze through the tiny microvasculature. Therefore, bloodborne materials can flow through the system until they can no longer move forward, lodging and obstructing flow distal to the obstruction.

Types and Causes of Emboli

There are five types of pulmonary emboli: thrombus, fat, amniotic, septic, and venous air.

Thromboembolism Almost all pulmonary emboli are thrombi, or blood clots. The major type of thromboembolism is venous thromboembolism (VTE) in the lower extremities, usually in the thigh or pelvic areas. Thromboembolism is discussed in detail later in this section.

Fat Embolism Fat embolism occurs when fat gains access to the venous circulation. Fat embolism may be quite common; however, life-threatening illness is rare and usually results from long-bone trauma or orthopedic surgery. Fat emboli are often small and may go undetected. When symptoms are present, they usually appear within 12 to 72 hours after the predisposing event. Major criteria for fat embolism syndrome include petechiae (e.g., over the anterior neck, chest, and face), dyspnea and tachypnea, hypoxemia, neurologic symptoms (e.g., confusion, drowsiness, or coma), and diffuse bilateral shadowing on chest radiography (Meyer & Schmidt, 2015). A person experiencing this form of embolus may also exhibit a fever, tachycardia, and other signs and symptoms. The pathophysiology of fat embolism is not completely understood; mechanisms of physical obstruction and an inflammatory process similar to ARDS are thought to be involved (Kwiatt & Seamon, 2013). As there is no specific treatment for fat embolism, the approach to care is supportive (Fedullo & Yung, 2015).

Amniotic Embolism Normally, the fetal membranes prevent amniotic fluid from gaining access to the maternal circulation. Amniotic emboli can develop during the birthing process when amniotic fluid mixes with maternal blood.

Emerging Evidence

- A novel therapy is showing promise for the treatment of severe asthma in patients over 18 years of age. Thermoplasty is the application of radiofrequency energy (heat) to reduce the amount of airway smooth muscle that lines bronchial airways (contributing to bronchospasm), thereby reducing airway constriction. The treatment is applied in several sessions by bronchoscopy. Studies to date have shown decreased asthma symptoms and exacerbations in some patients (Chakir et al., 2015; Sheshadri, Castro, & Chen, 2013).

- Prone positioning is not new and has been used for years as a therapy to improve oxygenation in severe ARDS. Prior research, however, has not demonstrated any significant improvement in survival. In a multicenter randomized controlled trial, Guérin et al. (2013) did demonstrate a reduction in mortality with early prone positioning versus standard supine care (16% versus 32.8%) in patients with severe hypoxemic ARDS. Of note, the protocol included prone position for 16 hours per day and was instituted early (within 36 hours) in centers with experience in this maneuver (Guérin et al., 2013).

- Administration of oxygen via a high-flow nasal cannula (HFNC), a technology that has been used in pediatrics, is now being evaluated for use in high-acuity adults. The technology allows oxygen flows up to 60 L/min, is administered through a blender to allow precise titration of oxygen percentage, adds high humidification of warm air, and is delivered through a large, soft nasal cannula. The system also generates positive end expiratory pressure (PEEP). Expected or observed benefits include increased patient comfort and reduced work of breathing, improved secretion removal, and improved ventilation and oxygenation. Additional research is needed to clarify which patients will benefit from HFNC: Possibilities include hypoxic respiratory failure (versus noninvasive ventilation by mask), postoperative patients, pulmonary edema, and palliative care (Spoletini, Alotaibi, Blasi, & Hill, 2015).

- Turning is a time-honored nursing intervention to prevent pulmonary complications of atelectasis and pneumonia. Studies comparing manual turning to continuous automated turning with specialty beds have shown improved outcomes with the specialty beds. In a randomized controlled trial comparing manual versus continuous automated lateral rotation to reduce preventable pulmonary complications in ventilator patients, Hanneman et al. (2015) found no statistically significant differences in preventable pulmonary complications or length of ICU stay. The authors noted that automated turning may be more effective at ensuring that patients were consistently turned. A study with a larger sample size is needed to be able to detect significant differences between groups (Hanneman et al., 2015).

Amniotic fluid embolism is not well understood, but three pathophysiologic mechanisms have been suggested: mechanical obstruction caused by amniotic material; cytokine release causing vasoconstriction, coagulopathy, and ARDS; and an anaphylactic-type syndrome resulting in shock (Thongrong et al., 2013). The patient presents with sudden-onset shock, severe hypoxemia, and disseminated intravascular coagulation (DIC), a potentially severe coagulopathy. Neurologic changes, including seizures, are also common. Care is supportive, focusing on oxygenation, cardiovascular support with vasopressors and inotropes, and blood products to correct the coagulopathy (Fedullo & Yung, 2015).

Septic Embolism Septic emboli are increasingly seen in association with intravenous (IV) drug use and central venous catheters. The emboli may arise from various sources including endocarditis, implanted devices, and periodontal disease. Two problems arise when infected, thrombotic material embolizes to the lung: pulmonary arterial obstruction followed by lung infection. Symptoms of septic pulmonary emboli include fever, cough, and hemoptysis (Stawicki et al., 2013). Prompt antibiotics and source control (e.g., removal of an infected central line) are treatment priorities (Fedullo & Yung, 2015).

Venous Air Embolism Venous air embolus (VAE) results from a bolus of air being introduced into the venous circulation. VAE is a rare but potentially lethal complication, usually resulting from iatrogenic procedures or trauma. The potentially catastrophic effects of air embolus can be better understood by visualizing venous flow into the heart. On introduction into the venous circulation, an air embolus (air bubble) follows venous flow into the right atrium, into the right ventricle, and then into the pulmonary artery. If the embolus is sufficiently large, it can become trapped at the pulmonary valve in the right ventricle, blocking venous blood from entering the lungs.

Common predisposing factors for development of air embolism include venous or arterial intravenous catheters, procedures in which the incision is higher than the heart, such as neurosurgery, head and neck surgery, and penetrating chest trauma (Meyer & Schmidt, 2015). Gordy and Rowell (2013) explain that surgical procedures and central venous cannulization pose the greatest risk. The exact volume required for a lethal air bolus is unknown, but volumes of 3 to 5 mL/kg can cause right-heart outflow obstruction, subsequent cardiovascular collapse, and death. For example, a lethal dose in a 150-pound (68-kg) adult male would be a bolus of 204 to 340 mL of air. Smaller volumes of air can move from the right heart into the pulmonary artery system, causing pulmonary vascular injury (e.g., vasoconstriction, pulmonary hypertension, injury to the capillary endothelium, and pulmonary edema).

Air embolism has a mortality rate of about 12% to 30%; thus, prevention is key (O'Dowd & Kelley, 2015). The clinical manifestations of VAE are similar to those of thromboembolism. Recommendations for treatment include steps to prevent further air entry, administration of 100% oxygen, and positioning on the left side in Trendelenburg position. This position encourages the embolus to float away from the pulmonary valve, thus allowing blood to move into the pulmonary artery. Air embolism associated with central venous catheters can be prevented with careful technique during insertion and removal (Cook, 2013).

Predisposing Factors of Venous Thromboembolism

Venous thromboembolism (VTE) is the term applied to both pulmonary embolism and deep vein thrombosis (DVT). VTE is a common, potentially preventable hospital complication and is the focus of national prevention strategies. More than 80% of pulmonary emboli (PEs) originate as deep vein thrombosis (DVT) in lower-extremity deep veins. Many high-acuity patients are at increased risk for development of venous thromboembolism. Three major factors, called Virchow's triad, place a person at risk for development of VTE:

- **Venous stasis.** *Venous stasis* refers to the slowing of blood flow. It most commonly results from significantly reduced mobility, such as with prolonged bed rest, severe illness, or major surgery, or from immobility states, such as with limb casts or paralysis. It can also develop when vein valves in the extremities are incompetent, as in severe varicose veins. People with polycythemia vera can also develop venous stasis because of thickening of the blood (hyperviscosity) from a significantly elevated red blood cell count.

- **Hypercoagulability.** Hypercoagulability is an abnormal tendency to form thrombi that can be inherited or acquired. Acquired causes include conditions such as cancer, oral contraceptive use, sepsis, and others.

- **Venous (endothelial) injury.** Endothelial injury can occur either directly or indirectly. It can result from such predisposing events as surgery, trauma, infection, and central venous catheters.

Box 12–5 lists the most common predisposing factors for development of venous thromboembolism.

In addition to individual symptoms, patients with PE can be classified according to the severity of their hemodynamic signs and symptoms. Table 12–8 summarizes one such classification system. Groups of symptoms may give clues as to the location or extent of the pulmonary embolus. Pleuritic chest pain and hemoptysis are associated with smaller peripheral emboli causing pulmonary infarction (Cohen, Dobromirski, & Gurwith, 2014).

BOX 12–5 Common Predisposing Factors for Thromboembolism

- Immobilization, paralysis, bed rest, prolonged travel
- Indwelling intravenous catheters
- Surgery, especially hip and knee and trauma
- Malignancy
- Pregnancy, contraceptives, and hormone replacement therapy
- Previous history of thrombophlebitis

SOURCE: Data from Meyer & Schmidt (2015) and Fedullo & Yung (2015).

Table 12–8 Three Categories of Pulmonary Embolus Presentation

Category	Percentage of Patients	Presentation and Hemodynamics	Risk of Death
Massive PE	5%	Shock, syncope, cardiac arrest	High risk
Submassive PE	20%–25%	Normal blood pressure with right ventricular dysfunction	Increased risk
Usual	Majority	Normal blood pressure, no RV dysfunction	Low risk

SOURCE: Data from Piazza (2013).

Pathophysiology of Pulmonary Embolism

The severity of pulmonary embolism depends on the degree of obstruction and the location of the embolus. Pulmonary embolism creates changes in both pulmonary and cardiovascular function. A clot in the pulmonary vasculature creates dead space, may cause bronchoconstriction, and leads to hypoxemia by complex mechanisms. Hemodynamic effects are related to acute pulmonary hypertension and possibly right-heart failure (Simko & Culleiton, 2013). Figure 12–4 illustrates some of the major pathophysiologic events associated with pulmonary embolism.

Signs and Symptoms of Pulmonary Embolism

Pulmonary embolism often is not easy to recognize or diagnose, particularly when the patient's health status is deteriorating rapidly. Although the presenting manifestations of PE are frequently described in general terms (see Box 12–6), not all episodes of pulmonary embolism present in the same way.

Diagnosis

Diagnosis of pulmonary embolism is frequently not made until autopsy. Patients may have no symptoms, or the presenting manifestations may not be recognized or may be misinterpreted. Diagnostic testing generally is initiated based on clinical suspicion, such as a positive history and presenting signs and symptoms. Prompt recognition is important: 30% of patients will die if not treated versus only 8% mortality with appropriate therapy (Tarbox & Swaroop, 2013). Tests are recommended to aid in diagnosis.

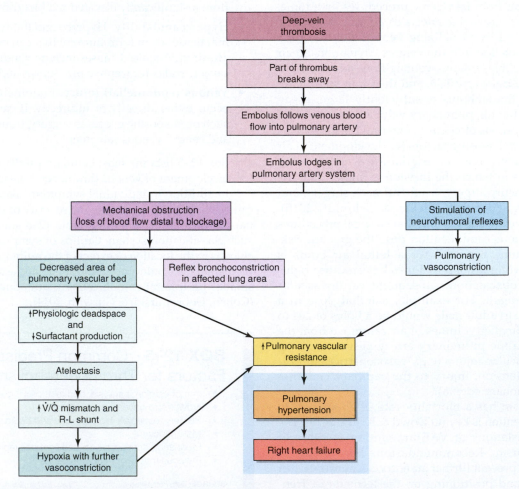

Figure 12–4 Pathophysiology of pulmonary embolus.

Clinical Probability Assessment Given the difficulty of diagnosing pulmonary embolus, screening tools have been developed to estimate the probability of PE in presenting patients. Two such tools are the Wells Score and the Geneva Score (York, Kane, Smith, & Minton, 2015). These pretests categorize patient risk as low, intermediate, or high probability. The scores are based on presence or past medical history of DVT or PE, immobility or surgery, cancer, vital signs, and other parameters. The higher the score, the higher the probability of pulmonary embolus. Based on the risk stratification, further diagnostic testing may be warranted or excluded.

D-dimer D-dimer is a type of fibrin degradation product (i.e., a product of fibrin clot breakdown) that increases in the blood following any thrombotic event in the body such as pulmonary embolus, venous thrombosis, or myocardial infarction. In patients with low or moderate pretest scores, a D-dimer assay may be performed to eliminate pulmonary embolism as a diagnosis. A normal (negative) D-dimer level strongly suggests that the patient has no detectable thrombolytic activity present in the body and therefore no active pulmonary embolism (Komissarova, Chong, Frey, & Sundaram, 2013). An elevated (positive) D-dimer level is indicative of the presence of thrombolytic activity, but the test is too nonspecific to indicate a precise location, and for this reason a normal D-dimer is not helpful in excluding the diagnosis of PE. This rationale limiting D-dimer as a diagnostic tool is because in patients with moderate to high clinical suspicion for PE and a normal D-dimer, the prevalence of PE is 5% or more (Kearon et al., 2006; Righini et al., 2008; Stein et. al., 2004; Stein et al., 2006). Because the D-dimer lacks specificity, it should not be used for patients with a high-risk Wells score (Huisman & Klok, 2013).

Contrast-enhanced CT Angiogram Technological developments in recent years have changed the recommendations for diagnostic testing for pulmonary embolism. A contrast-enhanced, spiral computed tomographic angiogram (also known as **CT angiography**) has now become the more common diagnostic test for patients with high suspicion of PE (Fedullo & Yung, 2015). The spiral CT angiography has advantages over the traditional $\dot{V}/\dot{Q}$ scan as a rapid test that may reveal other pulmonary pathology. Limitations of the contrast-enhanced CT angiogram include inability to detect very small emboli (subsegmental) in the lung periphery. Use is also limited in patients with contrast dye allergy, renal insufficiency, and an increasing appreciation for the significant radiation dose (Meyer & Schmidt, 2015).

Ventilation–perfusion ($\dot{V}/\dot{Q}$) Scan The $\dot{V}/\dot{Q}$ scan is a two-part test that provides information on ventilation and perfusion relationships in areas of the lung. An intermediate- or high-probability abnormal $\dot{V}/\dot{Q}$ scan result supports a diagnosis of PE but is not specific to this diagnosis. The $\dot{V}/\dot{Q}$ scan is a diagnostic option for patients with allergy to IV contrast and renal insufficiency when spiral CT scan is contraindicated. It also involves less radiation exposure and may be preferred with pregnant patients (Meyer & Schmidt, 2015).

Magnetic Resonance Imaging Gadolinium-enhanced magnetic resonance imaging (MRI) is a newer option for diagnosis of pulmonary embolism. The accuracy of the pulmonary MRI is similar to that of CT angiography. It involves less radiation exposure and presents an option for patients with contrast dye allergy (Fedullo & Yung, 2015).

Compression Ultrasound Evaluating the patient for deep vein thrombosis (DVT) is important because of the high percentage of PE attributed to DVT; thus, ultrasound of both lower extremities may be ordered to rule it out. This test is often performed if CT angiography or a $\dot{V}/\dot{Q}$ scan is nondiagnostic. A positive result suspicious of DVT occurs when the vein cannot be fully compressed. This test, in conjunction with unilateral lower extremity swelling, tenderness, redness, and a positive Homans sign, is strongly suggestive of DVT.

Chest Radiography Chest x-rays are frequently normal early in the course of a pulmonary embolus, and, depending on the severity of the PE, they may remain normal. Atelectasis, **pleural effusion** (abnormal accumulation of fluid in the intrapleural space), or pulmonary tissue abnormalities may be noted but are nonspecific for PE. For these reasons, chest radiographs are not considered a good diagnostic tool but may be helpful when accompanied by other tests. A chest radiograph is also useful in identifying other pathologies that may cause symptoms that are similar to pulmonary embolism (Fedullo & Yung, 2015).

Echocardiogram An echocardiogram may play a valuable role in the evaluation of right-heart function for patients with more severe disease, especially if they are too unstable to transport for other tests (Meyer & Schmidt, 2015). Abnormalities may include right ventricular (RV) dilation, decreased RV function, and tricuspid regurgitation (Thompson & Hales, 2015). Echocardiography may also provide information about other cardiopulmonary abnormalities when the diagnosis of PE in acutely ill patients is not clear (Fedullo & Yung, 2015).

Electrocardiograms Electrocardiograms (ECGs) are often normal and may indicate only sinus tachycardia. The ECG may show certain abnormalities such as ST/T wave changes that indicate right-heart strain and can be used to support a diagnosis of, but cannot specifically diagnose, PE (York et al., 2015).

Pulmonary Angiography   The angiogram has long been considered the definitive diagnostic test for pulmonary embolus because it can pinpoint the blockage(s). However, angiography is invasive, carries risks from contrast dye and bleeding, and has been largely replaced by newer technology (Meyer & Schmidt, 2015).

Arterial Blood Gases   Abnormal arterial blood gas (ABG) results typical of PE (low PaO_2 and $PaCO_2$, and elevated PaO_2) are nonspecific for pulmonary embolus. A normal PaO_2 cannot exclude the patient from a diagnosis of PE. However, ABG results are helpful in assessing the level of hypoxia present. Hypocapnia is typically seen with PE, except in patients with preexisting lung disease or on controlled mechanical ventilation (Meyer & Schmidt, 2015).

Management of Pulmonary Embolism

Proper management of pulmonary embolism is contingent on its diagnosis, which is often difficult. Table 12–9 summarizes the major medical options for treating pulmonary embolism.

Nursing Considerations   Prevention of pulmonary embolism is a priority of nursing care in all high-risk patients. Because DVT is the major cause of PE, management should center on interventions to prevent DVT. Preventive measures include early ambulation, anticoagulant therapy, antiembolism stockings, compression boots, elevation of the injured leg above heart level, and frequent assessment of the leg for signs of DVT. There may be no signs or symptoms; however, when present, they may include unilateral leg swelling, pain or tenderness, or cramping.

Pulmonary embolism is a potential complication (PC) rather than a nursing diagnosis; therefore, it requires a collaborative practice model. This means that, in addition to addressing any appropriate nursing diagnoses, the nurse also focuses on administering treatments as ordered by the healthcare provider monitoring for status changes, as well as monitoring for the therapeutic and nontherapeutic effects of prescribed treatments.

Table 12–9 Summary of Medical Treatment Options for Pulmonary Embolism

Medical Therapy	Treatment and Comments
General	Hospitalization recommended for anyone suspected of pulmonary embolism; consideration of outpatient treatment possible for select, low-risk patients Oxygen therapy and airway management (as required) Management of shock (as required)

Anticoagulant therapy	Time of initiation: immediately when PE is suspected while patients are awaiting testing
	Goal of treatment: rapid anticoagulation (within 24 hours) to prevent the formation of additional clot or additional PE
	Major risks: bleeding and heparin-induced thrombocytopenia
	Type
	• Heparin (either unfractionated heparin [UH] or low molecular weight heparin [LMWH])
	    Usually administered for 5 to 6 days; discontinued when international normalized ratio [INR] has been therapeutic for 2 consecutive days
	    LMWH may be ordered for home management (subcutaneously); caution with renal insufficiency
	• Unfractionated heparin (UH)
	    May be preferred for patients with renal dysfunction or obesity, who are unstable, or in a situation requiring rapid reversal
	    Loading dose followed by continuous IV drip
	    Use sliding-scale dose based on activated partial thromboplastin time (aPTT)
	    Draw aPTT every 6 hours
	• Low-molecular-weight heparin (LMWH)
	    Routine lab monitoring may not be required; may be indicated for patients with obesity, pregnancy, and renal dysfunction
	• Fondaparinux (Arixtra)
	    Routine lab monitoring may not be required
	    Lower risk for development of heparin-induced thrombocytopenia (HIT)
	    Caution in use with renal insufficiency
	• Warfarin
	    May also be initiated at same time as heparin therapy
	    Initiation may be delayed for high-acuity patients due to difficulty of reversal
	    Goal: maintain prothrombin time at INR 2–3
	    May be ordered for 3 to 6 months or indefinitely

Vena cava filter	Indications: situations in which patients cannot be anticoagulated (e.g., GI bleeding); major bleeding while on anticoagulation; recurrent PE on therapy Recent advancement: temporary removable filters
Thrombolytic therapy	Indication: circulatory collapse due to massive PE Risks: bleeding, especially intracranial hemorrhage

Embolectomy	Catheter embolectomy
	    Indication: massive PE with shock, thrombolytic therapy contraindicated
	Surgical embolectomy
	    Indication: massive PE with shock
	    If emergency thrombolytic therapy not successful, thrombolytic therapy contraindicated; requires cardiopulmonary bypass

SOURCE: Data from Meyer & Schmidt (2015) and Fedullo & Yung (2015).

The following interventions are appropriate for pulmonary embolism (not including potential interventions unique to air or fat embolism):

- Monitor for signs and symptoms of PE.
- Initiate shock protocols if manifestations of PE develop.
- Initiate O_2 therapy and monitor SpO_2 or SaO_2.
- Monitor labs: ABG, CBC, electrolytes, and BUN.

- Initiate thrombolytic therapy as ordered.
- Initiate and monitor heparin therapy as ordered following thrombolytic therapy.
- Monitor clotting times.
- Monitor closely for abnormal bleeding when the patient is receiving thrombolytics or anticoagulant therapy.

Section Four Review

1. Which type of embolism manifests as dyspnea, tachypnea, neurological symptoms, and petechiae?
   - A. Venous air
   - B. Amniotic
   - C. Thrombus
   - D. Fat

2. What is the most common predisposing factor for development of thromboembolism?
   - A. Immobility
   - B. Postsurgery status
   - C. Malignancy
   - D. Coronary artery disease

3. What is a common sign or symptom of PE?
   - A. Rhonchi
   - B. Pneumothorax
   - C. Dyspnea
   - D. Bradycardia

4. What is the major initial treatment for PE?
   - A. Thrombolytic therapy
   - B. Surgical embolectomy
   - C. Oxygen therapy
   - D. Anticoagulant therapy

Answers: 1. D, 2. A, 3. C, 4. D

Section Five: Acute Respiratory Infections

The lower respiratory tract is normally sterile. When the lung is exposed to pathogens, immune defenses are typically sufficient to resist infection. When host defenses are overwhelmed, microorganisms that gain access to the lung may cause infection, such as bronchitis or pneumonia.

Pneumonia

Pneumonia poses a serious health threat in the United States. It is a leading cause of death from infection and, combined with influenza, is the eighth most common cause of death (Heron, 2015).

Classification   Traditionally, pneumonia was classified according to the patient's location when the infection was contracted—for example, at home in the community (community acquired) or in the hospital (healthcare-associated). The typical microorganisms in these two categories were sufficiently different that antibiotic recommendations could be made based on the most likely pathogens. The categories were useful in guiding early and appropriate antibiotic therapy.

In recent years, it has been recognized that patient location and exposure have become more complex. Patients may not be hospitalized, yet they may be exposed to healthcare environments such as long-term care facilities or outpatient treatment centers. Potential organisms in these settings are different from community-acquired organisms in that they more closely resemble hospital bacteria and are often multidrug resistant. Within the hospital, the distinction is also made between patients on mechanical ventilation (ventilator-associated pneumonia) and nonventilated patients. New terminology has been developed to better describe categories of pneumonia (Table 12–10).

Microbiology and Pathogenesis   The type of pathogen responsible for pneumonia varies somewhat by the location of the exposure. For example, in the United States the typical community-acquired pneumonia (CAP) is most likely to be caused by *Streptococcus pneumoniae (pneumococcus)*. The incidence of pneumococcal pneumonia appears to be decreasing, however, attributed to increased use of the pneumococcal vaccine (Musher & Thorner, 2014). Other common community-acquired pathogens include *S. aureus* and *H. influenzae*. Atypical CAP pathogens include *Legionella, Mycoplasma pneumoniae*, and others. *S. pneumoniae* infection can be particularly severe and is the leading cause of severe pneumonia requiring admission to ICU (Wunderink & Waterer, 2014). Gram-negative organisms, although less common, can be the cause of pneumonia in certain high-risk patients, such as those with underlying lung disease (e.g., COPD and cystic fibrosis) and those receiving steroid treatment (Musher & Thorner, 2014). The common pathogens associated with VAP include *P. aeruginosa, S. aureus, Acinetobacter, Enterobacter*, and others (Kalanuria, Zai, & Mirski, 2014).

The spread of antibiotic-resistant strains of bacteria is a growing concern in the treatment of both community- and healthcare-associated pneumonia. The occurrence of

Table 12–10 Classifications of Pneumonia

Pneumonia Categories	Description
Hospital-acquired (nosocomial) pneumonia (HAP)	Develops 48 hours or more after admission to the hospital and was not incubating prior to admission Highest increase in morbidity or mortality of all healthcare-associated infections Increases length of hospital stay Highest incidence = ICU setting while on mechanical ventilation (see VAP)
Ventilator-associated pneumonia (VAP)	A subtype of HAP (American Thoracic Society and the Infectious Diseases Society of America, 2005) and more recently a subtype of ventilator-associated events (Centers for Disease Control & Prevention, n.d.) Develops at least 48 hours after intubation for mechanical ventilation and was not incubating prior to intubation Highest risk within first 5 days on mechanical ventilation Risk for developing pneumonia is 6 to 20 times greater in ventilated patients than in other hospitalized patients.
Healthcare-associated pneumonia (HCAP)	Pneumonia that occurs in a nonhospitalized patient who has the following risk factors: • Resident of long-term care facility • Hospitalized within 90 days • Long-term hemodialysis • Home infusion, chemotherapy, or wound care within previous 30 days
Community-acquired pneumonia (CAP)	Pneumonia present on admission in a patient not previously hospitalized or in outpatient treatment

SOURCE: Data from American Thoracic Society and the Infectious Diseases Society of America (2005), Magill et al. (2013), and Wunderink & Waterer (2015).

methicillin-resistant *S. aureus* (MRSA) pneumonia is on the increase. MRSA was previously only a healthcare-associated infection; however, a separate strain of community-acquired MRSA is now seen more frequently (Wunderink & Waterer, 2014). In the high-acuity hospital environment, MRSA pneumonia increases the risk of septic shock and death (Marrie & File, 2015). MRSA and MSSA (methicillin-susceptible *S. aureus*) are both necrotizing infections that cause destruction of lung tissue, abscesses, and **empyema** (abnormal accumulation of purulent fluid in the intrapleural space) (Strange, 2015) and are associated with increased mortality (Marrie & File, 2015).

To cause infection, organisms must gain access to the lung and overwhelm the defense mechanisms. Patients can become exposed to pathogens in a number of ways, including aspiration of oral flora or gastric contents (microaspiration or large volume), airborne spread, direct inoculation (e.g., via endotracheal tube), through the bloodstream, or spread from adjacent infections (e.g., abscess). Additional factors influence the incidence and severity of pneumonia. Older adults are particularly vulnerable to viral infection, as are immunocompromised patients (Wunderink & Waterer, 2015). Underlying chronic conditions (comorbidities) such as COPD and heart disease, as well as smoking and alcohol abuse, medications such as proton pump inhibitors and steroids, and poor dental hygiene are also risk factors (Remington & Sligl, 2014).

Clinical Presentation The classic signs and symptoms associated with pneumonia include acute onset of cough, fever, chills, purulent sputum, pleuritic chest pain, shortness of breath, and abnormal chest radiograph (Wunderink & Waterer, 2014). There is considerable variation in presentation, however, depending on the infecting pathogen and host factors. Older adults may present with fewer symptoms than younger patients (Marrie, 2015). A category of infections called atypical pneumonias (e.g., *Legionella*) may have a gradual onset over days, with fever, headache, gastrointestinal symptoms, and dry cough.

The severity of pneumonia varies greatly, as does the clinical presentation, impacting the decision of where to treat the patient (e.g., outpatient, general ward, ICU).

Patients with mild disease are frequently treated as outpatients with antibiotic regimens geared toward likely community-acquired pathogens. More serious symptoms or risk factors require hospital admission. Predicting which patients will need high-acuity care or are at risk of deterioration has proven to be challenging. Patients with severe CAP who are hypoxic and require intravenous antibiotics should be admitted to an ICU or high-acuity monitoring unit. The 2007 IDSA/ATS consensus guidelines identified two major criteria for direct admission to an ICU: septic shock requiring vasopressor support and requirement for mechanical ventilation (Mandell et al., 2007). The presence of either criteria requires ICU care. Pneumonia scoring systems have been developed to aid in accurate prediction of the site where patients should be treated (Mandell & Wunderink, 2015; Wunderink & Waterer, 2014).

The CURB-65 is one example of a simple guide for evaluating the severity of CAP. Other, more complex sets of criteria are available to aid in determining if the patient needs ICU admission, such as the Severe Community Acquired Pneumonia (SCAP) score, and the Pneumonia Severity Index (PSI) (Mandel & Wunderink, 2015; Sligl & Marrie, 2013; Yandiola et al., 2009). The CURB-65 criteria include five risk factors: confusion, urea nitrogen, respiratory rate, blood pressure, and age. Each criterion has a value of one point. The higher the score, the more severe the pneumonia. A score of 4 or greater is associated with increased mortality and hospitalization, and possible ICU admission should be considered. A P/F ratio of less than 250, low albumin, and multilobar chest radiograph involvement are also sometimes included in severe pneumonia criteria (Mandell et al., 2007; Mandell & Wunderink, 2015). Research is ongoing to develop serum biomarkers to aid in determining the severity of the disease (Wunderink & Waterer, 2015). Table 12–11 lists the CURB-65 criteria, which can be used to quickly evaluate the need for hospitalization and possible ICU (Sligl & Marrie, 2013).

Prevention of Pneumonia Prevention strategies aimed at decreasing the incidence of community-acquired pneumonia include influenza and pneumococcal vaccines and smoking cessation. The Centers for Disease Control & Prevention

Table 12–11 CURB-65 Severe Pneumonia Criteria

Criteria	Points
C – Confusion; altered level of consciousness	1
U – BUN (greater than 19.6 mg/dL)	1
R – Respiratory rate (30 or greater breaths/minute)	1
B – Blood pressure (SBP less than 90; DBP less than 60)	1
65 – Patient age is 65 or older	1

Additional criteria to consider: serum albumin less than 3 g/dL; P/F ratio less than 250; multilobar pneumonia on radiograph.)

(CDC) guidelines now require assessment of vaccination status and administration of vaccine to appropriate patients while in the hospital. Smoking is a risk factor for pneumonia; patients should be encouraged to stop smoking and offered educational materials (Sligl & Marrie, 2013).

Diagnosis Diagnostic testing is done to determine whether a patient has pneumonia and to identify the causative organism. Diagnosis of pneumonia presents several challenges depending on the organism involved. In many cases, the pathogen is never identified. Chest x-rays are important for establishing a baseline to monitor changes and for helping differentiate pneumonia from other pulmonary disorders. The following diagnostic and laboratory tests are used in this setting to help identify the pathogen involved and the severity of disease (Table 12–12).

Treatment Extensive guidelines have been written on the treatment of pneumonia (Wunderink & Waterer, 2015). These guidelines recommend elements of initial care that include chest radiograph, blood cultures, assessment of oxygenation, screening for pneumococcal infection and influenza, smoking history and cessation information, and recommendations for admission and antibiotic regimens.

Early and appropriate antibiotic therapies are important elements to improve patient outcomes in pneumonia (Lee, Giesler, Gellad, & Fine, 2016). The Centers for Medicare & Medicaid Services (CMS) guidelines specify that antibiotics should be given within 6 hours of diagnosis. Other recent recommendations specify treatment as soon as possible rather than a particular time frame. Critically ill patients in shock are the exception to this rule; those patients should be treated within 1 hour of diagnosis to

Table 12–12 Diagnostic and Laboratory Tests for the Diagnosis of Pneumonia

Routine Tests	Special Diagnostic Tests
Chest radiograph	Bronchoscopy
Sputum culture and gram stain	Thoracentesis
Blood cultures	Lung biopsy
Complete blood count	Serology for antigens and antibodies
Pulse oximetry, arterial blood gas	Computed tomography scan
	Urinary antigen assays
	Polymerase chain reaction

SOURCE: Data from Bartlett (2015a) and Wunderink & Waterer (2014).

improve survival (Wunderink & Waterer, 2014). Initial antibiotics are selected to cover likely organisms and high-risk infections. When microbiologic sensitivity data from cultures is available, the antibiotics are changed or narrowed as necessary to cover the identified pathogens.

Approximately 40% of patients with bacterial pneumonia develop pleural effusions (parapneumonic effusions). Such pleural effusions may become infected and pose two problems: continued sepsis and the risk of pleural thickening from the fibrotic, inflammatory process. Large pleural effusions associated with pneumonia require sampling of the pleural fluid and drainage, usually with a chest tube, if the fluid is considered high risk for infection (Strange, 2015).

Aspiration Pneumonitis and Aspiration Pneumonia

Aspiration plays a particularly important role as a complication of high-acuity illnesses; thus it is presented here in greater detail. Aspiration, the entry of oral secretions or gastric contents into the lower respiratory tract, is the cause of CAP in up to 15% of all cases (Prather et al., 2014) and causes two different aspiration syndromes: aspiration pneumonitis and aspiration pneumonia.

Aspiration Pneumonitis Aspiration of acidic gastric contents results in aspiration pneumonitis, an acute chemical lung injury. This injury is seen in states of decreased level of consciousness such as stroke, seizures, and drug overdose (Prather et al., 2014). Inflammation, not infection, results from aspiration as the acidic gastric juices trigger an inflammatory response that damages exposed airway tissues (Bartlett, 2015b).

Aspiration Pneumonia Aspiration pneumonia may result when oral secretions or colonized gastric secretions reach the lung. Gastric contents can become colonized with bacteria when the gastric pH is alkalinized (e.g., by acid-reducing medications or enteral feedings). Proton pump inhibitors are increasingly identified as a risk factor for aspiration pneumonia (DiBardino & Wunderink, 2015). It is estimated that 50% of healthy people aspirate small volumes of secretions while sleeping; however, because of effective lung-protective mechanisms, pneumonia does not normally occur. Pneumonia results when the volume of aspirate is greater, the aspirate contains pathogens, or the natural defenses are impaired.

Major risk factors for aspiration include decreased level of consciousness, an incompetent lower esophageal sphincter (e.g., gastroesophageal reflux disease [GERD]), elevated pressure or volume in the stomach, and neuromuscular diseases that alter glottic closure. Two additional risk factors are poor oral hygiene, which increases the bacterial load in oral secretions, and **dysphagia** (impaired swallowing) (DiBardino & Wunderink, 2015). The presence of tubes through the lower esophageal sphincter (LES), such as nasogastric or feeding tubes, prevents the LES from closing fully and may contribute to aspiration risk due to reflux of gastric contents. Anaerobic organisms, normally found in the oral cavity, are frequently implicated in aspiration pneumonia.

BOX 12–7 Clinical Features of Aspiration Syndromes

Aspiration Pneumonitis

- Acute onset:
  - Tachypnea
  - Dyspnea
  - Bronchospasm
  - Cyanosis
  - Cough
- Chest x-ray: Localized or diffuse opacities (ARDS)

Aspiration Pneumonia

- Presentation is that of bacterial pneumonias.

SOURCE: Data from Bartlett (2015a), DiBardino & Wunderink (2015), and Enfield & Sifri (2015).

These bacteria can cause necrosis and empyema and are typified by a putrid odor (Enfield & Sifri, 2015).

Clinical Manifestations of Aspiration   The exact clinical presentation depends on the type and volume of aspirate. The position of the patient at the time of aspiration will dictate where the pneumonia or pneumonitis develops (i.e., the part of the lung in which the aspirate settles). Box 12–7 lists some of the major clinical features of aspiration syndromes.

Prevention of Aspiration Syndromes   Reducing the incidence of aspiration requires a multidisciplinary approach (Quinn & Baker, 2015). In addition to identifying patients at risk, nurses must recognize signs of aspiration such as coughing, drooling, development of a hoarse voice, or gurgling sounds associated with eating (Macht, Wimbish, Bodine, & Moss, 2013). A witnessed aspiration event requires immediate airway suctioning (Bartlett, 2015b). Nurses must also be aware that some patients show no overt signs of aspiration; the only indication of an event may be oxygen desaturation, which may be obvious if the patient is wearing an SpO_2 monitor (Bartlett, 2015b). Assessment by a speech pathologist can identify measures such as positioning and food consistency to improve swallowing (Macht et al., 2013). Oral care in all at-risk patients reduces the incidence of aspiration pneumonia, as does elevation of the head of the bed at least 30 degrees (Quinn et al., 2014). Medications that can contribute to aspiration by impairing swallowing, such as sedatives and antipsychotics, should be avoided when possible (DiBardino & Wunderink, 2015).

Viral Pneumonias

When we think of pneumonia, we tend to focus on its bacterial forms. However, pneumonia caused by viruses, particularly the influenza virus, constitutes a significant percentage of pneumonia cases that occur each year, primarily during the winter season. With the development of improved testing for respiratory viruses, viral pneumonia is now more frequently recognized as a common etiology of community-acquired pneumonia (Wunderink & Waterer, 2015). Furthermore, emerging viral infections have the potential to become the world's next viral pandemics.

Influenza Viral Pneumonia   Viral pneumonia is a serious-to-severe complication of influenza, more commonly referred to as the flu. In 2013, more than 53,000 confirmed cases of influenza were documented, with 87% classified as influenza A viruses and 13% as influenza B viruses (Centers for Disease Control & Prevention, 2014). There are three types of influenza-related pneumonias:

- Primary viral pneumonia—caused by the influenza virus
- Secondary bacterial pneumonia—develops directly following influenza
- Mixed viral and bacterial pneumonia—concurrent infections

Primary viral pneumonia is a complication of influenza, usually type A. While it is the least common influenza-related pneumonia, it is the most severe and deadly of the three types.

Clinical Presentation and Diagnosis.   Primary viral pneumonia presents as flu that, rather than resolving after a few days, becomes progressively worse. The patient develops progressive dyspnea that begins several days after the onset of flu symptoms, a persistent fever, and eventual onset of cyanosis (Dolin, 2015). As with most pure viral infections, sputum is scanty but blood may be present due to sloughing of necrosed airway tissue. As the pneumonia progresses, the chest x-ray usually shows diffuse infiltrates that have a pattern similar to acute respiratory distress syndrome (ARDS). Older adults and patients with cardiac disease are at particular risk for primary viral pneumonia (Ramsey & Kumar, 2013). Diagnosis can be made on the basis of a confirmed influenza virus culture, the presence of antigens or elevated serum antibody titre, or by nucleic acid testing, especially the polymerase chain reaction (PCR) test (Marrie & File, 2015). Chest radiographic changes resemble pulmonary edema (Ramsey & Kumar, 2013).

Mixed viral and bacterial pneumonia is the most common complication of influenza. People with chronic respiratory or cardiac disease are at highest risk for developing the mixed type. The clinical presentation is one of a viral illness that improves, followed by a recurrence of fever, a cough, and progression to purulent sputum, more typical of bacterial pneumonia (Dolin, 2015). The chest x-ray appears patchier (more focal) than what is seen in primary viral pneumonia, a pattern more typical of bacterial pneumonia.

H1N1 Influenza Pneumonia   In April 2009, a novel form of the seasonal influenza—type A (H1N1)—was first detected. The virus is of swine origin and is believed to have originated in Mexico, rapidly spreading into the United States and internationally. As with many other seasonal influenza viruses, transmission is airborne, via large-particle droplets dispersed through coughing and sneezing. The incubation is short—1 to 7 days—and patients frequently report gastrointestinal symptoms of vomiting and diarrhea as well as respiratory symptoms (Ramsey & Kumar, 2013).

Risk factors for severe H1N1 pneumonia differ from those for seasonal influenza in that many patients are younger and previously healthy. Obesity and pregnancy have also emerged as risk factors. While most cases of H1N1 influenza are mild, severe respiratory failure can develop. In severe cases, chest radiographic changes resemble ARDS and patients require mechanical ventilation and aggressive oxygenation strategies (Napolitano, Angus, & Uyeki, 2014).

Prevention and Treatment   Given the potential for serious illness, widespread vaccination for influenza is recommended as a public health policy. Vaccination of healthcare workers is increasingly promoted to protect hospitalized patients (Nowalk, Lin, Raymund, Bialor, & Zimmerman, 2013). Although the prognosis for influenza pneumonia is poor, it has shown improvement with the advancement of antiviral drug therapy. Ideally, treatment with neuraminidase inhibitors, such as zanamivir (Relenza) or oseltamivir (Tamiflu), is initiated within 48 hours of symptom onset (Ramsey & Kumar, 2013). Other potential supportive therapies include those used for other etiologies of ARDS, such as prone positioning, extracorporeal membrane oxygenation (ECMO), and avoidance of fluid overload (Ramsey & Kumar, 2013).

Emerging Viral Infections   Historically, widespread outbreaks or pandemics of new or novel viral illnesses have caused unusually high mortality. Some of these new viruses have been found in other animal species but not in humans. Of particular concern is the development of viruses able to cross species and not only infect humans but also become transmissible via human-to-human contact. Two such viruses, H5N1 (avian) and SARS-CoV, have caused outbreaks in recent years. There is no vaccine or treatment for either virus.

Avian Influenza Pneumonia.   Worldwide, health organizations are closely monitoring the H5N1 virus as a potential pandemic virus. Currently few humans have contracted this virus, and the flu has developed primarily in humans with close direct contact with infected birds (Hui & Zumla, 2015). The concern is that while the H5N1 virus has bridged the species (human–bird) barrier, it will eventually mutate sufficiently to allow human-to-human transmission, thereby triggering rapid spread, as occurred with the SARS-CoV virus. Avian influenza can lead to viral pneumonia and has a poor prognosis and a high mortality rate. As with SARS-CoV, there is no vaccine or definitive treatment for avian influenza (Hui & Zumla, 2015).

Severe Acute Respiratory Syndrome (SARS).   **Severe acute respiratory syndrome (SARS)** was first described when it suddenly appeared in 2003 as an atypical pneumonia. The virus that causes SARS (SARS-CoV) is actually a novel form of coronavirus (CoV), which is a major cause of the common cold worldwide and usually affects the upper respiratory tract. The unique SARS-CoV is suspected to have originated as a nonhuman virus, possibly in bats and civet cats, that jumped to humans (Marrie & File, 2015). Fortunately, the SARS epidemic was short lived, lasting from November 2002 through May 2003, with 28 countries reporting a total of 8096 cases (McIntosh, 2015). Incidence is now low, and cases are isolated.

The world was caught unprepared for the sudden emergence of SARS; this is a good example of the potential seriousness of viral mutations that can spread not only quickly but lethally in pandemic proportions. The global outbreak was contained through the cooperation of multiple agencies. Lessons learned from SARS have application for other infectious diseases. These include the importance of public health preparation and response systems, strict implementation of infection control measures, and training of personnel (McIntosh, 2015).

Middle East Respiratory Syndrome.   Middle East respiratory syndrome (MERS) is another new coronavirus that appeared in 2012 in Saudi Arabia. By 2014, 688 cases had been reported with mortality rates of 35% to 50%. Thus, MERS appears to be less contagious but more lethal than SARS (Cunha & Opal, 2014).

Section Five Review

1. Which statement is correct regarding MRSA pneumonia in high-acuity clients?
   A. It causes a chronic, low-level infection.
   B. It increases the risk for death and septic shock.
   C. It has a low mortality risk.
   D. About 50% of cases require hospitalization.

2. What are the risk factors for aspiration? (Select all that apply.)
   A. Incompetent lower esophageal sphincter
   B. Age greater than 65 years
   C. Decreased level of consciousness
   D. Elevated gastric pressure
   E. Male gender

3. According to the CURB-65 severity-of-CAP criteria, which value is considered a risk factor?
   A. BUN of 15 mg/dL
   B. Hemoglobin of 9.8 mg/dL
   C. Respiratory rate of 28 breaths/min
   D. Systolic BP of 85 mmHg

4. Viral pneumonia typically presents in which way?
   A. Productive cough with thick, purulent sputum
   B. Progressive dyspnea and persistent fever
   C. Pleuritis and copious sputum
   D. Night sweats and harsh dry cough

Answers: 1. B, 2. (A, C, D), 3. D, 4. B

Section Six: Thoracic Surgery and Chest Tubes

The term *thoracic surgery* applies to procedures on the structures within the chest: heart, lungs, esophagus, and the five great vessels (superior vena cava, inferior vena cava, pulmonary artery, pulmonary vein, aorta). This section focuses on surgery involving the lungs. Disorders commonly treated with thoracic surgery include lung cancer, emphysema, localized infection of the lung and pleura (e.g., abscess, empyema), injuries, lung transplantation, and chest wall deformities.

Surgical entry into the thorax is called a thoracotomy. Thoracic surgery for lung resection is categorized by the amount of lung tissue removed, as follows:

- **Pneumonectomy**–removal of one entire lung and creation of a stump (the sutured end of a main bronchus)
- Removal of smaller portions of the lung:
  - **Lobectomy**–removal of one or more lobes of the lung
  - **Segmentectomy**–removal of one or more portions (segments) of a lobe
  - **Wedge resection**–removal of a small, wedge-shaped section of the peripheral portion of the lung

Pneumonectomy

Pneumonectomy is an old procedure dating back to 1931, when it was performed for traumatic injury. Today pneumonectomy is used primarily in the treatment of lung cancer. Despite surgical improvements, pneumonectomy remains a high-risk procedure, with mortality estimates of 2% to 12% for elective surgery but significantly higher rates when performed in an emergent situation such as trauma (Kopec & Irwin, 2015).

In the pneumonectomy procedure, the lung and vessels are removed. When thoracotomy is performed, opening the chest wall breaks the integrity of the negative pleural space; thus, the lung on the thoracotomy side collapses. Postoperatively, the cavity fills with serosanguineous fluid and, eventually, fibrotic tissue. Because there is no remaining lung to expand, a chest tube is not required; however, one may be placed to detect postoperative bleeding.

Potential complications associated with pneumonectomy include vocal cord dysfunction (nerve injury during the procedure), atrial arrhythmias, pulmonary edema, bronchopleural fistula and empyema resulting from the breakdown of the stump suture line, and postpneumonectomy syndrome. Pulmonary edema may result from the dramatic change in hemodynamics as the entire blood volume is directed through the pulmonary vessels of the remaining lung. Postpneumonectomy syndrome is a tracheal obstruction caused by abnormal shifting of the intrathoracic structures.

Thoracic Incisions

Thoracotomy incisions used in thoracic procedures vary, depending on the size and area to be resected. Posterolateral incisions extend from the scapula/spine to the anterior axillary line. This traditional incision allows extensive view of the chest cavity. Other approaches include anterior, median sternotomy (used in cardiac surgery) and the "clamshell" incision, used primarily in bilateral lung transplantation (Nason, Maddaus, & Luketich, 2014).

Video-assisted Thoracoscopic Surgery Video-assisted thoracoscopic surgery (VATS) is the thoracic equivalent of minimally invasive laparoscopic abdominal surgery. Performed with a scope and small incisions, VATS is used for both diagnostic and therapeutic procedures. Common diagnostic procedures in which VATS is used include sampling of pleural effusions and biopsy of lung tissue, nodules, and mediastinal nodes. VATS is also used to treat persistent pleural effusions and repair pneumothorax, as well as for lung resections. Advantages cited for the VATS procedure versus open thoracotomy include decreased pain, more rapid recovery of pulmonary function, and improved functional status postoperatively (Nason et al., 2014).

Postthoracic Surgery Management

Two important considerations for postsurgery management are the common issues of pain management and postoperative pulmonary hygiene to prevent complications.

Pain Management Postthoracic surgical pain is significant due to retraction of the ribs and, in some cases, rib dissection, muscle dissection, possible nerve injury, and chest tubes. Postoperative pain is controlled with patient-controlled analgesia (PCA) or epidural catheters. Pain control is especially important to prevent postoperative hypoventilation and impaired cough, which may result in atelectasis and respiratory failure.

Pulmonary Hygiene Optimizing pulmonary hygiene—always a concern after surgery—becomes an even greater priority following thoracic surgery. In addition to the incision and pain, these patients commonly have underlying lung disease. Assessment of preoperative function and sputum production are important to guide treatment and evaluate the effectiveness of therapy. Effective cough is essential for adequate airway clearance but causes pain. Pharmacologic control of pain must be balanced to avoid oversedation and respiratory depression.

Postthoracic surgery patients must be able to take a deep breath and generate an exhalation sufficiently strong to clear secretions. As described by Traver (1985) in a classic paper on airway clearance, two modifications of the standard cough may be helpful for patients with chest wall pain from the surgery. The first, the "cascade" cough, is a series of three to four coughs on one exhalation. Repeated several times, this technique moves peripheral secretions. Another modification is the "huff" cough, in which the patient coughs with the glottis open. This cough is a gentler maneuver and is effective for postoperative patients and patients with emphysema. Splinting the incisional area will also decrease pain with cough (Figure 12–5). An alternative splinting method—for example, for a lateral incision—is to use a folded towel wrapped around the chest. To splint, the patient crosses the hands and holds the end of the towel, pulling tighter during the cough. A modification for a

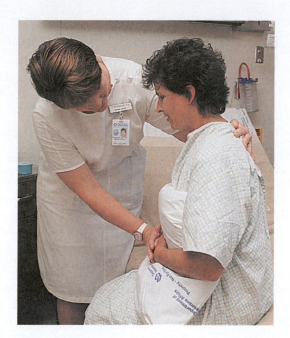

Figure 12–5 Splinting abdomen while coughing.

posterolateral incision is to use a folded sheet wrapped over the shoulder, across the incision in back, and under the arm. The ends of the sheet are pulled tightly with the cough to splint the incision.

Chest Drainage Management

The remainder of this section presents two cases that describe chest drainage principles and management.

Case 1: Nineteen-year-old TJ was thrown from his motorcycle onto the hood of a vehicle approaching from the opposite direction. He was stabilized at the scene by the rescue squad and rapidly transferred to a nearby hospital emergency department (ED). On arrival at the ED, a rapid assessment revealed the following: TJ was oriented and complaining of severe left chest pain. Chest contusions were noted on the left upper chest. He was tachypneic, with circumoral cyanosis noted. Chest auscultation revealed positive breath sounds on the right but negative breath sounds in the left upper lung field. A portable chest x-ray showed multiple left rib fractures and left hemopneumothorax. Preparations were made for immediate chest tube placement.

Case 2: MT, a 55-year-old woman, was admitted to the hospital with a diagnosis of exacerbation of COPD. She has been receiving intermittent positive pressure breathing (IPPB) therapy, oxygen at 2 L per nasal cannula, and a bronchodilator drug. This afternoon, MT suddenly developed sharp right-side chest pain and increased shortness of breath. During a rapid focused respiratory assessment, the nurse was unable to auscultate breath sounds in the right upper anterior lung field. A

portable chest x-ray showed a right upper-lobe pneumothorax. Chest drainage was initiated, with one chest tube inserted on the right side of MT's chest.

Chest Drainage Chest drainage is the active or passive removal of air or fluid from the intrapleural space of the lungs or from the mediastinal compartment. Chest drainage may be a short-term or intermittent therapy (e.g., aspiration of intrapleural air or fluid using a needle and syringe), or it may be relatively long-term therapy (e.g., treatment of pneumothorax or **hemothorax** [abnormal presence of blood in the intrapleural space] resulting from chest trauma).

Who Requires Chest Drainage? Both TJ and MT required chest drainage, but for different reasons. Chest drainage is used to treat thoracic problems that may be external or internal in origin. External origins include blunt chest trauma and traumatic or surgical entry into the intrapleural or mediastinal spaces that results in pneumothorax or hemothorax (Figure 12–6). Frequently both pneumothorax and hemothorax occur simultaneously (**hemopneumothorax**). TJ's case is an example of an external origin. Internal origins of pneumothorax include spontaneous rupture of a pulmonary **bleb** (a cyst that develops in the visceral pleura), procedural rupture of the visceral pleura, or barotrauma. Bleb rupture is most commonly found in patients with chronic lung diseases. Barotrauma-induced pneumothorax results from therapies that increase airway pressure and hyperinflate the alveoli. MT's case is an example of an internal origin. Common external and internal origins of pneumothorax are listed in Table 12–13. In addition to treating pneumo- or hemothorax, chest tubes may be inserted to drain severe pleural

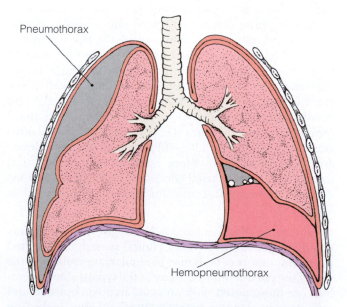

Figure 12–6 Pneumothorax and hemopneumothorax. Pneumothorax refers to air in the intrapleural space, and hemothorax refers to blood in the intrapleural space around the lung. A hemopneumothorax, such as depicted here, is a combined problem of having both air and blood in the intrapleural space.

Table 12–13 Origins of Pneumothorax

External Origins	Internal Origins
Thoracic surgery (e.g., open heart surgery)	Spontaneous bleb rupture
Penetrating chest trauma (e.g., knife or bullet)	Procedural rupture of visceral pleura (e.g., lung tissue biopsy)
Unintentional catheter entry into intrapleural space during central line placement	Barotrauma (e.g., mechanical ventilation, positive end expiratory pressure)
Chest contusion	

BOX 12–8 Summary of Common Clinical Findings of Pneumothorax

- Signs of chest trauma (external origin)
- Tachypnea, tachycardia (with possible onset of cardiac dysrhythmias)
- Shortness of breath
- Diminished or absent breath sounds on one side (or one area of lung)
- ABG: Decreased PaO_2 and SaO_2, respiratory alkalosis
- Sharp chest pain on one side of chest (may not be present initially)
- Signs of pneumothorax on chest radiograph, CT, or ultrasound

---

effusion or empyema if either condition is causing significant compression of lung tissue.

Pathogenesis of a Collapsed Lung The thorax and lungs exist as opposing forces—the thorax's natural state is expansion, whereas the lungs' natural state is collapsed. Normal lung inflation depends on the intactness of the two pleural linings, which act as a single unit because of a state of negative intrapleural pressure. Thus, as the thorax expands during inhalation, the lungs expand with it. Loss of negative intrapleural pressure, either of external or internal origin, results in the rapid collapse (atelectasis) of the affected lung tissue because the two pleura separate, allowing the opposing forces to come into play. The size of lung collapse depends on how much of the intrapleural space loses negative pressure. Table 12–14 summarizes the three major types of pneumothorax, including their pathophysiology and manifestations.

The size of the pneumothorax and the patient's symptoms are important considerations when determining whether chest drainage is required. A small pneumothorax without symptoms may be observed and not require drainage. Symptomatic patients or those with underlying lung disease will need either needle aspiration or chest tube insertion to manage the pneumothorax (Patel & McConville, 2015). Chest tube sizes vary from 10 to 40 French, the larger numbers indicating a larger diameter. Size selection depends on the indication for chest tube insertion. Traditional guidelines recommend small chest tubes (12F–24F) for air in the pleural space (pneumothorax), medium size (24F–36F) for pleural effusions, and large bore (36F–40F) for hemothorax (blood) and empyema (pus). More recent data indicate that smaller tubes can be used effectively for pleural effusions and are more comfortable for patients (Mahmood & Wahidi, 2013).

Common Clinical Findings Although TJ's case differs greatly from MT's in etiology, clinical presentation related to pneumothorax of both may be similar, depending on the size of the pneumothorax. Many of the typical clinical findings are those noted with an acute hypoxia episode and reflect normal compensatory mechanisms, including tachypnea, tachycardia, agitation, and confusion. If chest pain is present, shallow respirations with splinting may be noted. In addition, the presence of tachypnea is frequently associated with initial respiratory alkalosis. Box 12–8 provides a summary of common clinical findings.

Chest Tube Insertion The nurse frequently assists with insertion of chest tubes; hence, a brief description of necessary equipment and procedure is provided here. Equipment includes the following:

- Chest tube thoracotomy tray and drainage system
- Antiseptic solution
- Protective eyewear
- Local anesthetic (1% lidocaine)
- Sterile gowns, gloves, masks, caps, and drapes
- Chest tube (size dependent on indication)
- Suction source and tubing

Depending on the size of the pneumothorax and other circumstances, preparation for insertion may need to be rapid. It is important to prepare the patient for the procedure as thoroughly as possible based on the patient's condition. The nurse's role varies but often centers on obtaining (and possibly preparing) the necessary equipment, supporting the patient, and maintaining the patient in the appropriate position during the procedure. Box 12–9 summarizes common nursing activities in preparation for and during chest tube insertion.

The Procedure If a pneumothorax is present, the chest tube typically is inserted anteriorly at the level of the second intercostal space, which approximates the lung apex. If a hemothorax (or fluid) is present, the chest tube is typically inserted midaxillary at the fifth or sixth intercostal space to drain the base of the lung field (Kane et al., 2013). After the chest tube has been inserted, it is quickly connected to special extension tubing that joins with the collection chamber of the chest drainage system. The chest tube is then sutured to the patient to prevent unintentional removal. An occlusive dressing is applied (Figure 12–7). All connections are properly taped or banded (plastic strips tightly wrapped around connections) to prevent unintentional disconnection (Figure 12–8). The chest drainage system is placed and maintained below heart level at all times to ensure proper drainage. A chest x-ray is ordered immediately following the procedure to ensure correct tube placement.

Chest Drainage System Although many types of chest drainage systems are available, the most common is the

Table 12–14 Types of Pneumothorax

Type	Pathophysiology	Manifestations
(A) Spontaneous 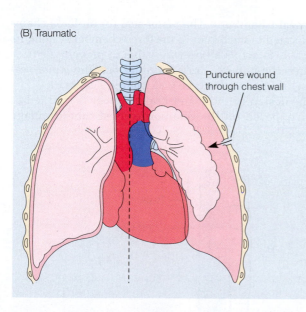	Rupture of a bleb on the lung surface allows air to enter pleural space from airways. • *Primary pneumothorax* affects previously healthy people. • *Secondary pneumothorax* affects people with preexisting lung disease (e.g., COPD).	• Abrupt onset • Pleuritic chest pain • Dyspnea, shortness of breath • Tachypnea, tachycardia • Unequal lung excursion • Decreased breath sounds and hyperresonant percussion tone on affected side
(B) Traumatic	Trauma to the chest wall or pleura disrupts the pleural membrane. • *Open* occurs with penetrating chest trauma that allows air from the environment to enter the pleural space. • *Closed* occurs with blunt trauma that allows air from the lung to enter the pleural space. • *Iatrogenic* involves laceration of visceral pleura during a procedure such as thoracentesis or central-line insertion.	• Pain • Dyspnea • Tachypnea, tachycardia • Decreased respiratory excursion • Absent breath sounds in affected area • Air movement through an open wound
(C) Tension 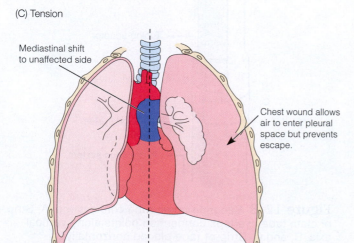	Air enters pleural space through chest wall or from airways but is unable to escape, resulting in rapid accumulation. Lung on affected side collapses. As intrapleural pressure increases, heart, great vessels, trachea, and esophagus shift toward the unaffected side.	• Hypotension, shock • Distended neck veins • Severe dyspnea • Tachypnea, tachycardia • Decreased respiratory excursion • Absent breath sounds on affected side • Tracheal deviation toward unaffected side

Image labels (A) Spontaneous: Normal lung; Pleural space

Image labels (B) Traumatic: Puncture wound through chest wall

Image labels (C) Tension: Mediastinal shift to unaffected side; Chest wound allows air to enter pleural space but prevents escape.

disposable self-contained system (Figure 12–9), sometimes referred to as a three-chamber system. It includes the collection, water-seal, and suction chambers. This unit essentially mimics the older three-bottle chest drainage systems; there are also one- and two-bottle systems (Figure 12–10).

Collection Chamber.   The collection chamber accepts air or fluid coming into the system through extension tubing directly attached to the patient's chest tube. The collection chamber is composed of several interconnected vertical towers that are marked in mL for ease of fluid volume measurement.

Water-seal Chamber.   The water-seal (or air-leak) chamber is located in the center of the three-chamber system. Its purpose is to act as a one-way valve to prevent air flow back into the patient. Prior to initial use, the water-seal chamber is filled with sterile water to the 2 cm mark.

The design of the water-seal chamber is simple but effective, based on the one-bottle chest tube drainage

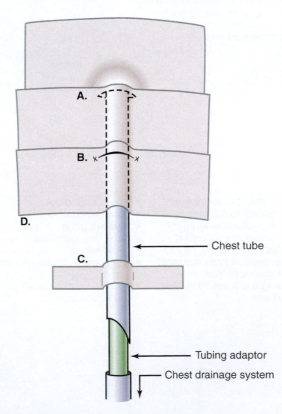

Figure 12–7 Securing the chest tube. A, Incision site. B, Tube sutured to patient. C, Tube stabilized with tape. D, Occlusive dressing.

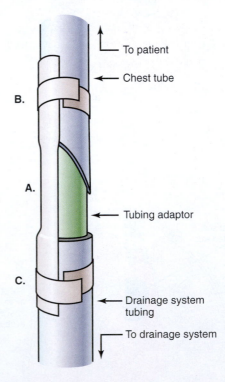

Figure 12–8 Securing chest tube connections. A, Strip of cloth tape overlaps connection points along vertical axis. B, and C, Strip of tape placed horizontally, overlapping vertical axis tape on both sides of connection.

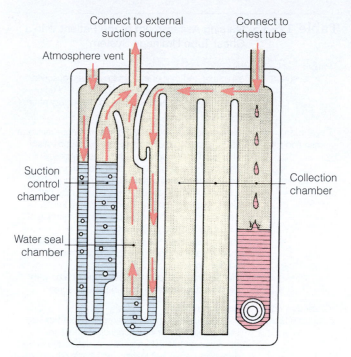

Figure 12–9 Disposable self-contained chest drainage system with wet suction control.

system is an effective method of managing simple pneumothorax.

Bubbling in the water-seal chamber indicates one of two things: (1) intermittent bubbling noted with pneumothorax suggests that air continues to be present in the intrapleural space, or (2) constant or vigorous bubbling may indicate an air leak in the system. If the chest tube drainage system is not attached to external suction, the water level in the water-seal chamber should move up and down with breathing. This is a normal phenomenon called tidaling.

Suction Chamber. The suction chamber regulates the amount of negative suction pressure being exerted on the intrapleural space. The amount of negative pressure is determined by the volume of water in the suction chamber. Typically, it is set at 20 cm H_2O in the adult. The suction chamber does not require attachment to external suction (e.g., wall suction) to work, but it is commonly added to make the system more effective. In the absence of external suction, the suction chamber does not bubble; however, if additional vacuum suction is used, continuous bubbling should be present. Vigorous bubbling in the suction chamber has no advantage and results in rapid evaporation, which requires more frequent refilling by the nurse. Gentle bubbling is all that is required.

Dry Chest Drainage Systems. Some chest drainage systems are "dry" in that they do not require water in the suction chamber. The amount of suction is regulated by a dial on the system and the wall suction. Depending on the design, this type of system may still require water in the water-seal chamber. Dry systems offer the advantage of easily adjusted levels of suction and are quiet (Kane et al., 2013).

Assessment of the Patient with a Chest Tube in Place
Assessing the patient with a chest tube includes assessing the patient and the chest tube and drainage system. In assessing the patient's status, vital signs and respiratory status are closely monitored, including chest auscultation and oxygenation status (e.g., level of consciousness, ABG, pulse oximetry [SpO_2], skin or mucous membrane coloring, and respiratory effort). Chest radiographs may be ordered to monitor the status of the pneumothorax. Chest

system. To understand how the water seal works, it may help to visualize a bottle filled with 2 cm (about 0.8 in.) of water (refer to Figure 12–10). The bottle is sealed with a tight lid with two holes punched into it. A long tube is inserted into the bottle through one of the holes, such that the distal tip is underwater (a water seal). The bottle is placed on the floor and the proximal end of the tube is kept at bed height. Air is drawn into the bottle through the tube because of negative gravity pull. As the air is pulled through the distal end of the tube, it bubbles through the water and escapes through the second hole in the lid. Air left in the bottle, however, cannot move back into the tube because of the presence of the water seal and negative gravity pull. Although it is no longer commonly used in the United States, the one-bottle

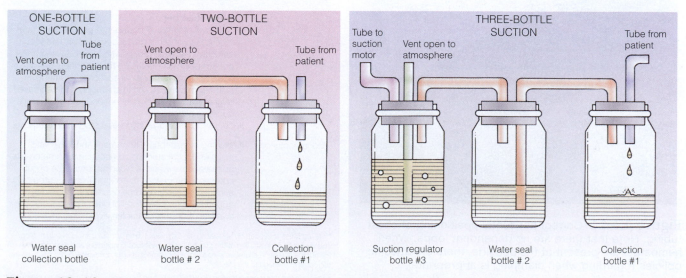

Figure 12–10 One-, two-, and three-bottle chest drainage or suction bottle systems.

tube–related pain is common and should be assessed frequently, with appropriate administration of analgesia.

Assessment of the chest tube and drainage system includes the dressing and site, position and patency of the extension tubing (Figure 12–11), type and amount of output draining into the collection chamber, and fluid levels and activities in the water-seal and suction chambers. Table 12–15 provides a summary of the assessment of the patient with a chest tube and drainage system.

Chest Tube Removal Nurses may assist with the procedure to remove chest tubes. Determining when a chest tube can be safely removed depends on the patient's requirement for chest drainage (e.g., pneumothorax, thoracic surgery). Box 12–10 outlines general guidelines for the decision to remove the tube.

Chest tube removal is a painful procedure. Premedication for anticipated pain is important and may be accomplished with a systemic narcotic, a local anesthetic patch, relaxation techniques, or ice packs (Muzzy & Butler, 2015). A sterile, occlusive dressing is applied as the chest tube is removed to prevent air entry into the pleural space (Patel & McConville, 2015).

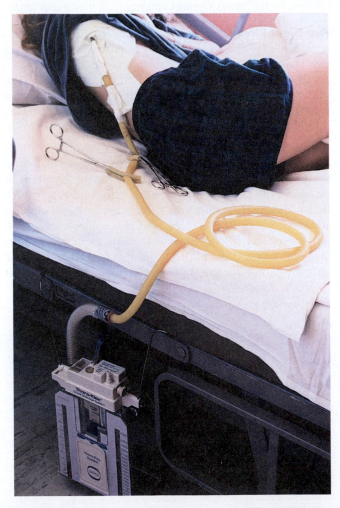

Figure 12–11 Correct horizontal positioning of chest tubing. Note that there are no dependent loops. When hemostats are present at the bedside, there are specific policies regarding when clamping is appropriate.

SOURCE: Ron May/Pearson Education, Inc.

Table 12–15 Nursing Assessment of the Patient with a Chest Tube Drainage System

Patient assessment	Vital signs Respiratory and oxygenation status (chest auscultation, level of consciousness, ABG, SpO_2, skin or mucous membrane coloring, and respiratory effort) Level of pain
Chest tube insertion site	Dressing should be occlusive, dry, and intact—reinforce as necessary (dressings may or may not be initially changed by the nurse based on hospital policy or physician or advanced practitioner orders). Note: Routine use of petroleum gauze around chest tube is no longer recommended due to the risk of skin maceration and loosening of suture knots. If dressing requires changing, assess appearance of tube insertion and suture sites. Monitor for excessive bleeding through the dressing. Palpate around dressing site for subcutaneous emphysema. If affected area is enlarging, mark edge of area with pen to further evaluate rate and size of spread.
Chest drainage system tube	**Extension tubing** Check all tubing connections to ensure that they are secured to avoid unintentional disconnection. Loop extension tubing horizontally on the bed to avoid excessive dependent looping, which may decrease drainage flow (see Figure 12–11). **Collection chamber** Routinely check blood or fluid output in the collection chamber. Assess volume and appearance (e.g., sanguineous, serosanguineous, serous, purulent). Be aware of expected volume of bleeding for the first 24 hours following surgery, and be alert for drainage above acceptable volume; a reverse appearance of drainage (serous → serosanguineous → sanguineous) is a potential hemorrhage complication. If clots are present, gently milking[a] the tubing will facilitate movement of clots into the collection chamber. Avoid stripping[b] the tubing. Routinely mark the volume on the outside of the collection chamber, indicating the time and date of the marking. **Water-seal chamber** Assess for the presence of abnormal (constant) bubbling as an indication of a system leak. Check water level to assure that it is at 2-cm level and refill if necessary. **Suction chamber** Check level of water in chamber to ensure that it is at 20 cm H_2O or other prescribed level and refill to prescribed level as required (to stop bubbling, temporarily pinch off the tubing that connects the drainage system to the external suction equipment). Check degree of bubbling in chamber, and decrease level of external suction as needed to create gentle bubbling action. For dry systems, verify suction level is set at ordered level.
Documentation	If charting by exception, document abnormal vital signs and respiratory or oxygenation parameter; site appearance; excessive bleeding; presence of subcutaneous emphysema; abnormal chest output, such as excessive volume or change in drainage appearance (e.g., reversal of drainage appearance, or other abnormal characteristics).

[a] *Milking* refers to repeatedly squeezing the extension tubing without using a pulling motion. This is usually done starting at the proximal end (chest tube connection) and working down toward the collection chamber to encourage movement of clots. Excessive or vigorous milking can result in damage to the pleura.

[b] *Stripping* is a vigorous squeezing or pulling motion on extension tubing to move an obstructing clot. Stripping can create excessive negative intrapleural pressure that damages the pleura.

BOX 12–10   Indications for Chest Tube Removal

- Patient status improved and stable
- Decreased chest tube drainage, usually less than 100 mL in 24 hours
- Air leak resolved
- Lung reinflated on chest x-ray and remains inflated without recurrent pneumothorax when system is on water seal

SOURCE: Data from Patel & McConville (2015).

Related Patient Potential Conditions   Potential complications (PC) may affect patients who require a chest tube, including the following:

- Anxiety
- Impairments in gas exchange and oxygenation
- Altered breathing and ventilation
- Pain
- Infection
- Bleeding

Section Six Review

1. A client with chest trauma has sustained a hemothorax, and preparations are made for chest tube placement. The chest tube will be inserted at which location?
   A. Anteriorly at level of second intercostal space
   B. Midaxillary at the fifth or sixth intercostal space
   C. Posterior-laterally at the second intercostal space
   D. Anteriorly at the fifth or sixth intercostal space

2. Internal-origin problems that may require chest tube insertion include which types of injury? (Select all that apply.)
   A. Barotrauma
   B. Penetrating chest trauma
   C. Procedural rupture of visceral pleura
   D. Chest contusion
   E. Bleb rupture

3. Pneumothorax is characterized by which common clinical findings? (Select all that apply.)
   A. Tachypnea
   B. Bradycardia
   C. Respiratory acidosis
   D. Shortness of breath
   E. Decreased PaO_2

4. What is the purpose of the water-seal chamber in a three-chamber chest drainage system?
   A. Facilitate drainage from the chest tube
   B. Prevent airflow back into the client
   C. Facilitate control of level of negative suction
   D. Prevent fluid from draining into the suction chamber

Answers: 1. B, 2. (A, C, E), 3. (A, D, E), 4. B

Section Seven: The Standard Respiratory Plan of Care

This section presents a standard respiratory plan of care that focuses on respiratory function. Patient outcomes reflect the relative nature of "normal" parameters as they apply to high-acuity patients, who often have chronic respiratory disorders in addition to the current acute health problem.

Three areas of potential concern for patients include the following complications:

- Breathing pattern and ventilation
- Gas exchange and oxygenation
- Airway clearance of secretions

Breathing Pattern and Ventilation

Problems with breathing pattern is characterized as inspiration and/or expiration that does not provide adequate ventilation (LeMone et al., 2015).

Expected Outcomes   Maintenance of an effective breathing pattern is evidenced by the following:

1. Normal respiratory rate, depth, and rhythm
2. ABGs and/or $PaCO_2$ within normal limits for patient
3. Bilateral chest excursion
4. No dyspnea

Independent Nursing Actions and Interventions

1. Assess for ineffective breathing patterns (report abnormals). Observe for changes in respiratory rate or rhythm:
   - Increasingly shallow, labored breathing
   - Increasing dyspnea
   - Increasingly abnormal $PaCO_2$, or pulse oximetry results
   - Increasingly irregular breathing pattern; abdominal paradox (abdomen moves in during inspiration rather than the normal pattern of expanding)
   - Increasing use of accessory muscles
2. Monitor for abdominal or chest pain.
3. Reduce level of abdominal or chest pain.

- Regularly administer pain medication, as ordered (observe for respiratory depression).
- Splint chest or abdomen with pillow or arms for coughing and deep-breathing exercises.

4. Encourage incentive spirometer use every 1 to 2 hours, as ordered.
5. Encourage slow, deep breaths (as appropriate).
6. Elevate head of bed to 45 degrees or level of comfort.
7. Turn (self or assisted) every two hours.
8. Plan activity and rest to meet patient's needs.

Impaired Oxygenation and Ventilation

Problems with oxygenation and ventilation are due to excessive or deficient oxygenation and/or the elimination of carbon dioxide at the alveolar–capillary membrane (LeMone et al., 2015).

Expected Outcomes Maintenance of normal gas exchange is evidenced by the following:

- ABGs within normal (acceptable) limits for patient
- Usual mental status
- Breathing unlabored (or baseline for patient)
- Respiratory rate 12 to 20/min (or usual rate for patient)
- Baseline heart rate for patient

Independent Nursing Actions and Interventions

1. Assess respiratory effort including rate, depth, and effort.
2. Assess lung sounds for decreased ventilation and adventitious sounds.
3. Assess for impaired gas exchange (report abnormals):
   - Change in mental status
     - Increased lethargy
     - Increased restlessness
     - Confusion
   - Accessory muscle use
   - Abnormal ABGs
     - Elevated $PaCO_2$ (above acceptable limits)
     - Decreased PaO_2 (below acceptable limits)
   - Decreasing pulse oximetry readings
4. Turn every 2 hours.
   - In patients with pneumonia or other unilateral pulmonary disorder, turning to the unaffected lung side may enhance oxygenation (improve $\dot{V}/\dot{Q}$ relationship), whereas turning to the affected side may cause oxygen desaturation.
5. Encourage incentive spirometer use every 1 to 2 hours.
6. Maintain a position of comfort, with the head of the bed elevated greater than 30 degrees (assist to tripod position, if desired).

7. Monitor effects of drug therapy, including oxygen therapy (refer to the "Related Pharmacotherapy: Agents Used for Treatment of Pulmonary Diseases" feature).
8. Encourage early ambulation.
9. Assist patient to sit up in chair.
10. Maintain supplemental oxygen as ordered to achieve oxygenation at desired level.
11. Schedule care and activity to allow rest periods to prevent fatigue.

Ineffective Ability to Clear Airway Secretions

Problems with reduced ability to clear airway secretions is common to patients with pneumonia and COPD and can be characterized as an inability to clear secretions or other impediments from the respiratory tract to maintain a clear airway (LeMone et al., 2015).

Expected Outcomes Maintenance of effective airway clearance is evidenced by the following:

- Normal or improved lung sounds
- Ability to generate effective cough and clear secretions
- Normal respiratory rate and depth

Independent Nursing Actions and Interventions

1. Assess for ineffective airway clearance:
   - Adventitious breath sounds
   - Ineffective cough
   - Increase in respiratory rate or depth
   - Color, viscosity, odor, and volume of secretions
   - Pulse oximetry or arterial blood gases
   - Complaint of dyspnea
2. Assist the patient to cough and deep-breathe every 1 to 2 hours.
   a. Place in optimal position (usually sitting)
   b. Use splinting with cough, if appropriate
   c. Alternate cough techniques (huff and cascade, assisted)
   d. Use incentive spirometer
3. Encourage fluid intake within appropriate limits for patient.
4. Perform tracheal suction as necessary.
5. Monitor for effects of drug therapy (expectorants, mucolytics; refer to "Related Pharmacotherapy: Agents Used for Treatment of Pulmonary Diseases" feature).
6. Monitor for and treat acute pain. Administer pain medications as needed.
7. Encourage self-care as tolerated.
8. Encourage activity and early ambulation.

Section Seven Review

1. Evaluation of the effectiveness of interventions to resolve a problem with breathing pattern and ventilation is best measured by which desired patient outcome?
   A. Usual mental status
   B. Normal or improved lung sounds
   C. Absent accessory muscle use
   D. Normal respiratory rate, depth, and rhythm

2. A client with right-sided pneumonia has impaired oxygenation and ventilation. Which position may enhance oxygenation?
   A. Any position of comfort
   B. Supine
   C. Side-lying on the unaffected side
   D. Side-lying on the affected side

3. Which assessments would suggest impaired oxygenation and ventilation? (Select all that apply.)
   A. Confusion
   B. Increased lethargy
   C. Decreased restlessness
   D. Increased PaO_2
   E. Decreased $PaCO_2$

4. Which nursing intervention would assist in maintaining effective clearance of airway secretions?
   A. Restricting fluids to 1 L/day
   B. Coughing and deep breathing every 1 to 2 hours
   C. Minimizing use of opioid analgesics
   D. Restricting activities

Answers: 1. D, 2. C, 3. (A, B, C), 4. B

Clinical Reasoning Checkpoint

Lilly T., 53 years old, is brought to the emergency department by the emergency squad. Lilly was reportedly driving home during an ice storm after eating dinner at a friend's house. Her vehicle went into a skid and crashed into a tree. She has multiple injuries; however, she was wearing a seatbelt. Lilly's medical history includes a 10-year history of severe COPD with cor pulmonale. Her social history is positive for a 30-year history of smoking between 1 and 1½ packs of cigarettes per day; she does not consume alcoholic beverages.

1. Explain the baseline arterial blood gas abnormalities you can anticipate on the patient's arrival at the ED, based on her history of COPD.

Clinical update: A rapid evaluation of Lilly's injuries shows a possible chest contusion, as bruising is noted on her right chest wall, where she likely hit the steering wheel. You auscultate her chest, finding no lung sounds in her right upper lobes. A portable chest x-ray confirms a right-sided pneumohemothorax. Chest tube insertion is ordered, and on completion of the procedure the tubing is attached to a chest drainage system that is connected to low wall suction.

2. Based on the fact that she has a pneumohemothorax, where will the patient's chest tube(s) be placed? Explain why.

3. The chest tubes have been inserted and are now connected to the drainage system. You are preparing to dress the tube insertion sites and stabilize the drainage tube system. (A) Describe the dressing that you will apply, (B) explain why you chose that type of dressing, and (C) discuss how you will stabilize the drainage tubes.

Clinical update: It is now day 1 postadmission. Lilly is in the trauma ICU. She has been breathing spontaneously, with oxygen at 28%. She responds appropriately to commands, although slowly. She has a nasogastric tube in place. You note that Lilly is becoming more tachypneic, her breathing appears more labored with each hour, she begins wheezing, and her mucous membranes appear cyanotic. A chest film is ordered, which shows diffuse opacities in her right lower lung field. It is decided that she may have an aspiration syndrome.

4. What risk factors does Lilly have for aspiration syndrome?

5. It is decided that Lilly has developed aspiration pneumonitis. Briefly explain how this form of aspiration differs from aspiration pneumonia.

Clinical update: Lilly's pulmonary status continues to deteriorate. An ABG is ordered (current O_2 level of FiO_2 of 0.28), showing pH 7.33, $PaCO_2$ 54 mmHg, PaO_2 78 mmHg, SaO_2 80%. Subsequently, her oxygen is increased to 0.4 (40%) with orders to observe her breathing carefully. After 1 hour, a second ABG is ordered, showing pH 7.32, $PaCO_2$ 51 mmHg, PaO_2 78 mmHg, SaO_2 80%. It is decided to intubate her and place her on ventilator support. Her FiO_2 is set at 0.5. An ABG is drawn 30 minutes after initiation of mechanical ventilation, showing pH 7.33, $PaCO_2$ 48 mmHg, PaO_2 76 mmHg, SaO_2 80%. A chest x-ray is ordered and shows bilateral diffuse infiltrates.

6. Examine the patient's ABG trends, focusing primarily on measures of oxygenation given her changes in FiO_2. What are your concerns at this time?

7. You decide that you want to estimate her degree of shunt by calculating her P/F ratio. You use her latest values, which are PaO_2 of 76 at an FiO_2 of 0.5. Calculate her P/F ratio and explain its significance.

8. Lilly's mechanical ventilator settings are reset based on a new diagnosis of ARDS. What are the general guidelines for tidal volume and PEEP? Include the rationale.

	Recommendations	Rationale
Tidal volume		
PEEP		

Chapter 12 Review

1. A client is admitted to the hospital with severe dyspnea and a productive cough. History reveals that the client has smoked one to two packages of cigarettes daily for the last 45 years and was diagnosed with COPD 10 years ago. A diagnosis of right lower lobe pneumonia is established. Based on this data, the nurse would plan care for a client who has which type of acute lung disorder?

   1. Restrictive disease
   2. Obstructive disease
   3. Respiratory failure
   4. Ventilatory failure

2. A client who has COPD is in a state of chronic respiratory insufficiency. Which assessment finding would the nurse attribute to that condition?

   1. BP 145/88
   2. Respiratory rate 10 breaths/min
   3. Temperature 99.8°F
   4. Pulse rate 63

3. A client who was severely injured in a motor vehicle crash 7 days ago has developed ARDS. The nurse has explained the concept of nonhydrostatic pulmonary edema to the client's family. Which statement by a family member would indicate understanding of this concept?

   1. Her disease has injured the membranes in her lung so that fluid is leaking into her lungs from the tiny blood vessels.
   2. The high blood pressure in the left side of her heart is forcing fluid from her blood vessels into her lung tissues.
   3. Infection in her lungs has harmed the small blood vessels there, causing blood to spill into the lung tissue.
   4. The small air sacs have been destroyed, which has allowed air to enter into the blood vessels.

4. A client whose left femur was surgically repaired 7 days ago has been on bedrest since surgery. This morning, the nurse is concerned with an acute change in the client's pulmonary status. Which factors of Virchow's triad would the nurse identify in this case, putting the client at risk for development of deep-vein thrombosis? (Select all that apply.)

   1. Venous stasis
   2. Increased temperature
   3. Hypercoagulability
   4. Venous injury
   5. Venous enlargement

5. A client who has had flu-like symptoms for the last few days presents in the emergency department with increasing shortness of breath. The client states that the cough "has become worse over the last few hours, and I am coughing up thick stuff." The nurse would ask assessment questions about which manifestations of post-influenza bacterial pneumonia? (Select all that apply.)

   1. Chills
   2. Chest pain
   3. Decreased temperature
   4. Dysphagia
   5. Diarrhea and vomiting

6. A client who has a right upper-lobe pneumothorax has had a chest tube for 2 days. While assessing the chest drainage system, the nurse notes continuous vigorous bubbling in the water-seal chamber. What should the nurse do?

   1. Decrease the amount of wall suction attached to the system
   2. Check all connections for a leak
   3. Check for subcutaneous emphysema
   4. Place the client on the left side

7. A client is hospitalized with chronic respiratory insufficiency. The nurse is developing a plan to address the problem of impaired oxygenation and ventilation. Which desired client outcome most accurately measures progress in addressing this problem?

   1. ABG within acceptable limits for client

   2. SaO_2 greater than 95%

   3. Usual mental status

   4. No cyanosis

8. A client is scheduled for chest tube removal today. How should the nurse plan to address pain control for this procedure?

   1. Place a warm, dry compress over the dressing site directly following the tube removal.

   2. Have the client take a deep breath and hold it during the procedure.

   3. Provide the client with a thorough explanation of the procedure before it begins.

   4. Administer a prn IV analgesic so that the drug's peak effect coincides with tube removal.

9. A client is at high risk for pulmonary embolus. The nurse would monitor this client for the development of which common clinical manifestations? (Select all that apply.)

   1. Dyspnea

   2. Chest pain

   3. Increased blood pressure

   4. Cough

   5. Hemoptysis

10. Brain natriuretic peptide (BNP) has been drawn to assess whether a client has heart failure or ARDS. What will the nurse expect the test to reveal if this client has heart failure rather than ARDS?

    1. No inflammatory cells

    2. High uric acid content

    3. High RBC content

    4. A value over than 100 pg/mL

Answers to questions found inside your textbook are available on the faculty resources site. Please consult with your instructor.

References

Albertson, T. E., Sutter, M. E., & Chan, A. L. (2015). The acute management of asthma. *Clinical Reviews in Allergy & Immunology, 48*(1), 114–125. doi:10.1007/s12016-014-8448-5

American Thoracic Society and the Infectious Diseases Society of America. (2005). Guidelines for the management of adults with hospital-acquired, ventilator-associated, and healthcare-associated pneumonia. *American Journal of Respiratory and Critical Care Medicine, 171*(4), 388–416.

ARDS Definition Task Force. (2012). Acute respiratory distress syndrome: The Berlin definition. *Journal of the American Medical Association, 307*(23), 2526–2533. doi:10.1001/jama.212.5669

ARDS Network. (2000). Ventilation with lower tidal volumes as compared with traditional tidal volumes for acute lung injury and the acute respiratory distress syndrome. *New England Journal of Medicine, 342*(18), 1301–1308.

Ashbaugh, D. G., Bigelow, D. B., Petty, T. L., & Levine, B. E. (1967). Acute respiratory distress in adults. *Lancet, 2*(7511), 319–323.

Bartlett, J. G. (2015a). *Diagnostic approach to community-acquired pneumonia in adults.* UpToDate. Retrieved December 28, 2016, from http://www.uptodate.com/contents/diagnostic-approach-to-community-acquired-pneumonia-in-adults?source=see_link

Bartlett, J. G. (2015b). *Aspiration pneumonia in adults.* UpToDate. Retrieved December 28, 2016, from http://www.uptodate.com/contents/aspiration-pneumonia-in-adults?source=search_result&search=aspiration+pneumonia&selectedTitle=1%7E150

Bernard, G. R., Artigas, A., Brigham, K. L., Carlet, J., Falke, K., Hudson, L., . . . Spragg, R. (1994). Report of the American-European consensus conference on acute respiratory distress syndrome: Definitions, mechanisms, relevant outcomes, and clinical trial coordination. Consensus Committee. *Journal of Critical Care, 9*(1), 72–81.

Burnham, E. L., Janssen, W. J., Riches, D. W., Moss, M., & Downey, G. P. (2014). The fibroproliferative response in acute respiratory distress syndrome: Mechanisms and clinical significance. *European Respiratory Journal, 43*(1), 276–285. doi:10.1183/09031936.00196412

Carlucci, M., Graf, N., Simmons, J. Q., & Corbridge, S. J. (2014). Effective management of ARDS. *The Nurse Practitioner, 39*(12), 35–40. doi:10.1097/01.NPR.0000454981.96541.e6

Centers for Disease Control & Prevention. (n.d.). Ventilator-associated pneumonia. Retrieved February 10, 2017, from https://www.cdc.gov/HAI/vap/vap.html

Centers for Disease Control & Prevention. (2014). Influenza activity—United States, 2013–14 season and composition of the 2014–15 influenza vaccines. *Morbidity and Mortality Weekly Report (MMWR), 63*(22), 483–490. Retrieved December 28, 2016, from http://www.cdc.gov/mmwr/preview/mmwrhtml/mm6322a2.htm

Chakir, J., Haj-salem, I., Gras, D., Joubert, P., Beaudoin, E. L., Biardel, S., . . . Laviolette, M. (2015). Effects of bronchial thermoplasty on airway smooth muscle and collagen deposition in asthma. *Annals of the American Thoracic Society, 12*(11), 1612–1618. doi:10.1513/AnnalsATS.201504-2080C

Chesnutt, A. N., & Matthay, M. A. (2015). Chapter 140: Acute respiratory distress syndrome: Pathogenesis. In M. A. Grippi, J. A. Elias, J. A. Fishman, R. M. Kotloff, A. I. Pack, R. M. Senior, & M. D. Siegel (Eds.), *Fishman's pulmonary diseases and disorders* (5th ed.). Retrieved December 27, 2016, from http://accessmedicine.mhmedical.com/content.aspx?bookid=1344&sectionid=81205381

Chiumello, D. A., Algieri, I., Brioni, M., & Babini, G. (2015). The prone position in the treatment of patients with ARDS: Problems and real utility. In D. Chiumello (Ed.), *Practical issues updates in anesthesia and intensive care* (pp. 1–13). Basel, Switzerland: Springer International Publishing. doi:10.1007/978-3-319-18066-3_1

Chudow, M., Carter, M., & Rumbak, M. (2015). Pharmacological treatments for acute respiratory distress syndrome. *AACN Advanced Critical Care, 26*(3), 185–191. doi:10.1097/NCI.0000000000000092

Chung, K. F., Wenzel, S. E., Brozek, J. L., Bush, A., Castro, M., Sterk, P. J., . . . Teague, W. G. (2014). International ERS/ATS guidelines on definition, evaluation and treatment of severe asthma. *European Respiratory Journal, 43*(2), 343–373.

Cohen, A. T., Dobromirski, M., & Gurwith, M. M. (2014). Managing pulmonary embolism from presentation to extended treatment. *Thrombosis Research, 133*(2), 139–148. doi:10.1016/j.thromres.2013.09.040

Cook, L. S. (2013). Infusion-related air embolism. *Journal of Infusion Nursing, 36*(1), 26–36. doi:10.1097/NAN.0b013e318279a804

Cunha, C. B., & Opal, S. M. (2014). Middle East respiratory syndrome (MERS): A new zoonotic viral pneumonia. *Virulence, 5*(6), 650–654. doi:10.4161/viru.32077

Curley, G. F., & Laffey, J. G. (2015). Future therapies for ARDS. *Intensive Care Medicine, 41*(2), 322–326. doi:10.1007/s00134-014-3578-z

Davidson, J. E., Harvey, M. A., Bemis-Dougherty, A., Smith, J. M., & Hopkins, R. O. (2013). Implementation of the Pain, Agitation, and Delirium Clinical Practice Guidelines and promoting patient mobility to prevent post-intensive care syndrome. *Critical Care Medicine, 41*(9), S136–S145. doi:10.1097/CCM.0b013e3182a24105

De Jong, A., Molinari, N., Sebbane, M., Prades, A., Futier, E., Jung, B., . . . Jaber, S. (2013). Feasibility and effectiveness of prone position in morbidly obese patients with ARDS: A case-control clinical study. *CHEST Journal, 143*(6), 1554–1561. doi:10.1378/chest.12-2115

Desai, S. V., McClave, S. A., & Rice, T. W. (2014). Nutrition in the ICU: An evidence-based approach. *CHEST Journal, 145*(5), 1148–1157. doi:10.1378/chest.13-1158

DiBardino, D. M., & Wunderink, R. G. (2015). Aspiration pneumonia: A review of modern trends. *Journal of Critical Care, 30*(1), 40–48. doi:10.1016/j.jcrc.2014.07.011

Dolin, R. (2015). *Clinical manifestations of seasonal influenza in adults.* UpToDate. Retrieved December 28, 2016, from http://www.uptodate.com/contents/clinical-manifestations-of-seasonal-influenza-in-adults?source=search_result&search=viral+pneumonia+adult&selectedTitle=3%7E48

Enfield, K. B., & Sifri, C. D. (2015). Chapter 127: Aspiration, empyema, lung abscesses, and anaerobic infections. In M. A. Grippi, J. A. Elias, J. A. Fishman, R. M. Kotloff, A. I. Pack, R. M. Senior, & M. D. Siegel (Eds.), *Fishman's Pulmonary Diseases and Disorders* (5th ed.). Retrieved December 28, 2016, from http://accessmedicine.mhmedical.com/content.aspx?bookid=1344&sectionid=81199180

Fanelli, V., Vlachou, A., Ghannadian, S., Simonetti, U., Slutsky, A. S., & Zhang, H. (2013). Acute respiratory distress syndrome: A new definition, current and future therapeutic options. *Journal of Thoracic Disease, 5*(3), 326–334.

Fedullo, P. F., & Yung G. L. (2015). Chapter 73: Pulmonary thromboembolic disease. In M. A. Grippi, J. A. Elias, J. A. Fishman, R. M. Kotloff, A. I. Pack, R. M. Senior, & M. D. Siegel (Eds.), *Fishman's pulmonary diseases and disorders* (5th ed.). Retrieved December 28, 2016, from http://accessmedicine.mhmedical.com/content.aspx?bookid=1344&sectionid=81192733

Flanders, S. A., & Zwerneman, K. (2014). Pulmonary embolism: Prevention, recognition, and treatment. *Nursing 2014 Critical Care, 9*(6), 14–20. doi:10.1097/01.CCN.0000455853.39879.c0

Fuller, B. M., Mohr, N. M., Drewry, A. M., & Carpenter, C. R. (2013). Lower tidal volume at initiation of mechanical ventilation may reduce progression to acute respiratory distress syndrome: A systematic review. *Critical Care, 17*(1), R11. doi:10.1186/cc11936

Girard, R., Baboi, L., Ayzac, L., Richard, J. C., Guérin, C., & Proseva Trial Group. (2014). The impact of patient positioning on pressure ulcers in patients with severe ARDS: Results from a multicentre randomised controlled trial on prone positioning. *Intensive Care Medicine, 40*(3), 397–403. doi:10.1007/s00134-013-3188-1

Gordy, S., & Rowell, S. (2013). Vascular air embolism. *International Journal of Critical Illness and Injury Science, 3*(1), 73. doi:10.4103/2229-5151.109428

Greenberg, S. B., & Vender, J. (2013). The use of neuromuscular blocking agents in the ICU: Where are we now? *Critical Care Medicine, 41*(5), 1332–1344. doi:10.1097/CCM.0b013e31828ce07c

Guérin, C., Reignier, J., Richard, J. C., Beuret, P., Gacouin, A., Boulain, T., . . . Ayzac, L. (2013). Prone positioning in severe acute respiratory distress syndrome. *New England Journal of Medicine, 368*(23), 2159–2168. doi:10.1056/NEJMoa1214103

Hanneman, S. K., Gusick, G. M., Hamlin, S. K., Wachtel, S. J., Cron, S. G., Jones, D. J., & Oldham, S. A. (2015). Manual vs automated lateral rotation to reduce preventable pulmonary complications in ventilator patients. *American Journal of Critical Care, 24*(1), 24–32. doi:10.4037/ajcc2015171

Hansen-Flaschen, J., & Siegel, M. D. (2015). *Acute respiratory distress syndrome: Clinical features and diagnosis in adults.* UpToDate. Retrieved December 27, 2016, from http://www.uptodate.com/contents/acute-respiratory-distress-syndrome-clinical-features-and-diagnosis-in-adults?source=search_result&search=ARDS%5C&selectedTitle=1%7E150

Hanson, C., Rutten, E. P., Rollins, C., & Dobak, S. (2015). Chapter 4: Nutrition and acute lung injury in critical care: Focus on nutrition care process. In R. Rajendram, V. R. Preedy, & V. B. Patel. (Eds.), *Diet and Nutrition in Critical Care* (Vol. 1, pp. 49–61). doi:10.1007/978-1-4614-7836-2_34

Heron, M. (2015). Deaths: Leading causes for 2011. *National Vital Statistics Reports, 64*(7), 1–96. U.S. Department of Health and Human Services, Centers for Disease Control and Prevention, National Center for Health Statistics National Vital Statistics System. Retrieved December 28, 2017, from http://www.cdc.gov/nchs/data/nvsr/nvsr64/nvsr64_07.pdf

Hudack, M. E. (2013). Prone positioning for patients with ARDS. *The Nurse Practitioner, 38*(6), 10–12. doi:10.1097/01.NPR.0000429897.48997.6e

Hui, D. S., & Zumla, A. (2015). Emerging respiratory tract viral infections. *Current Opinion in Pulmonary Medicine, 21*(3), 284–292. doi:10.1097/MCP.0000000000000153

Huisman, M. V., & Klok, F. A. (2013). Diagnostic management of acute deep vein thrombosis and pulmonary embolism. *Journal of Thrombosis and Haemostasis, 11*(3), 412–422. doi:10.1111/jth.12124

Jones, C. (2013). What's new on the post-ICU burden for patients and relatives? *Intensive Care Medicine, 39*(10), 1832–1835. doi:10.1007/s00134-013-3015-8

Kalanuria, A. A., Zai, W., & Mirski, M. (2014). Ventilator-associated pneumonia in the ICU. *Critical Care, 18*(2), 208. doi:10.1186/cc13775

Kalisch, B. J., & Xie, B. (2014). Errors of omission: Missed nursing care. *Western Journal of Nursing Research, 36*(7), 875–890. doi:10.1177/0193945914531859

Kane, C. J., York, N. L., & Minton, L. A. (2013). Chest tubes in the critically ill patient. *Dimensions of Critical Care Nursing, 32*(3), 111–117. doi:10.1097/DCC.0b013e3182864721

Kangelaris, K. N., Calfee, C. S., May, A. K., Zhuo, H., Matthay, M. A., & Ware, L. B. (2014). Is there still a role for the lung injury score in the era of the Berlin definition ARDS? *Annals of Intensive Care, 4,* 4. Retrieved December 28, 2016, from http://www.biomedcentral.com/content/pdf/2110-5820-4-4.pdf

Kearon, C., Ginsberg, J. S., Douketis, J., Turpie, A. G., Bates, S. M., Lee, . . . Gent, M. (2006). An evaluation of D-dimer in the diagnosis of pulmonary embolism: A randomized trial. *Annals of Internal Medicine, 144*(11), 812–821.

Koh, Y. (2014). Update in acute respiratory distress syndrome. *Journal of Intensive Care, 2*(2), 1–6. doi:10.1186/2052-0492-2-2

Komissarova, M., Chong, S., Frey, K., & Sundaram, B. (2013). Imaging of acute pulmonary embolism. *Emergency Radiology, 20*(2), 89–101. doi:10.1007/s10140-012-1080-x

Kopec, S. E., & Irwin, R. S. (2015). *Sequelae and complications of pneumonectomy.* UpToDate. Retrieved December 28, 2016, from http://www.uptodate.com/contents/sequelae-and-complications-of-pneumonectomy?source=search_result&search=pneumonectomy&selectedTitle=1%7E54

Krüger, W., & Ludman, A. J. (2014). *Core knowledge in critical care medicine.* Berlin, Germany: Springer-Verlag.

Kwiatt, M. E., & Seamon, M. J. (2013). Fat embolism syndrome. *International Journal of Critical Illness and Injury Science, 3*(1), 64. doi:10.4103/2229-5151.109426

Leatherman, J. (2015). Mechanical ventilation for severe asthma. *CHEST Journal, 147*(6), 1671–1680. doi:10.1378/chest.14-1733

Lee, J. S., Giesler, D. L., Gellad, W. F., & Fine, M. J. (2016). Antibiotic therapy for adults hospitalized with community-acquired pneumonia: A systematic review. *JAMA, 315*(6), 593–602.

LeMone, P. T, Burke, K. M., Bauldoff, G., & Gubrud, P. (2015). *Medical-surgical nursing: Clinical reasoning in patient care* (6th ed.). Hoboken, NJ: Pearson.

Linn, D. D., Beckett, R. D., & Foellinger, K. (2015). Administration of enteral nutrition to adult patients in the prone position. *Intensive and Critical Care Nursing, 31*(1), 38–43. doi:10.1016/j.iccn.2014.07.002

Macht, M., Wimbish, T., Bodine, C., & Moss, M. (2013). ICU-acquired swallowing disorders. *Critical Care Medicine, 41*(10), 2396–2405. doi:10.1097/CCM.0b013e31829caf33

Magill, S. S., Klompas, M., Balk, R., Burns, S. M., Deutschman, C. S., Diekema, D., . . . Lipsett, P. (2013). Executive summary: Developing a new, national approach to surveillance for ventilator-associated events. *Annals of the American Thoracic Society, 10*(6), S220–S223. doi:10.4037/ajcc2013893

Mahmood, K., & Wahidi, M. M. (2013). Straightening out chest tubes: What size, what type, and when. *Clinics in Chest Medicine, 34*(1), 63–71. doi:10.1016/j.ccm.2012.11.007

Makic, M. B. F., Rauen, C., Watson, R., & Poteet, A. W. (2014). Examining the evidence to guide practice: Challenging practice habits. *Critical Care Nurse, 34*(2), 28–45. doi:10.4037/ccn2014262

Mandell, L. A., & Wunderink, R. G. (2015). Chapter 153, Section 2, Clinical syndromes: Community acquired pneumonia. In D. L. Kasper, A. S. Fauci, S. L. Hauser, D. L. Longo, J. L. Jameson, & J. Loscalzo (Eds.), *Harrison's principles of internal medicine* (19th ed., pp. 803–809). McGraw-Hill Education.

Mandell, L. A., Wunderink, R. G., Anzueto, A., Bartlett, J. G., Campbell, G. D., Dean, N. C., . . . Whitney, C. G. (2007). Infectious Diseases Society of America/American Thoracic Society consensus guidelines on the management of community-acquired pneumonia in adults. *Clinical Infectious Diseases, 44*(Suppl 2), S27–S72.

Marrie, T. J. (2015). Chapter 128: Acute bronchitis and community-acquired pneumonia. In M. A. Grippi, J. A. Elias, J. A. Fishman, R. M. Kotloff, A. I. Pack, R. M. Senior, & M. D. Siegel (Eds.), *Fishman's pulmonary diseases and disorders* (5th ed.). Retrieved December 28, 2016, from http://accessmedicine.mhmedical.com/content.aspx?bookid=1344&sectionid=81199286

Marrie, T. J., & File, T. M. (2015). *Epidemiology, pathogenesis, and microbiology of community-acquired pneumonia in adults.* UpToDate. Retrieved December 28, 2016, from http://www.uptodate.com/contents/epidemiology-pathogenesis-and-microbiology-of-community-acquired-pneumonia-in-adults?source=search_result&search=pneumonia&selectedTitle=8%7E150

McIntosh, K. (2015). *Severe acute respiratory syndrome (SARS)*. UpToDate. Retrieved December 28, 2016, from http://www.uptodate.com/contents/severe-acute-respiratory-syndrome-sars?source=search_result&search=sars&selectedTitle=1%7E25

Meduri, G. U., Annane, D., Chrousos, G. P., Marik, P. E., & Sinclair, S. E. (2009). Activation and regulation of systemic inflammation in ARDS: Rationale for prolonged glucocorticoid therapy. *Chest, 136*(6), 1631–1643. doi:10.1378/chest.08-2408

Meyer, N. J., & Schmidt, G. A. (2015). Chapter 39: Pulmonary embolic disorders: Thrombus, air, and fat. In J. B. Hall, G. A. Schmidt, & J. P. Kress (Eds.), *Principles of critical care* (4th ed.). New York, NY: McGraw-Hill. Retrieved December 28, 2016, from http://accesssurgery.mhmedical.com/content.aspx?sectionid=80031468&bookid=1340&jumpsectionID=80031510&Resultclick=2

Mikkelsen, M. E. Lanken, P. N., & Christie, J. D. (2015). *Chapter 52: Acute lung injury and the acute respiratory distress syndrome*. In J. B. Hall, G. A. Schmidt, & J. P. Kress (Eds.), *Principles of critical care* (4th ed.). New York, NY: McGraw-Hill. Retrieved December 27, 2016, from http://accessmedicine.mhmedical.com/content.aspx?sectionid=80032725&bookid=1340&Resultclick=2

Monahan, L. J. (2013). Acute respiratory distress syndrome. *Current Problems in Pediatric and Adolescent Health Care, 43*(10), 278–284. doi:10.1016/j.cppeds.2013.10.004

Musher, D. M., & Thorner, A. R. (2014). Community-acquired pneumonia. *New England Journal of Medicine, 371*(17), 1619–1628. doi:10.1056/NEJMra1312885

Muzzy, A. C., & Butler, A. K. (2015). Managing chest tubes: Air leaks and unplanned tube removal. *American Nurse Today, 10*(5), 10–13. Retrieved December 28, 2016, from https://americannursetoday.com/wp-content/uploads/2015/05/ant5-Chest-Tube-420.pdf

Nakawah, M. O., Hawkins, C., & Barbandi, F. (2013). Asthma, chronic obstructive pulmonary disease (COPD), and the overlap syndrome. *The Journal of the American Board of Family Medicine, 26*(4), 470–477. doi:10.3122/jabfm.2013.04.120256

Napolitano, L. M., Angus, D. C., & Uyeki, T. M. (2014). Critically ill patients with influenza A (H1N1) pdm09 virus infection in 2014. *Journal of the American Medical Association, 311*(13), 1289–1290. doi:10.1001/jama.2014.2116

Nason, K. S., Maddaus, M. A., & Luketich, J. D. (2014). Chapter 19: Chest wall, lung, mediastinum, and pleura. In F. Brunicardi, D. K. Andersen, T. R. Billiar, D. L. Dunn, J. G. Hunter, J. B. Matthews, & R. E. Pollock (Eds.), *Schwartz's principles of surgery* (10th ed.). Retrieved December 28, 2016, from http://accessmedicine.mhmedical.com/content.aspx?bookid=980&sectionid=59610861

National Heart, Lung, and Blood Institute (NHLBI) Acute Respiratory Distress Syndrome (ARDS) Clinical Trials Network. (2006). Comparison of two fluid-management strategies in acute lung injury. *New England Journal of Medicine, 354*(24), 2564–2575. doi:10.1056/NEJMoa062200

Nowalk, M. P., Lin, C. J., Raymund, M., Bialor, J., & Zimmerman, R. K. (2013). Impact of hospital policies on health care workers' influenza vaccination rates. *American Journal of Infection Control, 41*(8), 697–701. doi:10.1016/j.ajic.2012.11.011

O'Dowd, L. C., & Kelley, M. A. (2015). *Air embolism*. UpToDate. Retrieved December 28, 2016, from http://www.uptodate.com/contents/air-embolism

Papazian, L., Forel, J., Gacouin, A., Penot-Ragon, C., Perrin, G., Loundou, A., . . . Roche, A., for the ACURASYS Study Investigators. (2010). Neuromuscular blockers in early acute respiratory distress syndrome. *New England Journal of Medicine, 363*(12), 1107–1116.

Patel, S. B., & McConville, J. F. (2015). Chapter 56: Thoracostomy. In J. B. Hall, G. A. Schmidt, & J. P. Kress (Eds.), *Principles of critical care* (4th ed.). Retrieved December 28, 2016, from http://accessmedicine.mhmedical.com/content.aspx?sectionid=80033265&bookid=1340&jumpsectionID=80033279&Resultclick=2

Perner, A., Citerio, G., Bakker, J., Bassetti, M., Benoit, D., Cecconi, M., . . . Azoulay, E. (2015). Year in review in Intensive Care Medicine 2014: II. ARDS, airway management, ventilation, adjuvants in sepsis, hepatic failure, symptoms assessment and management, palliative care and support for families, prognostication, organ donation, outcome, organisation and research methodology. *Intensive Care Medicine, 41*(3), 389–401. doi:10.1007/s00134-015-3707-3

Petrucci, N., & Lacovelli, W. (2004). Ventilation with lower tidal volumes versus traditional tidal volumes in adults for acute lung injury and acute respiratory distress syndromes. Cochrane Database of Systematic Reviews (2):CD003844.

Piazza, G. (2013). Submassive pulmonary embolism. *Journal of the American Medical Association, 309*(2), 171–180. doi:10.1001/jama.2012.164493

Prather, A. D., Smith, T. R., Poletto, D. M., Tavora, F., Chung, J. H., Nallamshetty, L., . . . Rojas, C. A. (2014). Aspiration-related lung diseases. *Journal of Thoracic Imaging, 29*(5), 304–309. doi:10.1097/RTI.0000000000000092

Putensen, C., Theuerkauf, N., Zinserling, J., Wrigge, H., & Pelosi, P. (2009). Meta-analysis: Ventilation strategies and outcomes of the acute respiratory distress syndrome and acute lung injury. *Annals of Internal Medicine, 151*(8), 566–576.

Quinn, B., & Baker, D. L. (2015). Comprehensive oral care helps prevent hospital-acquired nonventilator pneumonia. *American Nurse Today 10*(3), 18–22. Retrieved December 28, 2016, from https://americannursetoday.com/wp-content/uploads/2015/03/ant3-CE-Oral-Care-225.pdf

Quinn, B., Baker, D. L., Cohen, S., Stewart, J. L., Lima, C. A., & Parise, C. (2014). Basic nursing care to prevent nonventilator hospital-acquired pneumonia. *Journal of Nursing Scholarship, 46*(1), 11–19. doi:10.1111/jnu.12050

Ramsey, C. D., & Kumar, A. (2013). Influenza and endemic viral pneumonia. *Critical Care Clinics, 29*(4), 1069–1086. doi:10.1016/j.ccc.2013.06.003

Reilly, J. P., & Christie, J. D. (2015). Chapter 141: Acute lung injury and the acute respiratory distress syndrome: Clinical features, management, and outcomes. In M. A. Grippi, J. A. Elias, J. A. Fishman, R. M. Kotloff, A. I. Pack, R. M. Senior, & M.D. Siegel (Eds.), *Fishman's pulmonary diseases and disorders* (5th ed.). Retrieved December 27, 2016, from http://accessmedicine.mhmedical.com/content.aspx?bookID=1344&sectionID=81206199&jumpsectionID=111844807&CAClickthru=82699

Remington, L. T., & Sligl, W. I. (2014). Community-acquired pneumonia. *Current Opinion in Pulmonary Medicine*, 20(3), 215–224. doi:10.1097/MCP.0000000000000052

Righini, M., Le Gal, G., Aujesky, D., Roy, P. M., Sanchez, O., Verschuren F., . . . Perrier, A. (2008). Diagnosis of pulmonary embolism by multidetector CT alone or combined with venous ultrasonography of the leg: A randomised non-inferiority trial. *Lancet*, 371(9621), 1343–1352. doi:10.1016/S0140-6736(08)60594-2

Schivo, M., Phan, C., Louie, S., & Harper, R. W. (2013). Critical asthma syndrome in the ICU. *Clinical Reviews in Allergy & Immunology*, 48(1), 31–44. doi:10.1007/s12016-013-8394-7

Schwartz, D. R., Atul Malhotra, A., & Kacmarek, R. M. (2015). *Prone ventilation for adult patients with acute respiratory distress syndrome.* UpToDate. Retrieved December 27, 2016, from http://www.uptodate.com/contents/prone-ventilation?source=search_result&search=prone+ventilation&selectedTitle=1%7E7

Sheshadri, A., Castro, M., & Chen, A. (2013). Bronchial thermoplasty: A novel therapy for severe asthma. *Clinics in Chest Medicine*, 34(3), 437–444. doi:10.1016/j.ccm.2013.03.003

Siegel, M. D. (2015a). *Acute respiratory distress syndrome: Epidemiology, pathophysiology, pathology, and etiology in adults.* UpToDate. Retrieved December 27, 2016, from http://www.uptodate.com/contents/acute-respiratory-distress-syndrome-epidemiology-pathophysiology-pathology-and-etiology-in-adults?source=search_result&search=ARDS&selectedTitle=2%7E150

Siegel, M. D. (2015b). *Acute respiratory distress syndrome: Investigational or ineffective pharmacotherapy in adults.* UpToDate. Retrieved December 27, 2016, from http://www.uptodate.com/contents/acute-respiratory-distress-syndrome-novel-therapies-in-adults?source=search_result&search=ARDS&selectedTitle=5%7E150

Siegel, M. D. (2015c). *Acute respiratory distress syndrome: Supportive care and oxygenation in adults.* UpToDate. Retrieved December 27, 2016, from http://www.uptodate.com/contents/acute-respiratory-distress-syndrome-supportive-care-and-oxygenation-in-adults?source=search_result&search=ARDS&selectedTitle=3%7E150

Simko, L. C., & Culleiton, A. L. (2013). Pulmonary embolism: Know the signs, act fast, save lives. *Nursing Critical Care*, 8(5), 26–31. doi:10.1097/01.CCN.0000433812.63351.9f

Sligl, W. I., & Marrie, T. J. (2013). Severe community-acquired pneumonia. *Critical Care Clinics*, 29(3), 563–601. doi:10.1016/j.ccc.2013.03.009

Slutsky, A. S., & Ranieri, V. M. (2013). Ventilator-induced lung injury. *New England Journal of Medicine*, 369(22), 2126–2136. doi:10.1056/NEJMra1208707

Spoletini, G., Alotaibi, M., Blasi, F., & Hill, N. S. (2015). Heated humidified high-flow nasal oxygen in adults: Mechanisms of action and clinical implications. *CHEST Journal*, 148(1), 253–261. doi:10.1378/chest.14-2871

Stawicki, S. P., Firstenberg, M. S., Lyaker, M. R., Russell, S. B., Evans, D. C., Bergese, S. D., & Papadimos, T. J. (2013). Septic embolism in the intensive care unit. *International Journal of Critical Illness and Injury Science*, 3(1), 58. doi:10.4103/2229-5151.109423

Stein, P. D., Hull, R. D., Patel, K. C., Olsen, R. E., Ghali, W. A., Brant, R., . . . Katra, N. K. (2004). D-dimer for the exclusion of acute venous thrombosis and pulmonary embolism: A systematic review. *Annals of Internal Medicine*, 140(8), 589–602.

Stein, P. D., Woodard, P. K., Weg, J. G., Wakefield, T. W., Tapson, V. F., Sostman, H. D., . . . Buckley, J. D.; PIOPED II investigator group. (2006). Diagnostic pathways in acute pulmonary embolism: Recommendations of the PIOPED II investigators. *American Journal of Medicine*, 119(12), 1048–1055.

Strange, C. (2015). *Parapneumonic effusion and empyema in adults.* UpToDate. Retrieved December 28, 2016, from http://www.uptodate.com/contents/parapneumonic-effusion-and-empyema-in-adults

Tarbox, A. K., & Swaroop, M. (2013). Symposium: Embolism in the intensive care unit. *International Journal of Critical Illness and Injury Science*, 3(1), 69–72. doi:10.4103/2229-5151.109427

Terpstra, M. L., Aman, J., van Nieuw Amerongen, G. P., & Groeneveld, A. J. (2014). Plasma biomarkers for acute respiratory distress syndrome: A systematic review and meta-analysis. *Critical Care Medicine*, 42(3), 691–700. doi:10.1097/01.ccm.0000435669.60811.24

Thompson, B. T., & Hales, C. A. (2015). *Overview of acute pulmonary embolism in adults.* UpToDate. Retrieved December 28, 2016, from http://www.uptodate.com/contents/overview-of-acute-pulmonary-embolism-in-adults?source=search_result&search=pulmonary+embolism&selectedTitle=1%7E150

Thongrong, C., Kasemsiri, P., Hofmann, J. P., Bergese, S. D., Papadimos, T. J., Gracias, V. H., . . . Stawicki, S. P. (2013). Amniotic fluid embolism. *International Journal of Critical Illness and Injury Science*, 3(1), 51. Retrieved December 28, 2016, from http://www.ijciis.org/printarticle.asp?issn=2229-5151;year=2013;volume=3;issue=1;spage=51;epage=57;aulast=Thongrong

Traver, G. A. (1985). Ineffective airway clearance: Physiology and clinical application. *Dimensions of Critical Care Nursing*, 4(4), 198–208.

Villar, J., Fernández, R. L., Ambrós, A., Parra, L., Blanco, J., Domínguez-Berrot, A. M., . . . Kacmarek, R. M.; for the Acute Lung Injury: Epidemiology and Natural History (ALIEN) Network. (2015). A clinical classification of the acute respiratory distress syndrome for predicting outcome and guiding medical therapy. *Critical Care Medicine*, 43(2), 346–353. doi:10.1097/CCM.0000000000000703

Villar, J., Sulemanji, D., & Kacmarek, R. M. (2014). The acute respiratory distress syndrome: Incidence and mortality, has it changed? *Current Opinion in Critical Care, 20*(1), 3–9. doi:10.1097/MCC.0000000000000057

Weinberger, S. E., Cockrill, B. A., & Mandel, J. (2014). Chapter 28: Acute respiratory distress syndrome. In *Principles of pulmonary medicine* (6th ed.). Saunders, ISBN 978-1-4557-2532-8

Wiedemann, H. P., Wheeler, A. P., Bernard, G. R., Thompson, B. T., Hayden, D., deBoisblanc, B., . . . Harabin, A. L. (2006). Comparison of two fluid-management strategies in acute lung injury. National Heart, Lung, and Blood Institute Acute Respiratory Distress Syndrome (ARDS) Clinical Trials Network. *New England Journal of Medicine, 354*(24), 2564–2575.

Wilson, B. A, Shannon, M. T., & Shields, K. M. (2017). *Pearson nurse's drug guide.* Hoboken, NJ: Pearson.

Wunderink, R. G., & Waterer, G. W. (2014). Community-acquired pneumonia. *New England Journal of Medicine, 370*(6), 543–551. doi:10.1056/NEJMcp1214869

Wunderink, R. G., & Waterer, G. (2015). Chapter 65: Pneumonia. In J. B. Hall, G. A. Schmidt, & J. P. Kress (Eds.), *Principles of critical care* (4th ed.). New York, NY: McGraw-Hill. Retrieved December 28, 2016, from http://accessmedicine.mhmedical.com/content.aspx?sectionid=80034063&bookid=1340&Resultclick=2

Yandiola, P. P., Capelastegui, A., Quintana, J., Diaz, R., Gorordo, I., Bilbao, A., . . . Torres, A. (2009). Prospective comparison of severity scores for predicting clinically relevant outcomes for patients hospitalized with community-acquired pneumonia. *Chest, 135*(6), 1572–1579.

York, N. L., Kane, C. J., Smith, C., & Minton, L. A. (2015). Care of the patient with an acute pulmonary embolism. *Dimensions of Critical Care Nursing, 34*(1), 3–9. doi:10.1097/DCC.0000000000000082

Chapter 13
Determinants and Assessment of Cardiac Function

13.1 Apply knowledge of cardiopulmonary circulation to the assessment of cardiac function in the high-acuity patient.

13.2 Analyze cardiac anatomy and physiology as it relates to cardiac function and myocardial perfusion.

13.3 Examine cardiac output and how the determinants of heart rate, stroke volume, preload, afterload, and contractility compensate to maintain adequate cardiac output.

13.4 Analyze the relationships between arterial blood pressure, venous blood pressure,

cardiac output, and tissue perfusion, and examine how arterial blood pressure is regulated by the renin-angiotensin-aldosterone system, the kidneys, and the autonomic nervous system.

13.5 Evaluate the cardiac function of the high-acuity patient using data obtained from patient history, physical assessment, and diagnostic testing.

13.6 Differentiate the indications and nursing implications for common noninvasive and invasive cardiac diagnostic procedures.

This chapter focuses on essential anatomic and physiologic concepts that influence the function of the cardiovascular system, with particular focus on the heart. An understanding of these concepts will allow the nurse to apply them to a variety of clinical situations in order to understand assessment findings related to cardiovascular health and disease. The chapter includes core information that will enhance understanding of multiple chapters in the book, particularly Chapter 8: Basic Hemodynamic Monitoring, Chapter 9: Basic Cardiac Rhythm Monitoring, Chapter 14: Alterations in Cardiac Function, and Chapter 15: Alterations in Myocardial Tissue Perfusion.

We would like to acknowledge Dr. Darlene Welsh's contribution to the myocardial tissue perfusion portion of Section Two of this chapter.

Section One: Review of the Cardiopulmonary System

The cardiopulmonary system is composed of the heart, lungs, a vast network of blood vessels, and blood. Its purpose is to take in and deliver oxygen and nutrients to the organs and tissues and remove metabolic waste products for elimination from the body. This section focuses on the vascular portion of the cardiopulmonary system. Pulmonary gas exchange is presented in depth in Chapter 11: Determinants and Assessment of Pulmonary Function.

Cardiopulmonary Circuits

The cardiopulmonary vascular system consists of two interdependent major circuits: the pulmonary circuit and the systemic circuit (Figure 13–1).

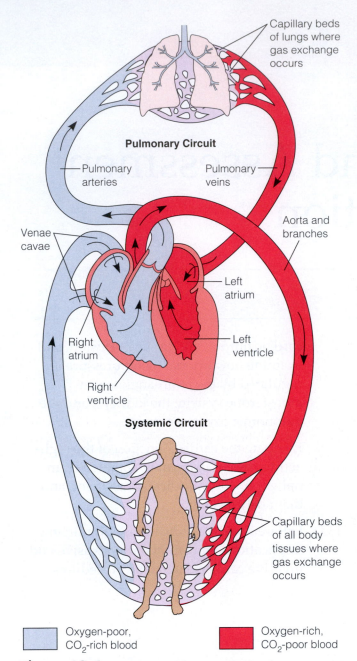

Capillary beds of lungs where gas exchange occurs

Pulmonary Circuit

Pulmonary arteries

Pulmonary veins

Venae cavae

Aorta and branches

Left atrium

Right atrium

Left ventricle

Right ventricle

Systemic Circuit

Capillary beds of all body tissues where gas exchange occurs

Oxygen-poor, CO₂-rich blood

Oxygen-rich, CO₂-poor blood

Figure 13–1 Pulmonary and systemic circuits.

Pulmonary Circuit The pulmonary circuit includes the right side of the heart, the pulmonary arteries, the lungs, and the pulmonary capillaries; it ends with the pulmonary veins where they join the left atrium. Its purpose is to facilitate pulmonary (external) gas exchange. Oxygen-poor blood coming into the right heart is pumped into the lungs through the pulmonary artery and into the pulmonary capillary beds, where gas exchange takes place. Oxygen-enriched blood then leaves the lungs through the pulmonary veins, which empty into the left atrium. The pulmonary circuit is a low-pressure system; it requires only sufficient pressures to pump blood through the lungs and into the left heart. The pulmonary veins have no valves. For this reason, if pressures in the left

heart increase (e.g., heart failure), blood can back up through the pulmonary veins and into the lungs, causing increased pulmonary vascular pressures and pulmonary edema.

Systemic Circuit The systemic circuit begins with the left side of the heart (left atrium) and ends with the superior and inferior venae cavae, where they join the right atrium. This circuit transports oxygen-enriched blood to the capillary beds of the organs and tissues for gas exchange. It delivers nutrients and transports metabolic waste products away from the organs and tissues for removal from the body, and it returns oxygen-depleted blood to the pulmonary circuit. The systemic circuit is a high-pressure system; the heart must pump using sufficient pressure to perfuse the organs and tissues (Hall, 2016).

Blood Vessels

Blood vessels are a vast network of conduits through which oxygen and nutrients are delivered to the tissues. Blood vessel walls are composed of one to three layers, called tunica. Vessels that move blood away from the heart are arteries, and those that move blood toward the heart are veins.

Blood Vessel Layers Blood vessels are composed of three layers: the tunica intima (interna), the tunica media, and the tunica externa (adventitia) (Figure 13–2).

Tunica Intima. The tunica intima (tunica interna) lines the inside of the vessel and is the only layer that directly interfaces with blood flowing through the vessels. It consists of **endothelium**, the squamous-cell epithelium that lines the entire circulatory system. Just below the endothelium are a subendothelial basement membrane and a thin connective tissue that is rich in elastic fibers (Cunningham, Brashers, & McCance, 2014). The smooth surface of the endothelium reduces friction and prevents clotting and damage to blood cells as blood flows by. The endothelial cells also produce several vasoactive substances that either constrict or dilate the arteries (Hall, 2016).

Tunica Media. The tunica media, or middle layer, is composed of smooth muscle with loose connective tissue and elastic fibers. This layer is thicker in arteries than in veins, which gives arteries the ability to constantly adjust the size of their lumen (the space within an artery) by vasoconstriction in response to sympathetic nervous system stimulation.

Tunica Externa. The tunica externa (tunica adventitia) is the outermost layer surrounding the vessel and is composed of connective tissue. Its functions are to protect and stabilize the vessels. Stabilization is provided by fibers in this layer that interlace with bordering tissues (Cunningham et al., 2014). The tunica externa is thicker in veins than in arteries.

Types of Blood Vessels The cardiovascular system consists of an intricate network of arteries, veins, and capillaries.

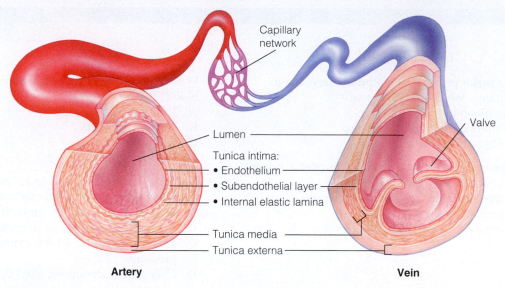

Figure 13–2 Structure of arteries, veins, and capillaries.

While all of these vessels transport blood throughout the body, each has some unique properties and functions.

Arteries. Arteries are blood vessels that transport blood away from the heart. They can be classified by diameter as large, medium, and small. Each size has a slightly different wall layer structure.

The large arteries are also known as *elastic* or *conducting arteries*. They comprise the major arteries, such as the aorta and its major branches and the trunk of the pulmonary artery. These arteries have a large tunica media that contains more elastic fibers than smooth muscle (Hall, 2016). The thick tunica media makes large arteries well suited for the constantly changing pulsatile pressures and blood volume coming from the heart, readily expanding and relaxing in response to the cardiac cycle.

The medium arteries, also known as *muscular arteries*, have a tunica media that contains more smooth muscle than elastic fibers. They deliver blood to the muscles and organs and are sometimes referred to as *distribution arteries* (Hall, 2016).

The *arterioles* are the smallest arteries and consist of only two layers, a tunica media and a tunica intima. The tunica media is thin, and depending on the size of the arteriole, it may have one or two smooth muscle layers (Hall, 2016). The arterioles are referred to as *resistance vessels* because they play a critical role in the regulation of blood flow and blood pressure.

Veins. With the exception of the pulmonary veins, the venous system collects blood from the periphery and brings it back toward the heart. Unlike the arteries, which must adapt to high pressures, veins are exposed only to low pressures; thus, venous walls are much thinner than arterial walls and require only a thin tunica media. Because veins have a thin, smooth-muscle tunica media, veins have

limited ability to constrict and dilate; however, this ability influences the venous return of blood to the heart. In the limbs, veins rely on a valve system, referred to as the venous muscle pump, to move blood in a forward direction toward the heart against gravity. As a person moves, the skeletal muscles in the limbs contract, exerting force against the veins and moving the blood toward the heart. Blood is prevented from flowing backward by the closing of the valves.

Veins can be classified by diameter as large, medium, and small. The large veins include the superior and inferior venae cavae and their immediate tributaries. The medium veins are of equivalent size to the medium arteries and, in the limbs, contain valves. The small veins, or *venules*, are transition vessels located between the capillaries and the medium veins.

Capillaries. Capillaries, the smallest structures of the vascular system, are composed of a single layer, the tunica intima, which consists of endothelium with a basement membrane. Capillaries form a complex interconnected network known as a *capillary bed* that links the arterioles with the venules. Capillaries interact with their adjacent (interstitial) environment by way of the selectively permeable endothelial membrane. Substances such as dissolved gases, solutes, and water rapidly diffuse through the endothelial cells while larger molecules shift through gaps or pores between the endothelial cells.

Capillaries begin with a precapillary sphincter that expands and constricts the entryway into the capillary to control the rate and volume of blood flow. Flow through the capillaries is not continuous; rather, the precapillary sphincters open and close in a cyclic fashion, resulting in intermittent blood flow and increasing the time available for the exchange of gases, fluids, and other molecules (Hall, 2016).

Section One Review

1. What is a major purpose of the pulmonary circuit?
   A. Maintain a low-pressure system
   B. Pump blood to the right heart
   C. Facilitate external gas exchange
   D. Provide nutrients to the lungs

2. Which statement is correct regarding the systemic circuit?
   A. It is a high-pressure system.
   B. It delivers oxygen-rich blood to the right heart.
   C. It begins at the right atrium.
   D. It is composed of arteries but not veins.

3. Which blood vessel layer interfaces directly with the blood?
   A. Tunica media
   B. Tunica adventitia
   C. Tunica externa
   D. Tunica intima

4. The large arteries are able to adjust their size in response to the cardiac cycle for which reason?
   A. The presence of a thick, smooth muscle layer
   B. An abundance of elastic fibers in the tunica media
   C. Their thin walls, which cannot withstand high pressures
   D. Chemical mediators secreted by the arteries, which alter vessel size

Answers: 1. C, 2. A, 3. D, 4. B

Section Two: Review of Heart Anatomy

This section reviews essential cardiac anatomy to facilitate understanding of the alterations in cardiovascular function experienced by high-acuity patients. The physiology of the cardiac conduction system is presented in detail in Chapter 9: Basic Cardiac Rhythm Monitoring and is therefore not covered in this section.

The heart is nestled within the mediastinum directly behind the sternum between the right and left lungs, with the majority of the heart apex lying in the left chest. It is protected by the anterior and posterior bony structures of the thorax (see Figure 13–3).

Heart Chambers

In simple terms, the heart is a four-chambered, two-pump system (right and left heart) that drives fluid (blood) through a complex network of pipes (blood vessels) for the purposes of facilitating gas exchange and cellular nutrition and transporting metabolic waste products. The right and left sides of the heart each have two chambers: an atrium and a ventricle. The upper chambers are called atria (singular: atrium), and the lower chambers are called ventricles. The atria act as a temporary holding tank for blood coming into the heart, while the ventricles eject blood forward out of the heart.

The right atrium accepts venous (oxygen-poor) blood coming into the heart from the superior and inferior vena cava and the coronary sinus. The right ventricle accepts the blood from the right atrium and ejects it into the pulmonary artery and then into the lungs. On the left side of the heart, the left atrium accepts arterial (oxygen-rich) blood from the lungs via the pulmonary veins. The left ventricle accepts blood from the left atrium and ejects it from the heart through the aorta to the organs and tissues. Figure 13–4 illustrates the four heart chambers and the blood flow through them.

Heart Wall Layers

The heart is essentially a muscle that is lined on the inside and outside by thin sheaths. It is composed of three distinct layers: the endocardium, myocardium, and epicardium (Figure 13–5).

Endocardium   The **endocardium** is the innermost layer of the heart and is continuous with the endothelium (inner layer) of the blood vessels; like the blood vessels, it is composed of squamous-cell epithelium. The endocardium is the only heart surface that directly interfaces with blood flowing through the chambers. This is important because the smooth endocardial surface allows blood to easily flow through the heart without clotting or traumatizing the red blood cells The direct contact with the blood, however, also makes the endocardium more susceptible to injury, such as colonization by bloodborne pathogens (e.g., endocarditis).

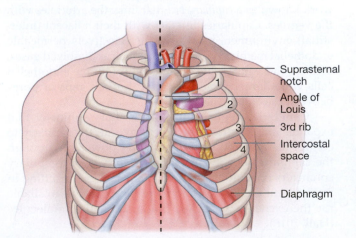

Figure 13–3 Diagram of heart in chest.

Suprasternal notch
Angle of Louis
3rd rib
Intercostal space
Diaphragm

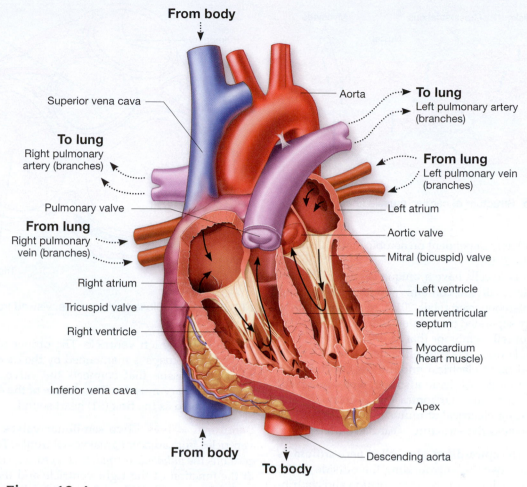

Figure 13–4 Blood flow through the chambers of the heart.

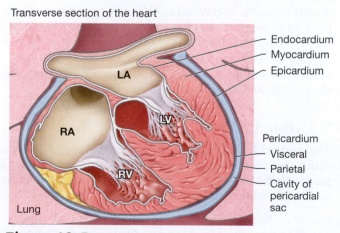

Figure 13–5 Layers of heart.

Myocardium   The thick middle layer, the **myocardium**, forms the bulk of the heart wall. It is composed of contractile muscle fibers, called *sarcomeres*, that are unique in the way they conduct electrical impulses. The thickness of the myocardium in each of the four heart chambers varies based on its workload. The walls of the atria are relatively thin compared to those of the ventricles because the atria do not have major pumping responsibilities.

The thickness of the right and left ventricular walls differs relative to the amount of work required to pump blood forward. The right ventricle pumps blood only into the lungs, which are part of a low-pressure system, about 20 mmHg (Hall, 2016). Pumping against low pressures results in a low workload for the right heart pump; thus, the right ventricle walls are relatively thin. The opposite is true for the left ventricle, which pumps blood to all the organs and tissues in the systemic circuit. The left ventricle is often referred to as the workhorse of the heart because it must provide adequate pumping power to perfuse organs and tissues. Such pumping power requires a high-pressure system, about 80–120 mmHg (Hall, 2016). Working in a higher-pressure environment increases the left ventricular workload; thus, the left ventricle wall is thick to accommodate the additional stress.

Cardiac Muscle Structure   Cardiac muscle has many similarities with skeletal muscle but also has unique characteristics (Hall, 2016). Like skeletal muscle, it is striated and contains identical myofibrils (basic muscle units), and muscle contraction involves shortening of the sarcomeres (segments of myofibrils). Cardiac muscle, however, has more mitochondria (to make energy via aerobic metabolism) and more myoglobin (to store oxygen) than does skeletal muscle. This is important because cardiac muscle

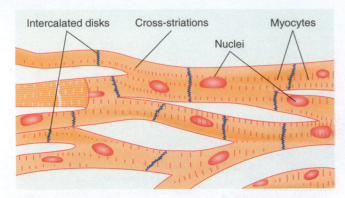

Figure 13–6 Structure of cardiac muscle fibers.

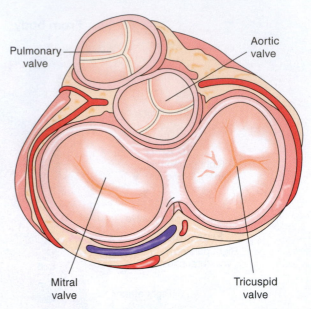

Figure 13–7 Closed heart valves, viewed from above.

is almost completely dependent on aerobic metabolism for energy (Banasik, 2015).

Cardiac muscle cells have a unique latticework structure whereby fibers divide, combine, and redivide, making them highly interconnected (Hall, 2016). Moreover, cardiac muscle cells are separated by an intercalated disk, which is a special type of cell membrane that facilitates fast travel of action potentials from one cell to the next. The interconnectedness and rapid electrical impulse transport system of the cardiac muscle results in a strong, well-organized, and relatively long muscular contraction in response to a sufficiently strong electrical stimulus. Figure 13–6 illustrates the interconnective structure of cardiac muscle fibers.

Epicardium   The **epicardium**, also called **pericardium**, is a tough fibrous covering surrounding the outside of the heart that helps maintain the heart in position and contributes to its structure. It consists of two overlapping layers: the *visceral pericardium*, which is attached to the heart, and the *parietal pericardium*, which overlaps the visceral pericardium, forming the pericardial sac that surrounds the heart (refer to Figure 13–5). The two layers create a potential space called the *pericardial cavity*, which contains approximately 30 to 50 mL of serous fluid. The pericardial fluid provides lubrication to reduce friction associated with the rhythmic contraction and relaxation of the heart.

Structure and Function of Heart Valves

Heart valves play a critical role in maintaining normal blood flow through the heart (see Figure 13–4). Their sole function is to promote blood flow in a forward direction, thereby preventing backflow (known as regurgitation). The heart valves are thin, paperlike, fibrous structures that open and close in response to changes in pressure gradients within the heart. There are two sets of valves: the atrioventricular (AV) valves and the semilunar valves.

Atrioventricular Valves   Two atrioventricular (AV) valves separate the atria from the ventricles and prevent the backflow of blood from the ventricles back into the atria. The right heart has the *tricuspid valve*, consisting of three flaps, or cusps, that open and close. It separates the right atrium from the right ventricle. The left heart has the *mitral valve*, which has two cusps (bicuspid) and separates the left

atrium from the left ventricle. The proper functioning of the AV valve cusps is maintained by the *chordae tendineae*, connective tissue that connects the valve cusps to the heart's papillary muscles. The closure of the AV valves can be auscultated as the first (S1) heart sound.

Semilunar Valves   Two semilunar valves separate the ventricles from adjacent great vessel trunks. The right heart contains the *pulmonic (or pulmonary) valve*, which is located at the junction of the right ventricle and the pulmonary artery. It prevents the backflow of blood from the pulmonary artery into the right ventricle. The left heart has the *aortic valve*, at the junction of the left ventricle and the aorta, which prevents the backflow of blood from the aorta into the left ventricle. In contrast to AV valves, semilunar valves have no supportive structures and are dependent on pressure gradients on either side of the valves for opening and closing. The closure of the semilunar valves can be auscultated as the second (S2) heart sound. Figure 13–7 illustrates the location and appearance of the heart valves.

Cardiac Cycle

The term **cardiac cycle** refers to the heart muscle activities associated with one complete heartbeat. There are two phases to the cardiac cycle, systole and diastole, and each of the four heart chambers experiences both phases.

Systole   **Systole** refers to the contraction of a heart chamber, whereby blood is ejected into either an adjacent ventricle (atrial systole) or into the pulmonary artery or aorta (ventricular systole). Chamber pressure increases during systole. The atrial contraction during systole, also called atrial kick, contributes about 20% of total ventricular blood volume (Hall, 2016). The atria contract slightly before the ventricles to allow the blood in the atria to be pushed into the ventricles, thereby contributing to total ventricular volume and increasing cardiac output. This delay in systole between the two chambers results from a 0.1-second delay of the electrical impulse when it arrives

Table 13–1 The Cardiac Cycle

Phase of Cardiac Cycle	Valve Activity	Description
Atrial systole	AV valves open. Semilunar valves close.	As atrial pressure increases to above that in the ventricles, the AV valves open. Both filled atria contract, adding 20%–30% volume to completely fill ventricles. There is insufficient pressure in the ventricles to force open the semilunar valves.
Atrial diastole	All valves close.	The empty atria relax and begin to refill. As pressure within the ventricles increases, the AV valves are forced to close. There is insufficient pressure in the ventricles to force open the semilunar valves.
Ventricular systole	AV valves close. Semilunar valves open.	Early: When there is sufficient pressure in the ventricles, the AV valves close; however, there is still insufficient pressure to force open the semilunar valves. Late: Pressure in the ventricles surpasses pressure in the pulmonary artery and aorta, forcing the semilunar valves to open. Ventricular blood is ejected from the heart during contraction.
Ventricular diastole (3 phases)	AV valves open. Semilunar valves close.	Early: As the ventricles empty, pressure decreases rapidly, closing the semilunar valves. As ventricular pressure drops below that in the adjacent atria, the AV valves open. This is a period of rapid ventricular filling. Middle: Only a small amount of additional blood passively enters the ventricles from the atria. This volume consists of blood that is draining into the atria from adjacent veins, flowing directly into the ventricles with the AV valves open. Late: The atria contract (atrial systole), forcefully pushing an additional 20% of blood volume into the ventricle just prior to ventricular systole.

SOURCE: Data taken partially from Cunningham et al. (2014) and Hall (2016).

at the atrioventricular (AV) node from the sinoatrial (SA) node (Hall, 2016).

Diastole   Diastole refers to the relaxation of a heart chamber, when blood fills the chamber in preparation for the next cardiac cycle and the coronary arteries fill with blood. Chamber pressure decreases during diastole. As soon as systole ends, blood passively flows back into the chambers from the adjoining vessels (vena cava on right and pulmonary veins on left), refilling the atria. In the ventricles, diastole occurs in three phases: early, middle, and late (Hall, 2016). Table 13–1 summarizes the cardiac cycle, including the phases of ventricular diastole and the associated status of the heart valves.

Mycocardial Tissue Perfusion

The coronary arteries begin in the ascending aorta, close to the aortic valve. They are the first vessels to receive cardiac output after blood is leaving the left ventricle. This location provides the heart with arterial blood that contains the richest oxygen concentration. Blood flow through the coronary arteries is about 225 mL per minute. Coronary blood flow increases three or four times in response to exercise to provide adequate nutrients and oxygen to the myocardium (Hall, 2016).

Anatomy of the Coronary Arteries

The main coronary arteries lie along the epicardial surface of the heart. There are four primary coronary arteries: the left main coronary artery (LMCA), left anterior descending artery (LAD), left circumflex artery (LCX), and right coronary artery (RCA) (Figure 13–8). The LAD and the LCX are branches of the LMCA after its bifurcation. The RCA predominantly supplies the right ventricle and atrium and gives rise to the posterior descending artery (PDA). The LAD supplies the anterior aspect of the left ventricle and

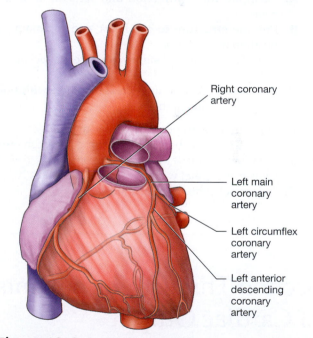

Right coronary artery

Left main coronary artery

Left circumflex coronary artery

Left anterior descending coronary artery

Figure 13–8 Coronary arteries.

septum, and the LCX supplies the lateral walls of the left ventricle. As the arteries cross the epicardial surface, small feeder arterioles penetrate the chamber walls, giving rise to a dense network of thousands of capillaries per square millimeter called *arteriosinusoidal channels*. This network of capillaries ensures that each cardiac muscle cell is in contact with a bordering capillary.

There are no connections between the large coronary arteries, but there are collateral channels between the smaller arterioles. Collateral circulation usually develops to compensate for chronic low-output heart disease, such as heart failure, over a long period and is seen in patients with chronic cardiovascular disease. These channels become important when the large arteries occlude. The collateral channels, if present, can enlarge to provide an alternate route for blood and oxygen to myocardial tissues, which can diminish or eliminate myocardial tissue damage from poor perfusion, as seen in myocardial infarction (Cunningham et al., 2014).

Regulation of Coronary Perfusion   Blood flow through the coronary arteries and perfusion of the myocardium is regulated primarily by aortic pressure. Blood flow through the coronary arteries is influenced by the anatomy and activity of the aortic valve due to the close proximity of the coronary arteries to the aortic valve. During systole, blood flow through the coronary arteries is diminished due to movement of the aortic valve. The majority of blood that perfuses the myocardium of the left ventricle flows through the coronary arteries during diastole (Cunningham et al., 2014). The coronary arteries fill with blood after the aortic valve closes during diastole (resting phase). Coronary blood flow is greatest just after closure of the aortic valve and gradually slows during diastole. Autoregulation maintains coronary perfusion pressure (CPP) at a fairly constant level within a mean arterial pressure range of 60 to 180 mmHg. During times of extreme stress this pressure may rise above the upper normal limit (Cunningham et al., 2014). This is one possible explanation for the increased incidence of plaque rupture during episodes of stress and elevated blood pressure.

Section Two Review

1. The endocardium has which major function?
   A. Facilitate the contraction and relaxation of the heart
   B. Provide structure to the heart and maintain its position in the chest
   C. Provide a protective surface for direct exposure to blood cells
   D. Provide lubrication to decrease friction with normal movements of the heart

2. What is a unique property of cardiac muscle?
   A. Contraction involves the shortening of sarcomeres.
   B. It has an abundant amount of myoglobin.
   C. Cells run parallel with few interconnections.
   D. It does not contain mitochondria.

3. What is the major purpose of the heart valves?
   A. Prevent the backward flow of blood
   B. Separate the heart chambers
   C. Directly contribute to cardiac output
   D. Increase cardiac contractility

4. How is the term *cardiac cycle* best defined?
   A. Blood flow through the heart during one complete heartbeat
   B. Electrical activities of the heart during one complete heartbeat
   C. Activities of the heart valves during one complete heartbeat
   D. Heart muscle activities during one complete heartbeat

Answers: 1. C, 2. B, 3. A, 4. D

Section Three: Determinants of Cardiac Output

Cardiac output (CO) is the amount of blood pumped by the heart each minute. It is a critical aspect of cardiovascular function in both health and illness. Knowledge of how CO changes in response to various physiologic conditions facilitates understanding of pertinent physical assessment findings when there is an alteration in CO.

Normal CO varies significantly for individuals depending on body size and body surface area (BSA); therefore, when CO is measured, it is corrected to account for BSA. BSA is calculated using the patient's height and weight. The correction is called the **cardiac index (CI)** and is calculated by dividing CO by BSA (Barrett, Barman, Boitano, & Brooks, 2016a). Extreme values of BSA in morbidly obese patients demonstrate the need to use CI rather than CO. For example, patient A is 70 inches (1.78 meters) tall and weighs 320 pounds (145 kg) (BSA of 2.5). Patient B is the same height as patient A but weighs 170 pounds (77 kg) (BSA of 2). Both patients have a "normal" CO of 5 L/min; however, when a CO of 5 L/min is indexed to BSA, patient A has a low CI of 2 L/min/m^2 while patient B has a CI of 2.5 L/min/m^2, which is within normal limits. This interpretation is based on normal values of 4 to 8 L/min for cardiac output and 2.4 to 4 L/min/m^2 for cardiac index.

Determinants of Cardiac Output

In all, there are four determinants of cardiac output (CO): heart rate (HR), preload, afterload, and contractility. Any condition or disease that affects one determinant will alter one or more other determinants in an effort to maintain a stable CO. Recall that the formula for calculating cardiac output is CO = HR × SV and that stroke volume (SV) is determined by the interplay of three of the determinants: preload, afterload, and contractility.

Heart Rate Heart rate is controlled by the heart's pacemaker sites, which are influenced by the interplay of the sympathetic and parasympathetic nervous systems. The sympathetic nervous system (SNS) causes the fight-or-flight reaction, in which the body's resources are mobilized to counteract a real or perceived threat. The cardiovascular effects of SNS stimulation include increased heart rate, increased contractility, and vasoconstriction. Stimulation of the parasympathetic nervous system causes the opposite effects: decreased heart rate, decreased contractility, and vasodilation.

Increasing the heart rate is the most effective mechanism for increasing cardiac output; however, this mechanism has limitations. A severe tachycardia causes stroke volume to decrease because the heart spends too little time in diastole (relaxation) and the ventricles do not have time to fill with blood. The faster the heart rate, the shorter the time spent in diastole. Reduced ventricular filling results in decreased preload and decreased stroke volume.

Stroke Volume The volume of blood pumped with each heartbeat is called the **stroke volume (SV)**. It is calculated as cardiac output (CO) divided by heart rate (HR), a simple calculation once CO is known. For example, given a normal heart rate of approximately 72 beats per minute (bpm, adult range 60–100) and CO of approximately 5 L/min, the usual stroke volume for an adult is 5000 mL/min divided by 72 bpm = 69 mL/beat or approximately 70 mL/beat.

A change in either heart rate or stroke volume alters CO. The interrelationship between these two factors maintains a normal CO (see Table 13–2), for example:

- If SV falls, HR increases to compensate and maintain CO. Conversely, if HR decreases, SV increases to compensate and maintain CO.
- If SV is held constant (remains the same), any change in HR results in an immediate change in CO. For example, if SV is stable at 70 mL and HR drops from 70 to 50 bpm, CO drops from 4.9 to 3.5 L/min. If HR increases from 70 to 100 bpm and SV remains at 70 mL, CO increases from 4.9 to 7 L/min.

Table 13–2 Relationship of Changes in Heart Rate or Stroke Volume to Cardiac Output

Heart Rate (HR)	Stroke Volume (SV)	Cardiac Output (CO)
↑	↓	↔
↓	↑	↔
↑	↔	↑
↓	↔	↓
↑↑*	↓	↓

*Severe tachycardia.

Of course, there is a limit to the capacity of the body to use these compensatory efforts to maintain cardiac output.

Preload. Preload is the amount of stretch in the myocardial fibers at the end of diastole and represents the volume of blood in the ventricle at the end of diastole. The greater the volume of blood in the ventricle, the greater the amount of stretch that the fibers experience. Preload is greatly affected by the volume of blood delivered to the heart from the venous system. If a large volume of blood returns from the venous system to the ventricle, the myocardial fibers are stretched so that they are far apart. This represents a high preload. If a small volume of blood returns from the venous system to the ventricle, there is less stretch and, therefore, less preload. High preload corresponds to high volume; low preload corresponds to low volume.

Within limits, the heart pumps the amount of blood it receives with each beat. This is known as the *Frank–Starling law* of the heart. In other words, as preload increases, so does stroke volume; as preload decreases, stroke volume falls. This law only applies within a certain range. Note in Figure 13–9A that until a critical point is reached, as preload increases, so does stroke volume—an optimal preload results in optimal stroke volume. Past this point, an increase in preload results in a decrease in stroke volume and contractility (Figure 13–9B). Too much

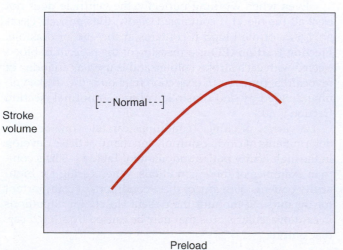

A

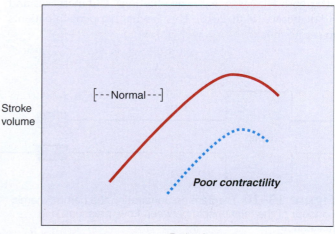

B

Figure 13–9 Graphs demonstrating the Frank–Starling law of the heart.

preload, such as occurs with fluid volume overload, causes excessive stretching of the myocardial fibers; the ventricles cannot effectively contract, resulting in a decreased stroke volume.

Afterload

Afterload is the resistance against which the ventricles pump blood. An optimal amount of resistance is necessary for the system to work properly. If afterload increases, stroke volume decreases because the ventricle is meeting increased resistance and cannot effectively pump out its volume. Most of the resistance the heart meets is related to the size of the arterioles—that is, whether they are vasoconstricted or vasodilated. If they are vasoconstricted, afterload to the ventricle increases and stroke volume decreases. If the vessels are vasodilated, afterload to the ventricle decreases and stroke volume increases. Other variables include the functionality of the semilunar (pulmonic and aortic) valves, which, if stenotic, are unable to fully open during systole, increasing afterload in the ventricles.

Imagine a system with a pump, a rigid tube, and a valve some distance from the pump, as shown in Figure 13–10. If the valve is half closed, the pressure in the tube increases as the rate of the liquid being pumped increases. If the pump runs very fast and the valve is partially closed, the pressure in the pipe is high. If, however, the pump output remains constant and the valve is opened completely, there is little pressure in the tube. This relationship among flow, resistance, and pressure is expressed in *Ohm's law*:

$$Pressure = Flow \times Resistance$$

Just as stroke volume and heart rate compensate to maintain cardiac output, flow and resistance compensate to maintain blood pressure (BP). Flow in the cardiovascular system is cardiac output (CO), resistance is afterload, and pressure is arterial blood pressure (ABP). Therefore, ABP is the product of CO and afterload. When afterload increases (e.g., vasoconstriction), CO decreases and BP increases. This is what happens to patients with hypertension. When afterload decreases (e.g., vasodilation), CO increases and BP decreases (Hall, 2016). This is what happens to patients in septic shock.

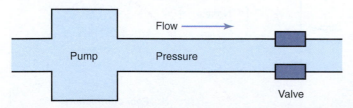

Figure 13–10 Diagram demonstrating the hemodynamic concept of the relationship between flow, pressure, and resistance

Contractility

Contractility is the ability of a muscle cell to become shorter, given a suitable stimulus. Clinically, in the context of heart function, it refers to the force of myocardial contraction and reflects the ability of the heart muscle to work independently of preload and afterload—that is, the heart's ability to function as a pump. If the heart contracts forcefully, it pumps out most of the blood in the ventricles. If the heart pumps weakly, it pumps out less blood. Many variables affect the force with which the heart muscle contracts; however, anything that enhances or diminishes the ability of myocardial fibers to contract significantly affects contractility.

The functioning of cardiac muscle is dependent on the coordinated interaction of multiple factors, including heart rate, velocity of cardiac muscle shortening, calcium, force, and muscle length. Increased calcium release allows for greater interaction between actin and myosin filaments, resulting in greater contraction. Cardiac muscle contraction depends on an influx of calcium; however, cardiac muscle does not store calcium, so serum calcium levels are important to monitor. It is important for the nurse to recognize that when a patient's serum calcium is low, contractility may be reduced. Intravenous replacement of calcium may be required to regain normal levels and increase contractility.

Factors that influence contractility are known as **inotropes**. Factors that increase myocardial contractility have a positive inotropic effect. Examples of positive inotropes include sympathetic nervous system stimulation, increased calcium release, and the administration of inotropic drugs. Factors that decrease contractility have a negative inotropic effect. Because hypoxemia decreases contractility, it is an example of a negative inotrope. In high-acuity settings, positive inotropic drugs are often used to augment cardiac output by improving myocardial contractility. Examples of positive inotrope agents include cardiac glycosides (e.g., digoxin), sympathomimetic agents (e.g., dopamine and dobutamine), and phosphodiesterase inhibitors (e.g., amrinone and milrinone).

Even when working perfectly, the ventricle does not eject all the blood it contains. Usually, the ventricle ejects only 60% of the blood it contains at the end of diastole. **Ejection fraction (EF)** is a measure of the percent of blood ejected with each stroke volume and is used as an index of myocardial function. The ejection fraction is the stroke volume divided by end diastolic volume. A normal ejection fraction is 60%.

A variety of clinical conditions can alter one or more determinants of cardiac output, and many of these develop in the high-acuity patient population. Table 13–3 lists common examples of these conditions. When caring for high-acuity patients with any of these conditions, it is important for the nurse to monitor the patient closely for alterations in cardiovascular status that may be caused by altered cardiac output.

Table 13–3 Conditions That Alter Determinants of Cardiac Output

CO Determinant	Trend	Factors	Examples of Clinical Conditions
Heart rate	Increased	SNS stimulation	Drug side effects Events or conditions perceived as threats Hospital environment: stimuli that activate SNS (e.g., pain, anxiety, sensory overstimulation, physiologic stressors)
		Rapid cardiac conduction	Tachycardias of any origin (e.g., sinus tachycardia, ventricular tachycardia)
	Decreased	Parasympathetic nervous system (PNS) stimulation Impaired or slowed cardiac conduction	Drug side effects, poisoning Straining during bowel movement (and other Valsalva maneuvers) Bradycardia of any origin (e.g., sinus bradycardia, AV blocks) Drug-induced bradycardia (e.g., beta blockers, calcium channel blockers)
Preload	Increased	Increased blood volume	Heart or kidney failure Fluid overload from IV therapy Increased aldosterone secretion Excess dietary sodium
	Decreased	Decreased blood volume	Hemorrhage, dehydration, diuretic use, severe ascites, generalized edema (e.g., severe hypoalbuminemia) AV valve stenosis (decreases ventricular filling) Venous vasodilation (blood pools peripherally; decreased blood returns to right heart)
		Rapid heart rate	Severe tachycardia (decreases ventricular filling time)
Contractility	Increased	Sympathetic nervous system (SNS) stimulation Drug effects	Refer to heart rate examples Epinephrine, norepinephrine, dobutamine, dopamine, digitalis
	Decreased	PNS stimulation Hypoxia or ischemia	Refer to heart rate examples Acute coronary syndrome, global hypoxia disorders (e.g., severe pulmonary disease)
		Myocardial disease Drug effects	Myocarditis, cardiomyopathy Depressant effects of many narcotic and anesthetic agents
Afterload	Increased	Arteriole vasoconstriction	Stimulation of SNS Drugs that vasoconstrict (epinephrine, norepinephrine)
		Semilunar valve failure	Pulmonic or aortic valve stenosis
	Decreased	Arteriole vasodilation	Depression of SNS Drugs that vasodilate (e.g., nitroglycerine) Septic shock, anaphylactic shock, or spinal cord injury

Section Three Review

1. A client has developed a heart rate of 150 bpm. This would have which effect on cardiac output?
   A. Increase
   B. Decrease
   C. No effect
   D. Unpredictable

2. A client with a normal heart has developed increased preload. This will result in which hemodynamic change?
   A. Increase in heart rate
   B. Decrease in contractility
   C. Increase in stroke volume
   D. Decrease in afterload

3. In a client with normal heart function, if blood pressure decreases and flow remains unchanged, peripheral resistance will change in which way to increase the blood pressure?
   A. It will decrease.
   B. It will increase.
   C. It will remain unchanged.
   D. It will fluctuate.

4. Which conditions, if present in the client, can result in decreased afterload? (Select all that apply.)
   A. Septic shock
   B. Depressed sympathetic NS
   C. Vasodilating drugs
   D. Aortic valve stenosis
   E. Hypertension

Answers: 1. B, 2. C, 3. B, 4. (A, B, C)

Section Four: Review of Blood Pressure

Blood pressure is the amount of pressure exerted against blood vessel walls by circulating blood as it is pumped throughout the body. Arterial blood pressure is a major factor in tissue oxygenation and perfusion and is closely tied to cardiac output. Keeping in mind that the source of arterial blood pressure begins with contraction of the left heart (circulatory pump), it stands to reason that the aorta, which is adjacent to the left ventricle, has the highest blood pressures while most distal venous vessels have the lowest pressures. Figure 13–11 depicts how normal blood pressure varies throughout the circulatory system.

The purpose of blood pressure is to circulate blood throughout the pulmonary and systemic circuits. There are two types of measurable blood pressure, arterial pressure (AP) and venous pressure (VP).

Arterial Blood Pressure

Arterial pressure is a function of peripheral resistance (PR) and cardiac output (CO) and is expressed as arterial BP = PR × CO (Barrett, Barman, Boitano, & Brooks, 2016b). This formula shows that anything that alters peripheral resistance or cardiac output must alter arterial blood pressure. Recall from Section Three that peripheral resistance (afterload) involves arterial tone (vasodilation or vasoconstriction of arterioles), whereas cardiac output involves heart rate and stroke volume.

Venous Blood Pressure

In Section One, venous circulation was presented as a low-pressure system. It is influenced by four factors: systemic filling pressure, adequacy of the venous (muscle) pump, venous peripheral resistance, and right atrial pressure.

Systemic Filling Pressure *Systemic filling pressure* refers to the amount of force that is available to return blood to the right side of the heart. The filling pressure is influenced by venous tone (how dilated or constricted the veins are) and blood volume; thus, venous vasoconstriction or increased blood volume increases filling pressure and increases venous blood return to the heart. The opposite is true as well: Venous vasodilation or decreased blood volume decreases filling pressure and therefore decreases venous blood return to the heart.

Venous Muscle Pump The adequacy of the venous muscle pump, described in Section One, is an important factor in determining venous blood pressure because if the venous valves are not working correctly (e.g., in a person who has varicose veins, is paralyzed, or is not active), blood pools in the extremities rather than moving forward to the heart. Less blood coming back into the right heart reduces the amount of blood available for gas exchange and decreases cardiac output.

Venous Peripheral Resistance When the lumen size of veins becomes reduced for any reason, the result is increased resistance to blood flow. Veins have a thin muscular-wall layer, limiting their ability to change size; however, their lumen size is heavily influenced by external factors such as pressure from muscles and organs, which can partially

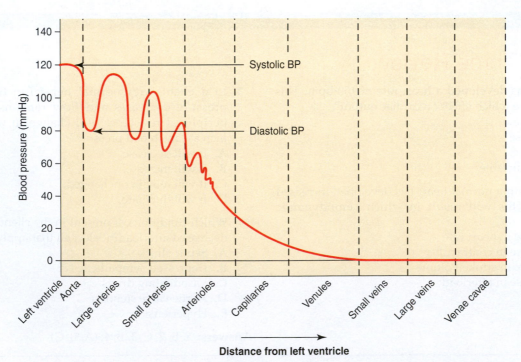

Figure 13–11 Normal blood pressures throughout the circulatory system. Note that the greater the distance from the left ventricle, the lower the pressure.

collapse adjacent veins. Moreover, any condition that increases intra-abdominal pressure (e.g., morbid obesity, ascites, or abdominal compartment syndrome) can result in complete or partial collapse of abdominal veins if the intra-abdominal pressure exceeds venous pressures (Hall, 2016).

Right Atrial Pressure   The pressure in the right atrium (RA) is the final influencing factor. At rest, the right atrial pressure is near zero; however, when the atrium contracts (systole), it causes a slightly negative pressure, which has a mild sucking or vacuum effect, pulling blood into the atrium from the vena cava. This action contributes to venous blood pressure, as well as cardiac output.

Regulation of Arterial Blood Pressure

Recall that arterial blood pressure is determined by peripheral resistance and cardiac output. Therefore, anything that causes peripheral vasoconstriction or vasodilation or that alters cardiac output will change blood pressure. It is important, then, to briefly consider the ways in which these factors are normally regulated by the body. There are three major regulatory systems: the renin-angiotensin-aldosterone system (RAAS), the kidneys, and the autonomic nervous system (ANS).

The Renin-angiotensin-aldosterone System   The renin-angiotensin-aldosterone system (RAAS) (Figure 13–12) influences arterial blood pressure through two mechanisms: vasoconstriction and water retention. The following is a brief review of how these two mechanisms affect blood pressure.

As blood pressure drops, so does perfusion to the kidneys, which triggers the release of renin, an enzyme produced by the kidneys. Renin triggers the release of angiotensin I, which converts to angiotensin II, a powerful vasoconstrictor that primarily targets the smooth muscles of arterioles, resulting in arteriole vasoconstriction and increased arterial blood pressure. Angiotensin II also stimulates the adrenal cortex to release aldosterone, a mineralocorticoid hormone that causes renal retention of sodium and water, resulting in increased circulating blood volume with subsequent increase in arterial blood pressure. When the actions of the RAAS have increased blood pressure sufficiently to regain normal kidney perfusion pressures, the RAAS shuts down (Eaton & Pooler, 2013).

The Kidneys   The kidneys alter blood pressure through the RAAS mechanism and through retention of water. Blood flow through the kidneys diminishes as arterial blood pressure drops, resulting in a reduced glomerular filtration rate (GFR). As GFR decreases, so does urine output, with resultant water retention, increased circulating blood volume, and increasing blood pressure. The close relationship between arterial blood pressure and urine output is clinically important because the nurse can monitor urine output trends as one indicator of adequate arterial blood pressure.

The Autonomic Nervous System   Both branches of the autonomic nervous system (ANS; sympathetic and parasympathetic) play active roles in regulating blood pressure through adjusting peripheral resistance and cardiac output. The sympathetic nervous system (SNS) increases CO by causing vasoconstriction, speeding up the heart rate, and increasing cardiac contractility, while the parasympathetic nervous system (PNS) decreases cardiac output by slowing the heart rate and decreasing cardiac contractility and vasodilation.

The autonomic nervous system is also responsible for the *baroreceptor reflex*, which is largely responsible for maintaining a steady-state blood pressure (BP). Baroreceptors are special nerve endings located in the walls of certain large vessels (e.g., aortic arch, aorta, vena cava, and carotid sinus) and the atria. These receptors are sensitive to changes in pressure at their locations. When pressure changes at a baroreceptor, it sends a signal to the medulla to trigger one of two actions: (1) If BP has fallen below the preset value, the medulla stimulates the heart rate to increase and the arterioles (and veins to a lesser extent) to constrict; or (2) if BP has risen above the preset level it will slow down the heart rate and trigger vessel dilation. Reflecting back on the two formulae presented at the beginning of this section, these actions alter cardiac output in two ways:

1. $BP = PR \times CO$ — any change in vessel tone (peripheral resistance, or PR) or BP changes CO

2. $CO = HR \times SV$ — any change in heart rate (HR) or stroke volume (SV) components (contractility, preload, and afterload) changes CO

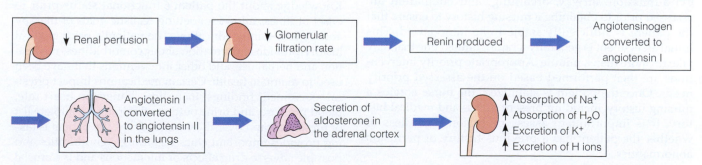

Figure 13–12 The renin-angiotensin-aldosterone system. Decreased blood volume and renal perfusion set off a chain of reactions leading to release of aldosterone from the adrenal cortex. Increased levels of aldosterone regulate serum K^+ and Na^+, blood pressure, and water balance through effects on the kidney tubules.

Section Four Review

1. Which formula correctly represents arterial blood pressure?
   A. $BP = HR \times SV$
   B. $BP = PR \times CO$
   C. $BP = CO / HR$
   D. $BP = CO / PR$

2. How is the term *systemic filling pressure* best defined?
   A. The amount of force available to return blood to the heart
   B. The degree to which veins are dilated
   C. The volume of blood pooled in the vessels
   D. The pressure in the right atrium during systole

3. Which statement correctly describes how the renin-angiotensin-aldosterone system (RAAS) alters blood pressure?
   A. Kidneys release angiotensin I, which causes the release of renin.
   B. The adrenal cortex releases renin.
   C. Angiotensin II stimulates the release of aldosterone.
   D. Renin triggers the adrenal medulla to release angiotensin I.

4. When baroreceptors sense a blood pressure that is below the individual's normal preset level, which set of actions is triggered?
   A. Increased heart rate, vasoconstriction
   B. Decreased heart rate, vasoconstriction
   C. Increased stroke volume and contractility
   D. Decreased stroke volume and contractility

Answers: 1. B, 2. A, 3. C, 4. A

Section Five: Assessment of Cardiac Function

In high-acuity patients with potentially severe hemodynamic issues, invasive or noninvasive means of monitoring hemodynamic status, including cardiac output, may be warranted. Chapter 8: Basic Hemodynamic Monitoring provides an overview of this type of complex monitoring; therefore, it is not covered in this chapter.

The key to accurately evaluating cardiac function lies in the assessment skills of the nurse. Assessment begins on admission. The nurse must obtain subjective data, conduct a complete physical assessment, interpret lab results, use bedside monitoring equipment effectively, and apply the data gained via various diagnostic procedures. The nursing process, particularly in high-acuity care, depends on a thorough assessment.

Patient History

On admission, airway, breathing, and circulation are assessed prior to obtaining a nursing history to ensure that the patient is sufficiently stable to be interviewed. This initial assessment is generally a rapid, limited one that may take no more than a minute. Appropriate priority interventions are then performed based on the assessed priority needs. Once the patient is stabilized, the nurse obtains a nursing history, including present illness and medical history. It is important to assess perfusion regardless of whether the patient has a previous history of perfusion abnormalities.

Present Illness and Medical History At the time of admission, the nurse may be interviewing the patient, a family member, or someone else. Eliciting a recent history of the present illness (i.e., the events leading up to this admission) provides the clinician with important data regarding the problem, possible etiologies, and the patient's ability to compensate for a cardiovascular stressor. Information about recent history also helps identify areas in which the patient may need external support in order to increase myocardial oxygen supply and decrease myocardial oxygen demand and thereby regain or maintain a state of compensation.

A detailed patient history at the time of admission helps determine the plan of care. By using interviewing techniques and therapeutic communication, the nurse obtains demographic data, family history (particularly of cardiovascular diseases), dietary information, functional status, and prior medical history. Demographic data include the patient's age, sex, race, and weight. Cardiovascular risk factors such as smoking history, exercise pattern, stress level, and obesity are assessed (D'Amico & Barbarito, 2016). Obesity (defined as body mass index of 30 kg/m² or greater in adults) is a known risk factor for coronary heart and cerebral vascular diseases (American Heart Association, 2016). Knowledge about the patient's functional status prior to onset of illness allows for setting realistic goals of therapy and patient–family education. The patient's prior medical history provides information about comorbidities, medication and herbal use, and other interventions that have been used to maintain health. Certain medications impact physical assessment findings, including changes in heart rate, blood pressure, and urine output. Obtaining a complete list of prescribed and over-the-counter drugs the patient is taking provides important clues regarding comorbidities and possible adverse drug effects or interactions and is a crucial first step in medication reconciliation.

Complaints of chest pain must be assessed and differentiated from pain of pulmonary or gastrointestinal origin

(Chyu & Shah, 2014). The mnemonic APQRST is helpful in organizing assessment data related to pain and eliciting information about (A) associated symptoms, (P) precipitating factors, (Q) quality, (R) radiation and region, (S) severity, and (T) timing and treatment strategies. These help the nurse determine the origin of the pain (Leeper, 2014). Pain may not always be present in patients with diminished myocardial perfusion. Individuals with diabetes mellitus, women, or older adults may not experience chest pain due to chronic neuropathy. Women may have atypical symptoms of myocardial ischemia, such as abdominal pain and fatigue.

A patient with a perfusion disorder may complain of **palpitations**, often described as a "skipping" or "thumping" of the heart. This symptom is related to the occurrence of premature cardiac beats. Palpation of the pulse will reveal premature beats. There will be irregular pulse amplitude because of the decreased blood volume associated with premature beats and the larger-than-normal volume of the beat immediately after the premature beat related to prolonged diastolic filling. The best way to detect premature beats is to obtain an electrocardiogram (ECG) and monitor the patient's cardiac rhythm.

A patient with a perfusion disorder may experience a change in level of consciousness related to a decreased cardiac output or blockage of cerebral circulation. A diminished level of consciousness, confusion, or agitation may be signs of decreased perfusion to cerebral tissue. The patient may experience **syncope**, a temporary loss of consciousness followed by complete, spontaneous recovery.

Nursing Physical Assessment

Techniques of physical assessment of cardiac function include inspection, palpation, and auscultation. Because of the rapid changes that can occur in the acute care setting, cardiac function is assessed frequently. By developing a systematic method of physical assessment, the nurse rapidly ascertains changes in hemodynamic status. Data obtained by technological means must be corroborated with physical assessments. Overreliance on monitoring equipment alarms may lead to complacency, and subtle physical changes may be missed.

Inspection Inspection of the precordium (the region of the thorax immediately in front of the heart) may demonstrate rhythmic movement associated with cardiac contraction. Abnormal movement may be visualized in the aortic, pulmonic, or tricuspid areas. Normal movement is found in the area of the mitral valve. This is the apical impulse. It is usually seen in the area of the left fifth intercostal space along the midclavicular line.

Peripheral Assessment. Inspection and palpation of the periphery can also indicate variations in the patient's cardiac output. Changes in skin color are a late sign of hemodynamic compromise, as is clubbing of the fingers. A cooling of the skin is brought about by the vasoconstriction of the arterioles as blood is shunted to the internal organs. A decrease in CO may be the cause. Cool distal extremities may be a useful marker of decreased CO. Delayed capillary refill is often associated with decreased CO; however, capillary refill as an indicator of the adequacy of CO is controversial. It may be useful as a marker of hypovolemia and poor myocardial function in children, but in older adult patients it may not be as useful.

Urine Output. The kidney is sensitive to changes in intravascular volume; therefore, urine output is frequently used to assess the adequacy of cardiac output. Theoretically, a decrease in CO results in a decrease in urine output. However, there are conditions in which urine output does

Emerging Evidence

- The use of Pooled Cohort Equations was recommended by the American College of Cardiology and the American Heart Association (ACC/AHA) in their updated cholesterol guidelines to estimate the 10-year risk of atherosclerotic cardiovascular disease (ASCVD). For decades, factors of age, sex, smoking, blood pressure, total cholesterol, high-density lipoprotein cholesterol, and use of antihypertensive medication were used to predict 10-year individual risk of ASCVD, to facilitate lifestyle changes, and to initiate lipid-lowering drug therapy. In addition to these long-standing variables that have calculated risk of acute coronary events, the Pooled Cohort Equations improve risk calculation by the inclusion of fatal or nonfatal stroke as an outcome endpoint and the inclusion of diabetes as an independent predictive risk factor. Inclusion of racial and geographical diversity in risk calculation has also improved predictions of ASCVD events among non-Hispanic white and African American men and women (Karmali, Goff, Ning, & Lloyd-Jones, 2014).

- Measurement of depressive symptoms and biomarkers of inflammation (tumor necrosis factor receptor I) should be considered as part of the overall cardiovascular assessment and care of individuals with heart failure. In a study of 145 patients with heart failure, when controlling for factors of age, body mass index, use of beta blockers, comorbid disease, and left ventricular ejection fraction, a higher level of the inflammatory biomarker was significantly ($p < .001$) associated with patient-reported severity of signs and symptoms of heart failure. When patients were stratified by depressed versus nondepressed (as measured by the Beck Depression Inventory II), the inflammatory biomarker (TNF-RI) was significantly ($p = .005$) associated with physical symptoms (dyspnea during day and when lying down, fatigue, chest pain, edema, sleeping difficulty, and dizziness) only among the nondepressed group. Patients who provided lower ratings of heart failure symptom severity reported higher social support and fewer comorbid conditions with lower levels of body mass index, and the inflammatory biomarker TNF (Heo, Moser, Pressler, Dunbar, Dekker, & Lennie, 2014).

- In a study of 90 patients, a higher troponin I level was associated with higher hospital mortality ($p = .01$) among ICU patients without acute coronary syndrome within 24 hours of admission. Patients with elevated cardiac troponin I levels had significantly higher frequencies of intubation ($p = .02$) and higher ICU mortality ($p = .01$) when compared to control group patients who did not have elevated troponin I levels (Liu, Shehu, Herrold, & Cohen, 2015).

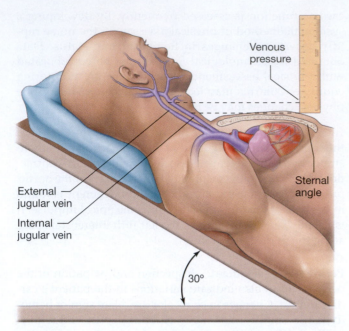

Figure 13–13 Measuring jugular vein pressure.

not reflect the adequacy of CO. These conditions may affect patients in compensatory shock states and older adults. Older adults may have chronic diseases and use medications that affect urine output.

Edema. The presence of peripheral edema may indicate too much preload to the right side of the heart. Edema associated with heart failure is generally located in the gravity-dependent areas of the body, such as the feet and lower legs and sacrum.

Jugular Vein Distention. Oscillations of the jugular veins are not normally observed when the chest is in an upright posture. Jugular venous distention (JVD) may indicate a fluid distribution problem and too much preload to the right side of the heart. The venous system is a low-pressure system, and it is sensitive to right atrial pressure. Retention of blood in the right side of the heart (as in heart failure or cor pulmonale) increases right atrial pressure and subsequently produces jugular vein distention as a result of backflow through the vena cava. In assessing for venous distention, the head of the bed is elevated 30 to 45 degrees. The patient's head is turned slightly away from the examiner. A penlight is used to shine a light tangentially across the neck (Figure 13–13).

Palpation Palpation gives the nurse a tactile indication of cardiac function. Rolling the patient onto the left side moves the heart closer to the surface of the body. Precordial palpation may produce a vibration, also known as a *thrill*. This may correspond to a murmur, valvular stenosis, or increased afterload. The point of maximal impulse (PMI) corresponds to the location of the apical impulse. Heaves and lifts also indicate ventricular hypertrophy on either side. On the periphery, palpation of pulses helps to assess cardiac output. Pulses should be of regular rate, strength, and rhythm. A hyperkinetic (bounding) pulse may indicate

increased CO because of thyrotoxicosis, fever, pain, or anxiety. A hypokinetic pulse may be the result of decreased CO, with causes such as dysrhythmias, damaged myocardium, or cardiomyopathy. Severely depressed cardiac function may cause **pulsus alternans**, or alternating weak and strong pulses in a regular rhythm.

Auscultation Auscultation is another technique for assessing cardiac output. Knowledge of the heart sounds associated with valvular dysfunction is essential. Recall that the function of heart valves is to provide a unidirectional flow of blood through the heart. With valve dysfunction, blood flow is turbulent or reduced, resulting in a decrease in CO.

Auscultation of the precordium must be systematic and performed using both the bell and the diaphragm of the stethoscope. The pattern of auscultation begins at the base of the heart, using the diaphragm in the area of the aortic valve, and proceeds to the pulmonic, tricuspid, and mitral valves in that order. The bell is used in a reverse sequence. Various extra heart sounds may be heard, such as high- and low-frequency murmurs, or extra systolic sounds, such as clicks and rubs. Heart murmurs heard during systole or diastole are evidence of turbulent blood flow and can result from stenotic or incompetent valves. Table 13–4 outlines the grading system used to classify murmurs.

Diastolic filling sounds may help determine why cardiac output is reduced. The S3 sound, heard early in diastole, is a ventricular filling sound caused by decreased ventricular compliance and is a sign of early heart failure. It is also known as **ventricular gallop**. S4 is also a ventricular filling sound but occurs late in diastole. It is heard during atrial contraction and is known as **atrial gallop**. It is a result of myocardial infarction, ventricular hypertrophy, and increased afterload. A **summation gallop**, when both S3 and S4 sounds are heard, is often indicative of severe heart failure. The presence of wet-sounding crackles (rales) on auscultation of the lungs indicates pulmonary edema. Severe pulmonary edema is associated with frothy, pink sputum production.

Auscultatory techniques can also be used on the peripheral vasculature system. Bruits along the carotid arteries may indicate areas of occlusion. These partial blockages represent potential compromise to the cerebral vasculature and account for some signs and symptoms also attributable to decreased cardiac output. Renal artery bruits may indicate renal artery stenosis, which leads to

Table 13–4 Grading System Used to Classify Murmurs

I/VI	Very faint
II/VI	Faint
III/VI	Loud; moderate in intensity
IV/VI	Loud; palpable thrill
V/VI	Loud enough to be heard with head of stethoscope partially off chest wall; palpable thrill
VI/VI	Loud enough to be heard with head of stethoscope completely off chest wall; palpable thrill

systemic hypertension. The resulting increase in afterload may compromise cardiac output.

Diagnostic Laboratory Tests

Numerous diagnostic lab parameters are used to assess cardiac function, which is adversely affected by myocardial damage.

Cardiac Markers   When myocardial cells die due to infarction, they release their intracellular contents, including enzymes, into local interstitium and then migrate into the circulation. Serum biomarkers specific for cardiac assessment include troponin-I (cTnI) and troponin-T (cTnT) as well as creatine kinase myocardial bands (CK-MB). Elevated serum levels are indicative of myocardial cell death.

Creatine Kinase.   Creatine kinase (CK) is an enzyme present in cells of the myocardium, skeletal muscles, and in a smaller quantity in the brain. CK is composed of three isoenzymes, including the myocardial band (MB,) which is specific for assessing myocardial cell damage. Elevation of CK-MB within the serum occurs 4 to 6 hours following myocardial damage from infarction. The highest elevation is expected around 18 to 24 hours postinfarction with a gradual return to normal limits within 3 to 4 days. Recurrent elevation of the CK-MB after the peak level is observed is associated with recurrence or extension of acute myocardial infarction (Kee, 2014). Because of the variability of when elevated levels appear following myocardial infarction, CK-MB and other cardiac enzymes are often obtained on a serial basis, every 6 to 8 hours following onset of signs or symptoms of acute myocardial infarction. The major limitation of CK-MB is that levels do not start to rise until 4 hours after the onset of myocardial damage. This can delay diagnosis and treatment of myocardial infarction. This is one of the reasons that troponin is considered the leading laboratory criterion for assessing myocardial infarction.

Troponin.   Troponin is the leading laboratory indicator to assess for myocardial damage and to assist with diagnosis of acute myocardial infarction (Hannibal, 2013). **Troponin** is a protein found in cardiac and skeletal muscle. It is part of a calcium-controlled protein complex that binds myosin and actin, the myofilaments that regulate contraction. The cardiac-specific troponin proteins include troponin-I (cTnI) and troponin-T (cTnT). Troponin-I is only present in the cardiac muscle, while troponin-T also exists in skeletal muscle. Elevated troponin can be detected in the blood as early as 1 to 3 hours after onset of symptoms of myocardial infarction. Troponin-I is elevated for 5 to 9 days following an infarction; troponin-T is elevated for as long as 10 to 14 days (Kee, 2014).

Positive troponin levels play an important role in diagnosis of acute myocardial infarction and prediction of the severity of patient outcomes postinfarction. While highly specific for diagnosing myocardial damage, elevated troponin values alone do not confirm myocardial infarction. Diagnosis of acute myocardial infarction also utilizes data from the electrocardiogram, acute symptoms, and patient history. Positive troponin levels are also found with other cardiac and systemic conditions, such as heart failure, cardiac inflammatory processes, chest trauma, cardiac interventional procedures, sepsis, renal failure, and neurovascular events (Newby et al., 2012).

Other Laboratory Tests   Other laboratory tests may be ordered to provide additional supportive data, including C-reactive protein, B-type natriuretic peptide, and lipid profile.

C-reactive Protein (CRP).   **C-reactive protein (CRP)** is a peptide released by the liver in response to systemic inflammation, infection, and tissue damage. It is a normal part of the inflammatory response, playing an important role in fighting infection or injury (Kee, 2014). In the absence of infection or injury, serum CRP levels should be negligible (normal range is 0–1 mg/dL in the healthy adult (Kee, 2014). Atherosclerosis is a chronic inflammatory process associated with increased serum CRP levels. This laboratory finding does not provide any additional diagnostic information in individuals with acute cardiac symptoms. Identification of increased serum CRP may be a more useful biomarker for preventive care. Elevation of CRP is recognized as an independent predictor of cardiovascular risk. However, routine screening of CRP is not recommended because the level can fluctuate significantly under a variety of circumstances, not just with atherosclerosis (Fedewa, Das, Forehand, & Evans, 2014).

B-type Natriuretic Peptide or Brain Natriuretic Peptide.   **B-type natriuretic peptide (BNP)** is a neurohormone released from the ventricular myocardium in response to fluid volume excess and increased intracardiac pressures (increased preload BNP is sometimes called "brain" natriuretic peptide because it was first discovered within pig brains but is present in humans only within the ventricles of the heart (Kee, 2014).

BNP is released as a compensatory response to progressively increased preload such as occurs with heart failure. The beneficial physiologic effects of BNP include suppression of the sympathetic nervous system, the renin-angiotensin-aldosterone system, and antidiuretic hormone (vasopressin) release. Sympathetic nervous system suppression results in venous and arterial vasodilation. With venous dilation, less blood is returned to the chambers of the heart and preload decreases. Decreased peripheral vascular resistance occurs with arterial vasodilation, causing a decrease in afterload and less work for the heart during systole. However, the effects stimulated by BNP are not adequate to overcome the fluid retention and vasoconstriction controlled by other hormonal actions in response to damaged myocardium (Miranda, Lewis, & Fifer, 2016).

The normal serum value of BNP is below 100 pg/mL or less than 100 ng/L (SI units), although in women age 65 and above, a level of up to 160 pg/mL may be within the normal range. Values above 100 pg/mL are diagnostic for heart failure (Kee, 2014). Increased BNP levels are positively associated with the extent of ventricular dysfunction. With severe cardiac disease, BNP levels can be increased 30-fold.

Lipid Profile. **Hyperlipidemia**, high levels of lipids in the blood, is associated with a high risk for coronary heart disease. High-risk lipids include elevated total cholesterol, increased low-density lipoprotein (LDL), decreased high-density lipoprotein (HDL), and elevated triglycerides. HDL is the "good" cholesterol (remember, H stands for "high"). LDL is the "bad" cholesterol (remember, L stands for "low"). Higher levels of HDLs than LDLs are desirable (Kee, 2014).

Assessment of Specific Components of Cardiac Output

Preload, like contractility and afterload, is difficult to assess at the bedside because the cardiovascular structures are embedded deeply in the chest, inaccessible for examination. Without special monitoring devices, the nurse must use indirect measures to estimate preload, contractility, and afterload.

Assessing Heart Rate Evaluating heart rate is relatively easy. A simple count of the radial pulse is useful for determining the number of heartbeats that are strong enough to reach the periphery. A count of the apical heart rate is useful to determine the total heart rate. Usually these two rates are equal, but there may be a deficit between the apical rate and the radial rate caused by irregular heart rhythms that result in stroke volume varying from beat to beat, which results in some beats being too weak to be felt at the radial artery (the **apical–radial pulse deficit**). For example, in a person complaining of dizziness, a radial pulse would give a better indication than an apical pulse of the adequacy of peripheral perfusion. It is recommended that the clinician use a 60-second counting interval when assessing a patient for the first time or if the patient is unstable, the cardiac rhythm is irregular, or treatment decisions are based on heart rate.

Assessing Preload Assessing ventricular preload is similar to assessing for fluid volume excess and fluid volume deficit, as seen in Table 13–5.

Right Ventricular Preload. Preload for the right ventricle is assessed by evaluating the systemic venous system. Increased preload to the right heart typically manifests as signs of too much fluid in the peripheral tissues and organs as fluid backs up from the right side of the heart.

Left Ventricular Preload. Preload for the left heart is assessed by evaluating the pulmonary venous system. Increased preload to the left heart typically manifests as signs of too much fluid in the pulmonary circulation as fluid backs up from the left side of the heart. No noninvasive assessments are currently available that specifically indicate diminished left ventricular preload. Usually, if the left heart has insufficient preload, the right heart has the same problem, and signs of diminished right ventricular preload are present. In some situations S1 and S2 may be muffled.

Assessing Contractility Contractility is difficult to measure indirectly by physical signs because so many other factors may alter the character of the pulse. Decreased contractility is usually determined by excluding other causes of poor cardiac output. Assessing the force of myocardial contraction (character of the pulse) through palpation of the radial pulse may provide clues regarding contractility as part of a broader assessment of cardiac output. Increased contractility demonstrates a bounding, vigorous pulse, whereas diminished contractility demonstrates a weak, thready pulse.

The mechanical events of the heart are synchronous between the right side and the left side, but they are not truly simultaneous. Events on the right side of the heart, including contraction of the atria and the ventricle, along with opening and closing of the tricuspid valve and the pulmonic valve with blood movement into the pulmonary artery, take slightly longer than the same mechanical activity within the heart's left side. This timing delay between the right and left side can produce a splitting of the S2 heart sound during inspiration. A splitting of S2 indicates that one ventricle is emptying earlier or later than the other. The splitting of S2 during inspiration is only physiologic and is a benign finding, especially in young individuals. This physiologic splitting is best heard in the second or third left intercostal space. This normal splitting is louder with inspiration but is not audible with expiration. However, S2 splitting during expiration is pathologic and likely due to a structural, mechanical, and/or electrophysiologic abnormality.

The **pulse pressure** is the difference between diastolic and systolic blood pressures. It reflects how much the heart is able to raise the pressure in the arterial system with each beat. Pulse pressure increases when stroke volume (SV) increases or in arteriole vasoconstriction. Pulse pressure drops with decreased SV or vasodilation (e.g., some shock states). The normal pulse pressure is approximately 30 to 40 mmHg. Within the restrictions noted, the pulse pressure can be a useful, objective, and noninvasive indicator of myocardial contractility.

Table 13–5 Assessments of Ventricular Preload

Right Ventricular Preload		Left Ventricular Preload	
Increased Preload	**Decreased Preload**	**Increased Preload**	**Decreased Preload**
Jugular vein distention (JVD)	Flat jugular veins	Dyspnea	Usually the same manifestations as decreased right preload
Ascites	Dry mucous membranes	Cough	Possible muffling of S1 and S2
Hepatic engorgement (enlarged, tender to palpation)	Orthostatic hypotension	S3, S4 heart sounds	
Peripheral edema	Poor skin turgor (immediate sign)		

Table 13–6 Assessments of Contractility

Increased Contractility	Decreased Contractility
Radial pulse: bounding and vigorous	Radial pulse: weak and thready
Increased pulse pressure	Pathologic splitting of S2 heart sound during expiration
	Decreased pulse pressure

Table 13–6 lists simple assessments that may reflect changes in contractility.

Assessing Afterload Indirect assessment of right ventricle afterload is difficult because of the location of the pulmonary arterial system deep in the chest. However, it is possible to assess the systemic arterial system for signs of increased or decreased afterload. Signs of altered afterload may be present in some patients, but not all. Remember again that all these determinants of cardiac output are interrelated, and it can be difficult to isolate individual factors at the bedside without invasive diagnostic tests.

Signs of increased systemic afterload include cool, clammy extremities. These signs may indicate that peripheral arterioles are constricted. Nonhealing wounds and thick brittle nails are indicators of chronic poor perfusion of the extremities. Signs of decreased systemic afterload include warm, flushed extremities, which may indicate peripheral vasodilation.

Section Five Review

1. The nurse is assessing a client who is complaining of chest pain, using the PQRST assessment format. The "S" in this mnemonic refers to which assessments?
   A. Timing and treatment strategies
   B. Associated symptoms
   C. Radiation and region
   D. Pain quality

2. Which cardiac enzyme appears in the blood within 3 hours of myocardial cell death?
   A. CRP
   B. BNP
   C. CK-MB
   D. Troponin

3. Decreased contractility is manifested by which signs?
   A. Bounding pulse
   B. Diminished pulse pressure
   C. Ascites
   D. Poor skin turgor

4. Which signs indicate possible increased afterload for the left ventricle?
   A. Cool, clammy extremities
   B. Thin, flexible toenails
   C. Liver engorgement
   D. Peripheral edema

Answers: 1. A, 2. D, 3. B, 4. A

Section Six: Cardiac Diagnostic Procedures

Numerous invasive and noninvasive diagnostic procedures evaluate cardiac function. A thorough investigation of cardiac status often requires a combination of diagnostic tests.

Noninvasive Procedures

Technology has increased the options for noninvasive diagnostic testing of cardiac structure and function. Common noninvasive procedures include electrocardiography and imaging techniques, alone or in combination with stress testing. With the growing number of diagnostic tests and their expanding availability, the American College of Cardiology Foundation and the American Heart Association established guidelines for the judicious and effective use of procedures to assess for cardiac risk (Goff et al., 2014). Noninvasive methods for cardiac diagnostic testing generally involve fewer patient risks, less discomfort, and lower costs when compared to invasive diagnostic procedures.

Electrocardiography The electrocardiogram (ECG) provides a graphic display for measuring the heart's electrical activity. It provides information about the rhythm, rate, and amplitude of the electrical impulse that travels through the specialized nerve fibers of the cardiac conduction system. Assessment of the heart's electrical conduction is important because it is the electrical impulse that stimulates the heart's mechanical actions. Electrocardiogram performance and interpretation are discussed in Chapter 15: Alterations in Myocardial Tissue Perfusion.

Chest Radiography A chest x-ray is used to view the size and position of the heart. An enlarged cardiac silhouette may be evidence of cardiac tamponade (excess fluid in the pericardial sac) or dilated cardiomyopathy. Pulmonary edema caused by decompensated heart failure may be visualized. No prior preparation is necessary for a chest x-ray, although it is important for the nurse to help the patient with proper positioning when the x-ray is obtained to ensure a high-quality film.

Echocardiogram The echocardiogram uses ultrasound to obtain graphic and audio recordings of sound waves bouncing off the heart's structures. There are two forms:

transthoracic echocardiogram and transesophageal echocardiogram (TEE). Echocardiograms are particularly useful for visualizing blood flow through the heart and the cardiac valves, localized cardiac wall motion, and pericardial effusion. Ultrasound technology can be used to assess and diagnose cardiomyopathies, valve dysfunction, septal wall abnormalities, cardiac tumors, and rupture of the ventricle wall or papillary muscle postinfarction. Hemodynamic data, such as an estimate of ejection fraction and cardiac output, can also be obtained. TEE is discussed under "Invasive Diagnostic Procedures."

Patients for whom echocardiography may provide useful diagnostic data include those with dyspnea, syncope, cardiac murmur, or ventricular or supraventricular dysrhythmias. The echocardiogram may also provide diagnostic findings in individuals with chest pain without abnormal ECG or cardiac enzymes (Ramos, 2014). An echocardiogram is recommended to assess for left ventricular hypertrophy in individuals with hypertension without visible signs or symptoms of heart disease (Goff et al., 2014).

Transthoracic echocardiograms are noninvasive tests that can be performed at the bedside or in the outpatient setting by a technician. The patient is usually placed in a semi-Fowler, left lateral, or supine position. The position is determined by the patient's overall condition and ability to tolerate the position, and the position that will give the best view of the structures to be visualized. Transducer gel applied on the skin helps to conduct sound waves. The transducer is then positioned on the chest. It emits ultrasound waves and receives a signal reflected back from structures of the heart and blood vessels. Continuous ECG is recorded along with the echocardiogram to correlate the timing of abnormal events with the cardiac cycle. Nursing responsibilities may include dimming of the lights in the room and ensuring patient privacy and warmth.

Stress Testing Stress testing is a common procedure for assessing the heart's response to increased oxygen demand. It can identify myocardial ischemia that may not be present at rest. The procedure involves exercise or a drug to stimulate, or stress, the heart. If the patient cannot tolerate exercise, stress to the heart muscle is stimulated with the administration of a vasodilator or dobutamine, a positive inotropic drug. Information about the heart's stress response always involves continuous ECG monitoring and could include echocardiography and/or injection of radioactive isotopes to assess for myocardial ischemia (Ramos, 2014).

Prior to the procedure, the patient may be anxious and may fear having a heart attack during the test. The patient should be assured of close monitoring during the procedure but should also be informed about the risks that can be as serious as acute myocardial infarction or death. The nurse conducting the exam must be familiar with cardiac dysrhythmias and emergency procedures and must ensure that emergency medications and a defibrillator are readily available.

The exercise-based stress test consists of the patient exercising on either a stationary bicycle or a treadmill.

During exercise, the myocardium's increased demand for blood supply provokes a compensatory response by the sympathetic nervous system. This sympathetic stimulation is intended to increase heart rate, stroke volume, and cardiac output. The rapid diversion of blood to the myocardium results from systemic vasoconstriction. In the presence of coronary artery blockages, impaired blood flow to the myocardium will lead to myocardial ischemia. Heart rate, blood pressure, and the ECG are closely monitored as the exercise workload is increased. The patient is reminded to let the nurse know if dizziness, chest pain, palpitations, or shortness of breath occurs. The test is discontinued when a predetermined heart rate is reached and maintained, signs of insufficient cardiac output appear, or ECG changes occur. Once the patient has returned to baseline hemodynamic status, he or she either returns to the hospital room or is allowed to go home. Some outpatients are admitted to the hospital for further diagnostic testing if results are unfavorable.

Absolute contraindications to stress testing include, but may not be limited to, myocardial infarction within the previous 2 days, unstable angina, congestive heart failure, aortic dissection, acute pulmonary embolus, and uncontrolled dysrhythmias. Relative contraindications to stress testing are already known blockage of the left coronary artery, acute anemia, tachydysrhythmias, and blood pressure above 200/110 mmHg (Fletcher et al., 2013).

Computed Tomography Computed tomography using multidetector methods obtains a series of x-rays of the heart during one breath-hold to provide images of the coronary arteries. Movement interferes with image resolution, so the patient must be able to cooperate during the procedure. The CT images are obtained during end-systole and mid-diastole when heart motion is at its lowest point. An antiarrhythmic drug is likely to be given to decrease heart motion by lowering the heart rate.

Cardiac CT is contraindicated with atrial fibrillation due to the heart's irregular motion. It is also not feasible for patients with surgical metal or implanted devices in the chest such as a pacemaker, defibrillator, and mechanical cardiac valves due to imaging artifact.

Cardiac CT can provide assessment of coronary artery calcium (CAC). Identification of calcium within the coronary artery (arteries) is always abnormal. Computer analysis of the CT images calculates a CAC score as a tool for predicting cardiac risk. Low cardiac risk is implied by a CAC score of 10 or less. Intermediate risk is within the range of a score between 11 and 399, and a score greater than 400 is considered very high risk for an acute cardiac event (Bunch, 2012).

Invasive Diagnostic Procedures

Common invasive procedures to evaluate cardiac function include transesophageal echocardiogram (TEE), cardiac catheterization, and electrophysiology study (EPS).

Transesophageal Echocardiogram (TEE) In preparation for the TEE procedure, an ultrasound probe is inserted orally into the patient's esophagus and advanced until it is close to the heart. The TEE provides a more definitive representation of the heart, producing images of intracardiac structures and the entire thoracic aorta. It produces high-quality images of both atrial chambers and is the procedure of choice to detect clots in the left atrium, atrial septal defects, infections on valve leaflets, and valve dysfunction.

Conscious (moderate) sedation is used with the TEE, so nursing care is much more involved than with a transthoracic echocardiogram. Prior to the procedure, the nurse reviews the patient's chart, obtains a detailed history, and inserts a peripheral intravenous catheter. Suction equipment should be available in case the patient vomits. During the procedure, the nurse administers sedation, monitors vital signs and pulse oximetry saturations every 3 to 5 minutes, adjusts fluid and oxygen, and documents the patient's condition. During and immediately after the procedure, the nurse monitors for complications, which include respiratory depression and aspiration. Movement of the probe in the esophagus may stimulate the vagus nerve, resulting in bradycardia or hypotension. Vital signs are monitored as the patient awakens from the procedure. The patient recovers in 1 to 2 hours. If the TEE is performed in an outpatient setting, the patient must be released to a responsible adult in case there are residual effects of the sedation.

Cardiac Catheterization

Cardiac catheterization, also called coronary angiography, remains the gold standard for assessment of coronary arteries. It is a powerful diagnostic tool used for a variety of reasons, such as determining the presence and extent of coronary artery disease, assessing left or right ventricular function, measuring intracardiac pressures, and evaluating valvular or other cardiac disorders. The catheterization can be performed on either the left or right side of the heart; however, left-heart catheterization is more common. Left-heart catheterization is performed primarily to determine the patency of the coronary vessels, but it can also be used to observe blood flow through the cardiac chambers and valves. Cardiac catheterization also provides access for interventions such as percutaneous transluminal coronary angioplasty, placement of stents within the coronary artery(ies), and intracoronary delivery of a thrombolytic drug (Smilowitz & Feit, 2016).

Preprocedure. The nurse in the preparation area is responsible for assessing the patient's knowledge and expectations regarding cardiac catheterization. This evaluation contributes to the patient teaching plan and helps to identify misunderstandings about the upcoming intervention. The nurse also reviews the patient's history and performs and documents a physical assessment along with vital signs. Special emphasis is given to the neurovascular status of the patient's extremities for postprocedural comparisons. Verifying or initiating intravenous access and securing electrocardiogram leads are also part of the nurse's preprocedure duties. A thorough review of the patient's medications and allergies is required. The dye used during this fluoroscopic procedure is iodine based, so inquiries concerning possible allergies to iodine

or seafood are imperative. History of allergy to clopidogrel (Plavix) should also be reported to the cardiologist because this drug is prescribed for patients receiving intracoronary stenting. The nurse should determine if the patient has taken aspirin or other nonsteroidal anti-inflammatory drugs (NSAIDs) due to the increased risk of bleeding, or sildenafil (Viagra) because it causes profound hypotension when taken with nitrates. If the patient has diabetes, particular attention is paid to verifying whether the patient has received the oral hypoglycemic drug metformin (Glucophage). Metformin should be omitted on the day of cardiac catheterization and for 48 hours afterward because it interacts with the contrast dye and increases the possibility of lactic acidosis. The nurse should also reinforce previous teaching that a flushing sensation and a metallic taste are common when the contrast medium is injected. Because this is an invasive procedure, the nurse verifies that the informed consent documentation is present and contains a current date as part of the patient's medical or health record.

Procedure. An interventional cardiologist, assisted by a nurse and a cardiovascular technician, performs the procedure. The nurse prepares the insertion site, monitors vital signs, cardiac rhythm and hemodynamics, and gives medications as ordered. Drugs for conscious (moderate) sedation could be administered and their effect monitored by a nurse anesthetist or anesthesiologist. The patient is instructed to report the onset of chest pain, breathing difficulty, or nausea during the procedure as these symptoms may be indicative of coronary artery reocclusion. The patient should also be assessed for anxiety or any pain experienced during the procedure.

Left-heart catheterization requires access to the arterial system. The most common insertion route is the femoral artery, although it is associated with the highest rate of bleeding complications and the need for the greatest restriction upon patient mobility. Other access sites include the radial or brachial artery. Radial artery access is used routinely in some centers due to decreased need for patient immobilization postprocedure and lessened risk of bleeding from the access site (Kern, 2013).

After conscious sedation and local anesthesia, a vascular sheath may be inserted. This provides a pathway for the smaller vascular catheter to be threaded in a retrograde fashion into the coronary arteries. The patient may be anticoagulated with heparin during the procedure to prevent stroke, which can occur during prolonged procedures from the embolization of clots that form on the interventional catheter. Femoral artery access complications can develop during the procedure, including laceration of the vessel, hematoma, pseudoaneurysm, and acute vessel closure or thrombus. It is imperative that the nurse and other team members monitor the patient's access site and distal pulses closely during the procedure to recognize early development of these and other complications.

If a lesion is discovered, a percutaneous transluminal coronary angioplasty is generally performed. Angioplasty is usually accompanied by the placement of a coronary stent at the site of the coronary obstruction. Multiple stents may be positioned at various sites within the coronary vasculature to help maintain long-term patency of the vessel.

Postprocedure. After the cardiac catheterization procedure, the patient remains in the cardiovascular lab for frequent nursing assessments until discharge to home or to the telemetry unit. The patient is monitored postprocedure for complications such as peripheral artery thrombosis or embolus, embolic stroke, contrast allergy, acute renal failure, or acute myocardial infarction. When the femoral artery is the access site, frequent inspection of the patient's flanks for signs of retroperitoneal bleeding is essential. Retroperitoneal bleeding is a potentially life-threatening complication that requires ongoing assessment and is difficult to diagnose.

Following the catheterization, it is important to minimize stress on the insertion site; therefore, the patient must keep the procedural leg straight, and the insertion site should be manually compressed when the patient coughs. A summary of the nursing care for this procedure can be found in the "Nursing Care: Pre- and Postprocedure Care of the Patient Undergoing Cardiac Catheterization" feature.

Electrophysiology Study (EPS)   The electrophysiology study (EPS) is an invasive procedure that evaluates the cardiac conduction system and helps classify cardiac arrhythmias. The findings from this study help to determine if the patient would benefit from further interventions, such as drug therapy, implanted pacemaker or implantable cardio-defibrillator, or ablation (destruction of tissue at the arrhythmia source).

The patient is usually given moderate sedation and analgesia. The electrophysiologist inserts a needle to access the vein or artery (often the femoral). Under fluoroscopy, electrode catheters are inserted into the heart. These catheters conduct electrical impulses to and from the heart to trigger abnormal heart rhythms; these dysrhythmias usually disappear after removal of the electrical stimuli. If a significant cardiac dysrhythmia is induced during the EPS that comes from a specific anatomic region, catheter ablation may be applied. Ablation destroys irritable cardiac tissue that is triggering the dysrhythmia. It is commonly performed with radio frequency energy; however, lasers, microwaves, freezing and ultrasound may also be used (Spragg & Tomaselli, 2015).

After completion of the procedure, the catheters are removed. Firm pressure is applied to the insertion site for 10 to 20 minutes to achieve hemostasis. The entire procedure can last 1 to 5 hours. Following the procedure, the patient must remain in supine position with the affected leg straight for 4 to 6 hours (per institution policy) to prevent bleeding from the insertion site.

Nursing Care
Pre- and Postprocedure Care of the Patient Undergoing Cardiac Catheterization

Expected Patient Outcomes and Related Interventions

Preprocedure

Outcome 1: The patient and family will indicate understanding of the procedure and postprocedure management.

Assess
- Patient and family knowledge about the procedure and postprocedure management

Interventions to educate the patient and family about the procedure
- Develop and initiate an individual teaching plan based on needs of patient and family and institutional cardiac catheterization policy and procedure. May include:
  - Steps of catheterization procedure
  - Conscious (moderate) sedation
  - Inform staff if having chest discomfort during procedure
  - Postprocedure management, including rationale
- Answer all questions from patient and family regarding the procedure
- Conduct patient and family teach-back of key information on cardiac catheterization following initial teaching, correcting misunderstandings
- Obtain signed informed consent for cardiac catheter and possible percutaneous coronary intervention (PCI)

procedure and locate it as per institution policy (e.g., in medical or health record, with patient)
- Document all patient and family teaching

Outcome 2: The patient's medical history and physical status will be evaluated prior to procedure.

Assess and compare to established norms, patient baselines, and trends
- Vital signs, medical history, preprocedure laboratory tests (per provider orders and/or institution policy), physical examination
- Status of peripheral pulses
- Known allergies, with particular emphasis on iodine, seafood, and x-ray dye allergies
- Current heart rhythm status (e.g., ECG, cardiac monitor assessments)
- Medication history, with emphasis on anticoagulants
- Previous experience with conscious (moderate) sedation (describe any prior complications associated with this sedation technique)

Interventions to ensure properly documented patient history and physical status
- Document findings in medical/health record
- Prior to leaving the waiting area for procedure, ensure that all precatheterization tests and information have been obtained and documented

Outcome 3: The patient will be free of complications during cardiac catheterization.

Assess and compare to established norms, patient baselines, and trends

Laboratory values related to clotting and coagulation
Intravenous access—patent and free flowing
Last dose of anticoagulant or antiplatelet aggregate therapy (e.g., no warfarin [Coumadin] within 48 hours of procedure)
Signs of allergic response to iodinated contrast media

Interventions to decrease risk of complications

Ensure adequate intravenous access or initiate new access
Ensure all allergies are documented and readily available for viewing, immediate treatment of allergic response to dye or other substances
Document findings in medical or health record

Administer related drug therapy and monitor for therapeutic and nontherapeutic effects

Administer 325 mg aspirin, as ordered

Postprocedure

Outcome: Patient will experience no postprocedure complications.

Assess and compare to established norms, patient baselines, and trends

Vital signs and pedal pulses as per institution policy (e.g., every 15 minutes for first 4 hours, every 30 minutes for 1 hour, then every hour for 2 hours)
Catheter insertion site for bleeding or hematoma formation
Cardiac rhythm

SOURCE: Data from Leeper (2014) and Leopold & Faxon (2015).

Pain level
Bilateral flanks for signs of retroperitoneal bleeding
Urine output
Neurologic status
Oxygenation status: lung sounds, pulse oximetry

Interventions to prevent postprocedure complications (refer to institution policy)

Keep patient supine for first hour postprocedure
Head of bed flat or no higher than 30 degrees (per institution policy)
Remind patient to keep procedural leg straight to reduce stress on catheter insertion site
Bed rest for 4 to 6 hours postprocedure
Femoral sheath removed when thrombin-time criteria met (e.g., 120 seconds)
Postremoval artery compression:
Per institution policy (e.g., manual pressure, C-clamp, FemoStop)
Observe for vascular complications with compression (ecchymosis, hematoma, oozing)
Apply pressure above (not directly on) insertion site sufficient to stop bleeding but not to cause absence of peripheral pulses
Notify provider of complication(s)
Document clinical findings and actions thoroughly

Potential Complications

- Bleeding
- Complications related to bleeding (e.g., hypotension, low cardiac output)
- Reduction in cardiac output
- Cardiac dysrhythmias

Section Six Review

1. The nurse preparing a client for cardiac catheterization must notify the cardiologist with which information?
   A. The diabetic client's fasting blood glucose is 244 mg/dL.
   B. The client reports an allergy to shellfish.
   C. The client's warfarin has been held for 5 days.
   D. The client complains of nervousness.

2. After a cardiac catheterization, the nurse must monitor for which primary complication?
   A. Bleeding
   B. Paresthesia
   C. Increased urine output
   D. Pain at the site of vascular access

3. Which statement is correct regarding transthoracic echocardiogram?
   A. It is an invasive procedure requiring an overnight stay in the hospital postprocedure.
   B. It is used to directly measure ejection fraction.
   C. It is used to evaluate structures within the heart, such as the septum and valves.
   D. It is the primary means of evaluating pulmonary artery pressures.

4. The electrophysiology study (EPS) is used for which purpose?
   A. To determine cardiac output
   B. To classify and locate cardiac arrhythmias
   C. To measure intracardiac pressures
   D. To evaluate blockages in the coronary artery system

Answers: 1. B, 2. A, 3. C, 4. B

Clinical Reasoning Checkpoint

Mrs. C is a 75-year-old patient who underwent a left total hip replacement today. Her past medical history is positive for obesity and myocardial infarction (3 years ago). Six hours after her surgery, she begins to experience shortness of breath. Crackles are heard throughout her lung fields. Her SpO_2 on 2 liters O_2 per nasal cannula had been 95% but is now 88%.

1. What additional physical assessment data would you obtain?

Clinical Update: You complete your focused assessment.

- BP 150/80 mmHg (within the patient's baseline); pulse 100 bpm, slightly weak and irregular; respiratory rate 28 bpm. Pulse oximeter is reading 88% on 2 liters of oxygen per nasal cannula. The probe is properly placed.

- Patient denies having chest pain and is not coughing up sputum. She states she feels as if she can't get in enough air. She appears to have significant increased work of breathing and is using her accessory muscles of inspiration.

- Auscultation of heart sounds reveals S1, S2, S3. Capillary refill is 3 seconds. JVD is elevated 4 cm above sternal angle while at 45 degrees.

- Assessment of extremities reveals they are cool to the touch and pink; pedal pulses +2 bilaterally; 3+ nonpitting edema is present.

- Intake and output (intraoperative and postoperative amounts): total 10,000 mL intake; 2000 mL urine output.

2. What are some abnormal findings based on the patient's history and physical? What is your interpretation of these findings?

3. Based on your focused assessment, what health problems, if any, do you suspect? Provide data to support your decision.

4. What additional cardiovascular diagnostic procedures might you anticipate that the provider will order?

Chapter 13 Review

1. The nurse is teaching about the layers of the arteries in a presentation on atherosclerosis. Which statement by a client would suggest the need for further teaching?
   1. The tunica intima is the middle layer and contains smooth muscle cells.
   2. The tunica externa provides protection and stabilizes the vessels.
   3. The tunica media allows arteries to adjust their size.
   4. The tunica adventitia is a thin layer that surrounds the blood vessels.

2. The nurse is monitoring a client's coronary perfusion pressures. Which findings would prompt the nurse to contact the primary care provider immediately? (Select all that apply.)
   1. CPP 30 mmHg
   2. CPP 40 mmHg
   3. CPP 50 mmHg
   4. CPP 60 mmHg
   5. CPP 70 mmHg

3. A 35-year-old client who is 6 feet tall and weighs 435 pounds is receiving inotropic medications to improve cardiac output. The client's heart rate at the beginning of the treatment was 62 bpm, and his temperature was 37.4°C. Which outcome measure would be the best to evaluate the efficacy of the medications?
   1. Cardiac output (CO)
   2. Cardiac index (CI)
   3. Stroke volume (SV)
   4. Heart rate (HR)

4. A client is being evaluated after accidentally overdosing on antihypertensive medication. Which clinical finding would the nurse anticipate?
   1. Low urine output
   2. Jugular vein distension
   3. Warm extremities
   4. Bounding pulses

5. A client with a history of palpitations reports feeling that her heart is skipping beats. Which assessment data warrants immediate intervention by the nurse?
   1. Heart rate of 60 bpm with regular rhythm
   2. S1 and S2 heart sounds present
   3. Patient report of feeling lightheaded
   4. S3 heart sound present

6. A client returns to the high-acuity unit after a cardiac catheterization. It is important for the nurse to question which order by the healthcare provider?

    1. Assess left groin insertion site for bleeding or hematomas.
    2. Assess bilateral pedal pulses.
    3. Ambulate as desired.
    4. Keep the client's left leg straight for 1 hour.

7. The nurse is caring for a client who has increased afterload. Which findings is the client most likely to exhibit? (Select all that apply.)

    1. Normal heart rate
    2. Decreased stroke volume
    3. Hypertension
    4. Hypotension
    5. Heart rate decreases

8. A client has decreased cardiac output from decreased myocardial contractility. The nurse would anticipate which treatment? (Select all that apply.)

    1. Digoxin
    2. Oxygen
    3. Calcium
    4. Dobutamine
    5. Furosemide

9. A client is admitted to the unit with multiple trauma resulting in significant blood loss. During assessment, the nurse notes low blood pressure and signs of low cardiac output. Based on these two findings, the nurse would expect which effect on the patient's peripheral resistance (PR)?

    1. PR will decrease.
    2. PR will increase.
    3. PR will remain the same.
    4. PR will fluctuate.

10. A client is admitted with unstable angina. Which information about this patient requires the most immediate action by the nurse?

    1. Elevation of the BNP
    2. S3 heart sounds
    3. Auscultation of a carotid bruit
    4. Elevation of serum troponin levels

Answers to questions found inside your textbook are available on the faculty resources site. Please consult with your instructor.

References

American Heart Association. (2016). Heart disease and stroke statistics: 2016 update. *Circulation, 133,* e38–e360. Retrieved February 12, 2017, from http://circ.ahajournals.org/content/circulationaha/133/4/e38.full.pdf

Banasik, J. L. (2015). Cardiac function. In L. C. Copstead & J. L. Banasik (Eds.), *Pathophysiology* (5th ed., pp. 398–417). Philadelphia, PA: Wolters Kluwer/Lippincott Williams & Wilkins.

Barrett, K. E., Barman, S. M., Boitano, S., & Brooks, H. L. (2016a). Chapter 30: The heart as a pump. In K. E. Barrett, S. M. Barman, S. Boitano, & H. L. Brooks (Eds.), *Ganong's review of medical physiology.* (25th ed.) Retrieved December 29, 2016, from http://accessmedicine.mhmedical.com/content.aspx?sectionid=97165586&bookid=1587&Resultclick=2

Barrett, K. E., Barman, S. M., Boitano, S., & Brooks, H. L. (2016b). Chapter 31: Blood as a circulatory fluid & the dynamics of blood & lymph flow. In K. E. Barrett, S. M. Barman, S. Boitano, & H. L. Brooks (Eds.), *Ganong's review of medical physiology* (25th ed.). Retrieved December 29, 2016, from http://accessmedicine.mhmedical.com/Content.aspx?bookId=1587&sectionId=97165676

Bunch, A. M. (2012). A systematic review of the predictive value of a coronary computed tomography angiography as compared with coronary calcium scoring in alternative noninvasive technique in detecting coronary artery disease and evaluating acute coronary syndrome in an acute care setting. *Dimensions of Critical Care Nursing, 31*(2), 73–83.

Chyu, K., & Shah, P. K. (2014). Chapter 244: Unstable angina/non-ST elevation myocardial infarction. In M. H. Crawford (Ed.), *Current diagnosis & treatment: Cardiology* (4th ed.). Retrieved December 29, 2016, from http://accessmedicine.mhmedical.com/content.aspx?bookid=331&sectionid=40727022&jumpsectionID=40750716

Cunningham, S. G., Brashers, V. L., & McCance, K. L. (2014). Structure and function of the cardiovascular and lymphatic systems. In K. L. McCance, S. E. Huether, V. L. Brashers, & N. S. Rote (Eds.), *Pathophysiology: The biologic basis for disease in adults and children* (7th ed., pp. 1083–1129). St. Louis, MO: Elsevier.

D'Amico, D., & Barbarito, C. (2016). *Health & physical assessment in nursing.* Boston, MA: Pearson.

Eaton, D. C., & Pooler, J. P. (2013). Chapter 7: Regulation of sodium and water excretion. In D. C. Eaton & J. P. Pooler (Eds.), *Vander's renal physiology* (8th ed.). Retrieved March 2, 2017, from http://accessmedicine.mhmedical.com/content.aspx?bookid=505&sectionid=42511986

Fedewa, M. V., Das, B. M., Forehand, R. L., & Evans, E. M. (2014). Area-level socioeconomic status, adiposity, physical activity, and inflammation in young adults, 2013. *Preventing Chronic Disease, 11*:140090. doi:10.5888/pcd11.140090

Fletcher, G. F., Ades, P. A., Kligfield, P., Arena, R., Balady, G. J., Bittner, V. A., . . . Williams, M. A. (2013). Exercise standards for testing and training: A scientific statement from the American Heart Association. *Circulation, 128*, 873–934. doi:10.1161 /CIR.0b013e31829b5b44

Goff, D. C., Lloyd-Jones, D. M., Bennett, G., Coady, S., D'Agostino, R. B., Gibbons, R., . . . Stone, N. J. (2014). 2013 ACC/AHA guideline on the assessment of cardiovascular risk: A report of the American College of Cardiology/American Heart Association Task Force on practice guidelines. *Circulation*, 129 (25 Suppl 2), S49–S73. doi:10.1161/01.cir.0000437741 .48606.98

Hall, J. E. (2016). *Guyton and Hall textbook of medical physiology* (13th ed.). Philadelphia, PA: Elsevier.

Hannibal, G. B. (2013). Interpretation of serum troponin elevation. *AACN Advanced Critical Care, 24*(2), 224–228.

Heo, S., Moser, D., Pressler, S. J., Dunbar, S. B., Dekker, R. L., & Lennie, T. A. (2014). Depressive symptoms and the relationship of inflammation to physical signs and symptoms in heart failure patients. *American Journal of Critical Care, 23*(5), 404–411.

Karmali, K. N., Goff, D. C., Ning, H., & Lloyd-Jones, D. M. (2014). A systematic examination of the 2013 ACC/AHA Pooled Cohort Risk Assessment Tool for Atherosclerotic Cardiovascular Disease. *Journal of the American College of Cardiology, 64*(10), 959–968. doi:10.1016/j.jacc.2014.06.1186

Kee, J. L. (2014). *Laboratory and diagnostic tests with nursing implications* (9th ed.). Upper Saddle River, NJ: Pearson.

Kern, M. J. (2013). *Cardiac catheterization techniques: Normal hemodynamics.* UpToDate. Retrieved December 29, 2016, from http://www.uptodate.com/contents/cardiac -catheterization-techniques-normal-hemodynamics

Leeper, B. (2014). Cardiovascular system. In S. M. Burns (Ed.), *AACN essentials of critical care nursing* (3rd ed., pp. 233–262). New York, NY: McGraw-Hill.

Leopold, J. A., & Faxon, D. P. (2015). Diagnostic cardiac catheterization and coronary angiography. In D. Kasper, A. Fauci, S. Hauser, D. Long, J. L. Jameson, & J. Loscalzo (Eds.), *Harrison's principles of internal medicine* (19th ed., chapter 272). Retrieved February 13, 2017, from http://accessmedicine.mhmedical.com.ezproxy.uky .edu/content.aspx?bookid=1130&sectionid=79742087

Liu, M., Shehu, M., Herrold, E., & Cohen, H. (2015). Prognostic value of initial elevation in cardiac troponin I level in critically ill patients without acute coronary syndrome. *Critical Care Nurse, 35*(2), e1–e10. doi: http://dx.doi.org/10.4037/ccn2015300

Miranda, D., Lewis, G. D., & Fifer, M. A. (2016). Heart failure. In L. S. Lilly (Ed.), *Pathophysiology of heart disease* (pp. 220–248). Philadelphia, PA: Wolters Kluwer.

Newby, L. K., Jesse, R. L., Babb, J. D., Christenson, R. H., De Fer, T. M., Diamond, G. A., . . . Weintraub, W. S. (2012). ACCF 2012 expert consensus document on practical clinical considerations in the interpretation of troponin elevations: A report of the American College of Cardiology Foundation task force on Clinical Expert Consensus Documents. *Journal of the American College of Cardiology, 60*(23), 2427–2463. doi:10.1016/j .jacc.2012.08.969

Ramos, L. M. (2014). Cardiac diagnostic testing: What bedside nurses need to know. *Critical Care Nurse, 34*(3), 16–28. doi:10.4037/ccn2014361

Smilowitz, N. R., & Feit, F. (2016). The history of primary angioplasty and stenting for acute myocardial infarction. *Current Cardiology Reports, 18*(5). doi:10.1007/s11886-015-0681-x

Spragg, D. D., & Tomaselli, G. F. (2015). Principles of electrophysiology. In D. L. Longo, A. S. Fauci, D. L. Kasper, S. L. Hauser, J. L. Jameson, & J. Loscalzo (Eds.), *Harrison's principles of internal medicine* (19th ed., chapter 273e). Retrieved February 13, 2017, from http://accessmedicine.mhmedical.com.ezproxy.uky .edu/content.aspx?bookid=1130&sectionid=79742140

Chapter 14
Alterations in Cardiac Function

Learning Outcomes

14.1 Describe the pathophysiology and treatment of patients with valvular heart diseases.

14.2 Apply knowledge of heart failure to the assessment and management of the high-acuity patient.

14.3 Demonstrate the ability to assess and manage care of patients with hypertension.

14.4 Apply knowledge of hypertensive crises to the assessment and management of the high-acuity patient.

14.5 Demonstrate the ability to assess and manage the patient with aortic aneurysm.

The cardiac system plays a pivotal role in pumping and transporting oxygen to tissues. As with any other organ, the heart is composed of various components that must work congruently in order to function optimally. Conceptually, the cardiac system is a sophisticated "plumbing system" where the heart is a pump that has valves to direct blood flow into the "pipes" (the vascular system). Pump, valve, or pipe dysfunction can lead to alterations in cardiac output. This chapter addresses these alterations in cardiac output, which include pump dysfunction (heart failure and cardiomyopathy), valve dysfunction (stenosis and regurgitation), and "pipe" dysfunction (hypertension and aortic aneurysms).

Section One: Valvular Heart Disease

Recall from Chapter 13 that the four heart valves allow forward blood flow, prevent **regurgitation** (or backward flow of blood), and open and close in response to changes in pressure gradients. The opening and closing of the valves during the cardiac cycle allows for forward unidirectional movement of blood through the four chambers of the heart. When valve dysfunction occurs, this forward unidirectional movement of blood flow through the heart is affected. The three major categories of valvular dysfunction are stenosis, regurgitation, and prolapse.

Valve Stenosis

Stenosis of a valve occurs when valve leaflets thicken, stiffen, or fuse together, causing the valve orifice to narrow and the valve to not fully open or close. This causes resistance of blood flow across the valve (Figure 14–1). The chamber before the valve is exposed to an increased afterload because flow through the valve requires more pressure. The blood from that chamber "backs up" to the preceding chamber. Stenosis of a valve may be caused by calcification, congenital factors, or rheumatic fever (Cary & Pearce, 2013). A summary of risk factors for the development of stenosis are listed in Table 14–1.

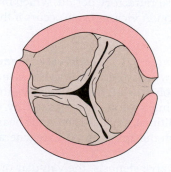

Thickened and stenotic valve leaflets

Figure 14–1 Stenosis of a heart valve.

Table 14–1 Risk Factors for the Development of Valve Disorders

	Risk Factors	
Valve Disorder	**Mitral Valve**	**Aortic Valve**
Stenosis	Acquired: rheumatic fever Age-related: degenerative valve changes of aging heart Women	Congenital: born with valve leaflet malformation Acquired: rheumatic fever Age-related: degenerative valve changes Men
Regurgitation	*Abnormalities of the leaflets:* • Rheumatic heart disease • Infective endocarditis • Collagen-vascular disease *Abnormalities of the annulus:* • Cardiomyopathy *Abnormalities of the chordae tendineae or papillary muscle:* • Ischemic heart disease • Mitral valve prolapse	Congenital: born with valve malformation Acquired: rheumatic heart disease Age-related: degenerative valve changes Calcification, infective endocarditis, trauma, Marfan syndrome

Mitral Valve Stenosis   Mitral valve stenosis (MS) is a narrowing of the mitral valve orifice that obstructs blood flow from the left atrium (LA) into the left ventricle (LV) during diastole. It is predominantly caused by rheumatic fever but may also occur as a congenital complication or secondary to collagen-vascular disease (Kusumoto, 2014). Left atrial pressure increases with MS and eventually causes an increase in pulmonary artery (PA) pressure and pulmonary vascular resistance (PVR) (Figure 14–2). Cardiac output (CO) can be normal with mild MS, but as the stenosis becomes more severe, the pressure gradient between the two left heart chambers increases and CO decreases. Furthermore, the right atrium (RA) must work harder to move blood forward, causing atrial enlargement and hypertrophy. With severe mitral valve stenosis, the patient develops a significantly increased pulmonary vascular pressure with elevated LA pressures eventually causing right-sided heart failure (Kusumoto, 2014).

An important factor to consider with MS is heart rate. During ventricular diastole the ventricle relaxes and fills. If a patient with mitral valve stenosis experiences a sudden increase in heart rate, diastolic filling time is shortened. This results in a substantial decrease in cardiac output and an increase in LA pressure, which leads to pulmonary congestion. Elevated LA pressures lead to left atrial enlargement and hypertrophy and changes in the LA electrical refractory period, which may precipitate atrial fibrillation. A vicious cycle occurs if the heart rate is not controlled.

Aortic Valve Stenosis   Aortic valve stenosis (AS) is a condition in which the aortic valve is narrowed and blood flow is obstructed from the left ventricle (LV) into the aorta during systole. It is caused by congenital or acquired conditions, such as rheumatic heart disease and aging. Through the aging process, degenerative calcifications occur.

In aortic valve stenosis, the valvular orifice narrows, increases the pressure gradient between the LV and aorta, and causes a backup phenomenon, which increases LA pressure. The LV end-diastolic pressure increases, and the LV hypertrophies (Figure 14–3). LA contractility increases

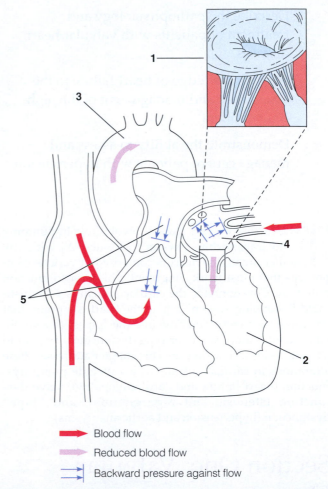

→ Blood flow

→ Reduced blood flow

⇒ Backward pressure against flow

Figure 14–2 Mitral valve stenosis. Narrowing of the mitral valve orifice (1) reduces blood volume to left ventricle (2) reducing cardiac output (3). Rising pressure in the left atrium (4) causes left atrial hypertrophy and pulmonary congestion. Increased pressure in pulmonary vessels (5) causes hypertrophy of the right ventricle and right atrium.

to eject volume against higher LV pressures. However, in the event of a loss of an effective atrial contraction, such as that which occurs with atrial fibrillation, cardiac output can decrease, producing light-headedness and syncope (O'Gara & Loscalzo, 2015a).

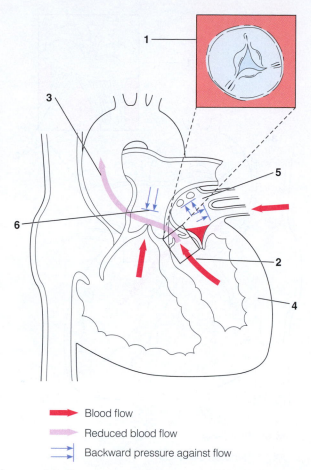

Blood flow

Reduced blood flow

Backward pressure against flow

Figure 14–3 Aortic valve stenosis. The narrowed aortic valve orifice (1) decreases the left ventricular ejection fraction during systole (2) and cardiac output (3). The left ventricle hypertrophies (4). Incomplete emptying of the left atrium (5) causes backward pressure through pulmonary veins and pulmonary hypertension. Elevated pulmonary artery pressure (6) causes right ventricular strain.

Valvular Regurgitation

Insufficient or incompetent valves that do not close completely are called regurgitant valves (Figure 14–4). This allows regurgitation of blood through the valve and back into the chamber that the blood just left. Risk factors for the development of regurgitant valves are summarized in Table 14–1.

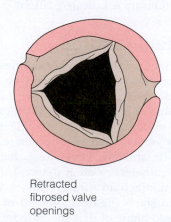

Retracted fibrosed valve openings

Figure 14–4 An incompetent or regurgitant valve.

Mitral Valve Regurgitation   **Mitral valve regurgitation (MR)** occurs when the mitral valve does not completely close and allows blood to flow back into the LA during ventricular diastole. This causes regurgitation of a portion of the ventricular stroke volume (SV) back into the LA and, if the regurgitant volume is significant, SV decreases (Figure 14–5). In an attempt to maintain an adequate SV, the LV pumps harder, increasing its workload, resulting in LV enlargement and hypertrophy. With prolonged severe MR, left-sided heart failure can develop.

Causes of MR are categorized into (1) abnormalities of the leaflets, (2) abnormalities of the annulus, or (3) abnormalities of the chordae tendineae or papillary muscle. When the leaflets are abnormal (especially with chronic rheumatic heart disease), they shorten, become more rigid and deformed, and retract. This causes the leaflets not to close properly during ventricular systole. The annulus or ring around the valve can either be dilated, calcified, or both. The annulus does not constrict properly during systole and regurgitation occurs. Finally, the supporting structures, the chordae tendineae, and papillary muscles can be damaged (O'Gara & Loscalzo, 2015b).

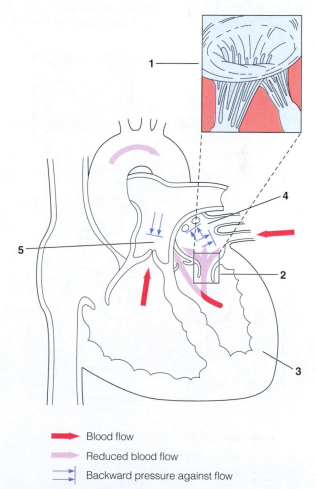

Blood flow

Reduced blood flow

Backward pressure against flow

Figure 14–5 Mitral valve regurgitation. The mitral valve closes incompletely (1), allowing blood to regurgitate during systole from the left ventricle to the left atrium (2). Cardiac output falls, to compensate, the left ventricle hypertrophies (3). Rising left atrial pressure (4) causes left atrial hypertrophy and pulmonary congestion. Elevated pulmonary artery pressure (5) causes slight enlargement of the right ventricle.

Aortic Valve Regurgitation **Aortic valve regurgitation (AR)**, which may also be called aortic insufficiency (AI), is caused by an incompetent aortic valve that allows blood to flow back into the left ventricle from the aorta during diastole. It occurs primarily as a result of rheumatic heart disease. The leaflets' structures are altered because of infiltration of fibrous tissue that causes the leaflets to retract and, therefore, they do not completely close during diastole.

With AR, regurgitation of part of the ventricular stroke volume back into the left ventricle leads to ventricular hypertrophy because more pressure is required to eject a larger stroke volume (Figure 14–6). Hypertrophy can compensate for increased left ventricular stroke volume in chronic AR, preventing clinical symptoms for years; however, acute AR can produce heart failure and pulmonary edema (O'Gara & Loscalzo, 2015a).

Valvular Prolapse **Valvular prolapse** is an abnormal condition in which heart valve (almost always the mitral valve) cusps balloon (bulge) up into the atrium during ventricular systole, making a "floppy" valve. **Mitral valve prolapse** is a type of mitral valve insufficiency that occurs when one or both of the mitral valve cusps bulge back into the LA during ventricular systole. Excess tissue in the valve

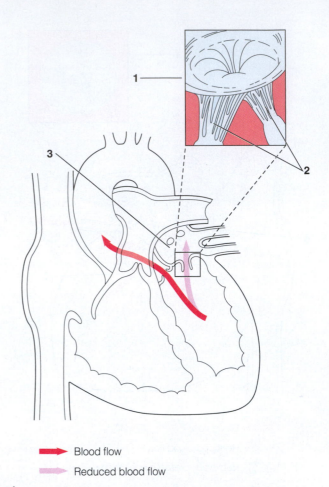

➡ Blood flow

➡ Reduced blood flow

Figure 14–7 Mitral valve prolapse. Excess tissue in the valve leaflets (1) and elongated chordae tendineae (2) impaired mitral valve closure during systole. Some ventricular blood regurgitates into the left atrium (3).

leaflets and elongated chordae tendineae impair mitral valve closure during systole (Figure 14–7). In an acute situation, such as a myocardial infarction and rupture of the papillary muscle, the left atrium and left ventricle cannot compensate for the volume overload. Elevated left heart pressures back up to the pulmonary vasculature, and acute pulmonary edema occurs. Prolapse is usually asymptomatic and may not be diagnosed except by chance during a routine physical exam. Mitral valve regurgitation is present in a small percentage of patients with severe mitral valve prolapse (O'Gara & Loscalzo, 2015b).

Infective Endocarditis

When valves have structural abnormalities, it increases their susceptibility to infection. **Infective endocarditis (IE)** is a disease caused by a microbial infection of the endothelial lining of the heart. The process begins with damage to the endothelium of a valve. Damage may be the result of congenital diseases, infection (e.g., rheumatic heart disease), or iatrogenic causes (e.g., the introduction of intracardiac catheters or other devices). The disrupted surface of the endothelium attracts platelets that adhere to the surface and starts the development of nonbacterial thrombi. The next phase of IE is the introduction of bacteria in the blood through portals of entry, such as wounds,

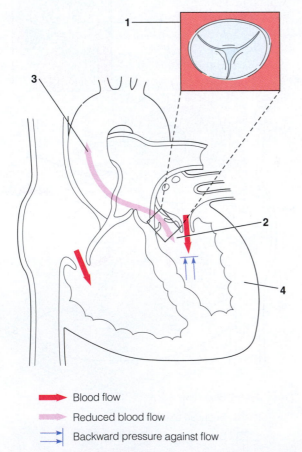

➡ Blood flow

➡ Reduced blood flow

⇉ Backward pressure against flow

Figure 14–6 Aortic regurgitation. The cusps of the aortic valve widen and fail to close during diastole (1). Blood regurgitates from the aorta into the left ventricle (2) increasing left ventricular volume and decreasing cardiac output (3). The left ventricle dilates and hypertrophies (4) in response to the increase in blood volume and work load.

biopsy sites, pacemakers, intravenous and arterial catheters, urinary catheters, or other invasive mechanisms, such as dental or gastrointestinal (colonoscopy) procedures. After bacteria enter the blood, they can colonize the heart valves, forming fibrin-encased growths of microorganisms called vegetations. Thrombus formation can also occur when blood flow is impaired. The vegetations and thrombi enlarge with time and increase valve dysfunction (Bloch, 2014). Some groups of patients are more susceptible to infective endocarditis, including those with preexisting heart disease, children, older adults, intravenous drug abusers, patients infected with human immunodeficiency virus, patients after cardiac surgery, and patients who require hemodialysis. These patients have weakened local and systemic defense mechanisms that may be unable to destroy the bacteria and stop the infectious process. The course of the disease can develop over months (subacute), or it can be very rapid, developing within a few days (acute). Several bacteria can cause infective endocarditis, but the more common species are *Streptococci* (*alpha-hemolytic* or *viridans*) and *Staphylococcus aureus*. *Streptococcus viridans* is found in the oropharyngeal and gastrointestinal flora and is a low-grade pathogen that is usually responsible for subacute endocarditis. Although all heart valves can be affected by this disease, aortic valve stenosis and mitral valve regurgitation most commonly occur as a result of infective endocarditis.

The treatment goal for infective endocarditis is aggressive administration of antibiotics for a minimum of 6 weeks. Timely administration of antibiotics is imperative so that adequate therapeutic levels can be maintained and the development of bacteria that are resistant to antibiotics is prevented. Three sets of blood cultures from different venipuncture sites identify the microorganisms prior to antibiotic therapy. The case mortality rate for endocarditis is approximately 25% with extended intravenous antibiotics and surgery to remove infected valves (Bloch, 2014).

Assessment and Diagnosis of Valvular Disorders

The assessment process starts with a thorough physical examination. Because turbulent blood flow is the result of valvular dysfunction, auscultation of the heart can reveal a murmur. The key to understanding the timing of murmurs in the cardiac cycle is to think about the valve position in relation to ventricular systole or diastole. Table 14–2 includes a summary of heart murmurs, their timing in the cardiac cycle, and characteristics.

The mitral valve is open during ventricular diastole, so the murmur of mitral valve stenosis occurs during diastole. The aortic valve is open during ventricular systole, so the murmur of aortic valve stenosis occurs during systole.

The opposite timing for murmurs applies for regurgitation. The mitral valve is closed during systole, so the murmur of mitral valve regurgitation occurs during systole. The aortic valve is closed during diastole, so the murmur of aortic regurgitation occurs during diastole.

With aortic valve stenosis, angina can occur from decreased blood flow through the coronary arteries because the opening of these arteries is located close to the aortic valve. If valvular dysfunction is severe, the patient

Table 14–2 Heart Murmurs Timing and Characteristics

Murmur	Cardiac Cycle Timing	Auscultation Site	Configuration of Sound	Continuity
Mitral valve stenosis	Diastole	Apical	S_2 — S_1	Rumble that increases in sound toward the end, continuous
Mitral valve regurgitation	Systole	Apex	S_1 — S_2	Holosystolic (occurs throughout systole), continuous
Aortic valve stenosis	Midsystolic	Right sternal border (RSB) 2nd intercostal space (ICS)	S_1 — S_2	Crescendo-decrescendo, continuous
Aortic regurgitation	Diastole (early)	3rd ICS, LSB	S_2 — S_1	Decrescendo, continuous
Tricuspid stenosis	Diastole	Lower LSB	S_2 — S_1	Rumble that increases sound toward the end, continuous
Tricuspid regurgitation	Systole	4th ICS, LSB	S_1 — S_2	Holosystolic, continuous

may develop syncope on exertion as a result of decreased cardiac output, which decreases blood pressure and cerebral perfusion and also may develop heart failure or pulmonary edema. Dyspnea, tachypnea, crackles in the lungs, tachycardia, and chest pain can be present. A chest radiograph may reveal pulmonary edema or an enlarged left atrium.

Another assessment tool that is helpful in the diagnosis of valvular disease is echocardiography. Transthoracic echocardiography (TTE) or transesophageal echocardiography (TEE) allows visualization of the valves as well as the size, thickness, and function of the atria and ventricles. Abnormal findings in the echocardiogram can be confirmed by cardiac catheterization. During this procedure, the valves can be thoroughly examined, and intracardiac pressures and pressure gradients across the chambers can be measured.

Collaborative Management

Patients who are asymptomatic with a valvular dysfunction usually do not require medical intervention. As the dysfunction becomes more severe, to increase ventricular filling time, the heart rate is controlled with drugs such as beta blockers (e.g., atenolol and metoprolol), calcium channel blockers (e.g., diltiazem and verapamil), and digoxin. The major therapeutic goal is to maintain normal sinus rhythm and avoid atrial fibrillation. If symptomatic atrial fibrillation occurs (causing loss of atrial kick), immediate treatment with cardioversion may be required. If heart failure (HF) occurs, diuretics and sodium restriction may be included in the treatment regimen. Other strategies for HF management in the presence of regurgitation include the use of angiotensin-converting enzyme (ACE) inhibitors and beta blockers. In severe HF cases, mechanical interventions such as biventricular pacing (cardiac resynchronization therapy [CRT]) or intra-aortic balloon counterpulsation may be used (O'Gara & Loscalzo, 2015b).

Percutaneous mitral balloon valvuloplasty (PMBV) in the cardiac catheterization lab by an experienced cardiologist can be used to treat mitral valve stenosis. With this procedure, a balloon is inserted into the left atrium after transseptal puncture and is positioned through the mitral valve. The balloon is inflated, resulting in stretching of mitral valve leaflets and separation of fused commissures, improving blood flow (O'Gara & Loscalzo, 2015b). Percutaneous aortic catheter balloon valvuloplasty is used in rare instances to treat older patients or pregnant women with aortic valve stenosis. This is primarily due to high valve restenosis and complication rates from the procedure (O'Gara & Loscalzo, 2015a).

When surgical valve replacement is indicated by severity of disease or symptoms, the valve can be replaced with a biologic or mechanical (artificial) valve. Mechanical valves last longer, but anticoagulation is required because the foreign material causes clot formation. The type of valve used depends on patient age and tolerance of anticoagulation. Anticoagulation is also required if chronic atrial fibrillation is present. Care of this patient population is similar to the percutaneous cardiac interventional patient. Advancement in surgical and medical management has decreased mortality and improved quality of life in patients with valvular disease. In some cases, minimally invasive surgery can be used to repair or replace damaged aortic or mitral valves. Others may require open heart surgery with cardiopulmonary bypass to replace a diseased cardiac valve (O'Gara & Loscalzo, 2015a).

Nursing Management

Nursing priorities include assessing and maintaining cardiac output, assessing for side effects of the disorder, preventing complications, administering pharmacologic therapies, and providing patient education.

Vital signs are carefully monitored because valvular stenosis and regurgitation disorders affect ventricular filling or emptying and result in decreased cardiac output, which can lead to hypotension and tachycardia. If a pulmonary artery catheter or other cardiac output measuring device is present, hemodynamic findings may include decreased cardiac output, elevated right atrial pressure, and increased afterload (systemic vascular resistance) (Leeper, 2014). These findings are associated with pulmonary congestion. Auscultation of heart sounds is performed regularly. Atrial fibrillation may be treated with antiarrhythmic medications such as amiodarone (January et al., 2014).

Failure of the heart to function as a pump results in decreased oxygen delivery to tissues and impaired tissue perfusion. An early sign of valve disease is dyspnea with exertion. The nurse monitors the patient's vital signs before and during activities. A change of heart rate of more than 20 beats per minute (bpm) or change in blood pressure of more than 20 mmHg with activity indicates activity intolerance. Other signs of activity intolerance include shortness of breath, chest pain, fatigue, diaphoresis, dizziness, or syncope. Physical exertion and self-care activities are gradually increased, and rest periods between activities are recommended because resting decreases oxygen demands of the heart. Using a shower chair during bathing saves valuable energy. A physical therapy consult is initiated to help the patient regain and maintain physical strength. Asymptomatic patients are counseled about exercise tolerance, the importance of adherence to medications, and the need for periodic exams with their primary care provider to monitor valve function.

Discharge planning includes education about the importance of monitoring blood pressure and heart rate. Because a therapeutic goal is to maintain a regular heart rate, the nurse educates the patient and family about monitoring pulse rate. They are observed for proper technique when practicing this skill. Patient education includes information about medications including mechanism of action and possible side effects.

Anticoagulation, the prevention of clot formation, is an important aspect of valvular heart disease treatment. Patients with atrial fibrillation, a previous history of a clot formation, or placement of a biological or mechanical valve have an increased risk for clot formation (Adams, 2016; Carnicelli, 2015). The most common drugs used for anticoagulation are heparin, aspirin, clopidogrel, and warfarin (Table 14–3). The patient is at risk for bleeding with anticoagulation therapy. Therefore, vigilant assessments of

Table 14–3 Common Drugs Used for Anticoagulation

Drug	Action
Aspirin	Inhibits the production of thromboxane A_2, which promotes platelet aggregation
Clopidogrel (Plavix)	Inhibits adenosine diphosphate binding to platelet receptors
Warfarin (Coumadin)	Antagonist to vitamin K
Heparin	Inactivates thrombin by binding to antithrombin III

serum coagulation studies, such as prothrombin time (PT), international normalized ratio (INR), and partial thromboplastin time (PTT), as well as hemoglobin and hematocrit, are necessary. When heparin is used, the PTT is the laboratory parameter used to guide therapy. If the patient is on

warfarin (Coumadin), an INR goal is set. The INR goal can range from 2 to 3 with 2.5 as an average value for therapeutic results (Adams, 2016).

The nurse must be cognizant of the INR goal for patient education and treatment purposes. Patients receiving anticoagulant therapy are monitored for signs of bleeding, such as unexplained bruises, bleeding gums, and blood in stools or urine. Patients who go home on anticoagulant therapy must receive patient education about monitoring for signs of bleeding, the need for drawing blood samples, taking the medication in the evening, and avoiding foods that have a high vitamin K content, such as liver and leafy green vegetables.

Follow-up treatment for valvular heart disease includes regularly scheduled physical examinations by a primary care provider and echocardiograms to check valve status and plan additional treatment.

Section One Review

1. If a client is on warfarin (Coumadin), which lab value guides the therapeutic goal?
   A. Activated clotting time
   B. Thrombin time
   C. Partial thromboplastin time
   D. INR

2. Which pathology is associated with narrowing of the orifice of the mitral valve and obstructed blood flow during diastole?
   A. Mitral stenosis
   B. Mitral regurgitation
   C. Aortic stenosis
   D. Infective endocarditis

3. Which clients are most susceptible to infective endocarditis?
   A. 45-year-old women
   B. 40-year-old men
   C. Clients who require hemodialysis
   D. Clients with type O blood

4. When a client has mitral regurgitation, which abnormal heart sound is detected?
   A. Diastolic murmur
   B. Systolic murmur
   C. S_3
   D. S_4

Answers: 1. D, 2. A, 3. C, 4. B

Section Two: Heart Failure

Heart failure (HF), a major health problem in our society today, is a clinical syndrome that results from any structural or functional cardiac disorder that decreases the ability of the ventricles to fill or eject.

Clinical Manifestations and Classification

Clinical manifestations of heart failure include dyspnea and fatigue that limit exercise tolerance and fluid retention that leads to pulmonary congestion and peripheral edema. Because not all patients have fluid volume excess at the time of evaluation, the term *heart failure* is considered a better description of this condition than the older term *congestive heart failure*. Symptoms of patients with heart failure result from impairment of ventricular function.

The New York Heart Association (NYHA) developed a classification of HF based on functional limitations. There are four classes (Yancy et al., 2013):

- Class I includes patients with cardiac disease who experience symptoms with activity that would limit those without disease.
- Class II includes patients with cardiac disease who experience symptoms with ordinary activity.
- Class III includes patients with cardiac disease who experience symptoms with less than ordinary activity.
- Class IV includes patients with cardiac disease who experience symptoms at rest.

There are two categories of heart failure: (1) heart failure with reduced ejection fraction, characterized by an ejection fraction (EF) less than or equal to 40%, and (2) heart failure with preserved ejection fraction, characterized

Table 14–4 Risk Factors for Heart Failure

Origin	Risk Factors
Cardiovascular disorders	Hypertension Coronary artery disease Valvular heart disease Peripheral vascular disease
Lifestyle choices	Illicit drug use Alcohol abuse
Infectious diseases	Rheumatic fever
Medication effects	Exposure to cardiotoxic agents (some chemotherapies)
Metabolic disorders	Diabetes

by an ejection fraction (EF) greater than or equal to 50% (Yancy et al., 2013).

Pathophysiology

Heart failure is a progressive disease that causes cardiac remodeling. The left ventricle dilates, hypertrophies, and becomes more spherical. The mechanism that causes heart failure is not clearly understood. Current theories support its development as the result of a sequence of events. Heart failure begins with a primary event that produces a loss of myocardium or excessive overload on the muscle. Many conditions increase the risk for heart failure as summarized in Table 14–4.

Whatever the cause, some cardiomyocytes are destroyed and other cells try to adapt by increasing their size and elongating. The cardiac muscle hypertrophies in order to sustain the increased workload. When the muscle can no longer maintain that workload, the left ventricle dilates in order to maintain stroke volume even though the ejection fraction has decreased. Compensatory neuro-hormonal mechanisms help achieve this adaptive response. Sodium and water retention occurs in an effort to increase preload and cardiac output. The renin-angiotensin-aldosterone system stimulates aldosterone release and increases sodium and water retention in addition to causing vasoconstriction. As cardiac output decreases, the sympathetic nervous system releases norepinephrine and vasopressin (antidiuretic hormone) to increase blood pressure, heart rate, and contractility. All these mechanisms help with short-term adaptation but have untoward long-term effects such as increased preload, afterload, or both (Bashore, Granger, Jackson, & Patel, 2017). A chronic increase in afterload eventually causes a decrease in cardiac output, which then leads to pulmonary congestion and peripheral edema. Prolonged increases in adrenergic activity lead to dysrhythmias (including tachycardias that heighten myocardial workload), decreased ventricular filling time, increased cardiac cellular activity, increased energy utilization, and cellular death.

Counter-regulatory hormones, atrial natriuretic peptide (ANP), and B-type natriuretic peptide (BNP) are released in response to distention of heart chambers. ANP is released in response to atrial distention, and BNP is released in response to ventricular distention. Both hormones cause vasodilation and induce diuresis and natriuresis, which is the loss of sodium (Barrett, Barman, Boitano, & Brooks, 2016).

Cardiomyopathy Cardiomyopathy is a severe myocardial disease that can produce heart failure. In advanced cardiomyopathy, symptoms of heart failure occur at rest, and the patient cannot perform activities of daily living. Causes of cardiomyopathy may be genetic or acquired, and sometimes the origins of the disorder are unknown (Yancy et al., 2013). The most common cause of heart failure is a specific type of dilation cardiomyopathy called *ischemic cardiomyopathy*, a type of failure that occurs secondary to coronary artery disease and hypertension (Lakdawala, Stevenson, & Loscalzo, 2015).

The disease progression is diffuse and can affect all heart chambers, although it may be more extensive in one chamber than others. Cardiomyopathies are classified into three major functional categories according to clinical and structural findings: dilated cardiomyopathy, hypertrophic cardiomyopathy, and restrictive cardiomyopathy (Bashore et al., 2017). The causes, pathophysiology, manifestations, and management of each of these cardiomyopathies are summarized in Table 14–5.

Dilated cardiomyopathy is primarily associated with left ventricular dilation and decreased ejection fraction (EF). Ischemic cardiomyopathy typically presents as this type of heart disease. **Hypertrophic cardiomyopathy** is associated with left ventricular hypertrophy that decreases the ability of the chamber to relax (diastolic dysfunction) and possibly a reduction in ventricular outflow. **Restrictive cardiomyopathy** is associated with a stiff noncompliant left ventricle that fills inadequately during diastole. Poor ventricular filling results in a low stroke volume and heart failure (Lakdawala et al., 2015). Depending on the type of cardiomyopathy, collaborative management may differ, but the same general principles of heart failure treatment continue.

Assessment and Diagnosis

A careful history and physical examination provide important information. Heart failure has multisystem effects. Dyspnea, orthopnea, and paroxysmal nocturnal dyspnea (PND) are classic respiratory symptoms of patients with HF. **Orthopnea** is the sensation of shortness of breath in the supine position, whereas PND is sudden dyspnea at night that may awaken patients. Both orthopnea and PND may be relieved by sitting or standing. Fatigue is another hallmark symptom. Jugular vein distention is a sign of fluid volume excess. Peripheral dependent edema may also be present as a sign of fluid volume excess, although it can also result from noncardiac causes. A third heart sound (S3) is an important assessment finding that is typically associated with increased end-systolic volumes and pressures that can occur in the presence of heart failure (Kusumoto, 2014).

The single most useful diagnostic test for heart failure is the echocardiogram due to the ability to differentiate heart failure with or without preserved left ventricular systolic function (Bashore et al., 2017). With these studies,

Table 14–5 Classifications of Cardiomyopathies

	Dilated	Hypertrophic	Restrictive
Causes	Usually idiopathic; may be secondary to chronic alcoholism or myocarditis Ischemic cardiomyopathy typically manifests as this class	Hereditary; may be secondary to chronic hypertension	Usually secondary to amyloidosis, radiation, or myocardial fibrosis
Pathophysiology	Scarring and atrophy of myocardial cells Thickening of ventricular wall Dilation of heart chambers Impaired ventricular pumping Increased end-diastolic and end-systolic volumes Mural thrombi common	Hypertrophy of ventricular muscle mass Small left ventricular volume Septal hypertrophy may obstruct left ventricular outflow Left atrial dilation	Excess rigidity of ventricular walls restricts filling Stroke volume may be low
Manifestations	Heart failure Cardiomegaly Dysrhythmias S_3 and S_4 gallop; murmur of mitral valve regurgitation	Dyspnea, anginal pain, syncope Left ventricular hypertrophy Dysrhythmias Loud S_4 Sudden death	Dyspnea, fatigue Right-sided heart failure Mild to moderate cardiomegaly S_3 and S_4 Mitral valve regurgitation murmur
Management	Management of heart failure Implantable cardioverter-defibrillator (ICD) as needed Heart transplantation	Beta blockers Calcium channel blockers Antidysrhythmic agents ICD, dual-chamber pacing	Management of heart failure Exercise restriction

an ejection fraction (EF) is obtained, and pericardial, valvular, or myocardial dysfunction is visualized A chest radiograph gives an estimate of heart size and pulmonary congestion. A 15-lead electrocardiogram (ECG) can demonstrate myocardial ischemia and infarction, ventricular hypertrophy, or dysrhythmia. However, the chest radiograph and electrocardiogram do not provide specific information to make the diagnosis of heart failure. Cardiac catheterization may also be needed to provide further information about coronary artery or valvular disease. B-type natriuretic peptide (BNP) or N-terminal pro-BNP (N-BNP) can be useful if the diagnosis of heart failure is uncertain. Normal BNP is less than 100 pg/mL and elevations above this level indicate left ventricular fluid volume overload (Bashore et al., 2017). It is important to remember that heart failure is a syndrome with many presentations, including decreased exercise tolerance, fluid retention, or symptoms of another cardiac or noncardiac disorder. Patients with chronic heart failure experience symptoms with exertion that can be evaluated through cardiopulmonary exercise testing. The severity of heart failure and associated symptoms can quickly change with acute exacerbations, resulting in hospitalization, complex treatment, and in some instances death.

Collaborative Management

The American College of Cardiologists and the American Heart Association established evidence-based guidelines for the management of HF (Yancy et al., 2013). Therapy is divided into four categories:

- Stage A includes patients at high risk for developing heart failure without structural heart disease or heart failure symptoms.

- Stage B includes patients with structural heart disease who have not developed heart failure symptoms.

- Stage C includes patients with structural heart disease with prior or current heart failure symptoms.

- Stage D includes patients with refractory heart failure requiring specialized interventions.

The focus of treatment for patients at high risk for heart failure is to control risk factors. Management of hypertension, diabetes, and hyperlipidemia reduces the risk of developing heart failure. Counseling patients on the hazards of recreational substances, such as tobacco, alcohol, and illicit drugs, provides a strong impetus for patients to reduce the use of these agents. Preventing atherosclerosis and coronary artery disease development is an important health promotion goal since ischemic heart disease is a major cause of heart failure.

Pharmacologic Therapy   Initial heart failure medication management focuses on the reduction of fluid volume excess and symptom relief with diuretics. A thiazide diuretic such as hydrochlorothiazide or metolazone may be used if symptoms are mild. With more severe symptoms of fluid excess, an oral loop diuretic such as furosemide or bumetanide may be used (Bashore et al., 2017). Combinations of diuretic therapy may also include an oral potassium sparing agent. First-line drug management for heart failure usually includes an angiotensin-converting enzyme (ACE) inhibitor or an angiotensin II receptor blocker (ARB) with a beta blocker to vasodilate, decrease afterload,

and decrease cardiac workload (Bashore et al., 2017; Yancy et al., 2013). This regimen controls the neurohormonal and sympathetic compensatory responses and decreases the occurrence of heart failure. Digoxin may be added to the regimen if the patient remains symptomatic with diuretic and ACE-inhibitor therapy or when the ventricular rate of atrial fibrillation must be controlled (Bashore et al., 2017).

Furosemide (Lasix) is the most common diuretic used to treat more severe fluid volume overload. If two diuretics are needed to obtain the desired response, the two drugs used may act differently in the nephron. For example, furosemide, a loop diuretic, inhibits resorption of sodium and chloride in the nephron, whereas metolazone (Zaroxolyn), a thiazide diuretic, increases the excretion of water, sodium, chloride, and other electrolytes (Wilson, Shannon, & Shields, 2016).

Related Pharmacotherapy
Agents for Treatment of Heart Failure and Hypertension

Beta Adrenergic Blocking Agents

Carvedilol (Coreg, Kredex)

Action and Uses
Alpha- and beta-adrenergic blocking activities that lower blood pressure. Alpha-1 blocking causes peripheral vasodilation and decreased peripheral vascular resistance. Decreases myocardial oxygen demand and lowers cardiac workload. Used in the management of hypertension and heart failure.

Dosages (Adult)
Heart failure: Initial PO dose of 3.125 mg 2 times/day for 2 weeks and double dose after 2 weeks as tolerated (max. dose 25 mg 2 times/day)
Post-MI with LV dysfunction: Initial PO dose of 6.25 mg 2 times/day and double dose as tolerated every 3 to 10 days (as required)
Hypertension: Initial PO dose of 6.25 mg 2 times/day; may increase by 6.25 mg 2 times/day (max. dose 50 mg/day)

Major Side Effects
Dizziness

Nursing Implications
Monitor for lessening of signs and symptoms of heart failure and improved blood pressure control
Monitor for orthostatic hypotension
Monitor liver function tests
Monitor digoxin levels with concurrent use; plasma digoxin concentration levels may increase
Educate patients to report any dizziness, faintness

Angiotensin-converting Enzyme Inhibitors

Captopril (Capoten)

Action and Uses
Lowers blood pressure by inhibition of angiotensin-converting enzyme. Interrupts conversion of angiotensin I to angiotensin II, a potent vasoconstrictor. Lowers peripheral vascular resistance by vasodilation. Used in hypertension and heart failure to decrease dyspnea and improve exercise tolerance.

Dosages (Adult)
Hypertension: 6.25 to 25 mg 3 times/day; increase to 50 mg 3 times/day if required (max. dose of 450 mg/day)
Heart failure: 6.25 to 12.5 mg 3 times/day; increase to 100 mg 3 times/day if required (max. dose of 450 mg/day)

Major Side Effects
Angioedema
Agranulocytosis
Maculopapular rash

Nursing Implications
Monitor blood pressure closely, especially after the first dose. Hypotension may occur 1–3 hours after the first dose. Advise the patient to remain on bed rest for 3 hours after the initial dose.
Before full therapeutic effect is achieved, 2 weeks of therapy may be required.
Mild skin eruptions may occur during first 4 weeks of therapy.

Angiotensin II Receptor Antagonists

Losartan (Cozaar)

Action and Uses
Selectively blocks the binding of angiotensin II to the angiotensin I receptors in vascular smooth muscle. Used for hypertension (produces vasodilation) and inhibition of aldosterone effects on sodium and water.

Dosages (Adult)
Hypertension: 25 to 50 mg PO in 1 or 2 divided doses (max. dose of 100 mg/day); if volume depleted, begin with 25 mg/day

Major Side Effects
Headaches

Nursing Implications
Monitor blood pressure; notify healthcare provider (HCP) for hypotension, patient complaints of dizziness or faintness.

SOURCE: Based on dosage information from Wilson et al. (2016).

ACE inhibitors, such as captopril (Capoten) and lisinopril (Zestril), are commonly administered during heart failure treatment as described in the Related Pharmacotherapy feature Agents for Treatment of Heart Failure and Hypertension. However, nurses must be aware of the two important contraindications to the use of ACE inhibitors: previous severe adverse reactions to ACE inhibitors and pregnancy. Patients with a systolic blood pressure less than 100 mmHg are at increased risk for significant hypotension when ACE inhibitors are administered. Low doses of ACE inhibitors should be administered with caution when beginning therapy in patients who present with a low systolic blood pressure, hypovolemia, prerenal azotemia, or hyponatremia. Patients should be routinely assessed for hypotension, impaired renal function, and electrolyte balance when ACE inhibitors are used (Bashore et al., 2017).

Angiotensin II receptor blockers (ARBs) may be used for patients who cannot tolerate ACE inhibitors. The ARB drugs can have clinical results similar to the ACE inhibitors. Figure 14–8 depicts how ARBs and ACE inhibitors work to block the renin-angiotensin-aldosterone system. ARBs do not have some of the adverse effects, such as cough, that are associated with ACE inhibitors (Wilson et al., 2016). Commonly used ARBs such as losartan (Cozaar) and valsartan (Diovan) may cause dizziness, stroke, or hypotension, which can impose additional treatments for adverse effects.

Beta blockers may be administered to patients who do not have fluid retention to reduce the sympathetic nervous response to heart failure. Some beta blockers, such as carvedilol (Coreg), are available in a controlled-release form, and these medications can be dosed once daily. Contraindications include hypersensitivity to the drug, cardiogenic shock, sinus bradycardia, advanced heart block without a pacemaker, and severe heart failure (Wilson et al., 2016). The nurse should notify the healthcare provider if the patient's heart rate is less than 50 beats per minute before administering beta blockers to determine the safety of delivering the medication.

Inotropic drugs increase contractility and improve cardiac output in severely decompensated heart failure. Dobutamine (Dobutrex) and dopamine (Intropin) are commonly used inotropic agents. Dopamine is usually administered in low doses, less than 5 mcg/kg/min, and for short durations of time to avoid adverse effects from increased afterload (Yancy et al., 2013). Digoxin is used to improve contractility when atrial fibrillation is present.

Another drug that may be used is nesiritide (Natrecor). This drug, given as an IV infusion, mimics brain natriuretic peptide (BNP) and causes vasodilation (Wilson et al., 2016). Other vasodilator medications include nitroprusside (Nitropress) and nitroglycerin (Tridil) intravenous infusions that are used to reduce afterload and preload in acute heart failure (Bashore et al., 2017).

Invasive Treatments Other procedural and surgical interventions have demonstrated some improvement in symptoms and are being used to prevent life-threatening dysrhythmias or improve cardiac output. Fast or ineffective cardiac rhythms that quickly cause decompensation or sudden death are controlled with an implantable cardioverter-defibrillator (ICD). Biventricular pacing, also called cardiac resynchronization therapy (CRT), is an intervention that synchronizes both right and left ventricular electrical activity and contraction and improves cardiac output.

Surgical interventions may include mitral valve replacement to decrease LV dysfunction. Coronary artery bypass surgery or percutaneous coronary intervention may be performed to improve cardiac muscle perfusion and contractility. Final surgical interventions include the placement of ventricular assist devices (VADs) and cardiac transplantation. These interventions are reserved for heart failure that is unresponsive to conventional medical treatment. Stem cell therapy, miniature mechanical assist devices, better hospital-to-home care, and novel prevention strategies are areas for future research with heart failure treatment and management (Yancy et al., 2013).

Nursing Management

The failure of the heart to function as a pump results in decreased cardiac output and impaired tissue perfusion. A major nursing goal is to decrease the patient's oxygen demands because oxygen supply is severely decreased. This goal is accomplished by ensuring adequate rest, administering medications as prescribed to decrease preload and improve contractility, assessing patient response to medications, and helping the patient manage the symptoms of this disease.

As the heart's pumping action fails, less oxygen is delivered to tissues and ineffective tissue perfusion results. Many of the nursing interventions listed for the patient with valve disease are pertinent for the patient with heart failure. Nursing assessments focus on astute observation of the patient for signs of decompensation and on monitoring vital signs for decreased cardiac output. The apical pulse may be palpated to the left of the mid-clavicular line because of left ventricular enlargement. Heart sounds are auscultated regularly. An early sign of heart failure is an S3 heart sound. Lung sounds are monitored for the development of

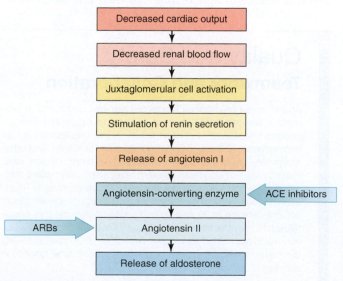

Figure 14–8 ACE inhibitors and ARBs block the renin-angiotensin-aldosterone system.

crackles. Cardiac rhythm, exercise tolerance, and kidney function are assessed for early signs of deterioration.

Continuous telemetry monitoring is recommended for patients in the high-acuity setting because beta blockers, digitalis, and other medications affect heart rate. Because digitalis and beta blockers slow the heart rate, patients are instructed on how to correctly take their pulse and when to call the healthcare provider if pulse parameters are violated.

The patient with heart failure may have activity intolerance and fatigue from a couple of sources. First, the disease process itself causes fatigue because of decreased oxygen delivery to peripheral tissues. Fluid volume excess in the lungs interferes with pulmonary gas exchange. Beta blockers also cause fatigue, a significant side effect that often causes patients to discontinue taking the drug. It is important for patients to know that the fatigue may disappear after the first several weeks of beta-blocker therapy. The patient is encouraged to rest between activities and to increase activity gradually. The nurse monitors the patient's activity tolerance by taking vital signs before, during, and after an activity.

Because fatigue is one of the major symptoms of heart failure, proper sleep and sleeping habits are very important to maintain quality of life. The nurse recognizes that these patients have sleep disturbances and obtains a brief sleep history, ensuring that other causes of sleep disturbances, such as depression or sleep apnea, are ruled out. The hospital environment is optimized to promote sleep using relaxation techniques, sleep protocols, and a quiet environment. Sleep disturbances are treated by (1) reviewing good sleep habits, (2) considering alternative practices such as relaxation, or cognitive or behavioral therapy, or (3) suggesting structured changes in sleep habits.

Careful monitoring of fluid status is important for patients with heart failure. The initial assessment of this patient population should include accurate measurement of height and weight, orthostatic blood pressure changes, and calculation of body mass index. Fluid status determination using jugular vein distension, breath sounds, and the degree of peripheral and central edema should be monitored. Diuretics can deplete circulating volume and cause hypovolemia and potassium and magnesium deficits. These electrolytes are replaced either by oral or IV supplements or food source supplementation. Potassium depletion is further exacerbated if digitalis is used with a diuretic. Decreased urine output can indicate a significant decrease in cardiac output and renal perfusion. Monitoring weight trends is also important in controlling fluid retention. Obtaining and recording daily weights is vital. Typically, a weight gain of 2.2 pounds (1 kg) equates to fluid retention of 1 liter. For discharge planning, the patient is given tools for recording daily weights and advised to call a healthcare provider if he or she gains 3 or more pounds (1.4 kg) in 24 hours. Dietary sodium restriction can decrease fluid retention and associated fluid volume excess symptoms in patients with heart failure.

Cardiogenic Shock

Patients with acute heart failure may experience cardiogenic shock when pumping failure is severe. The mean arterial pressure (MAP) is less than 65 mmHg, and the pulse will be weak and thready in this shock state. The mortality rate for hospitalized patients with cardiogenic shock is more than 50% (Hochman & Ingbar, 2015). Acute cardiogenic pulmonary edema occurs secondary to left ventricular failure. Treatment includes continuous monitoring, endotracheal intubation with mechanical ventilation, vasopressors such as norepinephrine (Levophed) or epinephrine, and positive inotropes including dopamine and dobutamine (Hochman & Ingbar, 2015). Vasopressor use should be limited to prevent the adverse effects of increased afterload. Diuretics may be used to reduce preload and pulmonary congestion. Intravenous fluids may be used to increase left ventricular filling pressures in cardiogenic shock; however, fluid resuscitation is contraindicated in pulmonary edema with shock. Cardiogenic shock is presented in more detail in Chapter 37.

Hospital Discharge

Because comprehensive discharge education is essential to heart failure treatment, instruction on self-care in the home should begin as soon as the patient's condition stabilizes. Patients and significant others should receive oral and written instructions on weight monitoring, diet, medications, symptom management, activity levels, and, when applicable, smoking cessation to achieve desired patient outcomes. It is important to address financial constraints that patients may have to ensure that they will be able to obtain medications and low-sodium foods after discharge. A social work consult may be necessary to identify post-discharge resources. The patient's advance directives, a discussion of future plans, and postdischarge follow-up arrangements should take place before discharge (The Joint Commission, 2013). A team approach to hospital treatment and home care is recommended. A description of team approach to heart failure care is described in the Quality and Safety: Quality and Safety Education for Nurses (QSEN) feature.

Healthcare providers and patients should engage in shared decision making as heart failure advances to ensure that palliative and end-of-life care incorporates patient values and goals. Palliative care, which is coupled with active medical treatment and is different than end-of-life care,

---

Quality and Safety
Teamwork and Collaboration

An NP (nurse practitioner) Model of Care was developed to promote a smooth transition from hospital to outpatient care for patients hospitalized with heart failure. Nurse practitioners led an interprofessional team of nurses, physicians, dieticians, and other healthcare professionals in the delivery of direct patient care. Patient care included heart failure management and patient education while hospitalized and in transition to outpatient care. Readmission rates for the patients receiving care through the NP Model of Care were 4% at 30 days ($n = 26$). Heart failure patients hospitalized 12 months before model implementation receiving usual care were readmitted at a higher rate: 26% at 30 days following discharge ($n = 85$). This reduction in readmission rates resulted in substantial cost savings for heart failure care.

SOURCE: Based on Kutzleb et al. (2015).

includes treatments that can reduce symptoms and improve quality of life (Sidebottom, Jorgenson, Richards, Kirven, & Sillah, 2015). End-of-life care may begin in the hospital and continue in the home when treatment options are exhausted.

Hospice care may be delivered with comfort as the ultimate goal. Care at the end of life may include the deactivation of implantable cardioverter-defibrillators (ICDs) and discontinuation of mechanical ventricular assist devices.

Section Two Review

1. Weight gain of greater than 3 pounds might indicate that a dosage increase is needed in a drug from which category?
   A. ACE inhibitors
   B. Diuretics
   C. Beta blockers
   D. Cardiac glycosides

2. It is time for a client's routine dose of an ACE inhibitor. The client's blood pressure is 75/45 mmHg. Which nursing action is MOST appropriate?
   A. Give the drug immediately; it will improve the client's blood pressure.
   B. Wait one hour and recheck the blood pressure.
   C. Notify the healthcare provider and ask if the dose should be held.
   D. Discuss the issue with your colleague.

3. The release of ANP and BNP typically causes which physiologic events?
   A. Myocardial infarction
   B. Hypertension
   C. Vasoconstriction and fluid retention
   D. Vasodilation and diuresis

4. A stiff noncompliant left ventricle with poor diastolic filling describes which condition?
   A. Restrictive cardiomyopathy
   B. Dilated cardiomyopathy
   C. Hypertrophic cardiomyopathy
   D. Stage II heart failure

Answers: 1. D, 2. C, 3. D, 4. A

Section Three: Hypertension

The focus on hypertension and its early detection, prevention, and treatment is a top priority in healthcare because hypertension contributes to an increased risk of myocardial infarction, heart failure, stroke, and kidney disease. Hypertension can lead to target organ damage in the patient who is hospitalized for a critical illness. **Target organ damage**, in this context, refers to dysfunction that occurs in organs affected by high blood pressure in the circulatory system. Cerebro- and cardiovascular consequences of hypertension can include left ventricular hypertrophy, angina or myocardial infarction, heart failure, stroke, and peripheral arterial disease. Hypertension can also produce organ damage that results in renal dysfunction and retinopathy. Hypertension can be found in the young, as well as older adults, and frequently patients do not have symptoms. Risk factors for the development of hypertension have been identified (Box 14–1).

Normal blood pressure is defined as a systolic blood pressure (SBP) less than 120 mmHg and a diastolic blood pressure (DBP) less than 80 mmHg (Kotchen, 2015). Prehypertension assists with earlier identification of those at risk for developing hypertension. Prehypertension is defined as a SBP of 120 to 139 mmHg and DBP of 80 to 89 mmHg. Definitions of the classifications of blood pressure are listed in Table 14–6. Healthcare providers routinely intervene to maintain an average blood pressure less than 140/90 in their patients, and in those with chronic illnesses such as diabetes and renal disease, the treatment goal may be less than 130/80 (Rosendorff et al., 2015).

BOX 14–1 Risk Factors for the Development of Hypertension

- Hypertension
- Cigarette smoking
- Obesity
- Physical inactivity
- Hyperlipidemia
- Diabetes mellitus
- Estimated glomerular filtration rate less than 60 mL/min
- Age (older than 55 for men, 65 for women)
- Family history of premature cardiovascular disease
- Obstructive sleep apnea

Table 14–6 Classification of Blood Pressure

Blood Pressure Classification	Systolic Blood Pressure (mmHg)	Diastolic Blood Pressure (mmHg)
Normal	Less than 120	And less than 80
Prehypertension	120 to 139	Or 80 to 89
Stage 1 hypertension	140 to 159	Or 90 to 99
Stage 2 hypertension	160 or greater	Or 100 or greater

Although research has focused on identifying the cause of primary or essential hypertension, the exact cause has not been identified (Mitrovic, 2014). Primary hypertension is the most common type of blood pressure elevation, accounting for 90% or greater of all hypertension cases. Secondary hypertension is related to renal artery stenosis, renal failure, hyperthyroidism, sleep apnea, and other pathologies (Mitrovic, 2014). Neurohormonal mechanisms appear to be important to the development of hypertension. The sympathetic nervous system plays a major role by releasing catecholamines that result in increased heart rate and vasoconstriction. The renin-angiotensin-aldosterone system also influences the development of hypertension by secreting aldosterone to promote sodium and water retention. Some patients have a genetic predisposition for oversensitivity to sodium with subsequent fluid volume excess and hypertension (Kotchen, 2015). Endothelin-1 (ET-1), a factor produced by endothelial cells in the renal medulla, has significant vasodilating properties and appears to contribute to the development of hypertension when ET-1 levels are low. A mechanism that can increase the stiffness of the vascular wall and produce hypertension with aging is the accumulation of collagen in the vascular walls (Zelman, Raymond, Holdaway, Dafnis, & Mulvihill, 2015).

Assessment and Diagnosis

The diagnosis of hypertension is based on measurement of blood pressure. Measurements are done on both arms and obtained on at least three different occasions before the diagnosis is made. Where blood pressure is measured affects its accuracy and significance (Weber et al., 2014). In general, home measurements of blood pressure predict patient outcomes better than assessments in the healthcare provider office or clinic.

Patient assessment is focused on detection or limitation of target organ involvement. An initial physical examination includes ophthalmoscopy with visualization of the optic fundi; auscultation of the carotid, abdominal, and femoral arteries for bruits; assessment of lower extremities for pulses and edema; a thorough exam of the heart, lungs, and abdomen (for enlarged kidneys); and a neurologic assessment (Kotchen, 2015; Weber et al., 2014).

Before initiating therapy, routine assessment includes an electrocardiogram, urinalysis, and serum evaluations of glucose, hematocrit, potassium, creatinine, calcium, and lipids. Once hypertension has been diagnosed, further testing may be indicated.

Collaborative Management

The ultimate goal of therapy is to lower the systolic blood pressure (SBP). Diastolic blood pressure usually decreases before SBP. Management centers on pharmacologic agents and lifestyle changes. For patients who are overweight or obese, the Dietary Approaches to Stop Hypertension (DASH) eating plan is implemented. This plan consists of a diet rich in calcium and potassium, sodium reduction, physical activity, and moderation of alcohol consumption. If these interventions do not achieve the target blood pressure, pharmacologic treatment is initiated.

Pharmacologic Therapies Pharmacologic treatment is evidence based and includes the use of several classes of drugs previously described in this chapter, including ACE inhibitors, angiotensin receptor blockers (ARBs), beta blockers (BBs), calcium channel blockers (CCBs), and thiazide-type diuretics. Thiazide diuretics are the basis of antihypertensive therapy. These diuretics are used either alone or in combination with another drug for initial therapy. For stage 1 hypertension, thiazide diuretics are most commonly prescribed. For stage 2 hypertension, a two-drug combination is usually needed (a thiazide diuretic and an ACE inhibitor, ARB, BB, or CCB). Direct renin inhibitors can also be used to treat hypertension. Aliskiren (Tekturna) is a potent renin inhibitor and has a long half-life that is favorable for once-daily dosing. The recommended daily dose is 150 mg, which can be increased up to 300 mg daily. Infrequent adverse effects include hyperkalemia, elevated uric acid, and gastrointestinal symptoms such as diarrhea (Wilson et al., 2016). Drug-resistant hypertension may be treated with combination therapy that includes an aldosterone-blocking medication such as spironolactone (Aldactone) or eplerenone (Inspra) (Sutters, 2017).

Hypertension along with certain comorbidities requires special consideration. In patients with ischemic heart disease, beta blockers and ACE inhibitors are commonly used (Rosendorff et al., 2015). Patients with heart failure attain good blood pressure control with diuretics, beta blockers, ACE inhibitors, ARBs, and, in some instances, aldosterone blockers. Decreased renal dysfunction and decreased risk for cardiovascular disease or stroke are benefits of ACE inhibitor and ARB use in diabetic patients (Rosendorff et al., 2015). Chronic kidney disease is treated aggressively and may require three or more types of drugs. When compared to beta blockers and ACE inhibitors, diuretics are more effective in controlling hypertension in African Americans, older individuals, the obese, and other groups with increased fluid volume and or decreased renin function (Sutters, 2017).

Nursing Management

A brief synopsis of the nursing management of hypertension is provided in the Nursing Care: The Patient with Hypertension feature.

Nursing management of patients with hypertension starts with accurate blood pressure measurement. The patient should be in a sitting or supine position for 5 minutes with the arm supported at heart level. An appropriately sized cuff is one that has at least 80% of the cuff bladder encircling the arm. Measurements are taken in both arms in an initial screening. In the acute care setting, noninvasive blood pressure machines are commonly used. All the same techniques in obtaining accurate blood pressure measurement are applied when using these machines. All blood pressure equipment is properly calibrated and checked at regular intervals. Patients and family are also instructed on how blood pressure is measured at home.

Patient Education Patient education is a major component in the nursing management of this patient population, and the goal is to increase adherence to the treatment

Nursing Care
The Patient with Hypertension

Expected Patient Outcomes and Related Interventions

Outcome 1: Blood pressure is controlled within acceptable limits

Assess blood pressure with consistency and accuracy

Measure blood pressure with an appropriate sized cuff.

Calibrate and properly maintain arterial lines if invasive monitoring is used.

Compare patient values to established norms and personal baselines.

Pharmacologic therapy to decrease blood pressure

Administer antihypertensive medications as ordered.

Monitor and treat side effects of pharmacologic therapy as warranted.

Treat electrolyte imbalances that may occur from antihypertensive therapy.

Monitor heart rate especially with beta-blocker use.

Nonpharmacologic therapies

Offer a diet that is rich in potassium and calcium and low in sodium.

Advise patient to avoid alcohol consumption.

Outcome 2: Target organ damage is minimized

Assess for changes in physical parameters

Auscultate for bruits, report new findings to primary care provider.

Monitor serum laboratory values, report and treat abnormals.

Assess and intervene for diminished pulses, decreased urine output, and changes in neurologic status.

Intervention

Administer pharmacologic therapies as ordered.

Replace electrolytes when levels are low.

Assist with further diagnostic testing such as renal or CT scans.

Outcome 3: Self-care principles are adopted

Provide instructions to patients and families on the following self-care strategies

Engage in physical activity as directed by primary care provider.

Maintain the preferred BMI, avoiding overweight and obesity.

Cease smoking.

Adhere to a low-sodium diet.

Adhere to medication regimen.

Routinely monitor blood pressure in the home.

Manage symptoms.

---

plan. Patients and families need significant training to manage this chronic condition. The nurse assists the patient with developing a medication administration schedule to promote adherence. It is essential that the patient and/or caregivers learn about medications, their actions, and side effects. For example, the potential side effects of drugs that block the sympathetic nervous system (angiotensin receptor blockers and beta blockers) can cause orthostatic hypotension, which is important for patients to know and avoid. The nurse instructs the patient to rise slowly from a supine position to avoid hypotension. Patients taking diuretics and their families also need to understand that diuretics can cause potassium, sodium, and magnesium depletions; consequently, these serum

Emerging Evidence

- Adverse reactions to the use of nifedipine immediate release (IR), a short-acting dihydropyridine calcium channel blocker, to treat hypertensive crisis were examined in a retrospective study of 122 patient cases. Researchers compared adverse events related to nifedipine use such as the need for cardiologist intervention, profound arrhythmia, stroke, myocardial infarction, and other endpoints in patients with (high risk) and without (low risk) a history of myocardial infarction, stroke, or arrhythmia. There were no differences in the adverse event composites for the two groups, and there were no cases of death. The recent decrease of nifedipine use for hypertensive crisis secondary to a concern for increased adverse events should be explored as the findings of this research suggest that nifedipine use may be a safer option for hypertensive crisis treatment than hypothesized by prescribing providers (*Means, Benken, & Tesoro, 2016*).

- Symptom clusters and associations between functional ability and mobility were examined in a sample of 117 patients with heart failure. Ten symptoms were grouped into clusters, and associations between clusters and functional status were described. Principal components analysis revealed three symptom clusters: sickness behavior (anxiety, depression, daytime functioning [sleepiness], cognitive dysfunction, and fatigue); discomforts of illness (shortness of breath, edema, pain), and gastrointestinal distress (loss of appetite, decreased hunger). Regression analysis revealed that functional limitations increase as discomforts of illness increase, and limitations increase at a faster rate when sickness behaviors are included in the equation. Symptom management may be an important strategy for promoting physical functioning among patients with heart failure. (*Herr et al., 2014*).

- A study of patients receiving open repair (*n* = 75) and endovascular aneurysm repair (EVAR) (*n* = 55) of an abdominal aortic aneurysm were evaluated on their aerobic fitness. Complication rates were identified in all study participants. Decreased anaerobic threshold measured by cardiopulmonary exercise testing and the use of open repair were associated with more cardiac complications (including myocardial infarction, unstable angina, arrhythmia). In addition, patients receiving the EVAR procedure had shorter hospital and critical care unit lengths of stay (*p* < 0.001) when compared to patients undergoing an open repair (*Barakat, Shahin, McCollum & Chetter, 2015*).

electrolytes must be monitored on a regular basis during hospitalization and after discharge. Patients must know how to correctly take their pulse to self-monitor for bradycardias that can occur with beta-blocker therapy.

Instructions on dietary sodium restrictions are part of routine patient education. Exercise programs may be introduced as part of the treatment plan using the expertise of other disciplines such as physical therapy.

Section Three Review

1. A client with a medical history of diabetes mellitus, hypertension, and coronary artery disease requiring bypass surgery is admitted with renal dysfunction. What may be the cause of the current condition?
   A. Target organ damage
   B. Chronic aldosterone secretion
   C. Release of endothelin-1
   D. Release of nitric oxide

2. Which dietary plan is most beneficial to a client with hypertension? (Select all that apply.)
   A. A diet rich in calcium
   B. Moderation of alcohol intake
   C. A diet rich in vitamin K
   D. A diet rich in sodium
   E. A diet rich in potassium

3. Which cuff most accurately measures blood pressure?
   A. Any cuff as long as it is an adult cuff
   B. A cuff that has at least 80% of the cuff encircling the arm
   C. A noninvasive machine cuff
   D. A cuff that is two thirds the diameter of the arm

4. Client education for those receiving angiotensin receptor blockers should prioritize information about what topic?
   A. Orthostatic hypotension
   B. Potassium intake
   C. Magnesium intake
   D. Weight changes

Answers: 1. A, 2. (A, B, E), 3. B, 4. A

Section Four: Hypertensive Crises

Hypertension is usually a chronic disease process associated with a slowly rising baseline blood pressure over a relatively long period of time, and the vascular system is able to adjust to the increasing pressures. A small percentage (less than 1%) of hypertensive patients develop an acute onset of severe hypertension that is significantly beyond their baseline levels—a hypertensive crisis. This section provides an overview of the types of hypertensive crises, their manifestations, and interventions.

Risk Factors for Development of Crises

There are no known specific risk factors to predict who will develop a hypertensive crisis. There are, however, common factors found in the patient history of those who develop crises. The typical profile of the person who develops a hypertensive crisis includes a history of hypertension that has not been well controlled, and either inadequate adherence to the prescribed drug regimen or inadequate treatment (Kotchen, 2015).

Pathophysiology

The pathophysiology underlying hypertensive crises is not well understood. It is believed that an acute increase in blood pressure causes additional stress on blood vessels, damaging the vessel endothelium. A cascade of physiologic events are triggered, such as activation of the renin-angiotensin-aldosterone system (RAAS), stimulation of the sympathetic nervous system, secretion of inflammatory cytokines, and activation of the coagulation cascade (Derhaschnig et al., 2013). The end result of these activities is vasoconstriction and thrombosis that result in hypoperfusion, tissue ischemia, and organ damage (Derhaschnig et al., 2013).

Autoregulation is another important factor in explaining organ damage associated with hypertensive crises, particularly in the brain, heart, and kidneys. Normally, organs are protected from large fluctuations in systemic blood pressure through autoregulation, which is the ability of an organ to maintain constant blood flow regardless of systemic blood pressure (Mitrovic, 2014).

People who develop hypertensive crises usually have chronic hypertension, which resets their "normal" autoregulation range to a higher baseline normal. In other words, in patients with chronic hypertension, the organs require a higher-than-normal mean arterial pressure to adequately meet their oxygenation needs. Clinically, this is important because reducing the patient's systemic blood pressure to within normal ranges may result in an insufficient perfusion pressure to the organs, and that can potentially result in organ ischemia and damage.

Types of Hypertensive Crises

Older terms used to describe hypertensive crises are accelerated hypertension and malignant hypertension; however, current literature tends to use the term hypertensive crises and divides the crises into two levels of severity: hypertensive urgency and hypertensive emergency. These designations are based on blood pressure and whether there is evidence of target organ (end-organ) damage. When a patient presents in a hypertensive crisis, it is crucial to rapidly establish whether it is an urgent or emergency situation because interventions are based on the severity of crisis. Table 14–7 provides comparative information on the two levels of hypertensive crisis.

Hypertensive Urgency Hypertensive urgency is defined as an arterial blood pressure greater than 180/110 mmHg without evidence of acute target organ damage (Nordquist, 2014). The recommended therapy is to administer oral antihypertensive agents to decrease the blood pressure gradually over a 24- to 48-hour period to a lower target blood pressure (which may not be within a traditional normal range). The slow rate of blood pressure reduction is recommended to decrease the chance of organ ischemia from a rapid blood pressure decline (Nordquist, 2014). The patient may present with minimal or no manifestations associated with the hypertension; however, headache, chest pain, vertigo, or other symptoms may be present (Salkic, Batic-Mujanovic,

Ljuca, & Brkic, 2014). Unless the patient has some underlying health issue that triggered the acute hypertension exacerbation, it is managed on an outpatient basis.

Hypertensive Emergency Hypertensive emergency is defined as an arterial blood pressure greater than 180/110 mmHg with evidence of acute target organ damage (Nordquist, 2014; Sutters, 2017). The major organs targeted for acute damage are the heart, brain, and kidneys. This is a medical emergency, and rapid reduction of blood pressure to lessen the degree of target organ damage is the highest priority. The patient is admitted to intensive care, and titratable intravenous antihypertensive agents are initiated (see Table 14–7). The choice of drug therapy will differ based on which organ is being targeted. The speed with which the blood pressure is reduced requires frequent monitoring to determine the effects of the reduction on organ perfusion. If aortic dissection is present, blood pressure will be reduced even more aggressively to try to halt the dissection progress (Nordquist, 2014).

Table 14–7 Comparison of Hypertensive Urgency and Emergency

	Hypertensive Urgency	Hypertensive Emergency
Blood pressure (inclusive criteria vary)	Greater than 180/110 mmHg Or diastolic BP greater than 120 mmHg	Same as hypertensive urgency
Target organ damage	No	Yes Brain: cerebral infarction, subarachnoid or intracerebral hemorrhage, hypertensive encephalopathy Heart/cardiovascular: acute MI, pulmonary edema, acute left ventricular failure, acute aortic dissection Kidneys: acute kidney failure
Manifestations	May be asymptomatic Headache, anxiety, epistaxis, dyspnea	Severe headache, neurologic deficit, vertigo Nausea and vomiting Chest pain Others: based on targeted organ
Treatment	Follow up as outpatient Alleviate pain and anxiety Oral antihypertensive agents Gradual decrease in blood pressure over 24–48 hours	Admit to ICU. Administer intravenous antihypertensive agents. BP reduction goals: • Reduce mean arterial blood pressure by approximately 20% in first half hour. Then goal is to achieve an approximate BP of 160/100 mmHg within 2–6 hours. • Exception: aortic dissection, rapidly reduce systolic blood pressure to less than 100 mmHg. Treat the damaged end-organ.
Antihypertensive therapy	Oral antihypertensives: clonidine, captopril, nifedipine	Titratable IV agents: • Adrenergic inhibitors: esmolol, labetalol, metoprolol • Vasodilators: nitroprusside, nitroglycerine, nicardipine • Diuretics: furosemide

SOURCE: Data from Kotchen (2015), Nordquist (2014), Salkic et al. (2014), and Sutters (2017).

Section Four Review

1. Common factors present in clients who develop a hypertensive crisis include which of the following? (Select all that apply.)
   A. History of heart failure
   B. Overuse of salt
   C. Inadequate adherence to prescribed drug regimen
   D. Positive history of hypertension
   E. History of frequent respiratory illness

2. The end result of the pathophysiologic processes associated with hypertensive crises includes which problems? (Select all that apply.)
   A. Vasoconstriction
   B. Bleeding tendencies
   C. Vasodilation
   D. Thrombosis
   E. Organ damage

3. Autoregulation of organ perfusion is altered in which way when a person has chronic hypertension?
   A. Organs require a lower pressure to be perfused.
   B. Autoregulation is reset to a higher baseline in organs.
   C. Organs adapt to higher pressures by vasodilating.
   D. Autoregulation of organs resets to a lower baseline pressure.

4. Which statement is correct regarding the difference between hypertensive urgency and hypertensive emergency?
   A. The blood pressure that defines hypertensive urgency is 160/110 or greater.
   B. Hypertensive emergency is treated with intravenous beta adrenergic blocking agents.
   C. In hypertensive urgency, blood pressure is reduced to a target level within 2 to 4 hours.
   D. A diagnosis of hypertensive emergency requires that target organ damage is present.

Answers: 1. (C, D), 2. (A, D, E), 3. B, 4. D

Section Five: Aortic Aneurysm

The incidence of aortic aneurysm and its complications have been on a steady rise as lifespan has increased. It is a silent disease that often becomes symptomatic only when the aneurysm ruptures or dissects. This section presents an overview of aortic aneurysm, its complications, and management.

Aneurysms

An **aneurysm** is an abnormal localized dilation of an artery that results from a weakened arterial wall. Aneurysms can occur throughout the body, but those of the aorta are relatively common and can be life-threatening.

Classification   Aortic aneurysms are classified by vessel wall involvement, shape, and location (LeMaire, Gopaldas, & Coselli, 2015).

By Vessel Wall Involvement.   When classified by the amount of vessel wall involvement, there are two types: True aneurysms are those in which all layers of the arterial wall (tunica intima, tunica media, and tunica externa) are involved, whereas pseudoaneurysms (false aneurysms) are those in which at least one layer of the wall is not involved (Figure 14–9). Pseudoaneurysms are usually a complication of an invasive intervention, such as artery catheterization or artery anastomosis.

By Aneurysm Shape.   There are two shapes characteristic of aortic aneurysm. A saccular aneurysm is one that involves only part of the vessel circumference, and a fusiform aneurysm involves the entire artery circumference (Figure 14–9) (Leeper, 2014). The fusiform shape is much more common than saccular.

By Aneurysm Location.   Aortic aneurysms can be located all along the aorta, from the ascending thoracic aorta through the trunk of the abdominal aorta. They are often referred to by their location, such as thoracic and abdominal aneurysms. Thoracic aneurysms are generally subcategorized by their specific location as ascending (most common thoracic location), transverse, or descending thoracic aneurysm (LeMaire et al., 2015). If the aneurysm involves both the lower thoracic aorta and the upper abdominal aorta, it is a

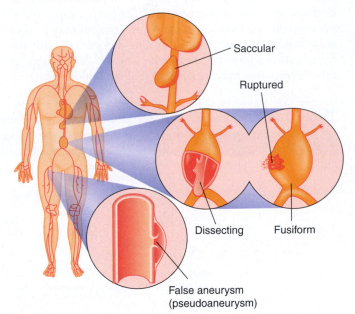

Figure 14–9 Classification of aneurysms.

thoracoabdominal aneurysm. The most common location for aortic aneurysm development is in the abdomen (abdominal aortic aneurysm [AAA]); and within the abdomen, the most common location is in the distal abdominal aorta beginning just below the junction of the renal arteries and ending near the junction of the aorta and iliac arteries.

Etiology and Risk Factors   Aneurysms are usually a complication of longstanding atherosclerosis; however, other etiologies include a genetic predisposition (positive family history of aneurysm), certain connective tissue disorders, traumatic injury, and infection (LeMaire et al., 2015; Mitrovic, 2014; Zelman, 2015). Specific genetic disorders that predispose the patient to aneurysm development are presented in the Genetic Considerations: Genetic Conditions Predisposing Aneurysm Development feature. Major risk factors for aneurysms are similar to those of atherosclerosis and include hypertension, smoking, age (greater than 60 years), men, and family history; furthermore, the prevalence is greater in Whites (Fuente, 2014).

Pathophysiology   Aneurysms are the result of degenerative atherosclerotic changes in the aorta. The middle layer of the arterial wall, the tunica media (thick middle muscle layer), slowly degenerates, which weakens the wall. Eventually, the affected wall becomes vulnerable to the effects

Genetic Considerations
Genetic Disorders Predisposing Aneurysm Development

- Marfan syndrome
- Loeys-Dietz syndrome
- Ehlers-Danlos syndrome
- Congenital bicuspid aortic valve
- Bovine aortic arch

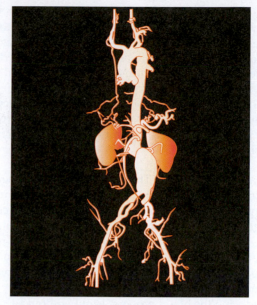

Figure 14–10 Depiction of a CT angiogram of an abdominal aortic aneurysm. Note the location of the aneurysm relative to the renal arteries (above) and iliac arteries (below).

of blood pressure being exerted against it, causing it to dilate. **LaPlace's law** (applied to blood vessels) helps explain why aneurysms grow. The law states that wall tension (T) is equal to the pressure (P) being exerted against the wall, multiplied by the wall radius (R), or $T = P \times R$; therefore, as an artery dilates, it increases the force on the arterial wall, which then causes more dilation. For this reason, once an aneurysm begins to grow, it will continue to do so, potentially leading to aortic rupture. The pressures in the aorta are the highest in the body, which explains why it is a major location for aneurysm development; this also explains why it is crucial to control the patient's blood pressure—to reduce the pressure (P) portion of the LaPlace's law equation.

Clinical Manifestation   In the absence of complications, aortic aneurysms are often asymptomatic or cause only minimal symptoms. Consequently they are often inadvertently discovered when the individual is undergoing diagnostic exams for other health problems. For this reason the patient may not be diagnosed with an aneurysm until it is large and impinging on some adjacent structure (e.g., an organ or nerve) or a complication arises such as rupture or dissection. Table 14–8 lists common manifestations associated with aortic aneurysms and their complications.

Diagnosis   Diagnostic imaging is the primary tool for diagnosing aortic aneurysms. Common tests include chest or abdominal radiograph, computed tomography (CT) scan, transesophageal or transthoracic echocardiography, and magnetic resonance imaging (MRI) (Figure 14–10) (LeMaire et al., 2015). Physical assessment is not considered a strong tool for diagnosing aneurysm because it relies on visualization or palpation of a pulsating mass. Visualization and palpation are not sensitive assessments for detecting aneurysms because patient weight is a factor. For example, in diagnosing abdominal aortic aneurysm, extremes of weight (either obesity or extreme thinness) can give false results—that is, obesity can result in a false negative assessment, whereas extreme thinness can result in a false positive one (Prince & Johnson, 2011).

Table 14–8 Clinical Manifestations of Aortic Aneurysms

Symptoms	Thoracic Aneurysm	Abdominal Aneurysm
General	Often asymptomatic Hoarseness (stretching of recurrent laryngeal nerves) Cough, dyspnea, wheezing (compression of trachea) Neck vein distention (superior vena cava obstruction) Heart failure (aortic insufficiency) Lump in throat sensation (compression of esophagus) BP difference of greater than 15 mmHg between right and left arms Peripheral pulses that differ between right and left sides	Often asymptomatic Abdominal pulsation Ischemia in extremities from thrombus formation Peripheral pulses may be weak or absent
Dissection	Primary symptom is pain: Acute onset of severe chest pain that may radiate to back Blood pressure: Hypertension is common; however, patients with type A dissection (ascending aorta) tend to be normotensive or hypotensive Other: syncope, heart failure, acute stroke or myocardial infarction, cardiac arrest	Rapid onset of severe pain in abdomen or back. Pain may migrate with path of extension. Peripheral neuropathy or paralysis
Rupture	Rapid onset of severe chest, back, abdominal, or flank pain; or atypical pain in trunk Hypotension (rupture into mediastinum or pleural cavity) Hematemesis (rupture into esophagus) Hemoptysis (rupture into airway)	Sudden onset of: • Severe pain in abdomen, flank, or back; may be described as ripping or tearing sensation • Syncope • Hypotension • Shock or sudden death

SOURCE: Data from Fuente (2014), Leeper (2014), and LeMaire et al. (2015).

Management Once discovered, aneurysms are monitored closely through regular diagnostic imaging to track changes in diameter. Treatment is based on the size and shape of the aneurysm with an assessment of the risk for rupture. The risk for rupture is low in abdominal aortic aneurysms (AAA) that are less than 5.5 cm in diameter with no recent changes in size. However, if the aneurysm increases in size by 0.5 cm every 6 months, the risk for rupture is high and repair is recommended (Gordon & Toursarkissian, 2014).

Medical Management. The goal of medical management is to keep the aneurysm small in size. This is primarily accomplished by aggressive blood pressure control through oral antihypertensive therapy, often using beta adrenergic blocking agents, and surveillance with regular follow-up assessments of the aneurysm size. The management plan may also include treatment of hyperlipidemia and smoking cessation.

Reducing the blood pressure is not without risk in this patient population since chronic hypertension is generally present. Pressure needs to be reduced to a level that provides maximum pressure relief to the aneurysm while maintaining adequate organ perfusion. Recall from Section Four that chronic hypertension resets autoregulation in the organs to a higher level; consequently, the organs require higher perfusion pressures than normal to remain perfused and oxygenated. Clinically, this requires that great care be taken when initiating antihypertensive therapy in the patient with chronic hypertension; therefore, the patient's vital signs and organ function status must be monitored closely as antihypertensive therapy is initiated.

Interventional Management. Procedural intervention is considered once the aneurysm has grown to a diameter of greater than 5 to 5.5 cm because of the high risk of rupture. There are two major repair interventions: surgical repair or endovascular aneurysm repair (EVAR).

Open Surgical Repair (OSR). The decision to repair an aortic aneurysm is largely made on the likelihood that the aneurysm is going to rupture. Surgical repair is a relatively high-risk procedure; therefore, surgery is reserved for when the risk of rupture outweighs the risk of the surgery. Repair of an abdominal aortic aneurysm has an estimated operative complication rate of 5% to 10% and a 2% to 4% intraoperative mortality rate (Rapp & Gasper, 2015). Potential complications include bleeding, renal failure, myocardial infarction, infection, loss of limb, bowel ischemia, and erectile dysfunction (Rapp & Gasper, 2015). For many years, the open surgical repair was the only available corrective method. Using this approach, the patient undergoes a laparotomy or left retroperitoneal incision and placement of a prosthetic graft, which is made of synthetic material such as Dacron (a type of polyester) or polytetrafluoroethylene (PTFE). The graft may be a straight tube that is sutured to the proximal and distal aorta or the proximal aorta alone, or it may be a bifurcated graft that attaches to the proximal aorta and the iliac arteries (see Figure 14–11). The aneurysm is left in place to prevent exposure of the graft to the gastrointestinal tract, and it may be wrapped around the graft to provide stability.

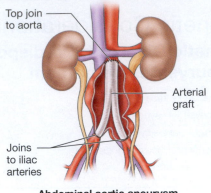

Figure 14–11 Repair of abdominal aneurysm.

Endovascular Aneurysm Repair (EVAR). EVAR is a less invasive procedure that is performed under fluoroscopic guidance. Using this approach, a catheter is inserted into the femoral artery, and a guide wire is threaded through the aorta to above the aneurysm. The endograft, a fabric-covered metallic stent, is then threaded into position and deployed (see Figure 14–12). The EVAR option can be used in individuals who meet specific vascular anatomic criteria and prefer to have a less invasive intervention (does not require an abdominal incision) with reduced recovery time (LeMaire et al., 2015). It is also used when the patient's general condition is poor, making OSR an undesirable option. Research suggests that the 30-day mortality and complication rates are lower with this procedure when compared to OSR; however, the mortality rates are similar 1 year following procedural or surgical intervention (Gordon & Toursarkissian, 2014). Two major advantages of EVAR over OSR are a short postprocedure recovery time and an earlier discharge from the hospital, often within 24 hours of the procedure.

Table 14–9 provides a list of complications associated with open surgical repair (OSR) and endovascular aneurysm repair.

Nursing Considerations Small aortic aneurysms are relatively common, and the high-acuity nurse is likely to care for a patient with an aortic aneurysm or with a medical

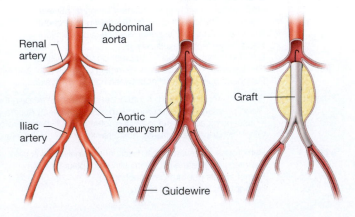

Figure 14–12 Endovascular stent graft.

Table 14–9 Complications of Interventional Management of Aortic Aneurysms

Open Surgical Repair (OSR)	Endovascular Aneurysm Repair (EVAR)
Acute myocardial infarction	Endoleaks
Ischemia of heart, lungs, or kidneys	Migration of endograft
Graft rejection	Thrombosis of limb
Para-anastomotic aneurysm	Mechanical graft issues (e.g.,
Graft-enteric erosions or fistula	fractures, separation, tears)
Occlusion of graft limb with lower limb	Graft infection
ischemia	

SOURCE: Data from Gordon & Toursarkissian (2014) and Rapp and Gasper (2015).

history of one. While medically managed patients are generally treated on an outpatient basis, the patient may require admission with another acute problem such as acute coronary syndrome. The patient also may be newly diagnosed with an aortic aneurysm after undergoing diagnostic testing for some unrelated problem. Regardless of the situation, the patient's aneurysm must be taken into consideration during the admission. Blood pressure must be carefully monitored, and with thoracic aneurysm, the nurse should measure BP in both arms to monitor for significant differences. Peripheral pulses are routinely checked with particular attention to differences between left and right pulses or a reduction in the strength of lower-extremity pulses. The nurse should also be aware of the common manifestations of aneurysm rupture and dissection to ensure that the development of either complication is rapidly recognized so that emergency interventions can be initiated.

Patient Education. When being medically managed, the patient needs to have a strong understanding of the disease and therapeutic plan. Blood pressure control and smoking cessation should be emphasized, as well as the need for regular surveillance of aneurysm size. Healthy lifestyle changes (diet, exercise, and stress management)

are important to reduce modifiable risk factors of atherosclerosis and to maintain aneurysm stability. The medication regimen, including therapeutic and nontherapeutic effects, and signs and symptoms of complications of aneurysm are critical for the patient and family to understand. The patient should also have a clear understanding of when to seek medical or emergency assistance.

Postsurgery Discharge Teaching. Discharge teaching should begin soon after surgery, usually while the patient is still in the critical care unit. Important teaching points include postdischarge activity, diet, medications, incision care, follow-up, and when to seek medical attention. Table 14–10 provides general discharge teaching appropriate to aneurysm surgery.

Aortic Aneurysm Emergencies

As aneurysms progress, they become more prone to two complications: aneurysm rupture and aortic dissection. Aneurysm dissection is most common in thoracic aneurysm, and rupture is more common in abdominal aneurysm. Both of these situations are life-threatening emergencies.

Aortic Rupture   Aneurysm rupture occurs when the pressure being exerted on the artery wall goes beyond the wall's tensile strength, just as a balloon bursts when it is blown up too large. The size of the aneurysm is the best indicator of the risk for rupture. An estimated 40% of aneurysms that are 5.5 to 6 cm or greater in size will rupture in 5 years if treatment is not initiated. In addition, the average length of survival without treatment under these circumstances is about 17 months (Rapp & Gasper, 2015).

Clinical Manifestations of Rupture. Recall that the patient is often asymptomatic prior to rupture. The most common symptom of rupture is rapid onset of severe pain

Table 14–10 Aortic Aneurysm Repair Discharge Teaching

Topic	Instruction Highlights
Activity	• Limit activity to slow walking. • Avoid climbing stairs or heavy lifting for 6 weeks. • Strength will return over time. • Do not drive for at least 1 week; can ride for short distances. • Endovascular repair: Elevate feet when sitting in chair and avoid prolonged sitting or standing.
Diet	• Resume normal diet (recommend low fat, low cholesterol). • Appetite will increase over time. • Take a mild laxative or a ready-to-use enema if required to regulate bowel movements.
Medications	• Take medications exactly as directed.
Incision	• Showering, rather than sitting in a tub, is recommended for the first week. • Do not get the incision wet for the first week or if the wound has any open area. • Check the incision daily for signs of infection. • Endovascular repair: Gently wash the incision site with soap and water while showering.
Follow-up	• Will be scheduled for periodic Doppler ultrasound studies; very important part of follow-up care • Will be scheduled for a follow-up appointment two to three weeks postprocedure
When to Seek Medical Attention	• With any signs of incisional infection • Contact provider for any of these: fever greater than 101°F, nausea or vomiting, breathing problems, pain in chest or arms, changes in lower extremities (loss of sensation, sudden development of coldness, paleness, or pain), problems urinating • Unusual bleeding

located in the chest, back, abdomen, or flank; however, the patient may present with atypical pain anywhere in the trunk, even the hips (Cotarlan & Austin, 2015). Impending rupture may be difficult to differentiate from other symptom origins such as acute coronary syndromes, myocardial infarction, or musculoskeletal pain (Mercer-Deadman, 2014). Rapid onset of shock develops as the patient hemorrhages into the extravascular spaces adjacent to the rupture site, and death is inevitable unless the patient has immediate emergency repair.

Collaborative Management.   Aneurysm rupture is a surgical emergency, and time is critical, making OSR the procedure of choice. Fluid resuscitation and blood replacement therapy are initiated to prevent hypovolemia and replace lost erythrocytes. Narcotics may be administered for pain. Postoperatively, the patient is admitted to the critical care unit, where blood pressure is tightly controlled to reduce pressure on the anastomosis sites and hemodynamic status is continuously monitored (Leeper, 2014). Mechanical ventilation may be continued to optimize oxygenation status until the patient is fully stabilized. Renal function is closely monitored to detect any kidney damage that might have occurred during the procedure. The patient will be placed on anticoagulant therapy to prevent clot formation from the presence of the prosthetic graft (Leeper, 2014).

Aortic Dissection   Aortic dissection refers to a potentially catastrophic event in which arterial blood enters the aorta tunica media, causing separation of the tunica media from the tunica intima. It is more common than aortic rupture, usually develops in the thoracic aorta, and has an extremely high early mortality rate.

Pathophysiology.   Aortic dissection often occurs in the right lateral wall of the ascending aorta where shear stress is high. The injury can be a circumferential or transverse tear of the intima. If the injury is in the descending thoracic aorta, an initial tear can cause a secondary dissection into the media, and hemorrhage into the intima may result in the formation of a false lumen (Creager & Loscalzo, 2015).

Tear in Tunica Intima.   Pressure being exerted against the tunica intima causes a tear through which arterial blood flows with pulsatile force. The force of the deviated blood flow creates a false lumen as the tunica media separates from the tunica intima, an activity known as dissection extension.

Vasa Vasorum Hemorrhage.   The vasa vasorum are small arteries that are embedded within the walls of large vessels such as the aorta, providing oxygen and nutrients to the large vessel walls. This theory suggests that rupture of the vasa vasorum causes hemorrhage within the wall of the aorta using pulsatile force that causes separation of the tunica media from the intima and creating a false lumen.

Dissection usually extends in an antegrade (forward) pattern from the point of origin—for example, beginning in the descending thoracic aorta and extending into the abdominal aorta. However, dissection can also extend in a retrograde (backward) pattern—for example, beginning at the transverse thoracic aorta and extending backward into the ascending aorta.

Table 14–11 Classification Systems for Aortic Dissection

DeBakey Classification	Stanford Classification
Type I: Origin: Ascending thoracic aorta Extension: At least to aortic arch	**Type A:** Involves ascending aorta
Type II: Origin: Ascending thoracic aorta Extension: None	**Type B:** Does not involve ascending aorta
Type III: Origin: Descending thoracic aorta Extension: Usually immediately distal to subclavian artery • IIIa extension: Above diaphragm • IIIb extension: Below diaphragm	

SOURCE: Data from LeMaire et al. (2015) and Mercer-Deadman (2014).

Classification.   Aortic dissection is classified by location using one of two major classification systems: the DeBakey or Stanford system (Mercer-Deadman, 2014). The DeBakey system divides aortic dissection into types I, II, and III (with two subclassifications of IIIa and IIIb) based on point of origin and extension. The Stanford system divides dissection into types A and B based solely on whether the ascending thoracic aorta is involved. Table 14–11 summarizes the two classification systems.

Clinical Manifestations.   The most common presenting symptom of aortic dissection is acute onset of severe pain that does not change in severity; however, the location may migrate along the extension path (Cotarlan & Austin, 2015). Additional pain descriptors that may be given by the patient include ripping, stabbing, tearing, or burning; however, in a small percentage of cases, no pain is present. The effect of dissection on blood pressure often depends on its location, with the most common finding being hypertension. In type A (ascending) dissection, the patient may be hypotensive on presentation related to aortic regurgitation, cardiac tamponade, or heart failure. Hypotension is considered an ominous finding and is associated with a high death rate. Clinical manifestations associated with aortic dissection are included in Table 14–10 (see When to Seek Medical Attention).

Diagnosis.   Rapid detection of aortic dissection is necessary to improve patient outcomes, yet the signs and symptoms of dissection are similar to those of multiple acute diseases, which makes a differential diagnosis more difficult (Cotarlan & Austin, 2015). The same diagnostic imaging tests that are used for diagnosing aneurysms are used for dissection; however, CT scan is a common test with echocardiogram as the backup tool when CT scan cannot be used. To improve the speed and accuracy with which dissection is diagnosed, risk score tools are available. One such tool is the Acute Aortic Dissection Diagnostic (ADD) Risk Score, which combines a diagnostic algorithm and risk score based on three high-risk categories: predisposing conditions, pain features, and examination features (Rogers et al., 2011).

Management   Treatment of aortic dissection requires rapid stabilization of the patient. Goals of therapy include rapid control of blood pressure, fluid management, anticoagulation, decreasing shear stress on the aorta, and pain control. Immediate surgical treatment is recommended for patients who present with type A dissection because it significantly improves patient outcomes; however, surgical repair is difficult because the walls of the aorta are extremely fragile and sutures can tear through it (Cotarlan & Austin, 2015). If dissection progresses to acute aortic rupture, severe pain and profound hypotension can occur and immediate life-saving emergency surgery is necessary (Creager & Loscalzo, 2015).

Nursing Considerations

Nursing care of the patient following surgical repair of aortic aneurysm, rupture, or dissection includes the prevention and management of complications and pain control (Leeper, 2014). The patient is returned to the critical care unit for frequent assessments and continuous cardiac and hemodynamic monitoring. The patient will most likely remain on the mechanical ventilator to optimize oxygenation during the immediate postoperative period. Control of postoperative pain can be a challenge because the wound pain associated with the repair procedure is often reported as severe. Blood pressure is tightly controlled to reduce stress on the operative site (Leeper, 2014). The nurse also monitors peripheral sensation and pulses to ensure that adequate circulation is getting to the extremities following the procedure. This is a critical assessment because vascular occlusion is a major complication associated with aortic procedures. Kidney function and neurological status are assessed to evaluate adequacy of circulation to the kidneys, brain, and spinal cord. The nurse will also closely monitor the patient for the development of complications.

Section Five Review

1. What is the most common location for aortic aneurysm development?
   A. Distal to the renal arteries
   B. Proximal to the diaphragm
   C. Ascending thoracic aorta
   D. Transverse thoracic aorta

2. Which of the following are known risk factors for development of aortic aneurysm? (Select all that apply.)
   A. Smoking
   B. Age older than 60
   C. Women
   D. History of peripheral arterial disease
   E. High carbohydrate diet

3. When aortic dissection occurs, blood flow is deviated in which way?
   A. Blood enters the aorta from the hemorrhaging vasa vasorum in the aorta wall.
   B. Blood flows out of the aorta into adjacent tissues such as the mediastinum.
   C. Blood enters the tunica media and separates it from the tunica intima.
   D. Blood enters the tunica externa and separates it from the tunica media.

4. Management goals that apply to both aortic rupture and dissection include which considerations? (Select all that apply.)
   A. Pain control
   B. Rapid control of hypertension
   C. Fluid management
   D. Prevention of complications
   E. Early return to oral nutrition

Answers: 1. A, 2. (A, B, D), 3. C, 4. (A, B, C, D)

Clinical Reasoning Checkpoint

A patient presents to the ED with complaints of chest pain and dizziness after climbing a flight of stairs. He has a past medical history of aortic valve stenosis. The nurse assesses vital signs and connects the patient to cardiac rhythm and pulse oximetry monitoring systems. The following data are available:

- Cardiac rhythm strip interpretation: uncontrolled atrial fibrillation with a ventricular rate of 146 contractions per minute
- Arterial oxygen saturation: 88%
- Mean arterial blood pressure: 70 mmHg
- Respiratory system: rate 32 breaths per minute, labored, crackles auscultated in bilateral, posterior lung fields

1. What is the pathophysiologic basis of chest pain and syncope in this patient?

2. Where is the best anatomic site to auscultate for the murmur of aortic valve stenosis, and where in the cardiac cycle would you expect to hear it?

3. Given these symptoms, it appears that the patient has significant valvular dysfunction. What interventions should the nurse perform?

4. The patient is scheduled to undergo an aortic valve replacement with a mechanical valve. Will this patient require anticoagulation therapy postprocedure?

5. Discuss what information the nurse should include in discharge teaching for this patient.

Chapter 14 Review

1. A client is admitted with newly diagnosed aortic valve stenosis. The nurse closely monitors this client for development of which cardiac dysrhythmia that may cause immediate decompensation?
   1. Premature ventricular contractions
   2. Premature atrial contractions
   3. Atrial fibrillation
   4. Sinus bradycardia

2. A client has been diagnosed with infective endocarditis. Which teaching information should the nurse provide to this client? (Select all that apply.)
   1. "You will probably be on antibiotic therapy for at least two weeks."
   2. "Infective endocarditis usually affects the muscle in the wall of your heart."
   3. "Most people who develop infective endocarditis are smokers."
   4. "It is very important that you take your antibiotics on time and according to the directions provided."
   5. "You will have several blood tests done to determine which antibiotic is necessary."

3. A client has been diagnosed with heart failure. How should the nurse explain this disorder to the client?
   1. "The fluid accumulated in your ankles makes it too difficult for your heart to pump blood effectively."
   2. "The two bottom pumping chambers of your heart are not working correctly."
   3. "The valves between the chambers of your heart are weak."
   4. "The large vessel leading from your heart is blocked."

4. A nurse is preparing to administer the client's daily dose of carvedilol (Coreg). What findings would indicate need to collaborate with the prescriber before administration? (Select all that apply.)
   1. Heart rate of 48 bpm
   2. Respiratory rate of 14 breaths/min
   3. Second degree AV block
   4. Presence of a dry cough
   5. Shortness of breath at rest

5. A client's blood pressure has measured 139/85 mmHg and 136/88 mmHg at the last two monthly appointments. What should the nurse tell the client about these blood pressure measurements?
   1. "Your blood pressure is normal."
   2. "Your blood pressure measurements fall in the pre-hypertension range."
   3. "You now have acute hypertension."
   4. "Since your hypertension is stable, no therapy changes are necessary."

6. Which food choices would the nurse interpret as indicating that the client understands dietary instruction for the management of hypertension? (Select all that apply.)
   1. Low-fat milk at lunch
   2. Wine at the evening meal and beer while watching television
   3. Potassium-bearing fruits such as bananas for breakfast
   4. Vitamin B–enriched cereal for breakfast
   5. Pretzels as an afternoon snack

7. A client has been diagnosed with hypertensive emergency. Which interventions would the emergency department nurse anticipate delivering? (Select all that apply.)
   1. Admitting the client to the hospital
   2. Titrating IV medications to control the blood pressure
   3. Interventions to slowly decrease the blood pressure
   4. Administration of oral medications
   5. Managing the client on an outpatient basis

8. A client is admitted to the emergency department in a hypertensive crisis. Which finding would indicate to the nurse that this is actually a hypertensive emergency?
   1. Client's systolic BP is 188 mmHg.
   2. Client complains of a headache.
   3. Client's diastolic BP is 118 mmHg.
   4. Client complains of chest pain.

9. A client with history of an abdominal aortic aneurysm (AAA) has been admitted for treatment of pneumonia. Which assessment finding would require the nurse to contact the client's primary healthcare provider immediately? (Select all that apply.)

    1. The client becomes suddenly hypotensive.
    2. The client reports a headache.
    3. The client's urine is cloudy.
    4. The client reports hip pain.
    5. There is new absence of pedal pulses in the left foot

10. A nurse is providing discharge instruction to a client whose abdominal aortic aneurysm (AAA) will be treated medically. Which topics should the nurse include in this instruction?

    1. Importance of smoking cessation
    2. Importance of keeping blood pressure in the hypotensive range
    3. How to palpate for changes in the diameter of the vessel
    4. How to monitor for blood in the urine

Answers to questions found inside your textbook are available on the faculty resources site. Please consult with your instructor.

References

Adams, M. P. (2016). Chapter 38: Pharmacotherapy of coagulation disorders. In M. P. Adams & C. Q. Urban (Eds.), *Pharmacology* (3rd ed.). Retrieved October 6, 2016, from https://bookshelf.vitalsource.com/#/books/9780133896848

Barakat, H. M., Shahin, Y., McCollum, P. T., & Chetter, I. C. (2015). Prediction of organ-specific complications following abdominal aortic aneurysm repair using cardiopulmonary exercise testing. *Anaesthesia, 70,* 679–685.

Barrett, K. E., Barman, S. M., Boitano, S., & Brooks, H. L. (2016). Chapter 38: Regulation of extracellular fluid composition & volume. In K. E. Barrett, S. M. Barman, S. Boitano, & H. L. Brooks (Eds.), *Ganong's review of medical physiology* (25th ed.). Retrieved October 12, 2016, from http://accessmedicine.mhmedical.com.ezproxy.uky.edu/content.aspx?bookid=1587&Sectionid=97166839

Bashore, T. M., Granger, C. B., Jackson, K. P., & Patel, M. R. (2017). Chapter 10: Heart disease. In M. A. Papadakis, S. J. McPhee, & M. W. Rabow (Eds.), *Current medical diagnosis and treatment, 2017.* Retrieved October 12, 2016, from http://accessmedicine.mhmedical.com.ezproxy.uky.edu/content.aspx?bookid=1843&sectionid=135705950#1132695457

Bloch, K. C. (2014). Infectious diseases. In G. D. Hammer & S. J. McPhee (Eds.), *Pathophysiology of disease: An introduction to clinical medicine* (7th ed.). Retrieved October 6, 2016, from http://accessmedicine.mhmedical.com.ezproxy.uky.edu/content.aspx?bookid=961&sectionid=53555685#1100857742

Carnicelli, A. (2015). Anticoagulation for valvular heart disease. American College of Cardiology. Retrieved October 6, 2016, from http://www.acc.org/latest-in-cardiology/articles/2015/05/18/09/58/anticoagulation-for-valvular-heart-disease

Cary, T., & Pearce, J. (2013). Aortic stenosis: Pathophysiology, diagnosis, and medical management of nonsurgical patients. *Critical Care Nurse, 33*(2), 58–73.

Cotarlan, V., & Austin, J. J. (2015). Chapter 42: Aortic dissection. In J. B. Hall, G. A. Schmidt, & J. P. Kress (Eds.), *Principles of critical care* (4th ed.). Retrieved February 6, 2017, from http://accessmedicine.mhmedical.com/content.aspx?sectionid=80031840&bookid=1340&Resultclick=2

Creager, M. A., & Loscalzo, J. (2015). Chapter 301: Diseases of the aorta. In D. Kasper, A. Fauci, S. Hauser, D. Longo, J. Jameson, & J. Loscalzo (Eds.), *Harrison's principles of internal medicine* (19th ed.). Retrieved February 6, 2017, from http://accesspharmacy.mhmedical.com/Content.aspx?bookid=1130&sectionid=79744168

Derhaschnig, U., Testori, C., Riedmueller, E., Aschauer, S., Wolzt, M., & Jilma, B. (2013). Hypertensive emergencies are associated with elevated markers of inflammation, coagulation, platelet activation and fibrinolysis. *Journal of Human Hypertension, 27*(6), 368–373.

Fuente, A. (2014). Chapter 29: Abdominal aortic aneurysm. In S. C. Sherman, J. M. Weber, M. A. Schindlbeck, & G. P. Rahul (Eds.), *Clinical emergency medicine.* Retrieved October 15, 2016, from http://accessemergencymedicine.mhmedical.com.ezproxy.uky.edu/content.aspx?bookid=991&Sectionid=57307924

Gordon, P. A., & Toursarkissian, B. (2014). Treatment of abdominal aortic aneurysms: The role of endovascular repair. *Association of perioperative nurses, 100*(3), 241–259.

Herr, J. K., Salyer, J., Flattery, M., Goodloe, L., Lyon, D. E., Kabban, C. S., & Clement, D. G. (2014). Heart failure symptom clusters and functional status—A cross-sectional study. *Journal of Advanced Nursing, 71*(6), 1274–1287. doi:101111/jan.12596

Hochman, J. S., & Ingbar, D. H. (2015). Cardiogenic shock and pulmonary edema. In D. Kasper, A. Fauci, S. Hauser, D. Longo, J. Jameson, & J. Loscalzo (Eds.), *Harrison's principles of internal medicine* (19th ed.). Retrieved October 13, 2016, from http://accessmedicine.mhmedical.com.ezproxy.uky.edu/content.aspx?bookid=1130&Sectionid=79745930

January, C. T., Wan, L. S., Alpert, J. S., Calkins, H., Cigarroa, J. E., Cleveland, J. C., . . . Yancy, C. W. (2014). 2014 AHA/ACC/HRS guideline for the management of patients with atrial fibrillation: A report of the American College of Cardiology/American Heart Association Task Force on Practice Guidelines and the Heart Rhythm Society. *Circulation, 130,* e199–e267. doi:10.1161/CIR.0000000000000041

Kotchen, T. A. (2015). Chapter 298: Hypertensive vascular disease. In D. Kasper, A. Fauci, S. Hauser, D. Longo, J. Jameson, & J. Loscalzo (Eds.), *Harrison's principles of internal medicine* (19th ed.). Retrieved October 13, 2016, from http://accessmedicine.mhmedical.com.ezproxy .uky.edu/content.aspx?bookid=1130&Sectionid=79743947

Kusumoto, F. M. (2014). Cardiovascular disorders: Heart disease. In G. D. Hammer & S. J. McPhee (Eds.), *Pathophysiology of disease: An introduction to clinical medicine* (7th ed.). Retrieved September 28, 2016, from http://accessmedicine.mhmedical.com.ezproxy.uky .edu/content.aspx?bookid=961&Sectionid=53555691

Kutzleb, J., Rigolosi, R., Fruhschien, A., Reilly, M. A., Shaftic, A. M., Duran, D., & Flynn, D. (2015). Nurse Practitioner Care Model: Meeting the health care challenges with a collaborative team. *Nursing Economics, 33*(6), 297–306.

Lakdawala, N. K., Stevenson, L., & Loscalzo, J. (2015). Cardiomyopathy and myocarditis. In D. Kasper, A. Fauci, S. Hauser, D. Longo, J. Jameson, & J. Loscalzo (Eds.), *Harrison's principles of internal medicine* (19th ed.). Retrieved October 12, 2016, from http:// accessmedicine.mhmedical.com.ezproxy.uky.edu /content.aspx?bookid=1130&Sectionid=79743046

Leeper, B. (2014). Chapter 19: Advanced cardiovascular concepts. In S. M. Burns (Ed.), *AACN: Essentials of critical care nursing* (3rd ed., pp. 475–505). New York, NY: McGraw-Hill.

LeMaire, S. A., Gopaldas, R. R., & Coselli, J. S. (2015). Thoracic aneurysms and aortic dissection. In F. Brunicardi, D. K. Andersen, T. R. Billiar, D. L. Dunn, J. G. Hunter, J. B. Matthews, & R. E. Pollock (Eds.), *Schwartz's principles of surgery* (10th ed.). Retrieved October 17, 2016, from http://accessmedicine .mhmedical.com.ezproxy.uky.edu/content.aspx?bookid =980&Sectionid=59610864

Means, L., Benken, S. T., & Tesoro, E. P. (2016). Safety of immediate release nifedipine. *Journal of Cardiovascular Pharmacology.* doi:10.1097/FJC.0000000000000425

Mercer-Deadman, P. (2014). Aortic dissections, aneurysms and ruptures: An emergency perspective. *Canadian Journal of Emergency Nursing, 37*(1), 18–22.

Mitrovic, I. (2014). Chapter 11: Cardiovascular disorders: Vascular disease. In G. D. Hammer & S. J. McPhee (Eds.), *Pathophysiology of disease: An introduction to clinical medicine* (7th ed.). Retrieved October 13, 2016, from http://accessmedicine.mhmedical.com .ezproxy.uky.edu/content.aspx?bookid=961&Sectio nid=53555692

Nordquist, E. K. (2014). Chapter 18: Hypertensive emergencies. In S. C. Sherman, J. M. Weber, M. A. Schindlbeck, & G. P. Rahul (Eds.), *Clinical emergency medicine.* Retrieved October 15, 2016, from

http://accessemergencymedicine.mhmedical.com .ezproxy.uky.edu/content.aspx?bookid=991&Sectio nid=55139125

O'Gara, P. T., & Loscalzo, J. (2015a). Chapter 283: Aortic valve disease. In D. Kasper, A. Fauci, S. Hauser, D. Longo, J. Jameson, & J. Loscalzo (Eds.), *Harrison's principles of internal medicine* (19th ed.). Retrieved September 28, 2016, from http://accessmedicine .mhmedical.com.ezproxy.uky.edu/content.aspx?bookid =1130&Sectionid=79742791

O'Gara, P. T., & Loscalzo, J. (2015b). Chapter 284: Mitral valve disease. In D. Kasper, A. Fauci, S. Hauser, D. Longo, J. Jameson, & J. Loscalzo (Eds.), *Harrison's principles of internal medicine* (19th ed.). Retrieved October 6, 2016, from http://accessmedicine .mhmedical.com.ezproxy.uky.edu/content.aspx?bookid =1130&sectionid=79742884

Prince, L. A., & Johnson, G. A. (2011). Chapter 63: Aneurysms of the aorta and major arteries. In J. E. Tintinalli, J. S. Stapczynski, D. M. Cline, O. J. Ma, R. K. Cydulka, & G. D. Meckler (Eds.), *Tintinalli's emergency medicine: A comprehensive study guide* (7th ed., pp. 453–458). Sydney, Australia: McGraw Medical.

Rapp, J. H., & Gasper, W. (2015). Chapter 34: Arteries. In G. M. Doherty (Ed.), *Current diagnosis & treatment: Surgery* (14th ed.). Retrieved February 6, 2017, from http://accesssurgery.mhmedical.com/Content.aspx?bo okId=1202&sectionId=71523863

Rogers, A. M., Hermann, L. K., Booher, A. M., Nienaber, C. A., Williams, D. M., Kazerooni, E. A., . . . Eagle, K. A. (2011). Sensitivity of the aortic dissection detection risk score: A novel guideline-based tool for identification of acute aortic dissection at initial presentation. Results from the international registry of acute aortic dissection. *Circulation, 123,* 2213–2218.

Rosendorff, C., Lackland, D. T., Allison, M., Aronow, W. S., Black, H. R., Blumenthal, R. S., . . . White, W. B. (2015). Treatment of hypertension in patients with coronary artery disease: A scientific statement from the American Heart Association, American College of Cardiology, and American Society of Hypertension. *Hypertension, 65,* 1372–1407. doi:http://dx.doi .org/10.1161/HYP.0000000000000018

Salkic, S., Batic-Mujanovic, O., Ljuca, F., & Brkic, S. (2014). Clinical presentation of hypertensive crises in emergency medical services. *Materia Socio Medica, 26*(1), 12–16.

Sidebottom, A. C., Jorgenson, A., Richards, H., Kirven, H., & Sillah, A. (2015). Inpatient palliative care for patients with acute heart failure: Outcomes from a randomized trial. *Journal of Palliative Medicine, 18*(2), 134–143. doi:10.1089/jpm.2014.0192

Sutters, M. (2017). Chapter 11: Systemic hypertension. In M. A. Papadakis, S. J. McPhee, & M. W. Rabow (Eds.), *Current medical diagnosis & treatment 2017.* Retrieved October 14, 2016, from http://accessmedicine .mhmedical.com.ezproxy.uky.edu/content.aspx?bookid =1843&Sectionid=135707761

The Joint Commission (TJC). (2013). Performance measures for advanced certification in heart failure finalized. Retrieved on October 13, 2016, from https://www .jointcommission.org/assets/1/6/JCP0613_HF.pdf

Weber, M. A., Schiffrin, E. L., White, W. B., Mann, S., Lindholm, L. H., Kenerson, J. G., . . . Harrap, S. B. (2014). Clinical practice guidelines for the management of hypertension in the community: A statement by the American Society of Hypertension and the International Society of Hypertension. *The Journal of Clinical Hypertension, 16*(1), 14–26.

Wilson, B. A., Shannon, M. T., & Shields, K. M. (2016). *Pearson nurse's drug guide 2016*. Hoboken, NJ: Pearson. Retrieved on October 13, 2016, from https://bookshelf .vitalsource.com/#/books/9780134070728 /cfi/6/8!/4@0.00:0.00

Yancy, C.W., Jessup, M., Bozkurt, B., Butler, J., Casey, D., Drazner, M. H., . . . Wilkoff, B. L. (2013). 2013 ACCF /AHA guideline for the management of heart failure: A report of the American College of Cardiology Foundation/American Heart Association Task Force on Practice Guidelines. *Circulation, 128*, e240–e327. doi:10.1161/CIR.0b013e31829e8776

Zelman, M. (2015). Chapter 5: Heredity and disease. In M. Zelman, J. Raymond, P. Holdaway, E. Dafnis, & M. L. Mulvihill (Eds.), *Human diseases: A systematic approach* (8th ed., pp. 88–121). Retrieved February 6, 2017, from https://bookshelf.vitalsource.com/# /books/9780133424775

Zelman, M., Raymond, J., Holdaway, P., Dafnis, E., & Mulvihill, M. L. (2015). Chapter 6: Diseases and disorders of the cardiovascular system. In M. Zelman, J. Raymond, P. Holdaway, E. Dafnis, & M. L. Mulvihill (Eds.), *Human diseases: A systematic approach* (8th ed., pp. 88–121). Retrieved from https://bookshelf .vitalsource.com/#/books/9780133424775

Chapter 15
Alterations in Myocardial Tissue Perfusion

⌄ Learning Outcomes

15.1 Describe the pathophysiology of atherosclerosis and coronary artery disease.

15.2 Identify risk factors for coronary artery disease and discuss collaborative interventions to reduce or manage the risk factors.

15.3 Differentiate types of angina and their assessment including stable angina, unstable angina, and variant angina.

15.4 Describe the diagnostic workup for alterations in myocardial tissue perfusion.

15.5 Describe the initial collaborative management of acute coronary syndromes, unstable angina, and myocardial infarction.

15.6 Explain the collaborative interventions commonly used to restore myocardial tissue perfusion.

This chapter focuses on disease processes that alter myocardial perfusion, signs and symptoms of altered myocardial perfusion, collaborative interventions used in the high-acuity setting to restore myocardial tissue perfusion, and the nursing care of patients who require these myocardial tissue reperfusion interventions.

Section One: Pathophysiology of Atherosclerosis and Coronary Artery Disease

Atherosclerosis, commonly referred to as "hardening of the arteries," accounts for a large percentage of deaths as a result of cardiovascular disease (CVD) in the United States and is the primary underlying cause of peripheral artery disease (PAD), coronary artery disease (CAD), and cerebrovascular disease. Atherosclerosis and its associated disorders are pervasive and affect both men and women. Approximately one of every three deaths in the United States is attributed to cardiovascular disease (Mozaffarian et al., 2015).

A normal artery consists of three concentric layers: the innermost layer is the tunica intima, the middle layer is the tunica media, and the outermost layer is the tunica adventitia (Figure 15–1A). Atherosclerosis is a chronic inflammatory disorder associated with injury to the intimal lining. It is a progressive disease characterized by formation of plaque in the intimal lining of medium and large arteries, including those in the aorta and its branches, the coronary arteries, and large vessels that supply the brain.

Although the precise mechanisms are unknown, atherosclerosis appears to begin with chronic injury or inflammation to the endothelial cells that line blood vessels. Collectively, all these endothelial cells are called the **endothelium**.

Sources of chronic injury and inflammation may include such things as hypertension, smoking, viruses, and

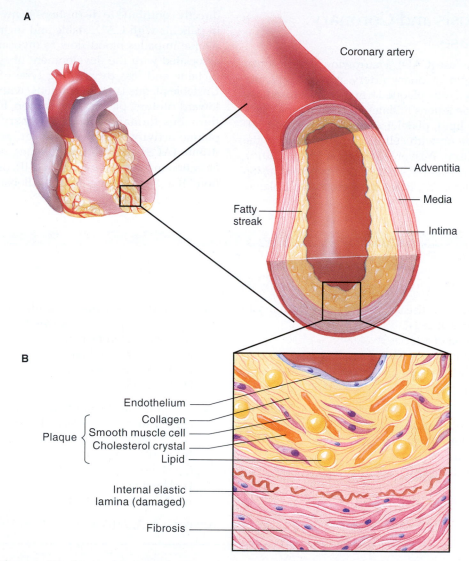

Figure 15–1 Atherosclerotic plaque development. Fatty streaks are lesions in the intimal lining that enlarge and protrude into the lumen of the artery. Plaque consists of cholesterol, phospholipids, collagen, and vascular smooth muscle cells.

high blood levels of cholesterol and glucose. These factors damage the endothelium, causing endothelial cells to separate. This allows monocytes from the bloodstream to enter into the intimal lining and become macrophages. Macrophages release substances that oxidize low-density lipoproteins (LDL) and are toxic to endothelial cells. This causes further endothelial cell dysfunction. Macrophages engulf LDL and become foam cells. A group of foam cells becomes the core of a fatty streak along the vessel wall (Figure 15–1). **Fatty streaks** are flat, thick, yellow lesions that can progressively thicken, enlarge, and protrude into the lumen of the artery.

As fatty streaks mature over several decades, they begin to develop into another type of atherosclerotic lesion called a **fibrous atheromatous plaque**. This is the basic lesion associated with atherosclerosis. Inside this lesion is an accumulation of lipids, collagen, scar tissue, and vascular smooth muscle cells (Mitrovic, 2014) (see Figure 15–1).

As these lesions grow, they become thicker and more complex. A fibrous cap forms on the top of the lesion, and in some instances the lesion enlarges and narrows the vessel lumen and reduces blood flow. Reduced blood flow to the coronary arteries leads to myocardial ischemia, a state in which oxygen demand exceeds supply, causing chest pain (angina pectoris).

Some atherosclerotic plaques advance to a more complicated lesion called an **atheroma**. Atheromas are calcified lesions that contain areas of hemorrhage, surface ulcerations, and scar tissue deposits. Decreased or sluggish blood flow past an atherosclerotic lesion combined with ideal blood clotting conditions, such as increased platelet aggregation, can produce a thrombus on the lesion (Kusumoto, 2014). The formation of this thrombus is dangerous because it not only further reduces blood flow but also can occlude the artery or break off to become an embolus.

Atherosclerosis and Coronary Artery Disease

Coronary artery disease (CAD), a narrowing of the internal space or lumen of a coronary artery, is most typically caused by atherosclerotic plaque formations. Hemorrhage or rupture of plaque lesions initiates an arterial repair process that includes lipid, platelet, cellular debris, and calcium deposition along with cellular inflammation in the affected artery (Wilson, Weaver-Agostoni, & Perkins, 2015). The end result is intimal thickening and further occlusion of the coronary artery. Two types of atherosclerotic plaque directly contribute to disruptions in myocardial blood flow in patients with CAD: stable and unstable plaque. Stable plaque impedes blood flow to myocardial tissues and is associated with the development of stable angina, a predictable and less-threatening type of cardiac ischemia. Unstable plaque is more ominous, with a greater tendency toward rupture, platelet aggregation, fibrin attraction, and thrombus formation in the coronary arteries. Unstable plaque activity can precipitate an **acute coronary syndrome (ACS)** such as unstable angina, non-*ST*-segment elevation myocardial infarction (MI), or *ST*-segment elevation MI in the patient with CAD (Bobadilla, 2016).

Section One Review

1. Atherosclerosis is a disease associated with injury to which structures or cells?
   A. Intimal lining of arteries
   B. Medial lining of arteries
   C. Fibrous atheromatous plaque
   D. Macrophages

2. Which factors are known sources of chronic endothelial cell injury? (Select all that apply.)
   A. Hypertension
   B. Vasodilation
   C. High cholesterol
   D. Smoking
   E. Viruses

3. Coronary artery disease is most commonly caused by which pathophysiologic event?
   A. Atherosclerotic plaque
   B. Vascular vasodilation
   C. Thrombus dissolution
   D. Platelet loss

4. Which medical conditions are considered acute coronary syndromes? (Select all that apply.)
   A. Unstable angina
   B. Aortic aneurysm
   C. Myocardial infarction
   D. Heart failure
   E. Pulmonary embolism

Answers: 1. A, 2. (A, C, D, E), 3. A, 4. (A, C)

Section Two: Etiologic Factors for Coronary Artery Disease

Risk factors that predispose the development of coronary artery disease (also called coronary heart disease) have been identified through epidemiologic research. Risk factors are categorized as either modifiable or nonmodifiable. **Modifiable risk factors** include those factors that can be altered through either lifestyle modification or medication. **Nonmodifiable risk factors** include those factors that, regardless of therapy, cannot be altered.

Nonmodifiable Risk Factors

Nonmodifiable risk factors for coronary artery disease are listed in Table 15–1. Increasing age is a nonmodifiable risk factor for CAD. In 2013, approximately 35% of deaths from all cardiovascular diseases, including the acute coronary syndromes, occurred before the age of 75 years in United States residents (Mozaffarian et al., 2015).

Table 15–1 Nonmodifiable and Modifiable Risk Factors for Coronary Artery Disease

Nonmodifiable	Modifiable
Age	Hyperlipidemia
Male	Hypertriglyceridemia
Diabetes mellitus type 1	Diabetes mellitus type 2
Genetic predisposition	Metabolic syndrome
	Hypertension
	Obesity
	Physical inactivity
	Smoking
	Diet

Men are at greater risk for developing atherosclerosis and coronary artery disease than premenopausal women. Estrogen may have some type of protective effect on endothelial cells. After menopause, the risk of atherosclerosis-related diseases increases in women. Coronary heart disease in a first-degree relative increases the risk for disease development because of genetic and environmental influences (Mozaffarian et al., 2015). Diabetes mellitus increases the risk of cardiovascular disease development and of death in the presence of cardiovascular disease in both genders (Mozaffarian et al., 2015).

Unfortunately, some risk factors, such as advanced age are nonmodifiable, and actions cannot be taken to change the specific risk; however, overall risk can be diminished by addressing the modifiable risk factors. For example, adherence to a comprehensive medical regimen for diabetes management is recommended to decrease cardiovascular disease risk in patients with diabetes mellitus.

Modifiable Risk Factors

Modifiable risk factors for coronary artery disease are listed in Table 15–1.

Hypercholesterolemia, or elevated serum cholesterol levels, is a major risk factor for atherosclerosis and coronary artery disease development. Cholesterol binds to protein as it is carried in the bloodstream, forming a molecule called a **lipoprotein**. There are different amounts, or densities, of proteins and cholesterol that form lipoprotein molecules. When a lipoprotein molecule contains a high amount of cholesterol and a low-density protein, it is called a **low-density lipoprotein (LDL)**. LDLs—which can be remembered by the mnemonic "**l**ess **d**esirable **l**ipoproteins"—are commonly referred to as "bad" cholesterol. When a lipoprotein molecule contains a small amount of cholesterol and a high-density protein, it is called a **high-density lipoprotein (HDL)**, or "good" cholesterol (to remember this, think of **h**ighly **d**esirable **l**ipoproteins). Atherosclerosis-producing cholesterol can accumulate in the intimal lining of arteries and promote formation of atherosclerotic lesions. Elevated serum cholesterol from a genetic etiology, familial hypercholesterolemia (FH), is described in the feature "Genetic Considerations."

In general, clinicians identify treatment goals on whether or not the cholesterol type is atherogenic (atherosclerosis producing). Two primary types of atherogenic cholesterol include non-high-density lipoprotein cholesterol (non-HDL-C) and low-density lipoprotein cholesterol (LDL-C). Routine assessment of changes in the lipid panel is recommended to determine cardiovascular disease risk. One additional blood test to measure atherosclerosis risk is the measurement of high-sensitivity C-reactive protein (CRP) levels, which can pinpoint the inflammation associated with

Table 15–2 Classification of Non-HDL-C and LDL-C Values

	Non-HDL-C (mg/dL)	LDL-C (mg/dL)
Very high	220 or greater	190 or greater
High	190–219	160–189
Borderline high	160–189	130–159
Above desirable	130–159	100–129
Desirable	130	Less than 100

SOURCE: Adapted from Jacobson et al. (2014).

atherosclerosis. The utility of CRP screening to guide treatments to reduce cardiovascular disease risk is sometimes questioned; many variables can impact accurate measurement. However, C-reactive protein levels greater than 3 mg/L may predict coronary complications or disease (Crawford, 2014). Non-HDL-C and LDL-C levels can be decreased by the use of cholesterol-lowering medications such as HMG Co-A reductase enzyme inhibitors, which are commonly referred to as the "statins" (Libby, 2015). Recommended levels for non-HDL-C and LDL-C are listed in Table 15–2.

Other diseases or attributes, including type 2 diabetes, metabolic syndrome, hypertension, and obesity, are additional risk factors for coronary artery disease (Libby, 2015; Mozaffarian et al., 2015). It is theorized that these conditions exacerbate chronic injury and inflammation, which damage endothelial cells and promote the development of atherosclerotic lesions. Control of these modifiable risk factors with medications and changes in healthcare behaviors can reduce the risk of coronary artery disease and the manifestations of acute coronary syndromes (Jacobson et al., 2014; Mozaffarian et al., 2015).

Modifiable risk factors that can be altered with lifestyle changes include physical inactivity, obesity, smoking, and diet. Components of cigarette smoke cause endothelial damage and vasoconstriction. Obese individuals (body weight greater than 30% above ideal weight) have higher rates of hypertension, hyperlipidemia, and diabetes. The cardiovascular benefits of exercise are well established; individuals who engage in regular exercise programs have a lower risk for cardiac diseases.

Collaborative Management of Risk Factor Reduction

Aggressive reduction and management of risk factors is crucial to reducing the incidence and progression of atherosclerosis and CAD. Identification of risk factors begins with obtaining a thorough health history. Laboratory testing to assess risk factors includes the measurement of serum cholesterol levels along with a lipid profile (e.g., non-HDL-C, LDL-C, HDL levels), fasting glucose, high-sensitivity CRP, and **homocysteine** levels. In addition, liver function tests are evaluated so that changes associated with the initiation of cholesterol-lowering medications can be assessed.

When people stop smoking, the risk of atherosclerotic heart disease is greatly reduced. Smoking cessation intervention is a high priority for preventing cardiovascular

Genetic Considerations
Familial Hypercholesterolemia

A rare variation of either the LDLR, APOB, or PCSK9 gene can result in extremely high low-density lipoprotein levels. This physiologic effect, called familial hypercholesterolemia (FH), increases the risk of myocardial infarction. About 1 in 200 to 500 people are affected with this anomaly. Careful management of serum lipid levels with cholesterol-lowering medications can increase survival and reduce morbidity in patients possessing this genetic variation.

SOURCE: McCarthy & Mendelsohn (2016).

disease. Educational material, counseling, and nicotine replacement therapies can be used to promote tobacco cessation.

People who are overweight or obese are encouraged to lose weight through a program that includes diet and exercise. Unless contraindicated, most individuals should participate in at least 150 minutes of moderate-intensity physical activity each week. American Heart Association (2016a, 2016b) dietary and nutritional goals for improved cardiovascular health are listed in Table 15–3.

Control of hypertension is vital to reducing atherosclerosis. Management strategies include a low-sodium diet, regular exercise, stress management, and compliance with medication regimens.

An integral part of reducing atherosclerotic disease progression is drug therapy to reduce serum cholesterol and LDL levels. Drug therapy must be used in combination with a diet that is low in fat and cholesterol. The first-line drugs used are the HMG Co-A enzyme inhibitors, or statins: lovastatin (Mevacor), pravastatin (Pravachol),

Related Pharmacotherapy

Antilipemic Agents

HMG Co-A Reductase Inhibitors

Lovastatin (Altoprev, Mevacor), atorvastatin (Lipitor), pravastatin (Pravachol), simvastatin (Zocor), fluvastatin (Lescol), rosuvastatin (Crestor)

Action and Uses

Increases the number of hepatic LDL receptors, thus increasing LDL uptake and catabolism of LDL and increasing HDL blood levels. Used as adjunct to diet to reduce LDL and triglycerides in patients with hypercholesterolemia and to prevent cardiovascular disease in patients with multiple risk factors.

Dosages (Adult)

Lovastatin: 20–40 mg 1–2 times/day
Atorvastatin: Initial dosing—10–40 mg daily (increase up to 80 mg/day as required)

Major Side Effects

Myalgias
Rhabdomyolysis

Nursing Implications

Lipid levels lower within 2–4 weeks after initiation of therapy or change in dosage.
Assess for muscle pain, tenderness, and, if present, creatine phosphokinase (CK) levels may be monitored.
Monitor liver function tests at 6 and 12 weeks after initiation or elevation of dose and periodically thereafter.

Bile Acid Sequestrants

Cholestyramine (Questran), colestipol (Colestid), and colesevelam (WelChol)

Action and Uses

Absorbs and combines with intestinal bile acids to form nonabsorbable complex that is excreted in the feces. Lowers LDL levels. Used as adjunct to diet therapy in management of hypercholesterolemia.

Dosages (Adult)

Cholestyramine: Hypercholesterolemia—4 g (PO) 2–4 times/day before meals and at bedtime (increase up to 24 g/day as required)

Major Side Effects

Constipation
Bloating
Gastrointestinal upset

Nursing Implications

Always dissolve powder before administration. Place contents with 120–180 mL preferred liquid. Permit drug to hydrate without stirring for 1–2 minutes, then stir until suspension is uniform.
Administer before meals.
Preexisting constipation may worsen in the older adult, women, and in those taking greater than 24 gm/day.

Fibrates

Gemfibrozil (Lopid) and fenofibrate (Tricor)

Action and Uses

Lowers plasma triglycerides by inhibiting their synthesis, reduces VLDL production; increases HDL levels. Used as adjunctive therapy to diet for patients with high triglyceride levels.

Dosages (Adult)

Gemfibrozil: 600 mg (PO) 2 times/day (take 30 min. before morning & evening meals). Increase up to 1500 mg/day as required.

Major Side Effects

Fatigue
Paresthesias
Arrhythmias

Nursing Implications

Assess for muscle pain, tenderness, weakness; if present, CK levels may be monitored.
Can increase the actions of hypoglycemic and anticoagulant medications.

Cholesterol Absorption Inhibitor

Ezetimibe (Zetia)

Action and Uses

Inhibits small intestine absorption of cholesterol; reduces storage of cholesterol in liver.

Dosages (Adult)

10 mg (PO) daily

Major Side Effects

Fatigue
Dizziness
Myalgias

Nursing Implications

Monitor for desired therapeutic response; decreases in serum cholesterol and LDL levels expected. Increases the action of cyclosporine.

Table 15–3 Dietary and Nutritional Goals for Cardiovascular Health

Factor	AHA Recommendations
Healthy diet	Include a variety of fruits and vegetables, whole grains, low-fat dairy products, skinless poultry and fish, nuts and legumes, and non-tropical vegetable oils. Limit saturated fat, trans fat, sodium, red meat, sweets, and sugar-sweetened beverages. Limit sodium to 1500 to 2400 mg/day.
Healthy body weight	Aim for Body Mass Index (BMI) of 18.5 to 25 kg/m^2

SOURCE: Data from the American Heart Association (2016a, 2016b).

simvastatin (Zocor), fluvastatin (Lescol), atorvastatin (Lipitor), and rosuvastatin (Crestor). These drugs lower LDL by creating more LDL receptors on liver cells. LDL receptors bring in LDL from the blood into liver cells where LDL is further broken down. Statins can reduce serum cholesterol levels by 50% (Adams, Holland & Urban, 2017). Other classes of cholesterol-reducing drugs include bile acid sequestrants (cholestyramine [Questran], colestipol [Colestid], and colesevelam [WelChol]); fibric acid derivatives (gemfibrozil [Lopid] and fenofibrate [Tricor]; and ezetimibe [Zetia]), which inhibits absorption of cholesterol at the small intestinal brush border (Adams et al., 2017; Wilson, Shannon, & Shields, 2016). These agents are summarized in the feature "Related Pharmacotherapy: Antilipemic Agents."

Section Two Review

1. Which lipoprotein contains a high amount of cholesterol and a low-density protein?
   A. High-density lipoprotein
   B. Low-density lipoprotein
   C. Hypercholesterolemia
   D. Lipoprotein A

2. The risk of atherosclerotic heart disease changes in which manner when people stop smoking?
   A. Does not change
   B. Decreases after 15 years
   C. Is greatly reduced
   D. Actually is greater

3. Desirable levels of non-HDL cholesterol are _____ mg/dL.
   A. less than 20
   B. 200 to 300
   C. at least 150
   D. 130 or less

4. In which way do statins work to reduce atherosclerotic disease progression?
   A. Increases LDL receptors on liver cells
   B. Increases HDL concentration
   C. Decreases total body cholesterol
   D. Sequesters cholesterol in bile

Answers: 1. B, 2. C, 3. D, 4. A

Section Three: Clinical Presentation of Impaired Myocardial Tissue Perfusion

The types of angina typically treated in the clinical setting include stable, unstable, and variant angina. A description of the different types of angina along with their assessments is included in this section.

Subjective Data

The classic presenting symptom of CAD is **angina pectoris**. Angina is chest pain that is usually precipitated by exercise and, with stable angina, is relieved by rest (Ohman, 2016). Angina is caused by an increase in myocardial oxygen demand and a decrease in myocardial oxygen supply as a result of partially occluded coronary arteries. When myocardial cells do not have an adequate oxygen supply for aerobic metabolism, they switch to anaerobic metabolism. The by-product of anaerobic metabolism is lactate. Lactate, an acid, irritates nerve endings and causes pain.

Patients may describe their angina as tightness, heaviness, or a viselike sensation in the chest. Angina may be accompanied by diaphoresis, shortness of breath, and lightheadedness. Patients will often report that the pain radiates to the left arm and hand, jaw, or shoulder. They also may report symptoms of nausea, shortness of breath, or fatigue.

There are three types of angina: stable angina, Prinzmetal's angina, and unstable angina. **Stable angina** is chest pain that is predictable. It occurs with increased physical activity. Often patients know they will get chest pain if they participate in a certain amount of activity. For example, a patient will state, "I get chest pain when I walk three blocks. I know I'm okay at two blocks, but three blocks does it." Stable angina is relieved by rest or nitroglycerin tablets. The typical sequence is activity, chest pain, rest, relief.

Prinzmetal's angina, or **variant angina**, is not common and is a unique form of angina: chest pain that occurs at rest and is not related to physical activity or heart rate. It often occurs at night and may be related to coronary artery spasms. The exact cause of these spasms is not known.

Unstable angina is chest pain that is not predictable. It occurs with rest or minimal activity, and it occurs with increased frequency and severity. Unstable angina requires immediate medical attention.

Time is an important variable to consider when assessing a patient complaining of angina symptoms. Immediate questions to consider include the time of onset of the pain, the activity that the patient was participating in when the pain began, and the length of the anginal episodes. Typically, stable angina begins gradually and peaks over a period of minutes as the precipitating activity continues. Chest pain that lasts several seconds or constant pain over a period of hours is not typical pain associated with altered myocardial tissue perfusion.

Quantifying the level of pain is important because treatment decisions are based on the initial intensity of the pain and the response of the patient to pain-relief interventions. Patients are asked to describe the pain using a numerical scale of 0 to 10, with 0 indicating no pain and 10 representing pain of maximum intensity. A pain rating of 0 is desirable when treating cardiac ischemia or injury.

Symptoms that are suggestive of cardiac ischemia but do not include angina are called **anginal equivalents**. These symptoms, occurring in a patient with high cardiac risk, include dyspnea, fatigue, lightheadedness, dizziness, or pain at another site, such as the jaw or arms. Patients reporting a history of exertional or resting dyspnea require close scrutiny because these symptoms strongly correlate with CAD.

When assessing a patient presenting with angina symptoms, it is helpful to employ the mnemonic PQRST as an assessment tool: precipitating factors (P), quality (Q), radiation and region (R), associated symptoms (S), and timing and treatment strategies (T). This is a systematic way to remember to ask appropriate questions when assessing a patient experiencing chest pain (Table 15–4).

Not all patients with altered myocardial tissue perfusion have classic anginal chest pain symptoms. Diabetics, women, and older adults are more likely to experience anginal equivalents or ischemia without chest pain (Boyle, 2014). Diabetics are especially prone to having silent ischemia and usually present with shortness of breath and fatigue. This is due to diabetes-related microvascular changes that manifest as neuropathies and decreased sensitivity to pain. It is important to remember that microvascular changes not only occur in the extremities and eyes but also in the blood vessels that supply the heart. Women are also more likely to experience anginal equivalents with complaints of fatigue or upper-arm weakness when compared to men. Some women with chest pain attribute their pain to heartburn. Overall, older people and women have a greater incidence of atypical symptoms of ischemia such as dyspnea and jaw pain (Ohman, 2016).

Table 15–4 Assessing Chest Pain

Pain Descriptor	Description	Examples
P	Provoked pain	Mowing the lawn, exercise, sexual activity
	Palliative factors	Nitroglycerine, watching TV, or rest and sleep
Q	Quality	Burning, tightness, heaviness, or viselike sensation in the chest
R	Region of pain	Located in center of chest, substernal, or left breast
	Radiation	Radiates to left arm, hand, jaw, or shoulder
S	Severity Symptoms	Scored from 0–10 Dyspnea, pallor, tachycardia, anxiety, fear, nausea, emesis, diaphoresis, sense of impending doom
T	Time factors	Time of onset, how long does it last, does it come and go? Does it occur in association with something else, such as eating?

Objective Data: Physical Assessment

A focused physical assessment of the cardiovascular and pulmonary systems precedes the history of the precipitating event and full patient history. Patients with CAD may or may not exhibit any outward signs of the disease. Their weight and vital signs may be within normal limits. An attempt should be made to correlate subjective data with physical signs.

Vital signs are reviewed to determine the presence of hypo- or hypertension and to assess for alterations in heart and respiratory rates. The overall appearance of the patient is noted, taking into account the patient's weight, skin color and tone, posture, and level of functional ability. The skin is examined for evidence of cyanosis and **xanthomas** (cholesterol-filled lesions commonly seen around the eyes). The color and temperature of the extremities are evaluated along with the intensity of the peripheral pulses. Peripheral edema is evaluated and graded according to the severity of pitting. Alterations in these findings may indicate peripheral vascular disease (PVD) or left ventricular dysfunction. PVD and left ventricular dysfunction (LVD) are commonly associated with CAD.

The chest and abdomen are inspected. Heart sounds are auscultated. Abnormalities in cardiac rhythm and rate and the presence of murmurs, rubs, or gallops are reported. Abnormal or additional heart sounds can be associated with left ventricular failure and fluid volume overload caused by an ischemic left ventricle. Respirations are assessed for depth and the presence of adventitious sounds. The abdomen is auscultated to evaluate the quality of bowel sounds and to screen for abdominal bruits. Abdominal bruits are associated with renal artery stenosis or abdominal aortic aneurysm development.

Section Three Review

1. Coronary artery disease (CAD) typically presents with which classic symptom(s)?
   A. Angina pectoris
   B. Chest pain without nausea
   C. Elevated lactate with chest pain
   D. Nausea, vomiting, heartburn

2. A client reports always having chest pain if he walks more than one block. The chest pain is relieved with rest and two nitroglycerin tablets. What type of angina pectoris does this patient have?
   A. Unstable
   B. Variant
   C. Stable
   D. Prinzmetal's

3. Which type of chest pain is not related to physical activity and often occurs at night?
   A. Unstable angina
   B. Prinzmetal's or variant angina
   C. Stable angina
   D. Silent myocardial ischemia

4. Renal artery stenosis may be evidenced by which clinical finding?
   A. Abdominal bruits
   B. Abdominal distention
   C. Decreased urine output
   D. Absent bowel sounds

Answers: 1. A, 2. C, 3. B, 4. A

Section Four: Diagnostic Tests for Alterations in Myocardial Tissue Perfusion

Tests for diagnosing alterations in myocardial tissue perfusion are described in this section. Test results are coupled with clinical presentation to determine the presence of myocardial ischemia.

Electrocardiogram

Several diagnostic tests can be used to evaluate the adequacy of myocardial tissue perfusion. The easiest and most cost effective test is the 12-lead electrocardiogram (ECG). Thousands of ECGs are performed each year to assess cardiac function. All patients who are evaluated for chest pain have a 12-lead ECG performed to document baseline cardiac rhythm and to assess for ischemic changes.

The 12 leads on the standard ECG are categorized as limb leads (leads I, II, III), augmented limb leads (aVR, aVL, aVF), and precordial leads (V_1 through V_6). Each lead overlies a specific area of the myocardium and provides an electrographic snapshot of electrical activity taking place in the heart (Goldberger, 2015; Goldich, 2014). Table 15–5 lists the anatomical regions of the myocardium and their corresponding leads.

The basic components of the ECG are depicted in Figure 15–2. The *ST* segment represents the early stage of ventricular recovery and corresponds with the plateau phase of the ventricular action potential. It begins at the end of the *QRS* complex and ends at the beginning of the *T* wave. The point where the *S* wave returns to the isoelectric line is described as the *J* point.

The *T* wave is a graphical representation of ventricular repolarization and should be isoelectric at its conclusion. Changes in the *ST* segment are sensitive electrographic indicators of ischemia and injury to the myocardium (Lancia et al., 2016). When blood flow is reduced or occluded to a region of the myocardium, depolarization changes take place. These changes manifest as abnormal changes in the *ST* segment (Figure 15–3A) and *T* waves (Figure 15–3B).

Table 15–5 Anatomical Regions of the Myocardium and Their Corresponding Leads

Anatomical Region	Coronary Artery	ECG Leads	Clinical Implications
Anteroseptal wall	LAD	V_1, V_2, V_3, V_4	Potential for significant muscle damage leading to pump failure and shock
Lateral wall	LCX	I, aVL, V_5, V_6	Often occurs in conjunction with anterior myocardial infarction
Inferior wall	RCA, LCX	II, III, aVF	Right ventricle damage in 30% of cases
Right ventricular infarction	RCA	V_{4R}, V_{5R}, V_{6R} *ST* elevation in V_1 II, III, aVF	Requires increased preload; use of nitrates may be contraindicated
Posterior wall	RCA	Tall *R* wave and *ST* depression in right precordial leads V_1 and V_2 V_7 to V_9 *ST* elevations	

SOURCE: Data partially from Boyle (2014), Goldberger (2015), and Goldich (2014).

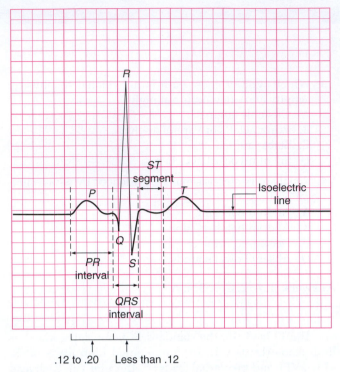

Figure 15–2 Components of a normal ECG.

Continuous *ST* segment monitoring provides valuable information for the management of patients with acute coronary syndromes or variant angina and for patients who receive thrombolytic therapy or a revascularization procedure. Current monitoring technology includes the ability to continuously monitor for *ST* segment changes in at least one precordial and one limb lead (Lancia et al., 2016). Elevation or depression of the *ST* segment can be detected with the monitoring system, alerting the nurse to potential cardiac ischemia or injury in the monitored patient. A 12-lead ECG may be necessary to confirm ischemia. The healthcare team can initiate early treatment measures when ischemic ECG changes are confirmed by the physician or advanced practice provider.

Myocardial regions and their corresponding leads are listed in Table 15–5. The nurse must be familiar with the leads to ensure rapid identification of which area of the myocardium may be ischemic or damaged. This is crucial because treatment options and potential conduction abnormalities differ depending on the myocardial region affected.

Proteins released by necrotic myocytes into the bloodstream are referred to as serum **cardiac markers**. When present in the blood, these markers signify myocardial muscle damage (Antman & Loscalzo, 2015). Cardiac markers include the troponins (cTn), creatine phosphokinase (CK), and creatine phosphokinase–myocardial bands (CK-MB). The cardiac markers appear in the blood at different times and, often, the higher the marker, the worse the cardiac muscle necrosis. Cardiac markers are summarized in Table 15–6.

CK is an enzyme found in brain, skeletal muscle, and cardiac muscle tissues. Therefore, elevations in CK levels can indicate tissue damage in any of these areas. The CK-MB is a subset of CK that is specific to cardiac muscle. A level greater than 6% is usually considered a positive indicator of cardiac muscle damage. The cardiac muscle troponins—troponin-I (cTnI) and troponin-T (cTnT)—are the most specific indicators of cardiac muscle damage. Troponins are proteins that are part of the actin–myosin unit. They are not normally in the blood unless there is damage to the actin–myosin units of cardiac muscle. Even a small amount of cardiac muscle damage can cause appearance of troponin in the blood.

Cardiac markers are obtained on most patients who seek treatment for chest pain that is suspicious for cardiac

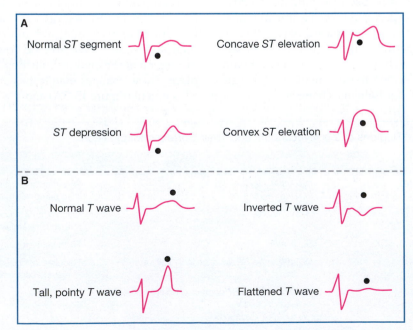

Figure 15–3 ECG ischemia and injury pattern. A, *ST* segment changes. B, *T* wave changes.

Table 15–6 Cardiac Biomarkers

Marker	Normal Level	Injury	Onset	Peaks	Duration
CK (U/L[a])	Male: 55–170 Female: 30–135	Elevated Elevated	4–6 hours	18–24 hours	3–4 days
CK-MB (%)	0–6	Greater than 6	4–6 hours	18–24 hours	3–4 days
cTnT (mcg/L[a])	Less than 0.2	Elevated	1–3 hours	10–24 hours	10–14 days
cTnI (mcg/L[a])	0.1–0.5	Greater than 2	1–3 hours	10–24 hours	5–9 days

[a] = SI units; CK = creatine kinase; CK-MB = creatine kinase–myocardial bands; cTnT = Cardiac troponin-T; cTnI = Cardiac troponin-I.
SOURCE: Data from Kee (2014).

origin. Blood sampling for cardiac markers occurs approximately every 6 hours to evaluate trends that signify continued or resolving myocardial damage. Serial levels help determine the extent of myocardial damage over time.

Exercise Stress Test

The exercise stress test (EST) is one of the most commonly used diagnostic tests available for the assessment of a patient who may have CAD. Exercise stress tests combine exercise (on a treadmill or bicycle) and continuous ECG monitoring to evaluate the patient for altered myocardial tissue perfusion. Patients with CAD may have a normal ECG at rest when myocardial oxygen supply meets myocardial oxygen demand. However, in some patients when myocardial oxygen demand increases (as with exercise), myocardial oxygen supply is not sufficient to meet this increased demand. This imbalance of myocardial oxygen demand and supply produces altered myocardial tissue perfusion and the resultant ECG changes.

Not all patients can exercise. Patients who cannot exercise may include those with arthritis, amputation, severe peripheral vascular disease, or chronic obstructive pulmonary disease. These patients undergo a pharmacologic stress test. An inotropic drug, such as dobutamine, is given to increase myocardial contractility and produce a cardiac workload similar to that which would occur with exercise.

Indications of myocardial ischemia during an EST include the development of angina, *ST* segment depression of 1 mm or more, failure to increase systolic blood pressure to 120 mmHg or more, or a sustained decrease of 10 mmHg or more with progressive increase in exercise. EST is less specific in young or middle-aged women than in men.

In preparation for the EST, the patient is instructed not to eat, smoke, or drink beverages containing caffeine for several hours prior to the test. Certain drugs, such as beta blockers, may be held for 24 hours prior to the procedure. Patients are instructed to wear comfortable shoes.

Echocardiography is an imaging technique used to assess the functional structures of the heart using ultrasound waves. Ultrasound waves are applied to the chest wall through a transducer and transect the heart at different planes, providing pictures of various cardiac structures. The echocardiogram identifies structural abnormalities of valves, the chamber size of the atria and ventricles, great vessels, and heart wall motion. Echocardiography can be done in conjunction with stress testing or performed at the bedside in the high-acuity unit.

During a stress echocardiogram the patient's ECG is monitored for abnormalities, and the myocardial walls are evaluated for ischemia-induced motion abnormalities. Myocardial wall motion abnormalities may include **hypokinesis** (decrease in movement), **akinesis** (lack of movement), or **dyskinesis** (movement in the opposite direction).

Myocardial Perfusion Imaging

Radionuclide myocardial perfusion imaging (MPI) is performed by injecting an intravenous nucleotide during peak exercise. Pictures are taken of the myocardial walls with a special type of camera. This procedure is very helpful in identifying specific areas of myocardial ischemia and damage, and ejection fraction is also calculated. The perfusion images help differentiate between exertional and resting myocardial perfusion abnormalities. Perfusion is reported as a fixed defect, a reversible defect, or being without defect (normal).

Section Four Review

1. Changes in which ECG waves are sensitive electrographic indicators of ischemia and injury to the myocardium?
   A. *ST* segment
   B. *U* wave
   C. *QRS* complex
   D. *P* wave

2. *T* wave inversion and *ST* segment depression are hallmarks of which condition?
   A. Classic heart failure
   B. Myocardial ischemia
   C. Conduction defect
   D. Good myocardial tissue perfusion

3. A CK-MB level greater than _____ is indicative of cardiac muscle damage.
   A. 2%
   B. 6%
   C. 10%
   D. 15%

4. For which reason may an exercise stress test be ordered?
   A. To assess the functional structures of the heart
   B. To induce the release of cardiac markers in the blood
   C. To evaluate the client's likelihood of having altered myocardial tissue perfusion
   D. To identify specific areas of myocardial ischemia and damage

Answers: 1. A, 2. B, 3. B, 4. C

Section Five: Impaired Myocardial Tissue Perfusion: Acute Coronary Syndromes

The initial diagnosis and collaborative management of acute coronary syndromes, unstable angina, and myocardial infarction are described in this section. The pharmaceutical management of these conditions is emphasized.

Diagnosis of Acute Coronary Syndromes

Coronary heart disease is commonly divided into two types of disorders: chronic ischemic heart disease and acute coronary syndromes (ACS). Chronic ischemic heart disease includes stable angina and variant angina (Section Four). Acute coronary syndromes represent a continuum of the atherosclerotic disease processes described in Section One and includes unstable angina and myocardial infarction.

Acute coronary syndromes are characterized by an imbalance between myocardial oxygen supply and demand. As blood flow is reduced, the affected myocardium becomes ischemic, leading to symptoms of angina. Thrombi that partially occlude arteries produce symptoms of unstable angina (UA). Total occlusion of the artery results in cell necrosis, release of cardiac markers, and MI distal to the occlusion.

Classification of ACS has changed based on a clearer understanding of plaque disruption and thrombus development. Not all patients with symptoms of chest pain are experiencing an acute MI, but many have a nonocclusive thrombus on preexisting plaque (Amsterdam et al., 2014). Current guidelines include the following diagnostic ACS criteria:

1. Patients with ECG changes suggestive of ischemia, but without the presence of serum biomarkers, are diagnosed as UA.

2. Patients with ischemic ST segment changes and the presence of elevated serum cardiac markers are diagnosed as having non-ST elevation myocardial infarction (NSTEMI) (Cannon & Braunwald, 2015).

3. Patients with ST segment elevation and the presence of elevated serum cardiac markers are diagnosed as having ST elevation MI (STEMI) (Antman & Loscalzo, 2015).

T wave inversion and ST segment depression in two or more contiguous leads are hallmarks of myocardial ischemia. In patients suspected of having ACS, symmetrical T wave inversion of 2 mm (0.2 mV) or greater strongly suggests acute ischemia. ST segments that are depressed from the baseline by 0.5 mm (0.05 mV) or greater and are horizontal or downsloping in two contiguous leads are also suggestive of ischemia. Nonspecific ST segment changes can complicate the picture of a patient presenting with symptoms suggestive of ACS.

ECG criteria indicative of acute myocardial infarction include T waves that are upright with increased amplitude and width or inverted T waves, ST segment elevation of 1 mm (0.1 mV) or greater, or depression of greater than 0.5 mm (0.5 mV) in two contiguous leads; and the presence of a new or presumably new left or right bundle branch block. Deep (larger than 25% of R wave) and wide (40 ms or greater) Q waves—pathologic Q waves—may also appear on the ECG with myocardial infarction.

Patients presenting with symptoms suggestive of ACS require a rapid assessment and ECG. Chest pain that suggests acute MI typically lasts longer than 20 minutes but less than 12 hours. Patients may describe the pain as crushing or gripping, or they may report chest heaviness and a sense of impending doom. UA is defined as having three possible presentations: symptoms of angina at rest (usually prolonged, greater than 20 minutes), new-onset angina with ordinary physical activity (such as walking one or two blocks), and increasing angina that has become more frequent and longer in duration. Some patients (often women, older adults, and diabetics) may not have chest pain but may present with exertional symptoms of jaw, neck, arm, or epigastric pain; fatigue; nausea; or unexplained worsening of exertional dyspnea.

Other diagnostic and prognostic tools are used to calculate the risk of death or myocardial infarction from an ischemic event and are used to guide treatment. Calculating the patient's risk of a major cardiac event (e.g., unstable angina, myocardial infarction, or cardiac intervention) or death following treatment for chest pain can be accomplished by determining GRACE, HEART, or TIMI risk scores (Poldervaart et al., 2016). Variables differ on tools used to quantify risk and may include predictors such as heart rate, systolic blood pressure, ST segment changes, the presence of positive cardiac enzymes, and age (Cannon & Braunwald, 2015; Poldervaart et al., 2016). Patients with higher risk scores realize more cardiac benefits from early invasive intervention than patients with lower scores.

Initial Collaborative Management

Nursing care priorities include relieving chest pain and reducing myocardial oxygen demand (see the feature "Nursing Care: The Patient with Angina"). Psychosocial support for the patient and family is important at this time because they are faced with the patient's potential mortality.

Medical management of ACS varies, depending on the initial 12-lead ECG findings, risk stratification, and evidence of elevated serum cardiac markers. In 2014, the American Heart Association and American College of Cardiology updated guidelines for the management of patients with UA and NSTEMI (Amsterdam et al., 2014). The current guidelines recommend that an initial ECG be obtained within 10 minutes of presentation to the emergency department (or in the high-acuity unit, an ECG should be obtained within 10 minutes of the patient complaining of chest pain). This ECG is used to differentiate patients with *ST* elevation (potential candidates for reperfusion) from UA and NSTEMI. Evidence supports that mortality is decreased and myocardium preserved when the decision to begin reperfusion therapy is made within 30 minutes of the patient's presentation.

Initial management of all patients with chest pain includes rapid triage to immediate care and placement in a treatment area established to manage such emergencies. After a 12-lead ECG is obtained, acetylsalicylic acid (ASA [aspirin]) is administered (Bobadilla, 2016). Aspirin inhibits platelet clot formation by decreasing the formation of thromboxane A_2. The American Heart Association recommends 162 to 325 mg of non-enteric-coated chewed aspirin for patients experiencing ACS symptoms unless contraindicated by allergy or other reasons (Amsterdam et al., 2014). Oxygen by nasal cannula is applied, and intravenous (IV) access is obtained. Supplemental oxygen raises the partial pressure of oxygen in the blood, supplying more oxygen to the ischemic myocardium. At the time that IV access is obtained, blood is drawn for serum cardiac markers.

Nitroglycerin may be administered sublingually for ongoing chest pain. Intravenous nitroglycerin may be given for the first 24 to 48 hours. Nitroglycerin, a fast-acting vasodilator, decreases ischemic pain by decreasing preload and afterload, and, subsequently, myocardial oxygen demand. If chest pain is not relieved with nitroglycerin, intravenous morphine is given. Morphine decreases pain through direct action on pain receptors, decreases anxiety, and causes vasodilation to further decrease myocardial workload. Morphine is administered intravenously in small doses (2–4 mg) and repeated every 5 minutes until chest pain is relieved. Repeated doses of morphine require the nurse to monitor the patient for respiratory depression. Use of a pulse oximeter aids in detection of impaired oxygenation associated with morphine administration.

If the preliminary ECG is normal or nondiagnostic (meaning there are no specific changes), the patient may be monitored in a chest pain unit. Here, serial serum cardiac markers and ECGs are obtained every 6 hours. The patient is "ruled out" for an MI if subsequent ECGs and serum cardiac markers remain unchanged for 12 to 24 hours. Most patients will undergo some form of noninvasive testing (stress test or noninvasive cardiac imaging) prior to discharge.

In addition to the therapies described here, patients with UA and NSTEMI are admitted to cardiac high-acuity units where they receive continuous ECG monitoring (telemetry). ECG monitoring with continuous *ST* segment monitoring technology is particularly helpful in monitoring these patients.

Pharmaceutical Management

Early pharmaceutical management of ACS should include oral beta blockers within the first 24 hours of treatment unless contraindicated by heart failure. Beta blockers decrease contractility, sinus node rate, and AV conduction by inhibiting catecholamine stimulation (Amsterdam et al., 2014). These actions decrease myocardial oxygen demand

---

Nursing Care
The Patient with Angina

Expected Patient Outcomes and Related Interventions

Outcome: Optimize myocardial tissue perfusion

Assess and compare to established norms, patient baselines, and trends
  Assess pain and anginal equivalents.
  Assess for nausea and vomiting.
  Perform focused cardiopulmonary assessment, including vital signs, heart sounds, lung sounds, peripheral pulses, skin color, and temperature; physical appearance during pain (shortness of breath, diaphoresis).
  Obtain 12-lead ECG if ordered.

Interventions to enhance myocardial tissue perfusion
  Elevate head of bed 30 degrees.
  Apply pulse oximeter.
  Continuous cardiac rhythm monitoring.
  Administer drugs as prescribed to control pain and anxiety.

Administer related drug therapy and monitor for therapeutic and nontherapeutic effects
  Acetylsalicylic acid (aspirin) unless contraindicated
  Morphine
  Nitrates (nitroglycerin)
  Oxygen

and increase the time in diastole, which extends the time for myocardial perfusion. Beta blockers such as sustained-release metoprolol, bisoprolol, or carvedilol should be considered (Amsterdam et al., 2014).

Pharmaceutical management may include an anticoagulation regimen including unfractionated heparin (UH) or low molecular weight heparin (LMWH), glycoprotein (GP) IIb/IIIa inhibitors, and, in many cases, drugs to inhibit platelet aggregation such as ticagrelor (Brilinta) or clopidogrel (Plavix) (Bobadilla, 2016). Heparin exerts its effect by inhibiting components of the coagulation cascade and increasing the inhibitory effects of antithrombin III. This results in inactivation of factors IIa, IXa, and Xa of the coagulation cascade and prevents new clot formation. Heparin is given as an initial bolus dose followed by a continuous infusion. Serum activated partial thromboplastin time (aPTT) is monitored at 6, 12, and 24 hours until the aPTT is maintained at 1.5 to 2.5 times the control value. Daily platelet counts should be monitored to detect a serious complication of heparin treatment: immune-mediated heparin-induced thrombocytopenia, type II HIT. The nurse should collaborate with the medical team to discontinue heparin and provide an alternative anticoagulation strategy when platelet counts dramatically decrease from type II HIT.

LMWH (enoxaparin) has also demonstrated excellent efficacy when used in conjunction with ASA in patients with UA and NSTEMI. Advantages to the use of LMWH include its subcutaneous delivery, safety, and administration without aPTT monitoring. Enoxaparin is dosed at 1 mg/kg every 12 hours in patients with UA or NSTEMI for up to 8 days. Another conservative anticoagulant medication is fondaparinux, the preferred anticoagulant for patients with increased risk of bleeding (Amsterdam et al., 2014).

In addition to ASA, thienopyridines, such as clopidogrel (Plavix), may be administered to patients with ACS. Clopidogrel blocks adenosine diphosphate (ADP)-induced platelet aggregation and is recommended for patients with UA and NSTEMI (Amsterdam et al., 2014). Adverse effects include gastrointestinal upset, neutropenia, and dyspnea.

Other antiplatelet medications, such as glycoprotein (GP) IIb/IIIa inhibitors, bind to IIb/IIIa platelet receptors, inhibiting platelet aggregation and new clot formation. GP IIb/IIIa inhibitors can be used with patients experiencing UA or NSTEMI. Currently available GP IIb/IIIa inhibitors include abciximab (ReoPro), tirofiban (Aggrastat), and eptifibatide (Integrilin) (Bobadilla, 2016). GP IIb/IIIa inhibitors are typically administered as a bolus dose followed by an infusion for 12 to 24 hours. Adverse effects include bleeding and thrombocytopenia. Complete blood counts are assessed at regular intervals, and patients are monitored for signs of bleeding.

Emerging Evidence

- The use of an automated peritoneal lavage system to produce and sustain therapeutic hypothermia in 46 patients experiencing cardiac arrest or acute myocardial infarction was described by researchers in a multicenter study. Researchers reported faster cooling times with the peritoneal lavage system when compared to the cooling times of other techniques that may enhance the neuroprotective effect of therapeutic hypothermia following cardiac arrest. Additional research is needed to compare patient outcomes related to the use of this system versus the use of other hypothermia techniques (*Polderman et al., 2015*).
- A sample of 466 women (69 Black and 397 White) undergoing coronary angiography used a symptom check list to identify their typical angina symptom experiences. Factor analysis and two-way analysis of covariance revealed that Black women reported more stomach symptoms, such as indigestion, and fewer chest symptoms—malaise, chest discomfort, and fatigue—than White participants. Atypical presentations may lead to delayed treatment and undesired outcomes for women experiencing cardiac ischemia (*Eastwood et al., 2013*).
- Patients (*n* = 158) were randomized into usual care (*n* = 79) or cognitive behavioral therapy (CBT) groups (*n* = 79) during medical center treatment for heart failure. Both groups received education on heart failure management. Instruments to measure depression, self-care concepts, and other variables were administered to all participants. Depression, fatigue, and anxiety scores were lower in the CBT group when compared to the usual care group 6 months after heart failure treatment. There were no differences in self-care variables between the groups. Patients who experience depression as part of their heart failure experience may benefit from CBT following hospital discharge (*Freedland, Carney, Rich, Steinmeyer, & Rubin, 2015*).

Section Five Review

1. Clients with ECG changes suggestive of ischemia, but without the presence of serum biomarkers, are diagnosed as having which coronary event?
   A. Unstable angina
   B. Non-*ST* elevation myocardial infarction
   C. *ST* elevation myocardial infarction
   D. Stable angina

2. Which ECG changes are indicative of an acute MI? (Select all that apply.)
   A. Hyperacute *T* waves
   B. *ST* segment elevation
   C. The presence of new left bundle branch block
   D. The loss of *P* waves
   E. Inversion of the *QRS*

3. Current guidelines recommend that an ECG be obtained within _____ of the complaint of chest pain in the high-acuity unit.
   A. 1 minute
   B. 10 minutes
   C. 30 minutes
   D. 1 hour

4. A client is ruled out for MI if which diagnostic findings are present?
   A. ECG and cardiac markers remain unchanged for 12 to 24 hours.
   B. Chest pain subsides within 30 minutes.
   C. There are no *ST* changes on the ECG.
   D. Serum cardiac markers return to normal after 6 hours.

Answers: 1. A, 2. (A, B, C), 3. B, 4. A

Section Six: Collaborative Interventions to Restore Myocardial Tissue Perfusion

Collaborative interventions to restore myocardial tissue perfusion are explained in this section. Thrombolytic therapy, percutaneous coronary procedures, and cardiac surgeries are described.

Reperfusion

As noted in Section Six, patients with chest pain, *ST* elevation greater than or equal to 1 mm (1 mv) in two contiguous leads, or new bundle branch blocks in the absence of ECG confounders are diagnosed with STEMI. Patients with STEMI have a high likelihood of thrombus-induced myocardial infarction. The initial collaborative management of patients presenting with STEMI, as mentioned in Section Six, includes rapid triage, administration of oxygen, ASA, nitroglycerin, analgesics, beta blockers, and anticoagulants (e.g., UH). The goals of these interventions are to promote myocardial reperfusion within 30 minutes and to prevent further myocardial tissue damage.

Rapid reperfusion of the affected artery reduces the amount of injury to the myocardium and preserves ventricular function. Maximum injury occurs approximately 6 hours after the initial occlusion of an affected artery. The amount of injury depends on the artery occluded and the location of the thrombus. Survival and quality of life are significantly improved if the function of the left ventricle is preserved. Left ventricular (LV) function is typically gauged by measuring the LV **ejection fraction (EF)**, which is the proportion of blood ejected from the left ventricle with each beat. The normal EF is greater than 50%. Ejection fraction values between 40% and 50% signify mildly depressed cardiac contractility, whereas more profound LV dysfunction, as in systolic heart failure, yields an EF of less than 40%.

Interventions to restore myocardial tissue perfusion include the administration of thrombolytic medications, percutaneous coronary intervention, and coronary artery bypass surgery.

Thrombolytic Therapy

Thrombolytic therapy includes the use of drugs that dissolve or lyse blood clots in the patient experiencing an acute *ST*-elevation MI. These drugs activate the **fibrinolytic** system to break up the blood clot and restore blood flow through the obstructed artery. This actually changes the course of an MI by reducing the area of infarction and decreasing mortality while increasing the likelihood that LV function will be preserved (Bashore, Granger, Jackson, & Patel, 2016).

Candidates for thrombolytic therapy include those whose time of onset of symptoms was less than 12 hours. Better survival outcomes are achieved in patients receiving thrombolytics within 2 to 3 hours of symptom onset. Contraindications for thrombolytics are typically categorized as absolute or relative, based on the degree of bleeding risk. Box 15–1 summarizes contraindications to thrombolytic therapy. The nurse should be aware that the literature is not conclusive regarding contraindications or their classification as absolute or relative. Risks and benefits must be carefully weighed. When the risks outweigh the benefits of thrombolytic therapy, other reperfusion therapies should be considered.

BOX 15–1 Contraindications to Thrombolytic Therapy*

Absolute
- Active internal bleeding
- Possible aortic dissection
- Intracranial neoplasm or previous hemorrhagic or other stroke
- Recent traumatic brain injury

Relative
- Severe, poorly controlled hypertension
- Dementia or other intracranial pathologies
- Active peptic ulcer
- Recent internal hemorrhage
- Pregnancy
- Recent major surgery or prolonged CPR
- Anticoagulant use
- Previous hypersensitivity response to thrombolytics

*Each thrombolytic agent provides product-specific contraindication information; consensus on absolute and relative contraindications has not been established for thrombolytic agents.

SOURCE: Data partially from Bashore et al. (2016).

Table 15–7 Percutaneous Coronary Interventions

Procedure	Description
Percutaneous transluminal coronary angioplasty (PTCA)	Cardiac catheterization with balloon catheter. Balloon is inflated in narrowing of coronary artery, which disrupts plaque and stretches vessel, increasing the internal diameter of artery; also called balloon angioplasty.
Coronary atherectomy Rotational atherectomy	Atherosclerotic plaques are removed by cutting the lesions away from the vessel wall with a high-speed rotational device.
Coronary stents	Metallic stents or cages that are placed in the coronary arteries following balloon angioplasty to decrease the likelihood of coronary artery restenosis.

SOURCE: Data from Faxon & Bhatt (2015).

Nursing responsibilities for the patient receiving thrombolytics include monitoring for evidence of bleeding, hemodynamic instability, reperfusion, and reocclusion. The risk for intracranial hemorrhage (ICH) is relatively low but increases in patients older than 65 years, in those with low body weight or hypertension, and in females. The first 24 hours after fibrinolytic administration holds the highest risk for intracranial hemorrhage. Routine neurologic checks are performed to detect evidence of a change in the level of consciousness. Change in level of consciousness is a very sensitive indicator of increased intracranial pressure secondary to intracranial hemorrhage. The nurse should closely monitor IV sites and wounds for evidence of bleeding, and pressure dressings may be required at IV removal sites. Hemodynamic instability may be an indication of hemorrhage or an allergic reaction to the thrombolytic agent.

Thrombolysis and reperfusion of the affected myocardium are indicated by resolution of *ST* segment elevation, pain resolution, and the occurrence of reperfusion arrhythmias, such as premature ventricular complexes or ventricular tachycardia. Antiarrhythmics, such as amiodarone, are necessary for sustained ventricular arrhythmias that influence hemodynamic stability. Continuous *ST* segment monitoring is useful in this setting to identify evidence of reperfusion. Reocclusion remains a problem with thrombolytics and occurs in 5% to 20% of patients. Reocclusion is indicated by reoccurrence of chest pain and *ST* segment elevation. Reocclusion most commonly occurs within the first 24 hours. Intravenous heparin, low molecular weight heparins, and GP IIb/IIIa inhibitors can be administered after thrombolytics or in combination with thrombolytics to minimize the incidence of reocclusion.

Patients not eligible for revascularization will typically be admitted to a high-acuity cardiac unit for observation and continued medical management. Patients who are not eligible for revascularization include those of advanced age with significant comorbidities such as end-stage kidney failure, severe chronic obstructive pulmonary disease, advanced cancer, or significant LV dysfunction. In these patients, the risks of the procedures outweigh the potential benefits. Patients admitted to the high-acuity unit may require short-term cardiovascular support with an intra-aortic balloon counter pulsation device or inotropic support for cardiogenic shock. Vital signs and fluid balance are closely monitored in these patients, and continuous ECG monitoring allows for prompt treatment of dysrhythmias.

Percutaneous Coronary Intervention

Percutaneous coronary intervention (PCI) is the procedure of choice for patients with STEMI. Descriptions of PCIs, including percutaneous transluminal coronary angioplasty (PTCA), coronary atherectomy, and coronary stenting, are presented in Table 15–7. Percutaneous coronary intervention is especially useful for patients who are older adults, not candidates for thrombolytics, or for those who have experienced reocclusion after receiving thrombolytic therapy. Guidelines recommend that hospitals performing PCI as a primary therapy in STEMI use experienced interventional cardiologists and operate within a multidisciplinary infrastructure for support and response to emergencies while providing a door-to-balloon time of less than 90 minutes (O'Gara et al., 2013).

Patients considered for PCI receive all the appropriate therapies used in the management of STEMI with the exception of thrombolytics. Thrombolytics are not necessary in the setting of acute PCI because their intended purpose is to lyse the thrombus. Anticoagulants such as aspirin, clopidogrel, prasugrel or ticagrelor may be administered prior to angioplasty to prevent new clot formation (Faxon & Bhatt, 2015). Unfractionated heparin, enoxaprin, or bivalirudin may be administered in the catheterization lab to prevent clot formation during the procedure. Bivalirudin (Angiomax), a direct thrombin inhibitor anticoagulant, can be used when the risk of bleeding is high (Faxon & Bhatt, 2015).

Percutaneous coronary interventions are performed in an angiography lab (Figure 15–4) under the direction of an

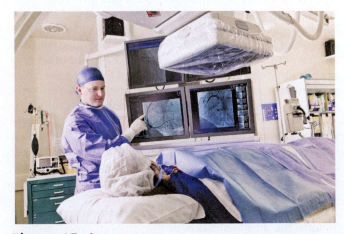

Figure 15–4 Angiography lab.
SOURCE: EPSTOCK/Shutterstock

interventional cardiologist who is trained to perform invasive cardiac procedures.

Preparing the Patient for PCI   Prior to the procedure, nursing responsibilities include continued monitoring of the patient's vital signs, timely medication administration, and patient and family education. Many institutions use standardized heart catheterization videos to instruct on the procedure and answer questions. A witnessed consent should be verified and placed in the chart. Some institutional protocols may include clipping of hair in the patient's groin area. Bilateral groin clippings are recommended in the event that the cardiologist is unable to access the femoral artery from one side or the other. The patient should have nothing to eat or drink after midnight, and the time of the patient's last meal is determined and documented. Renal function is assessed by examining blood urea nitrogen and serum creatinine levels. The baseline levels for these laboratory tests are used to assess for changes in renal function that can occur secondary to contrast dye use in coronary angiography or other procedures. Contrast-induced nephropathy, a decline in renal function after the administration of iodinated contrast medium, is a potential complication in patients undergoing a cardiac procedure that requires contrast dye. Strategies to prevent contrast-induced nephropathy include providing adequate hydration around the time of the procedure, withholding metformin in patients with diabetes, and administering intravenous sodium bicarbonate (Sinert & Peacock, 2016). Patients with contrast allergy are premedicated with an antihistamine such as diphenhydramine (Benadryl) and corticosteroids to help prevent allergic reactions to the dye (Brockow & Sanchez-Borges, 2014). Diabetic patients who have taken their oral hypoglycemic medications may require fingerstick glucose checks during the procedure. Diabetic patients should not take oral hypoglycemic agents (such as metformin) or metformin-containing products the day before, morning of, or for 48 hours after the procedure as it may cause kidney failure in combination with contrast dye. Oral anticoagulants such as warfarin (Coumadin) should also be stopped prior to PCI. Patients should void prior to being transported to the cardiac catheterization lab, and women may require an indwelling urinary catheter.

PCI Procedure   The procedure typically involves the insertion of an introducer catheter into the femoral or radial artery. A guiding catheter is inserted through the introducer, and the target vessel is engaged. The coronary anatomy is assessed using fluoroscopy with contrast dye administration, and the offending thrombus is located. Figure 15–5 shows how coronary artery stenosis looks using fluoroscopy.

A key decision at this point during the procedure is determining the best reperfusion strategies for the patient. Reperfusion interventions include removal of occlusions and performing balloon angioplasty, or transferring the patient to the operating room for emergent bypass surgery. Indications for surgery include severe left main coronary artery (LMCA) disease, LMCA-equivalent disease, and three or more proximal coronary artery obstructions.

The aspiration of a blood clot from a coronary artery, a thrombectomy, may be beneficial during PCI procedures

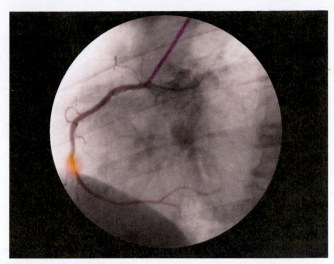

Figure 15–5 Stenosis of coronary artery identified by fluoroscopy during PCI.
SOURCE: Scott Camazine/Science Source

in selected cases (Levine et al., 2016). If the decision is made to proceed with a thrombectomy, the cardiologist crosses the occlusion with a guide wire and removes the thrombus. A thrombectomy device such as the AngioJet Ultra Coronary Thrombectomy System (Boston Scientific, 2016) may be used to remove the clot. The AngioJet Ultra system uses a catheter and high-pressure saline jets to create a vacuum effect that removes the thrombus. The lesion is then predilated with an angioplasty balloon (Figure 15–6).

Following the angioplasty, a coronary stent (a meshed hollow tube) is placed at the point of the blockage to maintain coronary artery patency. Figure 15–7 illustrates this procedure.

Bare-metal stents (BMS) or drug-eluting stents (DES) are commonly used to maintain coronary artery patency with PCI procedures. Balloon-expandable stents are placed into coronary arteries with a catheter that is inflated once the stent is properly positioned. The stent remains expanded in the vessel wall after the balloon is deflated and the catheter is removed. Cardiac stents are typically made of stainless steel or a cobalt chromium alloy.

Restenosis of the coronary artery and stent thrombosis are serious short- and long-term complications of stent placement. Restenosis, or narrowing of the internal wall of the stent, is caused by an exaggerated proliferation of smooth-muscle cell growth as a part of the healing process. Drug-eluting stents are less likely to cause restenosis than bare-metal stents; however, drug-eluting stents have higher rates of thrombosis than their bare-metal counterparts. Drug-eluting stents are coated with a polymer coating containing drugs such as everolimus, biolimus, and zotarolimus, which are released slowly over several months (Faxon & Bhatt, 2015), suppressing inflammation and **neointimal hyperplasia**, the overgrowth of cells in the internal stent wall. Patients who receive a drug-eluting stent may receive an anti-platelet drug such as clopidogrel for up to 1 year after stent placement to reduce the risk of thrombus formation (Amsterdam et al., 2014).

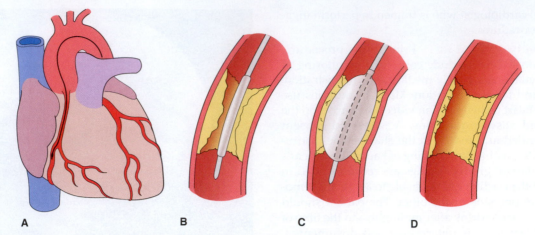

Figure 15–6 Balloon angioplasty. A, The balloon catheter is threaded into the affected coronary artery. B, The balloon is positioned directly at the site of the lesion. C, The balloon is inflated, compressing the lesion against the artery wall. D, The balloon is deflated and catheter removed, leaving a patent artery.

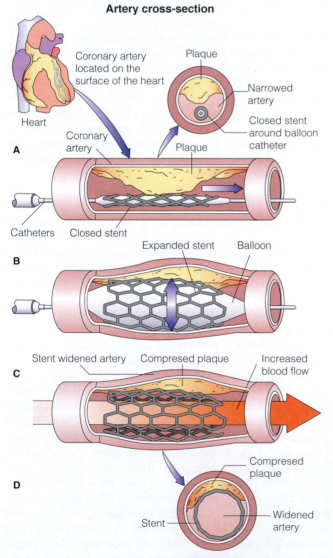

Artery cross-section

Coronary artery located on the surface of the heart

Heart

Plaque

Narrowed artery

Closed stent around balloon catheter

A

Coronary artery

Plaque

Catheters   Closed stent

Expanded stent   Balloon

B

Stent widened artery   Compresed plaque   Increased blood flow

C

Compresed plaque

D

Stent   Widened artery

Figure 15–7 Placement of the balloon-expandable intracoronary stent. A. The balloon catheter with the stent is threaded into the affected coronary artery. B. and C. The stent is positioned across the blockage and expanded. D. The balloon is deflated and removed, leaving the stent in place.

After the PCI, the catheters, guide wires, and introducer are removed and the patient is prepared for transport to a recovery area. Depending on the location of the insertion site, either direct pressure or closure devices are used to achieve hemostasis at the insertion site. An example of a currently available closure device is the Angio-seal VIP Vascular Closure Device (Terumo Interventional Systems, 2017). The Angio-seal device uses an anchoring device, a collagen plug, and suture to achieve arterial hemostasis. The Perclose ProGlide Suture-Mediated Closure System is another closure device that assists suturing and can be used for femoral artery closure following invasive cardiac procedures (Abbott Vascular, 2015). Internal or external vascular closure device use resulted in faster femoral artery hemostasis times in patients undergoing coronary angiography when compared to those receiving manual compression (Schulz-Schupke et al., 2014). Hemostasis of radial artery insertion sites can be achieved with a variety of direct pressure devices or manual compression.

Care of the Patient Post-PCI   Postprocedure management of the PCI patient includes monitoring frequent vital signs, the ECG rhythm strip, and assessing the access site for pain, swelling, or bleeding. Routine blood work typically includes a complete blood count, chemistry panel, and coagulation studies. Intravenous infusions may include a GP IIb/IIIa inhibitor and crystalloid solutions. GP IIb/IIIa inhibitors are continued for a minimum of 18 hours post-PCI unless contraindicated. Clopidogrel and ASA may be ordered to prevent new clot formation. Hydration with IV fluids continues until just prior to discharge if the patient is to go home the same day. If the patient is admitted to a high-acuity unit, IV hydration may continue for another 10 to 12 hours.

Patients whose access site was sealed using a closure device must remain flat for approximately 30 minutes. After this time, the head of the bed may be elevated to 30 degrees followed by ambulation in approximately 4 hours. Access sites closed with direct pressure require the patient to remain supine for approximately 6 hours with the affected leg in a straight position. Palpation of pedal pulses and observation of the access site for edema and bleeding are important nursing assessments that are made frequently after the procedure.

The most common postprocedure complications include chest pain, hypotension, and bleeding at the access site. Chest pain shortly after PCI can indicate acute coronary artery closure. If the patient complains of chest pain, the nurse obtains vital signs and an ECG, and notifies the cardiologist. Acute coronary artery closure requires a transfer of the patient to the cardiac catheterization lab for additional reperfusion procedures. Hypotension can be caused by bleeding at the access site, **retroperitoneal bleeding** from hematoma rupture or puncture of an artery in the groin, or a delayed IV contrast dye reaction. Patients are instructed to notify the nurse if they feel wetness or warmth around the affected leg, are dizzy or lightheaded, or experience backache. If the patient becomes hypotensive, tachycardic, or experiences an unexplained vagal episode, bleeding may be present, and the cardiologist is notified immediately. If a retroperitoneal bleed is suspected, a computed tomography scan is required to determine the extent of damage to the blood vessel. Treatment of retroperitoneal bleeding may include IV fluids or blood transfusions to support blood pressure, cessation of anticoagulation therapy, or surgical repair of the damaged artery.

Patient and family education is important prior to discharge and will include instruction on activity limitations, such as when to shower, drive, lift heavy objects, exercise, and access site care. Discharge medication education is also part of the patient–family teaching plan. Patients should receive a wallet card with information about their coronary stent when applicable, and they should be instructed to keep the card with them at all times. Signs and symptoms of post-PCI complications and provider information for follow-up care, including appointments and telephone numbers, should be discussed with patients and their families prior to discharge. Patients should be instructed to contact their nearest emergency department or licensed care provider if signs of infection from the access site, coronary artery reocclusion, arterial bleeding, or other unwanted complications occur.

Coronary Artery Bypass Surgery

Coronary artery bypass graft (CABG) has been performed in the United States since the late 1960s. Advances in surgical technique, cardiopulmonary bypass (CPB), conduit selection, and **cardioplegic** solutions have improved patient outcomes and have made the procedure available to a broader selection of patients. Mortality rates for 1, 3, and 5 years of 3%, 9%, and 17%, respectively, have been reported in patients requiring CABG surgery (Carr et al., 2015). Patients with renal dysfunction prior to surgery and those requiring dialysis for renal failure are at higher risk for complications including death following CABG surgery (Carr et al., 2015).

In the setting of ACS, CABG is performed after angiography has determined the anatomy of the coronary arteries and the location and extent of coronary artery blockage by atherosclerosis or thrombosis. Indications for CABG include severe left main coronary artery (LMCA) disease, proximal left anterior descending and proximal left circumflex stenosis,

and triple vessel disease (Leeper, 2014). In addition, CABG may be performed as a rescue procedure for acute restenosis or rupture of a coronary artery. Additional factors that influence the suitability of a patient for bypass include the size of the native coronary artery, muscle viability, left ventricular function, and the extent of disease distal to the stenotic lesion. The primary goal of CABG surgery performed under emergency conditions is prompt restoration of blood flow to the ischemic portion of the myocardium.

Coronary artery bypass grafting can be accomplished through the traditional method using cardiopulmonary bypass (CPB), which is referred to as on-pump coronary artery bypassing, or through an off-pump technique called off-pump coronary artery bypassing (OPCAB) (Leeper, 2014; Okada, Robertson, Saint, & Damiano, 2014). CPB is a technique used during surgery whereby blood is directed away from the vascular system and the nonbeating heart and is circulated through a system of reservoirs and pumps (Figure 15–8). The system that performs this function is referred to as extracorporeal circulation. The heart is stopped with a cardioplegia solution when CPB is used, and circulatory functions are performed through extracorporeal circulation. Blood that filters through the extracorporeal circulation bypass system undergoes oxygenation, filtration, and cooling and is returned to the systemic circulation. Moderate hypothermia is used during CPB to reduce myocardial oxygen demand and protect target organs from damage.

Off-pump coronary artery bypass (OPCAB) grafting can be performed through a median sternotomy or thoracotomy incision on a beating heart. This type of OPCAB is called a minimally invasive direct coronary artery bypass (MIDCAB). Another off-pump grafting technique, total endoscopic coronary artery bypass (TECAB), involves the use of a robotic device to perform the minimally invasive surgery. The TECAB procedure is difficult to learn, and operating times can be prolonged, making this a less desirable procedure by many surgeons (Okada et al., 2014). Off-pump surgeries appear to produce less postoperative bleeding than on-pump procedures; however, the off-pump surgical techniques can be technically challenging, and increased rates of adverse cardiac events have been noted in patients receiving off-pump versus on-pump procedures (Okada et al., 2014). A procedure to decrease healthcare team error during minimally invasive cardiac surgery is described in the feature "Quality and Safety."

Quality and Safety
Procedural Error Prevention

Physicians and other healthcare team members involved in a minimally invasive cardiac procedure, an atrial septal defect repair, noticed profound blood loss and hypotension in the patient during the surgical procedure. The patient was successfully resuscitated and did not display long-term effects on follow-up. A careful review of the case by an interprofessional team revealed that an open cannula in the superior vena cava resulted in unplanned blood loss into the cardiopulmonary bypass equipment. As a result, a procedural checklist was created to prevent similar mistakes in future procedures.

SOURCE: Based on Hussain et al. (2016).

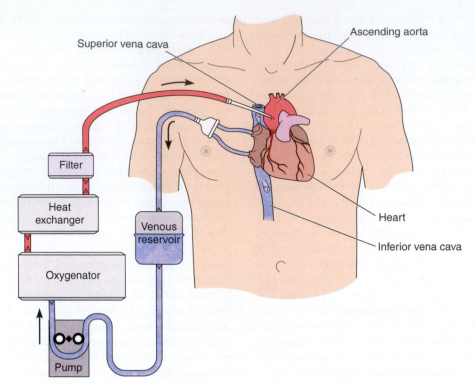

Figure 15–8 A diagrammatic representation of cardiopulmonary bypass.

When CPB is used for on-pump surgeries, monitoring of the bypass machine is under the control of a specially trained technician called a **perfusionist**. The perfusionist monitors the CPB machine and administers heparin and other medications to maintain anticoagulation and hemodynamic stability. Cardiopulmonary bypass is used exclusively for heart surgery. Factors associated with bypass that influence the patient's postoperative course include hypothermia, hemodilution, catecholamine release, hormone release, and platelet damage.

Bypass of the coronary artery lesion is performed under general anesthesia using blood vessels from the right or left internal mammary artery (RIMA, LIMA), saphenous vein grafts (SVGs), or a combination of both (Figure 15–9).

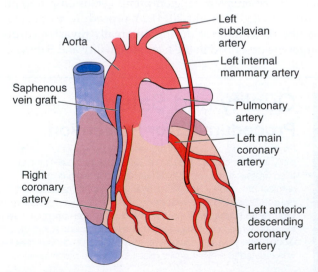

Figure 15–9 Coronary artery bypass grafting using the internal mammary artery and a saphenous vein graft.

The grafts are harvested from either the anterior chest wall (in the case of LIMA or RIMA grafts) or the saphenous veins of the legs. Many surgeons prefer the use of LIMA or RIMA grafts (depending on lesion location) because of the higher patency rates and their increased longevity (10 to 15 years). Alternate (but not commonly used) graft conduits include the gastroepiploic artery, inferior gastric artery, and radial artery. Great care is taken during the harvesting of the grafts to prevent injury to the vessel.

CABG surgery is classically performed as an on-pump procedure through a median sternotomy incision. In order to reduce the risk of myocardial ischemia, the heart is infused with a cold cardioplegia solution, which inhibits membrane depolarization and action potential propagation. This produces a temporary diastolic arrest (stopping the heart) that allows the surgeon to perform the delicate grafting procedure. The distal anastomoses are performed first so that cardioplegia solution may be infused into the vein graft. The proximal aortic anastomoses are performed as rewarming of the patient begins. The aortic cross-clamps are removed, and the rewarming process is completed. Once rewarming has taken place and the heart begins beating, the anastomoses sites are checked for leaks and final preparations are made for completion of the procedure. Epicardial pacing wires and mediastinal chest tubes are inserted. The sternotomy incision is closed using stainless steel wires after homeostasis is achieved. Usually five or six wire sutures secure the sternum prior to skin closure.

Dedicated surgery teams that include surgeons, anesthesiologists, perfusionists, nurses, and operating room and intensive care unit (ICU) staffs are available at hospitals that provide bypass surgery. This team approach provides the best outcomes for patients undergoing this procedure. Clinical pathways, patient care guidelines, and protocols are typically used to manage patients in the postoperative period. These patients are cared for by nurses who have received specialized education and training.

Care of the Patient Post-CABG Surgery Evidence-based nursing outcomes and the use of sound clinical judgment by healthcare professionals are essential to producing desired outcomes for hospitalized patients. While mortality from this surgery has decreased, length of stay has increased due to the increased survivability of those with multisystem complications who would have previously died. To achieve patient outcomes, it is important for the nurse to be knowledgeable of potential complications. The post-CABG patient is at an increased risk for infections such as ventilator-associated pneumonia (VAP) and central line or incisional infections. When the sternum is opened for CABG surgery, postoperative sternal infections can occur. Sternal infections can be superficial or deep with a separation of the sternum. The most effective strategy for preventing sternal infections and related complications is adequate stabilization of the sternum with wiring by the surgeon during CABG surgery (Simmons & Adam, 2015). The nurse should notify the healthcare provider of increased sternal pain, separation of skin in the sternum or unusual clicking noises with patient movement, as these may indicate sternal dehiscence and the need for additional intervention (Simmons & Adam, 2015). The risk of infection is significantly increased if patients have poor glucose control or diabetes. Increased risk for pressure ulcers exists from decreased mobility; other risks include postoperative delirium or confusion. There are order sets or bundles (e.g., VAP bundles) that have been developed to prevent some of these complications, and the order sets should be instituted as recommended by national guidelines and hospital protocols.

Management during the immediate postoperative period is aimed at optimizing cardiac output and tissue perfusion while preventing and treating complications. Postoperative care is frequently guided by unit protocols and guidelines. Nursing responsibilities include frequent and ongoing physical assessments of cardiopulmonary status, vital signs, intake and output, cardiac rhythms, and level of consciousness. Functioning of the gastrointestinal and renal systems is also assessed.

On arrival in the ICU, a nursing priority is to confirm a patent airway by assessing endotracheal tube placement and auscultating breath sounds. Ventilator settings are usually verified by a respiratory therapist. Ventilation management includes pulmonary hygiene, turning the patient every 2 hours, and suctioning. If there are no pulmonary complications postoperatively, the patient is extubated within a few hours of surgery.

Postoperative analgesia is usually accomplished with intermittent or continuous intravenous morphine. Epidural morphine or thoracic blocks with the infusion of 0.5% bupivacaine by way of a catheter placed in an intercostal space or the pleura can also be used to manage pain (Rosen, 2015; Ziyaeifard, Azarfarin, & Golzari, 2014).

Benzodiazepines may be administered to control anxiety. Level of consciousness, efficacy of pain management, respiratory functioning, and extent of sedation must be assessed when administering analgesic and sedative medications.

When the pleural space is opened for surgery, negative intrathoracic pressure must be restored postoperatively through the use of pleural chest tubes. Chest tubes are connected to wall or bulb suction and provide a mechanism for draining blood or pleural fluid. Depending on unit protocol, patients will return to the ICU with a central venous line and/or a pulmonary artery catheter. If a pulmonary artery catheter is in place, hemodynamic parameters, including mixed venous oxygen saturation, right atrial pressure, pulmonary artery pressure, pulmonary artery wedge pressure, cardiac output (CO), and cardiac index (CI), are obtained to assess adequacy of cardiac output and tissue perfusion. Continuous blood pressure monitoring is accomplished through the use of an arterial catheter. A tube for gastric decompression and a urinary catheter may be present; outputs must be closely monitored.

After the initial assessment, the nurse receives a report from a member of the operating room team. Key information is communicated about the length of time the patient was on CPB (when applicable), estimated blood loss, number of bypass grafts that were performed and where the grafts were harvested from, current medications, and blood products received. All medications infusing by IV route are assessed for accuracy; the medication type, concentrations of drips, and flow rates are confirmed for agreement with verbal report.

A 12-lead ECG and chest x-ray are obtained shortly after arrival at the ICU. Initial postoperative laboratory tests are obtained, which may include a complete blood count, coagulation studies, and electrolytes such as calcium, magnesium, and phosphorus. Vital signs are initially taken frequently to ensure that hemodynamic instability is detected early and promptly treated. Body temperature is monitored, and abnormals are treated to return the patient's temperature to normal.

The nurse must be vigilant in detecting problems in the postoperative period. Potential complications include bleeding from vascular grafts, cardiac arrhythmias, pain, anxiety, infection, and cardiac tamponade (Leeper, 2014). During the initial postoperative period, the patient is typically rewarmed to a temperature of 37°C (98.6°F) using a warming blanket. Care must be taken to avoid excessive peripheral rewarming, which can lead to vasodilation and cardiac decompensation. Hypovolemia and vasodilation lead to inadequate preload and low CO. Diuresis (greater than 2–3 liters/hour) can be significant during the initial postoperative period, which can contribute to hypovolemia and low CO. Patients undergoing bypass surgery typically gain several kilograms of body weight as a result of fluid shifts and neurohormonal activation. Prior to being taken off the bypass pump, the perfusionist may administer a diuretic. Aggressive volume resuscitation is the first step in obtaining fluid balance if hypovolemia becomes severe.

Low CO exists when the cardiac index (CI) is less than 2 L/min/m². Clinical manifestations of low CO include cool, clammy extremities, tachycardia, decreased urine output, and diminished pulses. Hypovolemia associated with bleeding may result from disruption of an anastomosis site or from coagulopathies. Drainage, from mediastinal tubes that are placed in the pericardial space to prevent cardiac tamponade, is monitored frequently for evidence of excessive bleeding that may require surgical exploration. Mediastinal chest tube drainage greater than 250 to 300 mL for the first 2 hours should be reported to the surgeon so the need for additional corrective surgery can be assessed (Butterworth, Mackey, & Wasnick, 2013). If coagulation abnormalities are present, they are promptly corrected by administering blood products. There are usually institutional protocols for intravenous potassium, calcium, and magnesium replacements.

Decreased CO in spite of increased preload may indicate impaired cardiac function. Impaired cardiac function can result from preexisting heart failure, perioperative MI, reperfusion injuries, or cardiac tamponade. Inotropic medications are used to treat impaired ventricular function and to facilitate fluid resuscitation. Medications to increase cardiac contractility, heart rate, or mean arterial pressure may be administered through continuous intravenous drip. These inotropic or vasoactive medications include dobutamine, dopamine, epinephrine, norepinephrine, and milrinone. All should be used with caution as they increase myocardial workload through inotropic properties (increase heart rate) and increased oxygen consumption and may induce myocardial ischemia.

Continuous ECG monitoring is required for the detection and treatment of postoperative dysrhythmias. Common causes of dysrhythmias include electrolyte disturbances, low oxygen levels and acid–base imbalances (Butterworth, Mackey, & Wasnick, 2013). Bradycardias including the heart blocks, atrial fibrillation or flutter, premature ventricular contractions, and nonsustained ventricular tachycardia are common dysrhythmias following cardiac surgery. An external pacemaker is usually in place, and the pacemaker settings for capture and sensitivity should be verified. Advanced cardiac life support (ACLS) guidelines are used to treat all dysrhythmias.

Cardiac tamponade is a life-threatening postoperative complication that may be associated with excessive mediastinal chest tube drainage. Cardiac tamponade is caused by bleeding into the pericardium, the membranous sac around the heart. The accumulating pressure of blood around the heart increases intracardiac pressures, impairs ventricular filling, and decreases CO. **Pulsus paradoxus** is one of the classic signs of cardiac tamponade. This is an exaggerated decrease (greater than 10 mmHg) of the systolic blood pressure during inspiration. **Beck's triad**, which includes an elevated right atrial pressure, hypotension, and muffled heart sounds, may be present (Simmons & Adam, 2015). Treatment of cardiac tamponade includes echo-guided drainage of blood from the pericardium, **pericardiocentesis**, or pericardial drainage in the operating room.

Elevated systemic vascular resistance and cardiac dysrhythmias can also exacerbate low CO states. When systemic vascular resistance is elevated, afterload is increased, which intensifies cardiac workload. Vasodilators, such as nitroglycerin and sodium nitroprusside, are used to vasodilate arteries to decrease afterload, which potentially eases cardiac workload. Caution must be taken to ensure that adequate preload exists prior to the administration of vasodilators to avoid unexpected hypotension.

Most patients are extubated within 24 hours of surgery. The pulmonary artery catheter, nasogastric tube, and urinary catheter are removed. Patient-controlled analgesia is initiated as the patient stabilizes. The patient receives aggressive pulmonary hygiene, including coughing and deep breathing exercises with incentive spirometry. Patients prepare for physical activity by dangling their feet over the side of the bed. Patients may get out of bed and sit in a chair. Diet is advanced as tolerated when the nasogastric tube is removed. At this time, if they are stable, patients are transferred from the ICU to a cardiac high-acuity unit.

Discharge planning is multidisciplinary and includes healthcare team members from physical therapy, occupational therapy, and nutritional support. Discharge planning along with patient and family education continue until the patient is discharged. Cardiac rehabilitation plans are made prior to discharge.

Education on self-care is a priority in this phase, although incorporating instruction into the hospital stay has become increasingly difficult due to the trend toward decreased lengths of stay. Audiovisual aids such as DVDs can be used to reinforce patient teaching for self-care. At-home management of postoperative incisions, diet, activity, medications, and symptoms should be included in the patient and family discharge instructions.

Section Six Review

1. Therapies to increase myocardial perfusion include which goals? (Select all that apply.)
   A. Reducing the area of infarction
   B. Containing the clot in a localized area
   C. Increasing the likelihood that LV function will be preserved
   D. Decreasing the likelihood of developing Q waves on ECG
   E. Decreasing oxygen use by the myocardium

2. Which assessment finding may indicate that reocclusion has occurred after thrombolytic therapy?
   A. Hypotension
   B. Chest pain
   C. Isoelectric ST segment
   D. Change in level of consciousness

3. Which statement best describes why clients require a chest tube after having CABG surgery?
   A. The lungs are injured during the operative procedure.
   B. There is a need to drain blood from the mediastinum.
   C. There is a need to keep pressure off the heart.
   D. The lungs require restoration of negative pleural pressure.

4. Which findings are signs of cardiac tamponade? (Select all that apply.)
   A. Muffled heart sounds
   B. Elevated right atrial pressures
   C. High peak pressures on the ventilator
   D. Pulsus paradoxus
   E. Hypotension

Answers: 1. (A, C, D), 2. B, 3. D, 4. (A, C, D, E)

Critical Reasoning Checkpoint

Mrs. O is a 65-year-old African American woman who was brought to the ED by her neighbor. She complained of substernal chest pain that began 2 hours earlier. She rates the pain as a 9 on a 10-point scale. She has a history of hypertension, diabetes mellitus type 2, hyperlipidemia, and obesity. Her mother was treated for hyperlipidemia before she died at age 55 from complications associated with an acute myocardial infarction.

1. What additional questions would you ask Mrs. O about her chest pain?

2. List at least four collaborative interventions that should be completed within 30 minutes of her arrival to the ED.

Clinical update: Her ECG reveals *ST* elevation. Serum cardiac markers were drawn, and the results are as follows: CK 170 U/L; CK-MB 7%; cTnT 0.5 mcg/L; cTnI 3.6 mcg/L.

3. What is your interpretation of these results?

4. Mrs. O is treated with a percutaneous coronary intervention. What complications should the nurse assess for in the immediate postprocedure period?

5. Identify Mrs. O's nonmodifiable and modifiable risk factors.

Chapter 15 Review

1. Atherosclerosis is an inflammatory disorder caused by chronic injury or inflammation to the endothelium. During client education which conditions does the nurse explain are sources of that injury? (Select all that apply.)
   1. Hypotension
   2. Tobacco smoke
   3. Hypercholesterolemia
   4. Hypoglycemia
   5. Low triglyceride levels

2. The nurse would monitor a client with which lesion most closely for the development of acute myocardial infarction?
   1. Stable plaque
   2. Unstable plaque
   3. Normal plaque
   4. Advanced plaque

3. Which laboratory result would the nurse interpret as indicating that the client is at greatest risk for developing atherosclerosis?
   1. Total cholesterol 180 mg/dL; LDL 80 mg/dL
   2. Total cholesterol 170 mg/dL; LDL 120 mg/dL
   3. Total cholesterol 210 mg/dL; LDL 140 mg/dL
   4. Total cholesterol 250 mg/dL; LDL 190 mg/dL

4. A client who has atherosclerosis is placed on the HMG Co-A enzyme inhibitor atorvastatin (Lipitor). Which outcome indicates to the nurse that the drug is having the desired effect? (Select all that apply.)
   1. Reduction in LDL levels
   2. Increase in HDL levels
   3. Reduced CRP levels
   4. Normalization of serum glucose levels
   5. Increase in triglyceride levels

5. The nurse is providing preprocedure education to a client scheduled for an exercise stress test (EST) at 0800. Which instruction should the nurse provide?
   1. "Take your beta-blocker medication at seven o'clock the morning of your exam."
   2. "Do not smoke for eight hours before your test."
   3. "You may have one cup of regular coffee without cream or sugar the morning of the procedure."
   4. "You should not eat or drink anything for at least 24 hours before the procedure."

6. A client walks up to the triage nurse's desk in the emergency department and says, "My chest is really hurting." What should be the nurse's first action?

   1. Ask the client when the pain started.
   2. Have the client sit down.
   3. Send the client's spouse to admit the client.
   4. Ask the client if there is a history of cardiac problems.

7. A client has a history of stable angina. How would the nurse expect this client to describe episodes of chest pain?

   1. "I have chest pain when I am resting. It's not related to physical activity."
   2. "My chest pain usually occurs with minimal activity."
   3. "I usually have chest pain when I am physically active, but resting makes it go away."
   4. "I've tried taking nitroglycerin tablets, but they don't help my chest pain."

8. A 60-year-old woman was just diagnosed with stable angina. Which information is important for the nurse to provide to this client? (Select all that apply.)

   1. Rest will not relieve your symptoms.
   2. You may not experience crushing chest pain.
   3. Your cardiac symptoms may include fatigue, upper arm weakness, or heartburn.
   4. Your cardiac symptoms may include dizziness or inability to think clearly.
   5. You should immediately contact your healthcare provider if you need to take nitroglycerin to control your chest pain.

9. A client with coronary artery disease experiences fatigue, shortness of breath, and heartburn after walking his dog. Which medication should the client take when he returns home?

   1. Lovastatin (Mevacor)
   2. Acetylsalicylic acid (ASA)
   3. Calcium carbonate (Tums)
   4. Theophylline (Theo-Dur)

10. A client is being monitored following thrombolytic therapy for coronary artery occlusion. The nurse notes a new 2-mm *ST* segment elevation from baseline on the client's cardiac monitor. What is the nurse's priority action?

    1. Assess the client and collaborate with the healthcare provider.
    2. Continue to monitor the client; this is a normal finding.
    3. Administer nitroglycerin as ordered.
    4. Adjust the sensitivity of the alarms.

Answers to questions found inside your textbook are available on the faculty resources site. Please consult with your instructor.

References

Abbott Vascular. (2015). Perclose ProGlide Suture-Mediated Closure System (ProGlide SMC). U.S. Food and Drug Administration. Retrieved November 10, 2016, from http://www.fda.gov/MedicalDevices/ProductsandMedicalProcedures/DeviceApprovalsandClearances/Recently-ApprovedDevices/ucm351099.htm

Adams, M. P., Holland, N., & Urban, C. (2017). Chapter 23: Drugs for lipid disorders. In M. P Adams, N. Holland, & C. Urban (Eds.), *Pharmacology for nurses: A pathophysiologic approach* (5th ed., pp. 325–341). Retrieved November 1, 2016, from https://bookshelf.vitalsource.com/#/books/9780134255378

American Heart Association. (2016a). *The American Heart Association's diet and lifestyle recommendations.* Retrieved November 1, 2016, from http://www.heart.org/HEARTORG/HealthyLiving/HealthyEating/Nutrition/The-American-Heart-Associations-Diet-and-Lifestyle-Recommendations_UCM_305855_Article.jsp#.WBjNMk0zXIU

American Heart Association. (2016b). *Master the scale.* Retrieved November 1, 2016, from http://www.heart.org/HEARTORG/HealthyLiving/WeightManagement/Weight-Management_UCM_001081_SubHomePage.jsp

Amsterdam, E. A., Wenger, N. K., Brindis, R. G., Casey, D. E., Ganiats, T. G., Holmes, D. R.,. . . Zieman, S. J. (2014). 2014 AHA/ACC guideline for the management of patients with non–ST-elevation acute coronary syndromes: A report of the American College of Cardiology/American Heart Association Task Force on Practice Guidelines. *Circulation, 130,* 344–426. doi:http://dx.doi.org/10.1161/CIR.0000000000000134

Antman, E. M., & Loscalzo, J. (2015). Chapter 295: ST-segment elevation myocardial infarction. In D. Kasper, A. Fauci , S. Hauser, D. Longo, J. Jameson, & J. Loscalzo (Eds.), *Harrison's principles of internal medicine* (19th ed.). Retrieved November 6, 2016, from http://accessmedicine.mhmedical.com.ezproxy.uky.edu/Content.aspx?bookid=1130&Sectionid=79743612

Bashore, T. M., Granger, C. B., Jackson, K. P., & Patel, M. R. (2016). Chapter 10: Heart disease. In M. A. Papadakis, S. J. McPhee, & M. W. Rabow (Eds.), *Current medical diagnosis & treatment 2017.* Retrieved November 6, 2016, from http://accessmedicine.mhmedical.com.ezproxy.uky .edu/content.aspx?bookid=1843&Sectionid=135705950

Bobadilla, R. V. (2016). Acute coronary syndrome: Focus on antiplatelet therapy. *Critical Care Nurse, 36*(1), 15–27.

Boston Scientific. (2016). The AngioJet Ultra Thrombectomy System. Retrieved November 10, 2016, from http://www.bostonscientific.com/en-US /products/thrombectomy-systems/angiojet-ultra -coronary-thrombectomy-system.html

Boyle, A. J. (2014). Chapter 8, Acute myocardial infarction. In M. H. Crawford (Ed.), *Current diagnosis & treatment: Cardiology* (4th ed.). Retrieved November 5, 2016, from http://accessmedicine.mhmedical.com.ezproxy.uky .edu/content.aspx?bookid=715&Sectionid=48214539

Brockow, K., & Sanchez-Borges, M. (2014). Hypersensitivity to contrast media and dyes. *Immunology and Allergy Clinics of North America, 34*(3), 547–564.

Butterworth, J. F., Mackey, D. C., & Wasnick, J. D. (2013). Chapter 56: Postanesthesia care. In J. F. Butterworth, D. C. Mackey, & J. D. Wasnick (Eds.), *Morgan & Mikhail's clinical anesthesiology* (5th ed.). Retrieved November 16, 2016, from http://accessmedicine .mhmedical.com.ezproxy.uky.edu/content.aspx?bookid =564&Sectionid=42800590

Cannon, C. P., & Braunwald, E. (2015). Chapter 294: Non-ST-segment elevation acute coronary syndrome. In D. Kasper, A. Fauci, S. Hauser, D. Longo, J. Jameson, & J. Loscalzo (Eds.), *Harrison's principles of internal medicine* (19th ed.). Retrieved November 6, 2016, from http://accessmedicine.mhmedical.com.ezproxy.uky .edu/Content.aspx?bookid=1130&Sectionid=79743570

Carr, B. M., Romeiser, J., Ruan, J., Gupta, S., Seifert, F. C., Zhu, W., & Shroyer, A. L. (2015). Long-term post-CABG survival: Performance of clinical risk models versus actuarial predictions. *Journal of Cardiac Surgery, 31*(1), 23–30.

Crawford, M. H. (2014). Chapter 6: Chronic ischemic heart disease. In M. H. Crawford (Ed.), *Current diagnosis & treatment: Cardiology* (4th ed.). Retrieved November 1, 2016, from http://accessmedicine.mhmedical.com .ezproxy.uky.edu/content.aspx?bookid=715&Sectio nid=48214537

Eastwood, J., Johnson, B. D., Rutledge, T., Bittner, V., Whittaker, K. S., Krantz, D. S., . . . Merz, C. N. B. (2013). Anginal symptoms, coronary artery disease, and adverse outcomes in black and white women: The NHLBI-Sponsored Women's Ischemia Syndrome Evaluation (WISE) Study. *Journal of Women's Health, 22*(9), 724–732.

Faxon, D. P., & Bhatt, D. L. (2015). Chapter 296: Percutaneous coronary interventions and other interventional procedures. In D. Kasper, A. Fauci, S. Hauser, D. Longo, J. Jameson, & J. Loscalzo (Eds.), *Harrison's principles of internal medicine* (19th ed.). Retrieved November 10, 2016, from http://accessmedicine.mhmedical.com.ezproxy.uky .edu/content.aspx?bookid=1130&Sectionid=79743772

Freedland, K. E., Carney, R. M., Rich, M. W., Steinmeyer, B. C., & Rubin, E. H. (2015). Cognitive behavior therapy for depression and self-care in heart failure patients. *Journal of the American Medical Association, Internal Medicine, 175*(11), 1773–1782. doi:10.1001 /jamainternmed.2015.5220

Goldberger, A. L. (2015). Chapter 268: Electrocardiography. In D. Kasper, A. Fauci, S. Hauser, D. Longo, J. Jameson, & J. Loscalzo (Eds.), *Harrison's principles of internal medicine* (19th ed.). Retrieved November 6, 2016, from http://accessmedicine.mhmedical.com.ezproxy.uky .edu/content.aspx?bookid=1130&Sectionid=79741703

Goldich, G. (2014). 12-lead ECGs Part II: Identifying common abnormalities. *Nursing, 44*(9), 30–36.

Hussain, S., Adams, C., Cleland, A., Jones, P. M., Walsh, G., & Kiaii, B. (2016). Lessons from aviation: The role of checklists in minimally invasive cardiac surgery. *Perfusion, 31*(1), 68–71.

Jacobson, T. A., Ito, M. K., Maki, K. C., Orringer, C. E., Bays, H. E., Jones, P. H., . . . Brown, W. V. (2014). National Lipid Association recommendations for patient-centered management of dyslipidemia: Part 1– executive summary. *Journal of Clinical Lipidology, 8*(5), 473–488.

Kee, J. L. (2014). *Laboratory and diagnostic tests with nursing implications* (9th ed.). Hoboken, NJ: Pearson.

Kusumoto, F. M. (2014). Chapter 10: Cardiovascular disorders: Heart disease. In G. D. Hammer & S. J. McPhee (Eds.), *Pathophysiology of disease: An introduction to clinical medicine* (7th ed.). Retrieved October 21, 2016, from http://accessmedicine.mhmedical.com .ezproxy.uky.edu/content.aspx?bookid=961&Sectio nid=53555691

Lancia, L., Toccaceli, A., Dignani, L., Lucertini, C., Petrucci, C., & Romano, S. (2016). Accuracy of EASI 12-lead ECGs in monitoring ST-segment and J-point by nurses in the coronary care units. *Journal of Clinical Nursing, 25*, 1282–1291. doi: 10.1111/jocn.13168

Leeper, B. (2014). Chapter 19: Advanced cardiovascular concepts. In S. M. Burns (Ed.), *AACN: Essentials of critical care nursing* (3rd ed., pp. 475–505). New York, NY: McGraw-Hill.

Levine, G. N, Bates, E. R., Blankenship, J. C., Bailey, S. R., Bittl, J. A., Cercek, B., . . . Zhao, D. X. (2016). 2015 ACC/ AHA/SCAI focused update on primary percutaneous coronary intervention for patients with ST-elevation myocardial infarction. *Journal of the American College of Cardiology, 67*(10), 1235–1250.

Libby, P. (2015). Chapter 291: The pathogenesis, prevention, and treatment of atherosclerosis. In D. Kasper, A. Fauci, S. Hauser, D. Longo, J. Jameson, & J. Loscalzo (Eds.), *Harrison's principles of internal medicine* (19th ed.). Retrieved November 1, 2016, from http://accessmedicine.mhmedical.com.ezproxy.uky .edu/content.aspx?bookid=1130&Sectionid=79743366

McCarthy, J. J., & Mendelsohn, B. A. (2016). Chapter 7: Heart disease. In J. J. McCarthy & B. A. Mendelsohn (Eds.), *Precision medicine: A guide to genomics in clinical practice.* Retrieved November 18, 2016, from http://accessmedicine.mhmedical.com.ezproxy.uky .edu/content.aspx?bookid=1930&Sectionid=140197690

Mitrovic, I. (2014). Chapter 11: Cardiovascular disorders: Vascular disease. In G. D. Hammer & S. J. McPhee (Eds.), *Pathophysiology of disease: An introduction to clinical medicine* (7th ed.). Retrieved October 21, 2016, from http://accessmedicine.mhmedical.com .ezproxy.uky.edu/content.aspx?bookid=961&Sectio nid=53555692

Mozaffarian, D., Benjamin, E. J., Go, A. S., Arnett, D. K., Blaha, M. J., Cushman, M., . . . Turner, M. B. (2015). Heart disease and stroke statistics—2016 update: A report from the American Heart Association. *Circulation, 132*, e1–323. doi:10.1161 /CIR.0000000000000350

O'Gara, P. T., Kusher, F. G., Ascheim, D. D., Casey, D. E., Chung, M. K., de Lemos, J. A., . . . Zhao, D. X. (2013). 2013 ACCF/AHA guideline for the management of ST-elevation myocardial infarction: Executive summary. A report of the American College of Cardiology Foundation/American Heart Association Task Force on Practice Guidelines. *Journal of the American College of Cardiology, 61*(4), 485–510.

Ohman, E. M. (2016). Chronic stable angina. *New England Journal of Medicine, 374*, 1167–1176. doi:10.1056 /NEJMcp1502240

Okada, S., Robertson, J. O., Saint, L. L., & Damiano, R. J. (2014). Chapter 21: Acquired heart disease. In F. Brunicardi, D. K. Andersen, T. R. Billiar, D. L. Dunn, J. G. Hunter, J. B. Matthews, & R. E. Pollock (Eds.), *Schwartz's principles of surgery* (10th ed.). Retrieved November 10, 2016, from http://accessmedicine .mhmedical.com.ezproxy.uky.edu/content.aspx?bookid =980&Sectionid=59610863

Polderman, K. H., Noc, M., Beishuizen, A., Biermann, H., Girbes, A. R. J., Tully, G. W., . . . Seidman, D. (2015). Ultrarapid induction of hypothermia using continuous automated peritoneal lavage with ice-cold fluids: Final results of the Cooling for Cardiac Arrest or Acute ST-Elevation Myocardial Infarction Trial. *Critical Care Medicine, 43*, 2191–2201.

Poldervaart, J. M., Langedijkb, M., Backus, B. E., Dekker, I. M. C., Sixe, A. J., Doevendans, P. A., . . . Reitsma, J. B. (2016). Comparison of the GRACE, HEART and TIMI score to predict major adverse cardiac events in chest pain patients at the emergency department. *International Journal of Cardiology, 227*. doi: http://dx.doi.org/10.1016/j.ijcard.2016.10.080

Rosen, J. E. (2015). Postoperative care. In G. M. Doherty (Ed.), *CURRENT diagnosis & treatment: Surgery* (14th ed.). Retrieved November 17, 2016, from http://accessmedicine.mhmedical.com.ezproxy.uky .edu/content.aspx?bookid=1202&Sectionid=71515676

Schulz-Schupke, S., Helde, S., Gewalt, S., Ibrahim, T., Linhardt, M., Haas, K., . . . Kastrati, A. (2014). Comparison of vascular closure devices vs manual compression after femoral artery puncture: The ISAR-CLOSURE randomized clinical trial. *Journal of the American Medical Association, 312*(9), 1981–1987. doi:10.1001/jama.2014.15305

Simmons, J., & Adam, L. A. (2015). Chapter 112: Principles of postoperative critical care. In J. B. Hall, G. A. Schmidt, & J. P. Kress (Eds.), *Principles of critical care* (4th ed.). Retrieved November 17, 2016, from http://accessmedicine.mhmedical.com.ezproxy.uky .edu/content.aspx?bookid=1340&Sectionid=80026410

Sinert, R., & Peacock, P. R. (2016). Chapter 88: Acute kidney injury. In J. E. Tintinalli, J. Stapczynski, O. Ma, D. M. Yealy, G. D. Meckler, & D. M. Cline (Eds.), *Tintinalli's emergency medicine: A comprehensive study guide* (8th ed.). Retrieved November 10, 2016, from http://accessmedicine.mhmedical.com.ezproxy.uky .edu/content.aspx?bookid=1658&Sectionid=109433339

Terumo Interventional Systems. (2017). Angio-Seal™ VIP Vascular Closure Device. Retrieved March 5, 2017, from http://www.terumois.com/products/closure/angio -seal-vascular-closure-devices/angio-seal.html

Wilson, B. A., Shannon, M., & Shields, K. (2016). *Pearson nurse's drug guide 2016* (3rd ed.). Retrieved November 1, 2016, from https://bookshelf.vitalsource.com/# /books/9780134070728

Wilson, S. A., Weaver-Agostoni, J., & Perkins, J. J. (2015). Chapter 20: Acute coronary syndrome. In J. E. South-Paul, S. C. Matheny, & E. L. Lewis (Eds.), *Current diagnosis & treatment: Family medicine* (4th ed.). Retrieved October 21, 2016, from http://accessmedicine.mhmedical.com.ezproxy.uky .edu/content.aspx?bookid=1415&Sectionid=77056211

Ziyaeifard, M., Azarfarin, R., & Golzari, S. E. J. (2014). A review of current analgesic techniques in cardiac surgery. Is epidural worth it? *Journal of Cardiovascular Thoracic Research, 6*(3), 133–140.

Chapter 16

Determinants and Assessment of Cerebral Function

Learning Outcomes

16.1   Describe selected anatomy and physiology of the brain, including cerebral tissue perfusion.

16.2   Explain the components of intracranial pressure (ICP), including the Monro-Kellie hypothesis, and cerebral perfusion pressure.

16.3   Assess cerebral tissue perfusion.

16.4   Describe diagnostic procedures used in acute brain injury.

his chapter provides a review of basic anatomy and physiology of the brain as well as the physiologic processes associated with intracranial pressure and cerebral tissue perfusion. The chapter also reviews neurologic assessments and common diagnostic procedures. Reviewing these essential concepts will enhance understanding of the material in subsequent neurological chapters.

Section One: Selective Neurological Anatomy and Physiology

The neurologic system is composed of two distinct but interacting systems: the central nervous system and the peripheral nervous system.

The Central Nervous System

The central nervous system (CNS) consists of the brain and spinal cord, which function to accept, interconnect, interpret, and generate responses to nerve impulses originating in other parts of the body (Figure 16–1). The CNS contains the majority of **axons** and **synapses**. An axon is a long slender projection of a nerve cell or neuron, that conducts electrical or chemical signals away from the neuron to effect a change in distant cells. Axons, also known as nerve fibers,

function to transmit information to different neurons, muscles, and glands. Axons make contact with other cells at junctions or spaces called synapses. The synapse permits a nerve fiber (axon) to pass an impulse or signal to another neuron. Information from one neuron flows to another neuron across a synapse, which is the space or junction that contains neurotransmitters (presynaptic end) and receptors (postsynaptic end). Areas with a high density of cell bodies are called gray matter; those primarily containing axons are referred to as white matter. Axons are generally covered in myelin, a lipid–protein composition, giving it a pale white color. Figure 16–2 shows two neurons connected by a synapse.

The brain is the control center for the CNS and has four specialized regions: cerebrum, diencephalon, cerebellum, and brainstem (Figure 16–3). Table 16–1 summarizes the functions of each of the brain's regions.

Cerebrum   The cerebrum is composed of the right and left hemispheres, which account for 60% of the brain's weight (LeMone, Burke, Bauldoff & Gubrud, 2015). The surface of the cerebrum is composed of gyri (ridges of tissue) with sulci (grooves or shallow depressions) and fissures (deeper depressions). A longitudinal fissure separates the hemispheres, and a transverse fissure divides the cerebrum from the cerebellum. Each cerebral hemisphere is divided into lobes (frontal, parietal, temporal, and occipital) and communicates with the opposite hemisphere via a collection of nerve fibers called the corpus callosum. Sensory tracts are ascending tracts and deliver information to

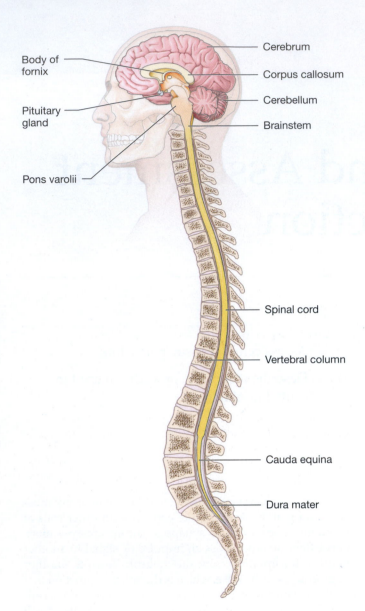

Figure 16–1 Brain and spinal cord.

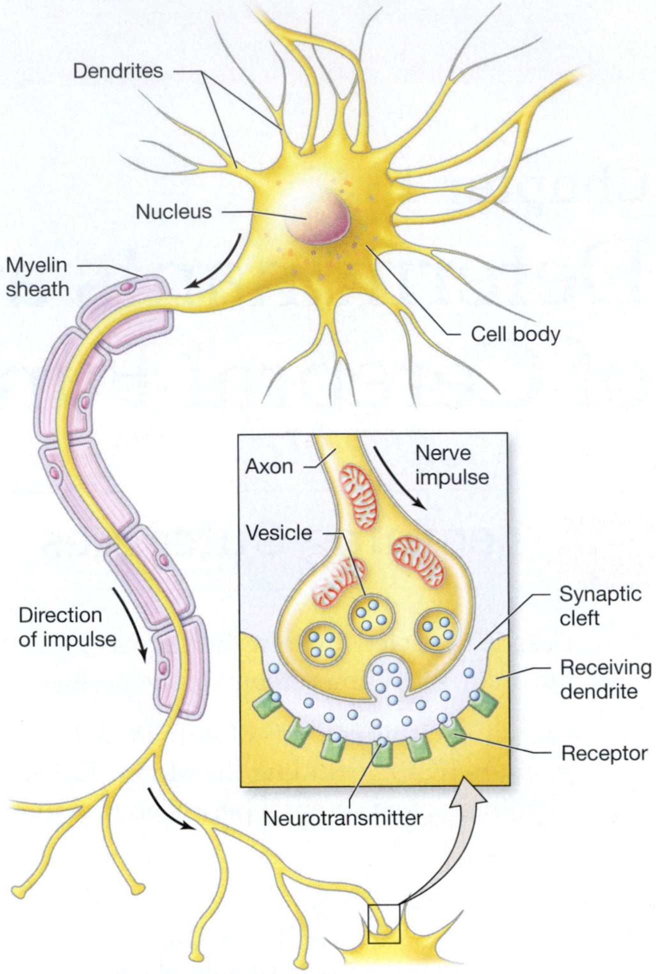

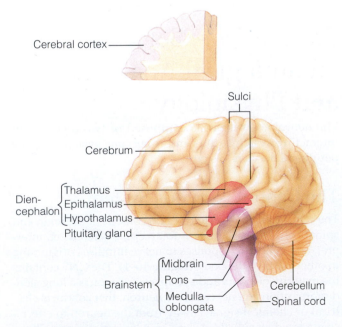

Figure 16–2 Neuron with synapse.

the brain from the periphery. Motor tracts are descending tracts that deliver information from the brain to the periphery. Motor tracts cross over at the medulla and control the opposite side of the body.

The cerebral cortex is the outer surface of the cerebrum (Figure 16–3), which consists of neuron cell bodies, unmyelinated fibers, neuroglia, and blood vessels. Each lobe of the cerebrum has a specific and unique function, as does each area of the cerebral cortex (Figure 16–4).

The **diencephalon**, located deep within the cerebrum and superior to the brainstem, consists of the thalamus, hypothalamus, pituitary gland, and epithalamus; the latter contains the pineal gland (Hickey, 2014; LeMone et al., 2015). The thalamus is the command center where all sensory impulses are sorted, processed, and relayed to the correct cortical region of the brain. The hypothalamus regulates temperature, water metabolism, thirst, appetite, emotional expressions, and the sleep–wake cycle. The optic chiasm is the location at which the optic nerves cross over each other before they enter the brain. The pineal gland is a

Figure 16–3 The four major regions of the brain.

Table 16–1 Functions of the Regions of the Brain

Region	Functions
Cerebrum	Interprets sensory input Controls skeletal muscle activity Processes intellect and emotions Contains skills memory
Diencephalon	Conducts sensory and motor impulses Regulates autonomic nervous system Regulates and produces hormones Mediates emotional responses
Brainstem	Conduction pathway Regulates respiration Regulates skeletal muscle function
Cerebellum	Processes cognitive information Provides information necessary for balance, posture, and coordination of muscular movement

small endocrine gland that secretes melatonin, a hormone that aids in regulating circadian rhythm (Shoja, Hoepfner, Agutter, Singh, & Tubbs, 2015).

Cerebellum   The cerebellum, located below the occipital lobe of the cerebrum in the posterior cranium, is the second-largest brain structure. The cerebellum is separated from the cerebrum by an extension of the dura mater called the **tentorium cerebelli**. Cerebellar functions include coordination of voluntary skeletal muscle movement, balance and postural stability, and fine motor movement (Crossman & Neary, 2015).

Brainstem   The **brainstem** contains the midbrain, pons, and medulla oblongata. The midbrain regulates auditory and visual functions and serves as the nerve pathway between the cerebral hemispheres and the lower (infratentorial) region of the brain. The pons, which lies just below the midbrain, consists mostly of fiber tracts that control respirations. The medulla oblongata controls heart rate, blood pressure, respirations, and swallowing.

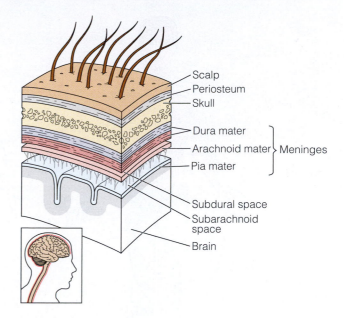

Figure 16–5 The anatomy of the meninges.

Meninges   The **meninges** are a protective connective tissue covering the brain and spinal cord. The meninges form the divisions that separate the lobes and structures of the brain, and contain the venous sinuses. There are three layers of meninges: the dura mater, the arachnoid mater, and the pia mater. The outermost layer is the dense dura mater ("tough mother"), which is rich in nerves and blood vessels and attaches to the inner surface of the skull. The middle layer is the delicate arachnoid mater ("spider mother"), which has no nerves or blood vessels but is composed of delicate connective fibers. Directly below the arachnoid mater is the subarachnoid space. The innermost layer is the pia mater ("tender mother"), which adheres to the brain and the spinal cord and is rich in nerves and blood vessels (Glickstein, 2014). Figure 16–5 displays the layers of the meninges.

Ventricles and Cerebral Spinal Fluid   The brain contains four **ventricles**, which are chambers that contain cerebral spinal fluid (CSF). Each cerebral hemisphere contains a ventricle, as does the midbrain, and the fourth ventricle is the central canal of the spinal cord. The CSF circulates between the ventricles via ducts.

CSF is a clear, colorless fluid that is produced by the choroid plexus, located within the ventricles. It is composed mainly of water but also contains small amounts of protein, sodium, chloride, potassium, bicarbonate, and glucose. Compared with plasma concentrations, CSF concentrations of these elements are lower. This information is helpful when interpreting CSF studies as alterations can indicate pathologic processes. The usual amount of circulating CSF ranges from 80 mL to 200 mL and is replaced several times daily as it is produced and reabsorbed in equal amounts (Marieb & Hoehn, 2013). CSF circulates from the hemispheres to the midbrain, then into both the spinal cord and the subarachnoid space before returning to the blood through the arachnoid villi located within the subarachnoid space. CSF serves to cushion and support

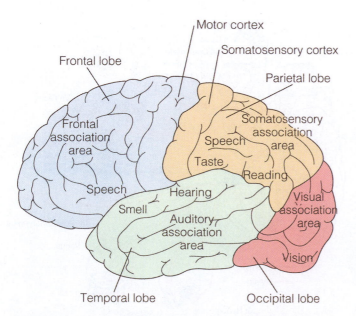

Figure 16–4 Lobes of the cerebrum and functional areas of the cerebral cortex.

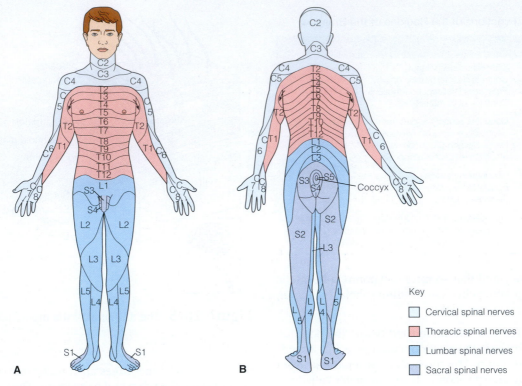

Figure 16–6 Dermatome map.

Key

- ☐ Cervical spinal nerves
- ☐ Thoracic spinal nerves
- ☐ Lumbar spinal nerves
- ☐ Sacral spinal nerves

the brain and spinal cord and protect them from trauma. It also provides homeostatic functions such as nourishing brain tissue, removing by-products of cellular metabolism, and monitoring carbon dioxide levels (Hickey, 2014; LeMone et al., 2015).

Spinal Cord   The spinal cord is centrally located within the spinal cavity of the vertebral column. It extends from the medulla to the level of the first lumbar vertebra and serves as a center for conducting messages to and from the brain and as a reflex center via ascending (sensory) and descending (motor) pathways.

The Peripheral Nervous System

The peripheral nervous system (PNS) functions as a link between the CNS and the organs and limbs. The PNS consists of nerves (cranial and spinal) and peripherally located sensory receptors (outside of the brain and spinal cord). Spinal nerves originate from the spinal cord and contain both sensory and motor fibers, which branch out and innervate the rest of the body. An area of skin innervated by a branch of a single spinal nerve is called a dermatome. Dermatomes (Figure 16–6) provide anatomic landmarks that are useful for locating spinal cord lesions. Cranial nerves (I through XII) originate in the brainstem and primarily innervate the head and neck regions with the exception of the vagus nerve, which innervates the chest and abdominal regions. Some of the cranial nerves are sensory only (I, II, and VIII), and others are mixed sensory and motor. Figure 16–7 shows the origination of the cranial nerves, and Table 16–2 lists the cranial nerves and their related functions.

   Reflexes are rapid, involuntary, predictable motor responses to a stimulus and are categorized as either somatic (result in skeletal muscle contraction) or autonomic (activate cardiac muscle, smooth muscle, or glands). Somatic reflexes mediated by the spinal cord are called spinal reflexes and can occur without impulses traveling to and from the brain. Examples of spinal reflexes are deep tendon reflexes and the withdrawal reflex in response to a noxious stimulus.

The Autonomic Nervous System   The autonomic nervous system (ANS) is a component of the peripheral nervous system and regulates the internal environment of the body. The

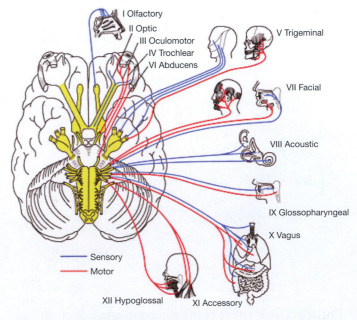

Figure 16–7 Cranial nerves.

Table 16–2 Cranial Nerves and Their Related Functions

Cranial Nerve	Related Functions
I. Olfactory	Sense of smell
II. Optic	Vision
III. Oculomotor	Eyeball movement Raising of upper eyelid Constriction of pupil Proprioception
IV. Trochlear	Eyeball movement
V. Trigeminal	Sensation of scalp, eyelid, nose, cornea Sensation of palate, cheek, top lip, lower eyelid, tongue, chin, chewing
VI. Abducens	Lateral movement of the eyeball
VII. Facial	Movement of facial muscles Taste
VIII. Acoustic	Equilibrium sense Hearing
IX. Glossopharyngeal	Swallowing and gag reflex Saliva secretion Taste Carotid artery receptors to regulate BP
X. Vagus	Swallowing Regulation of heart rate, respirations Digestion and taste Sensation from thoracic and abdominal organs Proprioception
XI. Accessory	Movement of head and neck Proprioception
XII. Hypoglossal	Movement of tongue for speech and swallowing

Table 16–3 Sympathetic and Parasympathetic Nervous System Effects on Target Organs, Systems, and Tissues

Organ, System, or Tissue	Sympathetic Effects	Parasympathetic Effects
Pupils	Dilated	Constricted
Glandular secretions	Inhibited	Stimulated
Heart rate and cardiac output	Increased	Decreased
Coronary arteries	Vasodilation	Vasoconstriction
Bronchial tone	Bronchodilation	Bronchoconstriction
Intestinal peristalsis	Decreased	Increased
Release of glucose by liver	Increased	Decreased
Urine output	Decreased	Increased
Vascular tone	Vasoconstriction	Vasodilation
Blood clotting	Increased	Decreased
Metabolic rate	Increased	Decreased
Mental alertness	Increased	Decreased
Other	Diaphoresis	Increased GI fluid secretion

known as the fight-or-flight response. The parasympathetic nervous system (PNS) aids in digestive functions, sexual arousal, and the body's normal resting state. Table 16–3 lists the effects of the SNS and the PNS on target organ systems and tissues.

ANS is controlled by stimulating the reticular formation in the brainstem, which then initiates reflexes to regulate heart rate, blood vessel diameter, and gastrointestinal function. The ANS further divides into the sympathetic and parasympathetic nervous systems. The sympathetic nervous system (SNS) mediates the stress response by preparing the body to respond to a stimulus that is perceived as harmful. This is

Cerebral Arterial Circulation

Cerebral arteries are structurally different from other arteries in that they are more delicate and, therefore, more susceptible to rupture in the event of intracranial hypertension. The brain is supplied by two major pairs of arteries: anteriorly by the right and left internal carotid arteries and posteriorly by the right and left vertebral arteries (Figure 16–8).

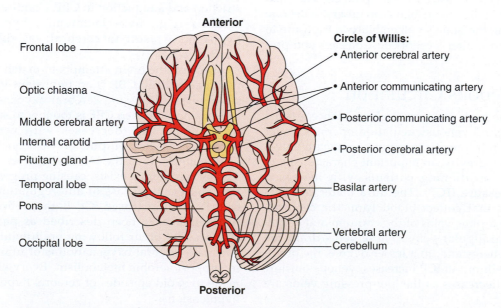

Figure 16–8 Major arteries serving the brain and the circle of Willis.

Together their branches unite within the brain to form the **circle of Willis**, a junction that provides collateral blood flow to either side of the brain. The internal carotid arteries supply the retinas and the anterior two thirds of the cerebrum via its branches: the middle cerebral artery, the anterior cerebral artery, and the anterior and posterior communicating arteries. The middle cerebral arteries (MCAs) are the largest branches of the internal carotids. They supply nearly the entire lateral surface of the frontal, parietal, and temporal lobes; the underlying white matter; and the basal ganglia. The MCAs are the most frequently affected arteries in acute ischemic stroke. The anterior communicating artery connects the anterior cerebral arteries, and the posterior communicating artery joins the posterior cerebral artery (PCA) to complete the circle of Willis. The circle of Willis serves as a protective mechanism because it provides collateral pathways in the event of a large cerebral vessel occlusion.

The vertebrobasilar system supplies the posterior portion of the cerebrum, cerebellum, and brainstem. The vertebral arteries originate from the subclavian arteries, enter the cranium, and join to form the single basilar artery at the pontine–medullary level. The vertebral arteries supply the lateral medulla and a portion of the cerebellum. The basilar artery supplies the pons and cerebellum. It divides at the junction of the pons and midbrain into the PCAs, which supply the midbrain, diencephalon, and inferior portion of the cerebrum. These major arteries are called conducting arteries, and their smaller branches, called penetrating arteries, penetrate into the depths of the brain. Penetrating arteries are frequently involved in small lacunar strokes or transient ischemic attacks

Within the cerebral circulation, the capillary system exhibits selective permeability, allowing it to function as a **blood–brain barrier**. This network of cells and membranes within the cerebral capillary system allows transport of lipids, glucose, amino acids, water, carbon dioxide, and oxygen, thus promoting a homeostatic environment. As a protective mechanism, the blood–brain barrier is impermeable to irritants such as urea, creatinine, proteins, some toxins, and most antibiotics. Brain injury can upset this delicate barrier, increasing the brain's vulnerability to exposure to substances that may alter level of consciousness and promote inflammation.

Cerebral Venous Circulation

Compared to the high-pressure, high-resistance arterial circulation, cerebral venous circulation operates under low-pressure conditions. Craniospinal veins are valveless and drain by gravity, an important characteristic to consider when positioning patients with increased **intracranial pressure (ICP)**. The dura mater contains venous sinuses that collect blood from the cerebral, meningeal, and diploic veins of the cranium and empty into the internal jugular veins. These veins drain the cerebral hemispheres and, to a lesser degree, the brainstem and cerebellum. As ICP increases, venous outflow from the brain decreases as the low-pressure veins are compressed.

Cerebral Oxygenation

Due to its limited glucose reserves and inability to store oxygen, the brain depends on a continuous supply of glucose, oxygen, and substrates. Cerebral metabolism varies regionally, with some areas of the brain being more metabolically active than others at any given time. **Cerebral blood flow (CBF)**, or blood flow to the brain, also varies regionally. The brain attempts to meet metabolic demands by locally increasing or decreasing CBF as needed. This localized matching of CBF with metabolism is achieved through the process of cerebral **autoregulation**. Autoregulation enables cerebral arterioles to alter blood flow within a cerebral perfusion pressure (CPP) limit (60 to 160 mmHg in adults) to promote a constant blood supply to the brain, regardless of systemic blood pressure fluctuations. In normotensive adults, cerebral blood flow is maintained at approximately 50 mL per 100 g of brain tissue per minute, provided CPP is in the range of 60 to 160 mmHg. Above and below this limit, autoregulation is lost and cerebral blood flow becomes dependent on mean arterial pressure in a linear fashion. In a person with functional autoregulation, as systemic blood pressure increases, cerebral arterioles constrict; conversely, as systemic blood pressure decreases, cerebral arterioles dilate, ensuring adequate cerebral perfusion. When CBF is inadequate to meet the brain's metabolic needs, a mismatch occurs, resulting in cerebral ischemia. Unable to maintain aerobic metabolism due to its limited glucose stores and inability to store oxygen, the brain is forced to convert to anaerobic metabolism. As lactate accumulates within the brain parenchyma, cerebral acidosis upsets the delicate equilibrium within the cranial vault.

Autoregulation enables the brain to maintain constant CBF despite changes in systemic metabolism and altered acid–base balance. An increase in basal metabolic rate (e.g., fever, pain) increases CBF, whereas a decrease in basal metabolic rate (e.g., sedation, paralysis, hypothermia) decreases CBF. Conditions that induce alkalosis (e.g., hypocapnia) result in cerebral vasoconstriction and a reduction in CBF. Conditions that induce acidosis (e.g., hyperlactatemia, hypercapnia, and hypoxemia) result in cerebral vasodilation and an increase in CBF.

Because the brain attempts to match CBF with cerebral metabolism, CBF is an important variable to consider when addressing cerebral oxygenation. Cerebral hypoxia occurs when CBF is too low to support cerebral metabolism. CBF decreases with cerebral edema, decreased cardiac output, or vasoconstriction. When CBF is higher than the metabolic needs of the brain, a state of **hyperemia** exists, causing progressive vasodilation and eventual loss of autoregulation, all of which contribute to increased ICP. Both cerebral hypoxia and hyperemia have been described as pathophysiologic changes that occur following brain injury. Maintaining adequate cerebral oxygenation is of utmost importance to support aerobic metabolism. Every effort should be made to avoid episodes of cerebral hypoxia or systemic hypotension.

Section One Review

1. Which structure is protective because it is the primary collateral pathway when major cerebral vessels are occluded?
   A. Circle of Willis
   B. Left internal carotid artery
   C. Right internal carotid artery
   D. Middle cerebral artery

2. Why are cerebral arteries more prone to rupture during hypertension?
   A. There are so many of them.
   B. They have autoregulation.
   C. They are thin and delicate.
   D. They are not protected by skeletal muscles.

3. Which statement about the venous circulation of the brain is correct?
   A. Craniospinal veins have valves.
   B. Craniospinal veins drain by gravity.
   C. It is a high-pressure system.
   D. It contains a high oxygen concentration.

4. The localized matching of CBF with cerebral metabolism occurs through which means?
   A. Autoregulation
   B. Anaerobic metabolism
   C. Luxury perfusion
   D. Cerebrospinal fluid

Answers: 1. A, 2. C, 3. B, 4. A

Section Two: Intracranial and Cerebral Perfusion Pressures

Two pressures within the cranial vault that significantly impact neurological status are intracranial pressure and cerebral perfusion pressure. Intracranial pressure (ICP) is the pressure exerted by the soft contents within the cranial vault against the rigid cranial bones. Cerebral perfusion pressure (CPP) is the amount of pressure utilized in providing blood flow to the brain. CPP is defined as mean arterial pressure (MAP) minus ICP.

Intracranial Pressure

The intracranial vault consists of a limited space within a rigid container. The contents of the intracranial vault include the brain, cerebral blood, and cerebrospinal fluid. The combination of the three intracranial component volumes forms the total intracranial volume and ICP.

Monro–Kellie Hypothesis The volume of each intracranial component remains relatively stable, with the following approximate volume percentages: brain, 80%; blood, 10%; and CSF, 10%. The Monro–Kellie hypothesis (or doctrine) states that a change in volume of any one of these components must be accompanied by a reciprocal change in one or both of the other components. If this reciprocal change is not accomplished, the net result is an increase in ICP.

Brain Volume. Brain volume is primarily composed of water, the majority of which is intracellular. Brain volume is regulated by the blood–brain barrier, which controls solutes and water attempting to enter cerebral circulation. Disruption of the barrier by trauma or metabolic abnormalities (e.g., drug overdose) results in increased brain volume. Fluid escapes from the intravascular space into the interstitial space of the brain parenchyma, resulting in cerebral edema. According to the Monro–Kellie hypothesis, there is limited space within the cranial vault; therefore, an increase in brain volume necessitates a compensatory decrease in either cerebral blood volume or CSF volume (or both) to maintain a normal ICP. If compensatory mechanisms are insufficient, ICP continues to increase.

Cerebral Blood Volume. Cerebral blood volume is the amount of blood in the cranial vault at any point in time. Cerebral blood volume is maintained at a constant level through cerebral blood flow (CBF). Recall from Section One that CBF is normally regulated by the process of pressure and chemical autoregulation. Conditions that affect cerebral blood flow and blood volume are summarized in Table 16–4.

Table 16–4 Conditions That Affect Cerebral Blood Flow and Cerebral Blood Volume

Increased CBF and CBV	Decreased CBF and CBV
Systemic hypertension	Systemic hypotension
Increase in body metabolic rate (fever, pain)	Decrease in body metabolic rate (sedation, paralysis, hypothermia)
Systemic acidosis (hypercapnia, ischemia)	Systemic alkalosis (hypocapnia) Cerebral edema Low cardiac output
Cerebral vasodilation	Cerebral vasoconstriction

CBF = cerebral blood flow, CBV = cerebral blood volume.

Cerebrospinal Fluid. Cerebrospinal fluid (CSF) is the third component of intracranial volume. Recall that CSF circulates in the subarachnoid spaces and spinal cord and is then resorbed into the venous system. Of the three components in the cranial vault, CSF is the most readily displaced and is absorbed into the external jugular veins. This explains why neck flexion or obstructive medical devices, such as tight endotracheal tube ties or cervical collars, can obstruct CSF outflow, as well as venous return, and increase ICP.

Normal ICP ranges from 0 to 15 mmHg. ICP greater than 15 mmHg in adults for more than 5 minutes is considered abnormally elevated. Treatment is required when ICP is greater than 20 mmHg. Transient elevations in ICP greater than 10 to 15 mmHg due to coughing or suctioning are considered normal if not sustained. It is important to understand that ICP is a dynamic variable and fluctuates constantly in response to changes in respiratory rate, body position, and activities such as coughing and sneezing. Whereas ICP is a fluctuating phenomenon, intracranial volume remains relatively stable by reciprocal compensation, the principle outlined in the Monro–Kellie hypothesis. In the adult, the combined volume of CSF, blood, and brain tissue measures approximately 1700 to 1900 mL. By decreasing the volume of one or more of the other brain components, the total brain volume remains stable.

As this principle states, reciprocal compensation can occur in any one of the three compartments. Although under normal circumstances the three intracranial components are kept in dynamic equilibrium, when ICP approaches 30 mmHg the components can no longer adapt to increases in volume. At this point, compliance is lost and ICP increases. This is considered a decompensated state in which normal autoregulation has failed (Zweifel, Dias, Smielewski, & Czosnyka, 2014). Box 16–1 illustrates the causes of increased intracranial pressure.

Cerebral Perfusion Pressure

Cerebral perfusion pressure (CPP) is defined as the pressure gradient associated with cerebral blood flow (CBF) that is necessary to supply an adequate amount of blood to the brain. CPP is calculated by finding the difference between mean arterial pressure (MAP) and ICP as shown in Box 16-2.

The average adult CPP is 80 mmHg, with a normal range between 70 and 100 mmHg (Hemphill, Smith, & Gress, 2015). Although what is considered an adequate CPP in the patient with acute neurologic injury remains controversial, the generally accepted recommendation is to maintain CPP greater than 70 mmHg to ensure adequate cerebral oxygenation. However, aggressive attempts to maintain CPP above 70 mmHg should be avoided, especially in the patient with impaired cerebral autoregulation, and a target CPP of 50 to 70 mmHg may be more appropriate (American College of Surgeons, 2015). Aggressive measures to maintain CPP greater than 70 mmHg, including vasopressors and IV fluids, increases the permeability of the pulmonary alveolar–capillary membrane, allowing increased accumulation of lung water, which can compromise gas exchange and increase risk for acute respiratory distress syndrome

---

BOX 16–1 Causes of Increased Intracranial Pressure

Cranial surgery

- Blood clot or hematomas
- Pneumocephalus (air)
- Cerebral edema

Increased CBF

- Increased BP
- Increased $PaCO_2$
- Decreased PaO_2
- Vasodilator drugs (nitroprusside, nitroglycerine)

Increased intra-thoracic or intra-abdominal pressure

- Coughing
- Straining (Valsalva)
- Suctioning
- PEEP
- Hip flexion

Decreased cerebral venous drainage

- Supine position with head of bed flat
- Neck flexion or rotation

BOX 16–2 Calculating Mean Arterial Pressure (MAP) and Cerebral Perfusion Pressure (CPP)

The following formula is used to calculate MAP:

$$MAP = (systolic\ BP + 2[diastolic\ BP])/3$$

CPP is calculated using the following formula:

$$CPP = MAP - ICP$$

(ARDS). ARDS results from indirect (extrapulmonary) lung injury in the setting of systemic inflammatory response to traumatic brain injury or multiple trauma (Fish & Talmor, 2017). Cerebral perfusion is decreased when ICP is high or MAP is low. Cerebral perfusion increases when ICP is low or MAP is high. If the ICP rises to the level of MAP, brain perfusion ceases and brain death results.

Consider the following scenario: Your patient has an ICP of 10 mmHg and a blood pressure of 120/80 mmHg. The calculation of CPP is as follows:

$$CPP = MAP - ICP$$
$$MAP = (SBP + 2[DBP])/3$$

The MAP is 93 because 120 + 2(80) = 280/3 = 93. The CPP in this situation would be 83 because 93 − 10 = 83. CPP is within normal range. Decreased CPP requires prompt recognition and treatment. Interventions for patients with decreased CPP include mechanisms to increase MAP and reduce ICP.

Section Two Review

1. According to the Monro–Kellie hypothesis, an increase in one intracranial compartment must be accompanied by which reciprocal action?
   A. Decrease in another compartment
   B. Increase in the blood–brain barrier
   C. Decrease in the blood–brain barrier
   D. Increase in another compartment

2. ICP remains relatively stable, and under normal conditions it is usually less than what amount?
   A. 5 mmHg
   B. 15 mmHg
   C. 30 mmHg
   D. 50 mmHg

3. What are the components within the cranial vault? (Select all that apply.)
   A. Blood
   B. Bone
   C. Brain tissue
   D. Cerebrospinal fluid
   E. Lacrimal fluid

4. Which situation would cause an increase in ICP?
   A. Decreased cerebral blood flow
   B. Decreased CSF production
   C. Increased cerebral venous drainage
   D. Increased intrathoracic pressure

Answers: 1. A, 2. B, 3. (A, C, D), 4. D

Section Three: Assessment of Cerebral Tissue Perfusion

Decreased cerebral perfusion pressure (CPP) requires prompt recognition. It is important to have a basic understanding of the techniques used to detect decreased cerebral tissue perfusion and increased intracranial pressure. This section describes a focused neurological assessment and provides an overview of the types of systems used for monitoring ICP and brain tissue oxygenation.

Level of Consciousness

Level of **consciousness** is the most important component of the neurologic assessment in the high-acuity patient. This assessment must be performed and documented in a reliable and consistent manner to provide an accurate transfer of information from clinician to clinician. Often a change in level of consciousness is the first sign of neurologic deterioration. In the high-acuity environment, assessment of level of consciousness is part of the recurring systems assessments performed by the nurse. The following are the common etiologies for impaired consciousness and their mnemonics:

Alcohol, **E**pilepsy, **I**nsulin, **O**piates, **U**remia (A-E-I-O-U)

Tumor, **I**njury, **P**sychological, **S**troke, **S**epsis (TIPSS)

Components of Consciousness There are two components of consciousness: arousal (alertness) and content (awareness).

Arousal. The term **arousal** refers to the component of consciousness concerned with an individual's ability to respond to environmental stimuli, such as opening the eyes to speech or turning the head toward a noise. Assessment of the arousal component of consciousness involves an evaluation of the **reticular activating system (RAS)**. The RAS is a diffuse collection of neuronal circuitry extending from the brainstem to the cerebral cortex and is vital for maintaining wakefulness

(Maldonato, 2014). Conditions that affect arousal do so by directly or indirectly depressing the brainstem structures and the reticular activating system. These conditions, if severe, could result in immediate loss of consciousness and produce coma. Any condition that impairs arousal will naturally impair content as well. Processes that impair arousal may include mass lesions that compress brainstem structures, medications that may temporarily depress the RAS, or any other process that involves the brainstem and/or cerebral hemispheres and produces a depressed level of consciousness. Table 16–5 lists the various labels or terms used to describe levels of consciousness (LOC). Labels like *comatose*, *lethargic*, and *stuporous* lend themselves to subjective interpretation, thus should be interpreted or used with caution because of the subjective interpretations.

The Glasgow Coma Scale (GCS) is the most frequently used assessment tool to identify changes in arousal. The scale assesses eye opening, verbal response, and best motor response to stimuli (Table 16–6). The scale ranges from 3 to 15, with a score of 15 indicating the best possible score for level of consciousness and 3 indicating the lowest score with the worst score. A score less than 8 is consistent with a significant alteration in level of consciousness (coma state) and severe brain injury. Any deterioration in the GCS score is significant and requires immediate provider notification to allow for early intervention and prevention of further neurologic decline. Certain patient conditions may affect the validity of the GCS. For example, patients with periorbital edema who are unable to open their eyes receive an eye opening response score of 1, which may or may not be valid. It is impossible to evaluate a verbal response for patients who are intubated or have a tracheostomy; they also receive a score of 1, which may not be a valid reflection of the patient's true level of consciousness (Munakomi & Kumar, 2015).

The first step is to determine what stimulus arouses the patient. First, address the patient by name. If the patient does not respond, shake an arm or shoulder gently. If no response is elicited, proceed from light pain to deeper pain in an attempt to elicit a response. If it is determined that a patient cannot comprehend and/or follow a simple command, the

Table 16–5 Terms Used to Describe Level of Consciousness

Full consciousness	Alert; oriented to time, place, and person; comprehends spoken and written words
Confusion	Unable to think rapidly and clearly; easily bewildered, with poor memory and short attention span; misinterprets stimuli; judgment impaired
Disorientation	Not aware of or not oriented to time, place, or person
Obtundation	Lethargic, somnolent; responsive to verbal or tactile stimuli but quickly drifts back to sleep
Stupor	Generally unresponsive; may be briefly aroused by vigorous, repeated, or painful stimuli; may withdraw (shrink away from) or localize (grab at) the source of stimuli
Semicomatose	Does not move spontaneously; unresponsive to stimuli, although vigorous or painful stimuli may result in stirring, moaning, or withdrawal from the stimuli, without actual arousal
Coma	Unarousable; will not stir or moan in response to any stimulus; may exhibit nonpurposeful response (slight movement) of area stimulated but makes no attempt to withdraw
Deep coma	Completely unarousable and unresponsive to any kind of stimulus, including pain; absence of brainstem, corneal, pupillary, pharyngeal, tendon, and plantar reflexes

use of noxious or painful stimuli is necessary to determine the patient's best motor response. It is important to vary the means of eliciting a response and to document the type of stimuli, location, and duration of time it was applied to illicit the response. If it becomes necessary to apply the stimulus for a longer time, a potential deterioration of the patient's neurological status should be suspected and appropriate actions taken (Hickey, 2014).

Central stimulation involves applying a painful stimulus to the central portion or trunk of the body to produce an overall body response. This type of stimulation tests the ability of the brain to respond to a noxious stimulus (Hickey, 2014). Examples of central noxious stimulation include but are not limited to the following:

- *Trapezius pinch*—administered by firmly squeezing or pinching the trapezius muscle
- *Sternal rub*—administered by applying firm pressure with an open hand to the sternum in a rubbing motion
- *Supraorbital pressure*—administered by pressing the thumb under the upper part of the ocular orbit; should be avoided in patients with facial fractures, frontal craniotomies, or glaucoma

It is important to note that pinching or twisting of the areolae to provide a noxious stimulus should be avoided.

Peripheral stimulation is delivered to the extremities, such as in the application of pressure to the nail beds. Response to this type of stimulus means that a functioning spinal cord exists or that the lesion is not complete (Hickey, 2014).

Central and peripheral stimulation are often combined during a neurological assessment, and the least noxious form of stimulation should be used first, proceeding to a more intense or increased stimulus until a response is noted. For example, the nurse would first call the patient's name and shake the arm, then apply nail bed pressure, and finally apply the trapezius pinch. This approach assesses two things: Is the patient responsive to verbal stimuli? If not, does the patient exhibit purposeful movement? Purposeful movement, such as removing the stimulus or withdrawing from the stimulus, indicates functioning of sensory pathways.

Abnormal posturing in response to a noxious stimulus indicates a dysfunction of either the cerebral hemispheres or the brainstem. **Decorticate posturing** (abnormal flexion) indicates cerebral hemispheric dysfunction. In response to painful stimuli, the upper arms move up toward the chest with the elbows, wrists, and fingers flexed. The legs extend with internal rotation and plantar flexion (feet extend downward; as shown in Figure 16–9A). **Decerebrate posturing** (abnormal extension) indicates brainstem dysfunction and is a more ominous sign. With decerebrate posturing, the arms pronate and extend straight out, wrists

Table 16–6 Glasgow Coma Scale

Category	Score	Response
Eye opening	4	Spontaneous—eyes open spontaneously without stimulation
	3	To speech—eyes open with verbal stimulation but not necessarily to command
	2	To pain—eyes open with noxious stimuli
	1	None—no eye opening regardless of stimulation
Verbal response	5	Oriented—accurate information about person, place, time, reason for hospitalization, and personal data
	4	Confused—answers not appropriate to question but correct use of language
	3	Inappropriate words—disorganized, random speech, no sustained conversation
	2	Incomprehensible sounds—moans, groans, and mumbles incomprehensibly
	1	None—no verbalization despite stimulation
Best motor response	6	Obeys commands—performs simple tasks, response on command; able to repeat performance
	5	Localizes to pain—organized attempt to localize and remove painful stimuli
	4	Withdraws from pain—withdraws extremity from source of painful stimuli
	3	Abnormal flexion—decorticate posturing spontaneously or in response to noxious stimuli
	2	Extension—decerebrate posturing spontaneously or in response to noxious stimuli
	1	None—no response to noxious stimuli; flaccid

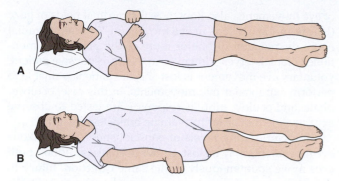

Figure 16–9 Decorticate and decerebrate posturing.
A, Decorticate (abnormal flexion)—upper arms move upward to the chest; elbows, wrists, and fingers flex; legs may extend with internal rotation; feet plantar flexed.
B, Decerebrate (abnormal extension)—arms pronate and extend straight out away from the chest; wrists and fingers flex; feet plantar flexed.

and fingers flex, and legs extend with plantar flexion (see Figure 16–9B). Patients may exhibit a "combination" of posturing, with components of both decerebrate and decorticate, depending on the level of the injury.

Content. Assessment of the content (cognitive) component of consciousness is an evaluation of the cerebral hemispheres. **Content**, a higher level of functioning than arousal, centers on the patient's orientation to time, place, and person. Content is sometimes referred to as awareness. The patient should respond to questions appropriately; any sign of disorientation may be the first indication of neurologic deterioration.

Conditions that impair content do so by widely affecting the cerebral hemispheres. Alterations are manifested by cognitive deficits such as memory impairment, disorientation, impaired problem-solving abilities, and attentional deficits. The degree of cognitive deficit is related to the location and size of the lesion. Lesions that affect small areas of the hemispheres usually do not produce a significant depression in the level of consciousness. Hemispheric strokes and small intracerebral hematomas and contusions result in localized deficits. Conditions that diffusely affect the hemispheres cause a significant depression in the level of consciousness and may result in coma. Anoxia, ischemia, metabolic alterations, ingested poisons, substance abuse, and psychiatric disturbances may all contribute to diffuse cerebral hemispheric dysfunction (Hickey, 2014).

The content of consciousness is assessed by noting behavior and verbal responses. The patient should be assessed for orientation and should know his or her name, the date, and where she or he is. The patient is considered disoriented if unable to answer the questions correctly. Testing for orientation also assesses short-term memory. Orientation can be assessed only if the patient is able to respond in some meaningful way, such as verbally, in writing, or by pointing to choices on a picture board. After assessing orientation, the ability to follow commands is assessed. Ask the patient to perform acts such as sticking out the tongue or holding up two fingers. This not only helps determine whether the patient is awake enough to respond but also whether he or she is aware enough to interpret and carry out the commands. Next, behavioral changes

are assessed by noting any restlessness, irritability, or combativeness. Although the following is not an all-inclusive list, such behavioral indicators can be caused by hypoxia, hypoglycemia, substance abuse or withdrawal, pain, or increased ICP (Hickey, 2014). In the high-acuity environment, the nurse must remain vigilant for behavioral changes that could indicate alterations in cerebral homeostasis.

The final component of content assessment is speech. Assessment of speech provides information about the functional relationship between the speech centers in the cerebrum and the cranial nerves, which can help localize the area of dysfunction. The patient's speech pattern is assessed for clarity. Slurred or garbled speech may indicate substance use, metabolic disturbance, stroke, or cranial nerve injuries. Content of speech is assessed for use of appropriate or inappropriate words. Confused patients may use inappropriate words. Patients with cranial nerve dysfunction may give appropriate responses; however, the speech pattern may be slurred. Patients may experience receptive, expressive, or global aphasia. Inability to understand written or spoken words is **Wernicke's** (receptive) **aphasia**. Inability to express language through speech or writing is called **Broca's** (expressive) **aphasia**. These aphasias are named for the region of the brain from which the aphasia originates. **Global aphasia** includes the inability to articulate or comprehend language (Chatterjee & Coslett, 2014).

In-depth Clinical Assessment

Beyond the assessment of arousal and content, a more in-depth neurological assessment includes assessments of pupillary and oculomotor reactions, vital signs, and cranial nerve reflexes.

Pupillary Reactions Pupillary reactions provide information about the location of lesions or mass effect from cerebral edema, resulting in increased ICP. Elevated ICP can cause compression of cranial nerves, resulting in abnormal pupillary reactions to light. Pupils are assessed for size, symmetry, shape, accommodation, and reaction to light. Pupil size is assessed using a standard pupil gauge (Figure 16–10). Pupils should be midline and equal in size. Abnormal pupil responses are shown in Figure 16–11. If both pupils are nonreactive (fixed)—meaning they do not constrict in response to a light source and are midline—damage to the midbrain is indicated. Remember that certain drugs (atropine, epinephrine) can dilate the pupils. Pupils that are constricted (nonreactive to light and pinpoint in size) can indicate a pons lesion or opiate drug overdose (Figure 16–11A). When both pupils are dilated (see Figure 16–11B) and fixed, emergency action is required, as this may be caused by severe anoxia or ischemia. A unilaterally dilated and fixed pupil may indicate compression of the oculomotor nerve (cranial nerve III; see Figure 16–11C) on the same side (ipsilateral) as the lesion.

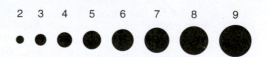

Figure 16–10 Pupil gauge in millimeters.

A

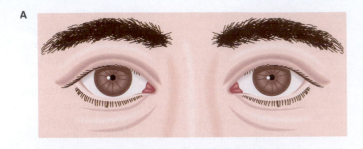

B

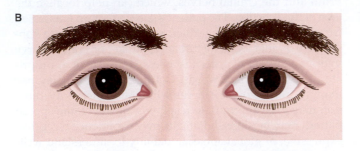

C

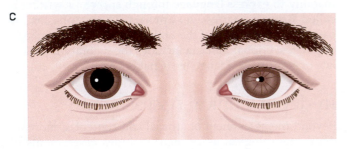

Figure 16–11 Abnormal pupil responses. A, Constricted (pinpoint). B, Dilated. C, Unequal.

Oculomotor Responses   Two reflexes used to determine brainstem integrity are the oculovestibular (caloric) and oculocephalic (doll's eyes) reflexes. Both reflexes involve cranial nerves III (oculomotor), IV (trochlear), VI (abducens), and VIII (acoustic). In the awake patient, it is easy to test these cranial nerves by asking the patient to perform a full range of eye movements, also known as the cardinal fields of gaze (Figure 16–12). Deficits in eye movements indicate a cranial nerve dysfunction of one or more of the previously mentioned cranial nerves. However, in the unresponsive patient, voluntary eye movement is lost and the patient is unable to perform extraocular eye movements. In this case, oculocephalic and oculovestibular responses are tested to observe eye movement in order to evaluate brainstem integrity.

In deteriorating levels of consciousness, spontaneous eye movements may be lost. Under normal conditions, both eyes move spontaneously in the same direction. Injury to the midbrain and pons impairs normal movement. **Doll's eye movements** (oculocephalic reflex) are reflexive movements of the eyes in the opposite direction of head rotation. This reflex is tested by holding the patient's eyes open and briskly turning the head from side to side, pausing at each side. If the patient has an intact brainstem, the examiner sees conjugate eye movement opposite to the side the head is turned, known as "full doll's eyes" (Figure 16–13). In cases of brainstem injury, the eyes will remain fixed in the midposition as the head is turned, and doll's eyes are absent. This test is contraindicated in patients whose cervical spine has not been cleared of injury.

Another reflex, the **oculovestibular reflex** (cold caloric test), may be performed when determining brainstem function. Instilling cold water into the ear canal causes **nystagmus** (involuntary, rapid, repetitive movements of the eyes) toward the stimulus. This reflex is absent when brainstem function is lost. The oculovestibular reflex is a sensitive indicator of brainstem function and central nervous system injury. Patients with an absent oculocephalic reflex may have a normal oculovestibular reflex; therefore, testing for the oculovestibular reflex always follows testing for the oculocephalic reflex. Testing the oculovestibular reflex is contraindicated if CSF or purulent drainage is leaking from the ear, or if there is perforation or a tear of the tympanic membrane.

Results of oculocephalic or oculovestibular testing are interpreted with caution because pharmacologic agents such as ototoxic drugs, neuromuscular blockers, and ethyl alcohol depress these reflexes.

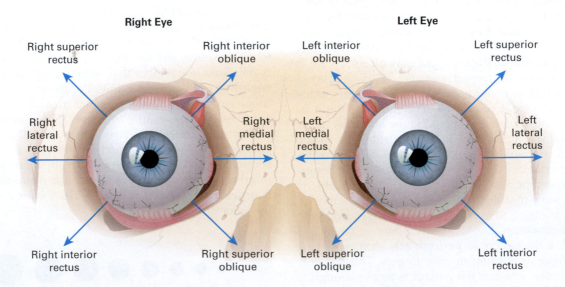

Figure 16–12 Cardinal fields of gaze.

Head in neutral position

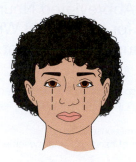

Eyes midline

Head rotated to patient's left

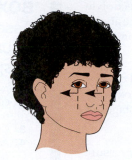

Doll's eyes present:
Eyes move right in
relation to head.

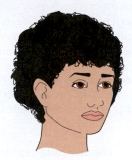

Doll's eyes absent:
Eyes do not move
in relation to head.
Direction of vision follows
head to left.

Figure 16–13 Testing the oculocephalic reflex (doll's eye movement). Absent doll's eye movements are characteristic of brainstem injury.

Vital Signs Routine parameters assessed in the high-acuity patient include respiratory rate and pattern, heart rate and rhythm, oxygen saturation, blood pressure, and temperature. Because the brainstem influences the cardiovascular and respiratory systems, changes in vital signs may indicate neurologic deterioration.

Respirations. Respiratory pattern provides valuable information because it correlates with the anatomic level of dysfunction. Respiratory rhythm and pattern, which are controlled by the medulla, are counted for 1 full minute before stimulating the patient. Common abnormal respiratory patterns observed in neurologically impaired patients are discussed in the following list and depicted in Table 16–7. As a nurse, remember that it is more important to describe the pattern than to fit the patient's respiratory pattern into a category. If the patient is mechanically ventilated, it is difficult to observe these patterns and would be extremely detrimental to the patient to remove ventilatory support for the purpose of assessing abnormal patterns. Deteriorating respiratory patterns are as follows:

- *Cheyne–Stokes respirations* are evidenced by a rhythmic waxing and waning in the depth of the respiration, followed by a period of apnea. This pattern indicates a bilateral lesion in the cerebral hemispheres, cerebellum,

midbrain, or, in rare circumstances, upper pons, and it may be caused by cerebral infarction or metabolic disease.

- *Central neurogenic hyperventilation* is evidenced by regular, rapid respirations (greater than 24) that increase in depth. Central neurogenic hyperventilation indicates a lesion in the low midbrain or upper pons and may be caused by infarction or ischemia of the midbrain or pons, anoxia, or tumors of the midbrain.

- *Apneustic breathing* is evidenced by prolonged inspiration with a pause at the point where the respiration is at its peak, lasting for 2 to 3 seconds. This may alternate with an expiratory pause. Apneustic breathing indicates a lesion in the mid or low pons that may be caused by infarction of the pons or severe meningitis.

- *Cluster breathing* is described as "clusters" of irregular breathing with periods of apnea that occur at irregular intervals. This pattern indicates a lesion in the low pons or upper medulla that may be caused by a tumor or infarction of the medulla.

- *Ataxic breathing* is completely irregular, with deep and shallow random breaths and pauses. Ataxic breathing indicates a lesion in the medulla that may be caused by a cerebellar or pons bleed, tumors of the cerebrum, or severe meningitis.

Table 16–7 Abnormal Respiratory Patterns

Pattern		Description
Cheyne-Stokes respirations	～∧∧∧∧∧—∧∧∧—	A regular crescendo–decrescendo pattern with increasing, then decreasing, rate and depth of respirations followed by a period of apnea
Central neurogena hyperventilation	∧∧∧∧∧∧∧∧∧∧∧∧∧	A sustained pattern of rapid, regular, deep respirations (hyperpnea)
Apneustic breathing	⊓_⊓_⊓_	Prolonged inspiration with a pause at full inspiration followed by expiration and a possible pause following expiration
Cluster breathing	‖‖‖_‖‖‖_‖‖	Clusters of several breaths with irregular periods of apnea between clusters
Ataxic breathing	∧_∧_∧∧_∧	Respirations that are completely irregular in pattern and depth with irregular periods of apnea

Remember that abnormal respiratory patterns may also be initiated by conditions such as acid–base and electrolyte imbalances, anxiety, pulmonary disease, or substance abuse, especially narcotics and anesthetic agents that depress the respiratory center (Urden, Stacy, & Lough, 2013).

Pulse. The pulse is assessed for rate, rhythm, and quality. Increased heart rate may indicate poor cerebral oxygenation. Decreased heart rate is present in the late stages of increased ICP.

Blood Pressure. The medulla regulates blood pressure based on input from special receptors that are sensitive to changes in oxygen, carbon dioxide, and pH in the blood (chemoreceptors) and blood pressure changes (baroreceptors). Mean arterial pressure must be maintained at a sufficient level to produce adequate cerebral tissue perfusion when ICP is elevated. Cerebral trauma is rarely associated with hypotension; on the contrary, cerebral trauma typically produces systemic hypertension. An important response to ischemia, known as the **Cushing's triad**, is a classic syndrome of increased ICP characterized by a specific change in vital signs evidenced by (1) an increase in systolic blood pressure, usually with a widening pulse pressure, (2) irregular respirations, and (3) bradycardia. The combination of an increase in systolic blood pressure and a decrease in the diastolic blood pressure is also known as *widening pulse* pressure. This response is activated when ICP rises to a point where it equals or exceeds MAP. Signs of a widening pulse pressure should alert the vigilant high-acuity nurse of impending brain herniation in the setting of severe intracranial hypertension (Hickey, 2014).

Temperature. The hypothalamus is the center for temperature regulation. Injury to or dysfunction of the hypothalamus produces alterations in body temperature. Hypothermia occurs as a result of spinal shock, metabolic coma, drug overdose (especially CNS depressants), and destructive lesions of the brainstem or hypothalamus. Hyperthermia occurs as a result of CNS infection, subarachnoid hemorrhage, hypothalamic lesions, or hemorrhage of the hypothalamus or brainstem. Temperature fluctuates widely and may exceed 106°F (41°C). Hyperthermia is treated promptly, as an increase in temperature and metabolic demand can lead to further cerebral hypoxia and secondary brain injury.

An abbreviated neurological assessment (Box 16–3) can be performed on patients in whom a neurological impairment is not suspected or diagnosed as well as in between more comprehensive neurological assessments. Manifestations of progressive deterioration in brain function are summarized in Table 16–8.

Cranial Nerve Reflexes Cranial nerve reflexes are protective reflexes indicative of brainstem functioning. The unresponsive patient is assessed for the presence of these reflexes, and if they are absent or decreased, measures must be taken to protect the patient from injury. The protective reflexes include (1) corneal reflex (blink), (2) gag reflex, (3) swallow reflex, and (4) cough reflex. The corneal reflex is assessed by touching the cornea, from the side, with a sterile wisp of cotton. The eye blinks rapidly if the reflex is intact. The gag reflex is assessed by touching the posterior tongue with a tongue blade. If intact, the patient gags. The cough and gag reflexes can also be assessed while suctioning the intubated patient. The swallow reflex

BOX 16–3 Abbreviated Neurologic Assessment for Patients in Whom a Neurologic Impairment Is Not Suspected

1. Assess LOC (response to auditory and/or tactile stimulus).
2. Obtain vital signs (blood pressure, pulse, respirations, pulse oximetry).
3. Check pupillary response to light.
4. Assess strength of hand grip and movement of extremities bilaterally.
5. Determine ability to sense touch or pain in extremities.

Table 16–8 Manifestations of Progressive Deterioration in Brain Function

Level of Consciousness	Pupillary Response	Oculomotor Responses	Motor Responses	Breathing
Alert, oriented to time, place, person	Equal, round, reactive to light	Eyes move as head turns	Purposeful movements; responds to commands	Regular rate, pattern
Responds to verbal stimuli; episodes of confusion, restlessness	Equal, round, reactive to light progressing to small, reactive	Caloric testing produces nystagmus	Purposeful movement in response to pain	Yawning, sighing
Requires continuous stimulation to rouse	Small, reactive, progressing to slowing response to light (sluggish)	Roving eye movements	Decorticate posturing	Cheyne–Stokes
Reflexive posturing to pain stimulus	Ipsilateral dilation; fixed (nonreactive)	Roving or no eye movements	Decerebrate posturing	Central neurologic hyperventilation
No response to stimuli	Bilateral dilation and fixation	No spontaneous eye movements; eyes fixed in midposition; absent doll's eyes. No eye movements to cold caloric testing	Flaccidity	Cluster or ataxic breathing; apnea

SOURCE: Data from Barker (2008).

can be initially assessed by observing the patient dry-swallowing or by instilling a small volume of water into the mouth and having the patient swallow repeatedly. During the swallowing, the patient may be observed for the ability to swallow, choking, changes in breathing, or the number of swallows over an established period of time (e.g., 30 seconds) (LeMone et al., 2015). Video fluoroscopy of swallowing may also be performed to determine the exact swallowing problem. In the mechanically ventilated patient, the swallow reflex is not routinely tested secondary to risk for aspiration.

Intracranial Pressure Monitoring

Intracranial pressure monitoring provides continuous, real-time ICP data, which can be used to direct medical or surgical therapy. The primary reasons for ICP monitoring are (1) to assist in calculating and maintaining adequate CPP and (2) to promote early detection and treatment of increased ICP. Continuous ICP monitoring allows titration of therapies to maintain adequate cerebral perfusion, subsequently preventing cerebral ischemia. ICP monitoring promotes the identification of impending brain herniation secondary to escalating ICP, determines the need for and impact of ICP treatment modalities, and aids in predicting patient outcomes. Although ICP monitoring provides meaningful clinical data in the patient with the potential for altered CPP, not all patients are appropriate candidates for ICP monitoring. Current guidelines recommend that ICP monitoring may be appropriate in (1) patients suffering from traumatic brain injury with a GCS of 8 or less with evidence of structural brain abnormalities on the initial head CT scan or (2) patients with evidence of altered cerebral tissue perfusion who have a normal head CT scan and two or more of the following: age greater than 40 years, unilateral or bilateral motor posturing, or systolic blood pressure less than 90 mmHg (American College of Surgeons, 2015; Moussazadeh, Stieg, & Mangat, 2017).

ICP Monitoring Devices Intracranial pressure (ICP) monitoring is classified by the anatomic placement of the internal

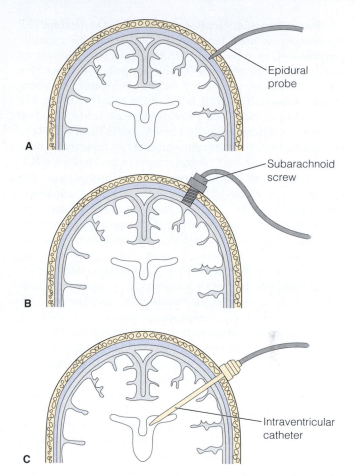

Figure 16–14 Types of intracranial pressure monitoring. A, Epidural probe. B, Subarachnoid screw. C, Intraventricular catheter.

monitoring device. Basic monitoring systems include intraventricular catheters, subarachnoid bolts, intraparenchymal catheters, and epidural probes (Figure 16–14). Each system has advantages and disadvantages for monitoring ICP (Table 16–9).

Table 16–9 Comparison of Intracranial Pressure Monitoring Sites

Site	Advantages	Disadvantages
Intraventricular	Gold standard Allows for therapeutic intervention by drainage of CSF Direct measurement of intraventricular pressure Highly accurate	Most invasive; carries high risk for hemorrhage, infection Contraindicated with coagulopathies or with small, misshapen, or collapsed ventricles
Subarachnoid	Less invasive than intraventricular Easy placement Low risk of infection Useful if ventricles cannot be cannulated Able to sample CSF	Unable to drain CSF May become obstructed with bone or tissue Decreased accuracy as time progresses Needs frequent recalibration Unreliable in setting of increased ICP
Intraparenchymal	Easy placement Low risk of infection Highly accurate	Unable to drain CSF Requires separate monitoring system Catheter fragile; may kink Cannot zero once in place Risk of hemorrhage, infection
Epidural probe	Easy placement Low risk of infection	Unable to drain CSF Cannot zero once in place Accuracy variable

Intraventricular monitoring, the gold standard for ICP monitoring, is used for both diagnostic and therapeutic purposes. This type of monitoring involves placing an intraventricular catheter (IVC) into the anterior horn of the lateral ventricle, preferably in the nondominant hemisphere. Diagnostically, it is the most reliable of the ICP monitoring devices and provides precise and consistent waveforms. Therapeutically, cerebrospinal fluid (CSF) can be drained from the intraventricular cavity, thereby decreasing the volume in the CSF compartment and reducing ICP. Drainage of CSF can be continuous or intermittent. The continuous drainage technique promotes automatic drainage of CSF by gravity into a closed buretrol system when the ICP exceeds a predetermined pressure. The predetermined drainage pressure is dialed into the buretrol, and the drain transducer is zeroed to atmospheric pressure using the foramen of Monroe as the anatomic landmark for the lateral ventricle. In most institutions, this landmark is considered to be level with the tragus of the ear. The intermittent drainage technique employs the same closed system as the continuous drainage technique, but it requires intermittent opening of a stopcock to allow CSF to drain into the buretrol when the ICP exceeds a predetermined limit, typically in the range of 20 to 25 mmHg (Hickey, 2014).

The IVC has several advantages. Because it is placed directly into the ventricle, it provides direct measurement of ICP and allows for drainage of CSF. However, because of its invasive nature, the IVC is not risk free. Because it is introduced through brain parenchyma directly into the ventricle, the risk of bleeding, neuronal destruction, and infection must be considered. Contraindications for placement of an IVC include patients with coagulopathies, small or collapsed ventricles, or severe generalized cerebral edema.

An alternative to the IVC is the subarachnoid bolt or screw. This type of monitoring device is used in patients with small, collapsed, or shifted ventricles and is placed into the subdural or subarachnoid space. The subarachnoid bolt provides some of the same monitoring capabilities as the IVC, such as measurement of ICP and evaluation of waveforms, although the waveform is easily dampened because fragments of bone and brain tissue may obstruct the tip of the bolt. Unlike the IVC, drainage of CSF is not possible because the ventricle is not cannulated.

Intraparenchymal monitoring devices are placed directly into the brain tissue via a bolt device, usually 1 cm below the subarachnoid space. These devices are easy to place, provide sharp and distinct waveforms, transmit accurate measurement of ICP, and carry a lower risk of infection. For these reasons, they are a desirable alternative to subarachnoid monitors. However, they are more costly, require a separate monitoring system, and do not have CSF drainage capabilities. An epidural probe is a small fiber-optic sensor that is placed through a burr hole and into the epidural space to monitor ICP. These catheters are easy to place and carry a low risk of infection (Moussazadeh et al., 2017).

ICP Waveforms   For all of the ICP monitoring devices previously mentioned, the catheters are connected to a

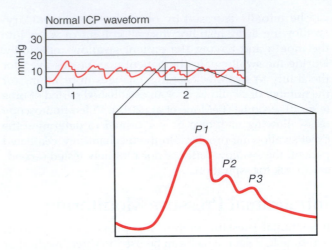

Figure 16–15 Three peaks of the ICP waveform. *P1*, percussion wave; *P2*, reflects brain compliance; *P3*, dicrotic wave. Normally, *P1* is the highest.

monitoring system that converts pressure impulses (waveforms) into an electronic display on a bedside monitor. The ICP waveform is derived from pulsations transmitted in the brain from intracranial arteries and veins. The high-acuity nurse must be able to identify physiologically normal ICP waveforms, recognize ominous waveforms, and correlate ICP waveforms with clinical symptoms and trends that may indicate elevated ICP. There are three peaks within each ICP waveform (Figure 16–15). The first peak is *P1*, which is referred to as the percussion wave. It has a sharp peak and originates from pulsations of the choroid plexus. The second peak, *P2*, reflects the compliance of brain tissue. If *P2* is as high as or higher than *P1*, a situation of decreased compliance is present. The third wave, *P3*, is the dicrotic wave.

There are three types of ICP pressure waveform patterns: *A waves*, *B waves*, and *C waves* (Figure 16–16).

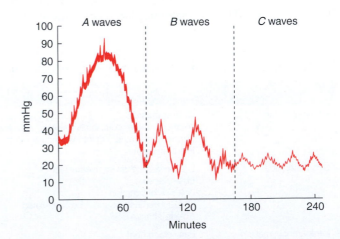

Figure 16–16 Three types of ICP pressure waveform patterns. *A* waves, spikes of sharp increases in ICP, are clinically significant; signs of neurologic deterioration may be present. *B* waves are oscillating waves that are normal except when elevated above 15 mmHg. *C* waves are small rhythmic waves that are normal.

A waves, or plateau waves, are clinically significant, as they typically occur when ICP is elevated. *A* waves are characterized by spikes of sharp increases in ICP that may be sustained in a plateau fashion for up to 20 minutes. Signs of neurologic deterioration may be seen with these waves (decreasing level of consciousness, pupillary changes, posturing). Plateau waves are significant, especially when the elevation in ICP decreases cerebral perfusion pressure (CPP). *B* waves, sharp oscillating waves, often precede *A* waves and occur every 30 seconds to 2 minutes. They are considered normal except when elevated to an amplitude of greater than 15 mmHg, indicating a state of low intracranial compliance. *C* waves are small rhythmic waves occurring every 5 to 8 minutes, varying with respirations and blood pressure fluctuations. *C* waves are considered physiologically normal.

Cerebral Oxygenation Monitoring

Although ICP and CPP monitoring provide an indirect assessment of cerebral tissue perfusion, they do not indicate the adequacy of cerebral oxygenation. Two types of cerebral oxygenation monitoring are available: jugular bulb oximetry and brain tissue oxygen monitoring.

Jugular Bulb Oximetry   Measurement of cerebral oxygen saturation via jugular vein bulb oximetry (SjO_2 or $SjVO_2$) is used to assess the relationship between cerebral oxygen supply and demand. The SjO_2 catheter is inserted by a specially trained provider in a similar manner to that of a central venous catheter. The fiber-optic catheter is typically inserted into the right internal jugular vein as this vein drains a greater proportion of blood from the sagittal sinus than does the left internal jugular; therefore, readings are more representative of global (versus local) brain oxygenation. After placement has been confirmed, catheter patency is maintained by connecting the SjO_2 catheter to a pressurized flush system consisting of a 250 to 500 mL bag of heparinized saline solution that produces, when under 300 mmHg of pressure, an average flow rate of 3 to 5 mL/hr to maintain catheter patency. No other fluids or medications should be infused through the SjO_2 catheter (Hiraki & Ushijima, 2015).

SjO_2 monitoring permits continuous measurement of cerebral venous oxygen saturation. The amount of oxygen extracted by cerebral tissue is reflected in the difference between the percentage of oxygen delivered to cerebral tissue (SAO_2 or SpO_2) and the percentage returning from cerebral tissue (SjO_2)—therefore, cerebral oxygen extraction (CEO_2) = SpO_2 − SjO_2. Normal CEO_2 is 30%, meaning that about 30% of the arterial oxygen in the brain is removed from the blood before leaving the brain.

The data provided by measuring SjO_2 can provide valuable information about the oxygenation status of the brain. For example, if the brain is receiving less oxygen than it needs, it extracts more oxygen from the cerebral circulation and SjO_2 is lower. If CBF is higher than the brain requires, less oxygen is extracted and the SjO_2 is higher. This information helps to determine therapies and interventions to improve cerebral oxygenation. The major advantage of using SjO_2 monitoring over simple ICP or CPP monitoring is that it can help determine if a given CPP is sufficient to satisfy cerebral metabolic demand (Slazinski, 2011a).

The nurse monitors for changes in SjO_2 measurements using an established set of parameters, such as noted below (Bhardwaj, Bhagat, & Grover, 2015; Hiraki & Ushijima, 2015):

- 55–75%: Indicates normal range
- Less than 50–55% : Reflects cerebral ischemia
- Greater than 75%: Reflects cerebral hyperemia (elevated brain blood volume) or death of brain cells (Dead tissue does not extract oxygen.)

If either cerebral ischemia or hyperemia persists for more than 15 minutes, the nurse should notify the provider (Chou & deMoya, 2010; Slazinski, 2011b).

Brain Tissue Oxygen Monitoring   Regional brain tissue oxygen monitoring ($PbtO_2$) provides continuous measurement of local brain tissue oxygen partial pressure and may be used as an adjunct monitoring modality along with ICP, SjO_2 and CPP. $PbtO_2$ monitoring requires insertion of an intracranial bolt system, a $PbtO_2$ probe, and use of a special $PbtO_2$ monitor. Normal $PbtO_2$ is greater than 20 mmHg. A $PbtO_2$ of 15 to 20 mmHg is accepted as the critical lower limit in patients with traumatic brain injury (TBI) and stroke. Brain tissue extracts oxygen from the hemoglobin into the brain tissue and is measured as partial pressure. Recommendation for placement of the brain tissue oxygen catheter is in the frontal white matter, 2 to 3 cm below the dura. A CT scan is recommended to verify correct placement.

Section Three Review

1. What does the Glasgow Coma Scale assess?
   A. Cranial nerves
   B. Arousal
   C. Abstract thinking
   D. Awareness

2. The nurse would expect to see which type of doll's eye movements if the patient has a brainstem injury?
   A. Eyes will remain fixed in the midposition as the head is turned.
   B. Eyes will conjugate opposite to the side to which the head is turned.
   C. Eyes will turn to the side opposite of where the head is turned.
   D. Eyes will turn to the same side to which the head is turned.

3. The rhythmic waxing and waning in the depth of respiration followed by a period of apnea is referred to as what?
   A. Central neurologic ventilation
   B. Apneustic breathing
   C. Cheyne–Stokes breathing
   D. Cluster breathing

4. Which findings are consistent with Cushing triad? (Select all that apply.)
   A. Increase in systolic blood pressure
   B. Unequal pupils
   C. Bradycardia
   D. Decrease in diastolic blood pressure
   E. Irregular respirations

Answers: 1. B, 2. A, 3. C, 4. (A, C, D, E)

Section Four: Diagnostic Procedures

Treatment of neurologic dysfunction is contingent upon accurate and timely diagnosis. A variety of diagnostic tests are available. Some of the more commonly performed diagnostic tests will be reviewed.

Computed Tomography Scanning

Computed tomography (CT) remains the initial imaging modality of choice in acute brain injury. A CT of the head (CTH) is useful for detecting a variety of pathological brain conditions, including primary injuries such as skull fractures, hematomas, and contusions; secondary injuries such as edema, mass effect, and herniation; as well as abscesses and tumors. CTH is minimally invasive, painless, produces rapid results, and has a high safety profile. In most clinical situations, CTH reduces the need for more invasive procedures, such as cerebral angiogram. CTH may be performed with IV contrast to enhance visualization of vascular structures. A xenon-enhanced CT can measure CBF quantitatively by measuring the uptake and clearance of xenon gas, which may be administered by inhalation or intravenously.

Magnetic Resonance Imaging

Magnetic resonance imaging (MRI) is a widely utilized imaging modality and is considered complimentary to CT by most providers. As with CTH, MRI can determine the anatomic location of a lesion, but MRI also offers superior visualization of soft tissue, providing more anatomic detail than CTH. MRI is more sensitive and specific for structural brain abnormalities and is superior for detecting white matter shearing, infarction, and ischemic tissue. Like CTH, MRI can also detect cerebral edema, bleeding, and abscess (Hickey, 2014). Because MRI has the ability to detect pathologic processes at an earlier stage than is possible with a CTH, it remains the procedure of choice for early diagnosis of cerebral infarction and brain tumors. As MRI employs magnetic fields to produce images, removal of all metal from the patient's body is essential. Most dental fillings, prostheses, and internal clips do not prevent the patient from having an MRI, but specific questions and concerns must be directed to the neuroradiologist. Obtaining an MRI study takes longer than a CTH; therefore, a CTH remains the procedure of choice when time is a factor, as in the case of stroke or TBI.

Positron Emission and Single Photon Emission Computed Tomography

Diagnostic procedures using tomography involve IV injection and tracking of radionucleotides to evaluate cerebral blood flow (Hickey, 2014). Two types are available: positron emission tomography (PET) and single photon emission computed tomography (SPECT). PET uses paired radiation-sensitive detectors, whereas SPECT uses unpaired detectors. Although PET studies are more costly than SPECT studies, both techniques are helpful in determining changes in CBF and metabolism during recovery. Areas of brain dysfunction and ischemia that are not detected by CT may be detected by these techniques and are helpful when determining prognosis following acute brain injury. CT and PET and SPECT scans are different but related imaging techniques. PET and SPECT scans use nuclear medicine imaging to produce a three-dimensional picture of functional processes in the body. PET scans provide metabolic information and complement CT and MRI scans, which provide anatomic information. PET scans involve injection of a radioactive tracer. CT scans outline bone and organs very well. PET and SPECT images show metabolic processes (blood flow, temperature) within the tissues and organs.

Transcranial Doppler

Transcranial Doppler (TCD) is a noninvasive tool that measures cerebral blood velocity in the branches of the circle of Willis. TCD is governed by the underlying principle that velocity depends on the pressure gradient between the two ends of a vessel, the radius of the vessel, and blood viscosity. Therefore, changes in velocity may reflect either change in CBF or in the diameter of a vessel. Diameter and flow do not always change concurrently, so providers should interpret studies with caution. Low velocity may reflect low flow or arterial dilation; high velocity may indicate high flow or vessel constriction. TCD is noninvasive and can be performed at the bedside, thus is ideal for use in the high-acuity environment. TCD is often used to monitor for cerebral vasospasm, intracranial lesions post-stroke, and to detect cerebral blood flow changes associated with elevated ICP. TCD may also be used during evaluation and determination of brain death (Escudero, Otero, Quindós, & Viña, 2015).

Evoked Potentials

Evoked potentials are recordings of cerebral electrical impulses generated in response to visual, auditory, or somatosensory stimuli. Stimulation of the visual or auditory sensory organs or the peripheral nerves evokes an electrophysiologic response that is extracted from continuous electroencephalography (EEG) monitoring. Evoked potentials are used to detect lesions in the cerebral cortex or ascending pathways of the spinal cord, brainstem, and thalamus. This test is so sensitive that it detects lesions that cannot be detected using other clinical or laboratory tests. Visually evoked potentials are elicited by a flashing light or changing geometric pattern, stimulating the visual center in the occipital lobe. The delay, known as the degree of latency, correlates with disease severity. Auditory evoked potentials are elicited by transmitting transient sounds, such as clicking noises, through earphones. They are useful to detect lesions in the central auditory pathway of the brainstem, to identify lesions that result in hearing disorders, and to assist in the diagnosis of acoustic tumors.

Somatosensory-evoked potentials are elicited by the application of a peripheral stimulus. The response to this stimulus and the degree of latency are measured. These are used to assist in the evaluation of the location and extent of brain dysfunction after brain injury. Testing for evoked potentials does not require an alert and cooperative patient and is not affected by anesthesia or sedation. Evoked potentials may be useful in predicting coma outcome. They are also especially useful during therapeutically induced comas (such as barbiturate coma) because the sensory pathways are not affected by barbiturates (Steiner, 2015).

Electroencephalography

Electroencephalography (EEG) allows recording of the electrical activity of the brain using electrodes attached to the scalp. Electrical impulses are detected and transferred to a device that interprets and converts the impulses into waveforms. Abnormal voltage fluctuations indicate seizures or space-occupying lesions, cerebral infarct, altered consciousness, and brain death. Absence of electrical activity provides evidence for clinical determination of brain death. An EEG may detect seizure activity in the brain when seizures are not clinically apparent. However, abnormal EEG findings do not identify the cause of the abnormality. It is important to note that significant pathology can be present even in the face of a normal EEG. Continuous EEG may be used in some high-acuity units to monitor patients with elevated ICP, seizure activity, and cerebral ischemia (Herman et al., 2015).

Cerebral Angiography

Cerebral angiography involves the injection of contrast material into cerebral arteries to visualize intra- and extracranial circulation. An angiogram traces blood flow through the cerebrovascular circulation and allows visualization of the size and patency of these vessels. Results can diagnose arteriovenous (AV) malformations, aneurysms, carotid artery disease, vasospasm, and venous thrombosis. Although angiography is useful in the evaluation of cerebral vasculature, it is an invasive procedure. Evaluation for the presence of allergy to the contrast medium is also warranted (Hickey, 2014). Postangiography monitoring in the

Emerging Evidence

- Patients with CT-positive traumatic brain injuries (TBI) are at increased risk of concurrent cervical spine fractures in comparison to patients with a CT-negative head injury, according to a large sample retrospective medical record review study by Thesleff, Kataja, Ohman and Luoto (2017). Medical records of 3023 patients were reviewed to identify patients whose cervical spine was CT-imaged within 1 week after primary head CT due to a clinical suspicion of a cervical spine injury (CSI) ($n = 1,091$); 24.7% ($n = 269$) had an acute CT-positive TBI, and of these, motor vehicle crashes 22.4% ($n = 244$) and falls 47.8% ($n = 521$) were the most frequent mechanisms of injury. Cervical spine fractures were found in 6.6% ($n = 72$) and dislocation and/or subluxation in 2.8% ($n = 31$) of the patients. Patients with acute traumatic intracranial lesions had significantly ($p = 0.04$; OR = 1.689) more cervical spine fractures (9.3%, $n = 25$) compared to head CT-negative patients (5.7%, $n = 47$). Head CT positivity was related to C6 fractures ($p = 0.031$, OR = 2.769). Patients with cervical spine fractures ($n = 72$) had altogether 101 fractured vertebrae, which were most often C2 (22.8%, $n = 23$), C7 (19.8%, $n = 20$), and C6 (16.8%, $n = 17$). TBI with acute intracranial lesions on CT have a higher risk for cervical spine fractures in comparison to patients with a CT-negative head injury. Although statistically significant, the difference in fracture rate was small. It is important to assess for spinal fractures in all patients with CT-positive TBIs (*Thesleff et al., 2017*).

- In a meta-analysis, Xie, Wu, Yan, Liu and Wang (2017) compared the effect of combined therapy (combination of brain tissue oxygen and standard intracranial pressure/cerebral perfusion pressure (ICP/CPP) with that of standard ICP/CPP guided therapy on mortality rate, favorable outcome, ICP/CPP, and length of stay (LOS). A systematic search in July 2016 of PubMed, EMBASE, Cochrane Library, ClinicalTrials.gov, and Web of Science for studies comparing combined therapy and standard ICP/CPP guided therapy yielded 362 studies, out of which 8 cohort studies and 1 RCT were included. Random-effect and fixed-effect models were used for pooled analyses for the primary outcomes of mortality and favorable outcome. Compared with standard ICP/CPP guided therapy, brain tissue oxygen combined ICP/CPP guided therapy improved long-term outcomes without any effects on mortality, ICP/CPP, or LOS (*Xie et al., 2017*).

high-acuity patient should include serial assessments for bleeding, ipsilateral reduction in or loss of peripheral pulses, changes in level of consciousness, vital sign abnormalities, and access site complications.

Magnetic Resonance Angiography

Magnetic resonance angiography (MRA) combines MRI with angiography for noninvasive visualization of cerebral vasculature (Pagana, Pagana, & Pagana, 2014). MRA is useful in the evaluation of carotid artery disease and in the identification of intracranial aneurysms, and it can be performed with or without contrast.

Lumbar Puncture

For the lumbar puncture (LP, or spinal tap) procedure, a needle is placed into the subarachnoid space, usually at the L4–L5 interspace or less commonly the L3–L4 interspace. CSF is removed and analyzed for the presence of blood or infection. In addition, CSF pressure can be obtained utilizing a sterile manometer. Medications may also be administered by this route. This procedure is contraindicated in patients with increased ICP, as the rapid shift in CSF can cause a low pressure shunt and lead to brain herniation. Complications of LP include herniation of the brainstem, infection, and headache (Schneider, 2013).

Section Four Review

1. CT scanning, rather than MRI, would be the initial procedure of choice for detecting which condition?
   A. White matter shearing
   B. The early stages of brain tumors
   C. Cerebral infarction
   D. Acute brain injury

2. What is PET scanning useful for evaluating?
   A. Cerebral blood flow
   B. Spinal fractures
   C. Skull fractures
   D. Anatomic location of a brain tumor

3. Which statement best describes evoked potentials?
   A. It is an invasive procedure.
   B. It is useful for imaging cellular metabolism.
   C. It is used in clinical research only.
   D. It evaluates a sensory response to a stimulus.

4. What does brain tissue oxygen monitoring ($PbtO_2$) measure?
   A. Generalized oxygen tension of gray matter
   B. Brain regional oxygen partial pressure
   C. Global brain oxygenation
   D. Regional cerebral electrical impulses

Answers: 1. D, 2. A, 3. D, 4. B

Chapter 16 Review

1. A client is diagnosed with a benign tumor in the medulla oblongata. The nurse would plan to assess this client for changes in which functions? (Select all that apply.)
   1. Heart rate
   2. Blood pressure
   3. Respirations
   4. Swallowing
   5. Balance

2. A client has developed cerebral edema from a metabolic disorder. Which nursing intervention would help this client maintain normal ICP?
   1. Encourage the client to cough every hour.
   2. Keep the client's neck in a neutral alignment.
   3. Position the client on the left side with two pillows.
   4. Maintain a patent peripheral IV site.

3. The client's blood pressure is 120/78 and ICP is 12. The client's CPP is _____.

4. A client becomes hypercapnic after being oversedated. The nurse acts quickly to reverse this situation to prevent which physiologic changes? (Select all that apply.)
   1. Increase in cerebral blood flow
   2. Systemic alkalosis
   3. Decrease in ICP
   4. Increase in cerebral blood volume
   5. Decrease in body temperature

5. A nurse is conducting initial assessment on a client who reports that he fell out of a tree while hunting. During the assessment, the client becomes unconscious, with arms pronating and extending straight out, wrists and fingers flexing, and feet plantar flexing.

The nurse calls for help because this client is exhibiting which posturing?

1. Trapezius
2. Decorticate
3. Decerebrate
4. Combination

6. A CT scan has been ordered for a patient who sustained a head injury playing football. A nurse who is new to the emergency department asks why an MRI was not ordered instead. Which responses, made by a seasoned ED nurse, are correct? (Select all that apply.)

1. "We can't do an MRI because the client has dental fillings."
2. "A CT is quicker."
3. "MRIs don't show bones as well."
4. "MRIs can't be done in emergent situations."
5. "We don't know if the client has been NPO."

7. A client presented to the emergency department with a Glasgow Coma Scale (GCS) score of 12. The nurse reassessed this client 15 minutes after arrival and assigned a score of 10. What action should the nurse take?

1. Plan to reassess the client in 10 minutes.
2. Check the client's vital signs for changes.
3. Collaborate with the ED physician immediately.
4. Assess the client using a different scale for comparison.

8. The nurse is monitoring a client's SjO$_2$. Which reading would require only documentation and continued monitoring?

1. 28%
2. 49%
3. 68%
4. 92%

9. Which changes would the nurse interpret as being part of Cushing triad? (Select all that apply.)

1. Systolic BP changes from 128 to 136.
2. Diastolic BP changes from 70 to 90.
3. Heart rate changes from 84 to 58.
4. Respiratory rate changes from 14 to 16.
5. Temperature increases from 37.4 to 37.8°C.

10. A nurse is assessing the client for presence of "doll's eyes." When the nurse turns the client's head side to side, the client's eyes move in the direction opposite of the movement. How would the nurse interpret this response?

1. This is a normal finding.
2. The client likely has brainstem injury.
3. This indicates nystagmus.
4. The client likely has a cerebellar injury.

Answers to questions found inside your textbook are available on the faculty resources site. Please consult with your instructor.

References

American College of Surgeons. (2015). Best practices in the management of traumatic brain injury. Retrieved March 25, 2017, from https://www.facs.org/~/media/files/quality%20programs/trauma/tqip/traumatic%20brain%20injury%20guidelines.ashx

Barker, E. (2008). Chapter 2: The adult neurologic assessment. In E. Barker (Ed.), *Neuroscience nursing: A spectrum of care* (3rd ed., pp. 58–63). St. Louis, MO: Elsevier/Mosby.

Bhardwaj, A., Bhagat, H., & Grover, V. K. (2015). Jugular venous oximetry. *Journal of Neuroanaesthesiology and Critical Care, 2*(3), 225–231.

Chatterjee, A., & Coslett, H. B. (2014). *The roots of cognitive neuroscience.* New York, NY: Oxford University Press.

Chou, S., & deMoya, M. (2010). Neurological trauma. In L. M. Bigatello (Sr. Ed.), *Critical care handbook of the Massachusetts General Hospital* (5th ed., pp. 534–540). Philadelphia, PA: Lippincott Williams & Wilkins.

Crossman, A. R., & Neary, D. (2015). *Neuroanatomy: An illustrated color text* (5th ed.). New York, NY: Elsevier Limited.

Escudero, D., Otero, J., Quindós, B., & Viña, L. (2015). Transcranial Doppler ultrasound in the diagnosis of brain death: Is it useful or does it delay the diagnosis? *Medicina Intensiva, 39*(4), 244–250.

Fish, E., & Talmor, D. (2017). The acute respiratory distress syndrome. In J. M. Oropello, S. M. Pastores, & V. Kvetan (Eds.), *Critical Care.* New York, NY: McGraw-Hill, 2016. Retrieved February 9, 2017, from http://accessmedicine.mhmedical.com.ezproxy.uky.edu/content.aspx?bookid=1944&sectionid=143516870

Glickstein, M. (2014). *Neuroscience: A historical introduction.* Cambridge, MA: The MIT Press.

Hemphill, J., III, Smith, W. S., & Gress, D. R. (2015). Neurologic critical care, including hypoxic-ischemic encephalopathy, and subarachnoid hemorrhage. In D. Kasper, A. Fauci, S. Hauser, D. Longo, J. Jameson, & J. Loscalzo (Eds.), *Harrison's principles of internal medicine* (19th ed., p. 2707). New York, NY: McGraw-Hill.

Herman, S. T., Abend, N. S., Bleck, T. P., Chapman, K. E., Drislane, F. W., Emerson, R. G., . . . Hirsch, L. J. (2015). Consensus statement on continuous EEG in critically-ill adults and children, Part I: Indications. *Journal of Clinical Neurophysiology, 32*(2), 87–95.

Hickey, J. V. (2014). *The clinical practice of neurological and neurosurgical nursing* (7th ed.). Philadelphia, PA: Lippincott Williams & Wilkins.

Hiraki, T., & Ushijima, K. (2015). Role of jugular venous oxygen saturation in neuroanesthesia. In H. Uchino, K. Ushijima, & Y. Ikeda (Eds.), *Neuroanesthesia and cerebrospinal protection* (pp. 163–171). New York, NY: Springer.

LeMone, P., Burke, K., Bauldoff, G., & Gubrud, P. (2015). *Medical-surgical nursing: Clinical reasoning in patient care* (6th ed.). Hoboken, NJ: Prentice Hall.

Maldonato, M. (2014). The ascending reticular activating system: The common root of consciousness and attention. In R. J. Howlett & L. C. Jain (Eds.), *Smart innovation, systems and technologies* (pp. 333–344). New York, NY: Springer.

Marieb, E. N., & Hoehn, K. (2013). *Human anatomy & physiology* (9th ed.). Upper Saddle River, NJ: Pearson Education.

Moussazadeh, N., Stieg, P. E., & Mangat, H. S. (2017). Intracranial pressure monitoring. In J. M. Oropello, S. M. Pastores, & V. Kvetan (Eds.), *Critical care.* New York, NY: McGraw-Hill.

Munakomi, S., & Kumar, B. M. (2015). Neuroanatomical basis of Glasgow Coma Scale—A reappraisal. *Neuroscience & Medicine, 6*, 116–120.

Pagana, K. D., Pagana, T. J., & Pagana, T. N. (2014). *Mosby's diagnostic and laboratory test reference* (12th ed.). St. Louis, MO: Elsevier/Mosby.

Schneider, V. F. (2013). Lumbar puncture. In R. Dehn & D. P. Asprey (Eds.), *Essential clinical procedures* (3rd ed., pp. 146–155). Elsevier: Edinburgh, UK.

Shoja, M. M., Hoepfner, L. D., Agutter, P. S., Singh, R., & Tubbs, R. S. (2015). History of the pineal gland. *Child's Nervous System, 32*, 583. doi:10.1007/s00381-015-2636-3

Slazinski, T. (2011a). Combination intraventricular/fiberoptic catheter insertion. In D. Lynn-McHale Wiegand (Ed.), *AACN procedure manual for critical care* (6th ed., pp. 809–815). St. Louis, MO: Elsevier/Saunders.

Slazinski, T. (2011b). Jugular venous oxygen saturation monitoring. In D. Lynn-McHale Wiegand (Ed.), *AACN procedure manual for critical care* (6th ed., pp. 816–825). St. Louis, MO: Elsevier/Saunders.

Steiner, L. A. (2015). ICU care: Surgical and medical management—neurological monitoring and treatment. In P. Vos & R. Diaz-Arrastia (Eds.), *Traumatic brain injury* (pp. 115–133). Hoboken, NJ: Wiley-Blackwell.

Thesleff, T., Kataja, A., Ohman, J., & Luoto, T. M. (2017). Head injuries and the risk of concurrent cervical spine fractures. *Acta Neurochirurgica (Wien).* doi:10.1007/s00701-017-3133-0 [Epub ahead of print]

Urden, L. D., Stacy, K. M., & Lough, M. E. (2013). *Critical care nursing* (7th ed.). St. Louis, MO: Mosby.

Xie, Q., Wu, H. B., Yan, Y. F., Liu, M., & Wang, E. S. (2017). Mortality and outcome comparison between brain tissue oxygen combined intracranial pressure/cerebral perfusion pressure guided therapy and intracranial pressure/cerebral perfusion pressure guided therapy in traumatic brain injury: A meta-analysis. *World Neurosurgery.* doi:10.1016/j.wneu.2016.12.097 [Epub ahead of print]

Zweifel, C., Dias, C., Smielewski, P., & Czosnyka, M. (2014). Continuous time-domain monitoring of cerebral autoregulation in neurocritical care. *Medical Engineering and Physics, 36*(5), 638–645.

Chapter 17
Mentation and Sensory Motor Complications of Acute Illness

 Learning Outcomes

17.1 Explain disorders of mentation and consciousness common to acute and critical illness.

17.2 Describe characteristics and management of delirium and coma.

17.3 Explain disorders of movement that occur with acute and critical illness, including polyneuropathy, myopathy, neuromuscular blockade, and related muscle weakness.

17.4 Describe characteristics and management of common seizure complications associated with acute and critical illness.

This chapter provides a broad overview of sensory motor complications that can occur in patients of acute and critical illness, focusing on assessment and management of the patient who experiences disruption of normal mentation, consciousness, and movement. Through the years, many terms have been used to describe cognitive dysfunction commonly associated with critical illness, including coma, acute confusional state, organic brain syndrome, acute organic reaction, cerebral insufficiency, brain failure, ICU psychosis, and septic encephalopathy (Harper, Johnston, & Landefeld, 2016). The terms *delirium* and *coma* are increasingly found in the scientific literature related to cognitive dysfunction in the critically ill patient and are a major focus of this chapter (Ropper, 2015).

Section One: Decreased Level of Consciousness, Abnormal Mentation, and Anxiety

Patients with prolonged periods of inactivity due to hemodynamic instability, mechanical ventilation, organ failure, pain, and/or prolonged deep sedation are at risk of developing decreased level of consciousness (LOC), abnormal mentation, neuromuscular complications, and sleep disturbances. Often early signs of serious illness, these conditions are associated with increased mortality, diaphragmatic and limb weakness, increased number of days requiring mechanical ventilation, and longer lengths of stay in the hospital and intensive care unit (ICU) (Friedrich et al., 2015; Pawley et al., 2015). Sepsis, which accounts for up to 50% of deaths in ICUs, is associated with development of decreased LOC and mentation disorder, commonly referred to as septic encephalopathy (or sepsis-associated encephalopathy [SAE]) (Mazeraud et al., 2016; Zampieri, Park, Machado, & Azevedo, 2011). Even so, impaired mentation often goes unrecognized and untreated (Ropper, 2015). Altered consciousness and delirium are two disorders of mentation that may occur in critically ill patients (Norbaek & Glipstrup, 2016; Ryan et al., 2013).

Alterations in Mentation

Alterations in mentation can range from subtle decreases in LOC to coma. Normal **mentation**, or mental activity, is characterized by an awareness of self and surroundings. The patient knows his or her name and is aware of the present surroundings. These patients have the ability to accurately perceive what is experienced in terms of sensory input and orientation to environment. Patients who have normal mentation have the ability to store and retrieve information. They are able to demonstrate memory, judgment, and reasoning in that they are able to process data to generate more meaningful information.

Mental processes include **consciousness** (wakefulness and responsiveness) and **cognition** (the ability to reason and think). For the purposes of this discussion, disorders of mentation will be classified as alterations in the LOC and alterations in cognitive ability.

Alterations in LOC The two components of consciousness are **arousal** (wakefulness) and **awareness** (responsiveness). Normal consciousness ranges from an unaroused and unaware state (sleep) to an aroused and aware state (wakefulness). Abnormal LOC may similarly be described with coma and brain death being an unaroused and unaware state. Coma is characterized by the absence of arousal and awareness and may be reversible. Brain death is similar to coma in that the individual is in an unarousable and unaware mental state, but it is irreversible, ending in death. Delirium and dementia are conditions where arousal is associated with varying degrees of awareness.

Alterations in Cognitive Function There are many causes of cognitive dysfunction or impaired mentation in patients who have not sustained a brain injury, including global brain disorders caused by multiple factors that may be infectious, ischemic, drug related, or metabolic (Box 17–1).

Agitation or Anxiety and Insomnia

Agitation or anxiety and insomnia are contributing factors to the development of delirium or cognitive dysfunction and altered mentation. Agitation and insomnia may be attributed to a variety of underlying physical or psychiatric disorders, and symptoms may be exacerbated by hospitalization for acute or critical illness. Possible causes of insomnia to consider include mood and anxiety disorders, substance abuse, commonly prescribed medications (e.g., beta blockers, steroids, bronchodilators), sleep apnea, hyperthyroidism, and nocturnal myoclonus (involuntary limb movements during sleep). Anxiety and agitation may be seen in depression, substance abuse, hyperthyroidism, and complex partial seizures (Barr et al., 2013; Reus, 2015).

Treatment for insomnia and agitation or anxiety includes the administration of benzodiazepines. Therapy

---

BOX 17–1 Causes of Impaired Cognitive Function in Acute and Critically Ill Patients

- Ischemic, thrombotic, or hemorrhagic stroke
- Drug or alcohol withdrawal
- Insomnia
- Anxiety
- Thiamine deficiency
- Toxins
- Water intoxication
- Hyperthyroid or hypothyroid
- Medications
- Central line infection
- Heart failure
- Hypoxia, hypercapnia (e.g., ARDS, pneumonia)
- Hyper- or hypotension
- Adrenal insufficiency
- Renal failure
- Liver failure
- Sepsis
- Hyper- or hyponatremia
- Hypercalcemia
- Hypophosphatemia
- Fat embolism

---

should be started at the lowest recommended dosage with intermittent dosing schedules. In older adults, it is important to remember that toxicity can occur in the presence of malnutrition, advanced age, hepatic disease, alcohol use, other central nervous system depressants, isoniazid, and cimetidine. Also, certain benzodiazepines with a longer half-life may contribute to an accumulation of active serum metabolites in older adult patients or those with liver disease. This accumulation of serum metabolites can contribute to the development of prolonged sedation, delirium, psychomotor impairment, and respiratory depression. Tolerance and physical dependence may develop after 2 to 4 weeks of therapy, resulting in the need for higher doses to achieve the same effects or withdrawal syndrome when the drug is stopped. Seizures and delirium are more likely to occur with sudden discontinuation of benzodiazepines. Flumazenil (Romazicon), a benzodiazepine antagonist, may be administered for overdose. Caution should be observed when administering flumazenil to patients with a known history of seizures (Barr et al., 2013; Reus, 2015).

Section One Review

1. Delirium may occur with sudden discontinuation of which class of drugs? (Select all that apply.)
   A. Opiate narcotics
   B. Benzodiazepines
   C. NSAIDs
   D. Diuretics
   E. H$_2$ blockers

2. Alterations in mentation refer to a client's inability to do what?
   A. Withdraw from pain
   B. Cough and gag
   C. Localize to noxious stimuli
   D. Recognize surroundings

3. Which disorders of mentation are common in the critically ill population?
   A. Delirium and altered level of consciousness
   B. Myopathy and polyneuropathy
   C. Neuromuscular weakness
   D. Anxiety and pain

4. Which condition most increases the risk of benzodiazepine toxicity?
   A. Diabetes
   B. Obesity
   C. Coronary artery disease
   D. Advanced age

Answers: 1. (A, B, C, E), 2. D, 3. A, 4. D

Section Two: Delirium and Coma

For multiple reasons, high-acuity patients are at increased risk for development of altered states of consciousness, such as delirium and coma. Delirium has been a focus of research over the past two decades, and we now have a better understanding of its etiology, risk factors, characteristics, and treatments. *Coma* is a term that labels an unconscious state. When coma becomes prolonged, the chances for a full recovery are bleak. It is important for the nurse to have an understanding of delirium and coma to facilitate early assessment and management.

Delirium

Delirium, the most common cognitive disorder in acute and critically ill patients, is considered one of six leading causes of preventable injury in those older than 65 years (Harper et al., 2016). Delirium develops in 18% to 64% of hospitalized patients, with higher rates reported for older adult patients (Josephson & Miller, 2015). Delirium develops in 56% to 80% of patients receiving mechanical ventilation and is predictive of a higher reintubation rate, which can add additional days to a patient's hospital stay (Barr et al., 2013; Salluh et al., 2015). The risk for the development of delirium is cumulative in that for each additional day spent in delirium, there is an increase in the risk of prolonged hospitalization or death (Girard, Jackson, et al., 2010; Salluh et al., 2015). Between 10% and 24% of patients experience persistent delirium that may be related to long-term cognitive impairment (Barr et al., 2013). Recent estimates of in-hospital mortality rates among delirious patients have ranged from 25% to 33%, a rate similar to that of patients with sepsis. Hospitalized patients with an episode of delirium have a fivefold higher mortality rate in the months after their illness compared with age-matched nondelirious hospitalized patients. Hospitalized patients have a longer length of stay, are more likely to be discharged to a nursing home, and are more likely to experience subsequent episodes of cognitive decline; as a result, this condition has significant quality of life and economic implications (Girard, Dittus, & Ely, 2016; Josephson & Miller, 2015).

Defining Delirium   **Delirium** is an acute confusional cognitive disorder characterized by attention deficits, fluctuating mental status, and either disordered thinking or an altered level of consciousness that develops over a short period of time (hours to days) and fluctuates over time (Josephson & Miller, 2015). The hallmark of delirium is its acute onset and/or fluctuating clinical course. This hallmark also distinguishes it from dementia, which develops slowly. Delirium is a dynamic state that is characterized by both hypoactive and hyperactive behaviors. It is common for patients to oscillate frequently between these two behaviors (Harper et al., 2016; Josephson & Miller, 2015). Although multiple pathophysiologic causes are thought to be involved in the development of delirium, most are considered to be related to imbalances in neurotransmitters that modulate cognition, behavior, and mood. The current consensus is to use the unifying term *delirium* and to categorize it as hyperactive, hypoactive, or mixed delirium. In addition, patients with sepsis are at risk for developing a distinctive type of delirium called septic encephalopathy.

Hyperactive Delirium.   Hyperactive delirium, often referred to as ICU psychosis, is less common than hypoactive delirium and is associated with a better overall prognosis. It is characterized by agitation and restlessness, and it is common for these patients to "pick" at their monitoring, feeding, or intravenous devices.

Hypoactive Delirium.   Hypoactive delirium is characterized by lethargy (rather than agitation), withdrawal, flat affect, apathy, and decreased responsiveness. This type of delirium is often referred to as *encephalopathy*. Hypoactive delirium, especially in older adults, is often missed as a diagnosis. There is a tendency to consider hyperactive delirium as the more common form, but that is not supported by the data. It is likely that this perception stems from the fact that patients with hyperactive delirium attract more attention due to their agitation and increased activity than those with hypoactive delirium. In fact, hypoactive delirium is estimated to be the most common form, is more deleterious for the patient in the long term, and remains unrecognized in 66% to 84% of hospitalized patients (Harper et al., 2016; Josephson & Miller, 2015; Ropper, 2015; Ryan et al., 2013). It is important that nurses assess for hypoactive delirium because of its worse prognosis. Some patients develop the clinical features of both hyperactive and hypoactive delirium. When this occurs, it is called *mixed delirium*.

Septic Encephalopathy.   **Septic encephalopathy** is a type of delirium that results from a non–central nervous system infection, or sepsis, and occurs in 50% to 70% of ICU patients (Hemphill, Smith, & Gress, 2015; Mazeraud et al., 2016). The encephalopathy can be an early sign of a septicemia, especially in the older adult population (Josephson & Miller, 2015). Sepsis itself is a major infection-induced syndrome that promotes failure of vital organs, such as lung, brain, liver, and kidney. Cognitive dysfunction can result from sepsis, systemic inflammatory response syndrome (SIRS), and multiple organ dysfunction syndrome (MODS) (Girard et al., 2016; Iacobone et al., 2009; Mazeraud et al., 2016; Zampieri et al., 2011).

A process that contributes to the development of septic encephalopathy is increased permeability of the blood–brain barrier. Inflammatory mediators can cross the blood–brain barrier and impair brain function, which may result in cerebral edema. Also, cerebral blood flow is decreased, which can contribute to cerebral ischemia. There may be multiple mechanisms by which septic encephalopathy develops, and the SIRS response to sepsis, rather than the infection itself, seems to be the cause. Septic encephalopathy may be the brain's expression of injury as part of a more widespread multiorgan injury associated with SIRS (Mazeraud et al., 2016; Zampieri et al., 2011).

Differentiating Delirium from Dementia Delirium and dementia are distinct mental disorders that are easily confused because of two overlapping clinical characteristics: attention deficits and abnormal thinking (refer to Figure 17–1). **Dementia** is characterized by slow, insidious onset of memory impairment that follows a long-term, progressive course over a period of months to years. It is irreversible, chronic in nature, and progressive. In contrast to delirium, dementia is not acute, nor does it have a fluctuating course. However, while they are separate altered consciousness states, delirium and dementia often can and do coexist. It is estimated that as many as two thirds of hospitalized patients with dementia may have a superimposed delirium, and acute onset of delirium can provoke further mental and functional decline and deterioration (Harper et al., 2016; Hemphill et al., 2015; Ropper, 2015; Salluh et al., 2010; Zaal & Slooter, 2012). Dementia is discussed in further detail in Chapter 4.

Etiology of Delirium Delirium may be precipitated by infectious or septic conditions or the adverse effects of drugs, or it may be of metabolic origin (e.g., metabolic encephalopathy). Box 17–2 lists general risk factors for the

---

BOX 17–2 Risk Factors for the Development of Delirium

Primary risk factor: Preexisting cognitive impairment (e.g., dementia)
Other risk factors:

- Older age
- Presence of acute systemic illnesses
- Medical comorbid diseases
- Use of benzodiazepines
- Sleep deprivation or loss of circadian rhythm
- Metabolic disturbances

---

development of delirium. Medications are perhaps the most prevalent modifiable risk factor for delirium in acute or critically ill patients, especially in the older adult population (Barr et al., 2013; Hemphill et al., 2015; Josephson & Miller, 2015; Ropper, 2015) . Opioid narcotics (e.g., morphine and fentanyl) and benzodiazepines (e.g., midazolam and lorazepam) are linked to the development of delirium (Barr et al., 2013; Pandharipande et al., 2006; Pandharipande et al., 2008). Box 17–3 lists medications associated with the development of delirium.

Sleep deprivation or loss of circadian rhythm is another potentially modifiable risk factor for the development of delirium (Knauert, Haspel, & Pisani, 2015; Pulak & Jensen, 2016). This is a common problem in critically ill patients due to excessive noise and lighting, patient care activities, metabolic consequences of critical illness, mechanical ventilation, and sedative and analgesic medications (Barr et al., 2013; Josephson & Miller, 2015; Salluh et al., 2010).

Dementia, advanced age, comorbidity, and depression are other risk factors that may predispose patients to the development of delirium (Girard et al., 2016). In addition, precipitating factors for delirium include preexisting hypertension, smoking, alcoholism, increased severity of illness scores, hypoxia, metabolic disturbances, electrolyte imbalances, withdrawal syndromes, acute infection, seizures, dehydration, hyperthermia, head trauma, vascular

---

Delirium is an acute change in level of

consciousness **OR** fluctuating behavior

over the past 24 hours **AND** difficulty

focusing or maintaining attention

AND EITHER

1. Disordered thinking or

2. Altered consciousness

Figure 17–1 Clinical characteristics of delirium.

BOX 17–3 Medications Associated with the Development of Delirium in Critically Ill Patients

- Alcohol
- Amiodarone
- Amphotericin B
- Aminoglycosides
- ACE inhibitors
- Atropine
- Benzodiazepines
- Beta blockers
- Cimetidine
- Corticosteroids
- Cephalosporins
- Cocaine
- Digitalis
- Isoniazid
- Lidocaine, bupivacaine
- Metoclopramide
- Metronidazole
- NSAIDs
- Opioids
- Phenytoin
- Penicillin
- Quinidine
- Ranitidine
- Trimethoprim-sulfamethoxazole

disorders, impaired vision or hearing, and immobilization (Barr et al., 2013; Josephson & Miller, 2015; Maldonado, 2013; Ryan et al., 2013).

Assessment and Management   The assessment and management of delirium should focus on identifying and treating the underlying cause. Assessment for delirium should occur early into a patient's hospitalization because delirium can develop within 24 hours of admission (Barr et al., 2013). Early detection and treatment are necessary if adverse effects of delirium are to be avoided. Patients who are mechanically ventilated are often sedated, making assessment particularly challenging. Early monitoring for delirium along with daily goals for sedation and analgesia are essential in creating a treatment plan that effectively manages pain and sedation and avoids overuse of agents known to cause delirium. The Confusion Assessment Method for the ICU (CAM-ICU) and the Intensive Care Delirium Screening Checklist (ICDSC) are the most valid and reliable delirium monitoring tools for adult ICU patients. The CAM-ICU has been validated and found to be reliable in mechanically ventilated patients (Barnes-Daly, Phillips, & Ely, 2017; Ely et al., 2001; Soja et al., 2008). Table 17–1 is an example of the CAM-ICU.

Prevention should be the major goal of care. Interventions are classified as physiologic, environmental, patient safety, and pharmacologic. Physiologic measures include identifying those at risk for delirium, early diagnosis, and treatment. An important physiologic intervention is correction of dehydration, metabolic disturbances, and oxygenation imbalances. Environmental interventions include early mobilization, adequate sleep and rest, and providing patients with eyeglasses and hearing aids when appropriate. Early mobilization and encouraging family and significant other visitation, positioning patients near a window, providing for TV or radio stimulation, and maintaining normal day and night light variations help the patient to remain oriented, rested, and free of delirium (Hu, Jiang, Zeng, et al., 2015; Needham et al., 2010). Music therapy interventions may have a beneficial effect

Table 17–1 Confusion Assessment Method–ICU Version (CAM-ICU)

Features	Score	Check if Present
FEATURE 1: ACUTE ONSET OR FLUCTUATING COURSE Is the patient different than his/her baseline mental status? **Or** Has the patient had any fluctuation in mental status in the past 24 hours as evidenced by fluctuation on a sedation scale (e.g., RASS, GCS) or previous delirium assessment?	If either question is Yes →	☐
FEATURE 2: INATTENTION **Letters Attention Test** **Directions**: Say to the patient, "*I am going to read you a series of 10 letters. Whenever you hear the letter 'A,' indicate by squeezing my hand.*" Read letters from the following letter list in a normal tone. **S A V E A H A A R T** or **C A S A B L A N C A** or **A B A D B A D A A Y** **Errors are counted when the patient fails to squeeze on the letter "A" and when the patient squeezes the examiner's hand on any letter other than "A."**	Number of Errors > 2 →	☐
FEATURE 3: ALTERED LEVEL OF CONSCIOUSNESS Present if the actual Richmond Agitation-Sedation Scale (RASS) score is anything other than 0 (zero). (**RASS scoring:** +4 Combative, +3 Very Agitated, +2 Agitated, +1 Restless, 0 Alert & Calm, −1 Drowsy, −2 Light Sedation, −3 Moderate Sedation, −4 Deep Sedation, −5 Unarousable)	RASS anything other than zero →	☐
FEATURE 4: DISORGANIZED THINKING **Yes/No Questions** 1. Will a stone float on water? 2. Are there fish in the sea? 3. Does one pound weigh more than two pounds? 4. Can you use a hammer to pound a nail? **Errors are counted when the patient incorrectly answers a question.** **Command** Say to patient: "Hold up this many fingers." (Examiner holds two fingers in front of patient.) "Now do the same thing with the other hand." (Examiner does not demonstrate this time.) If patient is unable to move both arms, for the second part of the command say to the patient, "Add one more finger." **An error is counted if patient is unable to complete the entire command.**	Combined number of errors > 1 →	☐
OVERALL CAM-ICU SCORE Features 1 PLUS 2 AND either Feature 3 OR 4 present = CAM-ICU positive	Criteria Met →	☐ CAM-ICU Positive (Delirium Present)
	Criteria Not Met →	☐ CAM-ICU Negative (No Delirium)

SOURCE: Adapted from Vanderbilt University Medical Center. (2016). Original copyright Ely et al. (2001).

on anxiety in mechanically ventilated patients by reducing respiratory rate and systolic blood pressure with possible beneficial impact on the use of sedatives and analgesics (Bradt, 2014).

Pharmacologic strategies center on optimizing the quantity and type of sedative and analgesic medications delivered to patients. Pharmacologic interventions for delirium have included using antipsychotics to manage symptoms; however, there is little evidence to support recommendation of antipsychotics (e.g., haldolperidol [Haldol] and quetiapine [Seroquel]) as a medication class of choice for delirium (Barr et al., 2013). In fact, no drug has been approved by the FDA to prevent or treat delirium. It is important to identify and treat all organ dysfunction and metabolic and electrolyte imbalances in order to reduce the risk for delirium. Current medications should be reviewed regularly for possible triggers to the development of delirium. Benzodiazepines and opioids, often used in the acute care setting to treat pain and anxiety, may worsen the patient's cognitive state or may increase agitation, contributing to delirium. While an appropriate dose of opioids may be needed to manage pain, the challenge is to determine the optimal dose for analgesia without causing delirium. Recent studies suggest that a benzodiazepine-sparing sedation strategy using an alternative sedative, such as dexmedetomidine (Precedex), may result in a decreased risk for delirium (Girard et al., 2016; Serafim et al., 2015). When compared with propofol, dexmedetomidine sedation reduced incidence, delayed onset, and shortened duration of postoperative days (POD) in older adult patients after cardiac surgery (Djaiani et al., 2016). Another retrospective study of patients admitted to the ICU found that sedation with dexmedetomidine compared to propofol resulted in a significant reduction in time on mechanical ventilation; however, no difference was seen in ICU or hospital length of stay (LOS), incidence of delirium, or mortality (Wanat, Fitousis, Boston, & Masud, 2014). Propofol has not been found to increase risk for delirium, but the research evidence on opioids and risk for delirium has been contradictory (Mu, Lee, & Joynt, 2015; Wanat et al., 2014; Zaal, Devlin, Peelan, & Slooter, 2015). Clearly, more research is needed, and all patients who receive continuous drip sedatives or opioids should be assessed for delirium and oversedation.

Antipsychotic drugs sometimes used in the treatment of delirium include haloperidol lactate for IV administration, and haloperidol decanoate for PO administration. Both are first-generation antipsychotic agents. Other drugs that are used off-label include risperidone (Risperdal) and quetiapine (Seroquel), both second-generation antipsychotic agents. The Modifying the Incidence of Delirium (MIND) study compared haloperidol, ziprasidone (Geodon), and a placebo in 101 medical and surgical critically ill patients and reported no differences in regard to delirium resolution or any other outcomes or safety concerns in the three treatment groups (Girard, Pandharipande, et al., 2010). Another study compared quetiapine to placebo in 36 adult ICU patients already determined to be delirious who had an as-needed haloperidol order and found that the patients who received quetiapine (Seroquel) added to as-needed haloperidol experienced a faster

resolution of delirium, less delirium, less agitation, and more somnolence (Devlin et al., 2010). Quetiapine, an antipsychotic, has been shown to reduce the duration of delirium in critically ill adults with hypoactive delirium when compared to no pharmacologic delirium treatment at all (Michaud, Bullard, Harris, & Thomas, 2015). Because of contradictory research findings, all patients receiving antipsychotics (haloperidol or any of the second-generation antipsychotics) should be routinely and systematically monitored for side effects, especially *QT* prolongation. In fact, a 2010 review of cases and FDA MedWatch study by Meyer-Massetti, Cheng, Sharpe, Meier, & Guglielmo (2010) resulted in an FDA alert that antipsychotic drugs are associated with increased incidence of torsades de pointes, a lethal arrhythmia that results from prolonged *QT* interval.

Box 17–4 summarizes the management of delirium. Drug management for treatment of delirium is summarized in the "Related Pharmacotherapy: Agents Used for Treating Delirium" feature.

Coma

Coma is a persistent state of unresponsiveness lasting for more than 6 hours from which a person cannot be aroused; it implies extensive brain injury (Ropper, 2015). On the level-of-consciousness continuum, it is the most severe state. Common causes of coma are cardiac arrest, stroke, or intracerebral hemorrhage. Other causes are infection, metabolic disorders (e.g., myxedema, hypoglycemic coma) and toxins (e.g., elevated BUN, ammonia, or drug overdose). In the critical care environment, coma sometimes is induced intentionally, usually using anesthetic, sedative, or hypnotic agents, such as propofol or dexmedetomidine or an opioid. A major goal of inducing coma in critically ill patients is to reduce organ injury. Its use is primarily reserved for cases in which more moderate therapies have failed to adequately reduce oxygen consumption. Drug-induced coma (deep sedation) has been associated with serious complications of critical illness, and moderate sedation protocols are recommended for use when possible (Barnes-Daly et al., 2017; Barr et al., 2013).

Coma is rarely permanent, but fewer than 10% of patients survive coma without some kind of significant disability. For ICU patients with prolonged coma, the outcome is grim. Outcomes of coma include full recovery with no long-term residual effects or recovery with residual damage that may include learning deficits, emotional instability, or impaired cognition and judgment. More severe outcomes include persistent vegetative state or brain death.

Persistent vegetative state (PVS) is a specific type of coma in which the patient continues to maintain the arousal component of consciousness but not awareness. It is characterized by periods of wakefulness in which the eyes are open and may appear to visually wander around the immediate environment (Ropper, 2015). The patient retains autonomic functions, such as swallowing, coughing, and yawning, and some movement of the head and limbs; however, there are no meaningful responses to the internal or

BOX 17–4   Management Principles for Delirium

Prevention

- Prevention and early identification is the best approach. All critically ill patients should be assessed for delirium using a validated tool (e.g., CAM-ICU, ICDSC) (Barr et al., 2013; Harper et al., 2016).
- Identify patients with risk factors for new onset or persistent delirium with daily discussion of delirium assessment scores (Barr et al., 2013; Harper et al., 2016).
- Delirium prevention strategies: Frequent reorientation, visible orientation cues (e.g., clock, calendar, window with clear view of outside); reduce sensory isolation by providing glasses or hearing aids for patients who normally wear them; optimize day and night cues (lighted room during day with activities to prevent napping; darkened, quiet room at night with periods of undisturbed sleep); encourage visitation throughout day by family and friends to reduce anxiety; allow objects from home to be placed where visible; allow wearing of home bedding and clothing (when feasible); encourage proper nutrition; music therapy interventions for mechanically ventilated patients (Bradt, 2014; Hemphill et al., 2015; Josephson & Miller, 2015; Knauert et al., 2015; Pulak & Jensen, 2016; Siddiqi et al., 2016).
- Monitor for optimal level of sedation daily, using a validated assessment tool such as the Richmond Agitation and Sedation Scale (RASS) and/or the Sedation-Agitation Scale (SAS); review sedation and analgesia therapy plan daily (Barr et al., 2013; Harper et al., 2016).
- Sedation strategies using nonbenzodiazepine sedatives (either propofol or dexmedetomidine) may be preferred over sedation with benzodiazepines (either midazolam or lorazepam) to improve clinical outcomes in mechanically ventilated adult ICU patients (Barr et al., 2013; Djaiani et al., 2016; Serafim et al., 2015; Wanat et al., 2014).
- Propofol or dexmedetomidine are preferred drugs when continuous infusions are needed for sedation in preference to benzodiazepines (Barr et al., 2013; Mu et al., 2015; Serafim et al., 2015).
- In mechanically ventilated patients ready for weaning: Both Spontaneous Awakening Trials (SAT) and Spontaneous Breathing Trials (SBT) focus on setting the time(s) each day to stop sedative medications, orient the patient to time and day, and conduct an SBT in an effort to liberate the patient from the ventilator; conduct daily SBT paired with sedation vacations (Barr et al., 2013).

Treatment

- Management is mostly supportive (e.g., treat underlying causes, reorient and reassure patient, avoid restraints, reevaluate the necessity of medications, avoid prolonged use of indwelling catheters (Barr et al., 2013; Harper et al., 2016; Hemphill et al., 2015; Josephson et al., 2015).
- Determine the cause of the delirium:
  For example: Toxins (e.g., medications [benzodiazepines, anticholinergics], drug abuse); metabolic abnormalities (e.g., hyperglycemia, electrolyte disturbances, abnormal body temperature, liver or kidney dysfunction); cerebrovascular disorders; infection or sepsis; hospitalization or immobilization; sensory deprivation (e.g., poor hearing, poor eyesight, lack of sleep, lack of meaningful touch) (Josephson & Miller, 2015; Zaal et al., 2015).
- Antipsychotic agents (e.g., haloperidol or quetiapine) are choices when drug treatment is required in patients with delirium (Michaud et al., 2015). It is important to monitor QT interval in patients who receive antipsychotic drugs (Meyer-Massetti et al., 2010).
- In ventilated patients in the ICU, dexmedetomidine and propofol should be considered over benzodiazepines if sedation is required (Barr et al., 2013; Djaiani et al., 2016; Harper et al., 2016; Serafim et al., 2015; Wanat et al., 2014).

---

external environments. The two most common causes of PVS are cardiac arrest and global cerebral hypoperfusion (Ropper, 2015). The prognosis for recovery from PVS that persists for more than several months is extremely poor. Families of patients with PVS may misinterpret the wandering eye movements and autonomic activities as being meaningful, giving false hope of eventual recovery. It is important for the healthcare team to provide information about PVS and the cause of the patient's "awake" behaviors, as well as to provide psychosocial support to family members.

Brain death is the irreversible loss of all brain and brainstem function (Kress & Hall, 2015). It most commonly results from severe brain injury (usually traumatic) causing global cerebral hypoperfusion. A diagnosis of brain death requires that the patient meet established brain death criteria that include tests to demonstrate the loss of all cerebral and brainstem function. Patients who are diagnosed with brain death are potential candidates as organ donors, making strict adherence to meeting diagnosis requirements extremely important.

Assessment and Management   The cause of coma is often immediately apparent, such as severe brain trauma, cardiac arrest, or known drug overdose (Ropper, 2015). However, the etiology is not always obvious and requires a thorough history and physical assessment with diagnostic laboratory and imaging studies to determine the cause. A battery of laboratory tests may be ordered to find possible chemical sources, such as drug overdose or metabolic toxins. Imaging studies of the brain help investigate potential physical or physiologic problems, such as a brain mass, cerebral edema, or hemorrhage. An electroencephalogram (EEG) may be taken to investigate possible seizure-related causes of coma. If infection is suspected, a lumbar puncture for CSF analysis may be performed.

A focused neurological assessment is warranted in comatose patients. The Glasgow Coma Scale (GCS) is a useful bedside measure of LOC trends. The GCS assesses three responses (eye, verbal, and motor responses) to an external stimulus. Patients who are in a coma state usually require noxious (painful) stimuli (e.g., sternal rub, nail-bed pinch) to elicit a measurable response. Documentation of the GCS score should include the score of each of the three components (eye, verbal, and motor responses) to make the results meaningful. The GCS scoring ranges from 3 to 15, and the lower the score, the more severe the brain dysfunction. As coma reverses, the GCS score increases.

A major goal in early management of the comatose patient is to prevent further deterioration of the neurologic system (Ropper, 2015). Coma is often reversible when treated quickly; therefore, it is crucial to identify and correct the underlying cause. For example, if coma is due to

Related Pharmacotherapy
Agents Used for Treating Delirium

Antipsychotic Agents

Haloperidol lactate (Haldol)
Risperidone (Risperdal)
Quetiapine (Seroquel)

Action and Uses

Haloperidol and risperidone block dopamine receptors; quetiapine blocks dopamine and serotonin receptors with some antihistamine activity. Used in the treatment of delirium, psychotic disorders, agitation; has antiemetic effects.

Dosages (Adult)

Haloperidol: Initial dose—1–2 mg (IV) every 2–4 hours, titrate to response assessing for prolonged *QT* interval; max. single dose 50 mg (max. daily dose 500 mg); continuous IV drip (off-label use)— data not provided.

Risperidone: 2 mg/day PO initially; may increase at every-24-hour intervals by 1–2 mg/day; recommended target dose: 4–8 mg/day PO daily or divide twice daily.

Quetiapine: (off-label use)—PO dose is to start at 25 mg at bedtime.

Major Adverse Effects

Prolonged *QT* interval (which may precipitate torsades), sedation, orthostatic hypotension, tardive dyskinesia (decreased with second-generation drugs), neuroleptic malignant syndrome, agranulocytosis, laryngospasm, hyperthermia, hyperglycemia; second-generation drugs may have less extrapyramidal side effects such as tardive dyskinesia. Seroquel is not as likely to prolong *QT* interval at lower doses; still should avoid using with other drugs or conditions known to prolong *QT* interval.

Nursing Implications

Monitor for therapeutic and nontherapeutic effects.

Older adults typically require lower initial doses.

Monitor with ECG for prolonged *QT* interval; avoid using with other drugs or conditions that prolong *QT* interval.

Monitor for neuroleptic malignant syndrome especially in those patients who take lithium or who have hypertension; discontinue the drug if symptoms occur.

Monitor for dyskinesia especially with higher doses and long-term therapy.

Monitor for extrapyramidal reactions as they are usually dose related.

FDA Black Box Warning: Issued regarding off-label use of antipsychotics for dementia in older adults as clinical trials show that these drugs may increase risk of death.

Monitor for hypotension during loading dose; reduction of loading dose may be required.

Monitor cardiovascular status continuously; notify medical care provider immediately of hypotension or bradycardia (more common in older adults).

Alpha2-adrenergic Agonist; Nonbarbiturate Sedative–Hypnotic Agent

Dexmedetomidine hydrochloride (Precedex)

Action and Uses

Stimulates alpha2-adrenergic receptors in the CNS (primarily in the medulla oblongata), causing inhibition of the sympathetic vasomotor center of the brain and resulting in sedative effects. Sedative properties utilized in intubating patients and for sedation during mechanical ventilator.

Dosages (Adult)

Adult: IV 1 mcg/kg loading dose infused over 10 min, then continue with infusion of 0.2–0.7 mcg/kg/h for up to 24 hr adjusted to maintain sedation; reduce initial dosage in hepatic or renal CrCl less than 30 mL/min.

Major Adverse Effects

Pain, infection. CV: hypotension, bradycardia, atrial fibrillation. GI: nausea, thirst. Respiratory: hypoxia, pleural effusion, pulmonary edema. Hematologic: anemia, leukocytosis. Urogenital: oliguria.

Nursing Implications

Monitor for hypertension during loading dose; reduction of loading dose may be required.

Monitor cardiovascular status continuously; notify prescriber immediately if hypotension or bradycardia occur.

Sedative–hypnotic Agent

Propofol (Diprivan)

Action and Uses

Sedative–hypnotic used in the induction and maintenance of anesthesia or sedation in patients who are mechanically ventilated.

Dosages (Adult)

Adult: IV 5 mcg/kg/min for at least 5 min, may increase by 5–10 mcg/kg/min q5–10 min until desired level of sedation is achieved (may need maintenance rate of 5–80 mcg/kg/min).

Major Adverse Effects

CNS: headache, dizziness, twitching, bucking, jerking, thrashing, clonic or myoclonic movements. Special senses: decreased intraocular pressure. CV: hypotension, ventricular asystole (rare). GI: vomiting, abdominal cramping. Respiratory: cough, hiccups, apnea. Other: pain at injection site.

Nursing Implications

Monitor hemodynamic status and assess for dose-related hypotension.

Take seizure precautions. Tonic–clonic seizures have occurred following general anesthesia with propofol.

Be alert to the potential for drug-induced excitation (e.g., twitching, tremor, hyperclonus), and take appropriate safety measures.

Provide comfort measures; pain at the injection site is quite common, especially when small veins are used.

SOURCE: Data from Wilson et al. (2016).

Emerging Evidence

- A Cochrane systematic review was undertaken to assess the effectiveness of interventions for preventing delirium in hospitalized non–intensive care unit (ICU) patients. Included in this review were randomized controlled trials (RCTs) of nonpharmacological and pharmacological interventions for preventing delirium in hospitalized non–ICU patients. Thirty-nine trials that recruited 16,082 participants, assessing 22 different interventions or comparisons, were reviewed. Strong evidence was found to support multicomponent interventions to prevent delirium in both medical and surgical settings with less robust evidence that they reduce the severity of delirium. Evidence about their effect on the duration of delirium is inconclusive. Monitoring the depth of anesthesia was shown to reduce the occurrence of delirium after general anesthetic. No clear evidence was found that a range of medications or other anesthetic techniques or procedures are effective in preventing delirium (*Siddiqi et al., 2016*).

- ICU environmental factors, such as noise and light, have been cited as important causes of sleep deprivation in critically ill patients. Previous studies indicated that using earplugs and eye masks can improve REM sleep in healthy subjects in a simulated ICU environment and improve sleep quality in ICU patients. This study aimed to determine the effects of using earplugs and eye masks with relaxing background music on sleep, as well as melatonin and cortisol levels, in ICU patients. Fifty patients who underwent a scheduled cardiac surgery and were expected to stay at least 2 nights in cardiac surgical ICU (CSICU) were included. They were randomized to sleep with or without earplugs and eye masks combined with 30-minute relaxing music during the postoperative nights in CSICU. Urine was analyzed for nocturnal melatonin and cortisol levels. Subjective sleep quality was evaluated using the Chinese version of the Richards-Campbell Sleep Questionnaire (a visual analog scale, ranging 0–100). This combination of nonpharmacological interventions is useful for promoting sleep in ICU adult patients; however, any influence on nocturnal melatonin levels and cortisol level may have been masked by several factors, such as the timing of surgery, medication use, and individual differences. Larger scale studies would be needed to examine the potential influences of these factors on biological markers and intervention efficacy on sleep (*Hu, Jiang, Hegadoren, & Zhang, 2015*).

- Researchers investigated the effectiveness and safety of implementing Awakening and Breathing Coordination, Delirium monitoring and management, and Early exercise and mobility (ABCDE) bundle into everyday practice in an 18-month prospective cohort, before-and-after study in five adult ICUs, one step-down unit, and one oncology and hematology special care unit in a tertiary medical center. The study included 296 adult patients (146 prebundle and 150 postbundle implementation). The postbundle group received the ABCDE bundle intervention. Critically ill patients who were managed with the ABCDE bundle spent three more days breathing without assistance, experienced less delirium, and were more likely to be mobilized during their ICU stay than patients treated with usual care (*Balas et al., 2014*).

an accumulation of metabolic toxins, such as blood urea nitrogen (BUN), interventions (e.g., dialysis) are taken to rapidly normalize the BUN and reverse the coma. The nurse meets the patient's supportive needs, such as airway, nutrition and elimination, and hygiene. During the initial management phase, the patient is often in a critical care setting on continuous cardiac monitoring. Mechanical ventilation may be required to protect the airway, promote oxygenation, and prevent hypoventilation. Intravenous access is needed to provide fluid and medications, and may also be used for hemodynamic monitoring. An enteral feeding tube may be inserted to provide nutrition support. In addition, the nurse plays an important role in communicating with the patient's family, providing status updates and explanations of tests and procedures as well as providing general psychosocial support.

Section Two Review

1. Which characteristics correctly describe delirium? (Select all that apply.)
   A. It is preventable.
   B. It has a slow insidious onset.
   C. It may lead to long-term cognitive impairment.
   D. It is associated with higher in-hospital mortality.
   E. It is a rare condition, but results are devastating.

2. Which client is least likely to develop delirium?
   A. A client with numerous comorbid illnesses
   B. A client who is receiving IV midazolam continuous infusion
   C. A client with preexisting cognitive impairments
   D. A client who is young

3. Which statements are correct regarding coma?
   A. Coma usually results in death.
   B. The altered consciousness state has lasted more than 6 hours.
   C. It is a completely irreversible condition.
   D. The most common cause is metabolic disturbances.

4. The consciousness state found in persistent vegetative state (PVS) is best described in which way?
   A. The client maintains the arousal component but not awareness.
   B. The client can only be aroused using highly noxious stimuli.
   C. The client has rare occurrences of awareness.
   D. The client usually shows improvement after 6–12 months.

Answers: 1. (A, C, D, E), 2. D, 3. B, 4. A

Section Three: Disorders of Movement

Sensory motor disorders of movement may occur in high-acuity patients. Immobilization and subsequent weakness are consequences of prolonged illness. Neuromuscular weakness disorders can produce severe, life-threatening complications that can impair function and quality of life following acute or critical care illness.

Critical Illness Polyneuropathy and Myopathy

A substantial number of patients admitted to the ICU because of an acute illness, complicated surgery, severe trauma, or burn injury will develop muscle weakness during the ICU stay that is referred to as intensive care unit acquired weakness (ICUAW). ICUAW may affect peripheral as well as respiratory muscles (Dres et al., 2017; Jung et al., 2016). ICUAW can be evoked either by critical illness polyneuropathy (CIP), by critical illness myopathy (CIM), or by both during the course of critical illness. These complications of acute and critical illness are associated with progressive and uncontrolled systemic inflammation, such as that which occurs with systemic inflammatory response syndrome (SIRS), severe sepsis, and multiorgan failure (Apostolakis, Papakonstantinou, Baikoussis, & Papadopoulos, 2015; Hermans & Van den Berghe, 2015; Osias & Manno, 2014; Santos et al., 2012; Zorowitz, 2016). Neuromuscular weakness disorders in the critically ill are relatively common and often go undetected because they are overshadowed by the more prominent clinical manifestations of the primary conditions. They contribute to immobility in the acute and critically ill population. ICUAW is associated with a high morbidity and mortality, and recent data reveal that ICUAW may also have longer-term consequences beyond hospitalization. For example, ICUAW may be an important contributor to the post intensive care syndrome (PICS) (Hermans et al., 2014; Needham et al., 2012). PICS includes the physical, mental, and cognitive dysfunctions that are part of the persisting disabilities, which extend beyond the acute hospitalization and have major impact on the quality of life of the growing population of ICU survivors. It is important to identify these disorders early (Hermans & Van den Berghe, 2015; Osias & Manno, 2014).

Patients with weakness acquired in the intensive care unit are often sedated and mechanically ventilated. Accurate sensory and motor examinations are often difficult to accomplish in these patients, making it difficult to get an accurate picture of the incidence and prevalence of ICUAW, CIP, and CIM. Some estimates published in the scientific literature note as many as 70% of patients with systemic inflammatory response syndrome (SIRS) or sepsis and multiple organ dysfunction syndrome will have evidence of polyneuropathy or myopathy, and often both disorders occur together in the same patient (Amato & Brown, 2015; Apostolakis et al., 2015; Dres et al., 2017; Zorowitz, 2016).

Risk Factors for Development ICUAW is most likely to develop in severely ill patients who have both SIRS and comorbidities. The onset of ICUAW can occur as early as 3 days after the diagnosis of sepsis or SIRS (Amato & Brown, 2015). ICUAW has also been associated with prolonged mechanical ventilation, malnutrition, coagulopathies, high-dose corticosteroids, the use of certain antibiotics (aminoglycosides such as gentamicin), use of neuromuscular blocking agents (NMBA; most notably pancuronium bromide), electrolyte disturbances, and elevated glucose levels (Amato & Brown, 2015; Friedrich et al., 2015; Hermans & Van den Berghe, 2015; Santos et al., 2012).

ICUAW is thought to be due to microcirculatory dysfunction or hyperinflammation that may cause damage to the motor neuron integrity (Amato & Brown, 2015; Friedrich et al., 2015; Hermans & Van den Berghe, 2015). Despite variability in reports of incidence of both polyneuropathy and myopathy, after a review of the research evidence, Pandit and Agrawal (2006) reported that both are present in 52% to 57% of patients in the ICU for 7 days or more and in 68% to 100% of patients with sepsis or SIRS, making this a significant event in the illness trajectory for patients who require high-acuity nursing care.

Critical Illness Polyneuropathy CIP is an acute axonal sensory–motor polyneuropathy that mainly affects the lower-limb nerves. It is often preceded by septic encephalopathy and is followed by difficulty in weaning from the ventilator. In these patients, a symptom of CIP is when a painful stimulus such as nail-bed pressure is applied, the patient may demonstrate facial grimacing but have reduced or absent movement of the affected limbs. There seems to be distal loss of pain, temperature, and vibration sensory abilities even in alert patients. Deep tendon reflexes are preserved in CIP. Autonomic function is preserved, which helps to distinguish this condition from other weakness syndromes such as Guillain-Barré syndrome. Onset of CIP is variable, occurring from 2 days to a few weeks after the onset of the inciting illness (Amato & Brown, 2015). Electrodiagnostic testing (with nerve conduction studies and electromyograms) is necessary to diagnose this disorder. There is no specific treatment; prevention involves anticipating this complication and promptly treating the predisposing condition. Van den Berghe et al. (2001) found that tight glucose control with intensive insulin therapy in adults receiving mechanical ventilation and admitted to the ICU can reduce the incidence of critical illness polyneuropathy by 44%. Complete recovery is expected in approximately half of cases (Hermans & Van den Berghe, 2015). Recovery can be complete within a few weeks in milder cases but can take months in severe cases.

Critical Illness Myopathy CIM is a spectrum of muscle disorders that present with diffuse weakness, depressed deep tendon reflexes, and mildly elevated creatine kinase levels (Amato & Brown, 2015). Electrodiagnostic testing reveals a myopathy, and muscle biopsy reveals atrophy with loss of the thick myosin filaments. CIM is associated with status asthmaticus in approximately one third of these patients. This association is thought to be more prevalent in patients who receive high-dose corticosteroid therapy. Also, neuromuscular blocking agent (NMBA) use is associated with CIM. Like CIP, there is no specific treatment for CIM, and most patients with this disorder make a full recovery within a few months. CIM, like CIP, prolongs mechanical ventilation and increases complications of immobility in high-acuity patients. Pulmonary complications are particularly problematic for patients with CIP and CIM. Pulmonary consequences of progressive neuromuscular weakness include decreased respiratory muscle strength, impaired cough and ability to clear secretions, increased risk of infection and airway obstruction, atelectasis and progressive hypoxemia, alveolar hypoventilation, and hypercapnia.

Management of these complications includes careful observation of oxygenation and ventilator status, pulmonary hygiene, tracheal intubation, supplemental oxygen, mechanical ventilation, and PEEP. As the neuromuscular weakness progresses, atelectasis and hypoxemia become prominent, followed by alveolar hypoventilation and progressive CO_2 retention. Hypoxemia is often a late finding. Early intubation and mechanical ventilation before the occurrence of respiratory failure are indicated.

Neuromuscular Blockade – Induced Paralysis

Neuromuscular blocking agents (NMBAs) are drugs that induce skeletal muscle paralysis and are most often used to immobilize patients during short procedures. In the critical care setting, it is sometimes necessary to paralyze the patient for a sustained period of time using NMBA therapy. NMBA use is reserved for life-threatening conditions in which there is a need to eliminate all skeletal muscle movement—for example, to decrease oxygen consumption, control mechanical ventilation (e.g., acute respiratory distress syndrome), or reduce intracranial pressure (Amato

& Brown, 2015). NMBAs are used only when analgesia and sedation have not been effective, or when needed to facilitate treatment. A major goal for neuromuscular blockade (NMB)–induced paralysis is to maximize oxygenation by preventing skeletal muscle movement.

Action   NMBAs work by binding to nicotinic acetylcholine receptors on the postsynaptic side of the neuromuscular junction. Depolarizing NMBAs like acetylcholine (ACh) produce a sustained postsynaptic depolarization that blocks subsequent muscle contraction. Nondepolarizing agents act by competitively inhibiting ACh-induced postsynaptic depolarization.

Nondepolarizing Agents   Multiple NMBAs are available for use in critical care, two of which are nondepolarizing agents: cisatracurium (Nimbex) and vecuronium (Norcuron). Cisatracurium is a rapid-acting agent with an onset of 1.5 to 3.3 minutes and a half-life of 22 minutes (Wilson et al., 2016). It has potential adverse effects of hypotension, bradycardia, and bronchospasm. Its clinical effect is not prolonged by hepatic or renal failure. Vecuronium is an immediate-acting agent with an onset of less than a minute and a half-life of 30 to 80 minutes (Wilson et al., 2016). Vecuronium has been associated, although rarely, with the major adverse effect of malignant hyperthermia. It can be used in patients with severe cardiac and renal dysfunction or asthma. These two drugs are profiled in the "Related Pharmacotherapy: Neuromuscular Blocking and Reversal Agents" feature.

Related Pharmocotherapy
Neuromuscular Blocking and Reversal Agents

Neuromuscular Blocking Agents (NMBA)

Cisatracurium (Nimbex)
Vecuronium (Norcuron)

Action and Uses

Nondepolarizing skeletal muscle relaxant; paralytic agent; requires ventilator support
Used for chemical paralysis to optimize mechanical ventilation, treat seizures

Dosages (Adult)

Cisatracurium: 0.15–0.2 mg/kg IV; maintenance dose is 0.03 mg/kg IV 40–50 minutes following initial dose of 0.15 mg/kg
Vecuronium: Load with 0.08–0.1 mg/kg IV push over 60 seconds with maintenance dose of 0.01–0.015 mg/kg IV push 20–45 min post initial loading dose; for continuous IV infusion, load with 0.0008–0.001 mg/kg/min IV starting 20 minutes post bolus with maintenance of 0.0008–0.0012 mg/kg/min

Major Adverse Effects

Cisatracurium
Vecuronium

Nursing Implications

Patient's respiratory muscles are paralyzed—requires intubation and mechanical ventilation prior to initiating therapy.

NM blockade does not treat anxiety or relieve pain—administer with a sedative and/or opiate.

SOURCE: Data from Wilson et al. (2016).

Monitor degree of paralysis using train-of-four peripheral nerve stimulation; administer at lowest possible doses.
Monitor BP, pulse; avoid hypotension.

NMBA Reversal Agents

Pyridostigmine bromide (Regonol)
Neostigmine

Action and Uses

Acetylcholinesterase inhibitor that increases the amount of available acetylcholine (ACh) so that ACh can compete with the neuromuscular blocking agent (NMBA) at the receptor sites. Reverse the paralytic action of NMBAs. Also used for treatment of myasthenia gravis. Pyridostigmine is an analog of neostigmine.

Dosages (Adult)

Pyridostigmine: 0.1–0.25 mg/kg (IV atropine or glycopyrrolate should immediately precede)
Neostigmine: 0.5–2.5 mg (administer slowly; repeat for a max total dose of 5 mg)

Major Adverse Effects

Most serious: bronchoconstriction
Most common: nausea and vomiting, miosis, excessive salivation and sweating

Nursing Implications

Monitor vegetative state closely and observe respirations.
Not usually used for reversal of sustained NMBA therapy (NMBA therapy is withdrawn for reversal).

Potential Complications The use of NMBAs to induce paralysis is associated with serious complications and should be used with caution. NMBAs are considered high-alert drugs that are to be used only by providers who have strong knowledge of the drugs and their appropriate use and management. Complications associated with NMBAs as a group include prolonged muscle weakness after the drug is discontinued, which may be due to residual drug effect with accumulation of active metabolites and delayed clearance, or a synergistic effect that occurs when the agents are given with corticosteroids or aminoglycosides. In addition, each NMBA has its own set of potential side and adverse effects that must be monitored for.

Aminoglycosides, antibiotics, hypothermia, hyperkalemia, and hypercalcemia potentiate the effects of NMBAs. Prolonged muscle weakness is associated with elevated serum creatine kinase levels, muscle fiber atrophy, and muscle fiber necrosis (Hemphill et al., 2015). NMBAs should be avoided in any patient who is receiving prolonged corticosteroid therapy as this increases the risk for extended weakness. The patient is also at increased risk for development of complications of immobility, such as deep vein thrombosis, pulmonary embolism, atelectasis, and pneumonia.

Nursing Considerations While NMBAs are highly effective for inducing and maintaining paralysis, they have no effect on pain sensation or anxiety. For this reason, NMBA therapy is typically given with a sedative or hypnotic (e.g., propofol or dexmedetomidine) and an analgesic (e.g., fentanyl or morphine). These adjunct drugs should be initiated before NMBA therapy begins. Adjunct drugs are profiled in the "Related Pharmacotherapy: Adjunct Sedation and Analgesia Agents" feature.

Related Pharmocotherapy
Adjunct Sedation and Analgesia Agents

Sedation

Central alpha-2 receptor antagonist
Dexmedetomidine (Precedex)

Action and Uses
A sedative or hypnotic used to provide ICU sedation (during initial intubation and mechanical ventilation); blocks central alpha-2 receptors; short-term clinical trials have shown this agent to decrease risk for duration of delirium episodes compared with benzodiazepines.

Dosages (Adult)
IV dose: Load with 1 mcg/kg over 10 minutes; maintenance dose 0.2–0.7 mcg/kg/hr continuous infusion

Major Adverse Effects
Hypotension, atrial fibrillation, bradycardia, use with caution in renal or hepatic impairment; use beyond 24 hours is associated with tolerance, tachycardia, pulmonary edema or pleural effusion.

Nursing Implications
Monitor for overdose symptoms (somnolence, confusion, sedation, diminished reflexes, coma, hypotension, and respiratory depression).
Monitor for hypertension during loading dose.

General anesthetic/sedative/hypnotic
Propofol (Diprivan)

Action and Uses
A general anesthetic used to provide ICU sedation (during initial intubation and mechanical ventilation); not associated with increased incidence of delirium at low doses.

Dosages (Adult)
IV dose: Initial dosing—0.005 mg/kg/min; maintenance dose—0.005–0.05 mg/kg/min with 0.005 mg/kg/min increment every 5 min

Major Adverse Effects
Respiratory depression, hypotension, bradycardia, tissue necrosis with extravasation; propofol infusion syndrome characterized by metabolic acidosis, hyperkalemia, rhabdomyolysis, cardiac or renal failure, hepatic enzyme elevation; drug-induced excitation.

Nursing Implications
Increased risk of microorganism growth. To avoid contamination: Discard vial if discoloration is present or particular matter noted; administer immediately after hanging infusion and must be completed within 6 hours of hanging.
Protect from light.
Shake well before use.
Control rate by using pump.
Monitor cardiac rhythm and hemodynamic status during and following administration.
Observe for drug-induced excitation (e.g., tremor or twitching).
May cause pain at injection site.

Analgesia
Fentanyl citrate (Duragesic, Sublimaze)
Morphine sulfate

Action and Uses
Fentanyl: Short-acting narcotic agonist with a duration of 30–60 minutes. Action is similar to that of morphine.
Morphine: Opioid analgesic that binds to endogenous opioid receptors.

Dosages (Adult)
Fentanyl: Moderate to severe pain: 50–100 mcg (IV) administered over 3–5 min
Morphine: 2.5–15 mg/70 kg every 2–4 hrs (IV) or continuous infusion of 0.8–10 mg/hr. Increase as needed to control pain

Major Adverse Effects
Fentanyl: Most serious—cardiac depression or arrest, respiratory depression or arrest. Most common—sedation, nausea.
Morphine: Most serious—anaphylactoid reaction, cardiac arrest, severe respiratory depression or arrest. Most common—constipation, nausea.

Nursing Implications
Fentanyl: Monitor vital signs (VS) closely and for signs of respiratory depression. Respiratory depression effects may last longer than analgesic effects.
Morphine: Respiratory rate of 12/min or less with miosis present suggests morphine toxicity; monitor VS closely and for signs of respiratory depression and hypotension.

SOURCE: Data from Wilson et al. (2016).

Assessing the patient's neurologic status using traditional bedside assessments is not meaningful during paralysis; however, it is important to monitor the level of paralysis to ensure that the patient is receiving the correct drug dose for optimal benefits. The level of paralysis is measured by applying a train-of-four (TOF) series of low-frequency (2 Hz) electrical impulses (current strength 50–90 milliamps) to the ulnar nerve at the forearm, and observe for adduction of the thumb. If there is an absence of thumb adduction, the level of neuromuscular blockade is excessive. The drug infusion is titrated to achieve one or two thumb twitches out of the four electrical impulses (Whetstone Foster, 2011).

Another method used to monitor the level of neuromuscular blockade is continuous airway pressure monitoring (CAPM), which uses a transducer cable, high-pressure tubing, and a transducer to display continuous airway pressures. CAPM can identify spontaneous diaphragmatic effort before any other signs of neurologic activity can be detected in patients with neuromuscular blockade. When continuous or prolonged neuromuscular blockade is indicated (occurs for more than 48 hours), the infusion should be stopped daily to assess for its continued need (Whetstone Foster, 2011). When excessive neuromuscular blockade has been identified, or when there is no longer a need for the therapy, paralysis from nondepolarizing agents can be reversed with administration of an anticholinesterase agent such as physostigmine (Antilirium) (Wilson et al., 2016).

Patients who are receiving NMBA require total comprehensive care. Prior to NMBA initiation, the patient must be intubated and mechanically ventilated using a mode that performs all of the breathing because the patient is not able to breathe independently. Nursing management during prolonged neuromuscular blockade also consists of protecting the airway, maintaining adequate ventilation, monitoring cardiac rhythm and blood pressure, treating pain and anxiety, protecting eyes, and maintaining skin integrity. All patients who receive neuromuscular blockade require prophylactic eye care (cannot blink); physical activity, including range-of-motion exercises; and deep-vein thrombosis (DVT) prophylaxis. Prophylactic eye care consists of keeping the eyes closed and covered with a soft eye pad, and includes use of eye lubricants or artificial tears. Skin should be observed for potential areas of breakdown, with frequent repositioning and consideration of pressure-reducing mattresses and surfaces. Continuous lateral rotation therapy (CLRT) with specialty beds that provide lateral rotation along with passive range of motion are strategies to prevent complications of immobility. Neuromuscular blockade does not provide sedation or amnesia, nor does it provide analgesia. Paralysis from neuromuscular blockade can be expected to be anxiety provoking because the sensation of paralysis can be frightening for the patient who is cognitively aware. Therefore, patients receiving NMBA therapy are also placed on a sedation or analgesia regimen.

Section Three Review

1. Critical illness polyneuropathy and myopathy are considered complications of which pathophysiologic complication?
   A. Systemic inflammation
   B. Endocrine imbalance
   C. Hemodynamic instability
   D. Diabetes

2. Which statements are true regarding intensive care unit acquired weakness (ICUAW)?
   A. It affects only peripheral muscles.
   B. It may be caused by critical illness polyneuropathy (CIP).
   C. It results in critical illness myopathy (CIM).
   D. It has few long-term consequences.

3. Which characteristics are present with critical illness myopathy (CIM)? (Select all that apply.)
   A. Severe confusion
   B. Decreased creatine kinase
   C. Preserved deep tendon reflexes
   D. Diffuse weakness

4. Train of four (TOF) testing is performed on patients receiving neuromuscular blocking agent (NMBA) therapy for which reason?
   A. To assess for pain
   B. To assess level of paralysis
   C. To assess for anxiety
   D. To assess degree of muscle strength

Answers: 1. A, 2. B, 3. D, 4. B

Section Four: Seizure Complications in High-Acuity Patients

Seizures occur when the brain's electrical system discharges in a disorganized fashion, disrupting normal functioning either focally or generally. High-acuity patients are at risk for acute development of seizures called new onset seizures, which are considered another sensory motor complication of critical illness. They occur in patients with no previous history of seizures. The incidence of new onset seizures in ICU patients is 0.8% to 3.5% (Zammit, Choi, & Rosengart, 2016). They are particularly common in neurointensive care units where brain injury (e.g., from trauma or stroke) is most commonly managed.

Table 17–2 Examples of Drugs Associated with New Onset Seizures

Issue	Drugs
INTOXICATION (Drugs that can precipitate seizure activity due to toxicity or hypersensitivity)	Amphetamines, ciprofloxacin, cocaine, imipenem, isoniazid, lidocaine, meperidine, penicillins, phencyclidine, theophylline, tricyclic antidepressants
WITHDRAWAL (Drugs that can precipitate seizure activity if withdrawn abruptly)	Barbiturates, benzodiazepines, ethanol, opiates

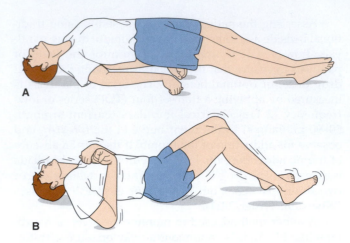

Figure 17–2 Tonic–clonic seizures. A, Tonic phase. B, Clonic phase.

Causes

New onset seizures can be the result of a drug intoxication, drug withdrawal (alcohol, sedative, or opioid), infections, brain trauma, ischemic injury of the brain, space-occupying lesions of the brain, or systemic metabolic derangements that can occur with hepatic or renal failure, sepsis, hypoglycemia, hyponatremia, or hypocalcemia. Toxic levels of or withdrawal from certain drugs can precipitate seizures (see Table 17–2).

Classification

Seizures are classified as being either generalized or partial. A generalized seizure is one in which the entire cerebral cortex is simultaneously activated; a partial (focal) seizure is one in which a localized area (epileptogenic focus) of the cortex is activated at onset of the seizure (Zammit et al., 2016). There are multiple subtypes of seizures under the generalized and partial classes, each with its own set of characteristics. Not all types of seizures have a motor component, and a seizure may involve only sensory aberrations or altered LOC. Two types of seizures that require rapid interventions in critical care are generalized tonic–clonic seizures and status epilepticus. They are the focus of this section.

Generalized Tonic–clonic Seizures Generalized tonic–clonic (formerly called grand mal or convulsion) seizures have an initial tonic phase that is associated with apnea and cyanosis. The tonic phase is followed by a clonic phase, during which the airway may become lost and respirations are labored (Lowenstein, 2015). The *tonic phase* is characterized by a sudden loss of consciousness and sharp tonic muscle contractions, during which muscles become rigid, arms and legs extend, and the jaw is clenched. The patient often develops apnea during this phase. The *clonic phase* is characterized by alternating contraction and relaxation of the muscles in all of the extremities, along with hyperventilation. The eyes often roll back, and there is increased lacrimation in the clonic phase. The *postictal period* occurs immediately following the seizure, which can be characterized by transient impairment of mentation and sensorium. The person slowly becomes more aware of the surroundings but does not remember the seizure. Figure 17–2 shows the phases of tonic–clonic seizures.

The adverse effects of generalized seizures include hypertension, lactic acidosis, hyperthermia, respiratory compromise, pulmonary aspiration or edema, rhabdomyolysis, self-injury, and irreversible neurological damage, especially if the seizure lasts for more than 30 minutes (Lowenstein, 2015).

Management of Acute Onset Seizures

It is important to identify any correctible etiology of the seizure and treat appropriately (e.g., correct electrolyte imbalance). If the seizure stops and the cause(s) is/are corrected, antiseizure medication may not be needed. However, if a tonic–clonic seizure lasts for longer than 5 to 10 minutes, drug management is needed because the risk for permanent neurological injury or refractory seizures increases the longer that the seizure persists.

Pharmacotherapy Several drug groups are effective for management of generalized tonic–clonic seizures, including benzodiazepines, phenytoins, and several other drug options such as barbiturates.

Benzodiazepines. Benzodiazepines are classified as anxiolytics and sedative–hypnotics, but they also have anticonvulsant capabilities. Intravenous benzodiazepines (e.g., lorazepam, diazepam) are effective in stopping the seizure 65% to 80% of the time (Lowenstein, 2015; Zammit et al., 2016). Lorazepam in a dose of 0.1 mg/kg IV is the treatment of choice over diazepam 0.15 mg/kg IV because it lasts longer, making recurrent seizures less likely to occur.

Phenytoins. Intravenous phenytoin should be administered with diazepam or, if the seizure is persistent, despite lorazepam administration. Fosphenytoin (Cerebyx) can be administered IV or IM and is preferred over phenytoin (Dilantin) because it can be delivered faster (maximum IV infusion rate of 150 mg/min) and thus produce more rapid suppression of seizures. Furthermore, fosphenytoin does not contain propylene glycol, which can cause cardiovascular depression. It is also compatible with dextrose solutions and, if infiltrated into the skin, will not cause skin necrosis as phenytoin does. Phenytoin is administered at a dose of 20 mg/kg in adults and 15 mg/kg for older adults, with a maximum infusion rate of 50 mg/min; therefore, it has a slower onset of action than fosphenytoin. Phenytoin administration can be associated with hypotension due to cardiac suppression from the propylene glycol that it contains. Phenytoin cannot be administered in dextrose-containing solutions; if infiltration occurs, it will cause tissue vesication and necrosis (Lowenstein, 2015; Zammit et al., 2016).

Other Drug Options. If seizures continue to persist despite administration of benzodiazepines, fosphenytoin, or phenytoin, administration of one or more of the following is needed: phenobarbital (20 mg/kg at 50 mg/min); propofol (3–5 mg/kg load, then 1–15 mg/kg/hr); midazolam (0.2 mg/kg load, then 0.05–2 mg/kg/hr); or pentobarbital (5–15 mg/kg load, then 0.5–10 mg/kg/hr). If propofol, midazolam, or pentobarbital is used, intubation and mechanical ventilation is required, as these drugs will suppress respiratory drive (Lowenstein, 2015; Zammit et al., 2016). Refer back to the "Related Pharmacotherapy: Adjunct Sedation and Analgesia Agents" feature for a profile of propofol and barbiturates.

Status Epilepticus

Status epilepticus refers to seizures that are continuous for more than 5 minutes or seizures that recur without a recovery of consciousness (Lowenstein, 2015). The most common cause of status epilepticus is a subtherapeutic plasma level of prescribed anticonvulsants. There are multiple less common causes, such as withdrawal from alcohol or drugs, CNS infection, cerebral hypoxia, brain trauma, and metabolic abnormalities (Lowenstein, 2015). Mortality is highest in this type of seizure activity because the patient is unable to breathe and is at risk of developing permanent neurologic damage within 20 minutes of onset, making this a medical emergency (Zammit et al., 2016).

Management of status epilepticus requires early recognition and rapid interventions, many of which occur simultaneously. Zammit et al. (2016) recommend the following therapeutic protocol:

- Within 5 minutes of onset, IV lorazepam (or diazepam) should be administered along with IV phenytoin (or fosphenytoin).

- If seizures do not cease within 30 minutes (refractory status epilepticus), other drug options should be initiated, such as IV phenobarbital (or valproic acid), IV propofol (or midazolam), or IV ketamine.

- Management also includes large-bore IV access, oxygen therapy and airway management, obtaining vital signs, pulse oximetry, and ECG. Priority laboratory tests include anticonvulsant drug blood levels, toxicology screen, ABG, electrolytes, glucose, and CBC. EEG monitoring should also be considered with refractory status epilepticus.

Drugs used for treating status epilepticus are profiled in the "Related Pharmacotherapy: Agents Used for Treating Status Epilepticus" feature.

Related Pharmacotherapy
Agents Used for Treating Status Epilepticus

Benzodiazepines

Lorazepam (Ativan)
Diazepam (Valium)
Midazolam (Versed)

Action and Uses

Anxiolytic, sedative–hypnotic agents with anticonvulsant capabilities. Midazolam is used for rescue treatment of seizures refractory to lorazepam and diazepam.

Dosages (Adult)

Lorazepam (IV): (First-line drug) 4 mg slow push at 2 mg/min, may repeat dose once if inadequate response after 10–15 min.
Diazepam (IV): (If lorazepam not available) IV/IM dose of 5–10 mg, repeat if needed at 10–15 min intervals up to 30 mg, then repeat if needed every 2–4 hrs.
Midazolam (IV): (For refractory status epilepticus) 1–2.5 mg, may repeat in 2 min; IV continuous infusion requires loading dose of

10–50 mcg/kg slow IV push or infusion over several minutes, may repeat every 10–15 min; maintenance dose of 20–100 mcg/kg/hr continuous infusion, titrate up or down 25%–50% to achieve desired effect.

Adverse Effects

Hypotension, respiratory depression, confusion, insertion-site redness. Diazepam will damage tissues if extravasation occurs.

Nursing Implications

Monitor respiratory rate, BP (avoid hypotension).
Monitor for arrhythmias.
Avoid extravasations.
Obese patients may have prolonged half-life with IV infusion of benzodiazepines.
Monitor for overdose symptoms (somnolence, confusion, sedation, diminished reflexes, coma, hypotension, and respiratory depression).
Monitor for hypertension during loading dose of dexmedetomidine.

Hydantoins

Phenytoin (Dilantin)
Fosphenytoin (Cerebyx)

Action and Uses

Anticonvulsants; increase the seizure threshold; alter cortical electrical discharge by reducing frequency and strength (voltage), thus limiting seizure spread. Used for treatment of seizure disorders. Fosphenytoin is a prodrug that converts to phenytoin. It stabilizes neuronal sodium channels and movement of calcium across neuronal cell membranes; stabilizes glial and neuronal Na^+/K^+ ATPase.

Dosages (Adult)

Phenytoin: Loading dose—10–15 mg/kg at 25–50 mg/min; THEN 100 mg IV/PO every 6–8 hr. **Administer IV dose slowly; not to exceed 50 mg/min (in older adult, administer no faster than 25 mg/min).**

Fosphenytoin (IV): Loading dose—15–20 mg PE/kg (PE = phenytoin sodium equivalents); infuse at 100–150 mg/min; maintenance dose: 4–6 mg PE/kg/day. If bolus dose given, administer at rate of 100–150 mg PE/min.

Major Adverse Effects

Phenytoin (IV): MUST be given at recommended rate to avoid potentially life-threatening cardiac dysrhythmias or cardiovascular collapse. Highly incompatible with other drugs—IV line should be flushed before and after use with normal saline and a dedicated IV line should be used for infusion. Extravasation can result in tissue sloughing. Also can cause agranulocytosis, aplastic anemia, Stevens-Johnson syndrome, and other dermatologic disorders.

Fosphenytoin (IV): MUST be given at recommended rate to avoid potential life-threatening adverse effects such as cardiovascular collapse or life-threatening cardiac dysrhythmias; agranulocytosis, aplastic anemia, toxic epidermal necrolysis.

Nursing Implications

Use with caution in patients with kidney or liver dysfunction, cardiac dysrhythmias.

Monitor ECG and respiratory patterns during and 10–20 min following administration.

Monitor closely for development of rash or other dermatologic signs and report immediately.

In diabetics—monitor glucose closely for development of hyperglycemia.

Monitor for purple glove syndrome, a local toxicity that includes edema, discoloration, and pain distal to the site of injection that may or may not be associated with extravasation, which can develop several days after injection.

Barbiturates

Phenobarbital sodium
Pentobarbital

Action and Uses

Anticonvulsant, sedative–hypnotic. Interferes with transmission of impulses in the cerebral cortex by inhibiting the reticular activating system. As an anticonvulsant, it limits seizure spread by increasing seizure threshold. Can be used during seizure emergencies such as status epilepticus.

Dosages (Adult)

Phenobarbital: 1–3 mg/kg/day in divided doses. For status epilepticus—15–18 mg/kg (IV) initially, then an additional 5 mg/kg.

Pentobarbital: Sedation or status epilepticus—10 mg/kg followed by 0.5–1 mg/kg, then adjust to lowest dose that gives desired effect. Control infusion rate to 50 mg/min or less.

Major Adverse Effects

Most serious—CNS depression, coma, death, agranulocytosis, respiratory depression, Stevens-Johnson syndrome. Most common—somnolence. Pentobarbital (additional effect)—laryngospasm.

Nursing Implications

Closely monitor patient receiving large doses for excessive CNS and respiratory depression.

Monitor VS at least every hour.

Monitor drug levels—serum levels greater than 50 mcg/mL can result in coma.

Paradoxical responses (e.g., marked excitation) can occur in special populations (e.g., older adult, debilitated person).

SOURCE: Data from Wilson et al. (2016).

Nursing Considerations

During the seizure, the goal is to prevent further injury. If in bed, hard objects such as the call bell should be temporarily moved away from the patient. If the patient's body is hitting the bed rails, the bed blankets or other readily available soft objects can be placed on the inside of the rail to buffer against injury. If the patient is on the floor, the head should be protected by placing something soft such as a pillow, blanket, or towel under it. No attempt should be made to place objects in the mouth or restrain the limbs during the seizure. The patient should be gently rolled to the side to allow secretions to clear the mouth and prevent aspiration. It is important for the nurse to time the seizure from beginning to end, estimate the length of time the patient was apneic, and take note of the exact progression of seizure activity. If a seizure lasts for longer than 5 minutes, the healthcare provider should be contacted immediately. Once the seizure is complete, the patient should be checked for injury, a set of vital signs including SpO_2 should be obtained, a rapid neuro check should be conducted, and the healthcare provider notified.

Nursing care for patients who suffer acute onset seizures in the acute care setting includes observing the injection site frequently during administration of phenytoin to prevent infiltration. Vital signs need to be continuously monitored during IV infusion and for an hour afterward. Watch for respiratory depression, hypotension, arrhythmias, or further neurologic compromise, such as decreased level of consciousness during IV administration of medications. Observe for signs and symptoms of an allergic reaction, such as rash or itching, burning or tingling, or glucose intolerance in diabetics. In order to prevent seizures, nurses must be vigilant in monitoring for and identifying any of the previously mentioned etiologies of acute onset seizures in acutely or critically ill patients. A summary of caring for the patient with seizures is found in the "Nursing Care: The Patient Who Experiences Seizures" feature.

Nursing Care
The Patient Who Experiences Seizures

Expected Patient Outcomes and Related Interventions

Outcome 1: Cessation of seizure activity

Assess and compare to established norms, patient baselines, and trends

Assess for changes in mental status and LOC, restlessness, drowsiness, lethargy, inability to follow commands.

Assess for seizure activity (onset, duration, characteristics).

Assess BP, HR, temperature, hemodynamics, and cardiac stability.

Monitor serum glucose, pH, lactic acid, creatine kinase, and myoglobin levels.

Administer related drug therapy and monitor for therapeutic and nontherapeutic effects

Anticonvulsant therapy (e.g., benzodiazepines, hydantoins)

Administer IV fluids or vasoactive medications to offset the effects of continued seizure activity or anticonvulsant drugs.

Interventions to prevent seizures

Treat hyperthermia with passive cooling or antipyretic.

Correct metabolic abnormalities (e.g., electrolyte imbalances, hyperglycemia, elevated ammonia).

Outcome 2: Maintain oxygenation

Assess and compare to established norms, patient baselines, and trends

Evaluate oxygenation and ventilation through the use of arterial blood gases and pulse oximetry.

Monitor for hemodynamic stability.

Monitor for apnea period during seizure.

Administer related drug therapy and monitor for therapeutic and nontherapeutic effects

Oxygen therapy to maintain SpO_2 of 92% or greater

Interventions to support oxygenation

Maintain an open airway using head-tilt or chin-lift maneuver.

Have suction and resuscitation equipment available and suction as needed.

Place in side-lying position during and directly following seizure to prevent aspiration of oral secretions.

Intubation may be needed with prolonged seizure activity.

Outcome 3: Freedom from injury

Assess and compare to established norms, patient baselines, and trends

Monitor patient's local environment for sources of potential injury should a seizure occur.

Following a seizure, assess for injury, including the oral cavity.

Interventions to prevent injury

Pad side rails of bed with rails up.

Have oxygen and suction source readily available.

Do not hold down limbs or restrain during seizure.

Loosen any restrictive clothing.

Do not force anything into the patient's mouth.

Keep area clear of sharp objects.

Allow the patient to sleep following seizure activity.

Document the duration and characteristics of the seizure activity as well as the postictal status of the patient.

Section Four Review

1. The tonic phase of a seizure is characterized by which occurrence? (Select all that apply.)
   A. Loss of consciousness
   B. Extension and rigidity of extremities
   C. Alternating contraction and relaxation of muscles
   D. Hyperventilation
   E. Clenching of the jaw

2. In a generalized tonic–clonic seizure, when is it most common for the patient to lose the airway?
   A. Clonic phase
   B. Tonic phase
   C. Postictal phase
   D. Patients rarely lose their airway with this type of seizure.

3. What advantage does fosphenytoin have over phenytoin?
   A. Fosphenytoin does not cause skin necrosis if infiltrated.
   B. Fosphenytoin can be delivered at a slower rate.
   C. Fosphenytoin contains propylene glycol.
   D. Fosphenytoin can be administered orally.

4. At which point does a seizure episode become status epilepticus? (Select all that apply.)
   A. If more than two seizures occur in 1 hour
   B. If seizures are continuous for more than 5 minutes
   C. If seizures recur without a recovery of consciousness
   D. If the patient loses consciousness during the seizure
   E. If seizures occur despite therapeutic-range medication levels

Answers: 1. (A, B, E), 2. A, 3. A, 4. (B, C)

Clinical Reasoning Checkpoint

Ms. T is an 82-year-old woman who was admitted from a long-term-care facility to the hospital with fever and chronic diarrhea. She is diagnosed with a urinary tract infection. On admission, she was pleasantly confused, oriented to name only, and following commands. Twenty-four hours after her admission, she became agitated, increasingly confused, and pulled out her lines.

1. Is Ms. T at risk for delirium? Why?

2. What are the risk factors for the development of delirium? What risk factors does the patient have?

3. What pharmacological treatment is indicated for delirium?

Clinical update: Ms. T's condition worsens as she is believed to have aspirated and developed pneumonia. Her chest x-ray now reveals bilateral interstitial infiltrates consistent with pulmonary edema and acute respiratory distress syndrome (ARDS). It becomes increasingly difficult to oxygenate her. She is orally intubated and placed on mechanical ventilation. She requires 100% FiO_2, PEEP, and neuromuscular blockade to maintain her oxygenation.

4. For patients such as Ms. T who are receiving neuromuscular blockade, what nursing interventions would be indicated?

5. What complications are patients who are paralyzed with neuromuscular blocking medications at risk for developing?

Chapter 17 Review

1. A client is hospitalized in ICU after a drug overdose. Which statement would the nurse interpret as indicating the client has normal mentation? (Select all that apply.)
   1. "Which part of the hospital am I in?"
   2. "I just want to die."
   3. "I should have swallowed the pills with bourbon."
   4. "Get that cat out of here."
   5. "My feet are cold."

2. A client reports feeling very anxious and not being able to sleep. The nurse anticipates initially administering a drug from which class to treat these disorders?
   1. Opiate narcotics
   2. Benzodiazepines
   3. Antidepressants
   4. Neuromuscular blockers

3. Which characteristics would the nurse attribute to delirium rather than dementia? (Select all that apply.)
   1. The client's mentation was clear until he was hospitalized last week.
   2. The client does not recognize his children.
   3. The client has periods of clarity that alternate with confusion.
   4. The client's family reports that his confusion has become steadily more pronounced over the last year.
   5. The client continually tries to get out of bed, stating "I've got to get off this train."

4. A nurse is concerned that a hospitalized client may be developing delirium. Which interventions are indicated? (Select all that apply.)
   1. Ask the family to bring the client's eyeglasses from home.
   2. Turn room lights down at night to encourage sleep.
   3. Maintain bed rest until mentation improves.
   4. Remove the television from the room.
   5. Review the client's medication list.

5. Which assessment finding would the nurse interpret as an indication that the client is developing critical illness polyneuropathy (CIP)?
   1. The client yawns at inappropriate intervals.
   2. The client's distal pain response is diminished.
   3. The client complains of a burning sensation in his feet.
   4. The client's deep tendon reflexes are diminished.

6. A client has critical illness myopathy (CIM). What information should the nurse provide the client's family?
   1. The treatment for CIM is expensive but not painful.
   2. A full recovery from CIM is probable.
   3. CIM will help the client wean from the ventilator more successfully.
   4. There is no definitive test for presence of CIM.

7. A client is to receive vecuronium for neuromuscular blockade. Which priority intervention should the nurse expect prior to initiating this drug?
   1. Patient should have an indwelling urinary catheter inserted.
   2. Patient should have a feeding tube inserted.

3. Patient should have no fewer than three patent intravenous sites.

4. Patient should be intubated and on mechanical ventilation.

8. A client with major injuries from a motor vehicle crash has been paralyzed with neuromuscular blockade. What other pharmaceutical agents should the nurse prepare to routinely administer?

   1. High-dose corticosteroids

   2. An analgesic

   3. An anticholinesterase agent such as physostigmine

   4. A sedative

   5. High-dose potassium supplementation

9. The nurse discovers a client having a seizure. What should be the nurse's initial action?

   1. Roll the client onto his or her side.

   2. Intubate the client immediately.

   3. Administer pentobarbital.

   4. Establish an IV line.

10. A client experiencing continued seizure activity is to be given propofol. The nurse should prepare for which other intervention?

   1. Administration of insulin

   2. Mechanical ventilation

   3. Placement of an oral airway

   4. Administration of a neuromuscular blocking agent

Answers to questions found inside your textbook are available on the faculty resources site. Please consult with your instructor.

References

Amato, A. A., & Brown, R. H., Jr. (2015). Muscular dystrophies and other muscle diseases. In D. Kasper, A. Fauci, S. Hauser, D. Longo, J. Jameson, & J. Loscalzo (Eds.), *Harrison's principles of internal medicine* (19th ed., p. 2707). New York, NY: McGraw-Hill. Retrieved from http://accessmedicine.mhmedical.com. ezproxy.uky.edu/content.aspx?bookid=1130&Sectio nid=79756769

Apostolakis, E., Papakonstantinou, N. A., Baikoussis, N. G., & Papadopoulos, G. (2015). Intensive care unit-related generalized neuromuscular weakness due to critical illness polyneuropathy/myopathy in critically ill patients. *Journal of Anesthesia, 29*(1), 112–121.

Balas, M. C., Vasilevskis, E. E., Olsen, K. M., Schmid, K., Shostrom, V., Cohen, M. Z., . . . Sullivan, J. (2014). Effectiveness and safety of the awakening and breathing coordination, delirium monitoring/management and early exercise/mobility bundle. *Critical Care Medicine, 42*(5), 1024–1036.

Barnes-Daly, M. A., Phillips, G., & Ely, E. W. (2017). Improving hospital survival and reducing brain dysfunction at seven California community hospitals: Implementing PAD guidelines via the ABCDEF Bundle in 6,064 patients. *Critical Care Medicine, 45*(2), 171–178.

Barr, J., Fraser, G. L., Puntillo, K., Ely, E. W., Gélinas, C., Dasta, J., . . . American College of Critical Care Medicine. (2013). Clinical practice guidelines for the management of pain, agitation, and delirium in adult patients in the intensive care unit. *Critical Care Medicine, 41*(1), 263–306.

Bradt, J. (2014). Music interventions for mechanically ventilated patients. *Cochrane Database Systematic Reviews, 12*, CD006902.

Devlin, J. W., Roberts, R. J., Fong, J. J., Skrobik, Y., Riker, R. R., Hill, N. S., . . . Garpestad, E. (2010). Efficacy and safety of quetiapine in critically ill patients with delirium: A prospective, multicenter, randomized, double-blind, placebo-controlled pilot study. *Critical Care Medicine, 38*(2), 419–427.

Djaiani, G., Silverton, N., Fedorko, L., Carroll, J., Styra, R., Rao, V., & Katznelson, R. (2016). Dexmedetomidine versus propofol sedation reduces delirium after cardiac surgery: A randomized controlled trial. *Anesthesiology, 124*(2), 362–368.

Dres, M., Dubé, B. P., Mayaux, J., Delemuzure, J., Reuter, D., Brochard, L., . . . Demoule, A. (2017). Coexistence and impact of limb muscle and diaphragm weakness at time of liberation from mechanical ventilation in medicine ICU patients. *American Journal of Respiratory and Critical Care Medicine, 195*(1), 57–66.

Ely, E. W., Inouye, S. K., Bernard, G. R., Gordon, S., Francis, J., May, L., . . . Dittus, R. (2001). Delirium in mechanically ventilated patients: Validity and reliability of the Confusion Assessment Method for the Intensive Care Unit (CAM-ICU). *Journal of the American Medical Association, 286*(21), 2703–2710.

Friedrich, O., Reid, M. B., Van den Berghe, G., Vanhorebeek, I., Hermans, G., Rich, M., & Larsson, L. (2015). The sick and the weak: Neuropathies, myopathies in the critically ill. *Physiological Reviews, 95*(3), 1025–1109.

Girard, T. D., Dittus, R. S., & Ely, E. W. (2016). Critical illness brain injury. *Annual Review of Medicine, 67*, 497–513.

Girard, T. D., Jackson, J. C., Pandharipande, P. P., Pun, B., Thompson, J., Shintani, . . . Wesley, E. (2010). Delirium as a predictor of long-term cognitive impairment in survivors of critical illness. *Critical Care Medicine, 38*(7), 1513–1520. doi:10.1097/CCM.0b013e3181e47be1

Girard, T. D., Pandharipande, P. P., Carson, S. S., Schmidt, G. A., Wright, P. E., Canonico, A. E., . . . MIND Trial Investigators. (2010). Feasibility, efficacy, and safety of antipsychotics for intensive care unit delirium: The MIND randomized, placebo-controlled trial. *Critical Care Medicine, 38*(2), 428–437.

Harper, G., Johnston, C., & Landefeld, C. (2016). Geriatric disorders. In M. A. Papadakis, S. J. McPhee, & M. W. Rabow (Eds.), *Current medical diagnosis & treatment 2016* (pp. 61–62). New York, NY: McGraw-Hill Education.

Hemphill J. C., III, Smith, W. S., & Gress, D. R. (2015). Neurologic critical care. In D. L. Kasper, A. S. Fauci, S. L. Hauser, D. L. Longo, J. L. Jameson, & J. Loscalzo (Eds.), *Harrison's principles of internal medicine* (19th ed., pp. 1777–1787). New York, NY: McGraw-Hill.

Hermans, G., & Van den Berghe, G. (2015). Clinical review: Intensive care unit acquired weakness. *Critical Care, 19*, 274.

Hermans, G., Van Mechelen, H., Clerckx, B., Vanhullebusch, T., Mesotten, D., Wilmer, A., . . . Van den Berghe, G. (2014). Acute outcomes and 1-year mortality of intensive care unit-acquired weakness: A cohort study and propensity-matched analysis. *American Journal of Respiratory and Critical Care Medicine, 190*, 410–420.

Hu, R. F., Jiang, X. Y., Hogadoren, K. M., & Zhang, Y. H. (2015). Effects of earplugs and eye masks combined with relaxing music on sleep, melatonin and cortisol levels in intensive care unit patients: A randomized controlled trial. *Critical Care, 19*(1), 115.

Hu, R. F., Jiang, X. Y., Zeng, Z., Chen, X. Y., Li, Y., Huining, X., & Evans, D. S. (2015). Non-pharmacological interventions for sleep promotion in the intensive care unit. *Cochrane Database of Systematic Reviews, 10*, CD008808.

Iacobone, E., Bailly-Salin, J., Polito, A., Friedman, D., Stevens, R. D., & Sharshar, T. (2009). Sepsis-associated encephalopathy and its differential diagnosis. *Critical Care Medicine, 37*(10 Suppl), S331–S336.

Josephson, S. A., & Miller, B. L. (2015). Confusion and delirium. In D. L. Kasper, A. S. Fauci, S. L. Hauser, D. L. Longo, J. L. Jameson, & J. Loscalzo (Eds.), *Harrison's principles of internal medicine* (19th ed., pp. 166–170). New York, NY: McGraw-Hill.

Jung, B., Moury, P. H., Mahul, M., de Jong, A., Galia, F., Prades, A., . . . Jaber, S. (2016). Diaphragmatic dysfunction in patients with ICU-acquired weakness and its impact on extubation failure. *Intensive Care Medicine, 42*(5), 853–861.

Knauert, M. P., Haspel, J. A., & Pisani, M. A. (2015). Sleep loss and circadian rhythm disruption in the intensive care unit. *Clinics of Chest Medicine, 36*(3), 419–429.

Kress, J. P., & Hall, J. B. (2015). Approach to the patient with critical illness. In D. L. Kasper, A. S. Fauci, S. L. Hauser, D. L. Longo, J. L. Jameson, & J. Loscalzo (Eds.), *Harrison's principles of internal medicine* (19th ed., pp. 1729–1735). New York, NY: McGraw-Hill.

Lowenstein, D. H. (2015). Seizures and epilepsy. In D. L. Kasper, A. S. Fauci, S. L. Hauser, D. L. Longo, J. L. Jameson, & J. Loscalzo (Eds.), *Harrison's principles of internal medicine* (19th ed., pp. 2542–2558). New York, NY: McGraw-Hill.

Maldonado, J. R. (2013). Neuropathogenesis of delirium: A review of current etiologic theories and common pathways. *American Journal of Geriatric Psychiatry, 21*(12), 1190–1222.

Mazeraud, A., Pascal, Q., Verdon, K. K., Herming, N., Chretien, F., & Sharshar, T. (2016). Neuroanatomy and physiology of brain dysfunction in sepsis. *Clinics in Chest Medicine, 37*(2), 333–345.

Meyer-Massetti, C., Cheng, C. M., Sharpe, B. A., Meier, C. R., & Guglielmo, B. J. (2010). The FDA extended warning for intravenous haloperidol and torsades de pointes: How should institutions respond? *Journal of Hospital Medicine, 5*(4), E8–E16.

Michaud, C. J., Bullard, H. M, Harris, S. A., & Thomas, W. L. (2015). Impact of quetiapine treatment on duration of hypoactive delirium in critically ill adults: A retrospective analysis. *Pharmacotherapy, 35*(8), 731–739.

Mu, J. L., Lee, A., & Joynt, G. M. (2015). Pharmacologic agents for the prevention and treatment of delirium in patients undergoing cardiac surgery: A systematic review. *Critical Care Medicine, 43*(1), 194–204.

Needham, D. M., Davidson, J., Cohen, H., Hopkins, R. O., Weinert, C., & Wunsch, H. (2012). Improving long-term outcomes after discharge from intensive care unit: Report from a stakeholders conference. *Critical Care Medicine, 40*, 502–509.

Needham, D. M., Korupolu, R., Zanni, J. M., Pradhan, P., Colantuoni, E., Palmer, J. B., . . . Fan, E. (2010). Early physical medicine and rehabilitation for patients with acute respiratory failure: A quality improvement project. *Archives of Physical Medicine and Rehabilitation, 91*(4), 536–542.

Norbaek, J., & Glipstrup, E. (2016). Delirium is seen in one-third of patients in an acute hospital setting: Identifications, pharmacologic and non-pharmacologic treatment is inadequate. *Danish Medical Journal, 63*(11), A5293. Retrieved March 20, 2017, from http://www .danmedj.dk/portal/page/portal/danmedj.dk /dmj_forside/PAST_ISSUE/2016/DMJ_2016_11/A5293

Osias, J., & Manno, E. (2014). Neuromuscular complications of critical illness. *Critical Care Clinics, 30*(4), 785–794.

Pandharipande, P., Cotton, B. A., Shintani, A., Thompson, J., Pun, B. T., Morris, J. A. Jr., . . . Ely, E. W. (2008). Prevalence and risk factors for development of delirium in surgical and trauma intensive care unit patients. *Journal of Trauma, 65*(1), 34–41.

Pandharipande, P. P., Shintani, A., Peterson, J., Pun, B. T., Wilkinson, G. R., Dittus, R. S., . . . Ely, E. W. (2006). Lorazepam is an independent risk factor for transitioning to delirium in intensive care unit patients. *Anesthesiology, 104*, 21–26.

Pandit, L., & Agrawal, A. (2006). Neuromuscular disorders in critical illness. *Clinical Neurology and Neurosurgery 108*, 621–627.

Pawley, E., Lishmanov, A., Schumann, S., Gala, G. J., van Diepen, S., & Katz, J. N. (2015). Delirium is a robust predictor of morbidity and mortality among critically ill patients treated in the cardiac intensive care unit. *American Heart Journal, 170*(1), 79–86, 86e1.

Pulak, L. M., & Jensen, L. (2016). Sleep in the intensive care unit. *Journal of Intensive Care Medicine, 31*(1), 13–23.

Reus, V. (2015). Mental disorders. In D. L. Kasper, A. S. Fauci, S. L. Hauser, D. L. Longo, J. L. Jameson, & J. Loscalzo (Eds.), *Harrison's principles of internal medicine* (19th ed., pp. 2708–2722). New York, NY: McGraw-Hill.

Ropper, A. H. (2015). Coma. In D. L. Kasper, A. S. Fauci, S. L. Hauser, D. L. Longo , J. L. Jameson, & J. Loscalzo (Eds.), *Harrison's principles of internal medicine* (19th ed.). New York, NY: McGraw-Hill Education.

Ryan, D. J., O'Ragan, N. A., Caoimh, R. O., Clare, J., O'Connor, M., Leonard, . . . Timmons, S. (2013). Delirium in an adult acute hospital population: Predictors, prevalence and detection. *British Medical Journal Open, 3*(1), e001772.

Salluh, J. I., Soares, M., Teles, J. M., Ceraso, D., Raimondi, N., Nava, V. S., . . . The DECCA (Delirium Epidemiology in Critical Care) Study Group. (2010). Delirium epidemiology in critical care (DECCA): An international study. *Critical Care, 14*, R210.

Salluh, J. I., Wang, H., Schneider, E., Nagaraja, N., Yenokyan, G., Damluji, A., . . . Stevens, R. (2015). Outcome of delirium in critically ill patients: Systemic review and meta-analysis. *BMJ 350*, h2538. doi:10.1136 /bmj.h2538

Santos, P. D., Teixeira, C., Savi, A., Maccari, J. G., Neres, F. S., Machado, A. S., & Rotta, F. T. (2012). The critical illness polyneuropathy in septic patients with prolonged weaning from mechanical ventilation: Is the diaphragm also affected? A pilot study. *Respiratory Care, 57*(10), 1594–1601.

Serafim, R. B., Bozza, F. A., Soares, M., do Brasil, P. E., Tura, B. R., Ely, E. W., & Sulluh, J. (2015). Pharmacological prevention and treatment of delirium in intensive care patients: A systematic review. *Journal of Critical Care, 30*(4), 799–807.

Siddiqi, N., Harrison, J. K., Clegg, A., Teale, E. A., Young, J., Taylor, J., & Simpkins, S. A. (2016). Interventions for preventing delirium in hospitalized non-ICU patients. *Cochrane Database Systematic Reviews, 3*, CD005563.

Soja, S. L., Pandharipande, P. P., Fleming, S. B., Cotton, B. A., Miller, L. R., Weaver, S. G., . . . Ely, E. W. (2008). Implementation, reliability testing, and compliance monitoring of the Confusion Assessment Method for the Intensive Care Unit in trauma patients. *Intensive Care Medicine, 34*(7), 1263–1268.

Van den Berghe, G., Wouters, P., Weekers, F., Verwaest, C., Bruyninckx, F., Schetz, M., . . . Bouillon, R. (2001). Intensive insulin therapy in critically ill patients. *New England Journal of Medicine, 345*, 1359–1367.

Vanderbilt University Medical Center. (2016). Confusion assessment method for the ICU (CAM-ICU): The complete training manual. Nashville, TN: Vanderbilt University.

Wanat, M., Fitousis, K., Boston, F., & Masud, R. (2014). Comparison of dexmedetomidine versus propofol for sedation in mechanically ventilated patients after cardiovascular surgery. *Methodist Debakey Cardiovascular Journal, 10*(2), 111–117.

Whetstone Foster, J. G. (2011). Peripheral nerve stimulators. In D. J. Lynn-McHale Wiegand (Ed.), *AACN procedure manual for critical care* (6th ed., pp. 303–312). Philadelphia, PA: Elsevier Saunders.

Wilson, B., Shannon, M., & Shields, K. (2016). *Pearson's nurse drug guide 2016*. Hoboken, NJ: Pearson.

Zaal, I. J., Devlin, J. W., Peelan, L. M., & Slooter, A. J. (2015). A systematic review of risk factors for delirium in the ICU. *Critical Care Medicine, 43*(1), 40–47.

Zaal, U., & Slooter, A. J. (2012). Delirium in critically ill patients: Epidemiology, pathophysiology, diagnosis and management. *Drugs 2012, 72*, 1457–1471.

Zammit, C., Choi, K., & Rosengart, A. (2016). Principles of neurosciences critical care. In J. M. Oropello, S. M. Pastores, & V. Kvetan (Eds.), *Critical care* (pp. 599–623). New York, NY: McGraw-Hill.

Zampieri, F. G., Park, M., Machado, F. S., & Azevedo, L. C. P. (2011). Sepsis-associated encephalopathy: Not just delirium. *Clinics, 66*(10), 1825–1831.

Zorowitz, R. D. (2016). ICU-acquired weakness: A rehabilitation perspective of diagnosis, treatment, and functional management. *Chest, 150*(4), 966–971.

Chapter 18
Acute Stroke Injury

Learning Outcomes

18.1 Define stroke and discuss the major classifications of stroke.

18.2 Explain the pathophysiology of stroke.

18.3 Identify the modifiable and nonmodifiable risk factors for stroke.

18.4 Analyze the manifestations of stroke and explain the rationale of various diagnostic tests used in the evaluation of stroke.

18.5 Apply the collaborative management of acute stroke.

18.6 Apply priority nursing interventions for the patient with acute stroke.

 troke is a potentially devastating neurologic event that often causes long-term cognitive and physical debilitation. This chapter focuses on the high-acuity patient who is experiencing an acute stroke with emphasis on acute management rather than rehabilitation. Initial management requires a collaborative team approach for quick diagnosis and treatment to minimize permanent neurologic deficits resulting from brain tissue infarction.

Section One: Definition and Classifications of Strokes

Stroke is an acute neurologic deficit that occurs when impaired blood flow to a localized area of the brain results in injury to brain tissue. The term *brain attack* has been advocated to raise awareness of the need for rapid emergency treatment, similar to what is done for heart attack. Stroke is the fifth-leading cause of death in the United States and a leading cause of serious long-term disability (Mozaffarian et al., 2015).

Major Classifications of Stroke

Strokes are commonly classified by cause as either ischemic or hemorrhagic (see Figure 18–1 and Table 18–1). *Ischemic*

strokes occur when blood supply to a part of the brain is suddenly interrupted and are, by far, the most common. *Hemorrhagic strokes* occur when there is bleeding into brain tissue or the cranial vault, such as what occurs with brain trauma, aneurysms, arteriovenous malformations, or hypertension, and they make up about 10% of all strokes (Aminoff, Greenberg, & Simon, 2015).

Ischemic Strokes   Ischemic strokes are caused by an interruption of cerebral blood flow by a thrombus or embolus. Atherosclerosis of cerebral arteries is one of the most common causes of ischemic stroke. Deposits of atherosclerotic plaque narrow vessel lumens and decrease cerebral blood flow. Plaque deposits in the intimal lining of arteries cause the internal elastic media to thin, weaken, expose the collagen layer, and create an opening in the vessel lining. Platelets become activated to adhere and aggregate in the tissue defect to close the opening. Formation of a platelet plug initiates the coagulation cascade, which results in the formation of a stable fibrin clot. This clot may remain at the site, eventually getting large enough to completely occlude the vessel, or it may break off and become an embolus.

Thrombotic Stroke.   A thrombotic stroke is caused by a blood clot that obstructs arterial blood flow to an area of the brain. Thrombotic strokes are more common in older persons and are frequently accompanied by evidence of atherosclerotic plaque deposits in the coronary (heart) or

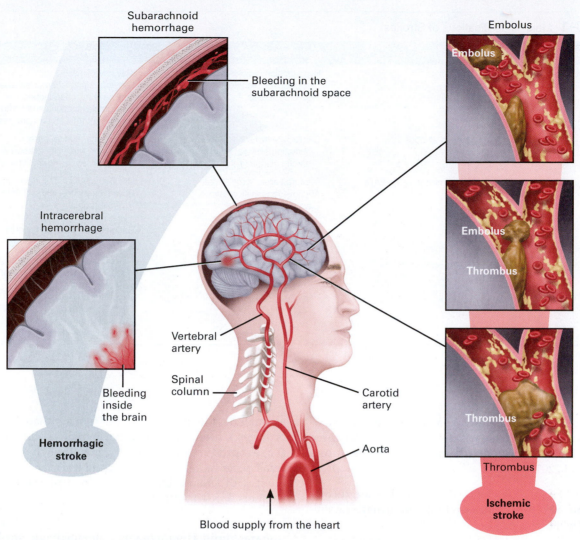

Figure 18–1 Classification of stroke: hemorrhagic and ischemic.

peripheral vasculature. They may occur at rest and are not associated with activity. Thrombotic strokes involving smaller vessels are referred to as *lacunar infarcts*. The infarcted areas leave behind small cavities (lacunae, or lakes). Lacunar infarcts occur in deep, penetrating arteries in a single region of the brain.

Embolic Stroke.   An embolic stroke is caused by a blood clot that travels from its original site outside the brain and becomes lodged in an artery that feeds the brain. Most emboli originate from a thrombus in the heart that develops with certain cardiac conditions (atrial fibrillation, rheumatic heart disease, recent myocardial infarction, or endocarditis). Emboli can also originate from rupture of atherosclerotic plaque. Embolic strokes usually occur suddenly when the person is awake and active.

Transient Ischemic Attack.   Interruption of cerebral blood flow can result in **transient ischemic attacks (TIAs)**.

These are brief episodes of focal neurologic deficits that usually resolve in a few minutes or hours and do not cause permanent brain injury. They are usually caused by an embolism coming from the heart or a major artery outside of the cranial arteries (Aminoff et al., 2015). Almost one third of the patients diagnosed with a TIA will have some evidence of brain injury when symptoms abate within 24 hours. As a result, treatments for TIA and ischemic stroke are similar (Kernan et al., 2014).

A stroke may be preceded by a TIA, much like angina precedes a myocardial infarction. Clinically, the patient may present with sudden unilateral dimness or partial loss of vision in one eye, weakness, numbness, tingling, severe headache, speechlessness, or unexplained dizziness. The symptoms are produced by inadequate perfusion to the brain, which can be caused by carotid stenosis (from atherosclerotic disease) or microemboli (from atherosclerotic plaques in major extracranial vessels). Transient ischemic attacks are warnings of an impending stroke

Table 18–1 Major Classifications of Strokes

Type of Stroke	Age	Risk Factors	Characteristics
Ischemic Stroke Thrombotic	Older adults	Hypertension, smoking, high cholesterol, diabetes mellitus, atherosclerosis	May have TIAs Develop during sleep or on awakening May have mild headaches Predictable locations and symptoms Intermittent attacks and progression
Embolic	Adults of all ages	Cardiac abnormalities: Atrial fibrillation, valvular heart disease, carotid plaque or thrombosis	No warning, sudden attack Symptoms vary with location Usually occur during daytime
Hemorrhagic Stroke Subarachnoid hemorrhage	Young, middle-aged adults	Ruptured aneurysms Arteriovenous malformations Brain tumors	Usually no warning, sudden attack Severe headache, nausea or vomiting, photophobia Hypertension Decreasing level of consciousness
Intracerebral hemorrhage	Older adults	Chronic hypertension Anticoagulant therapy	Usually no warning Gradual development Headache, nausea or vomiting, photophobia Hypertension Bloody cerebrospinal fluid (CSF) Decreased level of consciousness Motor–sensory deficits of face, arm, leg

and require immediate referral for treatment. Approximately 3% to 4% of patients with TIA or stroke will experience an initial or repeated ischemic stroke in the future (Kernan et al., 2014).

Hemorrhagic Strokes   Hemorrhagic strokes are further divided into two types: intracerebral hemorrhage or subarachnoid hemorrhage.

Intracerebral Hemorrhage.   Intracerebral hemorrhage is a type of hemorrhagic stroke that occurs when a cerebral blood vessel ruptures and blood accumulates in brain tissue, usually the basal ganglia, cerebellum, brainstem, or cortex. Intracerebral hemorrhage often occurs in older adults experiencing a sustained increase in systolic–diastolic blood pressure. The hemorrhage results in compression of intracerebral contents, cerebral edema, and spasm of adjacent blood vessels. Hypertension is a common cause of intracerebral hemorrhage; however, it can also be caused by a variety of other factors, including arteriovenous malformations, anticoagulant therapy, aneurysms, trauma, and erosions of blood vessels by tumors. Unlike ischemic strokes, which are preceded by TIAs, intracerebral hemorrhage appears suddenly without warning. A spontaneous intracerebral hemorrhage is the most common cause of a fatal stroke. Several conditions can cause a cerebral blood vessel to rupture, including degenerative changes, which damage the elastic layer of the artery; developmental defects, which cause a poorly developed arterial wall; high blood flow areas, which cause hemodynamic stress; and hypertension, which places greater stress on any areas of vascular weakness, thus increasing the risk for hemorrhage.

Primary intracerebral hemorrhage usually involves bleeding directly into the brain parenchyma; it may occur as small (less than 3 cm) or large (greater than 3 cm) hemorrhages. Chronic hypertension, one cause of these hemorrhages, produces gradual, degenerative changes in the small penetrating arteries, causing microaneurysms that burst with sudden increases in blood pressure (Ropper, Samuels, & Klein, 2014a).

Subarachnoid Hemorrhage.   Hemorrhagic strokes can occur due to a rupture of an aneurysm or due to trauma. Trauma-related hemorrhage is discussed in Chapter 19. An **aneurysm** is a weakening and dilatation of a vessel wall and is associated with long-term atherosclerosis and hypertension. Aneurysms are usually found at arterial bifurcations, where blood velocity is higher, causing arterial wall damage. In the brain, aneurysms are usually located in the circle of Willis (Figure 18–2). Rupture of an aneurysm in the circle of Willis causes hemorrhaging into the subarachnoid space and is called a subarachnoid hemorrhage (SAH)—a life-threatening event and an emergency situation. SAH develops suddenly without warning. The patient often complains of a sudden, severe, unilateral headache on the side of the bleed ("the worst headache of my life"), **nuchal rigidity** (neck pain or stiffness), and vomiting. SAH more commonly occurs in younger people than in older adults. Meningeal irritation by blood produces the severe headache and other meningeal signs, such as photophobia (intolerance to light) and nuchal rigidity. Hypertension is common. The cerebrospinal fluid (CSF) is usually bloody because the aneurysm ruptures in the subarachnoid space, where CSF flows. Following an SAH, a decrease in cerebral blood flow and transient loss of consciousness secondary to increased intracranial pressure (ICP) may occur.

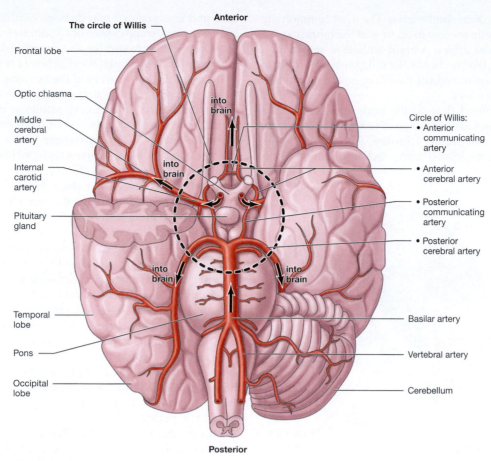

Figure 18–2 Major arteries serving the circle of Willis.

Section One Review

1. A client, age 33, experienced an episode of heaviness of the right arm and inability to speak that lasted for 3 minutes. Symptoms disappeared and function returned to normal. What category of stroke has this patient most likely experienced?
   A. Subarachnoid hemorrhage
   B. Transient ischemic attack
   C. Intracerebral hemorrhage
   D. Lacunar stroke

2. What are the major classifications of stroke?
   A. Subarachnoid and intracranial hemorrhage
   B. Thrombotic and embolic
   C. Ischemic and hemorrhagic
   D. TIA and embolic

3. Which conditions are associated with emboli formation? (Select all that apply.)
   A. Myocardial infarction
   B. Atrial fibrillation
   C. Brain trauma
   D. Endocarditis
   E. Low blood glucose

4. Which stroke event appears suddenly and without warning?
   A. Subarachnoid hemorrhage
   B. Ischemic strokes
   C. TIAs
   D. All strokes

Answers: 1. B, 2. C, 3. (A, B, D), 4. A

Section Two: Pathophysiology of Stroke

Recall from Section One that a stroke is characterized by neurologic deficits that occur when cerebral perfusion is diminished as a result of ischemic or hemorrhagic cerebral vascular events. The majority of strokes result from ischemic infarction and inadequate blood flow (Go & Worman, 2016; Powers & Jordan, 2015). Atherosclerosis of cerebral arteries is a process similar to that found in coronary arteries, whereby plaque formation and narrowing or occlusion of arteries results in enhanced platelet aggregation and clot formation. Formation of a blood clot superimposed on atherosclerotic plaque causes significant stenosis of cerebral arteries. The most common site for the atherosclerotic process to occur is at the bifurcation of the common carotid artery. A brain embolism results in a stroke when a clot, plaque, or platelet plug breaks off from an atherosclerotic lesion outside of the brain, enters the circulation, and blocks an artery.

Diminished blood flow to the brain impairs oxygen delivery to neurons. Cerebral ischemia can be focal, localized, or global, widespread (Smith, Johnston, & Hemphill, 2015). Global ischemia is associated with a lack of collateral blood flow and irreversible brain damage (within minutes). With focal ischemia, some degree of collateral circulation remains, allowing neurons to survive and neuronal damage to reverse after periods of ischemia. Focal ischemia is treatable because of the potential for recovery of the neurons. Figure 18–3 provides an illustration of brain tissue distal to the stroke event.

Impaired oxygen delivery results in impaired cellular function because the cells do not have enough oxygen to generate energy. Without oxygen, the cellular sodium–potassium pumps fail. This results in increased intracellular concentrations of sodium, chloride, and calcium. Accumulation of these intracellular electrolytes is toxic to intracellular structures, particularly the mitochondria. Severe or prolonged ischemia leads to cellular death.

In the evolution of a stroke there are usually two zones of affected neurons. In the central zone are neurons that are infarcted (dead), with permanent loss of function. Surrounding the infarcted zone is the ischemic **penumbra**, a zone of neurons that are minimally perfused but not totally ischemic (Figure 18–4). Although neurons within the penumbra are still alive, they are injured and have impaired functioning. The neurons in the penumbra remain potentially viable and are capable of responding to reperfusion therapy within a brief time window following the stroke. Ideally, reperfusion is undertaken within the first hour of injury (the "golden hour"); however, more realistically, it can still benefit the patient if performed within the therapeutic window of 4.5 hours after injury (Antoniello, 2014). When perfusion to neurons in the penumbra is reestablished within the therapeutic time window, many of the cells recover function; however, if perfusion is not reestablished before the neurons die, the central infarcted zone enlarges. Therefore, the fundamental goal of medical management is to restore cerebral blood flow and limit the size and extension of the infarcted zone.

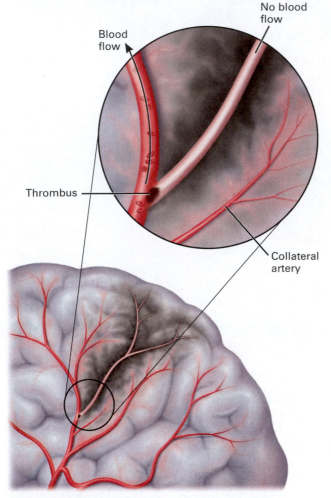

Figure 18–3 Ischemia, infarction, and collateral flow. Brain tissues distal to a rupture, thrombus, or embolus receive little or no perfusion and become ischemic and eventually infarct. When a thrombus forms slowly, collateral arteries may form to perfuse or partially perfuse the ischemic area of the brain.

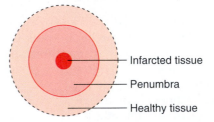

Figure 18–4 Ischemic penumbra. Surrounding the infarcted zone is the penumbra. In this zone are neurons that are minimally perfused but still viable and capable of responding to therapy. The goal of medical management is to limit the size of the infarct zone and reestablish perfusion to neurons in the penumbra zone.

Section Two Review

1. Impaired cerebral oxygen delivery results in what change?
   A. Failure of sodium–potassium pumps
   B. Aerobic metabolism
   C. Immediate cell death
   D. Cerebral vasodilation

2. The penumbra is defined as what zone?
   A. Infarct zone
   B. Zone of neurons that are minimally perfused
   C. Zone of healthy neurons
   D. Zone where ischemia is complete

3. What is the fundamental goal of medical management during cerebral ischemia?
   A. Limit sodium–potassium pumps
   B. Promote anaerobic metabolism
   C. Restore cerebral perfusion
   D. Prevent clot formation

4. Ideally, reperfusion of the penumbra occurs within which of the following time frames?
   A. 15 minutes
   B. 60 minutes
   C. 4 hours
   D. 8 hours

Answers: 1. A, 2. B, 3. C, 4. B

Section Three: Risk Factors for Stroke

Prevention of stroke is heavily dependent on the identification of risk factors. These risk factors, categorized as modifiable or nonmodifiable, are summarized in Table 18–2.

Modifiable Risk Factors

There are multiple risk factors for stroke that are considered modifiable, including blood pressure, cardiac disease, diabetes, dyslipidemia, and smoking.

Blood Pressure   Abnormal blood pressure is an important modifiable risk factor for stroke and is implicated in both ischemic and hemorrhagic strokes. Stroke prevention through hypertension management includes regular blood pressure screenings and treatment with lifestyle modifications and/or antihypertensive medications to maintain a blood pressure less than 140/90 (Meschia et al., 2014). Hypotension, particularly in older adults, may be a significant risk factor for cerebral ischemia if the hypotensive episode is sudden and profound, as may happen with the use of powerful antihypertensive agents, myocardial infarction, or bleeding. Dehydration also may lower blood pressure dangerously and decrease cerebral perfusion in older adults, who already have an age-related decline in cerebral blood flow.

Cardiac Disease   Cardiac disease is another important modifiable risk factor for stroke. Individuals with coronary heart disease, heart failure, left ventricular hypertrophy, or dysrhythmias (specifically atrial fibrillation) have a greater risk for stroke when compared with those without cardiac disease. Atrial fibrillation increases the risk for ischemic stroke four to five times above the typical risk due to the potential release of emboli from the left atrial area (Meschia et al., 2014). Therefore, cardiovascular risk reduction must be implemented to reduce coronary heart disease and, in turn, risk of stroke.

Diabetes Mellitus and Dyslipidemia   Other conditions that increase the risk for stroke are diabetes mellitus (DM) and dyslipidemia. Diabetes is associated with multiple chronic complications that are all independent risk factors for stroke, such as accelerated atherosclerosis, hypertension, dyslipidemia, and macrovascular disease (Powers, 2015). Dyslipidemia is a risk factor for atherosclerosis in both the coronary and cerebral vascular beds. Hypercholesterolemia is, therefore, another modifiable risk factor for stroke. Treating hyperlipidemia with antilipemic therapy, such as HMG-CoA reductase inhibitors (statins), reduces the risk of atherosclerosis and stroke in those with coronary artery disease and elevated total or low-density-lipoprotein cholesterol.

Smoking   Cigarette smoking plays an important role in development and progression of atherosclerosis (Libby, 2015). Cigarette smoking contributes to injury and dysfunction of the endothelium, which results in atherogenesis, as does dyslipidemia, diabetes, and hypertension. Smoking increases platelet activation and injures endothelium, thereby increasing the risk for thrombus formation. Cessation of smoking rapidly reduces the risk of cardiovascular disease and mortality, including the risk for stroke (Meschia et al., 2014; Mons et al., 2015).

Nonmodifiable Risk Factors

Nonmodifiable risk factors for stroke include age, sex, race and ethnicity, and genetic factors.

Age   The risk for stroke increases with age (Smith et al., 2015). Lifestyle modifications at any age, such as smoking cessation, weight control, and following dietary and activity recommendations, can decrease the overall risk for stroke (Mons et al., 2015; Niewada & Michel, 2016).

Sex   The risk for death from stroke in those who are 55 to 75 years of age is 20% to 21% in women and 14% to 17% in men (Mozaffarian et al., 2015). These sex-specific trends are not observed in younger populations. In 2013, 58% of U.S. deaths from stroke occurred in women, primarily due to higher numbers of older adult women in the population (Mozaffarian et al., 2015).

Table 18–2 Risk Factors for Stroke

Modifiable	Nonmodifiable
Hypertension and hypotension	Age
Cardiac disease	Sex
Dysrhythmias (atrial fibrillation)	Race or ethnicity
Coagulopathies	Genetic factors
Diabetes mellitus	Prior stroke or heart attack
Drug abuse Cigarette smoking Excessive alcohol consumption Cocaine	
Physical inactivity	
Hypercholesterolemia	

Race and Ethnicity Race and ethnicity are important stroke risks. Hispanics, American Indians, Alaska Natives, and African Americans have a higher risk than non-Hispanic Whites according to age-adjusted statistics (Meschia et al., 2014; Mozaffarian et al., 2015). Differences among these groups in the prevalence of risk factors for stroke, such as hypertension, obesity, and diabetes, may contribute to the variation in stroke rates. In addition, environmental influences including access to healthcare may also contribute to stroke rate differences among select groups (Meschia et al., 2014).

Genetic Factors A direct link between a single gene and strokes has not been supported; in fact, it is suspected that there may be different genetic factors for individual subtypes of stroke. A family history of stroke increases the risk by approximately 30% (Meschia et al., 2014). Several genetic changes—for example, variations in the 9p2, 4q25 and 16q22 chromosomes—are associated with increased risk for stroke (Meschia et al., 2014). According to Meschia and colleagues, a genetic stroke risk score that quantifies the combined impact of known risk factors (e.g., hypertension, hyperlipidemia, and diabetes) may be one method for identifying and reducing stroke risk in future generations. The clinical utility of determining a stroke risk score as part of the health screening process is under consideration by medical experts. Inherited metabolic conditions that can produce stroke in

Genetic Considerations
Inherited Conditions Linked to Stroke

- MELAS (mitochondrial myopathy, encephalopathy, lactic acidosis, and strokelike episodes)
- Homocystinuria
- Fabry disease
- Sulfite oxidase deficiency
- Tangier disease
- Familial hypercholesterolemia

SOURCE: Based on Ropper et al. (2014b).

children and young adults are listed in the "Genetic Considerations: Inherited Conditions Linked to Stroke" feature.

Despite knowledge of the importance of reducing risk factors for stroke, control of these factors is still inadequate because of poor patient compliance and adherence to behavior modifications, as well as decreased detection and treatment of stroke by healthcare providers. Further reductions in the incidence of stroke require improvements in the ability to identify, modify, and manage cerebral vascular risk factors.

Section Three Review

1. What is the most important modifiable risk factor for stroke?
   A. Age
   B. Hypertension
   C. Atrial fibrillation
   D. Diabetes mellitus

2. Which modifiable risk factors are associated with increased risk of stroke? (Select all that apply.)
   A. Cigarette smoking
   B. Heavy use of alcohol
   C. Physical inactivity
   D. Urban living
   E. Diabetes mellitus

3. Which statement regarding gender and risk for stroke is accurate?
   A. Women between ages 55 and 75 have a higher risk for stroke than do men of that age.
   B. Women have a higher risk for stroke than men at any age.
   C. Men between ages 55 and 75 have a higher risk for stroke than do women of that age.
   D. Men have a higher risk for stroke than women at any age.

4. Smoking increases risk of stroke in which ways? (Select all that apply.)
   A. Reduces oxygen-carrying capacity of the blood
   B. Contributes to dysfunction of the endothelium
   C. Increases platelet activation
   D. Causes hypertension
   E. Interferes with medication efficacy

Answers: 1. C, 2. (A, B, C, D, E), 3. A, 4. (B, C)

Section Four: Assessment and Diagnosis of Stroke

To understand assessment and diagnosis of stroke, it is important to have an understanding of the manifestations of stroke and the rationale for the diagnostic tests used in evaluation of acute stroke. A focused clinical assessment of the patient is important to establish a baseline and to assist in diagnosis and prognosis in terms of survival and functional recovery.

Assessment

When a stroke is suspected, a patient history and physical assessment should be conducted immediately. A focused bedside neurologic assessment is a key aspect of the initial physical exam and includes examining the head for possible

Table 18–3 Signs and Symptoms of Stroke Related to Vascular Territory Compromised

Vascular Territory Compromised	Signs and Symptoms
Carotid ischemia	Monocular vision loss Aphasia (dominant hemisphere) Hemineglect (nondominant hemisphere) Contralateral sensory or motor loss
Vertebrobasilar ischemia	Ataxia Diplopia Hemianopsia Vertigo Cranial nerve defects Contralateral hemiplegia Sensory deficits

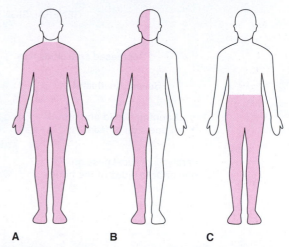

Figure 18–5 Types of paralysis. A, Tetraplegia (quadriplegia) is complete or partial paralysis of the upper extremities and complete paralysis of the lower part of the body. B, Hemiplegia is paralysis of one half of the body when it is divided along the median sagittal plane. C, Paraplegia is paralysis of the lower part of the body, usually below the waist or involving both lower extremities.

trauma and evaluating speech, level of consciousness (LOC), sensory and motor function, and cerebellar and cranial nerve functions (Go & Worman, 2016; Smith et al., 2015).

Manifestations of stroke vary according to the cerebral artery involved. About one third of patients who are having a stroke are aware of the symptoms; however, most bystanders who witness a stroke are not knowledgeable about the signs of stroke. The most common manifestation is numbness and weakness of the face and arm. Other manifestations may include difficulties with balance or speech and loss of vision in one eye (Go & Worman, 2016; Smith et al., 2015). Symptoms are usually sudden at onset and one sided. The specific stroke signs depend on the specific vascular territory compromised, as summarized in Table 18–3. Assessing the onset and progress of development of neurologic deficits is an important part of the assessment and diagnostic process.

It is important to assess the speed of onset and rate of progression of the neurologic deficits because it determines the type of stroke. In patients with ischemic stroke (e.g., thrombotic and embolic subtypes), the speed of onset of neurologic deficits is typically rapid; however, the speed at which signs and symptoms progress differs. The rate of progression in thrombotic strokes is relatively slow, with neurologic deficits progressing over minutes to hours or, rarely, over days. With embolic stroke, manifestations appear suddenly and cause immediate maximum neurologic deficits (Smith et al., 2015). The manifestations of hemorrhagic stroke appear suddenly and vary, depending on the location and extent of the bleeding, but may include headache, nausea, vomiting, seizures, **hemiplegia** (unilateral paralysis) (Figure 18–5), and loss of consciousness.

Several key physical assessment findings can be seen in a patient who has had a stroke, and the nurse must recognize them. If the patient is awake, the probability of a hemispheric stroke is high. Ptosis of the eyelid and cranial nerve III (oculomotor) involvement suggest that a posterior stroke may have occurred. Contralateral hemiparesis involving the face and limbs is indicative of a hemispheric (anterior or carotid) stroke. Assessment of extremity position and handgrips, arm drifts, and leg pushes for strength are imperative. The tone (flaccidity or spasticity) of the extremities is noted. Speech is assessed for coherency, content, and fluency. Orientation and the ability to follow

commands are assessed. Loss of consciousness raises suspicion of a posterior (vertebrobasilar) stroke or a bilateral hemispheric stroke. During the physical assessment, sensitivity to cognitive and perceptual–visual–spatial deficits and patient behavior manifesting as neglect or poor judgment is key in assessment findings. Cranial nerve abnormalities (III to XII) reflect brainstem involvement or a vertebrobasilar stroke. Cranial nerve assessment helps to establish a baseline against which to compare the patient's progress. Figure 18–6 illustrates many of the common general findings associated with stroke.

Determining Diagnosis and Recovery

A patient thought to be having a stroke requires prompt triage because time is crucial to prevent or at least minimize permanent brain tissue infarction. Treatment guidelines recommend that the patient be diagnosed and have a treatment plan in place within 60 minutes of arrival to the emergency department (Jauch et al., 2013).

Diagnosis Accurate diagnosis is based on a complete history and a thorough physical assessment with a focused neurologic exam. The goal of the exam is to quickly determine whether the stroke is ischemic or hemorrhagic because each requires different medical interventions. Important information to elicit includes any reports of recent medical or neurologic events (e.g., hemorrhage, surgery, trauma, myocardial infarction, or stroke) and medication history (e.g., antiplatelet or anticoagulant drugs). Particular attention is given to vital signs. An irregular heart rhythm may indicate atrial fibrillation. Hypertension increases the likelihood for intracranial hemorrhage.

Diagnostic Tests and Procedures Rapid diagnosis of a stroke is essential so that patients who meet the inclusion criteria (and do not meet the exclusion criteria) can receive thrombolytic therapy, the goal of which is to save damaged

GENERAL SIGNS AND SYMPTOMS OF STROKE

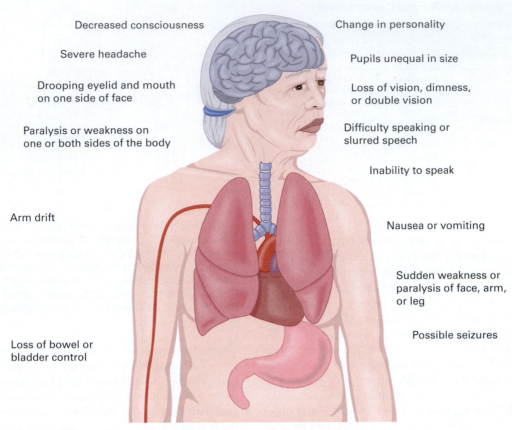

Decreased consciousness

Severe headache

Drooping eyelid and mouth
on one side of face

Paralysis or weakness on
one or both sides of the body

Arm drift

Loss of bowel or
bladder control

Change in personality

Pupils unequal in size

Loss of vision, dimness,
or double vision

Difficulty speaking or
slurred speech

Inability to speak

Nausea or vomiting

Sudden weakness or
paralysis of face, arm,
or leg

Possible seizures

Figure 18–6 General manifestations of stroke.

brain tissue and minimize permanent deficits. The time of symptom onset to administration of thrombolytic therapy (or time to needle) should be within a 3- to 4.5-hour window (Ropper et al., 2014a). A variety of tests and procedures are performed as soon as possible after arrival of the patient to the emergency department (ED) to determine the exact nature of the stroke. Table 18–4 lists some of the more common scans, ultrasonography, and angiography tests used for diagnosing strokes.

Imaging studies (e.g., CT scan or MRI) are used to determine the type, extent, and location of the injury. Specific MRI procedures, such as diffusion-weighted magnetic resonance techniques, can detect infarction within minutes of stroke onset (Ropper et al., 2014a). Lumbar puncture may be performed to detect blood in the CSF if subarachnoid hemorrhage (SAH) is suspected but not confirmed by CT scan. Transesophageal echocardiography detects cardiac and aortic causes of embolism. A 12-lead ECG is performed because cardiac abnormalities are prevalent among patients with stroke. A complete blood count, including platelets, prothrombin time (PT), international normalized ratio (INR), partial thromboplastin time (PTT), and fibrinogen, are evaluated to detect any coagulopathies and establish baselines for therapy. Serum electrolytes and blood glucose levels may be ordered to rule out other conditions that may mimic stroke, including hypoglycemia and severe electrolyte

Table 18–4 Scans, Angiography, and Ultrasonography Diagnostic Tests

Tests	Purpose
Computerized tomography (CT) scan of brain without contrast	Differentiate hemorrhagic from ischemic cause of stroke
Special CT scans (transcranial and extracranial contrast enhanced or single-photon-emission)	Establish the anatomical regions and structures involved; determine the cause of stroke
Cerebral vessel arteriography	Evaluate vessel structures, vasospasm, or stenosis; identify arterial occlusion or embolism
Magnetic resonance imaging (MRI) with angiography (MRA)	Gold standard to diagnose brain vascular lesions, dissections, and areas of infarction; produces angiographic images of the cervicocranial vasculature
Carotid duplex ultrasound	Used to screen patients for presence and degree of carotid stenosis as etiology of ischemic stroke
Transesophageal or transthoracic echocardiography (TEE or TTE)	Identifies cardiac sources of embolic ischemic stroke

Table 18–5 National Institutes of Health Stroke Scale (NIHSS)

Title	Responses and Scores	Title	Responses and Scores
Level of consciousness	0—Alert 1—Drowsy 2—Obtunded 3—Coma or unresponsive	Motor function (leg) a. Left b. Right	0—No drift 1—Drift before 5 seconds 2—Falls before 5 seconds 3—No effort against gravity 4—No movement
Orientation questions (two)	0—Answers both correctly 1—Answers one correctly 2—Answers neither correctly	Limb ataxia	0—No ataxia 1—Ataxia in one limb 2—Ataxia in two limbs
Response to commands (two)	0—Performs both tasks correctly 1—Performs one task correctly 2—Performs neither task correctly	Sensory	0—No sensory loss 1—Mild sensory loss 2—Severe sensory loss
Gaze	0—Normal horizontal movements 1—Partial gaze palsy 2—Forced deviation	Language	0—Normal 1—Mild aphasia 2—Severe aphasia 3—Mute or global aphasia
Visual fields	0—No visual field defect 1—Partial hemianopsia 2—Complete hemianopsia 3—Bilateral hemianopsia	Articulation	0—Normal 1—Mild dysarthria 2—Severe dysarthria
Facial movement	0—Normal 1—Minor facial weakness 2—Partial facial weakness 3—Complete unilateral palsy	Extinction or inattention	0—Absent 1—Mild (loss of one sensory modality) 2—Severe (loss of two modalities)
Motor function (arm) a. Left b. Right	0—No drift 1—Drift before 5 seconds 2—Falls before 5 seconds 3—No effort against gravity 4—No movement		

A lower score indicates better function.

SOURCE: Based on National Institutes of Health/National Institute of Neurological Disorders and Stroke (2017). *NIH Stroke Scale.* Retrieved March 28, 2017, from https://stroke.nih.gov /resources/scale.htm.

imbalances, which are a potential source of cardiac dysrhythmias. Arterial blood gases, drug screens, and a serum alcohol level may be obtained if indicated by history to detect possible causes of stroke. Doppler ultrasonography and duplex imaging are emergency noninvasive tests that are conducted when carotid artery disease is suspected.

Determining Degree of Recovery   The National Institutes of Health Stroke Scale (NIHSS) is widely used in the United States to assess neurologic outcome and degree of recovery (Table 18–5). A lower score indicates better neurological function. The complete questionnaire with instructions is available on the Internet. Evidence-based practice guidelines that facilitate stroke assessment across the continuum of care are available through healthcare professional organizations and national organizations (e.g., American Heart Association, Stroke Foundation).

Section Four Review

1. What is the most common manifestation of stroke?
   A. Numbness and weakness of the face and arm
   B. Monocular vision loss
   C. Aphasia
   D. Hemineglect

2. Headache, nausea, vomiting, and seizures are common manifestations of what kind of stroke?
   A. Thrombotic
   B. Embolic
   C. Hemorrhagic
   D. TIA

3. Which diagnostic test may be used to detect cardiac and aortic causes of embolism?
   A. CT scan
   B. MRI
   C. Transesophageal echocardiography
   D. Lumbar puncture

4. Sensory deficits are common symptoms of strokes that involve what vascular territory?
   A. Carotid ischemia
   B. Middle cerebral artery ischemia
   C. Vertebrobasilar ischemia
   D. Circle of Willis ischemia

Answers: 1. A, 2. C, 3. C, 4. C

Section Five: Acute Stroke Management

Acute medical and surgical management of stroke includes pharmacotherapy and surgery, depending upon the cause of the stroke and the complications that arise.

Medical Management of Strokes

Because most strokes are caused by an occlusion of a cerebral vessel, improvement and restoration of perfusion to the ischemic area are imperative. The concept of the penumbra is fundamental in treating ischemic strokes. Although a core of infarcted tissue is not salvageable, adjacent dysfunctional tissue is salvageable if circulation is promptly restored (Smith et al., 2015). Patients with acute ischemic stroke presenting to the ED within 24 to 48 hours of the onset of symptoms are given aspirin (initial dose 325 mg) to reduce stroke mortality and morbidity, provided contraindications, such as allergy and gastrointestinal bleeding, are absent and the patient has not or will not be treated with tissue plasminogen activator (Go & Worman, 2016).

Thrombolytic Therapy Intravenous tissue plasminogen activator (tPA or r-tPA) is strongly recommended for patients with acute ischemic stroke who meet specific criteria and who can be treated within 3 to 4.5 hours of onset of ischemic stroke (Jauch et al., 2013). In patients with acute ischemic stroke in whom treatment cannot be administered within 4.5 hours of symptom onset, intravenous tPA is not routinely recommended. An exception to the 4.5-hour time-limit rule is the patient with acute ischemic stroke due to occlusion of the proximal cerebral artery. In this situation tPA can be administered within 6 hours of symptom onset, by injecting it directly into the proximal cerebral artery (intra-arterial) at the clot site. Major indications and contraindications for use of tPA therapy for treatment of ischemic stroke are listed in Box 18–1.

The patient who receives tPA is usually admitted to an intensive care unit or stroke unit. When intravenous tPA therapy is initiated, a small dose is given as a bolus, followed by an IV infusion of the drug over an hour. During and after the infusion, the nurse performs frequent neurological assessments and evaluates the patient's blood pressure. During the infusion, if the patient develops nausea, vomiting, severe headache, or acute hypertension, the infusion is discontinued and the physician is notified immediately because these symptoms suggest development of an adverse drug effect that could be life-threatening. The "Related Pharmacotherapy: Thrombolytic Agents" feature provides a profile of tPA and includes an example of an assessment protocol during and directly following tPA therapy.

Other Priority Interventions In addition to thrombolytic therapy to reperfuse brain tissue, priority interventions in the first 24 hours of stroke care are management of oxygenation, blood pressure, serum glucose, dysrhythmias, and fever. Alterations in these parameters are associated with worse outcomes.

BOX 18–1 Indications and Contraindications for tPA Therapy

Indications

- Acute ischemic stroke within 4.5 hours from symptom onset
- Age older than 18 years

Contraindications

- Evidence of intracranial hemorrhage on pretreatment CT scan
- Suspicion of subarachnoid hemorrhage
- Recent stroke, intracranial or intraspinal surgery, or serious head trauma in the past 3 months
- Major surgery or serious trauma in the previous 14 days
- Arterial puncture at a noncompressible site or lumbar puncture in the last week
- Major symptoms that are rapidly improving or only minor stroke symptoms (NIHSS less than 4)
- History of intracranial hemorrhage
- Severe hypertension at the time of treatment
- Seizure at the stroke onset; active internal bleeding
- Intracranial neoplasm, arteriovenous malformation, or aneurysm
- Known bleeding disorder, including but not limited to the following:
  o Current use of anticoagulants or an international normalized ratio (INR) greater than 1.7 or a prothrombin time (PT) greater than 15 seconds
  o Administration of heparin within 48 hours preceding the onset of stroke and an elevated activated partial thromboplastin time at presentation
  o Platelet count less than 100,000 mm^3

Oxygenation. It is important to maintain oxygen saturation at greater than 94% by way of SpO_2 monitoring and, when necessary, supplemental oxygen (Go & Worman, 2016). Because aspiration often contributes to hypoxia, it is important to institute preventive measures such as elevation of the head of the bed to 30 degrees and evaluating ability to swallow before offering oral nutrition or liquids. Elevating the head of the bed to 15 degrees to 30 degrees also may decrease the risk of cerebral edema (Go & Worman, 2016).

Serum Glucose. Treating serum glucose levels under 60 mg/dL is important for determining if symptoms are the result of stroke or of hypoglycemia mimicking stroke (Go & Worman, 2016). Stress hyperglycemia is common and should be managed with rapid-acting insulin to decrease serum glucose if levels exceed 180 mg/dL (Bassily-Marcus & Khachaturova, 2016; Smith et al., 2015). To maintain an acceptable glucose level, an IV insulin infusion may be used since hyperglycemia can accelerate the ischemic processes of stroke.

Blood Pressure. Many patients who experience an ischemic stroke are hypertensive. The decision regarding when to treat the hypertension in the acute phase of ischemic stroke remains controversial. Collateral blood flow in the brain is dependent on the systemic blood pressure (SBP); therefore, if the SBP is reduced too much, collateral flow will decrease, worsening the ischemia in the penumbra

(Smith et al., 2015). Severe hypertension can contribute to the development of cerebral edema in acute ischemic stroke, increasing the risk for intracranial bleeding in patients who are treated with thrombolytic therapy. For these reasons, permissive hypertension may be allowed during the early phase of stroke treatment.

Permissive hypertension is an evidence-based treatment strategy in which higher than normal blood pressures are allowed for maintaining optimal cerebral blood flow. For example, one recommended permissive hypertension protocol consists of treating SBP of 220 mmHg or diastolic blood pressure (DBP) of greater than 120 mmHg; and if treatment is indicated, the blood pressure would be lowered by no more than 15% in the first 24 hours of stroke onset (Jauch et al., 2013; Go & Worman, 2016). However, if the patient is a candidate for thrombolytic therapy, BP should be treated if it exceeds 185/110 mmHg (Jauch et al., 2013). When treating severe hypertension is necessary, the preferred agents are labetalol, nicardipine, and nitroprusside (Jauch et al., 2013). In the days to weeks following a stroke, the goal should be for the patient to maintain a normal BP in order to reduce risk for recurrent stroke.

Conversely, hypotension following ischemic stroke should be avoided to prevent inadequate cerebral blood flow, which increases ischemia in the penumbra. Correction of hypotension with fluid administration or intravenous vasopressor medications should be instituted promptly. The goal is to administer sufficient fluids to achieve normal fluid volume (euvolemia) and normal BP only. Hemodilution and fluid volume overload are to be avoided, as it increases the risk of cerebral edema.

Fever.   Fever increases cerebral oxygen consumption, which can increase ischemia and injury to the penumbra (Smith et al., 2015). Fevers must be monitored frequently and managed aggressively in the acute stroke patient.

Dysrhythmias.   All patients admitted with acute stroke should have an admission ECG and continuous cardiac rhythm monitoring. The ECG may show atrial fibrillation, a risk factor for ischemic stroke or other dysrhythmias, or there may be evidence of recent myocardial ischemia or infarction present.

Invasive Procedure and Surgical Management of Strokes

There are a variety of invasive procedures and surgical options for treatment of stroke, including cerebral angioplasty, stent placement, craniotomy, aneurysm clipping, and carotid endarterectomy.

Angioplasty and Stent Placement   Cerebral angioplasty has been used to successfully reverse neurological deficits caused by atherosclerotic lesions in the cerebral arteries. This technique uses a balloon-tipped catheter to mechanically dilate vessels. Microballoon catheters are introduced via the femoral artery and directed to the major arteries at the base of the brain. Vascular stenting is an alternative to angioplasty. There are currently many different types of stents in various stages of clinical use and approval by the Federal Drug Administration, although additional clinical trials must be completed before widespread use can be recommended. Cerebral angioplasty or stenting carries the

---

Related Pharmacotherapy
Thrombolytic Agents

Tissue plasminogen activator, tPA (Alteplase)

Action and Uses
Thrombolytic—converts plasminogen to plasmin, leading to breakdown of fibrin clots. Used for acute ischemic stroke or thrombotic stroke.

Dosage (Adult)
0.9 mg/kg (IV) over 60 min with 10% of dose as an initial bolus over 1 min (max. dose: 90 mg)

Major Adverse Effects
Bleeding, anaphylaxis, cardiac dysrhythmias

Nursing Implications
Because of the increased risk for life-threatening intracranial bleeding, a head CT without contrast should be obtained before administration along with baseline labs (CBC, PT and PTT, fibrinogen, type and screen for blood).

Heparin, warfarin, and aspirin should not be coadministered for 24 hours following administration of this agent.

Venipunctures and invasive line placement should be avoided for 24 hours.

Example of protocol during and directly following tPA infusion:

- Assessment of neurological status and of vital signs (except temperature) should be performed every 15 minutes for the first 2 hours at the onset of tPA infusion, then every 30 minutes for 6 hours, then every 60 minutes for 16 hours (total of 24 hours).
- The frequency of blood pressure assessments may need to be increased if systolic blood pressure (SBP) is 180 mmHg or higher or diastolic blood pressure (DBP) is 105 mmHg or higher.
- The physician or supervising practitioner should be notified of any of the following:
  - SBP exceeds 185 or falls below 110 mmHg.
  - DBP exceeds 105 or falls below 60 mmHg.
  - Pulse is less than 50 or greater than 110 per minute.
  - Respirations are more than 24 per minute.
  - Temperature goes above 99.6°F.
  - For worsening stroke symptoms or deteriorating neurological status.
- Antihypertensive medications are given as required.

risks of intracerebral hemorrhage, injury to the vessel wall, and distal embolization. Following cerebral angioplasty, nursing assessments for neurologic and vital sign changes are done frequently until the patient is neurologically stable. In select patients with ischemic stroke, the administration of intravenous tPA in conjunction with clot removal using a "stent retriever" device may be effective (Powers & Jordan, 2015).

Craniotomy Emergency surgery is indicated for cerebellar infarction or hemorrhage with clinical evidence of brainstem compression and increased ICP, such as decreasing level of consciousness, restlessness, or cranial nerve palsies. Hemorrhage into the area of ischemic infarct is a common complication of stroke. The use of thrombolytic and antithrombotic agents and having significantly elevated blood pressure all increase the risk of hemorrhagic complications. Cerebellar lesions are critical because a hemorrhage or infarction can rapidly become life-threatening by compromising the brainstem. The size of the hemorrhage or infarction is a critical variable in medical management; and large hemorrhages or infarctions are more likely to cause brainstem compression and an urgent need for surgery. Management of intracranial hemorrhage is covered in Chapter 19.

Aneurysm Clipping Bleeding into the subarachnoid space, such as that which occurs with a ruptured aneurysm, requires immediate attention. Treatment, however, depends on the severity of neurological symptoms. Persons with no neurological deficits may require cerebral arteriography and early surgery. The surgical procedure, performed within 72 hours of the bleed, is known as an aneurysm clipping and involves opening the cranium (craniotomy) and inserting a metal clip around the aneurysm to prevent rebleeding. A major postoperative complication is cerebral vasospasm, which decreases perfusion to brain tissue. Vasospasm is prevented and treated with hypervolemia, hypertension, and hemodilution: triple H therapy. This combination of therapies is used to augment cerebral perfusion pressure (CPP) by raising systolic blood pressure, cardiac output, and intravascular volume to increase cerebral blood flow and minimize cerebral ischemia. Triple H therapy is maintained for the first 2 to 3 days postoperatively. Calcium channel blocking agents such as nimodipine (Nimitop) may be ordered to treat and prevent cerebral vasospasm in patients who have undergone an aneurysm clipping. Figure 18–7 shows an aneurysm clipping.

Carotid Endarterectomy For ischemic cerebrovascular disease, surgery may be performed to prevent recurring cerebral infarcts and TIAs. This procedure is done to remove the source of the occlusion and to increase cerebral blood flow to the ischemic area. A carotid endarterectomy is a surgical procedure to remove exposed occlusive atherosclerotic plaque from the carotid artery (Figure 18–8). Postoperative nursing care for the patient who has a carotid endarterectomy is summarized in Table 18–6.

Nursing Management

The nurse plays a major role in stabilizing, protecting, and managing care of the acute stroke patient.

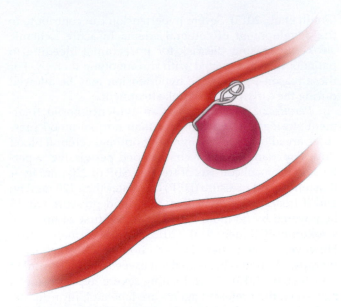

Figure 18–7 Aneurysm clipping.

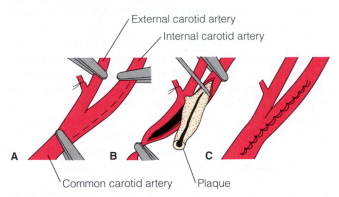

Figure 18–8 Carotid endarterectomy. A, The occluded area is clamped off and an incision is made in the artery. B, Plaque is removed from the inner layer of the artery. C, To restore blood flow through the artery, the artery is sutured or a graft is completed.

Initial Priorities When a stroke is suspected, airway, breathing, and circulation (the ABCs) are assessed. Impaired airway clearance may result from hemiplegia, dysphagia, a weak cough reflex, and immobility. This places the patient at high risk for hypoxemia, pneumonia, and aspiration. Continuous monitoring of breath sounds, breathing patterns, oxygen saturation, skin color, and arterial blood gases (ABGs) is important. The patient's ability to handle secretions is assessed. Intubation and mechanical ventilation are required for the patient who is comatose and has evidence of increased ICP. The patient may present with ineffective breathing patterns because of decreased level of responsiveness, aspiration, loss of protective reflexes, or a decrease in respiratory movements on the affected side. With inadequate ventilation, **hypercapnia** (abnormally elevated $PaCO_2$) occurs, causing cerebral vasodilation. This, however, diverts blood from the penumbra and contributes to an extension of the infarct. To prevent hypercapnia, the nurse monitors rate and rhythm of breathing, ABGs, and level of consciousness. Cardiovascular assessment includes frequent monitoring of vital signs (particularly blood pressure and heart rate) until the

Table 18–6 Caring for the Patient after Carotid Endarterectomy

Nursing Intervention	Rationale
Position patient on the nonoperative side, with head of bed elevated 30 degrees.	Elevation reduces operative site edema.
Maintain head and neck alignment; avoid rotating, flexing, or hyperextending head.	Proper alignment prevents additional tension or pressure on the operative side and facilitates blood flow.
Support the head during position change (teach patient to do the same).	Support prevents additional tension or stress on operative side; tension or stress may cause bleeding and hematoma formation.
Nursing assessments focus on early identification of complications, including hemorrhage, respiratory distress, cranial nerve impairment, and alterations in blood pressure.	The most common cause of respiratory problems is pressure on the trachea from hematoma formation. Cranial nerves may be stretched during surgery, leading to temporary deficits in cranial nerve function; assess for facial drooping, tongue deviation, hoarseness, dysphagia, or loss of facial sensation. Patients who have this procedure are at risk for developing unstable blood pressure as a result of denervation of the carotid sinus.

patient is stable. The heart rhythm is assessed for dysrhythmias. Peripheral and carotid pulses are palpated. Continuous telemetry identifies abnormal cardiac rhythms.

Activity As the patient's condition stabilizes, the activity level should increase and physical therapy should be started for strengthening, range of motion, and early mobilization to prevent joint contractures and muscle atrophy of limbs. These patients are at increased risk for falls, so involving physical therapy early helps to ensure patient safety when activity level is advanced. Ambulation and mobilization may also help to prevent pulmonary complications and improve mental status.

Nutrition Nutritional support and adequate fluid balance are important to offset malnutrition and dehydration, which can delay recovery, decrease cerebral perfusion, and increase the risk for venous thromboembolism (VTE). Dietary consultation should occur to ensure that caloric needs are met and to evaluate the patient's ability to swallow prior to initiation of oral food and fluids. Nutrition may be provided through an enteral route until the patient is safe to swallow or a percutaneous endoscopic gastrostomy is placed for long-term tube feedings.

Preventing Infection Pneumonia and urinary tract infection are two of the most common infections that complicate stroke recovery. Interventions aimed at preventing aspiration pneumonia as well as urinary tract infections are necessary. Patients should be monitored for the presence of infection and antibiotics started promptly as needed. Constipation and incontinence may occur, and nursing should manage these complications with a bowel regimen and bladder catheterization. Indwelling urinary catheters should be discontinued as soon as possible, with intermittent catheterization being instituted as early as possible.

Preventing Complications In patients with acute ischemic stroke or TIA, the use of aspirin therapy at a dose of 160 to 325 mg is recommended (Ropper et al., 2014a; Smith et al., 2015). In patients with acute ischemic stroke and restricted mobility, prophylactic use of anticoagulant medications, such as low-molecular-weight heparin (Lovenox) or heparin is recommended between days 2 and 4 following administration of thrombolytic agents. Clinical trials

support the superiority of low-molecular-weight heparin over unfractionated heparin for preventing VTE in patients with ischemic stroke (Winstein et al., 2016). Administration of these medications increases the risk of serious bleeding complications. (See the "Related Pharmacotherapy: Agents to Prevent Stroke Complications" feature). The administration of anticoagulants for VTE prophylaxis is currently contraindicated during the first 24 hours following treatment with tPA. Pneumatic compression devices are recommended for VTE prophylaxis early in acute stroke of all causes; compression stockings are no longer recommended (Winstein et al., 2016).

If the stroke was caused by an embolism from a cardiac source (e.g., cardiomyopathy or atrial fibrillation), chronic anticoagulation with warfarin (to maintain an INR of 2–3) or aspirin (325 mg/day) is indicated to decrease the risk for recurrent stroke. Aspirin in combination with warfarin (Coumadin) greatly increases the risk of intracranial hemorrhage; these drugs should not be given together. In noncardiac-related embolic strokes, patients should be started on a long-term antiplatelet regimen with aspirin (81–325 mg/per day) within 48 hours of stroke onset. In young patients without discernible risk factors for stroke, a hypercoagulation workup is warranted. Current recommendations for antiplatelet therapy and VTE prophylaxis in acute ischemic stroke patients are summarized in Box 18–2 (Jauch et al., 2013; Smith et al., 2015).

Seizures may develop in a small percentage of patients with ischemic stroke and are most likely to occur within 24 hours of stroke onset; however, there is no evidence to support the use of prophylactic administration of anticonvulsants after stroke (Jauch et al., 2013). Seizures are managed with benzodiazepines and anticonvulsant medications.

Severe cerebral edema may occur at a critical level, a complication known as malignant edema, within the first 24 hours following ischemic stroke reperfusion in patients with a large volume of damaged tissue (Jauch et al., 2013). Edema in the cerebellum region of the brain, which typically peaks within 3 to 4 days following cellular damage, may be life-threatening as it may lead to neurologic deterioration and respiratory failure. Management of cerebral edema and increased intracranial pressure is discussed in Chapter 19.

Related Pharmacotherapy
Agents to Prevent Stroke Complications

Anticonvulsants

(See "Related Pharmacotherapy: Agents Used for Treating Status Epilepticus", pages 479–480)

Antihypertensives

Nitroglycerine (Nitrostat IV)
Hydralazine (Apresoline)
Labetalol (Trandate, Propranolol)
Nicardipine (Cardene)

Action and Uses

Nitrate vasodilator—Reduces BP and angina by directly dilating arterioles (nitroglycerine).

Non-nitrate vasodilator—Reduces BP by directly dilating arterioles (hydralazine).

Alpha and beta adrenergic antagonist—Reduces BP by blocking alpha 1, beta 1, and beta 2 adrenergic receptors (labetalol).

Calcium channel blocker—Reduces BP by calcium channel blocking properties, resulting in depression of cardiac and vascular smooth muscle (nicardipine).

Dosages (Adult)

Nitroglycerine: (IV) Start with 5 mcg/min and titrate every 3–5 minutes until desired response (up to 200 mcg/min)

Hydralazine: 10–20 mg (IV) every 4–6 hours, may increase to 40 mg

Labetalol: 20 mg (IV) slowly over 2 minutes, with 40–80 mg every 10 minutes if needed up to 300 mg total or 2 mg/min continuous infusion (max: 300 mg total)

Nicardipine: Initiation of therapy in a drug-free patient: 5 mg/hr (IV) initially; increase dose by 2.5 mg/hr every 15 minutes (or faster) (max: 15 mg/hr); for severe hypertension: 4–7.5 mg/hr

Major Adverse Effects

Hypotension, tachycardia, dizziness, headache, lupus (hydralazine), bradycardia, bronchospasm (labetalol)

Nursing Implications

Labetalol—Avoid using in patients with asthma, AV heart block, and bradycardia.

Nicardipine—Do not abruptly discontinue this medication as it may result in cardiac ischemia and chest pain.

Monitor for hypotension; avoid sublingual route due to increased risk of hypotension.

Anticoagulants

Enoxaparin (Lovenox) (low molecular weight)
Heparin sodium
Warfarin (Coumadin)

Action and Uses

Anticoagulant—Prevention and treatment of venous thromboembolism and pulmonary embolism (enoxaparin and heparin); management of deep vein thrombosis (DVT) and pulmonary embolism; prevention of new emboli associated with carotid or vertebral dissections, prosthetic heart valve replacements and atrial fibrillation by interfering with vitamin K—dependent clotting factor synthesis (warfarin).

SOURCE: Data from Wilson et al. (2016).

Dosages (Adult)

Enoxaparin: Treatment of VTE and pulmonary embolus—1mg/kg subcutaneous every 12 hr or 1.5 mg/kg/day. Prevention of VTE in medical patients with severe mobility limitations—40 mg subcutaneous daily.

Heparin: Treatment of VTE—5000-unit (IV) bolus dose, then 20,000–40,000 units infused over 24 hours, dose adjusted to maintain desired aPTT; or 5000–10,000 units IV piggyback every 4–6 hours; subcutaneous 10,000–20,000 units followed by 8000–20,000 units every 8–12 hours; Prophylaxis of embolism subcutaneous 5000 units every 8–12 hours until patient is ambulatory.

Warfarin: PO/IV—usual dose 2–10 mg daily with dose adjusted to maintain a PT 1.2–2x control or INR of 2–3.

Major Adverse Effects

Bleeding, thrombocytopenia

Nursing Implications

Enoxaparin—Monitor for bleeding and thrombocytopenia.

Heparin—Monitor for bleeding, thrombocytopenia; trend aPTT levels and have protamine sulfate available as an antidote.

Warfarin—Not used in the acute phase of stroke management; PT/INR must be monitored; monitor for bleeding; requires intensive education regarding drug–food interactions and need for monitoring.

Antiplatelet Therapy

Acetylsalicylic acid (aspirin)
Clopidogrel (Plavix)
Dipyridamole (Persantine)
Ticlopidine (Ticlid)

Action and Uses

Antiplatelet aggregation; prolongs bleeding time, thereby reducing atherosclerotic events in high-risk patients; aspirin is also an antipyretic and analgesic.

Dosages (Adult)

Acetylsalicylic acid: Treatment of thromboembolic disorders—81–325 mg orally (PO) daily; TIA prophylaxis—650 mg PO twice daily

Clopidogrel: Secondary prevention after stroke, MI, and following stent placement—75 mg PO daily

Dipyridamole: Treatment and prevention of VTE disorders—150–400 mg/day PO in divided doses

Ticlopidine: Reduce risk of stroke or thrombotic event—250 mg PO twice daily with food

Major Adverse Effects

Bleeding, particularly in the gastrointestinal tract; GI irritation, thrombocytopenia, rash

Nursing Implications

Aspirin—Monitor for gastric irritation; use enteric-coated varieties and take with food

Clopidogrel—Monitor for gastrointestinal distress, heartburn, nausea, and bleeding; avoid administering with aspirin

Dipyridamole—Monitor for bleeding and thrombocytopenia

Ticlopidine—Monitor for gastrointestinal distress, heartburn, nausea; monitor for neutropenia, anemia, and thrombocytopenia, particularly during the first three months of therapy

---

BOX 18–2   Recommendations of Antiplatelet Therapy and VTE Prophylaxis

- Aspirin should be given as soon as possible after onset of stroke symptoms for most patients.
- The administration of aspirin, as an adjunct therapy, within 48 hours of the use of thrombolytic agents is recommended at a dose of 160 to 325 mg.
- Aspirin should NOT be used as a substitute for other acute interventions (tPA) for the treatment of acute ischemic stroke.
- No recommendation can be made about the urgent administration of other antiplatelet aggregating agents.
- The administration of VTE prophylaxis with heparin or low-molecular-weight heparin is recommended between days 2 and 4 following administration of thrombolytic agents in patients with restricted mobility.
- The administration of anticoagulants for VTE prophylaxis is currently contraindicated during the first 24 hours following treatment with tPA.
- Pneumatic compression devices are recommended for VTE prophylaxis early in acute stroke of all causes, but compression stockings are no longer recommended.

Emerging Evidence

- A review of 2027 acute ischemic stroke (AIS) cases from 16 emergency departments in the midwestern United States revealed that approximately 14% ($n = 283$) did not receive an accurate diagnosis in the emergency department (ED). Physician verification of AIS along with an examination of ICD-9 codes highlighted patients who were hospitalized due to ischemic stroke but were not accurately diagnosed in the ED. Length of hospital stay was 5 versus 3 days in those who were misdiagnosed ($p < 0.0001$). Decreased level of consciousness and younger age were linked to greater odds for a misdiagnosis (*Madsen et al., 2016*).
- Dysphagia was evaluated in a sample of 49 hospitalized stroke patients by speech and language pathologists (SLPs) and trained, experienced nurses. Nurses were able to identify 16 of 18 patients who were diagnosed with dysphagia by SLPs. The Nurse Dysphagia Screen guided the nurses' dysphagia assessments. The sensitivity (89%) and specificity (90%) of the screening tool in this study provide evidence that supports the tool's value for assessing dysphagia in the clinical setting (*Cummings et al., 2015*).
- A retrospective review of 2894 patient records from 84 ICU settings in the United States provided comparison data regarding the oxygenation status of mechanically ventilated patients with stroke over a 5-year time span. Higher rates of in-hospital mortality were documented in patients with hyperoxia ($PaO_2 > 300$ mmHg) when compared to those with hypoxia ($PaO_2 < 60$ mmHg) or normal oxygen levels by way of arterial blood gas analysis. As a result of these findings, the researchers recommended careful monitoring of patient oxygenation status as interventions were carried out to improve oxygen delivery and perfusion (*Rincon et al., 2014*).

Section Five Review

1. Which of the following is fundamental to the current approach to the treatment of ischemic strokes?
   A. Ischemic penumbra
   B. Infarcted area
   C. Cerebral edema
   D. Cerebral perfusion pressure

2. During administration of tPA, how frequently should neurological assessments initially be made?
   A. 12 hours
   B. 6 hours
   C. 1 hour
   D. 15 minutes

3. What is the rationale for ensuring adequate fluid balance in a client recovering from stroke? (Select all that apply.)
   A. Dehydration can delay recovery.
   B. Dehydration can decrease cerebral perfusion.
   C. Dehydration causes respiratory depression.
   D. Dehydration can increase risk for venous thromboembolism.
   E. Dehydration dramatically increases risk for stroke recurrence.

4. Which position is recommended postoperatively for a client who has had a carotid endarterectomy?
   A. Flat in bed
   B. Prone
   C. On the nonoperative side
   D. With neck extended and turned to operative side.

Answers: 1. A, 2. D, 3. (A, B, D), 4. C

Section Six: Hospital Management and Secondary Prevention in the Acute Phase

In the high-acuity setting, care of the patient with a stroke focuses on prevention and treatment of complications that may be neurological (e.g., secondary hemorrhage, space-occupying edema, or seizures) or medical (infections, pressure ulcers, deep vein thrombosis [DVT], hypertension, hypotension, aspiration, or pulmonary embolism).

Following a stroke, the patient may be placed in a special high-acuity unit in the hospital—the stroke unit—which is staffed with a multidisciplinary team. The core disciplines of the team include experts from medicine, nursing, physiotherapy, occupational therapy, speech and language therapy, and social work. The acute stroke unit admits patients quickly and continues treatment for several days, until transfer to a rehabilitation or nursing facility or to the patient's home. The use of standardized patient care guidelines or protocols can promote high-quality, safe care during the acute care and discharge phases of care (see the feature "Quality and Safety: Ischemic Stoke Care").

Peripheral Tissue Perfusion

Peripheral tissue perfusion can diminish related to interruption of flow and venous stasis from inactivity. A serious threat to the hemiplegic stroke patient is venous thromboembolism (VTE), a complication that includes deep vein thrombosis (DVT) and pulmonary embolism (PE). Stroke patients are at high risk for VTE because of hemiplegia; loss of vasomotor tone; venous stasis; edema in the paralyzed, flaccid limbs; and immobility. Dehydration places the patient at high risk for VTE. Hemiplegia or hemiparesis decreases muscle pump action for return of venous blood to the heart. Poor positioning (one extremity lying on another) or sitting for long periods in a chair can precipitate or exacerbate VTE formation. Subcutaneous unfractionated heparin, low-molecular-weight heparin, and heparinoids may be given for DVT prophylaxis for at-risk patients with ischemic stroke, as well as other nonpharmacologic measures, such as sequential compression devices, can also be used to prevent VTE (Jauch et al., 2013).

Compromised Physical Mobility

Physical mobility problems are related to motor and sensory deficits, particularly hemiplegia and impaired balance, changes in postural tone, and disinhibition of primitive reflex activity. Rehabilitation begins early after a stroke in an effort to increase independence. A multidisciplinary effort is required for maximum rehabilitation potential. Physical therapists assess motor function, plan exercise programs, and provide splints to prevent contractures. Occupational therapists assess the patient, provide a plan of therapy, and evaluate sensory and cognitive problems that interfere with functional independence. The physiatrist is a physician responsible for diagnosing and treating rehabilitative problems, such as spasticity and subluxation.

Following a stroke, a state of temporary disruption of neural processes related to motor function may occur, causing hypotonicity or flaccid hemiplegia. When a stroke causes hemiplegia, initially the patient's affected limbs are flaccid; later, tone is palpated in affected limb muscles and spasticity begins, with some resistance to movement. Spasticity results when reflex activity is released from cerebral inhibition after damage to the motor system. This spasticity is associated with an upper motor neuron lesion because the frontal cortex (motor centers) and/or corticospinal (voluntary motor) tracts are interrupted. Muscle spasticity, hypertonicity, resistance to passive stretch in joints, and abnormally brisk reflexes characterize upper motor neuron lesions. Depending on the stroke site, the patient can present with mild hemiparesis to severe hemiplegia, tetraplegia, ataxia, or involuntary movements.

Poststroke spasticity (excessive muscle tone) affects the antigravity muscles. In the lower limbs, these are the knee extensors and plantar flexors of the foot. In the upper limbs, these are the elbow flexors and wrist and finger flexors. The patient assumes a spastic hemiparetic posture, with the neck and trunk tilted toward the hemiparetic side; the shoulder pulled down and back; the elbow, wrist, and fingers flexed; and the arm adducted. The lower limb is extended, with the hip internally rotated and adducted, and the foot plantar is flexed with supination, inversion, and flexed toes. Because flexor muscles are stronger in the arms and extensors are stronger in the legs, the patient is prone to flexion contractures in the upper extremities and extension contractures in the lower extremities.

Maintaining functional abilities in the acute phase after stroke is an important component of patient care. Active and/or passive range of motion (ROM) exercises performed at least three or four times a day help prevent contractures. Proper body alignment is also important to prevent contractures. The patient is placed in positions that neutralize the abnormal hemiparetic posture (see Figure 18–9).

The patient is ready to ambulate when there is evidence of leg strength, some balance, and **proprioception**. Muscle tone is assessed regularly, and the patient is not asked to do an activity with the disabled limb until muscle tone is restored.

Quality and Safety
Ischemic Stroke Care

National guidelines for ischemic stroke care include the following:

- Intravenous tPA
- VTE prophylaxis
- Anticoagulation with atrial fibrillation or flutter
- Antithrombotic therapy
- Statins for lipid-lowering effects
- Patient education
- Determination of rehabilitation needs
- Smoking cessation measures
- Screening for dysphagia

SOURCE: Data from Elder el al. (2015); Jauch et al. (2013).

A

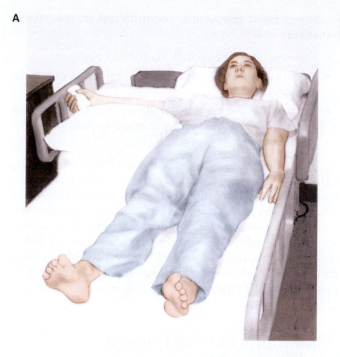

B

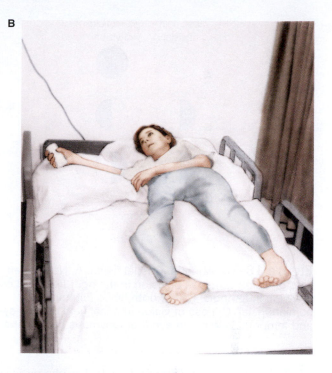

C

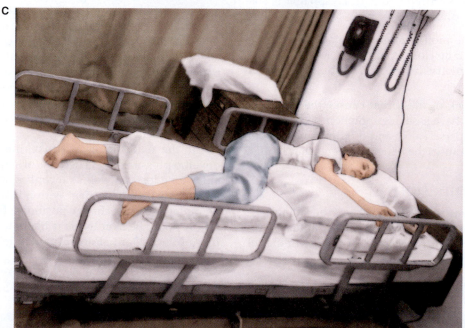

Figure 18–9 Positioning the stroke patient. A, Lying on back. B, Lying on affected side. C, Lying on unaffected side.

Altered Nutrition

Dysphagia, absent or diminished gag reflexes, facial paralysis, perceptual and cognitive deficits, hemiplegia (particularly affecting the dominant hand), an inability to perform bilateral hand tasks, and immobility all contribute to undernutrition. Absent gag reflexes and facial paralysis limit chewing and swallowing movements and increase the risk for aspiration. Perceptual deficits, such as impaired depth perception, agnosia, apraxia, hemianopsia (Figure 18–10), or neglect, may produce injury during eating.

During acute stroke, metabolic demands become greater while oral intake is often restricted. Clinically, the

patient may manifest a decrease in serum protein leading to a compromised immune state, weight loss, muscle weakness and atrophy, increased risk of pressure ulcers, higher morbidity and mortality, and a prolonged hospital stay. In well-nourished patients, nutritional support is started if no oral intake is anticipated for greater than 5 days. If the patient is malnourished on admission, as defined by a greater than 10% weight loss before critical illness, nutritional support is initiated promptly.

Early and rapid evaluation of swallowing is done as soon as possible. Dysphagia (difficulty in swallowing) is usually caused by lesions involving cranial nerves V (trigeminal), VII (facial), IX (glossopharyngeal), X (vagus),

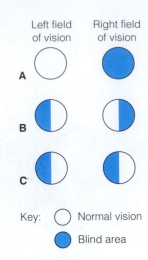

Left field of vision   Right field of vision

A

B

C

Key: ◯ Normal vision
       ● Blind area

Figure 18–10 Abnormal visual fields. A, Normal left field of vision with loss of vision in the right field. B, Loss of vision in temporal half of both fields (bitemporal hemianopsia). C, Loss of vision in nasal field of right eye and temporal field of left eye (homonymous hemianopsia).

XI (accessory), and XII (hypoglossal). Dysphagia is suspected when the following signs appear:

- Food put in the mouth causes the patient to choke, drool, have poor lip closure, engage in food pocketing, or have asymmetry of the mouth or a protruded tongue.

- Food in the back of the throat causes the patient to choke, aspirate, have nasal regurgitation, become weak, or develop a hoarse voice; and food passing through the esophagus causes the patient to regurgitate.

Urinary Elimination

Inadequate urinary elimination may be related to impaired mobility, cognitive impairment, aphasia, and preexisting elimination problems. Urinary elimination problems most frequently encountered in the stroke patient are as follows:

- Detrusor muscle hyporeflexia (flaccid bladder)
- Detrusor muscle hyperreflexia (uninhibited or spastic bladder)
- Detrusor muscle–sphincter dyssynergy (unsynchronized detrusor and sphincter muscles producing urinary retention)

After the acute phase of the injury has passed, the indwelling urinary catheter is removed and an intermittent catheterization program is implemented (every 4 hours) to ensure that the urine volume does not exceed 400 mL. For patients with bladder hyperreflexia, a voiding schedule is established with the patient and family based on previous patterns of voiding. When possible, diapers and long-term indwelling urinary catheter use should be avoided. Refer to Table 18–7 for a description of neurogenic bladder types.

Alterations in Skin Integrity

Sensation and skin integrity may be altered in the stroke patient related to loss of motor or vascular tone loss or the sense of touch, pressure, temperature, or sensation. Lesions in the parietal cortex or its afferent pathways produce a loss of primary sensations or **paresthesias**, placing the patient at risk for burns, bruises, and other forms of injury. Loss of proprioception or position sense may lead to falls. Loss of vision and hearing can cause injury, social isolation, and impaired learning. A care priority in these patients is to protect them from injury.

In the acute stages of stroke, the patient is prone to develop pressure ulcers because of sensory, motor, or vascular tone loss, as well as incontinence, parietal neglect, and spasticity. The patient with a hemisensory deficit or hemiplegia cannot change positions. In addition, if nutrition is poor, the skin tissue is likely to break down in the immobile patient. Perceptual deficits compound the

Table 18–7 Types of Neurogenic Bladder

Bladder Type	Features	Lesion Site	Effects on Patient	Nursing Approach
Detrusor hyporeflexia	Flaccid (large capacity)	Above the pons	Overflow incontinence Distended bladder High urine residual volumes	Monitor intake and output Observe for overdistention Intermittent catheterization Keep urine volume less than 400 mL
Detrusor hyperreflexia (uninhibited)	Spastic (small capacity)	Cerebral cortex, internal capsule, basal ganglia	Urinary frequency, urgency Bladder contractions or spasms Nocturia Low-volume voidings Incontinence (unable to reach toilet in time)	Voiding schedule every 2 hours or longer Monitor intake, output Encourage fluids Limit caffeine and evening fluids Upright position to void
Detrusor–sphincter dyssynergy (uncoordinated)	Spastic bladder and external sphincter that contract simultaneously (small capacity)	Pons, and pathways between pons and above sacral spinal cord	Small, frequent, or no voids Sensation of bladder fullness Dribbling, overflow incontinence High urine residual volumes Dysuria	Antispasmodics may be prescribed Consistent fluid intake Time voiding schedule Possibly intermittent catheterization within 5 minutes of voiding Observe for overdistention symptoms Keep residuals less than 75 mL Monitor intake, output

problem, particularly parietal neglect, when portions of the body are ignored.

To protect the patient from injury and to maintain skin integrity in hemiplegics or those who are experiencing neglect or denial, the patient and family must be alerted to the deficit and hazards related to the deficit. The skin should be inspected for adequate capillary refill, pallor, and hyperemia, and pressure should be avoided to the area should any of these signs appear. The patient is repositioned at least every 2 hours, and the skin is inspected with each reposition. The turning schedule is revised based on patient tolerance and skin integrity.

Unilateral Neglect

Unilateral neglect or perceptual hemineglect applies to a disorder of attention causing an inability to integrate and use perceptions in the contralateral side or space. The patient fails to respond to stimuli presented to the side contralateral to the brain lesion; therefore, that side is ignored but can be used if attention is drawn to it. Right brain damage produces this syndrome. Hemineglect is seen alone or in combination with **anosognosia** (unawareness) and left **homonymous hemianopsia** (hemineglect syndrome). Homonymous hemianopsia refers to loss of the same visual fields in both eyes, essentially causing right or left visual field blindness. When the visual field loss is on the same side as the loss of sensation and paralysis, the patient can experience hemineglect syndrome, whereby the patient completely ignores (neglects) the affected side of the body.

Patients with hemineglect syndrome can be assisted by increasing their awareness of their surroundings and by alleviating apprehension as to the source of the problem. When homonymous hemianopsia is present, the patient should be approached from the unaffected side, positioned so that the intact visual field is toward the action, provided with personal items arranged within the field of vision, and taught to scan the environment by turning the head vertically and horizontally. As the patient's apprehension decreases, awareness and attention can be stimulated by placing personal items toward the affected side to encourage awareness of and attention to that side. This is accomplished by careful positioning such that the patient's eyes are facing the affected side and by teaching the patient to handle, position, exercise, bathe, and dress the affected extremities with the patient's unaffected arm. Denial of illness usually resolves as the patient recovers.

Ineffective Verbal Communication

Patients with left hemispheric dysfunction caused by middle cerebral artery involvement experience expressive and receptive dysphasia because the speech centers or their pathways are involved in the lesion. Aphasia or dysphasia is a disorder of linguistic processing in which there is a disruption of translating thought to language. Literally, **aphasia** means a total inability to understand or formulate language. Language comprehension, speech expression, or writing ability may be lost. **Dysphasia** refers to difficulty with comprehending, speaking, or writing.

Wernicke's Aphasia   In Wernicke's aphasia, the patient receives auditory impulses but is unable to comprehend them. It is a receptive aphasia characterized by fluent, well-articulated speech with intact tone but inappropriate speech content that is unintelligible because of poor word choices. The patient makes up new words. Reading and speech comprehension, repetition of speech, and naming of objects are impaired. The patient is unable to write coherently. The goal of therapy for patients with Wernicke's aphasia is to develop an awareness of the language problem and to increase comprehension. Removing extraneous sounds and distractions, such as the television or radio, assist in getting the person's attention. The patient and nurse use nonverbal behavior to enhance communication. Keeping the conversation on one defined subject with one question at a time and avoiding multiple choices when communicating is helpful.

Broca's Aphasia   Broca's aphasia is an expressive aphasia characterized by nonfluent, telegraphic speech with outbursts of profanity, uninhibited speech, and word-finding difficulty, which reflects impaired memory for language. The patient uses nouns or phrases with pauses between words and lacks grammar. An awareness of speech errors is present, and speech production is labored and frustrating. A poor capacity for repetition and difficulty naming objects exist, although recognition of objects is present. Oddly, these patients can sing fluently because musical ability is intact in the nondominant hemisphere. Comprehension is usually intact, and responses are appropriate. Reading comprehension is variable, and writing ability is impaired, possibly because an associated right hemiparesis or hemiplegia is often found in these patients since Broca's area is located adjacent to the primary motor centers in the frontal lobe. The goal for the patient with Broca's aphasia is to establish reliable language output to express needs. This may be accomplished initially by asking the patient yes–no questions.

Global Aphasia   Global aphasia is a combination of Broca's and Wernicke's aphasias with an almost complete loss of comprehension and expression of speech. The lesion involves the frontal and temporal lobes. The patient has nonfluent speech and an inability to express his or her ideas in speech or writing. The goal for the patient with global aphasia is to improve the ability to communicate. The patient is taught to enhance communication with nonverbal gestures and facial expressions. The measures cited for both Wernicke's and Broca's aphasias are applicable with these patients as well.

Table 18–8 provides a summary comparison of expressive and receptive aphasias.

Dysarthria   **Dysarthria** is an impairment of the muscles that control speech. Hemispheric or brainstem strokes produce dysarthria, which is characterized by slurred, muffled, or indistinct speech. Uncoordinated, slow, monotone speech results if the cerebellum or basal ganglia are involved. Language comprehension and formulation are intact unless the patient also has aphasia. The goal of therapy is to strengthen the speech muscles in order to speak more clearly and fluently. Encouraging the patient to enunciate one word at a

Table 18–8 Comparison of Expressive and Receptive Aphasias

	Expressive (Broca's) Aphasia	Receptive (Wernicke's) Aphasia
Location of injury	Broca's area in frontal lobe, usually in left hemisphere	Wernicke's area located within temporal and parietal lobes
Normal function	Primary function is motor speech.	Primary function is translating thoughts into words.
Deficit description	Receives and comprehends auditory input but verbal responses (speech) are inappropriate Is aware of what they want to say but cannot say it correctly	Unable to comprehend language (receives auditory input but cannot comprehend it) Reading, writing, speech, and naming objects are impaired.
Characteristics	Understands what is being said and read Speech is nonfluent; may not be able to articulate words. Outbursts of uninhibited speech Difficulty with word finding Halting speech that lacks grammar	Unable to understand what is being said Speech is fluent, well articulated. Makes up new words Speech content is inappropriate. Difficulty naming objects Can sing fluently

time, particularly consonants, and increasing voice volume when it is low helps.

Inadequate Coping

Patients and their families are faced with multiple psychosocial stressors. The potential for ineffective coping is related to abrupt change in lifestyle, loss of roles, dependency, and economic insecurity. In addition, the family may have to assume new roles as care providers and relinquish jobs and salaries. They may be overwhelmed with medical bills or faced with nursing home placement of their loved one and subsequent guilt. Fears of another stroke, as well as inability to care for the patient at home, create more stress.

Other causes for ineffective coping are the emotional and cognitive impairments following a stroke. Emotional lability with inappropriate crying, laughing, or euphoria, or socially inappropriate behavior with an inability to interpret social cues of communication, creates stress for both the patient and family. Stroke patients with residual neurologic deficits are prone to severe depression.

Confusion and bewilderment may compound the problem. In terms of impaired cognition, there may be delayed processing, diminished learning and reasoning ability, and a short attention span. Memory deficits vary with the hemispheric involvement. If the nondominant hemisphere is involved, a memory deficit for performance may be seen; if the dominant hemisphere is involved, a memory deficit for language, word-finding difficulty, and naming problems surface. In addition, there are hemispheric differences in judgment. Patients with lesions in the left hemisphere are slow and cautious, and they underestimate their abilities. In contrast, patients with right hemispheric lesions may be prone to injury because they overestimate their abilities.

Clergy, friends, and family support groups may help assist the patient in coping and may provide comfort for both the patient and the family. Informing the patient that most recovery takes up to 6 months (and some even longer) may be helpful in preventing unrealistic expectations for recovery.

A positive body image is reinforced when the nurse focuses on the function that is left and not on what has been lost. Terms such as *affected* and *unaffected* are preferable to *good* and *bad* side. Reinforce independence early by involving the patient in decisions about family roles and care.

For the patient and family, multidisciplinary referrals may be necessary. Social workers, home health nurses, dieticians, occupational therapists, physiatrists, support groups, and voluntary and governmental agencies (e.g., Medicare) provide assistance. The American Heart Association and the National Stroke Association provide free and low-cost literature on stroke care developed by experts. These referral groups and services are essential for functional recovery and provide invaluable assistance in restoring the patient to a functional or complete recovery. Priority nursing interventions for the patient with acute brain attack are summarized in the "Nursing Care: The Patient with Acute Stroke" feature.

Other Sensory and Motor Deficits

There are several relatively common neurologic deficits that may involve both sensory and motor problems, including agnosia and apraxia.

Agnosia **Agnosia** is a cortical impairment that results in the inability to recognize or interpret familiar sensory information although there is no impairment of sensory input or dementia. The agnosias can be tactile, visual, or auditory (Table 18–9). Tactile agnosia (astereognosia) is the inability to recognize objects by touch, although tactile sensation is present. Visual agnosia is the inability to recognize or name familiar objects or faces although visual acuity is intact (e.g., the patient is unable to recognize utensils, toothbrush, clothes, or photographs). Auditory agnosia is the inability to recognize familiar sounds, such as a doorbell, telephone, horn, gun, or siren. When assessing for agnosias, the patient is asked to name objects and cite their purpose. The patient is asked to identify objects in the hands or to identify sounds, music, or songs with his or her eyes closed. When deficits are found, a referral is made to an occupational therapist (OT) who evaluates and establishes a rehabilitative program.

Nursing Care

The Patient with Acute Stroke

Expected Patient Outcomes and Related Interventions

Outcome 1: Prevent secondary brain injury and preserve neurologic function

Assess and compare to established norms, patient baselines, and trends

Obtain vital signs and perform neurologic assessment

Monitor BP, HR, hemodynamic and cardiac stability

Use the National Institutes of Health Stroke Scale (NIHSS) for detection of early changes suggesting cerebral edema or extension of stroke

ICP (less than 20 mmHg); CPP (60–70 mmHg)

Cerebral oxygenation ($SjVO_2$ at 55–75 mg/dl; $PbtO_2$ 20–24 mmHg)

Changes in mental status and level of consciousness (LOC), restlessness, drowsiness, lethargy, inability to follow commands, reflexes, and strength

Interventions to prevent secondary brain injury and preserve neurologic function

Position HOB at 30 degrees to promote venous drainage and prevent aspiration

Administer related drug therapy and monitor for therapeutic and nontherapeutic effects

Administer anticonvulsant agents to treat seizures

Diuretics, hypertonic saline, and sedation

Intravenous hydration—0.9% normal saline—initial rate 150–200 mL/hr

Outcome 2: Optimize oxygenation

Assess and compare to established norms, patient baselines, and trends

PaO_2, SaO_2, SpO_2, $PETCO_2$

Monitor breath sounds each shift

Interventions to improve oxygenation

Instruct to cough and deep breathe, and use incentive spirometry every 2 hours while awake

Assist with pulmonary hygiene as needed

Keep head of the bed at 30 degrees

Frequent oral care—plaque removal, moisturize mucous membranes to reduce bacterial load in the mouth so as to decrease risk for pneumonia

Sequential pneumatic compression devices

Administer related drug therapy and monitor for therapeutic and nontherapeutic effects

Oxygen to maintain SaO_2 or SpO_2 greater than 94%

VTE prophylaxis

Outcome 3: Stable hemodynamic status and cardiac rhythm

Assess and compare to established norms, patient baselines, and trends

BP, HR, hemodynamic parameters such as PAP, PCWP, CVP, CO/CI, stroke volume variability

Monitor cardiac rhythm

Systemic vascular resistance

Electrolyte levels

CK-MB, troponin levels

Interventions to maintain stable hemodynamic status and cardiac rhythm

Identify and treat dysrhythmias

Investigate and reverse underlying cause of hemodynamic instability

Manage BP carefully; avoid sharp drops in BP that could result in hypotension and cause an ischemic event

Administer related drug therapy and monitor for therapeutic and nontherapeutic effects

Administer medications per established advanced cardiovascular life support (ACLS) protocols as needed for rate or rhythm disturbances: amiodarone, diltiazem, adenosine, beta blockers

Outcome 4: Free from infection

Assess and compare to established norms, patient baselines, and trends

Monitor for infection and fever

White blood cell (WBC) count

Culture and sensitivity results

Observe for signs of infection in patients considered to be at increased risk: those with invasive lines, incisions, and those who require mechanical ventilation

Administer related drug therapy and monitor for therapeutic and nontherapeutic effects

Antibiotic therapy as ordered

Outcome 5: Fluid and electrolyte balance

Assess and compare to established norms, patient baselines, and trends

Monitor intake and output status

Electrolyte levels

Daily weights, CVP, PCWP, chest x-rays

Lung sounds

Administer related drug therapy and monitor for therapeutic and nontherapeutic effects

Electrolytes: potassium, calcium, phosphorous, sodium

Outcome 6: Maintain adequate nutrition, free from GI complications, free from aspiration

Assess and compare to established norms, patient baselines, and trends

Obtain admission weight and daily weights

Assess cranial nerve deficits, especially ability to swallow and gag reflex

Serum glucose levels

Indices of nutrition: C-reactive protein, albumin, prealbumin

Monitor nasogastric (NG) drainage and stool for occult or gross bleeding

Interventions to maintain nutritional needs and avoid GI complications

Test ability to swallow before initiating fluids or food orally (PO)

Start nutrition as soon as possible

Obtain consult for study to assess intake ability to swallow on admit and prior to initiating PO intake

Avoid dextrose-containing IV fluids

Administer GI/ulcer prophylaxis (H_2 blockers, proton pump inhibitors)

Monitor for coughing with eating or drinking as this may be indicative of dysphagia

Outcome 7: Maintain skin, mucous membrane integrity, and optimal joint mobility

Assess and compare to established norms, patient baselines, and trends

Skin and mucous membranes, joint mobility

Perform skin assessment using the Braden scale

Interventions to maintain skin integrity and joint mobility

Maintain a clean and dry environment

Utilize pressure-reducing surfaces

Provide active or passive range-of-motion (ROM) exercises each shift

Reposition every 2 hours

Order physical therapy and occupational therapy consults as soon as the patient has stabilized

Establish splinting routines for affected limbs to prevent contractures (foot and wrist drop)

Use protective padding of surfaces as needed

Mobilize the patient and/or get him or her out of the bed and into a chair as soon as stable

Consult with wound/ostomy nurse specialist for skin breakdown

Outcome 8: Maintain gastrointestinal and urinary elimination, free from complications

Assess and compare to established norms, patient baselines, and trends

Urine and stool output

Kidney function and effect of nephrotoxic agents

Neurogenic bowel and bladder complications—incomplete emptying, incontinence, retention, diarrhea, or constipation

Interventions to promote elimination and prevent complications

Monitor and treat urinary tract infection—remove indwelling urinary catheter as soon as the patient is able to participate

Fluids, fiber, and activity stimulate intestinal motility

Establishing a regular daily time for bowel movements in the upright position and in privacy promote normal bowel elimination

Administer related drug therapy and monitor for therapeutic and nontherapeutic effects

Stool softeners and/or fiber therapy

Antidiarrhea medications

SOURCE: Data from Evans et al. (2016); Jauch et al. (2013); LeMone et al. (2015); Mahanes (2015).

Table 18–9 Types of Agnosias and Apraxias and Associated Deficits

Type	Deficit
Agnosias	
Tactile	Inability to recognize objects by touch
Visual	Inability to recognize or name familiar objects or faces
Auditory	Inability to recognize familiar sounds
Apraxias	
Motor	Memory deficit for motor sequences affecting only upper limbs, although muscle and sensory function are intact
Ideomotor	Inability to perform a motor act on command even though the patient understands the act and has muscle and sensory function; can perform spontaneous, simple, isolated acts but not complex acts, such as writing or dressing
Ideational	Inability to perform activities automatically or on command
Constructional	Inability to copy, draw, or construct designs in two or three dimensions on command or spontaneously
Dressing	Inability to dress self because of a disorder in body schema, unilateral neglect, and/or spatial relations

---

Apraxia Apraxia is the inability to carry out a purposeful movement although movement, coordination, and sensation are intact. Several types of apraxias are summarized in Table 18–9. To assess for motor apraxia, the nurse observes the ability to initiate responses to motor commands, such as "Brush your teeth . . . comb your hair . . . put on your gown." The nurse notes the patient's ability to do spontaneous simple acts. Ideational apraxia is assessed by observing the patient's ability to perform spontaneous acts or acts on command, such as writing. The patient with ideational apraxia is unable to conceptualize the act and cannot perform a spontaneous act. Asking the patient to copy or draw a clock or daisy, or to build three-dimensional designs, such as a house or block, are requests used to assess the patient with constructional apraxia. Asking the patient to put on or remove a shirt, gown, or robe assesses dressing apraxia.

The effectiveness of therapy for ideomotor and ideational apraxia is uncertain. For ideomotor and ideational apraxia, the components of a motor sequence leading up to the entire activity need to be separated and taught in simple terms, with the therapist speaking slowly with clear directions. The patient with dressing apraxia is assisted by the use of labels to distinguish right and left, back from front, right side from wrong side, or by color-coding garments. For all apraxic patients, repetition, consistency, avoidance of distractions, and visual motor coordination exercises are useful.

Section Six Review

1. What are the causes of undernutrition in stroke clients? (Select all that apply.)
   A. Dysphagia
   B. Hemiplegia
   C. Perceptual deficits
   D. Hypometabolic state
   E. Immobility

2. Which statement about elimination problems in acute stroke client is true?
   A. Bowel incontinence is common.
   B. Indwelling urinary catheters are useful for clients with hyperreflexic bladders.
   C. Incontinence is usually stress related.
   D. Scheduled voiding programs can promote continence.

3. Which statement regarding the hemineglect syndrome seen in stroke clients is true?
   A. It usually occurs in dominant strokes.
   B. It can be accompanied by left homonymous hemianopsia.
   C. The client is paralyzed on one side of his or her body.
   D. The client has insight into the cause of the impairment.

4. Which finding is associated with Wernicke's aphasia?
   A. The client cannot speak.
   B. The client can speak, but the speech is halting.
   C. The client cannot comprehend the spoken word.
   D. The client cannot speak but can write coherently.

Answers: 1. (A, B, C, E), 2. D, 3. B, 4. C

Clinical Reasoning Checkpoint

Mrs. HA, a 45-year-old woman, is admitted to your unit with mental status changes. She came into the emergency department with complaints of having the "worst headache of her life." She rated her pain a 10 on a scale of 1 (no pain) to 10 (worst pain ever). She also reports the following symptoms: nausea, vomiting, photophobia, and increasing drowsiness.

Her medical history consists of migraine headaches that she experiences monthly. She reports that this headache is much worse than her usual migraine headache. She takes a calcium channel blocker for hypertension that she developed 6 years ago. She is a smoker (1½ packs per day for 20 years), and she is obese. Currently she continues to complain of headache (10/10).

You perform a physical examination and note that she has nuchal rigidity and a lopsided smile that give her face an asymmetrical appearance most notable on the right side. Her vital signs are normal other than her BP, which is hypertensive at 165/90. Other than her headache, she is neurologically intact. She continues to experience nausea and vomiting along with her headache. The healthcare providers suspect a stroke.

1. What diagnostic testing is indicated for this patient?

Clinical update: Her CT scan reveals diffuse subarachnoid blood and enlarged ventricles.

2. What pathophysiology underlies this stroke?
3. What should be the priorities of her care?
4. In three days, what will she be at increased risk of developing?

Chapter 18 Review

1. A client experienced an episode of vision loss and right-side weakness that lasted 4 hours before totally resolving. What information should the nurse provide to this client?

   1. "Your symptoms indicate that you have had a subarachnoid hemorrhage."

   2. "While these symptoms have resolved, your risk for a stroke is higher."

   3. "These symptoms often occur in older clients and are nothing to worry about."

   4. "Your stroke involved the occipital lobe and your vision will dim over the next few weeks."

2. A client suffered a stroke yesterday and has recovered partial function. The client's spouse says, "I don't understand what is happening. When my mother had a stroke, she was left in a coma for years before she died." What is the nurse's best response?

   1. "All strokes are different."

   2. "Each client responds differently."

   3. "There are different levels of damage done by strokes."

   4. "Your mother must have had some additional medical problems."

3. An 82-year-old African American man has a history of hypertension and type 1 diabetes, and he had a stroke two years ago. He is a smoker and admits to leading a sedentary lifestyle. What are this client's nonmodifiable risk factors for stroke?

   1. Being 82

   2. Being male

   3. Having diabetes

   4. Having a stroke history

   5. Smoking

4. A nurse's neighbor calls and reports that her 64-year-old husband is complaining about loss of vision in one eye after mowing the lawn on a hot Sunday afternoon. He is awake and alert and says the vision loss came on slowly over about an hour. What advice should the nurse give?

   1. "Have him lie down and cool off and see if his vision is better."

   2. "Call his physician's answering service and ask them to relay the information to the doctor."

   3. "Give him a cold drink, and I will be over as soon as I finish lunch to check on him."

   4. "Take him to urgent care or the emergency room."

5. A patient presents to the emergency department with one-sided facial numbness and drooping. Which priority questions will the triage nurse ask? (Select all that apply.)

   1. "Have you ever had these symptoms before this episode?"

   2. "What medications do you take?"

   3. "When was the last time you ate?"

   4. "Do you have numbness anywhere else in your body?"

   5. "Do you have any visual disturbances?"

6. A client is receiving an infusion of tPA for treatment of acute ischemic stroke. The nurse would immediately discontinue this infusion if the client manifested which assessment finding? (Select all that apply.)

   1. Nausea

   2. Severe headache

   3. Elevation of blood pressure to 180/100

   4. Atrial fibrillation

   5. Decrease in pedal pulse amplitude

7. A client being treated for an ischemic stroke has vital signs of temperature: 39.0°C (102.2°F), blood pressure 160/90 mmHg, heart rate 98 bpm, and respirations 16 bpm. What action should the nurse take? (Select all that apply.)

   1. Continue to monitor

   2. Treat the temperature according to protocol

   3. STAT page the provider regarding the blood pressure

   4. Increase the client's oxygen delivery

   5. Accept these vital signs as normal for the client after ischemic stroke

8. The wife of a client who had a stroke says, "I'll never be able to care for him at home unless he can help me. When will therapy start to help him with walking?" Which answer, made by the nurse, is most appropriate?

   1. "Most stroke clients don't rebuild enough strength to help with their care."

   2. "The physical therapist will make that determination, and I'm certain she will talk with you about it then."

   3. "When he has some leg strength and balance back, we will start helping him learn to walk again."

   4. "As soon as his vital signs are stable, we will start walking therapy."

9. A client was just admitted for treatment of stroke. Assessment reveals a well-nourished 63-year-old male with left-sided weakness, a weak gag reflex, and difficulty swallowing. The nurse would anticipate initiating nutritional support for this client if he is unable to take oral nourishment by which time?

   1. Within 24 hours of discontinuation of IV therapy

   2. Within 2 days of return of gag reflex

   3. Within 5 days of admission

   4. Within 12 hours of diagnosis

10. The nurse is caring for a client who has right-sided weakness and Broca's aphasia following a stroke that occurred 36 hours ago. Which assessment instruction should the nurse use with this client?

    1. "Tell me what you were doing immediately before your illness."

    2. "Can you see anything at all out of your bad eye?"

    3. "Lift your unaffected arm up as much as you can."

    4. "Describe the sensations you have in your good leg."

Answers to questions found inside your textbook are available on the faculty resources site. Please consult with your instructor.

References

Aminoff, M. J., Greenberg, D. A., & Simon, R. P. (2015). Stroke. In M. J. Aminoff, D. A. Greenberg, & R. P. Simon (Eds.), *Clinical neurology* (9th ed.). Retrieved November 26, 2016, from http://accessmedicine .mhmedical.com.ezproxy.uky.edu/content.aspx?bookid =1194&Sectionid=78430100

Antoniello, D. (2014). Chapter 23: Cerebrovascular disease. In B. A. Williams, A. Chang, C. Ahalt, H. Chen, R. Conant, C. Landefeld, C. Ritchie, & M. Yukawa (Eds.), *Current diagnosis & treatment: Geriatrics*, Retrieved November 29, 2016, from http://accessmedicine .mhmedical.com.ezproxy.uky.edu/content.aspx?bookid =953&Sectionid=53375647

Bassily-Marcus, A., & Khachaturova, I. (2016). Chapter 74: Controversies: Is glucose control relevant? In J. M. Oropello, S. M. Pastores, & V. Kvetan (Eds.), *Critical care.* Retrieved December 5, 2016, from http://accessmedicine.mhmedical.com.ezproxy.uky .edu/content.aspx?bookid=1944&Sectionid=143521451

Cummings, J., Soomans, D., O'Laughlin, J., Snapp, J., Jodoin, A., Proco, H., . . . Rood, D. (2015). Sensitivity and specificity of a Nurse Dysphagia Screen in stroke patients. *MEDSURG Nursing, 24*(4), 219–222.

Elder, K. G., Lemon, S. K., & Costello, T. J. (2015). Increasing compliance with national quality measures for stroke through use of standard order set. *American Society of Health-System Pharmacists, 72*, 56–60.

Evans, M. M., Miner, M. B., Harrison, G., Ferguson, J. M., Miller, A., & Favuzza, A. (2016). Ischemic stroke: A case study describing standards of care. *MedSurg Matters! 25*(5), 13–16.

Go, S., & Worman, D. J. (2016). Chapter 167: Stroke syndromes. In J. E. Tintinalli, J. Stapczynski, O. Ma, D. M. Yealy, G. D. Meckler, & D. M. Cline (Eds.), *Tintinalli's emergency medicine: A comprehensive study guide* (8th ed.). Retrieved December 5, 2016, from http://accessmedicine.mhmedical.com.ezproxy.uky .edu/content.aspx?bookid=1658&Sectio nid=109436585

Jauch, E. C., Saver, J. L., Adams, H. P., Bruno, A., Conners, J. J., Demaerschalk, B. M., . . . Yonas, H. (2013). Guidelines for the early management of patients with acute ischemic stroke: A guideline for healthcare professionals from the American Heart Association/ American Stroke Association, *Stroke, 44*, 870–947. doi:http://dx.doi.org/10.1161/STR.0b013e318284056a

Kernan, W. N., Ovbiagele, B., Black, H. R., Bravata, D. M., Chimowitz, M. I., Ezekowitz, M. D., . . . Wilson, J. A. (2014). Guidelines for the prevention of stroke in patients with stroke and transient ischemic attack: A guideline for healthcare professionals from the American Heart Association/American Stroke Association. *Stroke, 45*, 2160–2236, doi:10.1161/ STR.0000000000000024

LeMone, P., Burke, K., Bauldoff, G., & Gubrud, P. (2015). Chapter 42: Nursing care of patients with intracranial disorders. In P. LeMone, K. Burke, G. Bauldoff, & P. Gubrud (Eds.), *Medical-surgical nursing: Clinical reasoning in patient care* (6th ed., pp. 1352–1398). Hoboken, NJ: Pearson.

Libby, P. (2015). Chapter 291: The pathogenesis, prevention, and treatment of atherosclerosis. In D. Kasper, A. Fauci, S. Hauser, D. Longo, J. Jameson, & J. Loscalzo (Eds.), *Harrison's principles of internal medicine* (19th ed.). Retrieved December 4, 2016, from http://accessmedicine.mhmedical.com.ezproxy.uky .edu/content.aspx?bookid=1130&Sectionid=79743366

Madsen, T. E., Khoury, J., Cadena, R., Adeoye, O., Alwell, K. A., Moomaw, C. J., . . . Kleindorfer, D. (2016). Potentially missed diagnosis of ischemic stroke in the Emergency Department in the Greater Cincinnati/ Northern Kentucky Stroke Study. *Academic Emergency Medicine, 23*, 1128–1135. doi:10.1111/acem.13029

Mahanes, D. (2015). Neurologic system. In S. M. Burns (Ed.), *AACN essentials of critical care nursing* (3rd ed., pp. 311–336). New York, NY: McGraw-Hill Education.

Meschia, J. F., Bushnell, C., Boden-Albala, B., Braun, L. T., Bravata, D. M., Chaturvedi, S., . . . Wilson, J. A. (2014). Guidelines for the primary prevention of stroke: A statement for healthcare professionals from the American Heart Association/American Stroke Association. *Stroke, 45*, 3754–3832.

Mons, U., Muezzinler, A., Gellert, C., Schottker, B., Abnet, C. C., Bobak, M., . . . & Brenner, H. (2015). Impact of smoking and smoking cessation on cardiovascular events and mortality among older adults: Meta-analysis of individual participant data from prospective cohort studies of the CHANCES consortium. *British Medical Journal, 50*, h1551. doi:10.1136/bmj.h1551.

Mozaffarian, D., Benjamin, E. J., Go, A. S., Arnett, D. K., Blaha, M.J., Cushman, M., . . . Turner, M. B. (2015). Heart disease and stroke statistics—2016 update: A report from the American Heart Association. *Circulation, 132*, e1–323. doi:10.1161/ CIR.0000000000000350

National Institutes of Health/National Institute of Neurological Disorders and Stroke. (2017). NIH Stroke Scale. Retrieved March 28, 2017, from https://stroke .nih.gov/resources/scale.htm

Niewada, M., & Michel, P. (2016). Lifestyle modification for stroke prevention: Facts and fiction. *Current Opinion in Neurology, 29*, 9–13. doi:10.1097/ WCO.0000000000000285

Powers, A. C. (2015). Chapter 419: Diabetes mellitus: Complications. In D. Kasper, A. Fauci, S. Hauser, D. Longo, J. Jameson, & J. Loscalzo (Eds.), *Harrison's principles of internal medicine* (19th ed.). Retrieved December 1, 2016, from http://accessmedicine. mhmedical.com.ezproxy.uky.edu/content.aspx?bookid =1130&Sectionid=79753119

Powers, W. J., & Jordan, D. (2015). Chapter 84: Cerebrovascular disease. In J. B. Hall, G. A. Schmidt, & J. P. Kress (Eds.), *Principles of critical care* (4th ed.). Retrieved November 29, 2016, from http:// accessmedicine.mhmedical.com.ezproxy.uky.edu /content.aspx?bookid=1340&Sectionid=80036033

Rincon, F., Kang, J., Matlenfort, M., Vibbert, M., Urtecho, J., Athan, M.K., . . . Bell, R. (2014). Association between hyperoxia and mortality after stroke: A multicenter cohort study. *Critical Care Medicine, 42*(2), 387–396.

Ropper, A. H., Samuels, M. A., & Klein, J. P. (2014a). Chapter 34: Cerebrovascular diseases. In A. H. Ropper, M. A. Samuels, & J. P. Klein (Eds.), *Adams & Victor's principles of neurology* (10th ed.). Retrieved November 29, 2016, from http://accessmedicine.mhmedical.com.ezproxy.uky.edu/content.aspx?bookid=690&Sectionid=50910885

Ropper, A. H., Samuels, M. A., & Klein, J. P. (2014b). Chapter 37: Inherited metabolic diseases of the nervous system. In A. H. Ropper, M. A. Samuels, & J. P. Klein (Eds.), *Adams & Victor's principles of neurology* (10th ed.). Retrieved December 7, 2016, from http://accessmedicine.mhmedical.com.ezproxy.uky.edu/content.aspx?bookid=690&Sectionid=50910888

Smith, W. S., Johnston, S., & Hemphill, J., III. (2015). Chapter 446: Cerebrovascular diseases. In D. Kasper, A. Fauci, S. Hauser, D. Longo, J. Jameson, & J. Loscalzo (Eds.), *Harrison's principles of internal medicine* (19th ed.). Retrieved November 29, 2016, from http://accessmedicine.mhmedical.com.ezproxy.uky.edu/content.aspx?bookid=1130&Sectionid=79755261

Wilson, B. A., Shannon, M., & Shields, K. (2016). *Pearson nurse's drug guide* (3rd ed.). Retrieved December 7, 2016, from https://bookshelf.vitalsource.com/#/books/9780134070728

Winstein, C. J., Stein, J., Arena, R., Bates, B., Cherney, L. R., Cramer, S. C., . . . Zorowitz, R. D. (2016). Guidelines for adult stroke rehabilitation and recovery: A guideline for healthcare professionals from the American Heart Association/American Stroke Association, *Stroke, 47*, e98–e169. doi:10.1161/STR.0000000000000098

Chapter 19
Traumatic Brain Injury

 Learning Outcomes

19.1 Describe mechanisms of injury associated with brain and skull trauma.

19.2 Describe implications of decreased intracranial adaptive capacity.

19.3 Compare and contrast focal and diffuse brain injuries.

19.4 Discuss the assessment and diagnosis of traumatic brain injury.

19.5 Apply evidence-based practice principles to the collaborative management of traumatic brain injury.

19.6 Apply evidence-based principles to the nursing management of the patient with traumatic brain injury.

19.7 Describe sequelae associated with increased intracranial pressure.

This chapter outlines the pathophysiologic processes associated with the acute phase of traumatic brain injury and a collaborative management approach for improved patient outcomes. A review of Chapter 16: Determinants and Assessment of Cerebral Function, is recommended prior to beginning this chapter as it contains vital components of a basic neurologic assessment, as well as assessment findings indicative of acute neurologic deterioration and dysfunction commonly observed in acute brain injury. Securing a strong understanding of this foundational knowledge will enhance understanding of the complex pathologic processes, diagnostic tests, and procedures discussed here.

Traumatic brain injury (TBI), occasionally referenced as closed-head injury (CHI), is a neurologic insult resulting from a mechanical disruption of brain tissue from an external impact or injury to the head. TBI is both a closed or penetrating injury. The term *closed-head injury* is no longer preferred, as it distracts from the focal point of injury: the brain. TBI is a serious public health problem in the United States, contributing to a substantial number of deaths and cases of permanent disability annually. Each year, 1.6 million people have a TBI, and 284,000 of them require hospitalization; of those who are hospitalized, only 230,000 survive (Brain Trauma Foundation [BTF], 2012). Mortality for TBI approaches 54,000 per year (BTF, 2012; Centers for Disease Control and Prevention [CDC], 2010) and accounts for

2.4 million emergency department visits annually (CDC, 2010). An estimated 5.3 million Americans are living with disabilities from TBI (BTF, 2012; National Institute of Neurological Disorders and Stroke [NINDS], 2012). Direct medical costs and indirect costs such as lost productivity associated with TBI ranged an estimated $63.4 to $79.1 billion in the United States in 2013 (Ma, Chan, & Carruthers, 2014). These figures do not incorporate TBI victims treated in primary care settings. An estimated 25% of patients with TBI do not receive medical attention (Corrigan, Selassie, & Orman, 2010; Faul, Xu, Wald, &, Coronado, 2010). Finally, blasts are the leading cause of TBI among military personnel in war zones; veterans' advocates believe 150,000 to 300,000 Iraq veterans have suffered TBI (Bagalman, 2013).

Section One: Mechanisms of Brain Injury and Skull Fractures

TBI is a diagnosis with varying degrees of severity, ranging from mild (concussion) to severe (epidural hematoma or diffuse axonal injury). Understanding the mechanism of injury associated with TBI is essential to assessing and managing patients with these injuries.

Mechanisms of Injury

Three primary mechanisms of injury are associated with TBI: acceleration and deceleration, rotational, and penetrating (Figure 19–1). Mechanisms of injury are further explained in terms of immediate (primary) injury and delayed (secondary) injury.

Acceleration and Deceleration Injury   The most common mechanism of TBI is the result of acceleration and deceleration forces (Figure 19–1A). *Acceleration injury* occurs when a moving blunt object strikes the head, involving transfer of energy along a linear path. This type of injury is seen in victims of assault who have been hit in the head with a bat, baseball, or other moving object. The sudden acceleration causes brain injury at the site of impact with the skull. *Deceleration injury* occurs when an individual's head strikes an immovable object, such as the dashboard of a car or the ground during a fall. As the skull ceases

Mechanisms of Brain Injury

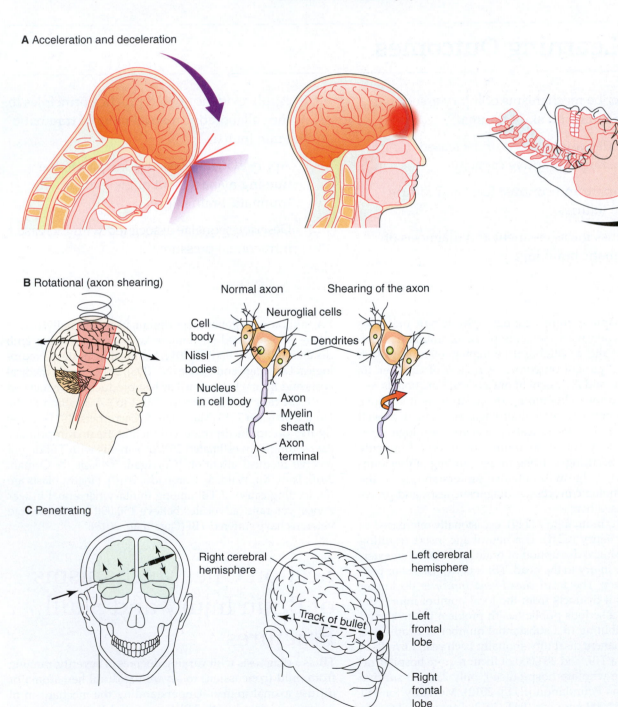

Figure 19–1   Mechanisms of brain injury. A, Acceleration and deceleration. B, Rotational (axon shearing). C, Penetrating.

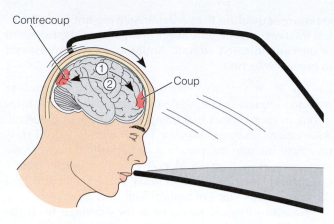

Figure 19–2 Coup–contrecoup brain injury.
(1) Following the initial (acceleration) injury (coup), (2) the brain rebounds within the skull and sustains additional (deceleration) injury (contrecoup) in the opposite part of the brain.

movement, the brain continues to move until it hits the skull. The force of rapid deceleration causes brain injury as it hits the bony wall of the cranium. Acceleration and deceleration injuries can occur together, as can be seen in a coup–contrecoup injury (Figure 19–2). Coup (acceleration) injury affects the cerebral tissue directly under the point of impact. Contrecoup (deceleration) injury occurs in a line directly opposite the point of impact. A coup–contrecoup injury results in more severe brain trauma.

Rotational Injury *Rotational injury* occurs when the force impacting the head transfers energy to the brain in a nonlinear fashion, whereby the head rotates on its axis (the neck), resulting in shearing forces being exerted throughout the brain and its axons (Figure 19–1B). An example of this type of mechanism occurs in boxing. When a boxer is punched in the side of the head, the force causes a rapid spinning (rotational) motion of the head and its contents, causing tearing of the axons in the brain. This type of injury is associated with diffuse axonal injury (DAI), discussed in Section Three.

Penetrating Injury Penetrating injury occurs when a foreign object invades the brain. The penetrating object may be a bullet, knife, or falling object (Figure 19–1C). The penetrating object may pass completely through the brain and exit on the opposite side, or it may bounce around the cranium causing multiple areas of injury. In addition to the obvious injury, some projectiles, such as bullets, may cause additional injury from shock waves transmitted throughout the brain.

Primary and Secondary Brain Injury **Primary injury** occurs from direct mechanical injury caused by the force of the impact from the traumatic event (e.g., a person's head striking the dashboard and injuring the brain during a motor vehicle crash) (Hickey, 2014; Osborn, Wraa, Watson & Holleran, 2014). The primary injury in this case is the immediate damage to neurons. Primary injury is immediate and often causes irreversible damage. **Secondary injury** occurs in response to the primary injury, arising from local tissue and systemic responses to the primary

injury. Secondary injury involves ischemia, neuronal death, inflammation, and cerebral swelling (Hickey, 2014; Osborn et al., 2014). Secondary injury increases the severity of primary injury, potentially extending the area of injury and worsening patient outcomes. Minimizing secondary injury is a major focus of TBI management.

Skull Fractures

Table 19–1 shows the four types of skull fractures that can occur with injury to the head: linear, depressed, open, and basilar skull fractures. All types indicate substantial force has been absorbed by the skull and underlying brain tissue injury may be present (see Figure 19–3).

Linear Skull Fracture Linear skull fractures are simple fissures in the skull with no bony fragmentation, and they are associated with minor traumatic injury. They are not typically obvious to the naked eye and are usually discovered during a computerized tomography (CT) scan of the head. Linear skull fractures are not life-threatening and are allowed to heal naturally without surgical intervention.

Depressed Skull Fracture In a depressed skull fracture, occurring with higher forces of impact, fragmentation of bone depresses into the cranial vault. Depressed skull fractures may be visible and palpable as an indentation of the skull, and they may be open or closed. The bony fragments may tear the underlying meninges of the brain and extend into brain tissue. Given the amount of force necessary to cause deformity of the skull, the probability of substantial brain injury in depressed skull fracture is high.

Medical interventions include surgical repair of the fracture and meninges, as well as the evacuation of any hematomas beneath the fracture.

Open Skull Fracture Open skull fractures are accompanied by a scalp laceration. These fractures are of particular concern because of the risk of infection associated with

Table 19–1 Types of Skull Fractures

Type	Description
Linear	A simple fracture involving the entire bony thickness without bone movement; considered the most benign type of skull fracture; associated with low-velocity blunt trauma; usually requires no interventions
Open	A fracture in which the scalp has been lacerated, creating a communication between the skull and the outside environment; in the presence of a depressed skull fracture the dura may be torn, exposing the brain to possible contamination
Depressed	A fracture in which a high-energy force depresses the skull inward; usually causes bone fragmentation (comminuted) with fragments potentially tearing through the dura and into brain tissue; an "open depressed fracture" if the scalp is lacerated to the bone, a "closed depressed fracture" if the scalp is intact
Basilar	A fracture that develops at the base of the skull; usually located in temporal or occipital regions; associated with a high-energy force; if dura is torn, can result in rhinorrhea (cerebrospinal fluid [CSF] draining from the nose) or otorrhea (CSF draining from the ear)

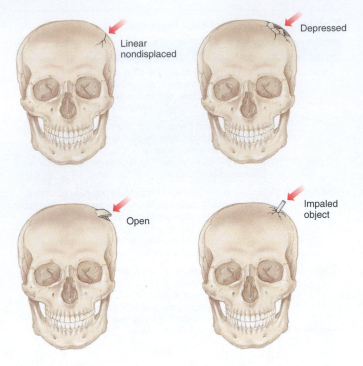

Figure 19–3 Types of skull fractures: linear, depressed (with bony fragmentation), open (with scalp laceration), and penetrating (impaled object).

exposure of the dura to a contaminated environment. Medical interventions include surgical repair and debridement of the contaminated wound. Antibiotics are administered to prevent infection.

Basilar Skull Fracture Basilar skull fractures, another common sequelae of high-impact brain injury, are fractures of one or more bones that compose the base of the skull. Assessment findings associated with a basilar skull fracture may include the presence of periorbital ecchymosis ("raccoon eyes"), mastoid ecchymosis ("Battle sign"), otorrhea, rhinorrhea, or facial nerve paralysis. Figure 19–4 illustrates major signs of basilar skull fracture.

Careful physical assessment for drainage from the nares and ear canals must be performed to detect the presence of cerebral spinal fluid (CSF) drainage. In the case of bloody drainage, one quick method to identify the presence of CSF is to look for the *halo sign*. Place a drop of the drainage onto a sterile 2 × 2 gauze. If the fluid contains CSF, a yellowish-colored ring will form around the drop of fluid, suggesting the drainage contains CSF. CSF drainage indicates a tear in the meninges. CSF may leak through the nose (**rhinorrhea**) or through the ear (**otorrhea**). Any drainage from the ear or nose should be tested with a glucose

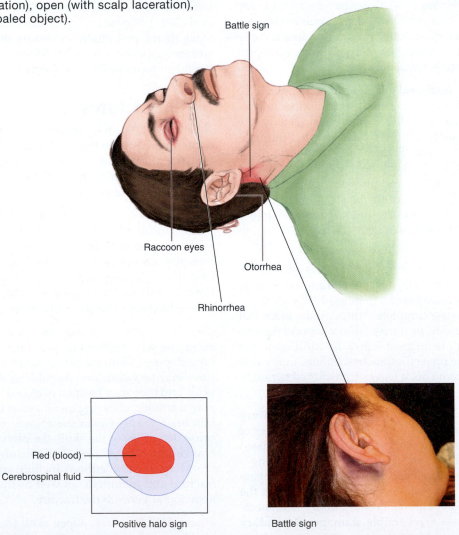

Figure 19–4 Signs of basilar skull fracture: Battle sign, raccoon eyes, otorrhea, rhinorrhea, positive halo sign.
SOURCE: Edward T. Dickinson, M.D.

reagent strip for the presence of glucose. Clear drainage that tests positive for glucose indicates the fluid is CSF. Medical management of basilar skull fracture includes allowing the CSF to drain and the dura to close on its own. If the injury does not heal within the first 1 to 2 weeks postinjury, surgical repair may be necessary. Sterile cotton gauze is placed in the ear or under the nose and requires changing when wet to prevent moisture stagnation and bacterial colonization, which would predispose the patient to infection (Hickey, 2014).

Nursing Considerations for Patients with Skull Fractures Nursing interventions when caring for patients who have sustained a skull fracture focus on routine neurologic assessments and pain management. The patient warrants close observation for patterns of neurologic deterioration, particularly during the initial 24 to 48 hours postinjury. Analgesia must be administered judiciously to patients with neurologic injury, as the administration of narcotics may obscure the neurologic exam and make it difficult to pinpoint the cause of mental status changes. Patients with an open skull fracture, particularly an open depressed fracture or basilar fracture should be monitored for signs and symptoms of infection associated with a disrupted meningeal layer. All dressings should be changed with aseptic technique in an effort to reduce the possibility of infection. Figure 19–5 illustrates trauma to the head and signs of a resulting injury to the brain.

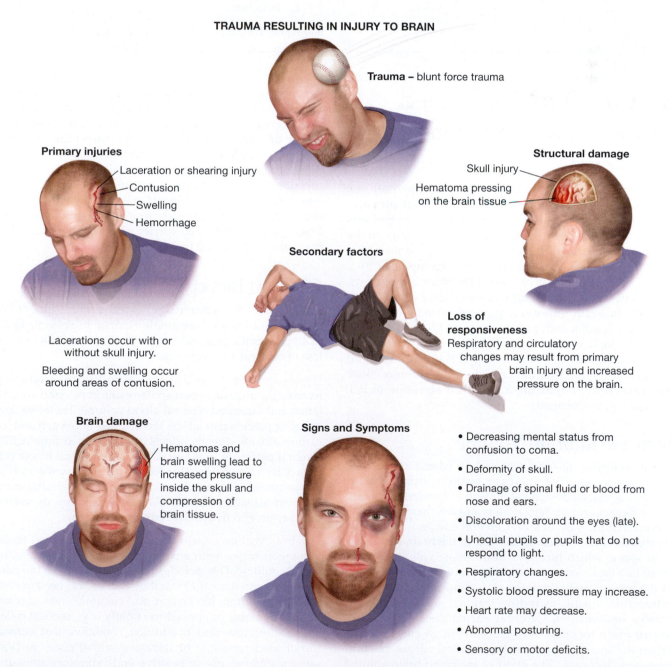

TRAUMA RESULTING IN INJURY TO BRAIN

Trauma – blunt force trauma

Primary injuries
Laceration or shearing injury
Contusion
Swelling
Hemorrhage

Lacerations occur with or without skull injury.

Bleeding and swelling occur around areas of contusion.

Structural damage
Skull injury
Hematoma pressing on the brain tissue

Secondary factors

Loss of responsiveness
Respiratory and circulatory changes may result from primary brain injury and increased pressure on the brain.

Brain damage
Hematomas and brain swelling lead to increased pressure inside the skull and compression of brain tissue.

Signs and Symptoms

- Decreasing mental status from confusion to coma.
- Deformity of skull.
- Drainage of spinal fluid or blood from nose and ears.
- Discoloration around the eyes (late).
- Unequal pupils or pupils that do not respond to light.
- Respiratory changes.
- Systolic blood pressure may increase.
- Heart rate may decrease.
- Abnormal posturing.
- Sensory or motor deficits.

Figure 19–5 Trauma to the head and resulting injury to the brain.

Section One Review

1. Acceleration and deceleration injuries are the result of what type of impact?
   - A. Cranial loading force
   - B. Penetrating trauma
   - C. Linear striking of head by a moving blunt object
   - D. Rotational movement of the brain in the skull

2. Which mechanism of injury commonly results in the tearing of axons in the brain?
   - A. Rotational
   - B. Acceleration
   - C. Deceleration
   - D. Penetrating

3. The administration of narcotics to a client with a traumatic brain injury may have which effect?
   - A. It will make the pain worse.
   - B. It may mask neurological changes in the client.
   - C. It allows the injury to heal quicker.
   - D. It may increase intracranial pressure.

4. Which problems can cause secondary injury? (Select all that apply.)
   - A. Hypoxia
   - B. Cerebral swelling
   - C. Inflammation of cerebral tissue
   - D. Skull fracture
   - E. Ischemia

Answers: 1. C, 2. A, 3. B, 4. (A, B, C, E)

Section Two: Decreased Intracranial Adaptive Capacity

When intracranial mechanisms fail to compensate for increases in intracranial volume, intracranial pressure (ICP) increases. According to the Monro-Kellie hypothesis (described in Chapter 16), ICP increases if a change in the volume of any one of the intracranial components (brain, blood, or cerebral spinal fluid) is not accompanied by a reciprocal change in one or both of the other components. Several conditions can cause an elevation in ICP: (1) an increase in brain volume (e.g., cerebral edema, space-occupying lesions such as a hematoma), (2) an increase in cerebral blood volume (e.g., hypercapnia, hypoxia), or (3) an increase in CSF. Increasing ICP impairs cerebral perfusion and oxygenation of brain cells and may cause **intracranial hypertension**, a sustained elevation in ICP that can be life-threatening.

Increase in Brain Volume

Space-occupying lesions and cerebral edema are the primary processes that increase brain volume. Space-occupying lesions develop as a result of tumors, abscesses, hemorrhages, and/or hematomas and are characterized as lesions that increase in size. Cerebral edema is caused by an abnormal accumulation of fluid in the brain's extracellular space, which increases brain tissue volume. It may occur in a localized or throughout a more generalized area of the brain. Cerebral edema may occur after any type of intracranial insult, including trauma, surgery, cerebral anoxia, or ischemia. Cerebral edema does not directly impair brain function until it results in an elevated ICP. When ICP increases as a result of cerebral edema, cerebral perfusion decreases. The effect of increased brain volume

depends on the rate of development. Slower growing lesions, such as chronic subdural hematomas (venous bleeding) or slow-growing tumors, may be tolerated for a longer time than, for example, an acute epidural hematoma (arterial bleeding), which develops quickly.

An intracranial tumor or cerebral edema that is compressing the surrounding areas of brain tissue causing (mass effect) a continued increase in volume without cerebral compensation eventually results in a shifting of brain tissue, or **herniation**, and carries a grave prognosis. Brain herniation is discussed in Section Seven.

Cerebral Blood Volume

Cerebral blood volume (CBV) is a dynamic value. CBV may increase under three circumstances: hypoxemia and/or hypercapnia, cerebral venous outflow obstruction, or loss of cerebral autoregulation.

Hypoxemia or Hypercapnia   Conditions producing hypoxemia and/or hypercapnia result in cerebral vasodilation and increased cerebral blood volume. Therefore, any systemic process that affects blood levels of oxygen and/or carbon dioxide directly affects cerebral blood flow (CBF), cerebral perfusion pressure (CPP), and cerebral blood volume (CBV). Conditions that may cause hypoxemia and/or hypercapnia include chronic respiratory insufficiency, hypoventilation, respiratory depression from oversedation, sepsis, and insufficient oxygen delivery.

Cerebral Venous Outflow Obstruction   Cerebral blood volume increases with any process that impedes cerebral venous outflow. This includes any mechanism that impedes jugular venous drainage from the head, such as head or neck rotation or flexion, hip flexion, and circumferential medical devices that may be applied too tightly (e.g., cervical collar, endotracheal tube ties). In addition, conditions that increase intrathoracic pressure or intra-abdominal pressure (Valsalva maneuver, use of positive end-expiratory pressure) also hinder jugular venous outflow and decrease venous return to the heart.

Loss of Cerebral Autoregulation   Autoregulation is a process whereby cerebral vessels have the capacity to dilate or constrict in response to changes in perfusion pressures. This process allows CBF to remain relatively constant despite changes in CPP. Autoregulation maintains adequate cerebral blood flow regardless of fluctuations in systemic blood pressure by altering cerebral vascular tone—as CPP increases, compensatory cerebral vasoconstriction occurs, and as it decreases, cerebral vasodilation occurs. However, autoregulation has its limits and only functions within certain hemodynamic parameters. Autoregulation requires a CPP within a range of 50 to 150 mmHg (Navi, Yap, Ahmad, & Gsosh, 2013) and a mean arterial pressure (MAP) range between 60 and 130 mmHg in adults. If the CPP or MAP values migrate outside of these homeostatic parameters, autoregulation is lost. Autoregulation becomes ineffective in prolonged ischemic conditions, sustained elevations in ICP, and sustained states of **hyperemia** (excessive cerebral blood flow). When autoregulation is lost, the cerebral blood vessels passively dilate, further insulting cerebral homeostasis by increasing CBV and ICP.

Cerebrospinal Fluid

When production of cerebrospinal fluid (CSF) increases, its circulation or flow is blocked, or its absorption decreases, then there is a net increase in the amount of CSF within the cranial vault. This net increase can increase the ICP. **Hydrocephalus** is a condition involving increased volume of CSF particularly within the ventricles of the brain. Hydrocephalus can increase the ICP. Normally, temporary increases in CSF volume can be compensated for through normal autoregulatory mechanisms that prevent sudden increases or decreases in ICP. Early or initial mechanisms include increasing CSF absorption, shunting CSF from the cerebral to the spinal subarachnoid space, or collapse of the cerebral

Table 19–2   Causes and Effects of Increases in Intracranial Volume, Cerebral Blood Volume, and CSF

Component	Causes	Predicted Effect on ICP
Intracranial volume	Space-occupying lesions Cerebral edema	Increased ICP Herniation is a late sign when autoregulation fails and increased ICP displaces structures within the cranial vault
Cerebral blood volume	Hypercapnia Hypoxemia Loss of autoregulation Venous outflow obstruction	Increased ICP Cerebral vasodilation Passive cerebral vessels Increased cerebral blood volume Herniation once autoregulation fails
CSF	Obstruction Decreased absorption Increased production	Increased ICP Hydrocephalus Herniation once autoregulation fails

veins and dural sinuses. Later compensatory mechanisms include decreasing CSF production, changes in cerebral blood volume through vasoconstriction or vasodilation, compression of the brain tissue, dispensability of the dura, and increasing venous outflow with shunting of venous blood out of the skull. Obstruction to CSF outflow can be caused by mass lesions or infection. Decreased CSF absorption can result from a subarachnoid hemorrhage or meningitis. If the cause of hydrocephalus is believed to be permanent, a surgical shunt is placed to improve CSF outflow. If the cause of hydrocephalus is considered to be a temporary condition, a ventricular drain may be inserted for intermittent or continuous drainage of CSF.

Table 19–2 summarizes the causes and effects of increased intracranial volume, cerebral blood volume, and CSF. Bear in mind that uncompensated increases in intracranial volume, cerebral blood volume, or CSF, if not treated, may result in increased ICP and subsequent brain herniation.

Section Two Review

1. Which condition is a common cause of increased cerebral blood volume?
   A. Subdural hematoma
   B. Hypotension
   C. Hypercapnia
   D. Meningioma

2. ICP can be increased by anything that does what?
   A. Increases intracranial volume
   B. Results in high compliance
   C. Results in low elastance
   D. Decreases carbon dioxide levels

3. Accumulation of CSF results in what condition?
   A. Herniation
   B. Cerebral dilation
   C. Hydrocephalus
   D. Seizures

4. What term describes the process whereby cerebral vessels have the capacity to dilate or constrict in response to changes in perfusion pressures?
   A. Autoregulation
   B. Shunting
   C. Herniation
   D. Dispensability

Answers: 1. C, 2. A, 3. C, 4. A

Section Three: Focal and Diffuse Brain Injuries

Traumatic brain injury comprises two distinct classifications: focal or diffuse. **Focal injuries** occur in a well-defined area of the brain. **Diffuse injuries** occur in several areas of the brain and may occur with concussion and diffuse axonal injury.

Focal Brain Injuries

Focal brain injuries are localized to the area of direct injury, which can range from a small contusion or bruise to a severe hematoma resulting from an intracranial hemorrhage. Focal brain injuries include cerebral hematomas and contusions. Focal brain injuries may be the result of a concentrated collection of blood from a blunt trauma or intracerebral bleed, a space-occupying brain lesion (e.g., tumor or abscess), or an object (e.g., projectile, missile such as a bullet).

Cerebral Hematomas   **Cerebral hematomas** represent a group of injuries associated with the accumulation of blood in the cranial vault. Hematomas occur as the result of injury to a cerebral vein or artery. There are several types of cerebral hematomas, and each is named according to its location in the cranium: subdural hematoma, epidural hematoma, subarachnoid hemorrhage, and intraparenchymal hematoma (Figure 19–6 shows three of these types). With high-impact injury, two or more types of cerebral hematomas may occur.

Subdural Hematoma.   **Subdural hematoma (SDH)** is the accumulation of blood between the dura and the arachnoid layers of the meninges (covering layers of the brain) (see Figure 19–7). SDH usually develops secondary to venous injury in the subdural space from tears in the bridging veins. The onset of symptoms in SDH is slower than if the bleeding were from an arterial source. SDH may occur as a result of mild brain trauma, particularly in the elderly

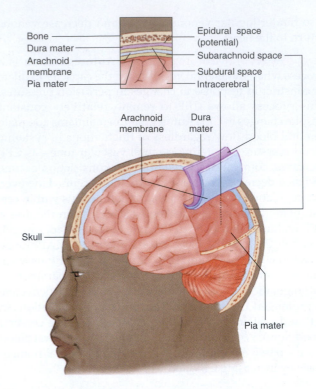

Figure 19–7 Meninges (covering layers) of the brain and the spaces within the intracranial vault.

and/or alcoholics who fall, or it can occur spontaneously (Wang, Kim, & Kim, 2013), which is more commonly associated with anticoagulant therapy (Gaist et al., 2017). The three categories of SDH are based on time of onset of manifestations: acute, subacute, and chronic. Assessment findings are determined by the rate and volume of blood accumulation in the subdural space, and a small SDH may remain asymptomatic.

Acute SDH.   With an acute SDH, manifestations develop less than 48 hours after the injury (Hickey, 2014). The manifestations of SDH vary widely from drowsiness to comatose, and symptoms typically progress rapidly (though not always), with most patients becoming drowsy or comatose immediately following the injury (Hickey, 2014). Other manifestations include unilateral headache, confusion, slowed thinking, or agitation.

Subacute SDH.   With a subacute SDH, manifestations develop 48 hours to 2 weeks after the injury because the expansion of the hematoma is over a longer time. Onset of neurologic deterioration may not occur for days or weeks. Typical manifestations include headache, mild contralateral hemiparesis, drowsiness, and confusion (Hickey, 2014; LeMone, Burke, Bauldoff, & Gubrud, 2015).

Chronic SDH.   With a chronic SDH, manifestations develop over the course of weeks after the injury (Hickey, 2014). Clinical manifestations are vague and are often attributed to other conditions, such as increasing dementia. The patient may complain of headache, lethargy, absentmindedness, and vomiting. Other serious manifestations that may be present with any type of SDH, given a sufficiently

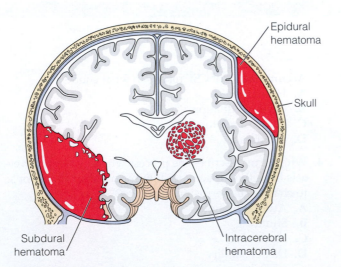

Figure 19–6 Three types of hematomas: epidural, subdural, and intraparenchymal.

large hematoma, include ipsilateral pupillary dilation, altered level of consciousness (LOC), seizures, visual field alterations (e.g., homonymous hemianopsia), or contralateral hemiparesis.

Surgical management of SDH involves surgical evacuation of the hematoma if there is radiological evidence of a midline shift of brain structures on CT or for symptomatic hematomas 1 cm in size in adults or greater than 5 mm in children (Halpern & Grady, 2015). Surgical evacuation techniques involve using burr holes or craniectomy, as well as possible placement of a subdural drain, which may remain in place for a few days postoperatively to ensure removal of all blood and to monitor for recurrence of the hematoma (Wright & Merck, 2016). Nursing priorities for SDH include monitoring LOC and performing regular and frequent focused neurologic assessments (Hickey, 2014; LeMone et al., 2015).

Epidural Hematoma. An **epidural hematoma (EDH)** occurs in the space between the dura mater and the skull. High impact to the temporal areas of the brain can induce an epidural hematoma. When the force of the impact is transferred to the brain, it shears local vessels, usually the middle meningeal artery. This results in a rapid accumulation of arterial blood between the skull and the dura mater. Patients with EDH may have a brief loss of consciousness immediately following the injury from the initial traumatic impact, followed by an episode of lucidity, and then a recurrent loss of consciousness as the growing hematoma exerts excessive pressure on the brain. This scenario is the classic presentation of EDH, but it is important to remember that not all patients with EDH will present with these symptoms. A fixed and dilated pupil on the same side (ipsilateral) as the impact may be present. An ipsilateral fixed and dilated pupil occurs because of compression of the parasympathetic fibers, which lie outside of CN III and are inactivated. Because an injured artery is most often the source of the hematoma, the rapid accumulation of blood makes it critical to identify and treat these injuries rapidly before intracranial pressure reaches a critical point and causes brain herniation.

Depending on the size of the hematoma and the clinical symptoms and manifestations, surgical management of the EDH involves surgical evacuation of the hematoma with possible cauterization of the vessel and potential placement of an intracranial pressure (ICP) monitor. Medical management might include osmotic diuretics to reduce ICP and airway protection or mechanical ventilation. These patients are typically admitted to the ICU for frequent neurologic checks and ICP monitoring (Wright & Merck, 2016). Nursing care of the patient with EDH focuses on frequent, detailed neurologic assessments. The nurse must observe for sudden changes in level of consciousness, which may be subtle initially if a complication has occurred. Presence of an ipsilateral (on the side of the injury) fixed and dilated pupil is an emergent and late finding, suggestive of rebleeding (Hickey, 2014).

Intraparenchymal Hematoma. Intraparenchymal hematoma **(IPH)** is the accumulation of blood in the parenchyma or tissue of the brain rather than between the meningeal layers. IPH most commonly results from uncontrolled hypertension, ruptured aneurysms, or trauma with a high-impact blow to the head. Manifestations vary according to the location of the hematoma and may include headache, decreasing LOC, ipsilateral pupil dilation, and contralateral hemiplegia. Surgical evacuation of an IPH is usually not possible, as the hematoma is deep within brain parenchyma. Medical management includes treatment of elevated intracranial pressure and optimization of cerebral perfusion pressure (CPP) (American College of Surgeons, 2015).

Contusion A **contusion** refers to the bruising of cerebral soft tissue and is considered a moderate-to-severe injury. It is commonly seen in traumatic brain injury and may begin locally but become more diffuse over time. Contusions cause macroscopic tissue and vessel damage that is detectable through CT or MRI scanning, though MRI is more sensitive. Contusions are associated with longer periods of unconsciousness and a more guarded prognosis, depending on the severity of injury (Wright & Merck, 2016).

Diffuse Brain Injuries

Diffuse brain injuries are those with more widespread involvement of the brain, including concussion, diffuse axonal injury, and subarachnoid hemorrhage.

Concussion Concussion, classified as a mild traumatic brain injury (mTBI), is caused by blunt trauma to the head. Cerebral damage occurs at the microscopic level and is not detectable through radiographic or other testing. The clinical presentation depends on the severity of the injury but includes an immediate transient period of unconsciousness (lasting up to 20 minutes) and short-term amnesia. However, if the concussion is particularly mild, the patient may not lose consciousness but may appear confused, dazed, or stunned. On presentation to the emergency department (ED), if the patient reports a loss of consciousness, posttraumatic amnesia, altered mental status, focal neurologic deficits, or exhibits clinical deterioration or evidence of skull fracture, further evaluation is warranted and a CT scan of the head should be ordered (American College of Radiology, 2013; Wright & Merck, 2016).

Although the term *mTBI* implies a relatively benign injury, concussion can have devastating effects, including the inability to function at preinjury levels. Post concussion syndrome (PCS) is a condition where concussion symptoms similar to those experienced on presentation to the ED persist for 3 months or more after the initial injury. PCS has been found to affect between 15% and 25% of patients with concussion 1 year after the initial injury (Eliyahu, Kirkland, Campbell, & Rowe, 2016).

Diffuse Axonal Injury **Diffuse axonal injury (DAI)** occurs when shearing forces disrupt the structure of neurons and their nearby blood vessels; however, DAI may be present without bleeding, making it difficult to visualize on CT or MRI. DAI typically results from high-speed acceleration, deceleration, or rotational injury that occurs with motor vehicle crashes. The mechanism of injury involves shearing off of the axons at the gray matter–white matter boundary or a rotational (twisting motion) movement of the brain within the skull that causes widespread axon shearing (Perez et al., 2014). The severity of injury can range from mild to severe. Although DAI is difficult to assess on a CT scan, the presence of multiple small, diffuse hemorrhages located at the boundary of white and gray matter is strongly suggestive (Wright & Merck, 2016). An MRI may provide a more conclusive diagnosis.

The outcome of the patient with DAI is unpredictable. Mild DAI can result in a comatose state lasting hours to days, followed by recovery with minimal residual neurologic damage. Mild DAI may contribute to postconcussive syndrome, which is experienced by many patients following a brain concussion. In more severe DAI, the prognosis is poor and is associated with high morbidity and mortality (Zheng, Chen, Li, & Cao, 2013).

Subarachnoid Hemorrhage **Subarachnoid hemorrhage (SAH)** is the accumulation of blood between the meningeal arachnoid layer and the pia mater surrounding the brain. It most commonly results from a ruptured cerebral aneurysm, with a major risk factor being uncontrolled hypertension. SAH can also occur as a result of TBI. Excess accumulation of blood within the subarachnoid space results in blood leaking into the cerebrospinal fluid. The bleeding associated with SAH can be focal with little consequence, or it can be massive and diffuse with subsequent intracranial hypertension (Wright & Merck, 2016).

Patients typically present with acute onset of a severe headache that may be described as being different from any previously experienced, as the worst headache the person has ever experienced, or as a "thunderclap" headache. The headache may be accompanied by altered LOC (possibly unconsciousness), diplopia, meningeal signs (e.g., nuchal rigidity, photophobia), or seizures. SAH is presented in more detail in Chapter 18.

Management of Diffuse Brain Injuries Diffuse brain injuries are not limited to a localized area, which can make them more difficult to detect and treat. Depending on the severity of the injury, the patient's recovery can be unpredictable. Management in the acute care phase includes diligent and frequent neurologic assessments and pain management. When moderate-to-severe injury is present (e.g., DAI) management may include interventions to prevent secondary injury, decrease ICP, increase CPP, stabilize vital signs, and prevent complications (American College of Surgeons, 2015). Discharge planning should be initiated in the early phase of recovery, as many patients require rehabilitation services. Management of traumatic brain injury is presented in more detail in the next section.

Section Three Review

1. A brief loss of consciousness followed by a period of being alert and oriented and then a loss of consciousness again is a typical presentation for which condition?
   A. Subdural hematoma
   B. Epidural hematoma
   C. Intracranial hematoma
   D. Subarachnoid hemorrhage

2. What is the term used to describe an accumulation of blood between the dura and the arachnoid layers of the meninges?
   A. Intracerebral hematoma
   B. Subarachnoid hemorrhage
   C. Epidural hematoma
   D. Subdural hematoma

3. Management of intraparenchymal hematoma may include which intervention?
   A. Anticoagulation
   B. Maintaining mean arterial pressure of 70 mmHg or less
   C. Emergent surgical evacuation
   D. Maximizing cerebral perfusion pressure (CPP)

4. Presence of dizziness, headache, and confusion for long periods of time after concussion is _____.
   A. always expected
   B. known as postconcussive syndrome
   C. caused by taking too much pain medication
   D. the result of something other than the concussion

Answers: 1. B, 2. D, 3. B, 4. B

Section Four: Assessment and Diagnosis

Systematic neurologic assessments can help to diagnose and identify the severity of injury, provide prognostic information to aid in predicting the likely outcome, and guide development of a plan for further evaluation and treatment. A variety of diagnostic tests are performed to determine the type, location, and severity of the injury.

Assessment

Information such as the mechanism of injury, the emergency care provided, and the patient's condition during transport (particularly regarding any episodes of hypoxemia or hypotension) should be obtained from the prehospital care providers upon arrival to the emergency department (ED).

Initial Assessments The initial neurologic assessment that occurs in the ED becomes the baseline against which subsequent serial neurologic examinations are compared in order to detect changes in the patient's condition. It is imperative for the initial neurologic exam to be performed by the care team to ensure both medical and nursing staff observe the same baseline neurologic exam. Any unfavorable change in the patient's neurologic condition, even the most subtle, may indicate neurologic decline and should be reported to the medical team immediately. In the ED, the primary assessment begins with the patient's airway, breathing, circulation, and vital signs, followed by the initial neurologic assessment, noting any deficits in function. In addition, the entire body is assessed for outward signs of injury.

The secondary assessment includes gathering a detailed history of the mechanism of injury, the prehospital care, and the patient's past medical history, including medications, allergies, surgeries, and comorbid conditions that may impact management of the patient's condition. A more extensive neurologic examination and a general systems assessment will be completed as interventions are carried out to ensure adequate ventilation, oxygenation, and perfusion.

Priorities for care in the initial stages of TBI include evaluation of the airway, breathing, and circulation, along with ongoing neurologic assessments to detect subtle deterioration. The severity of injury will also be determined to aid in the development of the treatment plan.

Determining Severity of Injury

The **Glasgow Coma Scale (GCS)** is an objective neurologic assessment tool that was originally developed to standardize measurement of the ability of the patient with a TBI to interact with the environment. It is also a major tool used for grading severity of TBI and is useful for trending changes in mental status over time (Munakomi & Kumar, 2015). The GCS includes three categories: eye opening, verbal response, and motor response to stimuli. The highest (best) total score is 15 and the lowest (worst) is 3, with a higher total score being an indication of less severe injury. Stimuli used to elicit GCS responses begin with the least noxious (e.g., voice commands, light shaking) and increase to more noxious (e.g., sternal rub, nail bed compression, trapezius muscle compression), stopping when a measurable response occurs. The GCS should be scored when initial resuscitation is finished and before any sedation is administered (Hickey, 2014). The GCS is described in more detail in Chapter 16.

Traumatic brain injuries range from mild to severe, with severity being determined by the patient's initial GCS score.

Mild Traumatic Brain Injury.

A mild TBI involves a GCS score of 13–15, with or without a loss of consciousness lasting up to 15 minutes. These patients may be seen in an ED and be discharged home with a caregiver to be monitored within the home for at least 24 hours. The recommendation for routine frequent awakening and pupillary assessments in the patient with a negative head CT and no loss of consciousness has become outdated (West et al., 2011). However, caregivers should be alerted for signs to observe that could indicate neurologic decline and would warrant immediate medical attention (Hickey, 2014).

Moderate Traumatic Brain Injury.

A moderate injury involves a GCS score of 9 to 12, accompanied by a loss of consciousness for up to 6 hours. These patients will require admission into the hospital because of their high risk for developing cerebral edema and increased intracranial pressure (ICP). Serial assessments to monitor neurologic and hemodynamic status and a CT scan will be performed to identify any acute intracerebral bleeding.

Severe Traumatic Brain Injury.

A patient has a severe traumatic brain injury if the GCS score is 8 or less on initial assessment, or if the patient's GCS deteriorates to that level within 48 hours of admission. These patients are critically ill and may need ventilator support and ICP monitoring, as well as measures to treat increased intracranial pressure (American College of Surgeons, 2015). In a retrospective review of 189 patients with severe TBI due to blunt head trauma and a GCS of 3, the mortality rate was 49.2%. Bilateral, fixed, and dilated pupils were associated with a 79.7% mortality rate (Chamoun, Robertson, & Gopinath, 2009).

Bedside Neurologic Assessment

Level of consciousness, motor function, pupillary response, respiratory function, and vital signs are all elements of the bedside serial neurologic assessments. The GCS is an important part of the bedside neurologic assessment because it evaluates several of these neurologic parameters, as previously discussed. In addition, pupils are assessed for size, shape, equality, reactivity, and symmetry. Pupil constriction to a light source assesses parasympathetic function, while pupillary dilation when the light source is removed assesses sympathetic response. If one or both of the pupils are slow to react to the light, a brainstem injury is suspected. If one or both pupils are blown (dilated and nonreactive to light), this is due to compression of CV III, the ocular nerve, from cerebral edema or herniation. The patient's vital signs and respiratory patterns are also closely monitored. Abnormal respiratory patterns must be reported and documented because pattern changes can indicate deterioration in neurologic status. Refer to Chapter 16 for a more thorough discussion of neurologic assessment.

A summary of nursing surveillance priorities during the acute phase of TBI is provided in Table 19–3.

Advanced Assessment Modalities

Direct assessment of cerebral tissue oxygenation has gained significant importance in the management of the patient with TBI. Brain tissue oxygenation monitoring is used to assist in determining an optimal CPP in the patient whose cerebral autoregulation is compromised (American College of Surgeons, 2015). Brain tissue oxygenation monitoring is discussed in further detail in Chapter 16. Current recommendations support maintaining $PbtO_2$ levels greater than 15 mmHg in the patient with TBI (American College of Surgeons, 2015).

Jugular venous oximetry (SjO_2) is a measure of cerebral oxygen saturation to assess the relationship between oxygen supply and demand, and it assists in determining if a given CPP is sufficient to satisfy cerebral metabolic demand. SjO_2 is discussed in further detail in Chapter 16. When utilized as an adjunct therapy in TBI, an SjO_2 decrease to less than 55% is associated with worsening outcomes (Prabhakar, Sandhu, Bhagat, Durga, & Chawla,

Table 19–3 Nursing Surveillance Priorities and Assessments

Priority	Assessments

Identify intracranial hypertension	Manifestations of increased ICP:
	    Decreasing GCS
	    Changes in vital signs occur with intracranial hypertension (bradycardia or tachycardia, irregular breathing patterns, hypertension, widening pulse pressure)
	    Cushing's triad (bradycardia, severe systolic hypertension with a widened pulse pressure, and irregular breathing) indicates brainstem ischemia and can signal impending herniation.
	Signs of increasing ICP or decreased CPP: vomiting, headache, lethargy, restlessness, changes in mentation
	Temperature. Fever may increase ICP.
	Fluid status, intake and output hourly, serum osmolality. Osmotic agents may precipitate heart failure and pulmonary edema.

Identify ineffective breathing patterns	Respiratory pattern for rate, depth, and rhythm Oxygenation: breath sounds, presence of cyanosis, hypoxia, restlessness, and use of accessory respiratory muscles, pulse oximetry and arterial blood gas levels Monitor for increased respiratory effort and distress Administer oxygen to keep SaO_2 greater than 92%

SOURCE: Hickey (2014); LeMone et al. (2015); Osborn et al. (2014).

2014). Advances in cerebral oxygen monitoring and aggressive treatment of cerebral hypoxia have reduced mortality and improved long-term outcomes after traumatic brain injury (Prabhakar et al., 2014).

Initial Diagnostic Tests and Procedures

Decreasing the time from onset of injury to initial treatment is a crucial factor in minimizing the extent of brain injury. For this reason, a prescriptive approach to initial diagnostic testing is warranted. Standardizing the initial diagnostic approach, including laboratory testing, imaging studies, and other diagnostic procedures, saves time and aids in the understanding of the type and severity of injury while decreasing unnecessary variance in practice.

Laboratory Tests   To prevent secondary brain injury, laboratory values are monitored to ensure early detection of cerebral hypoxia and impending ischemia. Arterial blood gases are analyzed, with particular attention to oxygenation and carbon dioxide levels. Laboratory monitoring includes a complete blood count with emphasis on hemoglobin, hematocrit, and platelets; a coagulation profile (prothrombin time, international normalized ration, partial thromboplastin time); electrolytes, BUN and creatinine,

liver function, and serum osmolality; and urinalysis and urine osmolality. In addition, a panel of blood tests may be obtained to screen the patient for substance use, such as alcohol or illicit substances (e.g., cocaine, heroin, oxycodone, or methamphetamine).

Imaging Studies   Upon a patient's arrival to the ED, a CT scan of the brain is typically the first-line imaging study performed as it can visualize skull fractures, as well as many soft-tissue injuries (e.g., lacerations or contusions), hemorrhages, or masses. An MRI may be performed if the CT scan is unable to adequately visualize an area of concern in the brain. If DAI is suspected and requires immediate diagnosis, MRI is a more sensitive modality for detecting that type of injury (Hickey, 2014; Wright & Merck, 2016).

Other Diagnostic Testing   A variety of other diagnostic tests may be performed during the acute phase of TBI treatment to further evaluate some aspect of the patient's neurologic deficits. These may include tomography or transcranial Doppler, which can detect changes in CBF; evoked potentials, which can detect lesions in the CNS; and electroencephalography (EEG), which can detect abnormalities in brain electrical impulses such as seizures or brain death. These and other diagnostic tests are presented in more detail in Chapter 16.

Section Four Review

1. The nurse is monitoring the neurologic status of a client admitted with concussion. The client's response to which statement would be most helpful in identifying a change in mental status?
   A. "Tell me your name."
   B. "Do you have a headache?"
   C. "Are you having trouble breathing?"
   D. "Squeeze my hand."

2. On admission to the ED, a client who has altered LOC after being struck on the head with a baseball bat has a variety of diagnostic tests ordered. Which test should be done first?
   A. Urine for WBCs
   B. CT scan
   C. Chest x-ray
   D. Serum electrolytes

3. A client is admitted to the hospital with a cerebral contusion. During the night, he develops a headache, vomits, and seems more lethargic. What are the appropriate actions for the nurse to take?
   A. Give the client pain medication to treat the headache and reassess in 1 hour.
   B. Give the client antinausea medication and reassess in 1 hour.
   C. Perform a neurological and pupillary assessment immediately.
   D. Assess the client's lung fields.

4. The nurse reports that a trauma client's pupils are "blown." What has the nurse assessed?
   A. Pupils are slow to react to light.
   B. Pupils are not equal.
   C. Pupils have been injured and are not assessable.
   D. Pupils are dilated and nonreactive to light.

Answers: 1. A, 2. B, 3. C, 4. D

Section Five: Collaborative Management of Traumatic Brain Injury

Early management of TBI is based on the severity of injury and focuses primarily on optimizing cerebral tissue perfusion and controlling intracranial pressure. Table 19–4 provides a list of immediate care priorities.

Approach to Cerebral Tissue Perfusion Management

The priority goals in treating TBI are to limit ischemic injury by aggressive prevention and treatment of hypoxia and hypotension and to minimize secondary injury. Decreased cerebral tissue perfusion is a complication of cerebral edema and intracranial hypertension, both of which commonly occur after traumatic brain injury. Decreased cerebral tissue perfusion requires prompt recognition and treatment. Treatment is aimed at reducing one or more of the three components within the cranial vault: blood volume, brain tissue volume, or CSF. Identifying and eliminating the cause of the increase in any of these components is a treatment priority. Interventions for

patients with decreased cerebral tissue perfusion include therapeutic strategies that increase MAP and reduce ICP because cerebral perfusion pressure (CPP) is equal to the difference between mean arterial pressure (MAP) and ICP (CPP = MAP – ICP).

Optimizing Cerebral Perfusion Pressure Cerebral perfusion pressure (CPP) and cerebral blood flow (CBF) are directly related. Recall from Section Two that CPP is the net pressure gradient causing blood flow to the brain (brain perfusion) and that an increase in CBF will increase CPP. CPP must be maintained within certain limits (60–160 mmHg) as abnormally low pressures cause brain tissue to have inadequate blood flow and abnormally high ICP. Chapter 16 provides a detailed description of CPP and how it is derived.

CPP is optimized by controlling blood pressure and temperature and promoting venous return, thereby normalizing ICP. Ideally, mean arterial pressure (MAP) is maintained at a level sufficient to maintain CPP greater than 60 mmHg (American College of Surgeons, 2015). Blood pressure and ICP values outside of acceptable ranges result in a loss of cerebral autoregulation and inadequate CPP. IV fluids and vasopressors are utilized to maintain optimal CPP and cerebral blood flow, preventing ischemia-related causes of ICP (American College of Surgeons, 2015). Providers must thoughtfully consider aggressive fluid

Table 19–4 Summary of the Immediate Care Priorities for Traumatic Brain Injury (TBI)

Type of TBI	Immediate Care Priorities
Concussion (mild injury)	Require observation for 1 to 2 hours in the ED. Discharge home with instructions for further observation to detect neurologic deterioration. Postconcussion syndrome may include persistent headache, dizziness, irritability, insomnia, impaired memory and concentration, and learning problems. May be admitted into the hospital for observation if there was associated loss of consciousness for more than 15 minutes.
Other acute TBIs (moderate–severe injury)	Assessment of airway, breathing, and circulation, with management of intracranial hypertension and restoration of cerebral tissue perfusion, are necessary to prevent secondary injury. Recognition and management of acute TBI during the prehospital period with transport to an ED is essential to optimal patient outcomes. Morbidity and mortality increase with hypotension (SBP less than 90 mmHg) and hypoxia (PaO$_2$ less than 100 mmHg), so fluids (usually 0.9% sodium chloride) are given to support a MAP ≥ 90 mmHg, and to maintain sodium and water homeostasis. Hypotonic solutions are avoided to prevent an increase in cerebral edema. ICP monitoring is initiated in comatose patients with GCS < 8 and if there is evidence of structural brain damage. Osmotic diuretics (mannitol) and hypertonic saline solutions are indicated for treating elevated ICP. They draw water from the extracellular space within brain tissue into the intravascular space, thereby decreasing edema and ICP. Neurosurgical intervention may be required to manage bleeding or remove space-occupying lesions, such as a hematoma.

SOURCE: Data from American College of Surgeons (2015); Carney et al. (2016); Wright & Merck (2016).

resuscitation, as it may increase the patient's risk for developing cardiopulmonary complications, such as pulmonary edema (Zhao et al., 2016).

Optimizing Oxygenation. Maintaining optimal cerebral oxygenation is essential in preventing secondary brain injury and promoting brain tissue healing. Key management strategies that assist in promoting cerebral oxygenation in the TBI patient include controlling body temperature, promoting venous return, and ensuring adequate systemic oxygenation (Hickey, 2014).

Controlling Body Temperature. The injured brain is sensitive to changes in body temperature, as hyperthermia increases cerebral metabolism. Under conditions of increased cerebral metabolism, CBF increases to meet increased tissue oxygenation requirements. To avoid this increase in cerebral metabolism and subsequent increase in CBF, hyperthermia must be prevented. Antipyretics and cooling blankets help control body temperature. Severe injury to the hypothalamus impairs thermoregulation and causes a subsequent neurogenic (or central) fever, which is unresponsive to antipyretics. In this situation, external cooling methods, such as cooling blankets or ice packs, are the primary therapy. It is important when cooling patients to avoid causing shivering. Shivering in patients with severe brain injury treated with induced normothermia is associated with decreased $PbtO_2$ (brain tissue O_2 partial pressure), which correlated with the intensity of cooling (Oddo et al., 2010).

Induced or therapeutic hypothermia (TH) is a neuroprotective therapy whereby the patient's body temperature is lowered (33–36°C; 91.4–98.6°F) to protect the injured brain tissue from secondary injury. TH therapy remains controversial and is not currently recommended as an initial TBI treatment. TH should be reserved for refractory intracranial hypertension, used after traditional attempts at decreasing ICP have failed. TH is considered to be neuroprotective, as it decreases the cerebral metabolic rate and oxygen consumption, decreases ICP, and increases CPP (American College of Surgeons, 2015; Carney et al., 2016; Cook, 2017; Urbano & Oddo, 2012).

Induction of TH typically requires a multimodal approach, including the use of both pharmacological agents and physical cooling techniques. Drug therapy during TH typically includes some combination of analgesic or sedative or anesthetic agents, such as fentanyl, propofol, and/or lorazepam, and a neuromuscular-blocking agent, such as pancuronium or cisatracurium. Cooling techniques can be external, internal, or a combination of both. For example, ice bags or cooling blankets applied at the groin, chest, axilla, and sides of the neck can be utilized for external cooling; while cold normal saline IV infusions (4°C; 39.2°F) can help reduce body temperature internally. Internal and external methods of cooling the patient may be applied simultaneously. Shivering is a major complication of hypothermia, as it increases metabolism and oxygen consumption, and therefore must be controlled. If the patient is receiving a neuromuscular blocking agent, shivering will not occur. Other drugs such as buspirone or magnesium may also be used to help control shivering (Urbano & Oddo, 2012).

The practical application of therapeutic hypothermia carries risks and requires a clinical management protocol that focuses on detection and control of complications, which may include pneumonia, atrial fibrillation, acidosis, shivering, and coagulopathies. When TH is discontinued, the patient proceeds through a critical rewarming period, which can cause hemodynamic instability and cardiac dysrhythmias. Rewarming may be done passively by removing cooling modalities, or it can be done actively, controlling the process by slowly increasing the temperature on the cooling unit over a set period of time (e.g., 6 to 8 hours) and maintaining a target temperature for several days. Institutions where TH is utilized should have an evidence-based protocol for TH induction, maintenance, and rewarming (Carney et al., 2016; Urbano & Oddo, 2012) .

Promoting Venous Return. Venous return from the brain can be promoted by ensuring optimal patient positioning. In the absence of contraindications (e.g., unstable spine), the patient is placed in a Semi-Fowler position with the head of the bed elevated at least 30 degrees. If the Semi-Fowler position is contraindicated, the patient may be positioned in Reverse-Trendelenburg at 30 degrees. These positions minimize jugular venous compression by promoting venous drainage, thereby decreasing ICP (Harris, 2016). It is important to assess the patient's response to head-of-bed elevations and to avoid hypotension, as this would increase the patient's risk for decreased CPP and cerebral ischemia.

Neck flexion and lateral head rotation restrict venous outflow from the brain and can contribute to increased ICP. Hip flexion of greater than 90 degrees increases intra-abdominal and intrathoracic pressure, reducing venous outflow and thus increasing ICP. These positions should be avoided because they promote venous congestion in the intracranial and abdominal compartments, which can lead to increased ICP (Carney et al., 2016). The patient's body is turned as a unit; head, neck, trunk, and lower extremities are turned in unison to avoid head and neck rotation. Patients who are alert are assisted to reposition in bed. Asking patients to help reposition by pushing with their legs initiates the Valsalva maneuver, which increases intrathoracic pressure and impedes venous return (Hickey, 2014).

Ensuring Adequate Systemic Oxygenation. Any patient with a Glasgow Coma Scale (GCS) score of 8 or less should receive an artificial airway to ensure optimal systemic oxygenation and ventilation. Mechanical ventilator settings are adjusted to maintain PaO_2 greater than 100 mmHg and $PaCO_2$ between 35 and 45 mmHg (American College of Surgeons, 2015). Sedation or neuromuscular blocking agents may be required to control the patient's breathing on the ventilator.

Therapeutic hyperventilation (increasing tidal volume and/or respiratory rate) has been used to produce vasoconstriction of the cerebral blood vessels to decrease CBV and ICP. Hyperventilation decreases blood levels of $PaCO_2$, thereby producing vasoconstriction and reduced cerebral blood flow. Current guidelines suggest a $PaCO_2$ range of 30 to 35 as target for therapeutic hyperventilation therapy, taking caution to avoid cerebral hypoxia (American College of

BOX 19–1   Clinical Management of Traumatic Brain Injury

- Intubation with avoidance of mechanical hyperventilation unless intracranial hypertension becomes refractory to initial therapies
- Optimization of oxygenation to maintain PaO_2 greater than 100 mmHg
- Cerebral edema management utilizing osmotic diuretics and/or hypertonic saline
- Control of cerebral metabolism with sedation, anticonvulsants, antipyretic therapies
- Maintenance of SBP > 90 mmHg
- Targeted fluid resuscitation to maintain MAP and achieve normal fluid balance

Surgeons, 2015). Optimal $PaCO_2$ may be determined by the use of additional neuromonitoring, such as $PbtO_2$ and $SjvO_2$ (American College of Surgeons, 2015).

Box 19–1 summarizes clinical management of the patient with a brain injury.

Leveled Approach to Intracranial Pressure Management

Traditional approaches to management of elevated ICP warranted strict notification and treatment for sustained elevations in ICP of greater than 20 mmHg for more than 5 to 10 minutes. Contemporary guidelines challenge the rigid ICP alert threshold of 20 mmHg and provide a range of 20 to 25 mmHg as a treatment trigger (Carney et al., 2016; Sorrentino, Diedler, & Kasprowicz, 2012). Treatment threshold and interventions for elevated ICP should be individualized, multifaceted, and involve a stepwise or tiered approach (Table 19–5). Many strategies that have already been presented in the discussion of management of cerebral tissue perfusion also apply to managing elevated ICP. Table 19–6 provides a summary of intracranial parameters for treatment of brain injury.

Tier One Interventions   First-level interventions to reduce elevated ICP include patient positioning strategies to prevent restriction of venous outflow from the brain, normothermia maintenance, CSF drainage, and minimization of systemic oxygen requirements. Unless contraindicated, the head of the bed should be elevated, and hyperextension, flexion, or rotation of the head and neck should be avoided. In addition, it is important to ensure that there is no compression of the jugular veins from circumferential endotracheal tube tape, ties, or a cervical collar that may be too tight. Hyperthermia increases cerebral metabolic demands, so fever should be treated expeditiously. Abdominal distention, agitation, and increased levels of positive end-expiratory pressure (PEEP) also increase ICP by increasing intrathoracic pressure and reducing venous outflow. Reducing environmental stimulation and providing pain control and sedation for agitation are additional measures to optimize cerebral oxygenation by decreasing cerebral metabolic demand. Although seemingly benign in nature, many standard

Table 19–5   Tiered Approach for Management of Elevated ICP

Level	Treatment Approach
One	Short-acting analgesic and sedative medications in intubated patients Normothermia maintenance Patient positioning with head-of-bed elevation to 30 degrees and midline neck alignment Intermittent ventricular drainage via external ventricular drain If ICP remains greater than or equal to 20–25, proceed to level two.
Two	Consideration of external intermittent ventricular drainage (if not already in place) Intermittent (not scheduled) CSF drainage Hyperosmolar therapy with hypertonic saline administration and loop diuretics (mannitol) PaO_2 goal ≥ 100 mmHg; $PaCO_2$ goal 30–35 mmHg Assessment of cerebral autoregulation and optimal CPP determination: If autoregulation absent, reduce CPP goal to a minimum of 50 mmHg to decrease ICP. Repeat CT imaging and neurologic examination are needed to guide management. If ICP remains greater than or equal to 20–25, proceed to level three.
Three	Neuromuscular blockade if positive response to loading dose Barbiturate or propofol coma if ICP responsive to loading dose Decompressive hemicraniectomy or bilateral craniectomy

SOURCE: Data from American College of Surgeons (2015).

nursing interventions, such as bathing or turning, can provide enough stimulation to elevate ICP and compromise cerebral blood flow and oxygenation. To avoid unnecessary elevations of ICP, nursing activities are spaced apart to allow recovery time for the patient (Hickey, 2014). If the team determines that the patient would benefit from analgesia and/or sedation, short-acting agents for sedation are preferred, paired with standardized sedation assessments (e.g., Richmond Agitation-Sedation Scale), and daily sedation withdrawal for opportunities to assess neurologic status and to avoid oversedation.

Table 19–6   Intracranial Parameters for Treatment of Traumatic Brain Injury

Parameter	Recommendation	Supportive Therapy

ABG:
  PaO_2
  $PaCO_2$
	≥100 mmHg
	Goal 35–45 mmHg
		Oxygen therapy with mechanical ventilation as needed
		May drive $PaCO_2$ to goal range of 30–35 mmHg to decrease ICP in absence of cerebral hypoxia

Blood pressure	Systolic pressure > 90 mmHg	IV fluids and vasopressors as needed
Cerebral perfusion pressure (CPP)	≥ 60 mmHg	IV fluids and vasopressor therapy as needed
Intracranial pressure (ICP)	Less than 20 mmHg	Treat ICP > 20–25 mmHg sustained for more than 5–10 minutes See Table 19–5: Tiered Approach for Management of Elevated ICP

SOURCE: Data from American College of Surgeons (2015); Sorrentino et al. (2012).

Tier Two Interventions Second-level interventions aimed at reducing ICP, optimizing CPP, and preventing secondary injury include intermittent cerebrospinal fluid (CSF) drainage, hyperosmolar therapy, and PaCO$_2$ manipulation with mechanical ventilation. Drainage of CSF requires placement of an external ventricular drain (EVD). The EVD allows direct monitoring of the ICP via an indwelling ventricular catheter, along with observation of the color and amount of CSF. It allows for therapeutic drainage of CSF to reduce ICP.

Diuretic Therapy. Diuretic therapy for TBI consists of intermittent administration of an osmotic diuretic such as mannitol (Osmitrol). Mannitol draws fluid from the intracellular and interstitial spaces into the vascular compartment, reducing blood viscosity and resulting in improved cerebral blood flow and decreased cerebral edema. The primary therapeutic goal of diuretic therapy is to decrease ICP. Mannitol use for ICP control may become less effective over time. Additional information about mannitol is included in the "Related Pharmacotherapy: Agents Used to Treat Traumatic Brain Injury" feature.

Fluid Volume Maintenance. The goal for fluid volume maintenance is to keep the patient in a state of euvolemia in order to optimize cerebral perfusion. Volume replacement strategies may include fluid boluses, maintenance fluids, and urine output fluid replacements. Intravenous fluids are usually isotonic to prevent gradient shifts across the blood–brain barrier in the TBI patient.

Hypertonic Saline Therapy. Hypertonic saline has been shown to prevent secondary injury and has several neuroprotective effects on injured brain tissue. It reduces cerebral edema by creating an osmotic gradient that promotes passage of intracellular fluid from swollen neuronal cells into the blood vessels. Hypertonic saline also possesses hemodynamic, vasoregulatory, and anti-inflammatory properties that help reduce secondary injury (Boone, Oren-Grinberg, Robinson, Chen, & Kasper, 2015). Nurses caring for patients receiving hypertonic saline or mannitol must closely monitor the patient's serum sodium levels and serum osmolality as extreme elevations in these values may result in neurologic injury and renal failure.

PaCO$_2$ Manipulation. Controlled hyperventilation may be necessary to manage refractory ICP. In the absence of cerebral hypoxia, a target PaCO$_2$ range of 30 to 35 mmHg may be appropriate to aid in reducing CBF and subsequently reducing ICP (American College of Surgeons, 2015).

Tier Three Interventions Third-level interventions to reduce ICP include neuromuscular blockade, propofol or barbiturate coma, and decompressive craniectomy. Skeletal muscle paralysis using a neuromuscular blocking agent may be necessary to optimize mechanical ventilation and prevent coughing, posturing, and severe agitation, which increase cerebral metabolism and lead to increased ICP. Treatment of increased ICP that is refractory to neuromuscular blockade may include the use of high-dose barbiturates or propofol.

These interventions induce a comatose state and significantly decrease cerebral oxygen requirements. Barbiturates decrease electrical activity in the brain and can decrease the production of CSF. Due to the induction of hypotension with both barbiturates and propofol, these agents must be used with caution. Patients must be adequately volume resuscitated at baseline, and only patients who respond to test doses of these therapies with a decrease in ICP should be considered (American College of Surgeons, 2015). If the patient experiences hypotension with either of these therapies, vasopressors and/or inotropes may be considered. During therapy, continuous EEG is utilized to ensure appropriate suppression of electrical activity within the brain.

Surgical interventions for the treatment of refractory-increased ICP may include decompressive craniectomy. When a decompressive craniectomy is performed, a portion of skull is removed to allow more space for the injured brain to expand during the acute phase of injury (Figure 19–8). By opening the cranial vault, ICP is reduced and ischemia prevented. Decompressive craniectomy is not, however, without risk and should only be utilized if interventions to decrease ICP in the previous tiers have failed. Complications from decompressive craniectomy include hemorrhage, infection, delayed wound healing, and CSF complications, such as a CSF leak and hydrocephalus. Also described in the literature as a complication of craniectomy is syndrome of the trephined, or "sinking flap syndrome," a condition in which the scalp sinks due to the lack of cranial bone to bear normal atmospheric pressure. This condition results in excess pressure on the cerebral cortex, which can inhibit brain healing or even potentiate neurologic decline (Kurland et al., 2015).

The "Related Pharmacotherapy: Agents Used to Treat Traumatic Brain Injury" feature summarizes drugs for treatment of TBI.

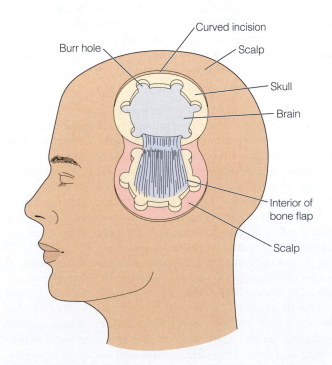

Figure 19–8 Craniectomy. In a craniectomy, a portion of the skull and overlying scalp is removed to allow access to the brain and may also decrease ICP.

Related Pharmacotherapy
Agents Used to Treat Traumatic Brain Injury

Osmotic Diuretic

Mannitol (Osmitrol)

Action and Uses

Reduces ICP by inducing diuresis; creates an osmotic gradient across the blood–brain barrier (BBB) and increases serum osmolality; pulls fluid out of brain cells and shifts it into the intravascular compartment.

Dosages (Adult)

Given as a 20% solution in bolus doses of 0.25–1 g/kg every 4–6 hours IV in patients who are euvolemic (well hydrated)

Major Adverse Effects

Hypotension, fluid and electrolyte imbalance, especially hypernatremia (hyponatremia in renal failure), hypokalemia, pulmonary edema, rebound increase in ICP

Nursing Implications

Monitor serum osmolality and intake and output.
Monitor closely serum and urine electrolytes and renal function.
Monitor vital signs closely; monitor ICP.
General therapeutic goals for hyperosmolar therapy: decreasing ICP, improving neurologic status, decreased cerebral edema
Therapeutic limitations: Treatment should be withheld if osmolar gap (difference between measured serum and calculated osmolalities) > 10 mOsm, serum sodium > 160 mEq, or serum osmolality > 320 mOsm (Layon, Gabrielli, & Friedman, 2013).

Hypertonic Saline

Action and Uses

Diuresis through action of atrial natriuretic peptide; restores resting membrane potential and cell volume; inhibits inflammation

Dosages (Adult)

Any saline solution with concentration higher than 0.9% (physiologic), infused at variable rates. Available preparations include 1.5%, 2%, 3%, 5%, 7%, and 23.4% NaCl.

Major Adverse Effects

Electrolyte abnormalities, fluid volume overload, rebound increase in ICP

Nursing Implications

Monitor serum sodium, serum osmolality, and renal function.
Monitor vital signs closely; monitor ICP.
General therapeutic goals for hyperosmolar therapy: a decreasing ICP, improving neurologic status, decreased cerebral edema

Antidiuretic Hormone (ADH)

Desmopressin (DDAVP)

Action and Uses

Reduces urine output and osmolality in patients with central diabetes insipidus by increasing resorption of water by kidney collecting tubules.

Dosages (Adult)

Diabetes insipidus: 2–4 mcg (IV or subcutaneously) in divided doses *or* 10–40 mcg/day (intranasally) in single or divided doses, *or* 0.05 mg orally twice daily initially, maintenance dose 0.1–0.8 mg/day in divided doses

Major Adverse Effects

Dose-related transient headache, dizziness, rhinitis, nausea, abdominal cramps, heartburn, facial flushing, shortness of air, pain or swelling at injection site

Nursing Implications

Monitor intake and output.
Daily weights
Assess for edema from severe water retention.
Monitor BP.
Monitor urine and plasma osmolality, serum sodium.

Sedative–Hypnotics and Sedatives

Propofol (Diprivan)
Midazolam (Versed) and lorazepam (Ativan)

Pain Medication

Morphine or fentanyl

Barbiturates

Pentobarbital, thiopental

Neuromuscular Blocking Agents

Atracurium (Tracrium), pancuronium (Pavulon), vecuronium (Norcuron)

Anticonvulsants

Phenytoin (Dilantin), fosphenytoin (Cerebyx), lorazepam (Ativan)

Emerging Evidence

- A systematic review of seven published articles (five prospective randomized trials, one prospective nonrandomized trial, and one retrospective cohort study) comparing efficacy of mannitol with hypertonic saline in TBI demonstrated that while both agents were effective in decreasing increased ICP, hypertonic saline decreased ICP more rapidly, achieved a greater degree of reduction, and was longer lasting than mannitol (*Boone et al., 2015*).

- In a prospective cohort study of 375 mild TBI (mTBI) or concussion patients with GCS of 13 to 15, 82% reported at least one lingering postconcussive symptom at both 6 months and 12 months postinjury. In addition, at 12 months postinjury 40.3% of patients had significantly reduced Satisfaction with Life scores, and 22.4% had still not returned to their baseline functional status (*McMahon et al., 2014*).

- In a study of 18 patients with severe TBI who were admitted to the ICU while requiring ICP monitoring and advanced neuromonitoring, noninvasive brain tissue oxygenation monitoring utilizing near-infrared spectroscopy and ultrasound technology (CerOx 3110) provided results comparable to invasive jugular venous oxygenation monitoring. Cerebral oxygenation values from the noninvasive monitor ($p < .001$) correlated only with SjO_2 measurements on the same side as the catheter (*Rosenthal, Furmanov, Itshayek, Shoshan, & Singh, 2014*).
- In a study of two independent cohorts of TBI cases and one control group without TBI, presenting to the ED, median brain-derived neurotrophic factor (BDNF) concentrations of circulating serum levels of BDNF were lower in the experimental groups versus the control group ($p = 0.0001$). In addition, mean-BDNF levels were lower in severe traumatic brain injury than in moderate traumatic brain injury, and lower in moderate traumatic brain injury than in mild injury ($p = 0.004$). Patients with very low levels of BDNF on the day of injury were also less likely to have completely recovered from their injury at 6 months. These findings suggest day-of-injury serum BDNF may be helpful in the diagnosis and prognosis for TBI (*Korley et al., 2016*).

Section Five Review

1. Controlling which factors will optimize cerebral perfusion pressure? (Select all that apply.)
   A. Pain
   B. Venous return
   C. Pulmonary vascular resistance
   D. Blood pressure
   E. Temperature

2. A client with a recent TBI is to receive mannitol 20% (IV) bolus doses of 0.50 g/kg every 4–6 hours. This drug reduces ICP through which action?
   A. Replaces lost fluid volumes to achieve a euvolemic state
   B. Inhibits inflammation via action of natriuretic peptide
   C. Increases resorption of water by the renal tubules
   D. Pulls fluid out of brain cells and into blood

3. Which statement is accurate regarding decompressive craniectomy?
   A. It is appropriate for all clients with secondary injury.
   B. It is used to treat intractable ICP elevation in some clients.
   C. It will reduce CPP.
   D. It will increase ICP.

4. A 42-year-old client with a severe acute traumatic brain injury has developed a fever. The nurse is aware that the fever should be reversed quickly for which reason?
   A. It decreases venous return from the brain.
   B. It often causes seizure activity.
   C. It increases the brain's metabolic needs.
   D. It may be caused by infection.

Answers: 1. (B, D, E), 2. D, 3. B, 4. C

Section Six: Nursing Management

Nursing care of the patient in the acute phase of TBI necessitates airway maintenance, hemodynamic support, and frequent, focused neurologic assessments. Patients with severe TBI often have advanced neurologic monitoring in place, requiring additional nursing expertise and targeted interventions.

Interventions to Reduce Secondary Injury Following TBI

Nurses play an integral role in preventing secondary injury following TBI. A number of nursing interventions aid in preventing or minimizing cerebral ischemia, including ongoing monitoring and assessment, rapid identification of neurologic or hemodynamic compromise, and timely intervention to correct clinical deterioration. These interventions are discussed in this section.

Optimizing Cerebral Perfusion Pressure and Cerebral Oxygenation Collaborative interventions to optimize CPP and cerebral oxygenation to reduce secondary injury have been presented in detail in Section Five, including promoting venous return by proper patient positioning; maintaining normothermia using antipyretics or cooling blankets; and performing interventions aimed at optimizing oxygenation and ventilation. In addition to the interventions previously discussed, nurses must take care to maintain adequate oxygenation while performing suctioning of the airway, as this intervention significantly increases oxygen demands. The nurse should pre-oxygenate the patient with 100% FiO_2 for 30 to 60 seconds prior to suctioning and should limit passage time of the suction catheter to 10 to 15 seconds or less (Wiegand, 2011), as ICP also increases when the patient coughs or gags.

Interventions to Manage ICP

Managing ICP is considered the cornerstone of nursing care for the patient with TBI. Timely recognition and intervention for elevated ICP are essential for preventing secondary injury and adverse patient outcomes. Basic information on ICP and ICP monitoring are included in Chapter 16. The material provided in this chapter focuses on care of the patient with TBI who has an ICP monitoring device in place.

A major advantage of placement of an intraventricular ICP monitoring device is that CSF can be diverted to decrease ICP. Patients who present with a GCS less than 8 with evidence of structural brain damage, or who present with GCS greater than 8 with evidence of structural brain damage, are ideal candidates for ICP monitoring. The determination of when to drain CSF must be carefully considered. Clinical neurologic assessment, ICP, and the patient's overall hemodynamic status are considered when determining when CSF diversion is appropriate. Current guidelines recommend treatment for ICP when it reaches the upper threshold of 20 to 25 mmHg (American College of Surgeons, 2015). Interpretation and treatment are corroborated by frequent clinical examinations and CPP monitoring. Clear, concise orders for CSF drainage should be maintained within the medical record, and the nurse should clarify any questions with the ordering provider.

The focus of nursing care of the patient with an ICP monitoring device is on maintenance of system integrity and prevention of complications.

Maintenance of System Integrity and Troubleshooting

One of the most important nursing interventions for any patient is to gather, document, and report accurate clinical data. The patient's plan of care is developed based on these data, and developing interventions based on inaccurate data can negatively impact outcomes. Ensuring that ICP monitoring systems are intact and that data are accurate (Table 19–7) is the primary responsibility of the nurse. A dampened, absent, or distorted waveform usually indicates that the ICP data are inaccurate. Any interference, such as air bubbles within the transducer or tubing; kinked tubing; loose connections; or catheter occlusion from blood, brain, or bone tissue, can produce a dampened waveform and inaccurate ICP readings. Technical malfunction within the external system, such as with monitoring equipment, also produces inaccurate data. Fiber optic cables are delicate and easily broken. If this occurs, the nurse should replace the cable and zero the transducer to

see if the ICP values improve. Often, the transducers used to convey the ICP data to the external monitor malfunction and must be replaced. When caring for patients with ICP monitoring technology, the nurse must have a clear understanding of the benefits and limitations of the systems used, troubleshooting scenarios that may arise, and how to obtain support from the manufacturer when needed (Hickey, 2014).

Prevention of Complications

Complications include those related to insertion, such as hemorrhage; overdrainage of CSF; and infection, particularly in the patient with an EVD.

Risk of Bleeding. Patients with coagulopathies are at higher risk for hemorrhage. Because hemorrhage is a space-occupying lesion, the patient's neurologic status must be carefully monitored before, during, and after insertion of the ICP monitoring device to detect neurologic deterioration. If an intraventricular device is inserted, the color of the CSF during subsequent assessments must be carefully observed and documented, as pink-tinged or bloody CSF is an indication of bleeding.

Risk for CSF Overdrainage. Overdrainage of CSF is a major complication of an intraventricular device, particularly an open system. To prevent overdrainage, the nurse observes unit standards for CSF drainage; accurately measures and positions the CSF drainage bag using the correct landmarks (typically using the foramen of Monro); and securely fastens the drainage bag at the prescribed level. CSF diversion may be prescribed in one of two ways: (1) the system may be closed and periodically opened for therapeutic CSF drainage or (2) the system may be open and drain CSF continuously. For a closed system, a prescribed amount of CSF is drained when the ICP is consistently elevated. Many factors transiently increase ICP, including environmental stimuli, patient positioning, and nursing care activities. Once these stimuli are eliminated, ICP may return to an acceptable level. If ICP remains elevated for several minutes, the appropriate nursing action is to institute CSF drainage.

For an open system, CSF drains continuously when the ICP exceeds a preset limit ordered by the provider and

Table 19–7 Troubleshooting System Integrity with ICP Monitors

Problem	Potential Source	Action
Dampened, absent, or distorted waveform	Catheter occlusion by blood, or by brain or bone tissue Air bubbles in system Loose connections Recalibration and zero referencing needed Kinked catheter or tubing Technical problem with transducer or pressure module Fiber optic cables broken Dislodgement of catheter	Systematically assess for problems Remove air from system Tighten all connections Recalibrate and zero Examine tubing for kinks Replace transducer or pressure module Replace fiber optic device Replace monitoring device
ICP values suspect	Recalibration and zero referencing needed Incorrect placement of catheter or transducer	Recalibrate and zero if fluid-filled system; replace device if fiber optic Verify correct placement of external transducer
Leakage of fluid from tubing	Loosened connections	Tighten all connections

dialed onto the drainage system by the nurse. While continuously draining, the transducer does not produce an accurate ICP reading, so the drain must be turned off at prescribed intervals to measure and document ICP.

Risk for Infection. Risk for infection is a concern for invasive neuromonitoring, with the duration of monitoring and the type of device used being risk factors. Sterile technique must be strictly observed during insertion of the ICP monitoring device. For fluid-filled systems, system sterility and integrity must be maintained at all times. All connection points are checked prior to insertion of the catheter and at regular intervals to ensure they are tight. Because fluid-filled systems require routine zero referencing and calibration, the risk of introducing pathogens into the system is increased. Care must be taken to re-zero and recalibrate in an aseptic manner. The insertion site is inspected for signs of infection on a routine basis. The appearance of the insertion site and duration (in days) of the monitoring device placement should be documented. Protocols for the care and maintenance of invasive neuromonitoring catheters vary by institution, but they typically include prescribed interventions for dressing changes, collection bag changes, and lab collection procedures for CSF analysis.

Interventions to Provide a Safe and Protective Environment

The following nursing interventions for patients with neurologic injury center on protecting the patient from injury, reorienting, and creating a safe and therapeutic environment. Patients with cognitive deficits become easily confused and agitated by external stimuli. Nurses must closely assess the patient's response to basic care interventions such as bathing and suctioning. Noise should be kept to a minimum, information presented simply and calmly, and the number of visitors limited. Clustering of care and minimization of sleep interruptions are essential in maintaining the patient's circadian rhythm and sleep–wake cycle. Patients with cognitive deficits often attempt to get out of bed and may pull out IV lines and catheters. Interventions such as maintaining the bed in the lowest position, utilizing side rails, and frequent rounding help keep the patient safe from injury. Frequent reorientation decreases confusion.

Major aspects of nursing management are summarized in the "Nursing Care: The Patient with Acute TBI and Increased ICP" feature. Also, refer to Table 19–3 for a summary of nursing surveillance priorities and interventions in Section Four of this chapter.

Nursing Care
The Patient with Acute TBI and Increased ICP

Expected Patient Outcomes and Related Interventions

Outcome 1: Treat or manage intracranial hypertension

Assess and compare to established norms, patient baselines, and trends.

Monitor for signs and symptoms of intracranial compromise.
ICP > 20–25 mmHg, CPP < 60 mmHg
Vital signs: SBP < 90 mmHg; bradycardia, sudden onset of hypertension; widening pulse pressure (increasing difference between systolic blood pressure [SBP] and diastolic blood pressure [DBP]); deteriorating breathing pattern
Cushing's triad (refer to Table 18–3) indicates brainstem ischemia and impending cerebral herniation.
Temperature: Impaired hypothalamic function can interfere with temperature regulation. Hyperthermia may increase ICP.
Pupils: abnormal pupil changes (e.g., pinpoint and sluggish; unequal; fixed and dilated)
Intake and output: fluid balance excess or fluid balance deficit; serum osmolality greater than 320 mOsm (osmotic diuretics may cause hypotension and decreased cardiac output)
Vomiting; headache; lethargy; restlessness; purposeless movements; changes in mentation; decreased eye opening, verbal, and motor response (early indicators of ICP changes)

Interventions to maintain normal ICP and prevent increased cerebral metabolism

Maintain euvolemia.
Intravenous fluid therapy or diuretic therapy as needed
Monitor for manifestations of fluid volume excess or deficit.

Facilitate venous drainage from the head.
Elevate head of the bed 30 degrees; neutral body positioning.
Control seizure activity.
Monitor for development of seizures; protect patient from injury.
Prevent overstimulation.
Observe closely for the effect of interventions on ICP; careful timing of activities and rest based on patient's tolerance; dark, quiet environment as needed; control or limit noxious stimuli.
Control body temperature.
Prevent hyperthermia: monitor temperature, cooling blanket, tepid baths
Hypothermia therapy (e.g., cooling blanket); prevent shivering

Administer related drug therapy and monitor for therapeutic and nontherapeutic effects.

Antipyretic agent as needed to control fever
Hyperosmolar therapy (e.g., mannitol or hypertonic saline) to decrease ICP
Sedatives, analgesics, neuromuscular blocking agents to control agitation and skeletal movements that increase ICP; barbiturate or propofol coma if stepwise interventions fail
Anticonvulsants to control seizure activity

Outcome 2: Optimize ventilation and oxygenation

Assess and compare to established norms, patient baselines, and trends.

Monitor for manifestations of inadequate cerebral oxygenation.
ICP readings for intracranial hypertension. Sustained elevations increase risk for herniation and death.

Cushing triad of bradycardia, irregular breathing pattern, and widening pulse pressure are signs of impending herniation.

Neurologic status, responsiveness, alertness, ability to follow commands, Glasgow Coma Scale

Unstable breathing pattern. Brain injuries may cause alterations in respiratory function; a decreased respiratory rate may be the result of depression of the medullary respiratory center within the brainstem. In general, an initial increase in ICP causes respirations to slow; as the ICP continues to increase, respirations become irregular with periods of tachypnea and bradypnea.

ABG: PaO_2 less than 100 mmHg, $PaCO_2$ less than 30–35 or greater than 45. If the patient is not intubated, prepare for oxygen administration and/or endotracheal intubation if respiratory distress occurs. Goal is to prevent hypoxia, maintain ventilation.

Hemoglobin (Hgb) less than 10 g, hematocrit (Hct) less than 32%

Interventions to optimize cerebral oxygenation

Administer oxygen at 2–4 L/min per nasal cannula; endotracheal intubation and mechanical ventilation if needed

Packed red blood cells to maintain adequate Hgb and Hct—monitor for therapeutic and nontherapeutic effects

Prevent pneumonia: aggressive pulmonary toilet, elevate head of bed 30 degrees, frequent oral care, turn every 2 hours.

Decrease cerebral metabolism (refer to Outcome 1).

Outcome 3: Prevent complications of immobility

Assess and compare to established norms, patient baselines, and trends.

Monitor for signs and symptoms of complications of immobility.

Deep vein thrombosis: swelling, redness or warmth of lower extremity

Contractures: increased resistance to passive range of motion

Intervene to prevent complications of immobility.

Deep vein thrombosis: anticoagulant therapy if appropriate; antiembolism stockings

Contractures: passive range-of-motion exercises; neutral body and limb positioning; physical therapy

Turn every 2 hours; logroll if spinal cord injury is present.

Early ambulation if feasible

Section Six Review

1. The nurse is assessing the integrity of a client's ICP monitoring system. Which system issues require corrective interventions? (Select all that apply.)
   A. Kinked tubing
   B. Fluid in the tubing
   C. Loose connections
   D. Air bubbles in the system
   E. Catheter is occluded by tissue

2. What are common complications in a client with an ICP monitoring device? (Select all that apply.)
   A. New-onset seizures
   B. Overdrainage of CSF
   C. Collapsed ventricles
   D. Bleeding
   E. Infection

3. Which intervention should the nurse perform to reduce the ICP in a client with an acute TBI?
   A. Flatten the head of the bed.
   B. Maintain the head and neck in neutral alignment.
   C. Suction the client every hour.
   D. Slightly hypoventilate the client.

4. What nursing intervention helps to prevent increased cerebral metabolism?
   A. Maintaining CPP less than 60 mmHg
   B. Vigorous suctioning of the client
   C. Spacing client care activities
   D. Keeping the client flat at all times

Answers: 1. (A, C, D, E), 2. (B, D, E), 3. B, 4. C

Section Seven: Complications Associated with Increased Intracranial Pressure

A significant number of complications may occur as a result of TBI. Complications that commonly occur in high-acuity patients with TBI include diabetes insipidus, syndrome of inappropriate antidiuretic hormone, cerebral salt wasting, seizures, brain herniation, and brain death. These conditions are primarily a result of elevated ICP. Any condition that causes increased ICP (e.g., cerebral edema from stroke; hydrocephalus from increased CSF production; space-occupying tumors or lesions; hepatic encephalopathy) places the patient at increased risk for development of these complications.

Neurogenic (Central) Diabetes Insipidus

Diabetes insipidus (DI) is a condition associated with improper water balance, which is maintained in the body in part because of the secretion of antidiuretic hormone (ADH) by the posterior pituitary gland. DI results from decreased secretion and action of ADH on the regulation of water balance. DI is characterized by polyuria and polydipsia, resulting from either inadequate ADH secretion (central or neurogenic DI) or from a decreased renal response to ADH (nephrogenic DI). Normally, ADH is secreted to prevent diuresis and loss of urine in times of physiological stress (such as hypotension) or in response to increased serum osmolality. In DI associated with TBI, the cause of DI is a loss or decrease in ADH secretion from disruption or damage to the hypothalamus or pituitary from impaired blood supply, or intracranial hypertension compressing these areas of the brain and resulting in polyuria. Any patient with TBI and increased intracranial pressure is at risk of developing central or neurogenic DI.

The range of onset for neurogenic DI due to cerebral injury is between 2 to 10 days following the initial injury (Capatina, Paluzzi, Mitchell, & Karavitaki, 2015). When elevated ICP is relieved, manifestations of DI usually lessen or dissipate. The earliest signs of neurogenic DI include large amounts of pale or clear urine and hypotension. Serum and urine samples are taken before and during a water deprivation test to determine if the cause of the DI is neurogenic or nephrogenic. The classic diagnostic profile of DI includes the production of large amounts (output often in excess of 300–600 mL/hour or 8–16 L/day) of dilute urine (specific gravity less than 1.005; urine osmolality less than plasma osmolality) with an associated increase in serum sodium (greater than 145 mEq/L) and serum osmolality (> 300 mOsm/L). Treatment of DI involves aggressive replacement of intravascular volume with intravenous (IV) fluids and the administration of synthetic antidiuretic hormone (ADH). Administration of ADH may be either in the form of a vasopressin infusion or desmopressin, administered orally or intranasally. Indications of improvement are decreased urine output and increased urine osmolality and specific gravity.

Syndrome of Inappropriate Antidiuresis Hormone

Syndrome of inappropriate antidiuretic hormone (SIADH) increases total body water because excess ADH secretion results in retention of water. The classic profile of SIADH includes the production of small amounts (< 400 mL/day) of concentrated (specific gravity > 1.020) urine with an associated decrease in serum sodium (dilutional hyponatremia). The presence of this hypo-osmolar state results in cellular edema, both systemically and intracerebrally. Cerebral edema increases intracranial pressure, potentiating

secondary injury. Treatment of SIADH involves restricting fluid intake to prevent further dilution of the serum (LeMone et al., 2015). Nursing interventions for the patient with SIADH include monitoring intake and output, neurologic status, and enforcement of fluid restriction.

Cerebral Salt Wasting

Cerebral salt wasting (CSW), also called neurogenic salt wasting, is similar to SIADH because patients present with low serum sodium and a low serum and urine osmolality. However, whereas SIADH represents a state of fluid overload, CSW is a state of hypovolemia. The mechanism of CSW is not well understood but may be related to secretion of atrial natriuretic factor (ANF), a type of peptide that opposes ADH and inhibits ADH release (Leonard et al., 2015). The end result is the loss of sodium into the urine, causing water to follow. It is important to differentiate CSW from SIADH, as restricting fluid in the CSW patient who is already volume depleted can be deleterious. The patient with CSW is treated with salt replacement via IV saline and oral salt tablets. CSW may be self-limiting, correcting itself over the course of 3 to 4 weeks, but in more severe cases, hypertonic saline and fludrocortisones (Florinef) may be used (Leonard et al., 2015). Table 19–8 provides a comparison of diabetes insipidus, syndrome of inappropriate ADH, and cerebral salt wasting.

Seizure Activity

Seizure activity is a complication of traumatic brain injury and can have lasting consequences, even after the patient appears to have returned to the neurologic baseline following TBI. Seizures can occur immediately with brain injury and are due to the direct disruption of cortical and subcortical neurologic function. Posttraumatic seizures are classified as early (occurring within 7 days of the injury) or late (occurring more than 7 days after the injury). Early-onset seizures are more likely due to neurochemical irritation and metabolic derangements. Late-onset seizures are thought to be related to scar tissue and inflammation. Risk factors for early- and late-onset seizures are listed in Table 19–9. There is a close correlation between injury severity and the incidence of seizures (Lucke-Wold et al., 2015). Early-onset seizures may cause increased intracranial pressure, hypoxia, and increased metabolic demands, in turn increasing the severity of secondary injury.

Table 19–8 Summary of Diabetes Insipidus, Syndrome of Inappropriate ADH, and Cerebral Salt Wasting

Value	Normal	DI (neurogenic)	SIADH	CSW
Urine output	1–1.5 L/day	Increased (diuresis)	Decreased (oliguria)	Increased (diuresis)
Urine specific gravity	1.005–1.030	Low	High	Low
Urine osmolality	300–1400 mOsm/L	Low	High	Low
Urine sodium	40–220 mEq/L/24 hr	Low	High	High
Serum ADH	1–5 pg/mL	Low	High	Normal or low
Serum osmolality	280–300 mOsm/L	High	Low	Low
Serum sodium	135–145 mEq/L	High	Low	Low
Fluid volume status	Euvolemia	Hypovolemia	Hypervolemia or euvolemia	Hypovolemia

Table 19–9 Risk Factors for Early and Late-onset Traumatic Seizures

Risk Factor	Early Onset	Late Onset
Acute intracerebral hematoma	X	
Acute subdural hematoma	X	
Loss of consciousness *or* Post-TBI amnesia longer than 30 minutes	X	
Loss of consciousness *or* Post-TBI amnesia longer than 24 hours		X
Age younger than 18 years	X	
Age older than 65 years		X
Severe, diffuse cerebral edema	X	
Skull fractures	X	X
Penetrating skull TBI	X	X
Neurologic deficits following TBI	X	X
Early-onset post-TBI seizures		X
Chronic alcoholism		X

X = risk factor known to increase the risk of seizures at specified time
TBI = Traumatic brain injury

SOURCE: Data from Beaumont (2010).

Table 19–10 Four Herniation Syndromes

Cingulate herniation	Lateral shift of brain tissue, usually as the result of a lesion in one of the cerebral hemispheres
Central or transtentorial herniation	Downward shift of one or both cerebral hemispheres, usually because of lesions in the frontal or parietal lobes
Uncal or lateral transtentorial herniation	Lateral and downward shift of brain tissue, usually the temporal lobe, as a result of lesions located most laterally, such as the middle fossa in the temporal lobe; causes compression of the oculomotor nerve, or cranial nerve III, evidenced by the classic sign of a unilaterally dilated pupil
Infratentorial or tonsillar herniation	Downward shift of brain tissue through the foramen magnum, which results in compression of the medulla and upper cervical spinal cord

Early-onset seizures should be managed with benzodiazepines (e.g., lorazepam) and anticonvulsants, such as phenytoin, carbamazepine, valproate, fosphenytoin, or levetiracetam. If seizures continue, higher doses of anticonvulsant agents may be ordered, and the patient should be intubated with initiation of continuous EEG monitoring. If seizures become prolonged or refractory to conventional anticonvulsant therapies, additional pharmacotherapy, such as continuous IV midazolam or propofol, may be warranted. For continued refractory seizures, it may be necessary to deeply sedate the patient using intravenous pentobarbital to induce coma. The goals of seizure treatment should be to prevent secondary brain injury, maintain patient safety, provide timely administration of anticonvulsant drugs, and support the patient's airway, breathing, and circulation. Seizure management is further detailed in Chapter 17.

Brain Herniation

Brain herniation is a catastrophic complication of traumatic brain injury caused by increased intracranial pressure. Pressure within the confines of the rigid intracranial vault increases as the space within the skull becomes filled with edematous brain tissue, an accumulation of blood, or a combination of both. As space becomes tight, the brain tissue shifts from its normal position in the cranial vault to an area of less pressure. The direction in which the brain herniates depends on the type and location of injury. There are four major forms of herniations: cingulate, central or transtentorial, uncal, and infratentorial.

Cingulate herniation occurs when one hemisphere of the brain is forced across the falx cerebri (the portion of the dura separating the hemispheres) into the space occupied by the contralateral (opposite) hemisphere. This usually occurs as a result of accumulation of blood on one side of the brain, as seen with subarachnoid hemorrhage. *Central or transtentorial herniation* occurs when cerebral swelling forces brain tissue to be displaced downward across the tentorium (the separation between the cerebrum and the cerebellum and medulla). *Uncal herniation* occurs when a lateral mass pushes the brain tissue centrally and forces the medial aspect of the temporal lobe into the tentorial notch. *Infratentorial herniation* occurs when brain tissue is forced into the foramen magnum onto the spinal cord. Herniation syndromes are described based on the end stage of the herniation (Table 19–10) and are depicted in Figure 19–9.

Herniation of any type is devastating as increased pressure is placed on the medulla, where basic functions needed to sustain life are located. During herniation, the nurse will see drastic deterioration patterns in the patient's neurologic status and vital signs. The classic vital sign changes are those of Cushing's triad (refer to Table 19–3). Another important sign of herniation is the classic pupillary pattern of development of unequal pupils with sluggish or no reaction to light and followed by bilateral fixed, fully dilated

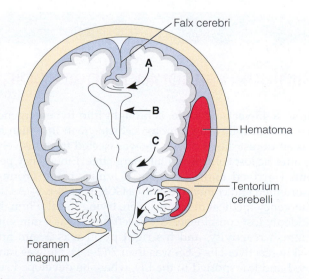

Figure 19–9 Forms of brain herniation. A, Cingulate. B, Central or transtentorial. C, Uncal or lateral transtentorial. D. Infratentorial.

pupils. Management of brain herniation requires emergent interventions to relieve the intracranial pressure, which may include emergency craniectomy. Prevention of herniation is critical to improving outcomes through close monitoring and control of intracranial pressure.

Brain Death

Brain death is an irreversible cessation of all brain activity, including brainstem function. The evolution of TBI to brain death can be both long and, at times, unexpected. Some patients may arrive in the ICU frequently for routine neurologic exams following a seemingly mild or moderate brain injury, and then they experience a rapid decline as a missed or new injury develops. Other patients may survive for weeks as healthcare providers battle elevated ICP

and associated injuries, only to succumb to total cerebral infarction. Brain death is suspected when there is no evidence of brainstem function for up to 24 hours in a patient with a normal temperature who is not under any influence of depressant drugs, paralytics, or alcohol. Signs of impending death include loss of the body's ability to maintain adequate blood pressure, profound bradycardia, and loss of basic neurologic functioning (e.g., fixed and dilated pupils and absence of reflexes). The nurse caring for the patient with suspected or confirmed brain death should provide emotional support to the family and access to a spiritual advisor, if so desired. It is not unusual for the body to continue to exhibit signs of movement after brain death has been established. The movements represent spinal reflexes only, and their significance must be explained to family members.

Section Seven Review

1. Treatment of diabetes insipidus (DI) includes which interventions? (Select all that apply.)
   A. Massive fluid resuscitation
   B. Fluid restriction
   C. Administration of vasopressin
   D. Administration of phenytoin

2. Syndrome of inappropriate ADH (SIADH) is treated with which intervention?
   A. Fluid restriction
   B. Fluid resuscitation
   C. Salt restriction
   D. Potassium replacement

3. Cerebral salt wasting (CSW) is treated with which intervention?
   A. Fluid restriction
   B. Administration of vasopressin
   C. Salt restriction
   D. Salt replacement

4. Which type of herniation results from lateral shift of brain tissue, usually as the result of a lesion in one of the cerebral hemispheres?
   A. Cingate
   B. Transtentorial
   C. Uncal
   D. Infratentorial

Answers: 1. C, 2. A, 3. D, 4. A

Clinical Reasoning Checkpoint

Mr. R, a 45-year-old male, is brought into the emergency department following a motor vehicle crash in which he was an unrestrained driver. He was ejected from his vehicle after he lost control and hit a large tree. Emergency personnel arrived and found Mr. R lying on the ground, disoriented and combative, with a GCS of 14 (4-6-4). As the emergency medical personnel were trying to calm him, he suddenly lost consciousness. His left pupil was 4 mm with sluggish reactivity, and his right pupil was 3 mm and briskly reactive. His GCS was then 7 (2-4-1). He was intubated and transported to the ED, where he developed seizurelike activity upon arrival. His pupils remained unequal, with right 4 mm and left 6 mm and both sluggish to light. His BP was 135/80, and HR was 60/minute. His

ventilator was delivering his breaths at an assist control mode at a rate of 16 breaths per minute.

1. Based on your initial assessment, what health problem, if any, do you suspect? Explain.
2. What diagnostic test(s) would be indicated for Mr. R at this time?

Clinical Update: Mr. R was sent for a CT scan, which revealed a left subdural hematoma (SDH), a small left temporal subarachnoid hemorrhage (SAH), a left temporal nondepressed skull fracture, and a left linear basilar skull fracture. He was transferred to the OR for evacuation of his subdural hematoma and then admitted to the neurosurgical

ICU. While on mechanical ventilation, his arterial blood gas was pH 7.34, $PaCO_2$ 45, PaO_2 188.

3. What aspects of his ABG might contribute to an increased ICP?

Clinical Update: Mr. R's vital signs are stable: HR 98, normal sinus rhythm (NSR), respiratory rate 18, BP 120/72, temperature 97°F, ICP 12, and CPP of 76–80. You note that he has bilateral periorbital ecchymosis (raccoon eyes). After 2 hours, he becomes agitated, able to localize to pain without eye opening, with no verbal response due to intubation. His pupils are now 4 mm and briskly reactive to light bilaterally.

4. What is the patient's current Glasgow Coma Scale?

5. What should the nurse monitor frequently?

Clinical Update: After 24 hours, Mr. R begins to have episodes during which his ICP increases to 32 and his CPP is 54. An external ventricular drain is placed.

6. What initial nonpharmacologic nursing interventions should be tried to reduce his ICP?

7. What is the benefit of the ventricular drain? What additional interventions could be used to help control his ICP?

8. What are the potential complications of traumatic brain injury?

Chapter 19 Review

1. A client is admitted after being struck in the right side of the head with a baseball bat. An MRI shows the presence of focal injury and diffuse axonal injury (DAI). Which mechanism of injury is likely to have occurred?
   1. Acceleration
   2. Deceleration
   3. Rotation
   4. Penetration

2. A client was admitted to the emergency department after a traumatic brain injury. Current assessment included a decrease in Glasgow Coma Scale by 1 point and development of a fixed and dilated pupil. What should the nurse do first?
   1. Plan to reassess the client in 15 minutes.
   2. Call the healthcare provider immediately.
   3. Continue to prepare the client for an ordered CT scan.
   4. Inform the family of the status changes.

3. A client fell on an icy sidewalk a week ago, striking the head on the curb. The CT scan reveals an accumulation of blood between the dura and the arachnoid covering of the brain. The nurse would prepare to care for a client with which diagnosis?
   1. Subdural hematoma
   2. Epidural hematoma
   3. Subarachnoid hematoma
   4. Intracerebral hematoma

4. A client sustained a brain injury when struck by a falling tree limb. Upon admission to the emergency department (ED), the client's Glasgow Coma Scale score was 10. What interventions will the ED nurse expect to manage? (Select all that apply.)
   1. Explanation of brain injury surveillance as discharge instructions
   2. Skull x-rays

   3. CT scan
   4. Hospital admission
   5. Placement of an indwelling urinary catheter

5. A client has an expanding epidural hematoma and is taken to the OR to have it evacuated. The client returns to the ICU ventilated and with an intraventricular catheter in place. According to American College of Surgeons Guidelines, what is the minimal cerebral perfusion pressure (CPP) desired to reduce secondary injury in this client?
   1. 50 mmHg
   2. 60 mmHg
   3. 70 mmHg
   4. 80 mmHg

6. A client who sustained a traumatic brain injury develops abrupt hypertension, bradycardia, and an irregular breathing pattern. The nurse immediately collaborates with the healthcare provider for which reason?
   1. The client needs additional pain medication.
   2. Anxiety is building that may cause additional problems.
   3. Herniation may be occurring.
   4. Brain death is occurring.

7. A client in the ICU who sustained a traumatic brain injury is being mechanically ventilated. Which nursing interventions should be implemented to manage increased intracranial pressure? (Select all that apply.)
   1. Position the client supine with head of bed flat.
   2. Preoxygenate the client if suctioning is needed.
   3. Keep the client's neck in a neutral position.
   4. Elevate the head of the bed by 30 degrees.
   5. Provide pain medication.

8. The nurse has attempted to control a client's increased intracranial pressure with tier one interventions, but the attempt has failed. The nurse discusses this situation with the neurosurgeon and anticipates which order?

   1. Preparing the client for an emergent decompressive craniectomy
   2. Administering hypertonic saline by IV bolus
   3. Administering DDAVP
   4. Aggressively hyperventilating the client

9. A 16-year-old football player sustained a mild concussion and was brought to the ED. Loss of consciousness lasted about 5 minutes. Which interventions would the nurse plan to provide for this client? (Select all that apply.)

   1. Observing the client in the ED for 1 to 2 hours
   2. Providing the parents with brain injury observation instructions before discharge
   3. Providing the nurse on the unit with a detailed client report when admitting the client to the hospital
   4. Discussing the possibility of postconcussive syndrome with the client and parents
   5. Administering IV mannitol (Osmitrol)

10. A 67-year-old client who is an alcoholic and smokes two packages of cigarettes a day sustained a skull fracture when he passed out and struck his head on a sidewalk. The client was released from the hospital 3 weeks ago with some lingering neurological deficits from the accident. Today, the client presents to the ED after having a seizure. The nurse admitting this client identifies which risk factors for late-seizure development in this client's history? (Select all that apply.)

    1. Age under 70 years
    2. Tobacco use
    3. Alcoholism
    4. Skull fracture
    5. Neurological deficit from the accident

Answers to questions found inside your textbook are available on the faculty resources site. Please consult with your instructor.

References

American College of Radiology. (2013). ACR appropriateness criteria: Headache. Retrieved March 17, 2017, from https://acsearch.acr.org/docs/69482/Narrative

American College of Surgeons, Trauma Quality Improvement Program. (2015). Best practices in the management of traumatic brain injury. Retrieved March 27, 2017, from https://www.facs.org/~/media/files/quality%20programs/trauma/tqip/traumatic%20brain%20injury%20guidelines.ashx

Bagalman, E. (2013). *Traumatic brain injury among veterans: CRS Report for Congress.* Congressional Research Service. Retrieved March 27, 2017, from http://www.ncsl.org/documents/statefed/health/TBI_Vets2013.pdf

Beaumont, A. (2010). Traumatic brain injury and seizures in the intensive care unit. In P. Varelas (Ed.), *Seizures in critical care: A guide to diagnoses and therapeutics* (2nd ed., pp. 119–136). New York, NY: Springer.

Boone, M. D., Oren-Grinberg, A., Robinson, T. M., Chen, C. C., & Kasper, E. M. (2015). Mannitol or hypertonic saline in the setting of traumatic brain injury: What have we learned? *Surgical Neurology International, 6,* 177.

Brain Trauma Foundation (BTF). (2012). TBI statistics. Retrieved September 20, 2016, from https://www.braintrauma.org/tbi-faqs/tbi-statistics

Capatina, C., Paluzzi, A., Mitchell, R., & Karavitaki, N. (2015). Diabetes insipidus after traumatic brain injury. *Journal of Clinical Medicine, 4*(7), 1448–1462.

Carney, N., Totten, A. M., O'Reilly, C., Ullman, J. S., Hawryluk, G., Bell, M. J., . . . Ghajar, J. (2016). *Guidelines for the management of severe traumatic brain injury* (4th ed.). Brain Trauma Foundation. Retrieved March 27, 2017, from https://braintrauma.org/uploads/03/12/Guidelines_for_Management_of_Severe_TBI_4th_Edition.pdf

Centers for Disease Control and Prevention (CDC). (2010). *Rates of TBI deaths by sex—United States, 2001–2010.* Retrieved March 27, 2017, from http://www.cdc.gov/traumaticbraininjury/data/rates_deaths_bysex.html

Chamoun, R. B., Robertson, C. S., & Gopinath, S. P. (2009). Outcome in patients with blunt head trauma and a Glasgow Coma Scale score of 3 at presentation. *Journal of Neurosurgery, 111*(4), 683–687.

Cook, C. J. (2017). Induced hypothermia in neurocritical care: A review. *Journal of Neuroscience Nursing, 49*(1), 5–11.

Corrigan, J., Selassie, A., & Orman, J. (2010). The epidemiology of traumatic brain injury. *Journal of Head Trauma Rehabilitation, 25*(2), 72–80. doi:10.1097/HTR.0b013e3181ccc8b4

Eliyahu, L., Kirkland, S., Campbell, S., & Rowe, B. H. (2016). The effectiveness of early educational interventions in the emergency department to reduce incidence or severity of post-concussion syndrome following a concussion: A systematic review. *Academic Emergency Medicine, 23*(5), 531–542. doi:10.1111/acem.12924

Faul, M., Xu, L., Wald, M., & Coronado, V. (2010). *Traumatic brain injury in the United States.* Atlanta, GA: Centers for Disease Control and Prevention, National Center for Injury Prevention and Control. Retrieved January 23, 2013, from http://www.cdc.gov/traumaticbraininjury/pdf/blue_book.pdf

Gaist, D., Rodriguez, L. A. G., Hellfritzsch, M., Poulson, F. R., Halle, B., Hallas, J., & Pottegard, A. (2017). Association of antithrombotic drug use with subdural hematoma risk. *JAMA 317*(8), 836–846.

Halpern, C. H., & Grady, M. (2015). Neurosurgery. In F. Brunicardi, D. K. Andersen, T. R. Billiar, D. L. Dunn, J. G. Hunter, J. B. Matthews, & R. E. Pollock (Eds.), *Schwartz's principles of surgery (10th ed.)*. New York, NY: McGraw-Hill. Retrieved March 10, 2017, from http://accessmedicine.mhmedical.com.ezproxy .uky.edu/content.aspx?bookid=980&sectionid =59610884

Harris, C. (2016). Neuromonitoring and assessment. *Critical Care Nursing Clinics, 28*(1), 1–136.

Hickey, J. V. (2014). *The clinical practice of neurological and neurosurgical nursing* (7th ed.). Philadelphia, PA: Lippincott Williams & Wilkins.

Korley, F. K., Diaz-Arrastia, R., Wu, A. H., Yue, J. K., Manley, G. T., Sair, H. I., . . . Schyner, D. M. (2016). Circulating brain-derived neurotrophic factor has diagnostic and prognostic value in traumatic brain injury. *Journal of Neurotrauma, 33,* 215–225.

Kurland, D. B., Khaladj-Ghom, A., Stokum, J. A., Carusillo, B., Karimy, J. K., Gerzanich, V., . . . Simard, J. M. (2015). Complications associated with decompressive craniectomy: A systematic review. *Neurocritical Care, 23*(2), 292–304.

Layon, A. J., Gabrielli, A., & Friedman, W. A. (2013). *Textbook of neurointensive care* (2nd ed.). New York, NY: Springer.

LeMone, P., Burke, K., Bauldoff, G., & Gubrud, P. (2015). Chapter 42: Nursing care of patients with intracranial disorders. In P. LeMone, K. Burke, G. Bauldoff, & P. Gubrud (Eds.), *Medical surgical nursing: Clinical reasoning in patient care* (6th ed., pp. 1382–1389). Hoboken, NJ: Pearson Education.

Leonard, J., Garrett, R. E., Salottolo, K., Slone, D. S., Mains, C. W., Carrick, M. M., & Bar-Or, D. (2015). Cerebral salt wasting after traumatic brain injury: A review of the literature. *Scandinavian Journal of Trauma, Resuscitation, & Emergency Medicine, 23,* 98.

Lucke-Wold, B. P., Nguyen, L., Turner, R. C., Logsdon, A. F., Chen, Y. W., Smith, K. E., . . . Richter, E. (2015). Traumatic brain injury and epilepsy: Underlying mechanisms leading to seizure. *Seizure, 33,* 13–23.

Ma, V. Y., Chan, L., & Carruthers, K. J. (2014). Incidence, prevalence, costs, and impact on disability of common conditions requiring rehabilitation in the United States: Stroke, spinal cord injury, traumatic brain injury, multiple sclerosis, osteoarthritis, rheumatoid arthritis, limb loss, and back pain. *Archives of Physical Medicine and Rehabilitation, 95,* 986–995.

McMahon, P. J., Hricik, A., Yue, J. K., Puccio, A. M., Inoue, T., Lingsma, H. F., . . . Vassar, M. J. (2014). Symptomatology and functional outcome in mild traumatic brain injury: Results from the prospective TRACK-TBI study. *Journal of Neurotrauma, 31,* 26–33.

Munakomi, S., & Kumar, B. M. (2015). Neuroanatomical basis of Glasgow Coma Scale—A reappraisal. *Neuroscience & Medicine, 6*(3), 116–120.

National Institute of Neurological Disorders and Stroke (NINDS). (2012). *NINDS traumatic brain injury information.* Retrieved March 27, 2017, from http:// www.ninds.nih.gov/disorders/tbi/tbi.htm

Navi, J., Yap, K. H, Ahmad, G., & Gsosh, J. (2013). Transcranial Doppler ultrasound: A review of the physical principles and major applications in critical care. *International Journal of Vascular Medicine, 2013,* 1–13.

Oddo, M., Frangos, S., Maloney-Wilensky, E., Andrew Kofke, W., Le Roux, P. D., & Levine, J. M. (2010). Effect of shivering on brain tissue oxygenation during induced normothermia in patients with severe brain injury. *Neurocritical Care. 12*(1), 10–16. doi:10.1007 /s12028-009-9280-2.

Osborn, K. S., Wraa, C. E., Watson, A. B., & Holleran, R. S. (2014). Chapter 21: Caring for the patient with an acute brain or cranial nerve disorder. In K. S. Osborn, C. E. Wraa, & A. B. Watson (Eds.), *Medical Surgical Nursing: Preparation for Practice.* Hoboken, NJ: Pearson Education.

Perez, A. M., Adler, J., Kulkarni, N., Strain, J. F., Womack, K. B., Diaz-Arrastia, R., & Marquez de la Plata, C. D. (2014). Longitudinal white matter changes after traumatic axonal injury. *Journal of Neurotrauma, 31,* 1478–1485.

Prabhakar, H., Sandhu, K., Bhagat, H., Durga, P., & Chawla, R. (2014). Current concepts of optimal cerebral perfusion pressure in traumatic brain injury. *Journal of Anaesthesiology Clinical Pharmacology, 30*(3), 318–327.

Rosenthal, G., Furmanov, A., Itshayek, E., Shoshan, Y., & Singh, V. (2014). Assessment of a noninvasive cerebral oxygenation monitor in patients with severe traumatic brain injury. *Journal of Neurosurgery, 120,* 901–907.

Sorrentino, E., Diedler, J., & Kasprowicz, M. (2012). Critical thresholds for cerebrovascular reactivity after traumatic brain injury. *Neurocritical Care, 16*(2), 258–266.

Urbano, L. A., & Oddo, M. (2012). Therapeutic hypothermia for traumatic brain injury. *Current Neurology and Neuroscience Reports, 12*(5), 580–591.

Wang, H. S., Kim, S. W., & Kim, S. H. (2013). Spontaneous chronic subdural hematoma in an adolescent girl. *Journal of Korean Neurosurgical Society, 53*(3), 201–203.

West, T. A., Bergman, K., Biggins, M. S., French, B., Galletly, J., Hinkle, J. L., & Morris, J. (2011). Care of the patient with mild traumatic brain injury: AANN and ARN clinical practice guideline series. Retrieved March 28, 2017, from http://www.aann.org/pubs /content/guidelines.html

Wiegand, D. L. (2011). *AACN procedure manual for critical care* (6th ed.). St. Louis, MO: Saunders.

Wright, D. W., & Merck, L. H. (2016). Chapter 257: Head trauma. In J. E. Tintinalli (Ed.), *Emergency medicine: A comprehensive study guide* (8th ed., pp. 1695–1707). New York, NY: McGraw-Hill.

Zhao, Z., Wang, D., Jia, Y., Tian, Y., Wang, Y., Wei, Y., . . . Jiang, R. (2016). Analysis of the association of fluid balance and short-term outcome in traumatic brain injury. *Journal of the Neurological Sciences, 364,* 12–18.

Zheng, X., Chen, M., Li, J., & Cao, F. (2013). Prognosis in prolonged coma patients with diffuse axonal injury assessed by somatosensory evoked potential. *Neural Regeneration Research, 8*(10), 948–954.

Chapter 20
Acute Spinal Cord Injury

Learning Outcomes

20.1 Explain anatomic features of the spinal cord and vertebrae, including unstable spinal cord injury.

20.2 Discuss spinal cord injury, including types of injury and primary and secondary injury.

20.3 Describe physical assessment techniques and diagnostic tests frequently used to identify the type and severity of spinal cord injury.

20.4 Discuss stabilization techniques used for spinal cord injuries.

20.5 Identify priority nursing assessments and interventions for the patient with a spinal cord injury in the acute care phase of recovery.

This chapter focuses on adult patients in the acute phase of spinal cord injury. During the initial phase following injury, the patient undergoes a cascade of fairly predictable pathophysiologic events based on the level and severity of injury. Gaining an understanding of these events and how they are assessed and managed will help the nurse to care for patients with this disorder in a high-acuity environment.

Section One: Spinal Cord Anatomy and Physiology

The vertebral (spinal) column performs two major functions: protection of the spinal cord and support of the body frame. The spinal cord transmits neural impulses from the brain to the rest of the body and also coordinates reflexes independent of the brain. This section provides a brief review of vertebral and spinal cord anatomy and neuronal function.

Vertebral Column

The spine is composed of 33 individual and fused vertebrae. There are 7 cervical (C), 12 thoracic (T), and 5 lumbar (L) vertebrae. The 5 sacral and 4 coccygeal vertebrae are fused in the adult. Each vertebra consists of a body (anterior) and

an arch (posterior). The arch section is composed of two pedicles that attach the arch to the body and two laminae that form the roof of the arch. The spinous process is located at the rear of the vertebra. In order to bear additional weight, vertebral bodies increase in size as they descend from C1 through L5.

As illustrated in Figure 20–1, the spine is composed of three columns: an anterior column that includes the anterior part of the vertebral body, a middle column that houses the posterior wall of the vertebral body, and a posterior column that includes the vertebral arch. If two or more of these columns are damaged, the injury is considered unstable. In an **unstable spinal injury** the vertebral and ligamentous structures are unable to support and protect the injured area.

Spinal Cord

The spinal cord runs through the center of the vertebral column through the spinal canal. It starts at the foramen magnum of the brain and ends at the first or second lumbar vertebra (Figure 20–2). The C1 through C7 spinal nerves exit above the correspondingly numbered vertebrae; however, the C8 spinal nerve exits below the C7 vertebra. The spinal nerves of T1 and below exit below the correspondingly numbered vertebra. The spinal nerves join complex networks after leaving the cord to innervate parts of the body. The brain and spinal cord are surrounded by a

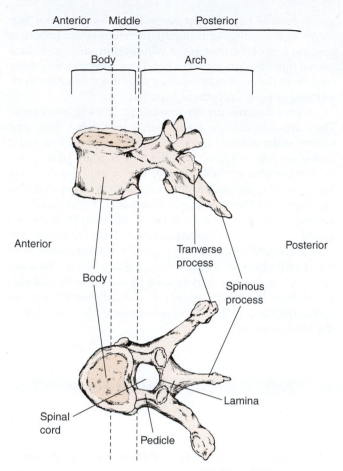

Figure 20–1 A lateral view and cross-section of a vertebra.

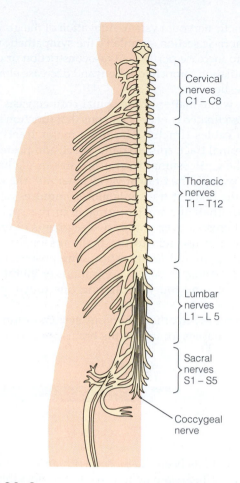

Figure 20–2 Distribution of spinal nerves.

protective, relatively tough membrane: the meninges. There are three meningeal layers: the dura mater (outermost), the arachnoid mater (middle), and the pia mater (innermost). Between the arachnoid mater and the pia mater is the sub-arachnoid space, which contains cerebrospinal fluid.

The primary vascular supply of the cervical spinal cord is the vertebral arteries. The anterior and posterior arteries supply the majority of the cord below this area. Any disruption in this vascular supply may damage the cord without direct physical trauma.

Spinal Cord Neuronal Function

The spinal cord consists of an outer region of white matter and an inner region of gray matter (Figure 20–3). The gray matter contains motor neurons that transmit motor impulses from the brain to the body, specifically the muscles (anterior column). It also serves as a relay station for sensory messages from the body to the brain (posterior column). In the first thoracic section through the second lumbar section of the cord, the gray matter gives rise to the

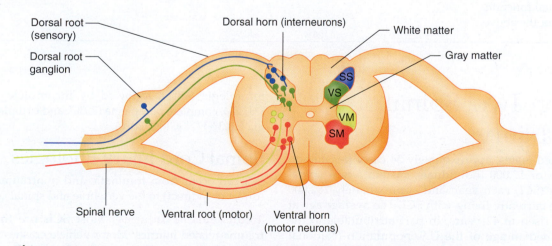

Figure 20–3 Structural components of the spinal cord (cross-sectional view).

sympathetic nervous system. Activation of the gray matter in the thoracic section stimulates the sympathetic nervous system to increase perfusion (vasoconstriction or dilation) and ventilation (bronchodilation) and decrease elimination and digestion.

The white matter of the spinal cord consists of insulated (myelinated) nerve-cell axons that function as transmission cables (tracts). The three major tracts are the corticospinal tract, spinothalamic tract, and posterior column. The corticospinal tract originates in the brain and crosses over in the brainstem to innervate the opposite side of the body. It transmits motor impulses or signals. The spinothalamic tract originates in the spinal cord, where it crosses over within two segments of entry into the cord and ascends to the thalamus in the brain. It transmits pain and temperature. The posterior column (dorsal columns) carries the sensations of vibration, proprioception, and touch, including fine touch, pressure, and texture.

The parasympathetic nervous system originates in a group of neurons located in the brainstem and in another group located between the second and fourth sacral segments of the cord. Parasympathetic stimulation produces specific responses that assist elimination, digestion, and sexual function, among other functions. Damage to specific regions of the cord may produce alterations in either sympathetic or parasympathetic function.

Motor neurons are responsible for muscle movement. They are classified in a two-tiered hierarchy: first- and second-order motor neurons. The cell bodies of first-order motor neurons are located in the motor center of the cerebral cortex and are called upper motor neurons (UMNs). These neurons do not leave the central nervous system and are responsible for voluntary movement. The cell bodies of second-order neurons are located in the brain stem and are called lower motor neurons (LMNs). These neurons connect to the UMNs through synapses in the brainstem or in the anterior horn of the spinal cord. The LMN axons leave the CNS as spinal nerves and synapse with muscles throughout the body. Damage to the anterior horn of the spinal cord severs the LMN connection to the brain below the level of injury.

Section One Review

1. A client has been diagnosed with an unstable spinal injury. Which statement correctly describes this specific type of injury?
   A. The reflex center for bowel function has been injured.
   B. The vertebral structures are unable to support the injured area.
   C. The client has multiple spinal fractures.
   D. The main blood supply to the spinal cord is disrupted.

2. The end of the spinal cord contains reflex centers for which function?
   A. Bowel function
   B. Bladder function
   C. Sexual function
   D. All of the above

3. Activation of the thoracic-section gray matter stimulates which structure?
   A. Sympathetic nervous system
   B. Parasympathetic nervous system
   C. Brainstem
   D. Spinothalamic tract

4. Which statement correctly describes lower motor neurons?
   A. Their cell bodies are located in the cerebral cortex.
   B. They are located only in the CNS.
   C. Their axons synapse with muscles.
   D. They work independent of the brain.

Answers: 1. B, 2. D, 3. A, 4. C

Section Two: Spinal Cord Injury

In the United States, approximately 54 cases per million population, or 17,000 individuals, sustain a new spinal cord injury (SCI) each year, and approximately 282,000 persons are currently living with SCI. The average age at injury has risen to 42 years, in part attributable to the increased median age of the U.S. population (National Spinal Cord Injury Statistical Center [NSCISC], 2016). The most frequent neurological level of injury is incomplete tetraplegia (45%), followed by incomplete paraplegia (21.3%), complete paraplegia (20%), and complete tetraplegia (13.3%) (NSCISC, 2016).

Spinal Cord Injury Etiologies

SCI can occur from traumatic and nontraumatic insults (direct or indirect) to the vertebrae and spinal cord.

Trauma-related Injuries   Most SCIs are the result of trauma-related injuries. Motor vehicle crashes account for 38% of SCI cases. The next most common cause is falls (30.5%), followed by acts of violence (13.5%, primarily gunshot wounds), and sports/recreation activities (9%) (NSCISC, 2016). After injury, pneumonia and septicemia are the most frequent causes of death. The mortality rate for septicemia has not changed in the past 40 years, with only a slight decrease in mortality due to respiratory diseases. Prognosis is poorest for individuals over the age of 50 with complete lesions at the time of injury. For severely injured persons, mortality rates are significantly higher during the first year after injury than in subsequent years.

Nontrauma-related Injuries   While some form of trauma accounts for the majority of SCIs, there are also important nontraumatic causes. Several conditions may produce narrowing of the spinal canal and subsequent SCI. Degenerative changes as a result of osteoarthritis in the spine predispose a person to hyperextension injuries. Ankylosing spondylitis (calcification of ligaments and soft tissue) and rheumatoid arthritis (inflammation causing osteoporosis and decreased mobility) are two causes of SCI. Space-occupying lesions (abscesses and solid tumors) may produce spinal cord compression. Lymphoma and multiple myeloma are two oncologic conditions associated with bone metastases. The first sign of spinal cord compression from tumor growth is usually a constant, dull back pain aggravated by coughing or sneezing. Leg weakness, urinary retention, and sexual dysfunction may also develop.

Acute spinal cord infarction is an uncommon but clinically significant disease. Onset often occurs suddenly, evolving over minutes. Typically there is sudden and severe back pain that radiates caudally along with weakness, tingling, and numbness distal to the point of cord injury. Vascular disease of the aorta is the most common cause of spinal cord infarction. Other risk factors include atherosclerosis, a vasculitic process such as syphilitica giant cell arteritis, cardiogenic embolism, hypoxia, sickle cell disease, polycythemia, vasoactive drug use (cocaine), and hypercoagulable states.

In regions where scuba and deep sea diving is a commercial or recreational activity, SCI may result as a complication of pressure decompression, whereby an inert gas embolism forms in the spinal cord and epidural vertebral venous plexus, resulting in spinal cord congestive infarction (Van Hoesen & Bird, 2012).

Spinal Cord Injury Classification

SCI may be described as **complete spinal cord injury** (loss of all voluntary motor and sensory function below the level of injury) caused by damage to the entire level of the spinal cord or as **incomplete spinal cord injury** (preservation of some sensory or motor function below the level of injury because of partial damage to the spinal cord). The injury is identified by vertebral level according to the International Standards for Neurological Classification of Spinal Cord Injury (ISNCSCI) developed by the American Spinal Injury Association (American Spinal Injury Association [ASIA], n.d.-a). Using the ASIA Impairment Scale (AIS) allows standardized examination and consistent assessment (see Figure 20–4)—for example, a C5 AIS B classification SCI is at the fifth cervical vertebrae with some sensation preserved below the level of the injury and minimum sensation

around the rectum (S4–S5). Of patients admitted to high-acuity units, 45.5% have complete SCI, and 43.6% have a complete SCI on discharge from rehabilitation. Fewer than 1% experience complete neurologic recovery by discharge from the hospital (NSCISC, 2015).

Complete Spinal Cord Injury   Complete SCI results in one of two conditions: paraplegia or tetraplegia. **Paraplegia** is the result of injury to the thoracolumbar region (T1–L1) that causes loss of motor and sensory function of the lower extremities. Upper-extremity function remains intact. **Tetraplegia** (also referred to as **quadriplegia**) is the result of injury to the cervical regions (C1–C8). Muscle function depends on the specific segments involved, but impaired function of the arms, trunk, legs, and pelvic organs may occur. Figure 20–5 compares the extent of paralysis with level of injury.

Incomplete Spinal Cord Injury   The alterations in function that occur as a result of an incomplete SCI vary greatly, depending on the amount and location of tissue damage and the level of injury. Damage to a UMN pathway results in loss of cerebral control over reflex activity below the lesion level. UMNs may become hyperactive to local stimuli, producing **spastic paralysis**, in which the muscles are affected by persistent spasms and exaggerated tendon reflexes. Damage to LMNs produces **flaccid paralysis**, characterized by weakness, loss of motor tone, and no reflexes. Types of incomplete SCIs are described in Table 20–1. Note that each syndrome has evidence of partially interrupted motor and sensory pathways.

Spinal Cord Injury Level   Spinal cord injuries are also identified based on where on the vertebral column the cord has been damaged. For example, in a C2 injury the cord is damaged at the level of the second cervical vertebrae; a T5 injury is located at the level of the fifth thoracic vertebrae.

Cervical Injuries.   The cervical region is the most vulnerable region of the spine because of its poor stability. Complete cord injuries at the C1 or C2 level are often fatal because the patient is unable to breathe spontaneously. Hyperflexion injuries of the cervical spine, especially C5 to C6, are associated with the rapid deceleration mechanism of injury; C4 and C5 injuries frequently occur in diving accidents.

Thoracic and Lumbar Injuries.   Great force is needed to produce T1 through T10 injuries because of the stability of the rib cage. The most common site of thoracic spinal injury is the T12–L1 junction. Flexion may occur with compression of the anterior aspects of the vertebrae. A fall onto the upper back can produce flexion along with rotation. Thoracic region injuries may result from vertical compression forces experienced during a fall onto the buttocks or feet. A patient with calcaneus fractures of the feet should be suspected of having thoracic vertebral or cord damage. The same forces producing thoracic injuries may be responsible for lumbar injuries. Violent flexion of the lumbar spine may occur when wearing a lap belt without a shoulder restraint (e.g., middle passenger in the rear seat) in a motor vehicle crash.

Muscle Function Grading

0 = total paralysis

1 = palpable or visible contraction

2 = active movement, full range of motion (ROM) with gravity eliminated

3 = active movement, full ROM against gravity

4 = active movement, full ROM against gravity and moderate resistance in a muscle specific position

5 = (normal) active movement, full ROM against gravity and full resistance in a functional muscle position expected from an otherwise unimpaired person

5* = (normal) active movement, full ROM against gravity and sufficient resistance to be considered normal if identified inhibiting factors (i.e. pain, disuse) were not present

NT = not testable (i.e. due to immobilization, severe pain such that the patient cannot be graded, amputation of limb, or contracture of > 50% of the normal ROM)

Sensory Grading

0 = Absent

1 = Altered, either decreased/impaired sensation or hypersensitivity

2 = Normal

NT = Not testable

When to Test Non-Key Muscles:

In a patient with an apparent AIS B classification, non-key muscle functions more than 3 levels below the motor level on each side should be tested to most accurately classify the injury (differentiate between AIS B and C).

Movement	Root level
Shoulder: Flexion, extension, abduction, adduction, internal and external rotation	
Elbow: Supination	C5
Elbow: Pronation	
Wrist: Flexion	C6
Finger: Flexion at proximal joint, extension.	
Thumb: Flexion, extension and abduction in plane of thumb	C7
Finger: Flexion at MCP joint	
Thumb: Opposition, adduction and abduction perpendicular to palm	C8
Finger: Abduction of the index finger	T1
Hip: Adduction	L2
Hip: External rotation	L3
Hip: Extension, abduction, internal rotation	
Knee: Flexion	
Ankle: Inversion and eversion	L4
Toe: MP and IP extension	
Hallux and Toe: DIP and PIP flexion and abduction	L5
Hallux: Adduction	S1

ASIA Impairment Scale (AIS)

A = Complete. No sensory or motor function is preserved in the sacral segments S4-5.

B = Sensory Incomplete. Sensory but not motor function is preserved below the neurological level and includes the sacral segments S4-5 (light touch or pin prick at S4-5 or deep anal pressure) AND no motor function is preserved more than three levels below the motor level on either side of the body.

C = Motor Incomplete. Motor function is preserved at the most caudal sacral segments for voluntary anal contraction (VAC) OR the patient meets the criteria for sensory incomplete status (sensory function preserved at the most caudal sacral segments (S4-S5) by LT, PP or DAP), and has some sparing of motor function more than three levels below the ipsilateral motor level on either side of the body.

(This includes key or non-key muscle functions to determine motor incomplete status.) For AIS C – less than half of key muscle functions below the single NLI have a muscle grade ≥ 3.

D = Motor Incomplete. Motor incomplete status as defined above, with at least half (half or more) of key muscle functions below the single NLI having a muscle grade ≥ 3.

E = Normal. If sensation and motor function as tested with the ISNCSCI are graded as normal in all segments, and the patient had prior deficits, then the AIS grade is E. Someone without an initial SCI does not receive an AIS grade.

Using ND: To document the sensory, motor and NLI levels, the ASIA Impairment Scale grade, and/or the zone of partial preservation (ZPP) when they are unable to be determined based on the examination results.

Steps in Classification

The following order is recommended for determining the classification of individuals with SCI.

1. Determine sensory levels for right and left sides.
The sensory level is the most caudal, intact dermatome for both pin prick and light touch sensation.

2. Determine motor levels for right and left sides.
Defined by the lowest key muscle function that has a grade of at least 3 (on supine testing), providing the key muscle functions represented by segments above that level are judged to be intact (graded as a 5).
Note: in regions where there is no myotome to test, the motor level is presumed to be the same as the sensory level, if testable motor function above that level is also normal.

3. Determine the neurological level of injury (NLI)
This refers to the most caudal segment of the cord with intact sensation and antigravity (3 or more) muscle function strength, provided that there is normal (intact) sensory and motor function rostrally respectively.
The NLI is the most cephalad of the sensory and motor levels determined in steps 1 and 2.

4. Determine whether the injury is Complete or Incomplete.
(i.e. absence or presence of sacral sparing)
If voluntary anal contraction = **No** AND all S4-5 sensory scores = **0** AND deep anal pressure = **No**, then injury is **Complete.** Otherwise, injury is **Incomplete.**

5. Determine ASIA Impairment Scale (AIS) Grade:

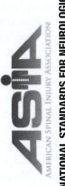

Is injury Complete?   If YES, AIS=A   and can record ZPP (lowest dermatome or myotome on each side with some preservation)

NO ↓

Is injury Motor Complete?   If YES, AIS=B

NO ↓

(No=voluntary anal contraction OR motor function more than three levels below the motor level on a given side, if the patient has sensory incomplete classification)

Are at least half (half or more) of the key muscles below the neurological level of injury graded 3 or better?

NO ↓   YES ↓

AIS=C   AIS=D

If sensation and motor function is normal in all segments, AIS=E

Note: AIS E is used in follow-up testing when an individual with a documented SCI has recovered normal function. If at initial testing no deficits are found, the individual is neurologically intact; the ASIA Impairment Scale does not apply.

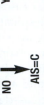

AMERICAN SPINAL INJURY ASSOCIATION

INTERNATIONAL STANDARDS FOR NEUROLOGICAL CLASSIFICATION OF SPINAL CORD INJURY

ISCOS
INTERNATIONAL SPINAL CORD SOCIETY

Figure 20-4 ASIA Impairment Scale.

SOURCE: American Spinal Injury Association: International Standard for Neurological Classification of Spinal Cord Injury, revised 2016; Atlanta, GA. Reprinted 2016.

**Levels of Injury and
Extent of Paralysis**

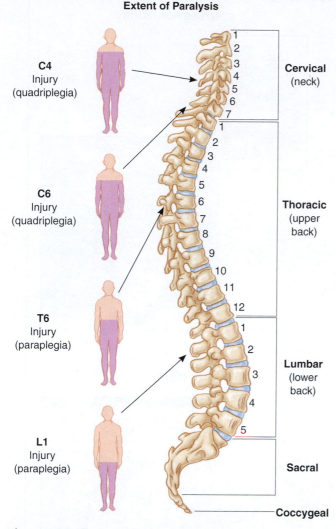

Figure 20–5 Spinal injury levels.

Table 20–1 Incomplete Spinal Cord Injury Syndromes
Cord Injury Syndromes

Syndrome	Functions Lost	Functions Present
Anterior cord	Motor function below level of injury, pain, temperature, touch	Proprioception, vibration, and pressure sense
Brown–Séquard	Loss of voluntary motor movement on same side as injury; loss of pain, temperature, sensation on the opposite side (below the level of injury)	Side of the body with the best motor control has little or no sensation
Central cord	Variable motor function of lower extremities, sensory deficit in upper extremities, often spastic	Motor, sensory pathways in lower extremities; some bladder, bowel function
Posterior cord	Proprioception, vibration sensation below the level of injury	Motor function, sense of pain and light touch

columns, and torn posterior muscles and ligaments cannot support the spinal column.

Hyperextension Injury. Hyperextension injuries are caused by a forward and backward motion of the head (e.g., rear-end collisions). With this injury, the anterior ligaments are torn and the spinal cord is stretched. A mild form of hyperextension injury is the whiplash injury.

Flexion–rotation Injury. A flexion–rotation injury is caused by excessive lateral (twisting) movement, usually of the head on its axis. This motion causes shearing and tearing of the posterior ligaments and rotation of the spinal column. Examples of rotation injuries include sports injuries and those incurred by nonbelted persons in a car hit broadside.

Compression Injury. A compression, or axial-loading, injury is caused by a vertical force along the spinal cord that fractures vertebral bodies and sends bony fragments into the cord. Compression fractures typically occur with diving into shallow water or jumping from tall heights and landing on the feet or buttocks.

Distraction Injury. A distraction injury occurs when the vertebrae and spinal cord are stretched excessively, pulling the structures apart. The major example of this type of injury is hanging.

Secondary Injury   Secondary SCI refers to the multifaceted pathological mechanisms that start after the primary SCI that can last from days to weeks. These secondary injuries can include edema, bleeding, and ischemic injury to the cord. There can be a breakdown of the blood–spinal cord barrier, neuroinflammation, oxidative stress, neuronal injury, and ischemic dysfunction (Anwar, Shehabi, & Eid, 2016). The 24-hour period immediately following SCI involves a series of pathophysiologic processes that cause cellular membrane destruction and are

Mechanisms of Injury

Like traumatic brain injuries, SCIs occur as a result of primary and secondary injury.

Primary Injury   Primary injury to the spinal cord occurs when excessive force is applied to the cord; it is the neurologic damage that occurs at the moment of impact. Primary SCIs are caused by violent motions of the head and trunk, fracture or dislocation of the vertebral column, and blunt or penetrating trauma. Mechanisms of injury include hyperflexion, hyperextension, flexion–rotation, and compression (axial loading). Figure 20–6 illustrates each of the primary mechanisms of injury.

Hyperflexion Injury. Hyperflexion injury is most often caused by a sudden deceleration of the motion of the head (e.g., head-on collision). This forcible bending forward dislocates anterior vertebrae, tears posterior ligaments, and compresses the cord. As described in Section One, the vertebral column is composed of three structural columns: anterior, middle, and posterior. An unstable spine results when loss of integrity occurs in two of the three structural

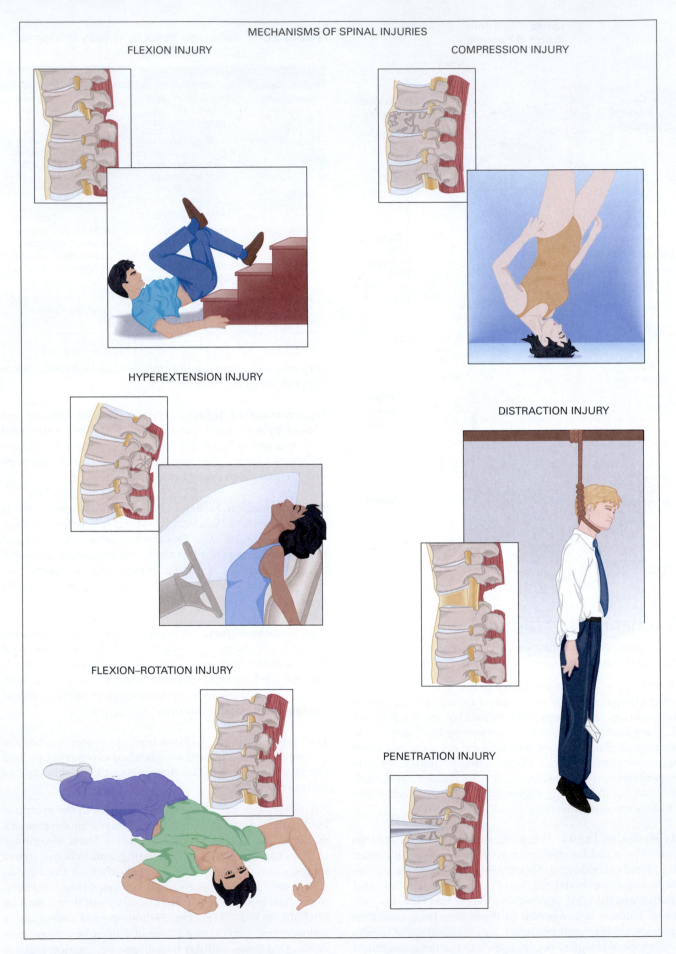

Figure 20–6 Mechanisms of spinal cord injury.

very similar to secondary injuries associated with traumatic brain injury.

Two pathophysiologic processes that contribute to secondary injury are intraparenchymal hemorrhage and ischemia and inflammatory processes.

Intraparenchymal Hemorrhage and Ischemia.   The initial trauma causes intraparenchymal hemorrhage, which immediately causes vasospasm of the superficial blood vessels. Blood flow to the spinal cord decreases instantly upon injury as a result of hypotension and the vasospasm-induced thrombosis. Thrombi in the microcirculation impede blood flow. Elevated interstitial pressure related to edema further impairs perfusion to the cord. Vasoconstrictive substances such as norepinephrine are released post injury, contributing to decreased circulation and cellular perfusion. The zone of ischemia can spread if perfusion to the cord is not restored.

Inflammatory Processes.   Changes in the vasculature cause an ischemia-reperfusion injury (IRI) that leads to endothelial dysfunction and changes in vascular permeability. The IRI triggers a full-blown inflammatory cascade from the activation of immune cells (microglia and astrocytes) and infiltrating leukocytes (neutrophils and macrophages). These cells release neurotoxins (proinflammatory cytokines, chemokines, free radicals, excitotoxic amino acids, and nitric oxide), all of which cause axon and neuronal loss (Anwar et al., 2016). With inflammation the cord swells within the bony vertebrae, and edema moves up and down the cord. A patient may exhibit symptoms as a result of the edema and not the initial injury. For example, a patient with a C4 injury may have edema up to the C2 level. Because edema can extend the level of injury for several cord segments above and below the affected level, the extent of injury may not be determined for several days, until after the cord edema has resolved.

Section Two Review

1. A client has been diagnosed with anterior cord syndrome. What does this syndrome represent?
   A. An upper motor neuron problem
   B. A lower motor neuron problem
   C. The best prognosis for recovery
   D. An incomplete cord injury

2. Whiplash is a mild form of which primary injury to the spinal cord?
   A. Hyperflexion
   B. Axial loading
   C. Hyperextension
   D. Rotation

3. Which region of the spine is most vulnerable to injury?
   A. Cervical
   B. Thoracic
   C. Lumbar
   D. Sacral

4. The events contributing to secondary injury of the spinal cord include which conditions? (Select all that apply.)
   A. Ischemia
   B. Edema
   C. Hypertension
   D. Inflammation
   E. Vasospasm

Answers: 1. D, 2. C, 3. A, 4. (A, B, D, E)

Section Three: Diagnosis and Assessment of Spinal Cord Injury

The diagnosis of SCI begins with a detailed history of events surrounding the incident, radiographic studies of the spine, and an assessment of sensory and motor function. Frequently, diagnostic testing of the SCI patient is completed in the emergency department. In situations in which SCI is suspected later in the hospitalization, diagnostic testing may be initiated in the high-acuity unit. Therefore, in order to prepare the patient and family, the nurse should be aware of the types of tests ordered and the information they provide.

SCI is frequently associated with traumatic brain injury. Therefore, the healthcare provider assumes that an unconscious patient has an SCI until it is ruled out. SCI should also be suspected in a patient with any maxillofacial injury and clavicle or upper rib fractures. Patients with an SCI should be transferred as soon as possible to a level I or II trauma center (Mistovich, Keith, & Brent, 2014). If prolonged time on a backboard is anticipated, the nurse should initiate measures to prevent skin breakdown and perform baseline skin assessment as soon as the backboard is removed.

Diagnostic Testing

A variety of diagnostic tests are performed to evaluate the location and extent of injury and to develop a therapeutic plan based on diagnostic findings.

Radiography Radiographic assessment documents the level of injury and provides information regarding the stability of the vertebral column. As soon as the patient is stabilized (airway, breathing, and circulation), x-rays of the spine are obtained. The risk for a cervical SCI should be considered high among patients with altered mental status, evidence of intoxication, suspected extremity fracture, focal neurological deficit, or spinal pain or tenderness. In patients with an SCI the entire spine should be imaged, and the nurse should be aware that bony images may be negative.

Computed Tomography Scan A computed tomography (CT) scan may be ordered after completion of x-rays if the spine is not well visualized or there are suspicious findings. A CT scan provides superior visualization of bony structures of the spine and identifies spinal fractures. The CT scan is an accurate method for detecting posterior and central column injuries, as well as cord impingement. If radiopaque contrast is used, the nurse must question the patient about dye and seafood allergies and any underlying kidney disease. Also, creatinine values should be obtained on admission and monitored throughout because rhabdomyolyis is common in acute traumatic SCI patients, causing renal dysfunction in half of them (Galeiras et al., 2016).

Magnetic Resonance Imaging Magnetic resonance imaging (MRI) should be performed at all levels of the cord for known or suspected SCI (Consortium for Spinal Cord Medicine, 2008; Mistovich et al., 2014). MRI identifies injuries to the spinal cord, ligaments, and disks. It is also used to detect tumors, inflammation, infection, degenerative disorders, and vascular disruptions in the spinal cord and brain. Noninvasive fields and radiofrequency waves are used to align protons (hydrogen atoms) in tissue. The computer reconstructs signals from the resonance or vibration of protons into video images based on signal intensity in order to diagnose specific lesions or abnormalities. MRI offers greater sensitivity to evaluate the tissues, including the actual spinal cord and ligaments for contusions, hematomas and edema, whereas CT scans are used to better evaluate the bony structures for fractures and dislocations.

Angiography Because of their anatomic location, the vertebral arteries within the cervical spinal column are predisposed to injury from cervical spine trauma. Rates of traumatic vertebral artery injury have increased as our screening methods have become more sensitive. Recent findings show vertebral artery injury in 17.2% to 25.5% in cervical spine trauma, with some literature reporting up to 70% in cervical spine fractures (deSouza, Crocker, Haliasos, Rennie, & Saxena, 2011). The majority of unilateral vertebral artery injuries are asymptomatic from this injury. It is imperative to identify the population of patients who are symptomatic from this injury because the pathophysiology of vertebral artery injury can include occlusion, dissection, thromboembolism, intimal damage, pseudoaneurysm, rupture, and arteriovenous fistula and transection. All of these injuries can cause secondary vasospasm (deSouza et al., 2011). Digital subtraction angiography is the gold standard to evaluate for vertebral artery injury. CT angiogram (CTA) is quick and easy to perform, and the ability to detect vertebral artery injury is improving, with some series showing up to 99% sensitivity (deSouza et al., 2011). The Congress of Neurological Surgeons and American Association of Neurological Surgeons (2013) recommends CTA as a screening tool in selected patients after blunt cervical trauma who meet the modified Denver Screening Criteria for suspected vertebral artery injury (VAI). The screening criteria include (1) presence of signs and symptoms of VAI: arterial bleeding, audible cervical bruit, expanding hematoma, focal neurological deficit, neurologic exam findings incongruous with CT scan results, ischemic stroke on secondary CT scan, and (2) presence of risk factors for VAI: high-energy transfer mechanism of injury with (a) Lefort II or III fracture, (b) cervical spine fracture patterns (subluxation, fractures extending into the transverse foramen, fractures of C1–C3, (c) basilar skull fracture, (d) diffuse axonal injury with GCS = 6, and (e) near hanging with anoxic brain injury (Cothren et al., 2005). CTA has a 0.14% to 1% risk for stroke (Kaufmann et al., 2007). This risk is highest in patients 55 years of age or older, those with cardiovascular disease, and those undergoing longer fluoroscopic times (10 minutes or longer) (Kaufmann et al., 2007).

Somatosensory-evoked Potentials Somatosensory-evoked potentials (SEPs) are used to prevent iatrogenic injuries during surgery. A change in SEP can alert the surgeon to changes in the spinal cord. In an extremity below the level of injury, a peripheral nerve is stimulated. The response of the cerebral cortex to this stimulation (evoked potential) is recorded using scalp electrodes. In complete SCI, SEPs are absent because the stimulus is not transmitted to the cortex.

Physical Assessment

Accurate assessment of motor, sensory, and reflex function is important for several reasons: to assist in diagnosis of the lesion, to provide a baseline with which to compare effectiveness of treatment, and to determine realistic functional goals. Sensory and motor function are assessed and documented. The International Standards for Neurological Classification of Spinal Cord Injury (ASIA, n.d.-a) are used to document sensory and motor function (Figure 20–7). This scale remains the most frequently used tool to evaluate SCI, should be completed within 72 hours of admission, and is recommended by the Congress of Neurological Surgeons (2013) in their Guidelines for the Management of Acute Cervical Spine and Spinal Cord Injuries (Hadley & Walters, 2013). Self-paced learning modules are available from the American Spinal Injury Association on how to administer the scale (American Spinal Injury Association [ASIA], n.d.-b).

Serial neurologic exams are performed hourly for at least the first 24 hours after SCI. The patient is monitored closely for respiratory failure in the first days following SCI. The nurse obtains baseline respiratory parameters (vital capacity, forced expiratory volume in 1 second [FEV1]) and arterial blood gases when the patient is first evaluated and at intervals until stable (Consortium for Spinal Cord Medicine, 2008).

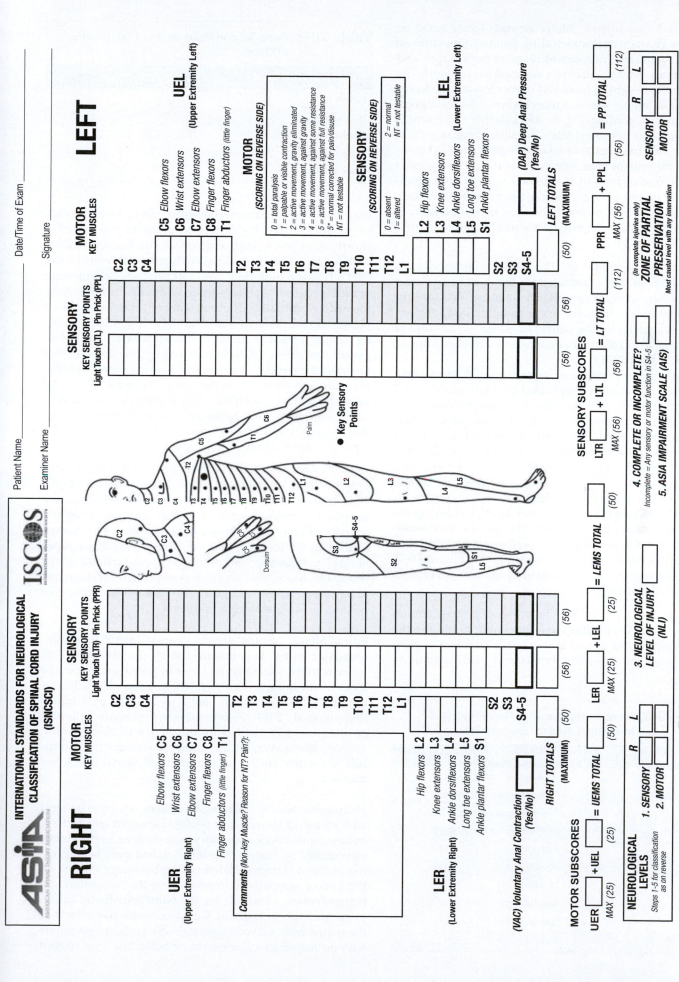

Figure 20–7 Standard neurological classification of spinal cord injury.

SOURCE: American Spinal Injury Association: International Standard for Neurological Classification of Spinal Cord Injury, revised 2016; Atlanta, GA. Reprinted 2016.

Assessing Motor Status Motor strength varies based on preinjury characteristics including gender, fitness level, and age. Voluntary movement requires both upper and LMN activity. Motor activity is assessed for strength. The examiner begins at the head and moves toward the lower body. The examiner assesses muscles based on the 5-point scale of muscle grading (Figure 20–4). Active movement is assessed against gravity. If this is possible, range of motion is assessed against partial resistance, then against full resistance. If the patient is unable to move the muscle against gravity, range of motion is assessed with gravity eliminated (the examiner eliminates gravity on the extremity and asks the patient to move the muscle being tested); if this is not possible, the muscle should be palpated for a contraction.

Assessing Sensory Status The most important data to collect in the sensory examination is the exact point on the patient where normal sensation is present. The sensory assessment moves from the lower to upper body regions because it is easier for the patient to recognize the onset of a sensory stimulus than the cessation of a stimulus (Ropper, Samuels, & Klein, 2014 .

Sensation is tested along dermatomes. A **dermatome** is a section of the body innervated by a particular spinal (or cranial) nerve (see the human form as depicted in Figure 20–7). A cotton swab is used to assess sensation (spinothalamic tract function). A pinprick is used to assess pain (posterior column function). The patient's eyes are closed. The examination begins distally and moves proximally (i.e., up to the neurologically intact area). Position sense (**proprioception**) is tested by moving the big toes and thumbs up and down and asking the patient to confirm the direction. The areas where sensation and pain are present are marked and dated on a dermatome diagram similar to that shown in Figure 20–7. Table 20–2 shows the relationship between nerve root and innervated area.

Assessing Reflex Activity The presence of deep tendon reflexes (Table 20–3) below the level of injury indicates the cord is coming out of spinal shock. The presence of perineal reflexes indicates that bowel and bladder training

Table 20–2 Relationship Between Nerve Root and Innervated Area for Sensory Testing

Nerve Root	Innervated Area
C5	Upper lateral arm
C6	Posterior aspect of thumb
C7	Posterior aspect of middle finger
C8	Posterior aspect of little finger
T4	Nipple line
T10	Umbilicus
L1	Groin
L2	Anterior thigh
S1	Sole of the foot
S3, S4, S5	Perineal

Table 20–3 Deep Tendon Reflexes and Their Source of Origin

Deep Tendon Reflex	Neural Origin
Biceps	C5
Supinator	C6
Triceps	C7
Knee (patellar)	L3
Ankle (Achilles)	S1

may be feasible. **Priapism** (persistent penile erection) may be present in males. It probably occurs at the moment of or shortly after injury and resolves spontaneously, usually within a few hours but occasionally up to 30 hours (Todd, 2011). This is a high-flow (arterial) priapism; a semi-erect or erect priapism is always associated with an AIS-A complete SCI (Todd, 2011). The anal wink reflex is initiated by a pinprick in the perianal area. A visual external anal sphincter contraction will occur if the reflex is present. The bulbocavernosus reflex (BCR) is initiated by placing a gloved finger in the patient's rectum and tugging on an indwelling urinary catheter or on the penis or clitoris. The rectal sphincter will contract if the reflex is present. The presence of the anal wink and bulbocavernosus reflexes indicate that the injury is an UMN injury and will determine the type of bowel training.

Assessing for Shock States The autonomic nervous system functions to maintain homeostasis within the body. With trauma to the spinal cord, autonomic dysfunction develops. The degree of dysfunction varies by level and severity of injury. Autonomic dysfunction is more extensive when the level of injury is higher. Two major types of shock may develop following severe cord trauma: spinal shock and neurogenic shock. It is important for the nurse to be able to rapidly recognize and differentiate these two potentially life-threatening problems.

Spinal Shock. **Spinal shock** occurs within 30 to 60 minutes after injury. It is manifested by the absence of all reflex activity, flaccidity, and loss of sensation below the level of the injury. This syndrome generally subsides within 24 hours but may last 7 to 20 days post injury (Ropper et al., 2014). Treatment is symptomatic. The end of this period is marked by the return of deep tendon reflexes, spasticity, and increased muscle tone. It is difficult to classify an SCI accurately until spinal shock has resolved.

Neurogenic Shock. **Neurogenic shock** occurs in patients with an injury above T6. It is often classified as a form of hypovolemic shock secondary to a relative hypovolemic state caused by massive vasodilation and peripheral pooling of blood. The associated pathophysiology centers on the loss of sympathetic control from the brainstem and higher centers, which allows the parasympathetic output to go unchecked. Without the vasoconstrictive effects of the sympathetic nervous system (SNS), vasodilation occurs with decreased vascular resistance below the level of cord injury. Blood pools in the lower extremities, significantly reducing venous return to the heart and cardiac output (CO). Consequently, the patient experiences hypotension, bradycardia, decreased CO, and hypothermia with the loss of the ability to sweat below the level of the lesion.

It is important that neurogenic shock be differentiated from other causes of hypovolemic shock (such as hemorrhage) because the treatment strategies differ. The critical clinical assessment that characterizes neurogenic shock is arterial hypotension in the presence of bradycardia and warm flushed skin (Mistovich et al., 2014). Treatment involves both fluid resuscitation and vasopressor medications. Chapter 36 presents neurogenic shock in further detail.

Section Three Review

1. A client has been admitted with a diagnosis of a possible C7 compression injury. A CT scan with contrast of the cervical spine is ordered. Which action should the nurse perform?
   A. Remove all metal objects.
   B. Supply in-line mobilization of the neck.
   C. Ask if the client is allergic to seafood or radiopaque dye.
   D. Prep the client's neck with povidone–iodine solution.

2. A client with an SCI has somatosensory-evoked potentials (SEPs) testing performed 2 days after admission to help establish a functional prognosis. What conclusion would the nurse draw if the client had no SEPs during the test?
   A. The SCI is complete.
   B. The SCI is unstable.
   C. An upper motor neuron lesion is present.
   D. A lower motor neuron injury is present.

3. Which type of testing can determine the exact point on the client where normal sensation is present?
   A. Dermatomes
   B. MRI
   C. Proprioception
   D. SEPs

4. Absent reflexes, flaccidity, and loss of sensation below the level of injury are signs of which condition?
   A. Priapism
   B. Autonomic dysreflexia
   C. Neurogenic shock
   D. Spinal shock

Answers: 1. C, 2. A, 3. A, 4. D

Section Four: Stabilization and Management of Spinal Cord Injury in the Acute Care Phase

Timely spinal cord alignment and stabilization maximize spinal cord recovery, minimize additional damage, and prevent late deformity. The spinal cord is stabilized using surgical or manual techniques. Stabilization in the high-acuity unit includes bed rest with log-rolling maneuvers and use of a hard cervical collar until the spine has been stabilized with surgery or traction.

Surgical Stabilization

The Consortium for Spinal Cord Medicine (2008) recommends a closed or open reduction as soon as is permissible on patients with bilateral cervical facet dislocation, a complete displacement of the anterior vertebral body usually resulting from a severe hyperflexion injury. Furthermore, with this type of dislocation injury, early surgical spinal canal decompression in the deteriorating SCI patient will

be considered. In practice, the majority of spine surgeons prefer to decompress within 24 hours, and very early decompression (within 12 hours) should be considered for a patient with an incomplete SCI (with the exception of central cord injury) (Fehlings, Rabin, Sears, Cadotte, & Aarabi, 2010).

A large international prospective cohort study, the Surgical Timing in Acute Spinal Cord Injury Study (STASCIS), showed that early decompression surgery (prior to 24 hours) versus late decompression is significantly associated with improved outcomes and reduced complication rates in adults aged 16 to 60 with cervical SCI (Fehlings et al., 2012). A Canadian cohort study also showed evidence that incomplete acute traumatic SCI patients who received surgery within 24 hours from injury had improved motor neurological recovery and reduced length of stay (Dvorak et al., 2015). Early surgical decompression was also shown to be more cost-effective than delayed surgical decompression (Furlan, Craven, Massicotte, & Fehlings, 2016). Clinically there is a growing consensus among spine surgeons favoring early surgical intervention (Congress of Neurological Surgeons and American Association of Neurological Surgeons, 2013).

During surgery, spinal segments are fused and spinal canal decompression is accomplished. Rods are inserted

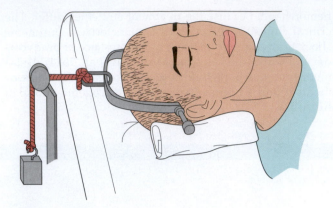

Figure 20–8 Cervical traction may be applied by several methods, including Gardner-Wells tongs.

to stabilize thoracic spinal injuries. External traction may be required postoperatively. Special braces, such as the Jewett orthosis, may be used postoperatively to maintain hyperextension when the patient is not supine. Surgery is reserved for patients not sufficiently aligned with manual stabilization.

Manual Stabilization

The spinal column may be immobilized through the use of manual fixation devices, including tongs, halos, and braces.

Skull Tongs Tong devices, such as Gardner-Wells or Vinke cervical tongs, may be used initially to reduce a fracture (Figure 20–8). Screws are implanted into the patient's skull a few centimeters above the ear using a local anesthetic. The patient feels pressure but usually not pain. Sequential weights are added to these devices. Ten pounds of traction is applied if an injury but no fracture is present. If a fracture is present, 5 pounds per interspace beginning with C1 to the level of lesion is applied. Muscle relaxants increase the efficacy of the traction.

Halo Device The halo device is an external fixation device (Figure 20–9). It keeps the spine aligned; prevents flexion, extension, and rotational movement of the head and neck, and it allows for early mobilization. The device is secured with four pins inserted in the skull—two in the frontal bone and two in the occipital bone. The halo ring is attached to a rigid plastic vest. Patients in these devices require special nursing interventions, which are summarized in Table 20–4.

Braces A hard cervical collar and a molded plastic body jacket (clamshell) brace may be sufficient for stabilization of some injuries. Braces, such as the Jewett orthosis, are most frequently used with thoracic and lumbar spine injuries.

Whether surgical or mechanical stabilization of the spine is used, the goals are the same: to align and stabilize the spine, minimize additional damage, and prevent late deformity. The methods, indications, goals, lengths of therapy, and precautions of various spine immobilization techniques are summarized in Table 20–5.

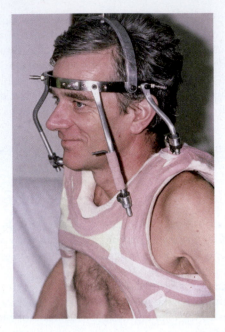

Figure 20–9 Example of external fixation (halo) device with vest.

SOURCE: Dr P. Marazzi/Science Source

Steroid Therapy

Methylprednisolone (MPSS) is a steroid that has been used post SCI to prevent secondary injury despite limited evidence. A Cochrane review was undertaken and included randomized controlled trials of the use of steroids in the setting of acute SCI (Bracken, 2012). Only eight trials were available at the time of this review, seven of MPSS. The studies measured neurologic recovery of motor function at 6 weeks, 6 months, and 1 year; mortality; and incidence of infections. The first National Acute Spinal Cord Injury

Table 20–4 Caring for the Patient in a Halo Vest

Intervention	Rationale
1. Tape a halo vest wrench on the front of the vest.	The fixation device must be taken off to remove the vest to expose the chest in the event CPR is required.
2. Inspect pins and traction bars for loose pins.	Maintain the integrity of the external system.
3. Do not pull the vest's struts to move or position the patient.	This can disrupt the integrity of the device and potentially damage the cord.
4. Assess motor function and sensation every 2 to 4 hours.	Early identification of neurologic deficits can be made.
5. Perform pin care per unit protocol and monitor pin sites for signs of infection.	Organisms can enter through the pin insertion sites.
6. Turn every 2 hours, inspect skin around vest edges.	Prevent skin breakdown. Prevent stasis complications.
7. Provide skin care.	Clean skin under vest with a moist cloth. Use a pillowcase to pull through vest from top to bottom to remove dead skin and debris and to monitor for any wound drainage.

Table 20–5 Methods, Indications, Goals and Lengths of Therapy, and Precautions of Various Spine Immobilization Techniques

Methods	Indications	Goal of Therapy	Length of Therapy	Precautions
CERVICAL SPINE (C-SPINE)				
Hard cervical collar (short term)—Philadelphia collar and Stiff-neck collar	Prehospital immobilization Uncleared c-spine	Preevaluation, presumptive SCI	Less than 48 hours	Ensure good collar fit Skin care Decubitus ulcers
Hard cervical collar (long term)—Miami-J collar and Aspen collar	Stable c-spine fracture Ligamentous injury	Hasten healing, diminish pain	8–12 weeks	Ensure good collar fit Worn continuously—provide second collar for washing Meticulous skin care
Soft cervical collar	Cervical strain, whiplash	Symptom management	Varies, depending on symptom severity	Limit use to avoid dependence (e.g., nighttime, riding in car only)
CERVICAL TRACTION				
Gardner-Wells tongs	Unstable malaligned c-spine fracture, dislocation, or ligamentous injury	Cervical reduction Bridge to operative therapy	Varies	Pin site care and assessment Reposition patient every 2 hours
Halo vest	Unstable c-spine fracture, dislocation, or ligamentous injury	Definitive cervical immobilization	8–12 weeks	Pin site assessment and care Decubitus ulcers beneath vest
Four poster or Yale brace	Stable c-spine injuries or adjunct to surgery for unstable c-spine injuries	Hasten healing, diminish pain	8–12 weeks	
THORACIC OR LUMBAR SPINE				
Hyperextension cast and thoraco–lumbar support orthotic (clamshell or tortoiseshell brace)	Stable thoracic or lumbar spine column fractures; anterior compression fracture with < 40% loss of height; burst fractures with no neurologic deficit, < 50% vertebral body involvement, < 30% canal compromise, angulation < 20 degrees	Hasten healing, diminish pain After spinal decompressive and stabilization surgery for support and comfort	8–12 weeks	Requires custom fit Meticulous skin care
Elastic thoraco–lumbar supports	Minor compression fractures or transverse process fractures Lumbar strain	Symptom management	Varies, depending on symptom severity	

SOURCE: Logan, Paul, *Principles of Practice for the Acute Care Nurse Practitioner*, 1st Ed., © 2000. Reprinted and Electronically reproduced by permission of Pearson Education, Inc., New York, NY.Nursing.

Study (NASCIS trial) (Bracken et al.,1984) did not find any beneficial effect of MPSS given at 1 gram per day for 10 days. In post hoc analyses completed for this review, which stratifies the patients according to those treated within 8 hours, there is some modest evidence of potential benefit in patients treated early. The second NASCIS trial (Bracken et al., 1990) found significantly increased neurologic recovery among patients treated with very-high-dose MPSS within 8 hours of injury. This treatment has become a standard therapy in many countries. As shown by this review, additional trials (Otani et al., 1994; Petitjean et al., 1998) support the conclusion that this regimen offers some neurologic benefit to some patients and is not associated with any significant increased risk of medical complication. A third NASCIS trial (Bracken et al., 1997) contrasted the NASCIS 2 treatment with MPSS with an extended 48-hour regimen, which was shown to further improve motor function and functional outcomes in patients whose initiation of steroid therapy could not start until 3 to 8 hours post SCI. Two trials—Glasser, Knego, Delashaw,

and Fessler (1993) and Pettersson and Toolanen (1998)— provide some supportive evidence for a role for MPSS in recovery from acute SCI. In the whiplash trial (Pettersson & Toolanen, 1998), the identical regimen of MPSS to that administered in NASCIS 2 was found to result in fewer disabling symptoms ($p = 0.047$), fewer sick days ($p = 0.01$) and a healthier sick leave profile ($p = 0.003$) at 6 months post injury. For patients treated with MPSS at the time of their discectomy for lumbar disc disease, their hospital stay was significantly shorter than patients not so treated (1.4 versus 4.0 days, $p = 0.0004$) (Glasser et al.,1993).

A systematic review of almost 2500 patients in 51 trials of the use of high-dose MPSS (any IV dose exceeding 15 mg/kg or 1 gm) versus placebo or nothing by Sauerland, Nagelschmidt, Mallmann, & Neugebauer, 2000) provides further reassurance of safety. High-dose MPSS was defined as any intravenous dose exceeding 15 mg/kg or 1 gram given as a single or repeated dose within a maximum of 3 days and discontinued afterward, and the trials included both traumatic SCI and elective spine surgery. No evidence was found for any increased risk of gastrointestinal bleeding ($RD = 0.3\%$, $p = 0.4$), wound complication ($RD = 1\%$, $p = 0.2$), pulmonary complications (for which MPSS was significantly protective $RD = -3.5\%$, $p = 0.003$) or death (also moderately protective $RD = -0.9\%$, $p = 0.10$). No evidence of harm was found when spine surgery alone was considered.

In summary, according to the Cochrane review, treatment of acute SCI with MPSS sodium succinate has been shown to enhance sustained neurologic recovery. Therapy must be started within 8 hours of injury using an initial bolus of 30 mg/kg by IV for 15 minutes followed 45 minutes later by a continuous infusion of 5.4 mg/kg/hour for 24 hours. Further improvement in motor function recovery has been shown to occur when the maintenance therapy is extended for 48 hours, especially in patients whose initial bolus steroid dose could only be given 3 to 8 hours after the injury (Bracken, 2012). There is a clear and critical need for more randomized trials to evaluate management of acute SCI.

Despite empirical evidence, best practice guidelines do not recommend routine use of steroids in the treatment of acute SCI. In 2013 the American Association of Neurological Surgeons (AANS) and Congress of Neurological Surgeons (CNS) released a consensus statement that the use of glucocorticoids in acute traumatic SCI is no longer recommended (Congress of Neurological Surgeons, 2013). In a study of acute traumatic SCI, 46 patients who received MPSS and 1555 who received no steroid treatment, complication rates have been significantly higher in the MPSS group, and this is why guidelines now recommend against its routine administration (Evaniew et al., 2015).

The Consortium for Spinal Cord Medicine (2008) concluded that there was not enough clinical evidence to definitively recommend using steroids in the treatment of acute SCI to improve functional recovery. In order to reduce deleterious side effects, the consortium also recommended that steroids used in the setting of acute SCI should be stopped as soon as possible in both neurologically intact patients and in those whose prior neurologic symptoms have resolved.

Steroid use is associated with a considerable amount of risk, including increased incidence of pneumonia, sepsis, gastrointestinal complications, electrolyte imbalances, and delayed wound healing. Therefore, the potential benefits of MPSS therapy must be weighed against the risks of complications. MPSS may be considered a treatment option but, due to a lack of conclusive evidence, should not be a standard of care in the treatment of acute SCI.

Section Four Review

1. A client is admitted to the unit with an unstable T2 SCI. The healthcare provider will place cervical traction in 6 hours. What is a priority nursing intervention?
   A. Administer pain medications as ordered.
   B. Place a hard cervical collar and perform log-rolling maneuvers.
   C. Shave and prep the client's head.
   D. Place a wrench at the client's bedside.

2. What is the best advantage of surgical stabilization?
   A. It decreases complications attributed to immobility.
   B. It secures the spine better than cervical tongs.
   C. It is cheaper.
   D. It is available to all clients with SCI.

3. Which nursing intervention is a priority for the client with a halo vest?
   A. Place an appropriate wrench on or near the client.
   B. Maintain the hard neck collar.
   C. Log-roll the client.
   D. Add sequential weights.

4. Which statement is true about the use of methylprednisolone for SCI?
   A. It must be given to all clients within 6 hours of injury.
   B. It is now contraindicated in all clients with SCI.
   C. It is considered a treatment option.
   D. High doses are better than low doses.

Answers: 1. B, 2. A, 3. A, 4. C

Section Five: High-Acuity Nursing Care of the Patient with a Spinal Cord Injury

During the acute care phase of recovery from SCI, there are priority nursing assessments and interventions that the nurse focuses on.

Alteration in Oxygenation and Ventilation from Problems with Gas Exchange and Abnormal Breathing Patterns

Respiratory complications are the most common cause of morbidity and mortality in acute SCI with an incidence of 36% to 83%, and 83% of the deaths in patients with acute cervical SCI are due to pulmonary dysfunction with pneumonia being the cause in 50% of the cases (NSCISC, 2016; Wong et al., 2012). As with any high-acuity patient, the nurse begins the patient assessment using the ABCs. The patient's airway and breathing may be compromised, particularly with a cervical cord injury. The nurse must be aware of the patient's prior medical history along with prior substance use. A history of smoking will significantly increase the patient's risk of respiratory complications. Patients with C1–C2 injuries will require mechanical ventilation because of loss of phrenic nerve innervation to the diaphragm. Those with injuries to C3–C5 will have varying degrees of diaphragm paralysis and need some ventilatory support; they may be able to be weaned from mechanical ventilation. Injuries below C6 have varying degrees of impaired intercostal and abdominal muscle function. Patients with these injuries experience compromise in respiratory protective reflexes, including coughing and sneezing. Even with aggressive care, 20% of patients with a cervical SCI will need a tracheostomy (Branco et al., 2011).

The number of respiratory complications during the acute hospital stay contributes significantly to the length of hospital stay and cost. Four factors—use of mechanical ventilation, pneumonia, the need for surgery, and use of tracheostomy—explain nearly 60% of hospital costs and may be as important a predictor of hospital cost as level of injury. Atelectasis (36.4%), pneumonia (31.4%), and ventilatory failure (22.6%) are the most common complications during the first 5 days after injury. Respiratory failure occurs on average 4.5 days after injury (NSCISC, 2016; Wong, Shem, & Crew, 2012). Oxygen saturation and end tidal CO_2 should be continually measured during the first few days after injury to monitor for respiratory distress.

Respiratory management goals are achieved through aggressive respiratory therapy and careful monitoring to identify and promptly treat actual and potential respiratory problems (see the "Quality and Safety Considerations for Potential Respiratory Problems" feature.) Humidified oxygen is administered via nasal cannula or face mask. The patient is taught to use an incentive spirometer and the assisted "quad" coughing technique, a maneuver in which a care provider performs an abdominal thrust and/or squeeze over the chest wall that is coordinated with either the patient's spontaneous breath or with an assisted breath. Contraindications to quad coughing are as follows: unstable spine in traction, internal abdominal complications, chest trauma such as fractured ribs, and a recently placed vena cava filter. The Cough Assist Mechanical Insufflation–Exsufflation device (cough assist machine) is an effective strategy to assist the SCI patient in mobilizing secretions that can be used when there is an unstable spine (Wong et al., 2012).

Best practice recommendations include obtaining initial laboratory assessments (ABGs, CBC, coagulation profile, comprehensive metabolic profile, cardiac enzyme profile, urinalysis, and toxicology screen). Respiratory function testing should be carried out on a periodic basis to monitor lung compliance, volumes, respiratory muscle strength, and need for mechanical ventilation. Respiratory care should include aggressive interventions to prevent and treat atelectasis, pneumonia, and aspiration (Congress of Neurological Surgeons and American Association of Neurological Surgeons, 2013; Consortium for Spinal Cord Medicine, 2008).

Chest physiotherapy may be performed depending on the patient's ability to tolerate this procedure and the level and extent of the SCI. The decision to suction the patient should be based on assessment findings because this procedure may stimulate the vasovagal response and lead to bradycardia. Mobilization of secretions is best obtained with frequent turning and position changes. However, this may not be possible because of the injury and the use of traction devices. The nurse should collaborate with the healthcare team to determine whether the use of a specialized bed is warranted.

Quality and Safety
Considerations for Potential Respiratory Problems

- Changes in ABGs and vital capacity signal respiratory insufficiency.
- When treating autonomic dysreflexia in a patient with an SCI, it is important to closely monitor for hypotension following administration of any antihypertensive medication (nifedipine, hydralazine, labetalol, and diazoxide).
- A distended bladder can be palpated over the lower abdomen above the symphysis pubis bone. Voiding frequently in small amounts may signal neurogenic bladder.

Cardiac Dysfunction

The patient with SCI is at high risk for developing cardiac dysfunction, specifically decreased cardiac output related to orthostatic hypotension, spinal and neurogenic shock, venous pooling, emboli, and bradycardia. In the acute care phase, cardiac output may be closely monitored by invasive and noninvasive means. Cardiac monitoring allows for early detection of bradycardia, which is a constant threat because of unopposed vagal stimulation of the heart in patients with SCI above T6. All patients with motor-complete cervical SCI develop bradycardia, 68% develop arterial hypotension, 35% require vasopressor treatment, and 16% experience a cardiac arrest. These conditions can be precipitated by endotracheal suctioning, or a simple position change (Oh & Eun, 2015). Bradycardia will typically peak in incidence at 4 days post injury (Hagen, 2015). Atropine should be kept at the bedside for immediate treatment of symptomatic bradycardia, although the use of enteral albuterol will significantly decrease the need for chronotropic agents (Evans et al., 2014). In a retrospective chart review of 18 patients with cervical SCI induced bradycardia, the patients who received treatment with enteral albuterol experienced fewer symptomatic bradycardic episodes and significantly fewer days on chronotropic agents than the patients who did not receive enteral albuterol (Evans, Duby, Berry, Schermer, & Cocanour, 2014).

Techniques, such as central venous pressure (CVP) to monitor cardiac preload, may be required. Use of IV fluids must be judicious when treating hypotension because too much fluid can precipitate pulmonary edema. Inotropic and/or vasopressor support may be required to maintain adequate cardiac output and tissue perfusion. A systolic blood pressure less than 90 mmHg is detrimental because it causes hypoperfusion to the cord; current guidelines recommend that mean arterial pressure (MAP) should be maintained 85 to 90 mmHg for the first 7 days post SCI (Congress of Neurological Surgeons and American Association of Neurological Surgeons, 2013). (See the "Emerging Evidence" feature.) Current research is investigating the outcomes of increased MAP. A systematic review of nine studies of mean arterial pressure and functional outcomes post traumatic SCI, failed to identify statistically significant relationships between MAP and functional outcome (Sabit, Zeiler, & Berrington, 2016).

Impaired Bladder and Bowel Function

Bladder and bowel dysfunctions are predictable in many spinal cord injuries, based on level of injury. Effective nursing management of bladder and bowel dysfunction is needed to prevent the development of complications.

Bladder Dysfunction   The degree of bladder dysfunction depends on the location and completeness of the SCI. Facilitation and inhibition of voiding is under three main centers: the sacral micturition center, the pontine micturition center, and the higher center (cerebral cortex). Patients with complete quadriplegia are typically unaware of bladder activity except through ancillary clues (e.g., sweating, chills). Because of the effects of spinal shock and the usual need for aggressive fluid replacement immediately after SCI, patients with acute SCI are best managed with an indwelling urinary catheter. Once fluid resuscitation is complete, intermittent catheterization should be instituted to prevent overdistention of the bladder (Cameron et al., 2010; Consortium for Spinal Cord Medicine, 2006). It is best to initiate a catheter-free status as soon as reflex activity returns, the patient is medically stable, and urine output averages 2 liters in 24 hours. Injuries above the T12 level result in upper motor neuron (UMN; hyperreflexic or spastic) bladder dysfunction.

Bowel Dysfunction   Bowel dysfunction also depends on the location and completeness of SCI. The bowel is innervated by the sacral segments of the spinal cord. The bowel is flaccid and areflexic in complete SCI or during spinal shock. With resolution of spinal shock, an injury above the conus or the distal tip (L2) of the spinal cord results in a UMN bowel or reflexic bowel. This reflex activity facilitates bowel evacuation because the nerve connection between the spinal cord and the bowel is intact.

The bowels are regulated by initiating the defecation reflex by inserting an irritant suppository and/or performing digital stimulation. Bowel training typically begins with bisacodyl (Dulcolax) suppository and/or digital stimulation. If the SCI is a lower motor neuron (LMN) lesion (below the sacral level), the bowel remains areflexic, and retention of stool becomes a problem. The defecation reflex has been damaged in the LMN lesion, and the rectum will be flaccid, increased problems with incontinence will occur, and the need will arise at times to manually evacuate the bowels.

Bowel care must also include monitoring the patient's diet and fluid intake. Timing the performance of the bowel routine with food intake (thereby incorporating gastrocolonic and anorectal reflexes into the bowel routine) is important. For example, following breakfast, gastric distention can activate bowel motility and cause morning defecation.

Injuries to the conus medullaris (at the L2) or cauda equine result in an LMN bowel or flaccid bowel. The loss of nerve connection between the spinal cord and the bowel

---

Emerging Evidence

- Neuroprotective intervention to preserve injured spinal cord tissues and reduce secondary insult are key. Current investigations include the following:
  - Hypothermia to decrease metabolic rate. The pending Acute Rapid Cooling Therapy for Injuries of the Spinal Cord (ARTIC) phase II/III is evaluating this therapy.
  - Riluzole, a sodium-channel blocker. Its use in amyotrophic lateral sclerosis has slowed progression of motor loss and improved survival. The Riluzole in Spinal Cord Injury Study (RISCIS) phase II/III is in trail and expected to complete in 2018.
  - Minocycline, a tetracycline-class antibiotic with anti-inflammatory properties. It inhibits tumor necrosis factor, microglial activation, and nitric oxide synthase. Minocycline in Acute Spinal Cord Injury (MASC) phase III trial is to be completed in 2018.
  - Magnesium use has been applied in neuroprotection of multiple central nervous system disorders. Results are pending from a phase I trial (Ahuja, Martin, & Fehlings (2016)).

- Urinary tract infection is the most common infection in the outpatient setting. The clinical dogma that healthy urine is sterile is being changed to a healthy urine microbiome that prevents infection (Fouts et al., 2012).
- Current study trials are investigating using oral *Lactobacillus* to aid in colonizing the bladder and preventing urinary tract infection (UTI) in people with SCI (Lee et al., 2016).
- Mean arterial pressure (MAP) after a traumatic SCI is maintained at 85 to 90 mmHg for 7 days. The goal is to increase intraspinal pressure (ISP). What may be more important is that MAP minus ISP equals spinal cord perfusion pressure (SCPP). Early bony decompression still keeps the swollen cord compressed against the dura. A phase II nonrandomized trial compares laminectomy and laminectomy plus expansion duroplasty. A probe is inserted intradurally during surgery at the injury site to monitor ISP. Dural decompression is postulated to allow better SCPP. In the future high-acuity nurses may need to monitor ISP and adjust pressure to improve SCPP (Saadoun & Papadopoulos, 2016).

causes slowed stool movement and lack of central coordinated peristalsis. A patient without a bulbocavernosus reflex is considered to have an LMN bowel and will not respond to digital stimulation. The patient will have more problems with constipation and a higher risk of incontinence due to the atonic external sphincter and lack of control of the levator ani muscle, which causes the lumen of the rectum to open (Krassioukov, Eng, Claxton, Sakakibara, & Shum, 2010).

Whether a patient has a reflexic or flaccid bowel, the nurse plays an integral role in the success of bowel care. Establishing routine daily bowel care helps ensure that the patient will leave the acute care setting and enter rehabilitation with a lower risk of severe constipation or incontinence.

Ineffective Temperature Regulation

Interruption in the communication between the spinal cord and the hypothalamus results in the loss of temperature regulation and control whereby the patient's temperature approaches that of the ambient environment. The presence of a fever is common following an acute SCI, with a mean incidence of 48.9% of patients with acute traumatic SCI at increased risk of fever because of thermoregulatory abnormalities arising from dysfunction of the autonomic system. Febrile complications of SCI have the following etiologies: infections (urinary tract, pulmonary, upper respiratory tract, soft tissues, gastrointestinal, and spinal abscess), deep venous thrombosis, pulmonary embolism, colitis, heterotopic ossification (HO), and drug fevers. The most common identifiable cause of fever is UTI (Savage et al., 2016).

With many possible causes of fever a source is frequently not found, and neurogenic fever is currently a diagnosis of exclusion, assigned after all possible alternative etiologies have been ruled out. The mechanism by which fever occurs after SCI is not fully understood. Based on a systematic review of seven studies, the incidence of neurogenic fever ranged from 2.6 to 27.8% with a mean incidence of 8.0% and a median incidence of 4.7% in patients with acute traumatic SCI (Savage, Oleson, Sidhu, Vaccaro, & Schroeder, 2016). More research is needed in this area, but it is important for the high-acuity nurse to closely monitor patients' temperature and provide appropriate cooling interventions.

Malnutrition

In the initial phase of recovery, paralytic ileus is common. A nasogastric tube prevents gastric distention. Alterations in metabolism occur after acute SCI, but the marked hypermetabolic response seen after acute traumatic brain injury appears to be blunted in SCI patients by the flaccidity of denervated musculature after SCI (Congress of Neurological Surgeons and American Association of Neurological Surgeons, 2013).

A nutrition consult is initiated as soon as possible to ensure that the patient's nutritional needs are met. The type of diet the patient receives depends on level of consciousness and the severity of associated injuries. Nursing care includes monitoring intake and weight, assessing electrolyte balance, and administering total parenteral nutrition or enteral feedings as ordered. The patient with dysphagia should be observed for coughing or choking when eating. Thickening food to allow formation of a food bolus is helpful, as is coordination with a speech therapist regarding swallow evaluation and special diet considerations.

Inability to Care for Self

Baseline and ongoing motor, sensory, and reflex assessments provide information about the patient's neurological progress. Rehabilitative goals are set and independence (to the degree possible) encouraged early. Bowel and bladder routines are initiated and ambulation supported as necessary. Table 20–6 outlines functional status based on level of SCI.

Table 20–6 Functional Status Based on Level of SCI

Level	Eating	Dressing	Bathing	Bowel/Bladder	Mobility
C1–C4	Dependent	Dependent	Dependent	Dependent	Electric wheelchair with breath, head, or shoulder controls; requires ventilatory support (partial or full)
C5	Independent with aids	Major assistance with aids	Wheelchair shower with major assistance	Major assistance with aids	Electric wheelchair with adapted hand controls
C6	Independent with aids	Minor assistance with aids	Independent in wheelchair shower	Independent with aids	Independent in manual wheelchair with hand controls; can use some manual wheelchair types
C7	Independent	Independent with aids	Independent wheelchair shower or tub with bath board	Independent with aids	Independent in manual wheelchair with hand controls
C8–T1	Independent	Independent	Independent in tub with bath boards	Independent with aids	Independent in manual wheelchair
T2–T12	Independent	Independent	Independent	Independent with aids	Independent in manual wheelchair
L1–L5	Independent	Independent	Independent	Independent	Optional use of knee, ankle, or foot orthoses
S1–S5	Independent	Independent	Independent	Independent	Independent with or without ankle or foot orthoses

Preventing Complications

Complications associated with the physical effects of SCI (Figure 20–10) can be classified into three broad categories of alterations in mobility, perfusion, and reflex activity.

Complications Related to Altered Mobility SCI significantly reduces the patient's mobility, thereby increasing the risk of potentially serious complications of immobility. Four particular areas of concern are skin breakdown, joint mobility, thromboembolism, and skeletal changes.

Skin Breakdown. Several factors contribute to skin breakdown in the patient with an SCI. Sensory and motor impairment results in areas of the skin subjected to prolonged

periods of pressure. The patient is unable to feel the discomfort or pain from pressure and change position independently. In addition to the usual areas of pressure development (sacrum, ischium, trochanter, and heels), the patient's ears, ankles, and occipital area of the head must be assessed for early indications of the development of pressure ulcers. Moisture exposure from sweating and from bladder or bowel incontinence also contributes to pressure ulcer formation. In a retrospective study of 94 SCI patients, hypotension was the strongest predictor of developing pressure ulcers (Wilczweski et al., 2012). Frequent repositioning and/or turning, while maintaining spinal precautions, every 2 hours are important to provide pressure relief. In addition, foot and heel protectors and specialty beds that

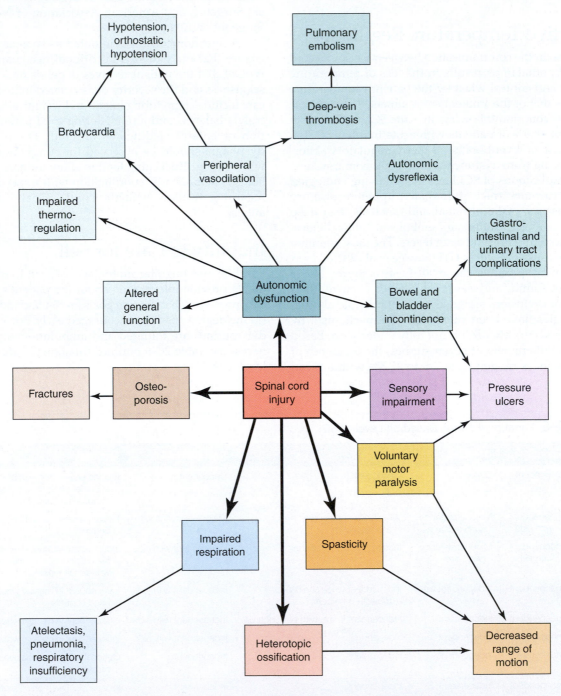

Figure 20–10 Schematic representation of the physical effects of spinal cord injury.

provide pressure reduction or relieving surfaces reduce the risk for skin breakdown. Routine daily or twice-daily inspection of all skin is important to identify areas at risk of breakdown.

Decreased Joint Mobility. This complication is preventable. The tendency to remain in one position for extended periods is greater when the patient is dependent on someone else to initiate movement. Spasticity may contribute to this problem by exaggerating responses to movement. Spasms can be used positively to enable use of some assistive devices. Deformity and contracture develop if joint mobility is not maintained through range of motion.

Thromboembolism. Venous thromboembolism (VTE)—deep vein thrombosis and pulmonary embolism—is the leading cause of mortality and morbidity following acute SCI. The major factors predisposing persons with acute SCI to VTE make up Virchow's triad: venostasis (due to failure of the venous muscle pump with paralysis), a transient hypercoagulable state, and frequent endothelial injury due to concomitant injuries, venous dilatation, and pressure on the veins. Persons with acute SCI have increased risk for VTE and demonstrate the highest incidence of VTE compared with the general population, especially during the first 3 months following the injury (Chung et al., 2014). The Consortium for Spinal Cord Medicine (2016) includes the following recommendations for prevention of venous thromboembolism in patients with SCI:

- Mechanical thromboprophylaxis with intermittent pneumatic compression devices (PCDs) with or without graduated compression stockings (GCSs) should be applied to improve venous return and prevent VTE in the lower extremities.

- Low molecular weight heparin (LMWH) should be used as thromboprophylaxis in the acute-care phase following SCI in the absence of active bleeding.

- Thromboprophylaxis should be continued for at least 8 weeks after injury in SCI patients with limited mobility

- Persons with chronic SCI who are hospitalized for medical illnesses or surgical procedures should receive thromboprophylaxis during the period of increased risk.

Heterotopic Ossification. Ectopic bone formation (overgrowth of bone) occurs below the level of the SCI, restricting joint mobility. The SCI patient is at significant risk of developing heterotopic ossification (HO). The onset of HO is typically within 4 to 12 weeks of injury, and although the diagnosis is not life-threatening, missing the diagnosis and allowing the extra-articular bone to grow can greatly affect the patient's ability to be independent.

Spinal Cord Injury-induced Immune Depression Syndrome (SCI-IDS). Infections are the leading cause of death in the acute phase following SCI and qualify as an independent risk factor for poor neurological outcome (Kopp et al., 2013). The high rate of infection among SCI patients is not completely explained by the long list of their risk factors that can explain frequent infections. Research is investigating to determine if SCI-IDS is neurogenic, causing deactivation of immunity. Natural killer (NK) cells comprise the main components of lymphocyte-mediated nonspecific immunity. Through their effector function, they play a crucial role combating bacterial and viral challenge (Laginha et al., 2016). In the high-acuity environment, nurses frequently focus on technology, but basic hygiene and infection prevention are important when treating a patient who has the potential of developing SCI-IDS. High-acuity nurses can be the best advocate for their patients and keep them from developing further complications by using and enforcing good universal precautions to prevent infections.

Pulmonary Dysfunction Patients with SCIs, especially high thoracic and cervical injuries, have a high incidence of pulmonary complications, including pneumonia, atelectasis, aspiration, and respiratory failure. Pneumonia is now one of the two leading causes of death in patients with SCI (NSCISC, 2015). There is a direct correlation between the level of injury diagnosed between the ASIA Impairment Scale (AIS) and the development of respiratory complications. In individuals with SCI who have neurological levels of C3 and above and are able to spontaneously breathe initially, ventilatory failure can occur 4.5 ± 1.2 days after injury and last for an average of 5 weeks (Wong et al., 2012). Atelectasis and pneumonia can develop due to weak respiratory muscle strength and inability to clear secretions. In addition, patients with a high-level injury usually require mechanical ventilation, which increases the risk for ventilator-associated pneumonia. Aspiration can result from vomiting stomach contents secondary to ileus development. Clinical manifestations may include development of adventitious breath sounds, a deteriorating pattern of pulse oximetry and arterial blood gas values, and changes in vital signs such as fever, tachypnea, tachycardia, and increased blood pressure. Preventing pulmonary complications requires aggressive pulmonary hygiene, as described earlier in this section, and implementation of a ventilator bundle.

Complications Related to CNS Dysfunction **Autonomic dysreflexia (AD)** is a potentially life-threatening complication that involves an exaggerated sympathetic response in patients with SCI at or above the T6 level. AD may occur any time after spinal shock resolves. The prevalence of autonomic dysreflexia in patients with SCI with injury above T6 is 48% to 90% (Hagen, 2015). AD occurs as a result of sympathetic nervous system (SNS) stimulation (typically noxious) below the level of SCI where CNS control of spinal reflexes is lost. Normally the CNS, through a negative feedback system, counteracts sympathetic overstimulation (vasoconstriction, increased heart rate) with opposing parasympathetic nervous system stimulation (vasodilation, decreased heart rate). In the patient with an SCI at T6 level or higher, the negative feedback loop is lost, and sympathetic overstimulation is no longer directly opposed by parasympathetic stimulation, allowing the SNS to predominate below the level of injury. The sympathetic response clinically manifests as hypertension due to vasoconstriction below the level of injury, along with sweating, piloerection (goose bumps), sudden headache, blurred vision, and anxiety.

Baroreceptors located in the neck vessels sense the rapidly increasing blood pressure and attempt to compensate by activating the parasympathetic nervous system, which can directly affect only vessels located above the level of injury. The parasympathetic response clinically manifests as vasodilation above the level of injury with visible flushing of the skin, pupil constriction, increased nasal secretions (resulting in stuffy nose), and a decreased heart rate (due to vagus nerve [CN X] stimulation).

The first priority of the nurse is to lower the blood pressure, usually with a short-acting antihypertensive agent, and then determine the cause of the AD. The patient's blood pressure should be measured every 2 to 3 minutes. The most common factors that produce AD are listed in Box 20–1. To lower the blood pressure, the nurse should immediately raise the head of the bed and loosen any binding or restrictive clothing. Because the most common cause of AD is bladder or bowel distention, the nurse should check the urinary catheter for occlusion, palpate the bladder for distention, and implement measures to relieve the bladder distention. If bladder distention is excluded, the bowel should be checked for impaction, and measures to remove the impaction or facilitate defecation should be implemented. Any potential irritant below the level of the SCI should be found and eliminated. If the patient has cause for pain, such as trauma or wound below the level of the SCI, medicating the patient for pain may stop the AD. If the AD cannot be controlled, medications to manage the hypertension should be administered. Refer to the "Related Pharmacotherapy: Agents Used for Treating Acute Traumatic Spinal Cord Injury" feature.

Complications Related to Abnormal Perfusion An overall drop in baseline arterial blood pressure (decrease of 20 mmHg SBP or 10 mmHg DBP within 3 minutes of being placed in an upright position) and bradycardia is called **orthostatic (postural) hypotension**. Patients with cervical or high thoracic SCI are often prone to it. Factors causing orthostatic hypotension include venous blood pooling in organs and lower extremities due to reduced sympathetic activity and loss of reflexive vessels, constriction below the level of injury, loss of lower extremity muscle function, reduced plasma volume from hyponatremia, and cardiovascular deconditioning from prolonged bedrest (Tom, Partida, Mironets, & Hou, 2016). These factors in combination with a quick position change result in a loss of consciousness. Therefore, initial attempts to mobilize the patient are done slowly. The nurse gradually raises the head of the bed and assesses the patient's tolerance to these position changes. An abdominal binder and compression hose are applied, and the patient dangles the feet on the side of the bed prior to moving to a chair. Medications to reduce orthostatic hypotension include ephedrine and midodrine.

Complications Related to Abnormal Reflex Activity There are three major complications associated with alterations in reflex activity in the SCI patient: bladder dysfunction, bowel dysfunction, and sexual dysfunction.

Bladder Dysfunction. Renal disease is a major cause of morbidity and mortality in individuals with SCI (NSCISC, 2015). The most common urologic complications of neurologic bladder following SCI are urinary tract infections (UTI), upper and lower urinary tract deterioration, and bladder or renal stones (Taweel & Seyam, 2015). Goals

BOX 20–1 Factors That Produce Autonomic Dysreflexia

- Bladder distention/spasm
- Bowel impaction
- Stimulation of anal reflex
- Labor
- Temperature change
- Ingrown toenails
- Tight, irritating clothes
- Urinary tract infection
- Decubitus ulcer
- Pain

of bladder management are bladder drainage, low-pressure urine storage, and voiding without urinary leakage, overdistention, or incontinence. Goals should also include maintaining an infection-free genitourinary system and prevention of complications (Consortium for Spinal Cord Medicine, 2006; Salameh, Mohajer, & Daroucihe, 2015).

Long-term use of urethral catheters can carry a high risk for UTI, urethritis, prostatitis, epididymitis, urethral erosion, bladder stones, and bladder cancer. In patients unable to perform intermittent catheterization independently, an indwelling catheter is typically used. A suprapubic catheter is a valuable option for management. In fact, 90% of patients prefer a suprapubic over a urethral catheter. Suprapubic catheterization also avoids complications of epididymitis and iatrogenic hypospadias (Taweel & Seyam, 2015; Salameh et al., 2015).

Clean intermittent catheterization (CIC) has been shown to have the lowest risk of complications (Goetz & Klausner, 2014) and is considered the gold standard. Although CIC can cause urethral trauma, false passages, urethral strictures, and infections, it is considered one of the safest forms of bladder management for the SCI patient. Bladder spasticity may lead to problems such as leaking between catheterizations or leaking around the indwelling catheter. Anticholinergic (antispasticity) agents may be required to prevent leaking.

Urinary tract infections are a common problem for the SCI patient. UTIs are frequently caused by organisms that colonize the bowel and perineum. There is an increased risk for antimicrobial-resistant bacterial UTI in patients treated with prophylactic antibiotics, according to a large systematic review of the literature (Taweel & Seyam, 2015). Routine nursing care should be performed to keep the catheter and perineum clean.

Bowel Dysfunction. Constipation is a common problem of SCI. Delayed colonic transit time is present in 32% of upper motor neuron bowel dysfunction and 36% of lower motor neuron bowel dysfunction and can worsen constipation (Vallès & Mearin, 2009). The addition of dietary fiber may actually cause colonic transit time to increase (Krassioukov et al., 2010). If a patient is experiencing constipation, the medication list should be evaluated. If possible the patient should be taken off opioids and other medications that could delay colonic transit time and contribute to the risk of constipation.

Related Pharmacotherapy
Agents Used for Treating Acute Traumatic Spinal Cord Injury

Neuropathic Pain Analgesics*

Gabapentin (Neurontin) and pregabalin (Lyrica)
Tricyclic Antidepressants (TCAs): (amitriptyline, desipramine, doxepin, imipramine, nortriptyline, clomipramine, and trimipramine; all are structurally similar)

Action and Uses

Gabapentin: A GABA neurotransmitter analog—however, it does not inhibit GABA uptake or degradation. It appears to interact with GABA cortical neurons, but its relationship to functional activity as an anticonvulsant is unknown. Used for adjunctive therapy for partial seizures with or without secondary generalization in adults, post-herpetic neuralgia, restless leg syndrome. Effective in controlling painful neuropathies.
Amitriptyline: Serotonin and norepinephrine reuptake inhibitor—restores neurotransmitter levels, which has an antidepressant effect. Off-label use for neuropathic pain.

Dosages (Adult)

Gabapentin: (unlabeled use): No recommended dosages provided
TCA: (unlabeled use): No recommended dosages provided

Major Adverse Effects

Most common: drowsiness, fatigue. Other: dizziness, sedation, orthostatic hypotension, constipation, weight gain, dry mouth, swelling. Rare: bone marrow depression.

Nursing Implications

Do not stop abruptly—withdraw over 1-week period.
Avoid taking antacids 2 hours before or after taking medications.
May require several weeks to achieve full effects.
Monitor for therapeutic and nontherapeutic effects.
Baseline and periodic monitoring of blood cell levels.
Monitor blood pressure—change positions slowly.
Monitor for constipation.

Skeletal Muscle Relaxants

Baclofen (Lioresal)
Diazepam (Valium)
Dantrolene (Dantrium)

Action and Uses

Centrally acting skeletal muscle relaxant that depresses at the level of the spinal cord. Baclofen stimulates the GABA receptors. Useful in treatment of muscle spasticity in neuromuscular disorders such as SCI and multiple sclerosis. Benzodiazepines are also used for treating spasms, anxiety, and sleep problems in spinal cord–injured patients. Dantrolene acts directly on relaxing the skeletal muscle.

Dosages (Adult)

Baclofen: 5 mg (PO) 3 times/day. Increase by increments of 5 mg/dose every 3 days as required; max dose of 80 mg/day
Diazepam: 5 to 10 mg (IV/PO) every 3 to 4 hours as needed
Dantrolene: 25 mg (PO) 1 time/day; increase to 25 mg 2 times/day to 4 times/day. May increase dose every 5 to 7 days to max dose of 100 mg 2 to 4 times/day.

Major Adverse Effects

Most common: Drowsiness

Nursing Implications

Cautious use in presence of hepatic or renal dysfunction

Interacts with other drugs that depress CNS, including alcohol
Can increase serum glucose, AST, and alkaline phosphatase levels
Should not be stopped suddenly—results in withdrawal symptoms that can be severe

Antidepressants

Tricyclic antidepressants (as previously described)
Selective serotonin reuptake inhibitors (SSRIs): Lexapro, Prozac, Zoloft, Paxil, Celexa, Luvox (structurally different but same mechanism of action)

Action and Uses

Depression is commonly noted in SCI patients. Antidepressants are commonly used for short-term therapy and may be required for long-term therapy. The dual role of amitriptyline as an effective analgesic as well as an antidepressant may be advantageous in this patient population.
SSRIs are more selective in preventing reuptake of serotonin and have less side effects.
Both classes are equally effective, but TCAs may be more effective for severe depression.

Dosages (Adult)

25–75 mg/day. May increase up to 150–300 mg/day (gradually)

Stool Softeners/Laxatives

Bisacodyl (Dulcolax) suppository
Docusate sodium (Colace)

Action and Uses

Bisacodyl: Increases fluid volume in intestines and stimulates peristalsis
Docusate sodium: Allows fats and water into stool through lowering the surface tension of stool; softens stool, making it easier to pass

Dosages (Adult)

Bisacodyl: PO 5–15 mg as needed; PR 10 mg as needed
Docusate sodium: PO 50–500 mg/day; PR 50–100 mg added to enema fluid

Major Adverse Effects

Most common: cramping, nausea, diarrhea
Fluid and electrolyte imbalances are possible

Nursing Implications

Important to establish a daily bowel program
Laxative therapy used when needed if poor results on bowel program
Observe for development of ileus

Anticoagulants

Enoxaparin (Lovenox)

Action and Uses

Low molecular weight heparin contains antithrombotic properties—antifactor Xa and antithrombin. Used to prevent deep vein thrombosis.

Dosages (Adult)

Prophylactic: 30 mg subQ BID
Treatment dose: 1mg/kd subQ BID

Major Adverse Effects

Potentially life-threatening—angioedema, hemorrhage

Nursing Implications

Should be initiated within 72 hours of SCI

Should have baseline studies of coagulation

Monitor platelet count

Monitor for bleeding

Anti-inflammatory

Methylprednisolone (Solu-Medrol)

Action and Uses

A synthetic corticosteroid with strong anti-inflammatory action used for reducing inflammation and edema in SCI

Dosages (Adult)

During the first hour following injury, give 30 mg/kg IV over 15 minutes; next 23 hours following injury, give 5.4 mg/kg/hour IV infusion**

Major Adverse Effects

No major common side effects (SEs) for short-term use

Nursing Implications

For acute nonpenetrating SCI within 8 hours of trauma but not recommended for SCI over 8 hours after injury or for penetrating SCI

Blood Pressure Agents

Antihypotensives
  Ephedrine
  Fludrocortisone (Florinef)
  Midodrine (ProAmatine)
Antihypertensives
  Nifedipine (Procardia)
  Nitroglycerine

Action and Uses

Antihypotensives: Stimulate the sympathetic nervous system, thereby increasing contractility and cardiac output. Used when nonpharmacologic therapies are not successful in controlling orthostatic hypotension in patients with SCI. Mineralocorticoids for hypotension work by expanding the intravascular volume.

Antihypertensives: Through various mechanisms cause vasodilation that results in decreased blood pressure. Used in SCI as a treatment for autonomic dysreflexia to rapidly reduce blood pressure.

Dosages (Adult)

Antihypotensives

Ephedrine: PO 25 mg 1 to 4 times/day; IV 10–25 mg slow IV and repeat in 5–10 min if needed (max. dose 150 mg/24 hr)

Fludrocortisone: 0.1 to 0.2 mg PO daily to BID. Max dose 1 mg/day.

Midodrine: 10 mg 3 times/day (PO) during day. Separate doses by at least 3 hours; last dose no later than 4 hours before bedtime (HS); max. dose 20 mg/dose

Antihypertensives

Nifedipine: 10–20 mg 3 times/day (PO); extended release 30–60 mg 1 time/day; max. dose 180 mg/day

Nitroglycerine: Unlabeled use; no recommendations provided

Major Adverse Effects

Antihypotensives: tachycardia, hypertension, tremors, nervousness, and restlessness

Antihypertensives: dizziness, hypotension, flushing, diarrhea, headache

Nursing Implications

Antihypotensives: Give 45 minutes to 1 hour before raising head of the bed or assuming a sitting position; midodrine dose may need to be adjusted for renal dysfunction

Antihypertensives: When administering nitroglycerine ointment, place ointment on the patient's forehead for quick access and absorption.

Monitor blood pressure and heart rate

Find and relieve cause of dysreflexia episode. Assess for bladder distention, bowel impaction, pain, other factors that could be causing inflammation (refer to Box 20–1).

*Opioid analgesia (e.g., morphine or fentanyl) is ordered for nonneuropathic pain.

**Methylprednisolone drug doses from Aminoff & Kerchner (2011), Bracken (2012), and Sayer, Kronvall, & Nilsson (2006). All other drug dosages from Wilson, Shannon, & Shields (2017).

A paralytic (adynamic) ileus is a bowel obstruction resulting from a loss of intestinal peristalsis in the absence of any mechanical (physical) obstruction. This condition is common during the initial days following injury and usually subsides spontaneously within 5 days of injury (Sisto, Druin, & Sliwinski, 2008). Impaired extrinsic innervation affects neuromuscular structures, which may contribute to decreased bowel motility (den Braber-Yonker, Lammens, van Putten, & Nagtegaal, 2017). Clinical manifestations include gastric and abdominal distention and absent bowel sounds. Management includes early insertion of a nasogastric tube with gastric decompression until bowel sounds return.

Sexual Dysfunction. Although it may not be a priority in the acute care phase post-SCI, the patient or a significant other may ask questions about sexual function after an injury to the spinal cord. Sexual function is still possible for all patients with SCI. Men may have reflexogenic erections, but up to 95% of men with spinal cord injuries will experience ejaculatory problems (Hess & Hough, 2012). Fatherhood is a possibility because, in some patients, ejaculation can be stimulated using special techniques. In addition, sperm can be harvested, and the sperm can then be used for insemination purposes. Men should be referred at some point to a urologist for information on new erectile and fertility treatments.

It is important to maintain an open discussion with the SCI patient and consider using a treatment framework, such as the Permission, Limited Information, Specific Suggestions, and Intensive Therapy (PLISSIT) model, for education (Consortium for Spinal Cord Medicine, 2010). For both men and women, achieving arousal and orgasm may take longer after SCI; however, research has shown that the presence of an SCI does not preclude the ability to do so (Consortium for Spinal Cord Medicine, 2010). Menses may be disrupted for several months post injury, but after menses returns, pregnancy is still possible. The major risk is autonomic dysreflexia, which can occur during labor and delivery (Consortium for Spinal Cord Medicine, 2010).

Psychosocial Issues Acute SCI is the result of sudden trauma. Within moments, a formerly independent, fully functioning person experiences sudden immobility and faces enormous adjustments in social, economic, and personal roles and relationships. Hope is an important concept and emotion that the high-acuity nurse must foster in the new SCI patient. In a study of 242 participants with SCI, the best predictors of hope are proactive coping, self-esteem, and perceived social support, whereas disability acceptance did not predict hope (Phillips, Smedema, Fleming, Sung, & Allen, 2016). The role of spirituality in facilitating adjustment and resilience after SCI is also an important factor (Jones, Simpson, Briggs, & Dorsett, 2016). Rather than the nurse focusing on the patient's acceptance of an injury, ensuring that the patient's social support group is recognized early and that spirituality is addressed can foster the best chance of hope for a newly injured SCI patient.

Rehabilitation of the patient with an SCI is an ongoing process that moves from intensive care through intermediate care to rehabilitation and then community-based and home care. Nursing interventions are necessary at all points in the process to prevent the complications of altered physical mobility and body functions and to teach the patient and family measures that promote independence in self-care. Discharge planning should begin following the initial injury while the patient is in intensive care. Advance planning will better ensure continuity of care when the patient returns home.

In a study of 15 SCI patients and their families, factors that help the patient adjust to SCI include faith, learning to accept the injury as a part of life, focusing on one's abilities, and getting out socially (DeSanto-Madeya, 2009). Adaptation depends on personality, coping style, and life experiences. Self-esteem, body image, and role performance are affected. Educational level, employment status, income, and social support systems can influence post injury quality of life.

The aim of nursing is to alleviate suffering, as well as to promote health, courage, and hope in individuals when they are potentially or actually suffering from an illness. The focus of patients' hope following their SCI ranges from a focus on the hope of recovering from their injury and for their condition to improve to a focus on the hope of being "just fine" and to preserving their current level of function following rehab (Lohne, 2008). In a qualitative study of 10 patients' experiences of hope following SCI, patients focused on the hope of improvement during the time following their SCI and up to 2 to 3 years after they completed their rehabilitation, at which time they focused their hope more on the hope of being "just fine" (Lohne, 2008).

Neuropathic Pain Neuropathic pain (also referred to as phantom or central pain) is frequently experienced by the patient with SCI. This pain is described as a burning, stabbing, shooting, aching, numbness and/or tingling, or electric shocklike pain that occurs at, just above, or below the level of injury. Neuropathic pain is common, with the prevalence of below-level pain after SCI being 34% and at-level pain 42% (Loh et al., 2016).

A meta-analysis review of pharmacological treatment of pain after SCI showed the following evidence (Mehta, McIntyre, Janzen, Loh, & Teasell, 2016):

- The best evidence supports the use of anticonvulsant, gabapentin (Neurontin), and pregabalin (Lyrica) as being effective at treating post-SCI neuropathic pain.
- Antidepressants may be effective but only among patients with comorbid depression.
- Local anesthetics remain an effective option for short-term pain relief.
- Cannabinoids, intrathecal baclofen, and botulinum toxin remain the most supported treatments for nociceptive- or spasticity-related pain.

Nursing care appropriate in the acute care phase for the patient with an SCI is summarized in the "Nursing Care: The Patient with Acute Spinal Cord Injury" feature.

Nursing Care
The Patient with Acute Spinal Cord Injury

Expected Patient Outcomes and Related Interventions

Outcome 1: Maintain pulmonary oxygenation and ventilation

Assess and compare to established norms, patient baselines, and trends.
Monitor for signs of pulmonary dysfunction.
Monitor ABGs, breath sounds, respiratory pattern and rate.
Monitor temperature, sputum color and consistency, pulmonary function tests, pulse oximetry.

Intervene to maintain pulmonary oxygenation and ventilation
Quad assist cough.
Suction as needed.
Deep breathing, incentive spirometer.

Reposition every 2 hours.
Elevate head of bed 30 degrees.
Maintain intake and output (for adequate hydration).

Administer related drug therapy and monitor for therapeutic and nontherapeutic effects.
Administer oxygen therapy as ordered.

Outcome 2: Optimize cardiac output

Assess and compare to established norms, patient baselines, and trends.
Monitor for signs of decreased cardiac output.
Monitor heart rate and rhythm, mentation, blood pressure (keep MAP greater than 90 mmHg).
Maintain extremities for warmth, capillary refill, pulses.
Balance intake and output.

Interventions to maintain cardiac output

Continuously monitor cardiac function.

Slowly elevate head of bed to prevent orthostatic hypotension.

Administer related drug therapy and monitor for therapeutic and nontherapeutic effects.

Administer intravenous fluids as ordered.

Deliver vasopressors as ordered.

Outcome 3: Maintain normal elimination

Assess and compare to established norms, patient baselines, and trends.

Monitor for signs of altered urinary and bowel elimination.

Balance intake and output.

Measure residual urine after voiding (< 400 mL residual is desired).

Watch bowel elimination pattern (regular pattern, soft stool desired).

Interventions to maintain normal urine and bowel elimination

Begin intermittent urinary catheterization when intake is less than 2 L/day.

Record bowel movements.

Adhere to bowel elimination schedule.

Administer related drug therapy and monitor for therapeutic and nontherapeutic effects.

Administer stool softeners as ordered.

Outcome 4: Maintain normal skin integrity

Assess and compare to established norms, patient baselines, and trends.

Monitor for signs of altered skin integrity.

Monitor for redness, edema, skin breakdown especially over pressure points (e.g., elbows, sacrum, coccyx, ischium, trochanters, heels, lateral malleolus).

Interventions to maintain normal skin integrity

Determine need for specialized bed (based on patient needs and hospital policy).

Turn every 2 hours; log-roll if appropriate.

Inspect bed for foreign objects.

Remove wrinkles from bedding underneath patient.

Maintain body in neutral position.

Outcome 5: Free from thrombus formation and pulmonary embolus

Assess and compare to established norms, patient baselines, and trends.

Monitor for signs of deep vein thrombosis (DVT) and pulmonary embolus (PE).

Monitor for DVT: swelling, redness, warmth in leg, fever.

Monitor for PE: Sudden shortness of breath, decreased SpO_2, pain on breathing, bloody secretions.

Interventions to prevent DVT and PE

Use compression devices on lower limbs (for at least the first 2 weeks post injury).

Keep well hydrated.

Administer related drug therapy and monitor for therapeutic and nontherapeutic effects.

Administer low molecular weight heparin as ordered.

Outcome 6: Maintain normal nutritional state

Assess and compare to established norms, patient baselines, and trends.

Monitor signs of altered nutrition.

Monitor for weight and muscle mass loss.

Monitor serum albumin and prealbumin.

Monitor for development of ileus

Monitor for GI bleeding (stress ulcer).

Interventions to maintain nutritional state

Arrange for early nutrition consult.

Use feeding tube as ordered. Check for proper tube tip placement.

Administer related drug therapy and monitor for therapeutic and nontherapeutic effects.

Administer histamine-blocking agent or proton pump inhibitor as ordered.

Outcome 7: Free from infection

Assess and compare to established norms, patient baselines, and trends.

Monitor for signs of infection.

Monitor for fever.

Monitor for urine color and clarity.

Monitor for skin and mucous membranes.

Monitor for sputum color and consistency, lung sounds.

Interventions to prevent infection

Carefully clean urinary catheter and meatus with soap and water.

Outcome 8: Minimize anxiety of patient and family.

Assess and compare to established norms, patient baselines, and trends.

Monitor for signs of anxiety.

Monitor for expressions of anxiety, concerns

Interventions to minimize anxiety

Provide psychological support to patient and family.

Make appropriate referrals (e.g., social worker, chaplain).

Section Five Review

1. Which SCI requires long-term mechanical ventilation?
   A. C1–C2
   B. C6–C7
   C. T1–T5
   D. All clients with SCI require long-term mechanical ventilation.

2. The main cause of complications or death post-SCI is related to which condition?
   A. Sepsis
   B. Respiratory complications
   C. Autonomic dysreflexia
   D. Bradycardia

3. A client is admitted to the unit with a C8 SCI. Which statement is true about recovery after this injury?
   A. The client will be able to eat independently.
   B. The client will be independent with dressing.
   C. The client will require an electric wheelchair.
   D. The client will require major assistance with bowel and bladder issues.
   E. The client will require major assistance for bathing.

4. Which sign indicates autonomic dysreflexia?
   A. Heart rate: 60 beats per minute
   B. Blood pressure: 220/120
   C. Priapism
   D. Poikilothermia

Answers: 1. A, 2. B, 3. (A, B), 4. B

Clinical Reasoning Checkpoint

It is the start of your 12-hour shift. You are assigned to Daniel R., a 25-year-old male injured in a diving accident 3 days ago. He dove into a sandbar at a remote river; alcohol was positive in the trauma toxicology screen, negative for other substances. He was diagnosed with a C4 burst fracture and a C4 ASIA A injury. The initial CT of his head was negative for any bleed. He had a posterior spinal fusion from C3 to C5 on the day of injury and is immobilized in a cervical collar. He has remained in sinus rhythm. Over the last 24 hours his forced vital capacity (FVC) and forced expiratory volume in 1 second (FEV_1) have been steadily decreasing. Last night his SpO_2 dropped to 82% and would only maintain at 90% with high concentrations of oxygen via a reservoir nasal cannula. Trauma anesthesia was called, and Daniel was endotracheally intubated with a fiber-optic scope. He has remained in normal sinus rhythm overnight with pulse oximetry remaining at or above 98%. You are completing your assessments, as follows:

- Vital signs: temp 99.8, HR 6/min, BP 100/72, with SpO_2 of 98%
- Pulmonary assessment: Breath sounds are diminished in the bases (right worse than left) with coarse rhonchi.
- Abdominal assessment: Bowel sounds are diminished, and abdomen is palpable but slightly distended.

- Peripheral perfusion assessment: Lower leg pulses are strong bilaterally; no redness, warmth, or swelling noted. No compression devices are present.
- Skin assessment: A purple discolored area is noted on the coccyx.

1. Examine Daniel's peripheral perfusion and skin assessments. What orders (medical and nursing) should be considered based on these findings?

2. Based on Daniel's presentation, what mechanism of injury is likely to be associated with his SCI, and what other associated injuries are likely to be present?

3. It has now been 48 hours since the injury. What are the priorities of caring for him now?

4. Describe interventions that Daniel will likely require to minimize complications of prolonged immobilization.

Clinical update: It is now 1 month post SCI, and Daniel exhibits reflex activity. He calls you to his room and complains of a severe headache. You note flushing and decide to take his BP. It is 180/95. Normally his BP is around 112/68. His pulse is 60. You remember that since yesterday he no longer has an indwelling urinary catheter for bladder training.

5. What is occurring, and what should you do about it?

Chapter 20 Review

1. A client arrives in the emergency department under full spinal cord injury precautions after being involved in a motor vehicle crash as an unrestrained driver. He has a C5–C6 fracture that involves the posterior wall of the vertebral body and bilateral lamina. The nurse will plan care for which type of fracture?
   1. Stable spinal fracture
   2. Subluxed spinal fracture
   3. Compression spinal fracture
   4. Unstable spinal fracture

2. A client presents with a complete spinal cord injury at T4, sustained when the client was shot in a robbery. The nurse prepares to care for a client with which impairment?
   1. Paraplegia
   2. Quadriplegia
   3. Tetraplegia
   4. No impairment

3. A client has sustained a spinal cord injury. The nurse asks the client to close her eyes while the nurse moves the big toe up and down, having the client state the direction in which the toe moves. What is the nurse assessing with this technique?

    1. Priapism
    2. Proprioception
    3. Dermatomes
    4. Sensation

4. A client who sustained a C4–C5 fracture subluxation has been placed in Gardner-Well tong traction with 20 pounds of weight. The client is alert and oriented and complaining of neck pain and spasms. Which nursing intervention should be implemented?

    1. Remove 10 pounds of weight from the traction apparatus.
    2. Administer PRN muscle relaxants.
    3. Report this unusual finding to the surgeon immediately.
    4. Place a pillow under the client's neck with ice bags to the side.

5. A client sustained a C4 spinal cord injury 3 weeks ago. This morning the client's BP is 204/110, heart rate is 45, and the client is complaining of a headache. What should the nurse do immediately? (Select all that apply.)

    1. Administer antihypertensive medications immediately.
    2. Encourage the client to rest and plan to recheck blood pressure in 30 minutes.
    3. Elevate the head of the bed.
    4. Check for a source of noxious stimuli.
    5. Order a stat 12-lead ECG.

6. A client is diagnosed with a lower motor neuron lesion. The nurse uses this information to plan care for which condition?

    1. Permanent loss of bladder function
    2. Flaccid paralysis
    3. Contralateral motor weakness
    4. Spastic paralysis

7. A client who has a spinal cord injury has been admitted to the ICU. Which factors, associated with the development of decreased cardiac output, are essential for the nurse to monitor? (Select all that apply.)

    1. Orthostatic hypotension
    2. Neurogenic shock
    3. Venous pooling
    4. Bradycardia
    5. Atelectasis

8. A client sustained an injury to the right side of the neck 3 years ago that resulted in Brown-Séquard syndrome. The nurse admitting the client to the hospital for an elective surgery would expect which assessment findings? (Select all that apply.)

    1. Loss of voluntary motor movement on the right
    2. Loss of temperature sensation on the left
    3. Inability to feel pain on either side
    4. Loss of voluntary motor movement on the left
    5. Loss of sensation on the right

9. The nurse is talking with the family of a client who was just admitted to the emergency department after a swimming accident that resulted in neck fracture and spinal cord injury. The family asks if the client will be paralyzed. Which response by the nurse is indicated?

    1. "We won't know how to classify the fracture until she is out of spinal shock."
    2. "Right now she is in neurogenic shock, so we are not concerned about the extent of the injury."
    3. "We have to wait until the autonomic dysreflexia passes before we will know."
    4. "Spinal cord injuries always result in some form of paralysis."

10. A client who has a spinal cord injury at T4 is to be moved out of bed today. Which nursing intervention should be done first?

    1. Recheck the mobility order, as these clients are generally on complete bed rest.
    2. Raise the head of the bed and reassess the client's status.
    3. Set the client up quickly to dangle on the side of the bed.
    4. Help the client ambulate to the bedside chair.

Answers to questions found inside your textbook are available on the faculty resources site. Please consult with your instructor.

References

Ahuja, C. S., Martin, A. R., & Fehlings, M. (2016). Recent advances in managing a spinal cord injury secondary to trauma. *F1000Research*, *5*, 1017. doi:10.12688 /f1000research.7586.1

American Spinal Injury Association (ASIA). (n.d.-a). *International Standards for Neurological Classification of Spinal Cord Injury (ISNCSCI)*. Retrieved March 14, 2017, from http://asia-spinalinjury.org/wp-content/ uploads/2016/02/International_Stds_Diagram_ Worksheet.pdf

American Spinal Injury Association (ASIA). (n.d.-b). *ASIA e-Learning Center*. Retrieved May 1, 2017, from http://asia-spinalinjury.org/learning

Aminoff, M. J., & Kerchner, G. A. (2011). Nervous system disorders. In S. J. McPhee & M. A. Papadakis (Eds.), *Current medical diagnosis and treatment* (50th ed., pp. 976–978). New York, NY: McGraw-Hill Professional.

Anwar, M. A., Shehabi, T. S., & Eid, A. H. (2016). Inflammogenesis of secondary spinal cord injury. *Frontiers in Cellular Neuroscience, 10*. doi:10.3389/fncel.2016.00098

Bracken, M. B. (2012). Steroids for acute spinal cord injury. *Cochrane Database Systematic Reviews, (3)*, CD001046. doi:10.1002/14651858.CD001046.pub2

Bracken, M. B., Collins, W. F., Freeman, M. J., Wagner, F. W., Silten, R. M., Hellenbrand, K. . . . Perot, P. L. (1984). Efficacy of methylprednisolone in acute spinal cord injury. *JAMA, 25*(1), 45–52.

Bracken, M. B., Shepard, M. J., Collins, W., Holford, T. R., Young, W., Baskin, D. S., . . . Maroon, J. (1990). A randomized controlled trial of methylprednisolone or naloxone in the treatment of acute spinal cord injury: Results of the second national acute spinal cord injury study. *New England Journal of Medicine, 322*(20), 1405–1411.

Bracken, M. B., Shepard, M. J., Holford, T. R., Leo-summers, L., Aldrich, E. F., Fazl, M., . . . Young, W. (1997). Administration of methylprednisolone for 24 or 48 hours or tirilazad mesylate for 48 hours in the treatment of acute spinal cord injury. Results of the Third National Acute Spinal Cord Injury Randomized Controlled Trial. National Acute Spinal Cord Injury Study. *Journal of American Medical Association, 277*(20), 1597–1604.

Branco, B. C., Plurad, D., Green, D. J., Inaba, K., Lam, L., Cestero, R.,. . . Demetriades, D. (2011). Incidence and clinical prediction of tracheostomy after cervical spinal cord injury: A national trauma database review. *Journal of Trauma, Injury, and Critical Care, 70*(1), 111–115.

Cameron, A., Wallner, L., Tate, D., Sarma, A., Rodriguez, G., & Clemens, J. (2010). Bladder management after SCI in the United States 1972–2005. *The Journal of Urology, 184*(1), 213–217.

Chung, W. S., Lin, C. L., Chang, S. N., Chung, H. A., Sung, F. C., & Kao, C. H. (2014). Increased risk of deep vein thrombosis and pulmonary embolism in patients with spinal cord injury: A nationwide cohort prospective study. *Thrombosis Research 133*(4), 579–584. doi:10.1016/j.thromres.2014.01.008. Epub 2014 Jan 11

Congress of Neurological Surgeons and American Association of Neurological Surgeons. (2013). Guidelines for the management of acute cervical spine and spinal cord injuries. *Neurosurgery, 60*, 1–259. doi:10.1227/01.neu.0000430319.32247.7f

Consortium for Spinal Cord Medicine. (2006). Bladder management for adults with spinal cord injury: A practice guideline for healthcare providers. *Journal of Spinal Cord Medicine, 29*(5), 527–573.

Consortium for Spinal Cord Medicine. (2008). Early acute management in adults with spinal cord injury: A clinical practice guideline for health-care professionals. *Journal of Spinal Cord Medicine, 31*(4), 403–479.

Consortium for Spinal Cord Medicine. (2010). Sexuality and reproductive health in adults with spinal cord injury: A clinical practice guideline for health-care professionals. *Journal of Spinal Cord Medicine, 33*(3), 281–336.

Consortium for Spinal Cord Medicine. (2016). *Prevention of venous thromboembolism in individuals with spinal cord injury: Clinical practice guideline for health care providers* (3rd ed.). Paralyzed Veterans of America. Retrieved March 14, 2017, from http://www.pva.org/media/pdf/CPG_thrombo_fnl.pdf

Cothren, C. C., Moore, E. E., Ray, C. E. Ciesla, D. J., Johnson, J. L., Moore, J. B., & Burch, J. M. (2005). Screening for blunt cerebrovascular injuries is cost-effective. *American Journal of Surgery, 190*, 845–849.

den Braber-Yonker, M., Lammens, M., van Putten, M., & Nagtegaal, I. D. (2017). The enteric nervous system and the musculature of the colon are altered in patients with spina bifida and spinal cord injury. *Virchows Archive, 470*(2), 175–184. Retrieved April 4, 2017, from https://link.springer.com/article/10.1007/s00428-016-2060-4.doi:10.1007/s00428-016-2060-4

DeSanto-Madeya, S. (2009). Adaptation to spinal cord injury for families post-injury. *Nursing Science Quarterly, 22*(1), 57–66.

deSouza, R. M., Crocker, M. J., Haliasos, N., Rennie, A., & Saxena, A. (2011). Blunt traumatic vertebral artery injury: A clinical review. *European Spine Journal, 20*(9), 1405–1416. doi:10.1007/s00586-011-1862-y

Dvorak, M. F., Noonan, V. K., Nader, D. Fisher, C. G., Finkelstein, J., Kwon, B. K., . . . the RHSCIR Network. (2015). The influence of time from injury to surgery on motor recovery and length of hospital stay in acute traumatic spinal cord injury: An observational Canadian Cohort Study. *Journal of Neurotrauma, 32*(9), 645–654. doi:10.1089/neu.2014.3632

Evaniew, N., Noonan, V. K., Fallah, N., Kwon, B. K., Rivers, C. S., & Dvorak, M. F. (2015). Methylprednisolone for the treatment of patients with acute spinal cord injuries: A propensity score-matched cohort study from a Canadian multi-center spinal cord injury registry. *Journal of Neurotrauma, 32*(21), 1674–1683. doi:10.1089/neu.2015.3963

Evans, C. H., Duby, J. J., Berry, A. J., Schermer, C. R., & Cocanour, C. S. (2014). Enteral albuterol decreases the need for chronotropic agents in patients with cervical spinal cord injury–induced bradycardia. *Journal of Trauma and Acute Care Surgery, 76*(2), 297–302. doi:10.1097/ta.0000000000000118

Fehlings, M., Rabin, D., Sears, W., Cadotte, D., & Aarabi, B. (2010). Current practice in the timing of surgical intervention in spinal cord injury. *Spine, 35*(21 Suppl.), S166–S173.

Fehlings, M. G., Vaccaro, A., Wilson, J. R., Singh, A., Cadotte, D. W., . . . Rampersaud, R. (2012). Early versus delayed decompression for traumatic cervical spinal cord injury: Results of the Surgical Timing in Acute Spinal Cord Injury Study (STASCIS). *PLoS ONE, 7*(2). doi:10.1371/journal.pone.0032037

Fouts, D. E., Pieper, R., Szpakowski, S., Pohl, H., Knoblach, S., Suh, M., . . . Groah, S. L. (2012). Integrated next-generation sequencing of 16S rDNA and metaproteomics differentiate the healthy urine microbiome from asymptomatic bacteriuria in neuropathic bladder associated with spinal cord injury. *Journal of Translational Medicine, 10*(1), 174. doi:10.1186/1479-5876-10-174

Furlan, J. C., Craven, B. C., Massicotte, E. M., & Fehlings, M. G. (2016). Early versus delayed surgical decompression of spinal cord after traumatic cervical spinal cord injury: A cost-utility analysis. *World Neurosurgery, 88*, 166–174. doi:10.1016/j.wneu.2015.12.072

Galeiras, R., Mourelo, M., Pertega, S., Lista, A., Ferreiro, M. E., Salvador, S., . . . Rodriguez, A. (2016). Rhabdomyolysis and acute kidney injury in patients with traumatic spinal cord injury. *Indian Journal of Critical Care Medicine, 20*(9), 504–512. doi:10.4103/0972-5229.190370

Glasser, R. S., Knego, R. S., Delashaw, J. B., & Fessler, R. G. (1993). The perioperative use of corticosteroids and bupivacaine in the management of lumbar disc disease. *Journal of Neurosurgery, 78*(3), 383–387.

Goetz, L. L., & Klausner, A. P. (2014). Strategies for prevention of urinary tract infection in neurogenic bladder dysfunction. *Physical Medicine and Rehabilitation Clinics of North America, 25*(3), 605–618.

Hadley, M. N., & Walters, B. C. (2013). Introduction to the guidelines for the management of acute cervical spine and spinal cord injuries. *Neurosurgery, 72*(Suppl 2) 5–16. doi:10.1227/NEU.0b013e3182773549

Hagen, E. M. (2015). Acute complications of spinal cord injuries. *World Journal of Orthopedics, 6*(1), 17–23. doi:10.5312/wjo.v6.i1.17

Hess, M. J., & Hough, S. (2012). Impact of spinal cord injury on sexuality: Broad-based clinical practice intervention and practical application. *The Journal of Spinal Cord Medicine, 35*(4), 211–218. doi:10.1179/2045772312y.0000000025

Jones, K., Simpson, G. K., Briggs, L., & Dorsett, P. (2016). Does spirituality facilitate adjustment and resilience among individuals and families after SCI? *Disability and Rehabilitation, 38*(10), 921–935. doi:10.3109/09638288.2015.1066884

Kaufmann, T. J., Huston, J., Mandrekar, J. N., Schleck, C. D., Thielen, K. R., & Kallmes, D. F. (2007). Complications of diagnostic cerebral angiography: Evaluation of 19,826 consecutive patients. *Radiology, 243*(3), 812–819. doi:10.1148/radiol.2433060536

Kopp, M. A., Druschel, C., Meisel, C., Liebscher, T., Prilipp, E., Watzlawick, R., . . . Schwab, J. M. (2013). The SCIentinel study—prospective multicenter study to define the spinal cord injury-induced immune depression syndrome (SCI-IDS)—study protocol and interim feasibility data. *BMC Neurology, 13*(1). doi:10.1186/1471-2377-13-168

Krassioukov, A., Eng, J., Claxton, G., Sakakibara, B., & Shum, S. (2010). Neurogenic bowel management after spinal cord injury: A systematic review of evidence. *Spinal Cord, 48*(10), 718–733.

Laginha, I., Kopp, M. A., Druschel, C., Schaser, K., Brommer, B., Hellman, R. C., . . . Schwab, J. M. (2016). Natural killer (NK) cell functionality after human spinal cord injury (SCI): Protocol of a prospective, longitudinal study. *BMC Neurology, 16*(1). doi:10.1186/s12883-016-0681-5

Lee, B. B., Toh, S., Ryan, S., Simpson, J. M., Clezy, K., & Kotsiou, G. (2016). Probiotics [LGG-BB12 or RC14-GR1] versus placebo as prophylaxis for urinary tract infection in persons with spinal cord injury [ProSCIUTTU]: A study protocol for a randomised controlled trial. *BMC Urology, 16*(18). doi:10.1186/s12894-016-0136-8

Loh, E., Guy, S. D., Mehta, S., Moulin, D. E., Bryce, T. N., Middleton, J. W., . . . Wolfe, D. (2016). The CanPain SCI clinical practice guidelines for rehabilitation management of neuropathic pain after spinal cord: Introduction, methodology and recommendation overview. *Spinal Cord, 54*, S1–S6. doi:10.1038/sc.2016.88

Lohne, V. (2008). The battle between hope and suffering: A conceptual model of hope within a context of SCI. *Advances in Nursing Science, 31*(3), 237–248.

Mehta, S., McIntyre, A., Janzen, S., Loh, E., & Teasell, R. (2016). Systematic review of pharmacologic treatments of pain after spinal cord injury: An update. *Archives of Physical Medicine and Rehabilitation, 97*(8), 1381–1391.e1. doi:10.1016/j.apmr.2015.12.023

Mistovich, J. J., Keith, J., & Brent, Q. (2014). *Prehospital emergency care* (10th ed.). Hoboken, NJ: Pearson. Retrieved March 30, 2017, from https://www.vitalsource.com/products/prehospital-emergency-care-joseph-j-mistovich-keith-j-v9780133775501

National Spinal Cord Injury Statistical Center (NSCISC). (2015). *The 2015 annual statistical report for the spinal cord injury model systems.* Retrieved October 15, 2016, from https://www.nscisc.uab.edu/PublicDocuments/reports/pdf/2015%20NSCISC%20Annual%20Statistical%20Report%20Complete%20Public%20Version.pdf

National Spinal Cord Injury Statistical Center (NSCISC). (2016). *Spinal cord injury facts and figures at a glance.* Retrieved October 15, 2016, from https://www.nscisc.uab.edu/Public/Facts%202016.pdf

Oh, Y., & Eun, J. (2015). Cardiovascular dysfunction due to sympathetic hypoactivity after complete cervical spinal cord injury. *Medicine, 94*(12). doi:10.1097/md.0000000000000686

Otani, K., Abe, H., Kadoya, S., Nakagawa, H., Ikata, T., & Tominaga, S. (1994). Beneficial effect of methylprednisolone sodium succinate in the treatment of acute spinal cord injury. *Sekitsui Sekizui, 7*, 633–647.

Petitjean, M. E., Pointillart, V., Dixmerias, F., Wiart, L., Sztark, F., Lassie, P., . . . Dabadie, P. (1998). Traitement medicamenteux de la lesion medullaire traumatique au stade aigu. *Annales françaises d'anesthèsie et de reanimation, 17*, 115–122.

Pettersson, K., & Toolanen, G. (1998). High-dose methylprednisolone prevents extensive sick leave after whiplash injury. A prospective, randomized, double-blind study. *Spine, 23*(9), 984–989.

Phillips, B. N., Smedema, S. M., Fleming, A. R., Sung, C., & Allen, M. G. (2016). Mediators of disability and hope for people with spinal cord injury. *Disability and Rehabilitation, 38*(17), 1672–1683. doi:10.3109/09638288. 2015.1107639

Ropper, A. H., Samuels, M. A., & Klein, J. P. (2014). Chapter 44. Diseases of the spinal cord. In *Adams & Victor's principles of neurology* (10th ed.). New York, NY: McGraw-Hill. Accessed March 11, 2017, from http://accessmedicine.mhmedical.com.ezproxy.uky .edu/content.aspx?bookid=690&sectionid=50910896

Saadoun, S., & Papadopoulos, M. C. (2016). Spinal cord injury: Is monitoring from the injury site the future? *Critical Care, 20*(1). doi:10.1186/s13054-016-1490-3

Sabit, B., Zeiler, F. A., & Berrington, N. (2016). The impact of mean arterial pressure on functional outcome post trauma-related acute spinal cord injury: A scoping systematic review of the human literature. *Journal of Intensive Care Medicine.* doi:10.1177/0885066616672643

Salameh, A., Mohajer, M. A., & Daroucihe, R. O. (2015). Prevention of urinary tract infections in patients with spinal cord injury. *CMAJ: Canadian Medical Association Journal, 187*(11), 807–811. doi:10.1503/cmaj.141044

Savage, K., Oleson, C., Sidhu, G., Vaccaro, A., & Schroeder, G. (2016). Neurogenic fever after acute traumatic spinal cord injury: A qualitative systematic review. *Global Spine Journal, 6*(06), 607–614. doi:10.1055/s-0035-1570751

Sauerland, S., Nagelschmidt, M., Mallmann, P., & Neugebauer, E. A. (2000) Risks and benefits of preoperative high dose methylprednisolone in surgical patients: A systematic review. *Drug Safety, 23*, 449–461.

Sayer, F. T., Kronvall, E., & Nilsson, O. G. (2006). Methylprednisolone treatment in acute spinal cord injury: The myth challenged through a structured analysis of published literature. *Spine Journal, 6*(3), 335–343.

Sisto, S. A., Druin, E., & Sliwinski, M. M. (2008). *Spinal cord injuries: Management and rehabilitation.* St. Louis, MO: Elsevier.

Taweel, W. A., & Seyam, R. (2015). Neurogenic bladder in spinal cord injury patients. *RRU Research and Reports in Urology, 7*, 85–99. doi:10.2147/rru.s29644

Todd, N. V. (2011). Priapism in acute spinal cord injury. *Spinal Cord, 49*(10), 1033–1035. doi:10.1038/sc.2011.57

Tom, V., Partida, E., Mironets, E., & Hou, S. (2016). Cardiovascular dysfunction following spinal cord injury. *Neural Regeneration Research, 11*(2), 189–194. doi:10.4103/1673-5374.177707

Vallès, M., & Mearin, F. (2009). Pathophysiology of bowel dysfunction in patients with motor incomplete spinal cord injury: Comparison with patients with motor complete spinal cord injury. *Diseases of the Colon and Rectum, 52*(9), 1589–1597.

Van Hoesen, K. B., & Bird, N. H. (2012). Diving medicine. In P. S. Auerbach (Ed.), *Wilderness medicine* (6th ed., pp. 1520–1549). St. Louis, MO: Elsevier.

Wilczweski, P., Grimm, D., Gianakis, A., Gill, B., Sarver, W., & McNett, M. (2012). Risk factors associated with pressure ulcer development in critically ill traumatic spinal cord injury patients. *Journal of Trauma Nursing, 19*(1), 5–10.

Wilson, B. A., Shannon, M., & Shields, K. (2017). *Pearson Nurse's Drug Guide 2017.* Hoboken, NJ: Pearson, VitalSource Bookshelf Online.

Wong, S., Shem, K., & Crew, J. (2012). Specialized respiratory management for acute cervical spinal cord injury: A retrospective analysis. *Topics in Spinal Cord Injury Rehabilitation, 18*(4), 283–290. doi:10.1310 /sci1804-283

Chapter 21
Determinants and Assessment of Gastrointestinal Function

Learning Outcomes

21.1 Describe the gastrointestinal tract, including anatomic structure, physiologic functions, blood supply and innervation, and laboratory assessments.

21.2 Explain how mechanisms within the gastrointestinal tract protect the integrity of the gut.

21.3 Describe the liver, including anatomic structure, physiologic functions, blood supply and innervation, and laboratory assessments.

21.4 Discuss the exocrine pancreas, including anatomic structure, physiologic functions, blood supply and innervation, and laboratory assessments.

21.5 Determine the diagnostic tests used to evaluate gastrointestinal, liver, and pancreatic function.

21.6 Apply the components of a focused nursing gastrointestinal database.

This chapter provides a review of foundational information needed to understand the alterations in gastrointestinal, liver, and pancreatic function addressed in Chapters 22, 23, and 24. It focuses on the major organs of the digestive system: the gastrointestinal tract, liver, and exocrine pancreas. Each system is profiled, with a review of normal anatomic structures, physiologic functions, blood supply and innervation, and associated laboratory assessments. A brief overview of general gastrointestinal assessments and diagnostic tests is also provided. Nursing assessments and other considerations specific to disease states of the gastrointestinal tract, liver, or pancreas are presented in individual chapters focusing on those organs.

Section One: The Gastrointestinal Tract

The gastrointestinal system includes the gastrointestinal tract, which consists of the mouth, pharynx, esophagus, stomach, small intestine, and large intestine. The gastrointestinal tract is essential in providing nutrition to the body through the processes of ingestion, mechanical processing, digestion, secretion, and absorption.

Anatomic Structures

The anatomy of the gastrointestinal (GI) tract includes the upper and lower GI or digestive systems (Figure 21–1). The upper portion includes the oral cavity, the teeth and tongue, the salivary glands, the pharynx, and the esophagus. The lower GI tract includes the small intestine (duodenum, jejunum, ileum) and large intestine (cecum colon, rectum, anus).

Mouth The mouth, or buccal cavity, is lined with mucous membranes and is enclosed by the lips, cheeks, palate, and tongue (Figure 21–2). The lips and cheeks are skin-covered muscle whose function is to keep food in the mouth during chewing. Inside the mouth is the boney **hard palate** in the roof of the mouth, which provides a surface against which the tongue forces food during chewing. The muscular **soft palate** extends from the hard palate to the back of the mouth

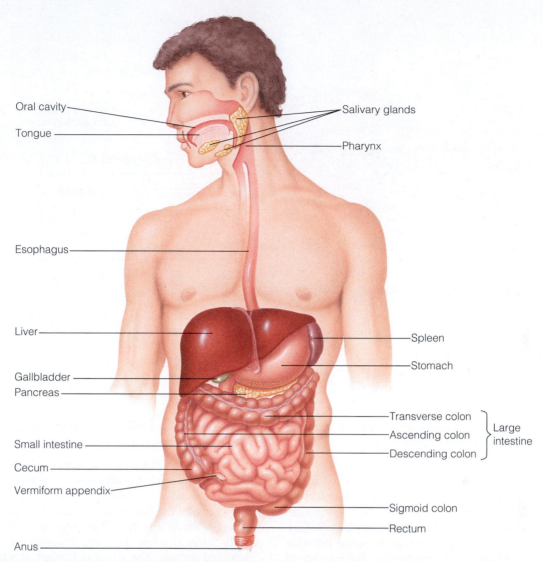

Figure 21–1 Organs of the gastrointestinal tract and accessory digestive organs.

and includes the uvula. When food is swallowed, the soft palate rises as a reflex to close off the oropharynx. The **tongue** is a muscle and is responsible for mixing the food with saliva during chewing, forming the food into a bolus (mass), and assisting with licking and swallowing. The tongue also contains papillae that house taste buds. Saliva, produced by salivary glands, provides moisture to the food bolus and contains enzymes (amylase) that begin the breakdown of food for digestion. The teeth function to grind and tear food into smaller parts. The muscular pharynx consists of the oropharynx and the laryngopharynx, both passageways for food and fluids into the esophagus through peristalsis. Peristalsis is the involuntary alternating waves of muscular contraction and relaxation. Mucous glands are in the mucosa of the pharynx and provide fluid to facilitate passage of food during swallowing (Barrett, 2014).

Esophagus The esophagus extends approximately 17.5 inches (45 cm) from the lower incisor teeth and serves as a passageway for food from the pharynx to the stomach. It is a muscular tubelike structure with the capacity to contract and release during peristalsis, which facilitates the movement of food toward the stomach. The mucosal lining is made up of stratified squamous epithelium and changes to columnar epithelium at or near the gastroesophageal junction. The **lower esophageal sphincter (LES)**, also known as the cardiac sphincter, is not formed from a distinct muscle but is a structure with high resting muscle tone at the distal end to prevent gastroesophageal reflux (Barrett, 2014).

Stomach The stomach is located in the upper-left abdominal quadrant. It begins at the terminal end of the esophagus just below the LES, where it receives food from the esophagus. The stomach is divided into three major parts: the fundus, the body, and the antrum (Figure 21–3). The **fundus** is the upper part of the stomach, just to the left of the LES, and appears as a bulge that bumps up against the diaphragm. The **body**, the largest part of the stomach, is located just beneath the fundus and ends at the antrum. The **antrum** is the base of the stomach, ending at the pyloric sphincter, which separates the stomach from the duodenum. The stomach wall is composed of the **mucosa**, the innermost lining; the **submucosa**, a layer that contains blood and lymphatic vessels; the **muscularis**, a three-layer muscle set; and the **serosa**, the outermost

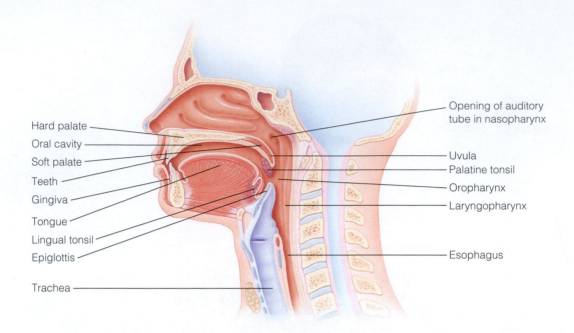

Figure 21–2 Structures of the mouth, the pharynx, and the esophagus.

lining (Figure 21–4). The size of the stomach changes based on the volume of contents within it. At rest it is small, containing only about 50 mL of fluid (Barrett, 2014).

Small Intestine The small intestine is composed of the duodenum, the jejunum, and the ileum. The small intestine extends from the pylorus of the stomach to the ileocecal valve, with a total length of approximately 16 to 20 feet. The mucosal and submucosal layers of the small intestine are arranged in folds and function to slow the passage of chyme through the small intestine to maximize digestion and absorption. Fingerlike projections called **villi** cover the intestinal folds. Each villus is covered with tiny, absorptive, fingerlike projections called **microvilli** that

collectively with the villi make up the brush border of the small intestine (Barrett, 2014).

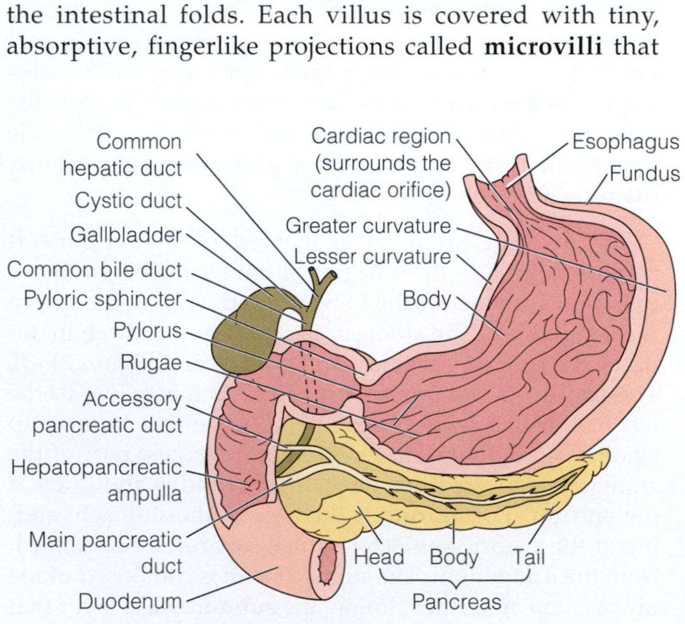

Large Intestine The large intestine is a hollow, muscular, tubular structure that originates at the terminal ileum at the ileocecal valve and extends to the anus. The ileocecal valve prevents the backflow of feces from the large intestine to the small intestine. The large intestine is approximately 5 feet (1.5 meters) long. It consists of the cecum, colon, and rectum. The colon is further divided into four segments: ascending, transverse, descending, and sigmoid. The absorption of water and electrolytes is largely completed in the ascending colon. It absorbs approximately 1 liter of water and electrolytes daily (Barrett, 2014).

When food is consumed, distention of the stomach leads to an immediate increase in colonic contractions, referred to as the **gastrocolic reflex**. The action of the large intestine, called **haustral churning**, moves the intestinal contents back and forth slowly in a kneading motion. This churning motion allows time for absorption of water to occur. As the rectum fills with stool, the defecation reflex is initiated (Barrett, 2014).

Physiologic Functions

Each structure of the digestive system plays a distinctive part in the digestive process, and each structure has specific physiologic functions that contribute to the process.

Stomach The stomach has a number of functions, including food storage, digestion, and propulsion. The stomach receives food via the esophagus. In preparation for accepting the food, the gastric wall relaxes through the influences of two hormones, **cholecystokinin (CCK)** and **gastrin**. Once in the stomach, peristaltic waves mix the food material with

Figure 21–3 The anatomic structures of the stomach, pancreas, and gallbladder.

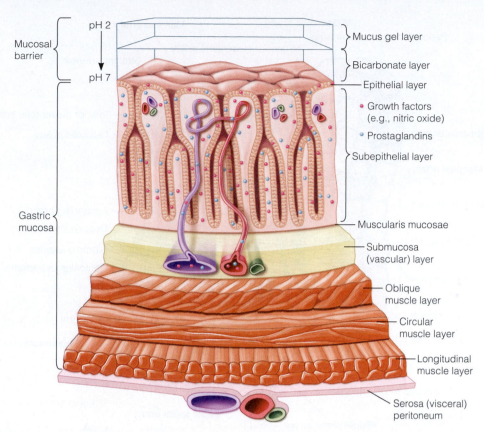

pH 2

pH 7

Mucosal barrier

Gastric mucosa

Mucus gel layer

Bicarbonate layer

Epithelial layer

• Growth factors (e.g., nitric oxide)

• Prostaglandins

Subepithelial layer

Muscularis mucosae

Submucosa (vascular) layer

Oblique muscle layer

Circular muscle layer

Longitudinal muscle layer

Serosa (visceral) peritoneum

Figure 21–4 Layers of the stomach wall and mechanisms for maintaining mucosal integrity.

the digestive juices (gastric acid and pepsin) to form **chyme**. While chyme is being formed, it is also being moved through the stomach toward the pyloric sphincter. The peristaltic action facilitates the emptying of the chyme into the duodenum, where it continues through the GI tract for further processing and elimination of waste.

The gastric body is richly supplied with gastric glands that contain **parietal cells** and **chief cells**. Parietal cells secrete **hydrochloric acid** and **intrinsic factor (IF)**, and chief cells secrete **pepsinogen**. Intrinsic factor is an important protein that is necessary for the absorption of vitamin B_{12} in the small intestine; without IF, pernicious anemia results. Pepsinogen is a precursor of pepsin, an enzyme that aids in protein digestion. The vagus nerve releases acetylcholine and stimulates gastrin secretion from G-cells within the antrum of the stomach. Gastrin and acetylcholine stimulate the release of histamine, which increases gastric acid production by stimulating H2 receptors on parietal cells within the gastric body. The gastric mucosa is protected from the caustic damaging effects of gastric acid and pepsin by a protective mucous and bicarbonate layer called the mucosal barrier. The health of this barrier is promoted by prostaglandins, which stimulate mucus and bicarbonate secretion and inhibit acid secretion.

Small and Large Intestines The primary function of the small intestine is absorption of nutrients and water. The small intestine secretes hormones that have stimulatory and inhibitory effects that help regulate digestion (Table 21–1).

These hormones include cholecystokinin, secretin, and gastric inhibitory peptide. Cholecystokinin (CCK) is secreted in response to the presence of fat, protein, and an acidic pH. The role of CCK is to stimulate secretion of pancreatic digestive enzymes that play an important role in the digestion of fat and protein, to increase contractility of the gallbladder so that bile is released into the duodenum to aid in the absorption of fats, and to inhibit gastric motility to slow the digestive process so that absorption can take place (Barrett, Barman, Boitano, & Brooks, 2016).

Table 21–1 Intestinal Hormones

Hormone	Secretion Stimulus	Action
Secretin	Secreted in response to acidic chyme and alcohol entering the duodenum	Stimulates release of bile, pancreatic enzymes, bicarbonate, water, and the action of CCK
Cholecystokinin (CCK)	Secreted in response to the presence of fat, protein, and acidic chyme in the duodenum	Stimulates release of pancreatic digestive enzymes; increases contractility of gallbladder; inhibits gastric motility
Gastric inhibitory peptide (GIP)	Secreted in response to carbohydrates and fat	Inhibits gastric acid secretion and motility; stimulates insulin secretion

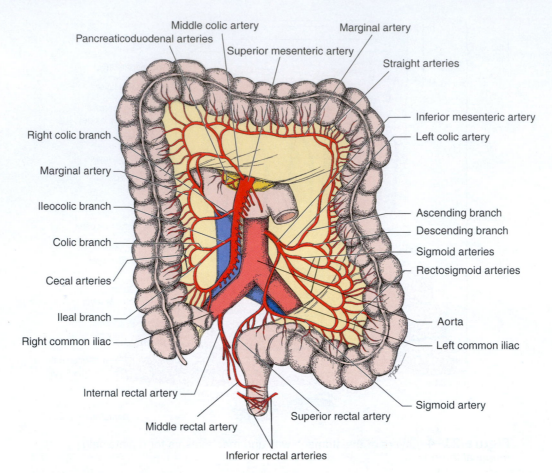

Figure 21–5 Arterial blood supply to the intestines.

When gastric acid comes into contact with the intestinal mucosa, it stimulates the release of the hormone **secretin**. Secretin further stimulates the release of alkaline pancreatic bicarbonate and water, raising the pH of chyme in the duodenum. This alkalinity is important because pancreatic digestive enzymes are active only in an alkaline environment. **Gastric inhibitory peptide (GIP)** is a hormone that is secreted in the presence of carbohydrates and fats within the small intestine. It facilitates the digestion of fats and carbohydrates by inhibiting intestinal motility and the secretion of gastric acid. GIP also stimulates insulin secretion. The inhibition of gastric acid contributes to the action of secretin to maintain the alkaline environment necessary for pancreatic **proteolytic** enzymes (those that break down proteins) to metabolize proteins and fats (Barrett et al., 2016).

The primary functions of the large intestine are the completion of water and nutrient absorption, the manufacture of certain vitamins, the formation of feces, and expulsion of the feces from the body. Digestion that occurs in the large intestine results from bacterial rather than enzymatic action. Normal flora residing in the large intestine break down dietary cellulose and synthesize folic acid, vitamin K, riboflavin, and nicotinic acid.

Blood Supply

The entire GI tract receives arterial blood from branches that arise from the abdominal (descending) aorta (AA). The celiac trunk (a large arterial branch located just below the diaphragm) divides into three smaller arteries (left gastric, splenic, and common hepatic), which distribute blood to the stomach and duodenum (Figure 21–5). The superior and inferior mesenteric arteries divide off from the AA to distribute blood to the proximal two thirds of the large intestine and the distal one third of the large intestine respectively (Table 21–2) (Barrett et al., 2016).

The major veins that drain blood from the stomach and intestines are the superior and inferior mesenteric veins and the gastric veins (Table 21–3). The GI tract is an important part of splanchnic circulation and the hepatic portal system, which are described in Section Three.

Table 21–2 Arterial Blood Supply of the Digestive System

Artery	Area Supplied with Blood
Left gastric	Stomach and esophagus
Hepatic to right gastric	Stomach
Gastroduodenal	Duodenum, gallbladder, stomach
Cystic	Gallbladder
Splenic	Stomach, spleen, pancreas
Superior mesenteric	Ascending colon, cecum, ileum, jejunum, transverse colon
Inferior mesenteric	Rectum, sigmoid colon, transverse colon, descending colon

Table 21–3 Venous Branches and Drainage Sites

Portal Vein Branch	Drainage Site
Gastric	Esophagus, stomach
Splenic	Duodenum, esophagus, gallbladder, stomach, pancreas
Superior mesenteric	Ascending and transverse colon, small intestine
Inferior mesenteric	Descending and sigmoid colon, rectum

Innervation

The GI tract receives sympathetic nervous system (SNS) innervation via the splanchnic nerves that branch off the spinal cord at the level of the low thoracic and high lumbar (T5–L2) segments (Figure 21–6). The splanchnic nerves are routed into several collateral ganglia, which, as postganglionic nerves, directly innervate the target mesenteric organs. Activation of the SNS inhibits most GI system functions to reroute blood to more vital organs during periods of stress. Activation of the SNS decreases gastric and intestinal motility and causes contraction of the sphincters. In general, secretions within these organs are decreased.

Parasympathetic innervation to the GI tract comes from cranial nerve (CN) X, the vagus nerve, and from S2 through S4. Parasympathetic stimulation of the organs within the GI tract is responsible for stimulating normal GI functions, such as processing of food, propulsion of contents through the GI tract, and absorption of nutrients. Parasympathetic stimulation increases gastric and intestinal motility and secretions (Barrett et al., 2016).

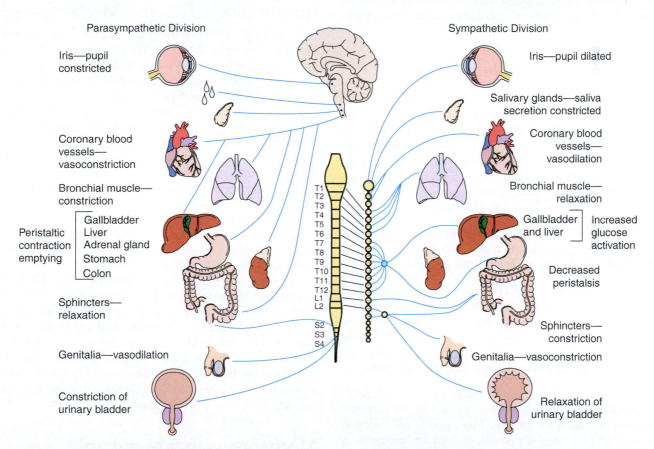

Figure 21–6 Parasympathetic and sympathetic divisions of the autonomic nervous system.

Section One Review

1. What is the largest portion of the stomach?
   A. Fundus
   B. Body
   C. Antrum
   D. Pylorus

2. The gastric parietal cells secrete which substance?
   A. Gastrin
   B. Pepsinogen
   C. Hydrochloric acid
   D. Mucus

3. The cystic artery supplies which gastrointestinal organ?
   A. Gallbladder
   B. Stomach
   C. Duodenum
   D. Esophagus

4. Which effect does the sympathetic nervous system have on the gastrointestinal system?
   A. Decreases gastric motility
   B. Increases intestinal motility
   C. Causes contraction of the sphincters
   D. Increases secretions from the stomach

Answers: 1. B, 2. C, 3. A, 4. A

Section Two: Gut Defenses

Mechanisms within the GI tract (or gut) are designed to protect its integrity. The GI system has two major mechanisms of defense: nonimmunologic and immunologic. The GI system plays a major role in the body's defense against bacteria, viruses, parasites, and other toxic pathogens.

Nonimmunologic Defense Mechanisms

The GI tract is exposed to potential contamination from the external environment through consumption of food and fluids on a daily basis, yet few pathogens introduced into the GI tract result in infection. This is primarily due to protection of the GI tract by nonimmunologic defense mechanisms: salivary secretions, gastric acidity, the mucosal barrier, peristalsis, and commensal bacteria.

Salivary Secretions Saliva contains defense proteins such as immunoglobulins that are active against foreign antigens and against bacteria ingested with food.

Gastric Acidity The acid environment of the stomach (pH lower than 4) is unfavorable for pathogen growth. This environment inhibits bacteria from entering the small intestine, where the pH must remain 7 or greater to allow the pancreatic proteolytic enzymes to become active and participate in the digestive process (Barrett et al., 2016).

Mucosal Barrier Pathogens that survive the gastric acidity have difficulty invading and colonizing the mucosa. There are two reasons for this. First, goblet cells secrete mucus that provides a protective barrier, preventing potential pathogens from adhering to the epithelial surface. Second, the epithelial mucosal cells are joined together by tight junctions that make it difficult for pathogens to move through to invade and colonize the underlying tissue.

Peristalsis Peristaltic motility further inhibits pathogen attachment to the intestinal mucosa by pushing contents along, reducing the amount of time pathogens can invade and colonize, preventing stagnation of the chyme, and preventing reflux of duodenal contents back up into the stomach.

Commensal Bacteria Commensal bacteria, or normal microflora, reside in the ileum and large intestine and limit the proliferation and adherence of potentially harmful bacteria. Commensal bacteria prevent the overgrowth of pathogenic species such as *Bacteroides fragilis*, an anaerobic bacteria, and *Escherichia coli*, an aerobic bacteria.

Immunologic Defense Mechanisms

Immunologic defense is provided by the **mucosa-associated lymphoid tissue (MALT)**, which includes the **gut-associated lymphoid tissue (GALT)** located primarily in the digestive system and small bowel, as well as in the urogenital and conjunctiva mucosa. MALT also includes the lymphoid tissue located in the respiratory system, known as the **bronchial- and tracheal-associated lymphoid tissue (BALT)**. The GI tract is a major defense organ, with 70% to 80% of all immunologic secreting cells located within the intestinal wall and about 25% of the intestinal mucosa composed of lymphoid tissue. GALT includes the tonsils, lymph tissue within the intestinal wall, and the appendix. These tissues produce immunoglobulins and immunocytes that migrate to the GI tract, tear ducts, and salivary glands to defend against pathogen penetration of epithelial surfaces (Barrett et al., 2016).

Peyer's patches are a component of GALT found throughout the small bowel, specifically the ileum. The patches have two lymphoid constituents: B cell follicles and parafollicular T-cell areas. The mucosal Peyer's patches also contain M cells of epithelial origin that have phagocytic functions. Small-bowel physiology continues to be studied intensely, with relevance to fields as diverse as vaccine development, food allergies, tumor immunology, and infectious diseases (Barrett et al., 2016).

Mechanisms that Maintain Mucosal Integrity

Superficial epithelial cells secrete mucus and bicarbonate, which aid in maintaining a pH gradient between the lumen and the mucosa to protect the underlying epithelial tissues from damage by gastric acid and pepsin. Mucosal blood flow is also an important mechanism in maintaining mucosal integrity. Prostaglandin provides important protection to the mucosal barrier by stimulating secretion of bicarbonate, increasing blood flow to the mucosa, and stimulating mucus secretion. Risk factors for disruption of intestinal mucosa include shock, trauma, intestinal obstruction, protein malnutrition, and total parenteral nutrition (Barrett et al., 2016).

Section Two Review

1. Commensal bacteria are part of which mechanism in the gut?
   A. Humoral defense mechanism
   B. Nonimmunologic defense mechanism
   C. Gut-associated lymphatic tissue
   D. Immunologic defense mechanism

2. How does peristalsis promote gastrointestinal health?
   A. By pushing intestinal contents along the GI tract and preventing reflux
   B. By creating an acid environment that is unfavorable to pathogen growth
   C. By secreting substances that are active against foreign antigens
   D. By covering the epithelial surface with mucus

3. What is a function of the mucosal coating?
   A. Maintains an acid environment
   B. Activates protective digestive enzymes
   C. Provides a physical barrier against invasion by pathogens
   D. Interferes with bacterial replication

4. What is the initial nonimmunologic defense mechanism against antigens?
   A. Salivary secretions
   B. Intestinal peristalsis
   C. *Escherichia coli* bacteria
   D. Peyer's patches

Answers: 1. B, 2. A, 3. C, 4. A

Section Three: The Liver

The liver is the largest of the abdominal organs and has many important functions, including metabolic and hematologic regulation and production of bile.

Anatomic Structures

The liver is located in the right-upper quadrant of the abdominal cavity and lies directly beneath the diaphragm. The anterior upper border of the liver is roughly parallel to the fifth right intercostal space and a lower border that runs obliquely upward from the right ninth to the left eighth costal cartilage. The liver has two major lobes—the right lobe and the left lobe—which are divided by the falciform ligament. The right lobe can be further divided into the caudate and quadrate lobes. The liver is enclosed in the visceral **peritoneum** and covered with a connective tissue structure known as Glisson's capsule. The capsule subdivides into branches called septa that extend into the liver parenchyma to form individual liver lobules. The liver can be divided into eight functionally distinct segments, each with its own set of blood vessels and bile ducts.

The **lobule** is the functional unit of the liver. It is shaped like a cylinder and surrounds a central vein in spokelike fashion, with portal triads (sheathlike structures containing a portal vein, hepatic artery, and bile duct) at the corners of the hexagonal lobule (Figure 21–7). Each lobule is composed of hepatic cellular plates that radiate out

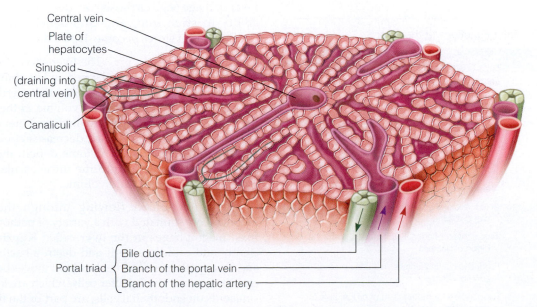

Figure 21–7 The liver lobule. The bile duct (represented in green) is one part of the bile canaliculus, the network of channels containing bile.

of the central vein. The hepatic cells (hepatocytes) secrete **bile**, which flows into the bile **canaliculi**, small spaces or canals that run through the hepatocytes separating the hepatic cellular plates. From the canaliculi the bile flows into terminal bile ducts located in the portal triad septa or spaces lying between adjoining lobules. The septa contain the portal venules, which provide blood flow from the portal veins.

Physiologically, it is useful to understand the liver architecture in terms of the portal-to-central direction of blood flow. The portal venules supply the blood that flows by the hepatic cellular plates and ultimately into the central vein of the lobule. The physiologic structure of the lobule allows continuous exposure of the hepatic cells to blood. Blood enters the **sinusoids** from the portal vein and hepatic artery. It is helpful to think of the sinusoid as a type of blood vessel that serves as a location and conduit for oxygen-rich blood from the hepatic artery and the nutrient-rich blood from the portal vein (Barrett et al., 2016).

Physiologic Functions

The liver performs a variety of crucial functions, including metabolism, regulation of circulating blood volume, filtering, clotting, and drug and chemical detoxification. Table 21–4 provides a summary of these functions.

Metabolic Functions The liver plays a crucial role in fat, carbohydrate, and protein metabolism because of its ability to synthesize, convert, degrade, or store these nutritional substances. In addition, the liver is important in maintaining normal levels of fat-soluble vitamins and iron in the body.

Fat Metabolism. The liver synthesizes phospholipids and cholesterol. Through oxidation of fatty acids, the liver can supply the body with massive amounts of energy. The liver produces and excretes bile. Bile salts, a major component of bile, are necessary for normal digestion. In the intestines, bile salts assist in the absorption of fat products, such as fatty acids, cholesterol, and fat-soluble vitamins. Bile salts also assist in the breakdown of fat molecules through a detergentlike action.

Carbohydrate Metabolism. The liver plays a major role in maintaining normal blood glucose levels. Glucose is stored in the liver as glycogen, which is converted back into glucose as needed by the body through the process of **glycogenolysis**. The liver also converts amino acids to glucose through the process of **gluconeogenesis**.

Protein Metabolism. Protein metabolism is essential to life. The liver not only synthesizes the majority of the body's proteins but also degrades amino acids for energy use through the process of deamination. The major by-product of deamination is *ammonia*, which is toxic to tissues. The liver converts ammonia into **urea**, a nontoxic substance. Urea diffuses from the liver into the circulation for urinary excretion. When liver failure occurs, ammonia cannot be converted to urea and levels build rapidly in the blood.

Vitamin- and Mineral-related Functions. Adequate levels of bile are needed for absorption in the small intestine of the fat-soluble vitamins A, D, E, and K. Should the production of bile become deficient, fat absorption decreases and the levels of these vitamins become significantly reduced. The liver requires vitamin K to produce clotting factors. If the level of vitamin K is low, clotting-factor production will be reduced. The liver also plays a crucial role in the early steps of the conversion of vitamin D into its active product—1,25-dihydroxycholecalciferol—which controls the concentration of calcium.

The liver is the major storage center for iron. Approximately 10% of iron is bound to ferritin within hepatocytes and is released when iron levels are depleted (Barrett et al., 2016). Iron is an important part of hemoglobin synthesis; more than half the body's iron is located in hemoglobin. Liver damage (e.g., cirrhosis) can decrease the hepatocytes' ability to store iron, and iron-deficiency anemia can develop if iron stores become depleted.

Blood Volume Reservoir The liver serves as a reservoir for blood. Its massive vascular bed and its ability to expand and compress provide a large potential overflow receptacle. During states of high fluid volume in the right heart, the liver is able to accept approximately 1 liter of the excess volume by distending, which decreases circulating fluid volume. In states of fluid volume deficit, the liver compresses, shifting blood into the intravascular space and increasing circulating fluid volume.

Blood Filter Blood flowing through the intestines becomes contaminated with a variety of pathogens. Special fixed macrophages in the liver called **Kupffer cells** efficiently and rapidly engulf and destroy bacteria, viruses, and other pathogens before the blood moves back into general circulation. The Kupffer cells, which are located in the sinusoids on endothelial cells, are part of the tissue macrophage system (also called the reticuloendothelial system). This important system consists of mobile macrophages,

Table 21–4 Major Functions of the Liver

General Function	Comments
Metabolic	Fat metabolism—massive energy source; produces bile Carbohydrate metabolism—maintains normal blood glucose Protein metabolism—synthesis of proteins and deamination of amino acids; converts ammonia to urea Vitamins and minerals—major role in absorption of fat-soluble vitamins (A, D, E, and K); major storage area for iron
Blood volume reservoir	Able to distend and compress to alter circulating blood volume
Blood filter	Tissue macrophages, Kupffer cells, purify the blood of bacteria
Blood clotting factors	Produces clotting factors, including prothrombin and fibrinogen
Drug metabolism and detoxification	Responsible for metabolism of drugs; able to deactivate potentially harmful substances and ready them for excretion in a harmless form

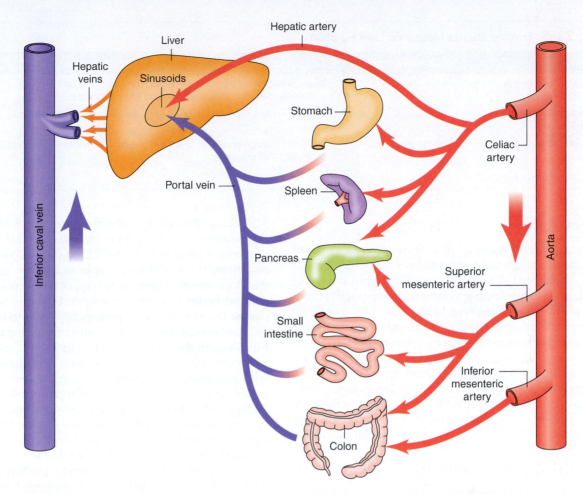

Figure 21–8 Splanchnic circulation. Includes blood flow through the liver, spleen, pancreas, stomach, and intestines (large and small).

which move freely through the tissues, and fixed macrophages, which are attached to tissues. Fixed macrophages, such as the Kupffer cells, are able to detach from their tissue when stimulated to carry out their phagocytic activities. The Kupffer cells also filter out foreign particles and old cells.

Blood Clotting Factors   The liver is responsible for the formation of most blood clotting factors. The normal formation of clotting factors requires synthesis of vitamin K by bacteria in the large intestines. When vitamin K synthesis is hindered, the formation of clotting factors is inhibited, leading to bleeding tendencies. The liver also produces fibrinogen, a protein that forms fibrin threads and blood clots due to the action of thrombin.

Drug Metabolism and Detoxification   The liver plays a major role in the metabolism of fat-soluble drugs. Through biotransformation, it changes potentially harmful drugs into less harmful or biologically active substances that are then excreted by the kidneys. The liver also has the ability to detoxify harmful endogenous substances.

Splanchnic Circulation

The portal venous and arterial circulatory systems of the viscera are collectively called the **splanchnic circulation**

(*splanchnic* refers to the abdominal [visceral] organs) (Figure 21–8). The liver is richly supplied with both arterial and venous blood. It receives arterial blood supply from the abdominal aorta (AA) by way of the common hepatic artery branch of the celiac trunk. Blood leaves the liver through the hepatic portal vein, which connects to the inferior vena cava.

Almost all venous blood draining from the abdomen returns to the heart through the inferior vena cava; however, it does not access the vena cava directly. Venous circulation from the digestive organs is part of the *hepatic portal system*, which acts as a gatekeeper—that is, the blood draining from the visceral organs flows through the liver before moving into the general circulation. The hepatic portal system allows the liver to absorb and store nutrients, as well as process and excrete substances such as metabolic waste products and toxins moving into the general circulation.

Approximately 30% of cardiac output flows through the liver and viscera. Blood enters the liver at a rate of about 1800 mL/min (fasting) or greater (after eating) through the hepatic artery and portal veins (Barrett et al., 2016). The exact volume of blood flowing into the liver is determined primarily by the volume of blood flow through the spleen and GI tract, both of which are parts of the splanchnic circulation.

Table 21–5 Enzyme Studies Measuring Liver Function

Enzyme	Normal Range	Comments
Alanine aminotransferase (ALT, SGOT)	5–35 units/L	More specific to liver than to other organs; the ratio of AST/ALT is usually > 1 in alcoholic cirrhosis and liver congestion and < 1 in acute hepatitis.
Aspartate aminotransferase (AST, SGOT)	0–35 units/L	Rises with damage to kidneys, heart, pancreas, and brain, as well as liver
Alkaline phosphatase (Alk phos)	20–90 units/L	Rises with damage or disease of kidneys and bone as well as liver; a sensitive measure of biliary tract obstruction

SOURCE: Data from Kee (2014).

Innervation

The liver receives sympathetic nervous system (SNS) innervation through the splanchnic nerves, which branch off the spinal cord at vertebral levels between the lower thoracic and higher lumbar vertebrae. Sympathetic stimulation to the viscera reduces blood flow and metabolic activities (decreased energy requirements). The liver releases stored energy reserves by converting glycogen to glucose. Sympathetic stimulation effects on the viscera are important in times of crisis for short-term survival. The parasympathetic nervous system (PNS) innervation comes through cranial nerve (CN) X, the vagus nerve. In the liver, excess glucose is stored as glycogen and blood flow and metabolic activities are increased (Kibble & Halsey, 2015).

Laboratory Assessment

An important part of assessing liver function is obtaining a laboratory panel of serum enzymes, proteins, bilirubin, and clotting measures. This panel is often referred to as a *liver function panel* or *liver function tests* (*LFTs*).

Liver Enzymes   Serum enzymes that are commonly included in LFTs are alanine aminotransferase (ALT), aspartate aminotransferase (AST), and alkaline phosphatase (Alk phos, ALP). These enzymes are not specific to liver cells, so abnormal levels can occur with a variety of other organ disorders. For this reason, **isoenzymes**, which are more specific to the liver, are often measured. These include LDH isoenzymes (LDH$_4$ and LDH$_5$), 5'-nucleotidase (5'NT), and gamma glutamyltransferase (GGT) (Kee, 2014). Refer to Table 21–5 for more information on specific enzymes and Table 21–6 for more detailed information on the isoenzymes.

Bilirubin   **Bilirubin** is the end-product of hemoglobin degradation, which occurs in the spleen and liver. It is the pigmented portion of heme. Through the oxidation process, heme is turned into bilirubin and is then released into the bloodstream. There are two types of bilirubin: fat soluble and water soluble. Fat-soluble bilirubin has not yet passed through the liver (prehepatic). Prior to undergoing a conversion in the liver, it is called **unconjugated bilirubin**. Once in the liver, bilirubin is first split from albumin molecules by the hepatocytes, then conjugated (joined) with glucuronic acid. In this conjugated state, it becomes water soluble and is called **conjugated bilirubin**. It is transported as bile from the liver into the intestines. From the intestines, most of the bilirubin is excreted through the feces. A small amount is excreted through the urine (**urobilinogen**). Very little conjugated bilirubin remains in the circulation to return to the liver; therefore, when bilirubin is measured, it is primarily the unconjugated (prehepatic) level that is being measured.

Bilirubin is a yellow pigment that is responsible for the brown color of stool. When the normal elimination of bilirubin is obstructed, causing bilirubin levels to increase, a yellowish discoloration (called **jaundice**) is evident in body fluids, the skin, the sclera, and the mucous membranes. Jaundice usually is not evident until the total bilirubin level exceeds 3 mg/dL (Kee, 2014).

Bilirubin testing is done by measuring the total bilirubin, the indirect and direct levels, as well as urobilinogen. Conjugated (or "direct") bilirubin (posthepatic, water soluble) is measured using a direct method because it requires no modifications before being measured. Unconjugated (or "indirect") bilirubin (prehepatic, fat soluble) is measured using an indirect method because it must be altered to a water-soluble state with a solvent before it can be measured.

Table 21–6 Isoenzymes for Evaluation of Liver Function

Isoenzyme	Normal Range	Comments
Lactate dehydrogenase isoenzyme 5 (LDH$_5$)	6%–16%	The LDH$_5$ isoenzyme is much more specific to the liver than the LDH enzyme.
Alkaline phosphatase isoenzyme 1 (ALP$_1$)	42–136 WI	The ALP$_1$ is specific to the liver and can increase significantly with liver injury.
5'-nucleotidase (5'NT)	Less than 17 U/L	5'N when measured with ALP is important in differentiating liver disease from bone disease.
Gamma glutamyl transferase (GGT)	Males: 9–69 units/L Females: 4–33 units/L	GGT is fairly specific to hepatobiliary tissues; it is, however, also present in pancreatic and renal cells; elevated GGT is present in the serum of alcohol abusers.

SOURCE: Data from Kee (2014).

Table 21–7 Bilirubin Testing

Type	Normal Values	Comments
Total bilirubin	0.1–1.2 mg/dL	Measures both conjugated and unconjugated bilirubin Elevations seen with biliary obstruction
Indirect (unconjugated)	0.1–1 mg/dL	Measures prehepatic, unconjugated bilirubin; elevations associated with viral hepatitis and other disease processes where lysis of red blood cells occurs
Direct (conjugated)	0.1–0.3 mg/dL	Measures posthepatic conjugated bilirubin; elevations associated with multiple intrahepatic and bile duct dysfunctions
Urobilinogen	Negative in freshly voided urine	Measures posthepatic urobilinogen in the urine; elevations associated with early or recovery phase liver cell damage Antibiotics may decrease levels

SOURCE: Data from Kee (2014).

Urobilinogen is measured as a sensitive test for hepatic damage. It may increase before serum bilirubin levels increase. In early hepatitis or mild liver cell damage, the urine urobilinogen level increases despite an unchanged serum bilirubin level. However, with severe liver failure, the urine urobilinogen level may decrease because less bile is produced. This test might be ordered along with a urinalysis. Table 21–7 provides a summary of bilirubin laboratory testing.

Clotting Measures   The liver has an important role in maintaining normal coagulation because it produces fibrinogen, prothrombin, vitamin K–dependent clotting factors essential to the coagulation cascade. If liver function becomes compromised and these substances can no longer be synthesized in adequate quantities, the patient is at increased risk for serious bleeding complications. Two common blood tests used to measure the two coagulation pathways are prothrombin time and partial thromboplastin time.

Prothrombin Time and International Normalized Ratio. The prothrombin time (PT) measures the extrinsic coagulation pathway. Prothrombin (factor II of the coagulation cascade) is produced by the liver and is dependent on vitamin K, which is also produced by the bacteria in the intestinal tract. Prolonged PTs may be seen with chronic liver disease (e.g., cirrhosis) or vitamin K deficiency. Normal PT is 10 to 13 seconds (Kee, 2014). Unfortunately, the traditional measurement of PT can vary depending on the lab analysis method used. For this reason, the preferred measure is the international normalized ratio (INR), particularly when the patient is being anticoagulated. The normal range of INR during anticoagulation therapy is 2 to 3 (Kee, 2014). INR is particularly recommended for monitoring long-term warfarin therapy once the dose has been stabilized.

Partial Thromboplastin Time.   Partial thromboplastin time (PTT) measures the intrinsic coagulation pathway. It is more sensitive than PT in measuring clotting abnormalities in all factors except VII and VIII. Elevations of PTT are seen with severe liver disease or with heparin administration. Normal values are 60 to 70 seconds (Kee, 2014). Activated partial thromboplastin time (aPTT) is an even more sensitive indicator than PTT in the detection of defects in the clotting factors. It differs from PTT in that the reagent contains an activator. Normal aPTT is 20 to 35 seconds (Kee, 2014).

Serum Ammonia   Elevations of serum ammonia levels indicate that the liver is not adequately converting ammonia to urea for elimination in the urine. The normal range for serum ammonia levels is 15 to 45 mcg/dL (Kee, 2014). Elevated levels can lead to the development of hepatic encephalopathy, a complication of liver failure.

Serum Albumin   The liver synthesizes albumin and many other proteins; thus, as liver function decreases, protein levels also decrease. Serum albumin is a good indicator of general protein levels. The half-life of albumin is relatively long (several weeks), so it is a poor marker of acute hepatic injury but can be an indicator of long-standing illness, malnutrition, or disease. The normal range is 3.5 to 5 g/dL (Kee, 2014).

Section Three Review

1. What is the primary substance in bile?
   A. Bile salts
   B. Bilirubin
   C. Cholesterol
   D. Electrolytes

2. What is the major by-product of amino acid deamination?
   A. Bilirubin
   B. Ammonia
   C. Fatty acids
   D. Glucose

3. The action of which factor is responsible for the blood filtering capabilities of the liver?
   A. Kupffer cells
   B. Immunoglobulins
   C. Ammonia
   D. Bile

4. The blood volume flowing through the liver represents what percentage of cardiac output?
   A. 15%
   B. 20%
   C. 25%
   D. 30%

Answers: 1. A, 2. B, 3. A, 4. D

Section Four: The Exocrine Pancreas

The pancreas is a multifunctional organ, having both endocrine and exocrine functions. Its exocrine functions are an integral part of the digestive process. The endocrine pancreas is covered in detail in Chapter 31.

Anatomic Structures

The pancreas is located in the upper abdominal cavity, lying in a horizontal position (Figure 21–9). It is a soft, elongated, flattened gland 5 to 8 inches (12 to 20 cm) in length. In an adult, it normally weighs between 70 and 110 grams. It has three divisions: the head, the body, and the tail. The head lies adjacent to the duodenum, within its curve. The pancreatic body lies directly behind the stomach, and the tail is adjacent to the spleen (Kibble & Halsey, 2015).

The pancreatic exocrine cells comprise almost the entirety (about 98%) of the pancreatic tissue. The functional exocrine unit of the pancreas is the **acinus**, which can be spherical or tubular or even irregular in form. The acinus is composed of cells that synthesize, store, and secrete digestive enzymes, as well as a network of ductal cells that secrete alkaline fluids with important digestive functions. Acini are clustered into larger units called pancreatic lobules. The lobules are separated from each other by septa (Figure 21–10).

Once released, the pancreatic digestive enzymes flow into the duodenum (refer to Figure 21–9 and Figure 20–10A) through a connecting network of ducts, eventually terminating at the main pancreatic duct, called the duct of Wirsung. This duct runs through the center of the organ from head to tail and joins with the common bile duct, sharing the same opening into the duodenum at the ampulla of Vater. Located at the junction of the common bile duct and the duodenum, the sphincter of Oddi controls the rate of pancreatic enzyme and bile flow into the duodenum (Barrett et al., 2016).

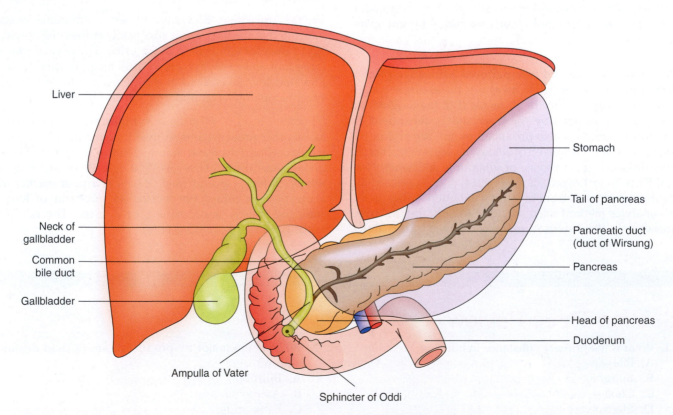

Liver

Stomach

Tail of pancreas

Pancreatic duct (duct of Wirsung)

Neck of gallbladder

Common bile duct

Pancreas

Gallbladder

Head of pancreas

Duodenum

Ampulla of Vater

Sphincter of Oddi

Figure 21–9 Structures and anatomical location of the pancreatic–biliary system.

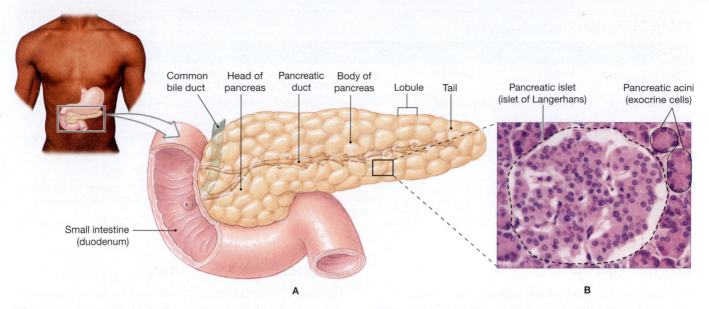

Figure 21–10 The pancreas. A, Pancreatic anatomic structures. B, Acinus, the pancreatic exocrine functional unit.

Physiologic Functions

The pancreas is rather unique in that it has both endocrine and exocrine functions. The endocrine functions consist primarily of the secretion of the two major hormones that maintain glucose homeostasis: insulin and glucagon. The exocrine functions of the pancreas directly influence the GI system and accessory organs.

The pancreas normally secretes approximately 1.5 liters of enzyme fluid daily. These enzymes are secreted in their inactive form and are activated in the duodenum for the digestion of fats, starches, and proteins. Pancreatic secretions are composed of water, bicarbonate, electrolytes (specifically potassium and sodium), and digestive enzymes. In a healthy person, pancreatic secretions are clear, colorless, isotonic, protein rich, and alkaline.

There are four major stimuli of pancreatic secretion: gastrin, cholecystokinin (CCK), secretin, and acetylcholine. The acidic pH of the chyme that enters the duodenum from the stomach stimulates mucosal secretion of secretin and CCK. These two hormones are essential in the regulation of intestinal pH; both are regulatory hormones responsive to a negative feedback system. Secretin and CCK are also stimulated by stomach acids, amino acids, and fatty acids. Gastrin, secretin, and CCK stimulate the pancreatic acinar cells and are responsible for the release of large quantities of pancreatic enzymes. Acetylcholine is secreted by parasympathetic, vagal, and cholinergic nerve endings located throughout the gut. Vagal influence stimulates secretion of pancreatic enzymes, which are then placed in temporary storage in the acini, awaiting a transport mechanism to move them into the intestines (Barrett et al., 2016).

The release of secretin is stimulated by a drop in pH to less than 4.5. When the intestinal pH becomes too acidic, secretin stimulates the pancreas to secrete large quantities of bicarbonate and water. Bicarbonate raises the intestinal pH, protecting the mucosa. Pancreatic enzymes work best within a pH level that is neutral to slightly alkaline. The alkaline pH of the small bowel is important for deactivating pepsin, which protects the delicate intestinal mucosa and facilitates normal digestive enzyme processes. In contrast, cholecystokinin is secreted from the mucosal epithelial cells in the first segment (proximal portion) of the small intestine (duodenum), and stimulates delivery into the small intestine of digestive enzymes from the pancreas and bile from the gallbladder. Cholecystokinin uses vagal mechanisms (activation of acetylcholine and its release) to stimulate acinar cells to release digestive proteolytics (Barrett et al., 2016).

Pancreatic Enzymes   Normal digestion depends on the digestive enzymatic activities of the pancreatic enzymes (Table 21–8). The proteolytic pancreatic enzymes (trypsin, chymotrypsin, and elastase) make up about 90% of pancreatic digestive enzymes and are responsible for breaking down proteins. The lipolytic pancreatic enzyme, **phospholipase A**, breaks down phospholipids into fatty acids (Kibble & Halsey, 2015). This enzyme may contribute to the development of pulmonary complications (acute respiratory distress syndrome [ARDS]) by decreasing surfactant in the lungs (Elder, Saccone, & Dixon, 2012). The pancreatic amylolytic enzyme, amylase, breaks down starch into sugars.

Pancreatic Self-protective Properties   Without some protective mechanism, these enzymes are capable of digesting pancreatic and other tissues, a process called **autodigestion**. Under normal circumstances, mechanisms are in place to prevent autodigestion. Pancreatic proteolytic enzymes are produced in an inactive, precursor form, remaining inactive while in the pancreas (refer to Table 21–8 for the precursor names). For example, a trypsin inhibitor (secreted by the acinar cells) maintains trypsin in its inactive state in the pancreatic ducts and cells (Kibble & Halsey, 2015).

Table 21–8 Major Pancreatic Enzymes

Enzyme	Target	Precursor Name	Comments
Trypsin	Proteins	Trypsinogen	Most abundant proteolytic enzyme; activated in intestinal mucosa by enterokinase or by preexisting trypsin
Elastase	Proteins	Proelastase	Activated by trypsin; breaks down elastic tissue; can break down blood vessel walls
Chymotrypsin	Proteins	Chymotrypsinogen	Activated by trypsin; splits (via hydrolyzing) proteins into peptones
Amylase (pancreatic)	Carbohydrates	—	Splits glycogen, starches, and other carbohydrates, with the exception of cellulose, into disaccharides (primarily)
Lipase	Fats	—	Requires bile salts; splits fats into monoglycerides and fatty acids
Phospholipase A	Fats	—	Activated by trypsin or bile salts; splits phospholipids into fatty acids; breaks down cell membranes and is capable of causing pancreatic and fat tissue necrosis and reduction in lung surfactant levels

Blood Supply

The pancreas is part of the splanchnic circulation, as described in the previous section. Arterial blood supply comes from the splenic artery, the common hepatic artery of the celiac trunk, and the superior mesenteric artery. The pancreas is part of the hepatic portal system, with venous blood leaving the pancreas through the portal, splenic, and superior mesenteric veins.

Innervation

The SNS innervation of the pancreas stems from the splanchnic nerves and PNS innervation coming from cranial nerve (CN) X, the vagus nerve, as was described with liver innervation. Stimulation of the SNS exocrine pancreas inhibits the acinar cells, which reduces the secretion of digestive enzymes. When the PNS is stimulated, acinar cells are stimulated to increase secretion of the enzymes.

Laboratory Assessment

A variety of diagnostic tests are used to assess pancreatic function. Each provides the practitioner with different information; tests that directly stimulate the pancreas are the most sensitive.

Pancreatic Enzymes   Pancreatic enzymes can be found in a variety of body fluids. Blood tests are used to evaluate the function of the pancreas. Levels of two pancreatic enzymes, amylase and lipase, can be measured in the serum. **Amylase** can be detected in the urine, serum, ascitic fluid, pleural fluid, and as an isoenzyme. Amylase is often used as a screening test for pancreatitis in patients with acute abdominal pain or back pain; however, there are multiple other causes of elevation of this enzyme. Amylase can be identified in the urine when the serum levels may be normal because renal clearance of the enzyme can be elevated in an acute pancreatic event. A normal value for amylase is 30 to 170 units/L (Kee, 2014).

Table 21–9 Measures of Pancreatic Function

Laboratory Test	Normal Values	Comments
Serum		
Amylase	30–170 units/L	In acute pancreatitis, serum levels peak 4–8 hours after onset, then fall to normal within 48–72 hours; low levels usually indicate pancreatic insufficiency.
Isoamylase P (pancreatic)	30%–55%	Elevated in acute pancreatitis
Lipase	14–280 units/L	Elevated only in pancreatitis, markedly in acute cases and with biliary tract disease; remains increased after amylase returns to normal
Total calcium	8.2–10.2 mg/dL	High total calcium levels occur in malignancy of liver, pancreas, and other organs.
Ionized calcium	4.65–5.28 mg/dL	Ionized calcium is useful in tracking the course of cancer disorders and acute pancreatitis.
Triglycerides	50–250 mg/dL	Patient must fast for 12 hours before specimen is drawn; levels are increased in cirrhosis, diabetes mellitus, hypertension, and hyperlipoproteinemia.
Glucose	65–110 mg/dL (fasting)	Patient must fast for 12 hours before specimen is drawn.
Stool		
Fat	Less than 6 g/24 hr	Levels greater than 6 g/24 hr is suggestive of decreased absorptive ability and indicative of pancreatic exocrine insufficiency as in chronic pancreatitis.
Urine		
Amylase	2 hour: 2–34 units 24 hour: 24–408 units	These values are 6–10 hours behind serum values; low levels indicate pancreatic insufficiency.

SOURCE: Data from Kee (2014).

Lipase levels in the serum will be elevated if pancreatic inflammation is present. As with amylase, lipase can be elevated for multiple reasons. Lipase is currently the best enzyme to identify acute pancreatitis. A normal value for lipase is 14 to 280 units/liter (Kee, 2014).

Exocrine Pancreatic Function Testing Exocrine pancreatic function tests provide the most reliable indication of pancreatic function. Table 21–9 provides a summary of major pancreatic function tests and normal ranges.

Secretin Stimulation Test. The secretin stimulation test measures the ability of the pancreas to respond to secretin. **Secretin** is a hormone made by the small intestine. Secretin stimulates the pancreas to release a bicarbonate-rich fluid that neutralizes stomach acid and aids in digestion. This test may be performed in patients with diseases that affect the pancreas to determine the activity of the pancreas. During the test, a tube is inserted through the mouth (or nose) into the esophagus, through the stomach, then into the upper part of the small intestine. Secretin is administered and the contents of the duodenal secretions are aspirated and analyzed over a period of about 2 hours.

Elastase Test. The fecal elastase test is another test of pancreas function. The test measures the levels of **elastase**, an enzyme found in fluids produced by the pancreas that digests proteins. In this test, a patient's stool sample is analyzed for the presence of elastase.

Section Four Review

1. The sphincter of Oddi primarily serves which purpose?
   A. Controls the rate of pancreatic enzyme flow into intestines
   B. Controls the activation of the pancreatic enzymes
   C. Regulates the level of intestinal secretin
   D. Regulates the rate of bicarbonate secretion

2. How is the pH of pancreatic secretion best described?
   A. Acidic
   B. Moderately acidic
   C. Neutral
   D. Alkaline

3. What is the most abundant pancreatic enzyme?
   A. Chymotrypsin
   B. Lipase
   C. Trypsin
   D. Elastase

4. How is the pancreas protected from autodigestion?
   A. By bicarbonate and water
   B. By the presence of the hormone secretin
   C. By protective pancreatic cell wall coverings
   D. By the production of enzymes in their inactive states

Answers: 1. A, 2. D, 3. C, 4. D

Section Five: Diagnostic Tests

Multiple diagnostic studies and laboratory tests are used to evaluate the GI system and accessory organs. Many of the radiographic studies require a contrast medium; therefore, the patient's allergy status must be known, as severe hypersensitivity reactions can occur in sensitive people.

Diagnosing disorders of the GI system and accessory organs can be challenging because the complex disease status of the high-acuity patient may mask the development of GI or accessory organ complications. Symptoms often are vague initially and may have an insidious onset; thus, early manifestations may be overlooked in the presence of other high-priority health concerns. Diagnostic studies, either invasive or noninvasive, are often required to definitively diagnose an acute problem.

Diagnostic and Laboratory Tests of the GI System

Many diagnostic tests are available for evaluating the status of the GI system, such as radiographic exams, CT scans, MRIs, and others.

Radiographic Exam The radiographic exam or flat-plate x-ray of the abdomen is helpful in diagnosing intra-abdominal problems such as intestinal obstruction, rupture, masses, abnormal fluid or air levels, and the presence of foreign bodies. An upper GI series with contrast medium is another type of radiographic exam. The contrast medium (barium) allows visualization of any abnormalities. Visualization of the GI tract aids in the diagnosis of tumors, masses, hernias, obstructions, ulcers, fistulas, and diverticular disease. To prevent serious allergic reactions, it is important to ask about the patient's allergy history prior to administration of the contrast medium. Following the test, the patient should be assessed and monitored to ensure that the contrast is expelled, with interventions if needed.

Computed Tomography Scan The computed tomography (CT) scan is another test allowing visualization of the abdomen, retroperitoneal structures, masses, abscesses, and abnormal fluid or air levels, which might be visible if perforation has occurred. This noninvasive exam requires the patient to ingest a barium contrast solution prior to the exam. The nurse should provide specific instructions on expelling the barium contrast.

Ultrasound Sonography Ultrasound sonography allows visualization of abdominal and retroperitoneal soft-tissue structures to diagnose fluid or air pockets, abscesses, and masses, and to observe movement (i.e., peristalsis, gastric emptying). This procedure may take place at the patient's bedside. Transducing gel is applied to the skin, and mild pressure is applied with a transducer. Adipose tissue, air, and barium may diminish ultrasound wave transmission.

Magnetic Resonance Imaging

A magnetic resonance imaging (MRI) scan is used to assess abdominal and retroperitoneal structures for masses, abscesses, and fluid or air pockets. Internal metal objects or foreign bodies are a contraindication to MRI; all external metal objects and dental appliances must be removed. It is very important that the patient lie still for this test; therefore, he or she must be able to cooperate.

Nuclear Scan

A nuclear scan allows visualization of organs, GI motility, and bleeding. An intravenous contrast medium is administered; an allergy history should be obtained to reduce the risk of allergic reaction. Nonuniform radioactive uptake in tissues often indicates disease. A nuclear scan is contraindicated in pregnancy, breastfeeding, or recent nuclear exposure. All metal must be removed from patients prior to a nuclear scan.

Angiography

Angiography allows visualization of blood flow in selected vascular beds. Obstructed or bleeding vessels can be identified with this test. A contrast medium is administered intravenously; an allergy history is important.

Endoscopy

Endoscopy allows inspection of internal surfaces of organs. It includes a series of diagnostic tests for the GI system using a flexible scope with a fiber-optic light and lens system. Removal of tissue for testing (biopsy)—as well as some treatments, such as sclerotherapy, suction, and cauterization of bleeding vessels—may be performed during endoscopy of the upper or lower GI tract. Common endoscopic tests are summarized in Table 21–10.

Gastric Tonometry

Gastric tonometry is an invasive monitoring technique that allows the assessment of gut perfusion in critically ill patients. This technique uses a special nasogastric tube with a balloon sensor that is inserted into the stomach to measure the carbon dioxide (CO_2) level of the gastric mucosa, which rises when the GI tract is underperfused (Figure 21–11). Tonometry provides an early warning of reduced gastric perfusion, which can occur when a patient is hypovolemic or in shock. During a period of hypoperfusion, the GI tract is one of the first organ systems to suffer reduced blood flow. A decrease in the delivery of oxygen-rich blood to the gut mucosa results in anaerobic metabolism. Tonometry measures the changes in the pH and CO_2 levels of the gut, which are indicative of GI tract perfusion.

Conditions that alter the intramucosal pH and CO_2 levels include (1) acid entering and bicarbonate refluxing back into the stomach from the duodenum, (2) enteral feeding that refluxes into the stomach, and (3) continuous aspiration of the stomach by a sump-style nasogastric tube.

If any of these conditions exist, the gastric tonometry results should be questioned (Lee, 2012).

Sublingual Capnometry

Sublingual capnometry is a simple, noninvasive technology that provides immediate measures of partial pressure of sublingual carbon dioxide ($PslCO_2$). It measures sublingual perfusion, requires a special CO_2 probe to be placed beneath the tongue, and provides an alternative to invasive gastric tonometry monitoring for splanchnic perfusion. Sublingual capnometry provides intermittent measurements that require trending rather than a continuous measurement of CO_2 trends. The presence of orogastric or nasogastric tubes does not appear to affect the accuracy of the results. Enteral feedings do not need to be stopped to obtain measures. Additional studies in human subjects are necessary to support the clinical usefulness of this technology (Zuckerbraun, Peitzman, & Billiar, 2014).

Additional Pancreatic Diagnostic Studies

Multiple studies are available to determine if pancreatic structure is intact and functioning properly. Standard abdominal x-ray films are a good starting point for diagnosis; however, many patients with pancreatitis have normal abdominal films. Computed tomography (CT) scans can provide detailed visualization of the pancreas and can also identify other possible causes of elevated pancreatic enzymes. A CT scan can identify complications of pancreatic disease such as fluid around the pancreas, an abscess, or a collection of tissue, fluid, and pancreatic enzymes.

Further investigation of the pancreas to evaluate the pancreatic and bile ducts can be accomplished by magnetic resonance imaging (MRI). This is known as **magnetic resonance cholangiopancreatography (MRCP)**. Abdominal ultrasound can provide information regarding swelling, inflammation, calcification, pseudocysts, and lesions of the pancreas.

Endoscopic Retrograde Cholangiopancreatography (ERCP)

Endoscopic retrograde cholangiopancreatography (ERCP) provides visualization of the pancreatic–biliary duct system. This test can provide diagnostic data in 60% to 85% of pancreatitis cases. In an ERCP, a healthcare provider (HCP) threads a tube down the esophagus, into the stomach, then into the small intestine. Contrast dye is used to help the HCP see the structure of the common bile duct, other bile ducts, and the pancreatic duct on an x-ray (Conwell & Banks, 2016).

Endoscopic Ultrasound

Endoscopic ultrasound is another invasive test in which a probe attached to a lighted scope is placed down the patient's throat and into the stomach. Sound waves show images of organs in the abdomen. Endoscopic ultrasound may reveal gallstones and can be helpful in diagnosing severe pancreatitis when an invasive test such as ERCP might make the condition worse. Pancreatic biopsy is the definitive test for inflammation.

Table 21–10 Diagnostic Tests of the Gastrointestinal System

Test	Purpose & Indication	Related Nursing Considerations
Esophagus, Stomach, and Intestines		
Upper GI series (barium swallow)	Performed to diagnose esophageal varices, inflammation, ulcerations, hiatal hernia, foreign bodies, polyps, diverticula, and tumors of the esophagus, stomach, and duodenum. The patient drinks an oral contrast (Gastrografin) prior to the test, and the movement of the contrast medium is visualized with fluoroscopic x-ray.	Instruct patient not to eat, drink fluids, or smoke for 8–12 hours before the test. Oral medications and narcotics are withheld for 8–12 hours pretest. During posttest period, ensure that the patient eliminates the barium by taking laxatives and increasing fluid intake.
Magnetic resonance imaging (abdominal MRI)	Performed to identify the source of gastric bleeding and tumors, as well as to stage colon cancer.	Instruct patient to lie completely still during the exam. Assess for metal implants (pacemakers, clips on brain aneurysms), body piercings, tattoos, presence of shrapnel or bullets. Transdermal patches should be removed. Contraindicated in pregnancy.
Upper GI endoscopy (esophagogastroduodenoscopy [EGD]), gastroscopy	Performed to directly visualize the lining of the esophagus, stomach, and duodenum via fiber-optic endoscope to assess for tumors, ulcerations, inflammation, or varices. Indicated for upper GI bleeding.	Performed at least 2 days after a barium swallow or upper GI series. Remove patient's dentures. Ensure that patient has not had food or drink for 6–8 hours before the procedure. Local anesthetic is applied to the throat when sedation is administered; may cause bloating, belching, flatulence. Following procedure, patient should be assessed for difficulty swallowing; epigastric, substernal, or shoulder pain; fever; vomiting blood; and black tarry stools.
Ultrasound (abdominal)	Performed to identify abdominal masses, ascites, and disorders of the appendix; involves application of conducting jelly to transmit high-frequency sound waves.	Ensure that patient eats a fat-free meal the evening before the test, then does not eat, drink, smoke, or chew gum for 6 hours prior to the test. Performed at least 2 days apart from an upper GI series.
Lower GI endoscopy (colonoscopy, sigmoidoscopy, proctoscopy, anoscopy)	Performed to evaluate lower GI bleeding. Allows visualization of large intestine, sigmoid colon, rectum, and anus, or from the colon up to the ileocecal valve, to identify tumors, polyps, and inflammation. Aids in tissue biopsy and/or removal of polyps.	Ensure that the patient undergoes a bowel prep (clear liquid diet) and bowel preparation (citrate of magnesia, laxatives, or polyethylene glycol) and/or remains NPO for 8 hours before the test. Explain that sedation is used for the procedure. Following the test, patient may experience flatulence or gas pains. Assess patient for fever, chills, abdominal pain, rectal bleeding, or discharge.
Small-bowel series	Performed to diagnose abnormalities of the small intestine; involves the patient drinking oral contrast; may be done in conjunction with an upper GI series or barium swallow.	Requires that the patient not eat 8 hours pretest or drink fluids 4 hours pretest. Patient should increase oral fluid intake and/or take laxatives to facilitate evacuation of the barium contrast medium; stools will be white for up to 72 hours posttest or until all the barium is evacuated.
Stool specimen, stool culture	Collected for gross and microscopic examination to identify blood, pus, mucus, fat, WBCs, parasites, and/or enteric pathogens.	The stool sample should be fresh, in a sterile container. If the female patient is menstruating, be sure to note this on the laboratory request.
Gallbladder, Pancreas, and Liver		
Ultrasound (abdominal, hepatobiliary, gallbladder)	Detects abdominal tumors, cysts, and ascites fluid; allows visualization of the biliary ducts; detects subphrenic abscesses, gallstones, cysts, tumors, and cirrhosis	Instruct the patient not to eat or drink for 8–12 hours pretest.
Computed tomography (CT)	Noninvasive procedure to evaluate disorders of the gallbladder, pancreas, and liver.	No special preparation is needed unless intravenous contrast is used, in which case patient should be assessed for allergies to contrast medium.
Endoscopic retrograde cholangiopancreatography (ERCP)	Involves insertion of a fiber-optic endoscope for direct visualization of GI structures, to retrieve gallstones from distal common bile duct, to dilate strictures, and to perform tissue biopsy. Contrast dye is injected into GI structures to allow visualization.	Ensure that patient does not drink fluids or eat for 8 hours pretest. Assess patient for allergy to iodine, seafood, or x-ray dye. Assess gag reflex prior to giving food or fluids following procedure. Be aware that oral hypoglycemic agents are contraindicated with iodine-containing contrast.
Magnetic resonance cholangiopancreatography (MRCP)	Noninvasive; performed to evaluate the biliary and pancreatic ducts	See information for abdominal MRI.
Liver biopsy	Performed to diagnose cancer or detect a cyst or cirrhosis. Using ultrasound, a biopsy needle is inserted into the liver and guided to the pathologic site.	Assess use of anticoagulants. Withhold aspirin and ibuprofen for a week before the test. Foods and fluids are withheld 4–6 hours pretest. Measure baseline vital signs, PT/PTT, and platelet counts. Vitamin K is often administered. Patient lies on right side for 1–2 hours postprocedure so that pressure is applied on the insertion site. Assess dressing frequently for evidence of bleeding. Tell patient that right shoulder pain may occur posttest.

SOURCE: Data from LeMone et al. (2015).

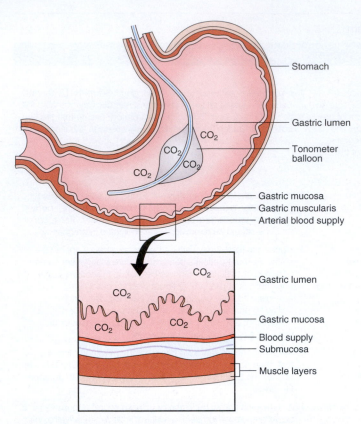

Figure 21–11 Gastric tonometry. A special gastric tube with a balloon on the distal end is inserted into the stomach to measure the CO_2 level of the gastric mucosa. Gastric CO_2 (PrCO$_2$) rises when the mucosa is hypoperfused.

Laboratory Assessment for Acute GI Bleeding, PUD, and Intestinal Obstruction

Acute GI bleeding includes the following laboratory testing:

- *Complete blood count (CBC)* with platelets, hemoglobin and hematocrit—Helpful to determine the extent and effects of blood loss and if thrombocytopenia is present. The hemoglobin and hematocrit may not indicate the extent of blood loss because plasma is lost along with blood cells.

- *Blood type and crossmatch*—Necessary to prepare for transfusion of blood products.

- *Serum electrolytes, osmolality, blood urea nitrogen (BUN)*—Imbalances can result from blood cell and plasma loss, as well as protein digestion of blood as it passes through the GI system.

- *Liver function and coagulation studies*—Measured to help determine the cause of bleeding.

Peptic Ulcer Disease

- *Fecal H. pylori antigen test* and the *urea breath test*—Noninvasive measures of detecting *H. pylori*. Proton pump inhibitor (PPI) medications must be discontinued for at least 7 days prior to either of these tests because PPI medications can interfere with test results.

Diarrhea

- *Stool specimen analysis and culture*—Indicated to identify infectious source of diarrhea.

- *Serum electrolytes, osmolality and arterial blood gas analysis*—Used to assess and monitor for dehydration, electrolyte and acid–base balance. Elevated osmolality indicates water loss and fluid volume deficit.

Intestinal Obstruction

- *Complete blood count*—Leukocytosis indicates inflammation, perforation, or possible bowel strangulation.

- *Serum amylase*—Levels are elevated with inflammation and may indicate severe obstruction and possible strangulation.

- *Serum osmolality* and *electrolyte levels*—Reflect fluid and electrolyte losses from vomiting and fluid accumulation within the bowel lumen. Hypovolemia is associated with elevation in osmolality. Hypokalemia and hypochloremia may occur because of vomiting or with nasogastric suction of gastric contents.

- *Arterial blood gases*—Can reflect acid–base disturbances, specifically metabolic alkalosis due to loss of hydrochloric acid with severe vomiting associated with bowel obstruction.

Emerging Evidence

- Little is known about how diet might contribute to the pathogenesis of pancreatitis. A prospective analysis of 145,886 African Americans, Native Hawaiians, Japanese Americans, Latinos, and Whites in the Multiethnic Cohort was undertaken to characterize dietary factors that are associated with risk of pancreatitis. Patients with pancreatitis were identified from hospitalization claim files from 1993 through 2012 and were categorized as having gallstone-related acute pancreatitis (AP) (n = 1210), AP not related to gallstones (n = 1222), or recurrent AP or suspected chronic pancreatitis (n = 378). Diet information was obtained from a questionnaire administered when the study began. Associations between dietary factors (saturated fat, cholesterol, and red meat consumption) and pancreatitis were observed mainly for gallstone-related AP. Interestingly, dietary fiber protected against

AP related and unrelated to gallstones. Coffee drinking protected against AP not associated with gallstones (*Setiawan et al., 2016*).

- Studies of whether cigarette smoking increases the risk of developing pancreatic cancer have produced conflicting results in a meta-analysis to provide quantitative pooled risk estimate of the association between cigarette smoking and risk of developing pancreatitis. Twenty-two studies that investigated the association of cigarette smoking with pancreatitis were included in the review. Summary relative risks (RRs) with 95% confidence intervals (CIs) were pooled using a random-effects model. The evidence suggests a positive association of cigarette smoking with the development of pancreatitis. It is possible that smoking cessation may be a useful strategy for the management of pancreatitis (*Ye, Lu, Huai, & Ding, 2016*).

Section Five Review

1. A 46-year-old male is admitted to the acute care unit for acute onset of abdominal pain. He has a history of pancreatitis. Which diagnostic test would be a good starting point for diagnosis of this client's abdominal pain?
   A. Plain abdominal x-ray
   B. Magnetic resonance cholangiopancreatography
   C. Upper gastrointestinal series with contrast
   D. Endoscopic ultrasound

2. The quality of abdominal ultrasound may be diminished by the presence of which factor?
   A. Metal clips in the abdomen
   B. Excessive adipose tissue
   C. Client's inability to stay still
   D. Allergy to contrast

3. Gastric tonometry measures which physiological parameter?
   A. Pressure in the stomach
   B. Gastric perfusion
   C. Motility of the intestine
   D. Patency of cardiac sphincters

4. Sublingual capnometry can be used as a noninvasive alternative to which test?
   A. Ultrasound
   B. CT scan
   C. Gastric tonometry
   D. MRI

Answers: 1. A, 2. B, 3. B, 4. C

Section Six: Nursing Assessment

Acute GI disorders that involve GI bleeding or hepatic or pancreatic dysfunction require nursing care centered on health promotion, assessment, and identification of priority nursing diagnoses and interventions. Obtaining a thorough database is important on admission for those patients who present with acute GI dysfunction, and it provides the foundation upon which collaborative nursing care is based.

Focused Nursing Database

When a patient is admitted to the acute care setting with GI complaints, it is important to first obtain a history of the precipitating events leading up to the admission (including signs and symptoms) and then perform a focused assessment. The nurse also obtains a full nursing database to elicit pieces of the patient's history that could aid the diagnostic process and possibly affect the outcome of the hospitalization. As with all patients, a general history should be taken to include past medical and surgical history.

A current medication list should be obtained so the high-acuity healthcare team members can be aware of preexisting conditions for which the patient has been taking prescribed and over-the-counter drugs. In addition, the nurse should elicit information about when each drug was last taken, as some drugs may cause adverse effects if not taken within the correct timeframe. The nurse should also ask which drugs were taken prior to admission. If the patient is agreeable, it is often helpful to

ask a family member or significant other to assist with the history-taking process. The family history also should be taken, as some GI and accessory organ disorders are hereditary.

A focused health maintenance history should be taken that focuses on diet and eating patterns, appetite, weight fluctuations, and skin healing problems. Baseline data should be obtained regarding mental status, ability to communicate, and presence of pain. It is also important with every admission to discuss with the patient and family their value–belief pattern in order to prepare for future needs.

Abdominal Assessment

A focused abdominal assessment should be completed by the nurse to evaluate the patient who presents with signs of alteration in GI, hepatic, or pancreatic function. The

Genetic Considerations
Family History

When conducting the health assessment, it is important for the nurse to question for the presence of genetic disorders or diseases with a genetic component. The nurse should ask about family members with known abnormalities of copper accumulation, hypercholesterolemia, problems with fat metabolism, obesity, Crohn disease, celiac disease, Gaucher disease, or history of cancer of any organ associated with the GI system. If the patient has a family history of any of these disease processes, it may be necessary to refer them for genetic counseling and evaluation (LeMone et al., 2015).

steps of abdominal assessment include inspection, auscultation, percussion, and palpation. During inspection, the abdomen is examined for abnormal contour, alteration in skin, pulsations, and peristalsis. It is important to have good lighting for visual examination of the abdomen. Next, the abdomen is auscultated with the stethoscope over all four quadrants. Listen for bowel sounds for at least 5 minutes if they are hypoactive or absent. Bowel sounds should be auscultated before the next two steps, which may alter the GI contents. Next, the abdomen is percussed. Percussion helps to assess the amount of gas and fluid present. The nurse percusses over all four quadrants and likely will hear tympany and/or dullness. Finally, palpation is performed to evaluate for tenderness, organs, masses, and any abnormality. Any abnormal findings should be immediately reported to the HCP so that a full abdominal examination and necessary interventions can be initiated.

Box 21–1 provides a summary of important information to obtain during a focused GI system assessment.

BOX 21–1   Focused Gastrointestinal Nursing Assessment

The Nursing History

- Points to elicit include the following:
  - Onset of problem: When did it start? Was it gradual or quick? What was the person doing when it started?
  - Duration of problem: How long does it last? Does it come and go?
  - Quality and description of problem: What does the problem feel like (using adjectives)?
  - Severity of problem: How badly does the problem bother the person?
  - Location of problem: Where is the problem isolated? Does it radiate or spread?
  - Precipitating factors: What brought on the problem?
  - Alleviating factors: What relieves the problem?
  - Associated symptoms: What other symptoms bother the person?
- Previous medical history
- Family history
- Surgical history
- Current medication list
- Psychosocial factors that affect the patient
- Cultural factors that affect the patient

The Physical Examination

- Abdominal assessment
  - Ask patient to empty bladder unless he or she has a Foley catheter.
  - Provide appropriate privacy.
  - Warm hands and stethoscope before use.
  - Inspect abdomen first. Look for contour, shape, masses, bumps, abnormal colors.
  - Auscultate abdomen. Listen in all four quadrants for at least 2 minutes, noting quality and quantity of sounds.
  - Percuss abdomen. Dullness will be heard over solid organs, tympany over air and gas.
  - Palpate abdomen in all four quadrants. Include light and deep touch.
- General
  - Obtain vital signs and baseline assessment and document in nursing database.
  - Prepare patient and family for further diagnostic testing and medication use.

Section Six Review

1. When obtaining a focused GI history, which question specifically focuses on precipitating factors of symptoms?
   A. When did the symptoms start?
   B. What brought the problem on?
   C. What does the problem feel like?
   D. How long does it last?

2. Just before beginning an abdominal assessment, what should the nurse do?
   A. Ask the client to attempt a bowel movement.
   B. Palpate the abdomen first, before inspecting or auscultating.
   C. Listen to bowel sounds for at least 30 seconds in each quadrant.
   D. Ask the client to empty his or her bladder unless an indwelling urinary catheter is in place.

3. In the first step of abdominal assessment, which skill is used?
   A. Inspection
   B. Palpation
   C. Auscultation
   D. Percussion

4. Which client history finding may require a referral for genetic counseling?
   A. Mother had hyperemesis during pregnancy
   B. Brother has Crohn disease
   C. Grandmother had gallbladder extraction
   D. Grandfather abuses alcohol

Answers: 1. B, 2. D, 3. A, 4. B

Clinical Reasoning Checkpoint

A 48-year-old female is admitted to the acute care unit with acute-onset abdominal pain. The nurse is preparing to obtain a baseline assessment.

1. What are some questions that need to be answered regarding the patient's appearance? What nonverbal clues should the nurse look for?

2. Are vital signs an important first step after the appearance has been observed?

3. It is important to determine if there are postural changes in the BP and HR. If the supine BP is normal, does this rule out postural changes?

4. Why is it important to assess the patient's temperature?

Clinical update: The nurse is ready to perform a selective history. Diagnosis is often dependent on a careful history addressing the onset of the pain, how it has progressed, any associated symptoms, and the past medical history of the patient.

5. What is important information to assess with regard to the location of the pain?

6. What other characteristics of pain are worth noting during the history section of the physical exam?

7. What associated symptoms should the nurse ask about?

Chapter 21 Review

1. A client has developed weakness of the cardiac sphincter following blunt trauma to the chest and abdomen. The nurse would attribute which assessment finding to this weakness?
   1. The client's heart rate varies with inspiration.
   2. The client has developed esophageal reflux.
   3. The client becomes constipated easily.
   4. The client has intermittent periods of jaundice.

2. The client is found to have a deficit of intrinsic factor (IF) secretion. What disorder is likely to occur?
   1. Anemia
   2. Indigestion
   3. Gastroesophageal reflux
   4. Constipation

3. An arteriogram reveals a clot in the client's superior mesenteric artery. The nurse would expect changes in which organs? (Select all that apply.)
   1. The liver
   2. The small intestine
   3. The stomach
   4. The esophagus
   5. The transverse colon

4. A client with an eating disorder refuses to eat anything that has not been boiled because "food is full of bacteria." Which nursing statement may help this client cope with this concern?
   1. "People have been eating uncooked food for centuries without any problems."
   2. "As long as you wash the food well, there will be no problems."

3. "Your saliva and gastric acids are designed to kill bacteria."
   4. "We all breathe in germs all the time, and that is no different than eating them."

5. Laboratory results reveal that a client has very decreased serum amylase. The nurse would monitor the client for intolerance to which food?
   1. Butter
   2. Red meat
   3. Potatoes
   4. Chicken

6. Which laboratory results would the nurse evaluate as indicating damage to the liver? (Select all that apply.)
   1. ALT of 135 units/L
   2. AST of 25 units/L
   3. ALP_1 of 280 IU/L
   4. Triglycerides of 225 mg/dL
   5. Alk phos of 80 units/L

7. A client is being discharged after having an upper GI endoscopy this morning. What instructions should the nurse provide? (Select all that apply.)
   1. "Do not eat anything for at least 8 hours."
   2. "Call the healthcare provider's office if you have any difficulty swallowing that is more serious than a minor sore throat."
   3. "You should expect your stools to be darker in color and sticky for the next few days."
   4. "You may experience belching and a bloated feeling for a few hours after you get home."
   5. "Call the healthcare provider's office if you have any fever."

8. A client is being discharged after having a small bowel series. Which information would the nurse provide?

   1. "You should sleep in an upright position in a recliner tonight."
   2. "Your stools may be white for the next two or three days."
   3. "You should avoid acidic foods for a week or so."
   4. "Your throat may be sore for a few days."

9. A nurse is conducting an assessment of a client admitted with a gastrointestinal illness. Which client statements would the nurse report to the client's healthcare provider? (Select all that apply.)

   1. "I have gained ten pounds over the last couple of years."
   2. "I have always enjoyed eating meat, but it just doesn't taste good to me anymore."
   3. "I can't get this bruising on my arm to go away."
   4. "I just started a new diet and have lost ten pounds."
   5. "I have noticed that I get constipated more often than I once did."

10. A client is scheduled for a liver biopsy. What instruction should the nurse provide?

    1. Do not eat or drink anything for 12 hours before the test.
    2. Do not use aspirin for 7 days before the test.
    3. Eat a soft diet for 5 days before the test.
    4. Take two ibuprofen with a small sip of water 2 hours before the test is scheduled.

Answers to questions found inside your textbook are available on the faculty resources site. Please consult with your instructor.

References

Barrett, K. E. (2014) Chapter 1. Functional anatomy of the GI tract and organs draining into it. In K. E. Barrett (Ed.), *Gastrointestinal physiology* (2nd ed.). New York, NY: McGraw-Hill. Retrieved December 10, 2016, from http://accessmedicine.mhmedical.com.ezproxy.uky.edu/content.aspx?bookid=691&Sectionid= 454313 99

Barrett, K. E., Barman, S. M., Boitano, S., & Brooks, H. L. (2016). Overview of gastrointestinal function & regulation. In K. E. Barrett, B. M. Barman, S. Boitano, & H. L. Brooks (Eds.), *Ganong's review of medical physiology* (25th ed.). New York, NY: McGraw-Hill. Retrieved December 10, 2016, from http://accessmedicine.mhmedical.com.ezproxy.uky.edu/content.aspx?bookid=1587&Sectionid=97165 032

Conwell, D. L., & Banks, P. A. (2016). Chronic pancreatitis. In N. J. Greenberger, R. S. Blumberg, & R. Burakoff (Eds.), *CURRENT diagnosis & treatment: Gastroenterology, hepatology, & endoscopy* (3rd ed.). New York, NY: McGraw-Hill. Retrieved December 10, 2016, from http://accessmedicine.mhmedical.com.ezproxy.uky.edu/content.aspx?bookid=1621&Sectionid105184743

Elder, A. S., Saccone, G. T., & Dixon, D. L. (2012). Lung injury in acute pancreatitis: Mechanisms underlying augmented secondary injury. *Pancreatology, 12*(1), 49–56.

Kee, J. L. (2014). *Laboratory and diagnostic tests with nursing implications* (9th ed.). Upper Saddle River, NJ: Pearson.

Kibble, J. D., & Halsey, C. R. (2015). Gastrointestinal physiology. In J. D. Kibble, & C. R. Halsey (Eds.), *Medical physiology: The big picture.* New York, NY: McGraw-Hill. Retrieved December 10, 2016, from http://accessmedicine.mhmedical.com.ezproxy.uky.edu/content.aspx?bookid=1291&Sectionid=75577353

Lee, R. K. (2012). Intra-abdominal hypertension and abdominal compartment syndrome: A comprehensive overview. *Critical Care Nurse, 32*(1), 19–32.

LeMone, P., Burke, K., Bauldoff, G., & Gubrud, P. (Eds.). (2015). *Medical surgical nursing: Critical thinking in patient care* (6th ed.). Hoboken, NJ: Pearson.

Setiawan, V. W., Pandol, S. J., Porcel, J., Wei, P. C., Wilkens, L. R., Le Marchand, L., . . . Monroe, K. R. (2016). Dietary factors reduce risk of acute pancreatitis in a large multiethnic cohort. *Clinical Gastroenterology and Hepatology, 15*(2), 257–265. e3. doi:10.1016/j.cgh.2016.08.038

Ye, X., Lu, G., Huai, J., & Ding, J., (2016). Impact of smoking on the risk of pancreatitis: A systematic review and meta-analysis. *PLoS One, 10*(4), e0124075. doi:10.1371/journal.pone.0124075. eCollection 2015

Zuckerbraun, B. S., Peitzman, A. B., & Billiar, T. R. (2014). Shock. In F. Brunicardi, D. K. Andersen, T. R. Billiar, D. L. Dunn, J. G. Hunter, J. B. Matthews, & R. E. Pollock (Eds.), *Schwartz's principles of surgery* (10th ed.). New York, NY: McGraw-Hill. Retrieved December 10, 2016, from http://accessmedicine.mhmedical.com.ezproxy.uky.edu/content.aspx?bookid=980&Sectionid=59610846

Chapter 22
Alterations in Gastrointestinal Function

 Learning Outcomes

22.1 Describe the incidence and clinical manifestations associated with acute gastrointestinal (GI) bleeding.

22.2 Discuss the etiology and pathophysiology of acute upper GI bleeding due to ulcers.

22.3 Discuss the etiology and pathophysiology of acute upper GI bleeding due to stress-related mucosal disease and nonulcer etiologies.

22.4 Explain the etiology and pathophysiology of acute lower GI bleeding.

22.5 Describe the nursing diagnoses and management of acute GI bleeding.

22.6 Describe the etiology, pathophysiology, and management of acute intestinal obstruction and paralytic ileus.

22.7 Describe the etiology, pathophysiology, and management of intra-abdominal hypertension and abdominal compartment syndrome.

This chapter presents the pathophysiologic processes involved in acute gastrointestinal (GI) dysfunction and management of the patient with acute GI bleeding, problems in motility, and intestinal ischemia. It is recommended that normal GI anatomy and physiology be reviewed in Chapter 21 prior to reading this chapter to enhance understanding of the material.

Section One: Incidence and Clinical Manifestations of Acute GI Bleeding

GI bleeding is a common and major medical problem, despite advances in diagnosis and treatment.

Incidence and Mortality

Despite a gap in recent epidemiological studies to determine the incidence of all-cause acute GI bleeding, it is estimated that this disorder is responsible for more than 400,000 hospitalizations in the United States per year, with a mortality rate of 5% to 10% (Abougergi et al., 2015;

McQuaid, 2017). The incidence per year of upper GI bleeding is 100 per 100,000 people, and it is estimated that an additional 100,000 to 150,000 patients per year develop upper GI bleeding during hospitalizations for other reasons, particularly patients who take nonsteroidal anti-inflammatories (NSAIDs) and antiplatelet drugs (Kim, Sheibani, Park, Buxbaum, & Laine, 2014; McQuaid, 2017). GI bleeding manifests itself in one or more of the following clinical scenarios: (1) bleeding is from the upper GI tract; (2) bleeding is from the lower GI tract; (3) bleeding is occult (unknown to the patient); and (4) bleeding is obvious but the site (whether the upper or lower GI tract) is obscure (Hreinsson, Kalaitzakis, Gudmundsson, & Björnsson, 2013; McQuaid, 2017). GI bleeding can range in severity from a very slow occult blood loss to a sudden, massive hemorrhage.

The overwhelming majority (75%–80%) of patients with bleeding ulcers stop bleeding spontaneously. However, despite progressive advances in diagnosis, treatment, and prevention of *H. pylori*–related peptic ulcer disease (PUD) and the use of proton pump inhibitors (PPIs) in patients at higher risk for development of stress ulcers, the mortality from acute upper GI bleed (UGIB) remains near 4% for young persons and as high as 15% in older adults (Hreinsson et al., 2013; McQuaid, 2017).

Etiology and General Manifestations of Upper GI Bleeding

More than 90% of upper GI bleeding cases are caused by peptic ulcer, erosive gastritis, Mallory-Weiss tears, or esophagogastric varices (Laine, 2015). Other etiologies of UGIB include tumors, arteriovenous malformations, and stress ulcers. Sometimes the presenting diagnosis for GI bleeding is anemia, with symptoms ranging from syncope, angina, and dyspepsia to increasing weakness and fatigue (Laine, 2015). Table 22–1 summarizes the causes of upper GI bleeding.

The amount and degree of upper GI bleeding vary. When an ulcer erodes through an artery or vein, the bleeding can be profuse. The manifestations of GI bleeding depend on the source, the rate of bleeding, and comorbid disease. Severe GI bleeding may seriously aggravate coronary artery disease, hypertension, diabetes mellitus, pulmonary disease, and renal failure, and it often presents as shock. Lesser degrees of bleeding may present as orthostatic changes in pulse (a change of greater than 10 beats per minute) or blood pressure (a drop of 10 mmHg or greater) secondary to compensatory baroreceptor stimulation and vasoconstriction that prevent a greater drop in pulse and BP (Laine, 2015). Baroreceptors sense the decrease in BP when the patient sits up or stands, and this stimulates an increase in heart rate and vasoconstriction that prevents a drop in BP. The most common cause of death in GI hemorrhage is the exacerbation of the underlying disease rather than intractable hypovolemic shock from exsanguinations (McQuaid, 2017). However, if unrecognized or treated too late, GI hemorrhage can lead to hypovolemic shock and ultimately death.

Etiology and General Manifestations of Lower GI Bleeding

Lower GI bleeding occurs at a rate of 20 per 100,000 people. Hematochezia, the most common presenting symptom, can be described as bloody diarrhea, blood, and/or clots from the rectum. Hematochezia can result from bleeding anywhere in the GI tract; 10% of patients who present with hematochezia have an upper GI source of bleeding (Laine, 2015; McQuaid, 2017). The mortality rate for lower GI bleed (LGIB) is about 5% (McQuaid, 2017). Most cases of LGIB resolve spontaneously, but with a 10% to 40% chance of rebleed. Between 5% and 50% of patients have persistent rebleeding and require surgical hemostasis (Laine, 2015).

Table 22–1 Causes of Upper GI Bleeding

Etiology	Occurrence (Percentage of Total Upper GI Bleed Cases)
Peptic ulcers	50
Gastritis	10–15
Varices	10–15
Esophagitis	15
Mallory-Weiss tear	5–10
Arteriovenous malformation	5

SOURCE: Data from Laine (2015).

Clinical Manifestations of Upper and Lower GI Bleeding

GI blood loss may be acute (sudden or massive with hypovolemia) or chronic (slow and often unnoticed by the patient). Acute GI bleeding may present in one of several ways:

- **Occult blood**—blood that is present in the GI tract but not really visible. Occult bleeding is often detected by chemical testing of a stool or nasogastric specimen, in a process known as *hemoccult* or *guaiac testing*.
- **Hematemesis**—vomiting of bright red blood or blood that looks like coffee grounds. This bleeding is often brisk and is likely proximal to the ligament of Treitz in the upper GI tract.
- **Melena**—black, tarry, foul-smelling stools passed after a GI bleed, usually from an upper GI source. However, the small intestine or right colon may also be the source.
- **Hematochezia**—bright red blood or maroon stool from the rectum, usually the result of lower GI bleeding or massive upper GI bleeding. Severe hematochezia is associated with an upper GI source of bleeding.

Chronic GI bleed may present as recurrent episodes of melena or hematochezia. Patients may have no signs or symptoms of acute blood loss (occult bleeding) but may present with manifestations associated with anemia, such as fatigue, dyspnea, lightheadedness or syncope, and low red blood cell (RBC) count and hemoglobin (Laine, 2015; McQuaid, 2017). In addition, the patient is typically iron deficient and demonstrates positive fecal occult blood testing.

Section One Review

1. Where is the section of the GI tract that is involved in an upper GI hemorrhage located?
   A. Proximal to the ligament of Treitz
   B. Proximal to the ileocecal valve
   C. Distal to the pyloric sphincter
   D. Distal to the duodenal bulb

2. How does the mortality rate for acute lower GI bleeding compare to that for acute upper GI bleeding?
   A. It is twice as high.
   B. It is lower.
   C. It is about the same.
   D. It is slightly higher.

3. What is a characteristic of acute lower GI bleeding?
    A. Commonly of arterial origin
    B. Usually resolves spontaneously
    C. Massive 80% of the time
    D. Always occult

4. Clients with occult GI bleeding often present with which manifestations?
    A. Nausea and vomiting
    B. Mental status changes
    C. Headache and abdominal pain
    D. Fatigue and syncope

Answers: 1. A, 2. C, 3. B, 4. D

Section Two: Acute Upper GI Bleeding Due to Peptic Ulcer Disease

Peptic ulcer disease (PUD) is the most common cause of upper GI bleeding. Ulcers range in size from several millimeters to several centimeters and are characterized by mucosal damage extending through the muscularis mucosae layer of the GI tract. Peptic ulcers occur in the portion of the GI tract exposed to acid–pepsin secretion, which includes the stomach and the proximal duodenum. Approximately 500,000 people develop PUD in the United States each year (Kanotra et al., 2016; Laine, 2015). The incidence of PUD is declining, likely as a result of better PUD prophylaxis and decreasing rates of *H. pylori* infection (Lew, 2016). Mortality from PUD is quite low; however, persons suffer substantial pain as a result of the chronic nature of this disease. Interestingly, PUD is the most common cause of upper GI bleeding in critically ill patients. It accounts for approximately 40% of patients admitted to an intensive care unit (ICU) specifically for bleeding and 50% of patients who develop upper GI hemorrhage during their stay but are admitted for some other reason (Lew, 2016; McQuaid, 2017).

Risk Factors

Traditional theories on the cause of peptic ulcer disease have focused on acid hypersecretion or the inability of the gastric mucosa to secrete mucus for protection. It is now known that acid hypersecretion is not the primary mechanism by which ulceration occurs. Under normal circumstances, a balance exists between hostile and protective mucosal factors (Figure 22–1). The cause of mucosal injury in PUD is usually multifactorial and relates to an imbalance in protective and hostile factors in the stomach and duodenum. The two most common causes of PUD are *H. pylori* infection and NSAIDs. Both of these factors disrupt the mucosal defense barrier, making it susceptible to the damaging effects of gastric acid and pepsin. Table 22–2 summarizes the more common alterations in protective and hostile factors. Because so many patients are prescribed antiplatelet medications (e.g., Plavix), it is important for the nurse to be aware of which patients are on antiplatelet therapy and are at increased risk for GI bleeding.

***H. pylori* Infection**   The bacterium *Helicobacter pylori* (*H. pylori*) is a gram-negative rod that can be cultured from the stomachs of the majority of patients with peptic ulcer disease (e.g., 90% of duodenal ulcers and 75% of gastric ulcers) (Elie-Turenne, Cregar & Brewster, 2012; Laine, 2015; Lew, 2016). *H. pylori* can survive and even thrive in the high-acid environment of the stomach through its ability to secrete the enzyme urease, which splits urea (which is abundant in gastric secretions) into ammonia and carbon dioxide, ammonia being a weak base and carbon dioxide a strong base. Ammonia and carbon dioxide then react with the acids to produce a neutralized environment for *H. pylori* to thrive. These bases form an alkaline cloud around the bacterium, protecting it from the low-pH gastric environment. The mechanism by which *H. pylori* impairs mucosal integrity is poorly understood. The organism is responsible for

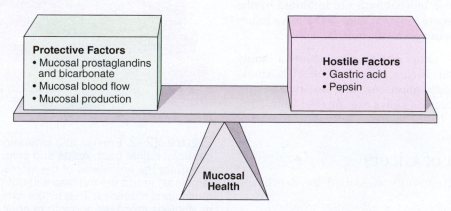

Figure 22–1 Normal balance between physiologic protective and hostile factors of gastrointestinal mucosal health.

Table 22–2 Alterations in Protective and Hostile Factors of Gastrointestinal Mucosal Health

Factors	Alterations
Decreased Protective Factors	
Mucosal prostaglandins & bicarbonate	Inhibited by NSAIDs (COX-1 inhibitors)
Mucosal blood flow	Decreased with inhibition of mucosal prostaglandins and severe stress
Mucus production	Decreased with inhibition of mucosal prostaglandins and tissue ischemia
Increased Hostile Factors	
Gastric acid	Corrosive activity when exposed to mucosa; acid hypersecretion possibly present
Pepsin	Corrosive activity when exposed to mucosa; promotes lysis of clot
H. pylori infection	Invades mucosa, activating cytokines and establishing and maintaining inflammatory response
NSAIDs (COX-1 inhibitors)	Inhibit production of mucosal prostaglandins; reduced gastric protection: decreased bicarbonate, decreased mucus production, increased acid secretion, decreased blood flow to submucosa
Antiplatelet drugs	Inhibits platelet aggregation; reduces blood clotting ability in the event of bleeding
Alcohol	Gastric irritant; stimulates production of gastric acid; direct mucosal injury in large doses; when used with NSAIDs, intensifies injury
Stress	High levels of physiologic stress results in shunting of blood flow from GI tract to more vital organs resulting in reduced blood flow, tissue ischemia, mucosal injury, reperfusion injury, and tissue acidosis ("Curling ulcers").
Traumatic brain injury and increased intracranial pressure	In patients with increased intracranial pressure, altered vagus nerve stimulation can cause hypersecretion of gastric acid; severe burns also commonly result in hypersecretion ("Cushing ulcers").

SOURCE: Based on Kasper et al. (2017); McQuaid, (2016); Saltzman (2016b).

the production of cytotoxins and mucolytic enzymes (e.g., protease) that erode the mucous barrier and trigger an inflammatory response, all of which make the mucosa more susceptible to acid damage.

NSAIDs   Among patients receiving long-term NSAID therapy, 15% to 30% develop ulcers at one time or another. NSAID-induced ulcers are more common in older adults (Del Valle, 2015; Lew, 2016). Other factors that may increase the risk of NSAID-induced ulcers include a previous history of peptic ulcer disease, corticosteroid use, and high doses of NSAIDs. Also, the incidence is slightly higher in women (Del Valle, 2015; Laine, 2015; McQuaid, 2017). NSAIDs compete with prostaglandin receptor sites in the gastric mucosa. NSAIDs inhibit the production of prostaglandins, particularly prostaglandin E, by blocking COX enzymes. Prostaglandin E is linked to mucosal repair and maintenance of mucosal integrity. When these prostaglandin-supported defense mechanisms are inhibited by the action of NSAIDs, severe inflammation and erosive injury to the gastric mucosa can occur (Barrett, 2014).

Other Risk Factors   Other risk factors include a family history of peptic ulcer disease, the use of NSAIDs, smoking, and genetic predisposition. Smoking also increases the risk of ulcer recurrence and slows healing (Del Valle, 2015; Lew, 2016).

Classification of Ulcers

Peptic ulcers are commonly classified by depth and location.

Ulcer Depth   Ulcers are often classified by how deeply into the wall they have penetrated and include erosion,

acute ulcer, or chronic ulcer (see Figure 22–2). Erosion is a superficial injury that is confined to the mucosal layer; an acute ulcer has penetrated through the mucosa and

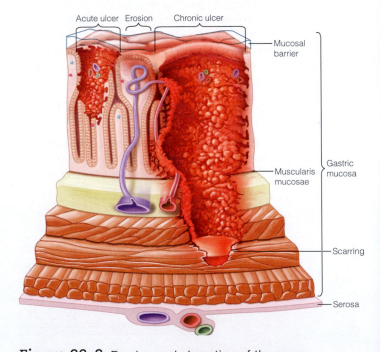

Figure 22–2 Erosion and ulceration of the upper gastrointestinal tract. Acute and chronic ulcers may penetrate the entire wall of the stomach. Superficial ulcers (erosions) erode the mucosa without penetrating the muscularis mucosae. True ulcers extend through the muscularis mucosae and into deeper layers of the GI wall, damaging blood vessels and potentially penetrating the entire wall.

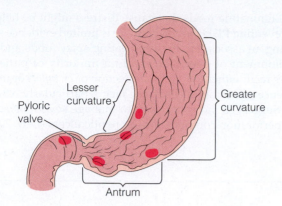

Figure 22–3 Common sites of peptic ulcers.

submucosa; and a chronic ulcer (sometimes called a perforating ulcer) has penetrated into the muscularis layer. A chronic ulcer can perforate the serosa, exposing the sterile abdominal cavity to GI contents, which can result in peritonitis.

Ulcer Location There are two types of peptic ulcers, based on location: gastric ulcers (prepyloric) and duodenal ulcers (postpyloric). Figure 22–3 illustrates common sites of peptic ulcers.

Gastric Ulcers. Gastric ulcers are more common in older adults but may also affect younger people. Long-term NSAID use is a risk factor for the development of these ulcers. Gastric ulcers tend to be chronic, usually involving branches of the left gastric artery, and can produce severe hemorrhage if erosion into the arterial wall occurs.

Duodenal Ulcers. Duodenal ulcers constitute the majority of peptic ulcers (about 75%) (Del Valle, 2015; Lew, 2016). The most frequent sites for duodenal ulcers are the gastric pylorus and the first portion of the duodenum, where the pH is still acidic. Duodenal ulcers can develop at any age but are most common among young adults, especially those with type A blood who smoke, abuse alcohol, and report a family history of peptic ulcers.

Common Clinical Manifestations

Pain is the most common manifestation of peptic ulcer disease. It is generally located in the upper abdomen in the epigastric area and is usually an intermittent rather than steady pain. Timing of pain onset can vary based on the exact ulcer location; however, in general, the most common is burning stomach pain. Other manifestations, seen more often in persons with gastric ulcer, may include pain during the meal, nausea, vomiting, anorexia, and weight loss (Del Valle, 2015; Lew, 2016). If a gastric ulcer is located in the pyloric canal (the narrow region of the stomach that opens through the pylorus into the duodenum), the symptoms are often associated with obstruction (e.g., bloating, nausea, vomiting) (Del Valle, 2015; Lew, 2016). Duodenal ulcer pain is typically relieved by eating food because the pyloric sphincter closes; pain occurs 2 to 3 hours after eating, and the stomach pain is chronic intermittent pain.

If GI bleeding is present, it may be hidden (occult) or gross, evidenced as hematemesis, melena, or hematochezia.

Diagnosis and Treatment

Diagnosis of peptic ulcer disease is largely suggested by history and confirmed by visualization with fiber-optic endoscopy, the diagnostic tool of choice. Barium radiography is contraindicated in acute upper GI bleed because it interferes with subsequent endoscopy, angiography, or surgery (Lew, 2016). Determination of a duodenal or gastric ulcer by upper endoscopy or radiographic study should be followed by confirmation of *H. pylori* infection. Diagnostic tests for the presence of *H. pylori* include serologic testing, carbon-labeled urea breath tests, rapid urease assay (Clotest), and culture or histologic analysis of endoscopic biopsies (Lew, 2016).

General PUD Treatment Treatment of PUD involves combination antibiotic therapy (for eradication of *H. pylori*), proton pump inhibitors (PPIs) for acid secretion inhibition, prostaglandins to inhibit acid secretion and enhance the mucosal barrier (for patients on chronic NSAID therapy), bismuth subsalicylate for its antisecretory (salicylate) and antimicrobial (bismuth) actions, sucralfate (Carafate) to promote the mucosal barrier, and antacids to give symptomatic relief and raise gastric pH. In patients with a nasogastric or small-bore enteric feeding tube, the appropriate route of administration for sucralfate and antacids is through the nasogastric tube to allow for direct contact with the gastric mucosa. If the nasogastric tube is attached to suction, the suction must be interrupted for 30 to 60 minutes following administration of antacids.

H. pylori Infection Treatment *H. pylori*–associated ulcers often heal spontaneously, but acid-suppressive therapy accelerates healing and ameliorates symptoms. Four weeks of acid-suppressive therapy heals 70% to 80% of ulcers. Because persistent *H. pylori* infection is common, eradication therapy with two or more antibiotics

Genetic Considerations
Gastrointestinal Dysfunction

Helicobacter pylori infection is known to be associated with the pathogenesis of peptic ulcer disease (PUD). *H. pylori* virulence, determined by bacterial adhesions and gastric inflammation factors, is associated with an increased risk of PUD. However, differences in bacterial virulence factors alone cannot explain duodenal and gastric ulcer development. Presumably, both bacterial and host factors contribute to response. Host carriers of the high-producer alleles of the pro-inflammatory cytokines IL-1B, IL-6, IL-8, IL-10, and TNF-α who also carry low-producer alleles of anti-inflammatory cytokines have severe gastric mucosal inflammation, whereas carriers of the alternative alleles have mild inflammation. Recent reports have suggested that the PSCA and CYP2C19 ultra-rapid metabolizer genotypes are also associated with PUD. (Miftahussurur & Yamaoka, 2015).

plus a proton pump inhibitor medication is preferred. After successful *H. pylori* eradication, the risk of recurrent infection in most populations is small. Drug treatment for peptic ulcer disease is summarized in the "Related Pharmacotherapy: Peptic Ulcer Disease" feature. It is important to explain to the patient the importance of completing the entire course of therapy even if symptoms disappear.

Eliminating foods that cause distress might be helpful in preventing PUD; however, there is limited evidence supporting an association between eating spicy foods and the development of peptic ulcers. In a minority of patients, ulcers recur either owing to reinfection of *H. pylori* or in the presence of another ulcerogenic factor, particularly NSAID use. Surgery is indicated only to manage severe bleeding and perforation complications of peptic ulcers (Lew, 2016).

Related Pharmocotherapy
Peptic Ulcer Disease

H$_2$ Receptor Blocking Agents

Ranitidine (Zantac)

Famotidine (Pepcid)

Action and Uses
Reduces gastric acid secretion and increases gastric mucus and bicarbonate production, creating a protective coating on gastric mucosa.

Dosages (Adult)
Ranitidine (IV): Intermittent infusion—50 mg every 6–8 hrs diluted in 50–100 mL of compatible IV solution (e.g., NS, D5W, or LR); or 150 mg over 24 hrs continuous infusion at 6.25 mg/hr. Intermittent bolus—50 mg every 6–8 hrs. Dilute to a concentration not exceeding 2.5 mg/mL. Inject no faster than 4 mL/minute.

Major Adverse Effects
Usually well tolerated. Hypersensitivity is rare but potentially life-threatening.

Nursing Implications
Give oral doses with or without food. Give once-daily dose at bedtime.
Know that intravenous form may be added to total parenteral nutrition solutions.
Use cautiously in patients with impaired renal or hepatic function.

Antisecretory Agent

Misoprostol (Cytotec)

Action and Uses
Synthetic prostaglandin E analog; replaces prostaglandin lost due to NSAID therapy. Reduces gastric acid secretion and increases gastric mucus and bicarbonate production, creating a protective coating on gastric mucosa. Primary use is in prevention of NSAID-induced peptic ulcer disease.

Dosages (Adult)
200 mcg PO 3 times/day

Major Adverse Effects
Most common: diarrhea, abdominal discomfort
Other important: women—miscarriage, menstrual disorders, postmenopausal bleeding

Nursing Implications
Assess GI status, report significant adverse reactions.
Instruct patient to take with food.
Advise patient to report diarrhea, abdominal pain, and menstrual irregularities.
Tell patient drug may cause spontaneous abortion.

Caution patient not to take magnesium-containing antacids, which may worsen diarrhea.

Cytoprotective Agent

Sucralfate (Carafate)

Action and Uses
Combines with gastric acid to form protective coating on injured mucosal surface, inhibiting gastric acid secretion, pepsin, and bile salts. Action is almost exclusively local. Used for short-term ulcer treatment.

Dosages (Adult)
1 g (PO) 4 times/day with 1 dose before breakfast and 1 dose at bedtime.
Maintenance dose: 1 g (PO) 2 times/day

Major Adverse Effects
Most common: constipation

Nursing Implications
Monitor bowel pattern; report severe, ongoing constipation.
Monitor to prevent constipation: unless contraindicated, water intake should be increased to 8–10 glasses per day, increase dietary bulk, increase physical exercise.
Caution patient not to take within 30 minutes of antacids or other drugs.

Antacids

Aluminum carbonate (Gaviscon), calcium carbonate (Caltrate)

Action and Uses
Neutralizes excess gastric acid.

Dosages (Adult)
Aluminum carbonate (Gaviscon): Chew 2–4 tablets PO qid or 10–20 mL suspension PO qid
Calcium carbonate (Caltrate): 1–2 tablets every 2 hours PO or 5–10 mL suspension every 2 hours PO prn

Major Adverse Effects
Aluminum and calcium based: fecal impaction, constipation, abdominal cramping
Both: metabolic alkalosis

Nursing Implications
Tell patient that taking too much medication can cause systemic problems.
Advise patient to avoid the herb oak bark and not to take with milk.
Advise patient that some antacids interfere with action of many common drugs; do not take other oral medications within 30 minutes of taking antacids.

Proton Pump Inhibitors (PPIs)

Esomeprazole (Nexium)

Omeprazole (Prilosec)

Pantoprazole (Protonix)

Lansoprazole (Prevacid)

Rabeprazole (Aciphex)

Action and Uses

As a group: inhibit activity of proton pump in gastric parietal cells, decreasing gastric acid production; along with antibiotics, cause *H. pylori* eradication; reduce risk of duodenal ulcer recurrence.

Dosages (Adult)

Esomeprazole: 40 mg PO/IV every day

Omeprazole: 20 mg PO every 12 hours

Pantoprazole: 40 mg PO/IV every day

Lansoprazole: 15–30 mg PO every day

Rabeprazole: 20 mg PO every day

Major Adverse Effects

Generally minor: headache, nausea, diarrhea, rash, and abdominal pain. Should not be taken when pregnant or lactating or for more than 2 months.

Nursing Implications

General implications include:

Concurrent use with diazepam, phenytoin, CNS depressants, and warfarin may cause increase in blood levels of these drugs.

Give oral forms of medications before meals.

If patient has difficulty swallowing the delayed-release capsule, open it and sprinkle contents onto small amount of soft food, such as applesauce or pudding. Do not crush or let patient chew drug.

When giving oral suspension, empty packet contents into container with 2 tbsp. water. Stir contents well, and have patient drink immediately. Do not give oral suspension through nasogastric tube (NG).

When putting contents of delayed-release capsule through NG tube, open capsule and mix granules with 40 mL of apple juice. Then rinse tube with additional apple juice to clear.

Advise patient to minimize GI upset by eating frequent servings of food and drinking plenty of fluids.

H. pylori Eradication Therapy

Action and Uses

Eradication of *H. pylori*; combination therapy is preferred over single antibiotic therapy related to high risk for development of resistance.

Dosages (Adult)

Consists of a combination of antibiotics, PPIs, and bismuth compound:

Metronidazole (Flagyl) 500 mg PO bid–tid

Tetracycline (Sumycin, Achromycin) 500 mg PO qid

Levofloxacin (Levaquin) 300 mg PO bid

Doxycycline (Vibramycin) 100 mg PO bid

Nitazoxanide (Alinia) 1 gm PO bid

Amoxicillin (Amoxil) 1 gm PO bid

Clarithromycin (Biaxin) 500 mg PO bid

Triple Therapy:

PPI or bismuth compound *plus* two antibiotics, given for 7–14 days

Quadruple Therapy:

PPI plus combination of bismuth compound, metronidazole, and tetracycline given for 4–10 days *or* the combination of levofloxacin, doxycycline, and nitazoxanide given for 10 days

Sequential Therapy:

10 days of PPI plus amoxicillin during days 1–5 and a combination of clarithromycin and metronidazole during days 6–10

Major Adverse Effects and Nursing Implications

Multiple, depending on the combination used. Refer to specific drugs in drug resoruce of choice.

Discontinuation of all NSAIDs is recommended when treating PUD.

Section Two Review

1. What is the most common cause of upper GI bleeding?
   A. Esophageal varices
   B. Arteriovenous malformation
   C. Peptic ulcer disease
   D. Stress gastritis

2. A 35-year-old male is diagnosed with PUD. His father had a gastric ulcer. He smokes one pack of cigarettes per day, takes a diuretic to treat his hypertension, and is obese (310 pounds at 6 feet tall). He takes aspirin every day for his arthritis. How many risk factors for PUD does this person have?
   A. Two
   B. Three
   C. Four
   D. Five

3. What is the cause of peptic ulcers?
   A. Disruption of the mucosal barrier
   B. Hypersecretion of pancreatic enzymes
   C. Underproduction of bicarbonate
   D. Colonization of bacteria within the GI tract

4. Which statement correctly reflects the general timing of duodenal ulcer symptoms?
   A. They have no relationship to eating.
   B. They tend to occur 2 to 3 hours after eating.
   C. They tend to occur 6 to 8 hours following eating.
   D. They follow an inconsistent pattern.

Answers: 1. C, 2. B, 3. A, 4. B

Section Three: Acute Upper GI Bleeding Due to Non-ulcer Etiologies

Acute upper GI bleeding can occur in the absence of PUD from several major sources, including stress, gastritis, varices, and tears at the gastroesophageal junction.

Stress-related Mucosal Disease

For many years, the link between critical illness and the development of mucosal injury has been recognized. Stress-related mucosal disease (SRMD) is an acute form of peptic ulcer disease related to severe illness or major trauma. SRMD encompasses two types of injury: (1) superficial, diffuse erosions and (2) stress ulcers, which are deeper, discrete lesions. It has been estimated that at least 75% of critically ill patients have evidence of mucosal injury within the first 24 hours postadmission to ICU (Barrett, 2014; Laine, 2015; Mills & Stappenbeck, 2013).

Pathophysiology Ischemia related to illness or trauma causes disruption of the mucosal barrier. As with peptic ulcer disease, stress-related mucosal disease is believed to be caused by an imbalance in hostile and protective factors in the stomach and duodenum. The high-acuity patient, particularly in the critical care setting, is at significant risk for developing decreased protective factors and increased hostile factors (see Table 22–2).

Prevention and Treatment Early in the critically ill patient's ICU stay, it is common practice to initiate GI prophylactic measures to prevent stress-related mucosal disease (SRMD). Drug groups commonly chosen for GI prophylaxis include histamine-2 receptor blockers and proton pump inhibitors. If GI bleeding occurs and is found to be caused by stress ulceration, intravenous PPI and/or histamine-2 receptor blocker medication is administered.

Acute Erosive or Hemorrhagic Gastritis

Acute gastritis is inflammation of the stomach. Acute erosive or hemorrhagic gastritis involves transient inflammation of the gastric mucosa. Common causes of erosive gastritis include *H. pylori*, NSAIDs, alcohol, and acute stress. Uncommon causes of gastric mucosal erosion include radiation, viral infections, caustic ingestion, and direct trauma (e.g., irritation from nasogastric tubes). The role of NSAIDs in precipitating acute gastritis is inhibition of prostaglandin synthesis, essentially the same as in peptic ulcer disease. Chronic alcohol ingestion can result in inflammation of the gastric mucosa, and the inflammation can progress to erosions and hemorrhage. Episodes of upper GI bleeding as a result of this alcohol-induced gastritis are usually mild. The risk for bleeding significantly increases if a person continues to drink alcohol while on long-term NSAID therapy.

Clinical Manifestations The most common clinical manifestation of erosive gastritis is upper GI bleeding, which presents as hematemesis, "coffee ground" emesis, bloody aspirate in a patient receiving nasogastric suction, or melena. Because erosive gastritis involves superficial lesions, bleeding is not as rapid as with a lesion that extends deeper into the mucosa and may erode into a blood vessel. The slow loss of blood can be noted in continuously decreasing hemoglobin and hematocrit levels. Gastritis is often asymptomatic but may cause epigastric pain, nausea, vomiting, and bleeding. GI bleeding as a result of gastritis is usually not severe except in the critically ill. Diagnosis of gastritis is accomplished by direct visualization with endoscopy.

Prevention and Treatment The incidence of gastritis can usually be reduced or prevented if the gastric pH level is maintained above 4. This can be accomplished with the prophylactic administration of histamine receptor antagonists, proton pump inhibitors, or oral antacids to all at-risk patients to raise the gastric pH above 4 (Laine, 2015). Sucralfate, given orally, is also effective in reducing the risk for bleeding. Early enteral feeding has been advocated as a means of lowering the incidence of bleeding in acutely ill persons. Treatment is aimed at prophylaxis, but histamine-2 receptor agonists (H2RAs), PPIs, and sucralfate are used for both treatment and prophylaxis (Buendgens, Koch, & Tacke, 2016).

Once significant GI bleeding from gastritis occurs (in about 2% of ICU patients), the mortality rate is more than 60% (Laine, 2015; Saltzman, 2016). Severe bleeding from a localized lesion may be treated with endoscopic sclerotherapy to cauterize the lesion. Diffusely bleeding lesions may respond to vasopressin administered intravenously or intra-arterially into a bleeding vessel. Vasopressin (also known as antidiuretic hormone [ADH]) is a potent stimulator of smooth muscle, particularly that of capillaries and arterioles. Vasopressin manages GI bleeding by vasoconstriction of the splanchnic vessels, which reduces blood flow through the bleeding vessel. It exerts its vasoconstricting effects systemically; therefore, untoward side effects of abdominal cramping, angina, hypertension, dysrhythmias, and headache may occur. Surgical resection of the involved portions of the stomach is indicated if bleeding does not respond to more conservative treatment.

Conservative treatment for NSAID-induced gastritis includes discontinuation of the drug, reduction to the lowest effective dose, or administration with meals. Patients with persistent gastritis or those who are at increased risk of developing gastric mucosal injury should be treated with sucralfate, histamine receptor antagonists, or proton pump inhibitors. Misoprostol can be administered along with NSAID therapy to prevent ulcer formation. Misoprostol is a synthetic prostaglandin E analog that replaces the protective prostaglandins consumed with prostaglandin-inhibiting therapies (e.g., NSAIDs). Misoprostol is reserved for use with long-term NSAID therapy in high-risk patients (Laine, 2015; Saltzman, 2016). If the patient has adequate renal function, switching the patient to a COX-2 inhibitor NSAID may prevent NSAID-induced gastritis. Alcohol-induced gastritis usually responds well to cessation of alcohol intake and antiulcer therapy.

Esophageal and Gastric Varices

Upper GI bleeding from esophageal or gastric varices is associated with cirrhosis, portal hypertension, and portal or splenic vein thrombosis. Bleeding from esophagogastric varices is usually massive and occurs without warning. Portal hypertension causes the development of collateral venous pathways, called *varices*, in the esophagus and stomach. Hepatic cirrhosis as a result of alcohol abuse is the most common cause of variceal bleeding in the United States. An in-depth discussion of cirrhosis and esophageal varices is presented in Chapter 23: Alterations in Liver Function.

Mallory-Weiss Tears

A Mallory-Weiss tear is a small laceration in the mucosa at the gastroesophageal junction, although a small percentage occur in the esophageal mucosa. Mallory-Weiss tears are commonly thought to be caused by retching or vomiting; however, only about 30% of patients report a history of vomiting prior to acute hematemesis (McQuaid, 2017; Saltzman, 2016). High-risk patients are those with a history of alcohol abuse. Bleeding from a Mallory-Weiss tear often presents with mild-to-massive hematemesis. Bleeding stops spontaneously in 80% to 90% of patients, and rebleeding is rare (Saltzman, 2016; Shah, 2016). Diagnosis is confirmed by upper GI endoscopy. If acute intervention is required, the tear is endoscopically visualized and the bleeding is stopped using therapies such as thermocoagulation or sclerosing injection (Saltzman, 2016).

Arteriovenous Malformation

An arteriovenous malformation (AVM), sometimes referred to as an angiodysplasia, is a small, abnormal mucosal or submucosal blood vessel that has a tendency to bleed. AVMs can occur in both the upper and lower GI tracts, but they are most commonly located in the cecal region of the lower GI tract. The cause of AVMs is unknown but appears to be genetic. Once GI bleeding from an AVM occurs, recurrent GI bleeding, chronic anemia, or severe acute GI bleeding is the usual clinical course (Laine, 2015; McQuaid, 2017). AVM can be associated with chronic renal insufficiency or renal failure; valvular heart disease, specifically aortic stenosis; and heart failure (Laine, 2015). Upper GI bleeding as a result of an AVM is most commonly diagnosed by upper GI endoscopy. Definitive treatment of the underlying or concomitant conditions (e.g., valvuloplasty or kidney transplantation) can cure bleeding AVMs. Endoscopic sclerotherapy is used palliatively because new AVMs can continue to develop in high-risk patients.

Section Three Review

1. How is the primary treatment for stress-related mucosal disease (SRMD) best described?
   A. It is prophylactic, using antiulcer therapies.
   B. It consists of flushing the stomach with vasopressin to stop the bleeding.
   C. It combines endoscopic visualization with coagulation therapy.
   D. It is reactive; SRMD is treated symptomatically.

2. Stress-related mucosal disease (SRMD) begins to develop in most critically ill clients within how many hours of admission to an ICU?
   A. 12
   B. 24
   C. 36
   D. 48

3. Which drug is often prescribed for high-risk clients on long-term NSAID therapy to prevent the development of ulcers or SRMD?
   A. Neomycin
   B. Misoprostol
   C. Sucralfate
   D. Antacids

4. GI bleeding as a result of a Mallory-Weiss tear often presents with which manifestation?
   A. Hematemesis
   B. Hematochezia
   C. Melena
   D. Pain

Answers: 1. A, 2. B, 3. B, 4. A

Section Four: Acute Lower GI Bleeding

Lower GI bleeding is anatomically defined as bleeding beyond the ligament of Treitz. It accounts for about 20% of major GI bleeding and is less common and generally less severe than upper GI bleeding. There are about 20 to 27 hospitalizations annually per 100,000 adults in the United States due to lower GI bleeding; it is most common in the older adult population (mean age 63–77 years) (Aoki et al., 2015; Shah, 2016).

The two most common causes of acute lower GI bleeding are diverticulosis and arteriovenous malformations. Other common causes are ischemic colitis, internal hemorrhoids, rectal ulcers, and neoplasms. Less frequent causes of lower GI bleeding include ischemic bowel disease and inflammatory bowel disease. Table 22–3 summarizes the

Table 22–3 Causes and Characteristics of Lower GI Bleeding

Cause	Characteristics
Diverticulitis	Sustained, dark, occasionally massive bleeding throughout the colon
Inflammatory bowel disease (e.g., Crohn disease, ulcerative colitis)	Intermittent bleeding, mixed with frequent bowel movements
Perianal disorders (e.g., hemorrhoids, fissures)	Bright red blood per rectum, intermittent with bowel movements
Carcinoma	Occult bleeding with intermittent melena, right colon tumors
Arteriovenous malformation	Intermittent, both dark and bright red bleeding, clots, coming from cecal area
Ischemic colitis (due to mesenteric vascular insufficiency or *Clostridium difficile* infection)	Intermittent, both dark and bright red blood per rectum, and diarrhea if *Clostridium difficile* infection is present

SOURCE: Data from Saltzman & Lee (2016).

most common causes and characteristics of lower GI bleeding.

Bleeding stops spontaneously in 80% to 90% of patients, with a risk of recurrence in 10% to 40%. Unlike upper GI bleeding, the majority of lower GI bleeds are slow and intermittent and do not require hospitalization. About 10% to 20% of acute lower GI bleeding cases do not resolve spontaneously and, therefore, require high-acuity nursing. The overall mortality rate of lower GI bleeding is 10% to 20% (Laine, 2015; Saltzman & Lee, 2016). As with upper GI bleeding, those who begin lower GI bleeding as outpatients have a significantly lower mortality rate (3.6%) than those who develop lower GI bleeding as inpatients (23%) (Laine, Yang, Chang & Datto, 2012; Saltzman & Lee, 2016).

Diverticular Bleeding

Diverticular disease is the most common etiology of major lower GI bleeding. Diverticula (singular: diverticulum) are small outpouchings (herniations) in the bowel wall caused by weakness in the wall of the descending or sigmoid colon (Figure 22–4). Risk factors include age older than 60 years and chronic constipation. Complications of diverticular disease include diverticulitis (inflammation or infection) and rupture. Diverticular bleeding occurs in fewer than 20% of people with the disease and is self-limiting in most cases; however, it can also be massive and life-threatening. About 25% of these cases rebleed, requiring surgical intervention or angiography with intra-arterial infusion of vasopressin (Laine, 2015; Saltzman & Lee, 2016; Shah, 2016).

Inflammatory Bowel Disease

Inflammatory bowel diseases (IBDs), which include ulcerative colitis and Crohn disease, are chronic disorders of the GI tract. They are usually diagnosed by colonoscopy and biopsy. Ulcerative colitis is largely confined to the mucosa and submucosa, but in Crohn disease, the disease extends through the intestinal wall from mucosa to serosa. Bloody diarrhea is the most common symptom of IBD and is a major feature of ulcerative colitis. The degree of bleeding is usually light to moderate but can be massive. Significant bleeding is much more common with ulcerative colitis than with Crohn disease. In very rare instances (about 4% in ulcerative colitis and 1%–2% in Crohn disease), life-threatening bleeding can result when the underlying inflammation ulcerates into adjacent arteries. The treatment of bleeding associated with IBD consists of managing the underlying disorder with drugs such as amino-salicylates and corticosteroids (Laine, 2015; Saltzman & Lee, 2016). If the bleeding is uncontrollable by medical means, then surgical resection of the affected portion of the bowel is necessary.

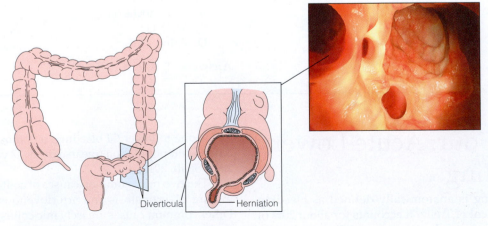

Figure 22–4 Diverticula of the colon.

SOURCE: Juan Gaertner/Shutterstock

Neoplasms and Polyps

Colorectal cancers are primarily associated with occult bleeding; however, massive bleeding occurs in 5% to 20% of cases (Laine, 2015). Bleeding from neoplasms is usually slow, chronic, and self-limiting. Only rarely is there acute blood loss of significant proportions from a neoplasm. In these cases, bowel resection and tumor excision are indicated. Bleeding is relatively common for up to a month following surgical removal of polyps.

Arteriovenous Malformations

Bleeding from an arteriovenous malformation (AVM) is usually slow and chronic and can be occult. Patients usually present with weakness, fatigue, dyspnea on exertion, and guaiac-positive stools. Bleeding from an AVM is rarely massive. A typical bleeding episode requires minimal blood transfusion, usually less than 2 to 4 units of blood, and is not often associated with hypotension unless the patient is an older adult or has multiple other comorbid conditions. Older adults have an increased risk of severe blood loss from this type of GI bleed.

Arteriovenous malformations are angiodysplastic lesions that are usually small, superficial, multiple, and located in the right colon, although lesions can occur throughout the intestinal tract and are often numerous. The cause of AVMs is not clear, but they appear to be associated with cardiac disease, low-flow states, and the aging process. Bleeding occurs from weakened, friable vessel wall lesions caused by chronic tension and dilation of the blood vessels most commonly located in the cecal area of the intestine.

In cases in which the bleeding does not stop spontaneously, arterial embolization is performed with various agents such as intra-arterial infusion of vasopressin or gelatin sponge, microcoils, and polyvinyl alcohol particles. Vasopressin can control bleeding in about 91% of all cases, but complications such as dysrhythmias, pulmonary edema, hypertension, and ischemia occur in about 10% to 20% of cases where vasopressin is administered (Laine, 2015; Saltzman & Lee, 2016).

Ischemic Bowel Disease

Ischemic bowel disease can be defined as ischemia of the colon caused by an interruption of the colonic blood supply. It may result from occlusion of a major artery, small-vessel disease, venous obstruction, low-flow states (e.g., cardiogenic shock), or intestinal obstruction. Intestinal ischemia can develop postoperatively following vascular bypass or colon resection with anastomosis. In older adults, risk factors for developing ischemic bowel disease include atherosclerosis, atrial fibrillation, and hypotension. Older adults are most commonly affected, although younger patients with diabetes, pancreatitis, heart disease, sickle cell disease, or systemic lupus erythematosus are also at risk.

Bleeding from ischemic bowel disease is often associated with anticoagulant use (25% of all bleeding cases) (Laine, 2015; McQuaid, 2017; Saltzman & Lee, 2016). The bleeding is usually intermittent, with mixed dark and bright red blood, and clots may be visible from the rectum. Fever and abdominal pain are usually present. Lower GI endoscopy reveals purple discoloration of the bowel, often in the presence of erosion and ulceration. Radiographic x-rays are nonspecific but may reveal abnormal air pockets if perforation is present. Barium contrast studies reveal characteristic "thumbprints," suggesting a necrotic process. Arterial or venous occlusion of the mesenteric vasculature should be suspected and ruled out when ischemia of the bowel is included in the differential diagnosis.

Treatment of ischemic bowel disease involves restoration of blood circulation to the intestines and might include fluid resuscitation, optimization of cardiac output, and treatment of any underlying disease. Antibiotics may be required for infections. Resection of the affected bowel may be necessary for fulminant disease or severe bleeding. Patients with ischemic bowel disease often have other medical problems, including multiple organ failure, and therefore have a mortality rate of about 50% (Saltzman & Lee, 2016).

Section Four Review

1. Diverticula are found in which structure?
   A. Stomach
   B. Small intestine
   C. Colon
   D. GI tract

2. Sustained, dark red, lower GI bleeding from the large intestine is a characteristic of which condition?
   A. Bleeding diverticula
   B. Bleeding hemorrhoid
   C. Bleeding tumor
   D. Bleeding angiodysplasia

3. Ulcerative colitis is defined as what type of process?
   A. Malignant process
   B. Infectious process
   C. Ischemic process
   D. Inflammatory process

4. Treatment of ischemic bowel disease may include which measure?
   A. Steroid administration
   B. High-dose narcotics
   C. Fluid resuscitation
   D. Enemas until clear

Answers: 1. C, 2. A, 3. D, 4. C

Section Five: Management of Acute Gastrointestinal Bleeding

Caring for patients with acute GI bleeding is complex and requires close assessment and monitoring of the patient's condition and progress. Collaborative management of physiological problems and concern for the patient's psychosocial response to the acute illness are priorities for the nurse. Because fear and anxiety often accompany acute GI bleeding, patients and their significant others need information and support during this time. Nurses coordinate plans for ongoing care based on accurate and ongoing nursing assessment.

Patients who are experiencing acute GI bleeding must be approached in a systematic manner. This approach should be collaborative and include (1) initial assessment, (2) resuscitation, (3) definitive diagnosis, and (4) treatment.

In collaboration with the healthcare provider, the nurse's role includes the following:

- Assessing the severity of blood loss
- Administering prescribed crystalloids and colloids for fluid replacement
- Assisting in determining the cause of the bleeding
- Planning and implementing treatment
- Managing the ongoing plan of care and monitoring progress
- Providing supportive care and education to the patient and significant others because any bleeding experience is potentially life-threatening

Initial Assessment

To assess the severity of blood loss, the nurse must determine hemodynamic stability. Evidence of instability includes decreased blood pressure or orthostatic hypotension, altered level of consciousness, and decreased urine output (which is suggestive of fluid volume deficit). Evidence of hemodynamic instability in the presence of hematemesis, hematochezia, or melena should be considered an emergency until proven otherwise, and admission to an intensive care unit (ICU) or intermediate-care unit (IMC) is recommended. The following are guidelines for admission to an ICU:

- Clearly documented frank hematemesis
- Coffee-ground emesis and either melena or hematochezia
- Hemodynamic instability (hypotension, tachycardia, or orthostatic hypotension)
- A continued drop in hemoglobin and hematocrit
- A significant unexplained increase in the BUN when GI bleeding is suspected (increased BUN suggests fluid volume deficit or metabolism of blood within the GI tract)

Resuscitation

Patients in shock require care in an intensive care unit (ICU). Careful and continuous assessment of the physiologic status is necessary. Resuscitation is the primary goal of early management in the hemodynamically unstable patient and mandates the maintenance of intravascular volume and tissue oxygenation. Arterial pressure through an indwelling line, pulse, and respiratory rate should be monitored continuously. Blood specimens for type and crossmatching, CBC, PT/PTT, and chemistries should be obtained. Nasal oxygen and pulse oximetry are warranted especially in older adults or in patients with a history of cardiac or pulmonary disease. Close nursing assessment of level of consciousness and oxygenation status is important in the acute phase. Endotracheal intubation should be considered for decreased level of consciousness, shock, massive bleeding, or if the patient is unable to protect their own airway. The nurse should have emergency intubation and oxygen equipment ready for use if needed. Vital signs, orthostatic blood pressure changes, and urine output are valuable clinical indicators of perfusion and blood volume. An indwelling catheter should be placed to monitor urine output because this is an indirect measure of perfusion. There is ongoing debate as to the indications for using the flow-directed pulmonary artery catheter (PAC), also known as a Swan-Ganz catheter, in the ICU. A recent Cochrane analysis showed that the use of a PAC did not alter mortality, length of stay, or cost for adult ICU patients (Rajaram et al., 2013). The reviewers found that most patients in the ICU can be safely managed without the use of a PAC. However, in shock with significant ongoing blood loss, fluid shifts, and underlying cardiac dysfunction, a PAC may be useful. The PAC is placed percutaneously via the subclavian or jugular vein through the central venous circulation and right heart into the pulmonary artery. There are ports both proximal in the right atrium and distal in the pulmonary artery to provide access for infusions and for cardiac output measurements. Right atrial and pulmonary artery pressures (PAPs) can be measured, and the pulmonary capillary wedge pressure (PCWP) serves as an approximation of the left atrial pressure. A PAC with an oximeter port offers the additional advantage of online monitoring of the mixed venous oxygen saturation, an important index of overall tissue perfusion. In resuscitation from shock, it is critical to restore tissue perfusion and optimize oxygen delivery, hemodynamics, and cardiac function rapidly. Determinations of oxygen content in arterial and venous blood, together with cardiac output and hemoglobin concentration, allow calculation of oxygen delivery, oxygen consumption, and oxygen-extraction ratio. A reasonable goal of therapy is to achieve a normal mixed venous oxygen saturation (65%) and arteriovenous oxygen extraction ratio (O_2ER normal is 22%–32%) (Maier, 2015). In addition, an elevated plasma lactate level is a measure of anaerobic metabolism and reflects inadequate tissue perfusion. Serial (every 4 hours) serum lactate levels should be obtained during the resuscitation period with a goal of a lactate level of less than 5 mEq/L (Vincent & De Backer, 2013).

Volume resuscitation is accomplished with crystalloid (normal saline or lactated Ringer's) at a rate to maintain a systolic blood pressure higher than 90 mmHg through at least two large-bore IV lines. If, after 2 to 3 liters of crystalloid infusion, the patient remains unstable, an infusion of blood products (packed red cells or whole blood) should be considered. Vasoconstricting drugs (vasopressors) are generally not indicated because hypovolemia is usually the cause of the hypotension. Packed red cells are transfused for massive bleeding to keep the hematocrit higher than 28% to 30% and the hemoglobin greater than 7 gm/dL (Maier, 2015). Patients with cardiac or pulmonary disease may require transfusion to a higher hematocrit (higher than 30%). Transfusions of whole blood may be considered in massively bleeding patients because they provide increased colloid osmotic pressure, thus decreasing the patient's total fluid requirements. O-negative blood can be used until the patient's blood has been crossmatched. A blood warmer should be considered for rapid fluid or blood administration to prevent hypothermia. Each unit of blood should elevate the hematocrit by three points. Fresh frozen plasma is considered for patients who have a coagulopathy (increased PT or PTT) or who have been on Coumadin therapy. If the patient has thrombocytopenia, platelet transfusion should be considered to maintain the platelet count above 50,000/mm^3 (Laine, 2015; McQuaid, 2017; Saltzman, 2016).

For patients with persistent bleeding, therapeutic intervention is necessary. This intervention can be pharmacotherapy, mechanical (balloon) tamponade (Sengstaken–Blakemore tube), endoscopic therapy (sclerotherapy), or surgery. Once blood volume is restored, the patient is monitored for evidence of further bleeding (e.g., tachycardia, decreased blood pressure, hematemesis, bloody or tarry

Table 22–4 Interventions for Severe GI Hemorrhage with Evidence of Hemodynamic Instability or Persistent Bleeding

Intervention	Effects
Vasopressin	Decreases portal pressure by vasoconstricting splanchnic arteries Untoward effects include decreased coronary blood flow and increased blood pressure
Somatostatin	Decreases portal pressure by vasoconstriction of splanchnic circulation
Octreotide	A synthetic analog of somatostatin; has same action as somatostatin
Mechanical tamponade	Provides tamponade to actively bleeding gastric or esophageal varices (use is restricted to bleeding esophageal or gastric varices)

SOURCE: Data from McQuaid (2016).

stools). Specific therapy depends on the bleeding site (refer to previously discussed etiologies of GI bleeding for specific treatments). Table 22–4 provides a summary of interventions for severe GI hemorrhage.

Definitive Diagnosis

Finding the source of the GI bleeding should be undertaken as soon as the patient has been stabilized. Early specialty consultation is essential for patients with GI bleeding. Patients with upper GI bleeding are usually seen by a gastroenterologist, and patients with lower GI bleeding are usually evaluated by a general surgeon. An example of a diagnostic approach to the patient with GI bleeding is provided in Figure 22–5.

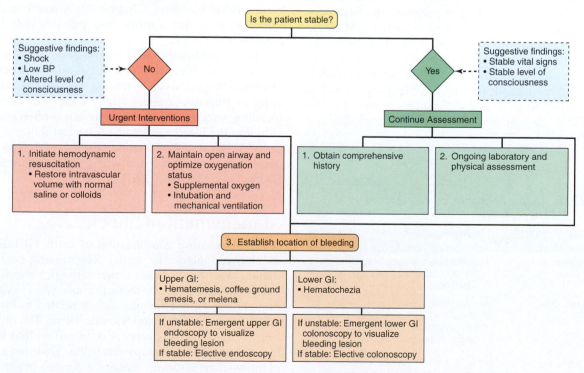

Figure 22–5 Diagnostic approach to the patient with GI bleeding.

Table 22–5 Endoscopic Interventions in GI Hemorrhage

Intervention	Description
Endoscopic injection sclerotherapy	Sclerosing agent is injected into bleeding vessel.
Endoscopic electrocoagulation	Direct electric current is applied to bleeding lesion = fibrosis.
Endoscopic laser therapy	Direct application of heat is used to coagulate bleeding lesion.
Endoscopic heater probe	Direct electric current is applied to coagulate bleeding lesion.

SOURCE: Data from McQuaid (2016).

Treatments

Multiple treatment options are available for the control and correction of GI bleeding, including endoscopic interventions, arterial angiotherapy, sclerotherapy, and surgery.

Endoscopic Interventions   Bleeding peptic ulcers, gastritis, Mallory-Weiss tears, and arteriovenous malformations are often diagnosed with endoscopy. Using a special flexible fiber-optic scope, structures in the GI tract can be viewed directly. A tiny camera provides visualization on a video screen. In some cases, therapeutic interventions to stop bleeding can be performed during the endoscopy. Table 22–5 provides a summary of endoscopic interventions.

Arterial Angiotherapy   Arterial angiography can be used to control massive bleeding from peptic ulcers in patients who are considered poor surgical risks. Selective arterial infusion of vasopressin is used to control massive or persistent bleeding in patients who have peptic ulcer disease, stress ulcers, erosive gastritis, Mallory-Weiss tears, and arteriovenous malformation. Selective catheterization of the bleeding artery is required for infusion of vasopressin. Arterial embolization is an alternative to arterial vasopressin; the bleeding vessel is selectively catheterized, and a coagulant is placed in the vessel. Table 22–6 summarizes arterial angiotherapy interventions.

Table 22–6 Arterial Angiotherapy Interventions in GI Hemorrhage

Intervention	Description
Selective arterial infusion of vasopressin	Requires selective catheterization of the bleeding artery for infusion of vasopressin
Arterial embolization	An alternative to arterial vasopressin where the bleeding vessel is selectively catheterized, and a coagulant is placed in the vessel

SOURCE: Data from Laine (2015); McQuaid (2016); and Saltzman & Lee (2016b).

Sclerotherapy   Sclerotherapy is the use of a chemical (called a sclerosant) to stop the bleeding and harden (sclerose) a blood vessel to prevent rebleeding. It is a strategy used to treat actively bleeding GI vessels, particularly bleeding esophageal varices. The chemicals used are usually sodium tetradecyl sulfate (Sotradecol) or sodium morrhuate (Scleromate). Vital signs should be taken before and after the procedure. Postprocedure, the patient requires close monitoring for signs of rebleeding and other complications, such as aspiration pneumonia, esophageal scar tissue contraction (which can cause partial obstruction), infection, and esophageal perforation.

Surgery   Surgery is considered for severe hemorrhage or recurrent bleeding when other, less invasive interventions have not been successful or when the patient's condition warrants immediate surgical repair.

Treatments of Specific GI Bleeding Problems

Bleeding from esophageal or gastric varices requires ICU admission. These patients require endotracheal intubation and early endoscopy. Sclerotherapy should be performed as soon as a diagnosis of variceal bleeding is confirmed. Rebleeding occurs in 10% to 20% of cases following sclerotherapy (McQuaid, 2017). Intravenous vasopressin or octreotide (somatostatin analog) may be used as an alternative to sclerotherapy (or concomitantly) to reduce portal pressures. Balloon tamponade therapy is an effective temporary method to stop variceal bleeding while awaiting more definitive therapy. Shunt surgery or transjugular intrahepatic portosystemic shunt (TIPS) should be considered if the risk is high for recurrent variceal bleeding. Chapter 23: Alterations in Liver Function provides a more in-depth discussion of the treatment of varices.

Bleeding Mallory-Weiss tears that do not stop spontaneously and bleeding arteriovenous malformations (AVMs) of the colon can be treated with therapeutic endoscopy or selective arterial angiotherapy. In diverticular bleeding, selective arterial vasopressin is often effective in stopping the bleeding. Selective arterial therapy requires catheterization of the bleeding vessel for infusion of vasopressin. Surgery is needed when the bleeding is severe (Laine, 2015; McQuaid, 2017).

Management of Shock

A life-threatening complication of acute GI bleeding is shock (hypovolemic or septic). Key nursing goals for the patient with hypovolemic (hemorrhagic) shock include maintenance of adequate tissue perfusion and oxygenation, prevention of fluid volume deficit related to blood loss, and optimization of hemodynamic status. The nurse must first see that venous access is achieved so that fluid and blood resuscitation therapy can begin. Ensuring adequacy of intravenous infusions remains a nursing priority for the

Table 22–7 Common Patient Conditions Related to Acute GI Problems

Problem Statement	Etiologic Factors
GASTROINTESTINAL BLEEDING	
Hypovolemia	Blood loss; NPO status; vomiting; diarrhea
Hypoperfused tissues: cerebral, cardiac, pulmonary, renal, peripheral, mesenteric	Hypovolemia and decreased oxygenation secondary to anemia, hypotension, shock
Hypoxemia	Hypovolemia, anemia
Anxiety	Fear of bleeding, threat of death
Inability to protect airway	Hematemesis and potential changes in level of consciousness
Malnutrition	Decreased appetite secondary to bowel irritability; NPO
Pain	Bleeding and discomfort
Diarrhea	Decrease in intestinal transit time secondary to cathartic effects of blood in GI tract
Acute confusion	Hypoxia secondary to anemia
Infection	Immune suppression; intestinal ischemia or infarction secondary to hypotension and shock
Fatigue	Anemia, decreased oxygenation
Deficient knowledge	Precipitating factors; therapeutic procedures or interventions; discharge information

duration of the treatment of shock. To maintain adequate gas exchange and tissue perfusion, the nurse should do the following:

1. Ensure an open airway and administer supplemental oxygen.
2. Initiate continuous monitoring for cardiac dysrhythmias.
3. Prepare for insertion of a central venous or pulmonary artery catheter and record and monitor cardiac filling pressures once placement has been achieved.
4. Prepare the patient for emergent surgical intervention to control bleeding.

The major nursing assessments and interventions specific to the care of the patient at risk for hypovolemia as a result of GI bleeding are summarized in the "Nursing Care: The Patient at Risk for Hypovolemia Due to Acute GI Bleeding" and "Nursing Care: The Patient with Gastrointestinal Bleeding" features. These interventions also apply to the patient who is in shock secondary to sepsis.

Related Nursing Diagnoses

Nursing diagnoses that are appropriate for patients diagnosed with GI bleeding are listed in Table 22–7.

Nursing Care

The Patient at Risk for Hypovolemia Due to Acute GI Bleeding

Expected Patient Outcomes and Related Interventions

Outcome: Maintain normal fluid volume status.

Assess and compare to established norms, baselines, and abnormal trends.

Signs and symptoms of shock; abnormal vital signs, decreased urine output, abnormal hemodynamic measures (PAP, CVP, PAWP, CI, CO, SVR), decreased SaO_2 (oxygen saturation), diminished peripheral pulses, restlessness, agitation; cool, pale, or moist skin, elevated serum lactic acid levels

Fluid status: intake and output (urine output, gastric drainage)

Electrolyte levels (may become altered from fluid loss or fluid shifts)

Hemoglobin, hematocrit, RBC, coagulation studies (PT, PTT), renal function (BUN, serum creatinine)

Gastric pH: consult with physician or practitioner about specific pH range and antacid administration.

Tests of gastric drainage, emesis, or stools for occult blood

Adverse reaction to blood products

Institute measures to regain or maintain normal fluid volume.

Consult with physician or practitioner about replacing fluid losses based on assessment findings.

Administer replacement fluids and blood products as directed.

PAP: pulmonary artery pressure; CI: cardiac index; CO: cardiac output; SVR: systemic vascular resistance; CVP: central venous pressure; RBC: red blood count; PT: prothrombin time; PTT: partial thromboplastin time; BUN: blood urea nitrogen.

Nursing Care
The Patient with Gastrointestinal Bleeding

Expected Outcomes and Related Interventions

Outcome 1: Maintain hemodynamic stability.

Assess and compare to established norms, baselines, and trends.

Monitor vital signs continuously for changes indicating hypovolemic shock.

Hypotension, tachycardia

Monitor hemodynamic parameters, which may include central venous pressure, cardiac output, and cardiac index to evaluate the patient's status and response to treatment

Monitor intake and output closely, including all losses from the GI tract.

Check stools and gastric drainage for occult blood.

Notify provider of sudden changes in laboratory findings, including serial hemoglobin and hematocrit.

Assess for the extent of blood loss.

Institute continuous cardiac monitoring to evaluate for possible dysrhythmias, myocardial ischemia, or adverse effects of treatment.

Institute measures to regain or maintain hemodynamic stability.

Assist with insertion of central venous catheter to evaluate hemodynamic status.

Initiate fluid resuscitation as ordered.

Obtain a type and crossmatch for blood component therapy.

Administer blood component therapy (usually packed red blood cells and fresh frozen plasma) as ordered.

Outcome 2: Maintain adequate oxygenation.

Assess and compare to established norms, baselines, and trends.

Assess level of consciousness frequently.

Assess breathing and circulation.

Monitor cardiac and respiratory status closely.

Monitor arterial blood gases.

Institute measures to regain or maintain adequate oxygenation.

Initiate actions to increase oxygen supply.

Ensure a patent airway.

Administer supplemental oxygen as ordered.

Anticipate possible need for endotracheal intubation and mechanical ventilation.

Initiate actions to decrease oxygen demands.

Treat fevers.

Keep patient quiet and comfortable.

Outcome 3: No further signs of bleeding.

Assess and compare to established norms, baselines, and trends.

Monitor vital signs and hemodynamic status (refer to outcome 1).

Institute measures to regain or maintain adequate oxygenation.

Assist with or insert NG tube.

Perform lavage as ordered to clear any blood or clots.

Administer antisecretory medications as ordered to reduce gastric acid secretion.

Prepare for possible endoscopic repair or surgery.

Encourage smoking cessation and avoidance of alcohol.

Section Five Review

1. To assess the severity of blood loss, what should the nurse determine?
   A. Respiratory status
   B. Hemodynamic status
   C. Level of consciousness
   D. Degree of impairment

2. In a client who has had a GI bleed, an increased BUN suggests fluid volume deficit or which other condition?
   A. Onset of acute renal failure
   B. Systemic inflammatory response
   C. Acute infectious process
   D. Metabolism of blood in the intestines

3. How is volume resuscitation generally accomplished in the client with an acute GI bleed?
   A. Intravenous crystalloid infusion
   B. Vasoconstricting drugs
   C. Blood transfusion
   D. Normal saline via a nasogastric tube

4. Which condition is a life-threatening complication of acute GI bleeding?
   A. Renal failure
   B. Abdominal aorta aneurysm
   C. Shock
   D. Pancreatitis

Answers: 1. B, 2. D, 3. A, 4. C

Section Six: Acute Intestinal Obstruction

Intestinal obstruction refers to failure of intestinal contents to pass through the bowel lumen.

Acute intestinal obstructions are relatively common complications that develop following surgery or as a result of gastrointestinal disease.

Types of Acute Intestinal Obstruction

Acute small-bowel obstruction and paralytic ileus both involve intestinal obstruction and have many common features; however, their etiologies differ. For this reason, they are described separately in this section. Large-bowel obstruction will also be described.

Acute Small-bowel Obstruction **Obstruction** of the small intestine is a common surgical complication, often the result of adhesions that develop following abdominal surgery. Other causes of obstruction can be mechanical, such as with incarcerated hernias, volvulus, intussusception, and tumors (Figure 22–6) or functional or adynamic as in paralytic ileus. Small-bowel obstructions represent 15% of hospital admissions for acute abdominal pain. Approximately 300,000 operations are performed every year in the United States for obstruction. Mortality rate overall is approximately 5%. Most obstructions involve actual occlusion of the intestinal lumen (mechanical or physical), resulting in distention, gas, and fluid accumulation proximal to the obstruction. Intestinal obstructions can be either partial or complete. Partial obstructions are often managed nonoperatively. Complete obstructions carry more risk of morbidity and can result in strangulation. Mechanical obstruction refers to physical blockage of luminal contents. This occurs in either the small bowel (80% of cases) or the large bowel (20% of cases). The most common cause of mechanical obstruction is adhesions from prior abdominal surgery (50%), followed by malignancy (20%), hernias (10%), inflammatory bowel disease (5%), and volvulus (3%) (Price & Orthober, 2016).

Swallowed air is the major cause of the distention. Bacterial fermentation within the lumen of the intestine produces other gases (methane) that contribute to distention. Inflammation soon develops and leads to transudation of fluid from the extracellular space into the intestinal lumen and peritoneal cavity. The inflammatory process causes large amounts of fluid and sodium to accumulate within the intestine (mass effect), which contributes to distention and edema of the intestinal wall proximal to the obstruction. Fluid and electrolytes are trapped within the obstructed bowel and leak out (third-space) into the peritoneum and surrounding tissues, further disturbing electrolyte and fluid balance. Fluid losses may be so severe that hypotension results, which can lead to cardiovascular collapse unless the condition is recognized and treated. As bowel contents are prevented from forward flow, increased secretions result in overdistention, which causes bowel wall edema and reduced lymphatic and venous outflow. This is referred to as strangulation and can progress to bowel ischemia, necrosis, perforation, and peritonitis. In severe cases, perforation of the intestinal wall can occur, with spillage of the bowel contents into the peritoneal cavity (McQuaid, 2017; Price & Orthober, 2016).

In severe cases of bowel obstruction, the intestine can become strangulated. **Intestinal strangulation** occurs when the intestine becomes so twisted that circulation is interrupted. Strangulation can result in necrosis, perforation, and sepsis. The mortality rate from strangulated obstructions approaches 30%. Corrective surgery is generally the treatment of choice to prevent ischemic bowel problems. Up to 40% of small-bowel obstructions become strangulated, most commonly from volvulus, adhesions, and hernias. Appropriately treated, simple obstruction has a low mortality rate (less than 2%), whereas strangulation is associated with a high mortality rate (up to 25% if surgery is delayed). When the obstruction is located in the colon, it usually stems from a malignant tumor (McQuaid, 2017; Price & Orthober, 2016).

Large-bowel Obstruction

Neoplasms are the most common cause of large-bowel obstruction. Large-bowel obstruction should prompt an evaluation for a neoplasm. Other etiologies of large-bowel obstruction are diverticulitis, stricture formation, and fecal impaction. Diverticulitis may lead to mesenteric edema and secondary obstruction. Stricture formation can occur with chronic inflammation and scarring. Fecal impaction is a common problem in older or debilitated adults and may present with symptoms of colonic obstruction. Another cause of large-bowel obstruction is sigmoid volvulus. Older, bedridden, or psychiatric patients who are taking anticholinergic medication are most at risk for volvulus. A history of constipation may precede the development of volvulus (Price & Orthober, 2016).

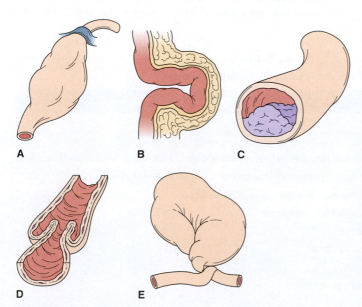

Figure 22–6 Selected causes of mechanical obstruction. A, Adhesions. B, Incarcerated hernia. C, Tumor. D, Intussusceptions. E, Volvulus.

Acute Paralytic Ileus In contrast to mechanical obstruction, functional obstruction (e.g., adynamic ileus) occurs when intestinal contents fail to pass because of disturbances in gut motility. Paralytic ileus (adynamic ileus) involves bowel obstruction resulting from a loss of intestinal peristalsis in the absence of any mechanical (physical) obstruction. It is commonly seen in hospitalized persons and can occur anywhere along the GI tract as a complication of trauma, handling of the bowel during surgery, electrolyte disturbances (hypokalemia, hypocalcemia, and hypomagnesemia), intestinal ischemia, peritonitis, or sepsis. In addition, multiple medications can reduce gastric motility (e.g., opioids, anticholinergics, and phenothiazines) and contribute to the development of paralytic ileus. Ogilvie syndrome involves paralytic ileus of the colon. This is a severe form of ileus that often arises in bedridden patients who have serious systemic illnesses (Price & Orthober, 2016).

Clinical Findings in Intestinal Obstruction

The clinical findings associated with acute intestinal obstruction center around an abnormal abdominal assessment. Laboratory and radiologic examinations, along with history and physical findings, aid in diagnosing intestinal obstruction.

Clinical Manifestations The hallmark clinical manifestation of intestinal obstruction is abdominal distention. Small-bowel obstruction is characterized by cramping and periumbilical pain that occurs in waves, with periods of relative comfort in between. Vomiting, possibly profuse, soon follows the onset of pain and is usually bilious, with a large quantity of mucus. Electrolyte imbalances and intraluminal loss of fluids occur, with dehydration soon following. Visible peristaltic waves may be observed on the abdomen, and high-pitched tinkles are auscultated during the painful spasms. The abdomen may be tender to palpation. If rebound tenderness develops, the nurse should observe for signs and symptoms of shock as a result of perforation. Symptoms of colonic paralytic ileus (Ogilvie syndrome) include abdominal distention and diminished bowel sounds without pain (McQuaid, 2017; Price & Orthober, 2016).

Laboratory Findings Hematology, electrolyte, and chemistry studies will reflect inflammation, fluid, and electrolyte imbalances that may develop as a result of intestinal obstruction. Mild leukocytosis (greater than 15,000) is common, whereas white blood cell (WBC) elevations from 15,000 to 25,000 may occur with strangulation and perforation (Jacobs, 2015). Serum BUN, creatinine, sodium, and osmolality levels become elevated as fluid and electrolytes leak out of the obstructed bowel and translocate into the intestinal lumen. Increases in serum amylase levels are common.

Radiologic Findings Radiology films are taken with the patient in upright, flat, and side-lying positions. Distended bowel loops will reveal air–fluid levels in a ladder-like pattern. Distention is more pronounced within the colon in patients with paralytic ileus. Direct visualization and barium studies may help to confirm the diagnosis (Jacobs, 2015).

Treatment

It is imperative to identify those patients at risk for developing a bowel obstruction or motility problem, such as paralytic ileus: those with dysfunction of multiple body systems and older adult, postoperative, and/or bedridden patients. Initial therapy is directed toward fluid resuscitation and stabilization of the patient. Oral food and fluids are withheld, and a nasogastric tube (Salem Sump) is inserted and attached to low, intermittent suction to relieve vomiting and decompress abdominal distention. Colonoscopy with decompression is sometimes useful in Ogilvie syndrome. Isotonic intravenous fluid should be administered to treat dehydration. Electrolyte losses should be replaced and

Table 22–8 Common Patient Conditions Related to Acute Paralytic Ileus and Intestinal Ischemia

Condition	Etiologic Factors
Paralytic Ileus	
Hypoventilation	Abdominal distention
Hypovolemia	Vomiting, distention, electrolyte imbalance, hypovolemia (loss of flulids and electrolytes due to stasis of bowel contents)
Risk for hypoperfusion (bowel)	Decreased oxygenation to tissues secondary to bowel strangulation, perforation, and/or shock
Risk for infection or sepsis	Perforation, strangulation, bowel ischemia → infarction → necrosis → sepsis
	Absent bowel sounds; NPO; electrolyte loss; constipation
Acute pain	Distention; intestinal angina; perforation
Patient education needs	Illness, treatments, procedures, and outcome
Intestinal Ischemia	
Acute pain	Intestinal angina; distention; infarction; peritonitis
Infection or sepsis	Infarction → necrosis → sepsis
Hypovolemia and electrolyte imbalance	Electrolyte imbalance; NPO; vomiting; diarrhea; third-spacing; shock if perforation occurs
Patient education needs	Illness, treatments, procedures, and outcome

monitored by the nurse. The extent of fluid resuscitation is best guided by the urine output, although in older adults or those with cardiopulmonary disease, central venous pressure monitoring is the best means of determining fluid volume needs. The nurse should closely monitor the patient's urine output with an indwelling urinary drainage catheter. If the patient demonstrates peritoneal signs (boardlike abdominal distention with severe pain) and strangulation is suspected, broad-spectrum antibiotics should be considered to provide anaerobic and gram-negative coverage. Early surgical consult is advised in high-risk patients. All cases of complete obstruction require surgical resection of the affected bowel (Jacobs, 2015; McQuaid, 2017). Common patient conditions with etiological factors for patients diagnosed with paralytic ileus and acute intestinal ischemia are listed in Table 22–8.

Section Six Review

1. If a client with a small-bowel obstruction develops rebound tenderness with boardlike distention, what should the nurse suspect?
   A. Constipation
   B. Perforation
   C. Ogilvie syndrome
   D. Retroperitoneal bleeding

2. Which substance frequently accumulates in the bowel proximal to the actual bowel obstruction, resulting in distention?
   A. Fluid
   B. Blood
   C. Stool
   D. Pus

3. What is the condition in which the bowel "twists" itself to such an extent that circulation is interrupted?
   A. Peritonitis
   B. Perforation
   C. Strangulation
   D. Peristalsis

4. What is the mortality rate for strangulation?
   A. less than 2%
   B. 50%
   C. 80%
   D. 30%

Answers: 1. B, 2. B, 3. C, 4. D

Section Seven: Intra-abdominal Hypertension and Abdominal Compartment Syndrome

Intra-abdominal hypertension (IAH)—abnormally high pressure within the abdominal cavity—has a prevalence of 50% in the critically ill population and has been identified as an independent risk factor for death (Ho & Barie, 2016). **Abdominal compartment syndrome (ACS)** is a rare but life-threatening condition resulting from an acute expansion of abdominal contents. Increased abdominal pressure (IAP) causes IAH, which impairs blood flow to multiple organs and causes tissue ischemia and organ failure. It is important to recognize patients who are at risk for ACS and identify early signs of increased abdominal pressure so that appropriate treatment can be initiated.

IAH/ACS Continuum

The terms *intra-abdominal hypertension* and *abdominal compartment syndrome* are sometimes used interchangeably, but it is generally accepted that the two represent a continuum of pathophysiologic changes. The World Society of the Abdominal Compartment Syndrome (WSACS) defines levels of IAH/ACS as depicted in Table 22–9 (Kirkpatrick et al., 2013).

- Intra-abdominal hypertension—a sustained or repeated pathological elevation of IAP of 12 mmHg or greater
- Abdominal compartment syndrome—intra-abdominal hypertension greater than 20 mmHg, causing end-organ dysfunction that is improved by abdominal decompression (Kirkpatrick, 2013).

These critical pressure levels can vary by 1 to 2 degrees between patients.

IAH/ACS Etiology

Intra-abdominal hypertension can result from a variety of chronic and acute causes, including the accumulation of

Table 22–9 Grades of IAH

Grade	IAP (mmHg)
I	12–15
II	16–20
III	21–25
IV	Greater than 25

SOURCE: Data from World Society of the Abdominal Compartment Syndrome. (2013).

BOX 22–1 Risk Factors for Development of IAH and ACS

- Abdominal aortic aneurysm rupture
- Abdominal trauma
- Acute pancreatitis
- Hepatic transplantation
- Ileus
- Intestinal obstruction
- Intra-abdominal or retroperitoneal hemorrhage
- Massive volume resuscitation
- Pregnancy
- Severe ascites
- Shock states

fluid, pregnancy, blood clots, or third-spacing of fluid into the peritoneal cavity. Sudden elevations of increased abdominal pressure are usually associated with abdominal surgery or trauma. Box 22–1 lists disorders that are known to increase the risk for development of intra-abdominal hypertension (IAH) and abdominal compartment syndrome (ACS). Patients who are at greatest risk include those with abdominal trauma who are postoperative for repair of the injuries. Because the abdomen functions as a single compartment, an increase in its contents (e.g., from fluid accumulation) may cause an elevation in IAP, leading to IAH. Other conditions that place patients at increased risk for developing IAH/ACS include ruptured abdominal aortic aneurysm, bowel obstruction, hemorrhagic pancreatitis, ascites, and intra-abdominal neoplasm. Therapies such as intra-abdominal packing during surgery, pneumatic antishock garments, and gas insufflation of the abdominal cavity during laparoscopic procedures are also associated with ACS. In nonsurgical patients the most common cause of IAH/ACS is bowel edema and distention (Hecker et al., 2016; Kirkpatrick et al., 2013).

Multisystem Effects of Intra-abdominal Hypertension

Multiple organ systems are affected by intra-abdominal hypertension. The GI tract is affected first by rising abdominal pressure, which compromises perfusion to the intestinal mucosa. The intestinal mucosa becomes ischemic, allowing bacteria to translocate into the bloodstream and predisposing the patient to systemic inflammatory response syndrome (SIRS) and sepsis. GI signs and symptoms of abdominal compartment syndrome include increased gastric carbon dioxide level, decreased arterial pH, and elevated serum lactic acid. These abnormalities may indicate intestinal ischemia (Schlichting & Schmidt, 2015). Table 22–10 provides a summary of the effects of IAH/ACS on major body systems.

Measurement of Intra-abdominal Pressure

If the patient develops signs of organ system dysfunction and is at risk for the development of IAH or ACS, it is important to consider ACS as a complication. The sequelae of ACS are often life-threatening, and many clinicians advocate using routine, noninvasive abdominal pressure monitoring for all critically ill patients at risk for developing IAH/ACS. Physical examination and serial measurements of abdominal girth are not sensitive or specific enough to detect IAH.

Abdominal distention does not always equate to IAH, just as the absence of a distended abdomen does not always indicate the absence of IAH (Hecker et al., 2016).

Table 22–10 Effects of Increased Intra-abdominal Pressure/Abdominal Compartment Syndrome on Body Systems

Body System	Effects of Increased Intra-abdominal Pressure	Potential Outcomes
Cardiovascular	Increased thoracic pressure because of increased pressure on diaphragm	Hemodynamic changes Elevated SVR, CVP, and RAP Tachycardia (compensatory) Decreased CO Hypotension (late sign)
Pulmonary	Decreased lung excursion and expansion because of increased diaphragmatic pressure	Decreased lung compliance Hypercapnia Hypoxemia Elevated PIP
Renal	Decreased renal blood flow because of elevated IAP and decreased CO, which decreases GFR and increases renal ischemia	Oliguria Azotemia Prerenal failure
Neurologic	Decreased cerebral perfusion pressure (CPP) because of elevated ICP, which results from decreased venous drainage from the head	Increased ICP Altered level of consciousness
Gastrointestinal	Decreased blood flow to abdominal organs which results in tissue hypoxia, conversion to anaerobic metabolism, and generation of free radicals, and lactic acidosis	Small-bowel ischemia Translocation of bacteria from gut Sepsis Further increase in intra-abdominal pressure Multiple organ dysfunction

SVR = systemic vascular resistance; CVP = central venous pressure; RAP = right atrial pressure; CO = cardiac output; PIP = peak inspiratory pressure; IAP = intra-abdominal pressure; GFR = glomerular filtration rate; ICP = intracranial pressure

Measurement of transurethral bladder pressure is a valid indirect measure of intra-abdominal pressure (Hecker et al, 2016; Katsios et al., 2013). Although the most accurate and direct technique for measuring increased abdominal pressure would be to insert a catheter directly into the peritoneal cavity, this invasive procedure requires tube placement in the abdomen, increasing the risk of bowel injury or peritoneal contamination.

Alterations in intra-abdominal pressure are indirectly reflected by changes in bladder pressure (Hecker et al., 2016). When the bladder is filled with approximately 20 mL to 25 mL of fluid, virtually no pressure is exerted on the bladder wall, enabling it to act as a passive diaphragm capable of transmitting abdominal pressure without imparting additional pressure from its own musculature.

Methods of IAP Measurement   Two methods of measuring intra-abdominal pressure using a urinary bladder catheter are the transducer and fluid manometer methods. It is important to ensure that the urinary catheter is draining freely and the bladder is empty for either method.

Transducer Method.   The transducer method uses a conventional transducer monitoring system, which is connected to the patient's urinary catheter drainage system. With the patient supine and the head of the bed flat, 20 to 25 mL of saline are injected through a catheter port into the bladder over 10 to 15 seconds and allowed to dwell for 30 seconds so that the bladder detrusor (detrusor urinae) muscle can relax and an accurate pressure can be measured. The pressure transducer that is connected to the urinary catheter should be calibrated and maintained at the level of the patient's pubis. The resulting bladder pressure waveform is viewed on a monitor screen (Figure 22–7). The measurement is obtained at end expiration (which corresponds to the trough on the ventilated patient's respiration waveform, and the peak in the nonventilated patient's respiration waveform). Commercial kits are available for the transducer method.

Fluid Manometer Method.   The fluid manometer method or U-tube technique uses the urinary catheter as a manometer and is used primarily for screening. As with the transducer technique, the patient should be positioned supine with the head of the bed flat. In this method, 20 to 25 mL of normal saline are instilled into the urinary catheter's aspiration port and the urinary catheter is raised above the patient, allowing a U-shaped loop to develop. The catheter is held at a 90-degree angle to the patient's pelvis, and the height of the fluid in the tubing above the pelvis is measured to determine the pressure reading (Hecker et al., 2016; Saltzman & Lee, 2016). The advantage of the manometer method is that it can be used to measure intra-abdominal hypertension outside of the ICU; however, this method may be associated with increased risk of infection.

Normal bladder pressure is 0 mmHg. After abdominal surgery, bladder pressures between 0 and 15 mmHg are not uncommon. Higher pressures indicate the onset of intra-abdominal hypertension (the precursor to abdominal compartment syndrome) and may be associated with early organ system pathophysiology (Hecker et al., 2016; Saltzman & Lee, 2016).

Treatment of IAH/ACS

Grading the severity of IAH/ACS may be helpful in determining appropriate management. Some patients tolerate an IAP of 15 mmHg, but in others this degree of elevation may be associated with symptoms of hypoperfusion. Treatment focuses on decompression and preserving cardiopulmonary and renal function. Interventions vary with the severity of the intra-abdominal pressure elevation (Ho & Barie, 2016).

Mild IAH/ACS   For mild intra-abdominal hypertension (IAP of 10–15 mmHg), elevating the head of the bed helps to minimize pressure on the diaphragm, allowing maximum lung expansion. Maintaining a state of normovolemia at this time is a management goal (Ho & Barie, 2016).

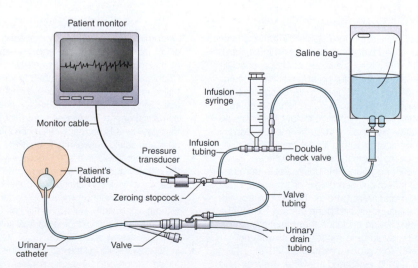

Figure 22–7 Intra-abdominal pressure measurement of bladder pressure using a transducer system; 20–25 mL of saline are infused through the catheter into the bladder. The bladder pressure is displayed as a waveform on a monitor screen.

In addition, assisting the patient to turn, cough, breathe deeply, and use an incentive spirometer will help to improve alveolar ventilation, reduce the risk of atelectasis, and prevent ventilation–perfusion mismatch (shunt) (Ho & Barie, 2016).

Moderate ACS If moderate abdominal compartment syndrome develops (IAP of 16–25 mmHg), the patient should be transferred to an intensive care unit for closer monitoring. Sedation or neuromuscular blockade to chemically paralyze and sedate the patient may be indicated. If the patient is hemodynamically unstable (e.g., demonstrating low cardiac output or hypotension), fluid resuscitation may be indicated (Regli et al., 2015). It is important to ensure that a surgical service is consulted early in the course of treatment in case surgical decompression using a laparotomy procedure is required. It should be noted that there have been no randomized clinical trials to support the use of routine abdominal decompression through midline laparotomy for treatment of abdominal compartment syndrome (Kirkpatrick, 2013).

Severe ACS Severe abdominal compartment syndrome (IAP greater than 25 mmHg) requires urgent surgical decompression of the abdominal cavity and may require reexploration of the abdomen (Hecker et al., 2016; Ho & Barie, 2016). In cases of trauma, the abdomen is sometimes left open after exploratory laparotomy to prevent ACS; however, even with this preventive measure, abdominal pressure may still rise to a dangerous level.

The abdominal perfusion pressure (APP) is a better marker of intra-abdominal organ perfusion than IAP alone. Calculation of APP is similar to that for cerebral perfusion pressure: $MAP - IAP = APP$. The APP should be maintained at greater than 60 mmHg in patients with IAH or ACS. In fact, any patient admitted to a critical care unit or in whom new organ failure develops should be screened for risk factors. One third of patients have IAH at the time of admission into a medical–surgical ICU, and the condition develops in another one third after admission (Ho & Barie, 2016).

Surgical decompression of the abdomen, if necessary for severe ACS, involves a risk for hypotension once the abdomen is opened. This hypotension may be caused by reperfusion, and researchers recommend volume resuscitation with fluids containing mannitol and sodium bicarbonate immediately before and during decompression surgery, which may prevent unstable dysrhythmias (Saltzman & Lee, 2016; Regli et al, 2015).

Complications of ACS

Complications of abdominal compartment syndrome may include reperfusion asystole, which occurs when by-products from ischemic areas circulate to the heart, causing acidosis-related impairments of cardiac electrical activity. Resuscitation equipment and emergency medications should be available in the event asystole occurs. The physician may order an intravenous infusion of sodium bicarbonate and mannitol to prevent this phenomenon.

Pulmonary embolism is a complication associated with reperfusion. The nurse should monitor for signs and symptoms of pulmonary embolism, such as dyspnea, pleuritic chest pain, and signs of shock. Oxygen administration, evaluation for and administration of thrombolytic drugs, and anticoagulants may be required if pulmonary embolism occurs.

Nursing Implications

Unless complications occur, abdominal decompression usually improves the patient's condition. If the ACS treatment is effective, end points of therapy will include decreased ventilation pressures, increased oxygenation,

Emerging Evidence

- In a Cochrane review of transfusion thresholds and other strategies for guiding allogenic red blood cell transfusion in 31 trials, involving 12,587 participants, across a range of clinical specialities (e.g., surgery, critical care), transfusing at a restrictive hemoglobin concentration of between 7 to 8 g/dL decreased the proportion of participants exposed to RBC transfusion by 43% across clinical specialities. In this systematic review, there was no evidence that a restrictive transfusion strategy impacts 30-day mortality or morbidity compared with a liberal transfusion strategy. Data were insufficient to inform the safety of restrictive transfusion policies in clinical subgroups, including acute coronary syndrome, myocardial infarction, neurologic or traumatic brain injury, acute neurologic disorders, stroke, thrombocytopenia, cancer, hematologic malignancies, and bone marrow failure. The findings from this review provide evidence that transfusions with allogeneic RBCs can be avoided in most patients with hemoglobin thresholds above 7 to 8 g/dL (*Carson et al., 2016*).
- Yang and colleagues (2017) evaluated the effectiveness and safety of proton pump inhibitors (PPIs), explored the association between effectiveness and potential influential factors, and investigated the comparative effect of different PPIs in a meta-analysis of randomized controlled trials comparing different classes of PPIs, or comparing PPIs with placebo, H_2 receptor antagonists (H_2RAs) or misoprostol in NSAIDs users. MEDLINE, EMBASE, and the Cochrane Library were searched to identify the randomized controlled trials. Analyses were based on 12,532 participants from 31 trials. PPIs are effective and safe in preventing peptic ulcers and complications in a wide spectrum of patients requiring NSAID therapy. There is no major difference in the comparative effectiveness and safety between different PPIs (*Yang et al., 2017*).
- In a systematic review and meta-analysis of randomized trials of the efficacy and safety of proton pump inhibitors (PPIs) for stress ulcer prophylaxis in critically ill patients, PPIs were superior to H_2RAs in preventing clinically important and overt GI bleeding, without significantly increasing the risk of pneumonia or mortality. Their impact on *Clostridium difficile* infection is yet to be determined (*Alshamsi et al., 2016*).
- In patients requiring long-term low-dose acetylsalicylic acid (ASA) for protection against cardiovascular events, combining the ASA with 20 mg of the proton pump inhibitor esomeprazole significantly reduced the incidence of peptic ulcers (*Lyseng-Williamson, Burness, & Scott, 2012*).

and improved cardiovascular and renal function. After surgery, nursing care consists of maintaining the patient's oxygenation and hemodynamic stability; caring for the abdominal wound; monitoring for infection; and measuring fluid intake and output, including wound drainage, to determine the patient's fluid requirements. The patient may require mechanical ventilation, aggressive volume resuscitation, and vasopressor and inotropic drugs. Management of the patient with ACS is challenging. It is critical for the nurse to recognize the signs of ACS early, so that prompt treatment can be initiated to avoid organ failure and death.

Section Seven Review

1. At which intra-abdominal pressure, if sustained, would a client first be diagnosed as having intra-abdominal hypertension on the IAH/ACS continuum?
   A. 5 mmHg
   B. 10 mmHg
   C. 12 mmHg
   D. 25 mmHg

2. Which client represents the population with the highest risk of developing abdominal compartment syndrome?
   A. Client with chronic obstructive pulmonary disease
   B. Client who is status postmyocardial infarction
   C. Client who is postoperative for repair of a liver laceration
   D. Client who is status post–hip replacement

3. Which statement correctly reflects the effects of abdominal compartment syndrome (ACS) on right arterial pressure and cardiac output?
   A. Right arterial pressure and cardiac output are decreased.
   B. Right arterial pressure and cardiac output are increased.
   C. Right arterial pressure and cardiac output are normal.
   D. Right arterial pressure is increased; cardiac output is decreased.

4. The nurse is preparing to obtain an IAP measurement using the transducer method. In which position should the nurse place the client in preparation for measuring the IAP?
   A. HOB elevated 30 degrees
   B. HOB flat
   C. High Fowler postion
   D. Trendelenburg position

Answers: 1. C, 2. C, 3. D, 4. B

Clinical Reasoning Checkpoint

Kenneth T, a 34-year-old salesman, presents at the emergency department with complaints of upper right abdominal pain and hematemesis. His medical history is negative for coronary heart disease and diabetes. He informs you that he has had several previous episodes of epigastric pain over the past 2 years. While he is talking, he suddenly tells you that he feels as if he is going to vomit. He promptly vomits 300 mL of bright red emesis with clots into a basin. His vital signs suggest that he is experiencing hypovolemia (low BP, tachycardia). He is quickly transferred to the ICU with a preliminary diagnosis of acute GI bleed. Acute GI bleed resuscitation is initiated on admission to the ICU. A gastroenterologist consultation is ordered.

1. Two major goals of resuscitation of acute GI bleeding are maintenance of intravascular volume and maintenance of tissue oxygenation. What interventions are likely to be performed to meet each goal?

2. Kenneth's bleeding persists, and the gastroenterologist decides to perform an endoscopic intervention. On investigation, a bleeding artery is found and sclerotherapy is performed. Kenneth's wife asks you what sclerotherapy is. Explain it to her in simple terms.

3. Once Kenneth has been stabilized, he is tested for *H. pylori* infection and the test comes back positive. He asks you to explain how having an infection is related to having an ulcer. How will you answer him in simple terms?

Chapter 22 Review

1. A client presents to the emergency department with complaints of fatigue. Testing reveals anemia secondary to a gastrointestinal bleed. The client says, "How could that be true? I have never seen blood in my stools." What is the nurse's best response? (Select all that apply.)
   1. "You must just have not noticed it."
   2. "Sometimes the blood is occult, which means you can't see it."
   3. "The blood may have made your stools black, not red."
   4. "The stools have to be tested to determine if blood is present."
   5. "If your stools are dark and sticky, it may be due to the presence of blood."

2. A 45-year-old man is diagnosed with a duodenal ulcer. He asks, "Now that I have an ulcer, what comes next?" What is the nurse's best response?
   1. "Most peptic ulcers heal with medical treatment."
   2. "People who have gastric ulcers have to accept that they will have pain when they eat."
   3. "Early surgery is usually advised, especially for duodenal ulcers."
   4. "If ulcers are untreated, cancer of the stomach will develop."

3. A client has been admitted to the ICU for treatment of trauma to his lower extremities. Which prescription would the nurse anticipate to prevent stress-related mucosal disease (SRMD)? (Select all that apply.)
   1. NSAID (Toradol)
   2. A proton pump inhibitor (Prilosec)
   3. Aluminum carbonate (Gaviscon)
   4. Antispasmodic (Levsin)
   5. H_2 blocker (Cimetidine)

4. The nurse is conducting a physical assessment of a client diagnosed with ulcerative colitis. Which finding would the nurse evaluate as indicating the most serious complication of this disease?
   1. Decreased bowel sounds
   2. Loose, blood-tinged stools
   3. Abdominal distention
   4. Pain on palpation

5. A client who has a history of ulcerative colitis has been hospitalized for repair of a fractured humerus. A combination of which findings would prompt the nurse to collaborate with the healthcare provider regarding a transfer to the ICU? (Select all that apply.)
   1. The client vomits coffee-ground material.
   2. The client's BUN drops.
   3. The client's stool is hemoccult positive.
   4. The client is tachycardic.
   5. The client is hypotensive.

6. A client who has a history of esophageal varices is vomiting blood. Which initial intervention does the nurse anticipate?
   1. Administration of an antiemetic
   2. Endotracheal intubation
   3. Laboratory analysis of the emesis
   4. STAT chest x-ray

7. A client has been diagnosed with a bowel obstruction. Which nursing intervention is indicated?
   1. Rapid initiation of parenteral feeding
   2. STAT soapsuds enema
   3. Insertion of a nasogastric tube
   4. Digital evacuation of stool mass

8. A client with suspected bowel obstruction has had flat and upright x-rays of the abdomen. Which findings would the nurse evaluate as supporting the potential diagnosis? (Select all that apply.)
   1. Distended bowel
   2. Air–fluid levels in the bowel
   3. Inability to visualize the bowel
   4. A ladderlike pattern in bowel loops
   5. Presence of air outside the bowel

9. A client has developed intra-abdominal hypertension (IAH). The nurse monitors for findings associated with which complication?
   1. Bacterial translocation
   2. Increased peristalsis
   3. Increased production of mucus
   4. Decreased production of carbon dioxide

10. A client has been diagnosed with mild intra-abdominal hypertension (IAH). Which intervention is indicated?
    1. Position the client with head flat in bed.
    2. Discourage any activity that will increase pressure, such as coughing or breathing deeply.
    3. Restrict fluids.
    4. Encourage use of incentive spirometry.

Answers to questions found inside your textbook are available on the faculty resources site. Please consult with your instructor.

References

Abougergi, M. S., Travis, A. C., & Saltzman, J. R. (2015). The in-hospital mortality rate for upper GI haemorrhage has decreased over 2 decades in the United States: A nationwide analysis. *Gastrointestinal Endoscopy, 81*(4), 882–888.e1.

Alshamsi, F., Belley-Cote, E., Cook, D., Almenawer, S. A., Alqahtani, A., Perri, D., . . . Alhazzani, W. (2016). Efficacy and safety of proton pump inhibitors for stress ulcer prophylaxis in critically ill patients: A systematic review and meta-analysis of randomized trials. *Critical Care, 20*(1), 120. doi:10.1186/s13054-016-1305-6

Anvari, E., Nantsupawat, N., Gard, R., Raj, R., Nugent, K. (2015). Bladder pressure measurements in patients admitted to a medical intensive care unit. *American Journal of the Medical Sciences, 350*(3): 181–185.

Aoki, T., Nagata, N., Niikura, R., Shimbo, T., Tanaka, S., Sekine, K., . . . Uemura, N. (2015). Recurrence and mortality among patients hospitalized for acute lower gastrointestinal bleeding. *Clinical Gastroenterology and Hepatology, 13*(3), 488–494e1. doi:10.1016/j.cgh.2014.06.023.Epub 2014 Jul3. [PMID:24997327].

Barrett, K. E. (2014). Chapter 6: Intestinal mucosal immunology and ecology. In K. E. Barrett (Ed.), *Gastrointestinal physiology* (2nd ed.). New York, NY: McGraw-Hill. Retrieved April 17, 2017, from http://accessmedicine.mhmedical.com.ezproxy.uky.edu/content.aspx?bookid=691&Sectionid=45431405

Buendgens, L., Koch, A., & Tacke, F. (2016). Prevention of stress-related ulcer bleeding at the intensive care unit: Risks and benefits of stress ulcer prophylaxis. *World Journal of Critical Care Medicine, 5*(1), 57–64. doi:10.5492/wjccm.v5.i1.57.eCollection 2016

Carson, J. L., Stanworth, S. J., Roubinian, N., Fergusson, D. A., Triulzi, D., Doree, C., & Hebert, P. C. (2016). Transfusion thresholds and other strategies for guiding allogeneic red blood cell transfusion. *Cochrane Database of Systematic Reviews, 12*(10), CD002042.

Del Valle, J. D. (2015). Peptic ulcer disease and related disorders. In D. L. Kasper, A. Fauci, S. Hauser, D. Longo, J. Jameson, & J. Loscalzo (Eds.), *Harrison's principles of internal medicine* (19th ed.). New York: McGraw-Hill. Retrieved January 3, 2017, from http://www.accessmedicine.mhmedical.com.ezproxy.uky.edu/content.aspx?bookid=1130&sectioned=79747602

Elie-Turenne, M., Cregar, C., & Brewster, S. (2012). Gastrointestinal bleeding. In D. A. Farcy, A. Flaxman, J. P. Marshall, W. Chiu, & W. C. Chiu (Eds.), *Critical care emergency medicine*. Retrieved January 27, 2016, from http://www.accessemergencymedicine.com/content.aspx?aID=55812126

Hecker, A., Hecker, B., Hecker, M., Riedel, J. G., Weigand, M. A., & Padberg, W. (2016). Acute abdominal compartment syndrome: Current diagnostic and therapeutic options. *Langenbecks Archives of Surgery, 401*(1), 15–24.

Ho, V. P., & Barie, P. S. (2016). Acute abdominal dysfunction. In J. M. Oropello, S. M. Pastores, & V. Kveta (Eds.), *Critical care.* New York, NY: McGraw-Hill. Retrieved January 05, 2017, from http://accessmedicine.mhmedical.com.ezproxy.uky.edu/content.aspx?bookid=1944&Sectionid=143518051

Hreinsson, J. P., Kalaitzakis, E., Gudmundsson, S., & Björnsson, E. S. (2013). Upper gastrointestinal bleeding: Incidence, etiology and outcomes in a population-based setting. *Scandinavian Journal of Gastroenterology, 48*(4), 439–447.

Jacobs, D. O. (2015). Chapter 355: Acute intestinal obstruction. In D. Kasper, A. Fauci, S. Hauser, D. Longo, J. Jameson, J. Loscalzo (Eds.), *Harrison's principles of internal medicine,* (19th ed.) New York, NY: McGraw-Hill. Retrieved May 5, 2017, from http://accessmedicine.mhmedical.com.ezproxy.uky.edu/content.aspx?bookid=1130&sectionid=79748236.

Kanotra, R., Ahmed, M., Patel, N., Thakkar, B., Solanki, S., Tareen, S., . . . Das, A. (2016). Seasonal variations and trends in hospitalizations for peptic ulcer disease in the United States: A 12-year analysis of the nationwide in-patient sample. *Cureus, 8*(10), E854.

Katsios, C., Ye, C., Hoad, N., Piraino, T., Soth, M., & Cook, D. (2013). Intra-abdominal hypertension in the critically ill: Interrater reliability of bladder pressure measurement. *Journal of Critical Care, 28*(5), 886. E1-6.

Kim, J. J., Sheibani, S., Park, S., Buxbaum, J., & Laine, L. (2014). Causes of bleeding and outcomes in patients hospitalized with upper gastrointestinal bleeding. *Journal of Clinical Gastroenterology, 48*(2), 113.

Kirkpatrick, A. W., Roberts, D. J., De Waele, J., Roman, J., Malbrain, M. L. N. G., De Keulenaer, B., . . . The Pediatric Guidelines Sub-Committee for the World Society of the Abdominal Compartment Syndrome. (2013). Intra-abdominal hypertension and the abdominal compartment syndrome: Updated consensus definitions and clinical practice guidelines from the World Society of the Abdominal Compartment Syndrome. *Intensive Care Medicine, 39*(7), 1190–1206.

Laine, L. (2015). Gastrointestinal bleeding. In D. L. Kasper, A. Fauci, S. Hauser, D. Longo, J. Jameson, & J. Loscalzo (Eds.), *Harrison's principles of internal medicine* (19th ed.). New York, NY: McGraw-Hill. Retrieved January 3, 2017, from http://accessmedicine.mhmedical.com.ezproxy.uky.edu/content.aspx?bookid=1130&Sectionid=79726350

Laine, L., Yang, H., Chang, S. C., & Datto, C. (2012). Trends for incidence of hospitalization and death due to GI complications in the United States from 2001 to 2009. *American Journal of Gastroenterology, 107*(8), 1190–1195. doi:10.1038/ajg.2012.168

Lew, E. (2016). Peptic ulcer disease. In N. J. Greenberger, R. S. Blumberg, & R. Burakoff (Eds.), *CURRENT diagnosis & treatment: Gastroenterology, hepatology, & endoscopy (3rd ed.).* New York, NY: McGraw-Hill. Retrieved January 3, 2017, from http://accessmedicine .mhmedical.com.ezproxy.uky.edu/content.aspx?bookid =1621&Sectionid=105183277

Lyseng-Williamson, K. A., Burness, C. B., & Scott, L. J. (2012). Fixed-dose acetylsalicylic acid/esomeprazole: A guide to its use to prevent cardiovascular events and reduce peptic ulcer risk. *Drugs and Therapy Perspectives, 28*(6), 10–14.

Maier, R. V. (2015). Approach to the patient with shock. In D. L. Kasper, A. Fauci, S. Hauser, D. Longo, J. Jameson, & J. Loscalzo (Eds.), *Harrison's principles of internal medicine* (19th ed.). New York, NY: McGraw-Hill. Retrieved January 4, 2017, from http://accessmedicine .mhmedical.com.ezproxy.uky.edu/content.aspx?bookid =1130&Sectionid=79745783

McQuaid, K. R. (2017). Gastrointestinal disorders. In M. A. Papadakis, S. J. McPhee, & M. W. Rabow (Eds.), *Current medical diagnosis & treatment 2017.* New York, NY: McGraw-Hill. Retrieved January 4, 2017, from http:// accessmedicine.mhmedical.com.ezproxy.uky.edu /content.aspx?bookid=1843&Sectionid=135709704

Miftahussurur, M., & Yamaoka, Y. (2015). *Helicobacter pylori* virulence genes and host genetic polymorphisms as risk factors for peptic ulcer disease. *Expert Review of Gastroenterology & Hepatology, 9*(12), 1535–1547. http:// dx.doi.org.ezproxy.uky.edu/10.1586/17474124.2015.10 95089

Mills, J. C., & Stappenbeck, T. S. (2013). Gastrointestinal disease. In G. D. Hammer & S. J. McPhee (Eds.), *Pathophysiology of disease: An introduction to clinical medicine* (7th ed.). New York, NY: McGraw-Hill. Retrieved January 3, 2017, from http://accessmedicine .mhmedical.com.ezproxy.uky.edu/content.aspx?bookid =961&Sectionid=53555694

Price, T. G., & Orthober, R. J. (2016). Bowel obstruction. In J. E. Tintinalli, J. Stapczynski, O. Ma, D. M. Yealy, G. D. Meckler, & D. M. Cline (Eds.), *Tintinalli's emergency medicine: A comprehensive study guide* (8th ed.). New York, NY: McGraw-Hill. Retrieved January 4, 2017, from http://accessmedicine.mhmedical.com .ezproxy.uky.edu/content.aspx?bookid=1658&Sectio nid=109430820

Rajaram, S. S., Desai, N. K., Kalra, A., Gajera, M., Cavanaugh, S. K., Brampton, W., . . . Rowan, K. (2013). Pulmonary artery catheters for adult patients in intensive care. *Cochrane Database of Systematic Reviews,* (2), CD003408. doi:10.1002/14651858.CD003408.pub3

Regli, A., De Keulenaer, B., De Laet, I., Roberts, D., Dabrowski, W., & Malbrain, M. (2015). Fluid therapy and perfusional considerations during resuscitation in critically ill patients with intra-abdominal hypertension. *Anaesthesiology Intensive Therapy, 47*(1), 45–53.

Saltzman, J. R. (2016). Chapter 31: Acute upper gastrointestinal bleeding. In N. J. Greenberger, R. S. Blumberg, & R. Burakoff (Eds.), *CURRENT diagnosis & treatment: Gastroenterology, hepatology, & endoscopy* (3rd ed.). New York, NY: McGraw-Hill. Retrieved January 3, 2017, from http://accessmedicine.mhmedical.com .ezproxy.uky.edu/content.aspx?bookid =1621&Sectionid=105185120

Saltzman, J. R., & Lee, L. S. (2016). Chapter 32: Acute lower gastrointestinal bleeding. In N. J. Greenberger, R. S. Blumberg, & R. Burakoff (Eds.), *CURRENT diagnosis & treatment: Gastroenterology, hepatology, & endoscopy* (3rd ed.). New York, NY: McGraw-Hill. Retrieved January 4, 2017, from http://accessmedicine .mhmedical.com.ezproxy.uky.edu/content.aspx?bookid =1621&Sectionid=105185390

Schlichting, A., & Schmidt, G. A. (2015). Abdominal compartment syndrome. In J. B. Hall, G. A. Schmidt, & J. P. Kress (Eds.), *Principles of critical care* (4th ed.). New York, NY: McGraw-Hill. Retrieved January 5, 2017, from http://accessmedicine.mhmedical.com.ezproxy.uky .edu/content.aspx?bookid=1340&Sectionid=80026616

Shah, P. (2016). Gastrointestinal hemorrhage (upper and lower). In J. M. Oropello, S. M. Pastores, & V. Kvetan (Eds.), *Critical care.* New York, NY: McGraw-Hill. Retrieved January 3, 2017, from http://accessmedicine .mhmedical.com.ezproxy.uky.edu/content.aspx?bookid =1944&Sectionid=143518107

Vincent, J. L., & De Backer, D. (2013). Circulatory shock. *New England Journal of Medicine, 369,* 1726.

Yang, M., He, M., Zhao, M., Zou, B., Liu, J., Luo, L. M., . . . Lei, P. G. (2017). Proton pump inhibitors for preventing non-steroidal anti-inflammatory drug induced gastrointestinal toxicity: A systematic review. *Current Medical Research and Opinion, 25,* 1–8. doi:10.1080/030079 95.2017.1281110

Chapter 23
Alterations in Liver Function

Learning Outcomes

23.1 Explain acute liver failure (ALF), including definitions, and identify common causes of ALF.

23.2 Discuss acute liver failure in terms of diagnostic approach and specific treatment strategies.

23.3 Identify the complications of acute liver failure and their treatment.

23.4 Discuss the acute complications of chronic liver disease.

23.5 Describe the nursing considerations for the high-acuity patient with liver failure.

ultiple factors can result in acute failure of liver function, a life-threatening complication of liver injury. The primary focus of this chapter is acute liver failure (ALF): its etiology, pathophysiologic processes, diagnosis, clinical presentation, and collaborative management. The chapter also presents a discussion of acute complications of chronic liver failure, using a systematic approach that concludes with nursing considerations for this patient population.

Section One: Introduction to Acute Liver Failure

Acute liver failure (ALF), previously called fulminant liver failure, is a life-threatening condition that occurs when there is catastrophic damage to a previously normal liver. Although these terms are still used interchangeably, the acronym ALF is used throughout this chapter.

Defining Acute Liver Failure

Acute liver failure is clinically defined by coagulation abnormalities, with an international normalized ratio (INR) greater than 1.5; the onset of encephalopathy in someone who has no previously known hepatic cirrhosis; and a duration of less than 26 weeks (Kumar & Qamar, 2015). ALF can be further categorized based on the amount of time between the development of jaundice and the development of hepatic encephalopathy as hyperacute

(less than 7 days), acute (7–21 days), or subacute (more than 21 days) (Sargent, 2010).

It is estimated that there are up to 2,800 cases of ALF reported each year in the United States. Mortality rates were previously as high as 85%, depending on the cause, but now, with the availability of liver transplantation and improved medical management, up to 80% of patients may survive (Foston & Carpentar, 2010; Larson, 2010).

Causes of Acute Liver Failure

The underlying cause of ALF can be identified in only 60% to 80% of cases (Larson, 2010). Causes are categorized as drug induced, infectious, vascular, metabolic, and miscellaneous.

Drug Induced Drug-induced ALF is either a dose-dependent or an idiosyncratic reaction to a medication. Table 23–1 lists common drug causes of ALF.

Acetaminophen toxicity is the leading cause of ALF in the United States; up to 49% of ALF cases are attributed to acetaminophen overdose (Hung & Nelson, 2016). Large-volume acetaminophen consumption, typically greater than 10 grams per day, can be intentional or unintentional, especially when people are taking two or more drugs that contain acetaminophen. The metabolism of acetaminophen is a multistep process that includes a toxic metabolite (N-acetyl-p-benzoquinone imine [NAPQI]) that is further broken down by glutathione in the liver. When large amounts of acetaminophen are ingested, glutathione stores in the liver can be depleted, allowing the accumulation of this toxic metabolite that causes damage to the hepatocytes.

Table 23–1 Drugs That Can Lead to the Development of ALF

Dose dependent	Idiosyncratic	Herbal
Acetaminophen	Halothane	Kava kava
Carbon tetrachloride	INH	Germander
Amanita phalloides (death cap mushroom)	Rifampin	Gum thistle
	Valproic acid	Ma huang
Tetracycline	NSAIDs	Skullcap
Ecstasy	Amiodarone	Comfrey
	Phenytoin	
	Sulfonamides	
	Statins	

Acetaminophen toxicity is characterized by extremely high liver enzymes and should be suspected when a patient presents with an alanine aminotransferase (ALT) level of greater than 1,000 units/mL (Kumar & Qamar, 2015). The risk of acetaminophen toxicity is increased in people who abuse alcohol, are taking drugs that induce the cytochrome P450 system, or are anorexic.

The clinical findings of acetaminophen toxicity change over time. Early symptoms include nausea and vomiting, which may appear to improve at 48 hours. Within 3 to 4 days after ingestion, jaundice and elevated ALT and AST enzyme levels are seen. With early identification and treatment, ALF caused by acetaminophen toxicity can be treated and reversed; however, with a delay in treatment, permanent liver damage occurs, and survival without a liver transplant is unlikely.

Viral Infections   Viral infections are the leading cause of ALF in the developing world. Five common viruses target the liver: hepatitis A (HAV), hepatitis B (HBV), hepatitis C (HCV), hepatitis D (HDV), and hepatitis E (HEV). However, only some of these viruses significantly increase the risk of developing ALF. Other viral infections that can lead to ALF include cytomegalovirus (CMV), Epstein–Barr virus (EBV), and herpes simplex virus (HSV), as well as parvovirus B19 and yellow-fever viruses; however, development of ALF from these viruses is rare.

Hepatitis A Virus.   While ALF from HAV is rare in the general population, certain populations are at higher risk (e.g., older adults, women, persons with preexisting liver disease) (Kumar & Qamar, 2015). HAV is primarily transmitted through the fecal–oral route. It is frequently associated with epidemics and is spread mainly through contaminated water or food, such as raw or partially cooked shellfish. HAV is usually a mild, fairly benign, and self-limiting infection that results in immunity following acute illness and rarely leads to ALF. However, in adults and particularly older adults or those with underlying chronic liver disease, HAV can be more severe, with a higher mortality rate (Bernal et al., 2010). It is not associated with development of chronic hepatitis. Two vaccines against HAV have been approved in the United States. Vaccination is recommended for high-risk populations (e.g., healthcare and childcare workers, travelers to areas of the world where HAV is endemic, and persons who are immunosuppressed).

Hepatitis B Virus.   HBV is the cause of the majority of ALF associated with viral infection, particularly when there is an associated superinfection with HDV (Kumar & Qamar, 2015). HBV is transmitted through contaminated blood serum or body fluids. The at-risk population for HBV is similar to the HIV at-risk group, and it is considered a significant sexually transmitted disease (STD). HBV is a major cause of acute and chronic hepatitis and cirrhosis, as well as a precursor to hepatocellular carcinoma. The prevalence of HBV has decreased over the past 15 to 20 years because of the rise in safe sexual practices in response to the HIV epidemic, as well as the development and wide distribution of HBV vaccine. Hepatitis B is seen in all age groups. It occurs throughout the world and is endemic in many parts of the world; however, it is less prevalent in the United States.

Hepatitis C Virus.   Hepatitis C rarely leads to the development of ALF; however, it is a major cause of chronic hepatitis, cirrhosis, and hepatocellular carcinoma. It is transmitted primarily through blood and blood products.

Hepatitis D Virus.   The Delta hepatitis virus, or HDV, like HBV is a bloodborne virus transmitted through direct contact with blood from an infected person. HDV co-infects with and requires the helper function of HBV for its replication and ability to cause pathology. HDV can infect a person simultaneously with HBV (co-infection) or superinfect a person already infected with HBV (superinfection). Because HDV relies on HBV, the duration of HDV infection is determined by the duration of (and cannot outlast) HBV infection. HDV is cleared if HBV is cleared (Dienstag, 2015).

Hepatitis E Virus.   HEV is the most common cause of ALF in India, China, and Southeast Asia and should be considered in patients who have recently traveled to these areas (Bernal, Auzinger, Dhawan, & Wendon, 2010). HEV is transmitted by contaminated water and oral–fecal routes. In the United States, HEV rarely leads to the development of ALF.

Vascular   Vascular causes of ALF are those that interfere with the liver's blood supply. There are several ways in which blood supply can be altered, as follows:

- **Shock liver**—This condition develops when a patient has been hypotensive and there is reduced blood flow to the liver.
- **Heart failure**—An alteration in blood flow to the liver can lead to a backflow of blood or fluid, resulting in liver engorgement. This can occur in acute right-sided heart failure, when blood and fluid back up into the systemic circulation, thereby engorging the liver.
- **Vascular obstruction**—Acute liver failure can result from acute cases of Budd-Chiari syndrome, which is characterized by blood flow obstruction to the hepatic veins due to blood clots and which prevents the normal outflow of blood from the liver.

Metabolic   Three main metabolic causes of ALF have been recognized: HELLP syndrome in pregnancy, Reye syndrome, and Wilson disease.

- **HELLP**—HELLP syndrome is a complication of pregnancy that is identified by Hemolysis, Elevated Liver enzymes, and a Low Platelet count. The cause of HELLP syndrome is not known but may be related to preeclampsia.

- **Reye syndrome**—Reye syndrome is a severe, often fatal disease that can cause encephalopathy and liver injury or failure (Grosser & Smyth, 2011). Although it can occur in any age group, it occurs most commonly in children. There is no known cause for Reye syndrome, but it is associated with the use of aspirin and other salicylate-containing products. Although all organs are affected, the liver and the brain suffer the most damage.

- **Wilson disease**—Wilson disease is a genetic, inherited disorder that leads to an accumulation of copper in the body's tissues, particularly the liver and the nervous system. The buildup of copper in the liver can be slow and progressive, leading to cirrhosis; however, in a small number of patients, ALF is the initial presentation of Wilson disease.

Miscellaneous   Miscellaneous causes of ALF include autoimmune hepatitis and malignancy, as well as idiosyncratic complications of other conditions. Mushroom poisoning, most often seen with *Amanita phalloides*, which is typically found in the Pacific Northwest and the Appalachian Mountains, also falls into this category.

Pathophysiologic Basis of Acute Liver Failure

Regardless of the underlying cause, ALF occurs when a large number of hepatocytes have been damaged and destroyed. This destruction of hepatocytes prevents the liver from performing the many functions necessary to keep the body in homeostasis. Recall that the liver synthesizes important proteins (e.g., albumin) and coagulation factors. With the development of ALF, liver synthesis of protein is quickly disrupted, and the liver is unable to produce the clotting factors necessary for coagulation. This is manifested by a prolongation of the prothrombin time (PT) by 4 seconds or more, with an INR of 1.5 or higher (Foston & Carpentar, 2010).

The liver is also unable to clear the toxins from the blood, as it does when functioning normally. Although the exact cause remains unknown, a buildup of toxins is one theory behind the development of hepatic encephalopathy. The increased INR and the development of encephalopathy are the hallmark signs of ALF.

Section One Review

1. Acute liver failure is defined as the presence of encephalopathy and which lab abnormality?
   A. Total bilirubin greater than 5.0 mg/dL
   B. International normalized ratio greater than 1.5
   C. Platelet count less than 50,000/mm³
   D. Sodium level less than 130 mEq/L

2. Which drug is the major cause of ALF in the United States?
   A. Acetaminophen
   B. Halothane
   C. Isoniazid
   D. Carbon tetrachloride

3. In clients with subacute ALF, what is the timeframe of development of jaundice to development of encephalopathy?
   A. Less than 7 days
   B. 1–2 weeks
   C. Longer than 21 days
   D. Longer than 30 days

4. Which hepatitis virus infection most commonly leads to the development of ALF?
   A. Hepatitis A virus
   B. Hepatitis B virus
   C. Hepatitis C virus
   D. Hepatitis D virus

Answers: 1. B, 2. A, 3. C, 4. B

Section Two: Diagnosis and Treatment Strategies

When a patient presents with clinical findings suggesting acute liver failure, it is essential that the diagnosis be rapidly confirmed and aggressive therapy initiated. This is particularly important with drug-induced ALF, as time from ingestion is a critical factor.

Diagnosis of Acute Liver Failure

Whenever a patient is admitted to the hospital with ALF, an extensive workup needs to be done to determine the underlying cause and severity of the disease. Determining the cause is extremely important because for some causes of ALF specific treatments can reverse the process. Identifying the severity of the disease process and extent of damage to the liver helps to determine the need for, and timing

Table 23–2 Laboratory Evaluation of Hepatic Function and Abnormal Trends

Test	Normal Range	Comments
Transaminase levels		
Alanine aminotransferase (ALT)	10–35 units/mL	Elevation of transaminase levels indicates injury to hepatocytes. ALT is a more specific indicator
Aspartate aminotransferase (AST)	0–35 units/L	of liver damage as AST levels can increase with damage to cardiac or muscle cells.
Canalicular enzymes		
Alkaline phosphatase (ALP)	20–130 units/L	Elevation of canalicular enzymes is an indication of injury or damage to the bile ducts.
Γ-glutamyltranspeptidase (GGT)	0–45 units/L	ALP levels can increase with injury to the bone or intestine. GGT can aid in determining elevation in ALP related to liver injury.
Bilirubin		
Total	0.1–1.2 mg/dL	End-product of hemoglobin degradation; increased total bilirubin with decreased direct
Indirect (unconjugated)	0.1–1 mg/dL	bilirubin levels suggests hepatic dysfunction. Elevations in direct bilirubin usually
Direct (conjugated)	0.1–0.3 mg/dL	indicate a posthepatic biliary problem.
Synthetic function		
Albumin	3.5–5 g/dL	Hypoalbuminemia is seen more commonly in chronic liver disorders such as cirrhosis; other conditions causing decreases include malnutrition, nephrotic syndrome, and other disorders.
Prothrombin time (PT)	10–13 seconds	Elevated PT/INR is the abnormal trend seen in liver dysfunction or acute liver failure.
International normalized ratio (INR)	2–3	Five times normal is refractory to vitamin K is poor prognostic sign.
Other		
Ammonia	15–45 mcg/dL	Produced by protein metabolism by intestinal bacteria, it is detoxified in liver; elevations develop with liver dysfunction; high levels contribute to mental status changes (e.g., hepatic encephalopathy).

SOURCE: Data from Kee (2013).

of, liver transplantation. Blood work includes routine chemistry values, as well as liver function tests (LFTs), serum amylase and lipase, complete blood count (CBC), PT/INR, hepatitis serologies, and autoimmune markers. Table 23–2 lists liver function lab tests and the abnormal trends associated with ALF.

The patient should also have a type and screen; a toxicology screen, including acetaminophen level; arterial blood gas; and lactate level. Women of childbearing age should have a pregnancy test. An ammonia level should also be drawn, preferably from an arterial blood sample, if access is available. Patients who might be referred for transplantation should also have their HIV status determined. The nurse may also be asked to send blood, urine, and sputum cultures because patients with ALF do not always exhibit classic signs and symptoms of infection.

Diagnostic testing may include a computed tomography (CT) scan or ultrasound, which can identify any abnormalities of the abdomen or liver and blood flow. This will also allow for estimation of liver size, which can be helpful for the patient who might ultimately be referred for liver transplantation. Because there is a high risk of cerebral edema in patients with ALF, a CT scan of the head may also be done.

Specific Treatment Strategies Based on Diagnosis

For some of the causes of ALF, there are specific treatment options available.

Acetaminophen Toxicity　Initially, decontamination of the GI system is necessary. Activated charcoal and placement of a nasogastric (NG) tube (Hung & Nelson, 2016) are used. In acetaminophen toxicity, N-acetylcysteine (NAC) has been the mainstay of therapy. For the best chance of reversing the effects of acetaminophen toxicity, NAC must be administered as soon as possible after drug ingestion. It can be administered orally or through a nasogastric tube as a 140 mg/kg loading dose followed by 70 mg/kg every 4 hours, for a total of 17 doses (Hung & Nelson, 2016). It is extremely important that each dose be given on time to optimize the antidote effect.

Because patients cannot always tolerate the oral dose due to its taste and odor of rotten eggs, NAC is frequently given as a continuous IV infusion. The IV dose is 150 mg/kg over 15 minutes as a loading dose, followed by 6 mg/kg/hour (Lee, Larson, & Stravitz, 2011). There is controversy over how long the infusion of NAC should continue, and some providers continue the infusion until there is improvement of liver function, the patient undergoes a transplant, or the patient dies. NAC is frequently started on any patient presenting with ALF, regardless of the underlying cause.

***Amanita phalloides* Mushroom Toxicity**　Patients who are thought to have ingested *Amanita phalloides* are treated with penicillin G in the United States. Intravenous doses range from 300,000 to 1 million units/kg/day. Silibinin, an active component of milk thistle (*Silybum marianum*), 30 to 40 mg/kg/day either PO or IV, is also administered; however, silibinin is not an approved drug in the United States and must be obtained from Europe through an emergency application (Lee et al., 2011). Silymarin is an antioxidant that may block toxins from binding to the cell membrane receptors of hepatocytes, providing a protective function (Abenavoli, Capasso, Milic, & Capasso, 2010).

Herpes Simplex Virus　Although rare, patients suspected of having ALF secondary to herpes simplex virus should be treated with acyclovir 5 to 10 mg/kg IV every 8 hours for a minimum of 1 week. Pregnant women with ALF related to HELLP syndrome are treated with delivery of the fetus, usually by Cesarean section. Patients with Budd-Chiari syndrome may be treated by placement of either a transjugular intrahepatic portosystemic shunt (TIPS) or surgical shunt (Canbay et al., 2011).

Section Two Review

1. Which statements are TRUE concerning the diagnosis of ALF? (Select all that apply.)
   A. Blood work includes chemistry and hematology values.
   B. CT scan of the head may be ordered.
   C. An arterial ammonia level is preferred.
   D. A liver biopsy is done to confirm the diagnosis.
   E. Urine pregnancy tests will be inaccurate.

2. Which medication can reverse the effects of acetaminophen toxicity?
   A. Acyclovir
   B. N-acetylcysteine
   C. Penicillin G
   D. Rifaximin

3. Which drug, although not approved for use in the United States, can be obtained for emergency use to treat poisoning by *Amanita phalloides*?
   A. Rifaximin
   B. Protamine sulfate
   C. Acyclovir
   D. Silibinin

4. What is the definitive treatment for women with ALF related to HELLP syndrome?
   A. N-acetylcysteine therapy
   B. Delivery of the fetus
   C. Charcoal decontamination of the gastrointestinal track
   D. Acyclovir treatment

Answers: 1. (A, B, C), 2. B, 3. D, 4. B

Section Three: Complications and Treatment Strategies

A number of life-threatening complications can occur with ALF, including hepatic encephalopathy, cerebral edema, coagulopathy, hypoglycemia and electrolyte abnormalities, infection, cardiopulmonary abnormalities, and acute kidney injury.

Hepatic Encephalopathy

Hepatic encephalopathy (HE) is one of the defining characteristics of ALF. While the exact cause of HE is unknown, it is understood that the more severe the HE in patients with ALF is, the worse the outcomes (Lee et al., 2011).

Levels of Severity   There are four levels of HE, which reflect increasing severity: grades I through IV. The grade of HE is determined by clinical evaluation.

Grade I.   In grade I encephalopathy, patients exhibit mild personality changes that are frequently recognized as abnormal by family and close friends. A reduced attention span and lack of coordination are typical. There can also be a disruption of sleep/wake patterns.

These patients, while they may be managed on a hospital ward, need close monitoring for any deterioration in their mental status. Frequent neurologic evaluations should include the patient's ability to perform simple calculations, such as serially subtracting 7 starting at 100, as well as orientation to person, place, and time.

Grade II.   Patients with grade II HE become disoriented and may be incontinent of urine and stool. They may be

more lethargic but do arouse spontaneously. Their speech may be slurred and confused. These patients also exhibit asterixis, a bilateral flapping tremor most often seen in the wrist with dorsiflexion (Figure 23–1). A patient who exhibits a unilateral tremor should be evaluated for a brain lesion unless there is an underlying neuromuscular disorder. These patients can experience a rapid deterioration in mental function and should be transferred to an intensive care unit (ICU) where they can be more closely monitored.

Grade III.   Patients who have grade III or IV HE should be in an ICU and frequently must be intubated and mechanically ventilated for airway protection and support of ventilatory function. In grade III HE, patients are stuporous but can still be aroused with noxious stimulation. Prior to intubation, their speech is incoherent, and they show marked confusion. These patients may also exhibit noticeable and nearly continuous asterixis.

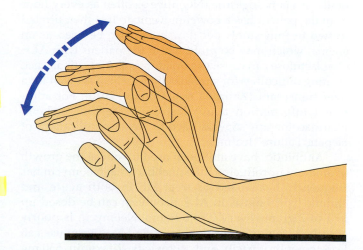

Figure 23–1 Asterixis.

Table 23–3 Summary of Hepatic Encephalopathy

Grade	Clinical Manifestations
I	Mild personality changes, decreased attention span
II	Asterixis with dorsiflexion, disorientation, lethargy, impaired ability to do simple computations
III	Stuporous but arousable with noxious stimulation, incoherent speech, noticeable asterixis, marked confusion
IV	Comatose, unresponsive to stimulation

SOURCE: Data from Hassanein et al. (2017).

Grade IV. With a decline to grade IV HE, patients become comatose. It may or may not be possible to elicit asterixis with dorsiflexion of the wrist. Grade IV HE can be further classified as IVa, in which patients still respond to noxious stimuli and may exhibit decerebrate posturing, and IVb, in which patients no longer respond to noxious stimuli and are flaccid (Larson, 2010).

Table 23–3 provides a summary of the clinical manifestations of hepatic encephalopathy.

Ammonia Although there is no lab test that evaluates HE and its severity, ammonia levels may be used as a surrogate marker. Ammonia, a by-product of protein metabolism, is normally converted to urea by the liver (Kee, 2013). When liver failure occurs, serum ammonia accumulates and may contribute to hepatic encephalopathy because of neurotoxic properties. Specific ammonia levels are not associated with a particular grade of HE; however, an arterial ammonia level of greater than 200 mcg/dL has been associated with brain herniation. It is important to reduce the ammonia level and closely monitor for any neurological changes (Lee et al., 2011).

Treatment Lactulose is a mainstay of treatment for HE. Lactulose helps to acidify the colon, which reduces absorption of ammonia by favoring the formation of the nonabsorbable NH_4^+ from NH_3, trapping NH_3 in the colon and effectively reducing plasma NH_3 concentrations. Lactulose also has a cathartic effect that helps to eliminate ammonia from the body. In ALF, 45 mL of lactulose can be given orally or via nasogastric (NG) tube as often as every hour until the patient has a bowel movement. It is then titrated to two to four stools per day. It can also be used as an enema, which may be preferred in the patient with ALF. Oral lactulose can cause gas buildup in the intestinal tract, creating difficulties for surgeons if the patient is taken for a liver transplant (Zafirova & O'Connor, 2010). For additional information about lactulose, see the "Related Pharmacotherapy: Agents Used to Treat Complications of Hepatic Failure" feature.

Antibiotics have also been used to reduce the growth of ammonia-producing intestinal bacteria. Neomycin has frequently been used to treat HE in both acute and chronic liver failure. In ALF, neomycin can be dosed up to 1 to 2 grams every 4 to 6 hours. Neomycin is poorly absorbed from the intestinal tract, and long-term use can lead to nephrotoxicity and ototoxicity. Rifaximin, 550 mg two times per day, is now being used more often for the treatment of HE. It is nonabsorbable and has fewer side effects than neomycin. Metronidazole, 250 mg every 12 hours, while not approved for the treatment of HE, may also be given to decrease intestinal bacterial growth (Zafirova & O'Connor, 2010). See the "Related Pharmacotherapy: Agents Used to Treat Complications of Hepatic Failure" feature for additional information on neomycin, rifaximin, and metronidazole.

Because electrolyte imbalances, acid–base disturbances, hypoxia, and hypovolemia can precipitate and contribute to the severity of HE, it is important to monitor and correct any abnormalities. Nutrition is also important in patients with ALF. Although an increase in dietary protein can contribute to HE, restricting protein intake has not been shown to decrease either the incidence or severity of HE. Patients should have full enteral nutritional support as tolerated (Zafirova & O'Connor, 2010).

Cerebral Edema

Cerebral edema is a potentially life-threatening complication of ALF, and the severity correlates to the severity of HE. The exact mechanism for the development of cerebral edema is not understood, but as HE worsens, the risk of cerebral edema increases, up to 35% in grade III HE and as high as 80% in grade IV HE (Larson, 2010). The greatest concern is the development of increased ICP and ultimately brain herniation.

Clinical Findings Monitoring for cerebral edema can be difficult in patients with ALF. The classic presentation of increased ICP is a pattern of progressive deterioration of brain function, characterized by increasing alterations in level of consciousness, pupils, oculomotor and motor responses, and breathing. Late signs of severe increased ICP, called Cushing's triad (systolic hypertension, bradycardia, and irregular respirations), are not always seen in this patient population. Changes in the size of the pupils and their reaction to light typically occur very late and can indicate the onset of brain herniation. If herniation occurs, the pupils become dilated and fixed.

Treatment Intracranial pressure monitoring may be employed to directly measure the cerebral pressure. If an ICP monitor is used, the cerebral perfusion pressure (CPP) should be monitored and maintained at greater than 50 to 60 mmHg while keeping the ICP less than 20 mmHg (Lee et al., 2011). The head of the bed should be elevated to 30 degrees, and stimulation of the patient should be limited. Mannitol, an osmotic diuretic, may be used, but its effect is limited, especially in patients who also have abnormal kidney function.

Adequate sedation is also important, and propofol is frequently used. It is short acting, which allows for neurologic evaluations soon after it is stopped; however, it can also cause hypotension, which will decrease CPP.

Hypothermia may also be used to decrease ICP, although it is still experimental in patients with ALF. Keeping the patient's temperature between 33°C (91.4°F) and 34°C (93.2°F) can be done to bridge a patient to liver transplantation. Hypothermia can increase the risk of infection and compound problems with coagulopathy and must be

Related Pharmacotherapy
Agents Used to Treat Complications of Hepatic Failure

Ammonia-Reducing Agents

Neomycin (Mycifradin)
Metronidazole (Flagyl)
Rifaximin (Xifaxan)

Action and Uses

Neomycin is an aminoglycoside-type antibiotic that interferes with bacterial protein synthesis; metronidazole is an amebicide that inhibits DNA synthesis in susceptible organisms. These agents suppress ammonia-producing intestinal bacteria to reduce hepatic encephalopathy. Neomycin is not typically used in the presence of hepatic failure but may be used for long-term treatment of encephalopathy.

Dosages (Adult) (specific to hepatic encephalopathy)

Neomycin: 4–12 g/day (PO) in four divided doses for 5 to 6 days
Metronidazole: 250 mg (PO) every 12 hours (off-label use)
Rifaximin: 550 mg (PO) 2 times/day

Major Adverse Effects

Nausea, vomiting, diarrhea
Stomatitis
Abdominal cramping
Neomycin specific: nephrotoxicity and ototoxicity
May cause falsely decreased AST/ALT
Other: flattening of T wave on ECG, impaired coordination

Nursing Implications

Administered orally
Monitor renal function (neomycin): report signs and symptoms of renal dysfunction.
Monitor for overgrowth of *Candida*.

Ammonia Detoxicant

Lactulose (Cephulac)

Action and Uses

Lactulose is a hyperosmotic laxative that causes an acidic pH when degraded, promoting NH_3 to NH_4. For treatment of hepatic encephalopathy, it prevents absorption of ammonia from the bowel and moves stool more rapidly, decreasing the amount of ammonia formed.

Dosages (specific to hepatic encephalopathy)

30–45 mL (PO) t.i.d. or q.i.d adjusted to produce two to four soft stools/day

Major Adverse Effects

Abdominal cramps
Flatulence, diarrhea

Nursing Implications

May be administered orally or rectally; drug must be in colon for laxative action to take place
Monitor intake and output balance.

Prevention of Hypoglycemia

Dextrose IV

Actions and Uses

Dextrose IV is used to maintain consistent glucose levels because liver failure interferes with gluconeogenesis.

Major Adverse Effects

Redness, swelling, burning at injection site
Hyperglycemia

Nursing Implications

Administered as continuous IV infusion
Can be given as $D_{10}W$ or $D_{50}W$
If administered too quickly can cause nausea

Prevention of Gastrointestinal Hemorrhage

Phytonadione (vitamin K, AquaMEPHYTON, Mephyton)

Actions and Uses

Vitamin K is useful in correcting abnormal clotting factors. Hepatic patients often have elevated International Normalized Ratio (INR) levels, which increases the risk for abnormal bleeding. Vitamin K promotes liver synthesis of clotting factors and therefore controls the coagulopathy of liver failure.

Dosages (specific to prothrombin deficiencies)

5–10 mg (PO or IV) to correct INR

Major Adverse Effects

Anaphylaxis
Cyanosis
Dyspnea
Hypersensitivity reaction

Nursing Implications

Administer intravenously, subcutaneously, or orally.
Dose depends on INR level.
Continue to monitor INR and PT level.

SOURCE: Data from Lee et al. (2011); Wilson et al. (2017); Zafirova & O'Connor (2010).

---

very closely monitored (Lee et al., 2011). Chapter 19: Traumatic Brain Injury provides an in-depth discussion of the management of increased ICP.

Coagulopathy

By definition, patients with ALF have an INR greater than 1.5 due to the liver's inability to produce clotting factors.

However, these patients do not experience the severity of bleeding abnormalities associated with chronic liver failure and cirrhosis.

Vitamin K can be given, 5 to 10 mg by mouth or IV, to try to correct the INR. Vitamin K should not be given intramuscularly because of the risk of bleeding into the muscle. Unless the patient is actually bleeding, or is to undergo an invasive procedure, there is no evidence to support transfusion of fresh frozen plasma (Lee et al., 2011). See the "Related Pharmacotherapy: Agents Used to Treat Complications of Hepatic Failure" feature for additional information on vitamin K.

Thrombocytopenia may also be seen in patients with ALF. If patients are not bleeding, it is not recommended to infuse platelets unless the count is lower than 10,000/mm^3. For invasive procedures, platelets are transfused to raise the platelet count over 50,000/mm^3 (Lee et al., 2011)

Hypoglycemia and Electrolyte Abnormalities

Hypoglycemia is common in ALF because the liver is unable to clear insulin from the blood or make glucose by gluconeogenesis. It is important to closely monitor glucose levels and treat hypoglycemia because low levels can adversely affect cerebral edema (Sargent, 2010). Patients should have a continuous IV infusion of 10% dextrose and may require 50% dextrose if glucose levels are extremely low. Electrolyte levels need to be closely monitored. It is common to see low phosphate, potassium, and magnesium levels in patients with ALF, and these electrolytes should be replaced as needed.

Infection

Patients with ALF are at increased risk for developing both bacterial and fungal infections. As mentioned earlier, these patients do not always exhibit typical symptoms of infection, such as temperature or white blood cell count elevation. It

may be necessary to intermittently send cultures of blood, urine, and sputum to monitor for any new infection.

The nurse needs to closely monitor the patient for any change in urine or sputum and for drainage from catheter sites. This requires that additional cultures be collected. Any infection could prevent a patient from receiving a liver transplant or could complicate the recovery if a transplant is performed, so the threshold is typically low for providers to begin antimicrobial therapy.

Cardiopulmonary Abnormalities

In ALF, hypotension is common, and patients frequently have a high cardiac output (CO) with a low systemic vascular resistance (SVR). A combination of intravascular volume replacement and vasopressor and inotropic support may be needed to maintain an adequate mean arterial pressure (MAP) of greater than 60 mmHg. If an ICP monitor is in place, the MAP should be kept high enough to maintain a CPP greater than 50 to 60 mmHg.

Patients who have progressed to grade III or IV HE should be intubated and mechanically ventilated. This is done to protect the airway, prevent aspiration, and support ventilation.

Acute Kidney Injury

Up to 50% of patients with ALF develop acute kidney injury (AKI) (Sargent, 2010). This risk is higher in patients with acetaminophen toxicity. Moreover, patients with ALF who develop AKI have worse outcomes. The cause of AKI is

Table 23–4 Complications and Management of Acute Liver Failure

Complication	Management
Hepatic encephalopathy	Enema for constipation Lactulose (PO, NG, rectal), 15–45 mL administered every 2 hours until stool output, and then as necessary to attain two to four soft stools per 24 hours Rifaximin, 550 mg (PO, NG) 2 times per day Neomycin, 1–2 g (PO, NG) every 4–6 hours Metronidazole 250 mg (PO every 12 hours) Intubation and mechanical ventilation
Cerebral edema	IV mannitol Elevate head of bed 20 to 30 degrees, decrease stimulation Intracranial pressure monitoring (ICP catheters may be placed in patients with grade III or IV.) Barbiturate-induced coma may be indicated if first-line interventions are inadequate.*
Coagulation abnormalities	Vitamin K, 5–10 mg (PO, NG, IV) Fresh frozen plasma, platelets as needed
Hypoglycemia	10% dextrose continuous IV infusion 50% dextrose IV, as required Monitor for low serum glucose and clinical manifestations of hypoglycemia.
Metabolic abnormalities	Monitor serum electrolytes and pH frequently. Correct electrolyte abnormalities. Administer bicarbonate, as necessary.
Infection	Surveillance cultures, blood, urine, and sputum Antibiotic therapy
Cardiopulmonary abnormalities	Volume replacement Vasopressor and/or inotropic infusion
Acute kidney injury	Fluid resuscitation if prerenal injury Renal replacement therapy if indicated

*Treatment for increased ICP and cerebral edema is presented in Chapter 19: Traumatic Brain Injury.

multifactorial and includes decreased perfusion of the kidneys related to low SVR and hypovolemia. It is important to closely monitor kidney function and avoid nephrotoxic agents such as aminoglycoside antimicrobials and intravenous contrast agents. If patients require support of renal function, continuous renal replacement therapy (CRRT) is preferred over intermittent hemodialysis because it has fewer cardiovascular and cerebral effects (Sargent, 2010).

Table 23–4 provides a summary of complications of acute liver failure and their management.

Emerging Evidence

- The effect of extracorporeal liver support using molecular adsorbent recirculating system (MARS) as a detoxifying therapy was evaluated on 64 patients with life-threatening acute liver failure. The MARS treatments were done as a bridge for liver transplantation or for liver function recovery. The investigators concluded that patients' clinical characteristics on starting MARS therapy were the main factors predicting survival, the MARS therapy was well tolerated by all patients, and it reduced hepatic toxins although the patients who received liver transplantation had improved 1-year survival (*Donati et al., 2014*).
- A retrospective review of data was performed on 1604 patients in the acute liver failure study group with regard to acute kidney injury. Review of the data revealed 70% of the patients with acute liver failure developed acute kidney injury. Renal replacement therapy was initiated on 30% of the acute kidney injury group. Only 4% of the renal replacement therapy group became dependent on dialysis. The data revealed acute kidney injury was a common occurrence in patients with acute liver failure but had a low incidence of chronic kidney disease (*Tujios et al., 2015*).
- A study of 102 liver failure patients who were removed from the transplant list or denied transplantation was evaluated for patient access to palliative care. Palliative care referral occurred for 11% of the patients. Patients who had been removed from the transplant list were infrequently referred for palliative care, although a high percentage had pain or nausea. Along with do not resuscitate, goals of care were rarely discussed (*Poonja et al., 2014*).

Section Three Review

1. Which grade of hepatic encephalopathy is associated with disorientation, slurred speech, and asterixis?
   A. Grade I
   B. Grade II
   C. Grade III
   D. Grade IV

2. Herniation of the brain occurs more frequently when arterial ammonia levels are:
   A. Less than 50 mcg/dL
   B. 50–100 mcg/dL
   C. 100–200 mcg/dL
   D. More than 200 mcg/dL

3. As a therapy for ALF, vitamin K can be administered through which routes? (Select all that apply.)
   A. Orally
   B. Subcutaneously
   C. Intramuscularly
   D. Intravenously
   E. Intradermally

4. Which statement is TRUE about infection in clients with ALF?
   A. Surveillance cultures can be important in clients with ALF.
   B. Use of antimicrobial medications may begin early.
   C. Infection can be identified by temperature and WBC count elevations.
   D. Viral infections are the greatest concern in clients with ALF.

Answers: 1. B, 2. D, 3. B, 4. B

Section Four: The High-Acuity Patient with Chronic Liver Disease

Chronic liver disease causes slow, progressive destruction of the liver with a clinical pattern of deteriorating liver function and the eventual onset of potentially life-threatening complications. This section presents an overview of complications of chronic liver disease that may be present on admission to a high-acuity setting.

Hepatic Encephalopathy

The evaluation and grading of HE in chronic liver failure is the same as for ALF. Although patients with chronic liver failure are typically on a daily medication regimen to prevent HE, in certain circumstances they can deteriorate to grade III or grade IV HE. If HE severity worsens, it may necessitate transfer of the patient to the ICU for intubation and mechanical ventilation because of the inability to protect the airway. Factors that contribute to HE in chronic liver failure are listed in Box 23–1.

In patients with chronic liver failure, lactulose is taken daily and titrated to two to four loose bowel movements per day to keep ammonia levels low. However, if HE worsens, the dose of lactulose may be increased or given by retention enema until the patient has a bowel movement. Unless the patient is being prepared for an imminent liver transplant, there is less concern related to gaseous distention of the bowel. Additional treatment strategies are the same as those for HE associated with ALF. These patients, however, do not have the same risk of developing cerebral edema and brain herniation, and treatment associated with increased ICP is rarely needed.

Esophageal Variceal Bleeding

Varices are dilated and tortuous vessels that can be found anywhere within the splanchnic circulation. However, they are most commonly found in the distal esophagus and stomach, where they are called esophageal varices. **Esophageal varices** are a complication of portal hypertension. Normally, there is only a pressure difference of 2 to 6 mmHg in blood flow from the portal vein system into the inferior vena cava. When there is damage to the liver lobules, which occurs in cirrhosis, there is resistance to the normal flow of blood through the portal system. As the resistance increases, so does the pressure difference, and when it is greater than 10 to 12 mmHg, there is significant portal hypertension (Figure 23–2) (Friedman, 2017). With this increase in pressure, collateral circulation develops between the portal and systemic circulations.

A rapid increase in pressure (e.g., coughing, vomiting, straining) can cause these dilated varices to rupture, which can cause a life-threatening hemorrhage. These patients must be cared for in the ICU as they require intubation and mechanical ventilation for airway protection and ventilator support, as well as volume resuscitation with crystalloids, blood, and blood products. An endoscopy may be performed by the gastroenterologist to visualize and treat the bleeding vessel. If the bleeding cannot be stopped, insertion of a Sengstaken–Blakemore tube (Figure 23–3) may be necessary to tamponade the bleeding vessels.

Once the bleeding has been controlled, steps are taken to reduce the risk of future esophageal bleeding. These may include medical management to decrease pressure in the portal circulation, or surgical portocaval shunt placement, which is more likely in patients not being considered for liver transplantation. Patients may also undergo a transjugular intrahepatic portosystemic shunt (TIPS) procedure, which shunts blood from the portal vein into the hepatic vein and inferior vena cava (see Figure 23–4). While

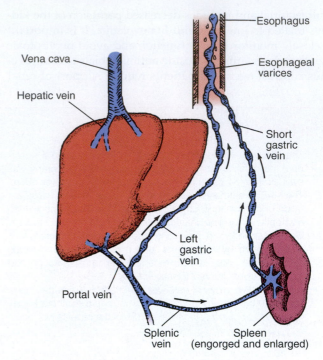

Figure 23–2 Portal hypertension.

this can decrease the pressure in the portal venous system, including varices, blood is shunted around the liver parenchyma, and the risk of worsening HE increases. The management of patients with esophageal varices is summarized in Table 23–5.

Ascites

Ascites is defined as an abnormal collection of fluid in the abdominal (peritoneal) cavity. Several factors can contribute

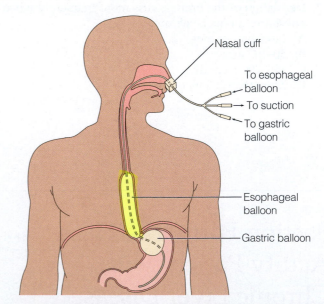

Figure 23–3 Sengstaken–Blakemore tube, a tamponade system used to stop bleeding esophageal varices. It consists of a tube, two balloons, and a distal suction port. The tube is inserted nasally and threaded into the stomach. The balloons are then inflated, one in the esophagus and one in the hiatus of the stomach, compressing the bleeding varices.

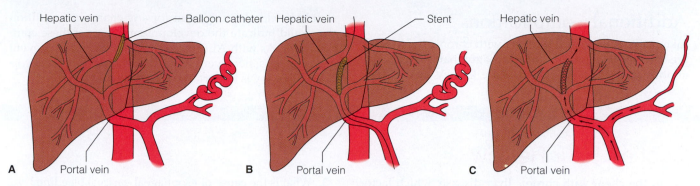

Figure 23–4 Transjugular intrahepatic portosystemic shunt (TIPS). **A,** Guided by angiography, a balloon catheter inserted via the jugular vein is advanced to the hepatic veins and through the substance of the liver to create a portacaval (portal vein-to-vena cava) channel. **B,** A metal stent is positioned in the channel and expanded by inflating the balloon. **C,** The stent remains in place after the catheter is removed, creating a shunt for blood to flow directly from the portal vein into the hepatic vein.

to the development of ascites in patients with chronic liver failure. Two important factors are portal hypertension and hypoalbuminemia. Portal hypertension increases the hydrostatic (water-pushing) pressure within the portal system, which can help to push fluid into the abdomen. Hypoalbuminemia, which occurs when the liver is unable to produce adequate amounts of albumin, leads to a decrease in oncotic (water-pulling) pressure within the vessels. This decrease in oncotic pressure leads to the shifting of fluid out of the intravascular space and the interstitium and peritoneal cavity.

When enough fluid accumulates within the peritoneal cavity, pressure can be exerted on the diaphragm, possibly compromising ventilation. There can also be leakage of fluid around the diaphragm that can then accumulate within the pleural space and cause a pleural effusion, called hepatic hydrothorax, further compromising ventilation

(Olson et al., 2011; Parks, Berkowitz, & Bechara, 2012). Pressure can also be exerted on the renal vessel, decreasing circulation to the kidneys, which can contribute to abnormal renal function. The volume of ascites can be so large that the patient may develop abdominal compartment syndrome.

In cases of ascites with compartment syndrome, the patient will need a large-volume paracentesis. A catheter is inserted into the abdominal cavity, and 4 or more liters of fluid are removed. The goal of volume removal is to improve ventilation, reduce dyspnea, and increase abdominal comfort (Wang, 2012), or to decrease the bladder pressure, which is a measurement of abdominal compartment syndrome, to less than 20 mmHg (Olson et al., 2011). Because removal of this much fluid can cause severe fluid shifts and hemodynamic compromise, the patient should receive 8 to 10 grams of albumin for every 1 liter of ascites that is removed (Olson et al., 2011; Wang, 2012).

Table 23–5 Management of the Patient with Esophageal Varices

Focus of Treatment	Interventions
Control bleeding	**IV vasopressin** Reduces splanchnic blood flow Initial dose of 20 units followed by continuous IV infusion of 0.4–0.6 units per minute **Octreotide** Reduces splanchnic blood flow, hepatic blood flow, and portal pressure Fewer systemic vasoconstrictive effects than vasopressin Initial dose of 50 mcg bolus followed by 50 mcg per hour by continuous IV infusion for 2–5 days **Nitroglycerin** May be given with vasopressin to decrease systemic vasoconstrictive effects (i.e., cardiac or mesenteric ischemia) **Fresh frozen plasma** A replacement of clotting factors Platelets may be ordered, although their efficacy is controversial
Aggressive correction of bleeding varices	**Sengstaken–Blakemore tube** or Minnesota tube placement (see Figure 23–3) **Portal systemic shunt surgery** Portocaval anastomosis Transjugular intrahepatic portosystemic shunt (TIPS) Distal splenorenal shunt
Preventive therapy	Therapy to reduce portal pressure: • Nonselective beta blockers (i.e., propranolol, nadolol) • Mononitrates (i.e., isosorbide mononitrate) • Elective shunt surgery • Endoscopic sclerotherapy • Endoscopic variceal banding (varix is isolated and banded, which results in ablation)

SOURCE: Data from Garcia-Tsao & Bosch (2010); McQuaid (2017); Olson et al. (2011).

Additional Complications

Like patients with ALF, patients with chronic liver failure are at a high risk of developing coagulopathy, electrolyte abnormalities, infection, and acute kidney injury. They should be closely monitored for any change in condition that could indicate the development of any of these complications. As with ALF, steps should be taken to prevent complications; however, if they occur, supportive and corrective therapy is undertaken.

Section Four Review

1. In the client with chronic liver disease, which factor contributes to the development of hepatic encephalopathy?
   A. Diarrhea
   B. GI bleeding
   C. Increased fat intake
   D. Elevated lipid levels

2. In the client with chronic liver disease, oral lactulose is given daily for which reason?
   A. To prevent hepatic encephalopathy
   B. To reduce the risk of infection
   C. To prevent esophageal variceal bleeding
   D. To reduce ascites

3. What is the cause of esophageal variceal bleeding?
   A. Systemic arterial hypertension
   B. Decreased synthesis of clotting factors
   C. Hypoperfusion of splanchnic circulation
   D. Increased portal hypertension

4. Which therapy would be considered to relieve severe abdominal ascites?
   A. Paracentesis
   B. TIPS procedure
   C. IV albumin
   D. Surgical intervention

Answers: 1. B, 2. A, 3. D, 4. A

Section Five: Nursing Considerations

The complex needs of patients experiencing acute liver failure require frequent monitoring of multisystem parameters and frequent evaluation of laboratory trends. Overall, the treatment strategies require collaborative management by interdisciplinary team members to optimize patient outcomes.

General Goals

Evaluation of hepatic function is performed through laboratory testing and other diagnostic procedures (noninvasive and invasive). The overall goals that drive the management activities are as follows:

- To determine and correct the underlying cause of ALF and prevent worsening of liver function
- To support organ function until the patient recovers or receives a liver transplant

Collaborative interventions to support the patient center around two goals: (1) promoting stable hemodynamic and ventilatory status and (2) preventing or minimizing secondary complications.

The nurse plays a crucial role in improving patient outcomes by being responsible for bedside assessment and analysis of the patient's status on a continual basis. A major focus of the nursing assessment involves monitoring the patient for the signs and symptoms of multisystem complications. The nurse facilitates the medical diagnostic process by preparing the patient and family for procedures, assisting with procedures, and monitoring the patient's status during and after procedures. The nurse also develops independent nursing diagnoses based on the patient's response to the illness rather than the illness itself. The following section provides a description of the part of a comprehensive nursing history and physical assessment that focuses specifically on hepatic function.

The Focused Nursing Database and History

On admission, it is crucial that the nurse obtain a comprehensive nursing database. The nurse especially focuses on data that may have a positive or negative impact on patient outcomes. General historical data the nurse should be sure to collect include preexisting medical conditions; surgeries; and recent history information, such as the events leading up to the patient's admission and a description of the patient's symptoms.

Focused Cognitive–Perceptual History Information regarding the patient's usual mental status, ability to communicate, and presence of discomfort or pain provides important baseline data.

Focused Value–Belief History Acute liver failure places the patient at significant risk. Information regarding the value–belief patterns of the patient and family can assist the healthcare team with planning appropriate supportive interventions. Value–belief patterns focus on the philosophical positions held by the patient and family that are used to guide personal decisions and choices. Major concepts include spirituality and quality-of-life beliefs.

The Focused Nursing Assessment

Assessment of the patient with ALF has two major focuses: (1) monitoring for potential complications and (2) monitoring the progress of the independent and collaborative nursing diagnoses. The following sections present some of the major assessments that may be obtained on an ongoing basis during an acute hepatic dysfunction episode to monitor the patient for potential complications.

Respiratory/Circulatory Assessment Hepatic failure can significantly alter cardiopulmonary function, primarily through severe second- and third-spacing of fluids with subsequent intravascular fluid volume deficit and decreased SVR. The nurse must monitor the patient for the following:

- Signs and symptoms of fluid volume deficit
- Edema, which may be generalized or may be present in the form of pulmonary edema
- Diminished or adventitious breath sounds (crackles in particular)
- Abnormal trends in blood pressure and pulse

Elimination Assessment The adequacy of renal function is closely monitored because of the risk for development of AKI. This is accomplished through observation of ordered laboratory tests (e.g., blood urea nitrogen [BUN] and creatinine) and evaluation of renal function by measuring intake and output balance and urine volume every 1 to 2 hours.

Neurologic Assessment The patient's neurologic status requires close monitoring throughout the duration of the acute illness because worsening HE increases the risk of cerebral edema, increased ICP, and herniation. The clinical manifestations of HE, as well as contributing factors, were described elsewhere in this chapter. The neurologic assessment should minimally include the following elements.

Focused Cognitive–Perceptual Assessment. The nurse assesses the patient's cognitive–perceptual status using the Glasgow Coma Scale (GCS). The GCS is a useful trending tool that assesses the arousal component of consciousness. An altered level of consciousness is an early finding in hepatic encephalopathy. The GCS specifically addresses eye opening, verbal response, and motor response.

Focused Muscular–Skeletal Assessment. The nurse assesses the patient's:

- **Coordination.** Coordination becomes increasingly impaired in the early stages of encephalopathy.
- **Reflexes.** Reflexes are brisk in grade II HE, a positive Babinski reflex may be seen in grade II HE, and by grade IV HE reflexes are decreased to absent.
- **Movement.** Asterixis (refer to Figure 23–1).

Focused Neurosensory Assessment. The nurse assesses for the presence of seizures, which may develop in the later stages of hepatic encephalopathy.

Gastrointestinal and Integumentary Assessment
Hepatic dysfunction is associated with a variety of GI and integumentary clinical manifestations. The majority result from the accumulation of hepatotoxins, third-spaced body fluids, coagulopathies, and decreased protein levels.

Focused GI Assessment. The nurse should assess for the following:

- Nausea and vomiting, anorexia
- Diarrhea or constipation
- Hepatic tenderness and enlargement on palpation

Focused Integumentary Assessment. The nurse should assess for the following:

- Jaundice
- Pruritus
- Edema

In addition, the skin can be assessed for several clinical manifestations of problems with coagulation, bleeding, and diminished proteins that usually occur with severe hepatic dysfunction, including the following:

- Evidence of poor wound healing
- Ecchymosis or petechiae
- Bleeding gums
- Pale mucous membranes and nail beds

The Nursing Care Plan

The nursing care plan of the patient experiencing either ALF or acute complications of chronic liver failure usually includes both collaborative problems and independent nursing diagnoses.

Frequently Occurring Collaborative Problems Collaborative problems include complications associated with ALF and chronic liver failure, including the following:

- Hepatic encephalopathy
- Esophageal varices
- Ascites
- Cerebral edema
- Coagulopathy
- Metabolic disorders (e.g., acid–base imbalance, electrolyte imbalances, insulin resistance)
- Infection
- Cardiopulmonary abnormalities (e.g., pulmonary effusions, dysrhythmias, cardiac dysfunction, cardiomyopathy)
- Acute kidney injury
- Hemorrhage
- Malnutrition

Frequently Occurring Nursing Interventions On completion of the nursing database, the nurse clusters data and develops a set of nursing differential diagnoses based on the available data. Additional critical data that may either support or eliminate each diagnosis should also be identified and obtained. Once the diagnoses have been established, the nurse is ready to develop a plan of care.

For the patient with ALF who is in a crisis period, a variety of independent and collaborative nursing interventions to address common patient conditions may be appropriate. The following is a partial list of these interventions:

- Interventions to optimize airway, breathing, and oxygenation/gas exchange
- Administration of fluid resuscitation to maintain euvolemia
- Initiation of mobility protocols to prevent complications of immobility
- Administration of oral, enteral, or total parenteral nutrition to meet metabolic demands
- Administration of pharmacologic and nonpharmacologic measures to optimize comfort and prevent anxiety or delirium
- Monitoring for and preventing infection

A summary of the nursing management of this patient population is provided in the "Nursing Care: The Patient with Acute Liver Failure" feature.

Nursing Care
The Patient with Acute Liver Failure

Expected Patient Outcomes and Related Interventions

Outcome 1: Absence of hepatic encephalopathy

Assess and compare to established norms, patient baselines, and trends.
Monitor patient for signs and symptoms of worsening hepatic encephalopathy:
Neurological status: altered mental status, lethargy, drowsiness, abnormal reflexes, asterixis, abnormal posturing, seizures
Nausea and vomiting
Monitor the results of ordered laboratory tests and report increasingly abnormal trends:
Arterial ammonia

Institute measures to reduce serum ammonia levels including drug therapy, and monitor for therapeutic and nontherapeutic effects.
Antibiotics to destroy intestinal ammonia-producing bacteria
Lactulose to prevent absorption and increase ammonia excretion through the bowel

Outcome 2: Absence of active bleeding

Assess and compare to established norms, patient baselines, and trends.
Monitor patient for signs and symptoms of bleeding.
Hematemesis, hematochezia
Vital signs: increasing or decreasing BP, increasing heart rate
Hemodynamic instability
Monitor the results of ordered laboratory tests and report increasingly abnormal trends.
Hemoglobin and hematocrit
RBC count
PT, INR

Institute measures to prevent or control bleeding.
Institute bleeding precautions.

Administer related drug therapy and monitor for therapeutic and nontherapeutic effects.
Vitamin K to reverse coagulopathy (Refer to the "Related Pharmacotherapy: Agents Used to Treat Complications of Hepatic Failure" feature.)
Fresh frozen plasma or platelets as ordered

Outcome 3: Improved hepatic function

Assess and compare to established norms, patient baselines, and trends.
Monitor: jaundice, generalized edema, pruritus.
Monitor nutritional status: hypoglycemia, nausea and vomiting, anorexia, constipation or diarrhea, caloric intake.
Monitor the results of ordered laboratory tests and report increasingly abnormal trends.
Liver function tests (LFT), including AST, ALT, alk phos, bilirubin, albumin, GGT, total protein
Serum or fingerstick glucose

Institute measures to improve liver function.
Nutrition consult
Supportive care

Administer related drug therapy and monitor for therapeutic and nontherapeutic effects.
Refer to information in the "Related Pharmacotherapy: Agents Used to Treat Complications of Hepatic Failure" feature.

Outcome 4: Maintains normal renal function

Assess and compare to established norms, patient baselines, and trends.
Monitor patient's renal status: BUN, creatinine, potassium, sodium.
Intake and output; notify provider if output less than 0.5 mL/kg/hr.

Institute measures to improve renal function.
Administer intravenous fluids
Administer vasopressor, inotropic, and oncotic agents.
Administer renal replacement therapy as ordered.

Administer related drug therapy and monitor for therapeutic and nontherapeutic effects.
Refer to information in the "Related Pharmacotherapy: Agents Used to Treat Complications of Hepatic Failure" feature.

Section Five Review

1. What is a major underlying goal that drives the majority of medical management activities for the client experiencing acute liver failure? (Select all that apply.)
   A. To promote stable hemodynamic status
   B. To prevent secondary complications
   C. To promote stable ventilatory status
   D. To prevent further deterioration of liver function
   E. To provide comfort as the client dies from this intractable disorder

2. The client with acute renal failure should have intake and output measurements at least how often?
   A. Every 15 minutes
   B. Every hour
   C. Every 2 hours
   D. Every 8 hours

3. How does hepatic failure alter cardiopulmonary function?
   A. It makes it more difficult for the client to breathe.
   B. It causes massive vasodilation of the peripheral vessels.
   C. It results in severe second- and third-spacing of fluids.
   D. It results in fluid volume overload.

4. What is the typical point at which urine output is considered adequate in the client in acute renal failure?
   A. 0.1 mL/kg/hr
   B. 0.5 mL/kg/min
   C. 0.5 mL/kg/hr
   D. 0.1 mL/kg/min

Answers: 1. B, 2. B, 3. C, 4. C

Clinical Reasoning Checkpoint

A 35-year-old male presents to the emergency department (ED) with a 2-day history of headache and increasing drowsiness. His past medical history is benign. In the ED the initial laboratory values are as follows: AST 530, ALT 325, alk phos 45, total bilirubin 3.0, INR 5.0. The patient's mental status deteriorates, and he becomes obtunded. His vital signs include BP 160/110 and HR 58, and his respiratory pattern is irregular. His wife reports that he has taken an entire bottle of acetaminophen over the past 2 days in an effort to relieve the constant severe headache he has been suffering.

1. What is your initial assessment?
2. What nursing interventions should be employed immediately?
3. What possible treatments are available for this patient?

Chapter 23 Review

1. A client presents in the emergency department and reports taking an intentional overdose of acetaminophen 3 days earlier. The client says, "I thought it would kill me, but I just got sick." What assessment finding would corroborate this client's report?
   1. The client is vomiting.
   2. The client has circumoral cyanosis.
   3. The client's ALT and AST enzymes are elevated.
   4. The client's BUN is elevated.

2. A client with a history of heart failure reports to the clinic complaining of tenderness at the right costal margin along with increasing shortness of breath. No other findings are reported. The nurse would ask assessment questions to determine if which common process is occurring?

   1. The client has developed gallbladder disorder.
   2. The client's appendix is inflamed.
   3. The client's liver is engorged.
   4. The client is constipated.

3. A client is prescribed N-acetylcysteine (NAC) as treatment of an acetaminophen overdose. Which nursing interventions are essential? (Select all that apply.)
   1. Send enough NAC home with the client for 18 total doses.
   2. Be certain to give each dose on time.
   3. Warn the client that the taste and smell are not pleasant.
   4. Plan to administer the medication intramuscularly.
   5. Start the medication as soon as possible after the prescription is written.

4. A client's total bilirubin is elevated. Which other lab result would the nurse expect if this client has liver failure?

   1. Increased direct bilirubin
   2. Decreased prothrombin time
   3. Increased alkaline phosphatase (ALP)
   4. Decreased ammonia

5. A client has been diagnosed with grade II hepatic encephalopathy. The nurse should expect which assessment?

   1. Comatose state
   2. Mild decrease in coordination
   3. Inability to maintain spontaneous respiration
   4. Intermittent asterixis

6. A client is receiving lactulose (Cephulac). Which findings would the nurse evaluate as indicating this medication is having the desired effects? (Select all that apply.)

   1. The client's serum ammonia level is dropping.
   2. The client is having two to four soft stools daily.
   3. The client's hemoglobin level has stabilized.
   4. The client has stopped vomiting.
   5. The client's urine output has increased to above 45 mL/hr.

7. A client hospitalized with chronic liver failure begins coughing up small amounts of blood. What nursing action is indicated?

   1. Give the client some warm salted water to rinse the mouth after every episode.
   2. Collaborate with the client's primary care provider immediately.
   3. Position the client flat in bed, rolled to the left side.
   4. Inspect the client's oral pharynx for ulcerations.

8. A client has had 6 liters of fluid removed by paracentesis. What intervention would the nurse expect?

   1. Administration of albumin
   2. Management of mechanical ventilation
   3. Oral fluid restriction
   4. NPO status

9. Which findings would the nurse expect when conducting a focused gastrointestinal assessment on a client with liver failure? (Select all that apply.)

   1. Tenderness under the right costal margin
   2. Absent bowel sounds
   3. Presence of diarrhea
   4. Report of anorexia
   5. Firm mass under the left costal margin

10. A client with acute liver failure has developed increasing ascites. Which client statement would alert the nurse that this situation is becoming dangerous? (Select all that apply.)

    1. "I feel so short of breath today."
    2. "I am not urinating as much as normal today."
    3. "I feel as if I can't take a deep breath."
    4. "I am not very hungry today."
    5. "I need pain medication because I have a headache."

Answers to questions found inside your textbook are available on the faculty resources site. Please consult with your instructor.

References

Abenavoli, L., Capasso, R., Milic, N., & Capasso, F. (2010). Milk thistle in liver disease: Past, present, future. *Phytotherapy Research, 24*(10), 1423–1432.

Bernal, W., Auzinger, G., Dhawan, A., & Wendon, J. (2010). Acute liver failure. *Lancet, 376,* 190–201.

Canbay, A., Tacke, F., Hadem, J., Trautwein, C., Gerken, G., & Manns, M. P. (2011). Acute liver failure: A life threatening disease. *Deutsches Ärzteblatt International, 108*(42), 714–720.

Dienstag, J. L. (2015). Acute viral hepatitis. In D. Kasper, A. Fauci, S. Hauser, D. Longo, J. Jameson, & J. Loscalzo (Eds.), *Harrison's principles of internal medicine* (19th ed.). New York, NY: McGraw Hill. Retrieved May 12, 2017 from http://accessmedicine.mhmedical.com .ezproxy.uky.edu/content.aspx?bookid=1130&sectio nid=79748507

Donati, G., Manna, G., Cianciolo, G., Grandinetti, V., Carretta, E., Cappuccilli, M., . . . Stefoni, S. (2014). Extracorporeal detoxification for hepatic failure using molecular adsorbent recirculating system: Depurative efficiency and clinical results in a long-term follow-up. *Artificial Organs, 38*(2), 125–134.

Foston, T. P., & Carpentar, D. (2010). Acute liver failure. *Critical Care Nursing Clinics of North America, 22*(3), 395–402.

Friedman, L. S. (2017). Liver, biliary tract, & pancreas disorders. In S. McPhee, M. Papadakis, & M. W. Rabow (Eds.), *CURRENT Medical Diagnosis and Treatment 2017* (56th ed.) New York, NY: McGraw-Hill. Retrieved October 4, 2016 from http://www.accessmedicine.com/content

Garcia-Tsao, G., & Bosch, J. (2010). Management of varices and variceal hemorrhage in cirrhosis. *New England Journal of Medicine, 362*(9), 823–832.

Grosser, T., & Smyth, E. (2011). Anti-inflammatory, antipyretic, and analgesic agents: Pharmacotherapy of gout. In L. L. Brunton, B. A. Chabner, & B. C. Knollmann (Eds.), *Goodman & Gilman's The pharmacological basis of therapeutics* (12th ed.). Retrieved October 4, 2016, from http://www.accessmedicine.com/content

Hassanein, T., Blei, A. T., Perry, W., Hilsabeck, R., Stange, J., Larsen, F. S., . . . Fontana, R. (2017). Performance of the hepatic encephalopathy scoring algorithm in a clinical trial of patients with cirrhosis and severe hepatic encephalopathy scoring algorithm. *The American Journal of Gastroenterology, 104*(6), 1392–1400. doi:10.1038/ajg.2009.160

Hung, O. L., & Nelson, L. S. (2016). Acetaminophen. In J. E. Tintinalli, G. D. Kelen, & J. S. Stapczynski (Eds.), *Tintinalli's emergency medicine: A comprehensive study guide* (7th ed.). Retrieved October 4, 2016, from http://www.accessemergencymedicine.com/content

Kee, J. L. (2013). *Laboratory and diagnostic tests with nursing implications* (9th ed.). Upper Saddle River, NJ: Pearson.

Kumar, S., & Qamar, A. A. (2015). Acute liver failure. In N. J. Greenberger, R. S. Blumberg, & R. Burakoff (Eds.), *CURRENT diagnosis & treatment: Gastroenterology, hepatology, & endoscopy* (3rd ed.). Retrieved October 4, 2016, from http://www.accessmedicine.com

Larson, A. M. (2010). Diagnosis and management of acute liver failure. *Current Opinion in Gastroenterology, 26*, 214–221.

Lee, W. M., Larson, A. M., & Stravitz, R. T. (2011). AASLD position paper: *The management of acute liver failure: Update 2011*. Retrieved January 25, 2013, from http://www.aasld.org/practiceguidelines/Documents/AcuteLiverFailureUpdate2011.pdf

McQuaid, K. R. (2017). Gastrointestinal disorders. In S. J. McPhee, M. A. Papadakis, & L. M. Tierney (Eds.), *Current medical diagnosis and treatment 2017* (56th ed.). New York, NY: McGraw Hill. Retrieved October 4, 2016, from http://www.accessmedicine.com

Olson, J. C., Wendon, J. A., Kramer, D. J., Arroyo, V., Jalan, R., Garcia-Tsao, G., & Kamath, P. S. (2011). Intensive care of the patient with cirrhosis. *Hepatology, 54*(5), 1864–1872.

Parks, C., Berkowitz, D. M., & Bechara, R. (2012). Pleural diseases. In S. C. McKean, J. Matloff, J. J. Ross, D. D. Dressler, D. J. Brotman, & J. S. Ginsberg (Eds.), *Principles and practice of hospital medicine*. Retrieved January 25, 2013, from http://www.accessmedicine.com/content.aspx?aID=56214905

Poonja, Z., Briscbois, A., Zaten, S. V., Tandon, P., Meeberg, G., & Karvellas, C. J. (2014). Patients with cirrhosis and denied liver transplantation rarely receive adequate palliative care or appropriate management. *Clinical Gastroenterology and Hepatology,12*(4), 692–698.

Sargent, S. (2010). An overview of acute liver failure: Managing rapid deterioration. *Gastrointestinal Nursing, 8*(9), 36–42.

Tujios, S. R., Hynan, L. S., Vazquez, M. A., Larson, A. M., Seremba, E., Sanders, C. M., & Lee, W. M. (2015). Risk factors and outcomes of acute kidney injury in patient with acute liver failure. *Clinical Gastroenterology and Hepatology, 13*(2), 352–359.

Wang, S. (2012). Paracentesis. In S. C. McKean, J. Matloff, J. J. Ross, D. D. Dressler, D. J. Brotman, & J. S. Ginsberg (Eds.), *Principles and practice of hospital medicine*. Retrieved January 25, 2013, from http://www.accessmedicine.com/content.aspx?aID=56201106

Wilson, B. A., Shannon, M. T., & Shields, K. (2017). *Pearson nurse's drug guide 2017*. Hoboken, NJ: Pearson Education.

Zafirova, Z., & O'Connor, M. (2010). Hepatic encephalopathy: Current management strategies and treatment, including management and monitoring of cerebral edema and intracranial hypertension in fulminant hepatic failure. *Current Opinion in Anaesthesiology, 23*(2), 121–127.

Chapter 24
Alterations in Pancreatic Function

Learning Outcomes

24.1 Describe the pathophysiologic basis of acute pancreatitis.

24.2 Analyze diagnostic data used in the determination of acute pancreatitis.

24.3 Demonstrate assessment of the patient with acute pancreatitis.

24.4 Explain the complications of acute pancreatitis.

24.5 Describe the medical management of a patient with acute pancreatitis.

24.6 Apply the concepts of nursing management for a patient with acute pancreatitis.

ancreatitis can present as an acute-onset or chronic disorder. This chapter focuses on the pathophysiology, assessment, and management of acute pancreatitis, which is more commonly seen in the high-acuity setting. While chronic pancreatitis is an important disease, it is generally managed in an outpatient setting unless there is a significant acute exacerbation of symptoms. Acute pancreatitis presents a challenge for the entire healthcare team because it can precipitate potentially life-threatening complications and cause intractable pain.

It is recommended that the pancreas sections of Chapter 21: Determinants and Assessment of Gastrointestinal Function, be reviewed prior to reading this chapter to enhance understanding of this material.

Section One: Pathophysiologic Basis of Acute Pancreatitis

Pancreatitis is inflammation of the pancreas, which results in injury to the pancreas. It can occur either as an acute or a chronic condition. In acute pancreatitis there is a sudden onset of pancreatic inflammation, which progresses to a generalized systemic inflammatory response syndrome

(SIRS). Acute pancreatitis is characterized by varying degrees of abdominal pain, pancreatic tissue edema, necrosis of pancreatic tissue, and possibly hemorrhage. There are two phases of acute pancreatitis: early (within the first week), characterized by the SIRS response, and late (after 1 week), when local complications are seen (Tenner, Baillie, DeWitt, & Vege, 2013). Severity ranges from mild to severe; however, the majority of patients develop a mild form called interstitial or edematous pancreatitis (Sarr et al., 2013). Mild acute pancreatitis is characterized by areas of fat inflammation in and around the pancreas accompanied by interstitial edema without organ failure or local or systemic complications. It is usually self limited, resolving within 5 to 7 days.

The more severe form of acute pancreatitis, often called necrotizing pancreatitis, occurs in approximately 15% to 25% of patients (Bell, Keane, & Pereira, 2015; De Waele, 2014). This may involve extensive necrosis in and around the pancreas, pancreatic cellular necrosis, and hemorrhage within the pancreas (see Figure 24–1). Moderately severe pancreatitis is associated with local or systemic complications without persistent organ failure. Severe pancreatitis is characterized by persistent (greater than 48 hours) single or multi organ failure. Determining the presence of pancreatic necrosis is of clinical importance as the morbidity and mortality are higher for these patients (Maheshwari & Subramanian, 2016). The mortality rate rises from less than 15% for all pancreatitis patients to more than 30% with

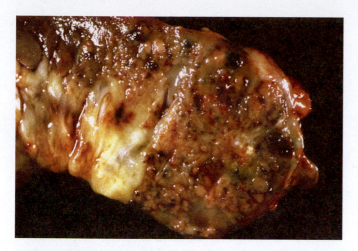

Figure 24–1 In acute pancreatitis, the pancreas appears edematous and is commonly hemorrhagic.

SOURCE: CNRI/Science Source

severe acute pancreatitis (Schub & Kornusky, 2015). Concurrent extrapancreatic infections have occurred in 33% of patients with acute pancreatitis while hospitalized; therefore, patients with acute pancreatitis require careful monitoring for early diagnosis and prompt treatment (Brown, Hore, Phillips, Windsor, & Petrov, 2014). Pregnant women with severe acute pancreatitis are at increased risk for preterm labor, premature delivery, and fetal loss (Ducarme, Maire, Chatel, Luton, & Hammel, 2014).

Acute pancreatitis is the leading cause of hospitalization for gastrointestinal disorders in the United States (Wu & Banks, 2013). Annual incidence ranges from 13 to 45 per 100,000 persons (Conwell, Banks, & Greenberger, 2015). Readmission is common for patients with acute pancreatitis, with rates as high as 34% (Vipperla et al., 2014). Recurring acute pancreatitis is most common when resulting from alcohol consumption (Talukdar & Vege, 2015). More severe forms of acute pancreatitis with local complications have been reported for alcohol-related pancreatitis versus biliary causes (Cho, Kim, & Kim, 2015). Table 24–1 lists the characteristics of mild, moderately severe, and severe pancreatitis.

Etiologies

There are multiple causes of acute pancreatitis. In the United States, gallstones and chronic alcohol abuse account for approximately 90% of cases (Valsangkar & Thayer, 2014). Gallstone-induced pancreatitis is the most common (40%–50% of cases in the United States) and is seen more often in women (Cucher, Kulvatunyou, Green, Jie, & Ong, 2014); alcohol-induced acute pancreatitis (15%–30% of cases in the United States) is more common in men (Cho et al., 2015). Gallstone-induced pancreatitis is caused by obstruction of the common bile duct by a lodged gallstone. The obstructing gallstone can either obstruct outflow of enzymes from the pancreatic duct or cause reflux of bile into the pancreatic duct. Either mechanism is believed to increase pancreatic ductal pressure and permeability, with resultant premature activation of pancreatic enzymes. Alcohol may induce acute pancreatitis by several mechanisms, including triggering spasms of the sphincter of Oddi, resulting in transient obstruction; changing the composition of pancreatic secretions, causing the formation of plugs within the pancreas; increasing the tendency for pancreatic secretion production; and triggering hyperresponsiveness of monocytes, which contributes to increased inflammation. Furthermore, alcohol metabolites cause direct injury to the acinar cells.

Medications may induce acute pancreatitis through an idiosyncratic response, a hypersensitivity response, or toxic metabolite, or a combination (Conwell et al., 2015). Hypercalcemia and significant hypertriglyceridemia are metabolic causes of acute pancreatitis. Idiopathic pancreatitis may develop during pregnancy, during administration of total parenteral nutrition, or following major surgery. Acute pancreatitis is also one of the major complications of AIDS. Endoscopic manipulation of the ampulla of Vater, such as may occur during endoscopic retrograde cholangiopancreatography (ERCP), endoscopic sphincterotomy (EST), or abdominal trauma, may also precipitate acute pancreatitis. Numerous genetic factors have been identified as causing premature activation of pancreatic precursors or modifying the severity of or the susceptibility to acute pancreatitis (Lipsett, 2011). Box 24–1 lists the major causes of acute pancreatitis.

Pathophysiology

Acute pancreatitis is an inflammatory disease with micro- and macrovascular failure. It occurs in three stages. First, trypsin and other enzymes in the pancreas are prematurely activated. The second stage is intrapancreatic inflammation, and the third is extrapancreatic or systemic injury.

Table 24–1 Characteristics of Severity of Acute Pancreatitis

Mild	Moderately Severe	Severe
• Short term	• Organ failure that resolves in 48 hours (transient), and/or	• Longer duration
• Pancreatic edema and swelling	• Local or systemic complications without persistent organ failure	• Persistent single or multi organ failure (greater than 48 hours)
• Localized inflammation		• Poor prognosis—associated with sepsis and multiple organ dysfunction
• No organ failure		
• No local or systemic complications		
• Reversible		
• Good prognosis		

SOURCE: Adapted from Banks et al. (2013).

BOX 24–1 Major Causes of Acute Pancreatitis

- Alcohol abuse*
- Biliary disease*: gallstones, microlithiasis, or biliary sludge; common bile duct obstruction
- Drug related: may include acid-suppressing medications, immunomodulators, diuretics, antimicrobials, nonsteroidal anti-inflammatory medications
- Genetic mutations
- Hypercalcemia
- Hypertriglyceridemia (greater than 1000 mg/dL)
- Idiopathic
- Infection
  Viral: mumps, coxsackievirus, cytomegalovirus (CMV), HAV, HBV, HIV/AIDS
  Bacterial: *Mycoplasma, Legionella, Salmonella*
  Fungal: *Aspergillus, Candida albicans*
  Parasitic: *Toxoplasma, Cryptosporidium*
- Inflammatory bowel disease
- Pancreas divisum
- Peptic ulcer disease
- Trauma related: blunt or penetrating abdominal trauma, post-ERCP, surgical trauma
- Toxins

*Most common

Regardless of the cause, acute pancreatitis develops when pancreatic enzymes—first trypsin and then the others—become prematurely activated by diverse stimuli within the pancreas, overwhelming normal regulatory mechanisms (Lankisch, Apte, & Banks, 2015). This premature activation results in the destruction of pancreatic tissue and surrounding (peripancreatic) tissues by its own activated digestive enzymes, a process called **autodigestion**.

Pathogenesis includes excessive leukocyte activation and transmigration, microcirculatory digestion of cellular membranes, vascular damage, coagulation necrosis, fat necrosis, interstitial hemorrhage, bacterial translocation, and/or acinar cell necrosis and apoptosis (Conwell et al., 2015). The inflammatory mediators lead to systemic inflammatory response syndrome (SIRS) and other complications. Intrapancreatic release of trypsin promotes further release of trypsin and activation of the precursors to phospholipase A, elastase, and carboxypeptidase into active enzymes and activates the kinin and complement pathways (Lipsett, 2011). **Phospholipase A** digests phospholipids on the cell membranes, and **elastase** digests the elastic tissue of vessel walls. Figure 24–2 shows the cascading effects of premature pancreatic enzyme activation. As vessel walls sustain increasing damage, both capillary and lymphatic vessels become injured, which results in hemorrhage, edema, pain, lymphocytic invasion, and hypotension. As the damage progresses, more acini are triggered to activate and secrete their digestive enzymes, which further increases autodigestive activities.

As part of the inflammatory process, kallikrein is activated by trypsin. **Kallikrein** is a basophil mediator of inflammation. It is responsible for causing bradykinin formation. Kallikrein causes vasodilation and increases the permeability of blood vessels, pain, and leukocyte invasion. Once kallikrein has been activated, systemic hypotension may lead to shock and multiple organ failure (such as acute respiratory distress syndrome and acute renal failure). The resultant local and distant effects of pathogenesis pose a risk for further tissue injury (Conwell et al., 2015). Thus, the initial local insult of acute pancreatitis may become a complex multisystem dysfunction disease process.

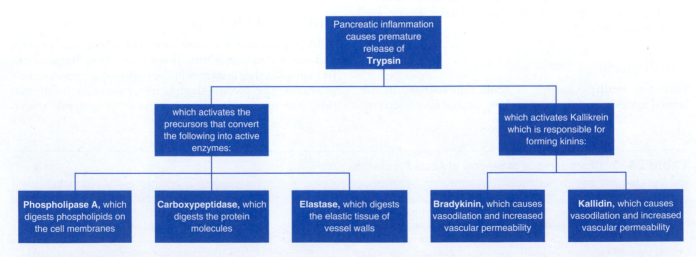

Figure 24–2 Cascading effects of premature pancreatic enzyme activation. These enzymes and kinins cause systemic capillary and lymphatic blood vessel damage, dilation, and permeability, which results in hemorrhage, edema, pain, lymphocyte invasion, and hypotension. As the damage progresses, more acini are triggered to activate and secrete their digestive enzymes, which further increases autodigestive activities. This cascade can progress to shock, acute respiratory distress syndrome, acute renal failure, and multiple organ failure.

Section One Review

1. What is a common cause of acute pancreatitis?
   A. Chronic alcohol abuse
   B. Steroid therapy
   C. Vascular disease
   D. Viral infections

2. Regardless of the etiology of acute pancreatitis, what is the primary pathophysiologic event?
   A. Hemorrhage
   B. Edema
   C. Autodigestion
   D. Pain

3. Premature activation of which pancreatic enzymes is thought to cause the most pancreatic damage?
   A. Trypsin, amylase
   B. Lipase, chymotrypsin
   C. Phospholipase A, elastase
   D. Elastase, amylase

4. How does alcohol affect the pancreas?
   A. Decreases enzyme secretion
   B. Depresses secretin secretion
   C. Inhibits the inflammatory response
   D. Causes spasm of the sphincter of Oddi

Answers: 1. A, 2. C, 3. C, 4. D

Section Two: Diagnosing Acute Pancreatitis

The initial clinical presentation of the patient with acute pancreatitis is similar to that of patients with a variety of other acute abdominal disorders. Diagnosing acute pancreatitis requires data from multiple sources, including laboratory tests and other diagnostic procedures. In addition, the patient history and physical assessment provide valuable information that will support or rule out a diagnosis of acute pancreatitis. The nursing history and assessment are presented in Section Three.

Generally a diagnosis of acute pancreatitis requires at least two of the following three criteria: (1) abdominal pain characteristic of acute pancreatitis, (2) serum amylase and/or lipase more than three times the upper limit of normal, and/or (3) characteristic findings of acute pancreatitis on abdominal imaging (Tenner et al., 2013). Contrast-enhanced computed tomography (CT) scan (previously the gold standard) and/or magnetic resonance imaging (MRI) are not necessary for all patients but should be used when the diagnosis is unclear or for patients who fail to improve clinically within the first 48 to 72 hours after hospital admission (Tenner et al., 2013). Box 24–2 lists clinical findings of acute pancreatitis.

Laboratory Assessment of Acute Pancreatitis

Laboratory testing is an important part of monitoring a patient for the development or progression of acute pancreatitis. Enzymes produced by the pancreas escape into the serum and urine when there is damage to the pancreatic parenchyma. The trends in pancreatic enzyme values are closely evaluated as an indication of disease progress. A variety of other laboratory tests may be ordered to further evaluate the pancreatitis, as well as the status of any multisystem involvement. A brief description of important laboratory assessments follows.

Pancreatic Enzyme Levels Pancreatic enzyme levels are usually measured in the serum and urine. Cellular enzymes leak into the blood when pancreatic tissue is injured, thereby increasing serum enzyme levels. The most commonly measured pancreatic enzymes are serum **amylase** and **lipase**.

Serum amylase levels rise within hours in the course of acute pancreatitis and can return to normal within as little as 3 days (Kee, 2014). Because serum amylase is nonspecific to the pancreas, it can increase for a variety of reasons. Therefore, altered serum amylase levels are examined in the context of other supportive clinical data. Amylase is secreted from both the salivary glands and pancreas, each with a distinct isoenzyme. Measurement of amylase isoenzyme P (P refers to pancreatic) is useful in ruling out nonpancreatic elevations in serum amylase.

BOX 24–2 Clinical Findings of Acute Pancreatitis

- Gastrointestinal:
  - Nausea and vomiting
  - Abdominal pain: acute onset of severe pain; location: epigastric and left upper quadrant (rarely in right upper quadrant); radiation to back possible; tenderness on palpation in epigastric area
  - Bowel sounds: decreased or absent
- Vital signs:
  - Fever, tachycardia; shock findings possible (hypotension, weak thready pulse, cold clammy skin)
- Laboratory:
  - Elevated pancreatic enzymes: amylase, lipase
  - Leukocytosis
- Other:
  - Positive Cullen or Turner sign
  - Jaundice (possible)

SOURCE: Data from Dooley et al. (2015) and Stevenson & Carter (2013).

The serum lipase level is considered the best pancreatic enzyme parameter (Dooley et al., 2015; Dupuis et al., 2013). Serum lipase levels rise later than amylase and remain elevated for approximately 1 to 2 weeks after serum amylase returns to normal (Dooley et al., 2015). Measuring lipase levels provides a longer period for trending values than that provided by serum amylase levels. While a range of nonpancreatic factors can cause hyperlipasemia, lipase levels retain a greater sensitivity for pancreatitis (Dupuis et al., 2013; Kee, 2014).

Other Laboratory Tests   A variety of laboratory tests may be helpful in evaluating acute pancreatitis and multisystem involvement, particularly the liver and gallbladder. Table 24–2 summarizes some of the major laboratory tests used in making a differential diagnosis of acute pancreatitis.

Diagnostic Tests

Diagnosis of acute pancreatitis requires data from a variety of sources. Frequently ordered major diagnostic tests include abdominal x-rays, ultrasound, computed tomography (CT) scan, endoscopic retrograde cholangiopancreatography (ERCP), magnetic resonance cholangiopancreatography (MRCP), and aspiration biopsy.

Abdominal and Chest Radiography   Radiographs of the abdomen and chest are used to exclude intestinal ileus, perforation, pericardial effusion, and pulmonary disease as causes of abdominal pain. The abdominal radiograph may be used initially as a quick means of revealing abdominal distention as well as gross abdominal abnormalities, such as an ileus. It is limited in its usefulness as a tool for diagnosing organ disorders. Chest films are valuable in

Table 24–2 Differential Laboratory Diagnosis of Acute Pancreatitis

Laboratory Test	Normal Values[a]	Trends	Trend Values	Comments
Serum				
Amylase	30–170 units/L	↑↑	> 500 units/L	Increases 2–12 hours post onset; peaks in 20–30 hours; may remain elevated 2–5 days; level does not correlate well with severity
Isoamylase P (pancreatic)	30–55%	↑	> 55%	Isoenzyme that is specific to pancreas
Lipase	14–280 units/L (SI units)	Rapid ↑	> 280 units/L	May remain elevated after amylase returns to normal
Glucose	70–110 mg/dL	Transient ↑	> 180 mg/dL	Secondary to islet cell malfunction; criteria used in absence of preexisting history of hyperglycemia
Calcium	9–11 mg/dL	↓	< 7.5 mg/dL	Due to saponification[b] of fat; also attributed to hypoalbuminemia (decreased availability of protein for calcium binding) due to malnutrition, especially in alcoholics
White blood cell count	4500–10,000/mcL	↑	> 15,000/mcL	Secondary to inflammatory process
Blood urea nitrogen	5–25 mg/dL	↑	> 45 mg/dL	Level remains elevated following correction of fluid volume deficit
Direct bilirubin (posthepatic)	0.1–0.3 mg/dL	↑	> 0.3 mg/dL	Associated with biliary obstruction
LDH	100–190 units/L	↑	> 350 units/L	Associated with biliary obstruction and pancreatitis; LDH4 isoenzyme is found in pancreas and other organs
C-reactive protein	< 1 mg/dL	↑	> 150 mg/L at 48 hours	Protein values are useful for severity assessment but may not be reflective within the first 48–72 hours. Levels rise in response to inflammation; not specific for pancreatitis.
Hematocrit	Male 40–54% Female 36–46%	↑	> 47% on admission or no improvement within first 24 hours	Hemoconcentration caused by dehydration may indicate possible pancreatic necrosis.
AST (SGOT)	8–35 units/mL	↑↑	> 250 units/mL	May see transient rise in acute pancreatitis; in acute extrahepatic obstruction, AST rises quickly to 10 times normal and remains elevated for 4–6 days.
Serum albumin	3.5–5 g/dL	↓	< 3.2 g/dL	Associated with protein deficiency
PaO₂	75–100 mmHg	↓	< 60 mmHg	Associated with pulmonary involvement
Stool				
Fat	2–7 g/24 hr	—	> 6 g/24 hr	Steatorrhea; stool is pale or gray, smells foul; caused by deficiency in pancreatic enzymes in bowel.

[a]Values may vary slightly according to the laboratory performing the test.

[b]Conversion of fat into a soap

SOURCE: Data from Kee (2014).

revealing pulmonary complications associated with acute pancreatitis, such as atelectasis and pleural effusion.

CT Scan A CT scan confirms diagnosis and is used to determine severity. A CT scan may not be needed in diagnosing mild cases of acute pancreatitis with classic pain and elevated amylase and lipase. Dynamic-contrast CT helps to distinguish interstitial from necrotizing pancreatitis. The CT scan provides a noninvasive means of viewing the structure of the pancreas, the bile ducts, and the gallbladder. Damaged pancreatic tissue and lesions can be visualized. Contrast-enhanced CT is currently considered one of the best tests for assessing pancreatic necrosis, excluding acute pancreatitis, and evaluating for the presence of local complications (Wu & Banks, 2013).

Ultrasound Ultrasound uses high-frequency sound waves rather than radiation. It provides a real-time view of the structure being tested. Ultrasound is particularly valuable in viewing the bile ducts and can identify gallstones more readily than the CT scan. In this way, an ultrasound on admission can assess for gallstones as the etiology of the pain rather than establish a diagnosis of acute pancreatitis. It may also visualize abnormal findings such as ascites and cholangiectasis. However, abdominal ultrasound is of limited usefulness when bowel gas is present (Quinlan, 2014). Endoscopic ultrasound (EUS) may be used to evaluate necrotic collections, detect gallstones or sludge in the gallbladder or common bile duct, and determine which patients may benefit from ERCP (Besselink, van Santvoort, & Gooszen, 2013; Quinlan, 2014).

Endoscopic retrograde cholangiopancreatography (ERCP) is an invasive endoscopic test that allows cannulation and direct viewing of the ampulla of Vater and the pancreatic and bile ducts. It requires injection of a radiographic contrast medium followed by a series of x-rays under fluoroscopy. ERCP is particularly useful in diagnosing obstructions. In addition, it provides the opportunity for direct removal of mechanical obstructions, such as a gallstone or pancreatic stone; stent placement to provide drainage through a stricture; sphincterotomy; and biopsy.

Magnetic resonance cholangiopancreatography (MRCP) uses magnetic resonance imaging to produce images used to evaluate the hepatobiliary tree. Because it is noninvasive and requires no contrast, MRCP has a decreased morbidity rate compared to ERCP. MRCP has greater accuracy than ERCP for diagnosing common bile duct stones (Bell et al., 2015). The usefulness of MRCP is limited by the inability to intervene with stone extraction, stent insertion, or biopsy and impaired visualization due to peripancreatic fluid collection.

Image-guided Aspiration Biopsy Aspiration biopsy involves the removal of a small plug of tissue using a syringe-and-needle technique. It is useful in diagnosing the severity of pancreatic tissue damage, diagnosing types of lesions, and draining pseudocysts. It is also helpful in distinguishing sterile necrosis from infected necrosis (Upchurch, 2014). Aspiration biopsy can be performed during ultrasound or CT scan, to enable visualization of needle placement.

Table 24–3 Scoring Systems for Determining Severity of Acute Pancreatitis

Ranson Criteria (48 hours after onset of symptoms)	APACHE II	CTSI (combination of CT grade score and % fat necrosis score)	BISAP
		CT Scan Grade Score	
Age > 55 years	Age > 55 years	A = normal pancreas	BUN > 25
WBC > 16,000 mm^3	WBC < 3000 or > 14,900 mm^3	B = pancreatic enlargement	Impaired mental status
Serum glucose > 200 mg/dL	RR < 12 or > 24; HR < 70 or > 109	C = pancreatic inflammation ± peripancreatic fat stranding	Age > 60 years
Serum LDH > 350 International Unit/L	MAP < 70 or > 109 mmHg	D = single peripancreatic fluid collection	Pleural effusion
Serum AST > 250 International Unit/mL	Rectal temperature < 36°C (96.8°F) or > 38.4°C (101.1°F)	E = ≥ 2 fluid collections ± retroperitoneal gas	Greater than or equal to SIRS criteria
HCT decrease > 10%	Chronic health problems	**Percent Fat Necrosis Score**	
BUN rise of > 5 mg/dL	Na$^+$ < 130 or > 149 mmol/L	0% necrosis	
Serum calcium < 8 mg/dL	K$^+$ < 3.5 or > 5.4 mmol/L	< 30% necrosis	
PaO$_2$ < 60 mg/dL	PO$_2$ < 70 or > 200 mmHg	30–50% necrosis	
Base deficit < 4 mEq/L	Cr < 0.6 or > 1.4 mg/100 mL	> 50% necrosis	
Estimated fluid sequestration > 6 L	HCT < 30% or > 45.9%		
	Glasgow Coma Score		
Additional acute health issues increase the risk of death.	pH < 7.33 or > 7.49 HCO$_3$ < 23 or > 31.9		
Associated mortality is based on number of risk factors.	Associated mortality is based on number of risk factors.		More variables are associated with higher mortality.

A higher incidence of risk factors results in higher scores, which are associated with increased severity and a worse prognosis.

SOURCE: Data from Bollen et al. (2012); Kuo et al. (2015); Park et al. (2013); and Ranson et al. (1974).

Predicting the Severity of an Episode of Acute Pancreatitis

A clinical severity scoring system is important in acute pancreatitis to identify patients who need high-acuity care. The highest incidence of organ failure occurs in patients with persistent SIRS (more than 48 hours) and may identify patients who require high-acuity care (Tenner et al., 2013). SIRS has a high sensitivity for predicting organ failure and mortality at admission and when persistent beyond 48 hours (Working Group IAP/APA, 2013). Several multifactorial scoring systems have been developed and tested to predict mortality. The Ranson criteria were used for many years to estimate mortality of patients with pancreatitis but require 48 hours for complete assessment. The Acute Physiology and Chronic Health Evaluation (APACHE II) scale estimates ICU mortality (not specific to pancreatitis) and is useful for assessing severity on admission. The modified computed tomography severity index (CTSI) based on contrast-enhanced CT findings and an update of the Balthazar criteria originally published in 1985 (Balthazar et al., 1985) distinguishes mild, moderate, and severe forms of acute pancreatitis and correlates with morbidity and mortality (Stevenson & Carter, 2013). The Bedside Index of Severity in Acute Pancreatitis (BISAP) may be helpful in the emergency department in predicting the severity and prognosis for acute pancreatitis (Kuo, Rider, Estrada, Kim, & Pillow, 2015).

In addition to scoring systems, individual factors may serve as predictors of severe acute pancreatitis, although no easily available and consistently accurate laboratory test has been found. BUN measurement has been shown to be an early and accurate predictor of mortality in acute pancreatitis and may assist in guiding early resuscitation efforts (De Waele, 2014). A C-reactive protein greater than 150 mg/dL 48 hours after hospital admission may indicate future development of pancreatic infection and mortality (De Waele, 2014). Obesity with BMI greater than 30, pleural effusion or pulmonary infiltration, increased serum creatinine, and increased hematocrit indicative of hemoconcentration are all associated with the development of severe necrotizing pancreatitis (Conwell et al., 2015; Kuo et al., 2015).

With all prognostic scoring systems, an elevated initial score or an elevated score at repeat testing indicates a higher risk of mortality. Increased severity of illness translates into the need for high-acuity care. There has been no consensus as to which scoring system should be used (Nesvaderani, Eslick, & Cox, 2015). Table 24–3 describes the factors included in selected severity scoring systems.

Section Two Review

1. Which laboratory tests are the primary ones obtained to help diagnose pancreatitis?
   A. Amylase and lipase
   B. Calcium and glucose
   C. LDH and AST
   D. Hematocrit and BUN

2. Severe acute pancreatitis usually has which effect on serum glucose?
   A. Severe hypoglycemia
   B. Transient hypoglycemia
   C. No effect
   D. Transient hyperglycemia

3. Which assessment data are associated with increased severity scores in acute pancreatitis? (Select all that apply.)
   A. Age > 45
   B. Increased BUN
   C. Base Excess > +4
   D. Decreased hematocrit
   E. Decreased PaO_2

4. What is the advantage of magnetic resonance cholangiopancreatography (MRCP) over endoscopic retrograde cholangiopancreatography (ERPC)?
   A. MRCP is noninvasive.
   B. MRCP can be used to guide stone extraction.
   C. MRCP is more accurate when stent insertion is necessary.
   D. MRCP is more useful with peripancreatic fluid present.

Answers: 1. A, 2. D, 3. (B, D, E), 4. A

Section Three: Nursing Assessment of the Patient with Acute Pancreatitis

The nursing assessment of a patient experiencing acute pancreatitis requires a thorough multisystem evaluation with particular focus on assessment of pain, the GI system, and inflammation.

Assessment of Pain

Pain is the most consistent complaint associated with acute pancreatitis and is a high-priority assessment. The classic pattern of pain is described as a sudden onset of sharp, knifelike, twisting and deep, upper abdominal (epigastric) pain that frequently radiates to the back and is often associated with nausea and vomiting (Bell et al., 2015). Pain intensity varies greatly from patient to patient. It may be described as vague and mild, or it may be excruciating, unbearable, and refractory to analgesic therapy. The intensity often reflects the degree to which the disease process has extended beyond the confines of the pancreas. If localized, the pain is usually vague and mild; however, if pancreatic proteolytic enzymes infiltrate extrapancreatic tissues (into the peritoneum), the pain becomes well defined and sharp, and the intensity increases significantly. The pain is believed to be a result of edema and distention of the pancreatic capsule, chemical burn of the peritoneum by pancreatic enzymes, and the release of kinin peptides or biliary obstruction. Initially, the patient's complaints of pain intensity may seem out of proportion to other clinical manifestations. The patient may report some degree of relief by leaning forward or assuming a knee to chest position and may report an increase in pain when doing activities that increase abdominal pressure (e.g., coughing).

Focused History and Assessment

The majority of the clinical manifestations of acute pancreatic dysfunction are of gastrointestinal origin; thus, while taking the nursing history, the nurse should particularly focus on obtaining a complete gastrointestinal history. Ask the patient about previous symptoms of gallstones, alcohol use, history of hypertriglyceridemia or hypercalcemia, family history of pancreatic disease, drug history (prescription and nonprescription), history of trauma, or the presence of an autoimmune disease. The remainder of this section presents the major signs and symptoms associated with acute pancreatitis.

Gastrointestinal Assessment   The presence of abdominal pain is a major finding in acute pancreatitis. Additional GI clinical manifestations include the following:

- Anorexia
- Upper abdominal tenderness without rigidity
- Abdominal distention
- Nausea and vomiting
- Diarrhea
- Increased intra-abdominal pressure
- Peritoneal signs (noted in severe cases):
  - Diminished or absent bowel sounds (ileus may develop)
  - Increased pain
  - Abdominal rigidity, guarding, rebound tenderness

Signs of Systemic Inflammation   Because pancreatitis is a highly inflammatory process, it is important to periodically assess the patient for any changes in the signs of inflammation, including the following:

- Leukocytosis
- Tachycardia
- Fever
- Decreased mental status or confusion
- Hypoxemia

Additional Assessments   In addition to the major clinical and inflammatory manifestations, a variety of other common or classic signs and symptoms are associated with the disease process.

Integumentary.   If the patient has hemorrhagic pancreatitis, two uncommon signs that are associated with severe acute pancreatitis and a higher mortality may be observed:

- **Cullen sign**, a bluish discoloration around the umbilicus
- **Grey Turner sign**, a bluish discoloration of the flank region

Other observations that may be noted by skin inspection are jaundice and edema. If the patient develops shock, the skin becomes mottled or pale, cold, and moist.

Cardiovascular.   Cardiac signs and symptoms usually present themselves in conjunction with the complication of shock. The nurse should observe the patient for the signs and symptoms of hypovolemic shock (tachycardia, hypotension, and orthostasis) and myocardial depression (decreased cardiac output with increased systemic vascular resistance).

Pulmonary.   Respiratory signs and symptoms include those typical of the following:

- Pleural effusion—adventitious breath sounds, particularly crackles (usually left sided)
- Respiratory insufficiency or failure
- Pneumonia and/or ARDS

Neurologic.   The nurse can rapidly trend alterations in level of consciousness by using the Glasgow Coma Scale (GCS). Common neurologic manifestations include confusion, restlessness, and agitation.

Renal.   Assess for the development of acute tubular necrosis. Monitor urine output, blood urea nitrogen (BUN), and creatinine levels. Observe urine color and consistency. As increased levels of bile are excreted through the urine, it develops a brownish color and may become foamy.

Hematologic.   The nurse should monitor the patient for clinical manifestations of disseminated intravascular coagulation.

Endocrine and Exocrine.   The nurse should closely monitor serum glucose, as pancreatitis affects both exocrine and endocrine pancreatic functions, which can cause wide fluctuations in glucose levels.

Electrolyte Imbalances.   Hypocalcemia may develop as a result of fat necrosis because serum calcium migrates to the extravascular space surrounding the pancreas where the fat necrosis is taking place. Two classic signs of hypocalcemia are these:

- **Chvostek sign.** The facial nerve is tapped directly in front of the ear. A positive sign is present when the

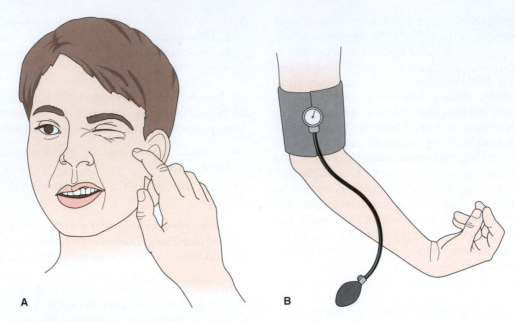

Figure 24–3 A, Positive Chvostek sign. B, Positive Trousseau sign.

facial muscles contract on the same side of the face as the tapping (Figure 24–3A).

- **Trousseau sign.** A blood pressure cuff is inflated on the upper arm to a level directly above the patient's systolic blood pressure for 2 minutes. A positive sign is present when the hand flexes (carpopedal spasm) in response to the test (Figure 24–3B).

In addition to hypocalcemia, the patient should be monitored for the hypokalemia and hypomagnesemia that may result from gastrointestinal loss and insufficient intake. Detailed information on the clinical manifestations of hypocalcemia, hypokalemia, and hypomagnesemia is available in Chapter 26: Alterations in Fluid and Electrolyte Balance.

Section Three Review

1. How is the classic pattern of pain typically described by the client with acute pancreatitis?
   A. Dull, diffuse, and poorly defined
   B. Sharp and confined to the epigastric area
   C. Well defined, dull, and localized in the flank area
   D. Sharp, knifelike, often radiating to the back

2. The intensity and description of pain associated with acute pancreatitis varies, often based on which factor?
   A. pH of the pancreatic enzymes
   B. Degree to which extrapancreatic invasion has occurred
   C. Pain threshold of the individual client
   D. Degree of release of myocardial depressant factor (MDF)

3. What are the peritoneal signs of acute pancreatitis? (Select all that apply.)
   A. Rebound tenderness
   B. Rigid abdomen
   C. Hyperactive bowel sounds
   D. Leukocytosis
   E. Guarding

4. The Cullen sign may be noted under which circumstance?
   A. Acute tubular necrosis
   B. Hemorrhage
   C. Hypovolemic shock
   D. Respiratory failure

Answers: 1. D, 2. B, 3. B, 4. B

Section Four: Complications of Acute Pancreatitis

Acute pancreatitis is considered a multisystem disease process. Complications are common and may be local and systemic. Both types of complications are mediated by active enzymes and cytokines released in the early phase (Conwell et al., 2015). Obesity is a risk factor for both local and systemic complications and increases the risk of severity and mortality (Premkumar, Phillips, Petrov, & Windsor, 2015). In its most severe form, acute pancreatitis may be complicated by the development of multisystem organ dysfunction syndrome (MODS). In severe acute pancreatitis with infected necrosis, the mortality is as high as 30% to 50% (Valsangkar & Thayer, 2014).

Local Complications

Peripancreatic fluid collections, acute necrotic collections, walled-off necrosis, and pseudocyst are local complications. The development of both pseudocyst and abscess usually requires 4 or more weeks from the initial clinical onset of acute pancreatitis. Peripancreatic fluid collections occur in the first 4 weeks and are associated with interstitial edematous pancreatitis without necrosis. These fluid collections are usually left to resolve on their own. Acute necrotic collections can be sterile or infected, are associated with necrotizing pancreatitis, and typically occur in the first 4 weeks. These can appear in the pancreas or in peripancreatic tissues. Walled-off necrosis can be infected or sterile and appear as encapsulated collections of necrosis in and around the pancreas replacing portions of the pancreas or peripancreatic tissues (Bell et al., 2015). Infected necrosis may require drainage and minimally invasive approaches are preferred over open surgical procedures (Tenner et al., 2013). A pancreatic **pseudocyst** is a cavity containing pancreatic enzymes, fluid, possibly blood, and little or no necrosis that is enclosed by a wall of fibrous or granulation tissue (Bell et al., 2015). Although not truly encapsulated, the pseudocyst is enclosed either by some type of adjacent tissue or by pancreatic tissue. Some pseudocysts resolve on their own; however, while they are present, they may become infected or rupture into the peritoneal cavity, which can precipitate peritonitis (Upchurch, 2014). In patients who fail to improve, a contrast-enhanced CT scan should be performed to evaluate for these complications (Wu & Banks, 2013).

In addition, abdominal compartment syndrome (ACS) is a serious complication of severe acute pancreatitis. Intra-abdominal hypertension and ACS can result from the aggressive fluid resuscitation, ascites, ileus, and the inflammatory response (De Waele, 2014; Malledant, Malbrain, & Reuter, 2015). Increased intra-abdominal pressure raises the diaphragm and leads to atelectasis and hypercapnia. Nasogastric decompression, rectal tubes, ultrafiltration, diuretics, and sedation may help to decrease the pressure depending on the cause (Working Group IAP/APA, 2013). Surgical decompression may be necessary.

Systemic Complications

The release of humoral mediators, such as **platelet activating factor (PAF)**, interleukins, neutrophils, tumor necrosis factor, anti-inflammatory mediators and cytokines, and the development of systemic inflammatory response syndrome (SIRS) may lead to complications that have the potential to interfere with virtually all of the body's functions (Stevenson & Carter, 2013).

Pulmonary Hypoxemia develops in the majority of severe acute pancreatitis patients within the first 2 days of onset. Respiratory insufficiency and failure are common complications and are attributed to the release of pancreatic enzyme phospholipase A, which destroys the phospholipid component of surfactant. The patient is at risk of developing pneumonia and/or pleural effusion and, in severe cases, acute respiratory distress syndrome (ARDS). Pleural effusions may result from enzyme-induced inflammation of the diaphragm, while atelectasis may result from decreased diaphragmatic excursion as a result of abdominal distention. Lung injury may be due to an array of systemic factors and the specific effects of pancreatic enzymes like proteases and phospholipase A_2 (Akbarshahi, Rosendahl, Westergren-Thorsson, & Andersson, 2012).

Cardiovascular Pancreatic enzymes released into the bloodstream can have devastating effects on the cardiovascular system through the release of myocardial depressant factor (MDF) and the development of hypovolemic shock. MDF is the result of pancreatic autodigestion by proteolytic enzymes and has a negative inotropic (contractility) effect on heart muscle, reducing cardiac output.

Hypovolemic Shock Vasoactive substances are released from damaged pancreatic tissue. Trypsin activates the powerful vasodilating and circulating enzyme kallikrein, which forms two plasma kinins (kallidin and bradykinin). These two substances are responsible for vasodilation, decreased systemic vascular resistance and for increased permeability of endothelial linings of vessels. As vessels become more porous, intravascular fluids shift into other compartments and into the retroperitoneal cavity, causing hypovolemia, third-spacing, and hypovolemic shock.

Hemorrhage is also a major cause of hypovolemic shock in hemorrhagic pancreatitis. When it is prematurely activated, the pancreatic enzyme elastase is able to break down duct and blood vessel elastic fibers, causing hemorrhage. Hemorrhage can also occur as a result of other complications, such as bleeding ulcers, varices, or tissue necrosis.

Renal Acute tubular necrosis (ATN), a type of renal failure, is a fairly common sequela in severe acute pancreatitis. It results from renal ischemia secondary to hypotension and hypoxemia. If fluid resuscitation is timely and adequate, the kidney damage may be decreased. When hypoxemia occurs, immediate respiratory support is necessary to avoid renal compromise.

Neurologic A decreased level of consciousness is a common problem in severe pancreatitis and is related to several potential etiologies, including analgesia and pancreatic encephalopathy. The alleviation of pain associated with acute pancreatitis requires large doses of opioids and possibly sedation. Cerebral function is altered by either of these therapies. The pathogenesis of pancreatic encephalopathy is unclear but may be related to both pancreatic and extrapancreatic factors.

Hematologic Disseminated intravascular coagulation (DIC) is associated with severe acute pancreatitis. It may be related to the systemic inflammatory response, leading to cytokine activation and coagulation activation and/or release of procoagulant material in the blood (Levi, Nagalla, & Schmaier, 2015). Table 24–4 summarizes the major systemic complications.

Table 24–4 Major Systemic Complications of Acute Pancreatitis

Body System or Function	Complications
Neurologic	Encephalopathy
Pulmonary	Hypoxia, respiratory failure, pneumonia, pleural effusion, atelectasis, acute respiratory distress syndrome (ARDS)
Cardiovascular	Hemorrhage, hypotension, shock, pericardial effusion, pericardial tamponade
Gastrointestinal	Bleeding, pancreatic pseudocyst
Renal	Acute renal failure
Metabolic	Hyperglycemia, metabolic acidosis, hypocalcemia
Hematologic	Vascular thrombosis, disseminated intravascular coagulation (DIC)
Infectious	Infected pancreatic necrosis, peritonitis, sepsis

Metabolic Hyperglycemia is a common clinical finding in acute pancreatitis. The transient elevation of glucose levels is partially attributed to damage to the alpha islet cells (Kee, 2014). High serum glucose levels and wide glucose level swings (glucose lability) are predictors for poor prognosis and place patients at higher risk for secondary infections (Valsangkar & Thayer, 2014). Metabolic acidosis may occur as a complication of severe acute pancreatitis, especially if renal failure develops (Kee, 2014).

Section Four Review

1. If a pseudocyst were to rupture into the peritoneal cavity, the client would most likely develop which condition?
   A. Septicemia
   B. Acute renal failure
   C. Paralytic ileus
   D. Peritonitis

2. In the acute pancreatitis client, hypovolemic shock usually results from which conditions? (Select all that apply.)
   A. Hemorrhage
   B. Third-spacing
   C. Renal failure
   D. Kallikrein release
   E. Vasodilation

3. Pulmonary complications are attributed to which pancreatic enzyme?
   A. Insulin
   B. Elastase
   C. Amylase
   D. Phospholipase A

4. The release of MDF by injured pancreatic tissue is believed to have what effect on the heart?
   A. Decreases cardiac output
   B. Decreases heart rate
   C. Increases blood pressure
   D. Increases cardiac output

5. Which intervention is useful in decreasing kidney damage associated with acute pancreatitis?
   A. Fluid resuscitation
   B. Pain control
   C. Early return to oral nutrition
   D. Emergent drainage of developing pseudocysts

Answers: 1. D, 2. (A, B, D, E), 3. D, 4. A, 5. D

Section Five: Medical Management

The medical management of the patient with acute pancreatitis may be either supportive or curative but is often a combination of both. Supporting the patient's hemodynamic and oxygenation status is essential while correction of the underlying problem is undertaken. If there is evidence of a mechanical obstruction, such as would occur with biliary tract obstruction (gallstones), a cholecystectomy should be performed. If the underlying problem is chemical inflammation, as in alcohol-induced pancreatitis, the problem is allowed to resolve itself and supportive therapy is provided.

Supportive Therapy

Medical management is based on prioritized goals, including stabilizing hemodynamic status, controlling pain, minimizing pancreatic stimulation, correcting the underlying problem, and preventing or treating complications. Antibiotics are generally not indicated unless there are signs of intra-abdominal infection. A summary of supportive management of the acute pancreatitis patient is listed in Table 24–5.

Table 24–5 Supportive Therapy for Acute Pancreatitis

Type of Support	Collaborative Management
Fluid resuscitation	This may consist of up to 10–20 L of fluid during the first 24 hours, as required. Fluids may be crystalloids or colloids. Lactated Ringers may be preferred over normal saline (0.9%). If hypoalbuminemic, consider albumin replacement. If hemoglobin less than 10 mg/dL, consider blood transfusion. Fresh frozen plasma or vitamin K may be ordered for coagulopathy.
Inotropic	When hypotension predominates, consider vasopressor therapy. When poor tissue perfusion predominates, consider dobutamine therapy to increase cardiac output.
Respiratory	If PaO₂ is less than 60 mmHg in the presence of high oxygen concentration, and/or respiratory rate is greater than 30/min, consider early intubation and mechanical ventilation with sedation and analgesia.
Renal	In the presence of impaired renal function, timely and adequate fluid resuscitation and respiratory support are essential to prevent permanent damage; some form of dialysis may be required.
Nutritional	Once hemodynamic stability has been achieved, nasojejunal enteral feeding is initiated. Total parenteral nutrition (TPN) is used when enteral feedings are not tolerated and nutritional support is needed. Monitor serum glucose closely, maintaining levels at approximately 150 mg/dL if possible. High doses of insulin may be necessary because of severe insulin resistance.

SOURCE: Data from Fitzpatrick (2014); Maheshwari & Subramanian (2016); and Tenner et al. (2013).

Goal 1: Stabilize the Patient's Hemodynamic Status
Hypovolemia must be identified and treated aggressively. Especially in the early phase of the illness, aggressive fluid resuscitation is critically important to provide micro- and macrocirculatory support. Hemodynamic stability is accomplished primarily through two types of interventions: fluid resuscitation and inotropic therapy. Fluid resuscitation includes crystalloids, plasma expanders, and possibly colloids. Fluid resuscitation should be enough to maintain hemodynamic stability, which is usually an initial several-liter fluid bolus followed by 250 to 500 mL/hour continuous infusion (Gardner & Berk, 2016). It is essential to closely monitor the patient's hemodynamic status as treatment progresses, with careful attention to signs of overhydration, such as pulmonary edema causing hypoxia. Hemodynamic status monitoring might include the following:

- Blood pressure, respiratory rate, pulse, and temperature
- Oxygen saturation
- Blood gas analysis for labored respirations or hypotension unrelieved with fluid bolus
- Pulmonary artery pressure
- Pulmonary artery wedge pressure
- Central venous pressure
- Cardiac output, cardiac index
- Intake and output (hourly), daily weights (to reflect fluid status)
- Hematocrit, serum blood urea nitrogen (BUN) levels, and creatinine

Goal 2: Control the Patient's Pain   Acute pancreatitis can be extremely painful. Controlling the level of pain is essential for comfort and to decrease secretion of pancreatic enzymes. Morphine has been theoretically implicated in increasing pressure in the sphincter of Oddi and potentially decreasing pancreatic and biliary flow into the small bowel,

but no studies confirm this (Ona, Comas, & Urrutia, 2013). There is no evidence to suggest an advantage of any particular type of medication (Fitzpatrick, 2014). Fentanyl, morphine, and hydromorphone remain effective pain relievers for patients with acute pancreatitis (Valsangkar & Thayer, 2014). Opiates are usually administered every 2 to 4 hours. Patients with severe pain who cannot take medications orally require the parenteral route of administration. Alternatively, a patient-controlled analgesia pump may be used.

Meperidine is not considered a drug of choice. Its major metabolite, normeperidine, can accumulate in the body and is neurotoxic, particularly in high-dose, long-term use in older adults and patients with reduced renal function. The neuroexcitatory toxic effects can cause central nervous system (CNS) irritability and seizures (Fitzpatrick, 2014). In addition, meperidine is known to interact with many drugs that may cause excessive and prolonged CNS depression, convulsions, or increased sedation (Wilson, Shannon, & Shields, 2016).

Goal 3: Minimize Pancreatic Stimulation   It is important to reduce the stimulation of pancreatic secretion as much as possible. Keeping the GI tract at rest minimizes pancreatic secretion and reduces pain. Organ rest needs to continue until serum amylase levels have returned to normal and pain has subsided. In mild pancreatitis, oral intake may be restored in 2 to 7 days, and nutritional support is not needed. In more severe cases, this may take up to 7 weeks. The supervising healthcare provider may order the following:

- Initial nothing-by-mouth (NPO) status
- Intravenous fluid hydration
- Placement of a nasogastric tube to intermittent suction (in the presence of paralytic ileus and/or frequent vomiting)
- Drug therapy, such as antacids, proton pump inhibitors, or anticholinergics (anticholinergics reduce GI motility)

Patients who are experiencing acute pancreatitis are especially hypermetabolic and hypercatabolic. They have extremely high nutritional demands but are often unable to consume nutrients orally for a prolonged period. Nutritional support is essential to improving the patient's outcome.

Enteral nutrition has been found to improve outcomes by decreasing the rate of systemic infection, need for surgical intervention, mortality rate, hospital length of stay, and multiple organ failure (Al-Omran, Albalawi, Tashkandi, & Al Ansary, 2010; Olah & Romics, 2014). Placing or maintaining a nasojejunal tube may be difficult and poorly tolerated in some patients so TPN should be used in these select cases. Nutritional support should be considered if oral nutrition is unlikely to resume within 5 days. Once abdominal pain has resolved and the patient regains an appetite, oral feedings can be reintroduced.

Goal 4: Provide Psychosocial Support Acute pancreatitis can be an anxiety-producing, extremely painful experience with an unpredictable outcome; and depending on the severity, the patient may require admission to a critical care unit. Survival of severe acute pancreatitis is associated with increased morbidity and mortality (Vipperla et al., 2014) and a decreased quality of life (Amann, Yadav, & Barmada, 2013; Balliet et al., 2012) related to continuing pancreatic dysfunction. The nurse should assess (and periodically reassess) the psychosocial needs of the patient and family throughout the hospitalization period. Based on the assessment, a multidisciplinary plan of care should be developed, initiated, and evaluated, making adjustments as required. Patient and family education should be ongoing and include simple explanations of the disease process, diagnostic procedures, and therapies. Family members usually desire frequent, simple updates on patient status and may benefit from assisting with basic patient care needs. Once the crisis has passed, patients with reversible risk factors, such as alcohol abuse or hypertriglyceridemia, should receive additional education about the risk factors and ways to decrease their risk of future episodes.

Curative Therapy

Curative therapies focus on relieving the underlying cause and preventing complications or aggressively treating any existing complications.

Goal 5: Correct the Underlying Problem Generally, medical interventions are more desirable than surgical ones. Some triggering events, such as binge alcohol abuse, may subside spontaneously if given sufficient rest time using supportive therapy. If the etiology is mechanical, however, the underlying problem can be corrected surgically. For example, if a patient has a biliary obstruction, such as a gallstone, a cholecystectomy may be performed to relieve the obstruction. Certain surgical procedures to relieve obstructions can be performed during an ERCP. Drug-induced acute pancreatitis should be considered after other etiologies are excluded. A high index of suspicion and a detailed medication history are crucial (Nesvaderani, Eslick, & Cox, 2015).

Goal 6: Prevent or Treat Complications It is imperative that complications be recognized early in their development and then treated aggressively. Close patient monitoring is a crucial part of meeting this goal. Medical interventions are based on correcting or supporting system complications as they develop. In addition to the various supportive therapies listed in Table 24–5, any of the following may be needed:

- Electrolyte replacement
- Insulin therapy
- Antibiotic therapy
- Antisecretory therapy with octreotide
- Arterial blood gases
- Oxygen therapy
- Pulmonary hygiene (e.g., incentive spirometry)
- Radiographic studies
- Cardiac monitoring
- Pulmonary artery flow-directed or central venous catheter
- Intra-abdominal pressure monitoring

CT-guided percutaneous aspiration with Gram stain and culture may be done when infected necrosis is suspected. Surgical drainage or debridement may be indicated if the patient develops infected pancreatic necrosis and is best accomplished using minimal invasive techniques if possible (Bell et al., 2015). Surgical incisions of pancreatic tissue may lead to the development of pancreatic fistulas, which can result in the entry of pancreatic juice into other tissues, causing further damage and new complications. Patients with subtotal or total pancreatic necrosis usually require a proton pump inhibitor on a daily basis as the bicarbonate secretion of the pancreas is severely diminished, putting the patient at risk for a duodenal ulcer.

Section Five Review

1. What is the highest priority in the management of a client with severe acute pancreatitis?
   A. Controlling pain
   B. Stabilizing hemodynamic status
   C. Minimizing pancreatic stimulation
   D. Correcting the underlying problem

2. Pain management of the client with acute pancreatitis would include which drug?
   A. Morphine sulfate
   B. Codeine
   C. Meperidine
   D. Ibuprofen

3. Anticholinergics may be ordered for the client with acute pancreatitis for which purpose?
   A. Reducing GI motility
   B. Reducing pain
   C. Increasing pancreatic stimulation
   D. Increasing gastric pH

4. The effective management of complications depends on which actions? (Select all that apply.)
   A. Close monitoring
   B. Early recognition
   C. Aggressive treatment
   D. Age of the client

Answers: 1. B, 2. A, 3. A, 4. A

Section Six: Nursing Care of the Patient with Acute Pancreatitis

Patients with acute pancreatic dysfunction experience a variety of signs and symptoms due to the systemic involvement of this condition. The following is a list of some of these systemic complications (Wilkinson & Barcus, 2017).

- *Cardiac output is decreased* due to circulating myocardial depressant factor, hypovolemia, vasodilation, abdominal compartment syndrome (ACS), and SIRS.

- *Hypovolemia* is common due to vomiting, decreased fluid intake, fever, diaphoresis, and fluid shifts that occur with SIRS.

- *Oxygenation and gas exchange* can be impacted due to abdominal pain with respiratory depressant effects of opioid therapy, decreased lung expansion, and inflammatory changes at the lung tissue level. These patients are at increased risk for development of acute respiratory distress syndrome (ARDS).

- *Acute epigastric or abdominal pain* is common and is due to irritation and edema of the inflamed pancreas, localized peritonitis, pancreatic capsule distention, and nasogastric suction (refer to the "Related Pharmacotherapy: Agents Used to Control Pain in Acute Pancreatitis" feature).

- *Nausea and vomiting* are related to stimulation of the vomiting center.

- *Impaired nutritional intake* is due to nausea, vomiting, anorexia, and impaired digestion secondary to decreased pancreatic enzymes and increased needs as a result of acute illness

- *Increased risk for infection* is from infected pancreatic necrosis and abscess formation, peritonitis, and sepsis.

- *Anxiety* is commonly related to acute illness; unfamiliar environment; discomfort; lack of understanding of diagnosis, diagnostic tests, and interventions; and fear of death.

- *Patient is at increased risk for injury* related to hypoxia, infection, hemorrhage, shock, encephalopathy, and acute tubular necrosis.

- *Electrolyte imbalance* is common and is related to vomiting, fluid imbalances, fat necrosis, and insufficient fluid and nutritional intake.

Nursing care of the patient with acute pancreatitis includes frequent focused assessments for the earliest signs

Related Pharmacotherapy
Agents Used to Control Pain in Acute Pancreatitis

Opioid Analgesics

Morphine
Hydromorphone (Dilaudid)
Fentanyl (Sublimaze)

Actions and Uses
Bind with opiate receptors in the central nervous system, altering the patient's perception of and emotional response to pain.

Dosages (Adult)
Morphine (IV): 2.5–15 mg/70 kg every 2–4 hrs or 0.8–10 mg/hr using controlled infusion device. If direct IV bolus: administer over 4–5 min.
Hydromorphone (IV): 1–2 mg every 2–3 hrs as needed. PCA: 0.2–0.4 mg by demand dose with lock out.
Fentanyl (IV): 50–100 mcg. If direct IV injection: administer over 3–5 min.

Major Adverse Effects
Most common: sedation, constipation, nausea
Potentially life-threatening: respiratory or cardiac depression or arrest

Nursing Implications
Monitor vital signs, respiratory rate and depth, level of sedation, and bowel function.
Pain associated with severe acute pancreatitis can be severe and intractable, making pain control difficult to attain.
Meperidine is avoided because of its toxic metabolites with their potentially severe adverse effects (seizures) but may be considered if patient is allergic to other opioids.
Be knowledgeable of equianalgesic dosing of these medications.
Reassess patient's response to analgesic within 30 to 60 minutes after administration.
Patient's ability to correctly use a patient-controlled analgesia (PCA) mechanism should be closely evaluated before this option is chosen. Critical illness may prevent appropriate use.

SOURCE: Based on Wilson et al. (2016).

and symptoms of the many potential complications identified in Section Four. Any increase in the patient's symptoms or the development of new abnormal findings is immediately communicated in a collaborative manner to other healthcare providers.

Nursing care is also impacted by the cause of the episode of acute pancreatitis. Prevention of the development of chronic pancreatitis and future episodes relies on the continuum of care. Patients whose acute pancreatitis is related to alcohol abuse are referred for alcohol cessation counseling. Patients whose acute pancreatitis is related to gallstones receive surgical consults and may undergo surgery during the current admission when the acute episode has resolved. Patients with drug-induced acute pancreatitis should be educated to avoid the causative medication when determined. Other causes of pancreatitis often require follow-up after resolution of the acute episode.

Nursing management of the patient experiencing an acute pancreatic dysfunction episode is summarized in the "Nursing Care: The Patient with Acute Pancreatitis" feature.

Nursing Care
The Patient with Acute Pancreatitis

Outcome 1: Optimize cardiac output

Assess and compare to established norms, patient baselines, and trends.

Intake and output, blood pressure, pulse; cardiac output, cardiac index, central venous pressure; daily weight; pulmonary artery wedge pressure

Abdominal compartment syndrome monitoring

Administer related drug therapy and monitor for therapeutic effects.

Intravenous fluids
Vasopressors
Inotropic drugs

Related interventions

Maintain oxygen therapy.
Position in semi to high Fowler position.
Assist patient to rest and conserve energy.
Avoid activities that create a Valsalva response.

Outcome 2: Optimize respiratory status

Assess and compare to established norms, patient baselines, and trends.

Respiratory rate, rhythm, and depth; lung sounds; coloring of mucous membranes and skin

Arterial blood gases; SpO2; mental status

Administer related drug therapy and monitor for therapeutic effects.

Oxygen therapy as ordered

Related interventions

Encourage use of incentive spirometer, ambulate as tolerated.
Provide suction when needed.
Turn every 2 hours.
Manage ventilatory support as needed.

Outcome 3: Fluid and electrolyte balance

Assess and compare to established norms, patient baselines, and trends.

Intake and output, blood pressure, pulse, breath sounds, daily weights, restlessness

Serum electrolyte levels

Administer related drug therapy and monitor for therapeutic effects.

Intravenous fluids
Electrolyte replacements as ordered

Related interventions

Monitor intake and output
Monitor cardiac output

Outcome 4: Pain control or relief of pain

Assess and compare to established norms, patient baselines, and trends.

Level of pain on pain rating scale

Administer related drug therapy and monitor for therapeutic effects.

Analgesics as ordered (refer to the "Related Pharmacotherapy: Agents Used to Control Pain in Acute Pancreatitis" feature for additional information)

Related interventions

Give nothing by mouth (NPO) during acute phase.
Assist the patient to use pain rating scale accurately.
Careful positioning of patient with head of bed elevated to semi-Fowler position and knees bent may help alleviate pain.
Support the patient's use of nonpharmacologic methods to control pain, such as relaxation, distraction, and imagery.

Outcome 5: Relief of nausea and vomiting

Assess and compare to established norms, patient baselines, and trends.

Nausea, vomiting, and dry heaves

Administer related drug therapy and monitor for therapeutic effects.

Antiemetic therapy
Pain medicine

Related interventions

Prevent or relieve gastric distention, nasogastric tube care as needed.
Restrict oral intake, NPO as needed.
Encourage deep slow breathing, change positions slowly, frequent oral hygiene.

Outcome 6: Optimize nutrition

Assess and compare to established norms, patient baselines, and trends.

Daily weights, serum albumin, prealbumin, serum total protein
Monitor for ileus formation; bowel sounds

Administer related drug therapy and monitor for therapeutic effects.

Parenteral or enteral feeding as indicated (feeding tube tip should be located below the ligament of Treitz)
Antiemetics as needed

Related interventions

Obtain nutrition consult.
Monitor patient response to each step in diet progression.

Emerging Evidence

- Prealbumin has been used as an indication of nutritional condition and the need for enteral nutrition. In a study of 101 patients with mild acute pancreatitis and 68 patients with severe acute pancreatitis, the authors looked at the combination of prealbumin and fibrinogen as a prealbumin/fibrinogen marker as a predictor of severity of acute pancreatitis. It was found that the prealbumin/fibrinogen ratio was decreased in patients with severe acute pancreatitis and therefore a high predictive value for severity of disease. The conclusion to the study was that "The prealbumin/fibrinogen ratio is a promising predictor of AP severity and prognosis" (*Yue et al., 2015*).
- Researchers investigated the contribution of smoking and alcohol intake on the risk of developing chronic pancreatitis (CP). Consecutive patients with CP who underwent secretin-enhanced magnetic resonance cholangiopancreatography were compared with consecutive patients without pancreatic disease who underwent secretin-enhanced magnetic resonance cholangiopancreatography for irritable bowel syndrome. Included in the study were 145 consecutive CP patients and 103 irritable bowel syndrome patients from 2010 to 2014. The authors confirmed in an Italian population that smoking and alcohol were co-factors in the development of CP. This study shows that alcohol intake and smoking habits are two of the most important risk factors for the development of CP (*Di Leo et al., 2017*).
- Researchers conducted a systematic review of randomized controlled trials to assess the benefits and harms of duodenum-preserving pancreatic head resection (DPPHR) versus pancreaticoduodenectomy (PD) in people with chronic pancreatitis for whom pancreatic resection is considered the main treatment option. Low-quality evidence suggested that DPPHR may result in shorter hospital stays than PD. Based on low- or very low-quality evidence, there is currently no evidence of any difference in the mortality, adverse events, or quality of life between DPPHR and PD (*Gurasamy, Lusuku, Halkias, & Davidson, 2016*).
- In a retrospective cohort study of 16,709 subjects aged 20 to 84 as the pneumococcal pneumonia group, and 66,836 subjects without a history of pneumonia as the non-pneumonia group, the authors found a 51% increased incidence of acute pancreatitis in patients who had pneumococcal pneumonia when compared to those who did not have pneumococcal pneumonia with a highest risk beginning in the first 3 months after diagnosis (*Lai, Lin, Liao, & Ma, 2015*).

Section Six Review

1. A nurse planning care for a client with acute pancreatitis will monitor closely for which problems? (Select all that apply.)
   A. Autonomic dysreflexia
   B. Electrolyte imbalances
   C. Inability to swallow
   D. Fluid volume decrease
   E. Cardiac output decrease

2. In developing a plan of care for the client with acute pancreatitis, the nurse plans to closely monitor respiratory status. Which factors may result in respiratory depression in this client? (Select all that apply.)
   A. Effects of pain medication
   B. Decreased lung expansion
   C. Paralysis of the diaphragm
   D. Inflammatory changes in the lung
   E. Hemorrhage into the pleural cavity

3. Which intervention would the nurse plan to treat the epigastric pain of a client in the acute phase of pancreatitis?
   A. Offering nothing by mouth
   B. Encouraging a soft-food diet
   C. Monitoring for therapeutic effects of gastric acid reduction
   D. Encouraging the client to assume a prone position to reduce pain

4. A nurse providing care for a client with acute pancreatitis is intervening to optimize the client's cardiac output. The nurse assists the client to assume which position?
   A. Prone in bed
   B. Left lateral recumbent with bed flat
   C. Semi to high Fowler
   D. Supine

Answers: 1. A, 2. (A, B, D), 3. A, 4. C

Clinical Reasoning Checkpoint

T. B., a 36-year-old male, arrives in the emergency department with complaints of acute-onset mid-epigastric pain that developed 24 hours ago. He describes his pain as sharp, radiating to his midback, and he rates it as a 9 on a 1–10 point scale, with 10 being the worst possible pain. The pain has been constant, unrelieved by position changes or ibuprofen. He is currently vomiting large amounts of bilious-looking fluid. T. B.'s medical history includes hypertension, for which he takes a thiazide diuretic. He reports drinking a couple of alcoholic cocktails per day, usually in the evening when he returns home from his job as a stockbroker. Physical exam findings are as follows:

- HR 142/min, BP 96/45, RR 32/min (light bibasilar crackles), and temp 37.8°C (100°F)
- SpO$_2$ 90%
- Abdomen tender to palpation, noticeably distended, diminished bowel sounds
- Intermittent nausea with vomiting

1. What risk factors does T. B. have for the development of pancreatitis?

Clinical update: Normal saline 0.9% infusion is administered at 150 mL/hr. His respiratory rate is 24/minute. Oxygen therapy is initiated at 2 L/min. Laboratory results are as follows:

- Amylase – 700 units/L
- Lipase – 1300 units/L
- WBC – 22,000/mm^3
- Ionized calcium – 3.1 mg/dL
- Potassium – 3.1 mEq/L
- BUN – 22 mg/dL

He is sent for a stat CT scan, and the results reveal that he probably has a biliary tract obstruction due to a gallstone. An abdominal ultrasound reveals that he has two large gallstones and retroperitoneal fluid collection consistent with biliary tract disease. He is transferred to an ICU because of his borderline hemodynamic status.

2. What is the rationale for the development of his borderline hemodynamic status?

Clinical update: On admission to the ICU, T. B. rapidly deteriorates, becoming hypotensive with a BP of 70/40, tachycardic with HR 192; his urine output decreases to less than 20 mL/hour. His SpO$_2$ continues to decrease despite supplemental oxygen delivered at 100% non-rebreather mask. An ABG is obtained with the following results: pH 7.30, PCO$_2$ 55, PaO$_2$ 52, SaO$_2$ 78%. A stat chest x-ray confirms a large pleural effusion with atelectasis. His shortness of breath worsens.

3. Based on his latest clinical update, what complications are occurring with T. B.?

4. What interventions are needed at this time?

Clinical update: Three days later, T. B. is still intubated, requiring mechanical ventilation. His hypoxia has worsened. His ventilator settings are as follows: TV 600, AC mode at a rate of 16, FiO$_2$ 100%, and PEEP 12 cm H$_2$O. His chest x-ray shows fluffy, white, bilateral infiltrates. He has a fever and elevated WBC and required deep sedation to keep his SvO$_2$ greater than 60%.

5. Based on these latest data, what complications is T. B. now experiencing?

6. What additional complications is he at risk for developing?

Chapter 24 Review

1. A 48-year-old woman has just been diagnosed with hemorrhagic pancreatitis. Which statement by the nurse is most accurate?
   1. "You will be over this problem in less than a week."
   2. "You will get well very quickly once the correct antibiotics are prescribed."
   3. "You may feel sick for a month or more, but no one dies from this disorder."
   4. "A common cause of this problem in women is gallbladder disease."

2. A client has experienced intermittent abdominal pain for the last 6 months and is being evaluated for possible pancreatitis. The nurse would expect serial serum lipase levels to be drawn rather than serum amylase levels for which reason?
   1. Serum lipase levels are more accurate.
   2. Serum lipase is more sensitive to pancreatitis.
   3. Serum lipase remains elevated for a longer period.
   4. Serum lipase requires no special analysis technique.

3. A client is being admitted to the hospital for treatment of hemorrhagic pancreatitis. The emergency department report indicates that the client has a positive Cullen sign. The nurse admitting the client would look for which manifestation?

   1. Decreased bowel sounds in the left upper quadrant
   2. Bruising over the high epigastric area
   3. Bluish discoloration around the umbilicus
   4. Decreased deep tendon reflexes in the lower extremities

4. The nurse is writing a plan of care for a client who was just admitted with acute pancreatitis. The nurse would include monitoring for which major pulmonary complications? (Select all that apply.)
   1. Influenza
   2. Pleural effusion
   3. Hypoxia
   4. Respiratory failure
   5. Pneumonia

5. Which intervention would the nurse expect to perform as the initial step in the medical management of severe acute pancreatitis?
   1. Administering pain medication every 2–4 hours
   2. Maintaining NPO status
   3. Giving IV fluids at 250 mL/hr
   4. Preparing the client for surgery

6. The nurse closely observes a client admitted with acute pancreatitis for respiratory complications related to ineffectiveness of breathing pattern. Which situations will increase the client's risk for this problem? (Select all that apply.)

   1. The client's abdominal pain is severe and difficult to manage.
   2. The client has a history of hepatitis C.
   3. The client is taking opioids for pain relief.
   4. The client's diaphragmatic excursion is diminished.
   5. The client's position of comfort is sitting up in bed.

7. A client is scheduled for an ERCP. Which information should the nurse provide for the client? (Select all that apply.)

   1. The procedure is not invasive.
   2. A radiographic contrast media will be injected.
   3. The procedure will be performed at the bedside under local anesthesia.
   4. The procedure provides access to both the gallbladder and the pancreas.
   5. There is a chance that mechanical obstructions can be removed during the test.

8. The nurse is concerned that a client diagnosed with pancreatitis may be developing hypocalcemia. How would the nurse perform the Chvostek sign to check for this complication?

   1. Tap the client's facial nerve in front of the ear.
   2. Perform deep palpation over the lower half of the client's abdomen.
   3. Inflate a blood pressure cuff placed on the client's upper arm.
   4. Check for a bluish discoloration on the flank.

9. A client who has been diagnosed with acute pancreatitis states, "I'm not a drinker, and I have never had problems with my gallbladder. Why did I end up having a problem with my pancreas?" Which other etiologies for pancreatitis should the nurse consider before responding?

   1. Using chewing tobacco
   2. Taking some prescription medications
   3. Being significantly underweight
   4. Drinking large amounts of carbonated beverages

10. A client who was admitted for treatment of pancreatitis 3 days ago continues to have very severe pain and nausea. An MRI done today reveals a pancreatic abscess. How does the nurse interpret this information?

   1. The client will be taken off the proton pump inhibitor.
   2. This client's risk for death is greatly increased.
   3. After the abscess is drained, the client will recover quickly.
   4. A pseudocyst is likely also present.

Answers to questions found inside your textbook are available on the faculty resources site. Please consult with your instructor.

References

Akbarshahi, H., Rosendahl, A. H., Westergren-Thorsson, G., & Andersson, R. (2012). Acute lung injury in acute pancreatitis—awaiting the big leap. *Respiratory Medicine, 106*(9), 1199–1210.

Al-Omran, M., Albalawi, Z. H., Tashkandi, M. F., & Al Ansary, L. A. (2010). Enteral versus parenteral nutrition for acute pancreatitis. *Cochrane Database of Systematic Reviews, 1,* CD002837.

Amann, S. T., Yadav, D., & Barmada, M. (2013). Physical and mental quality of life in chronic pancreatitis: A case-control study from North American Pancreatitis Study 2 cohort. *Pancreas, 42*(2), 293–300.

Balliet, W. E., Edwards-Hampton, S., Borckardt, J. J., Morgan, K., Adams, D., Owczarski, S., . . . Malcolm, R. (2012). Depressive symptoms, pain, and quality of life among nonalcohol-related chronic pancreatitis. *Pain Research and Treatment*. Retrieved April 23, 2017, at https://www.hindawi.com/journals/prt/2012/978646. doi:10.1155/2012/978646

Balthazar, E. J., Ranson, J. H., Naidich, D. P., Megibow, A. J., Caccavale, R., & Cooper, M. M. (1985). Acute pancreatitis: The role of imaging in diagnosis and management. *Radiology, 16,* 767–772.

Banks, P. A., Bollen, T. L., Dervenis, C., Gooszen, H. G., Johnson, C. D., Sarr, M. G., . . . Vege, S. S. (2013). Classifications of acute pancreatitis–2012: Revision of the Atlanta Classification and Definitions by International Consensus. *Gut, 62,* 102–111.

Bell, D., Keane, M. G., & Pereira, S. P. (2015). Acute pancreatitis. *Medicine, 43*(3), 174–181.

Besselink, M., van Santvoort, H., & Gooszen, H. G. (2013). Acute pancreatitis. In C. J. Yeo, J. B. Matthews, D. W. McFadden, J. H. Pemberton, & J. H. Peters, *Shackelford's surgery of the alimentary tract* (7th ed.). Philadelphia, PA: Elsevier Saunders.

Bollen, T. L., Singh, V. K., Maurer, R., Repas, K., van Es, H. W., Banks, P. A., & Mortele, K. J. (2012). A comparative evaluation of radiologic and clinical scoring systems in the early prediction of severity in acute pancreatitis. *American Journal of Gastroenterology, 107*(4), 612–619. doi:10.1038/ajg.2011.438

Brown, L. A., Hore, T. A., Phillips, A. R. J., Windsor, J. A., & Petrov, M. S. (2014). A systematic review of the extra-pancreatic infectious complications in acute pancreatitis. *Pancreatology, 14*(6), 436–443.

Cho, J. H., Kim, T. N., & Kim, S. B. (2015). Comparison of clinical course and outcome of acute pancreatitis according to the two main etiologies: Alcohol and gallstone. *BMC Gastroenterology, 15*(1), 87–93.

Conwell, D. L., Banks, P., & Greenberger, N. J. (2015). Acute and chronic pancreatitis. In D. L. Kasper, A. S. Fauci, S. L. Hauser, D. L. Longo, J. L. Jameson, & J. L. Loscalzo (Eds.), *Harrison's principles of internal medicine* (19th ed.). New York, NY: McGraw Hill Education.

Cucher, D., Kulvatunyou, N., Green, D. J., Jie, T., & Ong, E. S. (2014). Gallstone pancreatitis: A review. *Surgical Clinics of North America, 94*(2), 257–280.

De Waele, J. J. (2014). Acute pancreatitis. *Current Opinion in Critical Care, 20*(2), 189–195.

Di Leo, M., Leandro, G., Singh, S. K., Mariani, A., Bianco, M., Zuppardo, R. A., . . . Cavestro, G. M. (2017). Low alcohol and cigarette use is associated to the risk of developing chronic pancreatitis. *Pancreas, 46*(2), 225–229.

Dooley, N., Hew, S., & Nichol, A. (2015). Acute pancreatitis: An intensive care perspective. *Anaesthesia and Intensive Care Medicine, 16*(4), 191–196. http://dx.doi.org/10.1016/j.mpaic.2015.01.017

Ducarme, G., Maire, F., Chatel, P., Luton, D., & Hammel, P. (2014). Acute pancreatitis during pregnancy: A review. *Journal of Perinatology, 34*(2), 87–94.

Dupuis, C. S., Baptista, V., Whalen, G., Karam, A. R., Singh, A., Wassef, W., & Kim, Y. H. (2013). Diagnosis and management of acute pancreatitis and its complications. *Gastrointestinal Intervention, 2*(1), 36–46.

Fitzpatrick, E. (2014). Assessment and management of patients with biliary disorders. In J. L. Hinkle & K. H. Cheever (Eds.), *Brunner & Suddarth's textbook of medical-surgical nursing* (13th ed.). Philadelphia, PA: Wolters Kluwer, Lippincott Williams & Wilkins.

Gardner, T. B., & Berk, B. S. (2016). Acute pancreatitis. *Medscape: Drugs & Diseases, Gastroenterology.* Retrieved January 27, 2017, from http://emedicine.medscape.com/article/181364-overview#a3

Gurasamy, K. S., Lusuku, C., Halkias, C., & Davidson, B. R. (2016). Duodenum-preserving pancreatic resection versus pancreatic duodenectomy for chronic pancreatitis. *Cochrane Database of Systematic Reviews, 2,* CD011521. doi:10.1002/14651858.CD011521

Kee, J. L. (2014). *Laboratory and diagnostic tests with nursing implications* (9th ed.). Hoboken, NJ: Pearson.

Kuo, D. C., Rider, A. C., Estrada, P., Kim, D., & Pillow, M. T. (2015). Acute pancreatitis: What's the score? *Journal of Emergency Medicine, 48*(6), 762–770.

Lai, S.-W., Lin, C.-L., Liao, K.-F., & Ma, C.-L. (2015). Increased risk of acute pancreatitis following pneumococcal pneumonia: A nationwide cohort study. *International Journal of Clinical Practice, 69*(5), 611–617.

Lankisch, P. G., Apte, M., & Banks, P. A. (2015). Acute pancreatitis. *The Lancet, 386*(9988), 85–96. doi:10.1016/S0140-6736(14)60649-8

Levi, M. M., Nagalla, S., & Schmaier, A. H. (2015). Disseminated intravascular coagulation. Retrieved May 9, 2017, from http://emedicine.medscape.com/article/199627-overview

Lipsett, P. A. (2011). Acute pancreatitis. In J-L. Vincent, E. Abraham, P. Kochanek, F. A. Moore, & M. P. Fink, *Textbook of critical care* (6th ed.). Philadelphia, PA: Elsevier Saunders.

Maheshwari, R., & Subramanian, R. M. (2016). Severe acute pancreatitis and necrotizing pancreatitis. *Critical Care Clinics, 32*(2), 279–290.

Malledant, Y., Malbrain, M. L., & Reuter, D. A. (2015). What's new in the management of severe acute pancreatitis? *Intensive Care Medicine, 41*(11), 1957–1960.

Nesvaderani, M., Eslick, G. D., & Cox, M. R. (2015). Acute pancreatitis: Update on management. *Medical Journal of Australia, 202*(8), 420–423.

Olah, A., & Romics, L. (2014). Enteral nutrition in acute pancreatitis: A review of the current evidence. *World Journal of Gastroenterology, 20*(43), 16,123–16,131.

Ona, X. B., Comas, D. R., & Urrutia, G. (2013). Opioids for acute pancreatitis pain. *Cochrane Database of Systematic Reviews, 7,* CD009179. doi:10.1002/14651858.CD009179.pub2

Park, J. Y., Jeon, T. J., Ha, T. H., Hwang, J. T., Sinn, D. H., Oh, T.-H., . . . Choi, W.-C. (2013). Bedside index for severity in acute pancreatitis: Comparison with other scoring systems in predicting severity and organ failure. *Hepatobiliary and Pancreatic Diseases International, 12*(6), 645–650.

Premkumar, R., Phillips, A. R. J., Petrov, M. S., & Windsor, J. A. (2015). The clinical relevance of obesity in acute pancreatitis: Targeted systematic reviews. *Pancreatology, 15*(1), 25–33.

Quinlan, J. D. (2014). Acute pancreatitis. *American Family Physician, 90*(9), 632–639.

Ranson, J. H., Rifkind, K. M., Roses, D. F., Fink, S. D., Eng, K., & Spencer, F. C. (1974). Prognostic signs and the role of operative management in acute pancreatitis. *Surgery, Gynecology & Obstetrics, 139*(1), 69–81.

Sarr, M. G., Banks, P. A., Bollen, T. L., Dervenis, C., Gooszen, H. G., Johnson, . . . Vege, S. S. (2013). The new revised classification of acute pancreatitis 2012. *Surgical Clinics of North America, 93*(3), 549–562.

Schub, T., & Kornusky, J. (2015). Acute pancreatitis. CINAHL Nursing Guide. Retrieved from http://web.a.ebscohost.com/nrc/detail?vid=4&sid=c0ed90eb-fa14-4c66-91ce-b5e3b2a42e6b%40sessionmgr4002&hid=4204&bdata=JnNpdGU9bnJjLWxpdmUmc2NvcGU9c2l0ZQ%3d%3d#AN=T700324&db=nrc

Stevenson, K., & Carter, C. R. (2013). Acute pancreatitis. *Surgery, 31*(6), 295–303.

Talukdar, R., & Vege, S. S. (2015). Acute pancreatitis. *Current Opinion in Gastroenterology, 31*(5), 374–379.

Tenner, S., Baillie, J., DeWitt, J., & Vege, S. S. (2013). American College of Gastroenterology guideline: Management of acute pancreatitis. *American Journal of Gastroenterology, 108*(9), 1400–1415.

Upchurch, E. (2014). Local complications of acute pancreatitis. *British Journal of Hospital Medicine, 75*(12), 698–702.

Valsangkar, N., & Thayer, S. P. (2014). Acute pancreatitis. In J. L. Cameron & A. M. Cameron (Eds.), *Current Surgical Therapy* (11th ed.). Philadelphia, PA: Elsevier Saunders.

Vipperla, K., Papachristou, G. I., Easler, J., Muddana, V., Slivka, A., Whitcomb, D. C., & Yadav, D. (2014). Risk of and factors associated with readmission after a sentinel attack of acute pancreatitis. *Clinical Gastroenterology and Hepatology, 12*(11), 1911–1919.

Wilkinson, J. M., & Barcus, L. (2017). *Pearson nursing diagnosis handbook* (11th ed.). New York, NY: Pearson Education.

Wilson, B. A., Shannon, M. T., & Shields, K. T. (2016). *Pearson nurse's drug guide.* New York, NY: Pearson.

Working Group IAP/APA. (2013). IAP/APA evidence-based guidelines for the management of acute pancreatitis. *Pancreatology, 13*(4 Suppl 2), e1–e15.

Wu, B. U., & Banks, P. A. (2013). Clinical management of patients with acute pancreatitis. *Gastroenterology, 144*(6), 1272–1281.

Yue, W., Liu, Y., Ding, W., Jiang, W., Huang, J., Zhang, J., & Liu, J. (2015). The predictive value of the prealbumin-to-fibrinogen ratio in patients with acute pancreatitis. *International Journal of Clinical Practice, 69*(10), 1121–1128.

Chapter 25
Determinants and Assessment of Fluid and Electrolyte Balance

▽ Learning Outcomes

25.1 Discuss the composition and distribution of body fluids.

25.2 Describe the roles of the nervous and endocrine systems in the regulation of fluid balance.

25.3 Demonstrate assessment of the fluid status in high-acuity patients.

25.4 Compare and contrast the electrolytes sodium, chloride, calcium, potassium, magnesium, and phosphorus/phosphate.

25.5 Demonstrate assessment of the electrolyte balance in high-acuity patients.

aintenance of fluid and electrolyte balance is a major goal in improving the outcomes of high-acuity patients with complex health problems. Nurses monitor high-acuity patients for actual or potential alterations in fluid and electrolyte balance. This requires an understanding of the physiologic mechanisms that maintain fluid and electrolyte balance. Nursing observations are then interpreted within the context of the patient's history and pathological condition to determine if an alteration in fluid and electrolyte balance exists, and if so, to what degree. The high-acuity nurse uses critical thinking skills to determine the appropriate nursing action; this includes determining when a healthcare provider must be notified.

Section One: Body Fluid Composition and Distribution

Body fluids compose about 60% of body weight in the average adult male and about 50% in the adult female. The composition of body fluids is primarily water with electrolytes, glucose, urea, and creatinine. These fluids provide both an internal and external environment for the cells, playing crucial roles as a medium for metabolic reactions, a cushion to protect body parts from injury, and an influence on the regulation of body heat.

Total body water content is affected by age, gender, and body fat content. The percentage of body water decreases with advancing age. A greater percentage of body fluids is found in individuals with a small body surface area. The older adult's fluid balance is affected by alterations in thirst and nutritional intake, diminished renal function, chronic illness, and medications. The older adult is predisposed to developing fluid volume deficit related to decreased muscle mass, increased fat stores, and a reduction in the percentage of body fluids. Fat cells contain little water; therefore, obese individuals have a lower percentage of total body water. Women tend to have more body fat than men and therefore a lower percentage of total body water.

Fluid Compartments

Body fluids are found primarily in two compartments: the **intracellular** compartment (within cells) and the **extracellular** compartment (outside of cells) (Figure 25–1). Extracellular fluid is further divided into intravascular fluid (plasma within blood vessels), interstitial fluid (fluid that lies between cells or tissues), and transcellular fluid (cerebral

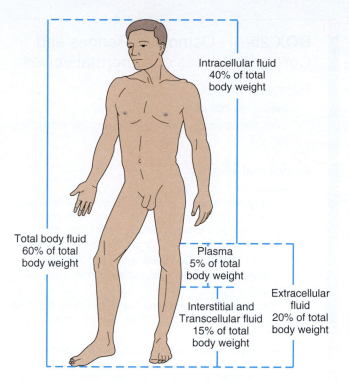

Figure 25–1 Water distribution in the adult male body.

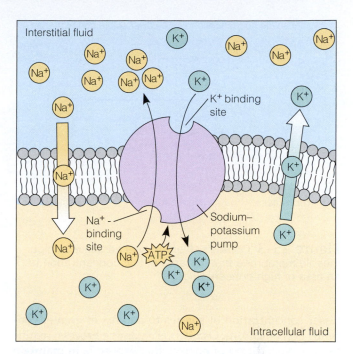

Figure 25–2 The sodium–potassium pump. Sodium and potassium ions are moved across the cell membranes against their concentration gradients. This active transport process is fueled by energy from ATP.

spinal fluid, peritoneal fluid, synovial fluid) (Patton & Thibodeau, 2016). Table 25–1 summarizes water distribution in the adult.

Intracellular Compartment The intracellular fluids (ICFs) are rich in potassium, phosphate, and protein and contain moderate amounts of magnesium and sulfate ions. Intracellular fluids provide the cells with nutrients and assist in cellular metabolism. The ICF volume is regulated by several important mechanisms. First, the presence of intracellular proteins attracts fluid into the cells. Second, negatively charged ions within the cells attract positively charged ions, such as sodium (Na^+) and potassium (K^+), which draws fluid into the cells. Without the counterregulating forces provided by the Na^+–K^+ pump, the cells would rupture and die. The sodium–potassium pump (Na^+–K^+) pump is located in the cell membrane (Figure 25–2). The pump requires adenosine triphosphate (ATP) for energy to actively move Na^+ from the cell into the extracellular fluid (ECF) and to move K^+ into the cell. Because water is attracted to Na^+ ions, more water accumulates in the extracellular compartment and ICF balance is maintained. Certain physiological conditions, including hypoxia, interfere

with the functioning of the pump. When the pump fails, Na^+ accumulates inside the cell, which causes retention of water inside the cell and accumulation of K^+ outside the cell.

Extracellular Compartment All body fluid outside the cells exists in the extracellular compartment and is referred to as extracellular fluid (ECF). Plasma, the fluid portion of the blood, is composed of water (about 90%), plasma proteins (about 7%), and other substances. Interstitial fluid functions as a transport medium between the blood and the body cells for nutrients, gases, waste products, and other substances. It also acts as a backup fluid reservoir that can rapidly provide fluid during situations in which there is vascular fluid loss (e.g., hemorrhage).

The interstitial compartment contains a spongelike substance called *tissue gel* that helps distribute interstitial fluid evenly. The gel is held together with collagen fibers. Tissue gel exerts force against the capillaries, which helps maintain fluids inside the capillaries. It also keeps free water from accumulating in the interstitial spaces. Transcellular fluid normally comprises about 1% of total ECF. It is located in the gastrointestinal and respiratory tracts, sweat glands, cerebrospinal fluid (CSF), and other tissues (e.g., pleural and pericardial spaces and peritoneal cavity).

Movement of Fluids

To understand intercompartmental fluid movement, it is crucial to first understand the concepts of osmosis and osmolality. The principle of **osmosis** explains the net diffusion or movement of water across the cell membrane (Figure 25–3). Fluid moves across a semipermeable (or selectively permeable) cell membrane from an area of

Table 25–1 Water Distribution in the Body (Adult)*

Location	Distribution
Total body weight	Females – 50% Males – 60%
Intracellular compartment	55%–75%
Extracellular compartment	25%–45%

*Approximate.

SOURCE: Adapted from Mount (2015).

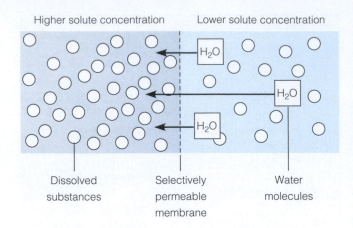

Figure 25–3 Osmosis. Fluid moves across a semipermeable membrane from an area of low concentration to an area of high concentration.

lesser concentration of solutes to an area of greater concentration of solutes. Osmosis is a passive process, requiring no expenditure of energy. Its purpose is to maintain fluid equilibrium between the fluid compartments. Water moves freely between the various fluid compartments; therefore, an alteration in one compartment produces a shift in body fluids in another compartment.

Osmolality Osmolality refers to the concentration of solute in body water and reflects a patient's hydration status. Measurement of the serum osmolality can be used as an approximation of the extracellular fluid status. Serum osmolality may be increased or decreased in various disease processes. Box 25–1 provides the normal parameters and lists examples of common causes of abnormal osmolality. The clinical manifestations of decreased serum osmolality are similar to those of fluid volume excess and

BOX 25–1 Osmolality Ranges and Common Causes of Abnormal Values

Ranges

Serum: 280–300 mOsm/kg

Urine: 50–1200 mOsm/kg/H_2O (average of 288–800 mOsm/kg H_2O)

Abnormal Values

Serum:

Decreased levels: fluid volume excess conditions (e.g., high fluid intake, syndrome of inappropriate antidiuretic hormone [ADH], syndrome of inappropriate antidiuretic hormone [SIADH], excessive 5% dextrose in water [D_5W])

Increased levels: fluid volume deficit conditions (e.g., dehydration, hyperglycemia, hypernatremia)

Urine:

Decreased levels: high urine output conditions (e.g., high fluid intake, acute kidney failure, diabetes insipidus [DI], diuretic therapy)

Increased levels: low urine output conditions (e.g., SIADH, dehydration, glycosuria related to hyperglycemia, Addison disease, high-protein diet); acidosis and shock

SOURCE: Data from Kee (2014).

hyponatremia. Those of increased serum osmolality are similar to those of fluid volume deficit and hypernatremia.

Starling Forces Through the processes of osmosis and diffusion, body fluids move between the interstitial and intravascular compartments. Four forces, called *Starling forces*, control this movement (Figure 25–4): capillary hydrostatic pressure, capillary oncotic pressure, interstitial

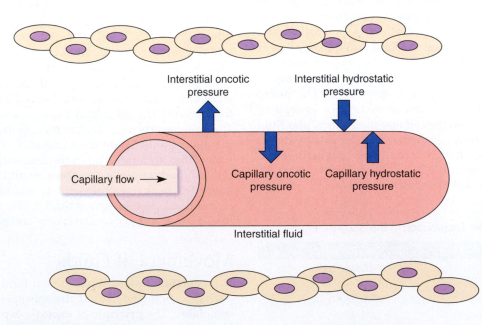

Figure 25–4 Starling forces. The forces of capillary hydrostatic pressure and interstitial oncotic pressure tend to shift fluid out of capillaries, and interstitial hydrostatic pressure and capillary oncotic pressure tend to shift fluid back into capillaries.

hydrostatic pressure, and interstitial oncotic pressure (Doig & Huether, 2014).

Capillary Hydrostatic Pressure. The pressure exerted by fluid moving through the capillaries to push fluid out of the capillary into the interstitial space is known as the capillary hydrostatic pressure. It is this pressure that is responsible for blood pressure. The majority of this movement occurs at the arterial end of the capillary, where the hydrostatic pressure is greatest (30–40 mmHg). The venous end of the capillary has a much lower hydrostatic pressure (10–15 mmHg), and fluid is resorbed into the capillary at this end.

Capillary Oncotic Pressure. The pressure exerted by plasma proteins as they flow through the capillary to draw fluid into the capillary is known as capillary oncotic (or colloidal osmotic) pressure. The plasma protein, albumin, is primarily responsible for this pressure.

Interstitial Hydrostatic Pressure. The pressure exerted by fluid in the interstitial space that pushes against the capillaries, opposing shifts of fluid out of the capillaries, is known as interstitial hydrostatic (or fluid) pressure.

Interstitial Oncotic Pressure. The pressure exerted by the small amount of proteins (primarily albumin) located in the interstitial space, which attracts fluid out of the capillaries and into the interstitium, is known as the interstitial (or tissue) oncotic pressure.

As can be seen, the opposing forces found in the capillaries and the interstitial spaces cause fluids to shift in and out of the capillaries, maintaining fluid balance between compartments and preventing excess fluid buildup in the interstitial spaces. In high-acuity patients, these forces can become unbalanced, causing abnormal fluid shifts or the trapping of intravascular fluid in the interstitium.

Section One Review

1. Older adult clients are predisposed to develop fluid volume deficit for which reasons? (Select all that apply.)
   A. Decreased muscle mass
   B. Decreased fat stores
   C. Alterations in nutrition
   D. Alterations in thirst
   E. Diminished renal function

2. What is the major function of tissue gel in the interstitial compartment?
   A. Shift fluid out of capillaries
   B. Provide a source of electrolytes
   C. Distribute fluid evenly
   D. Dispose of cellular waste products

3. Which statement is correct regarding low serum osmolality?
   A. It reflects fluid volume deficit.
   B. It reflects fluid volume excess.
   C. It is associated with dehydration.
   D. It is associated with hypernatremia.

4. Capillary hydrostatic pressure is the pressure exerted by which element?
   A. Plasma proteins in the capillaries
   B. Fluid in the interstitial spaces
   C. Plasma proteins in the interstitial spaces
   D. Fluid moving through the capillaries

Answers: 1. (A, C, D, E), 2. C, 3. B, 4. D

Section Two: Regulation of Fluid Balance

Two main mechanisms regulate and maintain body fluid homeostasis: thirst via hypothalamus regulation and excretion of body water through the kidneys via endocrine system regulation.

Hypothalamus Regulation of Fluid Balance

Under normal situations, most fluids are gained by drinking in response to stimulation of the thirst mechanism. **Thirst** is the awareness of the desire to drink that occurs in response to stimulation of **osmoreceptors** (neurons that detect changes in osmotic pressure) in the hypothalamus (Figure 25–5) (Huether, 2017). Thirst plays an important

role in maintaining fluid and electrolyte balance because it is the primary regulator of water intake. Osmoreceptors are stimulated under specific conditions: decreased blood volume, increased serum osmolality, and mouth dryness (Huether, 2017). The osmoreceptors also stimulate the posterior pituitary to release antidiuretic hormone (ADH), which increases water resorption into the plasma. The lateral area of the hypothalamus regulates body water, especially thirst and renal excretion of excess water. Thirst is decreased by a lower-than-normal serum osmolality, decreased angiotensin II, increased circulating blood volume or arterial blood pressure, and distention of the stomach. When thirst is triggered, the conscious person responds by drinking fluids.

Hypernatremia increases serum osmolality and stimulates osmoreceptors in the hypothalamus to initiate the thirst mechanism. Many high-acuity patients have altered levels of consciousness and therefore cannot experience the sensation of thirst. This is why hypernatremia is a common

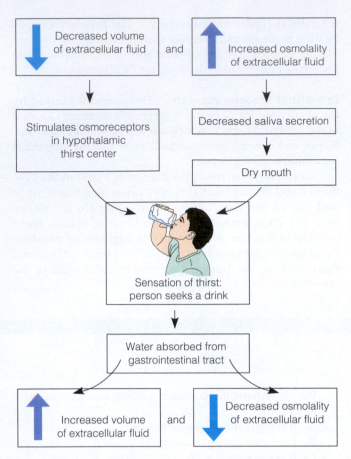

Figure 25–5 Factors stimulating water intake through the thirst mechanism.

electrolyte imbalance in high-acuity patients. In the high-acuity patient, fluids may be administered parenterally or by means of a gastrointestinal tube. Fluids are lost through the lungs, sweat glands, gastrointestinal fluids, and kidneys. Excess fluid can be lost during periods of tachypnea, fever, vomiting, diarrhea, or any condition that affects kidney function.

Clinical conditions that decrease the sense of thirst or the individual's ability to respond to thirst can decrease the circulating extracellular volume. Because the unconscious or high-acuity patient often cannot respond to thirst signals, the nurse needs to closely evaluate the patient's fluid status in the clinical setting using objective data obtained through physical assessment as well as urine and serum lab analysis data.

Arterial Baroreceptors Arterial **baroreceptors** (stretch receptors that detect pressure changes) are located in the arch of the aorta, carotid sinus, and pulmonary arteries (Doig & Huether, 2014). When baroreceptors sense a decrease in arterial blood pressure, they send a signal to the autonomic nervous system. The sympathetic nervous system responds to this signal by causing peripheral vasoconstriction. Vasoconstriction of renal arteries decreases glomerular filtration, which reduces urine output to increase circulating blood volume. The baroreceptors trigger opposite actions if they detect increased arterial blood pressure, causing vasodilation.

Endocrine Regulation

There are three major endocrine responses to decreased circulating blood volume: adrenocorticotropic hormone (ACTH), antidiuretic hormone (ADH), and the renin-angiotensin-aldosterone system (RAAS).

Adrenocorticotropic Hormone As part of the stress response, the hypothalamus sends a signal to the pituitary gland to release adrenocorticotropic hormone (ACTH). In response, ACTH stimulates the adrenal cortex to release aldosterone. Aldosterone is the most potent of the mineralocorticoids and is sometimes referred to as the salt-regulating hormone. Furthermore, aldosterone is regulated by the renin-angiotensin system, which responds to low sodium and water or increased potassium. It regulates water balance by facilitating sodium resorption in the renal distal tubules, collecting tubules, and collecting duct. As sodium is resorbed, potassium is excreted by the kidneys. The sodium resorption increases circulating blood volume by increasing water resorption. In this way, circulating blood volume and arterial blood pressure increase.

Antidiuretic Hormone When the hypothalamus osmoreceptors detect a change in the concentration of body fluid, it also sends a message to the posterior pituitary to either decrease or increase the release of antidiuretic hormone (ADH), which is vasopressin (Figure 25–6). For example, when serum osmolality increases, ADH increases

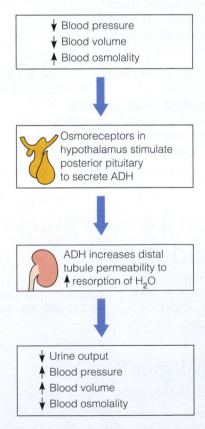

Figure 25–6 Antidiuretic hormone (ADH) release and effect. Increased serum osmolality or a fall in blood volume stimulates the release of ADH from the posterior pituitary. ADH increases the permeability of distal tubules, promoting water resorption.

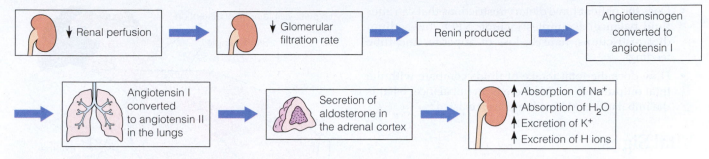

Figure 25–7 The renin-angiotensin-aldosterone system. Decreased blood volume and renal perfusion set off a chain of reactions leading to release of aldosterone from the adrenal cortex. Increased levels of aldosterone regulate serum K^+ and Na^+, blood pressure, and water balance through effects on the kidney tubules.

the permeability of the renal distal tubules and collecting ducts, allowing a large volume of water to be resorbed. This results in the expansion of the extracellular fluid, decreases serum osmolality, and improves arterial blood pressure and perfusion.

Renin-angiotensin-aldosterone System The renin-angiotensin-aldosterone system (RAAS) is a major contributor to blood pressure and intravascular fluid homeostasis

(Figure 25–7). When sodium is low, or potassium is high, or blood volume or blood pressure is low, the kidneys release renin, which acts on a plasma protein (renin substrate) to release angiotensin I. Angiotensin I is converted in the lungs to angiotensin II, a powerful vasoconstrictor. Angiotensin II stimulates the release of aldosterone and ADH from the adrenal cortex, which causes retention of sodium and water by the kidneys. This combination of actions results in a rapid increase in blood pressure, which improves perfusion.

Section Two Review

1. What is the primary regulator of water intake?
   A. Nervous system
   B. Endocrine system
   C. Renal system
   D. Hypothalamus

2. Which substance, released by the adrenal cortex, is known as the salt-regulating hormone?
   A. ACTH
   B. ADH
   C. Aldosterone
   D. Renin

3. When the hypothalamus senses a change in serum osmolality, it stimulates the posterior pituitary to release which substance?
   A. Renin
   B. Testosterone
   C. ADH
   D. ACTH

4. How is angiotensin II best characterized?
   A. Diuretic
   B. Vasoconstrictor
   C. Thirst trigger
   D. Sodium waster

Answers: 1. D, 2. C, 3. C, 4. B

Section Three: Assessment of Fluid Balance

A thorough assessment of the patient's fluid status focuses on looking for signs of fluid volume excess or deficit and includes vital signs, physical assessment, and evaluation of laboratory data. While assessment of fluid balance cannot be completely separated from assessment of electrolytes, this section primarily focuses on physical and laboratory assessments specific to fluid balance. Assessment of electrolyte balance is covered in Section Four.

History

A nursing history is an essential component of an assessment of fluid balance in the high-acuity patient. The following questions should be asked:

- Does the patient have an injury or disease process that can alter fluid balance? Examples include nausea, vomiting, diarrhea, recent surgery, placement of a nasogastric tube, diaphoresis, and hyperventilation.

- Is the patient receiving any medications that can alter fluid balance? Examples include diuretics, laxatives, nonsteroidal anti-inflammatory agents, glucocorticoids, and aminoglycosides.

- Does the patient have dietary restrictions that can alter fluid balance? Examples include NPO, low-sodium diet restrictions, nausea, loss of appetite, and tube feedings.
- How does the total intake of fluids compare with the total output of fluids? If there is an imbalance, what is the imbalance and how long has it existed?

Vital Signs

Changes in fluid balance are often reflected in alterations in vital signs, often as compensatory changes.

Temperature   Elevated temperature can result in excess loss of water and sodium through diaphoresis. Fever also increases the basal metabolic rate. Water is also lost through the lungs when a patient develops tachypnea, which often occurs with fevers.

Pulse   Tachycardia may be associated with decreased intravascular volume and hypomagnesemia and hypokalemia. Conversely, bradycardia can be associated with elevated serum levels of these electrolytes. Alterations in electrolytes can also produce cardiac dysrhythmias.

Respirations   Alterations in potassium balance and/or low magnesium levels can cause weakness of the respiratory muscles. Dyspnea with mild exertion or dyspnea at night may indicate pooling of fluid in the lungs. Severe acid–base disorders also can affect breathing patterns.

Arterial Blood Pressure   Arterial blood pressure and pulse together provide valuable information about a patient's fluid volume status. Orthostatic vital sign measurement can be used to assess for dehydration, blood loss, and the effects of antihypertensive medications. **Orthostatic (postural) hypotension** is defined as a drop in blood pressure of more than 20 mmHg or an increase in pulse greater than 20 bpm when going from a lying to sitting or sitting to standing position.

Physical Assessment

The physical assessment provides essential information that helps determine potential etiologies and the severity of abnormalities in the patient's fluid status.

Inspection   Inspection can reveal important data about fluid volume status. The patient's eyes may appear sunken if a fluid volume deficit is present, whereas a round, edematous face may indicate fluid volume overload or low serum proteins. The mouth should be inspected to determine if the oral tissues appear dry. If the patient is breathing through the mouth, fluids are lost through hyperventilation. The patient's tongue should also be checked for dryness. Tongue furrows may be a sign of fluid volume deficit.

Jugular venous pressure is an important parameter to assess for fluid volume status (Figure 25–8). Changes in fluid volume are reflected by changes in external jugular vein filling and can be used as an indicator of systemic venous pressure. The jugular vein on the right should be assessed because it is in close proximity to the right atrium.

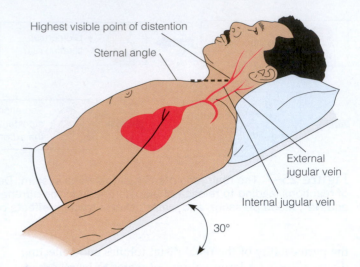

Figure 25–8 Assessing jugular venous pressure.

Hand veins provide important data on volume status. Place the patient's hand in a dependent position and observe for venous distention. Hypovolemia may be present if venous filling takes longer than 5 seconds. Distention should disappear within 5 seconds when the hand is elevated. Distention that does not clear within 5 seconds may indicate hypervolemia. Inspection of the extremities and the sacrum may reveal evidence of edema in bedridden patients and should be followed up with palpation to assess for pitting edema.

Palpation   Tissue turgor is assessed by pinching the skin on the forehead, sternum, or inner aspects of the thigh. In a patient with fluid volume deficit, the skin flattens more slowly after the pinch is released. Older patients, however, have reduced skin turgor as a result of less tissue elasticity. Therefore, this assessment is not used as a diagnostic tool for level of hydration in older adults. Tissue turgor also varies with race and nutritional status. Pitting edema leaves an impression on the skin with palpation.

Capillary Refill   Decreased capillary refill may be present in patients with hypovolemia. However, many physiologic factors can alter capillary refill, such as vasoconstriction of peripheral vessels, decreased cardiac output, anemia, cold temperatures, and cigarette smoking.

Abnormal Extravascular Accumulation of Fluids   Abnormal accumulations of fluid outside of the vascular system occur for a variety of reasons. Depending on the location of the abnormal fluid, these accumulations are referred to as second-spacing or third-spacing of fluids. If a hemodynamically significant volume of fluid escapes from the intravascular compartment into the second- or third-space, the patient is at high risk for developing hypovolemia or hypovolemic shock.

Second-spacing of Fluids.   **Edema** (second-spaced fluids) is an excess accumulation of fluid in interstitial spaces. Edema can be described in terms of certain characteristics, such as location, whether it is pitting or nonpitting, and amount of fluid weight gain.

Location. Determining whether the edema is localized or generalized provides important clues to its possible origin because pathologic conditions are usually associated with one or the other type of edema. Generalized edema is present all over the body and is seen primarily in the presence of decreased plasma proteins resulting from severe protein malnutrition. Localized edema results from a more localized pathologic condition, such as local inflammation and infection; however, generalized edema may develop secondary to a localized process that has expanded, causing widespread damage to the capillary endothelium. Examples of severe conditions in which this form of secondary generalized edema can occur are septic and anaphylactic shock.

Localized edema is confined to areas in which the causative condition is affecting the capillaries or lymph tissues (e.g., the area of inflammation, obstruction, or high capillary hydrostatic pressure). The edema associated with heart failure is considered localized because it is confined to gravity-dependent body areas (e.g., feet, lower legs, and sacrum). Pulmonary edema caused by left-sided heart failure is localized edema created by increased capillary hydrostatic pressure in the lungs as a result of elevated left-heart pressures.

Clinical Manifestations. The exact clinical manifestations associated with edema depend on its location. For example, a patient with pulmonary edema is at risk for developing pulmonary gas exchange problems, usually hypoxemia. A patient with cerebral edema is at risk for increased intracranial pressure, which can clinically present as a headache, deterioration in level of consciousness, and possible alterations in visual, motor, and respiratory status. Edema around a joint reduces range of motion or immobilizes the joint. Severe edema can compress capillary blood flow, causing tissue ischemia and pain.

Pitting or Nonpitting Edema. Pitting edema develops when the accumulation of fluid exceeds what can be absorbed by the interstitial tissue gel (Figure 25–9). Firm pressure applied to the edematous area displaces the interstitial fluid, causing a temporary pitting (Huether, 2017). It can be measured on a scale of 1 to 4 based on the depth and the length of time it takes for the indentation to disappear:

- 1+: 2 mm indentation, disappears rapidly
- 2+: 4 mm indentation, disappears in 10 to 15 seconds
- 3+: 6 mm indentation, disappears in 1 to 2 minutes
- 4+: 8 mm indentation, disappears in 2 to 5 minutes

Third-spacing of Fluids. Third-spacing is the shift of fluid from the intravascular compartment into a "third" (transcellular) space—usually a serous cavity, such as the pericardial or pleural sac and the peritoneal cavity. Normally there is no accumulation of serosal fluid in a serous cavity due to balanced Starling forces and a rich lymphatic network. Common causes of third-spacing are liver failure, myocarditis, pleuritis, and peritonitis. Clinically, third-spacing may manifest as ascites and pericardial and pleural effusions.

Clinical Manifestations. Assessment of third-spaced fluids is difficult because the serous cavities are deep structures, particularly the pericardial sac and pleural cavity. A thorough evaluation is necessary and may include a comprehensive physical examination, chest or abdominal radiography, electrocardiogram, and echocardiogram. **Ascites** (abnormal accumulation of fluid in the peritoneal cavity) can involve fluid shifts that are hemodynamically significant and can have an effect on breathing by compressing the diaphragm or forming a pleural effusion. For this reason, close evaluation of oxygenation status, arterial blood pressure, and serum albumin are important. In addition, daily weights and abdominal girth measurements provide valuable trending data. Pericardial effusion can also cause hemodynamic instability if cardiac tamponade develops because the patient can develop signs of circulatory shock as the heart becomes compressed.

Body Weight In the adult, peripheral edema develops when 5 L or more of fluid have accumulated in the interstitial spaces, and pitting edema develops with an accumulation of 10 L or more of interstitial fluid. Clinically, a weight gain or loss of 1 kg (2.2 lbs) represents a fluid gain or loss of

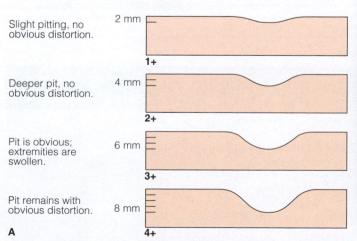

Slight pitting, no obvious distortion. — 2 mm — **1+**

Deeper pit, no obvious distortion. — 4 mm — **2+**

Pit is obvious; extremities are swollen. — 6 mm — **3+**

Pit remains with obvious distortion. — 8 mm — **4+**

A

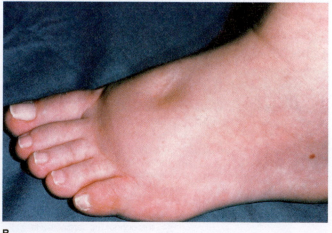

B

Figure 25–9 Evaluation of edema. A, Four-point scale for grading edema. B, 4+ pitting edema.

SOURCE: (A) LeMone et al. (2015). (B) Dr P. Marazzi/Science Source.

about 1 L. Evaluating daily weight trends provides valuable information on fluid status.

Auscultation　Auscultation of the heart and lungs provides important information about fluid status.

Heart.　Auscultation of the heart may reveal a third or fourth heart sound in patients with fluid volume overload. Tachycardia and hypotension may indicate fluid volume deficit. A pericardial friction rub may be heard and is a sign of an accumulation of fluid in the pericardial sac around the heart, a condition known as pericardial effusion. This is a complication that can occur in patients with kidney failure.

Lungs.　Auscultation of the lungs provides extremely valuable information in determining the presence of pulmonary edema. Pulmonary edema results from a shifting of fluid from the vascular space into the pulmonary interstitium, which in high-acuity patients may indicate heart failure (cardiogenic pulmonary edema) or acute respiratory distress syndrome (noncardiogenic pulmonary edema). Pulmonary crackles that do not clear with coughing may indicate fluid volume overload.

Percussion　Pain upon percussion of the flank area may indicate a urinary tract infection that has extended into the kidneys. Percussion of the abdomen can provide information about fluid volume status, particularly in patients with ascites. Patients with renal failure may have ascites as a result of increased capillary hydrostatic pressure and fluid volume excess. Patients with liver failure may have ascites related to decreased intravascular oncotic pressure as a result of decreased serum albumin. Patients with liver failure and ascites have decreased intravascular volume and actually have fluid volume deficit.

Hemodynamic Monitoring

Fluid balance disturbances are common in high-acuity patients, and frequent, accurate measurement of circulating fluid volume is sometimes needed to improve patient outcomes. Such measurements can be obtained through hemodynamic monitoring, including measurements such as central venous pressure (CVP), pulmonary artery wedge pressure (PAWP), cardiac output (CO) and cardiac index (CI), and mean arterial pressure (MAP). Table 25–2 provides basic information about each of these hemodynamic measurements; for a full discussion, see Chapter 8: Basic Hemodynamic Monitoring.

Urine Assessment

Urine volume and concentration provide important data about the patient's fluid status.

Urine Volume　Evaluating urine output in the high-acuity patient provides important, although nonspecific, information about fluid volume status. Multiple conditions alter the volume of urine output; thus, it cannot be used as a single marker of kidney function. Under normal conditions, a low urine volume suggests fluid volume deficit and a high urine volume suggests fluid volume excess. Table 25–3 summarizes a number of factors that alter the volume of urine output.

Urine Concentration　Urine concentration is measured in two ways: specific gravity and osmolality.

Urine Specific Gravity.　Urine specific gravity measures the ability of the kidneys to concentrate urine. Normal urine specific gravity is 1.005–1.030 (Kee, 2014). A specific

Table 25–3 Factors That Alter the Volume of Urine Output

Factor	Description
Circulatory volume status	Decreased cardiac output decreases renal blood flow, glomerular filtration rate, and urine output.
Hormonal influences	Renin-angiotensin-aldosterone system Antidiuretic hormone
Solute load	Urine volume is increased in conditions where there is increased solute load such as hyperglycemia, alcohol, elevated protein, or nitrogenous waste products
Decreased concentrating ability of the kidneys	Urine volume increases when the kidneys lose their ability to concentrate urine.

Table 25–2 Hemodynamic Implications of Fluid Disturbances

Measurement	Description	Normal Parameters	Effects of Fluid Disturbances Fluid Excess	Fluid Deficit
Central venous pressure (CVP)	Represents the filling pressure of the right atrium; measures right ventricle preload	2–6 mmHg	High	Low
Cardiac output (CO) and cardiac index (CI)	Cardiac output (CO) represents the amount of blood ejected from the heart each minute. Cardiac index (CI) is the cardiac output adjusted by body surface area (BSA), which corrects CO for body size, making it more accurate.	CO = 4–8 L/min CI = 2.4–4 L/min/m^2	High*	Low
Mean arterial pressure (MAP)	Represents the average arterial blood pressure throughout the cardiac cycle	70–90 mmHg	High	Low
Pulmonary artery wedge pressure (PAWP)	Represents left ventricular preload (pressure in the left heart just before the ventricle contracts)	4–12 mmHg	High	Low

*Exception: CO and CI will be low in the patient with cardiac pump failure.

gravity greater than 1.030 indicates concentrated urine, which results from conditions that cause fluid volume deficit (e.g., fever, dehydration, diabetes mellitus, diarrhea, or vomiting). A specific gravity of less than 1.005 can develop in conditions that cause fluid volume excess (e.g., high fluid intake, diabetes insipidus, and renal diseases in which the kidneys can no longer concentrate urine). However, urine specific gravity can be elevated out of proportion to the actual concentration in the presence of high urine concentrations of glucose, albumin, or radiocontrast dyes. Therefore, it is more accurate to measure urine osmolality in patients with glycosuria, proteinuria, or recent administration of radiocontrast dyes.

Urine Osmolality. Urine osmolality is the concentration of solutes in the urine. It can be directly measured and is more accurate than urine specific gravity as an indicator of the kidney's ability to concentrate urine (Kee, 2014). Normal urine osmolality is 200 to 800 mOsm/kg. Urine osmolality increases during fluid volume deficit as the kidneys hold on to water (urine output decreases). Urine osmolality decreases during fluid volume excess as the kidneys excrete more water (urine output increases).

Laboratory Assessment

Periodic evaluation of serum and urine laboratory data provides important information about fluid balance. Data trends are monitored to assess the patient for status improvement or deterioration.

Serum Labs A variety of serum laboratory tests evaluate fluid status. Many evaluate kidney function, which is closely aligned with fluid status. What follows are some of the major laboratory tests that indirectly reflect fluid status. Table 25–4 provides a summary of these tests, including normal ranges and major causes of abnormal levels. The laboratory assessment of electrolytes is covered in Section Five.

Blood Urea Nitrogen. Urea is an end-product of protein metabolism that is excreted by the kidneys. It is measured as blood urea nitrogen (BUN) and is useful as an indicator of glomerular filtration and kidney health. BUN levels are dependent on protein intake and nitrogen metabolism; therefore, factors other than kidney function alter serum levels and must be interpreted with caution. With renal dysfunction and a decrease in glomerular filtration rate (GFR), there is decreased excretion of BUN and therefore an increase in serum BUN levels; however, BUN can increase in the presence of normal kidney function.

Creatinine. Creatinine (Cr) is an amino acid compound located in skeletal muscle and subsequently metabolized in the liver. The normal range of serum creatinine is 0.5 to 1.5 mg/dL (Kee, 2014). It is released at a relatively constant rate, is freely filtered by the glomerulus, and is not resorbed or metabolized by the kidneys. Creatinine is affected by fewer conditions than is BUN and is therefore a better indicator of renal function. Creatinine levels increase in states of renal dysfunction.

Table 25–4 Serum Laboratory Assessments That Reflect Fluid Status

Lab	Description	Normal Parameters	Common Causes of Abnormal Low and High Values	
			Low Level	**High Level**
Blood urea nitrogen (BUN)	By-product of protein metabolism	5–25 mg/dL	Overhydration, severe liver disease, malnutrition, low protein intake	Dehydration, kidney injury, excessive protein breakdown or high protein intake, GI bleeding, multiple drugs
Creatinine	By-product of muscle breakdown; metabolized by the liver; released at a relatively constant rate and readily filtered by kidneys	0.5–1.5 mg/dL	Pregnancy	Kidney injury (acute or chronic), cancer, shock, heart disease (e.g., acute myocardial infarction [MI], heart failure), multiple drugs
BUN-to-creatinine ratio (BUN:Cr)	Normal ratio between serum BUN and creatinine	10:1–20:1 (average = 15:1)	Decreased ratio: liver disease, excessive IV fluid intake, overhydration, malnutrition, acute renal tubular necrosis	Increased ratio: hypovolemia, shock, GI bleeding, kidney injury (decreased kidney perfusion, glomerular disease), muscle or tissue injury, high intake of protein
Osmolality	Represents serum concentration (solute concentration per volume of a solution [body fluids])	280–300 mOsm/kg	Fluid volume excess or hemodilution; excessive 5% dextrose in water (D_5W) intake; SIADH	Fluid volume deficit or hemoconcentration (e.g., hypernatremia, dehydration, diabetes insipidus, hyperglycemia, kidney failure)
Anion gap (AG)	A measurement of the difference between positively charged ions (cations) and negatively charged ions; formula: $Na^+ - (Cl^- + HCO_3^-)$	10–17 mEq/L	Metabolic alkalosis: severe dehydration, elevations of cations (Na^+, Ca^{++}, Mg^{++}), diuretic therapy	Metabolic acidosis: lactic acidosis, ketoacidosis, kidney injury, multiple drugs
Albumin	Major plasma protein; synthesized by liver. Major role: maintenance of vascular osmotic pressure.	3.5–5 g/dL	Liver failure, severe malnutrition, kidney injury, others	Dehydration, severe diarrhea or vomiting

SOURCE: Laboratory data from Kee (2014), "Part One Lab Tests," pp. 1–453.

BUN-to-Creatinine Ratio. Blood urea nitrogen (BUN) and creatinine (Cr) are both by-products of protein metabolism that are excreted by the kidneys, and they normally maintain a predictable relationship with each other. The normal ratio of BUN to Cr is 10:1 to 20:1 (average 15:1) (Kee, 2014). A change in the ratio can be used to help identify the etiology of renal dysfunction.

Osmolality. Osmolality is expressed in milliosmoles (mOsm); normal serum osmolality in an adult is 280 to 300 mOsm/kg. Serum values of less than 240 mOsm/kg or more than 320 mOsm/kg are considered critically abnormal. A low serum osmolality suggests fluid volume excess or hemodilution, meaning there is more fluid than solute in the serum. A high serum osmolality suggests fluid volume deficit or hemoconcentration, meaning there is less fluid than solute in the serum. The following formula can be used to calculate serum osmolality:

$$\text{Serum Osmolality} = (\text{serum Na} \times 2) + \frac{\text{BUN}}{3} + \frac{\text{Glucose}}{18}$$

For example: Given that a patient's sodium (Na) is 140 mEq/L, blood urea nitrogen (BUN) is 20 mg/dL, and glucose is 250 mg/dL, it can be calculated that the serum osmolality is 301 mOsm/kg. This indicates that there are more particles than fluid in this patient's serum. This osmolality is slightly high, which suggests fluid volume deficit.

Clinically, serum osmolality can be used to determine the need for fluid replacement in the high-acuity patient.

Anion Gap. The anion gap is a calculation of the difference between the cations (sodium, potassium) and anions (chloride, bicarbonate). However, in common practice, potassium is ignored for calculation purposes as shown in the formula:

$$\text{Na}^+ - (\text{Cl}^- + \text{HCO}_3^-)$$

The anion gap can be used to determine the cause of metabolic acidosis. Normally the kidney conserves HCO_3^- and excretes H^+. In conditions where the glomeruli are damaged, metabolic acids (such as phosphoric and sulfuric acid) are retained, causing a widening of the gap. An increased anion gap reflects decreased excretion or increased production of acid products. Anion gap is increased with kidney injury because of decreased bicarbonate resorption and retention of acids.

Serum Albumin. Albumin is a plasma protein synthesized in the liver and represents the majority of the proteins carried in the blood. Normal blood levels are 3.5 to 5 g/dL (Kee, 2014). Recall from Section One that albumin is responsible for maintaining intravascular oncotic pressure; therefore, hypoalbuminemia (abnormally low serum albumin) can have a profound effect on fluid balance and is a frequent cause of generalized edema. The most common causes of hypoalbuminemia are chronic inflammation and malnutrition, both of which may be present in the high-acuity patient.

Urine Labs The urinalysis and creatinine clearance tests are additional laboratory tests that provide valuable screening information.

Urinalysis. Urinalysis involves simple observation and separate measurements using commercially available dipsticks. Urine pH is usually 5. Urine is generally acidic as a result of net acid excretion. Alkaline urine may be present in patients on a vegetarian diet or in the presence of an infection or acute tubular acidosis. Glucose may be present during pregnancy and in diabetes mellitus. Proteinuria occurs in the presence of glomerular basement membrane disease. The most common protein lost in the urine is albumin. Heme can be present in the urine and can indicate the presence of hemoglobin, myoglobin, or red blood cells.

Urine sediment is an important component in the assessment of renal disease. *Sediment* describes the cellular components in urine, which can include red blood cells, white blood cells, tubular cells, transitional cells, and squamous epithelial cells.

Creatinine Clearance. Creatinine clearance (CrCl) provides information about kidney function and is a reliable measure for estimating glomerular filtration rate (GFR). It is the amount of creatinine measured in the urine and the amount in the blood over a 24-hour period. As renal function decreases, CrCl decreases; a clearance of less than 40 mL/minute suggests significant renal dysfunction (Kee, 2014). It is estimated by obtaining a 12- or 24-hour urine specimen and a blood creatinine level and is calculated with the following formula:

$$\text{CrCl} = \frac{\text{Urine creatinine (mcg/dL)} \times \text{Urine volume (dL)}}{\text{Serum creatinine (mcg/dL)}}$$

Section Three Review

1. Elevated temperature can cause fluid volume deficit through which process? (Select all that apply.)
   A. Diaphoresis
   B. Tachypnea
   C. Vasoconstriction
   D. Diarrhea
   E. Increased metabolic rate

2. During a physical assessment, it is noted that the client has pitting edema around the ankles, with 4 mm indentation that disappears within 10 seconds. How should this be documented?
   A. 1+ pitting edema
   B. 2+ pitting edema
   C. 3+ pitting edema
   D. 4+ pitting edema

3. What is the normal BUN-to-Cr ratio?
   - **A.** 1:1
   - **B.** 1:5
   - **C.** 5:1
   - **D.** 10:1

4. An increased anion gap reflects which condition?
   - **A.** Increased serum osmolality
   - **B.** Increased renal excretion of sodium
   - **C.** Decreased excretion or increased production of acids
   - **D.** Inability of the kidneys to concentrate urine

Answers: 1. (A, B, E), 2. B, 3. D, 4. C

Section Four: Electrolytes

Electrolytes are electrically charged microsolutes found in body fluids. There are two types of electrolytes: **cations** (positively charged ions) and **anions** (negatively charged ions). Electrolytes play a vital role in many physiologic activities, including enzyme activities, muscle contraction, and metabolism. The three major extracellular electrolytes are sodium (Na), chloride (Cl), and calcium (Ca); the three major intracellular electrolytes are potassium (K), magnesium (Mg), and phosphorus (PO_4). Table 25–5 provides a summary of normal serum electrolyte ranges.

Sodium

Sodium (Na^+), the most abundant cation in the extracellular fluid, is responsible for water balance and is required for the normal transmission of impulses across muscle and nerve cells through the sodium-potassium pump mechanism. Sodium plays an important role in maintaining acid–base balance by combining with chloride or bicarbonate to increase or decrease serum pH.

Serum sodium is maintained within normal limits by two important mechanisms: secretion of antidiuretic hormone (ADH) by the hypothalamus and the release of aldosterone by the adrenal glands, which increases the resorption of sodium (Patton & Thibodeau, 2016). The amount of sodium in the diet varies widely because the supply is abundant in many (particularly processed) foods. When the serum sodium is high, fluid volume in the intravascular compartment increases. In response, the kidneys increase urinary excretion of sodium through enhanced filtering from the blood; inhibition of ADH prevents resorption of sodium by the kidneys; and aldosterone release is suppressed, enhancing urinary excretion of sodium. When the serum sodium is low, plasma volume is decreased. The kidneys sense the decreased volume and trigger the renin-angiotensin-aldosterone system, which causes increased sodium resorption, thus decreasing urine output and increasing fluid volume.

Sodium and Water Balance   Changes in sodium levels alter water balance; thus, the clinical manifestations of sodium alterations also reflect symptoms of water imbalance. Because water is drawn to sodium, an excess sodium level in the extracellular fluid pulls water from the intracellular spaces. This results in shrinking of the intracellular fluid compartment and expansion of the extracellular compartment. Such expansion may precipitate heart failure and pulmonary edema in patients whose renal or cardiovascular system cannot tolerate fluid shifts. When serum levels of sodium are low, water moves from an area of low sodium concentration (extracellular) to an area of high sodium concentration (intracellular). This causes excess volume in the intracellular compartment and fluid volume deficit in the extracellular compartment.

Chloride

Chloride (Cl^-) is the most abundant anion in the extracellular fluid. Chloride works with sodium in the regulation of body fluids by its influence on osmotic pressures within the interstitial and intravascular compartments. Serum chloride levels tend to closely follow sodium levels because chloride normally follows sodium in the body. Aldosterone regulates chloride levels indirectly by stimulating resorption of sodium in the kidney. Chloride assists in maintaining the resting membrane potential of cells and, with sodium, maintains osmolality of the extracellular fluid space.

The extracellular fluid acid–base status requires a balance between the total number of anions and cations within the fluid. Thus, the major cation (sodium) must be in balance with the two major extracellular anions (chloride and bicarbonate). To regulate this balance, chloride and bicarbonate maintain an inverse relationship, competing for sodium ions. For example, if a patient receives an excessive dose of sodium bicarbonate to treat metabolic acidosis, the presence of excess bicarbonate ions in the serum results in the exchange of bicarbonate with chloride ions, precipitating hypochloremia.

Calcium

Calcium (Ca^{++}) is located almost entirely within bone, with a small amount (1%) within cells and organelles and a miniscule amount (0.1%) in a dissolved state in the extracellular fluid. Calcium enters the body through diet and is absorbed in the small intestine; excess calcium is excreted through the stool and urine (Eaton & Pooler, 2013). Calcium is required for blood coagulation, neuromuscular contraction, enzymatic activities, and bone integrity. Calcium regulation

Table 25–5 Serum Electrolyte Normal Ranges

Electrolyte	Normal Range
Sodium (Na^+)	135–145 mEq/L (or mmol/L)
Chloride (Cl^-)	95–105 mEq/L (or mmol/L)
Calcium (Ca^{++})	2.3–2.8 mmol/L (9–11 mg/dL)
Potassium (K^+)	3.5–5.3 mEq/L (or mmol/L)
Magnesium (Mg^{++})	1.5–2.5 mEq/L (1.8–3 mg/dL)
Phosphate (PO_4^-)	1.7–2.6 mEq/L (2.5–4.5 mg/dL)

SOURCE: Normal ranges from Kee (2014).

is under the influence of parathyroid hormone (PTH), calcitonin, and calcitriol.

Although the small intestine and kidneys play a large role in calcium balance, the primary regulation of plasma calcium is accomplished by moving calcium into and out of bone (Eaton & Pooler, 2013). Consequently, despite variations in day-to-day ingestion and excretion of calcium, plasma levels stay relatively constant due to regulation provided by the skeletal system. PTH heavily influences calcium regulation by mobilizing calcium and increasing bone resorption, thereby increasing serum levels. PTH also increases calcium resorption in the renal tubules and facilitates rapid calcium shifts from bones into the extracellular fluids (Eaton & Pooler, 2013). Calcium is absorbed in the small intestine only under the influence of vitamin D that has been activated in the kidneys. Renal disease prevents activation of vitamin D, thus reducing the body's ability to absorb calcium.

PTH and calcitonin (a hormone produced by the thyroid) work in opposition to regulate calcium levels. When calcium levels are low, PTH is released, stimulating the conversion of calcidiol to calcitriol (the active form of vitamin D), which causes the small intestines to absorb more calcium. PTH also stimulates the release of calcium from bony tissues into the blood. When calcium levels are high, PTH secretion is suppressed as calcitonin is secreted by the thyroid, thereby inhibiting the release of calcium from bone into the blood, inhibiting calcium absorption in the small intestines, and increasing the elimination of calcium through urine (Eaton & Pooler, 2013).

Serum calcium can be measured in two different ways: as total calcium and as ionized calcium. These measurements evaluate body calcium in two different states: total calcium and ionized calcium.

Total Calcium Total calcium reflects calcium bound to proteins (primarily albumin) in the serum. Total calcium levels are influenced by the patient's nutritional state. Therefore, if a patient's serum albumin level is low (e.g., from malnutrition or liver dysfunction), serum calcium levels will also be low (Doig & Huether, 2014).

Ionized Calcium Approximately 50% of serum calcium exists in an ionized state (Kee, 2014). Ionized calcium represents the calcium that is used in physiologic activities and is crucial for neuromuscular activity; therefore, it is the ionized calcium levels, rather than total calcium, that should be monitored in high-acuity patients. The acid–base state of the patient influences calcium levels. An alkalosis state causes increased binding of ionized calcium (Ca^{++}) to albumin, thereby causing lower ionized calcium levels, which can precipitate the clinical manifestations of hypocalcemia (Doig & Huether, 2014). An acidotic state decreases binding of calcium to albumin, increasing ionized calcium levels, which can result in clinical manifestations of hypercalcemia.

Potassium

Potassium (K^+) is the major intracellular cation; almost all potassium is located within the cells. Proper distribution between the intracellular and extracellular fluid compartments, as well as effective renal excretion, is tightly controlled to maintain potassium homeostasis in the blood.

Although the concentration in the plasma is small, monitoring serum potassium is very important because the body is intolerant of abnormal serum levels. Potassium is readily found in many foods; thus, we normally consume sufficient quantities of potassium to meet daily requirements. Excess potassium is eliminated in the urine by the kidneys, and about 40 to 120 mEq of potassium is excreted daily in the urine (Doig & Huether, 2014).

Potassium is vital in maintaining normal cardiac and neuromuscular function because it affects muscle contraction. Potassium also influences nerve impulse conduction; therefore, abnormal serum potassium levels can produce potentially lethal cardiac conduction abnormalities, which could result in dysrhythmias and cardiac arrest. Potassium is vital to carbohydrate metabolism and plays an important role in normal cell membrane function. It is important in maintaining an acid–base balance because hydrogen ions in the vascular space exchange with potassium ions in the intracellular space.

Magnesium

Magnesium (Mg^{++}) is an intracellular electrolyte with a distribution similar to that of potassium. Magnesium ensures sodium and potassium transportation across cell membranes. It is needed for activation of certain enzymes required for normal protein and carbohydrate metabolism. Magnesium is crucial to many biochemical reactions and plays a significant role in nerve cell conduction. It is important in transmitting CNS messages and maintaining neuromuscular activity.

Magnesium balance is closely related to potassium and calcium balance. Magnesium enters the body through the diet and is predominantly excreted in feces, but a small amount is excreted in the urine. The kidneys, however, have a remarkable ability to conserve magnesium, and renal excretion is the only regulatory mechanism for plasma magnesium.

Phosphorus / Phosphate

Phosphorus is an intracellular mineral commonly found in many foods. In the body, its predominant form is phosphate (PO_4^-); it combines with calcium and, as calcium phosphate, is an essential component of the bones and teeth. It is also vital to normal neuromuscular function and is required for energy in the production of ATP. Phosphate also contributes to protein, fat, and carbohydrate metabolism and assists in the maintenance of acid–base balance.

The serum phosphorus level is under the influence of parathyroid hormone (PTH) and maintains an inverse relationship to calcium. The kidneys are essential to phosphorus regulation through resorption and excretion. When glomerular filtration decreases, phosphorus resorption increases, causing an elevation in serum levels. As glomerular filtration increases, phosphorus resorption diminishes, allowing more phosphorus to be excreted by the kidneys and reducing serum phosphate levels. Age-related changes in parathyroid function, along with decreased intake and impaired intestinal absorption, make mild hypophosphatemia common in the older high-acuity patient.

Emerging Evidence

- Pre– and post–serum potassium levels were measured in a sample of 142 ICU patients receiving potassium replacement therapy. Despite the well-known reliability of potassium chloride absorption, and even though 77% of the patients in this study had enteral route available, 7 out of every 10 potassium doses were administered intravenously. Data analysis revealed a comparable dose response with increases in serum potassium levels after the administration of enteral or intravenous supplements. Because the intravenous route carries substantially higher risk, intensive care patients may benefit from enteral, in place of intravenous, potassium replacements when feasible *(DeCarolis, Kim, Rector, & Ishani, 2016)*.

- A retrospective audit of the medical records of 594 ICU patients supports that fluid management in the ICU patient with sepsis and septic shock is time sensitive. "Early-goal directed therapy" (EGDT), introduced over 10 years ago, included in its protocol that fluid resuscitation should occur within 6 hours of the onset of sepsis. This study found that patients who received earlier resuscitation (within the first 3-hour block of time) survived in greater numbers than those who were resuscitated in the second 3-hour block of time *(Lee et al., 2014)*.

- Data from over 30,000 critically ill patients were subjected to secondary analysis to determine if the administration of calcium alone predicted 28- or 90-day mortality. The administration of calcium during an ICU stay was independently associated ($p < 0.05$), with improved 28-day survival in this sample of patients when data were examined with multivariate analysis techniques *(Zhang, Chen, & Ni, 2015)*.

Section Four Review

1. Chloride levels closely follow the levels of which other electrolyte?
   - **A.** K^+
   - **B.** Na^+
   - **C.** Ca^{++}
   - **D.** Mg^{++}

2. Calcium is absorbed in the intestines under the influence of which nutrient?
   - **A.** Phosphorus
   - **B.** Vitamin D
   - **C.** Sodium
   - **D.** Vitamin C

3. What is one cause of hyperkalemia?
   - **A.** Renal failure
   - **B.** Diuretics
   - **C.** Metabolic acidosis
   - **D.** Severe diarrhea

4. Magnesium plays a role in which physiologic functions? (Select all that apply.)
   - **A.** Na^+ and K^+ transport
   - **B.** Nerve cell conduction
   - **C.** Fluid regulation
   - **D.** Energy transfer
   - **E.** Carbohydrate metabolism

Answers: 1. B, 2. B, 3. A, 4. (A, B, C, E)

Section Five: Assessment of Electrolyte Balance

Assessment of electrolyte balance is primarily dependent on evaluation of serum and urine laboratory electrolyte test results. In addition, the nurse monitors the patient who is at risk for one or more electrolyte imbalances for abnormal signs and symptoms associated with specific electrolyte imbalances.

The nursing history necessary to investigate potential electrolyte imbalances is essentially the same as the history required for fluid imbalances (see Section Three), with particular emphasis on the disease processes or conditions that are known to place a patient at risk for electrolyte abnormalities (e.g., parathyroid tumor, diabetes mellitus, acid–base imbalances, prolonged immobility, Addison disease, malnutrition, vomiting or diarrhea). Obtaining a thorough drug history (prescription, as well as over-the-counter) can also provide valuable information on potential sources of electrolyte imbalances.

Physical Assessment

Physical assessment provides important clues to potential electrolyte imbalances; however, the findings produced through physical assessment are insufficient to conclusively determine which specific electrolyte imbalances (or multiple imbalances) may be present, as similar signs and symptoms are characteristic of several different imbalances. Specific clinical manifestations associated with individual electrolyte imbalances are presented in Chapter 26: Alterations in Fluid and Electrolyte Balance.

Vital Signs and Cardiovascular Assessments Taking vital signs, particularly arterial blood pressure and heart rate and rhythm, and comparing these data with the patient's normal ranges provides valuable information on the patient's fluid and electrolyte status. Abnormal levels of sodium, calcium, potassium, magnesium, or phosphate are known to potentially alter arterial blood pressure, heart rate and rhythm, and cardiac function. If abnormalities are noted, further investigation may warrant obtaining a 12-lead electrocardiogram (ECG). Life-threatening rhythm changes and dysrhythmias in the ECG and heart function are possible with significantly abnormal serum levels in calcium, potassium, and magnesium.

Neurologic Assessment Abnormal levels of most of the electrolytes can cause changes in mental status and level of consciousness, such as disorientation, confusion, agitation or lethargy, and seizures or coma. For example, hypokalemia (low serum potassium) and hyponatremia (low serum sodium) can cause confusion and lethargy, while hypophosphatemia (low serum phosphate) and hypocalcemia (low serum calcium) can precipitate disorientation, irritability, and seizures.

Neuromuscular and Musculoskeletal Assessments Alterations in electrolyte balance can produce neuromuscular as well as musculoskeletal changes that can be evaluated by checking deep tendon reflexes, muscle strength and tone, and sensation. For example, hypomagnesemia (low serum magnesium) and hypocalcemia can produce tetany. Testing for a positive **Chvostek sign** is simple to perform. The nurse taps the patient's face, directly in front of the ear (on the facial nerve) and observes for spasm or twitching of the cheek and/or lip on the side being stimulated (Doig & Huether, 2014). Spasm or twitching is a positive Chvostek sign. The **Trousseau sign** is another simple test that can be performed by the nurse to evaluate the patient for potential low calcium. The nurse places a blood pressure cuff on one arm and inflates the cuff to above the systolic pressure. If the test is positive, the patient's fingers will hyperextend with the thumb flexing toward the palm. Both tests are illustrated in Chapter 24: Alterations in Pancreatic Function. As part of the neuromuscular assessment, the patient should be asked about any abnormal sensations in the extremities, such as tingling or paresthesia, which are characteristic of hypophosphatemia and hypocalcemia.

Gastrointestinal Assessment Anorexia, nausea, vomiting, and diarrhea are commonly associated with abnormal levels of serum electrolytes. Vomiting and diarrhea were presented as important findings in fluid status assessment in Section Three. However, they are also potential sources of electrolyte loss as well as manifestations of some existing electrolyte imbalances (e.g., hyponatremia, hypokalemia, and hypophosphatemia). The patient who presents with severe vomiting or diarrhea is at risk for developing significant loss of electrolytes through emesis or stool, which may result in acid–base imbalances as well, through loss of acids (vomiting) or bases (diarrhea).

Laboratory Testing

Serum and possibly urine electrolytes should be obtained to identify specific electrolyte abnormalities and evaluate their severity by comparing patient data against normal parameters.

Serum Electrolytes Obtaining baseline serum electrolytes is typically done when admitted to the hospital (as is the case in the Clinical Reasoning Checkpoint about Mr. R). Periodic serum electrolyte levels are usually drawn throughout hospitalization, with frequency based on the individual patient's needs. Serum electrolytes are obtained using a 3- to 5-mL venous blood sample.

Urine Electrolytes Urine electrolytes are often measured by collecting a 24-hour urine specimen. Urine electrolytes are obtained for a variety of reasons, such as monitoring renal function, evaluating fluid and electrolyte balance, and determining urine electrolyte composition. They are also used for diagnostic purposes, such as for Addison disease and for evaluation of aldosterone disorders. One of the most common urinary electrolytes assessed is sodium. Urinary sodium is helpful in assessing volume status, hyponatremia, acute renal failure, and dietary compliance in patients on sodium-restricted diets.

Section Five Review

1. Which statement is correct regarding the use of the physical assessment in diagnosing electrolyte abnormalities?
   A. Physical assessment findings can point to a specific electrolyte problem.
   B. Physical assessment provides important clues to the presence of a general electrolyte problem.
   C. Most signs and symptoms of electrolyte problems are highly specific to each electrolyte.
   D. There is little correlation between physical signs and symptoms and electrolyte levels.

2. Which vital signs are most important to monitor in clients with potential or actual electrolyte abnormalities? (Select all that apply.)
   A. Temperature
   B. Blood pressure
   C. Respiratory rate
   D. Heart rate
   E. Heart rhythm

3. Hypokalemia and hyponatremia have which neurologic effects?
   A. Confusion and lethargy
   B. Irritability and coma
   C. Disorientation and seizures
   D. Hallucinations and tetany

4. Urinary sodium is helpful in assessing which condition?
   A. Chronic pancreatitis
   B. Acute renal failure
   C. Alcohol intoxication
   D. Gastrointestinal bleeding

Answers: 1. B, 2. (B, D, E), 3. A, 4. B

Clinical Reasoning Checkpoint

Donald R, age 75 years, was admitted to the hospital with severe dyspnea. He has a history of chronic alcohol abuse and cirrhosis. On admission, the nurse assesses the following: thin, chronically ill-appearing male. Blood pressure 108/62 mmHg, pulse 118/min, RR 26/min, temperature 36.6°C (97.8°F). He has 3+ pitting generalized edema. His abdomen is distended and tight. He has orthopnea and complains of shortness of breath. Mr. R states that he has been confined to his chair or couch for the past 2 weeks because of his breathing difficulty and general weakness.

1. Identify factors in Mr. R's history that affect his fluid and electrolyte balance. What additional data would be important to elicit?

2. Given Mr. R's vital signs, what changes would support the presence of orthostatic hypotension?

3. Mr. R has generalized edema. Compare and contrast the pathophysiologic causes of generalized versus localized edema.

Clinical update: Mr. R's serum laboratory results are Na 128 mEq/L, Ca^{++} 5.8 mg/dL, K^+ 5.2 mEq/L, osmolality 315 mOsm/L, BUN 40 mg/dL, and Cr 4 mg/dL.

4. Examine Mr. R's BUN and creatinine and calculate his BUN to Cr ratio. What is your interpretation of these results?

Chapter 25 Review

1. A client is severely dyspneic and is extremely weak. The physical exam reveals 3+ pitting generalized edema. This client's edema is an example of fluid located in which space?
   1. Intracellular
   2. Intravascular
   3. Interstitial
   4. Transcellular

2. A client who has cirrhosis from chronic alcohol abuse presents with a tightly distended abdomen and shortness of breath. Assuming that this distention is from ascites, the nurse conducts an assessment looking for which condition?
   1. Third spacing
   2. Heart failure
   3. Edema
   4. Peritonitis

3. A client is bleeding from a deep laceration. On admission, the client's blood pressure was 118/62 mm Hg, pulse was 118/min, RR 26/min, and temperature 97.8°F. Current blood pressure is 90/56. The nurse expects which assessment finding based on baroreceptor response to this drop in blood pressure?
   1. Increased urine output due to renal vasodilation
   2. Decreased heart rate due to decreased sympathetic nervous system response
   3. Less potassium excreted by the kidney due to ACTH suppression
   4. Cool, clammy extremities due to peripheral vasoconstriction

4. A client has 3+ generalized edema and has had a urine output of 25 mL/hr for the past 2 hours. The most current serum osmolality is 315 mOsm/kg. Based on these data, the nurse would suspect which condition?
   1. Renal failure
   2. Cerebral vascular accident
   3. Suppressed ADH release
   4. Intravascular fluid deficit

5. A client's serum osmolality is 320 mOsm/kg. The nurse would relate which assessment findings to this condition? (Select all that apply.)
   1. The lab result reports that serum sodium is elevated.
   2. The client is thirsty.
   3. The client is unconscious.
   4. The client's temperature is low.
   5. The client's face is round and swollen.

6. A client's urinalysis reveals alkaline urine. Which assessment questions should the nurse ask? (Select all that apply.)
   1. "Do you drink wine?"
   2. "How much water do you drink daily?"
   3. "Have you had symptoms of a urinary tract infection?"
   4. "Do you follow a vegetarian diet?"
   5. "Do you have diabetes?"

7. A client's serum potassium level is approaching 7 mEq/L. The nurse would be most concerned about changes in which body system?

   1. Cardiovascular
   2. Respiratory
   3. Neurologic
   4. Renal

8. A client's lab work reveals these electrolyte levels: sodium 133 mEq/L; chloride 110 mEq/L; calcium 8.6 mg/dL; potassium 4 mEq/L; magnesium 1.7 mEq/L; and phosphate 1.8 mEq/L. Which results would the nurse report as abnormal? (Select all that apply.)

   1. Sodium
   2. Chloride
   3. Calcium
   4. Potassium
   5. Magnesium and phosphate

9. A client's electrolyte measurement reveals hypophosphatemia and hypocalcemia. To which client situation would the nurse attribute those imbalances? (Select all that apply.)

   1. The client states, "Where am I? How did I get here?"
   2. The client's family reports marked increase in irritability over the last week.
   3. Paramedics report the client had a seizure enroute to the hospital.
   4. The nursing home report states the client has had diarrhea for the last 3 days.
   5. The client vomited soon after breakfast.

10. A client has urine electrolytes ordered. The nurse should prepare for which procedure?

    1. Obtaining a sterile voided specimen
    2. Collecting urine for 24 hours
    3. Catheterizing the client for a sterile specimen
    4. Obtaining a standard clean-catch specimen

Answers to questions found inside your textbook are available on the faculty resources site. Please consult with your instructor.

References

DeCarolis, D. D., Kim, G. M., Rector, T. S., & Ishani, A. (2016). Comparative dose response using the intravenous versus enteral route of administration for potassium replenishment. *Intensive and Critical Care Nursing, 36,* 17–23.

Doig, A. K., & Huether, S. (2014). The cellular environment: Fluids and electrolytes, acids and bases. In K. L. McCance, S. E. Huether, V. L. Brashers, & N. S. Rote (Eds.), *Pathophysiology: The biologic basis for disease in adults and children* (7th ed., pp. 103–134). St. Louis, MO: Elsevier Mosby.

Eaton, D. C., & Pooler, J. P. (2013). *Chapter 10: Regulation of calcium, magnesium, and phosphate.* In D. C. Eaton & J. P. Pooler (Eds.), *Vander's renal physiology* (8th ed.) Retrieved January 2, 2017, from http://accessmedicine.mhmedical.com/content.aspx?bookid=505&sectionid=42511989

Huether, S. (2017). Fluids and electrolytes, acids and bases. In S. E. Huether, L. L. McCance, V. L. Brashers, & N. S. Rote (Eds.), *Understanding pathophysiology* (6th ed., pp. 114–133). St. Louis, MO: Elsevier Mosby.

Kee, J. L. (2014). *Laboratory and diagnostic tests with nursing implications* (9th ed.). Hoboken, NJ: Pearson.

Lee, S. J., Ramar, K., Park, J. G., Gajic, O., Li, G., & Kashyap, R. (2014). Increased fluid administration in the first three hours of sepsis resuscitation is associated with reduced mortality. *Chest, 14*(4), 908–915.

LeMone, P., Burke, K. M., Bauldoff, G., & Gubrud, P. (2015). Chapter 15: Assessing the integumentary system. In P. LeMone, K. M. Burke, G. Bauldoff & P. Gubrud (Eds.), *Medical-surgical nursing: Clinical reasoning in patient care* (6th ed., pp. 376–389). Hoboken, NJ: Pearson.

Mount, D. B. (2015). *Chapter 63: Fluid and electrolyte disturbances.* In D. Kasper, A. Fauci, S. Hauser, D. Longo, J. L. Jameson, & J. J. Loscalzo (Eds.), *Harrison's principles of internal medicine* (19th ed.). Retrieved January 2, 2017, from http://accessmedicine.mhmedical.com/content.aspx?bookid=1130&sectionid=79726591

Patton, K. T., & Thibodeau, G. A. (2016). *Anatomy & physiology* (9th ed.). St. Louis, MO: Elsevier.

Zhang, A., Chen, K., & Ni, H. (2015). Calcium supplementation improves clinical outcome in intensive care unit patients: A propensity score matched analysis of a large database MIMC-II. *SpringerPlus, 13*(4), 594. doi:10.1186/s40064-015-1387-7

Chapter 26
Alterations in Fluid and Electrolyte Balance

Learning Outcomes

26.1 Apply knowledge of fluid volume deficit when caring for the high-acuity patient.

26.2 Demonstrate knowledge of fluid volume excess when delivering patient care.

26.3 Discuss alterations in sodium balance that affect patient care.

26.4 Apply knowledge of alterations in calcium balance when caring for the high-acuity patient.

26.5 Demonstrate understanding of alterations in potassium balance.

26.6 Apply knowledge of alterations in magnesium balance when delivering patient care.

26.7 Apply knowledge of alterations in phosphorus/phosphate balance.

Fluid and electrolyte balance is essential to maintaining physiologic homeostasis. The body is composed largely of fluids (about 50%–60% in adults). Fluids serve critical functions, such as acting as a solvent for metabolic chemical reactions; transporting nutrients, oxygen, and waste products; moistening and lubricating skin and mucous membranes; and regulating body temperature (Felver, 2013). Fluids are located in and constantly shift between the extracellular and intracellular compartments to carry out their functions.

Electrolytes are positively (cation) and negatively (anion) charged salts that are dissolved in the body's fluids and dispersed throughout the body in all compartments. Electrolytes play essential roles in electrical conduction, chemical reactions, production of energy, and regulation of body fluids. Imbalances in fluid or electrolytes can have profoundly negative effects on essentially all body systems. High-acuity patients, by virtue of their disease states, are at high risk for fluid or electrolyte imbalance, and these imbalances can result in serious or even life-threatening complications.

It is recommended that Chapter 25: Determinants and Assessment of Fluid and Electrolyte Balance be reviewed prior to beginning this chapter to enhance understanding of this material.

Section One: Fluid Volume Deficit

There are two major fluid compartments in the body: extracellular (composed of intravascular and interstitial fluids) and intracellular (composed of fluid within cells). Extracellular fluid (ECF) volume deficit is an abnormally low volume of body fluid in the intravascular and interstitial compartments from loss of sodium and fluid (Felver, 2013). This produces a state of extracellular dehydration, which can then cause intracellular dehydration as fluid shifts out of the cells to increase intravascular volume. For the purposes of this chapter, fluid volume deficit (FVD) refers to **hypovolemia**, an abnormally low circulating fluid volume, which is specific to the intravascular compartment.

Etiology

Many clinical problems can cause or contribute to the development of fluid volume deficit (FVD), which is a common and potentially serious problem in the high-acuity patient. These factors are summarized in Table 26–1.

Table 26–1 Factors That Produce Fluid Volume Deficit

Source of Fluid Loss	Related Factors
Gastrointestinal	Diarrhea, vomiting, nasogastric suction, fistulas, bleeding
Urinary	Drug therapy (e.g., diuretics), hyperglycemia, diabetes insipidus, diuretic phase of acute tubular necrosis (ATN)
Integumentary	Burns, diaphoresis, increased capillary permeability
Insensible	Hyperventilation, fever, hypermetabolism, tachypnea, mechanical ventilation
Other	Hemorrhage, wound drainage

As discussed in Chapter 25: Determinants and Assessment of Fluid and Electrolyte Balance, loss of extracellular fluid volume can be due to **third-spacing**, a unique fluid-shifting situation that can lead to significant FVD if the fluids are shifting into a serous cavity in conditions such as liver failure, pancreatitis, or peritonitis. The fluid shifts of third-spacing result from altered capillary membrane permeability secondary to tissue injury, ischemia, or inflammation, or they can develop because of increased hydrostatic pressure or decreased oncotic pressure in the intravascular space. The resulting trapped fluid is essentially unavailable for functional use within the body and may accumulate rapidly because of protein-rich contents, which causes increased tissue colloidal osmotic pressure, attracting more fluids.

Clinical Manifestations

Assessing the high-acuity patient for FVD is an important part of the daily nursing assessment, and patients with FVD require close monitoring. These patients have higher serum osmolality (greater than 300 mOsm/kg) due to

FVD. The critical (panic) value for hyperosmolality is 390 mOsm/kg or greater. Table 26–2 lists assessment data associated with fluid volume deficit.

Medical Treatment

The primary goals of medical treatment are to identify and control the source of fluid loss and to correct the deficit by replenishing fluids. Fluids can be replaced by intravenous (IV), oral, or enteral routes, depending on the severity of the FVD and the acuity level of the patient. Intravenous fluids are generally preferred for acute situations.

Intravenous Fluid Resuscitation Early and rapid fluid resuscitation with isotonic solutions is the cornerstone of management. There is still no clear consensus over the choice of resuscitation fluid. Colloids have not been shown to improve survival compared with crystalloids; thus, either may be used for volume resuscitation (Perel, Roberts, & Ker, 2013).

Intravenous fluids are classified according to their osmolality or tonicity. **Osmolality** refers to the number of milliosmoles (mOsm) per kilogram of solution. **Tonicity** refers to the effect the solution has on the extracellular fluid and intracellular fluid compartments and is sometimes used instead of osmolality (McClelland, 2014). Intravenous solutions are classified as isotonic, hypotonic, or hypertonic. The nurse should be aware of the reason a patient is receiving a particular IV fluid and what complications are associated with that fluid based on tonicity.

Isotonic Solutions. The term **isotonic** means that the osmolality of the solution on one side of a membrane is the same as the osmolality on the other side. Isotonic solutions have the same osmolality as body fluids (McClelland, 2014). The osmolality of isotonic fluid closely approximates normal serum plasma osmolality (solute concentration of body fluids, expressed in mOsm/kg). For this reason, a

Table 26–2 Nursing Assessment of Fluid Volume Deficit

Assessment	Parameter	Data
Physical assessment	Neurologic	Altered mental status, anxiety, restlessness, diminished alertness or cognition, possible coma
	Mucous membranes	Dry, decreased tongue size with longitudinal furrows
	Integumentary	Poor skin turgor, dry skin, pale or cool extremities
	Urinary	Decreased urinary output, oligura (severe FVD)
	Cardiovascular	Flat neck veins, decreased pulse volume and capillary refill, decreased venous filling
	Other	Thirst, weight loss (mild FVD = 2%–5%, moderate FVD = 6%–9%, severe FVD = greater than 10%), fatigue
Vital signs and hemodynamic pressures	HR, BP, temperature	Tachycardia, hypotension, orthostatic hypotension, hypothermia (isotonic FVD) or hyperthermia (dehydration)
	Central venous pressure (CVP) and pulmonary artery (PA) pressures	Decreased CVP and PA pressures, decreased CO
Laboratory data	Hematocrit (Hct), urine osmolality, specific gravity	Increased Hct, high serum osmolality, high urine specific gravity (increased concentration), increased BUN

steady osmolar state is maintained between intracellular fluid (ICF) and extracellular fluid (ECF); therefore, fluids do not shift from one compartment to another. Isotonic fluids (Figure 26–1A) are used when rapid ECF expansion is needed. The most common reason for administration of isotonic solutions, such as 0.9% normal saline (NS) or lactated Ringer's (LR) solution, is intravascular dehydration (intravascular FVD).

Hypotonic Solutions. **Hypotonic** solutions (e.g., 0.45% NS, and 0.2% NS, 2.5% dextrose) contain a lower concentration of particles than exists in the ICF and ECF. The low osmolality shifts fluid from the intravascular compartment into the intracellular compartments. Hypotonic fluids (Figure 26–1B) are used primarily in the treatment of cellular dehydration because they expand the intracellular volume. Hypotonic solutions must be used with caution, however, because their overuse causes cells (including blood cells) to expand and potentially burst, resulting in cellular destruction. Cellular overexpansion will result in increased intracranial pressure (ICP) and mental status deterioration; therefore, it is important to avoid administering hypotonic solutions to patients with neurological problems associated with increased ICP.

Hypertonic Solutions. **Hypertonic** solutions (e.g., $D_{10}W$ and 3% NS) have a high osmolality because they contain a higher concentration of particles than exists in the ICF and ECF. The high osmolality shifts fluids from the ICF and ECF into the intravascular compartment, expanding blood volume. Hypertonic solutions (Figure 26–1C) are used in the treatment of water intoxication (intracellular fluid volume excess). Water intoxication can be caused by administration of large amounts of electrolyte-free water, overuse of hypotonic solutions (e.g., 0.45% sodium chloride), elevated antidiuretic hormone (ADH) secretion, or renal failure.

Nursing Considerations

Patients with fluid volume deficits may experience diminished tissue perfusion and a decrease in cardiac

output when circulating volumes are low. Nursing interventions center on the treatment of contributing factors and may include measures to decrease vomiting, diarrhea, or fever; increasing oral fluid intake or administration of intravenous solutions; and monitoring of fluid and electrolyte status. Continuous intravenous fluids should be routinely assessed to ensure that the correct fluid type, rate, mechanism for delivery, and route are used for patient care. An example of a safety precaution for intravenous fluid delivery is described in the feature "Quality and Safety: Color Coding IV Tubing." Desired patient outcomes include pulse, blood pressure, central venous pressure (CVP), and pulmonary artery wedge pressure (PAWP) within acceptable ranges for the patient; normal serum osmolality; increased urine output with normal specific gravity; improved skin turgor; balanced intake and output; stable weight; moist mucous membranes; hematocrit and blood urea nitrogen (BUN) within acceptable limits; and absence of other dehydration manifestations.

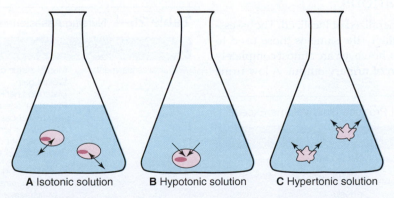

A Isotonic solution   **B** Hypotonic solution   **C** Hypertonic solution

Figure 26–1 Tonicity. A, Isotonic solutions (same osmolality as plasma, and IV fluids remain in intravascular space). B, Hypotonic solutions (lower osmolality than plasma, and IV fluids shift into the cells). C, Hypertonic solutions (higher osmolality than plasma, and IV fluids pull fluid from intracellular and extracellular compartments into intravascular compartment).

Section One Review

1. Where are third-spaced fluids most commonly located?
   A. Joints
   B. A serous cavity
   C. The cranial vault
   D. Interstitial fluid

2. Which statement is correct regarding extracellular FVD?
   A. It can lead to transcellular expansion.
   B. It can lead to intracellular expansion.
   C. It is associated with low serum osmolality.
   D. It is associated with high serum osmolality.

3. Which IV solution is commonly used for clients who have intravascular dehydration?
   A. Lactated Ringer's
   B. 0.45% normal saline
   C. 2.5% dextrose
   D. 3% normal saline

4. Which IV solution can cause cells to expand and burst, resulting in cellular destruction?
   A. 0.9% normal saline
   B. $D_{10}W$
   C. 0.45% normal saline
   D. Lactated Ringer's

Answers: 1. B, 2. D, 3. A, 4. C

Section Two: Fluid Volume Excess

Fluid volume excess (FVE), also called fluid overload or **hypervolemia**, produces a state of overhydration in the intravascular compartment. FVE results when both water and sodium are retained.

Etiology

Many high-acuity patients are at moderate to high risk for development of FVE. Common causes of FVE include such disorders as heart, liver, or kidney failure and overhydration secondary to excessive or too rapid delivery of IV therapy. FVE can also occur as a side effect of drugs such as corticosteroids. It is associated with fewer contributing factors than is FVD. These factors are summarized in Table 26–3.

Clinical Manifestations

Extracellular FVE can be generalized or localized. The assessment procedures are essentially the same as those used to assess for FVD. The findings, however, are almost completely opposite, with the exception of urinary output. A low urine output can be indicative of either a deficit or an excess. For example, a low urine output (< 0.5 mL/kg/hr) may be indicative of dehydration or kidney injury. Decreased urinary output in the patient with dehydration is a protective mechanism for the body to preserve volume. Decreased urinary output in the patient with kidney injury, however, causes fluid volume excess. Nursing assessment of the patient for FVE is summarized in Table 26–4. Altered serum laboratory values may include decreased hematocrit and hemoglobin, as well as a low serum osmolality, resulting from plasma dilution from excess extracellular fluid. The critical (panic) value for serum osmolality is 190 mOsm/kg or less.

Medical Treatment

The treatment for FVE is aimed at correcting the underlying cause and treating the manifestations. This is accomplished through restriction of sodium and water intake and administration of diuretics. Diuretics inhibit

Table 26–3 Factors That Produce Fluid Volume Excess

Source of Fluid Gain	Related Factors
Cardiovascular	Heart failure
Urinary	Renal failure (acute or chronic)
Hepatic	Cirrhosis Liver failure
Other	Cancer Thrombus Peripheral vascular disease Drug therapy (e.g., corticosteroids) High sodium intake Protein malnutrition

Table 26–4 Nursing Assessment of Fluid Volume Excess

Assessment	Data
Physical assessment	Mental status changes Weight gain Distended neck veins Periorbital edema, pitting edema over bony prominences Adventitious lung sounds, moist crackles Shortness of breath Generalized or dependent edema
Vital signs	Elevated blood pressure Elevated central venous and pulmonary artery pressures Increased cardiac output
Laboratory data	Decreased hematocrit (dilutional) Low serum osmolality Radiography: pulmonary vascular congestion, pleural effusion, pericardial effusion, ascites Low urine-specific gravity (decreased concentration)

Related Pharmacotherapy
Diuretics

Loop Diuretics

Furosemide (Fumide, Furomide, Lasix, Luramide)

Action and Uses

Inhibits resorption of sodium and chloride in the loop of Henle; decreases edema and intravascular volume.

Dosages (Adult)

Edema: 20–40 mg up to 600 g/day (IV) (administered in one or divided doses). May be given undiluted or dilute in D_5W, NS, or LR. Undiluted—administer no faster than 20 mg over 1–2 minutes.

Major Side Effects

Circulatory collapse
Hypokalemia

Nursing Implications

Monitor vital signs, especially during dosage adjustment.
Monitor for manifestations of hypokalemia.

Thiazide Diuretics

Hydrochlorothiazide (Apo-Hydro, Esidrix, Oretic, HCTZ, Urozide)

Action and Uses

Interferes with absorption of sodium ions across distal renal tubular segment to enhance excretion of sodium, chloride, potassium, bicarbonate, and water. Used in adjunct treatment of edema associated with heart failure, cirrhosis, and renal failure.

Dosages (Adult)

Edema: 25–200 mg/day (PO) in 1 to 3 divided doses
Hypertension: 12.5–100 mg/day (PO) in 1 to 2 divided doses

SOURCE: Based on Wilson et al. (2016).

Major Side Effects

Hyperglycemia
Hypokalemia

Nursing Implications

Monitor vital signs, especially during dosage adjustment.
Monitor for manifestations of hypokalemia.

Potassium-sparing Diuretics

Spironolactone (Aldactone, Novo-Spiroton)

Action and Uses

Competes with aldosterone for cellular receptor sites in distal renal tubule. Promotes sodium and chloride excretion without loss of potassium. Used for diuresis in cases of refractory edema due to heart failure or cirrhosis.

Dosages (Adult)

Edema: 25–200 mg/day (PO) in divided doses
Hypertension: 25–100 mg/day (PO) in 1 or divided doses, dose adjusted as needed

Major Side Effects

Hyponatremia
Hyperkalemia

Nursing Implications

Monitor serum electrolytes (sodium, potassium) during therapy.

---

sodium and water resorption and increase urine output and are commonly administered to patients with FVE. Diuretics are summarized in the "Related Pharmacotherapy: Diuretics" feature. Each diuretic drug group works on a different section of the kidney tubule.

Nursing Considerations

Fluid volume excess may result in impaired skin integrity, poor oxygenation of tissues due to impaired gas exchange, and symptoms secondary to fluid overload. Nursing interventions may include monitoring adherence to fluid or salt restrictions, administration of diuretics, or dialysis. Monitoring should also include daily weight, intake and output, and location and severity of edema, if present, as well as vital signs, chest x-ray, and possibly central venous pressures or pulmonary artery pressures. The desired patient outcomes for intravascular fluid excess include pulse, blood pressure, and central venous pressure (CVP) within acceptable ranges for the patient; lung sounds clear to auscultation; balanced intake and output; weight loss and resolution of edema; and hematocrit and blood urea nitrogen (BUN) within acceptable limits.

Section Two Review

1. Which assessments are consistent with fluid volume excess? (Select all that apply.)
   A. Weight loss
   B. Elevated central venous pressure
   C. Elevated blood pressure
   D. Sinus bradycardia
   E. Decreased hematocrit

2. Treatment for fluid volume excess may include restricting which intake? (Select all that apply.)
   A. Fluids
   B. Protein
   C. Carbohydrates
   D. Sodium
   E. Fats

3. Which drug inhibits resorption of sodium and chloride in the loop of Henle?
   A. Furosemide
   B. Spironolactone
   C. Hydrochlorothiazide
   D. No drugs work in this area.

4. Which client outcome would be appropriate for a client who is experiencing fluid volume excess? (Select all that apply.)
   A. CVP within normal range for client
   B. Weight gain of 2%–3%
   C. Balanced intake and output
   D. BUN within acceptable limits
   E. Pulse rate below 60 bpm

Answers: 1. (B, C, E), 2. (A, D), 3. A, 4. (A, C, D)

Section Three: Sodium Imbalances

Sodium is the major extracellular cation whose major function is regulation of body water. Therefore, imbalances in sodium result in fluid imbalances. Normal ranges and critical values of the electrolytes discussed in this chapter are listed in Table 26–5. Critical (or panic) values are laboratory measurements that are potentially life-threatening and require immediate attention.

Hyponatremia

Hyponatremia, or abnormally low serum sodium, occurs when the serum sodium level falls below 135 mmol/L and a critical value is 120 mmol/L or less (Kee, 2014; Mayo Clinic Laboratories, 2015).

Etiology Hyponatremia is the most common electrolyte disorder in hospitalized patients (Palmer, 2016), with many cases developing postadmission. Hyponatremia can result from excessive salt loss relative to water loss, excessive water gain in relation to salt gain, or both (Felver, 2013).

Excessive Salt Loss Relative to Water Loss. A variety of problems can cause an imbalance in salt and water excretion. Persistent hyponatremia can occur with continuous release of antidiuretic hormone (ADH) from the pituitary or ectopic production of ADH. This unregulated production of ADH is associated with the syndrome of inappropriate antidiuretic hormone (SIADH), which can result from head injury, malignant tumors, and certain drugs (Cho, 2017). Many diuretic agents, particularly thiazides,

block the resorption of salt (NaCl) in the distal convoluted tubules of the kidneys, causing it to be excreted (Felver, 2013). Water and electrolytes are not necessarily excreted in the same ratio as they exist in the blood, however; relatively more salt can be excreted than water, resulting in hyponatremia (and hypochloremia) (Lehne, 2016). Other possible causes include replacement of water without replacement of salt—for example, overuse of dextrose 5% in water (D_5W) intravenous fluid.

Excessive Water Gain Relative to Salt Gain. Hyponatremia can result from a net gain of water in the extracellular fluid compartment without an equivalent increase in sodium, which causes the plasma to become hypotonic. Normal-functioning kidneys are able to excrete about 16 to 20 liters of free water every day (Palmer, 2016). When the rapid ingestion or administration of large quantities of water exceeds the ability of the kidneys to excrete it, this form of hyponatremia can develop (Felver, 2013).

Clinical Manifestations The nature of hyponatremia onset (acute or chronic) influences the severity of symptoms. Rapid onset is associated with more severe symptoms because the body has less time to activate compensatory mechanisms; a slow onset is associated with less severe symptoms secondary to compensation. Clinical manifestations primarily reflect alterations in central nervous system function. Seizures and coma develop with a rapid decrease in sodium to less than 110 mEq/L. The most severe complication of hyponatremia is cerebral edema caused by intracellular swelling (Felver, 2013). Cerebral edema develops when sodium concentrations inside brain cells is greater than sodium concentration in the extracellular fluid due to hyponatremia. Osmotic forces pull water from the blood into the brain cells, resulting in cerebral edema. Hyponatremia is also associated with early changes in muscle tone because sodium plays a role in the transmission of neuromuscular impulses. The clinical manifestations of hyponatremia are summarized in Table 26–6.

Medical Treatment The treatment of hyponatremia depends on the cause; therefore, it is important to determine the underlying cause and correct it when possible. For example, if the patient has SIADH, water restriction is implemented. The aggressiveness with which the sodium imbalance is corrected depends on the severity of symptoms and duration of the imbalance (Palmer, 2016). Patients with severe hyponatremia may be given hypertonic fluids, such as 3% or 5% NaCl solution at a rate of 1 to 2 mL/kg/hr to raise the serum sodium by 1 to 2 mEq/hr, but this should be

Table 26–5 Laboratory Normal Ranges and Critical (Panic) Values*

Parameter	Normal Range	Critical (Panic) Values
Sodium (mmol/L)	135 to 145	≤ 120 or ≥ 160
Calcium (total) (mg/dL)	9 to 11	≤ 6.5 or ≥ 13
Potassium (mmol/L)	3.5 to 5.3	≤ 2.5 or ≥ 6
Phosphorus (mg/dL)	2.5 to 4.5	≤ 1
Magnesium (mg/dL)	1.8 to 3	≤ 1 or ≥ 9

*Normal laboratory ranges and critical values vary among agencies.
SOURCE: Data from Kee (2014); Mayo Clinic Laboratories (2016).

Table 26–6 Major Manifestations of Alterations in Sodium

Assessment	Hyponatremia	Hypernatremia
Cardiovascular	Hypotension	Severe: hypertension, tachycardia
Neurologic	Confusion, headache, lethargy, possible coma	Moderate: confusion, thirst Severe: restlessness, coma
Gastrointestinal	Anorexia, vomiting, diarrhea, cramps	Nausea and vomiting
Neuromuscular	Seizures, muscle cramps or spasms	Hyperreflexia, muscle twitching, seizures
Fluid balance	Deficit	Excess, edema

SOURCE: Data from Cho (2017).

limited to the initial phase of treatment. The overall correction should not exceed 10 to 12 mEq/L in 24 hours or 18 mEq/L in 48 hours; otherwise there is a risk of demyelination (Palmer, 2016). Conivaptan hydrochloride (Vaprisol) may be ordered. Conivaptan blocks ADH in the kidneys to cause excretion of water and retention of sodium (Wilson, Shannon, & Shields, 2016). Fluid restriction and reassessment of patient medications are also cornerstones of therapy. The "Related Pharmacotherapy: Sodium" feature provides a summary of intravenous sodium solution information.

Nursing Considerations The major manifestations of hyponatremia are related to central nervous system (CNS) dysfunction. Therefore, the nurse should focus assessments on CNS functions, and changes in the patient's mental status should be followed up immediately. If hypertonic fluids are given, the nurse must monitor the patient for pulmonary edema. The nurse should also closely monitor the patient's response to therapy, because correcting sodium levels too quickly can cause iatrogenic cerebral osmotic demyelination syndrome, causing neurological effects that are generally catastrophic and irreversible, such as loss of consciousness, cognitive changes, and paralysis (Cho, 2017).

Hypernatremia

Hypernatremia, abnormally elevated serum sodium, is clinically defined as a serum sodium level above 145 mmol/L, and a critical value is 160 mmol/L or higher (Kee, 2014; Mayo Clinic Laboratories, 2015). It develops when the extracellular volume of water is low relative to the amount of sodium ions available, causing sodium concentration. Hypernatremia results in the shift of water from the intracellular space into the extracellular compartment. The cells shrink and shrivel as fluid moves out of them, causing cellular dehydration; and the extracellular compartment becomes overloaded with water.

Etiology In the high-acuity patient, causes of hypernatremia include administration of sodium bicarbonate solutions to correct metabolic acidosis, renal water loss through a defect in the renal concentration system, the use of diuretics or diuresis from hyperglycemia (such as in diabetic ketoacidosis), gastrointestinal losses through nasogastric suction, water losses from fever, and drainage from open wounds.

Hypernatremia caused by excess water loss can result from renal dysfunction, profuse diaphoresis, or increased adrenocorticotropin hormone (ACTH) secretion (e.g., Cushing syndrome).

Clinical Manifestations As with hyponatremia, the clinical manifestations of hypernatremia are predominantly neurologic because brain cells are especially sensitive to sodium levels. However, in severe cases, multiple body systems are affected. If hypernatremia develops rapidly, cellular shrinkage also contributes to the neurologic symptoms. In addition, the patient will report extreme thirst if able to communicate. The clinical manifestations of hypernatremia are summarized in Table 26–6.

Medical Treatment Detection and treatment require recognition of symptoms, identification of underlying defects of water metabolism, correction of volume disturbances, and correction of serum sodium. The primary medical treatment for hypernatremia is water replacement. The

Related Pharmacotherapy
Sodium

Example Agents
0.9% NaCl, 0.45% NaCl, 0.25% NaCl, and 3% and 5% sodium solution (IV)

Action and Uses
Major intracellular cation, used in the sodium–potassium pump to maintain cellular homeostasis. Has a significant role in water balance and distribution between cells and vascular spaces. Used for sodium and volume replacement therapy.

Dosages (Adult)
Hyponatremia: No recommended doses. Treatment of severe hyponatremia depends on the underlying cause, whether patient is symptomatic, and severity of symptoms.

Major Side Effects
Cellular edema, confusion, seizures, coma

Nursing Implications
Monitor serum sodium values. Replace sodium carefully. Diuresis or sodium replacement performed too quickly can result in severe neurologic disturbances.
Weigh patients daily.
Monitor intake and output.

fluid volume deficit (FVD) may be corrected with administration of hypotonic IV fluids. The rate of correction depends on the rate of development and the presence of symptoms. It is recommended that half the water deficit be corrected in 24 hours while the neurologic status is monitored (Palmer, 2016). Diuretics may also be given to enhance sodium excretion.

Nursing Considerations The patient should be monitored for neurologic changes. This is especially important when administering water replacement, as changes in serum sodium or osmolality can cause rapid fluid and electrolyte shifts in the brain. The nurse should also monitor fluid volume replacement in intake and output, as well as the therapeutic and nontherapeutic effects of therapies.

Section Three Review

1. Hyponatremia is associated with which symptom?
   A. Edema
   B. Hyperreflexia
   C. Lethargy
   D. Restlessness

2. Clients with severe hyponatremia may require IV fluids. Which type of IV fluid would the nurse expect to be ordered to treat severe hyponatremia?
   A. Isotonic
   B. Hypotonic
   C. Hypertonic
   D. Lactated Ringer's

3. Hypernatremia can be caused by which conditions? (Select all that apply.)
   A. Hyperthyroidism
   B. Profuse diuresis
   C. Cushing syndrome
   D. Diabetes insipidus
   E. Fever

4. What is a sign or symptom of hypernatremia?
   A. Diarrhea
   B. Muscle twitching
   C. Stomach cramps
   D. Decreased muscle tone

Answers: 1. C, 2. C, 3. (B, C, D, E), 4. B

Section Four: Calcium Imbalances

Circulating blood normally contains very little calcium; the normal value range is 9–11 mg/dL (Kee, 2014). Calcium imbalances can result in complications primarily of the neurologic, skeletal, hematopoietic, and cardiovascular systems.

Hypocalcemia

Hypocalcemia, or abnormally low serum calcium, is defined as a total calcium level less than 9 mg/dL, with a critical value of 6.5 mg/dL or greater (Kee, 2014; Mayo Clinic Laboratories, 2015). Hypocalcemia is one of the most frequent electrolyte disturbances encountered in the high-acuity patient.

Etiology There are many potential causes of hypocalcemia, including hypoalbuminemia, trauma, acute kidney injury and chronic kidney disease, sepsis, hypoparathyroidism, hypomagnesemia, vitamin D deficiency, and the administration of citrate. Hypocalcemia can be induced by the administration of large amounts of stored blood because stored blood is preserved with citrate. When blood is administered, the citrate binds with calcium, which lowers ionized calcium. Other causes include decreased bone resorption, drug binding of calcium, decreased secretion of parathyroid hormone with or without hypomagnesemia, and hypocalcemia related to chronic kidney disease (Cho, 2017).

Clinical Manifestations Normally, calcium stabilizes neuromuscular cell membranes. When calcium is low, neuromuscular irritability increases, with multiple related signs and symptoms. In addition, cardiovascular manifestations include specific ECG changes (Table 26–7) (Cho, 2017).

Medical Treatment Medical management of hypocalcemia is aimed at correcting the underlying cause and restoring normal calcium balance. Severe, symptomatic hypocalcemia should be treated with intravenous calcium gluconate. A continuous calcium infusion is usually required, due to its short duration of action. Ten to 15 milligrams of calcium per kilogram body weight is added to 1 L of D_5W and infused over 4 to 6 hours. With subsequent serum calcium monitoring every 4 to 6 hours, the infusion rate is adjusted to maintain a serum calcium level at 7 to 8.5 mg/dL (Cho, 2017). The "Related Pharmacotherapy: Calcium" feature provides a summary of calcium therapy.

Nursing Considerations Hypocalcemia is commonly seen in the presence of other electrolyte disorders. For example, hypomagnesemia is common and should be corrected by calcium administration. It is hypothesized that magnesium deficiency may impair the release or activity of parathyroid hormone. If metabolic acidosis is present, hypocalcemia should be corrected first because the treatment of acidosis decreases the concentration of ionized calcium, which can precipitate problems such as tetany and cardiac arrest. Patients with hypocalcemia will have concomitant hyperphosphatemia, as calcium and phosphorus

Table 26–7 Major Manifestations of Alterations in Calcium

Body System	Hypocalcemia	Hypercalcemia
Cardiovascular	Hypotension, decreased myocardial contractility ECG changes: prolonged *QT* interval, long *ST* segment	Hypertension, cardiovascular calcification ECG changes: shortened *QT* interval, decreased *ST* segment, heart block, cardiac dysrhythmias (bradycardia, first- and second-degree heart block)
Neurologic	Irritability, reduced cognitive ability	Lethargy, depression, fatigue, impaired memory, emotional lability Severe: confusion, stupor, coma
Neuromuscular	Cramps (abdominal and extremities), paresthesias Severe: positive Chvostek or Trousseau sign, tetany, seizures	Muscle weakness
Gastrointestinal	—	Anorexia, constipation, peptic ulcer disease, abdominal discomfort
Skeletal	Bone fractures possible	Pathologic bone fractures, bone thinning (osteopenia, osteoporosis)
Other	Abnormal clotting	Kidney stones, polyuria, polydipsia

SOURCE: Data from Cho (2017).

are inversely related. The nurse should monitor the patient with hypocalcemia for signs and symptoms of decreased cardiac output, ECG changes, and neurologic and neuromuscular changes.

Hypercalcemia

Hypercalcemia, or abnormally elevated serum calcium, is defined as a serum calcium level above 11 mg/dL with a critical level of 13 mg/dL or higher (Kee, 2014; Mayo Clinic Laboratories, 2015). Hypercalcemia occurs when calcium enters the extracellular fluid more rapidly than it can be excreted by the kidneys.

Etiology   Primary hyperparathyroidism and malignancy account for more than 90% of the cases of hypercalcemia in ambulatory and non–critically ill patients. A small percentage of cases develop from immobilization, vitamin A or D intoxication, and lithium or thiazide diuretic use. Malignancy as a cause of hypercalcemia is complex and varies with the type of tumor, usually breast and lung cancers and multiple myelomas. Hyperparathyroidism accounts for about half of the cases of hypercalcemia, and it results from increased release of calcium from bone, augmented intestinal resorption, and renal resorption of calcium.

Calcium is absorbed in the intestines only under the influence of activated vitamin D (calcitriol); therefore, a high level of vitamin D in the body can lead to hypercalcemia from increased intestinal absorption. Hypercalcemia usually accompanies hypophosphatemia because calcium and phosphate levels shift in opposite directions (i.e., they maintain an inverse relationship).

Clinical Manifestations   The signs and symptoms of hypercalcemia generally are proportional to the serum calcium level. Serum calcium levels of 11.5 mg/dL rarely produce symptoms, but levels between 11.5 and 13 mg/dL may be associated with lethargy, anorexia, and nausea. Higher calcium levels are associated with more profound neurologic and neuromuscular changes. Hypercalcemia decreases neuromuscular excitability because it acts as a sedative at the myoneural junction. Altered GI motility associated with hypercalcemia results in delayed gastric emptying and vomiting; patients are predisposed to

Related Pharmacotherapy
Calcium

Example Agents

Calcium chloride, calcium gluconate

Action and Uses
Restores serum calcium levels in acute hypocalcemia, improves myocardial contractility. Calcium chloride contains more calcium than does calcium gluconate.

Dosages (Adult)
Calcium chloride (IV): Hypocalcemia: 0.5–1 g at 1–3 day intervals based on patient data. Hypocalcemic tetany: 4.5–16 mEq/kg 3–4 ×/day. CPR: 2–4 mg/kg (repeat in 10 min if needed).
Calcium gluconate (IV): Hypocalcemia: 2–15 g/day (divided or continuous dose). Hypocalcemic tetany: 1–3 g as needed;

may repeat every 6 hrs as needed (max. dose: 15 g/day). CPR: 2.3–3.7 mEq × 1 dose.

Major Side Effects
Cardiac arrest, hypotension, bradycardia with rapid infusion

Nursing Implications
Monitor ECG and BP closely during administration.
Can be irritating to veins when given in peripheral IV.
Can cause necrosis and sloughing of tissue if extravasation occurs.
Must be administered slowly when given IV (0.5–1 mL/min).
Calcium chloride is three times more potent than calcium gluconate; carefully check label.

SOURCE: Based on Wilson et al. (2016).

duodenal ulcer disease because of increased gastric acid secretion. Disturbed renal function from hypercalcemia can cause polyuria and polydipsia, and it is considered a form of nephrogenic diabetes insipidus that is usually reversible. Calcium exerts a positive inotropic effect on the heart and reduces heart rate similar to the effect of cardiac glycosides (e.g., digoxin).

The signs and symptoms of hypophosphatemia can accompany hypercalcemia, as their serum levels are inversely related. Alterations in phosphorus are presented separately in Section Seven.

Medical Treatment   Treatment focuses on correcting the underlying cause and reducing serum calcium levels. For example, hyperparathyroidism is managed by parathyroidectomy, and malignant tumors may be managed through surgical removal, chemotherapy, and radiation therapy. Strategies to lower serum calcium levels include the promotion of calcium elimination by the kidneys and the reduction of calcium resorption from the bone. Large volumes of IV fluids and diuretic therapy may be given to promote the elimination of calcium. Other drugs used to reduce calcium include bisphosphonates, calcitonin, and sodium phosphate or potassium phosphate.

Nursing Considerations   Patients with hypercalcemia may be at risk for injury as a result of a loss of calcium from bones (falls, pathological fractures). The nurse should be aware of patients at risk for hypercalcemia, increase patient mobilization if possible, and encourage the oral intake of fluids if possible or administer IV fluids as ordered if sufficient oral intake is not feasible. The nurse should also monitor the patient's diet to ensure that it contains sufficient fiber to prevent constipation. Furthermore, the increased risk of pathologic fractures warrants taking steps to reduce the risk of falls through careful environmental assessment and patient–family teaching regarding environmental and mobility safety.

Section Four Review

1. What are common causes of hypocalcemia in high-acuity clients? (Select all that apply.)
   A. Administration of large amounts of stored blood
   B. Hypoparathyroidism
   C. Acute pancreatitis
   D. Malignancy
   E. Sepsis

2. Rapid infusion of IV calcium can result in which manifestations? (Select all that apply.)
   A. Tachycardia
   B. Hypertension
   C. Cardiac arrest
   D. Hypotension
   E. Fever

3. Hypercalcemia can be caused by which factors? (Select all that apply.)
   A. Bone metastasis
   B. Hyperactivity
   C. Hypothyroidism
   D. Thiazide diuretics
   E. Hyperparathyroidism

4. Hypercalcemia increases the client's risk of complications from which factors? (Select all that apply.)
   A. Pathological fractures
   B. Falls
   C. Decreased mental status
   D. Cardiac dysrhythmias
   E. Seizures

Answers: 1. (A, B, E), 2. (C, D), 3. (A, D, E), 4. (A, B, C, D)

Section Five: Potassium Imbalances

Potassium is the major intracellular electrolyte, with a normal serum range of 3.5 to 5.3 mmol/L. The body does not tolerate significant alterations in serum potassium, and life-threatening cardiac complications can arise (as shown in Figure 26–2A).

Hypokalemia

Hypokalemia, or abnormally low serum potassium, is clinically defined as a serum potassium level below 3.5 mmol/L with a critical value of 2.5 mmol/L or less (Kee, 2014; Mayo Clinic Laboratories, 2015). When hypokalemia occurs, the body does not attempt to retain or resorb potassium.

Because the body does not compensate for potassium loss, it is essential that hypokalemia be rapidly detected and corrected through potassium supplementation. The body is intolerant of abnormal serum potassium levels, and critical derangements (either high or low) can result in cardiac dysrhythmias or cardiac arrest (Kee, 2014).

Etiology   High-acuity patients are at significant risk for development of hypokalemia, particularly related to compartment shifts, gastrointestinal loss, and therapies. Table 26–8 lists some of the major causes of hypokalemia.

Clinical Manifestations   Because potassium is important in nerve impulse as well as cardiac impulse conduction, muscle contraction, and cell membrane function, the signs and symptoms of imbalance reflect interference with these activities, such as paralysis and respiratory muscle weakness (Josephson & Samuels, 2015). Because potassium

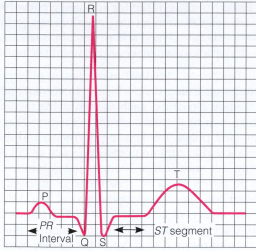

A Normal ECG

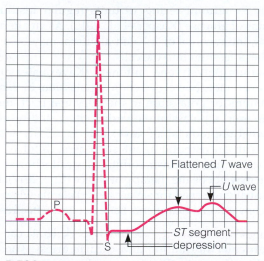

B ECG in hypokalemia

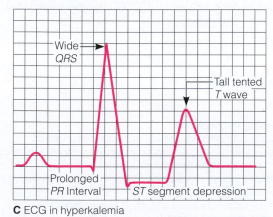

C ECG in hyperkalemia

Figure 26–2 The effects of changes in potassium levels on the ECG. A, Normal. B, Hypokalemia. C, Hyperkalemia.

affects the transmission of nerve impulses, hypokalemia can result in electrocardiogram (ECG) changes, including flattened or inverted *T* waves, the development of *U* waves, and depressed *ST* segment (Figure 26–2B). Cardiac disturbances can be especially significant in patients with hypertension, myocardial infarction, ischemia, or heart failure. In patients receiving digoxin therapy, low serum

Table 26–8 Major Causes of Potassium Abnormalities

Causes of Hypokalemia	Causes of Hyperkalemia
Loss of gastrointestinal secretions through vomiting, diarrhea, excessive nasogastric suction fluid loss, and fistulas Excessive excretion by kidneys Movement of potassium into cells (e.g., metabolic alkalosis) Prolonged fluid administration without potassium supplementation Excessive use of potassium-wasting diuretics without adequate potassium supplementation	Renal failure Adrenal insufficiency Insulin deficiency and resistance Rhabdomyolysis Severe burns Acidosis Drug induced (e.g., beta-adrenergic blockers, ACE inhibitors or angiotensin receptor blockers, potassium-sparing diuretics, cyclosporine, NSAIDs, and others)

SOURCE: Data from Cho (2017).

potassium levels can potentiate the action of digitalis (Mossop & DiBlasio, 2017). The clinical manifestations of hypokalemia are summarized in Table 26–9.

Medical Treatment   The major objective of hypokalemia treatment is to determine the cause and prevent emergencies such as severe cardiac dysrhythmias or respiratory muscle weakness. Urinary excretion of potassium should be measured by obtaining a 24-hour urine specimen. Hypokalemia is treated with oral or IV administration of potassium. The preferred route of replacement is oral unless the patient is having cardiac disturbances. The "Related Pharmacotherapy: Potassium" feature provides a summary of potassium therapy.

Nursing Considerations   The patient with hypokalemia should be monitored closely for dysrhythmias and the development of characteristic ECG changes. The nurse should monitor potassium levels and take action to prevent hypokalemia. The patient receiving digitalis should be assessed for symptoms of digitalis toxicity (e.g., vision changes, confusion, dizziness, vomiting, and cardiac dysrhythmias). Administration of potassium through a peripheral vein can be painful and cause irritation to the vein; it is

Table 26–9 Major Manifestations of Alterations in Potassium

Assessment	Hypokalemia	Hyperkalemia
Cardiovascular	ECG changes: flattened or inverted *T* waves, development of *U* waves, and depressed *ST* segment	ECG changes: progression from tachycardia to bradycardia to cardiac arrest is possible; prolonged *PR* interval; flat or absent *P* wave; slurring of *QRS*; tall peaked *T* wave; *ST* segment depression
Pulmonary	Respiratory muscle weakness	
Musculoskeletal	Muscle weakness or cramps	Muscle weakness or cramps
Gastrointestinal	Constipation or ileus	Nausea, vomiting, abdominal cramping, diarrhea
Acid–base		Metabolic acidosis

SOURCE: Data from Cho (2017).

preferable to administer potassium through a central venous catheter.

Hyperkalemia

Hyperkalemia, or abnormally elevated serum potassium, is clinically defined as a potassium level above 5.3 mmol/L with a critical value of 6.0 mmol/L or higher (Kee, 2014; Mayo Clinic Laboratories, 2015). Many high-acuity patients are at risk for development of hyperkalemia related to their disease process, disease complications, or therapies.

Etiology Severe kidney injury and acidosis are common risk factors for hyperkalemia in the high-acuity patient. In the presence of renal failure, the kidneys cannot excrete sufficient amounts of potassium, thus increasing serum levels. Acidosis contributes to hyperkalemia because excess hydrogen ions shift into the cells, forcing potassium out into the serum (Mount, 2015). Medications also can precipitate hyperkalemia. For example, beta-adrenergic blockers such as propranolol interfere with the entry of potassium into the cells. Captopril (ACE inhibitor) and nonsteroidal anti-inflammatory drugs (NSAIDs) exert an inhibitory effect on aldosterone secretion, which can cause hyperkalemia in patients with renal insufficiency. Table 26–8 lists common causes of hyperkalemia.

Manifestations Because potassium is important in nerve impulse conduction, muscle contraction, and cell membrane function, the signs and symptoms of imbalance reflect interference with these activities. Manifestations of hyperkalemia usually develop when serum potassium levels rise above 6.0 mEq/L. ECG changes associated with hyperkalemia include peaked T waves, and in severe hyperkalemia, absent P waves and a widened QRS pattern can occur (Cho, 2017) (see Figure 26–2(C)). The manifestations of hyperkalemia are summarized in Table 26–9. Care must be taken when a blood sample is taken for evaluating potassium levels, as a false elevation in serum potassium can occur if the blood sample is hemolyzed and potassium is released or if blood is drawn above a site where potassium is infusing.

Medical Treatment Medical management of hyperkalemia includes returning the potassium to normal and treating the underlying cause, such as identifying medications that are known to increase serum potassium (e.g., ACE inhibitors and potassium-sparing diuretics) and decreasing substances that contain potassium, such as potassium-containing salt substitutes. Urinary potassium excretion should be assessed. The treatment of hyperkalemia depends on how high the potassium level is and the presence of any emergent conditions. If ECG changes or dysrhythmias are present, intravenous calcium gluconate should be administered to stabilize the cardiac membrane. The next step is to drive the potassium back into the cells, usually by administering 10 units regular insulin and 50 grams of glucose (Kasper et al., 2016). As an alternative therapy, intravenous or inhaled albuterol may be used to shift the potassium into the cells.

Sodium polystyrene sulfonate (Kayexalate) may be given to promote bowel excretion of potassium by exchanging sodium for potassium in the intestinal tract, but it is slow to exert a potassium-lowering effect, and results are somewhat unpredictable. Kayexalate is usually administered with an osmotic agent such as sorbitol to cause osmotic diarrhea; however, sorbitol may cause bowel necrosis so it may not be the therapy of choice (Cho, 2017). Dialysis is usually reserved for severe hyperkalemia when other, more conventional treatments have not been effective.

Nursing Considerations Severe hyperkalemia can result in ventricular fibrillation and cardiac arrest. The nurse should notify the healthcare provider of elevated potassium laboratory values and ECG changes associated with

---

Related Pharmacotherapy

Potassium

Example Agents

Potassium chloride (Slow K, K-Dur, many others)
Potassium gluconate (Kaon, Kaylixir)

Action and Uses

Needed for adequate transmission of nerve impulses and cardiac contraction, renal function, and intracellular ion maintenance.

Dosages (Adult)

Potassium chloride (IV): Exact dose is based on patient's potassium level. Generally 3 mEq/kg or less with maximum dose of 400 mEq/day. Rate of delivery: no higher than 10 mEq/hr typically. In emergency, can deliver at higher rate but must closely watch cardiac rhythm status.

Major Side Effects

Cardiac dysrhythmias, cardiac arrest, peaked T waves, prolonged $P–R$ intervals, U waves, widened QRS complex

Nursing Implications

IV potassium chloride is NEVER administered undiluted.
Always invert IV bag several times when adding KCl to thoroughly mix it with IV solution before administering.
Monitor for dysrhythmias and ECG changes (particularly at higher doses).
Monitor potassium levels and report abnormalities.
Monitor intake and output.
Monitor cardiac status and hematologic parameters such as central venous pressure (CVP) and pulmonary pressures if monitoring directly.
IV administration can be painful in peripheral sites. Administer 10 mEq/hr. Administer 20 mEq/hr in central lines only.

SOURCE: Based on Wilson et al. (2016).

hyperkalemia. Measures to prevent hyperkalemia should be taken, such as identification of at-risk patients, regular evaluation of serum electrolytes, review of medications for effects on potassium, and monitoring diet for potassium content. In the presence of abnormal kidney function, the nurse should monitor blood urea nitrogen (BUN) and creatinine (Cr) because kidney failure is a major cause of hyperkalemia. The nurse should also monitor the patient's intake and output and report low urine output to the healthcare provider.

Section Five Review

1. For a client with hypokalemia, the nurse should monitor the ECG for which changes? (Select all that apply.)
   A. Presence of *U* waves
   B. Flattened *T* waves
   C. Peaked *T* waves
   D. Depressed *ST* segment
   E. Extreme bradycardia

2. What is a common side effect of the administration of potassium in a peripheral IV catheter?
   A. Burning pain
   B. Dysrhythmia
   C. Diarrhea
   D. Tissue necrosis

3. Hyperkalemia can be caused by which condition?
   A. Renal failure
   B. Potassium-wasting diuretics
   C. Metabolic alkalosis
   D. Severe diarrhea

4. The clinical findings of hyperkalemia include which set of signs and/or symptoms?
   A. Muscle weakness, *T* wave inversion on ECG
   B. Muscle twitching, *ST* segment depression on ECG
   C. Vomiting, peaked *T* wave on ECG
   D. Diarrhea, presence of *U* wave on ECG

Answers: 1. (A, B, D), 2. A, 3. A, 4. C

Section Six: Magnesium Imbalances

Magnesium is an intracellular electrolyte that plays a crucial role in ensuring that sodium and potassium are transported across cell membranes. It also plays an important role in nerve cell conduction. The normal range for magnesium is 1.8 to 3 mg/dL.

Hypomagnesemia

Hypomagnesemia, or abnormally low serum magnesium, is defined as a serum magnesium level of less than 1.8 mg/dL with a critical value of 1.2 mg/dL (Kee, 2014; Mayo Clinic Laboratories, 2015).

Etiology High-acuity patients are at moderate to high risk for development of hypomagnesemia. Common causes of hypomagnesemia include gastrointestinal or renal losses, surgery, trauma, infections or sepsis, burns, transfusions of blood preserved with citrate, alcoholism, and malnutrition. In addition, certain medications can cause hypomagnesemia, such as diuretics, aminoglycosides, amphotericin B, and cyclosporine (Cho, 2017). Hypoparathyroidism, with resultant hypocalcemia, can also cause hypomagnesemia because the regulatory mechanisms of magnesium and calcium are closely related.

Manifestations The signs and symptoms of magnesium imbalances are similar to those seen in calcium imbalances, altering CNS and neuromuscular and cardiac function. Hypomagnesemia is associated with ECG changes and ventricular dysrhythmias and seizures, coma, and death

(Cho, 2017). The clinical manifestations associated with hypomagnesemia are presented in Table 26–10.

Medical Treatment Medical management is directed at raising serum magnesium levels. Goals include preventing fatal cardiac dysrhythmias and resolving symptoms. The patient should be assessed for renal failure before administering magnesium because the kidneys are primarily responsible for its elimination. Intravenous administration is preferred in patients with severe hypomagnesemia (less than 1.2 mg/dL) or if neurologic changes or cardiac dysrhythmias occur. Infusion time is critical because magnesium distributes into tissues slowly and is rapidly excreted by the kidneys, with up to 50% of the infused magnesium lost in the urine (Cho, 2017). The "Related Pharmacotherapy: Magnesium" feature provides a summary of magnesium therapy.

Table 26–10 Major Manifestations of Alterations in Magnesium

Body System	Hypomagnesemia	Hypermagnesemia
Serum Mg level	Less than 1.8 mg/dL	Greater than 3 mg/dL
Cardiovascular	ECG changes: premature ventricular contractions, ventricular tachycardia and/or fibrillation, *T* wave flattening, decreased *ST* segment	Hypotension ECG changes: prolonged *PR* intervals, complete heart block, wide *QRS* complex, bradycardia, cardiac arrest
Respiratory		Depression
Neuromuscular	Tremors, tetany, Babinski response, confusion, disorientation	Absent deep tendon reflexes, lethargy, drowsiness

SOURCE: Data from Cho (2017).

Related Pharmacotherapy
Magnesium

Example Agents
Magnesium sulfate, magnesium oxide, magnesium citrate

Action and Uses
Significant role in the structure of bones and intracellular fluid component. Participates in numerous enzymatic reactions, many involving adenosine triphosphate (ATP). Important in neuronal control, neuromuscular transmission, and cardiovascular tone.

Dosages (Adult)
Magnesium sulfate (IV): seizures—1 g (repeat dose if needed). Severe hypomagnesemia—5 g to run over a 3-hr period.

SOURCE: Based on Wilson et al. (2016).

Major Side Effects
Impaired energy production and utilization of substrates
Dysrhythmias, *PR* and *QT* interval prolongation, widened *QRS* complex, *ST* segment depression.
Hypotension if administered too rapidly (IV).

Nursing Implications
Magnesium level is closely related to levels of calcium, phosphorus, and potassium.
Administer slowly according to directions.
Monitor blood pressure and EKG for changes.

Nursing Considerations The nurse should monitor patients with hypomagnesemia for the development of ventricular dysrhythmias, seizures, and neurologic deterioration. Hypokalemia is relatively common in patients with low magnesium levels because the kidneys are not able to conserve potassium when a magnesium deficiency exists. Hypocalcemia can occur in conjunction with hypomagnesemia because severe magnesium depletion interferes with parathyroid hormone, which is needed to return calcium levels to their normal ranges (Molina, 2013).

Hypermagnesemia

Hypermagnesemia, or abnormally elevated serum magnesium, results when magnesium levels rise above 3 mg/dL with a critical value of 9 mg/dL (Kee, 2014). This abnormality is not common but can occur with diminished renal excretion or excessive magnesium intake. Magnesium is primarily excreted by the kidneys, so patients with renal failure are at risk for hypermagnesemia. Consumption of large quantities of magnesium-containing antacids or laxatives can be a source of excessive intake.

Manifestations Hypermagnesemia diminishes neuromuscular transmission and can depress skeletal muscle function and cause neuromuscular blockade. Cardiovascular effects are due to the "calcium channel blocker effect" on cardiac conduction and the smooth muscle of blood vessels. Cardiac dysrhythmias that can develop include bradycardia, atrioventricular block, and asystole. Hypotension can develop due to the vasodilator effects of magnesium (Cho, 2017). The clinical manifestations associated with hypermagnesemia are presented in Table 26–10.

Medical Treatment The cause of hypermagnesemia should be identified and treated. Medications containing magnesium should be held; if the patient is in renal failure, the administration of magnesium should be avoided. In severe cases, dialysis may be required to remove magnesium. The neuromuscular and cardiac toxicity of hypermagnesemia can be antagonized by the administration of calcium chloride 500 mg or more at a rate of 100 mg per minute (Cho, 2017).

Nursing Considerations Hypermagnesemia may produce a decrease in cardiac output as a result of hypotension, bradycardia, and ECG changes. Nurses should be aware of patients at high risk for hypermagnesemia, such as those in renal failure. These patients should also be assessed for fluid volume excess and respiratory distress. Level of consciousness should be assessed, as well as low blood pressure and apnea. Magnesium-containing solutions should be avoided.

Emerging Evidence

- In a sample of 353 ICU patients, data were analyzed using logistic regression. Variables in the study were found to predict the presence, intensity, or distress of thirst. Thirst presence was reported by patients taking high doses of opioids, high doses of furosemide (Lasix), or presenting with low ionized calcium levels and other variables. Intensity of thirst was noted in patients who were not receiving oral fluids and in those with a GI diagnosis. Mechanical ventilation, the administration of hypertensive medications, and other factors were associated with increased thirst distress. The data from this study can guide clinicians as they identify and treat the discomfort and burden of thirst in critically ill patients (Stotts, Shoshana, Cooper, Nelson, & Puntillo, 2015).
- In a review of the Phillips eICU Research Institute database of over 7,000 patients with hyponatremia, approximately 48% did not receive correction for low serum sodium concentration. Patients with corrected serum sodium levels had lower mortality and longer survival than patients without correction. These findings illustrate the importance of correcting sodium imbalances in critically ill patients (Dasta et al., 2015).

Section Six Review

1. Magnesium balance is closely related to which other two electrolytes?
   A. Potassium and phosphorus
   B. Calcium and sodium
   C. Sodium and phosphorus
   D. Calcium and potassium

2. The symptoms of hypomagnesemia reflect which alteration?
   A. CNS hypoactivity
   B. Fluid compartment shifts
   C. Cardiac depressant effects
   D. Neuromuscular and CNS hyperactivity

3. Hypermagnesemia is associated with which symptom?
   A. Tetany
   B. Lethargy
   C. Tremors
   D. Positive Chvostek sign

4. Magnesium plays an active part in which physiologic functions? (Select all that apply.)
   A. Sodium transport
   B. Nerve cell conduction
   C. Fluid regulation
   D. Transference of energy
   E. Potassium transport

Answers: 1. D, 2. D, 3. B, 4. (A, B, E)

Section Seven: Phosphorus and Phosphate Imbalances

Phosphorus is an intracellular electrolyte that exists in the body primarily as phosphate, in combination with calcium as calcium phosphate. In addition to its importance to healthy bones and teeth, it is also vital to normal neuromuscular function and the production of adenosine triphosphate (ATP). The normal range for phosphorus is 2.5 to 4.5 mg/dL.

Hypophosphatemia

Hypophosphatemia is defined as a serum phosphorus level below 2.5 mg/dL with a critical value of 1 mg/dL or lower (Kee, 2014; Mayo Clinic Laboratories, 2015).

Etiology In the high-acuity patient, hypophosphatemia is associated with such disorders as gram-negative sepsis, cardiac surgery, malnutrition, acute respiratory alkalosis, diabetic ketoacidosis (lost through osmotic diuresis and through the administration of insulin, which drives phosphorus back into the cell), and alcoholism. Acute respiratory alkalosis can reduce plasma phosphate concentration as phosphate moves out of the blood and into the cells. The infusion of glucose and the effects of hormones such as insulin, glucagon, and cortisol can decrease plasma phosphate concentrations by its redistribution to the intracellular space.

Other conditions that can cause hypophosphatemia include hyperparathyroidism, certain renal tubular defects, metabolic alkalosis, disorders that cause hypercalcemia, and prolonged recovery from any catabolic state, such as starvation (Cho, 2017).

Manifestations Numerous cellular mechanisms require phosphate. Hypophosphatemia depresses cellular function, particularly of the hematologic and cardiovascular systems. This results in symptoms of impaired heart function and poor tissue oxygenation. Because phosphorus is essential to form part of ATP, it serves as a reservoir of energy in cells to fuel muscle contractility, neuronal transmission, electrolyte transport, and conversion of dietary nutrients into energy. Hypophosphatemia is associated with blood cell dysfunctions, as well as neurologic, neuromuscular, and cardiopulmonary problems. The clinical manifestations associated with hypophosphatemia are presented in Table 26–11.

Medical Treatment Medical management is directed at treating the underlying cause of the disorder and replacing serum levels. Plasma phosphate concentrations should be maintained within the normal range. Treatment of hypophosphatemia depends on the magnitude of the deficit and the presence and severity of symptoms. Asymptomatic mild hypophosphatemia can be treated with oral supplementation if the gastrointestinal tract is functional. Symptomatic or severe hypophosphatemia (less than 1 mg/dL) should be treated with intravenous phosphate (Cho, 2017). IV preparations include sodium phosphate and potassium phosphate. The "Related Pharmacotherapy: Phosphate" feature provides a summary of phosphate therapy.

Nursing Considerations Patients with hypophosphatemia should be monitored for muscle weakness, inadequate ventilation, and decreased energy stores. Weakness of the respiratory muscles can result in ineffective breathing patterns and may cause respiratory failure requiring mechanical ventilation. The choice of phosphate treatment depends on factors such as the patient's renal status. If the patient has renal failure, sodium phosphate may be the best choice for replacement. Phosphorus replacements should be infused slowly, usually over 4 to 6 hours. The nurse should be alert for symptoms of hypercalcemia, as phosphate and calcium are inversely related.

Table 26–11 Major Manifestations of Alterations in Phosphorus and Phosphate

Body System	Hypophosphatemia	Hyperphosphatemia
Cardiovascular	Diminished myocardial function Severe: heart failure	Hypotension, tachycardia ECG changes: prolonged *QT* interval and ventricular dysrhythmias
Gastrointestinal	Nausea and vomiting, anorexia	Diarrhea, nausea, abdominal cramping
Neurologic	Disorientation, irritability, coma Severe: Severe neurologic dysfunction	Altered mental state, delirium, coma Positive Chvostek and Trousseau signs, paresthesias
Neuromuscular	Weakness, numbness, and tingling Severe: seizures	Muscle cramping, tetany, seizures
Musculoskeletal	Pathologic fractures	—
Other (severe)	Respiratory failure or arrest, hemolysis, red blood cell, white blood cell and platelet dysfunction	—

SOURCE: Data from Cho (2017).

Hyperphosphatemia

Hyperphosphatemia is defined as a serum phosphorus level above 4.5 mg/dL (Kee, 2014; Mayo Clinic Laboratories, 2015) with a critical value of greater than 5 mg/dL. It is less common than hypophosphatemia in the high-acuity patient.

Etiology   Hyperphosphatemia is predominantly associated with advanced chronic kidney disease due to the inability to excrete the phosphate. Other causes include shifting of phosphorus from the intracellular space into the extracellular space and increased phosphorus uptake (Cho, 2017).

Clinical Manifestations   The clinical manifestations associated with hyperphosphatemia are similar to those of hypocalcemia because they are inversely related. These include signs of increased neuromuscular irritability and ECG changes. Common clinical manifestations of hyperphosphatemia are presented in Table 26–11.

Medical Treatment   Treatment of hyperphosphatemia is directed at lowering serum levels. Exogenous sources of phosphate, including enteral or parenteral nutrition and medications, should be reduced or eliminated. Agents that bind phosphate in the GI tract may be administered. Aluminum-containing agents were used in the past but are now avoided due to their proven toxicity. Currently, calcium-based salts are commonly used. An IV solution with saline can also be administered to promote renal excretion of phosphate if the patient has functional kidneys (Cho, 2017).

Nursing Considerations   Nursing care for the patient with hyperphosphatemia is directed at monitoring serum lab values and ECG rhythm status, as well as monitoring for improvements in neuromuscular status. Phosphate supplements, especially IV preparations, should be administered cautiously over several hours and the patient monitored for therapeutic and nontherapeutic effects. Patients should be instructed that phosphate-containing laxatives can cause phosphate poisoning and should be avoided.

The "Nursing Care: The Patient with Fluid and Electrolyte Disturbances" feature provides a summary of nursing considerations related to the topics covered in this chapter.

Related Pharmacotherapy
Phosphate

Example Agents
Sodium phosphate, potassium phosphate (IV)

Action and Uses
Important in cellular metabolism. Forms part of compounds that perform metabolic processes, such as adenosine triphosphate and 2,3-Diphosphoglycerate (2,3-DPG). Fuels muscle contractility, neuronal transmission, electrolyte transport, and conversion of dietary nutrients into energy, and facilitates release of oxygen to the tissues.

Dosages (Adult)
Potassium phosphate (IV): 0.08–0.16 mmol/kg (dilute in 500 mL of 0.45 NS) to run over 6 hrs

SOURCE: Based on Jang & Cheng (2014).

Major Side Effects
Muscle weakness, impaired cellular energy resources, impaired oxygen delivery to the tissues, respiratory failure, anemia, cardiomyopathy, and dysrhythmias

Nursing Implications
Replace phosphorus slowly (IV).
Monitor patients for respiratory distress.
Monitor the EKG for changes and dysrhythmias.
Watch for signs of calcium disturbances, as phosphorus and calcium are inversely related.

Nursing Care

The Patient with Fluid and Electrolyte Disturbances

Expected Patient Outcomes and Related Interventions

Outcome: No complications of fluid or electrolyte imbalances

Assess and compare to established norms, patient baseline, and trends.

Obtain thorough patient history:

Note any causes of potential fluid and electrolyte imbalances; any reports of thirst?

Review medications: Are there any that could contribute to fluid or electrolyte imbalance?

Review diet: Is the patient receiving adequate nutrition and fluids for maintenance of homeostasis?

Monitor laboratory results and compare to baseline labs.

Assess physical status:

Skin condition, wound healing, and moistness of mucous membranes

Assess lung sounds and heart sounds.

Note dysrhythmias or ECG changes from baseline.

Check capillary refill to assess volume status. Note the presence of edema or swelling, especially in extremities.

Note any signs of neuromuscular disturbances such as twitching, tetany.

Check vital signs. Note deviations from baseline in blood pressure, heart rate and rhythm, respiratory rate, rhythm, depth, and effort.

Weigh daily and monitor intake and output.

Note the color and character of urine, emesis, large amount of nasogastric output or wound drainage.

Measure central venous pressure or pulmonary artery pressures if indicated.

Interventions to prevent complications of fluid and electrolyte imbalances

Monitor all of the above on an ongoing basis and note trends.

Administer related fluid and drug therapy and monitor for therapeutic and nontherapeutic effects.

PO or IV fluids

Diuretic agents

Electrolyte supplements

Agents that decrease serum electrolyte levels (e.g., Kayexalate)

Section Seven Review

1. Hypophosphatemia is associated with which condition?
   A. Malnourished state
   B. Respiratory alkalosis
   C. Hypocalcemia
   D. Hyperthyroidism

2. Severe hypophosphatemia is associated with which symptom?
   A. Joint pain
   B. Muscle cramping
   C. Respiratory arrest
   D. Peptic ulcer disease

3. The clinical picture of hyperphosphatemia frequently reflects which other electrolyte abnormality?
   A. Hypermagnesemia
   B. Hypochloremia
   C. Hypernatremia
   D. Hypocalcemia

4. Severe hyperphosphatemia is associated with which ECG change?
   A. Tachycardia
   B. Bradycardia
   C. Flattened *T* waves
   D. Widened *QRS* complexes

Answers: 1. A, 2. C, 3. D, 4. A

Clinical Reasoning Checkpoint

Mrs. T has just been admitted to your telemetry unit. She is 82 years old and reports that she has been homebound for about a week with "the flu." She also reports that she had several days of nausea and vomiting and has not been eating or drinking much since she got sick. She informs you that she has a long history of "heart problems" and is taking a drug for heart disease and a diuretic daily but has not been able to take either because of her nausea. Mrs. T had a complete lab panel drawn on admission, and you have just been informed that her serum potassium level is 2.8 mEq/L. You go to her room to reassess her.

1. List at least two clinical findings consistent with hypokalemia for each of the assessments below:

   a. Neurologic:

   b. Cardiovascular:

   c. ECG changes:

   d. Gastrointestinal:

   e. Musculoskeletal:

2. Is Mrs. T at risk for cardiac emergency? Why or why not?

3. Should you be concerned about her potassium level because she has a history of coronary artery disease and is taking a drug for heart disease? Why or why not?

4. From her recent history, what are the most likely causes of her hypokalemia?

5. If Mrs. T is experiencing fluid volume deficit (FVD) from her vomiting, what would you anticipate her serum sodium level would be?

6. It is determined that Mrs. T is experiencing FVD. The provider orders a moderate fluid challenge. What type of IV fluid would the provider likely order?

   a. D_5W

   b. 0.9% normal saline

   c. Hypertonic saline

   d. 0.225% saline

Chapter 26 Review

1. A client is admitted with intravascular fluid deficit secondary to third spacing. The nurse would anticipate providing which type of IV fluid as the probable best choice for this client?

   1. A hypertonic solution

   2. An isotonic solution

   3. A hypotonic solution

   4. A colloid solution

2. A client is admitted with fluid volume excess (FVE). Which assessment findings would the nurse attribute to this problem? (Select all that apply.)

   1. Shortness of breath

   2. Orthopnea

   3. 3+ pitting edema

   4. Hypotension

   5. Tachycardia

3. A client has a serum sodium of 128 mEq/L. The nurse should monitor this client for which problem?

   1. Hypertension

   2. Tachycardia

   3. Prolonged QT interval on ECG

   4. Changes in muscle tone

4. A client has a total calcium of 8 mg/dL. The nurse should monitor this client for which problems? (Select all that apply.)

   1. Decreased cardiac output

   2. Abnormal clotting

   3. Constipation

   4. Pathological fractures

   5. Reduced mental abilities

5. A client's potassium is 3.3 mEq/L. The nurse should alert the technician monitoring the client's ECG to be watchful for which changes? (Select all that apply.)

   1. Inversion of the T wave

   2. Development of a U wave

   3. Depression of the ST segment

   4. Prolongation of the PR interval

   5. Absence of the P wave

6. Which client would the nurse most closely monitor for the development of hypermagnesemia?

   1. Client in renal failure

   2. Client with burns over 40% of the body

   3. Client taking digoxin

   4. Client with history of alcoholism

7. A client has a phosphate level of 1.5 mg/dL. The nurse would monitor this client for which musculoskeletal changes?

   1. Muscle spasm

   2. Joint pain

   3. Muscle weakness

   4. Muscle cramping

8. A client who requires IV potassium replacement therapy has a peripheral IV line. The nurse would be confident to administer which order without further collaboration with the prescriber?

   1. 10 mEq potassium IV push STAT

   2. 20 mEq potassium per hour by continuous IV

   3. 10 mEq potassium per hour by continuous IV

   4. 80 mEq potassium IVPB every 6 hours

9. Which assessment finding would the nurse evaluate as indicating successful treatment of the client with fluid volume excess (FVE)?

    1. Lungs are clear to auscultation
    2. Input exceeds output
    3. Edema remains at 2+
    4. Weight gain of 1 kg in 24 hours

10. A client has hyperphosphatemia. The nurse looks for manifestations of which other electrolyte imbalance in this patient?

    1. Hypokalemia
    2. Hypocalcemia
    3. Hypernatremia
    4. Hypermagnesemia

Answers to questions found inside your textbook are available on the faculty resources site. Please consult with your instructor.

References

Cho, K. C. (2017). Chapter 21: Electrolyte & acid-base disorders. In M. A. Papadakis, S. J. McPhee, & M. W. Rabow (Eds.), *Current medical diagnosis & treatment 2017*. Retrieved January 3, 2017, from http://accessmedicine.mhmedical.com/content.aspx?bookid=1843&sectionid=135714601

Cho, J., Chung, H. S., & Hong, S. H. (2013). Improving the safety of continuously infused fluids in the emergency department. *International Journal of Nursing Practice, 19*(1), 95–100.

Dasta, J., Sushrut, S. W., Lin, X., Boklage, S., Baser, O., Chiodo, J., & Badawi, O. (2015). Patterns of treatment and correction of hyponatremia in intensive care patient. *Journal of Critical Care, 30*(5), 1072–1079.

Felver, L. (2013). Fluid and electrolyte homeostasis and imbalances. In L. C. Copstead & L. L. Banasik (Eds.), *Pathophysiology* (5th ed., pp. 520–538). St. Louis, MO: Elsevier Saunders.

Jang, J. J., & Cheng, S. (2016). *The Washington manual of medical therapeutics* (34th ed.). Philadelphia, PA: Wolters Kluwer Health/Lippincott Williams & Wilkins.

Josephson. S., & Samuels, M. A. (2015). Chapter 463e: Special issues in inpatient neurologic consultation. In D. Kasper, A. Fauci, S. Hauser, D. Longo, J. Jameson, & J. Loscalzo, (Eds.), *Harrison's principles of internal medicine* (19th ed.). Retrieved January 17, from http://accesspharmacy.mhmedical.com/Content.aspx?bookId=1130&sectionid=79757040

Kasper, D.L., Fauci, A.S., Hauser, S.L., Longo, D.L., Jameson, J., & Loscalzo, J. (2016). Chapter 1: Electrolytes/acid-base balance. In D. Kasper, A. Fauci, S. Hauser, D. Longo, J. Jameson, & J. Loscalzo (Eds.), *Harrison's principles of internal medicine* (19th ed.). Retrieved January 3, 2017, from http://accessmedicine.mhmedical.com/content.aspx?bookid=1820&sectionid=127553582

Kee, J. L. (2014). *Laboratory and diagnostic tests with nursing implications* (9th ed.). Upper Saddle River, NJ: Prentice Hall.

Lehne, R. A. (2016). *Pharmacology for nursing care* (9th ed.). St. Louis, MO: Elsevier Saunders.

Mayo Clinic Laboratories. (2015). *Department of Laboratory Medicine & Pathology: Critical values/critical results list*. Retrieved March 7, 2017, from http://www.mayomedicallaboratories.com/test-catalog/appendix/criticalvalues/view.php?name=Critical+Values%2FCritical+Results+List

McClelland, M. (2014). IV therapies for patients with fluid and electrolyte imbalances. *Medsurg Nursing, 23*(5), 4–8.

Molina, P. E. (2013). Chapter 5: Parathyroid gland and Ca2+ and PO4- regulation. In P. E. Molina (Ed.), *Endocrine physiology* (4th ed.). Retrieved January 3, 2017, from http://accessmedicine.mhmedical.com/content.aspx?bookid=507&sectionid=42540505

Mossop, E., & DiBlasio, F. (2017). Chapter 58: Overdose, poisoning, and withdrawal. In J. M. Oropello, S. M. Pastores, & V. Kvetan (Eds.), *Critical care*. Retrieved January 17, from http://accessmedicine.mhmedical.com/content.aspx?bookid=1944&sectionid=143520164

Mount, D. B. (2015). Chapter 63: Fluid and electrolyte disturbances. In D. Kasper, A. Fauci, S. Hauser, D. Longo, J. Jameson, & J. Loscalzo, (Eds.), *Harrison's principles of internal medicine* (19th ed.) Retrieved January 3, 2017, from http://accessmedicine.mhmedical.com/content.aspx?bookid=1130&sectionid=79726591

Palmer, B. F. (2016). Fluid and electrolyte disorders. In T. E. Andreoli, I. J. Benjamin, R. C. Griggs, & E. J. Wing (Eds.), *Andreoli and Carpenter's Cecil essentials of medicine* (9th ed., pp. 299–313). Philadelphia, PA: Elsevier Saunders.

Perel, P., Roberts, I., & Ker, K. (2013). *Colloids versus crystalloids for fluid resuscitation in critically ill patients*. Cochrane Database of Systematic Reviews 2013, Issue 2. Art. No.: CD000567. doi:10.1002/14651858.CD000567.pub6. Retrieved January 2, 2017, from http://www.cochranelibrary.com/enhanced/doi/10.1002/14651858.CD000567.pub6

Stotts, N. A., Shoshana, R. A., Cooper, B. A., Nelson, J. E., & Puntillo, K. A. (2015). Predictors of thirst in intensive care unit patients. *Journal of Pain and Symptom Management, 49*(3), 530–538.

Wilson, B. A., Shannon, M. T., & Shields, K. M. (2016). *Pearson nurse's drug guide: 2016*. Hoboken, NJ: Pearson.

Chapter 27
Alterations in Kidney Function

⌄ Learning Outcomes

27.1 Explain the pathophysiology associated with the three types of acute kidney injury: prerenal, intrinsic, and postrenal.

27.2 Describe the diagnosis and assessment of acute kidney injury.

27.3 Explain the management of the patient with acute kidney injury.

27.4 Compare and contrast the types of renal replacement therapy used to treat acute kidney injury.

27.5 Prioritize nursing interventions when caring for the patient with acute kidney injury.

27.6 Discuss the clinical implications of caring for a patient with preexisting chronic kidney disease who is admitted with an unrelated acute illness.

By virtue of being admitted with a serious illness, the high-acuity patient has a moderate-to-high risk for development of kidney injury. This chapter focuses on the disease processes that alter renal function, signs and symptoms of altered renal function, and collaborative interventions used in the high-acuity setting to restore and support renal function. The majority of the chapter focuses on acute kidney injury, which is a relatively common complication of critical illness. Chronic kidney disease is presented to a lesser extent with the understanding that patients with preexisting chronic kidney disease often require hospitalization for an acute disease process, which requires that their comorbid conditions be taken into consideration when planning care.

Section One: Pathophysiology of Acute Kidney Injury

There are many clinical causes for acute kidney injury, including dehydration, sepsis, and the use of nephrotoxic agents or drugs (Lee & Vincenti, 2013; Singh, Singh, & Kari, 2017). The two major categories of kidney injury are acute and chronic. Acute kidney injury is a rapid-onset disease process that develops within a few hours of an insult and may be reversible with early identification and treatment. Approximately 10% to 30% of patients hospitalized in critical care areas will develop acute kidney injury (Hannon & Murray, 2015). This contrasts with chronic kidney disease (CKD), which comprises a group of renal disease processes in which renal excretory function becomes increasingly compromised over time (Lang, Zuber, & Davis, 2016). Chronic kidney disease is characterized by progressive and irreversible destruction of the kidneys that often progresses to end-stage renal disease within months to years of onset.

Acute Kidney Injury

Acute kidney injury (AKI), previously referred to as *acute renal failure*, is characterized by an abrupt decrease in renal function that is often first manifested by a rapid decrease in urine output. The term *acute kidney injury* is now the accepted nomenclature to more accurately reflect the broad range of severity associated with injury to the kidneys; however, the term *acute renal failure* may still be used when renal replacement therapy is necessary (Thornburg & Gray-Vickrey, 2016). Acute kidney injury is usually characterized by **oliguria**, a marked decrease in urine production and elevations of serum blood urea nitrogen (BUN) and creatinine (Cr); however, with early aggressive treatment and rapid reversal of the pathologic process, AKI can be prevented. Often these changes take place over a number of hours to days, are associated with a reduction in cardiac output, and are often reversible if identified and treated early.

Biomarkers have been identified that show promise of early detection of AKI. They are interleukin-18 (IL-18), neutrophil gelatinase-associate lipocalin (NGAL), and kidney injury molecule-1 (KIM-1) (Pearson Education, 2015). However, at this point they are not commonly relied upon, and so conventional markers such as BUN and creatinine are generally used to indicate the level and timing of insult in AKI. The association between the development of AKI and higher in-hospital mortality has been well established for decades with death rates from 50% to 80% despite aggressive treatment (Hannon & Murray, 2015).

Types of Acute Kidney Injury

Acute kidney injury is often categorized by the origin of the insult that caused the injury. *Prerenal*, *intrinsic* (or *intrarenal*), and *postrenal* are the descriptors commonly used to aid in understanding the underlying pathophysiology.

Prerenal Kidney Injury   Prerenal kidney injury is by far the most common cause of AKI and accounts for 60% of the cases of acute kidney injury (Perrin & MacLeod, 2013). If prerenal kidney injury is not treated adequately and corrected in a timely manner, it will result in intrinsic kidney injury (Perrin & MacLeod, 2013). Prerenal kidney injury refers to kidney dysfunction resulting from an absolute decrease in effective blood volume (e.g., hemorrhage, severe dehydration), relative decrease in blood volume (e.g., relative hypovolemia from vasodilation and peripheral pooling that causes an ineffective blood volume), or arterial occlusion (Lee & Vincenti, 2013). In other words, the initial insult is decreased renal perfusion that interferes with blood flow to the kidneys. Table 27–1 lists some of the more common causes of prerenal kidney injury.

Table 27–1 Common Causes of Acute Prerenal Kidney Injury

Underlying Cause	Examples of Insults
Absolute decrease in effective blood volume	Vascular: hemorrhage Skin: severe burns, diaphoresis Gastrointestinal: vomiting, diarrhea Renal: polyuria (e.g., diuretics or severe glycosuria) Endocrine: diabetes insipidus Fluid pooling (e.g., peritonitis, pancreatitis)
Relative decrease in blood volume (ineffective blood volume)	Decreased cardiac output: Heart failure Myocardial infarction Sepsis Shock states
Arterial occlusion	Thromboembolism
Drugs that alter renal perfusion or are nephrotoxic	Angiotensin-converting enzyme (ACE) inhibitors Angiotensin receptor blockers (ARBs) NSAIDs Amphotericin B Contrast agents Cyclosporine

SOURCE: Data partially from Adams & Urban (2017); Lee & Vincenti (2013); Perrin & MacLeod (2013).

Kidney injury develops as filtration pressures decline in the face of reduced renal blood flow, which causes glomerular filtration pressures also to fall. The normal adaptive response is activation of the renin-angiotensin-aldosterone system (RAAS), upregulation of the sympathetic nervous system, and stimulation of vasopressin secretion. Angiotensin II acts on the afferent and efferent renal arterioles, causing vasoconstriction. Structural (permanent) damage does not occur until the kidneys' adaptive responses fail to maintain a near-normal glomerular filtration rate (GFR).

Decreased Cardiac Output.   Inadequate cardiac output is the underlying pathophysiologic problem in the vast majority of prerenal kidney injury cases. The kidneys rely on adequate systemic arterial blood pressure to maintain a normal rate of glomerular filtration. They require a sufficiently high mean arterial pressure (MAP) to sustain a renal perfusion pressure that perfuses and oxygenates the kidneys. Generally, a MAP of 65 mmHg is considered renal protective. However, MAP ranges of 72 mmHg to 82 mmHg may be needed to prevent acute kidney injury in patients with septic shock (Badin et al., 2011). This has important assessment implications for the nurse, who will need to closely monitor the at-risk patient's systemic arterial blood pressure, MAP, and urine output as indicators of adequate renal blood flow. Failure to maintain an adequate MAP results in decreased renal perfusion pressure, loss of kidney autoregulation, and decreased GFR.

There are two major mechanisms by which inadequate cardiac output can precipitate prerenal kidney injury: intravascular volume depletion and decreased perfusion.

Intravascular Volume Depletion.   The volume of fluid within the intravascular compartment can be decreased through absolute fluid volume loss (e.g., hemorrhage or diabetes insipidus), relative fluid volume decrease (e.g., widespread vasodilation), or translocation of fluid (e.g., second- or third-spacing). In absolute fluid volume loss, fluid has been lost from the body; depending on the volume and the rate at which it is lost, cardiac output can become significantly reduced. In relative intravascular fluid volume decrease, the fluid volume does not alter significantly, but the size of the vascular bed has increased through massive vasodilation. Finally, volume depletion can occur when intravascular fluids shift or translocate out of the blood vessels and into other body compartments. In high-acuity patients, this can occur with such problems as severely low serum albumin, severe ascites, pancreatitis, or peritonitis.

Decreased Perfusion.   Both kidneys receive approximately 25% of the cardiac output, and they are able to tolerate a wide variation in blood flow without causing tissue damage. This blood flow to the kidneys supplies enough plasma for the precise regulation of GFR necessary to regulate blood volume and solute concentrations (Marieb & Hoehn, 2016). Intravascular volume depletion can precipitate prerenal kidney injury if there is a significant drop in cardiac output sufficient to compromise perfusion to the kidneys.

When cardiac output decreases, the kidneys rapidly respond through renal capillary vasoconstriction, which shunts blood away from the kidneys and increases blood supply to other, more critical core organs. In the short term, this adaptive response is helpful to overall system blood flow; however, if the state of low renal blood flow becomes prolonged, renal tissue ischemia results. The renal tubules are the most vulnerable to low-flow states because of their relatively high metabolic rate; thus, ischemic tubular epithelial damage occurs first. If the low blood flow state is prolonged, tubular epithelial cell necrosis occurs.

Arterial Occlusion. Arterial obstruction (e.g., blood clot or trauma to the renal artery) results in reduced renal perfusion distal to the obstruction and is another cause of prerenal kidney injury. The obstruction is a localized problem, but the effect on the kidney is similar to that of reduced cardiac output. As blood flow to the kidney diminishes, the glomerular filtration rate falls and the tubular epithelial cells become ischemic (Hannon & Murray, 2015). Nurses caring for a patient with renal arterial occlusion may notice symptoms such as flank pain, nausea, vomiting, fever, and hematuria. New onset of hypertension or an acute worsening of hypertension can be common findings in the older patient (LeMone, Burke, & Baldoff, 2015).

Drug-Induced Altered Glomerular Hemodynamics. Alteration of glomerular hemodynamics created by the actions of drugs is a third important cause of prerenal kidney injury. There are specific classifications of drugs that can significantly decrease renal perfusion, particularly in volume-depleted patients. Nonsteroidal anti-inflammatory drugs (NSAIDs) are a major drug-related cause of prerenal kidney injury. NSAIDs inhibit the synthesis of prostaglandins, which are important mediators of glomerular afferent arteriole vasodilation; therefore, by inhibiting the action of prostaglandins, NSAIDs decrease glomerular capillary pressure. It is well recognized that the use of an NSAID in a volume-depleted patient can lead to kidney injury via inhibition of prostaglandin synthesis (Adams & Urban, 2017). The use of NSAIDs should be restricted in those patients with evidence of reduced renal function. This is particularly true when NSAID use is considered in frail older adults, who often have some degree of preexisting renal insufficiency.

Intrinsic Renal Injury Intrinsic kidney injury (or intrarenal injury) is caused by problems that target the kidney parenchyma (renal tissue) where the injury occurs (e.g., acute tubular necrosis and acute interstitial nephritis) (Table 27–2). The most common form of intrinsic kidney injury is **acute tubular necrosis (ATN)**, accounting for 85% to 90% of AKI cases (Hannon & Murray, 2015). Acute tubular necrosis often develops in critically ill patients as a result of prolonged prerenal kidney injury secondary to ischemia or cytotoxins. Glomerular filtration rate is reduced for two reasons: kidney hypoperfusion and back-leak of filtrate through the damaged epithelium due to the presence of casts and debris that obstruct tubule lumen (Hannon & Murray, 2015; LeMone et al., 2015). Because ATN is associated with tissue destruction, the

Table 27–2 Common Causes of Acute Intrinsic (Intrarenal) Kidney Injury

Underlying Cause	Examples of Insults
Ischemia	Secondary to prerenal failure
Nephrotoxic agents	Aminoglycosides Contrast agents Ethylene glycol NSAIDs Amphotericin B
Rhabdomyolysis	Crush injuries, severe burns, compartment syndrome, severe exertion, seizure activity, certain drug side effects (HMG Co-A reductase inhibitors for hypercholesterolemia)
Intratubular obstruction	Cellular debris, myoglobin casts, uric acid crystals

incidence of permanent renal damage is high. To minimize the amount of permanent damage, it is crucial to diagnose the condition early and correct the underlying cause through aggressive treatment.

Other, less common etiologies of intrinsic kidney injury include vascular problems (e.g., vasculitis, disseminated intravascular coagulation, or malignant hypertension), acute glomerulonephritis, acute interstitial nephritis, drug allergies, heavy metal toxins, and infections (Hannon & Murray, 2015; LeMone et al., 2015, Perrin & MacLeod, 2013).

Drug-Induced Injury. The kidneys are responsible for the excretion of most drugs, which makes them a natural target for direct and indirect damage from drugs or their metabolites. Different drugs are known to target different kidney structures; for example, aminoglycosides and lithium are cytotoxic to the renal tubules, while NSAIDs and proton-pump inhibitors target the renal interstitium (Perrin & MacLeod, 2013). Aminoglycosides are major antibiotics in the treatment of serious gram-negative infections. Their increased use and nephrotoxicity have made them a frequent cause of AKI. AKI occurs in 10% to 26% of patients on aminoglycosides, even with careful dosing and therapeutic plasma levels (Adams & Urban, 2017). Refer to Table 27–2 for a partial list of nephrotoxic agents.

Radiographic diagnostic tests may require the use of contrast agents that are potentially nephrotoxic. Ensuring that the patient is well hydrated prior to use of a contrast agent is key in reducing this risk. Premedication with N-acetylcysteine may be given orally or intravenously before contrast administration. It acts as a free radical scavenger, counteracts vasoconstriction from contrast agents, and indirectly exhibits cytoprotective effects (Wilson, Shannon, & Shields, 2016).

Management Considerations. The risk for nephrotoxicity caused by many of these agents can be reduced by keeping the patient well hydrated while maintaining a stable hemodynamic status. Not all agents harm the kidneys to an equal extent. For example, the damage caused by aminoglycoside antibiotics results in mild tubular epithelial sloughing that is usually reversible if the drug is withdrawn promptly.

Strategies to reduce aminoglycoside toxicity include once-daily dosing, which has been shown to be of better or comparable efficacy to multiple doses per day, with a trend toward lower nephrotoxicity (Wilson et al., 2016).

Endogenous Intrinsic Kidney Injury. Hepatorenal syndrome and rhabdomyolysis are two important causes of endogenous intrinsic kidney injury.

Hepatorenal Syndrome. Hepatorenal syndrome, primarily a complication of advanced liver disease, causes severe renal insufficiency. **Azotemia** (elevated nitrogen wastes in the blood),without other underlying causes of kidney injury, is a common finding. Precipitating factors include gastrointestinal bleeding, excessive administration of diuretics, large-volume paracentesis, and infections. As the disease progresses, renal perfusion is increasingly reduced, and renal function worsens.

Rhabdomyolysis. Rhabdomyolysis is a syndrome characterized by damage to the striated muscle cells (traumatic or nontraumatic), which results in the release of damaged muscle cell contents into systemic circulation. In high-acuity settings, the most common cause is severe crush injuries seen in multiple-trauma patients. **Myoglobin** is a ferrous (iron) protein complex in striated muscle that is responsible for the muscle's ability to store oxygen. It produces the red color in muscle and, when released in large quantities, produces urine that is dark red in color. High levels of serum myoglobin are both directly and indirectly toxic to the renal tubular cell epithelium. The deleterious effects of circulating myoglobin are accentuated by the presence of hypovolemia and hypotension. As myoglobin comes into the glomeruli, the glomerular tubules can become obstructed with cellular debris, myoglobin, hemoglobin casts, or uric acid crystals. These particles block the tubular structure, contribute to intrarenal injury, and reduce renal performance (Waikar & Bonventre, 2015).

Table 27–3 Common Causes of Acute Postrenal Injury

Mechanical causes	Blood clots, calculi, tumors, prostatic hypertrophy, prostate cancer, urethral strictures
Functional causes	Diabetic neuropathy, neurogenic bladder, certain drugs (e.g., parasympatholytics)

Management of rhabdomyolysis includes identifying the cause and preventing kidney failure. Myoglobin is closely monitored through serum and possibly urine sampling. Fluid replacement to increase urine flow to protect the kidneys from myoglobin damage has been most commonly used in the prophylaxis of renal failure in rhabdomyolysis. After fluid resuscitation, a forced saline–mannitol or alkaline–mannitol diuresis is performed. Urine pH is monitored, and IV bicarbonate may be administered to maintain an alkaline urinary pH of at least 6.5, which reduces precipitation of myoglobin (called casts) in the renal tubules, thereby reducing the risk of obstruction by the casts.

Postrenal Kidney Injury Postrenal kidney injury develops when there is an obstruction to the outflow of urine from the kidneys after it has left the tubules (Hinkle, 2014). Urinary tract obstruction accounts for less than 5% to 10% of AKI cases. It is usually reversible and must be ruled out early in the evaluation. Because a single kidney is capable of adequate clearance, obstructive AKI requires obstruction at the urethra or bladder outlet, bilateral ureteral obstruction, or unilateral obstruction in a patient with a single functioning kidney. Obstruction is usually diagnosed by the presence of ureteral and renal pelvic dilation on renal ultrasound. The obstruction can be either mechanical or functional in origin (Table 27–3) (Hinkle, 2014). Bilateral obstruction precipitates renal injury resulting from backup pressure caused by the increasing volume of urine proximal to the obstruction.

Section One Review

1. Acute kidney injury that develops from hypovolemic shock would be classified as which type of injury?
   A. Prerenal
   B. Intrarenal
   C. Postrenal
   D. Intrinsic

2. Which drug category is a common cause of prerenal kidney injury?
   A. Antibiotics
   B. Cardiac glycosides
   C. Nonsteroidal anti-inflammatory drugs
   D. Antihypercholesterolemic drugs

3. A mean arterial pressure (MAP) below 65 mmHg may result in which condition?
   A. Increased renal perfusion and increased GFR
   B. Release of substances that produce local vasodilation
   C. Inadequate renal perfusion pressure
   D. Renal artery obstruction

4. Myoglobin release into the circulation is associated with which condition? (Select all that apply.)
   A. Skeletal muscle damage
   B. Intrinsic kidney injury
   C. Dark red urine
   D. Increased glomerular filtrate rate
   E. Seizure activity

Answers: 1. A, 2. C, 3. C, 4. A

Section Two: Diagnosis and Assessment of Acute Kidney Injury

The diagnosis of acute kidney injury requires obtaining initial baseline data, including a thorough health history, a physical assessment, and a battery of laboratory tests. Additional diagnostic exams may be needed to confirm the underlying cause of the injury, rule out possible causes, or evaluate other aspects of the disease process or its complications.

Diagnostic Considerations

A rapid onset of decreasing urinary output, increasing azotemia, and development or worsening of electrolyte imbalances (especially hyperkalemia) are highly suspicious for AKI and require immediate investigation. Diagnosis of AKI involves close scrutiny of the patient's past and recent medical history to investigate possible risk factors, a thorough physical examination, and a full range of serum and urine laboratory diagnostic tests. In rare instances, renal dysfunction may be due to an inherited pathology; therefore, a comprehensive workup including genetics and family background may be necessary. The "Genetic Considerations" feature lists examples of inherited renal syndromes and diseases.

Once the diagnosis is made, it is important to stage the severity of the injury. A consensus conference of the Acute Dialysis Quality Initiative group made recommendations to more clearly define and grade AKI and suggests the use of a classification system called RIFLE (i.e., **R**isk, **I**njury, **F**ailure, **L**oss, **E**nd-stage kidney disease). The RIFLE system provides standardized definitions and criteria for staging of patients with AKI. The RIFLE criteria (see Table 27–4) are based on changes in glomerular filtration rate (GFR), serum creatinine, and urine output over time (Hinkle, 2014).

Laboratory Diagnostic Tests The initial diagnosis of AKI relies heavily on laboratory tests that measure uremic toxins and renal function. Major laboratory values measuring AKI are summarized in Table 27–5. Note that serum and urine values often have an inverse relationship. Monitoring laboratory trends over time is important for evaluating the patient's kidney function status.

Blood Urea Nitrogen and Creatinine. Blood urea nitrogen (BUN) and creatinine are two important measurements of renal status.

Genetic Considerations
Inherited Kidney Diseases

- Chronic hereditary nephritis
- Cystic diseases—polycystic kidneys and medullary cystic disease
- de Toni-Debré-Fanconi syndrome
- Renal glycosuria
- Wilson disease

SOURCE: Lee & Vincenti (2013).

Table 27–4 RIFLE Criteria

	GFR Criteria	Urinary Criteria
Risk	Serum Cr increased by 1.5 times or GFR decreased by more than 25%	Urine output less than 0.5 mL/kg/hr for 6 hours
Injury	Serum Cr increased by 2 times or GFR decreased by more than 50%	Urine output less than 0.5 mL/kg/hr for 12 hours
Failure	Serum Cr increased by 3 times, or GFR decreased by 75%, or serum Cr at or above 4 mg/dL. Acute rise greater than or equal to 0.5 mg/dL	Urine output less than 0.3 mL/kg/hr for 24 hours or anuria for 12 hours
Loss	Complete loss of renal function for greater than 4 weeks	
End-stage kidney disease	Need for renal replacement therapy for more than 3 months	

Blood Urea Nitrogen. Glomerular filtration and urine-concentrating capacity is reflected by the concentration of urea in the blood. Urea is the major end-product of protein metabolism and is filtered in the glomerulus and eliminated in the urine (Pearson Education, 2015). Because urea is filtered at the glomerulus, the BUN levels increase as glomerular filtration decreases, often due to reduction in renal blood flow (Kee, 2014). The BUN is also affected by the individual's hydration status, level of catabolism, protein intake, gastrointestinal bleeding, drug therapy, and chronic liver disease. BUN is also impacted by an individual's

Table 27–5 Major Laboratory Values Measuring Kidney Function

Laboratory Test	Normal Adult Parameters	Abnormal Trend
Serum		
Blood urea nitrogen	5–25 mg/dL	Increased
Creatinine	0.5–1.5 mg/dL	Increased
Uric acid	Male: 3.5–8 mg/dL Female: 2.8–6.8 mg/dL	Increased
Potassium	3.5–5.3 mEq/L	Increased
Calcium	4.5–5.5 mEq/L	Decreased
Chloride	95–105 mEq/L	Increased
Phosphorus	1.7–2.6 mEq/L	Increased
Albumin	3.5–5 g/dL	Decreased
Urine		
Protein	2–8 mg/dL (or negative reagent test)	Increased
Creatinine clearance	85–135 mL/min*	Decreased
Uric acid	250–750 mg/24 hr (normal diet)	Decreased
Glucose	Absent	Positive

*Women and older adults have slightly lower values.

SOURCE: Normal ranges from Kee (2014).

muscle mass; therefore, caution must be used when evaluating the BUN of older adults, women, and malnourished populations. Based on all of these possible confounding factors that can alter BUN, it is not considered a reliable measure of glomerular filtration rate (GFR) (Tabloski, 2014).

Creatinine.   Creatinine, the end-product of muscle metabolism, is filtered in the glomerulus but does not undergo reabsorption in the tubule. Therefore, creatinine clearance slightly overestimates glomerular filtration but is close enough to be useful in clinical situations. Hence, an increase in the creatinine in the blood usually indicates a decrease in glomerular filtration as a hallmark of kidney disease (LeMone et al., 2015).

BUN-to-Creatinine Ratio.   The reabsorption of urea by the tubules can be increased or decreased while creatinine reabsorption remains constant, which helps to explain the reason that the BUN rises more rapidly than creatinine. Under healthy renal conditions, the BUN and creatinine maintain a ratio of 10:1 to 15:1. Since BUN levels increase more quickly than creatinine, an increase in this ratio to greater than 20:1 may indicate reduced renal blood flow, glomerular disease, or azotemia (Kee, 2014). In addition, a lower than normal ratio can occur with acute tubular necrosis. Although BUN values are nonspecific indicators of kidney injury, creatinine corresponds to the glomerular filtration rate because there is an inverse relationship between the GFR and the serum creatinine value. A doubling of the serum creatinine value corresponds to a decrease in glomerular filtration rate of about 50%.

Creatinine Clearance.   No single creatinine value corresponds to a given glomerular filtration rate in all patients; therefore, change in creatinine clearance is the most useful indicator of a change in glomerular filtration rate, and hence the presence of kidney injury (LeMone et al., 2015). The serum creatinine level is compared with the excretion of creatinine measured in a volume of urine produced over a specified amount of time. A decrease in the creatinine clearance rate indicates a decrease in glomerular function. A 24-hour collection of urine and a blood sample to measure serum creatinine are needed for this analysis (Kee, 2014).

Osmolality.   The osmolality of urine or of serum is a measure of the number of mOsm of solute concentration per kg (Marieb & Hoehn, 2016). Sodium is the major contributor to serum osmolality, and urea is the major constituent of urine osmolality. The relationship of urine and blood osmolality is monitored as an indicator of adequate renal function. When renal function is normal, the urine and blood (plasma) osmolality maintain a direct relationship with each other (i.e., as one rises, the other also rises). If renal perfusion becomes diminished, the urine osmolality becomes more elevated than does the blood osmolality, and urine specific gravity increases (Kee, 2014).

An increase in BUN, creatinine, or both combined with oliguria (urine output of 500 mL/day or less than 20 mL/hr) or **anuria** (no urine, as defined as less than 100 mL/day) are considered principle manifestations of renal failure.

Electrolyte Imbalances.   AKI causes imbalances of multiple electrolytes. Some of the imbalances are potentially life-threatening. Assessment of serum and urine electrolytes provides important information regarding renal status and alerts the nurse to potential complications based on abnormal values (Chapter 26). Electrolyte imbalances cause a wide range of functional problems, particularly in the neurologic, musculoskeletal, cardiovascular, and gastrointestinal systems. Of particular concern is the serum potassium level, which can rapidly increase as kidney injury progresses. Recall that potassium is the major intracellular electrolyte and the body is intolerant of significantly abnormal serum levels, which can cause lethal dysrhythmias.

Assessment Considerations

In the high-acuity patient, AKI is a relatively common complication that manifests as an abrupt reduction in kidney function within 48 hours. A steady decrease in hourly urine output is often the earliest clinical finding that alerts the nurse of possible AKI.

Urine Output: A Measure of Renal Function

Urinary output is an assessment made routinely and frequently in high-acuity settings, and it is not unusual for high-acuity patients to have significant imbalances in both fluid and electrolyte balance. Although the amount of urinary output is an important physiologic sign, it is influenced by multiple factors; therefore, it is vital for the nurse to remember all the reasons for an altered urine output, including decreased oral intake and excess fluid loss. Making a diagnosis of AKI based only on urine output, BUN, and creatinine is not sufficient because these values can become altered for other reasons (Tabloski, 2014). For example, oliguria and increased serum levels of BUN and creatinine are also a response by the kidney to changes in extracellular volume or to renal blood flow (LeMone et al., 2015). It is important, therefore, to determine whether a drop in urine output and elevated BUN and creatinine are due to water conservation associated with fluid volume deficiency (or some other nonkidney problem) or due to the inability of the kidneys to excrete water associated with AKI.

Health History   High-acuity patients are at moderate to high risk for developing AKI. There are known risk factors that significantly increase a patient's risk of developing acute kidney problems; data obtained from the health history can identify some of the risk factors related to past medical history. Risk factors for development of AKI are listed in Box 27–1. Advanced age, coronary artery disease, and benign prostatic hypertrophy can be additional risk factors for developing AKI (Pearson Education, 2015).

Physical Assessment   Assessment of the patient with AKI requires a multisystem assessment approach because kidney injury has profound physiologic effects on all body systems. As kidney injury progresses, the patient develops a multisystem clinical syndrome known as *uremia* (Figure 27–1).

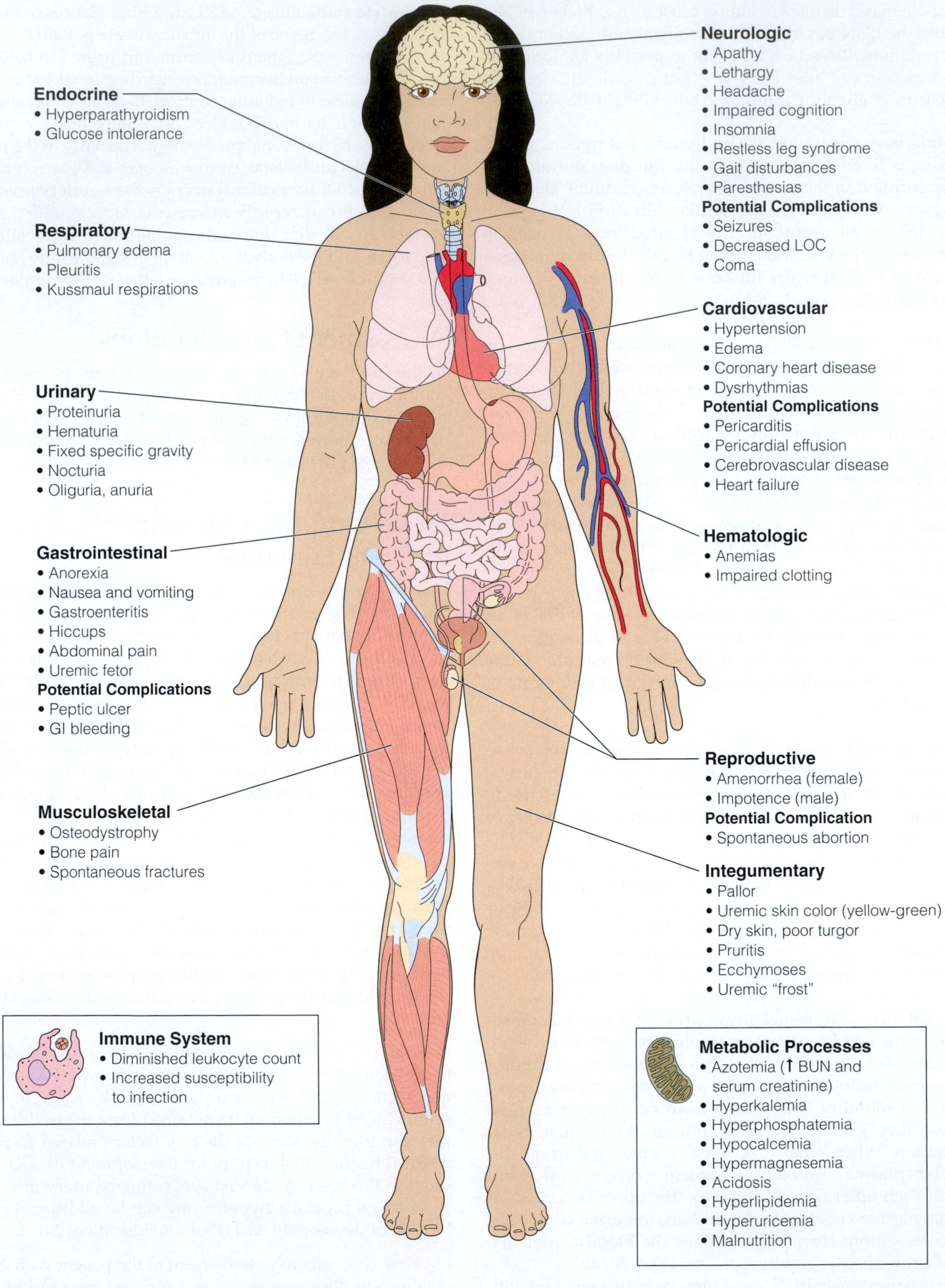

Neurologic
- Apathy
- Lethargy
- Headache
- Impaired cognition
- Insomnia
- Restless leg syndrome
- Gait disturbances
- Paresthesias

Potential Complications
- Seizures
- Decreased LOC
- Coma

Endocrine
- Hyperparathyroidism
- Glucose intolerance

Respiratory
- Pulmonary edema
- Pleuritis
- Kussmaul respirations

Cardiovascular
- Hypertension
- Edema
- Coronary heart disease
- Dysrhythmias

Potential Complications
- Pericarditis
- Pericardial effusion
- Cerebrovascular disease
- Heart failure

Urinary
- Proteinuria
- Hematuria
- Fixed specific gravity
- Nocturia
- Oliguria, anuria

Hematologic
- Anemias
- Impaired clotting

Gastrointestinal
- Anorexia
- Nausea and vomiting
- Gastroenteritis
- Hiccups
- Abdominal pain
- Uremic fetor

Potential Complications
- Peptic ulcer
- GI bleeding

Reproductive
- Amenorrhea (female)
- Impotence (male)

Potential Complication
- Spontaneous abortion

Integumentary
- Pallor
- Uremic skin color (yellow-green)
- Dry skin, poor turgor
- Pruritis
- Ecchymoses
- Uremic "frost"

Musculoskeletal
- Osteodystrophy
- Bone pain
- Spontaneous fractures

Immune System
- Diminished leukocyte count
- Increased susceptibility to infection

Metabolic Processes
- Azotemia ($\uparrow$ BUN and serum creatinine)
- Hyperkalemia
- Hyperphosphatemia
- Hypocalcemia
- Hypermagnesemia
- Acidosis
- Hyperlipidemia
- Hyperuricemia
- Malnutrition

Figure 27–1 Multisystem effects of uremia.

BOX 27–1   Risk Factors for the Development of Acute Kidney Injury

- Past history:
  - Renal problems
  - Hypertension
  - Diabetes mellitus
  - Proteinuria
- Recent:
  - Hypotensive episode
  - Exposure to nephrotoxic agents, heavy metals, or organic solvents
- Presence of:
  - Significant blood loss
  - Sepsis
  - Infection
  - Tumor or vascular obstruction

SOURCE: From Mehta et al. (2016).

The remainder of this section provides a brief overview of the more common multisystem effects of prolonged kidney failure on various body systems. The nurse plays a major role in monitoring the high-acuity patient for development or worsening of uremia, with prompt documentation and provider consultation when the patient's status deteriorates.

Uremia.   Uremia is defined as the clinical signs and symptoms of kidney failure that result from excess of protein metabolism end-products in the blood (Waikar & Bonventre, 2015; Zelman, Raymond, Holdaway, & Dafnis, 2015). Uremic signs and symptoms start to be detectable when at least two thirds of the total number of nephrons is functionally lost. Patients with AKI develop worsening uremia manifestations as kidney function deteriorates and physiologic alterations increase. Uremia can be difficult to confirm because many of its early clinical findings are those of other disorders seen in the critically ill, such as fluid overload, sepsis, inflammation, and vitamin deficiency. Moreover, other manifestations of uremia, such as fatigue, anorexia, nausea, vomiting, and neurologic changes, are common to many illnesses; their development may be difficult to distinguish as part of the uremic syndrome (LeBlond, Brown, Suneja, & Szot, 2015).

The pathophysiology associated with uremia stems primarily from the retention of protein metabolism end-products and from deranged hormonal and enzymatic homeostasis. The most pronounced physiologic alterations are found in the cardiovascular, neurologic, hematologic, and immunologic systems; consequently, these systems require more in-depth assessment.

Neurologic Effects.   AKI causes the accumulation of nitrogenous waste products and hydrogen ions from impaired renal excretion and metabolic acidosis. Both conditions cause a decrease in mental functioning. As uremic toxins build up in the brain tissue, neurologic encephalopathy causes confusion, delirium, and coma. The accumulation of toxins can slow peripheral nerve conduction and produce peripheral neuropathy, such as restless leg syndrome, and sensory neuropathies (Aminoff, Greenberg, & Simon, 2015). In addition, fluid volume excess caused by renal failure can precipitate cerebral edema, possibly increasing the intracranial pressure and altering the level of consciousness.

Cardiovascular and Pulmonary Effects.   The nurse should pay particular attention to the cardiopulmonary and renal systems to evaluate fluid and hemodynamic status. Hypertension is a common co-morbid condition in patients with kidney injury (Baumann, 2016). It is caused by systemic and central fluid volume excess and increased renin production. In the presence of renal ischemia, the renin-angiotensin-aldosterone system (RAAS) is triggered, resulting in increased blood pressure and increased renal blood flow. Increased effective circulating blood volume, fluid overload, and electrolyte imbalances are the basis of most cardiovascular symptoms. The presence of fluid volume excess may cause an exacerbation of heart failure symptoms such as hypertension, accompanied by peripheral and pulmonary edema due to salt retention (Bargman & Skorecki, 2015; Hung et al., 2014).

Patients with AKI require close monitoring for signs and symptoms of pneumonia. These patients are at increased risk for developing this complication as a result of fluid overload, decreased level of consciousness, weakness, decreased cough reflex, and decreased pulmonary macrophage activity.

Acid–Base Effects.   The inability of the kidneys to adequately excrete hydrogen ions and electrolytes causes them to accumulate in the body (Cho, 2017). The proximal tubule can reabsorb the bulk of the filtered load of bicarbonate, but this does not result in overall acid secretion. If there is accumulated acid in the body, the tubules must generate new bicarbonate to correct the acid–base imbalance. They do this by generating ammonia for eventual excretion. The resulting electrolyte imbalances with tubule dysfunction— most significantly, hyperkalemia—can precipitate cardiac dysrhythmias. The accumulation of hydrogen ions often presents a picture of metabolic acidosis for which the respiratory system may compensate with hyperventilation.

Gastrointestinal Effects.   Electrolyte imbalances and increasing levels of uremic toxins are the primary contributors to gastrointestinal (GI) manifestations. Urea in the digestive tract is broken down into ammonia and carbon dioxide. Elevated ammonia levels are destructive to the GI tract, causing increased capillary fragility and mucosal irritation that can cause small mucosal ulcerations. Common associated manifestations include GI pain, decreased appetite, and GI bleeding. Other common symptoms of GI injury include nausea, anorexia, bloating, and constipation or diarrhea, depending on GI motility status.

Hematologic Effects.   The kidneys produce erythropoietin in response to decreased oxygen delivery to the kidneys. Erythropoietin is necessary for red blood cell (RBC) production and also plays a role in maintaining healthy endothelium and promoting angiogenesis (development of new blood vessels). When kidney function deteriorates,

RBC production is compromised and the life span of the existing RBCs may decrease. Blood vessels are also at risk for injury, and the risk of blood clots increases. Platelet function is impaired, and platelet-to-platelet interactions cause impaired hemostasis. Uremic molecules interfere with von Willebrand factor proteins necessary for platelet adhesion to vascular walls. Therefore, the risk of bleeding problems increases (Adams & Urban, 2017). The combination of hematopoietic factors, GI irritation, and blood loss from hemodialysis all contribute to the development of anemia.

Integumentary Effects.   Because calcium and phosphate are not excreted by the kidneys, they may accumulate on the skin surface, causing dry skin. Hyperphosphatemia is associated with pruritus, which may be difficult to relieve (Bargman & Skorecki, 2015). Protein wasting seen in kidney injury, and most especially in renal failure, may cause thin hair and brittle nails. The patient's skin appears pale and may develop a yellow hue due to an increase in melanin caused by the kidneys' inability to excrete B-melanocyte-stimulating hormone. The sallow yellow skin coloring is different from the jaundice associated with liver disease (Bargman & Skorecki, 2015; Perrin & MacLeod, 2013). Bruising frequently results from dysfunctional platelets, as previously described. The development of uremic frost, a fine white layer of urate crystals that develops on the skin and a late-stage phenomenon of renal failure, is less common in acute care settings because of earlier treatment and more effective management. When uremic frost is present, the patient's skin will have the odor of urine.

Skeletal Effects.   Kidney disease is associated with abnormalities in bone and mineral metabolism and/or extraskeletal calcification secondary to the disease pathophysiology. The kidney is the primary site for phosphate excretion and the hydroxylation of vitamin D. Renal phosphate excretion is reduced. Patients develop hyperphosphatemia as a result of inadequate vitamin D levels. Phosphorus and calcium maintain an inverse relationship; therefore, serum calcium levels fall, resulting in increased secretion of parathyroid hormone (secondary hyperparathyroidism) (LeMone et al., 2015). Parathyroid hormone stimulates bone resorption to maintain calcium levels, which results in hypocalcemia and hyperphosphatemia. In long-term kidney dysfunction, the hypocalcemia results in hyperparathyroidism and significant renal osteodystrophy (Tabloski, 2014).

Urine Output.   Urine output was discussed under Diagnostic Considerations at the beginning of this section. Hourly monitoring of urine output is indicated in the unstable high-acuity patient, focusing on output trends and whether minimal hourly outputs are being maintained. Intake and output balance should be calculated each shift to evaluate whether significant imbalance, particularly fluid volume excess, is developing or worsening.

Section Two Review

1. A client with acute kidney injury is at higher risk for which pulmonary disorder?
   A. Asthma
   B. COPD
   C. Pneumonia
   D. Emphysema

2. The acidosis associated with kidney injury is directly related to which condition?
   A. Hypoventilation
   B. Excessive excretion of bicarbonate ions
   C. Decreased cardiac output
   D. Accumulation of hydrogen ions

3. Clients with long-term kidney dysfunction may develop which condition?
   A. Hyperparathyroidism
   B. Diabetes insipidus
   C. Thrombocytosis
   D. Hypoparathyroidism

4. Serum osmolality is determined in large part by which factor?
   A. Urea levels
   B. Sodium levels
   C. Potassium levels
   D. Creatinine levels

Answers: 1. C, 2. D, 3. A, 4. B

Section Three: Medical Treatment

The initial major goal of medical treatment is to take steps to prevent events known to precipitate kidney injury. However, this is not always possible, as the patient may be admitted to the hospital with preexisting risk factors for acute kidney injury (e.g., hemorrhage from trauma or GI ulceration), or drugs required to treat a current disease state may have an adverse effect that causes injury to the kidneys (e.g., aminoglycoside therapy for severe infection). A diagnosis of AKI requires prompt, aggressive interventions by the healthcare team to correct the underlying problem and support the body systems until renal function stabilizes.

Acute kidney injury may contribute to pathophysiologic complications in multiple body systems requiring individual and varied treatment plans. The four major potential complications routinely addressed are these:

- Fluid overload
- Metabolic imbalance (catabolism)
- Electrolyte/acid–base imbalance
- Infection

Treatment of Fluid Overload

Acute kidney injury that progresses to chronic renal disease can impact the maintenance of total water balance due to stimulation of the sympathetic nervous system and activation of the renin-angiotensin-aldosterone system (RAAS), leading to salt and fluid retention. Fluid overload can result in the development of heart failure and pulmonary edema, abdominal compartment syndrome, and intra-abdominal hypertension (Bargman & Skorecki, 2015; Perrin & MacLeod, 2013). Interventions focus on preventing fluid excess or, if overload is present, restoring optimal fluid balance. This can be accomplished with fluid restriction, diuretic therapy, and renal replacement therapy (presented in Section Four).

Fluid Restriction Fluid intake is restricted to the sum of measured output (urine, nasogastric [NG] drainage, fistula output) plus an estimate of insensible water loss (about 0.8 L to 1 L per day). Maintaining stringent fluid restrictions can be a nursing challenge because the volume of therapeutic fluid intake can be significant, including IV fluids, IV nutrition support (e.g., total parenteral nutrition, lipids), IV medications, and enteral feedings and medications with water flushes. Compliance with fluid restrictions requires frequent (possibly hourly) intake and output assessment and careful consideration of ways in which the volume of fluid intake can be minimized.

Diuretic Therapy Diuretics serve to remove excess fluid volume. Surgical patients and patients with sepsis or hypotension may receive large quantities of IV fluids. As these emergency situations are reversed and the patient is stabilized, the excess fluid used during resuscitation may be removed with diuretics. The type of diuretic is determined after consideration is given to the patient's needs, symptoms of volume overload, and electrolyte and acid–base status.

Loop diuretics, such as furosemide, continue to be the best and most commonly used medications to assist in maintaining fluid balance. Furosemide may have an important adjuvant role in maintaining fluid homeostasis in critically ill patients with AKI. Diuretic therapy may be prescribed in large intermittent doses or by a continuous and titrated intravenous drip. For example, furosemide, given IV bolus, is administered at a rate of 20 mg or less over 1 to 2 minutes, or it is given as a continuous IV infusion at a rate of 4 mg/min to avoid development of ototoxicity (Wilson et al., 2016).

Treatment of Metabolic Imbalance (Catabolism)

The high-acuity patient with AKI will develop hypermetabolic and hypercatabolic responses to stress or injury to some degree. As a result, these patients experience skeletal muscle breakdown, impaired amino acid transport into skeletal muscles, suppressed protein synthesis, depletion of body energy reserves, increased urea production, and peripheral insulin resistance. Protein intake is necessary for healing, but the provider typically limits the amount of protein to prevent azotemia. In patients who are highly catabolic and severely malnourished, the practice guidelines of the American Society for Parenteral and Enteral Nutrition (ASPEN) recommend amino acid intake of 10 g to 15 g/day (Connor, 2011).

Treatment of Electrolyte/Acid–Base Imbalance

Electrolyte imbalances are a frequent complication associated with acute renal failure. Two electrolytes that require especially close monitoring and management are potassium and sodium.

Hyperkalemia A critical elevation of serum potassium is a potentially lethal complication of AKI, as potassium is excreted in the kidneys (Mount, 2015). Treatment may include drug therapy or dialysis, and hyperkalemia should be managed according not only to ECG manifestations but also to serial potassium measurements and the patient's clinical picture.

There are three phases to treating symptomatic hyperkalemia: stabilizing the cardiac tissue membrane, shifting K^+ back into the cells, and removing excess K^+ from the body (Hinkle, 2014; Zelman et al., 2015). Because hyperkalemia can trigger life-threatening dysrhythmias, rapid stabilization of the cardiac tissue membrane is crucial. Intravenous calcium (calcium gluconate or calcium chloride) is recommended. Calcium therapy is administered with caution in patients receiving digitalis drugs because hypercalcemia, like hypokalemia, can result in digitalis toxicity. Several drugs can be used to drive potassium back into the cells, including nebulized albuterol, sodium bicarbonate, and a combination of insulin and glucose. Excess potassium can be removed from the body through the kidneys, using furosemide or through gastrointestinal excretion using the cation exchange agent sodium polystyrene sulfonate (Kayexalate). Hemodialysis may be ordered to clear a substantial amount of potassium rapidly, particularly when the hyperkalemia is accompanied by excess fluid volume (Hinkle, 2014; Mount, 2015). The "Related Pharmacotherapy: Cation Exchange Agent" feature provides additional information on Kayexalate.

Sodium Imbalances Serum sodium levels vary in the patient with AKI and should be monitored closely. Management depends on whether levels are normal, high, or low. Sodium administration in IV fluids should be chosen according to the patient's condition. Maintaining a balance of intake and output helps prevent or control hypernatremia. Maintenance IV solutions should contain more free water, such as 0.45% saline, to prevent hypernatremia and hyperchloremic acidosis (Adams & Urban, 2017). If renal function is sufficient, diuretic therapy may be ordered to lower sodium levels.

Related Pharmacotherapy
Cation Exchange Agent

Sodium Polystyrene Sulfonate
Kayexalate, SPS

Action and Uses
Removes potassium from the body by exchanging sodium ions for potassium in the large intestine; potassium-containing resin is then excreted in stool. Used to treat hyperkalemia.

Dosage (Adult)
PO: 15 g suspended in 70% sorbitol (or 20–100 mL of other fluid); 1–4 times/day
PR: 30–50 g/100 mL 70% sorbitol every 6 hr; deliver high in sigmoid colon as warm emulsion

Major Adverse Effects
Constipation
Fecal impaction

SOURCE: Based on Wilson et al. (2016).

FDA Safety Warning: Kayexalate has been shown to have drug–drug interaction with medications when taken at or near the same time as each other. This interaction has been shown to decrease the absorption of lithium and thyroxine. However, it is unclear if there are more drugs that could also be impacted by this interaction. Use caution when taking meds concurrently with Kayexalate; when possible separate ingestion of medications by 6 hours (U.S. Food and Drug Administration, 2015).

Nursing Implications
Can be given orally or rectally. Oral route is most effective.
If given rectally, administer at body temperature and introduce by gravity. Urge patient to retain enema at least 30 to 60 minutes, but as long as possible. Irrigate the colon after the enema solution has been expelled with 1 to 2 quarts of non-saline-containing flush solution.
Monitor serum electrolytes frequently.

Metabolic Acidosis Acid–base imbalances can become very severe in AKI, disrupting normal cellular functions. Acidosis increases the plasma potassium concentration by inducing a net shift of potassium from the cellular to the intravascular compartment in exchange for hydrogen. The injured kidneys are unable to remove excess hydrogen ions produced normally by metabolic activities, and the production and absorption of bicarbonate by the injured renal tubules are reduced. Metabolic acidosis is treated with dialysis, IV fluid administration, and possibly the judicious infusion of bicarbonate (Adams & Urban, 2017; Hannon & Murray, 2015).

Treatment of Infection

Sepsis is a leading cause of AKI, and sepsis-induced AKI is associated with high rates of mortality (Martensson & Bellomo, 2015). Renal blood flow declines after the development of sepsis or endotoxemia. This may result in a reduction of glomerular filtration; if hypoperfusion is severe and prolonged, it may also result in metabolic deterioration and diminished levels of high-energy phosphates, possibly causing cell death, tubular necrosis, and AKI (LeMone et al., 2015). Furthermore, infection is a major complication of AKI, particularly in patients requiring renal replacement therapy (Perrin & MacLeod, 2013). Prevention of sepsis through implementation of strict infection prevention and control procedures is vital. Early recognition of infection, identification of the specific pathogen, and careful antibiotic therapy are imperative. The choice of antibiotics should be carefully considered to avoid additional injury to the kidneys from nephrotoxic drug adverse effects, and adjustments to the dose may be required based on the severity of kidney dysfunction to prevent toxic drug levels. Evidence also supports therapies to enhance renal perfusion, avoid fluid overload, and treat venous congestion in the presence of sepsis. Specific focus is on possible anti-inflammatory drugs that would lessen the effects of sepsis on the kidneys and the use of various blood purification techniques (Martensson & Bellomo, 2015).

Emerging Evidence

- Rhabdomyolysis is a syndrome found in patients admitted into the ICU that can lead to AKI. One therapy used to lower the risk of irreversible kidney damage is renal replacement therapy (RRT). A review of the literature suggests that some hemofilter therapies are not effective at clearing the damaging myoglobin. Other alternative treatment options to preserve kidney function by clearing myoglobin, such as plasmapheresis, may be more effective (Petejova & Martinek, 2014).
- Pain, specifically chronic pain, impacts a large portion of the population, and treatment with opioids is a common choice by providers. In a nationally representative cohort of over 2 million U.S. veterans with normal glomerular filtration rates (GFRs), veterans with moderate to severe pain who were treated with opioids were found to have a greater risk of decreased renal function compared to those not reporting pain. The presence of pain along with opioid treatment was associated with lower GFRs, faster renal decline, and higher mortality (Ravel et al., 2016).
- The use of indwelling urinary catheters is common in ICU settings. However, their presence can increase the rate of catheter-associated urinary tract infections (CAUTIs) and sepsis. It is important for everyone on the healthcare team to take responsibility for the prompt removal of such catheters when they are no longer needed. Using a criteria-based reminder tool has the potential to promote appropriate catheter use and in one study resulted in a 48% decrease in the rate of CAUTIs (Chen et al., 2013).

Section Three Review

1. Which complications are routinely addressed in the client with AKI? (Select all that apply.)
   - **A.** Fluid overload
   - **B.** Acid–base imbalance
   - **C.** Anabolic processes
   - **D.** Infection
   - **E.** Dehydration

2. The hypercatabolic processes in clients with AKI make restriction of which nutrients an important consideration?
   - **A.** Carbohydrates
   - **B.** Fats
   - **C.** Proteins
   - **D.** Essential fatty acids

3. What is the major cause of death from AKI?
   - **A.** Hyperkalemia
   - **B.** Metabolic acidosis
   - **C.** Fluid volume excess
   - **D.** Sepsis

4. Sodium polystyrene sulfonate (Kayexalate) can be administered through which routes? (Select all that apply.)
   - **A.** Intravenous
   - **B.** Rectal
   - **C.** Oral
   - **D.** Intramuscular
   - **E.** Subcutaneous

Answers: 1. (A, B, D), 2. C, 3. D, 4. (B, C)

Section Four: Renal Replacement Therapy

Renal replacement therapy (RRT) is the major treatment option for acute renal failure that does not respond to medications and fluids. It is called RRT because it artificially replaces some of the functions of the kidneys. The primary functions of RRT include the removal of excess water and the removal of wastes (Udani, Koyner, & Murray, 2015). Renal replacement therapy does not correct renal impairment or perform the other native functions of the kidney, such as endocrine functions and the production of glutathione and erythropoietin, but it does serve to correct fluid, electrolyte, and acid–base imbalances and to remove waste products (Hinkle, 2014; Udani et al., 2015).

Renal replacement therapy involves the sequestration of blood on one side of a semipermeable membrane, movement of solute from a high to a low concentration gradient, or the movement of water utilizing a pressure gradient that "drags" solutes with it. Ultrafiltration is the removal of water from the blood. It moves fluid across a semipermeable membrane by an external pressure gradient.

Determining the Need for Renal Replacement Therapy

Early in the course of acute kidney injury, diagnostic studies are performed to determine the type of renal injury (e.g., diminished renal function secondary to shock state [prerenal] versus parenchymal tubular damage [intrinsic]) because therapeutic strategies differ based on etiologic factors. As an initial screening strategy, a diuretic challenge, using an osmotic diuretic or furosemide, or a fluid challenge, using a bolus of IV fluid, may be administered to differentiate between etiologies. For example, when a prerenal problem is present, the kidneys may be able to increase urine output when presented with a diuretic or fluid bolus because the kidney parenchyma may not yet have sustained significant damage. However, when an intrinsic kidney injury is present, the damage to the kidney structures may make them incapable of responding to the diuretic or fluid challenge. Therefore, if there is no response to the diuretic challenge, an intrinsic problem such as acute tubular necrosis would be seriously considered, and renal replacement therapy should not be delayed.

Types of Renal Replacement Therapy

There are three types of renal replacement therapy. Intermittent hemodialysis (IHD) and continuous renal replacement therapy (CRRT) are the two most efficient and commonly used treatments for AKI. The third type, peritoneal dialysis, is useful in the care of a patient with chronic kidney disease who has less severe kidney injury. Table 27–6 provides a comparison of these three treatment modalities.

Intermittent Hemodialysis Intermittent hemodialysis (IHD) provides efficient clearance of excess fluid and solutes, but too rapid removal may be destabilizing to the patient's hemodynamic and electrolyte status (LeMone et al., 2015). Intermittent hemodialysis rapidly removes water and wastes within 3 to 4 hours. Hemodialysis is usually performed three times a week.

Hemodialysis requires direct access into the vascular system. For short-term treatment, which is often used in the high-acuity patient, a double-lumen temporary-access catheter may be used. The two most common insertion sites are the internal jugular vein and femoral veins, accessed with a percutaneous insertion approach. The subclavian vein can also be used, but it carries a significant risk of stenosis or thrombosis and should be used as a last resort (Perrin & MacLeod, 2013). For long-term use, an internal arteriovenous fistula, shunt, or graft may be

Table 27–6 Comparison of Renal Failure Treatment Modalities

Factors	Intermittent Hemodialysis	Continuous Renal Replacement Therapy	Peritoneal Dialysis
Indications for use	Acute poisoning Acute/chronic renal failure Transfusion reaction Hepatic coma	Multiple organ dysfunction syndrome Sepsis Hemodynamic Instability Acute renal failure Inability to tolerate hemodialysis or peritoneal dialysis	Severe cardiovascular disease Hemodialysis not available Less rapid treatment appropriate Inadequate vascular access
Disadvantages	Requires vascular access and heparin Restricts activity level	Requires vascular access and anticoagulation Slow process Restricts activity level	Slower than hemodialysis Abdominal discomfort Risk of peritonitis
Contraindications	Coagulopathy Age extremes Hemodynamic instability	No absolute contraindications Not therapy of choice if rapid removal of fluid or substances is needed.	Adhesions of peritoneum or abdomen Peritonitis Recent abdominal surgery
Complications	Infection (primarily with tunneled catheter) Decreased cardiac output Cardiac arrhythmias Disequilibrium syndrome[a] Air embolism Disconnection hemorrhage	Infection Bleeding Infiltration Air embolism	Infection Decreased cardiac output Fluid overload Hyperglycemia Metabolic alkalosis Respiratory insufficiency Abdominal pain

[a]Symptoms of disequilibrium syndrome include a wide variety of neurological symptoms, such as hypertension, nausea and vomiting, seizures, and coma (Perrin & MacLeod, 2013).
SOURCE: Data from LeMone et al. (2015); Perrin & MacLeod (2013); and Zelman et al. (2015).

formed surgically. The site for these devices is usually the lower arm. Figure 27–2A and Figure 27–2B illustrate the fistula, graft, and temporary venous access. These accesses provide 200 to 400 mL/min blood flows, which are required for adequate dialysis (Callahan, 2015; Perrin & MacLeod, 2013). The extremity with the graft or fistula should be assessed for patency, and care should be taken not to reduce the blood flow through it. Simple measures to protect the access include taking blood pressures or drawing blood samples from the opposite extremity.

Intermittent hemodialysis "cleans" the blood by pumping it out of the patient via the venous access. The blood then passes through a dialyzer, which removes fluid and solutes, then returns the filtered blood back to the patient. The semipermeable membrane necessary for diffusion in hemodialysis is a thin, penetrable, synthetic material with small pores that allow the removal of water and small-molecular-weight substances such as urea and creatinine. Proteins and any drug that is bound to proteins cannot pass through the membrane because of their large molecular size (National Kidney Foundation, 2016).

In the hemodialyzer, the blood comprises the first fluid compartment and the dialysate the second. The **dialysate** is fluid used to remove or add solute to the plasma water, depending on the concentrations in the plasma and the dialysate. This process is termed *diffusive clearance* because the wastes diffuse from a high concentration to a lower one. It is more effective in removing small solutes such as urea and creatinine than larger solutes such as blood cells, bacteria, and proteins (Liu & Chertow, 2015). Dialysate fluid is a physiologic solution that can be altered to achieve certain electrolyte and acid–base goals. It includes bicarbonate and usually contains no potassium or only a small amount, as the goal is to remove potassium if the patient is

hyperkalemic (Zelman et al., 2015). Figure 27–3 illustrates the hemodialysis system.

Peritoneal Dialysis Peritoneal dialysis (PD) utilizes the patient's peritoneal membrane as the permeable membrane to remove wastes and water. A dialysate is infused through a catheter into the patient's abdomen for specific periods of time to "dwell," after which it is drained out of the patient. The selection of peritoneal dialysis versus hemodialysis is based on the severity of the renal failure, indications for therapy, and the patient's age and choice (Perrin & MacLeod, 2013). Peritoneal dialysis does not include the ability to remove precise amounts of water as intermittent hemodialysis and continuous dialysis do. Therefore, fluid loss is not predictable and may not be the best choice for those who need rapid or effective waste and water removal.

Continuous Renal Replacement Therapy Hemodynamic instability is a common complication of intermittent hemodialysis and may preclude or limit its use (Hinkle, 2014; Liu & Chertow, 2015). Continuous renal replacement therapy (CRRT) is a useful option in the patient with AKI who is critically ill and hemodynamically unstable. In contrast to intermittent hemodialysis, CRRT removes small volumes of fluid continuously (throughout a 24-hour day), which is more like natural kidney function. This prevents hemodynamic instability from rapid fluid volume changes. Continuous renal replacement therapy is used primarily in patients in the critical care setting because frequent assessments and ongoing monitoring are essential to the success of the treatment. Therapies include several different methods that clear excess fluid alone or fluid plus solutes, electrolytes, creatinine, and urea (Table 27–7).

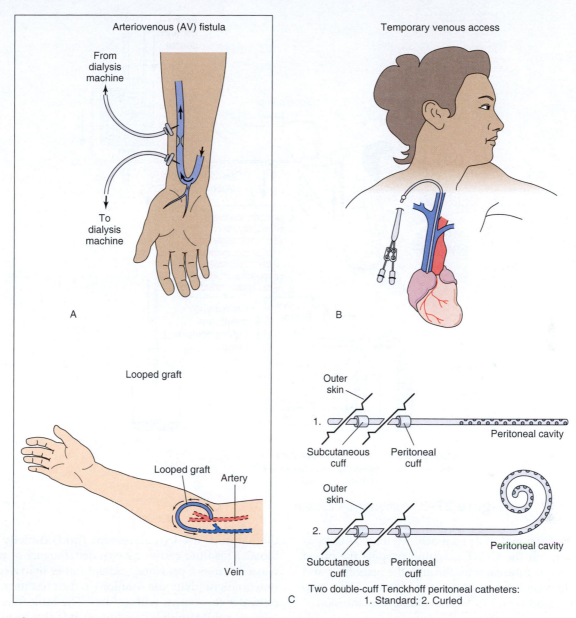

Figure 27–2 Types of renal dialysis access. A, The arteriovenous (AV) fistula and graft are used for long-term dialysis. B, A temporary venous access can be placed centrally or into the femoral vein for use in treating acute renal failure. C, The Tenckhoff catheter is used for peritoneal dialysis and is inserted through the lower abdominal wall.

SOURCE: From National Kidney and Urologic Diseases Information Clearing House (2004).

There are two forms of CRRT based on type of vascular access—arteriovenous and venovenous—and each type of access has its own risks and benefits (Pearson Education, 2015). Arteriovenous access CRRT does not require an external pumping device because it uses the patient's own arterial hemodynamics to move the blood; however, the rate of filtration depends on the patient's hemodynamic status. It requires cannulation of an artery, with all the inherent risks associated with arterial access devices (e.g., hemorrhage, embolism, limb ischemia). Venovenous access requires cannulation into a vein (e.g., internal jugular) and an external pumping device to move the blood. Because an external pump is used, the rate of flow is constant. Venovenous access also has potential risks, such as tube clotting, venous thromboembolism, and hemorrhage from disconnection. It is considered the safer, less risky CRRT alternative, and in

the critical care setting it is used more often than arteriovenous access (Pearson Education, 2015). For this reason, only venovenous access is profiled in this chapter.

The four major methods of venovenous CRRT are continuous venovenous hemofiltration (CVVH), continuous venovenous hemofiltration-dialysis (CVVH-D), continuous venovenous hemodiafiltration (CVVHDF), and slow continuous ultrafiltration (SCUF). Table 27–7 differentiates among these CRRT methods, and potential complications related to CRRT are identified in Box 27–2.

Continuous Venovenous Hemofiltration (CVVH). This form of CRRT uses a double-lumen catheter placed in a vein, usually a large vein such as the internal jugular, subclavian, or femoral vein. The equipment used in continuous therapies is typically specifically designed for it,

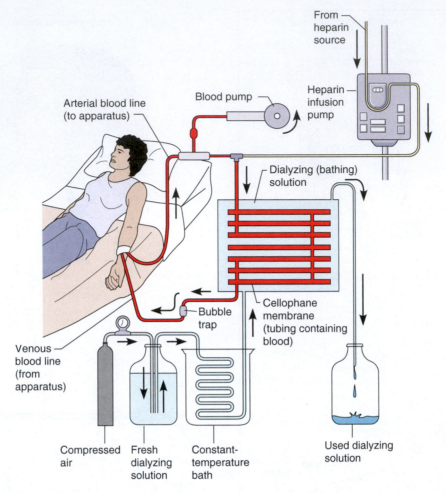

Figure 27–3 Hemodialysis system.

although conventional dialysis machines may be used as well. A pump on the CRRT machine propels the blood from one lumen of the catheter through the hemofilter and back into the vein through the second lumen. The pump controls the blood flow, fluid removal rate, and infusion of the solution used (replacement fluid) directly into the blood. This fluid causes a *convective clearance* of water and wastes. It uses a pressure gradient rather than a concentration gradient (dialysate solution), which has its main effect on water movement with solutes. The bulk flow of water "drags" solutes with it. In addition, it is able to remove not only small solutes but some middle-sized solutes as well (Liu & Chertow, 2015).

Continuous Venovenous Hemofiltration-Dialysis (CVVH-D).   This form of CRRT uses the same dialysate solution as is used in intermittent hemodialysis and works the same way. The solution is infused through the dialyzer in the opposite direction of the blood flow. The result is a diffusion of small wastes and water out of the dialyzer.

Table 27–7 Methods of Continuous Replacement Therapy

Method	Description
Continuous venovenous hemofiltration (CVVH)	Utilizes a double-lumen venous catheter and CRRT machine to remove fluids and small- and middle-molecular-weight solutes, then a replacement fluid to maintain electrolyte and acid balance
Continuous venovenous hemofiltration-dialysis (CVVH-D)	Utilizes a double-lumen venous catheter and CRRT machine to remove fluids and small-molecular-weight solutes using a dialysate solution
Continuous venovenous hemodiafiltration (CVVHDF)	Utilizes a double-lumen venous catheter and CRRT machine to remove fluids and small- and middle-molecular-weight solutes using both dialysate and replacement solutions
Slow continuous ultrafiltration (SCUF)	Uses venovenous access and continuous renal replacement therapy (CRRT) machine to circulate blood through hemofilter; primarily for water removal when waste products do not need to be removed or pH does not need correction

BOX 27–2   Potential Complications Related to CRRT

- Fluid imbalance
- Blood loss
- Hemofilter occlusion
- Infection
- Thrombosis
- Vascular occlusion

Continuous Venovenous Hemodiafiltration (CVVHDF). This form of CRRT uses the same equipment as other CRRT therapies but uses two solutions—replacement fluid and dialysate—to maximize the removal of wastes and water. One solution removes larger wastes, and the other removes smaller wastes.

Slow Continuous Ultrafiltration (SCUF). This form of CRRT also uses the same equipment, but the goal is the removal of water only, and no solutions are used. Because metabolic products are not cleared, its use is limited to fluid overload conditions such as heart failure.

Section Four Review

1. Which two activities are the primary functions of renal replacement therapy? (Select all that apply.)
   A. Addition of free fatty acids
   B. Removal of wastes
   C. Addition of nutrients
   D. Removal of excess water
   E. Removal of lipids

2. A client has been started on intermittent hemodialysis (IHD) to treat acute kidney failure. The nurse will closely monitor the client for which complications associated with IHD? (Select all that apply.)
   A. Infection
   B. Increased cardiac output
   C. Air embolism
   D. Acute myocardial infarction
   E. Hemorrhage

3. In peritoneal dialysis, which structure acts as the permeable membrane to remove wastes and water?
   A. Liver
   B. Peritoneal membrane
   C. Stomach
   D. Intestinal villi

4. Continuous renal replacement therapy has which major advantage over intermittent hemodialysis?
   A. Better retention of solutes
   B. Reduced loss of metabolic products
   C. Greater fluid removal
   D. Increased hemodynamic stability

Answers: 1. (B, D), 2. (B, D), 3. B, 4. D

Section Five: Nursing Care of the Patient with Acute Kidney Injury

Nursing care of the patient with acute kidney injury is complex because the patient is often acutely ill and unstable due to both the underlying cause of the renal impairment and the deranged renal function.

Managing Fluid Overload

Complications of AKI include hypervolemia, acute pulmonary edema, and a large cumulative positive fluid balance (Waikar & Bonventre, 2015). Therefore, nursing interventions focus on monitoring the patient for signs and symptoms of those complications. Prescribed fluids may be limited and their composition altered to adjust for changing serum electrolyte levels. A key nursing role is monitoring the patient's status and reporting changes to the supervising healthcare provider.

Fluid Restriction   Fluid restriction requires accurate assessment of the patient's intake and output balance. All output must be measured and carefully documented. When a patient is on fluid restriction, it is imperative that a decision be made about how to divide the free water requirement over a 24-hour period. To do this, the nurse must consider the timing of medication administration and meals to ensure that the fluid restriction is observed. Uremic patients may experience extreme thirst; oral fluids or ice chips in small quantities often increase patient comfort. Oral care is also an extremely important intervention to both minimize oral mucosal damage and increase patient comfort.

Diuretics   Any use of diuretic therapy requires accurate monitoring of intake and output (and intake/output balance), blood pressure, and serum electrolytes. The nurse should also monitor for hypovolemia and for signs and symptoms of electrolyte abnormalities based on the specific diuretic being used.

Renal Replacement Therapy (RRT)   Regardless of the specific RRT therapy used, the nurse must be competent at managing the specialized technology and providing the necessary education for the patient and the family. In the high-acuity setting, intermittent hemodialysis is often managed by a trained dialysis nurse or technician. Peritoneal dialysis and CRRT are often performed by a nurse who has received the appropriate training. For critically ill patients, IHD can be done at the bedside rather than off-unit and is usually managed by hemodialysis staff rather than a unit nurse.

Complications of Fluid Volume Excess   Fluid volume overload can contribute to the following complications:

- Symptoms secondary to fluid volume excess
- A decrease in cardiac output
- Alterations in gas exchange

- Electrolyte imbalances
- Skin integrity problems

Desired Outcomes   The patient will attain the following:

- Reduced edema or absence of edema
- Clear or improved lung sounds
- Absence of shortness of breath
- Weight trend toward baseline
- Blood pressure trending toward baseline
- Intact skin

Nursing Interventions   Monitor the patient for fluid volume excess and for evidence of heart failure and electrolyte imbalance. Inspect the skin, especially the extremities, for skin breakdown due to the presence of edema. Protect the extremity containing the graft or fistula by placing signs at the bedside that the patient has this type of dialysis access. Perform blood sampling and blood pressures in the opposite extremity to prevent a cessation of blood flow through the access while a tourniquet or blood pressure cuff is in place. Check for a bruit or a thrill with a stethoscope to determine if the access is patent and blood is flowing through it.

Managing Catabolic Processes

The underlying causes of the AKI are often associated with an accelerated metabolism and present unique problems for meeting the metabolic needs of the high-acuity patient. A hypercatabolic state requires protein intake; at the same time, the nitrogenous wastes from protein metabolism are not excreted efficiently with AKI and must be carefully monitored. The patient must have protein to heal. The desirable protein intake of patients receiving maintenance hemodialysis (MHD) or peritoneal dialysis (PD) appears to be approximately 1.4 to 1.8 g/kg/day with a maximum of 2.5 g/kg/day (Connor, 2011). Frequently, depending on the kidney injury, the provider will limit the amount of protein in feedings or diet to prevent excess accumulation of nitrogenous wastes.

Complications of Altered Catabolic Processes   Altered catabolic processes may produce the following:

- Inadequate nutrition
- Confusion
- Diarrhea
- Constipation
- Risk for bleeding

Desired Outcomes   The patient will attain the following:

- Weight trending toward baseline
- Serum protein (albumin, prealbumin) trending toward normal ranges
- Nitrogen balance
- Mental status trending toward baseline
- Stools of soft, formed consistency and usual frequency

Nursing Implications   Nursing implications include a focus on adequate nutritional support. The nurse should consider an early nutrition consult to establish estimated nutritional support needs for the patient. The diet should be restricted in protein, sodium, potassium, and fluids and should be high in carbohydrates, fats, and essential amino acids. To minimize the risk of infection, oral or enteral feeding routes are preferable to the IV route because they maintain the normal gut mucosal barrier, discourage bacterial translocation, and preserve the gut. Renal replacement therapy may be initiated if dietary restrictions are not sufficient to maintain acceptable nitrogenous waste levels (e.g., BUN and creatinine).

The patient's weight should be monitored daily with the understanding that rapid weight shifts are probably secondary to fluid retention. Serum protein and prealbumin levels should be monitored regularly to evaluate whether the patient's nutritional status is worsening or improving. The patient's mental status needs to be monitored at least every shift for onset of renal encephalopathy, which is associated with decreased creatinine clearance. Stool consistency and frequency are monitored, and orders are obtained as needed to attain or maintain adequate bowel evacuation patterns.

Managing Electrolyte and Acid–Base Imbalances

The two electrolytes of particular concern in patients with AKI are potassium and sodium. Potassium elevation is a consistent problem with the oliguria of AKI unless potassium intake is limited. Hyperkalemia is considered a clinical emergency because the cardiac dysrhythmias associated with hyperkalemia can lead to cardiac arrest. The nurse must be aware of the electrocardiographic clues of hyperkalemia; a prolonged QRS and tall, peaked T waves are the typical ECG changes seen with elevated serum potassium (Beasley, 2014). Hypokalemia may be seen with the use of potassium-wasting diuretics. Sodium levels may be either elevated or reduced in patients with renal insufficiency. More often, the patient with AKI will experience hypernatremia caused by water loss in excess of sodium loss. Alternatively, the use of diuretics prescribed to treat oliguria or a renal dysfunction in which there is sodium wasting in excess of volume loss can produce hyponatremia.

Metabolic acidosis associated with AKI results from the inability of the kidneys to excrete hydrogen ions and reabsorb bicarbonate ions (LeMone et al., 2015; Marieb & Hoehn, 2016). Early in the process of kidney injury, phosphate buffers are able to correct for acidosis in spite of reduced bicarbonate. As the dysfunction persists and phosphate buffers are unable to compensate, the serum pH falls and metabolic acidosis develops.

Complications of Electrolyte and Acid–Base Abnormalities

- A risk for injury
- A decrease in cardiac output

Desired Patient Outcomes   The patient will attain or maintain the following:

- Serum pH between 7.35 and 7.45
- Serum electrolytes within normal limits
- Normal cardiac rhythm

Nursing Implications The nurse should closely monitor the patient for clinical manifestations of electrolyte imbalances, especially sodium, potassium, calcium, phosphate, and magnesium. The patient's arterial blood gases are also monitored for metabolic acidosis (abnormally low pH and HCO_3). The patient should be on continuous cardiac monitoring with close surveillance of ECG pattern changes associated with electrolyte imbalances, particularly potassium and calcium. If any type of RRT is ordered to manage the patient's electrolyte and acid–base status, the nurse will need to alter the patient's plan of care accordingly.

Infection

Patients with acute renal failure are at risk for infection. The presence of severe infection can result in prerenal AKI because of the massive vasodilation and hypotension that develop in septic states (LeMone et al., 2015). In addition, the immunocompromised state associated with significant renal dysfunction increases the likelihood that the patient may acquire a nosocomial infection.

General Complications of AKI

- Infection
- Inability to engage in physical activity
- Hyperthermia
- Diminished perfusion of tissues
- Acute pain

- Anxiety
- Lack of knowledge about condition

Desired Patient Outcomes The patient will be free of infection as evidenced by the following:

- All invasive devices removed in a timely fashion
- WBC count within acceptable levels
- Absence of fever
- Negative cultures
- Wounds free of purulent drainage

Nursing Implications Nursing implications focus on monitoring the patient for signs and symptoms of infection. The nurse should strictly adhere to sterile procedure when performing or assisting with central line insertion, as well as scrupulous hand hygiene prior to and after patient care.

Major sources of infection in the patient with AKI include urinary tract infection, pneumonia, and septicemia from vascular catheters and skin or wound sources. Evidence-based practices and care bundles for vascular catheter insertion and care, minimizing ventilator-associated pneumonias, and sepsis care should be routine acute care practices. Antibiotic therapy requires dose adjustment based on the severity of renal impairment. If antibiotics are prescribed, the nurse monitors for therapeutic and nontherapeutic effects.

The "Nursing Care: The Patient Requiring Renal Replacement Therapy" feature provides additional information on care of the patient receiving some type of RRT.

Nursing Care
The Patient Requiring Renal Replacement Therapy

Expected Patient Outcomes and Related Interventions

Outcome 1: Fluid and electrolyte balance

Assess and compare to established normal patient baselines and trends.

Fluid—intake and output, weight, mean arterial pressure, breath sounds, jugular veins, extremities, hemodynamic monitoring values

Electrolytes—serum electrolyte levels, especially Na and K. Monitor ECG for electrolyte-related changes, dysrhythmias.

Kidney function—BUN, creatinine

Acid–base balance—arterial blood gases

Hemodynamics—Monitor vital signs and impact of treatment, volume of fluid dialyzed from patient and record

Assess for dialysis disequilibrium syndrome—headache, nausea, vomiting, altered level of consciousness, hypertension, seizures, coma

Administer related drug therapy and monitor for therapeutic and nontherapeutic effects.

Diuretics (e.g., furosemide [Lasix])

Cation exchange agents (e.g., sodium polystyrene sulfonate [Kayexalate])

Implement fluid restriction as ordered.

Outcome 2: Patient protected from possible harm

Assess and compare to established normal patient baselines and trends.

Hematologic:

Coagulation—Assess hourly ultrafiltration rate and patency of hemofilter and tubing hourly. Assess serum coagulation studies as ordered. Assess for bleeding at vascular access site or elsewhere.

Red blood cells—Monitor hemoglobin, red blood cell count and hematocrit, SaO_2 or SpO_2 to assess adequacy of gas exchange.

Infection—Assess vascular access device for signs and symptoms of infection. Assess white blood cell count, fever, cultures as ordered. Assess peak and trough levels of antibiotics as ordered.

Circulation—Check pulses and skin warmth and color at least once a shift. When appropriate to type of RRT venous access, check circulation and presence of a thrill or bruit in extremity that contains the dialysis access.

Administer related drug therapy and monitor for therapeutic and nontherapeutic effects.

Anticoagulants as ordered (e.g., heparin)

Antibiotics as ordered; doses may be adjusted to prevent renal toxicity.

Change hemofilter per unit protocol.

Protect vascular access device from dislodgement.

Section Five Review

1. Hyperkalemia associated with AKI may lead to which problem?
   A. Excessive thirst
   B. Cardiac arrest
   C. Skeletal muscle weakness
   D. Dysphagia

2. Dietary protein intake is monitored in clients with renal dysfunction for which reason?
   A. Dietary sources of protein include excess triglyceride levels.
   B. The client's weight must be controlled, and limiting protein is the easiest way to do this.
   C. Dietary protein intake increases nitrogenous waste products.
   D. The client requires twice the usual protein intake.

3. The nurse should expect which normal finding in an RRT access device?
   A. Bruit
   B. Murmur
   C. Irregular pulsation
   D. Coolness to touch

4. Which levels should the nurse routinely monitor to assess the nutritional status of a client with acute kidney injury? (Select all that apply.)
   A. Serum protein
   B. Prealbumin
   C. Albumin
   D. Urine glucose
   E. Weight

Answers: 1. B, 2. C, 3. A, 4. (A, B)

Section Six: Chronic Kidney Failure in the High-Acuity Patient

High-acuity patients may be admitted with preexisting chronic kidney disease, which must be taken into consideration when planning patient management. **Chronic kidney failure (CKF)** is defined as the gradual loss of renal function and affects nearly all organ systems. Individuals with CKD progress steadily toward end-stage renal disease (ESRD) (Watnick & Dirkx, 2017). Chronic kidney failure is the result either of a primary renal condition in which the kidneys are directly affected (e.g., polycystic kidney disease or glomerulonephritis) or of other diseases that produce a long-term renal insult (e.g., diabetes or hypertension). Risk factors for ESRD include heart disease, diabetes mellitus, smoking, hypertension, positive family history of kidney disease, obesity, and increasing age (Watnick & Dirkx, 2017; Zelman et al., 2015).

Pathophysiology of Chronic Kidney Disease

The renal excretory function in CKD is chronically compromised, and most, but not all, forms are progressive and irreversible. All forms of renal failure are characterized by a reduction in the glomerular filtration rate (GFR), reflecting a corresponding reduction in the number of functional nephrons (Watnick & Dirkx, 2017). Chronic loss of nephron function causes generalized wasting (shrinking in size) and progressive scarring within all parts of the kidneys. In time, overall scarring obscures the site of the initial damage. A variety of renal insults can cause CKD; however, the two leading causes are diabetes and hypertension (Mistovich,

Karren, Werman, & Hafen, 2014). Box 27–3 lists the common causes of CKD.

Stages of Chronic Kidney Disease   In 2002, the National Kidney Foundation (NKF) published *Classification of Stages of Chronic Kidney Disease,* presenting five stages based on GFR. This staging system continues to be widely accepted (Table 27–8), When revisited in 2016, these criteria were still valid, and no changes were made to the classifications.

Stage 1.   Stage 1, often referred to as *diminished renal reserve,* is characterized by the destruction of nephrons and compensatory hyperfiltration. Often the patient is asymptomatic, and the only clinical sign may be an elevated BUN. In this stage, the GFR is reduced to approximately 50% of normal function and the GFR is greater than 90 mL/min/1.73 m^2. The kidneys are at increased risk for nephrotoxicity from drugs, toxins, or other insults. Renal function laboratory tests are within normal ranges.

BOX 27–3   Common Causes of Chronic Kidney Disease

- Diabetes mellitus (leading cause)
- Hypertension (second leading cause)
- Disease may start in the tubules due to the following:
  - Systemic disease such as diabetes and hypertension
  - Autoimmune reactions and transplant rejection
  - Harmful actions of drugs or toxins
  - Infections
  - Mechanical damage
  - Ischemia
- Obstruction of the urinary tract

SOURCE: Data from LeMone et al. (2015).

Table 27–8 NKF Classification of Stages of Chronic Kidney Disease

Stage	Description	GFR (mL/min/1.73 m^2)
1	Kidney damage with normal or increased GFR	Greater than 90
2	Mild reduction in GFR	60–89
3	Moderate reduction in GFR	30–59
4	Severe reduction in GFR	15–29
5	Kidney failure	Less than 15 or dialysis

SOURCE: Based on National Kidney Foundation (2016).

Stage 2.   Stage 2, often referred to as *renal insufficiency*, occurs when the GFR is mildly reduced and mild symptoms such as blood or protein in the urine are present. The remaining functional nephrons attempt to compensate, but their effort is inadequate to clear the nitrogenous wastes. Parathyroid hormone secretion increases, and renal calcium reabsorption decreases. The GFR drops to 60–89 mL/min/1.73 m^2. The patient develops hypertension, anemia, and isosthenuria (a form of polyuria, or increased urine output, in which the urine has a low specific gravity similar to that of plasma because the kidneys can no longer concentrate it). Renal function laboratory tests reflect azotemia.

Stage 3.   Stage 3, sometimes referred to as *renal failure*, occurs as the GFR is reduced to 30–59 mL/min/1.73 m^2. The patient can experience left ventricular hypertrophy and anemia secondary to a decrease in erythropoietin production. The patient now exhibits manifestations of the onset of kidney failure, such as fatigue, fluid retention, changes in urine color, or muscle cramps, and laboratory tests reflect worsening renal functioning.

Stage 4.   In the fourth stage of CKD, the GFR drops to 15–29 mL/min/1.73 m^2. Serum triglycerides increase, and the patient experiences hyperkalemia, hyperphosphatemia, metabolic acidosis, fatigue, nausea, and bone pain. The patient also exhibits worsening manifestations of kidney failure, such as metallic taste, loss of appetite, numbness or tingling, and a further deterioration in laboratory results.

Stage 5.   Stage 5, usually referred to as *end-stage renal disease (ESRD)*, is true renal failure. The GFR is less than 15 mL/min/1.73 m^2, and the patient experiences severe uremic symptoms if not treated with dialysis. Renal function laboratory tests reflect total loss of renal function.

Diagnostic Features of Chronic Kidney Disease

Chronic kidney disease is diagnosed when one or both of the following conditions are present:

- Evidence of kidney damage lasting 3 months, as defined by structural or functional abnormalities of the kidney, with or without a decrease in glomerular filtration rate (LeMone et al., 2015).

- Glomerular filtration rate less than 60 mL/min/1.73 m^2 for at least 3 months, with or without kidney damage

The diagnosis and staging of CKD is heavily dependent on laboratory analysis, including GFR. As discussed in Section Two, two major laboratory tests that reflect kidney function—blood urea nitrogen (BUN) and creatinine—are the cornerstones of monitoring both acute and chronic kidney disease. Regardless of the underlying cause, both BUN and creatinine rise over time.

Manifestations of Chronic Kidney Disease

The systemic effects of CKD are wide-ranging and extend from those identified in AKI. CKD is associated with severe fluid and electrolyte imbalances primarily affecting sodium, potassium, calcium, and phosphorous. The patient increasingly displays the multisystem signs and symptoms of uremia as renal function deteriorates and uremic toxins build in the blood. Metabolic acidosis is common, particularly once the GFR falls below 15 to 30 mL/min (Cho, 2017). The acid–base imbalance seen in AKI continues as bicarbonate levels stabilize at 15 to 20 mEq/L and excess hydrogen ions are buffered by anions from bone. The laboratory findings of CKD are summarized in Table 27–9.

Cardiovascular Effects   Hypertension is a common feature of CKD and often progresses to heart failure if untreated. Atherosclerotic heart disease is the most common complication. Hypertensive nephropathy (kidney disease secondary to hypertension) is a glomerulopathy initiated by an increase in intraglomerular pressure that activates and damages glomerular cells (Pearson Education, 2015). Hyperlipidemia, a well-established risk factor for cardiovascular disease in the general population, is highly prevalent among patients with CKD and is estimated to be

Table 27–9 Laboratory Findings Associated with Chronic Kidney Disease

Lab Feature	Characteristics
Creatinine and BUN	Elevated as CKD progresses, with creatinine a more reliable indicator of renal function
Sodium	May be reduced as normal tubular reabsorption is reduced and urine excretion is increased; as CKD progresses, hypernatremia often predominates
Potassium	May be at or near normal levels as tubular secretion is increased; as CKD progresses and oliguria occurs, hyperkalemia is a principle feature and may be life-threatening
Calcium and phosphate	Reduced renal excretion of phosphate and decreased kidney synthesis of the active form of vitamin D; reduced vitamin D and elevated phosphate levels bind free calcium, causing hypocalcemia and resulting in hyperparathyroid activity and bone loss
Acid–base	Hydrogen ion excretion and bicarbonate resorption in the early stage progresses to metabolic acidosis in later stages

present in over 40% of patients with kidney failure. A loss of vessel elasticity associated with atherosclerosis and abnormal calcification of vessel walls contributes to macrovascular disease, ischemic heart disease, heart failure, stroke, and peripheral vascular disease (LeMone et al., 2015; McCullough & Roberts, 2016).

Pericarditis in end-stage renal disease is a significant complication of CKD (LeBlond et al., 2015). It is manifested secondary to azotemia or to inadequate dialysis or fluid overload. Pericarditis causes chest pain, a friction rub, and possible cardiac tamponade. Patients with CKD can develop uremic cardiomyopathy. Contributors to this condition are anemia, increased effective circulating blood volume, fluid overload, and hypertension. Among patients with CKD, 75% have left ventricular hypertrophy. This causes decreased cardiac systolic contraction and inhibits diastolic relaxation. Hyperphosphatemia is strongly associated with heart disease in patients with CKD (LeMone et al., 2015).

Hematologic Effects   The etiology of anemia in CKD is multifactorial. Chronic anemia is associated with a reduced production of the hormone erythropoietin, which is produced by the kidneys and stimulates the bone marrow to produce red blood cells. Inadequate production of erythropoietin is thought to be the most important factor in the pathogenesis of anemia in these patients. In addition to relative erythropoietin deficiency, shortened erythrocyte survival and the erythropoiesis inhibitory effects of accumulating uremic toxins also contribute to the anemia of CKD. Gastrointestinal blood loss and potential blood loss in dialysis treatment also can cause anemia (Wilkinson, 2014).

It is important to note that patients with CKD have abnormalities in the systemic homeostasis of iron, an essential component of red blood cells. Hemodialysis patients, in particular, are typically in negative iron balance, losing approximately 1 to 3 grams of iron as a consequence of repeated phlebotomy and due in part to blood trapping in the dialysis apparatus. Low available iron reduces the iron available to hemoglobin, and because oxygen molecules attach only to iron atoms on hemoglobin, oxygen delivery to the tissues is reduced.

Deficits in platelet function as the result of uremia contribute to bleeding abnormalities among patients with renal failure (Abrams, Shattil, & Bennett, 2016). The resulting coagulopathy is evidenced by easy bruising of the skin, nosebleeds, increased menstrual bleeding, and gastrointestinal bleeding in patients with uremia.

Gastrointestinal Effects   Anorexia-induced inadequate nutrient intake is an important cause of malnutrition in patients with CKD. A decline in protein and calorie intake typically becomes an issue once the GFR declines to less than 25–38 mL/min/1.73 m^2 (late stage 3/early stage 4 CKD). The causes of anorexia in CKD are multiple. The retention of uremic toxins and various comorbid conditions can lead to lowered appetite and a decrease in protein and energy intake, which is often compounded by the imposition of various dietary restrictions (LeMone et al., 2015). Elevated parathyroid hormone levels increase gastric acid production and are associated with complaints of

gastric distress and anorexia. As mentioned, the risk for GI bleeding is also increased in this chronically ill population due to coagulopathies and disruptions of the gastric mucosa.

Neurologic Effects   Central neurologic symptoms are nonspecific and progressive in the patient with CKD. These symptoms include sleep disorders, memory loss, impaired judgment, muscle cramps, and twitching, and they may progress to more severe manifestations of uremic encephalopathy such as confusion, delirium, seizures, and coma. Additional neurologic effects include restless leg syndrome and sensory neuropathies (Pearson Education, 2015). For those patients receiving hemodialysis, the neurologic risks are compounded by rapid fluctuations in electrolytes and acid–base balance.

Skeletal Effects   CKD is characterized by loss of bone mass due to secondary hyperparathyroidism. Excess parathyroid hormone (PTH) stimulates an increase in bone reabsorption of calcium, and the bones become brittle and can break easily. Decreased intestinal reabsorption of calcium secondary to a lack of conversion of vitamin D to its active form by the kidneys decreases serum calcium levels (Kibble & Halsey, 2015). Hyperphosphatemia develops as the kidneys fail to excrete it, and the resulting hyperphosphatemia stimulates parathyroid hormone secretion.

Immunologic Effects   The major immunologic issues associated with CKD result from impaired immunocompetence. Uremia negatively affects granulocyte and monocyte functions, significantly increasing the patient's susceptibility to infections. Infection is the second most common cause of death in individuals on dialysis (Perrin & MacLeod, 2013). The overall mortality rate in patients with CKD is 10 to 20 times higher than in the general population (LeMone et al., 2015).

Many physiological processes are affected by CKD, as summarized in Table 27–10.

Table 27–10 Physiologic Processes Affected by Chronic Kidney Disease

Processes	Characteristics
Sex hormones	Reduced estrogen in females with amenorrhea and inability to maintain pregnancy. In males, possible infertility from reduced testosterone and low sperm levels; possible impotence from vascular complications. Reduced libido in both genders.
Immune processes	Suppressed cell-mediated responses and reduced antibody production
Integumentary	Pale skin from anemia and yellow-brown hue due to pigment changes related to lipochrome and carotenoid deposits and crystallization of urea on the skin associated with uremia; dry skin and mucous membranes, decreased perspiration, and pruritus and resultant scratching may produce skin breaks
Carbohydrates, protein, and fat metabolism	Catabolic state and negative nitrogen balance, glucose intolerance associated with insulin resistance and reduced HDL, elevated LDL and triglycerides

Medical Treatment

Many of the medical treatments for CKD are targeted at the associated symptoms identified in this chapter. Medications and/or dialysis are commonly used for symptom management. Recall that in many CKD patients, poor absorption of dietary iron and inability to utilize the body's iron stores contribute to the anemia. Management of the anemia of CKD includes administration of recombinant human erythropoietin and iron supplementation. Parathyroid hormone can be suppressed through diet modifications and vitamin supplementation with 1,25 dihydroxycholecalciferol (vitamin D). Phosphate binders can be administered (primarily calcium and aluminum hydroxide antacids) to treat hyperphosphatemia and suppress parathyroid hormone secretion (Adams & Urban, 2017). Heart failure may be treated with cardioselective beta-blocking agents. Hypertension is treated with potassium-wasting diuretics, angiotensin-converting enzyme (ACE) inhibitors, and other pharmacologic vasodilator agents. An important aspect of the pharmacologic treatment of hypertension is the avoidance of medications that may cause harm in the presence of renal failure. The "Quality and Safety: Antihypertensive Medication Effects with Renal Failure" feature describes antihypertensive medications that can exert unwanted effects in patients with renal failure.

Dialysis   Patients admitted with late-stage CKD are usually already undergoing renal replacement therapy (intermittent hemodialysis or peritoneal dialysis) at home or at a dialysis center. These therapies continue while the patient is hospitalized; however, the patient who normally undergoes peritoneal dialysis may have to be moved to temporary intermittent hemodialysis during the acute illness phase if fluid and electrolyte status becomes severely imbalanced. Hemodialysis was discussed in a previous section of this chapter; an overview of peritoneal dialysis is presented here.

Peritoneal Dialysis.   Peritoneal dialysis (PD) uses the peritoneal cavity as the semipermeable membrane to remove waste, excess fluid, and electrolytes from the

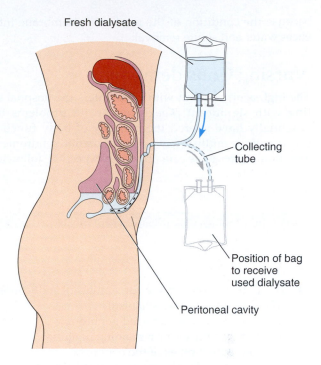

Figure 27–4 Peritoneal dialysis.

blood. A sterile peritoneal catheter is inserted into the peritoneal cavity with the proximal end extending out through the abdominal wall (Figure 27–4). The proximal end attaches to the dialysate tubing during treatments. As a prescribed volume and concentration of dialysate solution is instilled through this catheter using strict aseptic techniques, waste products and excess electrolytes in the blood cross the semipermeable peritoneal membrane into the dialysate. The dialysate fluid "dwells" in the peritoneal space for a prescribed amount of time to maximize this diffusion and is then drained.

Peritoneal dialysis comprises both diffusion and osmosis. Osmosis occurs as a high glucose concentration in the dialysate allows water to be pulled from the blood and into the peritoneal cavity during the dwell process. This process can be continuous with a prescribed instillation–dwell–drain sequence. It can also be intermittent, perhaps two or three times over the course of a day, or a cycling machine can make the process semiautomatic (Batsie, Mistovich, & Limmer, 2013).

The advantages of peritoneal dialysis include the fact that the patient can perform it on a regular basis, making the fluid and electrolyte shifts less dramatic than with intermittent hemodialysis. Peritoneal dialysis can be accomplished in the patient's home, and ambulatory patients can participate in work or relaxation activities while the process is ongoing. For the hemodynamically unstable patient, PD affords a less dramatic alteration in fluid balance, making it a safer alternative than intermittent hemodialysis. Disadvantages include a significant risk of infection from contamination of the peritoneal cavity, respiratory distress associated with the volume of fluid creating pressure against the diaphragm, and significant protein depletion from the blood into the peritoneal cavity and into the dialysate solution. PD is also not predictive of the precise fluid volume or solute that will be removed,

---

Quality and Safety
Antihypertensive Medication Effects with Renal Failure

- **Thiazide diuretics**—chlorthalidone (Thalitone) or chlorothiazide (Diuril)—Avoid if serum creatinine is greater than 2.5 mg/dL or creatinine clearance is less than 30 mL/minute, may worsen renal failure.
- **Aldosterone antagonists/potassium-sparing diuretics**—spironolactone (Aldactone)—Avoid if patient is at risk for elevated potassium level, potassium levels can increase.
- **Beta blockers, ACE inhibitors, and ARBs**—These drugs are less effective when used in conjunction with NSAIDs. (For additional drug information, see: Related Pharmacology, "Agents for Treatment of Heart Failure and Hypertension" in Chapter 14.)

SOURCE: Data from Gloe et al. (2016); Sinert & Peacock (2016); Trevor et al. (2015).

because the condition of the peritoneal membrane influences water and solute removal.

Nursing Considerations

The high-acuity patient with CKD enters the hospital setting with significant preexisting health problems that potentially have altered the majority of body functions because of the multisystem nature of uremic syndrome. At a minimum, the acute care nurse can expect the following:

- Dialysis will be required.
- Hypertension is likely.
- Fluid restriction and dietary restrictions of protein, sodium, potassium, and phosphate will be important.
- Hypoxia associated with anemia will be a focus.
- Increased risk of infection is a concern.
- GI disturbances and anorexia are common and can impact nutritional status.

Section Six Review

1. The kidneys compensate for significant reductions in GFR through which mechanism?
   A. Regeneration of damaged nephrons
   B. Hypertrophy of the remaining nephrons
   C. Hibernation reflex of the nephrons
   D. There are no compensatory mechanisms.

2. What is the leading cause of chronic kidney failure?
   A. Diabetes mellitus
   B. Renal calculi
   C. Hypertension
   D. Infection

3. Which findings suggest a client with chronic kidney disease may have developed pericarditis?
   A. Chest pain
   B. Increased serum potassium level
   C. Friction rub
   D. Hypotension
   E. Muffled heart sounds

4. A client with end-stage renal disease (ESRD) has been admitted for treatment of a different diagnosis. The nurse would expect which intervention due to the presence of ESRD?
   A. Encouraging fluid intake
   B. High-protein diet
   C. Sodium-restricted diet
   D. Potassium supplementation

Answers: 1. D, 2. A, 3. (A, C, E), 4. C

Clinical Reasoning Checkpoint

Mr. T, a 52-year-old long-distance trucker with a history of hypertension and peptic ulcer disease, presents to the ED with a 7-day history of severe vomiting and abdominal pain. Mr. T's weight is 80 kg. He states that during the previous week he has been able to eat very little food and tolerates only occasional sips of water. He has become progressively weaker and is dizzy as he tries to stand. He has not taken his antihypertensive medication (hydrochlorothiazide and metoprolol) for the past 3 days.

On physical exam, Mr. T appears acutely ill, very weak, and pale. He has tenting of the skin over the clavicles, dry mucous membranes, weak peripheral pulses, flat jugular veins, and bilateral upper-quadrant tenderness with palpation.

Parameter	Vital Signs (supine)	Vital Signs (sitting)
BP	96/50 mm Hg	72/38 mm Hg
HR	110/min/regular	140 min/regular
RR	24 bpm	
Temp	99°F	

An IV catheter was inserted 2 hours after his arrival in the ED, and an indwelling urinary catheter is inserted with a urine output of 150 mL. He last remembers voiding about 8 hours ago. His labs, drawn upon arrival in the ED, are as follows: Na 133 mEq/L, K 2.8 mEq/L, Cl 70 mEq/L, CO_2 42 mEq/L, glucose 72 mg/dL, creatinine 4.2 mg/dL, BUN 108 mg/dL, hematocrit 51%, hemoglobin 17 gm/dL, WBC 10.2×10^3.

1. What do Mr T's lab work and presenting features indicate?

Clinical Update: Mr. T was resuscitated with intravenous fluid and was taken to the operating room for surgical repair of a bleeding gastric ulcer. On postop day 1, Mr. T's urine output has decreased to 250 mL over the preceding 12 hours, and his lab results are as follows:

Electrolyte	ED admission # 1	Post-op day 1
Na	133 mEq/L	138 mEq/L
K	2.8 mEq/L	5.1 mEq/L
Cr	4.2 mg/dL	3.8 mg/dL
BUN	108 mg/dL	92 mg/dL
Hct	51%	31%
Hb	17 gm/dL	8.5 gm/dL
WBC	10.2×10^3	11×10^3

The nephrologist is called in for consult and recommends a fluid challenge.

2. What would be the purpose of administering fluids at this point?

3. What is your interpretation of Mr. T's BUN and creatinine?

Clinical Update: On postop day 3, Mr. T develops a temperature of 38.8°C (101.8°F), and his urine output remains low, at 20–25 mL/hour. A diuretic challenge was done after fluids were administered. He does not respond to diuretics. His weight is 8 kg above his preop weight. Some labs are indicated below.

Values	Postop day 1	Postop day 3
Na	138 mEq/L	135 mEq/L
K	5.1 mEq/L	5.3 mEq/L
Cr	3.8 mg/dL	4.7 mg/dL
BUN	92 mg/dL	102 mg/dL
Hct	31%	28%
Hb	8.5 gm/dL	7.8 gm/dL
WBC	11×10^3	14.6×10^3

A chest x-ray and physical exam indicate right lower-lobe (RLL) pneumonia.

4. Why is Mr. T at increased risk of pulmonary complications?

5. You are concerned about Mr. T's potassium level. What treatment might you expect the healthcare provider to prescribe?

Clinical Update: By postoperative day 6, Mr. T's respiratory infection and azotemia have worsened and his weight is now 14 kg above his preoperative weight. He is transferred to the critical care unit, intubated, and placed on mechanical ventilation. The nephrologist recommends RRT.

6. Would intermittent hemodialysis (IHD) or continuous RRT (CRRT) be most helpful to Mr. T?

Chapter 27 Review

1. A client who sustained severe injury in a motor vehicle crash presented to the emergency department with a blood pressure of 76/42 mmHg. Paramedics report that the client was pinned in the wreckage and that extrication took approximately 35 minutes. First blood pressure on scene was 86/50 mmHg. The nurse monitors this client for the development of renal failure of which origin?

   1. Postrenal
   2. Prerenal
   3. Intrinsic
   4. Perirenal

2. To prevent acute kidney damage, the medical team works to maintain a trauma client's mean arterial pressure (MAP) of at least:

   1. 65 mmHg
   2. 60 mmHg
   3. 100 mmHg
   4. 120 mmHg

3. A client was hospitalized 12 hours ago for observation after being injured in a fall from a ladder. Which assessment findings associated with AKI would the nurse communicate to the rest of the medical team immediately? (Select all that apply.)

   1. The client's urine output has been 20 mL for each of the last 2 hours.
   2. The client complains of a headache.
   3. The client is becoming more azotemic.
   4. The client's last potassium level was 4.8 mEq/L.
   5. The client's last blood glucose level was 132 mg/dL.

4. The nurse is reviewing laboratory results and would be most concerned about kidney damage if the client's serum report revealed which value?

   1. BUN 35 mg/dL
   2. Creatinine 4.3 mg/dL
   3. Potassium 4.5 mEq/L
   4. Phosphorus 2.4 mEq/L

5. A client with kidney failure had 980 mL of total output yesterday. The nurse would expect that fluid replacement therapy for this client today would be limited to _____ mL. (Fill in the blank.)

6. Which statement by the spouse of a client in renal failure would the nurse evaluate as indicating accurate knowledge of continuous renal replacement therapy?
   1. "With this therapy, it will be just like his kidneys were not damaged."
   2. "He will have to go to the dialysis center two or three times each week."
   3. "We will have to learn how much dwell time we should use."
   4. "He will probably have to stay in the critical care unit while on this therapy."

7. A nurse is administering 80 mg of IV furosemide to a client in renal failure. To avoid ototoxicity, how long should it take to inject this medication?
   1. 2 minutes
   2. 5 minutes
   3. 10 minutes
   4. 20 minutes

8. A nurse is assessing a client's venous access site used for dialysis. Which assessment finding would the nurse interpret as indicating this site is patent? (Select all that apply.)
   1. Presence of a thrill
   2. Presence of a pulse
   3. Presence of a bruit
   4. Presence of a visible lift
   5. Presence of an audible click

9. A client has been diagnosed with diminished renal reserve. Which symptoms would the nurse expect the client to report?
   1. Extreme fatigue
   2. No symptoms
   3. Itching of the skin
   4. Inability to concentrate

10. Which assessment finding would cause the nurse to suspect that a client in chronic kidney failure is developing pericarditis?
    1. Development of a friction rub
    2. BUN over 50 mg/dL
    3. Anorexia
    4. Development of a third heart sound

Answers to questions found inside your textbook are available on the faculty resources site. Please consult with your instructor.

References

Abrams, C. S., Shattil, S. J., & Bennett, J. S. (2016). Chapter 121: Acquired qualitative platelet disorders. In K. Kaushansky, M. A. Lichtman, J. T. Prchal, M. M. Levi, O. W. Press, L. J. Burns, & M. Caligiuri (Eds.), *Williams hematology* (9th ed.). Retrieved January 22, 2017, from http://accessmedicine.mhmedical.com.ezproxy.uky.edu/content.aspx?bookid=1581&Sectionid=108082231

Adams, M. P., & Urban, C. Q. (2017). *Pharmacology for nurses: A pathophysiologic approach* (5th ed.). Hoboken, NJ: Pearson.

Aminoff, M. J., Greenberg, D. A., & Simon, R. P. (2015). Chapter 10: Sensory disorders. In M. J. Aminoff, D. A. Greenberg, & R. P. Simon (Eds.), *Clinical neurology* (9th ed.). Retrieved January 19, 2017, from http://accessmedicine.mhmedical.com.ezproxy.uky.edu/content.aspx?bookid=1194&Sectionid=69192005

Badin, J., Boulain, T., Ehrmann, S., Skarzynski, M., Bretagnol, A., Buret, J., . . . Perrotin, D. (2011). Relation between mean arterial pressure and renal function in the early phase of shock: A prospective, explorative cohort study. *Critical Care, 15*, R135. **doi:**10.1186/cc10253

Bargman, J. M., & Skorecki, K. (2015). Chapter 335: Chronic kidney disease. In D. Kasper, A. Fauci, S. Hauser, D. Longo, J. Jameson, & J. Loscalzo (Eds.), *Harrison's principles of internal medicine* (19th ed.). Retrieved January 19, 2017, from http://accessmedicine.mhmedical.com.ezproxy.uky.edu/content.aspx?bookid=1130&Sectionid=79746512

Batsie, D. J., Mistovich, J. J., & Limmer, D. (2013). Genitourinary and renal disorders. In H. A. Werman (Ed.), *Transition series: Topics for the paramedic* (1st ed., pp. 245–249). Upper Saddle River, NJ: Pearson.

Baumann, B. M. (2016). Chapter 57: Systemic hypertension. In J. E. Tintinalli, J. Stapczynski, O. Ma, D. M. Yealy, G. D. Meckler, & D. M. Cline (Eds.), *Tintinalli's emergency medicine: A comprehensive study guide* (8th ed.). Retrieved January 19, 2017, from http://accessmedicine.mhmedical.com.ezproxy.uky.edu/content.aspx?bookid=1658&Sectionid=109388371

Beasley, B. M. (2014). *Understanding EKGs: A practical approach* (4th ed.). Upper Saddle River, NJ: Pearson.

Callahan, B. (2015). Elimination: Dialysis. In R. Bedard (Ed.), *Nursing clinical skills: A concept-based approach to learning* (2nd ed., pp. 250–257). Hoboken, NJ: Pearson.

Chen, Y., Chi, M., Chen, Y., Chan, Y., Chou, S., & Wang, F. (2013). Using a criteria-based reminder to reduce use of indwelling urinary catheters and decrease urinary tract infections. *American Journal of Critical Care, 22*(2), 105–114.

Cho, K. C. (2017). Chapter 21: Electrolyte & acid-base disorders. In M. A. Papadakis, S. J. McPhee, & M. W. Rabow (Eds.), *Current medical diagnosis & treatment 2017*. Retrieved January 22, 2017, from http://accessmedicine.mhmedical.com.ezproxy.uky.edu/content.aspx?bookid=1843&Sectionid=135714601

Connor, K. A. (2011). Nutrition and continuous renal replacement therapy. *Critical Connections*. Retrieved January 21, 2017, from http://www.sccm.org/Communications/Critical-Connections/Archives/Pages/Nutrition-and-Continuous-Renal-Replacement-Therapy-.aspx

Gloe, D., Kenneally, M., & Felicilda-Reynaldo, R. F. D. (2016). Medication therapy adjustments in patients with chronic renal failure. *Medical Surgical Nursing, 25*(5), 325–328.

Hannon, C., & Murray, P. T. (2015). Chapter 97: Acute kidney injury. In J. B. Hall, G. A. Schmidt, & J. P. Kress (Eds.), *Principles of critical care* (4th ed.). Retrieved December 28, 2016, from http://accessmedicine.mhmedical.com.ezproxy.uky.edu/content.aspx?bookid=1340&Sectionid=80037293

Hinkle, C. (2014). Chapter 15: Renal system. In S. M. Burns (Ed.), *AACN: Essentials of critical care nursing* (3rd ed., pp. 383–398). New York, NY: McGraw-Hill Education.

Hung, S. C., Kuo, K. L. Peng, C. H., Wu, C. H., Lien Y. C., Wang, Y. C., & Tarng, D. C. (2014). Volume overload correlates with cardiovascular risk factors in patients with chronic kidney disease. *Kidney International, 85*(3), 703–709. doi:10.1038/ki.2013.336

Kee, J. L. (2014). *Laboratory and diagnostic tests with nursing implications* (9th ed.). Upper Saddle River, NJ: Pearson.

Kibble, J. D., & Halsey, C. R. (2015). Chapter 6: Renal physiology and acid-base balance. In J. D. Kibble & C. R. Halsey (Eds.), *Medical physiology: The big picture*. Retrieved January 22, 2017, from http://accessmedicine.mhmedical.com.ezproxy.uky.edu/content.aspx?bookid=1291&Sectionid=75577039

Lang, J., Zuber, K., & Davis, J. (2016). Acute kidney injury. *Journal of the American Academy of Physician Assistants, 29*(4), 51–54.

LeBlond, R. F., Brown, D. D., Suneja, M., & Szot, J. F. (2015). Chapter 10: The urinary system. In R. F. LeBlond, D. D. Brown, M. Suneja, & J. F. Szot (Eds.), *DeGowin's diagnostic examination* (10th ed.). Retrieved January 19, 2017, http://accessmedicine.mhmedical.com.ezproxy.uky.edu/content.aspx?bookid=1192&Sectionid=68669084

Lee, B. K., & Vincenti, F. G. (2013). Chapter 34: Acute kidney injury & oliguria. In J. W. McAninch & T. F. Lue (Eds.), *Smith and Tanagho's general urology* (18th ed.). Retrieved January 21, 2017, from http://accessmedicine.mhmedical.com.ezproxy.uky.edu/content.aspx?bookid=508&Sectionid=41088111

LeMone, P. T., Burke, K. M., & Bauldoff, G. (2015). *Medical-surgical nursing: Clinical reasoning in patient care* (6th ed.). Hoboken, NJ: Pearson.

Liu, K. D., & Chertow, G. M. (2015). Dialysis in the treatment of renal failure. In D. Kasper, A. Fauci, S. Hauser, D. Longo, J. Jameson, & J. Loscalzo (Eds.), *Harrison's principles of internal medicine* (19th ed.). Retrieved January 22, 2017, from http://accessmedicine.mhmedical.com.ezproxy.uky.edu/content.aspx?bookid=1130&Sectionid=79746623

Marieb, E. N., & Hoehn, K. (2016). *Human anatomy and physiology* (10th ed., pp. 998–1022). San Francisco, CA: Pearson.

Martensson, J., & Bellomo, R. (2015). Sepsis-induced acute kidney injury. *Critical Care Clinics, 31*(4), 649–660. doi:http://dx.doi.org/10.1016/j.ccc.2015.06.003

McCullough, P. A., & Roberts, W. C. (2016). Influence of chronic renal failure on cardiac structure. *Journal of the American College of Cardiology, 67*(10), 1183–1185.

Mehta, R. L., Burdmann, E. A., Cerda, J., Feehally, J., Finkelstein, F., Garcia-Garcia, G., . . . Remuzzi, G. (2016). Recognition and management of acute kidney injury in the International Society of Nephrology 0by25 Global Snapshot: A multinational cross-sectional study. *Lancet, 387*(10032), 2017–2025. doi:10.1016/S0140-6736(16)30240-9

Mistovich, J. J., Karren, K. J., Werman, H. A., & Hafen, B. Q. (2014). *Pre-hospital emergency care.* Upper Saddle River, NJ: Pearson.

Mount, D. B. (2015). Chapter 63: Fluid and electrolyte disturbances. In D. Kasper, A. Fauci, S. Hauser, D. Longo, Jameson, J., & Loscalzo, J. (Eds.), *Harrison's principles of internal medicine* (19th ed.). Retrieved January 20, 2017, from http://accessmedicine.mhmedical.com.ezproxy.uky.edu/content.aspx?bookid=1130&Sectionid=79726591

National Kidney Foundation. (2016). Hemodialysis. Retrieved January 22, 2017, from https://www.kidney.org/atoz/content/hemodialysis

Pearson Education. (2015). *Nursing: A concept-based approach to learning* (vol. I, 2nd ed.). Hoboken, NJ: Pearson.

Perrin, K. O., & MacLeod, C. E. (2013). *Understanding the essentials of critical care nursing* (2nd ed.). Upper Saddle River, NJ: Pearson.

Petejova, N., & Martinek, A. (2014). Acute kidney injury due to rhabdomyolysis and renal replacement therapy: A critical review. *Critical Care, 18*(3), 224. Retrieved April 25, 2017, from http://ccforum.com/content/18/3/224

Ravel, V., Ahmadi, S., Streja, E., Sosnov, J. A., Kovesdy, C. P., Kalantar-Zadeh, K., & Chen, J. L. T. (2016). Pain and kidney function decline and mortality: A cohort study of U. S. veterans. *American Journal of Kidney Diseases, 68*(2), 240–246.

Sinert, R., & Peacock, P. R. (2016). Chapter 88: Acute kidney injury. In J. E. Tintinalli, J. Stapczynski, O. Ma, D. M. Yealy, G. D. Meckler, & D. M. Cline (Eds.), *Tintinalli's emergency medicine: A comprehensive study guide* (8th ed.). Accessed January 22, 2017, from http://accessmedicine.mhmedical.com.ezproxy.uky.edu/content.aspx?book'id=1658&Sectionid=109433339

Singh, A. K., Singh, A. T., & Kari, J. (2017). Chapter 239: Acute kidney injury. In S. C. McKean, J. J. Ross,

D. D. Dressler, & D. B. Scheurer. (Eds.), *Principles and practice of hospital medicine* (2nd ed.). Retrieved December 28, 2016, from http://accessmedicine.mhmedical.com.ezproxy.uky.edu/content.aspx?bookid=1872&Sectionid=146989547

Tabloski, P. A. (2014). *Gerontological nursing* (3rd ed.). Upper Saddle River, NJ: Pearson.

Thornburg, B., & Gray-Vickrey, P. (2016). Acute kidney injury: Limiting the damage. *Nursing Critical Care, 11*(5), 18–29. doi:10.1097/01.CCN.0000494764.37673.78

Trevor, A. J., Katzung, B. G., & Kruidering-Hall, M. (2015). Corticosteroids & antagonists. In A. J. Trevor, B. G. Katzung, & M. Kruidering-Hall (Eds.), *Katzung & Trevor's pharmacology: Examination & board review* (11th ed.). Retrieved January 22, 2017, from http://accessmedicine.mhmedical.com.ezproxy.uky.edu/content.aspx?bookid=1568&Sectionid=95703556

Udani, S. M., Koyner, J. L., & Murray, P. T. (2015). Chapter 98: Renal replacement in the intensive care unit. In J. B. Hall, G. A. Schmidt, & J. P. Kress (Eds.), *Principles of critical care* (4th ed.). Retrieved January 20, 2017, from http://accessmedicine.mhmedical.com.ezproxy.uky.edu/content.aspx?bookid=1340&Sectionid=80037439

U.S. Food and Drug Administration. (2015). Safety Alerts for Human Medical Products. Kayexalate (sodium polystyrene sulfonate): Drug Safety Communication–FDA Requires Drug Interaction Studies. Retrieved from https://www.fda.gov/Safety/MedWatch/SafetyInformation/SafetyAlertsforHumanMedicalProducts/ucm468720.htm

Waikar, S. S., & Bonventre, J. V. (2015). Chapter 334: Acute kidney injury. In D. Kasper, A. Fauci, S. Hauser, D. Longo, J. Jameson, & J. Loscalzo (Eds.), *Harrison's principles of internal medicine* (19th ed.). Retrieved December 28, 2016, from http://accessmedicine.mhmedical.com.ezproxy.uky.edu/content.aspx?bookid=1130&Sectionid=79746409

Watnick, S., & Dirkx, T. C. (2017). Kidney disease. In M. A. Papadakis, S. J. McPhee, & M. W. Rabow (Eds.), *Current medical diagnosis & treatment 2017*. Accessed January 22, 2017, from http://accessmedicine.mhmedical.com.ezproxy.uky.edu/content.aspx?bookid=1843&Sectionid=135715089

Wilkinson, J. (2014). *Pearson nursing diagnosis handbook with NIC interventions and NOC outcomes* (10th ed.). Upper Saddle River, NJ: Pearson.

Wilson, B. A., Shannon, M. T., & Shields, K. M. (2016). *Pearson nurse's drug guide: 2016*. Hoboken, NJ: Pearson.

Zelman, M., Raymond, J., Holdaway, P., & Dafnis, E. (2015). Diseases and disorder of the urinary system. In S. Breuer (Ed.), *Human diseases: A systematic approach* (2nd ed., pp. 198–21). Upper Saddle River, NJ: Pearson.

Chapter 28
Determinants and Assessment of Hematologic Function

Learning Outcomes

28.1 Explain the anatomy and physiology of the hematologic system.

28.2 Describe erythrocytes, the cells of oxygen transport.

28.3 Explain the characteristics and cells of innate (natural) immunity.

28.4 Discuss the characteristics and cells of adaptive (acquired) immunity.

28.5 Describe the characteristics of antigens and the antigen–antibody response.

28.6 Describe the origin and function of platelets and coagulation.

28.7 Apply the assessment of blood cells and coagulation to patient situations.

This chapter provides foundational information on the normal functioning hematologic system that will facilitate a deeper understanding of hematologic disorders presented in Chapters 29 and 30. High-acuity patients are at increased risk for a variety of problems involving the hematologic system. Hematologic disorders generally impact multiple body systems, potentially increasing morbidity and mortality.

Section One: Review of Anatomy and Physiology

The hematologic system consists of the blood cells (red blood cells, white blood cells, platelets) and plasma. The bone marrow and lymphatic system are also structures of importance to the hematologic system because of their critical roles in blood cell formation, storage, functions, and removal. This section provides a brief overview of the hematologic system; however, the various components of the system are presented in greater detail throughout the chapter.

Composition of Blood

The adult body contains about 5 liters of blood, which is primarily composed of plasma, plasma proteins, and blood cells. Blood transports oxygen, glucose, hormones, electrolytes, and cell wastes to and from the tissues. Plasma is a clear fluid that makes up 55% of the whole blood volume, with the remaining 45% composed of cells and other formed elements. The anatomic components of blood and their physiologic functions are summarized in Figure 28–1.

Blood cells are formed within the bone marrow, which consists of yellow marrow (primarily composed of fat) and red marrow. The red marrow is where blood cells are formed. By young adulthood, red marrow (and therefore blood cell formation) is confined to specific bones, including the skull, sternum, ribs, vertebrae, and the ends (epiphyses) of the humerus and femur.

Formation of Blood Cells

Blood cells comprise **erythrocytes** (red blood cells or RBCs); **leukocytes** (white blood cells or WBCs), which include neutrophils, eosinophils, basophils, lymphocytes, and monocytes; and **thrombocytes** (platelets) (see "Cells"

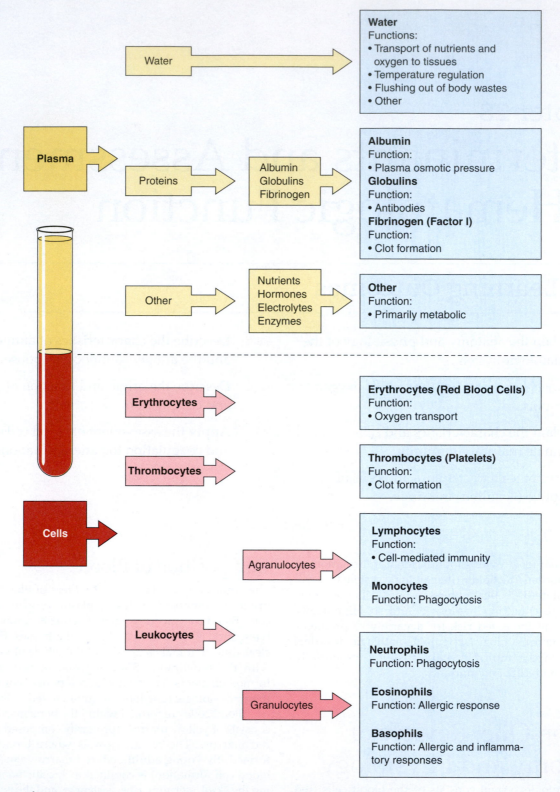

Figure 28–1 Major components of blood and their functions.

portion of Figure 28–1). These cells are constantly being replaced as they are used up (e.g., platelets forming a platelet plug in an injured vessel), are injured, or die naturally (**apoptosis**). Furthermore, increased numbers of specific blood cells may be required to meet a physiologic need, such as an increased WBC count during acute infection.

All types of blood cells are formed in the bone marrow from the same type of stem cells, called **pluripotential**

hematopoietic stem cells (PHSC). A PHSC divides into two cells when appropriately stimulated—one cell is a replacement PHSC and the other cell becomes a **committed stem cell**. Once formed, the committed cell begins to mature down a particular pathway of cell growth and differentiation (Figure 28–2). The term **cell differentiation** refers to the maturation process that a committed blood cell undergoes. It begins as an immature, undifferentiated

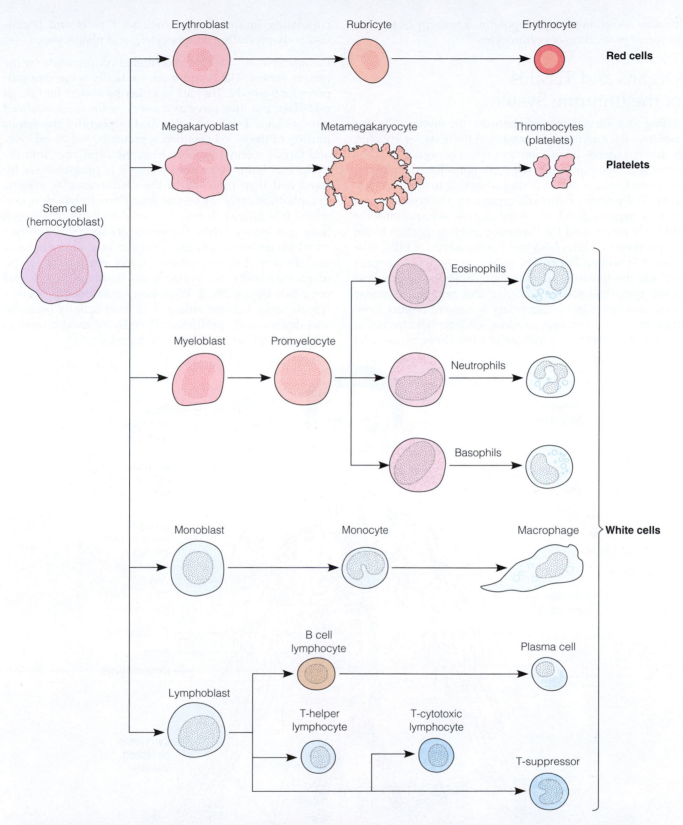

Figure 28–2 Blood cell formation from stem cells. Regulatory factors control the differentiation of stem cells into blast cells. Each of the five kinds of blast cells is committed to producing one type of mature blood cell. Erythroblasts, for example, differentiate only into RBCs; megakaryoblasts differentiate only into platelets.

(primitive) cell with no specific functions and ultimately becomes a mature, well-differentiated cell. A well-differentiated blood cell has two major characteristics—it has only one function, and it can no longer reproduce.

The cell maturation process requires special proteins, called growth inducers and differentiation inducers. Factors external to the bone marrow trigger the formation of these special proteins. For example, chronic hypoxia induces secretion of erythropoietin, a growth factor that increases production of erythrocytes.

Organs and Tissues of the Immune System

Acting as a surveillance mechanism, the immune system monitors the internal environment of the body for invasion by foreign agents. It is a complex system of organs and cells capable of distinguishing self from nonself, remembering previous invaders, and reacting according to needs as they arise. The primary lymphoid organs are the bone marrow and the thymus gland. The bone marrow is responsible for WBC formation, and the thymus gland is important to the preparation of T lymphocytes (T cells), a type of WBC (discussed in Section Four). The secondary lymphoid organs include the tonsils, adenoids, lymph nodes, spleen, and other lymphoid tissue. Cellular and humoral immune responses occur in the secondary lymphoid organs. Contributing to the immune response are lymphoid tissues in nonlymphoid organs (such as the intestinal tissue) and circulating immune cells, such as T cells and B cells (antibody-producing lymphocytes), and phagocytes.

Lymph System   The blood is filtered continuously by the lymph system. The lymph nodes actually serve two purposes for the body: They act as a filtering system for foreign materials, and they serve as a reservoir for the specialized immunologic T cells and B cells. Peripherally, the serous portion of the blood (excluding platelets, red blood cells, and large proteins) diffuses from the capillaries into the peripheral lymph channels, where it is progressively filtered and then returned to the cardiovascular system. Lymph ducts carry the serous fluid through lymph nodes, where it is filtered. It may be useful to think of a lymph node as a sponge, where the meshwork serves as a surface on which antigens and other foreign materials are arrested and destroyed or neutralized. Large clusters of lymph nodes are found in the axillae, groin, thorax, abdomen, and neck (see Figure 28–3). With many infectious processes, lymph nodes become enlarged as their activity increases and defense cells proliferate. T cells are most abundant here, although B cells can also be found.

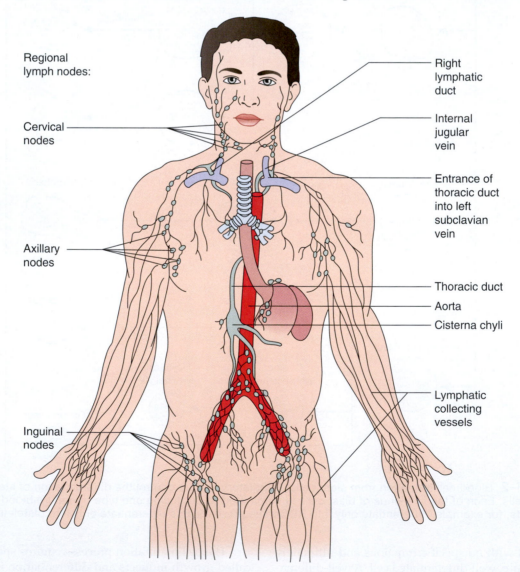

Figure 28–3 The lymphatic system. Lymph nodes are clustered in certain body areas such as the groin, neck, and axillae. They receive drainage from the lymph vessels.

Spleen   The spleen is a small organ about the size of a fist in the left upper quadrant of the abdomen. It is protected by the ninth, tenth, and eleventh ribs and usually is nonpalpable. The spleen serves three functions, only one of which is actually immune related. First, it is the site for the destruction of injured and worn-out red blood cells. Second, it is a reservoir for B cells, although T cells also are found there. Third, it serves as a storage site for blood that is released from distended vessels in times of demand. The spleen responds to primary bloodborne **antigens** (substances that can provoke an immune response), whereas the lymph nodes respond to antigens circulating in the lymph system.

Section One Review

1. What is the major single component of blood?
   A. Plasma
   B. Cell wastes
   C. Blood cells
   D. Glucose

2. A well-differentiated blood cell has which characteristics? (Select all that apply.)
   A. One function
   B. Clones itself
   C. Cannot reproduce
   D. No granules
   E. Immune to growth inducers

3. On appropriate stimulation, pluripotential hematopoietic stem cells (PHSCs) divide, forming one PHSC and one other cell type. What is the other cell type in the division?
   A. RBC
   B. WBC
   C. Committed stem cell
   D. Megakaryocyte

4. Which function is correct regarding the spleen?
   A. It destroys worn-out white blood cells.
   B. It filters out foreign materials.
   C. It produces the hormone thymosin.
   D. It is a reservoir for B cells.

Answers: 1. A, 2. (A, C), 3. C, 4. D

Section Two: Erythrocytes—the Cellular Component of Oxygen Transport

The erythrocyte (red blood cell or RBC), with its oxygen-bound hemoglobin, is a major factor in the delivery of oxygen to the tissues. Problems related to erythrocytes (e.g., too few or nonfunctional RBCs) can have deleterious effects on the patient's prognosis because without adequate available oxygen, wounds cannot heal, tissues become ischemic, and organs can become irreversibly damaged or die. Delivery of adequate amounts of oxygen to the tissues can mean the difference between life and death of an organ or a patient.

When compared to the total number of white blood cells and of platelets, red blood cells (RBCs) are by far the most plentiful of the blood cells. This quantity difference becomes readily apparent when looking at the laboratory blood cell counts: RBCs are measured in million per microliter (mcL), whereas white blood cells (WBCs) and platelets are measured in cells per mcL. Erythrocytes have a relatively long life span of approximately 120 days.

Erythropoiesis

The purpose of RBCs is to transport oxygen to the cells. Regulation is based on the level of tissue oxygenation, which is a function of tissue demands for oxygen and oxygen transport. Red blood cells arise from the myeloid cell line in the red bone marrow, and as reticulocytes they mature within the blood or spleen. Erythrocyte production (**erythropoiesis**) is tightly regulated through a feedback mechanism (Figure 28–4) controlled by the hormone **erythropoietin**, which is produced by the kidneys in response to decreased arterial oxygen tension and tissue hypoxia. Once stimulated into production, erythrocytes take 3 to 5 days to mature. The erythrocyte maturation process is illustrated in Figure 28–5.

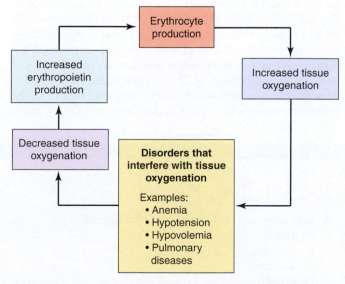

Figure 28–4 Erythrocyte production feedback loop.

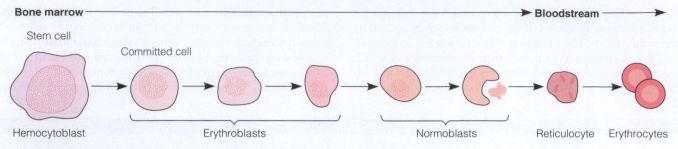

Bone marrow ⟶ Bloodstream ⟶

Stem cell

Committed cell

Hemocytoblast   Erythroblasts   Normoblasts   Reticulocyte Erythrocytes

Figure 28–5 Erythropoiesis. RBCs begin as erythroblasts within the bone marrow, maturing into normoblasts, which eventually eject their nucleus and organelles to become reticulocytes. Reticulocytes mature within the blood or spleen to become erythrocytes.

Production of normal RBCs requires adequate levels of certain nutrients, including protein, multiple vitamins, and minerals, such as the following:

- Amino acids to synthesize hemoglobin, which is protein based
- Vitamins B_6, B_{12}, folic acid, C, and E for normal RBC synthesis, development of DNA and RNA, and cell maturation
- Iron and copper for hemoglobin synthesis and strong plasma membrane

The need for maintaining adequate levels of these nutrients to optimize production and maturation of RBCs explains why it is crucial for the healthcare team to conduct a thorough nutritional assessment early in the course of hospitalization and then provide needed nutritional support. Attaining and maintaining nutritional balance has a powerful impact on tissue oxygenation and, therefore, on the patient's prognosis.

Hemoglobin

Hemoglobin (Hgb) is sometimes referred to as the respiratory protein because its function is to transport oxygen. The erythrocyte is uniquely structured to produce hemoglobin, which comprises the majority of the total weight of an erythrocyte. Hemoglobin production begins early in the RBC maturation process and ends on maturation. As its name suggests, hemoglobin has two components— heme (nonprotein) and globin (protein) (Figure 28–6). Each heme molecule contains one ferrous iron atom and one oxygen molecule (O_2). The oxygen molecule located in hemoglobin is attached only to the single iron atom in the molecule; thus, when there is deficient iron in the body

(e.g., iron-deficiency anemia), the oxygen-carrying capacity is significantly reduced. A heme molecule joins with a polypeptide chain to form a hemoglobin chain. It takes four linked hemoglobin chains to form one hemoglobin molecule. In a normal adult male, every 100 mL of blood contains about 15 grams of hemoglobin. Oxygen combines with hemoglobin loosely and reversibly. This means that oxygen can be loaded onto the hemoglobin, transported to the tissues, and then released from the hemoglobin to diffuse across the capillary membrane into the tissues.

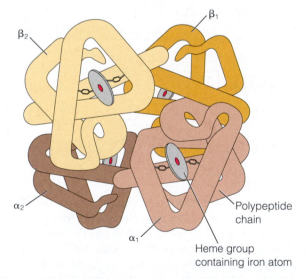

β_2 β_1

α_2 α_1

Polypeptide chain

Heme group containing iron atom

Figure 28–6 The hemoglobin molecule includes globin (a protein) and heme, which contains iron. Globin is made of four subunits: two alpha and two beta polypeptide chains. A heme disk containing an iron atom (red dot) nests within the folds of each protein subunit. The iron atoms combine reversibly with oxygen, transporting it to the cells.

Section Two Review

1. Erythropoietin is formed in which organ?
   - A. Lungs
   - B. Intestines
   - C. Kidneys
   - D. Spleen

2. Formation of new erythrocytes is regulated by the decreases in which physiologic process?
   - A. Alveolar oxygen tension
   - B. Tissue oxygenation
   - C. Cytokine stimulation
   - D. Stimulation of bone marrow

3. Why is adequate iron a crucial part of hemoglobin?
   A. It cements the hemoglobin chain together.
   B. It facilitates the release of oxygen to the tissues.
   C. The heme molecule attaches to it to make a chain.
   D. The oxygen molecule attaches to it.

4. The normal relationship between oxygen and hemoglobin is best described by which statement?
   A. Oxygen combines loosely and reversibly with hemoglobin.
   B. Oxygen bonds tightly with hemoglobin.
   C. Hemoglobin combines with iron to attract oxygen.
   D. The globin molecule of hemoglobin combines loosely with oxygen.

Answers: 1. C, 2. B, 3. D, 4. D

Section Three: Innate (Natural) Immunity

The purpose of the immune system is to discriminate between what is self (native and not potentially harmful) and nonself (foreign and potentially harmful) within the body and eliminate anything that is nonself. The immunity we experience is either natural (innate) or acquired (adaptive). Both types of immunity protect us from a hostile environment. This section focuses on innate immunity.

Innate (Natural) Immunity

Innate (natural) immunity is nonspecific, being composed of natural resistance and first-responder white blood cells that quickly recognize foreign cells and directly attack them. The term **nonspecific** refers to the general, nonadaptive natural protection. Nonspecific immunity is in contrast to specific (adaptive) immunity, which specifically targets a particular pathogen based on previous exposure to that pathogen (presented in Section Four). Examples of natural resistance include physical barriers to disease by means of the skin and mucous membranes and natural chemical barriers found in the gastrointestinal tract, respiratory tract, and genitourinary structures. Innate immunity is species specific—that is, human beings are immune to a variety of diseases to which certain animals are susceptible, and vice versa. For example, human beings are not vulnerable to feline leukemia, and cats are not susceptible to human immunodeficiency virus (HIV). Innate immunity is natural; human beings are born with specific immunities. Innate immunity is nonadaptive; therefore, natural resistance to a particular infectious agent is not improved with repeated exposure to the agent.

Phagocytosis   **Phagocytosis** is an important part of the innate immune response whereby invading foreign materials or injured cells are ingested and destroyed by phagocytic cells (phagocytes). The major phagocytic cells include neutrophils, monocytes and macrophages, and natural killer (NK) cells. Phagocytosis is a multistep process, including the following:

- **Chemotaxis**—the movement of phagocytic cells toward antigens as a result of some type of chemical stimulus

- **Engulfment**—the swallowing up of antigens by the phagocyte for the purpose of destruction or neutralization

- **Opsonization**—the modification of antigens to make them more susceptible to phagocytosis

Cytokines   Special secreted cellular proteins, collectively called **cytokines**, are another important part of innate immunity. Cytokines are regulators of the immune system, serving as chemical messengers for activation of components of the immune system. However, cytokine activities are not restricted to the immune system; they are important in regulation of many hematopoietic functions, such as hematopoiesis and inflammation. Cytokines vary widely as to their area of influence. For example, some cytokines activate cells only within their immediate environment, whereas others are able to activate cells at distant sites. Cytokine functions are redundant in that multiple cytokines perform the same function and may do so simultaneously. One major group of cytokines (called lymphokines) is produced by lymphocytes (T and B cells).

The many different types of cytokines help regulate the immune system, including **interleukins (IL)**, **interferons (INF)**, **granulocyte-macrophage colony-stimulating factors (GM-CSF)**, and **tumor necrosis factor (TNF)**. Many cytokines have multiple subtypes (e.g., more than 15 interleukins have been identified). Although interferons are pathogen nonspecific, they are species specific; thus, animal interferons offer little, if any, protection for human beings as vaccines. Table 28–1 summarizes the sources and functions of these four types of cytokines.

Cytokines are important in the normal inflammatory response, and they have also been associated with disease. For example, elevated levels of tumor necrosis factor (TNF), a proinflammatory cytokine, have been shown to play an active role in such diseases as rheumatoid arthritis, septic shock, and disseminated intravascular coagulation (Levinson, 2016). The use of cytokines for therapeutic reasons continues to be of interest, as is a research focus, particularly in the treatment of certain diseases such as cancer and HIV/AIDS. Granulocyte-macrophage colony-stimulating factor (GM-CSF) is sometimes administered to patients with leukopenia to shorten WBC recovery time following chemotherapy treatment.

Major Cells of Innate Immunity

The granulocytes (particularly neutrophils), the monocyte–macrophage system, and natural killer cells (agranular lymphocytes) are the major cells responsible for innate immunity.

Table 28–1 Major Cytokines

Cytokine	Sources	Functions
Interleukins (IL)	As a group, produced by WBCs, primarily T cells	Inflammatory mediator Lymphocyte activation, growth, and differentiation Attraction of neutrophils
Interferons (IF, IFN)	Originate from CD8 and some CD4 T cells, NK cells, and other cells.	Inhibit the synthesis of viral protein in their reproduction without inhibiting the host's protein synthesis in normal cell reproduction Macrophage activation Inflammatory mediator
Tumor necrosis factors (TNF)	Primarily produced by monocytes and macrophages and T cells	Proinflammatory regulators Endothelial activities Involved in programmed cell death (apoptosis) Death of tumor cells (hence the name)
Granulocyte-macrophage colony-stimulating factors (GM-CSF)	Primarily produced by T cells	Involved in the division and differentiation of neutrophils and monocytes Acts in the bone marrow in response to inflammation and infection A proinflammatory cytokine due to its ability to stimulate secretion of TNF alpha (TNFα) Different colony-stimulating factors influence the proportion of different cell types that are produced.

Neutrophils   The **neutrophil** is produced from the myelocyte cell line and is a type of *polymorphonuclear granulocyte* (Figure 28–2). The term **polymorphonuclear** refers to the presence of multiple nuclei and explains why neutrophils are commonly referred to as *polys* or *polymorphonuclear neutrophils* (PMNs). Neutrophils significantly outnumber all of the other types of leukocytes, making up 50% to 70% of the total leukocyte (WBC) count (Kee, 2014). The term **granulocyte** refers to cells with granules located within the cytoplasm (fluid within cells). The granules contain special enzymes that break down foreign and other substances. Neutrophils mature in the bone marrow and stay in reserve in the marrow for about 5 days before being sent into the general circulation. Once released from the bone marrow, they have a brief life span of 6 to 8 hours. The rapid turnover rate requires the bone marrow to dedicate a significant portion of its activities to reproduction of neutrophils.

Neutrophils are the immune system's first line of defense in the presence of an acute infection or inflammation. They are first at the scene, within 1 to 1.5 hours of an injury event. Neutrophils are responsible for the formation of pus that is produced when neutrophil-degrading enzymes are released, causing breakdown and liquefaction of local cells as well as foreign substances. **Pus** is a thin liquid residue that is an important visible indicator of inflammation. In the presence of significant neutropenia, the absence of pus can mask the presence of inflammation and infection, potentially leading to delayed assessment and diagnosis of infection.

Mononuclear Phagocyte System   The mononuclear phagocyte system, sometimes called the **reticuloendothelial system** or monocyte–macrophage system, refers to a group of immune cells and tissues, including monocytes, macrophages (mobile and fixed tissue), and certain endothelial cells found in the spleen, bone marrow, and lymph nodes. This powerful system plays a major role in phagocytosis, clearing the blood and tissues of pathogens.

Monocytes are large, single-nucleus cells that provide the second line of defense. Circulating monocytes are immature immune cells that do not actively participate in defense. They undergo maturational changes once they move into the tissues. During the maturation process, monocytes enlarge and develop a large number of **lysosomes** (sacs inside the cell containing digestive enzymes) in their cytoplasm. Lysosomes provide a digestive system to break down nutrients, bacteria, or other particles that are brought into the cell. After they have matured, the monocytes become powerful phagocytes called **macrophages**.

Monocytes act as long-term backup for neutrophils, arriving at the injury site within about 5 hours of an event, such as acute infection. Monocytes and neutrophils become the predominant cell types at the site of injury within 48 hours of the precipitating event. Monocytes live much longer than neutrophils, with a life span of 4 to 5 days, and under normal circumstances they circulate in the blood for about a day before taking up residence in a tissue, becoming tissue macrophages (histiocytes).

There are two types of macrophages: mobile and fixed. *Mobile macrophages* circulate in the blood supply and migrate out of the vessels into the tissues when required through the process of chemotaxis. *Fixed macrophages*, on leaving the circulation, affix themselves to tissues and remain there, waiting for pathogens to appear. When needed, fixed macrophages are able to break away from the tissue to initiate phagocytic activity. Tissue macrophages can remain in a fixed position for months or years until they are required to protect the tissue. Common examples of fixed macrophages include the Kupffer cells in the liver and the type I alveolar cells in the lungs. They play important roles in protecting the organs against pathogens (e.g., bacteria or viruses, sloughing tissue, or foreign particles).

Macrophages as Antigen-Presenting Cells.   Macrophages participate in the immune response as **antigen-presenting cells (APCs)** by processing the antigen and presenting a fragment of it in such a way as to increase its recognition and reaction by the B and T lymphocytes. By means of phagocytosis, the macrophage ingests and digests the antigen; in the process, a fragment of the altered antigen is released through the macrophage cell membrane, where it attaches to receptor sites on the surface of the macrophage. It is at these receptor sites that the interaction takes place between the invading antigen and T lymphocytes. The macrophage plays a critical role in the immune response to both the T lymphocytes and the B lymphocytes. By its production of interleukins, it is the link between the inflammatory response and the specific resistance of antibody production and cell mediation. The macrophage is primarily responsible for carrying antigens to the lymph tissue, where the B lymphocytes and T lymphocytes reside.

Migration Properties of Neutrophils and Macrophages.
Soon after initiation of the inflammatory response, the capillary endothelium becomes more permeable, allowing fluid to escape into the inflamed or injured area. The loss of fluid locally results in increased blood viscosity and increased concentration of cells in the local capillaries. When tissue becomes inflamed, a variety of chemicals, including chemical mediators and cytokines, are released at the site of injury. These chemical substances cause alterations of local capillary endothelial cells and stimulate leukocytes to increase their release of adhesion molecules.

Circulating neutrophils and monocytes require some means of recognizing where they are needed, and then they must have a means to transfer from the blood vessels to the injury site. This process of recognition and mobilization involves four steps: margination, diapedesis, migration, and chemotaxis, all of which play key roles in the processes of phagocytosis.

- **Margination**—the accumulation of circulating leukocytes and their adherence to the capillary wall near the site of injury
- **Diapedesis**—the process by which leukocytes that have undergone margination develop pseudopods (fingerlike projections) and squeeze out of the capillary using ameboid movement
- **Migration**—the movement (migration) of leukocytes to the site of injury via the chemotaxis process after they have escaped through the capillary wall
- **Chemotaxis**—the movement of leukocytes along an increasing concentration of chemical stimuli (chemotactic factors) toward an area of inflammation. The leukocytes follow the signal, traveling by ameboid action to the inflammatory site (Figure 28–7).

Natural Killer Lymphocytes Natural killer lymphocytes (NK cells) originate in the bone marrow, arising from the lymphocytic cell line. They are large in size and contain granules; thus, they are also known as large granulated lymphocytes or LGL. The NK cells make up only about 2% of the total WBC count. They are important in protecting the body from pathologic cells such as microbes, virus-infected cells, and cancer cells through cytolytic activities and secretion of cytokines (Trinchieri, Childs & Lanier, 2016). They do not require recognition of a specific antigen on target cells in order to attack and destroy them. When NK cells come into direct contact with a target cell, they chemically rupture the cell membrane of the target cell, leading to target cell death.

Complement System

The **complement system** is an immune mechanism that, once initiated, progresses through sequential stages, each contributing to the immune response and resulting in cellular destruction or cytolysis. The precursors to the complement pathways are normally circulating in the bloodstream. These precursors are activated only by specific agents, such as the immunoglobulins (Ig) immunoglobulin G (IgG) and immunoglobulin M (IgM). The complement system is instrumental in facilitating phagocytosis by making antigens more susceptible to digestion, lysis of antigen cell membranes, and attraction of phagocytes to the invading antigen. One fragment of the complement system (the C3b fragment) facilitates opsonization (antigen modification to enhance phagocytosis) by providing binding sites for the attachment of macrophages or neutrophils to the antigen.

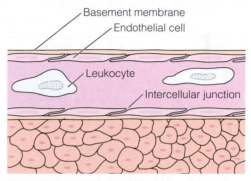

A Leukocytes in circulation

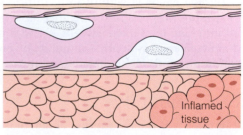

B Margination and pavementing

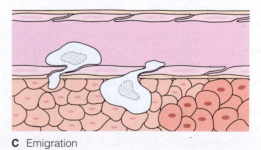

C Emigration

Figure 28–7 The process of leukocyte emigration at the site of inflammation. **A,** Normal blood flow with free movement of formed elements. **B,** As blood flow slows, leukocytes move toward the periphery of the bloodstream and begin to cling to capillary endothelium, a process known as margination and pavementing. **C,** Leukocytes emigrate from the vessel into inflamed tissues.

Section Three Review

1. What is one major function of macrophages?
   A. Presenting antigens to B cells and T cells
   B. Protecting against local mucosal invasion of viruses
   C. Triggering the complement system
   D. Interfering with the immune response

2. The primary purpose of the granules located within neutrophils is to initiate what action?
   A. Detect the presence of infection
   B. Break down foreign substances
   C. Stimulate the production of monocytes
   D. Initiate ameboid cell movement

3. The process by which circulating neutrophils and macrophages are able to squeeze out of a capillary to go to the site of injury is called _____.
   A. diapedesis
   B. chemotaxis
   C. margination
   D. translocation

4. Cytokines, as a group, perform which overall function?
   A. Directly destroy cancer cells
   B. Stimulate the bone marrow to produce lymphocytes
   C. Act as chemical messengers for immune system activation
   D. Regulate endothelial activities throughout the body

Answers: 1. A, 2. B, 3. A, 4. C

Section Four: Adaptive (Acquired) Immunity

Whereas innate (natural) immunity is a first-responder system, adaptive (acquired) immunity is a second-responder system. Adaptive immunity is a highly integrated process that is antigen specific—that is, it responds (adapts) to specific antigen exposure. Resistance to a particular infectious agent is significantly improved with repeated exposure to specialized cells that have been differentiated into long-term memory cells. T and B lymphocytes play a pivotal role in adaptive immunity by providing humoral immunity and cell-mediated immunity.

Humoral Immunity

Humoral immunity is the recognition of antigens and the production of specific antibodies in response to antigens. It provides a major defense against bacterial infections. The primary cell responsible for humoral immunity is the B lymphocyte (B cell).

B Lymphocytes The bursa-equivalent tissue in the bone marrow differentiates lymphocytes into B lymphocytes (B cells), where they are produced throughout life. Once released, most immature B cells are stored in the bone marrow, lymph nodes, and other lymphatic tissue; however, some circulate in the bloodstream.

On exposure to an antigen (via presentation by antigen-presenting cells [APCs]), mature B cells proliferate and differentiate into plasma cells and memory B cells. Plasma cells secrete protein-based antibodies called **immunoglobulins (Ig)**. Each plasma cell is specialized to produce only one type of antibody. This specificity is often described as a key-and-lock relationship since only a specific antigen (the key) can unlock a specific plasma cell to produce antibodies. On activation, each plasma cell produces identical cells capable of continuing production of antibodies in response to a specific antigen.

Immunoglobulins. The immunoglobulins are in the globulin fraction of the plasma protein and are commonly referred to as antibodies. Each has a distinct amino acid chain that creates its specificity to react with a particular antigen. Because of this basic protein matrix of antibodies, a person's nutritional status, particularly protein, is a major factor in determining the adequacy of the humoral immune system. Five classes of immunoglobulins have been identified, and each is active within a given course of events in the immune response. Each of the five immunoglobulins plays a particular role in the immune response (see Table 28–2).

Memory B cells live much longer than plasma cells and are largely responsible for long-term immunity (such as is seen with vaccinations), maintaining information about specific antigens, and accounting for the rapid recognition of "remembered" antigens on secondary exposure. They are produced in much smaller numbers than plasma cells but are a major characteristic of active immunity (Barrett, Barman, Boitano, & Brooks, 2016).

Primary and Secondary Response

Humoral immunity develops through a primary and secondary response pattern. During the **primary response**, there is a latency period—usually 48 to 72 hours after exposure—before the antibody is detectable in the serum. This is the time needed for the antigen to be recognized as nonself and specifically identified, after which antibodies form in response to the antigen's particular molecular makeup. When the latency period ends, a blood test will be positive for the presence of the antibody.

The **secondary response** occurs with subsequent exposure to the same antigen. B lymphocyte memory cells recognize the antigen almost immediately and initiate the

Table 28–2 Immunoglobulins in Adults

Immunoglobulin (percentage of total Ig)	Functions	Description
IgG (80%)	Antibacterial and antiviral activities	The chief immunoglobulin Produced on secondary exposure to an antigen The only immunoglobulin that is known to cross the placental barrier Responsible for protecting the newborn during the first few months of life
IgA (15%)	Protection of mucous membrane from invading pathogens	Found in large quantities in secretory body fluids such as tears, saliva, breast milk, as well as in vaginal, bronchial, and intestinal secretions Produced by B cells in Peyer's patches, tonsils, and other lymph tissue
IgM (4%)	Primary immunity; produced early in the immune response to most antigens; also important in activating the complement system	Found in body secretions Instrumental in forming natural antibodies (e.g., for ABO blood antigens)
IgD (0.2%)	Unknown; may influence B-cell maturation	A trace antibody found primarily in the blood
IgE (0.0002% units/mL)	Plays a role in allergy; levels elevate during hypersensitivity reactions (particularly type 1)	Exists in the body in miniscule quantities but is considered extremely powerful

SOURCE: Data from Kee (2014).

immune response with heightened antibody formation. If an antibody titer were to be drawn at this exposure, it would be higher than that of the primary exposure. The follow-up booster regimen of many vaccines, such as tetanus, takes advantage of this secondary response and boosts the titer of specific antibodies to a level that will prevent the disease should exposure occur. This is the rationale for administering a tetanus booster within 24 hours of a new puncture wound.

Cell-Mediated Immunity

Cell-mediated immunity is based on the activity and characteristics of the T lymphocyte (T cell). During this portion of the immune response, T cells and macrophages predominate, creating a direct attack on invading antigens. T-cell immunity provides protection from intracellular organisms (e.g., viruses, fungi, and parasites), cancer cells, and foreign tissue.

T Lymphocytes **T lymphocytes (T cells)** are formed in the bone marrow and travel to the thymus gland. The **thymus** is a flat, lobed organ located in the neck below the thyroid gland and extends into the upper thorax behind the sternum. During extrauterine life, the role of the thymus is to differentiate lymphocytes into various types of T cells. Reaching its peak size at puberty, the thymus steadily diminishes in size and composition until it is hardly distinguishable in adulthood. Its lymphoid tissue is gradually replaced by adipose tissue over a person's lifetime. T cells are marked by the thymus with specific surface antigens that characterize them and distinguish them from B cells. Mature, differentiated lymphocytes are released into the bloodstream, and they relocate in peripheral lymph tissue, where they await a call to action in body defense.

The T lymphocytes represent 70% to 80% of the total lymphocyte count and have a life expectancy of several years. There are different types of T cells, each playing a unique role in the body's defense. Subsets of mature T cells are identified by a nomenclature referred to as clusters of differentiation (CD). These clusters are actually surface antigens commonly known as **CD markers**. All T cells have CD4 or CD8 antigen on their cell surfaces but not both (McClanahan & Gribben, 2016). For example, helper T cells (T_H cells) bear a CD4 marker, and clinically the CD4 count can be measured as an indicator of immune status in disorders such as HIV/AIDS. The markers differentiate the various properties and functions of cells. Table 28–3 summarizes the major types of T cells, common abbreviations, associated CD markers, and their primary functions.

Cell-mediated immunity is one of the body's primary surveillance and attack mechanisms for protection from growth of malignant cells. Unfortunately, T-cell protection is not readily transferred from one individual to another, as humoral protection is. Cell-mediated immunity depends heavily on thymus and lymph node integrity, as well as on a nutritionally healthy body. As seen with nutrition and B-cell function, a poor state of nutritional health in a

Table 28–3 Major T Lymphocyte Types, CD Markers, and Functions

Type	CD Marker	Functions
T helper (T_H, T4 cell)	CD4	Orchestrate the activities of the other immune cells Interact with the mononuclear phagocytes and assist in the destruction of pathogens Interact with the B cells, assisting the B cells in division and production of antibodies
T suppressor (T_S cell)	CD8	Important in shutting down the immune response once a pathogen has been destroyed
T cytotoxic (T_C, killer, T8 cell)	CD8	Responsible for the destruction and lysis of infected host cells

high-acuity patient significantly increases the risk for complications related to infection. Clinically, it is the T cell that is also responsible for much of the rejection of transplanted organs and grafts phenomenon.

Passive and Active Acquired Immunity

Passive acquired immunity is a temporary form of immunity involving the transfer of antibodies from one individual to another or from some other source (laboratory cultures or other animals) to an individual. For example, a neonate does not yet have a mature immune system capable of efficient development of antibodies in response to invading agents but, rather, receives passive immunity from the mother in utero and from breast milk. Passive immunity can be transferred also through vaccination of antiserum, such as rabies; antitoxin, such as tetanus; or gamma globulin, which contains a variety of antibodies. One way to remember passive immunity is that a person who receives this type of immunity receives it as a gift—the recipient's own immune system is passive in the process. Passive immunity provides rapid but short-lived immunity and may be the treatment of choice for an individual with increased susceptibility to infection (e.g., immunocompromised state) who is inadvertently exposed to a pathogen. For example, for an organ transplant or HIV/AIDS patient who is exposed to chickenpox, passive immunity may be the treatment of choice.

Active acquired immunity develops on exposure to an antigen, such as the chickenpox virus, during which time antibodies are programmed to protect the body from illness with future exposures. These antibodies are quite specific, often providing lifetime immunity against another attack of the same antigen. Inoculation provides another means for development of active immunity through exposure to a specific antigen by introduction of a vaccine. Polio vaccine provides a lifetime of antibody protection without an actual illness occurring. Active immunity following exposure to a specific antigen does not provide immediate protection but develops over a period of days to weeks. However, the programming of specific antibodies provides heightened protection with subsequent exposures within a matter of minutes or hours.

Both passive and active immunity create levels of antibodies circulating in the body. Many of these levels can be monitored by venipuncture blood tests to determine full immunity to a particular disease. The result of testing the level of a particular antibody is called the *antibody titer*. The titer of the specific antibody is compared with a preestablished level thought to guarantee immunity. If the individual's titer is found to be lower than the preestablished norm, repeated immunization with the vaccine may be indicated. Antibody titer normally continues to rise for about 10 days to 2 weeks and generally peaks during recovery from most infectious diseases.

Section Four Review

1. A person who developed a case of chickenpox as a child is rendered immune from recurrence of the disease as an adult. This is an example of what type of immunity?
   A. Active acquired immunity
   B. Passive acquired immunity
   C. Innate (natural) immunity
   D. Species-specific immunity

2. What is the T lymphocyte that orchestrates activities of the other immune cells?
   A. Natural killer cell (NK)
   B. Cytotoxic T cell (T_C)
   C. Suppressor T cell (T_S)
   D. Helper T cell (T_H)

3. What can be said about an individual whose antibody titer is greater than the preestablished level of immunity?
   A. Requires reimmunization
   B. Transmits the disease as a carrier
   C. Demonstrates a specific antigen–antibody complex
   D. Demonstrates immunity from the disease in question

4. Which immunoglobulin makes up about 80% of the total immunoglobulins in the healthy human body?
   A. IgA
   B. IgE
   C. IgG
   D. IgM

Answers: 1. A, 2. D, 3. D, 4. C

Section Five: Antigens and the Antigen–Antibody Response

The environment in which we live is not a sterile one. On a daily basis we are exposed to potentially disease-producing organisms (pathogens), as well as potentially harmful substances from the external environment, through consumption, inhalation, and touch or through injury. Fortunately, the immune system provides active protection by which foreign substances are recognized (antigens) and destroyed (antigen–antibody response).

Antigens

Antigens are substances that are capable of triggering an immune response if they can be recognized by a B-cell antibody or T cell. The immune response can involve either humoral or cellular components of the immune system but commonly involves both. The degree to which an antigen stimulates an immune response is referred to as its *immunogenicity* or its immunogenic nature and is influenced by factors such as physical and chemical properties of the antigen, the relative foreignness of the antigen, and the person's genetic makeup. Antigens may be either foreign to the body, or they may be self-markers (self-antigens) or tumor markers (tumor-associated antigens).

Foreign Antigens Some foreign-body antigens are capable of causing disease and are called **pathogens** or pathogenic antigens. Many bacteria, viruses, parasites, and other microorganisms are pathogenic antigens, such as *Staphylococcus aureus*, *Mycobacterium tuberculosis*, herpes simplex, and HIV. Other antigens, such as vaccines, are foreign to the body but are not pathogenic. Vaccines induce a protective immunologic response by introducing a killed or weakened form of a virus or bacteria. Without causing the disease itself, these vaccines effectively stimulate a mild immune response as a protective mechanism against similar live microorganisms. A second example of a nonpathogenic antigen is a transplanted heart or kidney from a nonidentical twin donor. The cells making up the tissues of these organs are not disease producing but are recognized by the body as being foreign (nonself); thus, the transplanted organ can precipitate an immune reaction. Although the immune system is certainly capable of distinguishing self from nonself in its natural state, it is not able to determine that a foreign material is acceptable even if that material is beneficial to the well-being of the body as a whole. This is the scenario that occurs in organ transplant rejection.

Histocompatibility Antigens In addition to foreign materials being antigens, all nucleated cells in the body contain surface antigens, which are proteins found on the surface of a cell. Surface antigens are referred to as histocompatibility antigens or human leukocyte antigens (HLA). **Histocompatibility** refers to the ability of cells and tissues to live without interference from the immune system. Located on the sixth chromosome, the HLA proteins are coded by a group of genes called the **major histocompatibility complex (MHC)**. They exist in pairs (called haplotypes) on the surface of cells and are genetically determined. MHC molecules that are involved in intracellular communication for self-recognition are classified into two groups: MHC I (or class I) antigens and MHC II (or class II) antigens.

- **MHC I (Class I) Antigens.** Labeled HLA-A, HLA-B, and HLA-C, these are found on the surface of essentially all nucleated cells.
- **MHC (Class II) Antigens.** Labeled HLA-DR, HLA-DP, and HLA-DQ, these are primarily found on the cell surfaces of macrophages and B lymphocytes.

HLA antigens allow the immune system to distinguish self from nonself, functioning somewhat like fingerprints that are unique to the individual. Normally, the immune system is able to recognize its own HLA "fingerprint" as self, and the immune response is not triggered.

HLA antigens are inherited; thus, each full sibling in a family will have some combination of HLA inherited from both biological parents. The closer the HLA antigen combination matches between two people, the more the "fingerprint" is recognized as self. A multitude of combinations of pairings can occur; therefore, complete HLA matching is virtually impossible with the exception of identical twins. This has important implications in patients who will undergo organ transplantation. Because full siblings share the same biological parents, they have the best chance for a good organ donor/recipient HLA match. In contrast, a completely unrelated donor (e.g., a randomly chosen deceased donor) would have the lowest chance of a good HLA match. For this reason, immediate family members most often make the best kidney transplant donors because they are more likely to have a better matched tissue type. Identical twins, however, have the same histocompatibility pairings and are, therefore, perfect HLA matches. In the case of identical twins, a transplanted organ is recognized as having the same self-HLA fingerprint and is accepted into the recipient without an immune assault. In other words, the better the HLA match is between the donor and the recipient, the higher the probability for long-term transplantation success.

Tumor-associated Antigens Some human tumors have been found to display particular antigens (tumor-associated antigens) that distinguish normal cells from abnormally transformed cells. Identification of tumor-associated antigens has progressed rapidly with technological advances in tumor immunology. Tumor-associated antigens typically do not evoke an immune response (low immunogenicity) perhaps because they are recognized as self from early development during embryonic and fetal stages. Although many of these antigens occur naturally in small quantities, an elevation in the levels of a particular antigen type can be helpful in detecting potentially abnormal cells and tracking progression or regression of disease following treatment. For example, carcinoembryonic antigen (CEA) becomes elevated in a variety of adenocarcinomas of the colon, lung, breast, and pancreas; alpha-fetoprotein (AFP) is frequently elevated in patients with testicular and hepatic cancer; and serum elevations of prostate-specific antigen (PSA) have been found in occurrences of prostatic cancer. Serum elevations of tumor-associated antigens are also possible with several nonmalignant disease states, which prevent them from being diagnostic tools; however, they may be of value as initial screening tools.

Antigen–Antibody Responsiveness

Recall that immune responsiveness may be either specific or nonspecific. A specific response requires the recognition of a particular antigen and involves the production and action of a programmed antibody for that antigen. Normally, an antibody circulates in the bloodstream until it encounters an appropriate antigen to which it can bind. Such binding results in antigen–antibody complexes, or immune complexes. The process of binding is such that the antibody binds to specifically conformed antigenic

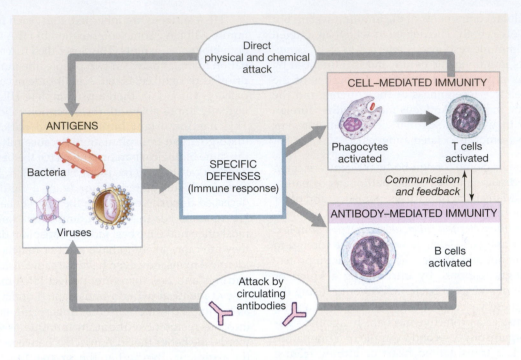

Figure 28–8 An overview of the immune response.

SOURCE: Martini et al.; Bledsoe, Bryan E.; *Anatomy and Physiology for Emergency Care*, 2nd ed., © 2008. Reprinted by permission of Pearson Education, Inc., Upper Saddle River, New Jersey.

determinant sites on the antigen, which effectively prevents the antigen from binding to receptors on host cells. The overall effect is protection of the host from antigen infection or penetration.

An antigen–antibody reaction can have several consequences for the invading agent. The reaction can cause agglutination (clumping of the cells), neutralization of the antigen toxin (e.g., a bacterial toxin), cell lysis (destruction of the antigen), enhanced phagocytosis of the antigen by other cells, opsonization, or activation of the complement system. Figure 28–8 illustrates how the immune system responds (cell-mediated and humoral immunities) to a specific antigen.

Antigen Entry Site

The location at which an antigen enters the body is an important consideration; it must have an appropriate portal of entry to survive and proliferate. For example, the gastrointestinal (GI) tract is a common portal of entry for antigens through intentional oral intake of many substances, including foods and fluids (that may or may not be contaminated), as well as unintentional pathogen exposure through hand-to-mouth contamination. When antigens enter the GI tract, many are readily destroyed or neutralized by salivary and other digestive enzymes and gastric acid in the stomach, rendering them incapable of causing disease. However, some antigens are resistant to the protective GI secretions, and if allowed to enter the GI system, they can proliferate rapidly, creating a pathologic state. The portal of entry also helps determine the strength or virulence of the antigen. For example, an antigen that is neutralized by digestive enzymes in the gastrointestinal tract might be quite virulent if it enters the body through the genitourinary tract or the respiratory tract, where digestive enzymes are not normally found.

Section Five Review

1. What is the purpose of histocompatibility antigens?
   A. Stimulate antibody production
   B. Muster an attack against foreign antigens
   C. Present foreign antigens to phagocytes
   D. Distinguish self from nonself

2. What is the name for antigens that precipitate disease states?
   A. Immunoglobulins
   B. Pathogens
   C. Human leukocyte antigens
   D. Histocompatibility antigens

3. Which statement is correct regarding tumor-associated antigens?
   A. They are highly recognizable as foreign or pathogenic.
   B. They escape immune recognition early in tumor growth.
   C. An antigen is called tumor necrosis factor (TNF).
   D. Elevations of alpha-fetoprotein (AFP) suggest lung cancer.

4. Which statements regarding an antigen's portal of entry are correct? (Select all that apply.)
   A. Saliva in the mouth destroys many antigens.
   B. Digestive enzymes neutralize many antigens.
   C. Site of entry helps determine virulence of the antigen.
   D. Strength of an antigen is independent of portal of entry.
   E. Each antigen has only one portal of entry.

Answers: 1. D, 2. B, 3. B, 4. (A, B, C)

Section Six: Hemostasis

The hematologic system is sometimes referred to as a fluid organ with the blood vessel walls providing its organ borders. Correct functioning of an organ requires that its borders remain intact. Vascular integrity is maintained through two closely interwoven mechanisms: hemostasis and blood coagulation.

Platelets: The Cell Component of Hemostasis

Platelets are tiny cell fragments composed of cytoplasm that shed from megakaryocytes, a type of blood cell produced in the bone marrow. Megakaryocyte production, and therefore platelet production, is primarily regulated by thrombopoietin, a regulatory hormone produced by the liver. Mature platelets survive about 10 days, and the majority circulate in the blood while a lesser percentage are stored in the spleen. Platelets continuously shift between the circulating blood and the spleen. The normal platelet count in an adult is 150,000 mcL to 400,000 mcL (Kee, 2014).

Hemostasis is defined as prevention of blood loss. Platelets play a crucial role in initial hemostasis by creating a **platelet plug** to seal off leaking vessels. The internal structures of platelets contain a variety of coagulation-related proteins and enzymes that influence the clotting process. Under normal circumstances, platelets circulate freely throughout the vascular system as inactive, smooth, disk-shaped particles. Normally, the vessel endothelium maintains platelets in an inactive state by secreting substances such as nitric oxide and prostacyclin I_2. When vessel endothelial injury occurs, special activating factors are produced, such as thrombin and platelet-activating factor, which stimulate platelet hemostatic activities. On activation, the platelets undergo significant changes. First they rapidly reshape themselves, developing pseudopods along the vessel's endothelial surface, and adhere to the damaged subendothelium. Second, as the platelets accumulate at the injury site, they aggregate (clump together) to form a cohesive mass, called a *platelet plug*. Once the platelet plug is formed, it is stabilized and consolidated by fibrinogen, forming a fibrin clot. Platelet plugs are particularly effective in rapid repair of small vascular leaks. Figure 28–9 depicts platelet plug formation and blood clotting.

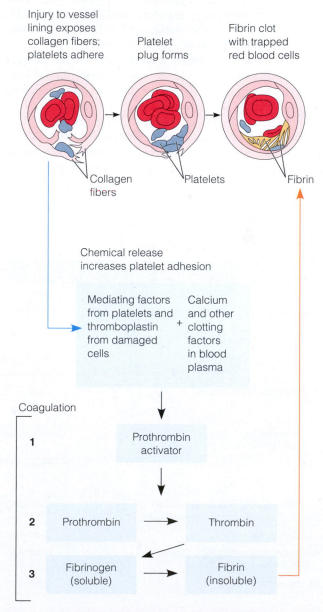

Figure 28–9 Platelet plug formation and blood clotting. The flow diagram summarizes the events leading to fibrin clot formation.

Coagulation

While platelets play a major role in maintaining hemostasis by providing a platelet plug to seal off an injured vessel, they are only one aspect of hemostasis. The platelet plug provides rapid reduction or complete closure of an injured vessel by forming a simple plug. The injury then requires a more stable and permanent repair through formation of a thrombus, which is the function of the coagulation cascade—a complex series of chemical events. The following is a brief overview of coagulation.

The Coagulation Cascade   The coagulation process is dependent on the presence of adequate numbers of coagulation factors (plasma proteins, calcium ions, and phospholipids). Once triggered into action, a specific sequence of chemical reactions occurs that results in a clot made of fibrin strands. Table 28–4 provides a list of the coagulation factors, where they are synthesized, and their purpose. The liver is the major source of most of the factors, and many require vitamin K for synthesis by the liver.

There are several different models of how the coagulation cascade works. The classic model (Figure 28–10) visualizes two coagulation pathways that join into a common pathway (Kibble & Halsey, 2014). In this model, coagulation is triggered by either (1) the direct exposure of blood to subendothelial vascular tissue (collagen), known as the **intrinsic pathway**, a slow process, or (2) blood is exposed to extravascular tissues, known as the **extrinsic pathway**, a rapid process. The pathways join into a common pathway, which results in clot formation. The normal clot formation cascade maintains homeostasis by balancing stimulating and inhibiting factors.

Clot Retraction and Dissolution   Hemostasis does not end with formation of the fibrin clot. Shortly after the clot has formed, it contracts (called retraction). This action draws the torn vessel walls into closer proximity, reducing leakage. Clot retraction is largely a function of platelets, which contain contractile proteins in their cytoplasm similar to those of muscle cells (Smyth, Whiteheart, Italiano, Bray, & Coller, 2016).

If the clotting process were allowed to continue without restraint, the clot would continue to grow and the vessel would become blocked off, resulting in loss of blood flow distal to the clot. When the clot has finished forming, it begins to alter in one of two ways. First, it can dissolve (called dissolution). A blood clot contains lytic plasma proteins (plasminogen) that when activated becomes plasmin. Plasmin is a powerful protein-busting (proteolytic) enzyme that destroys clotting factors contained in the clot. The plasminogen-to-plasmin conversion results from the slow release of tissue plasminogen activator (tPA) by the injured vessel endothelium. Second, the clot can form connective tissue to patch the injury. To form a patch, fibroblasts invade the clot within several hours following the injury and eventually form fibrous tissue.

Table 28–4 Coagulation Factors

Coagulation Factor	Source	Purpose
I – Fibrinogen	Liver	Precursor of fibrin
II – Prothrombin	Liver; requires vitamin K	Precursor of thrombin
III –Thromboplastin (tissue factor, TF)	Found throughout tissues	Conversion of prothrombin to thrombin
IV – Ionized calcium (Ca^{++})	Absorbed in GI tract from food sources	Required throughout coagulation cascade
V – Proaccelerin (labile factor)	Liver	Increases formation of thromboplastin (factor III); triggers prothrombin–thrombin conversion
VII – Proconvertin (stable factor)	Liver; requires vitamin K	Increases prothrombin–thrombin conversion
VIII – Antihemophilic factor (AHF)	Reticuloendothelial cells	Required for prothrombin–thrombin conversion and production of thromboplastin (factor III)
IX – Plasma thromboplastin component (PTC, Christmas factor, antihemophilic factor B)	Liver; requires vitamin K	Required for synthesis of thromboplastin
X – Stuart factor	Liver; requires vitamin K	Important in formation of thromboplastin
XI – Plasma thromboplastin antecedent (PTA, antihemophilic factor C)	Unknown	Required in formation of plasma–thromboplastin
XII – Hageman factor	Unknown	Stimulates factor XI to continue clotting process; during fibrinolysis it converts plasminogen–plasmin
XIII – Fibrin-stabilizing factor (FSF)	Unknown	Assists in stabilization of fibrin in forming a strong blood clot

SOURCE: Data from Kee (2014).

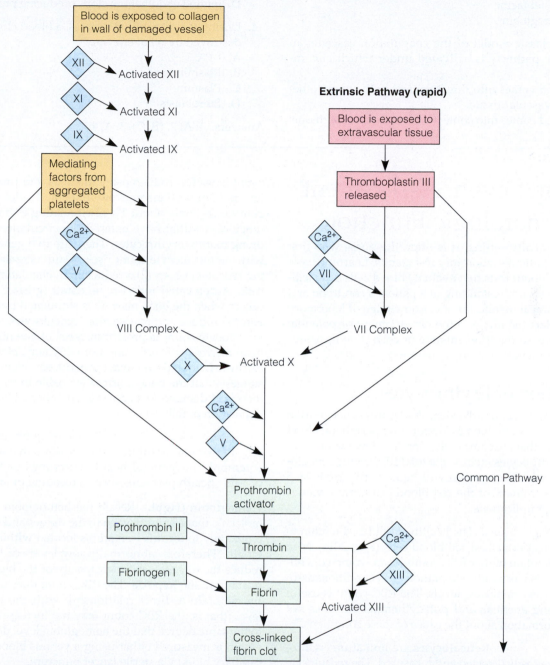

Figure 28–10 Clot formation. Both the slower intrinsic pathway and the more rapid extrinsic pathway activate factor X. Factor X then combines with other factors to form prothrombin activator. Prothrombin activator transforms prothrombin into thrombin, which then transforms fibrinogen into long fibrin strands. Thrombin also activates factor XIII, which draws the fibrin strands together into a dense meshwork. The complete process of clot formation occurs within 3 to 6 minutes after blood vessel damage.

Section Six Review

1. Platelet production is regulated by which substance?
   A. Thrombopoietin
   B. Platelet factor
   C. Erythropoietin
   D. Prostacyclin I_2

2. When not needed, platelets circulate through the vascular system in an inactive state that is maintained by which endothelial products? (Select all that apply.)
   A. Thromboplastin
   B. Prostacyclin I_2

C. Nitric oxide (NO)
D. Platelet factor
E. Hemoglobin

3. In the classic model of the coagulation cascade, an intrinsic pathway is activated under which circumstances?
   A. Blood comes into direct contact with subendothelial vascular tissue.
   B. Blood comes into contact with extravascular tissue.

C. Platelets secrete thromboplastin at the site of injury.
D. Injured endothelium stops producing prostaglandin.

4. During the dissolution process, a blood clot is directly destroyed by what enzyme?
   A. t-PA
   B. Plasminogen
   C. Plasmin
   D. Fibroblasts

Answers: 1. A, 2. (B, C), 3. A, 4. C

Section Seven: Assessment of Hematologic Function

In the high-acuity setting, it is often the nurse who first reviews the patient's laboratory test results. Learning basic information about tests that evaluate blood cells can facilitate the nurse's understanding of a patient's condition and causes of clinical manifestations. Knowledge of laboratory tests may alert the nurse to the development of potential complications so that preventative or corrective measures can be implemented in a timely manner.

Evaluation of Erythrocytes

Basic information about the size, shape, and concentration of erythrocytes is obtained by performing peripheral blood smears. Tests that are commonly monitored by the nurse to evaluate erythrocytes include the total RBC count, reticulocyte count, and hemoglobin and hematocrit. Table 28–5 provides a summary of the red blood cell normal values and nursing implications.

Red Blood Cell Count The healthy adult has 4 million to 6 million cells per mcL of red blood cells (Kee, 2014). Men normally maintain higher RBC counts than women or children. Table 28–5 lists common pathological conditions associated with abnormal RBC levels. The RBC count is useful in diagnosing anemias and polycythemias but does not provide information about the cause of these conditions.

Reticulocyte Count **Reticulocytes** are immature erythrocytes that are easily detected and measured. The reticulocyte

count is useful in diagnosing anemias and provides basic information on bone marrow function. Under normal circumstances, only about 1% of circulating erythrocytes are reticulocytes that have entered the circulation to replace dying mature erythrocytes. There are two general reasons why the reticulocyte count rises: (1) an increase in circulating reticulocytes, or (2) a reduction in circulating red blood cells. An elevated reticulocyte count (greater than 1.5%) occurs when the bone marrow is stimulated by erythropoietin to produce and release more reticulocytes. An elevated reticulocyte count is present in types of anemia where the bone marrow is functioning normally (e.g., blood loss and extrinsic hemolytic anemias). A reduced reticulocyte count suggests that the bone marrow is unable to respond to the increased demand (e.g., aplastic anemia and bone marrow depression or failure).

Hemoglobin and Hematocrit Hemoglobin and hematocrit are two important measures of RBCs that are obtained commonly for general health screenings or to diagnose possible health problems such as bleeding or anemia.

Hemoglobin (Hgb). Recall that hemoglobin is a protein molecule that carries oxygen to the tissues and that oxygen binds only to ferrous iron atoms located within the hemoglobin. Therefore, abnormally low levels of hemoglobin reduce the oxygen-carrying capacity of the blood and can result in tissue hypoxia. The RBC count does not necessarily maintain a direct relationship with the hemoglobin level (that is, the RBC count may not increase or decrease to the same degree that the hemoglobin level does). Hemoglobin is measured either using a venous blood sample or capillary blood via sterile lancet puncture.

Table 28–5 Normal Erythrocyte Values and Nursing Implications

Type	Adult Reference Values	Nursing Implications
Red Blood Cell (RBC) Count	M: 4.6–6 mil./mcL Fe: 4.0–5 mil./mcL	*Blood specimen information:* • Lavender-top tube (contains anticoagulant); venous blood sample • No preparatory food or fluid restrictions
Reticulocyte Count	0.5%–1.5% of total RBCs	*Abnormally low erythrocyte values:*
Hemoglobin	M: 13.5–17.0 g/dL Fe: 12–15.0 g/dL	• Assess for potential cause(s): Hemodilution (overhydration), anemias (e.g., iron-deficiency, aplastic), hemorrhage, and chronic kidney disease • Assess for clinical manifestations of potential causes
Hematocrit	M: 40%–54% Fe: 36%–46%	*Abnormally high erythrocyte values:* • Assess for cause(s): Hemoconcentration (dehydration), polycythemia vera, leukemias, and cor pulmonale

SOURCE: Data from Kee (2014).

Hematocrit (Hct). The hematocrit is a concentration measurement. It is the volume (in milliliters) of packed red blood cells in 100 mL of blood and is stated as a percentage. The hematocrit is measured using the same sampling methods as hemoglobin, and both are usually measured simultaneously. It should not, however, be sampled from the same arm in which the patient is receiving intravenous fluids due to hemodilution effects (Kee, 2014).

Other Erythrocyte Evaluations Additional RBC test results that provide important diagnostic information include RBC size and color and erythrocyte sedimentation rate.

RBC Size and Color. Measurement of **mean corpuscular volume (MCV)** evaluates the size (volume) of the RBCs. Determining the MCV is useful in differentiating types of anemias, many of which are associated with abnormal RBC size. The three MCV categories include **microcytic** (smaller than normal), seen in iron deficiency anemia; **normocytic** (normal size), seen in blood-loss anemia; and **macrocytic** (larger than normal), seen in vitamin B_{12} anemia. Evaluating the color of RBCs is also useful in determining types of anemias. Normal RBC color (**normochromic**) is pinkish-red in the outer two thirds of the disk and very pale in the center third (central pallor), reflecting the presence of adequate levels of hemoglobin. In certain anemias (e.g., iron-deficiency) the central pallor extends beyond its one-third border, giving the RBC a pale or **hypochromic** appearance, which indicates a lower than normal hemoglobin level. RBC size and color are often both altered in certain types of anemia. For example, iron-deficiency anemia causes RBCs to become microcytic and hypochromic, while vitamin B_{12} anemia is associated with macrocytic and normochromic RBCs. Hypochromic cells can also be normal if they are immature RBCs that have not yet taken in all of their hemoglobin.

Erythrocyte Sedimentation Rate (ESR). The erythrocyte sedimentation rate (ESR) is also a measurement of interest to the high-acuity patient. The ESR (commonly referred to as sed rate or sedimentation rate) measures how rapidly RBCs settle in unclotted blood. It is a nonspecific screening measure of inflammation or infection; however, elevated levels also result from a variety of other problems. No food or fluid restrictions are required in preparation for measuring ESR.

A venous sample in a lavender-top tube is required. The blood specimen must be maintained in a vertical position. It should be taken immediately to the laboratory since the longer the specimen is allowed to stand, the higher the sedimentation rate will be. Certain drugs (e.g., methyldopa, Dextran, and others) should be held until after the specimen is collected to avoid false readings. When ESR is abnormal, more specific diagnostic testing is indicated for making a differential diagnosis. ESR is measured in millimeters per hour (mm/hr) and increases with aging. Abnormally high ESR is associated with acute myocardial infarction, cancer, hepatitis, and rheumatic-type problems, such as rheumatic fever or rheumatoid arthritis. Abnormally low levels may be seen in patients with heart failure, angina pectoris, or polycythemia vera (Kee, 2014).

Evaluation of Leukocytes

Although a simple WBC count is often adequate for general screening purposes, it is not sufficient for gaining an in-depth understanding of the patient's infectious or inflammatory status. This information is obtained through the WBC differential count. The differential cell count breaks out the constituent cells of the WBCs. The high-acuity nurse most commonly monitors total WBC, neutrophils, lymphocytes, and monocytes, which make up over 80% of the total white cell count. Table 28–6 provides a summary of normal leukocyte values and nursing implications.

Neutrophils Neutrophils are measured in the serum as a percentage of mature versus immature cells. Mature neutrophils are called **segmented cells (segs)** (referring to a segmented nucleus). An immature neutrophil is often called a **band (stab)** (referring to the band- or horseshoe-shaped nucleus). When called into action, the bone marrow produces neutrophils at a faster rate to meet the increased demand. During periods of extremely high neutrophil production (e.g., severe infection), the bone marrow releases a higher percentage of immature bands (this clinical finding is referred to as a shift to the left) (Figure 28–11). The neutrophil count increases in response to inflammatory disorders (including cancer), acute bacterial infections, and tissue necrosis. An abnormally low neutrophil count (neutropenia) can occur under circumstances involving increased destruction or decreased production of neutrophils. Neutrophil counts are monitored closely in critically ill patients,

Table 28–6 Normal Leukocyte Values and Nursing Implications

Type	Adult Reference Values*	Nursing Implications
White Blood Cells (WBC) Count	4,500–10,000 mcL	*Blood specimen information:*
Differential Counts: Neutrophils	50%–70%	• Lavender-top tube (contains anticoagulant); venous blood sample
		• No preparatory food or fluid restrictions
Lymphocytes	25%–35%	*Abnormal leukocyte values:*
Monocytes	4%–6%	• Assess for potential cause(s): Refer to each cell type in text
		• Assess for clinical manifestations of infection (fever; increased heart rate; wound redness, heat, and exudate)
		• Monitor trends closely as an indication of resolution or progression of underlying disease state

*Differential counts are measured as percentages of total WBC count.
SOURCE: Data from Kee (2014).

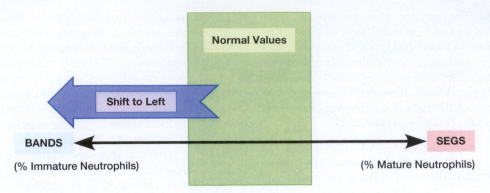

Figure 28–11 Neutrophil shift to the left, in which a higher percentage of bands are released by the bone marrow.

as severe neutropenia significantly increases mortality and sudden elevations strongly suggest acute infection.

Lymphocytes Recall that lymphocytes are the key cells of cell-mediated immunity. The lymphocyte count includes the total number of lymphocytes rather than differentiating them into B cells and T cells. Increased levels occur with viral infections (e.g., infectious mononucleosis and hepatitis), chronic infections, and lymphocytic leukemia. Abnormally low levels are associated with many diseases, such as cancers, leukemia, aplastic anemia, and multiple sclerosis (Kee, 2014).

Monocytes Monocytes and macrophages are key cells in innate immunity. Elevated levels of monocytes are associated with viral infections, a variety of cancers, parasitic diseases, certain forms of anemia, and monocytic leukemia. Two examples of disorders with abnormally low levels of monocytes are aplastic anemia and lymphocytic leukemia (Kee, 2014).

Evaluation of Hemostasis

In the high-acuity setting, the most common tests measuring some aspect of hemostasis are tests of clotting times, such as prothrombin time or International Normalized Ratio (INR), partial thromboplastin time, and platelet count. Furthermore, certain hematologic disorders require other types of coagulation testing. For example, disseminated intravascular coagulation (DIC), a coagulopathy that arises as a complication of critical illness, requires evaluation of clotting times and factor I (fibrinogen), fibrin split products, plasminogen, and others. Table 28–7 provides a summary of major measurements of hemostasis in the adult.

Platelet Count The number of platelets (thrombocytes) is measured using the platelet count. It is usually measured as part of the complete blood cell (CBC) count. Recall that platelets are necessary to provide initial clotting (platelet plug) when a vessel is injured. Therefore, any disorder or drug that interferes with platelet levels can result in prolonged bleeding.

Tests of Clotting Multiple tests measure some aspect of blood clotting, such as bleeding time, prothrombin time or INR, partial thromboplastin time, D-dimer, and fibrin split products.

Bleeding Time. A useful test of platelet function is the bleeding time, a test that is performed when a platelet abnormality is suspected. Bleeding time is a measurement of the time it takes for a small puncture wound to stop bleeding. To measure the bleeding time, a blood pressure cuff is inflated to 40 mmHg on one arm and left inflated during the procedure. A small puncture wound is made in that arm's forearm. Blood is blotted every 30 seconds until bleeding stops. A stopwatch is used to measure the length of time from the moment of skin puncture until bleeding stops. The test is contraindicated if the patient is taking aspirin or an anticoagulant (Kee, 2014). Bleeding time is prolonged with thrombocytopenia, platelet abnormalities, DIC, and a variety of hematologic disorders.

Prothrombin Time (PT) and INR. Prothrombin time (Pro-Time or PT) is a measure of factor II: prothrombin, which is synthesized by the liver. Recall that factor II is activated in the common pathway of the coagulation cascade and is one of the final steps in forming a fibrin clot (refer to Figure 28–10). It is frequently used to evaluate the anticoagulant status of patients on warfarin therapy. In patients who are on warfarin anticoagulant therapy, it is now recommended that prothrombin time be documented as an INR value because the ratio is an internationally standardized measure of long-term warfarin anticoagulant therapy. When warfarin therapy is being initiated, INR should not be used until the patient has been stabilized on the drug (about 1 week of therapy) as results can be misleading (Kee, 2014). Many diseases and drugs can alter prothrombin time; therefore, the patient's medical and medication history are important to consider when interpreting PT.

Partial Thromboplastin Time (PTT) and Activated Partial Thromboplastin Time (aPTT). The PTT and aPTT tests can be used as a screening test for factors VII, XIII, and platelets (Kee, 2014). Both tests are more sensitive to minor coagulation deficiencies than is the prothrombin time (PT) test, and the aPTT test is even more sensitive than the PTT. Both are useful in monitoring heparin anticoagulant therapy and in evaluation of clotting factor deficiencies.

D-dimer. D-dimer, or fibrin degradation fragment, is a measure of fibrin degradation, confirming that fibrin split

Table 28–7 Measures of Hemostasis in the Adult

Test	Adult reference value	Nursing Implications
Platelet Count	150,000 mcL to 400,000 mcL	*Blood specimen information:* • Lavender-top tube *Abnormally low platelet level:* • Assess for potential cause(s): thrombocytopenia (idiopathic), bone marrow depression, cancer, leukemias, DIC*, chronic kidney disease, drug related • Assess for clinical manifestations of potential causes *Abnormally high platelet level:* • Assess for potential causes(s): polycythemia vera, acute blood loss, metastatic cancer, trauma
Bleeding Time	1 to 9 minutes	*Blood specimen information:* • No collection tube required • Stopwatch required *Abnormally elevated bleeding time:* • Assess for potential cause(s): thrombocytopenia, abnormal platelets, leukemia, DIC, aplastic anemia, clotting factor deficiencies • Assess for clinical manifestations of potential causes
Prothrombin Time (PT)	10–13 seconds Desired levels in warfarin therapy: 1.5–2 times control (sec.)	*Blood specimen information:* • Blue-top tube (sodium citrate anticoagulant) or black-top tube (sodium oxalate anticoagulant) *Abnormally elevated PT:* • Assess for potential cause(s): clotting factor deficiencies, liver disease, leukemias, drug related • Assess for clinical manifestations of potential causes
INR (measure of PT)	Target in warfarin therapy: 2–3 Target in mitral valve replacement: 2.5–3.5	Refer to PT
Partial Thromboplastin Time (PTT) and Activated PTT (aPTT)	PTT: 60–70 seconds aPTT: 20–35 seconds Anticoagulant Therapy: 1.5–2.5 × control (sec.)	*Blood specimen information:* • Blue-top tube *Abnormally elevated PTT or aPTT:* • Assess for potential cause(s): clotting factor deficiencies, liver disease, leukemias, drug related • Assess for clinical manifestations of potential causes
Fibrin Split Products (FSP)	2 mcg/mL–10 mcg/mL	*Blood specimen information:* • Blue-top tube *Abnormally elevated FSP:* • Assess for potential cause(s): DIC, septicemia, tissue damage (massive), liver necrosis, acute kidney failure, acute leukemias, burns, other • Assess for clinical manifestations of potential causes
D-dimer (Fibrin degradation fragment)	Negative	*Blood specimen information:* • Blue-top tube *Abnormally elevated value:* • Assess for potential cause(s): thrombolytic therapy, DIC • Assess for clinical manifestations of potential causes

*DIC = disseminated intravascular coagulation

SOURCE: Data from Kee (2014).

products (FSP) are present (Kee, 2014). It is a nonspecific test that provides evidence that one or more clots are being broken down somewhere in the body. D-dimer is a useful tool in diagnosing disseminated intravascular coagulation (DIC) and may be of use in ruling out pulmonary embolism or other thrombosis. D-dimer values also increase as a result of fibrinolytic therapy, such as tissue plasminogen activator (tPA) treatment for acute myocardial infarction.

Fibrin Split (Degradation) Products. Fibrin split products (FSP), also referred to as fibrin degradation products, are a measurement of anticoagulation caused by the breakdown of clots via the clot dissolution portion of the coagulation process. The split products of fibrin act as anticoagulants. When FSP is elevated, prolonged bleeding

results; thus FSP is frequently used in emergency hemorrhage situations, such as in severe trauma or shock (Kee, 2014). It is also useful in diagnosis of DIC.

Evaluation of Bone Marrow

The bone marrow aspiration (biopsy) is used to rule out, confirm, or make a differential diagnosis of a disorder involving the bone marrow. It is often performed after suspicious cells are found in the peripheral blood. The biopsy is usually performed by needle aspiration and is usually taken from the iliac crest in an adult but may also be taken from the sternum. The bone marrow is examined for the presence, number, and type of abnormal cells, or the absence of normal cells. When assisting with a bone

Emerging Evidence

- In a study of patients hospitalized with sepsis ($n = 157$), participants were randomized into placebo or control groups to determine the effect of Shenfu injections (SFI, a pharmaceutical used in Chinese medicine) on immunology measures and patient outcomes. Groups received the Shenfu injections or a placebo every day for 7 consecutive days along with usual therapies. When compared to the placebo group, the SFI group demonstrated increased CD4 and CD8 T-cell levels, decreased lengths of ICU stay, and other benefits. The use of SFI as an adjunct therapy during sepsis or septic shock treatment may be enhanced cellular immunity of patients experiencing sepsis (*Zhang et al., 2016*).
- Red blood cell distribution width (RDW) measures the variation in the volume of erythrocytes (width of curve of distribution) in the circulating bloodstream. Researchers found that elevated RDW values were associated with systemic inflammatory response syndrome (SIRS) development in cardiac surgical patients receiving extracorporeal circulation. Retrospective medical record review revealed that patients receiving the same treatments who did not develop SIRS had lower RDW values (odds ratio for RDW levels exceeding 13.5%; 95% confidence limits of 1–1.3; $p < 0.04$). Because the RDW is a component of a routine complete blood count, this parameter may be a useful predictor of SIRS in cardiac surgery patients (*Ozeren et al., 2015*).
- In a sample of 1,495 patients with septic shock, the risk of death by day 28 increased when the platelet count was equal to or less than $100,000/mm^3$ within the first 24 hours of shock presentation. This risk increased as the decrease in platelet count became more severe (hazard ratio, 1.65; 95% CI, 1.31–2.08 for a platelet count below $50,000/mm^3$ vs. $> 150,000/mm^3$; $p < 0.0001$). Monitoring platelet counts may be one strategy to identify risk for septic shock in an effort to provide early intervention (*Thiery-Antier et al., 2016*).

marrow aspiration, the nurse should ensure prior to the procedure that the patient has received an explanation of the procedure, has had all questions answered, and has signed the appropriate consent form. Following the procedure, vital signs should be monitored as ordered, and the patient's aspiration site should be observed for bleeding. An analgesic may be needed to relieve postprocedure discomfort.

Section Seven Review

1. What does an elevated reticulocyte count indicate in the presence of anemia?
   A. Red blood cells are being destroyed prematurely.
   B. Bone marrow is depressed.
   C. Red blood cells are being sequestered in the spleen.
   D. Bone marrow is functioning correctly.

2. An elevated monocyte (monocytosis) level is associated with what condition?
   A. Early bacterial infection
   B. Aplastic anemia
   C. Hemolytic anemia
   D. Viral infections

3. Which cell component of the WBC differential count is normally the highest in percentage?
   A. Lymphocytes
   B. Monocytes
   C. Basophils
   D. Neutrophils

4. The D-dimer is a measure of which of the following?
   A. Presence of fibrin split products
   B. Platelet function
   C. Plasminogen activation
   D. Factor II

Answers: 1. B, 2. D, 3. D, 4. A

Clinical Reasoning Checkpoint

Angela M, a 28-year-old middle-school teacher, is brought to the urgent treatment center by her husband with complaints of fever, chills, and a productive cough of 2 days duration. Following appropriate evaluation, she is diagnosed with right lower lobe pneumonia. Her husband, Mark, is currently recovering from cancer chemotherapy for treatment of Hodgkin disease. His most current complete blood cell count shows evidence of moderate bone marrow depression.

1. Assuming that Angela has an intact immune system, describe neutrophils and explain their role in destroying her bacterial pneumonia.

2. In order to combat Angela's pneumonia, the immune cells have to be able to move to the site of the infection.

Explain how this is accomplished by describing margination, diapedesis, migration, and chemotaxis.

3. As the nurse interviewing and assessing Angela, do you have any concerns about her husband, Mark?

4. While you are interviewing Angela, Mark asks you to give him some advice. He tells you that he has been having frequent nosebleeds that are difficult to stop. Considering his recent history, why might he be having epistaxis (nosebleeds)?

5. Assume for a moment that Mark has thrombocytopenia. Briefly describe the role of platelets in hemostasis.

Chapter 28 Review

1. A client with breast cancer presents for chemotherapy for 4 days and says, "I think I am getting the flu. My throat hurts so badly, and I coughed so hard yesterday that I threw up some blood." The nurse would be most concerned that chemotherapy may be destroying which cells?
   1. Pluripotential hematopoietic stem cells
   2. Stem cells committed to the myeloid line
   3. Macrophage precursor stem cells
   4. Lymphoblast cells

2. A client's red blood cell (RBC) count is significantly lower than normal. The nurse should assess this client for problems associated with which process?
   1. Nutrient transport
   2. Bone marrow stimulation
   3. Iron transport
   4. Tissue oxygenation

3. A client who is receiving chemotherapy has a white blood cell differential of WBC 2,000/mcL, neutrophils 600/mcL (30%), and monocytes 400 (2%). The nurse receiving these results interprets them to suggest what about the client's innate immunity?
   1. There is insufficient data to make any inference regarding innate immunity.
   2. The innate immunity is adequate.
   3. The innate immunity is deficient.
   4. Without T cell values, no inference can be made.

4. A 27-year-old female preschool teacher has continued to work while undergoing successful treatment for breast cancer. Today the client presents to the chemotherapy clinic to report that one of the students in her class has confirmed chickenpox. Since the client has never had chickenpox, gamma globulin is administered. What is the primary rationale for this intervention?
   1. The client's age puts her at risk for shingles if exposed to the varicella virus.
   2. Cancer makes it more likely that the client will contract the virus.
   3. Women who wish to have children should avoid having chickenpox.
   4. The client is in an immunodeficient state due to chemotherapy.

5. A nurse is reinforcing teaching associated with an impending kidney transplant. Which client statements would the nurse evaluate as indicating a need for additional teaching? (Select all that apply.)
   1. "It would have sure been good if I had been born an identical twin."
   2. "My body needs this new kidney so much that I am sure it won't be rejected."
   3. "My body will recognize that the new kidney is from someone else."
   4. "Getting a kidney transplant will cause me to be immune from anything the donor was immune to."
   5. "Transplants can cause antigen–antibody responses in my body."

6. A 36-year-old female client presents to the emergency department with uncontrollable epistaxis. The nurse is most concerned with which findings from the CBC that was drawn? (Select all that apply.)
   1. WBC count = 4,625/mcL
   2. RBC count = 5.2 million/mcL
   3. Platelet count = 45,500/mcL
   4. Hemoglobin = 10.2 g/dL
   5. HCT = 38%

7. A client's hemoglobin has dropped from 11.4 g/dL to 9.8 g/dL. Based on this change, the nurse would anticipate managing which client problem?
   1. Shortness of breath with activity
   2. Fever and infection
   3. Bleeding and bruising
   4. Gastrointestinal pain

8. A client is diagnosed with thrombocytopenia and a platelet count of 45,000/mcL. Bleeding times are drawn for evaluation. What would the nurse anticipate to be the results of these studies?
   1. Bleeding times would be shorter than normal.
   2. Bleeding times would be normal.
   3. Bleeding times would be slightly longer than normal.
   4. Bleeding times would be significantly prolonged.

9. A client had a recent coronary artery bypass surgery. Today, the client's erythrocyte sedimentation rate (ESR) is elevated. The nurse interprets this finding as indicating which process is occurring?

1. The client is dehydrated.

2. There is premature death of RBCs occurring.

3. The client has an active inflammatory process.

4. A viral infection may be developing.

10. Which evaluation of MCV and RBCs would the nurse anticipate in an otherwise healthy 17-year-old client who has an acute hemorrhage from a gunshot wound? (Select all that apply.)

1. Normochromic

2. Hypochromic

3. Normocytic

4. Microcytic

5. Macrocytic

Answers to questions found inside your textbook are available on the faculty resources site. Please consult with your instructor.

References

Barrett, K. E., Barman, S. M., Boitano, S., & Brooks, H. L. (2016). Chapter 3: Immunity, infection, & inflammation. In K. E. Barrett, S. M. Barman, S. Boitano, & H. L. Brooks (Eds.), *Ganong's review of medical physiology* (25th ed.). Retrieved March 23, 2017, from http://accessmedicine.mhmedical.com.ezproxy.uky.edu/content.aspx?bookid=1587&sectionid=97162342

Kee, J. L. (2014). *Laboratory and diagnostic tests with nursing implications* (9th ed.). Upper Saddle River, NJ: Pearson.

Kibble, J. D., & Halsey, C. R. (2014). Blood. In J. D. Kibble & C. R. Halsey (Eds.), *Medical physiology: The big picture.* Retrieved March 23, 2017, from http://accessmedicine.mhmedical.com.ezproxy.uky.edu/content.aspx?bookid=1291&sectionid=75576369

Levinson, W. (2016). Chapter 58: Cellular basis of the immune response. In W. Levinson (Ed.), *Review of medical microbiology and immunology* (14th ed.). Retrieved March 22, 2017, from http://accessmedicine.mhmedical.com.ezproxy.uky.edu/content.aspx?bookid=1792&sectionid=120720848

McClanahan, F., & Gribben, J. (2016). Chapter 76: Functions of T lymphocytes: T-cell receptors for antigen. In K. Kaushansky, M. A. Lichtman, J. T. Prchal, M. M. Levi, O. W. Press, L. J. Burns, & M. Caligiuri (Eds.), *Williams hematology* (9th ed.). Retrieved March 23, 2017, from http://accessmedicine.mhmedical.com.ezproxy.uky.edu/content.aspx?bookid=1581&sectionid=108068314

Ozeren, M., Aytacoglu, B., Vezir, O., Karaca, K., Akin, R., & Sucu, N. (2015). Usefulness of elevated red cell distribution width for predicting systemic inflammatory response syndrome after extracorporeal circulation. *Perfusion, 30*(7), 580–586.

Smyth, S. S., Whiteheart, S., Italiano, J. E. Jr., Bray, P., & Coller, B. S. (2016). Chapter 112: Platelet morphology, biochemistry, and function. In K. Kaushansky, M. A. Lichtman, J. T. Prchal, M. M. Levi, O. W. Press, L. J. Burns, & M. Caligiuri (Eds.), *Williams hematology* (9th ed.). Retrieved March 23, 2017, from http://accessmedicine.mhmedical.com.ezproxy.uky.edu/content.aspx?bookid=1581&sectionid=108078506

Thiery-Antier, N., Binquet, C., Vinault, S., Meziani, F., Boisramé-Helms, J., & Quenot, J. (2016). Is thrombocytopenia an early prognostic marker in septic shock? *Critical Care Medicine, 44*(4), 764–772.

Trinchieri, G., Childs, R. W., & Lanier, L. L. (2016). Chapter 77: Functions of natural killer cells. In K. Kaushansky, M. A. Lichtman, J. T. Prchal, M. M. Levi, O. W. Press, L. J. Burns, & M. Caligiuri (Eds.), *Williams hematology* (9th ed.). Retrieved March 23, 2017, from http://accessmedicine.mhmedical.com.ezproxy.uky.edu/content.aspx?bookid=1581&sectionid=108068511

Zhang, N., Liu, J., Qiu, Z., Yiping, Y., Zhang, J., & Tianzheng, L. (2016). Shenfu injection for improving cellular immunity and clinical outcome in patients with sepsis or septic shock. *American Journal of Emergency Medicine, 35*(1), 1–6.

Chapter 29
Alterations in Red Blood Cell Function and Hemostasis

Learning Outcomes

29.1 Describe anemia, including the types, etiology, pathophysiology, clinical manifestations, and management.

29.2 Explain sickle cell disease, including the etiology, pathophysiology, clinical manifestations, complications, diagnosis, and management.

29.3 Discuss polycythemia, including the types, etiology, pathophysiology, clinical manifestations, complications, diagnosis, and management.

29.4 Describe thrombocytopenia, including the types, etiology, pathophysiology, clinical manifestations, complications, diagnosis, and management.

29.5 Explain disseminated intravascular coagulation, including the etiology, pathophysiology, clinical manifestations, diagnosis, and management.

29.6 Demonstrate nursing assessment of the patient with actual or potential problems of erythrocytes or hemostasis.

 igh-acuity illnesses are associated with problems involving red blood cells (RBCs) or hemostasis (coagulopathies). These problems may be related to the patient's reason for admission or as a complication of disease, therapy, or acute critical illness. It is, therefore, important that the high-acuity nurse have an understanding of the underlying disorders of RBCs and hemostasis.

This chapter presents hematologic disorders of the RBCs, platelets, and hemostasis. It focuses on the pathophysiology, clinical manifestations, and management of acute anemias, thrombocytopenias, and disseminated intravascular coagulation. It is recommended that the Chapter 28 content focusing on RBCs, platelets, and coagulation be reviewed prior to beginning this chapter to facilitate understanding of the content.

Section One: Acute Anemias

Anemia is not a disease; rather, it is an important sign of some underlying disorder. The term **anemia** refers to a reduction of or dysfunction in **erythrocytes** (also known as

red blood cells, or RBCs). It can be clinically expressed in terms of reduced levels of RBCs, hematocrit (Hct), or hemoglobin (Hgb). Anemia in adults is present in males when hemoglobin is less than 13.5 g/dL (hematocrit below 41%) and in females when hemoglobin is less than 12 g/dL (hematocrit below 36%) (Damon & Andreadis, 2017). High-acuity level illnesses are associated with multiple acute-onset types of anemias, including acquired aplastic, hemolytic, and acute blood loss anemias, and anemia of inflammation and its subtype, anemia of critical illness. Some anemias are acquired, while others are congenital. A list of selected inherited anemias is provided in the feature Genetic Considerations.

Types of Acute Anemias

Anemias are classified in a variety of ways. One common classification system is the mechanism by which the anemia occurs, including decreased RBC production, increased RBC destruction, and increased blood loss.

Anemias of Decreased Production of RBCs RBC proliferation is a tightly regulated and sequential maturation

Genetic Considerations
Inherited Anemias

- Sickle cell disease
- Beta and alpha thalassemias
- Fanconi anemia
- Hereditary hemolytic anemia
- Diamond-Blackfan anemia

SOURCE: Data from American Society of Gene & Cell Therapy (2017) and Jameson & Kopp (2015).

process in the bone marrow. Under certain circumstances, however, production becomes depressed. This can result from inadequate intake or absorption of certain vitamins or minerals, particularly iron (iron-deficiency anemia), or vitamin B_{12} and folic acid (megaloblastic anemias), which result in chronic forms of anemia. Decreased RBC production can also result from acute-onset bone marrow depression secondary to chemotherapy, infection, or primary bone marrow failure (e.g., aplastic anemia). Kidney failure also causes this type of anemia because the RBC-producing hormone erythropoietin is secreted by the kidneys; as kidney function fails, so does production of erythropoietin.

Aplastic anemia is a rare but serious clinical syndrome characterized by a significant reduction in the formation of all blood cells in the bone marrow, resulting in **pancytopenia** (abnormally low numbers of all blood cell types) and hypocellular bone marrow. The presence of pancytopenia makes aplastic anemia unique because the anemia portion of the disease is only one aspect of a larger problem that also includes thrombocytopenia (low platelet count) and leukopenia (low white blood cells, or WBCs). Aplastic anemia is most commonly an acquired disease, although there are rare inherited forms. Most cases are of idiopathic origin; however, it can develop secondary to certain therapies, such as chemotherapy or radiation therapy for cancer. Table 29–1 provides a summary of some of the more common etiologies of acquired aplastic anemia.

Table 29–1 Potential Etiologies of Acquired Aplastic Anemia

Potential Causes	Examples
Idiopathic	No known cause (majority of cases)
Autoimmune related	Rheumatoid arthritis
Adverse effects of therapies: drugs or ionized radiation	Antineoplastic agents: cytotoxic antibiotics, alkylating agents and antimetabolites Sulfonamides (e.g., sulfadiazine), anticonvulsants (e.g., phenytoin), chloramphenicol, cimetidine, phenylbutazone, gold Total body radiation therapy (such as in preparation for hematopoietic stem-cell transplantation)
Toxins	Benzene, chlorinated hydrocarbons
Viruses	Epstein-Barr virus, HIV

SOURCE: Data from Segel & Lichtman (2015).

Diagnosis and Treatment. Diagnosis of aplastic anemia focuses on blood cell counts (pancytopenia accompanied by a low reticulocyte count) and bone marrow biopsy. On evaluation of the test results, disease severity is graded on a scale that ranges from moderately severe to very severe. At its most severe, aplastic anemia is a relentless disease with rare spontaneous remissions, and if left untreated the prognosis is poor, with most patients dying within 6 months of onset. Even with effective treatment, life expectancy is often only a few years.

Treatment focuses on three general areas: supportive, hematopoietic stem-cell transplantation (HSCT), and immunosuppression. Supportive therapies include removal of the probable cause (e.g., discontinue offending drug or toxin exposure); blood transfusions to replace RBCs and platelets if severely low levels are present; and protection from infection if severe neutropenia exists (e.g., protective environment, possible antibiotic therapy). Allogenic HSCT is the definitive treatment for severe aplastic anemia, particularly in younger patients. If the patient is a candidate for HSCT, blood transfusions will be limited, with no transfusions coming from potential stem-cell donors; this reduces the risk of hypersensitivity reactions and potential stem-cell rejection. Immunosuppressive therapy is used when hematopoietic stem-cell transplantation is not planned. It is aimed at inhibiting T-cell activity and may include antithymocyte globulin (ATG) or antilymphocyte globulin (ALG), steroid therapy, and possibly other immunosuppressant agents. HSCT is described in detail in Chapter 39.

Nursing Considerations. While taking the history of a patient who may have aplastic anemia, the nurse includes questions that target possible exposure to known etiologies. The physical exam focuses on signs and symptoms of anemia, thrombocytopenia, and infection. The patient is closely monitored, evaluating trends in blood cell laboratory results, as well as monitoring for development of complications associated with aplastic anemia (tissue oxygenation problems, bleeding, and possibly infection). The nurse can anticipate administering therapies as ordered and monitoring for therapeutic and nontherapeutic effects. Certain protective measures are implemented if blood cell levels become critically low, including oxygen therapy and thrombocytopenia and neutropenia precautions. Nurses should assess for complications associated with general anemias and those specific to pancytopenia. For pancytopenia, patients should avoid over-the-counter medications that have antiplatelet qualities (e.g., aspirin). Nurses should also monitor for signs and symptoms of infection and bleeding. Complications from blood loss may include decreased cardiac output or fluid volume deficit, which may lead to shock. If a blood transfusion is ordered, the nurse must have a clear understanding of the processes for transfusion and the necessary assessments to perform. Patient and family teaching includes providing education regarding the diagnosis, diagnostic procedures, and interventions (such as thrombocytopenic or neutropenic precautions) that are associated with the blood disorder.

Anemias of Increased Destruction of RBCs
The term **hemolytic anemia** refers to all anemias that are caused by

Table 29–2 Etiologies of Acquired Hemolytic Anemia in Adults

Etiology	Examples	Mechanisms of Injury
Drugs	Sulfonamides Methyldopa	Immune-based injury through destruction and breakdown of targeted RBCs in a sensitized person. Destruction may be from attachment of drug or immune complexes to RBC membranes or autoantibody destruction.
Autoimmune	Autoimmune-induced hemolytic anemia (AIHA)	Unknown triggering mechanism. Involves production of autoantibodies against RBCs. Autoimmune reaction may at times result from an infectious agent, such as infectious mononucleosis.
Infectious agents	*Clostridium perfringens* Malaria (*Plasmodium* parasite)	Some bacteria produce toxins and other substances that hemolyze cells. Parasite (*Plasmodium*) enters RBC and reproduces, RBC ruptures, and disease spreads to other RBCs.
Physical agents	Severe burn injury Artificial heart valve trauma	Extreme heat makes RBCs fragile and causes them to fragment. Fragmented cells (schistocytes) are filtered by the spleen, and serum RBC levels drop significantly. Artificial heart valve fragments RBCs as blood flows through valve.
Microangiopathy	Disseminated intravascular coagulation (DIC) Thrombotic thrombocytopenic purpura/hemolytic uremic syndrome (TTP/HUS)	Fragmentation of RBCs as they move through small blood vessels.

SOURCE: Data partially from Rose & Berliner (2016).

premature destruction of RBCs, either intravascularly or within the reticuloendothelial system. In adults, problems associated with hemolytic anemia most commonly result from extrinsic (acquired) problems; however, there are also rarer intrinsic (e.g., congenital) etiologies. Sickle cell disease is a subtype of hemolytic anemia that has important implications for high-acuity care because of its potential for life-threatening complications. It is presented in detail in Section Two of this chapter.

The acquired hemolytic anemias are often categorized by the agent that causes the RBC destruction, including drugs, infectious agents, physical agents, and conditions associated with microangiopathy. The immune system plays an important role in many types of hemolytic anemias. Antibodies or complement (or sometimes both) coat the red blood cell membrane, causing premature death of the cell. The antibodies can be autoimmune induced (from self), isoimmune induced (from another person), or drug induced (e.g., sulfonamides). Table 29–2 provides major etiologies of hemolytic anemias and their mechanisms of injury.

Diagnosis and Treatment.   Diagnosing acquired hemolytic anemia initially requires tests that help discriminate it from other forms of anemia. A complete blood cell count is performed and typically shows decreased RBCs with increased levels of reticulocytes. Anemia in the presence of elevated reticulocyte counts suggests that the bone marrow is working correctly. A peripheral blood smear may show RBC fragmentation (**schistocytes**). A bilirubin is drawn to evaluate the blood for products of hemolysis. Hyperbilirubinemia would be anticipated with the patient presenting with possible jaundice and an underlying pallor. Hemoglobinuria and significantly elevated lactic dehydrogenase (LDH) enzyme are important indicators of intravascular hemolysis activity. Palpation of the spleen may show splenomegaly if RBCs are being sequestered or destroyed in the spleen (Luzzatto, 2014). A direct Coombs (antiglobulin) test may be ordered to check for antiglobulin antibodies on the

RBCs. Once a diagnosis of hemolytic anemia is made, additional testing will be performed to determine the exact etiology.

The treatment of hemolytic anemias depends on the underlying cause. For example, if the etiology is drug induced, the drug is discontinued. If the immune system is the underlying cause, treatment may include initial doses of glucocorticoids and, if needed, initiation of longer term immunosuppressant therapy to attempt to induce remission. Blood transfusion may be required in a critically ill patient if the hemoglobin falls below 8 g/dL (Damon & Andreadis, 2017). Treatment of sickling crisis is presented in Section Two.

Nursing Considerations.   The nurse focuses the patient history on possible etiologies of the anemia. The physical exam centers attention on clinical findings of anemia and hyperbilirubinemia (e.g., jaundice), as well as the manifestations of the underlying problem. The patient's urine color is assessed for hemoglobin, which is red-brown in color, and serum RBC count and bilirubin trends are monitored closely. The nurse will administer therapies as ordered and monitor for therapeutic and nontherapeutic effects.

Acute Blood Loss Anemia   Anemia caused by blood loss is a common problem with high-acuity patients. Blood loss can be acute (rapid onset) or chronic (slow, insidious onset) and can involve gross or occult bleeding. These two sets of factors largely determine the patient's clinical presentation. Presented here are problems of acute blood loss seen in high-acuity patients.

Trauma is a major cause of acute blood loss. Acute blood loss is also associated with surgery and acute gastrointestinal (GI) bleeding. The clinical manifestations of acute blood loss are usually more severe than those associated with chronic blood loss because of the body's inability to muster sufficient compensatory mechanisms in an acute situation. The effects of acute blood loss can be classified into stages of hemorrhage (Table 29–3).

Table 29–3 Patient Signs Associated with Stages of Hemorrhage

Class	Blood Loss	Vasoconstriction	Skin	Vital Signs		
				HR	SBP	RR
I	< 15%	↑	Normal to slightly cool and pale	↑	→	→
II	15%–30%	↑↑	Pale, clammy, and cool	↑↑	→	↑
III	30%–40%	↑↑↑	Severely cool and pale	↑↑↑	↓	↑↑
IV	> 40%	↑↑↑↑ or ↓↓	Severely cold, pale, mottled	↑↑↑↑ or ↓↓	↓↓↓	↓

HR = heart rate; SBP = systolic blood pressure; RR = respiratory rate; ↑ = increase; → = normal; ↓ = decrease.
SOURCE: Data from Wilson & Clebone (2014).

Diagnosis and Treatment. During acute bleeding, early laboratory studies can be deceptive. Hemoglobin and hematocrit do not initially reflect anemia because plasma and cells are equally lost. As bleeding continues, fluid begins to shift from the extravascular spaces into the intravascular space. This fluid shift causes dilution of the remaining blood cells. In addition, as fluid resuscitation is initiated, the intravascular space is loaded with fluids, which further increases the dilutional effect. The end result is a significant reduction in serum Hgb and Hct. The full extent of the bleed cannot be evaluated using Hgb and Hct values until 48 to 72 hours after the acute bleed. The reticulocyte count becomes elevated within several days of the bleeding event as the bone marrow begins to produce and release the immature RBCs at a rapid rate.

Treatment of blood loss anemia is largely based on the Hgb level. As with other forms of anemia, the underlying problem is corrected when possible or at least controlled. The hemodynamic status of the patient is supported as needed through blood product and/or fluid resuscitation and vasopressors. The objectives of fluid and blood resuscitation include the following:

- restoring intravascular volume sufficient for perfusion of critical organs,
- maintaining oxygen-carrying capacity for adequate cellular oxygen delivery, and,
- correcting coagulopathies (Somand & Ward, 2016).

If fluid and colloid resuscitation do not adequately restore volume, intravenous vasopressors may be considered. Blood products such as packed red cells or whole blood are reserved for treatment of shock that has not been corrected by crystalloid therapy. Transfusion should be considered when the Hgb is less than 8 in young healthy persons (Somand & Ward, 2016).

Nursing Considerations. The nurse assesses the patient for the clinical manifestations of anemia. If hospital protocol allows, periodic stool and nasogastric (NG) drainage guaiac testing may provide valuable information regarding stress ulcer occult bleeding. Occult bleeding is a common phenomenon in high-acuity patients, particularly those in the critical care units, through development of gastrointestinal erosions called *stress ulcers*. The nurse should be suspicious of CBC results that show a slow down-trending of RBC and

Hgb values. The nurse monitors the vital signs for compensatory increases in heart rate and changes in skin color and temperature. Should gross bleeding develop, frequent vital signs with close trending of blood pressure, pulse, mean arterial pressure, and urine output are warranted, and the healthcare provider must be notified immediately of the changing clinical situation. Pertinent patient and family teaching includes discussion about the importance of notifying a healthcare provider if overt blood loss is present.

Anemia of Inflammation Anemia of inflammation (AI) is a commonly occurring and mild-to-moderate form of anemia that develops with many disorders that acutely or chronically activate the immune system. Some of the major inflammatory and infective disorders that have an AI component include rheumatoid diseases, cancers, systemic inflammatory response syndrome (SIRS), and sepsis. In relatively healthy individuals, it is usually a benign condition; however, in the critically ill, it can result in comorbid complications and is an important component of anemia of critical illness.

The primary characteristic of AI is reduced production of RBCs in the presence of low serum iron and reduced iron-binding capacity despite adequate iron stores. In other words, there is a maldistribution of iron with inadequate supplies being delivered to the bone marrow, resulting in iron-deficient erythropoiesis (Adamson & Longo, 2015). The pathophysiologic processes involved in anemia of inflammation are not fully understood but are believed to involve the relationship of proinflammatory cytokines (such as Interleukin-6 [IL-6] and tumor-necrosis factor alpha [TNFα]) to **hepcidin**, the major iron-regulating hormone produced in the liver. In the presence of inflammation or infection, immune cells secrete proinflammatory cytokines, which play crucial roles in the inflammatory response. Some of these cytokines are also known to regulate hepcidin levels. The action of hepcidin is to hold iron intracellularly (in storage), causing a reduction in serum iron levels; thus, elevated hepcidin levels result in low serum iron and normal iron stores. Ultimately, lower serum iron makes less iron available to bind to hemoglobin, causing decreased oxygen delivery to the tissues. Figure 29–1 shows the possible relationship of inflammation to low serum iron counts.

Diagnostic laboratory testing will show elevated hepcidin and low serum iron levels. Examination of RBCs will usually show normal-looking RBCs unless the inflammatory state is prolonged. Treatment focuses on correcting the

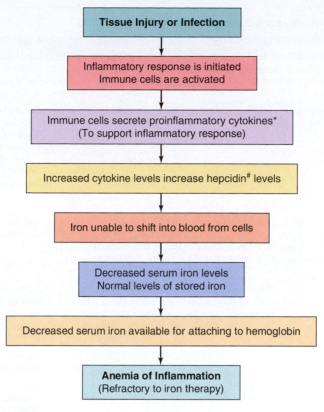

*(e.g., Interleukin-6 [IL-6])
Hepcidin, a hormone produced by the liver that inhibits release of iron from stores into the blood

Figure 29–1 Anemia of inflammation (AI).

underlying problem. Erythropoietin and iron drug therapy may be considered.

Anemia of Critical Illness.   The majority of critically ill patients develop anemia within 2 to 3 days postadmission to the intensive care unit (ICU). The underlying cause is multifactorial with the pathophysiology of anemia of inflammation as only one piece of a complex puzzle. Additional factors are unique to critical illness, such as the underlying disease process, blood loss, bone marrow suppression, and sequestration of RBCs in the spleen (see Box 29–1). One factor, iatrogenic blood loss through frequent diagnostic blood sampling, was studied heavily in the late 1990s into the mid 2000s and continues to be examined. In a retrospective study of 479 patients who were not anemic during admission, researchers found that between admission and discharge 49% developed hospital-acquired anemia (Kurniali et al., 2014).

Interventions to reduce the degree of anemia of critical illness include treatment of the underlying cause, diagnostic blood sampling conservation techniques, and stress ulcer prophylaxis. Blood cell transfusions are no longer routinely recommended in anemic patients. A transfusion may be indicated for patients with cardiovascular or pulmonary symptoms when the hemoglobin drops to less than 8 g/dL (Kasper et al., 2016).

Clinical Manifestations of Anemia

The patient's clinical manifestations usually reflect both the underlying disorder and the anemia. For example, a person with end-stage kidney disease will have manifestations related to anemia, plus any additional manifestations resulting from severe kidney dysfunction. Some of the anemias also have their own specific manifestations. For example, sickle cell disease (SCD) has many unique symptoms related to microvascular occlusion. In aplastic anemia, the decreased RBC level is just one part of a pancytopenia problem. If pancytopenia is present, the patient will also develop the clinical manifestations of deficiencies in the other blood cell types.

When caring for the patient with anemia, the ongoing nursing assessment focuses on the patient's oxygenation

BOX 29–1   Factors That May Contribute to Anemia of Critical Illness

- Underlying disease process
- Persistently elevated hepcidin levels (anemia of inflammation)
- Acute blood loss (e.g., postsurgery, trauma-related hemorrhage, GI hemorrhage)
- Occult blood loss (stress-related mucosal injury)
- Iatrogenic loss through frequent diagnostic blood sampling
- Hemolysis
- Bone marrow suppression (disease related or drug induced)
- Splenic sequestration of blood cells

Table 29–4 Pathophysiologic Basis of the Clinical Manifestations of Anemia

Alteration	Pathophysiologic Basis	Signs and Symptoms
Decreased oxygen affinity	The decreased affinity of oxygen to hemoglobin improves oxygen extraction from available hemoglobin to maintain adequate delivery and maintain tissue oxygenation.	A right shift on oxyhemoglobin-dissociation curve Decreased P_VO_2 and S_VO_2
Tissue hypoxia	Hypoxia-related symptoms develop if hypoxia becomes severe (oxygen supply and demand imbalance).	General—Fatigue (common) Pulmonary—Dyspnea on exertion (or at rest) Cardiovascular—Angina Peripheral vascular—Intermittent claudication, night muscle cramps Neurologic—Headache, lightheadedness Gastrointestinal—Abdominal cramping, nausea
Compensatory		
• Selective increased tissue perfusion	As a compensatory mechanism, selective increased tissue perfusion develops through selective vasoconstriction that shunts blood from nonvital areas of the body to priority organs. In acute anemia, blood is shunted from mesenteric and iliac beds. In chronic anemia, blood is shunted from skin and kidneys.	Pale skin and mucous membranes Urine output usually normal
• Increased cardiac output (in absence of increased BP)	The heart works harder to deliver oxygen: a hyperdynamic cardiac output. Blood pressure does not increase because blood viscosity is reduced (fewer RBCs), and peripheral vascular resistance becomes lower due to selective vasodilatation.	Tachycardia Systolic flow murmur Severe anemia: Angina, high-output heart failure, cardiomegaly are possible.
• Increased pulmonary function	Develops with severe anemia	Tachypnea Decreased A–a gradient Severe state: Exertional dyspnea and orthopnea
• Increased RBC production	Production of erythropoietin maintains an inverse relationship with the hemoglobin concentration to maintain a balance of RBC production with RBC loss.	Stress reticulocytosis—Increased number and proportion of reticulocytes Increased bone marrow discomfort

Key: P_VO_2 = partial pressure of venous oxygen; S_VO_2 = saturation of venous oxygen.
SOURCE: Data from Luzzatto (2014).

status. This is because the clinical manifestations of anemia, regardless of the cause, are primarily attributable to one problem—*impaired oxygen transport*, which affects all body systems. Additional manifestations may be present related to the rate of onset of the anemia, the hematocrit level, and the underlying cause. Table 29–4 summarizes the physiologic basis of major manifestations of anemia.

Impaired oxygen transport causes tissue hypoxia. During an anemia episode, some degree of hypoxia is necessary to stimulate the various compensatory mechanisms.

Nursing Care
The Patient with Anemia

Expected Patient Outcomes and Related Interventions

Outcome: Maintain adequate oxygenation.

Assess and compare to established norms, patient baselines, and trends.
Monitor for signs and symptoms of anemia and reduced oxygenation.
Cardiopulmonary: Tachycardia, systolic flow murmur, angina; tachypnea, orthopnea, dyspnea, low SpO_2
Peripheral vascular: Intermittent claudication, nighttime muscle cramps
Neurologic: Impaired thought processes, headache, dizziness
Integumentary and skeletal: Pale mucous membranes, skin pallor, cyanosis, cold sensitivity, bone marrow discomfort
Gastrointestinal: Anorexia, abdominal cramping, nausea
Laboratory tests: Low RBC, high reticulocyte count, low hemoglobin and hematocrit; low PaO_2, SaO_2

Investigate potential etiologies of anemia.
Obtain thorough nursing history including dietary, recent and chronic illnesses, medications, environmental exposure.

Administer related drug therapy and monitor for therapeutic and nontherapeutic effects.
Oxygen therapy, synthetic erythropoietin therapy.
Nutritional supplements to support RBC development as ordered (e.g., iron, vitamin B_{12}, folic acid)

Intervene to support adequate oxygenation.
Decrease energy expenditure.
Alternate rest and active periods.
Maintain comfortable room temperature for patient (prevent chilling).
Maintain normothermia (reduce fevers, warming blankets if hypothermic).
Assist with physical activities as needed.
Administer oxygen at 2–4 L/min per nasal cannula, as ordered.

SOURCE: Data partially taken from Adamson & Longo (2015).

Two factors determine the severity of clinical manifestations: the rate of anemia onset and the underlying cause. While taking the patient history, it is important to include questions that investigate these two factors. When a mild-to-moderate anemia develops slowly, the person often remains asymptomatic as long as the body is not stressed (by increasing oxygen demand). Given a slow-enough onset, a person may remain relatively asymptomatic (if sedentary) with a Hgb as low as 7 or 8 g/dL (Adamson & Longo, 2015). When the onset of anemia is rapid (e.g., hemorrhage), there is insufficient time for adequate compensatory mechanisms to be activated, which can potentially result in severe hypoxemia and tissue ischemia.

Grading Anemias   Anemias are graded by degree of severity (mild to severe). Such grading systems help quantify the severity of anemia based on the Hgb level, which is helpful in making treatment decisions. Clinically, the patient's assessment data will reflect the severity of the anemia, particularly when severe anemia is present. Anemia is graded 0 (normal) to 4 (life-threatening) and is categorized by levels of hemoglobin.

Nursing Considerations   The high-acuity nurse needs to be mindful of any risk factors that a patient may have for development of anemia, particularly in the critical care environment. Care of the patient with anemia centers on treating the underlying cause and improving oxygenation. Regardless of the cause, the nurse will largely focus on monitoring the patient's oxygenation status and supporting tissue oxygenation. Major assessments and interventions that apply to the anemic patient are provided in the "Nursing Care: The Patient with Anemia" feature.

Section One Review

1. The clinical manifestations of the anemias are primarily attributable to what function?
   A. Decreased cardiac output
   B. Impaired oxygen transport
   C. Decreased blood volume
   D. Impaired bone marrow function

2. The severity of symptoms associated with anemia largely depends on what?
   A. Type of anemia
   B. Total blood volume
   C. Speed with which it develops
   D. Degree of bone marrow involvement

3. Which form of anemia usually involves pancytopenia?
   A. Aplastic
   B. Hemolytic
   C. Megaloblastic
   D. Iron deficiency

4. Anemia of inflammation (AI) is characterized as a low serum-iron level in the presence of what?
   A. Adequate bone marrow iron stores
   B. Increased iron-binding capacity
   C. Chronic bleeding
   D. Premature death of RBCs

Answers: 1. B, 2. C, 3. A, 4. A

Section Two: Sickle Cell Disease—A Disorder of Abnormal RBCs

To understand sickle cell disease, it is important to have a basic understanding of the types of hemoglobin. Full-term newborns are born with RBCs that contain 60% to 80% fetal hemoglobin (Hb F). Hemoglobin A (Hb A, adult hemoglobin) nearly replaces all fetal hemoglobin by age 6 to 12 months. Hb F amounts to less than 1% of total hemoglobin by adulthood (Kee, 2013). Sickle cell disease refers to a group of inherited disorders characterized by abnormal hemoglobin and called "sickle hemoglobin" or hemoglobin S (Hb S), that develops rather than Hb A to replace fetal hemoglobin. Sickle cell disease results from an autosomal recessive mutation in the β-globin gene, whereby the sixth amino acid (glutamic acid) is replaced by another (valine) (Natrajan & Kutlar, 2015). There are variations of the disease based on inheritance patterns (Figure 29–2). This section focuses on the most severe form, sickle cell disease,

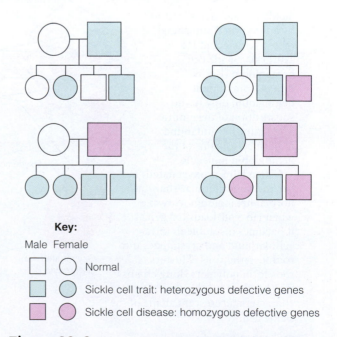

Key:

Male   Female

☐ ◯ Normal

☐ ◯ Sickle cell trait: heterozygous defective genes

☐ ◯ Sickle cell disease: homozygous defective genes

Figure 29–2 The inheritance for sickle cell disease.

Table 29–5 Two Major Forms of Sickle Cell Disease

Type	Description
Sickle Cell Disease	Hemoglobin = predominantly Hb S (75%–95%) Inheritance pattern: homozygous (inherit Hb S from both parents [HbSS]) Most severe form of disease
Sickle Cell Trait	Hemoglobin = Hb A/S (a mixture of Hb A and Hb S) Inheritance pattern: heterozygous (Hb S inherited from one parent, and Hb A [normal] inherited from other parent) Carrier state Rarely develop clinical manifestations

which has a homozygous inheritance pattern. Table 29–5 provides a brief summary of two major forms of the disease, sickle cell disease (the most serious form) and sickle cell trait (the carrier form).

Epidemiology

Sickle cell disease is most prevalent in Africa, the Mediterranean, the Middle East, and India (Natrajan & Kutlar, 2015). In the United States, the disease is primarily found in the African American population, affecting 1 in 365 African American births and 1 in 16,300 Hispanic American births (Centers for Disease Control [CDC], 2016). The fact that the disease is most prevalent in countries where malaria is endemic suggests that the sickle cell mutation may have resulted as a genetic adaptation against malaria (*Plasmodium falciparum* infection), which requires oxygen to survive. People with sickle cell disease (SCD) in the United States have a life expectancy greater than 50 years. The increased life expectancy is related to early diagnosis, close monitoring, and parental education (Williams-Johnson & Williams, 2016).

Pathophysiology of Sickle Hemoglobin

Sickle cell disease is a type of hemolytic anemia in which the hemoglobin S has a significantly shortened life span. In a normal, well-oxygenated state, sickle hemoglobin (Hb S) functions normally. The problem arises when the PaO_2 and SaO_2 decrease, producing a deoxygenated state. The relative hypoxic state causes the Hb S to polymerize, forming rodlike fibrous polymers (Janz & Hamilton, 2014). The realignment of polymers is what gives the RBC its sickled shape (see Figure 29–3). While sickled, RBCs take on two important characteristics: The polymer realignment makes the RBC membrane stiffer, and the RBC membrane becomes sticky. These altered characteristics result in sickled cells adhering to the endothelial walls, clumping together, and slowing down or obstructing blood flow in the small capillaries. Together, these two characteristics cause microvascular occlusion, the major characteristic of sickle cell disease. When the underlying cause of the hypoxic event is relieved, most of the sickled cells return to their normal shape; however, with the severe form, a significant number (up to 30% of Hb S) cannot revert back to normal and are destroyed by the spleen. Over time, the pooling of abnormal cells in the spleen causes ischemia, infarction, and eventual destruction of the spleen (**autosplenectomy**). Loss of the spleen significantly increases the risk for development of infections.

Hemoglobin S and Red Blood Cell Sickling

Sickle cell anemia is caused by an inherited autosomal recessive defect in Hb synthesis. Sickle cell hemoglobin (Hb S) differs from normal hemoglobin only in the substitution of the amino acid valine for glutamine in both beta chains of the hemoglobin molecule.

When Hb S is oxygenated, it has the same globular shape as normal hemoglobin. However, when Hb S off-loads oxygen, it becomes insoluble in intracellular fluid and crystallizes into rodlike structures. Clusters of rods form polymers (long chains) that bend the erythrocyte into the characteristic crescent shape of the sickle cell.

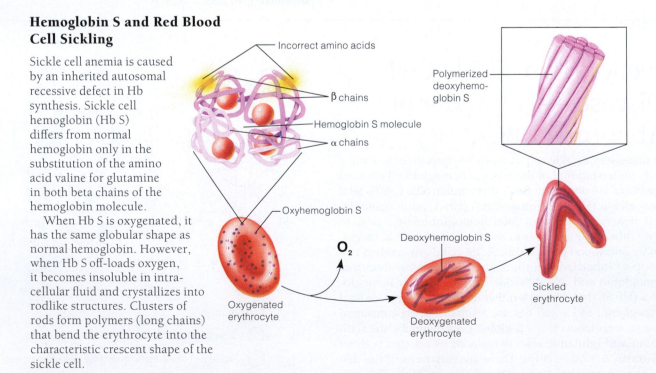

Figure 29–3 The polymerization process of Hb S.

The Sickle Cell Disease Process

Sickle cell disease is characterized by episodes of acute painful crises. Sickling crises are triggered by conditions causing high tissue oxygen demands or that affect cellular pH. As the crisis begins, sickled erythrocytes adhere to capillary walls and to each other, obstructing blood flow and causing cellular hypoxia. The crisis accelerates as tissue hypoxia and acidic metabolic waste products cause further sickling and cell damage.

Sickle cell crises cause microinfarcts in joints and organs, and repeated crises slowly destroy organs and tissues. The spleen and kidneys are especially prone to sickling damage.

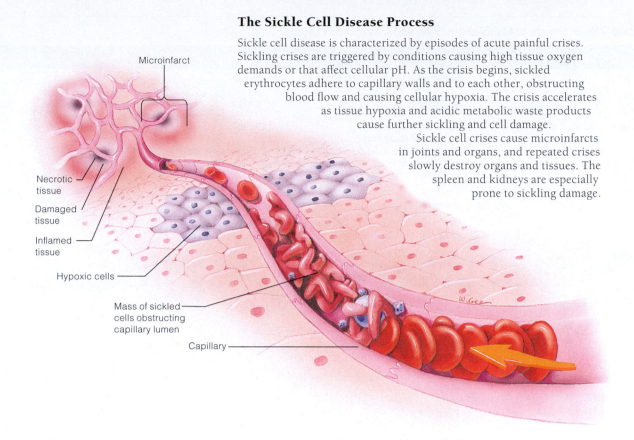

Figure 29–4 Vaso-occlusion caused by sickled cells.

Clinical Manifestations and Complications

The clinical manifestations of sickle cell disease develop between the ages of 6 months and 1 year, when Hb S becomes the predominant RBC type. Chronic anemia and intermittent episodes of microvascular occlusion (sickling crisis or vaso-occlusive crisis) become the sources of most of the manifestations of the disease. The damage caused by vaso-occlusive crises is cumulative and over time results in permanent damage to targeted tissues and organs (see Figure 29–4). The major manifestations associated with microvascular occlusion include moderate to severe pain (referred to as "painful crisis"), tenderness of the affected area, tachycardia, and fever. The location of pain depends on the location of the vaso-occlusion (frequently in the abdomen, back, chest, arms, legs, or knees). The painful crisis lasts anywhere from a few hours to several weeks.

Individuals with sickle cell disease maintain a mean hemoglobin of about 8 g/dL with a significantly elevated reticulocyte count owing to increased erythropoiesis (Jackups, Sanfilippo, Wang, & Blinder, 2014). Associated laboratory values that may be present include elevated reticulocyte count and elevated bilirubin level (related to RBC destruction). Jaundice may develop as bilirubin levels rise.

Sickle cell disease deaths are primarily related to recurrent vascular occlusion problems. The most common cause of death in adults with SCD is a pulmonary vaso-occlusive crisis called acute chest syndrome. Other causes of death include stroke, organ failure, and infection (Bunn, 2017). Table 29–6 provides a summary of the effects (complications) of micro-obstruction and infarction of some of the organs targeted by vascular occlusion in sickle cell disease.

Diagnosis and Treatment   Sickle cell disease is relatively easy to diagnose. A hematologic family history (mother and father) should be obtained. A positive family history of sickle cell disease in any of its forms is an important indicator of increased sickle cell disease risk for any child born to that family. Two major blood tests for Hb S include the following:

- Sickle cell screening test (e.g., Sickledex test)—A screening blood test that is read as positive or negative for Hb S. A hemoglobin electrophoresis should be ordered if the screening test is positive for hemoglobin S (Kee, 2013).

- Hemoglobin electrophoresis—Ordered when the sickle cell screening test is positive. It is a blood test that detects abnormal hemoglobin types in the red blood cell. This test confirms sickle cell disease, characterized by the S-shaped hemoglobin (Kee, 2013).

Hematopoietic stem-cell transplant is the only curative treatment option. Transplants from a sibling donor result in the best outcome for SCD (Shenoy, 2013). Supportive

Table 29–6 Effects of Micro-obstruction and Infarction on Organs

Ischemic Organ/Tissue	Results
Brain	Stroke (most common in children; often hemorrhagic)
Retina	Hemorrhage, retinopathy Retinal detachment
Lungs	Acute chest syndrome • A type of acute lung injury • Presentation: chest pain, tachypnea, fever, cough, oxygen desaturation, chest infiltrates Pulmonary hypertension and cor pulmonale (common cause of death in adults) Pulmonary embolism
Liver	Infarction Hepatitis (secondary to transfusions)
Spleen	Infarction and destruction (usually within 18–36 months of age) Loss of the spleen increases susceptibility to microbial infections
Kidneys	Papillary necrosis with isosthenuria Global renal necrosis Renal failure in adults (a common adult cause of death)
Bones and joints	Aseptic necrosis (especially humeral and femoral heads) Bone infarctions Chronic arthropathy Osteomyelitis, septic arthritis Hand–foot syndrome (dactylitis: painful inflammation and infarction of digits) Osteopenia, osteoporosis
Male genitalia	Priapism with possible tissue infarction Permanent impotence
Integument	Lower leg stasis ulcers

SOURCE: Data from Natarajan & Kutlar (2015).

Table 29–7 Sickling Crises Triggers and Patient Preventative Teaching

Sickling Triggers	Teaching Implications
Infection and fever	Contact healthcare provider immediately if illness is febrile (temperature greater than 38.5°C). Vaccinate against pneumococcal infection (preventative). Possible prophylactic antibiotic therapy
Temperature extremes	Avoid exposure to severe temperatures. Dress warmly during cold weather and when in cold air-conditioned rooms. Avoid swimming in cold water.
Anxiety or stress	Avoid stressful or anxiety-producing situations; stress-reduction techniques.
Excessive exercise	Regular low-to-moderate exercise is encouraged. Avoid exercise that is tiring. Consult provider before beginning new types of exercise. Drink more fluid with exercise.
Hypoxia (including sleep apnea)	Avoid conditions associated with reduced oxygen concentrations: • Fly only in pressurized aircraft cabins. • Avoid high-altitude geographic areas. Consult with healthcare provider before taking a trip to high-altitude area to discuss risks. Supplemental oxygen may be required. • Consult provider if snoring or sleep apnea is part of medical history. • Avoid decongestants such as pseudoephedrine that cause vasoconstriction. Optimize RBC production: folic acid supplement.
Smoking	Smoking cessation education
Dehydration	Stay well hydrated. Increase fluid intake in dry, hot climates. Drink at least 8 glasses per day.

SOURCE: Data partially from Jackups et al. (2014) and Brousse et al. (2014).

treatment includes antibiotic and analgesic (often opioid) drug therapies, intravenous fluids, and blood transfusions. The major pharmacologic therapy for treatment of sickle cell disease is the antisickling agent hydroxyurea (see the "Related Pharmacotherapy: Hydroxyurea" feature). See Box 29-2 for National Guideline recommendations for the treatment of SCD crisis.

Nursing Considerations   General supportive goals for managing sickle cell disease include providing disease-related education to the patient and family, preventing anemia complications, providing psychological support, and encouraging genetic counseling. A major focus of patient and family education is on avoiding sickling crises triggers as the tissue-damaging effects of the crises are cumulative and result in end-organ damage or destruction. If the spleen has been removed, prophylactic antibiotics may be ordered prior to any invasive procedures (e.g., dental procedures). Vaccinations against *H. influenza* and pneumococcal pneumonia are usually recommended, as respiratory infection is a major source of morbidity and mortality in this patient population. Table 29–7 lists common factors that can trigger a sickling crisis and patient preventative education. The "Nursing Care: The Patient with Sickle Cell (Sickling) Crisis" feature provides a summary of the nursing management of the patient experiencing sickling crisis.

BOX 29–2 National Guidelines for the Treatment of Sickle Cell Disease Crisis

- Rapid initiation of opioids for treatment of severe pain associated with a vaso-occlusive crisis
- Use of incentive spirometry in patients hospitalized for a vaso-occlusive crisis
- Use of analgesics and physical therapy for treatment of avascular necrosis
- Hydroxyurea therapy for adults with three severe vaso-occlusive crises during any 12-month period
- Preoperative transfusion therapy to increase hemoglobin levels to 10 g/dL
- Maintain sickle hemoglobin levels of less than 30% prior to the next transfusion during long-term transfusion therapy.
- In a vaso-occlusive crisis, administer oxygen for a saturation < 95% on room air.

SOURCE: Data from Yawn et al. (2014).

Related Pharmacotherapy
Hydroxyurea

Antisickling/Antimetabolite

Hydroxyurea (Hydrea, Droxia)

Action and Uses

Hydroxyurea inhibits DNA synthesis through RNA reductase inhibition, but it does not interfere with RNA synthesis. Its primary use is for cancer therapy. Hydroxyurea oral treatment has been found to decrease and prevent complications of SCD. This medication increases the number of fetal hemoglobin (Hb F), increases blood flow, and reduces vaso-occlusion. There has been a reduction in mortality with long-term use. It has also been shown to reduce hospitalizations, transfusions, and frequency of painful episodes (Yawn et al., 2014). It is considered to be a major advancement in the treatment of sickle cell disease.

Dosages (Adult)

Initial dosing: 15 mg/kg/day (PO); increase by 5 mg/kg/day as needed with maximum dosage of 35 mg/kg/day (or toxicity occurs)

SOURCE: Data from Natarajan & Kutlar (2015).

Major Adverse Effects

Generally well tolerated
Most common: Neutropenia—mild and reversible
Potentially life-threatening: Suppression of bone marrow

Nursing Implications

Monitor CBC and platelet count closely.
Monitor kidney and liver function periodically.
Teach patient and family:
 Cannot take during pregnancy due to teratogenic nature of drug
 Signs and symptoms of bone marrow suppression (neutropenia and thrombocytopenia)
 Signs and symptoms of infection

Nursing Care
The Patient with Sickle Cell (Sickling) Crisis

Expected Patient Outcomes and Related Interventions

Outcome 1: Optimize hydration

Assess and compare to established norms, patient baselines, and trends.
 Intake and output balance
 Monitor for S & S of fluid volume deficit.

Administer related drug therapy and monitor for therapeutic and nontherapeutic effects.
 Intravenous hydration—dextrose 5%/0.5% normal saline; initial rate 150–200 mL/hr

Encourage good oral hydration.
 Drink at least 8 glasses of water/day.

Outcome 2: Optimize oxygenation

Assess and compare to established norms, patient baselines, and trends.
 PaO_2, SaO_2, SpO_2

Administer oxygen at 2–4 L/min per nasal cannula.

Outcome 3: Control pain (in painful crises)

Assess and compare to established norms, patient baselines, and trends.
 Location and level of pain

Administer related drug therapy and monitor for therapeutic and nontherapeutic effects.

    Example emergency department painful crisis analgesic protocol:

        Morphine sulfate (IV)—start at 0.1–0.15 mg/kg, or Hydromorphone (IV)—0.015–0.02 mg/kg

    Other analgesics:

        NSAIDs, acetaminophen, aspirin

Investigate and reverse underlying cause of crisis.

SOURCE: Data from Natarajan & Kutlar (2015).

Outcome 4: Rapid diagnosis and treatment of infections

Assess and compare to established norms, patient baselines, and trends.

    Monitor for infection and fever.

Administer related drug therapy and monitor for therapeutic and nontherapeutic effects.

    Antibiotic therapy: e.g., cephalosporin and erythromycin

Treat suspected infections (high risk for salmonella, osteomyelitis, and pneumococcal infections).

Section Two Review

1. In a healthy baby, hemoglobin F (Hb F) is replaced by which type of hemoglobin at about 6 months of age?
   A. Hemoglobin A (Hb A)
   B. Hemoglobin B (Hb B)
   C. Hemoglobin C (Hb C)
   D. Hemoglobin S (Hb S)

2. When sickle hemoglobin (Hb S) experiences a deoxygenated state, what is the result?
   A. Release of iron from hemoglobin
   B. Stiff fibrous polymers develop
   C. Inability of oxygen to attach to iron
   D. Destruction of normal RBCs by the spleen

3. To what does the term *painful crises* in clients with sickle cell disease refer?
   A. Loss of a digit from tissue necrosis
   B. Sequestration of blood in the liver and spleen
   C. The result of microvascular occlusion
   D. Failure of the bone marrow to meet the high demands for new RBCs

4. The antimetabolite hydroxyurea (Hydrea) is useful in treating sickling disease for which reason?
   A. It reduces Hb S.
   B. It increases Hb F.
   C. It increases the reticulocyte count.
   D. It increases vascular adhesion.

Answers: 1. A, 2. B, 3. C, 4. B

Section Three: Polycythemia: A Disorder of Excessive RBCs

Polycythemia refers to the production and presence of an abnormally high number of red blood cells (erythrocytosis). There are two major forms of polycythemia: primary and secondary. This section provides a brief overview of primary polycythemia and focuses on secondary polycythemia, a more common disorder frequently seen in certain high-acuity patient populations.

Primary Polycythemia (Polycythemia Vera)

Polycythemia vera (PV), an acquired form of primary polycythemia, is a rare clonal myeloproliferative disease involving the pluripotential hematopoietic stem cells. It involves excessive production of all three blood cell types, but the degree of RBC proliferation is particularly severe. PV is a chronic disease that exists on a continuum from mild to severe but tends to worsen over many years. It is a disorder of older age and affects more men than women. The cause is unknown, but certain risk factors have been

identified, such as chemical exposure or a mutation in the JAK2 gene, which results in an overproduction of blood cells. The disease is characterized by a large increase in the RBC mass (red cell volume), elevated hematocrit, hypervolemia, increased blood viscosity, and splenomegaly from pooling of RBCs.

The major clinical manifestations of PV (shown in Box 29–3) result from the extreme RBC proliferation. The life span of patients with PV varies, depending on the severity of the disease and prevention of thrombotic complications. Treatment usually includes phlebotomy,

---

BOX 29–3 Common Manifestations of Polycythemia

- Headache, vision disturbances, dizziness, weakness, tinnitus
- Hypertension
- Plethora (ruddy [red] colored: face, ears, mucous membranes, hands, and feet)
- Night sweats
- Manifestations of chronic tissue hypoxia (e.g., digital ischemia)
- Elevated erythropoietin (EPO) levels
- Thromboses, arterial or venous (e.g., abdominal vessels)

SOURCE: Data from Adamson & Longo (2015).

myelosuppression therapy, and aspirin therapy. The overall treatment goal is to prevent thrombo-hemorrhagic complications. The target hematocrit should be less than 45% in PV (Tefferi & Barbui, 2017).

Secondary Polycythemia

Secondary polycythemia, or *erythrocytosis*, is a sign of some underlying pathology or environmental factor. In the high-acuity patient, secondary "appropriate" polycythemia frequently occurs as a compensatory response to chronic tissue hypoxia. Compensatory secondary polycythemia can result from the following:

- Environmental factors (e.g., living at a high altitude)
- Chronic cardiac or pulmonary diseases (e.g., congenital heart disease or COPD)
- Smokers who have an increased level of CO

In the presence of chronic tissue hypoxia, the kidneys produce more erythropoietin (EPO), which then stimulates the bone marrow to produce more RBCs (erythrocytosis). The elevated RBC count results in increased oxygen-carrying capacity of the blood and, ultimately, increased oxygen to the tissues. Some diseases can cause an "inappropriate" secondary polycythemia, whereby EPO is secreted without tissue hypoxia stimuli. Such is the case with some erythropoietin-secreting renal tumors.

Clinical Manifestations The clinical manifestations of secondary polycythemia are frequently those of the patient's underlying disease rather than the polycythemia. When symptoms are present, they reflect the elevated red cell mass (volume of RBCs), hyperviscosity (thickness of blood), and thrombosis. Smoking-related polycythemia is generally asymptomatic; however, there is increased risk for thrombotic episodes that may be more related to smoking than the polycythemia. Not all secondary polycythemias are mild. For example, some renal and cardiovascular problems significantly increase the risk for thrombotic episodes, hypertension, and heart failure (Prchal, 2016). Box 29–4 lists possible complications of severe polycythemia.

BOX 29–4 Complications of Polycythemia

- Thrombotic episodes
- Transient ischemia attacks (TIA) and ischemic strokes (major arterial complications)
- Acute myocardial infarction
- Deep vein thrombosis (DVT)
- Pulmonary embolus
- Hepatic vein thrombosis
- Ischemia of the digits
- Bleeding (gingival bleeding, easy bruising, GI bleeding, hemorrhage)
- Angina, heart failure
- Pulmonary hypertension

Diagnosis and Treatment The distinct hematologic features of secondary polycythemia include elevations in serum hemoglobin or hematocrit, an increase in red cell mass greater than 25% above the mean, and a subnormal serum erythropoietin level (Adamson & Longo, 2015). The absence of elevations in leukocytes or platelets helps differentiate it from primary polycythemia. Obtaining a thorough history is crucial to diagnosing secondary polycythemia as the diagnosis may stem from congenital abnormalities or acquired factors. Acquired factors of secondary polycythemia are either hypoxia driven or oxygen independent. Cardiac or pulmonary disease, smoking, hypoventilation from sleep apnea, and renal artery stenosis are examples of hypoxia-driven factors (Tefferi & Barbui, 2017). Certain medications, malignant tumors, or other tumors are examples of oxygen-independent factors (Tefferi & Barbui, 2017). An arterial blood gas confirms chronic hypoxemia if that is the underlying cause. A carboxyhemoglobin level may be drawn if smoking-related polycythemia is suspected. Contemporary treatment of secondary polycythemia focuses on eliminating or reducing the underlying problem. Symptom relief from aspirin or phlebotomy may be used to keep the patient comfortable (Longo, 2016).

Section Three Review

1. What are the two major features of polycythemia?
   - **A.** Elevated red cell mass and hematocrit
   - **B.** Larger-than-normal erythrocytes
   - **C.** Polymerization of red blood cells
   - **D.** Premature destruction of red blood cells

2. Polycythemia vera is a myeloproliferative hematopoietic disorder that affects which client population the most?
   - **A.** Younger women
   - **B.** Older women
   - **C.** Younger men
   - **D.** Older men

3. What is the underlying cause of secondary polycythemia?
   - **A.** Depletion of erythropoiesis
   - **B.** Myeloproliferative disease
   - **C.** Chronic tissue hypoxia
   - **D.** Chronic obstructive pulmonary disease

4. What is a major complication of severe polycythemia?
   - **A.** Thrombosis and tissue ischemia or infarction
   - **B.** Bleeding peptic ulcer
   - **C.** Eventual onset of leukemia
   - **D.** Chronic obstructive pulmonary disease

Answers: 1. A, 2. D, 3. C, 4. A

Section Four: Thrombocytopenia: A Problem of Hemostasis

Platelets, or thrombocytes, are cellular components of hemostasis. They play a crucial role in early hemostasis by forming a platelet plug at the site of a new vascular injury, and they also activate the coagulation cascade. **Thrombocytopenia** refers to an abnormally low platelet count. While there are rare forms of inherited thrombocytopenia, it is predominantly an acquired disorder and much more likely to be seen in the high-acuity patient population. For this reason, this section focuses only on acquired types of thrombocytopenia.

Underlying Processes

There are three major underlying processes (see Table 29–8) that result in acquired thrombocytopenia, including decreased platelet production, increased platelet destruction, and platelet sequestration. Acute hemorrhage also results in thrombocytopenia through loss of blood cells from the body. The most common cause of acquired thrombocytopenia is drug-induced adverse effects that can either decrease production or increase destruction of platelets. Examples of drugs that have been associated with development of thrombocytopenia are provided in Table 29–9.

Problems of Decreased Production Any disorder, therapy (including drug or radiation), or chemical that injures or suppresses the bone marrow results in temporary or permanent reduction in **megakaryocytes** (cells that produce thrombocytes). Problems of the bone marrow reduce production of all blood cells, with thrombocytopenia being only one aspect of a pancytopenia problem. Diseases that impair thrombopoiesis (formation of platelets) also decrease platelet production. For example, the liver produces thrombopoietin, a hormone that regulates megakaryocyte production; consequently, in severe liver disease, thrombopoietin

production decreases and thrombocytopenia develops. Megaloblastic anemias provide a second example of impaired thrombopoiesis. These anemias result from deficiencies in essential components of blood cell development, such as folic acid and vitamin B_{12} deficiencies, and are usually chronic forms of anemia.

Problems of Increased Destruction Premature destruction of platelets most commonly results from a drug-induced, immune-mediated, antibody–platelet antigen response; however it can also be caused by autoimmune disorders or infections (Thomas, 2015). Many drugs (see Table 29–9), foods (e.g., tahini), beverages (e.g., quinine in tonic water, alcohol), and herbal remedies are known or suspected of targeting thrombocytes (Shaffer & Santen, 2016). Two major types of thrombocytopenia that fall into this category are immunologic thrombocytopenic purpura (ITP) and heparin-induced thrombocytopenia (HIT).

Table 29–9 Examples of Drugs Associated with Thrombocytopenia

Type of Agent	Examples
Antibiotic, antiviral	Acyclovir Penicillin (e.g., ampicillin, methicillin) Sulfa-containing (e.g., trimethoprim or sulfamethoxazole)
Anticonvulsant	Carbamazepine, phenytoin, valproic acid
Anticoagulant	Heparin
Antidysrhythmic	Amiodarone, procainamide, quinidine
Cardiovascular agents	Captopril, digoxin, amiodarone, atorvastatin, simvastatin
Analgesic agents	Aspirin, ibuprofen, indomethacin, naproxen, acetaminophen
Cancer chemotherapy	All agents that cause general bone marrow suppression (e.g., alkylating agents)
Diuretic	Furosemide, hydrochlorothiazide
Histamine blocking	Cimetidine, ranitidine

SOURCE: Data from Konkle (2015) and Leavitt & Minichiello (2016).

Table 29–8 Processes Involved in Acquired Thrombocytopenia

Underlying Process	Mechanisms	Examples of Causes
Decreased platelet production	Bone marrow injury or suppression Impaired thrombopoiesis	Aplastic or megaloblastic anemia Chemical or radiation exposure Leukemia Drug induced (e.g., cancer chemotherapy) Viral infections (e.g., HIV) Nutritional deficiency
Increased platelet destruction	Autoantibodies coat and destroy platelets	Autoimmune diseases (e.g., rheumatoid arthritis and systemic lupus erythematosus) Disseminated intravascular coagulation (DIC) Drug induced (e.g., heparin, many others)
Platelet sequestration	Enlarged spleen traps platelets, reducing number in circulation	Cirrhosis Sickle cell disease (SCD) Lymphoma, leukemia Heart failure

SOURCE: Data from Leavitt & Minichiello (2016).

Table 29–10 Summary of Immunologic Thrombocytopenic Purpura and Heparin-induced Thrombocytopenia

	Immunologic Thrombocytopenic Purpura (ITP)	Heparin-Induced Thrombocytopenia (HIT)
Pathogenesis	Immune-mediated (IgG) destruction of platelets; involves formation of platelet autoantibodies that attack and destroy platelets	Formation of antibody–heparin–PF4 complexes that activate platelets causing clumping and thrombosis
Characteristics	Normal bone marrow Thrombocytopenia Normal spleen No identifiable cause	Onset 5–10 days post initiation of heparin (primarily unfractionated) Thrombocytopenia, typically no lower than 20,000/mcL Not associated with severe bleeding Risk for thrombosis can be prolonged (antibodies may take up to 100 days to completely exit body)
Laboratory findings	Low platelet count Negative lab results for other identifiable causes	Detectable antiheparin–PF4 antibodies Positive IgG-specific ELISA assay Positive platelet activation assay
Treatment options	Based on platelet count and whether bleeding is present Treatment options: • Steroid therapy (prednisone) • Immune anti-D antibody • Intravenous gamma globulin • Rituximab (anti B-cell antibody) considered for refractory ITP • Splenectomy if unresponsive to steroid therapy	Discontinue heparin and initiate alternative anticoagulant, usually direct thrombin inhibitor (e.g., argatroban, or lepirudin). Warfarin is not recommended; however, if being used at time of HIT diagnosis, vitamin K is initiated. Monitor closely for thromboses. Heparin is usually contraindicated for future use if it can be avoided but may be safe for brief use.

SOURCE: Data from Konkle (2015) and Weitz (2015).

Immunologic Thrombocytopenic Purpura. Immunologic thrombocytopenic purpura (ITP) is a rare autoimmune condition with the acute form most commonly seen in children. In adults, it usually develops in young women as a chronic disorder of autoimmune origin with formation of platelet autoantibodies. Moreover, ITP is more likely to develop in conjunction with a preexisting autoimmune disorder, such as systemic lupus erythematosus (SLE). Typically, in response to premature platelet destruction, the bone marrow increases thrombocyte production as a compensatory mechanism. Patients with ITP may not develop bleeding problems because the platelets in circulation continue to function normally. However, bleeding risks should be reduced as much as possible for patients with ITP. This should include avoiding antiplatelet medications, concentrating on fall risk, managing BP, and maximizing treatment of exacerbating comorbid conditions (Shaffer & Santen, 2016). Table 29–10 provides a summary of ITP, including treatment options.

Heparin-induced Thrombocytopenia. Heparin-induced thrombocytopenia (HIT) is a drug-induced form of thrombocytopenia in which activated platelets become aggregated (clumped) and are removed from the circulation. It is a complication of heparin (primarily unfractionated) anticoagulant therapy. The pathogenesis of HIT involves formation of immune complexes, as follows:

• Heparin has a high affinity for **platelet factor 4 (PF4)**, a platelet protein. Heparin and the PF4 protein bind, forming a *heparin–PF4 complex* that the immune system recognizes as foreign, and antibodies (IgG) are produced against it.

• The IgG antibodies bind with the *heparin–PF4 complexes* creating new *antibody–heparin–PF4 complexes* that subsequently activate circulating platelets. As a result, the activated platelets initiate prothrombotic activities that lead to formation of thrombi, which

leads to increased platelet consumption and a decrease in platelet count (Weitz, 2015).

Many patients receiving heparin therapy develop antibodies to *heparin-PF4 complexes* without developing thrombotic problems; of that group only a small fraction develop HIT. However, in the fraction that develops HIT, about 50% develop thrombosis (Konkle, 2015). In severe cases, patients can develop vaso-occlusive complications such as venous thromboembolism (VTE), pulmonary embolism, stroke, acute myocardial infarction, or other arterial or venous thrombotic events. Table 29–10 summarizes HIT, including treatment options.

Problems of Platelet Sequestration About one third of the platelets are located in the spleen. These sequestered platelets can respond when needed to bleeding or infection (Henry & Longo, 2015). In certain disease states associated with development of splenomegaly, vast numbers of platelets can become trapped in the spleen, which significantly reduces the numbers in the circulating blood.

Clinical Findings

Regardless of the underlying cause, the clinical presentation of thrombocytopenia is bleeding. This usually manifests as bleeding from the gums, bruising, or epistaxis (LeBlond, Brown, Suneja, & Szot, 2015). In general, risk of bleeding from minor trauma or surgery begins at a platelet count of 20,000 to 50,000 cells/mcL, and the patient is at risk for spontaneous bleeding at a platelet count of less than 20,000 cells/mcL. When the platelet count is less than 10,000 cells/mcL, the patient is at risk for spontaneous intracranial hemorrhage (LeBlond et al., 2015). Thrombocytopenia typically manifests itself as petechiae and purpura on the skin and mucous membranes with epistaxis and gingival bleeding as common findings. Other signs are hematuria, menorrhagia, and cutaneous bleeding.

Diagnosis and Treatment

Thrombocytopenia is clinically defined as a platelet count of less than 150,000 cells/mcL. Diagnosis is initially made through evaluation of the patient's complete blood count (CBC) with differential count. If other blood cells in the CBC are abnormally low, the bone marrow may be evaluated. If the CBC is normal, except for the low platelet count, a peripheral blood smear is obtained to directly view the platelets for evaluation of shape, size, and presence of fragments. A thorough medical history, including recent illnesses, and a physical exam are needed to explore potential etiologies. A complete drug history (prescription, nonprescription, and herbal remedies) is of great importance as drugs are the most common etiology. Moreover, nonprescription drugs, such as aspirin, nonsteroidal anti-inflammatory drugs, and some herbal supplements, may affect platelet function and bleeding time.

Treatment usually focuses on relieving the underlying cause rather than directly treating the thrombocytopenia unless the platelet count is sufficiently low to create a significant risk for bleeding. Treatment of immunologic thrombocytopenic purpura (ITP) and heparin-induced thrombocytopenia (HIT) is specific to those disease processes (refer to Table 29–10). General therapy options used to treat thrombocytopenia include corticosteroids to decrease the immune-mediated destruction; synthetic thrombopoietin (e.g., romiplostim [Nplate]) to stimulate platelet production; or splenectomy to relieve platelet sequestration problems if more conservative therapy is not sufficient. Transfusion of platelets or blood is not usually indicated unless active bleeding is present or the patient is at extremely high risk for bleeding.

Nursing Considerations

Protection from bleeding is a major concern in patients with severe thrombocytopenia. The patient is monitored for the typical signs of thrombocytopenia-related bleeding,

Quality and Safety
Thrombocytopenic Precautions

- Toothettes for oral care
- No flossing
- Electric shaver only
- Gentle nose blowing and coughing
- Avoid invasive procedures: enemas, rectal thermometers, suppositories, needlesticks
- No tourniquets
- No tampons
- Assessment for fall risk
- No aspirin or aspirin products
- Avoid constipation

such as petechiae and purpura, epistaxis, gingival bleeding, prolonged bleeding from skin wounds, stools that are bloody or tarry, brown or red urine, or menorrhagia (LeBlond et al., 2015). The patient, family, and staff are made aware of appropriate thrombocytopenia precautions that best ensure patient safety from bleeding (see the "Quality and Safety: Thombocytopenic Precautions" feature). Severe thrombocytopenia warrants close monitoring of the patient for signs of internal bleeding, particularly for intracranial hemorrhage (Shaffer & Santen, 2016). Invasive procedures are avoided if the patient is severely thrombocytopenic; however, if a procedure must be performed, platelet transfusions may be considered prior to the procedure. Patients that need vascular or neurological surgery should receive platelets to maintain concentrations over 100,000 (Thomas, 2015).

In a collaborative plan of care, the nurse is responsible for assessing factors that may be contributing to the thrombocytopenia. The nurse should monitor laboratory trends and manifestations associated with excessive bleeding, including hemorrhage. Patient safety should also be maintained throughout thrombocytopenic precautions.

Emerging Evidence

- Agents inhibiting polymerization of abnormal hemoglobin have numerous effects on adhesion and inflammation in sickle cell disease. Several novel therapies are targeting neutrophils, platelets, and inflammatory pathways in sickle cell disease. Medications targeting inflammation via modulation of coagulation and inflammatory cytokines, as well as oxidant stress and nitric oxide bioavailability, are being evaluated (*Zhang, Xu, Manwani, & Frenette, 2016*).
- In a study to define biomarkers of sepsis-induced DIC, blood samples from 82 patients admitted to a university hospital emergency department, with one or more markers of systemic inflammatory response syndrome (SIRS) criteria, included 11 serum biomarkers that assess inflammatory processes. Statistical techniques revealed two biomarkers from the 11-item panel that predicted the severity of sepsis-induced DIC in patients. A biomarker panel that included presepsin and protein C predicted the severity of sepsis-induced DIC with serum levels linked to categorization of mild,

moderate, and severe DIC. Higher levels of presepsin (greater than 900 pg/mL) and lower levels of protein C (less than 45%) were associated with severe sepsis-induced DIC. Presepsin and protein C may be useful in point-of-care testing to determine the severity of sepsis-induced DIC in critically ill hospitalized patients (*Ishikura et al., 2014*).
- Thrombopoietin is the main regulator of platelet production. Thrombopoietin receptor agonists (TRAs) are the most recent class of drugs for the treatment of immunologic thrombocytopenic purpura (ITP). This class of medication activates the thrombopoietin receptor and is associated with not only an increase in platelet counts but also a reduction in the number of bleeding events. New research with TRAs illustrates they have high efficacy and are well tolerated. A review of the literature suggests that approximately 30% of patients receiving these medications may achieve a sustained remission with safe or normal platelet counts off therapy (*Provan & Newland, 2015*).

Section Four Review

1. Thrombocytopenia is clinically defined as a platelet count of fewer than _____ cells/mcL.
   - **A.** 50,000
   - **B.** 100,000
   - **C.** 150,000
   - **D.** 200,000

2. What is an example of a disorder that causes thrombocytopenia from decreased platelet production?
   - **A.** Leukemia
   - **B.** Sickle cell disease
   - **C.** Heart failure
   - **D.** Rheumatoid arthritis

3. What causes the paradoxical thromboembolism associated with heparin-induced thrombocytopenia (HIT)?
   - **A.** Activated platelet prothrombotic activities
   - **B.** Heparin–platelet complexes
   - **C.** Accumulation of leukocytes
   - **D.** Red blood cell aggregation

4. Planning thrombocytopenia precautions for a client with severe thrombocytopenia would include which options? (Select all that apply.)
   - **A.** Aspirin for headaches
   - **B.** Electric shaver only
   - **C.** Vigorous coughing and deep breathing
   - **D.** No enemas or suppositories
   - **E.** Toothettes for oral care

Answers: 1. C, 2. A, 3. B, 4. (B, D, E)

Section Five: Disseminated Intravascular Coagulation: A Problem of Hemostasis

Acute disseminated intravascular coagulation (DIC), also called consumptive coagulopathy, is a systemic activation of the coagulation cascade. It is a complication of some underlying acute condition, such as sepsis, which is the most common (30%–50%) cause (Levi & Seligsohn, 2015). Box 29–5 lists underlying disorders associated with acute DIC in adults. The development of severe acute DIC is a critical setback for the patient because it significantly increases mortality. The widespread deleterious effects of DIC can result in multiple organ dysfunction syndrome (MODS).

The Coagulation Cascade and DIC

The normal coagulation cascade maintains homeostasis by balancing clot stimulating and inhibiting factors, with clot formation being activated and controlled locally rather than systemically. It is theorized that some underlying disorder (e.g., sepsis) injures and activates endothelial cells. Once activated, endothelial and mononuclear cells produce proinflammatory cytokines that, in turn, activate the clotting cascade (Bunn & Furie, 2017). Platelet activation, clot formation, and fibrinolysis are three important homeostatic activities of the normal coagulation process, but in the presence of DIC they are an integral part of the pathology of DIC.

Platelet Activation Platelets respond to vessel injury by becoming sticky and adhering to injured endothelium. Upon adherence, the platelets are stimulated to degranulate and release their mediators, resulting in local vasoconstriction, increased adherence of nearby platelets, and activation of more chemical mediators, all of which leads to rapid platelet plug formation. The injured vascular endothelium releases prostacyclin (a prostaglandin), which counteracts the effect of platelet mediators. This action limits (and localizes) vasoconstriction, platelet aggregation, and degranulation to the area of injury.

Clot Formation and Fibrinolysis The coagulation cascade converts prothrombin to thrombin, which then converts fibrinogen to fibrin and stimulates platelet aggregation. Fibrin binds platelets, white blood cells, and red blood cells when a clot is formed and functions to stabilize the clot. Following clot stabilization, tissue plasminogen activator (tPA) dissolves the clot by activating plasminogen to convert to plasmin. The plasmin digests fibrinogen and fibrin in the clots and in the circulation, restoring homeostasis.

DIC is a coagulation paradox—excessive systemic clotting develops with subsequent depletion of platelets and clotting factors, ultimately resulting in excessive bleeding. Platelet activation is widespread, and massive numbers of circulating platelets are consumed, eventually exhausting the available supply and thereby causing thrombocytopenia and bleeding. The thrombin level becomes excessive, which contributes to clot formation.

BOX 29–5 Underlying Disorders Associated with Acute DIC in Adults

- Bacterial and viral sepsis
- Trauma or burns
- Brain injury (gunshot)
- Heat stroke
- Snakebites
- Aortic aneurysm
- Transfusion reaction
- Severe liver disease (cirrhosis and fulminant hepatic failure)
- Solid tumors and leukemias
- Pregnancy complications (e.g., abruptio placentae, amniotic fluid embolism, HELLP syndrome)

SOURCE: Data from Levi & Seligsohn (2015).

Table 29–11 Clinical Manifestations of Disseminated Intravascular Coagulation

Basis of Findings	Clinical Manifestations
Bleeding related	**Superficial bleeding:** • Petechiae, ecchymoses • Bleeding or continuous oozing from arterial lines, catheters, and injured tissues **Internal bleeding:** • GI tract, lungs, and CNS (potentially life-threatening)
Thrombosis related	**Superficial:** • Cyanosis or ischemia, or gangrene of fingers, nose, and ears **Signs of organ ischemia or dysfunction:** • Renal: oliguria or anuria, azotemia, hematuria • Pulmonary: transient hypoxemia, pulmonary hemorrhage, acute respiratory distress syndrome (ARDS) • CNS: delirium, coma, cerebral hemorrhage, meningeal irritation • Hepatic: jaundice • Skin: necrosis, gangrene

SOURCE: Data from Levi & Seligsohn (2015).

Development of diffuse microthrombi (small vessels) and thrombi (medium to large vessels) can compromise the blood supply to organs and result in organ ischemia or necrosis, with the lungs and kidneys being the most common targets of diffuse injury (Levi & Seligsohn, 2015).

Clinical Findings of DIC

Not all cases of disseminated intravascular coagulation are severe. Some are mild, discovered only on laboratory data. Mild cases are often self-limiting and require no interventions. In severe cases, the clinical manifestations reflect the volume of blood being lost, organ-related manifestations, and the signs and symptoms of the underlying disease. Bleeding is often the first and most obvious sign of DIC with oozing seen from partially healed puncture wounds, old intravenous insertion sites, or incision sites. Extensive ischemic organ dysfunction results from microthrombi formation—for example, renal ischemia may result from microthrombosis of the afferent glomerular arterioles. The lungs may develop a range of problems from mild (transient hypoxemia) to severe (acute

respiratory distress syndrome [ARDS] or hemorrhage). The cerebral vasculature is at risk for ischemic problems or hemorrhage; therefore, changes in mental status are monitored closely. Infectious disease and prolonged hypotension contribute to hepatocellular dysfunction, which results in jaundice as bilirubin levels increase. Finally, shock is a possible complication resulting from either DIC or from the underlying pathology (Levi & Seligsohn, 2015). In severe cases of DIC, the patient can develop *purpura fulminans*, which is extensive large ecchymotic areas and hemorrhagic bullae (Koo, Nia, & Czernik, 2017). Table 29–11 summarizes some of the more common clinical findings associated with DIC.

Laboratory Studies

There is no specific laboratory test that definitively diagnoses DIC; rather, diagnosis requires close evaluation of the patient's clinical condition and laboratory results. The exact group of laboratory tests needed to diagnose and monitor DIC is not universally agreed upon; however, it usually includes a platelet count and tests of clotting time, fibrin, and fibrinogen. Table 29–12 lists some of the common adult DIC coagulation laboratory screening tests. In most cases, there may be changes of three or more parameters plus a decreased platelet count (Levi & Seligsohn, 2015).

Treatment

Morbidity and mortality are not usually related to DIC but, rather, to the underlying disease. Therefore, vigorously treating the underlying disease is imperative to correct DIC and restore the patient's vital functions. Volume replacement and correction of hypotension improve blood flow. Instituting supportive measures for the pulmonary, cardiac, and renal systems improves oxygenation, cardiac output, and fluid and electrolyte balance. Blood components, such as platelets, cryoprecipitate, and fresh-frozen plasma, may be administered if the patient is depleted of hemostatic factors, bleeding, or preparing for surgery. Thrombocytopenia is not generally treated with the administration of concentrated platelets unless the patient is actively bleeding or requires an invasive procedure and has a platelet count of less than 50,000 (Levi & Seligsohn, 2015). Hypofibrinogenemia can be treated by administering cryoprecipitate, and fresh-frozen plasma (FFP) may be

Table 29–12 Adult Disseminated Intravascular Coagulation Diagnostic Tests

Test	Trends Suggestive of DIC	Comments
Bleeding time	Prolonged	Useful in determining abnormal function of platelets
Platelet count	Decreased	Reflects increased destruction of platelets
Prothrombin time	Prolonged	Tests anticoagulant therapy
aPTT	Prolonged	Detects clotting factors and platelet disorders
Fibrinogen	Decreased	A deficiency of fibrinogen results in bleeding
Fibrin degradation product (FDP) and D-dimer	Significantly elevated	Increased FDP usually indicative of DIC caused by severe injury or trauma; D-dimer confirms presence of FDP.

SOURCE: Data from Kee (2013) and Levi & Seligsohn (2015).

ordered if the patient is depleted of coagulation factors. Heparin therapy has been shown to be of potential benefit in some cases of chronic DIC; however, in acute cases it has not demonstrated a significant reduction in mortality and may aggravate bleeding (Levi & Seligsohn, 2015). Currently, there is research interest in finding new potential therapies for treating some aspect of DIC, such as treating the underlying disease or reducing the severity of DIC. One such therapy is recombinant human soluble thrombomodulin (rhTM), a thrombin-binding agent. Early evidence suggests that in cases of sepsis-related DIC, use of rhTM may reduce in-hospital mortality among adult mechanically ventilated patients (Yamakawa et al., 2013).

Nursing Considerations

Early recognition and aggressive management of the underlying problem may improve outcomes; therefore, patients who are at risk for development of DIC should be monitored closely for bleeding and microthrombosis-related clinical manifestations. Care of the patient with DIC is primarily supportive. The nurse will closely monitor for early signs of complications, with particular focus on kidney, lung, and neurologic function, as well as for internal bleeding. Many nursing diagnoses may apply to the patient with DIC since bleeding and microthrombosis can develop in multiple body systems.

Section Five Review

1. In the presence of DIC, platelets are affected in which way?
   A. They lose their adherence qualities.
   B. They massively collect in the spleen, destroying it.
   C. They do not take part in the coagulation cascade.
   D. They activate throughout the microcirculation, exhausting the supply.

2. DIC is called a coagulation paradox because of what reason?
   A. Platelets are being destroyed while fibrinolysis is occurring.
   B. Coagulation factors are being produced at the same rate as platelets.
   C. Excessive clotting develops that ultimately results in excessive bleeding.
   D. Too much thrombin is produced while platelet production is decreased.

3. When working with a client at risk for development of DIC, the nurse would be suspicious if which assessment is noted?
   A. Harsh, nonproductive cough
   B. Oozing from around an old IV insertion site
   C. Complaints of severe generalized itching
   D. Development of hives and urticaria

4. What is the most important first step in treating DIC?
   A. Initiate heparin therapy
   B. Aggressive cryoprecipitate therapy
   C. Initiate large doses of fresh-frozen plasma
   D. Vigorous treatment of the underlying disease

Answers: 1. D, 2. C, 3. B, 4. D

Section Six: Nursing Assessment of the Patient with Problems of Erythrocytes or Platelets

Assessment of the patient with a problem of erythrocytes or platelets should include gathering data on the possible etiology, as well as assessing the effects of the disorder on major body systems. This section provides an overview of a focused nursing assessment and common nursing diagnoses that will facilitate development of a plan of care.

The Focused Nursing Assessment

Performing an assessment of the patient with a hematologic problem involving erythrocytes or platelets requires a multisystem approach. Focused assessments should be performed on the neurologic, cardiopulmonary, gastrointestinal, renal, and integumentary systems.

Focused Neurologic Assessment The neurologic status of the patient can change related to tissue hypoxia, bleeding, or clotting. The nurse's neurologic assessment may include determining level of consciousness (LOC), pupillary checks, cranial nerve assessment, and monitoring for increased intracranial pressure. The patient's state of consciousness is a sensitive indicator of tissue oxygenation; thus, in the presence of severe anemia (oxygen transport problem), LOC should be closely monitored. Cranial bleeding may manifest itself as headache, weakness, altered LOC, pupillary changes, altered cranial nerve functions, or symptoms of increased intracranial pressure.

Focused Cardiopulmonary Assessment Hematologic problems can cause significant alterations in the hemodynamic and oxygenation status of the high-acuity patient. In the presence of anemia, infection, bleeding, or clotting, the nurse can anticipate development of dysrhythmias or compensatory vital signs, such as tachycardia, tachypnea, and changes in blood pressure. Blood pressure may rise with oxygenation problems or may fall with hypovolemia from bleeding. The patient may develop dyspnea or orthopnea associated with tissue hypoxia. Sputum should be checked for occult blood in patients with bleeding problems. If the hematologic problem (e.g., DIC or severe thrombocytopenia) causes increased risk for hemorrhage, vital signs and hemodynamic parameters should be monitored closely for hypovolemic shock.

Focused Gastrointestinal Assessment Hepatomegaly and splenomegaly are associated with several hematologic disorders; thus, the nurse should palpate for their presence. Patients with bleeding disorders should have all gastrointestinal secretions closely monitored for occult or gross bleeding. Intestinal bleeding is also associated with cramping, diarrhea, and melena.

Focused Renal Assessments Patients with bleeding problems should have their urine routinely tested for occult blood. If hemoglobin is free in the urine, hemoglobinuria develops, with its characteristically port-wine–colored urine. Urine output should also be monitored for oliguria and anuria. Nurses may also see an elevation in BUN-to-creatinine ratio in patients with problems of erythrocytes or hemostasis.

Focused Integumentary Assessments In the patient with anemia, monitoring the skin, nail beds, and mucous membranes for the presence and degree of cyanosis is important. If the patient develops thrombocytopenia, the skin and mucous membranes should be examined for petechiae, purpura, and ecchymoses. Patients experiencing hemolytic anemia should be monitored for jaundice because of excessive bilirubin from RBC destruction. The jaundice may also be accompanied by pruritus.

Nursing Considerations

A plan of care is developed around the manifestations and complications associated with each disorder. These can be divided into four major underlying problems:

- Tissue hypoxia
- Hypertension
- Stasis of blood flow
- Bleeding

Tissue Hypoxia Impaired oxygen transport associated with the anemias causes varying degrees of tissue hypoxia, depending on the severity of the anemia. Fatigue is due to decreased energy production. A lack of energy may cause abnormalities in breathing. Activity intolerance stems from an oxygen supply-and-demand imbalance. A decreased oxygen-carrying capacity of the blood may cause an altered tissue perfusion. Individuals with tissue hypoxia sometimes experience acute pain and may have a higher risk for injury. Potential complications associated with tissue hypoxia include organ ischemia and infarction.

Hypertension Hypertension is a common finding in polycythemia related to increased intravascular volume and increased RBC mass. Individuals with hypertension are at risk for decreased tissue perfusion along with acute pain, which manifests as a headache. Potential complications associated with hypertension include stroke, heart failure or myocardial infarction, renal dysfunction, and others.

Stasis of Blood Flow Stagnant blood flow is particularly associated with polycythemia (extreme erythrocytosis). Venous stasis may cause altered tissue perfusion. Stasis of blood flow places the patient at risk for thrombus and thromboembolism complications.

Bleeding The bleeding related to decreased platelet count (thrombocytopenia) is primarily caused by aplastic anemia, leukemia, and chemotherapy. Patients with excessive bleeding may experience a fluid volume deficit due to intravascular fluid volume loss. The decreased intravascular volume may also cause decreased cardiac output.

Section Six Review

1. The compensatory vital sign changes associated with anemia, infection, and bleeding result in which parameter change?
   A. Elevated temperature
   B. Increased heart rate
   C. Decreased respiratory rate
   D. Decreased blood pressure

2. What conditions often result in hypertension in the client with polycythemia?
   A. Tissue hypoxia and pain
   B. Pain and infection
   C. Increases in RBC mass and intravascular volume
   D. Weakened heart and renal function

3. Polycythemia puts the client at risk for which complication?
   A. Bleeding
   B. Thrombus
   C. Hypertension
   D. Hypotention

4. The activity intolerance created by some of the hematologic disorders is specifically related to what condition?
   A. Intravascular fluid volume loss
   B. O_2 supply-and-demand imbalance
   C. Decreased systemic blood flow
   D. Inadequate secondary defenses

Answers: 1. B, 2. C, 3. B, 4. B

Clinical Reasoning Checkpoint

MP, a 32-year-old male, is in the trauma intensive care unit (TICU) as the result of a motorcycle–tree crash. MP has multiple fractures and contusions. On ICU day 7, MP's status begins to deteriorate, and it is determined that he has developed sepsis. On ICU day 8, the nurse notes petechiae on MP's trunk. In addition, oozing of blood is noted from several discontinued intravenous insertion sites and suture lines. The nurse suspects that MP may be developing disseminated intravascular coagulation (DIC) and contacts the intensivist. The following labs are ordered: bleeding time, platelet count, PT and aPTT, factor I (fibrinogen), fibrin degradation product (FDP), and D-dimer.

1. Briefly explain the basis for the nurse's suspicion that MP has developed DIC.

2. For each lab ordered by the intensivist: (a) indicate whether the value would be abnormally elevated or decreased if MP has DIC, and (b) explain the rationale for the abnormality.

Lab Test (units)	(a) Elevated or Decreased	(b) Reason for Abnormality
Bleeding time (minutes)		
Platelet count (cells)		
Prothrombin (PT) (seconds)		
Factor I (fibrinogen) (mg/dL)		
FDP (fibrin degradation product) (mcg/dL) and D-dimer (mg/dL)		

3. MP develops oliguria (abnormally low urine output) and azotemia (elevated serum nitrogen waste products) as a result of his DIC. Briefly explain the significance of this problem and how it can result from DIC.

4. MP's platelet count is 45,250, and his latest laboratory values show that he has significant hypofibrinogenemia. What interventions can the nurse anticipate in response to these values?

5. While providing supportive therapy for MP, what is the most important goal for treating his DIC?

Chapter 29 Review

1. A client who is diagnosed with idiopathic aplastic anemia has a reticulocyte count of 30,000/mcL. This count suggests which problem?

   1. Overproduction of RBCs in bone marrow
   2. Small, pale RBCs
   3. Bone marrow depression or failure
   4. RBCs are being rapidly hemolyzed

2. A 16-year-old African American male is brought into the emergency department with a chief complaint of severe chest pain after playing basketball. The client's medical history is positive for sickle cell disease (SCD). What, if any, is the probable relationship between the client's playing basketball and the onset of his pain?

   1. A high level of activity could have precipitated a deoxygenation episode.
   2. Air pollution where he was playing may have triggered an allergic response.
   3. He drank two caffeinated drinks while playing; the caffeine could have triggered a crisis onset.
   4. His playing basketball and the onset of his chest pain probably had no relationship.

3. A nurse is collecting historical information from a client diagnosed with secondary polycythemia. Which findings would possibly be implicated in this disorder? (Select all that apply.)

   1. The client has lived at high altitude for several years.
   2. The client smokes one package of cigarettes per day.
   3. The client donates blood three or four times per year.
   4. The client works as a computer analyst.
   5. The client has a history of sleep apnea.

4. A client has developed heparin-induced thrombocytopenia (HIT). While planning an explanation of this disorder for the client, the nurse considers which pathophysiology?

   1. Activation of cytokines (such as interleukins) by heparin, resulting in inappropriate activation of the coagulation cascade
   2. Formation of platelet–heparin–PF4 complexes that trigger increased levels of fibrinogen in the blood
   3. Activation of platelets by heparin–Fc receptor complexes resulting in prothrombotic activity
   4. Formation of antibody–heparin–PF4 complexes with subsequent activation of platelets by the antibody portion of the complexes

5. In order to best ensure a positive client outcome, the nurse anticipates which collaborative management of the client who has disseminated intravascular coagulation (DIC)?

    1. Close titration of IV fluid rate to optimize cardiac output

    2. Platelet replacement therapy through transfusions

    3. Measures to decrease the risk of vascular occlusions

    4. Aggressive treatment of the underlying problem

6. A nurse is providing care to a client who has been hospitalized for recurrent gastrointestinal bleeding. Which neurological assessment would be most significant for this nurse to monitor?

    1. Pupillary response

    2. Assessment of cranial nerves

    3. Level of consciousness

    4. Presence of headache

7. It is suspected that a client is experiencing hemolytic anemia secondary to exposure to a toxin at work. The nurse would expect which findings from the client's laboratory studies? (Select all that apply.)

    1. A decrease in RBCs

    2. A decrease in bilirubin levels

    3. A slight decrease in LDH levels

    4. No blood in the urine

    5. An increase in reticulocyte levels

8. A client in sickling crisis asks, "Why does this hurt so much?" Which nursing reponse is indicated?

    1. "When your sickled blood cells are destroyed by your spleen, they release bilirubin, which damages your tissues, resulting in pain."

    2. "A substance called bradykinin is released from your red blood cells when they are damaged. That substance causes muscle pain."

    3. "The sickled cells block the very small vessels in your tissues and keep them from getting enough oxygen. That causes pain."

    4. "We know that sickle cell disease is very complex, but no one has discovered exactly why the pain occurs."

9. A nurse is providing discharge education for a client diagnosed with polycythemia vera. Which teaching points should the nurse include? (Select all that apply.)

    1. "Be sure to report any easy bruising or bleeding of your gums."

    2. "Be certain to have your eyesight tested every six months."

    3. "If you develop pain in your chest or shortness of breath, contact your healthcare provider."

    4. "Avoid foods that have high carbohydrate levels, such as potatoes, pasta, or breads."

    5. "Do not drink alcohol."

10. A client developed thrombocytopenia while receiving heparin therapy. The heparin has been discontinued. Which anticoagulant therapy would the nurse expect to start for this client?

    1. Lepirudin (Refludan)

    2. Warfarin (Coumadin)

    3. Acetylsalicylic acid (aspirin)

    4. Hydroxyurea (Hydrea)

Answers to questions found inside your textbook are available on the faculty resources site. Please consult with your instructor.

References

Adamson, J. W., & Longo, D. L. (2015). Chapter 77: Anemia and polycythemia. In D. L. Kasper, A. S. Fauci, S. L. Hauser, D. L. Longo, J. L. Jameson, & J. Loscalzo (Eds.), *Harrison's principles of internal medicine* (19th ed.). Retrieved January 25, 2017, from http://accessmedicine.mhmedical.com.ezproxy.uky.edu/content.aspx?bookid=1130&sectionid=79727787

American Society of Gene & Cell Therapy. (2017). Blood disorders and anemias. Retrieved March 6, 2017, from http://www.asgct.org/general-public/educational-resources/gene-therapy-and-cell-therapy-for-diseases/blood-disorders-and-anemias

Brousse, V., Makani, J., & Rees, D. C. (2014). Management of sickle cell disease in the community. *British Medical Journal*, 348, g1765. doi:10.1136/bmj.g1765

Bunn, H. (2017). Chapter 9: Sickle cell disease. In J. C. Aster & H. Bunn (Eds.), *Pathophysiology of blood disorders* (2nd ed.). Retrieved February 22, 2017, from http://accessmedicine.mhmedical.com.ezproxy.uky.edu/content.aspx?bookid=1900&sectionid=137395019

Bunn, H., & Furie, B. (2017). Chapter 16: Acquired coagulation disorders. In J. C. Aster & H. Bunn (Eds.), *Pathophysiology of blood disorders* (2nd ed.). Retrieved February 24, 2017, from http://accessmedicine.mhmedical.com.ezproxy.uky.edu/content.aspx?bookid=1900&sectionid=137395412

Centers for Disease Control and Prevention (CDC). (2016). Sickle cell disease. *Data and statistics*. Retrieved February 17, 2017, from https://www.cdc.gov/ncbddd/sicklecell/data.html

Damon, L. E., & Andreadis, C. (2017). Chapter 13: Blood disorders. In M. A. Papadakis, S. J. McPhee, & M. W. Rabow (Eds.), *Current medical diagnosis & treatment 2017.* Retrieved February 15, 2017, from http://accessmedicine.mhmedical.com.ezproxy.uky.edu/content.aspx?bookid=1843&sectionid=135708533

Henry, P. H., & Longo, D. L. (2015). Chapter 79: Enlargement of lymph nodes and spleen. In D. Kasper, A. Fauci, S. Hauser, D. Longo, J. Jameson, & J. Loscalzo (Eds.), *Harrison's principles of internal medicine* (19th ed.). Retrieved February 24, 2017, from http://accessmedicine.mhmedical.com.ezproxy.uky.edu/content.aspx?bookid=1130&sectionid=79727886

Ishikura, H., Nishida, T., Murai, A., Nakamura, Y., Irie, Y., Tanaka, J., & Umemura, T. (2014). New diagnostic strategy for sepsis-induced disseminated intravascular coagulation: A prospective single-center observational study. *Critical Care, 18*(1), R19. http://doi.org/10.1186/cc1370

Jackups, R., Sanfilippo, K., Wang, T., & Blinder, M. (2014). Hematologic disorders and transfusion therapy. *The Washington manual of medical therapeutics* (34th ed.). Philadelphia, PA: Wolters Kluwer.

Jameson, J., & Kopp, P. (2015). Chapter 82: Genes, the environment, and disease. In D. Kasper, A. Fauci, S. Hauser, D. Longo, J. Jameson, & J. Loscalzo (Eds.), *Harrison's principles of internal medicine* (19th ed.). Retrieved February 24, 2017, from http://accessmedicine.mhmedical.com.ezproxy.uky.edu/content.aspx?bookid=1130&sectionid=79728075

Janz, T., & Hamilton, G. (2014). Chapter 121: Anemia, polycythemia, and white blood cell disorders. In J. Marx (Ed.), *Rosen's emergency medicine* (8th ed., pp. 1586–1605). Retrieved May 23, 2017, from https://www.clinicalkey.com/#!/browse/book/3-s2.0-C20101679059

Kasper, D. L., Fauci, A. S., Hauser, S. L., Longo, D. L., Jameson, J., & Loscalzo, J. (2016). Chapter 8: Transfusion and pheresis therapy. In D. Kasper, A. Fauci, S. Hauser, D. Longo, J. Jameson, & J. Loscalzo (Eds.), *Harrison's manual of medicine* (19th ed.). Retrieved January 25, 2017, from http://accessmedicine.mhmedical.com.ezproxy.uky.edu/content.aspx?bookid=1820&sectionid=127553783

Kee, J. L. (2013). *Laboratory and diagnostic tests with nursing implications.* Upper Saddle River, NJ: Pearson.

Konkle, B. A. (2015). Chapter 140: Disorders of platelets and vessel wall. In D. A. Kasper, S. Fauci, D. Hauser, J. Longo, J. Jameson, & J. Loscalzo (Eds.), *Harrison's principles of internal medicine* (19th ed.). Retrieved January 25, 2017, from http://accessmedicine.mhmedical.com.ezproxy.uky.edu/content.aspx?bookid=1130&sectionid=79732426

Koo, B., Nia, J. K., & Czernik, A. (2017). Chapter 47: Skin complications. In J. M. Oropello, S. M. Pastores, & V. Kvetan (Eds.), *Critical care.* Retrieved February 22, 2017, from http://accessmedicine.mhmedical.com.ezproxy.uky.edu/content.aspx?bookid=1944&sectionid=143518968

Kurniali, P. C., Curry, S., Brennan, K. W., Velletri, K., Shaik, M., Schwartz, K. A., & McCormack, E. (2014). A retrospective study investigating the incidence and predisposing factors of hospital-acquired anemia. *Anemia.* Retrieved February 27, 2017, from http://dx.doi.org/10.1155/2014/634582

Leavitt, A. D., & Minichiello, T. (2016). Disorders of hemostasis, thrombosis, & antithrombotic therapy. In M. Papadakis, S. J. McPhee, & M. W. Rabow (Eds.), *Current medical diagnosis & treatment 2017.* Retrieved February 24, 2017, from http://accessmedicine.mhmedical.com.ezproxy.uky.edu/content.aspx?bookid=1843&sectionid=135709357

LeBlond, R. F., Brown, D. D., Suneja, M., & Szot, J. F. (2015). Nonregional systems and diseases. In R. F. LeBlond, D. D. Brown, M. Suneja, & J. F. Szot (Eds.), *DeGowin's diagnostic examination* (10th ed.). Retrieved February 22, 2017, from http://accessmedicine.mhmedical.com.ezproxy.uky.edu/content.aspx?bookid=1192&sectionid=68665331

Levi, M., & Seligsohn, U. (2015). Chapter 129: Disseminated intravascular coagulation. In K. Kaushansky, M. A. Lichtman, J. T. Prchal, M. M. Levi, O. W. Press, L. J. Burns, & M. Caligiuri (Eds.), *Williams hematology* (9th ed.). Retrieved February 22, 2017, from http://accessmedicine.mhmedical.com.ezproxy.uky.edu/content.aspx?bookid=1581&sectionid=108084280

Longo, D. L. (2016). Chapter 45: Anemia and polycythemia. In D. Kasper, A. Fauci, S. Hauser, D. Longo, J. Jameson, & J. Loscalzo (Eds.), *Harrison's principles of internal medicine* (19th ed.). Retrieved April 4, 2017, from http://accessmedicine.mhmedical.com.ezproxy.uky.edu/content.aspx?bookid=1820&sectionid=127554643

Luzzatto, L. (2014). Chapter 129: Hemolytic anemias and anemia due to acute blood loss. In D. Kasper, A. Fauci, S. Hauser, D. Longo, J. Jameson, & J. Loscalzo (Eds.), *Harrison's principles of internal medicine* (19th ed.). Retrieved February 15, 2017, from http://accessmedicine.mhmedical.com.ezproxy.uky.edu/content.aspx?bookid=1130&sectionid=79731477

Natarajan, K., & Kutlar, A. (2015). Chapter 49: Disorders of hemoglobin structure: Sickle cell anemia and related abnormalities. In K. Kaushansky, M. A. Lichtman, J. T. Prchal, M. M. Levi, O. W. Press, L. I. Burns, & M. Caligiuri (Eds.), *Williams hematology* (9th ed.). Retrieved January 25, 2017, from http://accessmedicine.mhmedical.com.ezproxy.uky.edu/content.aspx?bookid=1581&sectionid=108061089

Prchal, J. T. (2016). Chapter 34: Clinical manifestations and classification of erythrocyte disorders. In K. Kaushansky, M. A. Lichtman, J. T. Prchal, M. M. Levi, O. W. Press, L. J.Burns, & M. Caligiuri (Eds.), *Williams hematology* (9th ed.). Retrieved July 20, 2017, from http://accessmedicine.mhmedical.com.ezproxy.uky.edu/content.aspx?bookid=1581&sectionid=94303608

Provan, D., & Newland, A. C. (2015). Current management of primary immune thrombocytopenia. *Advances in Therapy, 32*(10), 875–887. doi:10.1007/s12325-015-0251-z

Rose, M. G., & Berliner, N. (2016). Chapter 47: Disorders of red blood cells. In T. E. Andreoli, I. J. Benjamin, R. C. Griggs, & E. J. Wing (Eds.), *Andreoli and Carpenter's Cecil essentials of medicine* (9th ed., pp. 502–514). St. Louis, MO: Elsevier/Saunders.

Segel, G. B., & Lichtman, M. A. (2015). Chapter 35: Aplastic anemia: Acquired and inherited. In K. Kaushansky, M. A. Lichtman, J. T. Prchal, M. M. Levi, O. W. Press, L. I. Burn, & M. Caligiuri (Eds.), *Williams hematology* (9th ed.). Retrieved February 24, 2017, from http://accessmedicine.mhmedical.com.ezproxy.uky.edu/content.aspx?bookid=1581&sectionid=94303673

Shaffer, R. W., & Santen, S. A. (2016). Chapter 233: Acquired bleeding disorders. In J. E. Tintinalli, J. Stapczynski, O. Ma, D. M. Yealy, G. D. Meckler, & D. M. Cline (Eds.), *Tintinalli's emergency medicine: A comprehensive study guide* (8th ed.). Retrieved February 24, 2017, from http://accessmedicine.mhmedical.com.ezproxy.uky.edu/content.aspx?bookid=1658&sectionid=109416452

Shenoy, S. (2013). Hematopoietic stem-cell transplantation for sickle cell disease: Current evidence and opinions. *Therapeutic Advances in Hematology, 4*(5), 335–344. doi:10.1177/2040620713483063

Somand, D. M., & Ward, K. R. (2016). Chapter 13: Fluid and blood resuscitation in traumatic shock. In J. E. Tintinalli, J. Stapczynski, O. Ma, D. M. Yealy, G. D. Meckler, & D. M. Cline (Eds.), *Tintinalli's emergency medicine: A comprehensive study guide* (8th ed.). Retrieved February 22, 2017, from http://accessmedicine.mhmedical.com.ezproxy.uky.edu/content.aspx?bookid=1658&sectionid=109385029

Tefferi, A., & Barbui, T. (2017). Polycythemia vera and essential thrombocythemia: 2017 update on diagnosis, risk-stratification, and management. *American Journal of Hematology, 92*(1), 94–108. doi:10.1002/ajh.24607

Thomas, K. (2015). Chapter 90: Bleeding disorders. In J. B. Hall, G. A. Schmidt, & J. P. Kress (Eds.), *Principles of critical care* (4th ed.). Retrieved January 25, 2017, from http://accessmedicine.mhmedical.com.ezproxy.uky.edu/content.aspx?bookid=1340&sectionid=80036628

Weitz, J. I. (2015). Chapter 143: Antiplatelet, anticoagulant, and fibrinolytic drugs. In D. L. Kasper, A. S. Fauci, S. L. Hauser, D. L. Longo, J. L. Jameson, & J. Loscalzo (Eds.), *Harrison's principles of internal medicine* (19th ed.). Retrieved February 22, 2017, from http://accessmedicine.mhmedical.com.ezproxy.uky.edu/content.aspx?bookid=1130&sectionid=79732627

Williams-Johnson, J., & Williams, E. (2016). Chapter 236: Sickle cell disease and hereditary hemolytic anemias. In J. E. Tintinalli, J. Stapczynski, O. Ma, D. M. Yealy, G. D. Meckler, & D. M. Cline (Eds.), *Tintinalli's emergency medicine: A comprehensive study guide* (8th ed.). Retrieved February 22, 2017, from http://accessmedicine.mhmedical.com.ezproxy.uky.edu/content.aspx?bookid=1658&sectionid=109386508

Wilson, C. T., & Clebone, A. (2014). Chapter 1: Initial assessment and management of the trauma patient. In C. S. Scher (Ed.), *Anaesthesia for trauma new evidence and new challenges*. New York, NY: Springer.

Yamakawa, K., Ogura, H., Fujimi, S., Morikawa, M., Ogawa, Y., Mohri, . . . Shimazu, T. (2013). Recombinant human soluble thrombomodulin in sepsis-induced disseminated intravascular coagulation: A multicenter propensity score analysis. *Intensive Care Medicine, 39*, 644. doi:10.1007/s00134-013-2822-2

Yawn, B. P., Buchanan, G. R., Afenyi-Annan, A. N., Ballas, S. K., Hassell, K. L., James, A. H., . . . John-Sowah, J. (2014). Management of sickle cell disease: Summary of the 2014 evidence-based report by expert panel members. *Journal of the American Medical Association, 312*(10), 1033–1048. doi:10.1001/jama.2014.10517

Zhang, D., Xu, C., Manwani, D., & Frenette, P. S. (2016). Neutrophils, platelets, and inflammatory pathways at the nexus of sickle cell disease pathology. *Blood, 127*(7), 801–809. doi:https://doi.org/10.1182/blood-2015-09-618538

Chapter 30
Alterations in White Blood Cell Function and Oncologic Emergencies

⌄ Learning Outcomes

30.1 Discuss the etiology, pathophysiology, clinical manifestations, and management of neutropenia.

30.2 Explain hypersensitivity responses, including types I through IV and drug induced.

30.3 Describe autoimmunity and management considerations for patients with an autoimmune disease.

30.4 Discuss the etiology, pathophysiology, clinical manifestations, and management of acute leukemias.

30.5 Apply knowledge of oncologic emergencies and nursing implications to clinical practice.

30.6 Discuss human immunodeficiency virus (HIV) infection and its nursing implications in high-acuity patients.

30.7 Relate the effects of aging, malnutrition, stress, and trauma on the functions of the adult immune system.

30.8 Demonstrate competency in the assessment and care of the immunocompromised patient.

This chapter presents alterations of leukocyte (white blood cell) function that patients in high-acuity settings are likely to experience. Many of these alterations—such as leukemia, HIV/AIDS, neutropenia, and hypersensitivity responses—are usually managed outside of a high-acuity setting, often on an outpatient basis. However, when complications arise, these alterations can precipitate physiologic crises, requiring intensive treatment in a high-acuity environment. The chapter also provides an overview of oncologic emergencies—potentially life-threatening crises that can result from cancer chemotherapy. This chapter builds on foundational knowledge about white blood cells and associated laboratory tests presented in Chapter 28; therefore, it is recommended that the reader review normal WBC function before beginning this chapter.

Section One: Neutropenia

Neutrophils are white blood cells (WBCs) that are first-line responders to pathogenic invasion and account for about 60% of circulating WBCs. Bone marrow takes 10 to 14 days to mature a neutrophil; once released into the circulation, the neutrophil lives only 6 to 8 hours. Neutropenia is a reduction of these first responders, placing the patient at risk for infections and sepsis.

Neutropenia (granulocytopenia) refers to an abnormally low level of neutrophils—below 50% (1000/mcL) of the total WBC count. Neutropenia is not a disease; rather, it is an important symptom of an underlying problem. The neutropenic person is at a high risk for developing an infection, and the lower the neutrophil count, the higher the risk. The absolute neutrophil count (ANC) is the most

Table 30–1 Neutropenia Classification

Absolute Neutrophil Count	Severity of Neutropenia
1000 to 1500/mcL	Mild
500 to 999/mcL	Moderate
Less than 500/mcL	Severe
Less than 100/mcL	Profound

SOURCE: Data from Stapczynski (2016) and White & Ybarra (2014).

Table 30–2 Clinical Presentation of Agranulocytosis in Adults

Type of Data	Presentation
History	Rapid onset of malaise, fever, chills Stomatitis, pharyngitis with painful swallowing Patient report of recent new drug use, exposure to chemicals or physical agents, recent viral or bacterial infection, or preexisting autoimmune disease
Physical	High-grade fever of at least 100.9°F (38.3°C) or a fever of 100.4°F (38°C) or higher for at least 1 hour Tachycardia, tachypnea Hypotension if septic shock is present Oral examination: swollen, painful gums; mouth ulcers Integument: skin infections with edema (usually without redness or pus formation)
Lab studies	Absolute neutrophil count (ANC): less than 500 cells/mcL

SOURCE: Data from Gibson and Berliner (2014); Stapczynski (2016); and White and Ybarra (2014).

accurate measure of the total number of neutrophils. It is calculated as the number of WBCs multiplied by the sum of the percentage of polymorphonuclear neutrophils (PMNs) (mature) and the percentage of band (immature) neutrophils (ANC = WBC × [PMNs + bands]). **Agranulocytosis** is the alteration that occurs when ANC is less than 500/mcL. The degree of neutropenia can vary; defining parameters for severity are presented in Table 30–1. The cause of neutropenia can be intrinsic (primary, usually caused by a genetic mutation) or acquired (secondary, from some underlying disease or medication). The focus of this section is on acquired neutropenia, which is relatively common in high-acuity illnesses. As neutrophil counts decrease to less than 500/mcL, the risk for severe infection increases (White & Ybarra, 2014).

Underlying Causes

Neutropenia is usually an acquired complication that is associated with either premature destruction or decreased production of neutrophils.

Premature Neutrophil Destruction   Premature death of neutrophils is most commonly associated with a drug-induced hypersensitivity response. Certain drugs (e.g., some antibiotics) can cause development of drug–antibody immune complexes, which then attach to and destroy neutrophils. Neutropenia can also result from an isolated autoimmune process, or it can result as a complication of another autoimmune disorder, such as systemic lupus erythematosus (SLE). Furthermore, the spleen is capable of entrapping neutrophils and destroying them; this sometimes occurs with disorders that cause splenomegaly.

Decreased Neutrophil Production   Decreased production of neutrophils can occur by direct injury to the bone marrow (e.g., aplastic anemia), by overcrowding of normal bone marrow components from infiltration of malignant cells (e.g., leukemia), or by bone marrow suppression from cancer chemotherapy or irradiation. It can also result from severe nutritional deficits (e.g., starvation) and vitamin B_{12} or folate deficiency, chemical exposure, or infectious agents such as a virus. Drugs that are associated with a high incidence of agranulocytosis (severe neutropenia) defined above as an absolute neutrophil count (ANC) of less than 500 cells/mcL, include certain antibiotics, antifungals, antiinflammatory agents, antithyroid drugs, psychotropic agents, antiepileptics, cardiovascular drugs, and some diuretics (Gibson & Berliner, 2014). Table 30–2 summarizes the history and clinical presentation typical of the adult patient with agranulocytosis.

Clinical Manifestations

Neutropenia causes altered responses to inflammation and infection because neutrophils are the first line of internal defense against infection and play a crucial part in the inflammatory process. The source of the infection is usually from the person's own normal skin or gastrointestinal flora because the body is host to a variety of pathogens, both externally and internally. Under normal circumstances, these pathogens remain harmless, but in conditions such as neutropenia they can invade the body and cause serious and sometimes life-threatening infections.

The clinical manifestations associated with infection are altered to the degree that the neutrophil count is compromised. In mild-to-moderate cases of neutropenia, a normal inflammatory response to infection occurs (redness, swelling, heat, and fever) with exudate formation. These signs and symptoms become significantly blunted or disappear when the ANC drops below 500 cells/mcL. Fever is an exception, as it is produced by proinflammatory cytokines that come from most of the leukocytes, rather than requiring sufficient numbers of neutrophils. Thus, with severe neutropenia, fever may be the only remaining sign of inflammation and infection. A moderate fever that lasts for more than 1 hour may become the primary sign—often no higher than 100.4°F (38°C) if leukopenia is present. The absence of overt inflammation makes diagnosis of acute infections difficult. For example, a patient could have severe bacterial pneumonia for 3 or 4 days before the lungs develop sufficient exudate that it is evidenced in the sputum and is visible on a chest x-ray. The presence of fever associated with severe neutropenia (febrile neutropenia) is a critical event that must be treated immediately (Stapczynski, 2016). The clinical presentation of patients with agranulocytosis is fairly predictable; and without appropriate therapy, the patient usually develops sepsis.

Related Pharmacotherapy
Severe Neutropenia or Agranulocytosis

Granulocyte-Colony Stimulating Factors (G-CSF)

Filgrastim (Neupogen); long-acting form, pegfilgrastim (Neulasta)

Action and Uses

A growth factor cytokine (granulocyte-colony stimulating factor [G-CSF]) primarily stimulates increased proliferation and differentiation of neutrophils in the bone marrow, and it enhances phagocytic and cytotoxic functions of existing neutrophils. It is useful for reduction of severity and shortening recovery time from severe neutropenic episodes, including agranulocytosis. It is also used for speeding postcancer chemotherapy neutrophil recovery.

Dosages (Adult)

IV: 5 mcg/kg/day via infusion over 30 minutes; if needed, increase by 5 mcg/kg/day for maximum of 30 mcg/kg/day
Subcutaneous: 5 mcg/kg/day as single dose; if needed, increase by 5 mcg/kg/day for maximum of 20 mcg/kg/day

Major Adverse Effects

Most common: bone pain, fever, and fatigue

SOURCE: Data from Wilson et al. (2016).

Nursing Implications

Obtain a health history, including current infections.
Do not administer the G-CSF within 24 hours before or following cytotoxic chemotherapy because this will decrease the effectiveness of the chemotherapy.
Obtain baseline CBC with differential count, renal and liver function tests, uric acid levels and ECG; follow-up 2 times/week regarding CBC and to monitor recovery; monitor platelet count.
Discontinue filgrastim if ANC rises to greater than 10,000 cells/mm^3.
Assess for presence and level of bone pain.
Monitor temperature, neutrophil count, and any signs of infection.
Filgrastim is administered IV or SC daily; pegfilgrastim is administered once.
Drug vial precautions: Store in refrigerator. Enter a single vial only once; each vial is one dose only; discard vial after 6 hours if left at room temperature. The drug may warm to room temperature prior to administration—but no longer than 6 hours (measures to minimize contamination and bacterial growth).

Management

Early identification and aggressive treatment of the underlying cause of the neutropenia is imperative. Investigation of the cause may include antibody testing, bone marrow testing, or discontinuing a suspicious drug. Empiric antibiotic therapy is often initiated, with close attention being placed on monitoring for secondary infections. A granulocyte-colony stimulating factor (G-CSF) drug, either filgrastim (Neupogen) or its long-acting form, pegfilgrastim (Neulasta), may be administered to try to stimulate the bone marrow to increase production of neutrophils. G-CSF therapy has significantly improved patient recovery from an episode of agranulocytosis (Gibson & Berliner, 2014). For a summary of G-CSF therapy, refer to the "Related Pharmacotherapy: Severe Neutropenia or Agranulocytosis" feature. Nursing management of the immunosuppressed patient is discussed in Section Eight of this chapter.

Section One Review

1. What is the most common cause of premature destruction of neutrophils?
   A. Environmental toxins
   B. Autoimmune disorder
   C. Drug–antibody reaction
   D. Bacterial infection

2. Decreased production of neutrophils results from which type of insult?
   A. Splenomegaly
   B. Hypersensitivity response
   C. Circulating immune complexes
   D. Bone marrow suppression

3. What is usually the primary symptom of infection when severe neutropenia is present?
   A. Pus formation
   B. Fever
   C. Local edema
   D. Local erythema

4. What is one of the most common adverse effects of the drug filgrastim (Neupogen) used to stimulate proliferation and differentiation of neutrophils?
   A. Bone pain
   B. Nausea
   C. Headache
   D. Stomach upset

Answers: 1. C, 2. D, 3. B, 4. A

Section Two: Disorders of Hyperactive Immune Response: Hypersensitivity

Some immune responses can cause an excessive or inappropriate reaction referred to as **hypersensitivity** (Crowley, 2013). Hypersensitivity disorders are classified by cell involvement and include types I, II, III, and IV. Types I, II, and III involve humoral (antibody-mediated) immunity associated with specific immunoglobulins (antibodies), and type IV response is T-cell mediated. Many hypersensitivity responses manifest themselves with mild to moderately distressful symptoms, such as watery eyes, sneezing, and nasal congestion. Strong hypersensitivity responses, however, are capable of triggering a severe response—for example, anaphylactic shock response, severe transfusion reaction, or allergic asthma response.

Type I (Allergic) Hypersensitivity Response

The **type I (allergic) hypersensitivity response** is also referred to as allergic response or anaphylactic response and involves the binding of IgE to receptors on mast cells. **Mast cells** are large granule-containing tissue cells that are located in connective tissue throughout the body. The heaviest concentration of mast cells is in the skin and mucous membranes (e.g., gastrointestinal, genitourinary, and respiratory tracts), which places them in close proximity to the sites where antigens are most likely to appear (where the internal body interfaces with the external environment). Mast cells contain potent mediators, such as histamine, heparin, and leukotriene that, when stimulated, trigger strong vascular smooth muscle and hematologic actions. Table 30–3 lists the major mediators and some of their activities.

The type I response requires repeated exposures—a sensitization (priming or *primary response*) phase and subsequent exposure. When a person initially encounters an allergen–antigen (e.g., pollen), IgE binds to Fc receptors on the mast cells, which sensitizes the cells (e.g., pollen would trigger IgE antibodies to bind with Fc receptors on the mast

cells in the respiratory tract). The mast cells are now primed for an allergic response. With subsequent exposure to the same allergen–antigen, the allergic response (antigen–IgE–mast cell) interaction is triggered (called the secondary response), causing rapid degranulation of the primed mast cells and release of mediators and chemotactic factors—and the person becomes symptomatic. Figure 30–1 illustrates the type I IgE-mediated hypersensitivity response. The type I response can affect tissues at the local or systemic level.

Local Type I　Allergic asthma and allergic rhinitis (hay fever) are especially noteworthy examples of a local type I response. Type I allergies tend to be atopic—that is, a particular type of allergy tends to have a genetic predisposition. Common allergic rhinitis is a fairly benign process (local symptoms of stuffy and runny nose, sneezing, and watering eyes), whereas other local type I disorders, such as allergic asthma, can cause severe, even life-threatening symptoms. In allergic asthma, the chemical mediators cause smooth muscle constriction in the bronchioles, and histamine release results in edema of the bronchial tissues. The combination of bronchiolar constriction and bronchial edema, when severe, may require emergency treatment to prevent death by asphyxiation. Antihistamines may be used to block the effect of histamine release, but corticosteroids often are administered to suppress the entire immune response. Another example of local type I response that is of particular interest to healthcare professionals is latex glove allergy, which can cause mild to severe allergic reactions.

Systemic (Anaphylaxis) Type I　**Anaphylaxis** is a severe type I hypersensitivity response caused by the massive systemic release of the same mediators that are triggered in a local type I reaction. Common type I anaphylaxis-triggering allergens are drugs and insect venom. Less common allergens are food proteins (e.g., peanuts, shellfish). Of significance is that the reaction lacks a genetic predisposition, making its occurrence unpredictable, and it may be fatal in response to prior sensitization to a minute amount of allergen.

The symptoms of anaphylaxis develop rapidly following exposure—within minutes—and simultaneously in multiple organs in response to an allergen capable of stimulating the immune system. In anaphylaxis, mast cells trigger widespread release of histamine and other mediators, which then cause widespread edema and vascular

Table 30–3　Major Mediators of Type I Hypersensitivity Response

Mediators	Major Activities
Preformed (Primary) mediators[a] • Histamine • Chemotactic factors (eosinophil chemotactic factor of anaphylaxis [ECF-A] & neutrophil chemotactic factor [NCF])	Capillary dilation, increased vascular permeability, smooth muscle constriction, bronchoconstriction, mucous secretion Eosinophil and neutrophil recruitment to site of inflammation
Secondary mediators[b] • Leukotrienes • Prostaglandins • Platelet activating factor (PAF)	Increased vascular permeability, stimulation of leukocyte adherence to endothelium, platelet activation Increased vascular permeability, smooth muscle contraction, vasodilation; activation of local nerve endings, causing pain Same as leukotrienes

[a] Primary mediators: preformed; released immediately following mast cell degranulation

[b] Secondary mediators: newly formed; synthesized following activation of mast cells

SOURCE: Data from Owen et al. (2013).

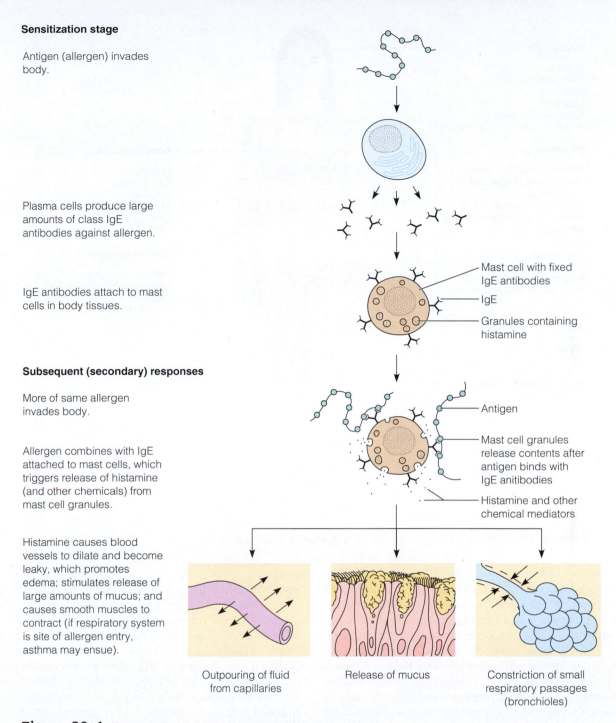

Sensitization stage

Antigen (allergen) invades body.

Plasma cells produce large amounts of class IgE antibodies against allergen.

IgE antibodies attach to mast cells in body tissues.

Mast cell with fixed IgE antibodies

IgE

Granules containing histamine

Subsequent (secondary) responses

More of same allergen invades body.

Allergen combines with IgE attached to mast cells, which triggers release of histamine (and other chemicals) from mast cell granules.

Antigen

Mast cell granules release contents after antigen binds with IgE anitbodies

Histamine and other chemical mediators

Histamine causes blood vessels to dilate and become leaky, which promotes edema; stimulates release of large amounts of mucus; and causes smooth muscles to contract (if respiratory system is site of allergen entry, asthma may ensue).

Outpouring of fluid from capillaries

Release of mucus

Constriction of small respiratory passages (bronchioles)

Figure 30–1 Type I IgE-mediated hypersensitivity response.

congestion. Complement is also activated, further stimulating histamine release and triggering a widespread inflammatory response. Anaphylaxis typically involves the cardiovascular, respiratory, cutaneous, and gastrointestinal systems. Urticaria, or hives, are the result of histamine release from the IgE–mast cell interaction in which receptors in cutaneous blood vessels cause the characteristic redness and swelling. Urticaria alone is not life-threatening but heralds the presence of an anaphylactic response. Assessment should include assessing the patient for upper airway edema with the risk of asphyxiation and irreversible shock. Gastrointestinal involvement is related to smooth muscle contraction and edema of the mucosa, resulting in cramplike

pain, nausea, and diarrhea. Similar responses can occur within the uterus, causing cramplike pelvic pain and a risk of spontaneous abortion. Figure 30–2 illustrates the effects of anaphylaxis, including clinical manifestations.

Anaphylactic shock is the extreme result of mediator-induced generalized vasodilatation with relative hypovolemia and increased vascular permeability causing rapid loss of plasma into interstitial spaces. This shift of fluid causes hypovolemic shock with profound hypotension, decreased cardiac output, myocardial ischemia, and widespread organ death. Furthermore, edema and bronchoconstriction of the airway can compromise airway patency, causing asphyxia.

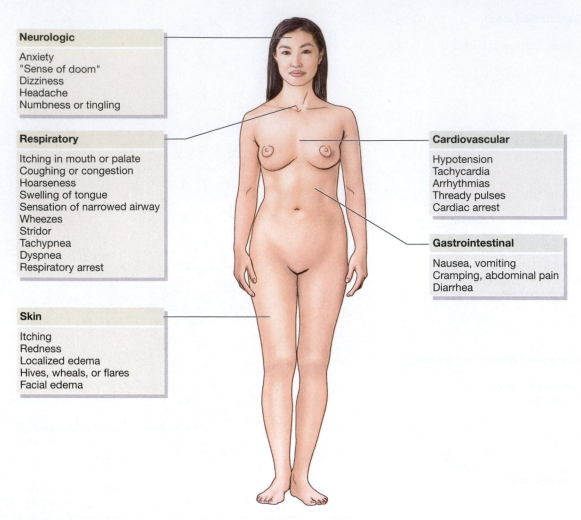

Neurologic

Anxiety
"Sense of doom"
Dizziness
Headache
Numbness or tingling

Respiratory

Itching in mouth or palate
Coughing or congestion
Hoarseness
Swelling of tongue
Sensation of narrowed airway
Wheezes
Stridor
Tachypnea
Dyspnea
Respiratory arrest

Skin

Itching
Redness
Localized edema
Hives, wheals, or flares
Facial edema

Cardiovascular

Hypotension
Tachycardia
Arrhythmias
Thready pulses
Cardiac arrest

Gastrointestinal

Nausea, vomiting
Cramping, abdominal pain
Diarrhea

Figure 30–2 The physiological effects of systemic anaphylaxis.

Treatment of systemic anaphylaxis must be instituted immediately and includes intravenous fluids to reverse the relative hypovolemia and the administration of epinephrine to stimulate vascular vasoconstriction and bronchodilation. Epinephrine may be administered through intramuscular (preferred) or intravenous routes, depending on anaphylaxis severity. Laryngeal edema may require tracheostomy when edema precludes endotracheal airway placement. Oxygen and injectable antihistamines should be administered. The patient should be kept warm if shock is suspected. Glucocorticoids may be used for severe or prolonged reactions because they reduce the immune response and stabilize the vascular system. Other symptoms, such as gastrointestinal cramping and urticaria, respond well to antihistamines. After the patient has fully recovered, diagnostic skin testing may be ordered to identify the offending allergen.

Type II (Cytotoxic) Hypersensitivity Response

A **type II (cytotoxic) hypersensitivity response** (Figure 30–3) is referred to as a cytotoxic (or hemolytic) reaction, meaning that it destroys cells. The immunoglobulins IgM and IgG react directly with cell-surface antigens, activating the complement system and producing direct injury to the cell surface. Cellular membranes are disrupted, and target cells such as erythrocytes (red blood cells [RBCs]), thrombocytes (platelets), and leukocytes (white blood cells [WBCs]), are destroyed. Transfusion reaction is a major example of this type of hypersensitivity. Other examples include Rh incompatibility in the neonate, drug reaction–induced hemolytic anemia, and hyperthyroidism caused by Graves disease.

Hemolytic Transfusion Reaction   Transfusion reactions can be subclassified as (1) febrile (fever and chills), whereby recipient antibodies act against donor white blood cells; (2) hypersensitivity reaction, whereby recipient antibodies attack donor blood proteins; or (3) hemolytic reaction, a type II cytotoxic response.

In a hemolytic transfusion reaction, preexisting antibodies in the recipient's serum target and attach to the ABO antigens on donor blood RBCs, which activates the complement cascade. As the immune system is activated, phagocytes destroy the donor RBCs, causing release of hemoglobin into the circulation. The released hemoglobin follows the general circulation and eventually flows into the renal glomeruli. Hemoglobin fragments can obstruct

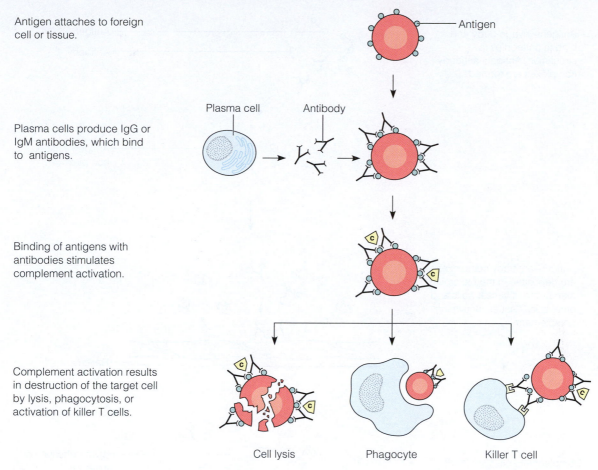

Antigen attaches to foreign cell or tissue.

Plasma cells produce IgG or IgM antibodies, which bind to antigens.

Binding of antigens with antibodies stimulates complement activation.

Complement activation results in destruction of the target cell by lysis, phagocytosis, or activation of killer T cells.

Cell lysis   Phagocyte   Killer T cell

Figure 30–3 Type II cytotoxic hypersensitivity response.

renal tubular blood flow, increasing the risk of oliguria and renal shutdown.

Symptoms of a hemolytic transfusion reaction are likely to occur within the first 2 to 5 minutes of initiation of the transfusion. Clinical manifestations that suggest this type of reaction include the sensation of heat and redness at the infusion site, nausea, headache, back pain, chills, fever, and a sense of chest heaviness with difficulty breathing. Tachycardia, hypotension, and death can follow if the transfusion is not interrupted immediately and treatment begun to reestablish cardiovascular stability. Immediate response protocols should be implemented when a transfusion reaction is suspected. The transfusion must be stopped immediately and blood samples sent to evaluate the reaction.

Type III (Immune Complex-mediated) Hypersensitivity Response

The **type III (immune complex-mediated) hypersensitivity response** involves formation of antigen–antibody complexes in the circulation. Once formed, the complexes follow the blood flow and eventually deposit themselves either in tissues (e.g., kidneys, joints, and skin) or on vessel walls, setting off the inflammatory response. The resulting tissue damage is not caused by the antigen–antibody complexes; rather, it results from altered blood flow, increased vascular permeability, and destruction by inflammatory cells secondary to activation of the inflammatory response by complement. The IgG and IgM antibodies are the major immunoglobulins involved in the type III response.

A combination of type III and type VI hypersensitivity may be seen in chronic organ transplant rejection, whereby the graft becomes compromised due to inflammation and altered blood flow, which slowly destroys the transplanted organ. This type of response is also often responsible for lung, joint, and skin damage in autoimmune disorders, such as systemic lupus erythematosus (SLE) and kidney damage in glomerulonephritis. Type III hypersensitivity can manifest as a local type III response (Arthus reaction) or as a systemic response (serum sickness).

Arthus Reaction   The Arthus reaction, or Arthus vasculitis, is localized to the skin and occurs when antigen–antibody complexes form in vessel walls, triggering an inflammatory response in the vessels (vasculitis). The reaction onset is relatively rapid, usually within 1 to 10 hours of exposure. The clinical manifestations are those caused by the inflammatory response, whereby the vessels become more permeable, allowing fluid to leak out and thereby causing edema. Neutrophils are attracted to the area of inflammation and attempt to destroy the complexes,

Antigens invade body and bind to antibodies in circulation. Antigen–antibody complexes are formed.

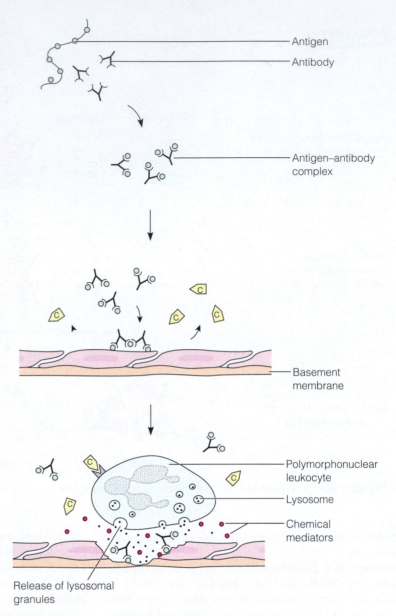

Antigen ————

Antibody ————

Antigen–antibody complex ————

Antigen–antibody complexes are deposited in the basement membrane of vessel walls and other body tissues, activating complement.

Basement membrane ————

Complement activation leads to release of inflammatory chemical mediators. Infiltration of polymorphonuclear leukocytes (PMNs) is followed by release of lysozymes. Tissue damage may be extensive.

Polymorphonuclear leukocyte ————

Lysosome ————

Chemical mediators ————

Release of lysosomal granules ————

Figure 30–4 Type III immune complex-mediated hypersensitivity response.

causing tissue damage. Other local vessel activities include localized hemorrhage and clotting; if severe, localized tissue necrosis can result.

Serum Sickness   Serum sickness is the systemic form of a type III hypersensitivity response. The onset of symptoms is slow, increasing over a week or more. The antigen–antibody complexes flow in the circulation and deposit in target tissues, usually the kidneys (glomeruli), joints, or blood vessels. The tissue destruction is the same as described in the Arthus response.

Figure 30–4 illustrates the type III immune complex-mediated hypersensitivity response.

Type IV (Delayed) Hypersensitivity Response

Cell-mediated **type IV (cell-mediated) hypersensitivity response** is a delayed response involving primarily T lymphocytes in the absence of antibody activity. In this response, sensitized T cells attack the antigen, releasing lymphokines, which then attract and activate macrophages. The macrophages cause localized inflammation and edema. Tissue injury and destruction are the hallmarks of the type IV hypersensitivity response, most notably through direct cellular destruction by T-cell toxins, lysosomal enzymes, or phagocytosis following activation by the release of cytokines and lymphokines. Figure 30–5 illustrates the type IV response.

Local reaction to a type IV response can be demonstrated in the induration of a positive tuberculin test or contact dermatitis, such as poison ivy. Clinical examples include graft or acute organ transplant rejection in which the HLA antigen is the principal target (graft-versus-host and host-versus-graft diseases). Furthermore, some autoimmune disorders have a type IV response component—for example Hashimoto thyroiditis, rheumatoid arthritis, and type 1 diabetes mellitus.

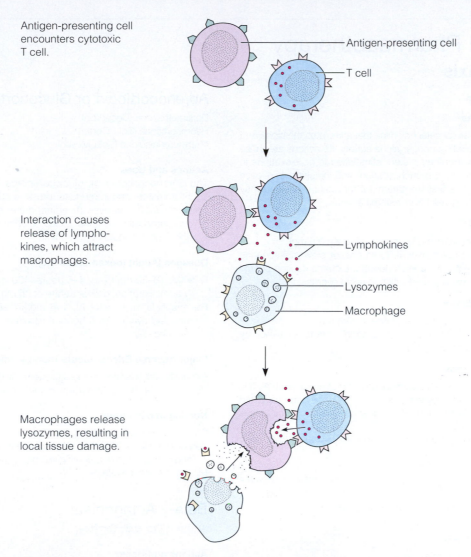

Antigen-presenting cell encounters cytotoxic T cell.

Antigen-presenting cell

T cell

Interaction causes release of lympho-kines, which attract macrophages.

Lymphokines

Lysozymes

Macrophage

Macrophages release lysozymes, resulting in local tissue damage.

Figure 30–5 Type IV delayed hypersensitivity response.

Drug-induced Hypersensitivity Reactions

Many drugs are capable of triggering a hypersensitivity reaction through one of the mechanisms previously described. Reactions can be classified as immediate, immune complex–dependent, or delayed. Immediate reactions reflect a type I anaphylactoid-type response whereby mediators are released through activation of tissue mast cells or circulating basophils. Penicillin, NSAIDs, quinolones, platinum-containing chemotherapy, and contrast dyes are known to trigger this type of response. Type II reactions are uncommon and involve antibody-mediated cell destruction—for example, drug-induced hemolytic anemia. Immune complex–dependent reactions reflect a systemic type III response (serum sickness) with manifestations increasing over a number of days as immune complexes are deposited. This is particularly noted with use of monoclonal antibodies or similar agents. A drug-induced hypersensitivity response can also be a delayed type IV response in which T cells act against the drug antigen (Pichler, 2014).

Management of Hypersensitivity Responses

The severity of symptoms varies widely in hypersensitivity reactions. Often, no therapy is required when symptoms are mild to moderate and of short duration (e.g., mild poison ivy or hay fever). When treatment is desired or required to reduce or eliminate a particular hypersensitivity response, the drug therapy typically ordered includes antihistamines, glucocorticoids, or both. The delivery method of these agents may vary, as well. For example, an oral (or injection) preparation of a glucocorticoid likely would be ordered for a systemic or severe hypersensitivity drug-induced reaction, whereas a topical preparation would be ordered for a mild contact dermatitis. If the patient is experiencing a systemic anaphylactic reaction, emergency measures using a combination of epinephrine and antihistamine are generally required. A summary of the drug interventions associated with anaphylaxis is provided in the "Related Pharmacotherapy: Anaphylaxis" feature.

Related Pharmacotherapy
Anaphylaxis

Epinephrine

Actions and Uses

Epinephrine is a natural catecholamine that stimulates the alpha and beta receptors with stronger alpha activity. Its actions are those of sympathetic nervous system stimulation (e.g., elevations in systolic BP, HR, CO; bronchodilation; and inhibition of release of histamine). It is first-line treatment for anaphylaxis and may provide temporary relief from asthma attacks.

Dosages (Adult)

IM (preferred route): 0.01 mg/kg (maximum dose 0.5 mg)

IV: 50 to 100 mcg bolus over 1–3 minutes, or slow maintenance infusion if patient deterioration persists. Extreme caution should be used when diluting medication to avoid overdosing.

Major Adverse Effects

Most common: palpitations, nervousness, tremors

Potentially life-threatening: acute myocardial infarction, pulmonary edema, ventricular fibrillation

Nursing Implications

Be aware of correct dosage, dilution, and rate of administration. It is recommended that lowest dose be used initially and repeated until desired effect is attained. If higher dose is required, increase the dose gradually.

Do not remove the epinephrine injection from the carton until ready to administer to the patient.

Protect from light at all times.

Follow institutional guidelines for diluting and administering accurate dosage.

Monitor VS and cardiac rhythm every 5 minutes.

Antihistamines

Diphenhydramine HCL (Benadryl)

Actions and Uses

Antihistamines block histamine release by competing for the histamine receptor sites. They are useful for temporary relief of allergic symptoms and are used in anaphylaxis as adjunct therapy with epinephrine. Epinephrine should be administered first.

Dosages (Adult)

PO: 25–50 mg t.i.d. or q.i.d (300 mg/day maximum). Oral administration: give with food or milk.

IV or IM: 10–50 mg every 4–6 hours (400 mg/day maximum). For IV administration, deliver at rate of 25 mg or less over 1 minute. Intramuscular administration: give injection deep into large muscle mass and alternate injection sites.

Major Adverse Effects

Most common: drowsiness, tachycardia, dry mouth

Potentially life-threatening (rare): hypersensitivity (cardiovascular collapse, anaphylactic shock)

Nursing Implications

Check for known hypersensitivity to antihistamines.

Cautious use in older adults—dose may require adjustment to decrease adverse effects.

SOURCE: Data from Wilson et al. (2016).

Adrenocorticoid or Glucocorticoids

Dexamethasone (Decadron)

Hydrocortisone (Solu-Cortef)

Methylprednisolone (Solu-Medrol)

Actions and Uses

The adrenocorticoid or glucocorticoids have powerful anti-inflammatory and immunosuppressive actions. They are useful as adjunct therapy with epinephrine in treatment of acute hypersensitivity reactions, including anaphylaxis. In anaphylaxis, epinephrine should be given first.

Dosages (Adult) (dexamethasone)

IV or IM: 10–50 mg every 4–6 hours (400 mg/day maximum). For IV administration, deliver at rate of 25 mg or less over 1 minute.

For anaphylactic shock—IV: 1–6 mg/kg (single dose) or 40 mg repeated every 2 to 6 hours if required; or 20 mg bolus, then 3 mg/kg/day

Major Adverse Effects (acute therapy only)

Generally well tolerated in the short term; hyperglycemia, euphoria

Potentially life-threatening (rare): hypersensitivity reaction possible

Nursing Implications

Check for known hypersensitivity.

Can be given IM or IV with anaphylaxis. Be aware of dosage, dilution, and rate of administration if given IV.

Monitor for desired effects.

Beta-2 Antagonists

Albuterol (Proventil, Ventolin)

Actions and Uses

Beta-2 antagonists act on the beta-2 receptors of smooth muscles of the airway, resulting in bronchodilation. They also have an inhibitory action on histamine release from the mast cells. Inhaling albuterol is useful as adjunct therapy to open the airways during an anaphylaxis reaction.

Dosages (Adult)

Bronchospasm—Inhaled: 1–2 inhalations every 4–6 hours; PO: 2–4 mg 3–4 times/day or 4–8 mg sustained release 2 times/day

Major Adverse Effects

Most common: tremor, palpitations

Potentially life-threatening: hypersensitivity possible

Nursing Implications

Monitor for desired effects of improved ventilation.

Important interaction: Can potentiate effects of epinephrine.

Section Two Review

1. What causes a true type I hypersensitivity response?
   A. A histamine precursor causing anaphylaxis
   B. Antigen–IgE–mast cell interaction
   C. Antigen–antibody complexes deposited in vessel walls
   D. Massive number of destroyed red blood cells

2. Type III hypersensitivity reactions are often characterized by which of the following?
   A. Specific target cells
   B. Widespread multiorgan involvement
   C. Rapidly progressing symptoms
   D. Relatively low-risk patterns

3. Which statement is correct regarding the type IV cell-mediated hypersensitivity response?
   A. It involves primarily antibody activity.
   B. It does not harm body tissues.
   C. T-cell activity is responsible.
   D. It directly interacts with cell surface antigens.

4. A client has developed a drug-induced hypersensitivity response in which immune complexes have deposited themselves into the client's tissues. This is an example of which type of response?
   A. Type I
   B. Type II
   C. Type III
   D. Type IV

Answers: 1. B, 2. B, 3. C, 4. C

Section Three: Disorders of Hyperactivity Immune Response: Autoimmunity

Autoimmunity is an intolerance of the immune system to one's own body tissue (self-antigens) that can involve abnormal activation of B cells, T cells, or the complement system. For reasons not fully understood, the immune system incorrectly recognizes self as foreign and initiates a destructive response against targeted tissues. Characteristic of most autoimmune disorders is B-cell hyperactivity. Any of the four types of hypersensitivity responses may be involved; however, types II and III are the most common. Many diseases are now attributed to an autoimmune response, and many others are suspected. Table 30–4 provides a list of common autoimmune diseases that target specific body systems or tissues. Other autoimmune diseases, such as systemic lupus erythematosus (SLE), affect multiple body systems where immune complexes are deposited.

Many autoimmune disorders seem to have a genetic predisposition; however, not all family members develop the autoimmune disease. It is theorized that many autoimmune diseases may require some type of stimulus or environmental trigger to be activated, such as a virus or chemical substance, for the disease to become evident. An example of such a stimulus is exposure to UV rays of the sun, which can trigger SLE. In addition to a positive family history, aging and gender are two important risk factors. The occurrence of autoimmune diseases increases with age, possibly related to the decreased effectiveness of the immune system. Women develop autoimmune disorders more frequently than men; the reason for this is unknown but may be hormone related.

Table 30–4 Common Autoimmune Diseases That Target Specific Body Systems or Tissues

System or Tissue	Disease
Pulmonary	Goodpasture disease
Cardiovascular	Cardiomyopathy
Gastrointestinal	Ulcerative colitis Crohn disease Pernicious anemia Inflammatory bowel disease (IBD)
Endocrine	Graves disease (thyroid gland) Type I diabetes mellitus (pancreas) Addison disease (adrenal gland) Partial pituitary deficiency (pituitary gland) 21-hydroxylase deficiency
Renal	Immune-complex glomerulonephritis
Neuromuscular	Multiple sclerosis Myasthenia gravis Rheumatic fever
Connective tissue	Systemic lupus erythematosus (SLE) Scleroderma (progressive systemic sclerosis) Rheumatoid arthritis Ankylosing spondylitis
Hematologic (blood and blood vessels)	Autoimmune hemolytic anemia Autoimmune thrombocytopenic purpura Polyarteritis nodosa Antiphospholipid antibody syndrome
Eyes	Acute anterior uveitis Sjogren syndrome
Skin	Scleroderma Dermatomyositis Psoriasis Alopecia areata

SOURCE: Data from Mandel (2015).

Currently, most autoimmune diseases are of idiopathic (unknown) origin; however, multiple complex mechanisms are likely involved. One major theory is molecular mimicry, which helps explain the development of rheumatoid heart disease and the consequent damage to heart valves (Cunningham, 2014). The cell-wall proteins of certain microbes (e.g., group A beta-hemolytic *streptococcus*) structurally resemble those of specific normal cells in the body, such as the heart valves. In response to development of strep throat or rheumatic fever, the immune system musters its attack, forming antibodies against the bacteria. The antibodies destroy the initial strep infection but also misidentify the similar (twin) proteins on the normal cells of the heart valves and shift their attack to those cells, causing valve damage.

Immunosuppression is a common therapeutic goal in treating autoimmune disorders. Immune-mediated tissue damage may be suppressed through drug-induced, radiation-induced, or surgically induced immunodeficiency. Treatment of organ-specific autoimmune disorders involves metabolic control (such as insulin replacement therapy for type I diabetes mellitus), whereas treatment of systemic disorders includes anti-inflammatory or immunosuppressive medications.

Systemic Lupus Erythematosus

Systemic lupus erythematosus (SLE) is an excellent example of an autoimmune disease. It is an inflammatory condition characterized by autoantibodies that develop against nuclear antigens (Bartels & Muller, 2016). Systemic lupus erythematosus affects multiple body systems and organs, developing along a continuum of severity from mild to life-threatening. There are two major disease patterns of almost equal frequency: relapsing–remitting disease (the classic "flare" pattern) and continuously active disease. SLE is not a common disease; the annual incidence from the 1970s to 2000s is estimated to be 1 to 10 cases per 100,000 people per year (Jarukitsopa et al., 2015). It primarily targets young non-White women of childbearing age; however, it is also seen in males, white females, and older adults. The incidence is significantly higher in African Americans, Hispanics, and Asians.

Onset of SLE has been associated with a variety of environmental triggers, the most well known being exposure to ultraviolet light. In addition, a variety of drugs (e.g., isoniazid, hydralazine, and procainamide) are known to trigger a drug-induced form of the disease; however, the disorder usually resolves upon discontinuation of the drug. Triggers, such as Epstein-Barr virus, stress, surgery, and pregnancy, have been implicated in lupus flares.

Pathophysiology   The cause of SLE is not fully understood but appears to be multifactorial, including genetic predisposition (HLA related), hormonal and environmental factors, and dysregulation of the immune system (Bartels & Muller, 2016). Estrogens seem to foster the development of SLE, perhaps by enhancing immune system activation, which results in autoimmune pathology (Young et al., 2014). SLE is thought to have a strong type III hypersensitivity response component in which antigen–antibody complexes deposit in the epithelial lining of blood vessels (causing widespread vasculitis) and tissue surfaces. These deposits create occlusions and inflammation, both of which cause local damage with edema, hemorrhage, or clotting and an accumulation of neutrophils. Occlusion leads to tissue death and scar tissue formation, which eventually impairs the function of affected organs, such as kidney, lungs, heart, brain, skin, joints, and the digestive tract.

Clinical Findings and Diagnosis   Nearly all patients with SLE experience general symptoms of malaise, fatigue, fever, weight loss, joint pain, and skin manifestations (rashes and patches). SLE can attack any organ in the body, with the most common affected systems being the vascular, cardiopulmonary and renal systems. The multisystem nature of the disease results in an unpredictable clinical presentation as specific manifestations depend on which body system is being targeted.

Emerging Evidence

- Cognitive and behavioral disturbances may be seen with systemic lupus erythematosus (SLE) impacting outcomes including quality of life for SLE patients. Some studies are being designed to evaluate the impairments. In a study of 17 subjects age 18 years or older who fulfilled the ACR revised criteria for SLE, Mackay et al. (2015) investigated whether or not SLE disease that resulted in repeated neurotoxin exposure was associated with abnormal regional glucose metabolism. Subjects with long-term SLE demonstrated hypometabolism in the prefrontal cortices, and all subjects with SLE demonstrated hypermetabolism in two areas: the hippocampus and the orbitofrontal cortex, which correlates with changes in memory and mood. Measuring resting brain metabolism improves assessment and attribution of these alterations of the central nervous system (*Mackay et al., 2015*).

- A qualitative study explored patients' perceptions regarding HIV mass screening and identified barriers to implementing screening for patients seeking healthcare. Twenty-four semi-structured individual interviews were conducted in France at a general practice clinic. Barriers included issues with sexuality, criticism of public policies, and HIV beliefs and perceptions (*Fernandez-Gerlinger, Bernard, & Saint-Lary, 2013*).

- A randomized, controlled, prospective study of 46 patients undergoing hematopoietic stem-cell transplantation (HSCT) was conducted to determine if rates of infection and the nutritional status of patients having a hematopoietic stem-cell transplant differed in groups with and without dietary restrictions. Data were collected at the beginning of the conditioning regimen. There were no significant differences in rates of infection or nutritional status between the two groups of patients (*Lassiter & Schneider, 2015*).

Diagnosis can be difficult and frustrating. When SLE is suspected, drug-induced etiology is first ruled out through close examination of the patient's drug regimen. No single laboratory test is specific to the diagnosis of SLE. The most common laboratory test performed is the antinuclear antibody (ANA), which is used for screening for autoimmune disease; however, ANA is not specific for SLE and can be elevated with other autoimmune diseases, such as scleroderma and rheumatoid arthritis. However, obtaining an ANA titer is important as a rule-out test because the absence of an elevated titer provides strong evidence that SLE is not present. Complement levels are also measured and may show low levels of C3 and C4 (Bartels & Muller, 2016). Diagnosis is commonly based on criteria established by the American Rheumatism Association (American College of Rheumatology, 1997), which requires that four or more criteria out of a possible eleven be present to establish a diagnosis of SLE. These criteria are a combination of laboratory and organ function findings (see Box 30–1).

Management and Prognosis   Treatment of SLE depends on the severity of the illness and the body systems being affected by an autoimmune attack. Lupus arthritic and dermatologic symptoms are usually controlled with a regimen of nonsteroidal anti-inflammatory drugs (NSAIDs) and antimalarial therapy (hydroxychloroquine [Plaquenil]). Liver and kidney function need to be monitored in patients on long-term NSAID therapy because of a known increased risk for organ toxicity in SLE patients; patients taking hydroxychloroquine should have yearly eye exams to monitor for development of drug-induced ophthalmologic complications (Bartels & Muller, 2016). Low-dose corticosteroid therapy is commonly used if symptoms cannot be controlled by more conservative therapy (Bartels & Muller, 2016).

Use of high-dose corticosteroid therapy is reserved for treatment of a potentially life-threatening autoimmune attack on affected organ systems (e.g., CNS, hematologic, and renal). When high-dose corticosteroid therapy is used, the dose is reduced to minimize long-term effects when the patient goes into remission. Uncontrolled lupus flares are often treated with immunosuppressive agents such as azathioprine (Imuran), cyclophosphamide (Cytoxan), mycophenalate mofetil (MMF), or methotrexate (Rheumatrex). Immunosuppressant therapy may also be initiated as alternative therapy to corticosteroids when the steroid dose cannot be reduced or adverse effects become severe (Bartels & Muller, 2016).

In the United States, survival at 10 years following diagnosis is about 90% (Bartels & Muller, 2016; Centers for Disease Control and Prevention, 2017a). Cause of death varies, depending on where the patient is in the course of the disease. Within the first few years of disease onset, death most commonly results from active disease-related injury to body systems or organs (e.g., heart, kidneys, or CNS system) or infection (a complication of immunosuppression therapy). In later years of the disease, the underlying cause of death is accelerated atherosclerosis, which causes premature coronary artery disease and hypertension with associated complications of heart attacks, strokes, and kidney disease.

Nursing Implications   When a patient with a history of SLE is admitted to a high-acuity environment, the nurse needs to be aware of the implications for care that this secondary diagnosis brings with it. The potential multisystem damage associated with the SLE disease process (particularly to the heart, lungs, and kidneys) makes it potentially one of the more complex chronic illnesses to manage simultaneously with an acute illness or trauma. It can have a significant impact on the prognosis of a high-acuity patient, making patient outcomes less predictable and management significantly more complex.

The nursing history should include assessment of the underlying SLE condition, including severity and pattern, baseline health status, medical history, and medication regimen. The physical assessment should include a full head-to-toe evaluation of body systems, and frequent reevaluation is necessary to recognize status changes quickly. The nurse will monitor vital signs and laboratory values closely for trends that indicate deterioration in organ function, with particular focus on heart, lung, and kidney function. If the patient has been on long-term steroid therapy, additional evaluation of potential adverse effects of therapy should be done, including evaluation of immunosuppression.

Prior to discharge, the patient's (and family's) understanding of the disease should be evaluated and supplemental education provided. Table 30–5 provides a list of topics included in teaching the patient with SLE. The nurse should be available for questions, to provide reassurance, and to encourage discussion of fears and anxieties.

BOX 30–1   Revised Criteria for Diagnosis of Systemic Lupus Erythematosus (American Rheumatism Association)

Systemic Involvement

- Arthritis
- Hematologic disorder (hemolytic anemia, leukopenia, or thrombocytopenia)
- Immunologic disorder (positive LE cell prep, anti-DNA antibodies, or anti-Sm antibodies, or false positive serologic test to syphilis)
- Neurologic disorder (seizures or psychosis)
- Renal disorder (persistent proteinuria or cellular casts)
- Serositis (pleuritis or pericarditis)

Other

- Antinuclear antibody (elevated titer)
- Discoid rash
- Malar rash (facial butterfly erythema)
- Oral ulcers (mouth or nasaopharyngeal)
- Photosensitivity (rash on skin exposed to sunlight)

SOURCE: Data from American College of Rheumatology (1997).

Table 30–5 Systemic Lupus Erythematosus Patient Teaching

Topic	Related Information
Knowledge about the disease	Etiology, description, manifestations, diagnosis, general management
Avoidance of known flare triggers: • Sunlight and ultraviolet light exposure • Smoking • Echinacea	Wear hat, long-sleeved shirt, and pants. Use umbrella. Cease smoking. Read cold remedy labels and avoid use.
Healthy lifestyle: • Regular exercise and rest • Immunizations • Healthy diet	Influenza vaccine yearly; pneumococcal vaccine every 5 years Low-fat diet
Other teaching needs: • Drug regimen (e.g., antimalarial, antilipemic, antihypertensive, glucocorticoid, NSAID) • Maintaining bone health if on long-term steroid therapy • Hormonal replacement therapy • Cancer screening (age appropriate)	Purpose of each drug, importance of taking drugs as ordered, effects and side effects, possible toxic effects Use of calcium and vitamin D supplements Use of hormone replacement therapy (HRT) may increase risk of flares. There is some evidence that there may be increased risk for cancer.

SOURCE: Data from Bartels & Muller (2016).

Section Three Review

1. Autoimmunity is most accurately described as a problem of which process?
   A. Loss of self-tolerance of body tissues
   B. T lymphocyte attack on self-antigens
   C. Development of antigen–antibody complexes
   D. Antibodies attacking tissue in absence of infection

2. What does the theory of molecular mimicry propose as a possible mechanism for development of autoimmunity?
   A. An imbalance occurs between T helper cells and T suppressor cells, causing excessive T helper cell activity.
   B. Enzymes secreted by some bacteria target certain normal body tissues, resulting in cellular destruction.
   C. Cell wall proteins of certain microbes are structurally similar to those on certain normal body cells.
   D. Certain viruses secrete proteins that fool the immune system into targeting normal cells.

3. How best can the course of systemic lupus erythematosus be characterized?
   A. A steady increase in intensity of symptoms
   B. A peak of symptoms followed by a slow decline to remission
   C. Symptom remission at the onset of old age
   D. Individual variation of symptom presentation and intensity

4. Disorders thought to be autoimmune in etiology include which of the following? (Select all that apply.)
   A. Chronic bronchitis
   B. Ulcerative colitis
   C. Breast cancer
   D. Diabetes mellitus (type 1)
   E. Pernicious anemia

Answers: 1. A, 2. C, 3. D, 4. (B, D, E)

Section Four: Acute Leukemia

Leukemia is a malignant process in which there is a transformation of hematopoietic cells, causing unregulated clonal growth. This proliferation of malignant leukocytes results in the accumulation of abnormal (leukemic) cells in the bone marrow and a decreased production of normal blood cells. Leukemias are categorized broadly as either acute or chronic, with different illness trajectories, prognoses, and approaches to treatment. Acute leukemias are characterized by aggressive proliferation of immature lymphoid or myeloid blast cells. Examine Figure 28–2 in Chapter 28 to review the early stage of blast cells in cell development. Chronic leukemias are characterized by production of mature, differentiated cells of either lymphoid or myeloid lineage that do not function normally. Chronic leukemias have a more insidious long-term clinical course than the acute leukemias. The patient with acute leukemia is much more likely to be admitted and treated in a high-acuity setting with complications of the disease. This section provides an overview of the acute forms of leukemia, including etiology, types, clinical manifestations, and management.

The exact causes of leukemia are unknown. It is believed that there may be multiple factors involved in the development of each of the different types, including environmental and genetic factors. There is an increased incidence of leukemia with certain chromosomal abnormalities, for example, in children with Down syndrome. Certain chemical and drug exposures are associated with its development (e.g., benzene, chloramphenicol, and some antineoplastic agents), as is radiation exposure that may occur following nuclear disasters or radiation treatment for malignancies.

Types of Acute Leukemia

There are two types of acute leukemia: acute lymphocytic (lymphoblastic) leukemia (ALL) and acute myelogenous (myelocytic) leukemia (AML). In essence, while the number of white blood cells is markedly elevated (leukocytosis), the functional ability of these mutated cells is severely impaired by their lack of maturation. With either type of acute leukemia, the uncontrolled production of malignant cells in the bone marrow suppresses and essentially crowds out the normal blood cells, which leads to progressive **pancytopenia** (abnormally low levels of all blood cell types). If left untreated, the patient rapidly succumbs to complications of pancytopenia, particularly infection or hemorrhage.

Acute Lymphocytic (Lymphoblastic) Leukemia   Acute **lymphocytic leukemia (ALL)** is primarily a disease of childhood; however, there is a second peak during middle age (Kotter & Banasik, 2013). ALL is associated with proliferation of lymphoblasts (immature lymphocytes) from the B-cell lineage or, less commonly, the T-cell lineage (Kotter & Banasik, 2013). The leukemic cells fail to mature or differentiate any further than the stage at which they are produced; therefore, they cannot carry on normal immune functions. The leukemic cells infiltrate other normal tissues, such as the liver, spleen, and lymph nodes.

Acute Myelogenous (Myelocytic) Leukemia   Acute **myelogenous leukemia (AML)** is primarily a disease of adulthood with the median age at onset being 64 years (Kotter & Banasik, 2013). AML accounts for the majority of the acute leukemias, with approximately 80% of patients in this category (Siegel, Miller, & Jemal, 2015). It is characterized by a proliferation of malignant blast cells from the myeloid stem-cell lineage. There are multiple subtypes of AML as the disease can involve any or all of the cells in the myeloid lineage (erythroblasts, megakaryoblasts, monoblasts, or myeloblasts). Blast cells are not programmed to die; thus, malignant blast clones can produce malignant cells indefinitely. The bone marrow must have more than 20% blast cells to qualify for AML (Kotter & Banasik, 2013). Cells rapidly accumulate in the bone marrow and then infiltrate into other tissues. An examination of peripheral blood and the bone marrow in AML will show a predominance of myeloblastic cells and possibly Auer rods. **Auer rods** are abnormally large granule-containing needlelike rods in the cytoplasm that are most commonly found in blast cells taken from the bone marrow and blood from patients with AML.

Clinical Manifestations

The initial clinical presentation of a person at the onset of acute leukemia is often dramatic and can include complaints

Table 30–6 Clinical Manifestations of Leukemia

Category	Common Clinical Manifestations
Pancytopenia	Leukopenia (immunodeficiency) • Frequent infections • Fever Thrombocytopenia (bleeding tendencies) • Epistaxis, bleeding gums • Petechiae and ecchymosis Erythrocytopenia (anemia) • Pale mucous membranes • Fatigue, activity intolerance, malaise • Intolerance to cold • Tachycardia, tachypnea
Malignant cell expansion	Bone • Bone tenderness or pain Vascular system • Leukocytosis and leukostasis • Impaired circulation (particularly brain and/or lungs)
Infiltration	CNS • Headache, nausea, and vomiting • Seizures, coma • Papilledema, cranial nerve palsies Liver and spleen • Hepatomegaly and splenomegaly • Abdominal discomfort • Worsening thrombocytopenia or pancytopenia

SOURCE: Data from Schiffer (2015).

of fever, fatigue, bruising, bleeding, bone pain, and persistent or frequent infections (Kotter & Banasik, 2013). The major clinical manifestations of the leukemias can be categorized into two groups: those that are caused by pancytopenia and those that are caused by expansion and infiltration of malignant cells into other tissues. Table 30–6 provides a summary of manifestations.

Pancytopenia Manifestations   Recall that leukemia causes overcrowding in the bone marrow, resulting in decreased production of all normal blood cell types. As the red blood cell count decreases, the person with leukemia becomes increasingly anemic, demonstrating all of the manifestations of anemia, including tissue hypoxia. As the normal leukocyte count decreases, the patient becomes increasingly immunodeficient and at high risk for development of infections. However, the typical clinical picture associated with infection may be diminished or absent if significant neutropenia is present. Infection and hemorrhage are the most common causes of death with acute leukemia. Fever is commonly related to infection and increased metabolism of the malignant cells. Finally, as platelet numbers decrease, the patient develops bleeding problems, particularly petechiae and ecchymosis on the skin, as well as epistaxis and bleeding gums.

Cell Expansion and Infiltration

As the malignant cells proliferate in the bone marrow, their expanding volume increases the pressure inside the bone. The increased pressure results in complaints of bone tenderness. Malignant cells that infiltrate into the central nervous system (CNS) can cause multiple CNS-related manifestations, such as nausea and vomiting, headache, seizures, lethargy, papilledema, and possible cranial nerve palsies (Schiffer, 2015). Infiltration of malignant cells into the spleen and liver gives rise to splenomegaly and hepatomegaly, which can cause general abdominal discomfort and worsening pancytopenia, particularly thrombocytopenia.

Diagnosis and Prognosis

Diagnosis of the exact type and subtype of leukemia requires thorough clinical evaluation. However, the blast cells collected from the peripheral blood are often so primitive that determining whether the malignant cell clones are of myelocytic or lymphocytic origin may be difficult (Kotter & Banasik, 2013). It is critical that the leukemic cells be correctly identified and characterized to allow for planning of appropriate treatment. A definitive diagnosis requires bone marrow biopsy and aspiration with analysis of the cells. Identification is accomplished by immunophenotyping and molecular analysis (cytogenetics) (Schiffer, 2015). Other common blood tests include a complete blood count (CBC) with differential and peripheral blood smears.

Leukemias are classified to aid in diagnosis, treatment, and prognosis. Several classification and staging systems have been developed over the years. The French–American–British (FAB) classification system was developed to differentiate ALL, AML, and myelodysplastic syndromes by morphology. It remains the most commonly used classification system in the clinical setting and provides invaluable morphologic guidance in diagnosing acute leukemia.

The prognosis depends on the age of the patient and the exact subtype of acute leukemia. In children, acute lymphocytic leukemia (ALL) is considered highly curable. In regard to overall long-term survival, acute myelogenous leukemia (AML) has a worse prognosis than ALL, with an estimated number of new cases of 21,380 each year and an estimated number of deaths of 10,590 annually (American Cancer Society, 2017). Successful AML remissions are being achieved in 60% to 70% of adults, and more than 25% of AML patients are anticipated to survive 3 or more years (National Cancer Institute, 2017). Treatment is based on the identification of AML subtypes, which are described in the "Genetic Considerations" feature.

Management

In general, acute leukemias are initially managed by treating complications of pancytopenia, initiating chemotherapy,

and implementing supportive measures to minimize risk of infection. The primary goals of acute leukemia therapy are to eliminate the malignant cells, restore normal hematopoiesis, and produce complete remission. This is typically achieved through aggressive chemotherapy, which may require multiple courses of treatment that may last for 2 years. The optimal treatment approach depends on the patient's age, overall clinical status, presence of comorbidities, and the cytogenetic and molecular profile of the patient's leukemia type (National Cancer Institute, 2017).

Induction Chemotherapy   The initial phase of chemotherapy is referred to as *induction*, which lasts for approximately 1 week. Induction therapy aims at creating a state of complete remission—the absence of leukemic cells in the bone marrow and peripheral blood. Patients may stay in the hospital for about a month until the blood counts recover and it is safe for the patient to be discharged. While in the hospital, many patients are given intravenous antibiotics, and blood products may be ordered to support the patient through the therapy.

Consolidation Chemotherapy   Induction therapy may be followed by consolidation chemotherapy, which aims to solidify the remission response and eradicate any remaining leukemic cells. It frequently includes the same chemotherapeutic agents used during induction but at lower doses and for shorter durations.

Maintenance Chemotherapy   The final phase of chemotherapy is called *maintenance* chemotherapy, which is primarily required for treatment of ALL. During this phase, the patient may receive prophylactic treatment of the CNS because ALL frequently recurs in the spinal fluid. Drugs are injected into the cerebrospinal space (intrathecally), which is typically done through a lumbar puncture but may also be given through an Ommaya Reservoir, which is a round-shaped port that is placed under the scalp.

Hematopoietic Stem-Cell Transplantation   Hematopoietic stem-cell transplantation (HSCT) may be the curative treatment of choice, particularly in patients with AML or relapsed ALL. Hematopoietic stem-cell transplantation, or bone marrow transplantation, is an intensive therapy used to eradicate hematological malignancy from the bone marrow and promote the return of a normally functioning immune system. HSCT can be used for a variety of disorders, including leukemia, multiple myeloma, autoimmune disorders such as systemic lupus erythematosus, and aplastic anemia. In some disorders it is the only potentially curative therapeutic option. Other treatments for acute leukemias include radiation, targeted therapy, and biological therapies. In adult AML, clinical trials are focused on targeted therapies while ALL clinical trials focus on examining the effectiveness of biological therapies (National Cancer Institute, 2017).

Nursing Implications

Nurses play a major role in the interdisciplinary team caring for the acute leukemia patient who is experiencing symptoms of the disease and side effects of treatment. Goals of nursing care include vigilant assessment,

Genetic Considerations
Subtypes of AML

Subtypes of AML are identified by the World Health Organization (WHO) using clinical features, morphology, cytogenetic data, or molecular structures to differentiate the groups. Consistently reoccurring genetic abnormalities are identified, and treatments are adjusted based on the subtype of AML identified. Subtype example: AML with t (8;21)(q22;q22); *RUNX1-RUNX1T1*[b] (Marcucci & Bloomfield, 2015).

prevention of infection, delivery of therapy and evaluation of its effects, and management of disease and treatment-associated complications. During the active stage of acute leukemia, the patient's condition may become extremely unstable, warranting close monitoring for pancytopenia or other complications that can arise (discussed in Section Five). The nurse needs to be aware that development of small status changes may be heralding in an early-stage complication; therefore, rapid recognition of physiologic changes and timely interventions are crucial. Meticulous care of invasive lines and catheters, skin and oral hygiene, protection against trauma, and reduction of oxygen demand (related to anemia) are all essential components of nursing care in patients with pancytopenia. The psychosocial needs of the patient and family must also be attended to through explaining therapies and procedures, answering questions, patient education, and providing emotional support throughout the patient's stay.

Section Four Review

1. Acute myelocytic leukemia (AML) differs from acute lymphocytic leukemia (ALL) in that AML involves which of the following?
   A. More than one type of blood cell
   B. A predominance of mature blood cells
   C. Red blood cells
   D. Plasma cell proliferation

2. Most acute lymphocytic leukemia cases involve proliferation of what type of immature cells?
   A. Plasma cells
   B. T cells
   C. B cells
   D. Megakaryocytes

3. Acute myelocytic leukemia has which unique feature?
   A. Normal platelet and RBC levels
   B. The presence of Auer rods in the cytoplasm
   C. A high degree of curability
   D. Primarily seen in young children

4. A "complete remission" is obtained when there are no leukemic cells in which body parts?
   A. Lymph nodes and bone marrow
   B. Lymph nodes and peripheral blood
   C. Bone marrow and lymph nodes
   D. Bone marrow and peripheral blood

Answers: 1. A, 2. C, 3. B , 4. D

Section Five: Oncological Emergencies

A significant number of patients with cancer develop oncological emergencies, potentially life-threatening complications related to the cancer, cancer therapy, or comorbid conditions. Cancer-related complications include spinal cord compression, superior vena cava syndrome, and leukostasis. Cancer treatment often includes drug regimens that are toxic to organs, cause severe immunosuppression, or overwhelm the body's homeostasis mechanisms. Many of these iatrogenic problems can become life-threatening and, therefore, medical emergencies. This section provides an overview of oncological emergencies, highlighting some of the more common ones. Table 30–7 provides a summary of the major oncological emergencies discussed, including a brief description and common clinical manifestations.

Tumor-related Emergencies

Malignant solid tumors grow in an uncontrolled fashion, compressing adjacent soft tissues and potentially causing a mechanical obstruction. In addition, in certain forms of leukemia, massive numbers of circulating WBCs can obstruct blood flow. Three major examples of tumor-related emergencies include spinal cord compression, superior vena cava syndrome, and leukostasis.

Spinal Cord Compression   Oncology patients who have back pain should be evaluated for possible spinal cord compression (SCC). Tumors may cause SCC through direct extension or by metastatic disease in the vertebral column. Edema and diminished blood supply to the spinal cord can lead to paresis and paralysis. Symptoms may include pain, motor weakness, and sensory deficit. Diagnosis is made by magnetic resonance imaging (MRI). If an MRI is contraindicated or not available, a CT myelography can be used. Spinal precautions should be implemented in patients with spine instability or neurologic symptoms until bony and neurologic stability is ensured. Treatment options for SCC may include surgery, chemotherapy, radiation, and medications. Corticosteroids are given to decrease spinal cord edema and are the first-line treatment, or the patient can be treated with a combination of radiation and steroid therapy. A laminectomy or spinal fusion may be required if the symptoms are rapidly progressing or if the tumor is resistant to radiation.

Superior Vena Cava Syndrome   Superior vena cava (SVC) syndrome refers to a group of clinical manifestations that result from obstruction of the SVC through development of a thrombosis, through tumor invasion of the vena cava, or by external compression of SVC by the tumor (Nickloes et al., 2016). Malignant disease of the upper lobe of the right lung or mediastinum is by far the most common cause of the syndrome, which results in venous engorgement due to decreased venous drainage in the upper trunk. Two factors determine the patient's clinical

Table 30–7 Summary of Oncologic Crises

Crisis	Description	Manifestations
Tumor related		
Spinal cord compression	Edema and ischemia to cord caused by pressure exerted by tumor in vertebral column.	Back pain and tenderness, paresis, paralysis
Superior vena cava (SVC) syndrome	Obstruction of blood flow through SVC into the right atrium from tumor that results in impaired venous drainage in the trunk and venous engorgement	General: facial swelling, shortness of breath, headache, confusion, dizziness, upper body swelling Gradual development: may be asymptomatic or mild symptoms Rapid development (rare): hemodynamic instability, increased intracranial pressure, seizures, airway distress
Leukostasis	Obstruction of blood flow in microvasculature caused by leukocyte microthrombi By definition, requires a leukocyte count of at least 50,000 cells/mcL. A count higher than 100,000 cells/mcL is a medical emergency.	Symptoms depend on location of occlusion. Lungs: respiratory distress and dyspnea. Brain: altered level of consciousness ranging from mild confusion to coma. Heart: chest pain, possible myocardial infarction. Kidneys: decreased renal function.
Therapy related		
Heart	Cardiotoxic effects of some chemotherapeutic agents (e.g., paclitaxel, antimetabolites, alkylating agents) Radiation therapy: can injure any heart structure; results in pericarditis, pericardial effusions, pericardial constriction	Dysrhythmias, cardiac ischemia, heart failure, shock, pericarditis. Patient may present with irregular pulse, chest pain, peripheral and/or pulmonary edema. Cardiac tamponade is possible.
Lungs	Pulmonary toxic effects of certain chemotherapeutic agents (e.g., ALTRA, bleomycin, mitomycin-C) Radiation therapy: injures tissue, causing pneumonitis and fibrosis	Acute respiratory distress syndrome (ARDS), pulmonary fibrosis, interstitial lung disease, veno-occlusive disease. Patient may present with increasing respiratory distress, chest pain, hypoxemia.
Liver	Toxic effects due to the liver's major role in breakdown of drugs, making it a target for toxic effects	Decreased liver function: Elevated liver enzymes, bilirubin Decreased serum albumin, protein, prolonged bleeding Jaundice
Intestines	*Neutropenic enterocolitis* (necrotizing enteritis): Chemotherapy-induced damage to intestinal wall with subsequent bacterial invasion. Develops with severe neutropenia (less than 1,000 cells/mm^3). Commonly seen in acute leukemia and also associated with cytotoxic chemotherapy.	Fever Right upper quadrant (RUQ) abdominal pain and abdominal distention Diarrhea (bloody or watery) Nausea and vomiting
Urinary bladder	*Hemorrhagic Cystitis* Results from severe bladder irritation secondary to chemotherapy or radiation	Urinary frequency, hematuria, dysuria Bladder hemorrhage
Other Crises		
Sepsis	Can result from therapy-induced immunosuppression that increases risk for development of opportunistic pathogens Risk increases as leukocyte count (particularly neutrophils) decreases.	Standard sepsis criteria
Tumor lysis syndrome	Results from escape of a massive load of intracellular metabolites into the circulation with death of cancer cells within 48–72 hours of chemotherapy. Usually associated with leukemia or lymphoma therapy.	Elevated serum: uric acid, phosphorus, potassium Abnormally low serum: calcium Possible renal failure
Hypercalcemia	Results from increased bone resorption by osteoclasts and decreased renal excretion causing elevated levels of circulating calcium	Nausea, vomiting, anorexia, abdominal pain, polyuria, weakness, fatigue, seizures, coma Heart block and cardiac dysrhythmias possible

SOURCE: Data from Niederhubur et al. (2014).

presentation: the speed at which the obstruction develops and the degree of venous blood flow compromise. If the development of SVC syndrome is gradual, collateral circulation has time to develop, and the patient may experience only mild symptoms; however, if the development is rapid, the patient can present in a crisis state (Nickloes et al., 2016). As soon as SVC syndrome is suspected, an MRI or CT scan is obtained to confirm the diagnosis.

Therapeutic treatment depends on the cause of the obstruction and may consist of radiation therapy or combination chemotherapy, depending on the type of cancer.

A stent may be placed if the syndrome is a recurrent problem. If thrombosis caused the syndrome, thrombolytic therapy and follow-up anticoagulation therapy may be ordered.

Leukostasis Leukostasis (or hyperleukocytosis) refers to partial or complete obstruction of blood flow resulting from excessive numbers of circulating leukocytes (peripheral blast count of more than 100,000 cells/mcL) and is potentially fatal at extreme elevations (Inoue, 2016). It is primarily associated with acute myelogenous leukemia (AML) that results from uncontrolled proliferation of leukocytes. The massive load of blast cells in the circulation increases the blood viscosity and aggregation (clumping) of leukemic cells, leading to sluggish blood flow through the capillaries. The end result is impaired capillary circulation and end-organ damage with the brain and lungs most commonly affected (Inoue, 2016). Neurologic symptoms include headache, dizziness, and altered level of consciousness ranging from mild confusion to deep coma. Pulmonary manifestations include hypoxemia, respiratory distress, and respiratory failure. Kidney and heart manifestations may also develop if microcirculation is affected in those organs. Treatment consists of hydrating the patient to decrease the concentration of circulating cells, removing leukocytes from the circulation through apheresis therapy, and administration of the antineoplastic agent, hydroxyurea, which rapidly reduces the high blast cell count (Inoue, 2016).

Therapy-related Emergencies

Cancer chemotherapeutic agents are considered to be the most toxic drug group. They have the potential of curing the malignancy; however, the risks of adverse effects are great. Many potentially severe complications are associated with chemotherapy. Multiple cancer chemotherapeutic agents have organ toxicity as a major adverse effect; thus, effective treatment of the cancer may severely injure one or more organs as a result of that therapy. Moreover, radiation therapy, another common form of cancer therapy, can cause significant organ and tissue injury. The following are some of the more common therapy-related organ system complications that, when severe, can be potentially life-threatening.

Intestinal   **Neutropenic enterocolitis** (necrotizing enteritis, typhlitis, or ileocecal syndrome) is a necrotizing infectious process that affects the bowel in acute leukemia patients who are receiving remission-induction cytotoxic chemotherapy. Risk factors for development may include cytotoxic chemotherapy, myeloproliferative neoplasms, and bone marrow or solid organ transplant. The pathogenesis of neutropenic enterocolitis is believed to involve chemotherapy-induced intestinal wall damage in the presence of neutropenia (neutrophil count of less than 1,000), whereby bacteria (e.g., *E. coli* or *Pseudomonas aeruginosa*) are able to shift through the injured gut wall to colonize and damage the mucosal layer (Sultan & Vasudeva, 2016). It is characterized by inflammation, injury, and ulceration of the mucosal layer of the small and large intestines, with the cecum being a common site of injury. The patient's severely immunosuppressed state allows bacterial invasion of the damaged mucosal layer that can eventually result in transmural intestinal wall damage, perforation, and possible peritonitis.

The severity of neutropenic enterocolitis varies along a continuum that ranges from mild to life-threatening. Typically the patient presents with a trio of symptoms: fever, abdominal pain, and diarrhea (watery or bloody) in the presence of chemotherapy-induced neutropenia; however, nausea and vomiting and abdominal distention are often present (Sultan & Vasudeva, 2016). Diagnostic procedures may include plain abdominal radiographs; barium enema;

and abdominal CT scan or ultrasonography, which allows visualization of the characteristic edema and thickening of the affected bowel walls. Treatment in mild cases is conservative and usually includes placement of a nasogastric tube for gastric decompression, IV fluid replacement therapy, and broad-spectrum antibiotic therapy. Surgical resection of the affected bowel is reserved for severe cases that have become life-threatening (e.g., hemorrhage, intra-abdominal abscess) (Sultan & Vasudeva, 2016).

Urinary Bladder   Chemotherapy and radiation can cause severe bladder irritation, resulting in urinary frequency, hematuria, and dysuria. In its severe form, it can cause gross bleeding and is known as **hemorrhagic cystitis**. Two chemotherapy agents, cyclophosphamide and ifosfamide, produce a liver metabolite, acrolein, which is a urotoxin (Basler & Stanley, 2016). The incidence of hemorrhagic cystitis has been significantly reduced with preventive therapy that includes patient hydration and prescribing the drug mesna (Mesnex, Uromitexan), which binds with acrolein to prevent bladder problems (Basler & Stanley, 2016). Treatment for hemorrhagic cystitis includes evacuating any clots and continuous bladder irrigation until the bleeding has stopped. A cystoscopy may be performed to evaluate the bleeding further. In severe cases a hypogastric artery embolization, open cystotomy, or a total cystectomy may be required.

Heart   Cardiac toxic effects such as dysrhythmias, cardiac ischemia, heart failure, cardiomyopathy, and pericarditis have been associated with a variety of cancer chemotherapeutic agents. For example, paclitaxel (Taxol) can cause asymptomatic bradyarrhythmia or ventricular tachycardia, and the antimetabolite 5-Fluorouracil (5-FU) is known to rarely cause cardiac ischemia. The anthracyclines (e.g., Daunorubicin) are known to cause heart failure and cardiomyopathy; however, development depends on the cumulative dose of the drug. Alkylating agents such as Cytoxan are known to cause severe myocarditis and exudative pericarditis.

Radiation therapy can cause cardiac damage that may manifest in a delayed fashion, even years following therapy (Marks, Constine, & Adams, 2015). Radiation may affect any structure of the heart, such as the myocardium or pericardium. Three major syndromes are associated with radiation therapy, including acute pericarditis, pericardial effusion, and pericardial constriction. When severe, pericarditis and pericardial effusion can cause cardiac tamponade, which is a life-threatening emergency. Patients often present with a low-to-normal arterial blood pressure with positive jugular vein distention and distant heart sounds (Marks et al., 2015). Therapy depends on the severity of the problem. If symptoms are mild, the patient may require only continued observation; however, if tamponade is present, emergency removal of pericardial fluid is required to relieve the pressure on the heart, and a pericardial drain may be required. Significant restrictive pericarditis damage may require surgical stripping of the affected pericardium.

Lungs   A number of cancer chemotherapeutic agents are known to potentially cause pulmonary damage. Development of acute respiratory distress syndrome (ARDS) has been associated with all-trans-retinoic acid (ALTRA), a drug used to treat acute promyelocytic leukemia, and bleomycin, which is known for causing pulmonary fibrosis (Camus, 2017). Interstitial lung disease may be a delayed effect of treatment, with symptoms sometimes appearing months later. Pulmonary veno-occlusive disease is a known complication of antineoplastic treatment using bleomycin, mitomycin-C, and HSCT drug regimens. Radiation therapy targeting the lungs also increases the risk of certain pulmonary complications, including radiation pneumonitis and fibrosis, the severity of which depends on the percentage of lung irradiated and the dose of radiation received. Common treatments include discontinuance of the drug and administration of corticosteroids. Treatment of pulmonary veno-occlusive disease may require discontinuing the offending drugs and administration of vasodilator therapy (Huertas et al., 2011).

Liver Hepatotoxicity has been associated with HSCT and bone marrow transplantation and multiple chemotherapeutic drugs. Because the liver is the primary source of drug metabolism, it is at high risk for toxicity problems with cancer chemotherapy agents. L-asparaginase and antimetabolite medications are particularly associated with liver damage, and interferon and retinoic acid therapies also have been reported to cause hepatotoxicity. Hepatotoxicity may initially present as decreased liver function, which may be noted first in abnormal liver-profile laboratory results. Treatment may require dose reduction or discontinuance of a particular offending agent.

Other Oncologic Treatment Emergencies

While chemotherapeutic agents and radiation directly injure organs, other treatment-related complications cause injury indirectly, either during or after completion of therapy. Some of the more common treatment-induced crises include sepsis, tumor lysis syndrome, and hypercalcemia. The remainder of this section provides a brief overview of these crises.

Sepsis Patients receiving cancer treatment have a high risk of acquiring opportunistic infections resulting from therapy-induced immunosuppression, which significantly increases the risk for the development of sepsis. Leukemia and HSCT or bone marrow transplant patients are especially at high risk when their marrow has been ablated, causing severe neutropenia. The severely neutropenic patient is predisposed to invasion by bacteria, viruses (e.g., herpes simplex), and fungi (e.g., *candida* and *aspergillosis*); even normally low virulent agents may cause a life-threatening infection. To further complicate matters, multiple infections may develop simultaneously. Disseminated fungal infections may lead to other life-threatening infections that may not respond to the standard treatment. Patients with bacteremia are placed on intravenous antibiotics, which should continue at least until the neutrophil count has sufficiently recovered. Acyclovir may be ordered prophylactically or for treatment of the herpes virus. Granulocyte-colony stimulating factor (G-CSF) may be prescribed to encourage rapid leukocyte recovery.

Tumor Lysis Syndrome Tumor lysis syndrome (TLS) is usually associated with treatment for leukemia and lymphoma but can result from other cancers. As cancer treatment destroys tumor cells, the intracellular metabolites from the destroyed cells spill out into the circulation at a rate that exceeds the kidneys' ability to excrete them, causing potentially life-threatening elevations in serum metabolite levels (Ikeda & Jaishankar, 2016). Common clinical findings include hyperuricemia, hyperphosphatemia, hyperkalemia, and hypocalcemia. Unless properly treated with intravenous hydration and loop diuretics, TLS can result in kidney failure and subsequent death. Antigout drugs, such as allopurinol or rasburicase (Elitek), are used to decrease uric acid levels and protect the kidneys. Hemodialysis is an effective treatment to rid the body of the excess metabolites if other treatment has failed. Hyperphosphatemia is treated by placing the patient on a restrictive diet, using oral phosphate binders and, in extreme cases, hemodialysis (Ikeda & Jaishankar, 2016).

Hypercalcemia Hypercalcemia is one of the most common cancer-related metabolic emergencies. It develops due to two factors: osteoclastic (bone breakdown) activities and decreased calcium excretion in the urine. Calcium leeches from the bones through osteoclastic activities, releasing calcium into the general circulation and increasing serum calcium levels. If renal urinary excretion of calcium is insufficient to counterbalance the increased serum calcium load, hypercalcemia develops. The treatment for hypercalcemia includes volume expansion with normal saline to improve renal function and decrease calcium resorption. Bisphosphonates, such as pamidronate and zoledronic acid, inhibit osteoclastic activity and bone resorption. Calcitonin decreases calcium by inhibiting bone resorption and increasing renal excretion. Dialysis may be needed if the patient is unable to tolerate volume expansion. Treatment for the cancer is the ultimate treatment for malignancy-associated hypercalcemia (Horwitz, 2014).

Nursing Implications

The nurse who is managing the care of a patient with cancer must be vigilant in monitoring for possible complications that may develop and must be familiar with the exact chemotherapeutic regimen to predict the type of toxicities involved. A thorough multisystem physical assessment is warranted with particular focus on the known high-risk organs. For example, when the patient has been receiving cardiotoxic agents, monitoring will include vital signs, heart sounds, periodic 12-lead ECG, evaluation of cardiac markers, and general cardiac assessment; when the patient is receiving a known pulmonary toxic agent, monitoring will include a thorough pulmonary assessment, including respiratory rate, rhythm, lung sounds, and periodic pulse oximetry readings. Organ function is also monitored through collection and trending of appropriate laboratory data. For example, if the patient is receiving a renal toxic agent, the serum blood urea nitrogen (BUN), creatinine, and potassium are closely monitored. Patient education on the therapeutic and nontherapeutic effects of the drug regimen is crucial to best ensure that the patient knows when to contact the provider regarding changes in status.

Section Five Review

1. The neutropenic client who presents with fever and hypotension suggests which oncologic complication?
   A. Hypercalcemia
   B. Superior vena cava syndrome
   C. Sepsis
   D. Spinal cord compression

2. A client with tumor lysis syndrome (TLS) may receive which initial treatment?
   A. Intravenous fluids and loop diuretics
   B. Radiation
   C. IV antibiotics
   D. Corticosteroids

3. The term leukostasis refers to which event?
   A. Infiltration of brain and lungs by blast cells
   B. Inability of leukocytes to move out of bone marrow
   C. Loss of vision or stroke caused by stagnant blood flow
   D. Impaired circulation as a result of capillary congestion by blast cells

4. The hypercalcemia that develops in some clients with cancer results from which underlying problem?
   A. Calcium-based chemotherapeutic agents
   B. Increased bone resorption by osteoclasts
   C. Ionic exchange of potassium with calcium
   D. Spontaneous bone fractures

Answers: 1. A, 2. A, 3. D, 4. B

Section Six: HIV Disease—A Disorder of Immunodeficiency

The immune system can be subject to inadequate development, disease, and injury from illness or treatments that can result in impaired immune activity. Such a situation is called an **immunodeficiency state**. Immunodeficiency results from an acute or chronic loss of function of one or more components of the immune system. Human immunodeficiency virus/acquired immunodeficiency disease syndrome (HIV/AIDS) is the most common disease associated with secondary (acquired) immunodeficiency. This section provides a broad overview of HIV/AIDS, including the epidemiology, transmission, viral invasion, cellular characteristics of HIV disease, progression of the disease, clinical manifestations, treatment approaches, and nursing implications.

Epidemiology and Transmission

First recognized in the United States in 1981, HIV/AIDS was initially thought to be a disease solely affecting homosexual males, but it occurs in heterosexual groups and all races and ethnic groups. The global pandemic continues, especially in sub-Saharan Africa and Southeast Asia. There is also increasing concern with the rapidly growing number of HIV-infected women. HIV infection is a chronic illness that requires long-term medical management to obtain optimal health and reduce the spread of infection (Centers for Disease Control [CDC] and Prevention, 2016a). Many patients with HIV infections require intensive medical and nursing care during the course of their disease. With newer antiviral therapies and early treatment of HIV, the lifespan of those infected with HIV approaches the lifespan of those without the disease when patients adhere to the prescribed treatment regimen (Katz, 2017).

HIV is transmitted predominantly through infected blood and body secretions, generally excluding saliva and tears. The HIV virus is fragile and cannot survive outside of the body; thus it requires direct contact—such as secretion–secretion, secretion–blood, or blood–blood—for transmission to occur. Modes include sexual contact, via the blood contact, contaminated needles, and mother–infant transmission either intrapartum, during the birth process, or through breast milk. In the United States, the CDC estimates that 1.2 million people have HIV. A decrease in incidence has been reported with an average of 50,000 new cases each year down from 130,000. The most common categories of transmission include male-to-male sexual contact (63%), heterosexual contact (25%), and intravenous drug use (11 %) (CDC, 2016b). Transmission through contaminated blood products was once considered a significant risk factor for transmission of HIV in the United States; however, it is now extremely rare, owing to use of sophisticated cross-matching and antibody screening precautions. Nonetheless, the risk of contaminated blood product remains a significant concern in countries where screenings are not as readily available. Blood product considerations to prevent HIV infection through contamination are identified in the "Quality and Safety: HIV Virus Exposure" feature. Individuals who require specific blood components (such as factor VIII and frequent plasma replacement) may be at increased risk because of the large numbers of donors needed to produce adequate quantities of these components.

The quantity of virus that enters the blood is also of major importance. Successful transmission requires a sufficient viral load—the higher the initial viral load, the higher the risk of developing HIV infection. Measuring viral load can assess medication effectiveness and is useful in the early diagnosis of infection (Katz, 2017).

Quality and Safety
HIV Virus Exposure

- Units of whole blood or packed red blood cells, platelets, leukocytes, or plasma can transmit the HIV virus when contaminated.
- Approximately 90% of patients exposed to HIV-infected blood products will become infected.
- Avoiding the use of blood products that are positive for HIV nucleic acid and antibodies to HIV-1 and HIV-2 can diminish the risk of infection through blood transfusions.

SOURCE: Data from Fauci & Lane (2015).

Pathophysiology

HIV is a type of retrovirus, carrying genetic information in ribonucleic acid (RNA) rather than in deoxyribonucleic acid (DNA). There are two forms of HIV: HIV-1 is the major cause of AIDS globally, and HIV-2 has been isolated in West Africa and currently is rarely found in the United States (Katz, 2017). The HIV-2 virus is less virulent, is less transmissible, and creates lower proportions of infected cells; however, it is still capable of causing AIDS.

Viral Invasion   The HIV virus is attracted to a subset of T lymphocytes, the helper T cells (T_H, $CD4^+$). On contact with the T cell, the virus binds to its cell surface at the $CD4^+$ T-cell receptor site and penetrates the T-cell membrane. Through an enzyme called reverse transcriptase, the viral RNA is copied as a double-stranded DNA and inserted into the host cell chromosome, where it may remain dormant. When the T cell is activated to reproduce, the viral genetic information is programmed to produce more of the virus within the $CD4^+$ cell, eventually destroying the infected cell and allowing massive numbers of viral copies to escape the dead T cell and move on to infect nearby T cells. Viral load and $CD4^+$ T-cell counts are reflective of viral activity and disease progression. Reverse transcriptase is highly error prone and may produce multiple mutations during each viral replication, which can make targeted therapy difficult. Most antiviral drugs currently being tested or used in treatment regimens work by inhibiting the action of reverse transcriptase or by inhibiting the protease enzyme that is needed at a later stage of the HIV's course. Figure 30–6 illustrates how HIV infects and destroys T helper cells.

Cellular Characteristics of HIV Disease   The immunodeficiency state that eventually develops with HIV infection involves elements of both cell-mediated and humoral-mediated immunodeficiency (Katz, 2017). The cellular immune deficiency characterizing HIV disease is manifested by markedly depressed T lymphocyte functioning, with a reduction of helper T cells (T_H, $CD4^+$), impaired cytotoxic T-cell (T_C, $CD8^+$) activity, and increased suppressor T cells (T_S, $CD8^+$). By selectively invading and infecting T cells (particularly T_H cells), the HIV virus damages the very cells whose function it is to orchestrate the identification and destruction of the virus as antigen. Eventually, the individual's supply of functional T_H cells becomes depleted. The humoral response in producing antibodies is less directly affected by the HIV virus. B-cell production does not seem to be decreased, but the induction and regulation of the humoral response may be affected by the lack of T-cell regulators (e.g., T_H and T_S cells), subsequently depressing B-cell responses to new antigen challenges.

Progression of HIV Infection

The progression of HIV disease in adults is monitored and categorized by the grouping of clinical manifestations or on $CD4^+$ T-cell levels, both of which reflect disease progression. For ease of discussion, HIV disease progression can be grouped into three general stages: early, progressive, and overt AIDS.

Early-stage HIV Disease   Early-stage HIV disease can be separated into two periods: an acute viral syndrome and a clinical latency (window) period.

Acute Viral Syndrome.   Within about 2 to 4 weeks of exposure to the virus, transient flu-like or mononucleosis-like symptoms may coincide with a burst of viral growth in the plasma, causing fever, swollen glands, rash, and joint and muscle pain and fatigue (AIDS.gov, 2015). About 70% of patients develop symptoms during this acute phase (Carpenter, Chan-Tack, & Bartlett, 2015). The virus is not lying dormant; rather, it is actively replicating, thereby increasing the serum viral load. If the blood is tested for HIV during this time, the results would be positive for HIV but negative for antibodies (seronegative). Eventually, during this period, sufficient antibodies develop against the virus to be measurable in the blood, an event called **seroconversion** (Carpenter et al., 2015).

Clinical Latency (Window) Period.   The time from the initial infection to the development of symptoms and the appearance of antibodies is referred to as the clinical latency period or the asymptomatic stage; however, mild symptoms may be present as the window period progresses. In untreated patients, it usually lasts about 10 years; with treatment, it can last much longer. During this time, the virus continues to replicate and may be transmitted to others, but the individual's immune system keeps the viral count sufficiently low to maintain control over the disease.

Progressive HIV Disease and AIDS   Eventually, the latency period ends (heralded by an increasing HIV viral load with a subsequent decline in $CD4^+$ [T_H] cell levels), and the patient develops symptoms. The clinical manifestations associated with HIV/AIDS worsen as the active disease progresses, and the potential for infection increases as the immune protection afforded by the $CD4^+$ cells becomes increasingly compromised. Eventually, the infected individual meets the AIDS-defining criteria.

Defining characteristics of AIDS were established in 1981 by the Centers for Disease Control and Prevention (CDC, 1992). The CDC defines AIDS thus:

- Seropositive HIV infection with
- A $CD4^+$ T cell count of less than 200 cells/mL, OR
- The presence of at least one AIDS-defining illness (regardless of $CD4^+$ count)

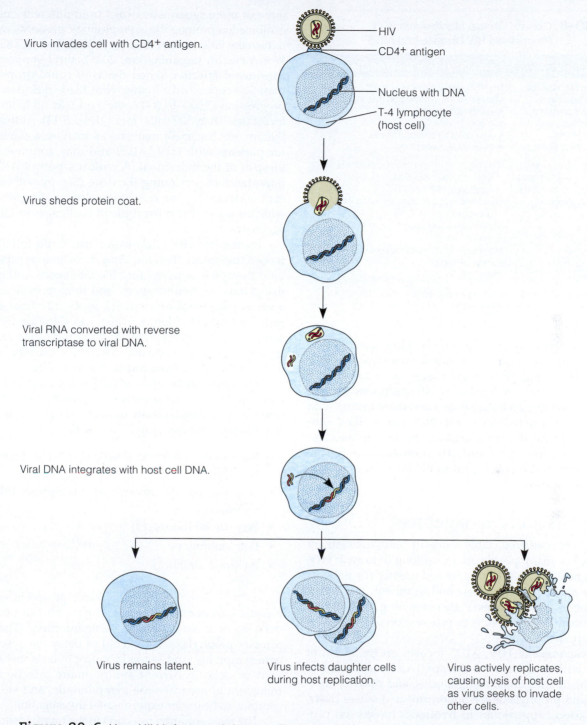

Virus invades cell with CD4+ antigen.

HIV
CD4+ antigen
Nucleus with DNA
T-4 lymphocyte (host cell)

Virus sheds protein coat.

Viral RNA converted with reverse transcriptase to viral DNA.

Viral DNA integrates with host cell DNA.

Virus remains latent.

Virus infects daughter cells during host replication.

Virus actively replicates, causing lysis of host cell as virus seeks to invade other cells.

Figure 30–6 How HIV infects and destroys T helper cells.

The most common AIDS-defining illnesses in the United States are *Pneumocystis jiroveci* pneumonia (PJP), cytomegalovirus (CMV), and *Mycobacterium avium-intracellulare* complex (MAC).

Clinical Manifestations

The clinical presentation of HIV/AIDS patients varies, depending largely on which opportunistic infections are present. Some of the more common general clinical manifestations of progressive disease and AIDS are summarized in Table 30–8. Eventually, the patient dies of complications of end-stage AIDS, which is usually uncontrollable infection.

Diagnosis of HIV

Laboratory testing to diagnose HIV infection relies predominantly on the presence of the p24 antibody. P24 is a major protein found in HIV that is capable of triggering a detectable immune system response to HIV. When HIV exposure is suspected, a screening test using the HIV-1/2 antigen–antibody combination immunoassay is used to

Table 30–8 General Clinical Manifestations of
Progressive HIV Disease and AIDS

Disease Phase	Common Clinical Manifestations
Progressive HIV disease (CD4$^+$ is less than normal but greater than 200 cells/mcL, with absence of any AIDS-defining illness.)	No AIDS-defining illness present Manifestations variable and may include: • Lymphadenopathy • Mouth lesions • Anemia or thrombocytopenia • Neurological symptoms
Overt AIDS (CD4$^+$ is less than 200 cells/mcL and may have the presence of one AIDS-defining illness)	Wasting syndrome (10% or greater weight loss; may also include fevers, general weakness, diarrhea) Neurological symptoms: dementia, tremors, encephalitis Malignancies and opportunistic infections or conditions Increasing debilitation and severe fatigue Lymphadenopathy Pharyngitis

SOURCE: Data from CDC, 2016c; Katz, 2017; Selik et al., 2014

identify the presence of an antibody. However, a false-positive result can occur as a result of cross-reactive antibodies to HLA antigens, hepatic disease, gamma globulin injections, and some malignancies. All specimens that are reactive or positive on initial assay need more testing with an immunoassay that differentiates HIV-1 from HIV-2 antibodies. Specimens that are reactive or positive to the combination immunoassay but are nonreactive to the differentiation test then proceed to the HIV-1 nucleic acid testing (CDC, 2014).

Prognosis and Management

To date, there is no predictable course of curative treatment for AIDS, but many people are living long lives with HIV. The prognosis of HIV has improved greatly for patients that have access to medical care and treatment. The majority of patients (70%), however, are not getting medical care and treatment, which results in progression of the disease (CDC, 2016a).

Management of HIV/AIDS focuses on treatment of the HIV with antiretroviral therapy (ART); treatment of opportunistic infections, malignancies, and other complications; and prophylaxis for opportunistic diseases (Katz, 2017). Various approaches to treatment have been proposed and tested. Restoration of immune function has been attempted by bone marrow transplant, transfusions of white blood cells, and interferon treatments. Unfortunately, the newest healthy cells are quickly infected by the virus. The structure of HIV is so variable (much like the variations of flu virus) that a medication formulated against one genetic mutation of the virus may not provide protection against another.

Antiviral Therapy Pharmacologic approaches using combination antiretroviral therapy rather than monotherapy have been successful in maintaining viral load suppression and in treating AIDS as a long-term chronic disease in adults. Antiretroviral therapy (ART) can reduce the viral replication but cannot kill the virus. With ART,

three or more synergistic drugs from different classes are combined to prolong the asymptomatic phase, as well as to reduce the viral load in the overt AIDS phase (CDC, 2017b; World Health Organization, 2016). Viral suppression is considered effective when the viral count drops to less than 500 copies/mL. Rising viral load indicates disease progression (5,000–10,000 copies/mL), as do falling CD4$^+$ levels (less than 500 cells/mcL) (Kee, 2014). Antiretroviral therapy has become a mainstay of treatment management for patients with HIV/AIDS and may continue for the lifespan of the individual. A critical aspect of ART is the importance of continuing the drug therapy without interruption to reduce the risk of developing drug resistance, which is one of the most difficult challenges in HIV management.

Incomplete HIV suppression can result in HIV resistance to treatment; therefore, long-term, uninterrupted antiviral therapy is required for HIV inhibition. Antiretroviral drugs have numerous short- and long-term side effects, such as peripheral neuropathy, gastrointestinal distress, rash, and hyperlipidemia, which can significantly impact compliance. In combination, the antivirals can be extremely toxic to organs and bone marrow; thus, close monitoring of organ and bone marrow function is necessary.

The ideal combination of ART is not clear, but the current standard of care involves a regimen of using at least three drugs simultaneously from at least two of the following different pharmacologic classes (Katz, 2017):

- Nucleoside and nucleotide reverse transcriptase inhibitors (NRTI)
- Non-nucleoside reverse transcriptase inhibitors (NNRTI)
- Protease inhibitors (PI)
- Entry inhibitors
- Integrase inhibitors

Drug Prophylaxis Drug prophylaxis protocols for opportunistic infections of HIV/AIDS have shown promise in delaying or avoiding symptomatic infections. The goal of primary prophylaxis is to avoid or delay the onset of disease symptoms, and secondary prophylaxis seeks to prevent or delay recurrent symptomatic infection. Other treatment approaches are symptomatic, and still others continue to be under experimental investigation.

The most common infection in the immunosuppressed HIV patient is *Pneumocystis jiroveci* pneumonia (PJP) and its recurrence. This pneumonia was originally called *Pneumocystis carinii* pneumonia (PCP); however, the name was changed to denote the specific form found in humans. PJP was one of the first opportunistic infections to be identified as an AIDS-defining illness. Since its prevalence in the AIDS population has been followed, it continues to be the most life-threatening opportunistic infection to both adult and pediatric AIDS patients, with its virulence increasing as the T$_H$ cell (CD4$^+$) count falls below 200 cells/mcL in the adult. The infected patient presents with fever, fatigue, and weight loss months before actual respiratory symptoms develop. Coughing, shortness of breath, hypoxemia, and abnormal pulmonary function studies contribute to the clinical picture of progressive illness. Prophylaxis therapy for PJP is indicated when the CD4$^+$ cell count falls below 300 cells/mcL in the adult HIV-1 patient. Typical preventive and treatment therapy for PJP includes trimethoprim-sulfamethoxazole (TMP-SMX; Bactrim, Septra) or an aerosol of pentamidine.

Prevention of other opportunistic infections such as toxoplasmosis, tuberculosis, *Mycobacterium avium* complex (MAC), cytomegalovirus (CMV), and fungi is crucial, and with the advent of ART, the need for prophylaxis therapy is largely guided by the patient's CD4$^+$ count (Katz, 2017). High-priority vaccine recommendations include pneumonia and influenza. Other vaccines, such as measles, mumps, and rubella (MMR) and chickenpox (varicella zoster), may be contraindicated because of their imposed risk as live viruses. Granulocyte stimulants, such as filgrastim (Neupogen), may be given to counteract the neutropenia related to antiretroviral therapy or to the HIV itself.

Nursing Implications

To provide the best care, high-acuity nurses need to be knowledgeable about HIV, the disease process, and complications that may arise. Patients who are positive for HIV can require acute-care hospitalization for many reasons that may be unrelated to their HIV status, such as trauma or surgery. However, they may require admission to the hospital after becoming acutely ill with an opportunistic infection, a malignancy, or another disease-related complication, or if they require intravenous therapy. Respiratory distress, high fevers, or acute mental status changes are common clinical admission complaints. On admission, early evaluation of the patient's immune status is crucial as HIV can cause a profound immunoincompetent state. If the patient's immune status meets the AIDS criteria, nursing management needs to include activities that protect the patient's immunocompromised state (see Section Eight).

The CDC (2016c) recommends routine screening of all people who come into any healthcare setting. For this reason, admission to the hospital with an acute illness and subsequent routine blood testing may be the point at which the patient becomes aware of an HIV-positive status. The nurse should be prepared to support the patient and caregivers who are coping with HIV/AIDS along the illness trajectory. Counseling should be offered at the time of screening and should continue as needed to meet individual patient needs. Despite advances in the management of HIV/AIDS, it remains an illness with a significant symptom burden, both physically and emotionally, and, unfortunately, lingering societal stigma. Not all patients with HIV/AIDS have access to care or the expensive drugs needed to manage their illness, and this reality, along with the growing numbers of infected individuals, will present challenges for our global healthcare community.

HIV Exposure in the Healthcare Professional   Although relatively few healthcare professionals are at risk for HIV, treatment approaches and protocols for occupational exposure to needlesticks, blood and body fluids, or contaminated instruments have been developed. Postexposure prophylaxis protocols include determining the source and severity of the exposure, determining the HIV status of the source, and recommendations for treatment. It is important to remember that the HIV virus is fragile, is easily destroyed by chemical disinfectants, and cannot survive outside of the human body. A basic postexposure prophylactic (PEP) regimen begins within hours (not days) after exposure and includes antiretroviral therapy (ART) for 4 weeks (CDC, 2016c). The most up-to-date PEP recommendations and protocols can be found on the CDC website.

Section Six Review

1. Which statement best characterizes HIV/AIDS?
   A. Symptoms result from opportunistic disease pathology.
   B. HIV invades cells only through the bloodstream.
   C. Clinical manifestations are in a characteristic and predictable sequence.
   D. HIV is a stable, nonmutating virus.

2. Which fluids are known to be modes of transmission for HIV? (Select all that apply.)
   A. Tears
   B. Semen
   C. Plasma
   D. Saliva
   E. Breast milk

3. Which are AIDS-defining illnesses? (Select all that apply.)
   A. Epstein-Barr Virus
   B. CMV
   C. MAC
   D. Rubella (measles)
   E. PJP

4. Which adverse effects often result in noncompliance with antiretroviral drug therapy for HIV/AIDS? (Select all that apply.)
   A. Peripheral neruopathy
   B. Gastrointestinal distress
   C. Rash
   D. Hyperlipidemia
   E. Hair loss

Answers: 1. A, 2. (B, C, E), 3. (B, C, E), 4. (A, B, C, D)

Section Seven: Aging, Malnutrition, Stress, Trauma, and the Immune System

The immune system has a remarkable ability to protect against many insults; however, it is also a vulnerable system that is significantly altered by factors such as aging, malnutrition, stress, and trauma. In high-acuity patients, one or all of these factors may be present or may develop during hospitalization. Alone, each factor can alter patient outcomes; in combination, the results can be devastating, significantly increasing patient morbidity and mortality.

Aging

The functioning of the immune system declines with age, a phenomenon known as immunosenescence (Azar & Ballas, 2017). The thymus gland, where T lymphocytes mature and differentiate, begins to atrophy early in life and continues to shrink until a person reaches middle age. Although T lymphocytes continue to be produced, their maturation and differentiation into the various types of T cells (e.g., T helper cells) decreases. This places the older patient at higher risk for increased frequency and severity of infections accompanied by a decreased ability to resolve the infection. Macrophages continue to function throughout life; however, the length of time it takes them to clear the pathogens increases significantly with age. The ability of the immune system to discriminate between antigens that are "self" from those that are "nonself" also declines with aging, which increases the incidence of autoimmune diseases by middle age and older. In addition, the immune system also becomes significantly less efficient at recognizing and destroying mutated (tumor) cells, which at least partially accounts for the increased incidence of cancer in the older adult. The B-cell response to antigens also declines in cell numbers and efficacy with aging. Production of the immunoglobulin IgM decreases; however, production of IgA and IgG increases, possibly related to autoantibody responses to self-antigens.

Malnutrition

Although nutritional deficiencies can occur at any age, older adults, particularly those who are frail, are at particular risk. Many factors contribute to the development of malnutrition in this patient population, including decreased appetite, loss of social supports, decreased ease of access to grocery stores, and impaired functional status. The possibility of malnutrition should be considered by the nurse whenever an acutely ill older adult is admitted because it can have a profound impact on the immune system and subsequently on the patient's overall prognosis.

Basic components of calorie and protein intake play key roles in the formation and integrity of T cells and immunoglobulins (antibodies). Malnutrition contributes to immunocompromise by causing impaired response of lymphocytes to pathogens, to vaccines, and to components of defense. Zinc plays a major role in the structure and function of both B cells and T cells and in collagen synthesis for wound healing. As a co-factor, zinc is required for the normal function of lymphocytes in their production of enzymes. Although zinc deficiencies are rare in those with regular diets, there can be significant loss through the gastrointestinal tract with malabsorption syndromes or inflammatory bowel disease. It also can be lost through the skin in burn victims. Vitamins such as A, E, pyridoxine, folic acid, and pantothenic acid serve as co-factors in enzyme production and, in malnourished states, can affect the function of both T cells and B cells.

Malnutrition is also believed to contribute to development of sepsis as the malnourished gut atrophies and becomes more permeable to bacteria. When bacteria seep out of the gut, immune system mediators are released, such as tumor necrosis factor (TNF), and they are capable of triggering systemic lymphocyte activity. Tumor necrosis factor is believed to be largely responsible for precipitating multiple organ dysfunction syndrome (MODS). Prevention of gut atrophy in the acutely ill patient by implementing early enteral feedings can greatly reduce the risk of sepsis by reducing circulating immune mediators and subsequent multiple organ dysfunction in the critically ill patient.

Stress and Trauma

Stress affects the immune system primarily through the effects of cortisol, a glucocorticoid hormone secreted by the adrenal glands. During periods of physical or psychological stress, the adrenal glands secrete more cortisol in response to perceived need. Cortisol is necessary to maintain homeostasis during stress; however, it has a direct suppressing effect on the immune system by inhibiting production of two interleukins (IL-1 and IL-2) that are necessary for normal T-cell production. Furthermore, elevated levels of cortisol result in increased serum glucose levels to provide the stressed body with more energy; hyperglycemia is known to alter leukocyte function.

Trauma, both intentional (such as surgery or anesthesia) and unintentional (such as burns, motor vehicle crashes, and falls), suppresses T-cell and B-cell activity and compromises immune function. Trauma can cause cellular dysfunction, characterized by decreased chemotactic and phagocytic activities and decreased antibody and lymphocyte levels. Impaired T-cell activity and depressed lymphokines have been linked to multiple organ system dysfunction and poor clinical outcomes in the trauma patient. The high-acuity trauma patient enters the intensive care unit already immunosuppressed because of a stress response to the injury, hemorrhage, and shock. Subsequent malnutrition, organ dysfunction, hypoxia, and multiple invasive procedures all create a potential scenario of vulnerability to pathogens.

Nursing Implications

The nurse assesses each newly admitted high-acuity patient for the presence of potential risk factors that alter immune system function, such as age, nutritional state, sources of physiologic and psychological stress, and trauma. A thorough nursing history and physical examination upon admission establishes the patient's baseline status against which subsequent assessments can be trended. Monitoring blood test results that measure immune, nutrition, and metabolic status (e.g., glucose, CBC with differential, liver function panel, and kidney function panel) adds important information on the patient's overall immune and metabolic health status. Frequent head-to-toe assessments and periodic reevaluation of the patient's laboratory trends facilitate rapid recognition of emerging problems. An aggressive approach must be taken to gain control of the patient's nutritional status through early nutrition consultation and nutritional support to ensure that the patient receives necessary nutrient requirements to meet often hypermetabolic needs during acute illness. In the presence of hyperglycemia, the patient may require implementation of an insulin therapy protocol to maintain a euglycemic state.

Section Seven Review

1. What is the function of zinc in the competent immune system?
   A. It is required for normal lymphocyte function.
   B. It protects B cells from being destroyed by macrophages.
   C. T cells require zinc for production of gamma globulin.
   D. Macrophages are composed primarily of zinc.

2. What effect does the normal aging process have on the immune system?
   A. B-cell function in general is particularly depressed.
   B. T-cell functioning begins to deteriorate.
   C. Autoantibodies begin to diminish with increasing age.
   D. The immune system becomes hypervigilant to invading organisms.

3. In the acutely ill adult, which nutritional loss is a critical factor in immune system integrity?
   A. Iron
   B. Vitamin C
   C. Complex carbohydrate chains
   D. Protein

4. Stress primarily affects the immune system through the effects of which substance?
   A. Lymphokines
   B. Interleukin
   C. Cortisol
   D. Epinephrine

Answers: 1. A, 2. B, 3. B, 4. C

Section Eight: Care of the Immunocompromised Patient

Care of the immunocompromised patient begins with a thorough assessment, with particular focus on the patient's immune and nutrition status. Nursing management includes frequent monitoring of immune and nutrition status, monitoring for infection, and protecting the patient from infection.

Focused Assessment

The physical examination for level of immunocompetence primarily reflects the patient's nutritional status because the proper functioning of the immune system depends on nutritional status. If the patient is malnourished, the immune status will be negatively affected. Physical assessment techniques and critical thinking must focus on seeking evidence of infection, either acute or chronic. This includes assessing for skin lesions, open wounds, the presence of adventitious breath sounds and abnormal sputum, enlarged liver or spleen, and palpable lymph nodes or masses.

The patient history gives important clues to possible altered immunocompetence. Healthcare providers should obtain medical history data from patients who may be immunocompromised with a focus on the following information:

- Complaints of fever, fatigue, weakness, swollen glands, lightheadedness, visual disturbances
- Loss of appetite
- Weight loss
- Slow wound-healing history
- Unexplained rashes, mouth sores, or oral patches
- Presence of increased levels of stress, infection, malignancy, or autoimmune disease
- History of exposure to infectious diseases
- Changes in menstrual patterns

- Unusual bleeding or bruising (reflective of platelet dysfunction)
- Recent use of immunosuppressant drugs
- Allergy history
- Burn injury
- Exposure to work environment chemicals
- At-risk factors for development of HIV/AIDS
  - Homosexual orientation or sexual partner of homosexual orientation
  - Transfusion of blood or blood products
  - IV illegal drug user or sexual partner of drug user
  - Child born of mother with AIDS
- Family history of autoimmune disorders or cancer

SOURCE: Data from Carpenito-Moyet (2014).

Immunocompetence Assessment

The high-acuity patient is at high risk for development of immunocompromise secondary to prolonged stress, severe infections, malnutrition, diabetes, and other problems. The nurse must monitor the patient for critical cues that suggest altered immune function. Some of these major critical cues include the presence of the following:

- Fever
- Poor wound healing
- Joint pain
- White oral patches
- Level of consciousness and mental status changes
- Abnormal complete blood count (CBC) with differential
- Abnormal coagulation studies
- Recurrent, prolonged, or severe infections
- Secondary infections
  - Other at-risk factors, such as splenectomy, diabetes mellitus, chronic alcohol abuse, malnutrition, or renal failure
- Immunosuppressive drug therapy, such as corticosteroids or cytotoxic drugs

Laboratory Findings   Laboratory testing is the major diagnostic tool for determining immune status. Tests may include the WBC with differential and total lymphocyte count (TLC) as well as tests establishing nutritional status, such as serum albumin or prealbumin. These tests are used as screening tests for general immune status. The nurse monitors these levels for abnormal trends.

A variety of cell-specific and disorder-specific laboratory tests are available if further evaluation of immunocompetence is necessary. Immunoglobulins, T cells, and B cells can be measured both quantitatively and functionally. Skin testing may be ordered to evaluate cellular immunocompetence. Protein and immunoglobulin levels through electrophoresis can help detect diseases associated with excess or deficient immune function. The ELISA can show exposure to HIV, to rheumatoid factor, and to lupus cells (Kee, 2014).

Collaborative Management

The goals for care of the immunocompromised patient include the goals appropriate to the malnourished patient. Additional goals include reestablishing immunocompetence and preventing and treating complications.

1. **Laboratory testing.** Various tests may be ordered to evaluate immune status. Initially, a CBC with differential count is usually obtained. Because many of the cell-specific blood tests are not commonly performed and are both expensive and time-consuming to obtain or measure, the nurse should confirm nursing responsibilities and expectations regarding the tests before drawing samples or having them drawn.

2. **Drug therapy.** Two types of drugs have a direct impact on the immune system: immunosuppressive therapy agents and agents that enhance immunity. Immunosuppressants decrease immune function. Uses include control of chronic inflammatory problems and prevention of organ transplant rejection. Examples of immunosuppressant drugs are steroids and cyclosporin A. Drugs that enhance immune function include immunotherapy agents, primarily used in cancer therapy; monoclonal antibodies, which act against specific antigens; and interleukin, a lymphokine used to enhance immune responses.

3. **Environmental protection.** Severe leukopenia places the patient at high risk for infection. The severely immunocompromised patient is placed in a controlled environment. Hospitals have protocols establishing the exact nature of the environmental protection. A private room is ordered. Some hospitals have special high-efficiency particulate air (HEPA) filter rooms that filter airflow of possibly contaminated air into the protected patient's room.

Independent Nursing Interventions

When caring for the immunocompromised patient, the nurse's role centers around monitoring for and preventing infection, regaining or maintaining adequate nutrition, and meeting the psychosocial needs of the patient and family. Remember that the severely neutropenic (agranulocytosis) patient will not be able to muster a normal immune response, which significantly alters the clinical findings. For example, the inability to form pus (a by-product of normal neutrophil activity) significantly reduces common infection findings, such as the following:

- Cloudy urine
- Purulent sputum and adventitious breath sounds
- Purulent wound drainage

Patient and family teaching to prevent and recognize infection is essential. Monitoring for infection should focus

Nursing Care

The Immunodeficient Patient

Expected Patient Outcomes and Related Interventions

Outcome 1: No evidence of infection[a]

Assess and compare to established norms, patient baselines, and trends.

Monitor patient every 2–4 hours for any signs and symptoms of infection.

Fever in the immunosuppressed patient—a persistent fever of 100.5°F (38°C) or higher for more than 1 hour may be the only sign of infection (severe neutropenia).

Signs and symptoms of inflammation, such as pain, redness, heat, or swelling (some or all of these may be absent if neutrophils are too low).

Skin or mucous membrane lesions: Check all skin folds, mouth, and perianal area; check wounds, mucous membranes, and skin-fold areas for yeast invasion (white patches).

Gastrointestinal lesions: Check all stools for occult blood; monitor for diarrhea or constipation.

Genitourinary problems: Check urine for color, odor; monitor patient for pain or fever.

Respiratory: Monitor for adventitious breath sounds, cough, dyspnea, pain; early in the course of a pulmonary infection, the patient may only develop dyspnea, tachypnea, and fever.

Invasive line or tube sites: Observe all sites closely for signs or symptoms of actual or potential infection.

Institute measures to protect the patient environmentally.

Place in private room; keep door closed.

Screen all persons coming into contact with patient for signs and symptoms of infection; apply mask if respiratory infection is suspected or confirmed.

Use excellent hand hygiene before contact (gloves recommended).

Maintain strict aseptic technique for all sterile procedures.

Minimize foods and objects brought into the room from the outside environment: Fresh fruits and vegetables may need to be washed or peeled before being taken into the room; flowers and vases with standing water may be restricted.

Special cleaning with disinfectants is recommended daily for the room.

Provide ongoing protection against development of infection.

Monitor hydration status every shift.

Turn every 1 to 2 hours.

Skin care:

Thorough daily bathing

Keep skin clean and lubricated at all times.

Keep linens clean and wrinkle free.

Perform pulmonary exercises every 4 hours.

Incentive spirometry, deep breathing

As ordered: percussion, postural drainage, vibration (percussion is contraindicated if coagulopathy exists)

Minimize invasive procedures: no rectal temperatures or enemas and no injections.

Protect against injury by instructing patient as follows:

No straining

No sharp objects: use electric razor

Report any signs and symptoms of infection.

Brush teeth with very soft bristle brush or toothette at least every 4 hours.

Meticulous central line care (if present)

Wash all raw fruits or vegetables.

Institute measures that foster drug regimen compliance.

Clarify the critical importance of regimen to prevent development of drug resistance.

Tailor medication regimen to patient lifestyle.

Direct observation, as needed

Help patient and family plan ahead for changes in routine.

Administer related drug therapy and monitor for therapeutic and nontherapeutic effects.

G-CSF (Filgrastim) or pegfilgrastim therapy (cytokine therapy to decrease severity of symptoms and increase rate of neutrophil recovery from moderate-to-severe neutropenia)

Antibiotic therapy, as ordered (for rapid control of infections)

Outcome 2: Maintain nutritional status

Assess and compare to established norms, patient baselines, and trends.

Examine oral mucous membranes, tongue, and pharynx for fungal growths, ulcers, redness, and swelling at least every shift (more often if pain, ulcers, or fungal growths are present).

Assess for presence and level of oral pain at least every shift and before meals (more often if pain is present).

Administer related drug therapy and monitor for therapeutic and nontherapeutic effects.

Saline and sodium bicarbonate mouth rinses every 3–4 hours

Nystatin oral rinse or other antifungal medication every 6 hours (q.i.d.) for oral fungal infection. If esophagitis is also present, nystatin can be swished and swallowed.

Use mouth moisturizers as needed.

Anesthetic throat lozenges, gels, or gargles

Perform actions to minimize oral pain at mealtime.

Mouth care before mealtime

If having problems with intake, may provide a liquid or soft food diet with frequent small meals.

[a] Finding evidence of infection may be extremely difficult in severely immunosuppressed patients, as any signs and symptoms of infection may be delayed, subdued, or completely absent, making this goal a particular challenge for the caregiver.

on the mucous membranes, skin, and lungs, which are the most common sites of infection in this patient population.

Oral complications associated with severe neutropenia negatively impact the patient's ability to take in nutrition. Common oral complications include infection-related fungal infection, mouth ulcers, and **mucositis** (inflammation of any or all of the oral mucous membranes [i.e., tongue, gums, pharynx, lips, and cheeks]).

The "Nursing Care: The Immunodeficient Patient" feature provides a summary of the nursing care related to infection and oral complications for a patient with immunodeficiency, including neutropenia.

Section Eight Review

1. Which are common client complaints associated with altered immunocompetence? (Select all that apply.)
   A. Abnormal bleeding
   B. Pain
   C. Swollen glands
   D. Fatigue
   E. Mouth sores

2. A severely immunocompromised hospitalized client should receive which types of environmental protection? (Select all that apply.)
   A. Screening visitors for infection
   B. No visitors
   C. Wearing sterile gloves for dressing changes
   D. Placement in semiprivate room with door closed
   E. Placement in private room

3. Which nursing actions provide ongoing protection against development of infection in a client with neutropenia? (Select all that apply.)
   A. Restricting client's fluid intake
   B. Turning client every 1 to 2 hours
   C. Bathing client every day
   D. Encouraging client's use of incentive spirometer hourly
   E. Administering acetaminophen p.o.

4. What is one of the most common sites of infection in the immunocompromised client?
   A. Gastrointestinal tract
   B. Urinary tract
   C. Skin
   D. Eyes

Answers: 1. (A, C, D, E), 2. (A, C, E), 3. (B, C, D), 4. C

Clinical Reasoning Checkpoint

Jason Q, a 36-year-old heterosexual male, comes into the hospital walk-in patient department seeking medical attention for breathing complaints, fevers, and malaise. His past medical history is positive for HIV, diagnosed about 10 years ago. Jason states that he is a recovered heroin addict who frequently took part in IV needle or syringe sharing in the early 1990s. He entered a drug rehabilitation program in 1995 and, with the exception of occasional marijuana smoking, denies any illegal drug use since his rehabilitation. Jason reports that he smokes 1 to 1.5 packs of cigarettes per day and drinks "one or two beers" in the evening. He is divorced and lives in the basement apartment of his parents' home. He also reports that he has unintentionally "lost a lot of weight," going from about 180 pounds to 165 pounds in 6 to 8 months.

1. Explain how and when Jason likely contracted the HIV infection, based on his brief history.

2. Assuming that Jason does have HIV disease, what does his presentation today suggest about the progress of his disease (based only on what little we know about him at this time)?

3. To evaluate the current status of Jason's HIV disease: (a) What labs would you want to obtain and (b) Why would you obtain them?

Clinical Update: Jason's CD4$^+$ count is drawn, and the result is 152 cells. His respiratory assessment includes dyspnea, light bilateral crackles, nonproductive cough, chills, and fever. A portable chest film shows bilateral pulmonary infiltrates.

4. Based on what you now know about Jason's situation, what do these data suggest?

5. Jason's HIV disease is primarily an immunodeficiency of CD4$^+$ and CD8$^+$ cells. Describe these two types of cells and how their dysfunction can eventually cause Jason's AIDS.

Chapter 30 Review

1. A 32-year-old client presents with complaints of recurrent fever, chills, and malaise. The client reports just completing radiation therapy for ovarian cancer. CBC with differential reveals WBC 2,600, PMN 15%, and bands 20%. Based on this report, the nurse calculates that the client has neutropenia of which severity?

   1. Mild
   2. Moderate
   3. Severe
   4. Profound

2. A client has been diagnosed with arthus vasculitis. To learn more about caring for this client, the nurse would research which type of hypersensitivity response?
   1. Type I
   2. Type II
   3. Type III
   4. Type IV

3. Systemic lupus erythematous (SLE) is being considered as the diagnosis for a client. An antinuclear antibody (ANA) is drawn and is negative. How should the nurse interpret this finding?
   1. The diagnosis of SLE is likely correct.
   2. The client's symptoms must be related to rheumatoid arthritis rather than SLE.
   3. The client's symptoms must be occurring for some reason other than SLE.
   4. The client has been exposed to scleroderma at some time in the recent past.

4. An 18-year-old presents with high fever, history of repeated respiratory infection, and exhaustion. A complete blood count (CBC) reveals pancytopenia. After additional diagnostic work, the client is diagnosed with acute lymphoblastic leukemia (ALL). How would the nurse explain the etiology of the pancytopenia to the client and his family?
   1. "The leukemic cells are crowding out the normal cells in your bone marrow."
   2. "Your bone marrow is failing."
   3. "Your body is making too much fatty tissue in your bone marrow."
   4. "Your blood cells are being killed by antigen–antibody complexes."

5. A client calls the chemotherapy clinic and says, "My back is hurting so much this morning, I don't know if I can ride in the car to my treatment." How should the nurse respond?
   1. "It will be fine if you wait until tomorrow to come in for your treatment."
   2. "I'm going to discuss your pain with your provider, and I will call you back shortly."
   3. "You get some rest today, and I will call to check on you tomorrow."
   4. "Do you have enough pain medication or should we call your pharmacy?"

6. While cleaning under a client's bed, a housekeeper stuck her finger with a needle. The source of the blood on the needle and how long the needle had been on the floor were not clear. Which information should the employee health nurse provide for this housekeeper? (Select all that apply.)

1. "If you start feeling bad, we will begin medications to reduce your risk of developing AIDS."
2. "You can expect to take antiretroviral therapy for at least one year."
3. "HIV viruses cannot live long outside the body."
4. "The HIV-AIDS virus is easily killed with regular household disinfectants."
5. "We will investigate the clients who have been in that room and will start you on medication if any of them had HIV or AIDS.

7. A client who has massive trauma is admitted to the ICU. Which pathophysiologic event associated with trauma would cause the nurse to intervene to protect the client's immune system?
   1. Zinc levels become dangerously high when extensive muscle trauma occurs.
   2. Extreme stress, such as is experienced in trauma, increases cortisol, which suppresses immune function.
   3. T-cell and B-cell activity is increased.
   4. Dehydration from trauma creates an imbalance between humoral and cell-mediated immunity.

8. A client has significant immunosuppression. The nurse monitors this client for which early signs of pulmonary infection? (Select all that apply.)
   1. Dyspnea
   2. Tachypnea
   3. Chest pain
   4. Adventitious breath sounds
   5. Fever

9. Which nursing interventions should the nurse provide for a client who is immunosuppressed? (Select all that apply.)
   1. Provide fresh fruits and vegetables with each meal.
   2. Change the water in flower vases every day.
   3. Screen visitors for respiratory infections.
   4. Keep the room door open for frequent observation.
   5. Monitor hydration status closely.

10. The nurse should suspect an infection in an immunodeficient client if the client's temperature remains at or exceeds which level for more than an hour?
    1. 100°F (37.8°C)
    2. 100.5°F (38°C)
    3. 101°F (38.3°C)
    4. 101.5°F (38.6°C)

Answers to questions found inside your textbook are available on the faculty resources site. Please consult with your instructor.

References

AIDS.gov. (2015). *Stages of HIV infection.* Retrieved February 9, 2017, from https://www.aids.gov /hiv-aids-basics

American Cancer Society. (2017). *Facts and figures 2017.* Retrieved April 8, 2017, from https://www.cancer.org /content/dam/cancer-org/research/cancer-facts-and -statistics/annual-cancer-facts-and-figures/2017 /cancer-facts-and-figures-2017.pdf

American College of Rheumatology. (1997). *1997 update of the 1982 American College of Rheumatology revised criteria for classification of systemic lupus erythematosus.* Retrieved April 7, 2017, from http://www.rheumatology .org/Portals/0/Files/1997%20Update%20of%20 1982%20Revised.pdf

Azar, A., & Ballas, Z. K. (2017). Immune function in older adults. *UpToDate.* Retrieved April 8, 2014, from https:// www.uptodate.com/contents/immune-function-in-older- adults

Bartels, C. M., & Muller, D. (2016). *Systemic lupus erythematosus.* Retrieved February 9, 2017, from http://emedicine.medscape.com/article/332244- overview#a3

Basler, J., & Stanley, D. (2016). *Hemorrhagic cystitis.* Retrieved February 9, 2017, from http://emedicine .medscape.com/article/2056130-overview

Camus, P. (2017). *The drug-induced respiratory disease website.* Retrieved April 17, 2017, from http://www .pneumotox.com/drug/view/280

Carpenito-Moyet, L. J. (2014). *Nursing care plans: Transition patient and family centered care.* Philadelphia, PA: Wolters Kluwer.

Carpenter, R. J., Chan-Tack, K. M., & Bartlett, J. (2015). *Early symptomatic HIV infection.* Retrieved August 29, 2015, from reference.medscape.com/article /211873-overview

Centers for Disease Control and Prevention (CDC). (1992). Revised classification system for HIV infection and expanded surveillance case definitions for AIDS among adolescents and adults. *Morbidity and Mortality Weekly Report, 41* RR 17–19. Retrieved March 29, 2008, from http://www.cdc.gov/mmwr/preview/mmwrhtml /00018871.htm

Centers for Disease Control and Prevention and Association of Public Health Laboratories. (2014). *Laboratory testing for the diagnosis of HIV infection: Updated recommendations.* Retrieved April 8, 2017, from https://www.cdc.gov/hiv/pdf/HIVtestingAlgorithm Recommendation-Final.pdf

Centers for Disease Control and Prevention (CDC). (2016a). *Understanding the HIV care continuum.* Retrieved February 11, 2017, from https://www.cdc .gov/hiv/pdf/library/factsheets/cdc-hiv-care -continuum.pdf

Centers for Disease Control and Prevention (CDC). (2016b). *Today's HIV/AIDS epidemic.* Retrieved February 11, 2017, from https://www.cdc.gov/nchhstp/newsroom/docs/ factsheets/todaysepidemic-508.pdf

Centers for Disease Control and Prevention (CDC). (2016c). *About HIV/AIDS.* Retrieved February 11, 2017, from https://www.cdc.gov/hiv/basics/whatishiv.html

Centers for Disease Control and Prevention (CDC). (2017a). *Lupus detailed fact sheet.* Retrieved April 7, 2017, from https://www.cdc.gov/lupus/facts /detailed.html

Centers for Disease Control and Prevention (CDC). (2017b). *Prevention benefits of HIV treatment.* Retrieved February 9, 2017, from https://www.cdc.gov/hiv/ research/biomedicalresearch/tap

Crowley, L. V. (2013). *An introduction to human disease: Pathology and pathophysiology correlations.* Burlington, MA: Jones and Bartlett Learning.

Cunningham, M. W. (2014). Rheumatic fever, autoimmunity and molecular mimicry: The streptococcal connection. *International Reviews of Immunology, 33*(4), 314–329. http://doi.org/10.3109/08830185.2014.917411

Fauci, A. S., & Lane, H. (2015). Chapter 226: Human immunodeficiency virus disease: AIDS and related disorders. In D. Kasper, A. Fauci, S. Hauser, D. Longo, J. Jameson, & J. Loscalzo (Eds.), *Harrison's principles of internal medicine* (19th ed.). Retrieved February 13, 2017, from http://accessmedicine.mhmedical.com.ezproxy .uky.edu/content.aspx?bookid=1130&sectionid =79738808

Fernandez-Gerlinger, M. P., Bernard, E., & Saint-Lary, O. (2013). What do patients think about HIV mass screening in France? A qualitative study. *BioMedCentral Public Health, 13,* 526. doi:10.1186/1471-2458-13-526

Gibson, C., & Berliner, N. (2014). How we evaluate and treat neutropenia in adults. *Blood, 124*(8), 1251–1258.

Horwitz, M. J. (2014). *Hypercalcemia of malignancy.* Retrieved August 30, 2015, from http://www.uptodate .com/contents/hypercalcemia-of-malignancy

Huertas, A., Girerd, B., Dorfmuller, P., O'Callaghan, D., Humbert, M., & Montani, D. (2011). Pulmonary veno- occlusive disease: Advances in clinical management and treatments. *Expert Review of Respiratory Medicine, 5*(2), 217.

Ikeda, A. K., & Jaishankar, D. (2016). *Tumor lysis syndrome.* Retrieved February 11, 2017, from http://emedicine .medscape.com/article/282171-overview

Inoue, S. (2016). *Leukocytosis.* Retrieved February 11, 2017, from http://emedicine.medscape.com /article/956278-overview?imageOrder=1

Jarukitsopa, S., Hoganson, D. D., Crowson, C. S., Sokumbi, O., Davis, M. D., Michet, C. J., . . . Chowdhary, V. R. (2015). Epidemiology of systemic lupus erythematosus and cutaneous lupus erythematosus in a predominantly white population in the United States. *Arthritis Care & Research, 67*(6), 817–828.

Katz, M. H. (2017). Chapter 31: HIV infection & AIDS. In M. A. Papadakis, S. J. McPhee, & M. W. Rabow (Eds.), *Current medical diagnosis & treatment 2017.* Retrieved February 13, 2017, from http://accessmedicine .mhmedical.com.ezproxy.uky.edu/content.aspx?bookid =1843&sectionid=135754355

Kee, J. L. (2014). *Laboratory and diagnostic tests with nursing implications* (9th ed.). Upper Saddle River, NJ: Pearson Prentice Hall.

Kotter, M. L., & Banasik, J. L. (2013). Malignant disorders of white blood cells. In L. Copstead & J. Banasik (Eds.), *Pathophysiology* (5th ed., pp. 214–231). St. Louis, MO: Elsevier.

Lassiter, M., & Schneider, S. M. (2015). A pilot study comparing the neutropenic diet to a non-neutropenic diet in the allogeneic hematopoietic stem cell transplant population. *Critical Journal of Oncology Nursing, 19*(3), 273–278.

Mackay, M., Tang, C. C., Volpe, B. T., Aranow, C., Mattis, P. J., Korpff, R. A., . . . Eldeberg, D. (2015). Brain metabolism and autoantibody titres predict functional impairment in systemic lupus erythematosus. *Lupus Science & Medicine, 2*(1). doi:10.1136/lupus-2014-000074

Mandel, A. (2015). *Types of autoimmune disease.* Retrieved August 22, 2015, from http://www.news-medical.net/health/Types-of-Autoimmune-Disease.aspx

Marcucci, G., & Bloomfield, C. D. (2015). Chapter 132: Acute myeloid leukemia. In D. Kasper, A. Fauci, S. Hauser, D. Longo, J. Jameson, & J. Loscalzo (Eds.), *Harrison's principles of internal medicine* (19th ed.). Retrieved February 13, 2017, from http://accessmedicine.mhmedical.com.ezproxy.uky.edu/content.aspx?bookid=1130&sectionid=79731765

Marks, L. B., Constine, L. S., & Adams, M. J. (2015). *Cardiotoxicity of radiation therapy for malignancy.* Retrieved August 30, 2015, from http://www.uptodate.com/content/cardiotoxicity-of-radiation-therapy-for-malignancy

National Cancer Institute. (2017). *Leukemia: Health professional version.* Retrieved April 8, 2017, from https://www.cancer.gov/types/leukemia/hp

Nickloes, T. A., Long, C., Mack, L. O., Kallab, A. M., Dunlap, A. B., & Gandhi, S. S. (2016). *Superior vena cava syndrome.* Retrieved February 11, 2017, from http://emedicine.medscape.com/article/460865-overview

Niederhubur, J. E., Armitage, J. O., Doroshow, J. H., Kastan, M. B., & Tepper, J. E. (2014). *Abeloff's clinical oncology.* Philadelphia, PA: Churchill Livingstone.

Owen, J. A., Punt, J., & Stranford, S. A. (2013). *Kuby immunology.* New York, NY: WH Freeman.

Pichler, W. J. (2014). *Drug allergy: Classification and clinical features.* Retrieved August 21, 2015, from http://www.uptodate.com/contents/drug-allergy-classification

Schiffer, C. A. (2015). *Clinical manifestations, pathologic features, and diagnosis of acute myeloid leukemia.* Retrieved August 22, 2015, from http://www.uptodate.com/contents/clinical-manifestations-pathologic-features-and-diagnosis-of-acute-myeloid-leukemia

Selik, R. M., Mokotoff, E. D., Branson, B., Owen, S. M., Whitmore, S., & Hall, H. I. (2014). Revised surveillance case definition for HIV infection—United States, 2014. *Centers for Disease Control and Prevention, Morbidity and Mortality Weekly Report (MMWR).* Retrieved February 9, 2017, from https://www.cdc.gov/mmwr/preview/mmwrhtml/rr6303a1.htm

Siegel, R. L., Miller, K. O., & Jemal, A. (2015). Cancer statistics. *CA: A Cancer Journal for Clinicians, 65*(1), 5–29. doi:10.3322/caac.21254

Stapczynski J. (2016). Emergency complications of malignancy. In J. E. Tintinalli, J. Stapczynski, O. Ma, D. M. Yealy, G. D. Meckler, & D. M. Cline (Eds.), *Tintinalli's emergency medicine: A comprehensive study guide* (8th ed.). Retrieved April 6, 2017, from http://accessmedicine.mhmedical.com.ezproxy.uky.edu/content.aspx?bookid=1658&sectionid=109386926

Sultan, K., & Vasudeva, R. (2016). *Neutropenic enterocolitis.* Retrieved February 11, 2017, from http://emedicine.medscape.com/article/183791-overview

White, L., & Ybarra, M. (2014). Neutropenic fever. *Emergency Medicine Clinics of North America, 32*(3), 549–561.

Wilson, B. A., Shannon, M. T., & Shields, K. M. (2016). *Pearson nurse's drug guide 2016.* Hoboken, NJ: Pearson.

World Health Organization. (2016). *HIV/AIDS fact sheet.* Retrieved February 13, 2017, from http://www.who.int/mediacentre/factsheets/fs360/en

Young, N. A., Wu, L., Burd, C. J., Friedman, A. K., Kaffenberger, B. H., Rajaram, M. V. S., . . . Jarjour, W. N. (2014). Estrogen modulation of endosome-associated toll-like receptor 8: An IFNα-independent mechanism of sex-bias in systemic lupus erythematosus. *Clinical Immunology, 151*(1), 66–77.

Chapter 31
Determinants and Assessment of Nutrition and Metabolic Function

∨ Learning Outcomes

31.1 Analyze and explain normal metabolism concepts, including anabolism and catabolism, aerobic and anaerobic, and energy.

31.2 Apply the primary functions of carbohydrates, lipids, and proteins as the body's fuel sources to the systematic assessment of the high-acuity patient.

31.3 Analyze neuro-endocrine factors that influence nutrition and metabolism during stress from acute illness.

31.4 Identify components of a focused nutrition, metabolic nursing history, and physical assessment.

31.5 Analyze the laboratory assessment of endocrine, nutritional, and metabolic status.

31.6 Determine appropriate physiologic studies used to measure endocrine, nutrition, and metabolic status.

cute illness and critical illness both cause significant physiologic stress that makes the patient vulnerable to the development of malnutrition and altered metabolic function, which negatively affects health status and may increase mortality (Maday, 2017). Nutritional intake can be altered by anything that impairs appetite or interferes with ingestion in addition to the disruption of the metabolism and absorption of nutrients, vitamins, and minerals. Chronic disease conditions, acute illness, and surgical interventions can further contribute to endocrine dysfunction that may alter metabolism. Nutritional and endocrine status should be evaluated in order to identify those who are malnourished or at risk for thyroid, adrenal, or glycemic imbalance due to hormonal, endocrine, or nutritional response to critical illness.

Nurses play a crucial role in the assessment and management of nutrition and metabolic function in the high-acuity patient. They can contribute to the interdisciplinary team's plans by identifying sources of stress for the patient and determining the proper interventions needed to improve nutritional status to facilitate recovery.

Section One: Metabolism

The energy required to maintain life is generated by chemical processes occurring throughout the body that involve transformation of nutrients. Collectively, these processes are called *metabolism*, which means state of change. Metabolism can be further classified as anabolic, catabolic, aerobic, and/or anaerobic.

Anabolism and Catabolism

Anabolism is a constructive metabolic process whereby simple molecules are converted into more complex molecules. It involves the synthesis of cellular components, contributing to tissue building. Anabolic events require energy much as would be needed to build something.

Catabolism is the process by which complex nutrients and body tissues are broken down into more basic elements, such as glucose, fatty acids, and amino acids, for the purpose of generating energy necessary to maintain bodily functions. Anabolic and catabolic processes both require enzyme catalysts that bind to nutrients, which are called substrates, and undergo enzymatic processes required for their use as fuel (Else & Hammer, 2013). Anabolism and catabolism are ongoing processes and, under normal circumstances, occur simultaneously to varying degrees. When a person is faced with a critical illness, catabolism predominates, creating systemic inflammation. Thus, catabolism is associated with many complications of critical illness, such as infection, the dysfunction of multiple organ systems, prolonged length of stay, and mortality (McClave et al., 2016).

Aerobic and Anaerobic Metabolism

Production of energy is a highly organized process. Nutrients are transformed into energy for immediate use or for storage inside the cell mitochondria for later use. Energy is used or stored in the form of **adenosine triphosphate (ATP)**, which is the major source of energy for all cells in the human body. Energy is generated from two distinct physiologic pathways—aerobic and anaerobic metabolism.

Aerobic Metabolism The Krebs (citric acid) cycle or the electron transport chain (through a series of biochemical sequence of reactions) are the two methods involved in **aerobic metabolism** to form ATP. The site where aerobic metabolism occurs is called the cell mitochondria. When the body's supply of oxygen is adequate, the oxidation of nutrients (carbohydrates, lipids, and proteins) occurs in the mitochondria. The pyruvate, which is the product of glycolysis (the breakdown of glucose), moves into the mitochondria to be processed in the Krebs (citric acid) cycle, ultimately forming 38 molecules of ATP and other end-products (carbon dioxide and water). Carbon dioxide and water normally are harmless and easily excreted from the body; however, excess retention of either of these substances can result in acid–base and fluid excess problems. The electron transport chain, however, produces an even greater amount of ATP than the Krebs cycle. Through a series of catalyzed reactions, hydrogen atoms are oxidized to form hydrogen ions and water. This process releases large amounts of energy, which is used to convert adenosine diphosphate (ADP) to ATP. This is where the body gets its energy to do work (Dwyer, 2014). Figure 31–1 shows a simplified concept of the aerobic (oxidative) pathway.

Anaerobic Metabolism Not all cells contain mitochondria, so not all are capable of aerobic metabolism. Cells without mitochondria receive their energy by the oxidation of glucose to pyruvate, which is then converted to ATP. The process of glucose oxidation in the cytoplasm is called *glycolysis*. Under circumstances in which there is decreased or delayed oxygen delivery to the cells (even those containing mitochondria), glycolysis is used for energy production and is referred to as **anaerobic metabolism**, or the Cori cycle. This form of metabolism produces significantly less ATP for energy compared to aerobic metabolism (Dwyer, 2014).

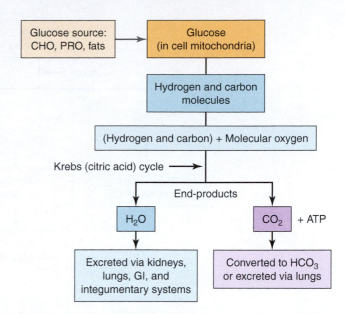

Figure 31–1 Simplified illustration of aerobic (oxidative) pathway. More than 90% of metabolism occurs using the aerobic pathway. The end-products of water and carbon dioxide are normally eliminated from the body.

Nicotinic acid dehydrogenase (NAD^+), an oxygen-reducing coenzyme, is required for anaerobic glycolysis. Maintaining adequate levels of NAD^+ depends on oxygen. When the supply of oxygen is inadequate, the energy of glucose can be released by the process of anaerobic glycolysis. During the anaerobic process, two ATP molecules are produced, in addition to pyruvate and lactic acid by-products. Pyruvate is converted to lactic acid by NAD^+, which is then available to participate in further energy synthesis. Most body cells can use lactic acid as an energy source in the short term; however, vital organs such as the brain and the nervous system have extremely limited capabilities to extract lactic acid as a fuel source (Dwyer, 2014). Figure 31–2 shows a simplified concept of the anaerobic (glycolytic) pathway.

The anaerobic metabolic pathway is inefficient as an energy source but is reversible with the reestablishment of an adequate oxygen supply. Anaerobic metabolism is partially a compensatory mechanism that allows energy production to proceed whenever energy demands exceed the oxygen supply, such as during exercise. Anaerobic metabolism, however, is intended only to be temporary and cannot sustain life indefinitely. High-acuity patients are at increased risk of developing anaerobic metabolism because of periods of severe or sustained decreases in oxygen delivery to the tissues. Therefore, maintaining adequate perfusion and oxygen delivery is critical for supporting aerobic metabolism; it prevents ischemia at the cellular level, subsequent organ failure, and possibly even death (Joosten, Alexander, & Connesson, 2015).

Elevated serum lactate levels are indicative of inadequate cellular oxygenation. Measuring serum lactic acid (or lactate) level is useful as an indicator of the severity and duration of anaerobic metabolism, which develops during states of inadequate ventilation and/or perfusion (e.g., shock states, cardiac arrest). A normal arterial serum lactic acid level is 0.5–2 mmol/L compared to the normal venous level, which is 0.5–1.5 mmol/L (Nicoll, Mark Lu, & McPhee, 2017).

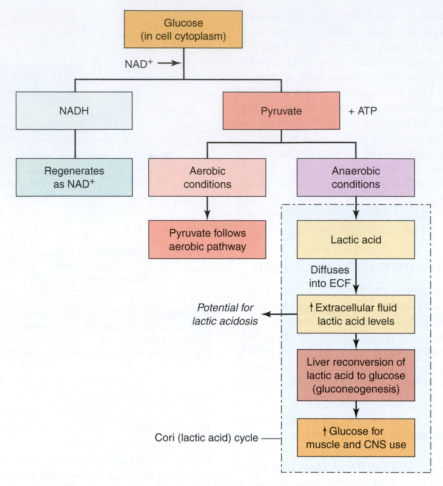

Figure 31–2 Simplified illustration of anaerobic (glycolytic) pathway. The anaerobic pathway is reversible when oxygen becomes available. Severe anaerobic conditions, such as cardiac arrest or shock, can lead to lactic acidosis.

Energy

The ability to do work is called **energy**. Heat is generated in the conversion of nutrients to energy. Energy is measured in a unit called a *calorie*, which is the amount of energy needed to raise the temperature of 1 gram of water by 1 degree Celsius. Because a calorie is such a minute quantity, energy measurement within the body is usually described in terms of a kilocalorie (1000 calories). A kilocalorie (kcal) is the amount of energy required to increase the temperature of 1 kg (1000 g) of water by 1 degree Celsius (Dwyer, 2014).

The majority of the energy needed by the body (about 40%) is used to maintain ion gradients across cell membranes. Approximately one third of all energy generated by the mitochondria in the cells is utilized by the **sodium–potassium pump (Na⁺/K⁺ pump)** to actively transport sodium and potassium ions across the cellular membrane's ion gradient. The central nervous system functions and the synthesis of proteins in the body each require about 20% of the body's energy expenditure. Other essential functions such as oxidation of nutrients, breathing, and cardiac contractility (pumping mechanism) consume the rest of the energy expenditure. Furthermore, any physical activity requires a greater than normal amount of energy than what is required to maintain normal homeostatic mechanisms in a resting state (Dwyer, 2014).

Section One Review

1. How is catabolism best described?
   - **A.** Metabolism occurring in the absence of oxygen
   - **B.** Metabolism occurring in the presence of oxygen
   - **C.** Breakdown of complex nutrients into more basic nutrients
   - **D.** Building of cells and tissues from nutrients

2. Which part of the cell is the site of aerobic metabolism?
   - **A.** Mitochondria
   - **B.** Cell membrane
   - **C.** Cytoplasm
   - **D.** Nucleus

3. Which lab test is frequently used as an indicator of anaerobic metabolism?
   A. Total lymphocyte count
   B. Lactic acid (lactate)
   C. Arterial blood gas
   D. Blood urea nitrogen

4. High-acuity clients are at risk for significant anaerobic metabolism because of what factor?
   A. NPO status
   B. Increased energy requirement
   C. Severe or sustained decrease in oxygen delivery
   D. Fluid volume overload

Answers: 1. C, 2. A, 3. B, 4. C

Section Two: Nutrition: The Source of Energy

Nutrition is a complex process by which an organism takes in and uses the nutrients in food for the purpose of providing energy for metabolism. This includes the growth, maintenance, and repair phases of metabolism. Nutrition involves ingestion (taking in food), digestion (breaking down food into absorbable substances), absorption (taking up substances from the GI tract into the bloodstream), and metabolism (transformation of substances into energy). **Nutrients**, the elements and compounds necessary for the nutrition process, are divided into two basic categories: macronutrients and micronutrients. **Macronutrients** consist of carbohydrates, proteins, and lipids (fats). **Micronutrients** include vitamins (both fat soluble and water soluble), minerals, and trace elements. Adequate intake of both macronutrients and micronutrients is essential to restore health and to promote healing in the high-acuity patient (Dwyer, 2014).

Carbohydrates

Carbohydrates are composed of carbon, hydrogen, and oxygen. Carbohydrates are introduced into the body in various forms of sugars or starches, which are converted into glucose. Carbohydrates are the preferred fuel source for most tissues and are necessary to supply energy for basic cellular functions. Heat produced during the oxidation of carbohydrates is used to maintain body temperature.

Excess glucose that is not needed for cellular activities is stored as glycogen in the liver and muscle cells through a process called **glycogenesis**. Excess glucose is converted to either glycogen or fatty acids (triglycerides) and stored for later conversion back into glucose when energy is needed. Often, reserved energy is required during times of physiologic stress. To meet this demand the stored glycogen is converted to glucose and is maintained within a steady range in the body to provide an immediate energy source. This transformation of glycogen back into glucose is called **glycogenolysis**. Stored glycogen may also be released in response to increased circulating levels of epinephrine, norepinephrine, vasopressin, and angiotensin II, which are hormones that are rapidly released during physiologic stress. Glycogen stores are depleted rapidly in the high-acuity patient who experiences intense or prolonged physiologic stress, such as occurs with surgery, trauma, infection, or organ failure.

Glucose metabolism is regulated by two pancreatic hormones, insulin and glucagon. Insulin is secreted by beta cells and is necessary for transport of glucose into cells. Under normal circumstances, ingestion or infusion of glucose causes an increase in insulin release from the beta cells. Comparatively, glucagon is secreted by the alpha cells and is released in response to falling blood glucose levels, stimulating conversion of stored glycogen into glucose.

Approximately 25% of the body's glucose supply is used by the brain and nervous system. Although maintenance of blood glucose within a narrow range is essential for preservation of central nervous system (CNS) functioning, the brain cannot store or synthesize glucose as a fuel source. Instead, the CNS relies primarily on glucose extraction from the bloodstream. The brain can use ketone bodies (derived from fat metabolism) as a fuel source; however, this does not supply enough energy for the brain to maintain its essential cellular functions (Dwyer, 2014; Molina, 2013a).

Adequate carbohydrate intake prevents proteins from being used as a fuel source. Proteins can provide energy, but they are not optimal sources because proteins are needed primarily for other cellular functions. Carbohydrates supply 4 kilocalories (kcal) of energy for each gram ingested and normally provide 40% to 60% of daily caloric requirements (Dwyer, 2014). Carbohydrate metabolism is altered during periods of physiologic stress, leading to hyperglycemia as part of the *metabolic stress response*.

Proteins

Proteins are composed of various combinations of amino acids and contain nitrogen in addition to carbon, hydrogen, and oxygen. Formation of proteins requires metabolism of carbohydrates and lipids as the principle substrate for energy to support protein synthesis for cellular growth/healing. Proteins have many complex functions at the cell membrane and are essential for the formation and maintenance of all cells, tissues, and organs. Proteins also play a role in many of the body's transport mechanisms, such as transmission of nerve impulses. Proteins are considered the body's building blocks because they contribute to the structure of genes, enzymes, hormones, antibodies, hemoglobin of red blood cells, bone matrix, muscles, and organs. Maintenance of osmotic pressure and appropriate blood pH also depend on an adequate protein supply. Proteins are categorized according to their location in the body:

- *Visceral proteins* are found within internal organs. Prealbumin, albumin, and transferrin (plasma proteins) are frequently measured in laboratory tests as indicators of protein status and overall nutritional status.

- *Somatic proteins* are found in accessory and skeletal muscles.

Protein synthesis and degradation are ongoing and opposing processes in the body. Under usual circumstances,

Table 31–1 Summary of Macronutrients

Nutrient	Caloric Value (kcal/gram)	Percentage of Recommended Total Daily Intake	General Functions
Carbohydrates			
Basic unit: glucose	Enteral: 4 Parenteral: 3.4	About 40%–60%	• Maintenance of body temperature • Supply energy for basic cell functions
Proteins			
Basic unit: amino acids	4	15%–20%	• Many complex functions at cell membrane • Essential for formation and maintenance of all cells, tissues, and organs • Contribute to structure of muscles, organs, antibodies, enzymes, and hormones • Important role in transport mechanisms • Important in maintenance of osmotic pressure and blood pH
Lipids (fats)			
Basic unit: fatty acids	9	No more than 30%	• Primary source of fuel reserve • Body insulation • Structural protection for some organs (e.g., kidneys)

the overall content of proteins in the body is relatively steady. However, under stress conditions, protein catabolism (or breakdown) is increased. In the high-acuity patient, inadequate protein intake can quickly lead to malnutrition, prolonged wound healing, decreased resistance to infection, and even death. Similar to carbohydrate metabolism, protein metabolism is influenced by hormones. For example, protein synthesis is enhanced by growth hormone (GH) and diminished by low levels of insulin.

When carbohydrate availability is not adequate to meet the body's energy requirements, proteins are broken down into their amino acid components. Amino acids enter the Krebs cycle to produce ATP (energy). Proteins supply 4 kcal of energy per gram. Average, healthy adults require about 15% to 20% of their nutrient intake as proteins (Dwyer, 2014). This amount increases considerably under conditions of physiologic stress. Protein malnutrition also leads to atrophy of the gut mucosa and is a factor in the development of bacterial translocation. Impairment of skin integrity, delayed wound healing, and loss of skeletal muscle mass result from protein malnutrition.

Lipids

Lipids are also referred to as fats. At the cellular level, lipids contribute to the structure of the cell membrane. Lipids are the primary source of stored (reserve) energy and are readily available if needed in the form of triglycerides, phospholipids, and cholesterol for later use as an energy source.

Lipids provide 9 kcal of energy per gram, more calories than any other nutrient (Dwyer, 2014). Functionally, lipids are similar to carbohydrates because their availability as an energy source can save proteins from being broken down.

As with the other macronutrients, lipid synthesis and reserves are influenced by insulin, which is needed for the transport of glucose into fat cells. Only small quantities of stored fat are found in the circulating blood. Most fat is stored in adipose tissue and the liver. The liver can produce lipids from glucose or amino acids through a process called **lipogenesis**. This occurs when there are more carbohydrates present than required for energy or for glycogen storage in the liver. Under normal conditions, lipogenesis is the preferred metabolic process for lipid production. During stress, lipolytic (lipid breakdown) metabolism predominates, which increases the availability of fatty acids for adenosine triphosphate (ATP) and consequent energy (Barrett, Barman, Boitano, & Brooks, 2016; Hall, 2016; Janson & Tischler, 2012).

Lipids are a source of essential nutrients and aid in the absorption of the fat-soluble vitamins A, D, E, and K. Stored lipids provide insulation for the body in the form of subcutaneous fat and also provide structural protection for some organs, such as the kidneys. The American Heart Association recommends limiting daily fat intake as follows: no more than 7% of saturated fat, no more than 1% of trans fat, and less than 300 mg of cholesterol or less than 30% of total fat intake. Total fat intake in the United States, however, generally exceeds this recommendation, being approximately 34% (Dwyer, 2014). Table 31–1 summarizes information on the macronutrients.

Section Two Review

1. Which of the following are micronutrients?
   A. Minerals
   B. Carbohydrates
   C. Proteins
   D. Fats

2. Glucose metabolism is regulated by which two hormones?
   A. Epinephrine and norepinephrine
   B. Glycogen and glucagon
   C. Insulin and vasopressin
   D. Glucagon and insulin

3. Which nutrient provides the greatest number of calories per volume?
   A. Carbohydrates
   B. Fats
   C. Visceral proteins
   D. Somatic proteins

4. Which organ is most dependent on maintenance of normal blood glucose levels?
   A. Heart
   B. Lungs
   C. Kidney
   D. Brain

Answers: 1. C, 2. D, 3. B, 4. D

Section Three: Endocrine Influence on Metabolism

Along with nutrition, the nervous and endocrine systems are necessary for regulation of the dynamic homeostasis and equilibrium among the various cells, tissues, organs, and systems of the body. Just as the nervous system communicates via nerve impulses, the endocrine system communicates via the various hormones secreted by the endocrine glands to regulate functions; these functions include metabolism, growth, fluid and electrolyte balance, and energy production. Hormones from the pituitary, thyroid, adrenal, and parathyroid glands and the endocrine function of the pancreas (see Figure 31–3) have a role in adaptation to altered internal and external environmental changes associated with stress and acute illness. Table 31–2 summarizes the hormones secreted by the glands and their target organ and feedback mechanism.

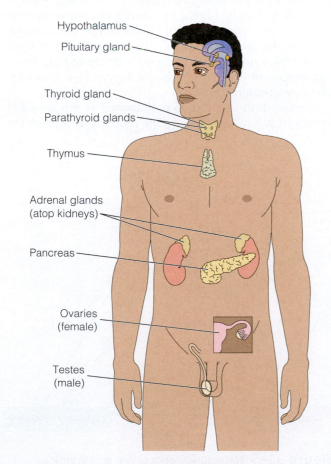

Figure 31–3 Location of major endocrine glands.

Endocrine Glands and Hormones

The *pituitary gland* is located just beneath the hypothalamus of the brain (see Figure 31–3). It responds to regulatory hormones secreted by the hypothalamus. This gland has two parts: the anterior pituitary and the posterior pituitary. Both parts are involved in the regulation of many body functions through the many hormones that they secrete. Adrenocorticotropic hormone (ACTH), which is secreted from the anterior pituitary, plays an important role in the physiologic response to stress by causing the adrenal gland to secrete cortisol. The posterior pituitary secretes antidiuretic hormone (ADH), which acts on the kidneys to promote conservation of water.

The *thyroid gland* is a butterfly-shaped gland whose primary function is to regulate metabolism. It is positioned anterior to the upper part of the trachea and just inferior to the larynx. Thyroid hormones are secreted in response to secretion of thyroid-stimulating hormone (TSH) from the anterior pituitary gland. The secretion of TSH and thyroid hormones have a negative feedback relationship. Thus, if enough thyroid hormone is produced, then the anterior pituitary gland will stop secreting TSH. The thyroid gland also secretes calcitonin, a hormone that regulates calcium levels in the blood. Calcitonin precursors are reliable markers of systemic inflammation. Calcitonin can serve as a marker for sepsis as it is believed to be a mediator of the inflammatory response. Figure 31–4 shows the thyroid gland and its location relative to the trachea. The four parathyroid glands are located on the surface of the lobes of the thyroid gland and secrete parathyroid hormone (PTH). PTH regulates serum calcium and phosphate levels (Molina, 2013b).

The adrenal glands sit on top of the kidneys and consist of an inner medulla and an outer cortex. The adrenal medulla produces and secretes catecholamines (epinephrine and norepinephrine), the fight-or-flight hormones that are released in response to sympathetic nervous system (SNS) stimulation. Catecholamines are major contributors to the physiologic response to stress, which is described later in this section. The adrenal cortex secretes corticosteroid hormones, which are classified into two groups: mineralocorticoids and glucocorticoids. The release of mineralocorticoids (aldosterone) is regulated by the renin-angiotensin-aldosterone system (RAAS) in response to decreased blood pressure or serum sodium level. Activation of the RAAS results in water and sodium retention to increase circulating blood volume (refer to Chapter 25 for more detail on RAAS). The major glucocorticoid is cortisol, which affects carbohydrate metabolism by regulating glucose use in body tissues and mobilizes fatty acids from adipose tissue for energy production in times of stress.

Table 31–2 Hormones, Target Organs, and Feedback Mechanisms

Gland	Major Hormones Secreted	Major Functions
Pituitary (Anterior)	Tropic hormones: Adrenocorticotropic hormone (ACTH) and thyroid-stimulating hormone (TSH) Somatotropic hormone: Growth hormone (GH)	ACTH: Targets adrenal cortex; regulates cortisol release TSH: Regulates thyroid gland activity GH: Targets liver, muscle, and bone; has diverse anabolic functions that affect many body tissues
Pituitary (Posterior)	Antidiuretic hormone (ADH) (other names: oxytocin, arginine vasopressin [AVP])	Regulates water balance
Thyroid	Thyroid hormone: Thyroxine (T4) is converted to triiodothyronine (T3) at the target tissues. Calcitonin	Maintains metabolic rate and tissue growth; T3 and T4 are secreted in response to thyroid stimulating-hormone (TSH). Maintains serum calcium and phosphate levels
Parathyroid	Parathyroid hormone (PTH)	Maintains serum calcium levels along with calcitonin
Adrenal cortex	Mineralocorticoids (aldosterone) Glucocorticoids (cortisol)	Promotes sodium and water reabsorption, thereby increasing circulating blood volume. Regulates metabolism of carbohydrates, fats, proteins. Activates anti-inflammatory responses to stressors. When levels are low, hypothalamic secretion of corticotropin-releasing hormone (CRH) stimulates the anterior pituitary release of ACTH, thus stimulating the adrenal cortex secretion of cortisol.
Adrenal medulla	Catecholamines (epinephrine and norepinephrine)	Mimic direct SNS stimulation Increases HR, BP, constricts blood vessels, dilates bronchioles, increases respiratory rate and metabolism, promotes hyperglycemia in response to stress

SOURCE: Data from Hall (2016).

Physiologic Response to Stress

When the body is stressed, compensatory processes are initiated to restore and maintain homeostasis. The physiologic response to stress involves the nervous system, the endocrine system, and the immune system, all of which are interrelated. Figure 31–5 shows the bidirectional communication via neurochemical links among the nervous, endocrine, and immune systems in response to stress. The body responds to a stressor by demonstrating changes in heart rate, breathing, and blood pressure. Metabolism may be altered by a series of neuroendocrine responses to stress, trauma, or infection. The immune system can also be suppressed during times of physiologic stress, which may inhibit the body's ability to fight infection or recover from critical illness. Figure 31–6 illustrates the body's response to stress.

Stress stimulates the hypothalamus to release CRH (corticotropin-releasing hormone), which stimulates the

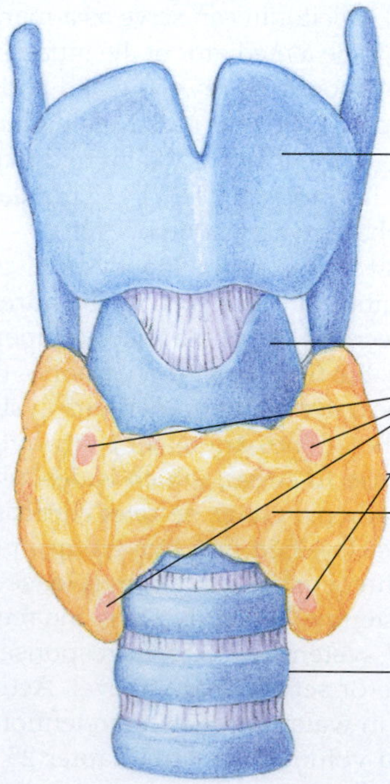

Figure 31–4 The thyroid gland.

SOURCE: Debbie Maizels/Dorling Kindersley, Ltd.

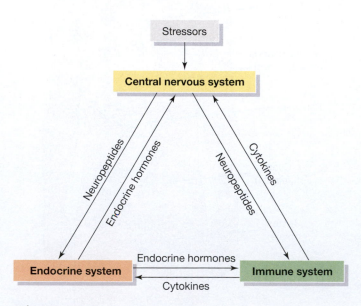

Figure 31–5 Neurologic, endocrine, and immune response to stress.

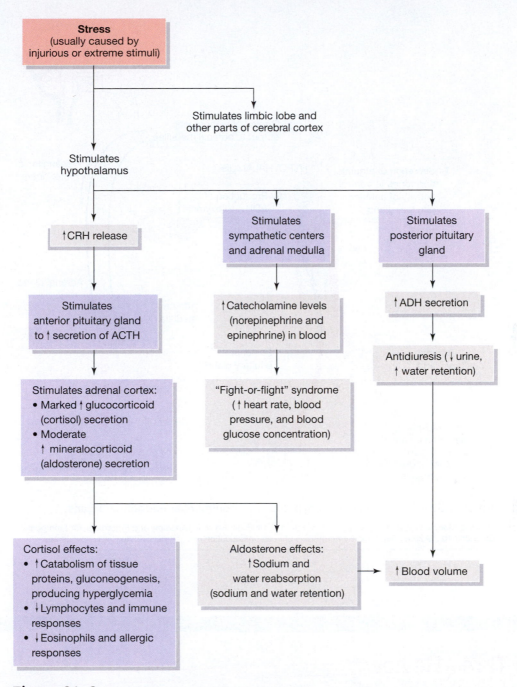

Figure 31–6 The body's response to stress.

anterior pituitary gland to increase secretion of ACTH (adrenocorticotropic hormone). This then stimulates the adrenal gland to secrete cortisol and aldosterone. Cortisol release increases catabolism of proteins and gluconeogenesis for energy production, but it also influences T-cell proliferation of the immune system to support mobilization and distribution of immune-boosting cells to areas of infection or injury. Chronic stress can suppress the immune system, making persons with chronic stress vulnerable to infection. Aldosterone release increases sodium and water reabsorption so that blood volume is increased to the same sites of infection or injury.

Stress-induced stimulation of the hypothalamus also stimulates the SNS and the adrenal glands to increase catecholamine levels. Catecholamine release increases the rate and force of cardiac muscle contractions, and it increases blood pressure and blood glucose levels, allowing more efficient transport of oxygenated blood. Catecholamines also stimulate the release of ACTH from the pituitary, which in turn stimulates the adrenal cortex to release cortisol. Furthermore, catecholamines constrict blood vessels in the skin, mucous membranes, and kidneys, and they dilate blood vessels in skeletal muscles, coronary arteries, and pulmonary arteries. Simultaneously, the hypothalamus stimulates the posterior pituitary gland, resulting in increased antidiuretic hormone (ADH) release, which along with aldosterone, increases water retention to increase circulating blood volume (Molina, 2013a). Figure 31–7 illustrates how the hypothalamus interacts with the pituitary and adrenal glands.

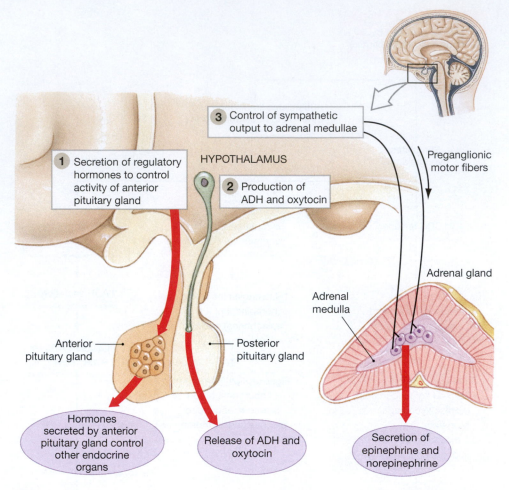

Figure 31–7 Mechanisms of hypothalamic control over endocrine organs.

SOURCE: Martini, Frederick H.; Bartholomew, Edwin F.; Bledsoe, Bryan E.; *Anatomy and Physiology for Emergency Care,* 2nd ed., © 2008. Reprinted by permission of Pearson Education, Inc., Upper Saddle River, New Jersey.

Section Three Review

1. The anterior pituitary produces and secretes which hormone that plays an important role in the physiologic response to stress?
   A. Adrenocorticotropic hormone (ACTH)
   B. Antidiuretic hormone (ADH)
   C. Thyroid-stimulating hormone (TSH)
   D. Parathyroid hormone (PTH)

2. The adrenal medulla secretes which hormone when stimulated by the sympathetic nervous system?
   A. Aldosterone
   B. Cortisol
   C. Epinephrine
   D. Adrenocorticotropic hormone

3. In the physiologic response to stress, which hormone is secreted by the hypothalamus to stimulate the anterior pituitary gland?
   A. Adrenocorticotropic hormone (ACTH)
   B. Corticotropin-releasing hormone (CRH)
   C. Aldosterone
   D. Antidiuretic hormone (ADH)

4. Catecholamines have which effect on the cardiovascular system? (Select all that apply.)
   A. Decrease systemic blood pressure
   B. Increase heart rate
   C. Decrease cardiac contractility
   D. Vasodilate coronary arteries
   E. Decrease uptake of glucose into cells

Answers: 1. A, 2. C, 3. B, 4. (B, D)

Section Four: Focused Nutritional History and Physical Assessment

Nutrition is fundamental to a healthy neuro–metabolic–endocrine response to acute and critical illness. The endocrine glands and the hormones that they regulate form the communication network linking all body systems. A strong nutritional and endocrine assessment is an important part of the evaluation of high-acuity patients. History and physical assessment data identify a patient's current nutrition/metabolic status, provide a baseline with which to compare the effectiveness of therapies, and identify patients who may be at risk for complications related to their nutritional status and inability to meet metabolic demands. Malnutrition present at baseline can be easily identified by assessing for a 10% unintentional weight loss in the past 3 to 6 months, reported decreased nutrient intake, and a BMI less than 18.5, indicating the patient is underweight. A BMI greater than 30 indicates obesity (Hiesmayr, 2012). Assessment of the patient's history is a key role of the nurse and can start the evaluation of the nutritional status to determine whether a patient's metabolic response is related to illness, nutritional status, endocrine imbalance, or a combination of all. These assessments allow the nurse to plan and initiate proper nutritional support to meet metabolic demands. This may include consultation of dieticians and nutritional support specialists, such as speech language pathologists, to diagnose the causes of malnutrition in the critically ill patient. Because nurses are often the first line of defense, they can help to initiate recommendations set forth by the American Society for Parenteral and Enteral Nutrition (ASPEN), which recommends that patients who are critically ill begin nutritional support within 24 to 48 hours of admission to the hospital (Aldeguer, Wilson, & Kohli-Seth, 2017; McClave et al., 2016; Mueller, 2012;). The rationale for this recommendation is to support gastrointestinal tract integrity so that translocation of bacteria may be prevented (McClave et al., 2016).

The influence of an illness or injury on a person's metabolic state is often difficult to predict. Some diseases such as acute pancreatitis or inflammatory bowel disease, and injuries such as traumas and burns, place acutely ill patients at high risk for malnutrition (McClave et al., 2016). Moreover, a patient's prehospitalization nutritional status can strongly influence the metabolic response to acute illness and the identification and treatment of existing malnutrition. For example, patients with comorbid disorders, such as chronic obstructive pulmonary disease or liver disease, are often admitted to the hospital in a poor state of nutrition. In such cases, the additional physiologic stress of the acute illness places the patient at significant risk for further deterioration of nutritional status and complications during the hospitalization.

Medical and Nutritional History

A nutritional history is directed toward identifying underlying mechanisms that put patients at risk for nutritional depletion or excess. These mechanisms include inadequate intake, impaired absorption, decreased utilization, increased losses, and increased requirements for nutrients.

Typical food intake and preferred choices are reviewed for caloric density, protein content, and micronutrient concentration. Social, cultural, ethnic, and religious traditions may be considered as they may impact choices, consumption, access, preparation, and storage of food. Social history—including a history of smoking, use of illicit drugs or alcohol, dietary supplements, herbal supplements, appetite suppressants, and laxatives—provide insight into a patient's nutritional status (White et al., 2012).

General components of the nutritional history include the following:

- History of food and fluid intake
- Barriers to normal food consumption
- Alterations in gastrointestinal anatomy and nutrient absorption
- Recent weight changes

Complex nutritional assessment scales have been developed that incorporate anthropometric measurements and laboratory studies (Jensen, Compher, Sullivan, & Mullins, 2013). Whereas such precise indices of nutritional status may be helpful, simple clinical evaluation (a history of weight loss, dietary habits, and knowledge of underlying disease) provides a good working assessment. Of the widely available clinical measures of nutritional status, the most useful data often are clinical history, absolute lymphocyte count, cholesterol, and serum protein levels at the time of admission (Jensen et al., 2013; White et al., 2012). Furthermore, in the critically ill adult, gastrointestinal tract integrity, the patient's comorbid conditions, and risk factors for aspiration should be considered when assessing nutritional status (McClave et al., 2016).

A comprehensive nutritional assessment includes medical history, physical examination, medication history, anthropometric measurements, and laboratory data. The resulting nutritional data are then used for documenting the baseline subjective and objective nutritional parameters, determining risk factors, identifying specific deficits, and establishing needs so that a plan can be developed to meet metabolic demands. Geriatric considerations include the presence of chronic diseases that affect nutritional intake or endocrine function. Potential drug interactions with nutrients should also be assessed in all geriatric patients.

Physical Assessment Physical assessment begins with subjective assessment, determining if the patient is alert and oriented, has an adequate gag reflex, and has the ability to swallow. The patient who is sedated or intubated but has a functioning gastrointestinal tract is a candidate for enteral nutrition by an alternate route, such as with a small-bore feeding tube. If the patient is hemodynamically unstable, enteral nutrition is usually withheld until vasopressor agents are no longer required for hemodynamic support (McClave et al., 2016). Additional assessments include muscle or adipose tissue loss, the appearance of wasting associated with chronic disease, and retention of fluid as evidenced by peripheral edema, which may be related to a protein deficit (Jensen et al., 2013).

Anthropometric Measurements

Anthropometrics is the assessment of height, weight, and waist circumference used to measure the body muscle mass and fat reserves. Serial anthropometric measurements can provide evidence of recovery from uncomplicated malnutrition and illness (Heimburger, 2014; Jensen et al., 2013; Jensen, Hsiao, & Wheeler, 2012).

Precise measurements of body composition, including body fat, require technically sophisticated methods, which are not practical in acute care clinical settings. Still, simple measurements of skinfold thickness, height, and weight can be acquired. Skin calipers are used to obtain an indirect measurement of subcutaneous fat thickness, using the triceps or subscapular region (see Figure 31–8). Many variables exist in the acute care setting—such as a lack of necessary training or equipment to perform anthropometric measurements, or the presence of wounds, dressings, and edema—and they may make this type of measurement difficult for the bedside nurse to obtain.

Height and Weight   Accurate measurement of height and weight is the cornerstone to assessment of body composition. Height is measured with a measuring rod while the patient is standing upright or lying supine. Under circumstances in which a head-to-toe measurement is not possible, height can also be measured by arm span method, which correlates with height at maturity. The arm span method is obtained by extending both arms out from the body and measuring the distance between the longest fingertips of each hand (Jensen et al., 2012). Height is used to determine ideal or desirable body weight and is an important factor in determining energy requirements.

Body weight is one of the most useful nutritional parameters to follow in patients who are acutely or chronically ill. Unintentional, rapid weight loss during illness often reflects loss of lean body mass (muscle and organ tissue). This can be an ominous sign as it indicates use of vital body protein stores for metabolic fuel (catabolism). In the high-acuity setting, a precise weight may be difficult to obtain for several reasons. Body water disturbances, electrolyte imbalances, and endocrine abnormalities are extremely common and cause rapid weight fluctuations. Also, intentional diuresis from the administration of medications such as diuretics or from endocrine imbalances can make it difficult to obtain a precise dry body weight.

Body weight measurements are usually taken at the same time each day, using either a standing weight or a bed or sling weight; however, in the high-acuity patient, use of such scales often does not reflect the patient's true weight. This inaccuracy is partially due to the relative inaccessibility of the patient who is connected to multiple pieces of equipment, has various lines or tubes, dressings, casts, orthopedic traction, or other devices in place. In such cases, weight measurement becomes relative—that is, current weights are compared to previous weights and the patient's "usual" weight, if possible, to identify obvious weight gains or losses. An increase or decrease in weight of as little as 2 pounds may indicate a gain or loss of up to a liter of fluid.

Ideal Body Weight and Body Mass Index   Once a body weight is obtained, it should be compared to **ideal body weight (IBW)** and body mass index (BMI). An IBW is the expected weight of an individual based on age, sex, and height. IBW is often determined by the Hamwi rule of thumb method (Hamwi, 1964). In this method, males are given 106 lbs (48 kg) for the first 5 ft of height (1.5 m) and an additional 6 lbs (2.7 kg) for each inch (2.54 cm) over 5 ft. Females are given 100 lbs (45 kg) for the first 5 feet and an additional 5 lbs (2.3 kg) for each inch over 5 ft. Adjustments are made for a large frame by adding 10% of body weight, and subtracting 10% for a small frame (McClave et al., 2016).

The reference standard for normal body weight is **body mass index (BMI)**, which is a widely accepted estimate for obesity but can also be helpful in the assessment of undernutrition. The BMI calculates body mass by using a formula (see Box 31–1). BMIs of less than 18.5 are considered underweight, 18.5 to 24.9 are normal, 25 to 29.9 are overweight, and greater than 30 are obese. Obesity can further be classified into class I (BMI of 30–34.9) indicating low risk for disease, class II (BMI of 35–39.9) indicating moderate risk for disease, and class III (BMI greater than 40) which is the highest risk for disease development. Risk for disease development includes cardiovascular disease, hypertension, and type II diabetes mellitus (National Heart, Lung, and Blood Institute, 2016). Comparatively, a BMI of less than 18 indicates malnutrition, and if less than 16, severe malnutrition (Jensen et al., 2012; Jensen et al., 2013; Heimburger, 2014).

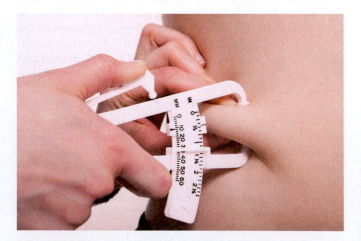

Figure 31–8 Measuring subcutaneous fat thickness with calipers.
SOURCE: Kisiel/123RF.com

BOX 31–1   Calculating Body Mass Index (BMI)

Metric Calculation:
    BMI = Wt. (in kg)/Ht. (in meters^2)

U.S. Customary Units Calculation:
    BMI = (Wt. [in lbs] × 703)/Ht. (in inches^2)

Obesity and Malnutrition Obesity in the high-acuity patient can place the patient at risk for complications of malnutrition such as insulin resistance and loss of lean muscle mass at a faster rate than the nonobese critically ill patient. Patients who are obese, or have a BMI greater than 30 should initiate feeding when critically ill within 24 to 48 hours, much like underweight or average-weight patients. A high BMI is commonly mistaken for adequate nutrition and is an area about which the nurse can advocate for the patient if early feeding is not initiated. Measurements of metabolic syndrome and preexisting comorbidities may further contribute to malnutrition. Assessment of metabolic syndrome includes blood pressure measurement, waist circumference, total cholesterol, serum glucose, and triglyceride levels (McClave et al., 2016).

Section Four Review

1. Which measurement is an acceptable substitute for measuring a client's height with a measuring rod?
   A. Family member report of the client's height
   B. Estimation based on length of the bed compared to client height
   C. Measurement of arm span
   D. Measurement of leg length doubled

2. An IBW is best described in which way?
   A. The expected body weight
   B. The desired body weight
   C. A variation due to the effects of illness
   D. A predictor of health outcomes

3. A BMI of 33 indicates which condition?
   A. Underweight
   B. Normal weight
   C. Overweight
   D. Obesity

4. A BMI of 18 indicates which condition?
   A. Underweight
   B. Normal weight
   C. Overweight
   D. Obesity

Answers: 1. C, 2. A, 3. D, 4. A

Section Five: Laboratory Assessment of Endocrine and Nutritional and Metabolic Status

A patient's nutritional and metabolic status strongly influences the acute and critical care illness and outcomes. It is imperative, therefore, for the nurse to have a basic understanding of the laboratory tests commonly used to assess the patient's overall metabolic/nutritional status. Common laboratory tests include albumin, prealbumin, transferrin, total lymphocyte count (TLC), and serum electrolytes. Serum albumin, prealbumin, and transferrin are indicators of visceral protein status. Abnormally low levels of these plasma proteins indicate that muscle has been catabolized for energy, which can result in serious multiple organ system complications.

In addition, laboratory assessment of the thyroid and adrenal glands can be used to identify patients who are at risk of impaired metabolic response from thyroid or adrenal imbalance in the presence of acute and critical illness. It is important to assess imbalances in these hormones because relative adrenal insufficiency and disrupted thyroid hormone balance can occur in critically ill patients. Complications related to resuscitation and recovery once the acute phase of illness has passed are possible, and the treatment of these imbalances should be initiated to support the metabolic response to stress.

Albumin

Albumin, a plasma protein, is the major protein produced in the liver, with more than 60% located in the extravascular space. There it is crucial for maintenance of intravascular volume because of its influence on blood osmotic pressure. Albumin is frequently measured in high-acuity patients and is often used by clinicians as a primary indicator of overall nutritional status. **Hypoalbuminemia**, or low serum albumin levels, correlates with increased occurrence of clinical complications, such as the development and progression of an acute kidney injury and other poor patient outcomes (e.g., unintended intubation, increased days of mechanical ventilation, and higher mortality in postoperative orthopedic patients) (Aldebeyan, Nooh, Aoude, Weber, & Harvey, 2016). More specifically, malnutrition in the form of protein-energy deficits has been found to be a predictor of mortality within 30 days of hospitalization for patients admitted for an acute or critical illness (Jellinge, Henriksen, Hallas, & Braband, 2014; Lyons, Whelan, Bennett, O'Riordan, & Silke, 2010; Mogensen et al., 2015).

Serum albumin levels must be interpreted cautiously because albumin has a 15- to 20-day half-life and is influenced by hydration status and hepatocellular injury. In patients who receive fluid resuscitation, low serum albumin levels are likely to be dilutional and not an accurate indicator of the actual albumin level. In patients with advanced liver disease, severely damaged hepatocytes can no longer synthesize albumin, resulting in hypoalbuminemia. These factors make albumin levels of little value for assessing acute changes in nutritional status, but the levels are valuable for tracking long-term changes in protein status. Albumin, therefore, should not be used as an indicator to detect early malnutrition or effectiveness of nutritional support during acute illness. Abnormally low albumin values may be detected in patients with liver or renal disease even when protein intake is adequate.

Prealbumin

Transthyretin, better known as **prealbumin**, is a protein that is extremely helpful in the nutritional assessment of the high-acuity patient. As an indicator of nutritional status, prealbumin is a transport protein that binds retinol-binding protein and thyroxin, a thyroid hormone. The half-life of prealbumin (48–72 hours) is significantly shorter than that of albumin, making prealbumin a more reliable indicator of acute changes in catabolism than serum albumin. Prealbumin is not influenced by hydration, renal, or liver status to the same extent as albumin. Periodic monitoring of prealbumin provides an indication of the effectiveness of nutrition support and the overall catabolic state. Prealbumin should increase within 4 to 8 days if a patient is receiving adequate nutritional support.

Transferrin

Transferrin is a plasma protein that binds to iron and transports it to cells. Transferrin may be more useful than albumin for tracking responses to nutritional therapies because its half-life is 8 to 10 days. The accuracy of transferrin as a nutritional indicator depends on the patient's underlying iron level, and its use as an indicator of adequacy of nutrition in the high-acuity patient may be limited because of other blood-related factors, such as blood loss anemia or blood transfusions.

BOX 31–2   Calculating Daily Nitrogen Balance

Formula: Nitrogen balance = nitrogen in (g/24h)/6.25 – nitrogen out + 4 gm/24hr

Where: Nitrogen in = gram of protein received during the 24 hours of UUN collection, divided by the constant 6.25; and nitrogen out = grams of protein excreted in the urine as measured by the UUN plus insensible loss, estimated at 4 g

SOURCE: Data from Heimburger (2014).

Nitrogen Balance

In the high-acuity patient, nitrogen balance may be evaluated as an indicator of protein status because 1 gram of nitrogen is equivalent to 6.25 grams of protein. Simply defined, **nitrogen balance** is the difference between nitrogen output and nitrogen intake. If a patient takes in more nitrogen than is lost (output), the patient is in a *positive nitrogen balance*; however, if a patient loses more nitrogen than is taken in, the patient is in a *negative nitrogen balance*.

Nitrogen balance is measured by a test called the urine urea nitrogen (UUN) test. Calculation of nitrogen balance first requires collection of a 24-hour urine specimen with an accurate account of urinary output during the collection time. Furthermore, the urine must be chilled, either in a specimen refrigerator or on ice throughout the 24-hour period. Because nitrogen is a component of protein, it is also necessary to know the patient's protein intake during the time of the UUN collection.

Nitrogen balance can be calculated once the UUN is reported by the laboratory. Box 31–2 provides the equations needed to calculate nitrogen balance. Four grams of nitrogen are often added to the UUN test to account for nitrogen losses that are not captured by urine collection alone (e.g., stool,

---

Emerging Evidence

- Glutamine (GLN) is an important pharmaconutrient in the body's response to critical injury and stress by attenuating inflammation and supporting metabolic function. Glutamine directly protects cells and tissue from injurious effects of inflammation. Data support GLN as an ideal pharmacologic intervention to prevent or treat multiple organ dysfunction syndrome after sepsis or other injuries in the intensive care unit population. A large and growing body of clinical data shows that in well-defined critically ill patient groups GLN can be a lifesaving intervention (Weitzel & Wischmeyer, 2010). In a Cochrane systematic review of 53 studies including 4671 patients with critical illness or undergoing elective major surgery, there was moderate evidence to support the addition of GLN to nutritional support for the high-acuity patient to reduce infection rate and days of mechanical ventilation. There was low-quality evidence for decreased length of hospital stay. There was no effect on risk of mortality or length of ICU stay (Tao et al., 2014).

- Thiamine is a vitamin that plays a significant role in the body's metabolism. Often, the high-acuity patient can be affected by thiamine deficiency. In a report evaluating three cases of severe lactic acidosis in patients who received parenteral nutrition (PN) with no vitamin supplementation, treatment with thiamine was associated with restored acid–base balance, hemodynamic stability, and disappearance of neurologic disturbances. The active form of thiamine is important to the oxidative process of pyruvate in the Krebs cycle. Without thiamine, energy production of the body may slow down. This contributes to a growing body of evidence that supports that thiamine replacement can be used to treat anaerobic metabolism (Giacalone et al., 2015).

- Nutritional deficiencies, although rare, can cause depressed myocardial functioning resulting in a reduced left ventricular ejection fraction. Cobalt is a metal that has many uses. Interestingly, cobalt is used in medical prosthetics and such other devices as coronary artery stents and dental implants. It is noted that excess cobalt in the body may interfere with the contractility of the heart by inhibiting the transport and use of calcium into cardiac myocytes (cobalt binds to calcium), creating a depressive effect. Traditionally, cobalt-induced cardiomyopathy has been rare, but new cases have been identified in patients with metal-containing hip prostheses that are not working appropriately. Patients at risk who have a metal hip prosthesis include those patients with thiamine deficiencies (common with alcoholism), low protein intake, and a medical history of hypothyroidism (Packer, 2016).

skin, enterocutaneous fistula drainage, excessive wound drainage). The major disadvantage of using the UUN level to assess protein need is that it is not valid in renal failure. Urinary nitrogen output is expected to be low in renal failure because the kidneys are unable to excrete nitrogenous waste. The UUN can be used to calculate the amount of protein needed. For a patient who is stressed and in a catabolic state, the goal of protein administration should be to provide a positive nitrogen balance. A positive nitrogen balance is typically obtained when the body's requirements for carbohydrates and lipids are met; an increase in protein alone is not sufficient to reach a positive nitrogen balance (Marino, 2014).

Vitamin and Mineral Assays

Low serum levels of vitamin A, zinc, and magnesium are common in acutely ill hospitalized patients. Fat-soluble vitamin (A, D, E) and mineral (iron, folic acid) deficiencies should be assessed if a patient has a digestive and/or absorptive disorder. If these or other micronutrient deficiencies are suspected, a variety of serum and red blood cell assays are available to assist with nutritional assessment. Commonly available assays include vitamin A, vitamin E, thiamine, folate (serum and red blood cell), vitamin B_{12}, zinc, magnesium, and phosphorus.

Total Lymphocyte Count

Many cells of the immune system, such as antibodies and lymphocytes, contain a significant amount of protein. Proper functioning of the immune system depends on an adequate total protein level. Measurement of the **total lymphocyte count (TLC)** provides some quantification of the effect of protein loss on immune system functioning. The total lymphocyte count is an easily obtained indicator of overall immune status and adequacy of protein. This indicator is considered most reliable when white blood cell and lymphocyte counts are relatively stable; therefore, a TLC should be interpreted with caution in the high-acuity patient experiencing hypermetabolism or infections.

The total lymphocyte count should be about 20% to 40% of the total white blood cell (WBC) count. Although many disease states and treatments affect immunocompetence, poor nutrition is a major contributor to immunosuppression. Malnutrition causes immunosuppression by depressing neutrophil chemotaxis and total lymphocyte count. It also delays hypersensitivity reactivity and may cause complete **anergy** (absence of a reaction) to antigen skin testing. A total lymphocyte count of less than 1500 mm^3 is indicative of impaired immune function. Total lymphocyte count can be calculated using the formula in Box 31–3.

Table 31–3 provides a summary of laboratory values pertinent to the nutritional/metabolic assessment of the high-acuity patient.

BOX 31–3 Calculating Total Lymphocyte Count

Formula: $TLC = \dfrac{\% \text{ lymphocytes} \times WBC}{100}$

Table 31–3 Laboratory Assessment of Adult Nutrition, Thyroid, and Adrenal Status

Nutritional Status	
Test	**Normal Levels**
Blood urea nitrogen (BUN)	5–25 mg/dL
Serum creatinine	0.5–1.5 mg/dL
Albumin	3.5–5 g/dL
Prealbumin (transthyretin)	17–40 mg/mL
Transferrin	200–430 mg/dL
Vitamin E	5–20 mcg/mL
Thiamine	10–60 ng/mL
Folate	3–16 ng/mL
Vitamin B_{12}	200–900 pg/mL
Zinc	60–150 mcg/dL
Magnesium	1.5–2.5 mEq/L
Phosphorous	1.7–2.6 mEq/L
Thyroid and Adrenal Hormones	
Test	**Normal Value**
Calcium Ionized calcium	4.5–5.5 mcg/L 4.25–5.25 mg/dL
Potassium	3.5–5.3 mEq/L
Glucose	60–110 mg/dL
Sodium	135–145 mEq/L
Cortisol (free serum)	8:00 a.m.–10:00 a.m.: 5–23 mcg/dL 4:00 p.m.–6:00 p.m.: 3–13 mcg/dL
Cosyntropin (ACTH) Stimulation Test	Normal response: cortisol level doubles in response to ACTH stimulation. Failure of cortisol levels to rise indicates adrenal insufficiency.
T3 (free or triiodothyronine)	80–200 ng/dL
T3 resin uptake (serum)	25–35 relative percentage uptake
T4 (thyroxine)	4.5–11.5 mcg/dL
TSH (thyroid-stimulating hormone)	0.35–5.5 µIU/mL*

*µIU, microinternational units.
SOURCE: Data from Kee (2014) and Nicoll et al. (2017).

Anergy Screen

Cell-mediated immunity is one of the body's defense mechanisms that is most affected by malnutrition. Delayed cutaneous hypersensitivity screening, also referred to as skin testing, is a simple method for evaluating cell-mediated immunity status. A test dose of a known antigen, such as tuberculin, *Candida*, mumps, or *Trichophyton*, is administered intradermally. The individual's ability to respond to this immunologic challenge is evaluated 24 and 48 hours after administration. If cellular immunity is intact, an induration of 5 mm or larger should be observed at the injection site. This indicates sufficient immunity of the patient. If no skin reaction occurs, the patient is considered to be anergic, which means that cellular immunity may have been negatively affected by malnutrition (Forbes & Watt, 2016).

Section Five Review

1. A low serum albumin can be caused by which circumstances? (Select all that apply.)
   A. Liver disease
   B. Acute malnutrition
   C. Chronic malnutrition
   D. Kidney disease
   E. Hydration status

2. Which lab value is the best indicator of current nutritional status?
   A. Prealbumin
   B. Albumin
   C. Transferrin
   D. BUN

3. A urine urea nitrogen (UUN) has been ordered on a client. The nurse can expect to take which action regarding this order?
   A. No action by the nurse is required.
   B. Collect the urine over a 24-hour period.
   C. Obtain a urine specimen by in-and-out catheterization.
   D. Maintain the urine specimen at room temperature.

4. The total lymphocyte count (TLC) is useful in estimating which of the following?
   A. Nitrogen balance
   B. Iron stores
   C. Vitamin A, zinc, and magnesium levels
   D. Immune system function

Answers: 1. (A, C, D, E), 2. A, 3. B, 4. D

Section Six: Physiologic Studies of Nutrition and Metabolic Status

The goal of nutritional support in the high-acuity patient is maintenance of nutritional status to avoid catabolism during periods of metabolic stress associated with acute and critical illness. Accurate estimates of nutritional requirements and early interventions help prevent complications associated with underfeeding and overfeeding. The calculation of the patient's caloric, protein, and fluid requirements is often accomplished by obtaining a nutritional consultation from a registered dietician or nutritionist. Nurses should be familiar with the effects of metabolic stress on the body and how it alters nutritional requirements so that they may have input into decisions about nutritional plans and be prepared to implement the nutritional interventions created.

A simple estimation of caloric requirements is to calculate 25 kcal/kg/day for a well-nourished, nonstressed individual with a normal albumin level. This individual would have a nitrogen requirement of 0.8–1 gram of protein/day. The fluid requirement would be 1 mL of fluid per calorie. Patients in high-acuity settings have additional stressors and disease states, which alter this basic formula and can lead to an increased need for calories, protein, and fluids (Heimburger, 2014).

Oxygen Consumption and Energy Expenditure

Oxygen consumption ($\dot{V}O_2$) and energy expenditure are indicators of the metabolic state and can be assessed by various methods. In-depth discussion of energy expenditure is beyond the scope of this chapter, but a basic understanding of the measurement is beneficial to the nurse caring for the high-acuity patient.

Oxygen consumption and energy expenditure can be measured directly by calorimetry or calculated using the Fick equation (Box 31–4). As oxygen consumption cannot occur without energy expenditure, any event or situation that increases cell and tissue oxygen demands will increase energy expenditure accordingly. Fever, shivering, infection, and pain are examples of events that increase metabolic oxygen demands in acutely ill patients. Nurses have a unique opportunity to vigilantly monitor for early detection of signs of increased oxygen demands and provide prompt intervention to minimize oxygen consumption.

Calorimetry **Direct calorimetry** measures whole body heat production while the individual is isolated in a chamber or a room specifically equipped for this procedure, which makes it impractical for use in the clinical setting. **Indirect calorimetry** offers a practical approach to bedside measurement of oxygen consumption, nutrient oxidation,

---

BOX 31–4 Fick Equation for Oxygen Consumption

Formula: $\dot{V}O_2 = (CaO_2 - CvO_2) \times 10$

Where: $\dot{V}O_2$ is tissue oxygen consumption; CO is cardiac output; CaO_2 is arterial oxygen content (hemoglobin $\times$ 1.34 $\times$ arterial oxygen saturation [decimal]); and CVO_2 is mixed venous oxygen content (hemoglobin $\times$ 1.34 $\times$ venous oxygen saturation [decimal]).

SOURCE: Data from Heimburger (2014).

and energy expenditure. An indirect calorimeter is also called a "metabolic cart." This portable unit (about the size of a portable cardiac monitor) estimates the resting energy expenditure (REE) by measurement of respiratory gas exchange. An indirect calorimetry measurement procedure takes 15 to 20 minutes and can be performed on patients receiving mechanical ventilation or breathing room air. Patients receiving oxygen therapy at less than 45% will have more accurate results.

Indirect calorimetry measures the amount of oxygen consumed ($\dot{V}O_2$) and the amount of carbon dioxide produced ($\dot{V}CO_2$) From these numbers, the metabolic cart calculates the daily amount of oxygen consumed and carbon dioxide produced, determining energy expenditure. Normal values are established based on gender, height, weight, age, and activity level. Indirect calorimetry is the most accurate method for determining energy requirements. It measures a patient's actual energy expenditure in order to determine precise needs of the patient. Therefore, indirect calorimetry allows for individualized nutrition therapy, while it prevents over- or underfeeding (Heimburger, 2014).

Respiratory Quotient. The **respiratory quotient (RQ)** is another valuable parameter provided by indirect calorimetry. The RQ is the ratio of carbon dioxide produced to oxygen consumed in a given time. The normal value of approximately 0.85 indicates that the individual is using about an equal amount of carbohydrates, fats, and proteins for energy. A positive, direct correlation exists between glucose utilization and RQ (the greater the amount of glucose being used, the higher the RQ). For example, an RQ above 1.0 indicates that the patient is receiving too many carbohydrates (i.e., overfeeding), and an RQ below 0.70 indicates inadequate nutrition (i.e., underfeeding). Because glucose breaks down to carbon dioxide, excess carbohydrate intake can potentially result in carbon dioxide retention (hypercapnia) with subsequent increased work-of-breathing, which can potentially impair weaning from mechanical ventilation in the high-acuity patient (Aldeguer et al., 2017).

Fick Equation. Because indirect calorimetry is not available in all facilities, the Fick equation offers an acceptable substitute if the blood is drawn over 30 seconds and no air bubbles are introduced into the specimen. The Fick equation (Box 31–4) requires blood gas analysis of arterial and venous blood. There are two disadvantages of using the Fick method: (1) It represents the oxygen consumption for only one moment in time, and (2) errors in calculation of the cardiac output can occur, which will alter the accuracy of the oxygen consumption value obtained.

Oxygen Extraction

While at rest, the amount of oxygen delivered (DO_2) via arterial blood for consumption by the body's tissues is normally approximately 1000 mL/min. The tissues extract about 20% to 40% of this available oxygen, which

---

> ### BOX 31–5 Harris–Benedict Equation
>
> **Male:** $66 + (13.7 \times \text{weight [kg]}) + (5.0 \, (\text{height [cm]}) - (6.8 \times \text{age})$
>
> **Female:** $655 + (9.6 \times \text{weight [kg]}) + (1.8 \times \text{height [cm]}) - (4.7 \times \text{age})$

equates to about 250 mL/m^2/min of oxygen. After gas exchange occurs at the capillary bed, about 750 mL/m^2/min of oxygen is returned to the venous blood, which makes the normal oxygen saturation of venous blood (SvO_2) about 60% to 80%. Oxygen consumption can increase considerably in the high-acuity patient; therefore, a higher amount of oxygen may be extracted from arterial blood, which corresponds with a decreased venous oxygen return (or decreased SvO_2). Monitoring of SvO_2 can provide important data regarding the amount of additional oxygen extracted from the blood and may help the nurse identify any changes in aerobic or anaerobic metabolic trends. SvO_2 can be continuously monitored at the bedside using a special thermodilution fiberoptic catheter.

Harris–Benedict Equation

There are over 200 equations for predicting energy needs, and many are population specific. The **Harris–Benedict equation** is one of the more commonly used formulas to calculate resting energy expenditure (REE) (Harris & Benedict, 1919). This formula is different for each gender and requires knowledge of the patient's height in centimeters, weight in kilograms, and age in years. The Harris–Benedict equation is given in Box 31–5.

The Harris–Benedict equation assumes that the patient is within the range of ideal weight relative to height. Ideal weight for adult males and females is 100 pounds for a height of 5 feet. For males, the weight allowance is 6 pounds for every inch above 5 feet. For females, the ideal weight allowance is 5 pounds for every inch above 5 feet. For patients above their ideal weight, a calculation is made for an adjusted weight to be used in the Harris–Benedict equation. Adjusted weight is obtained from the calculation in Box 31–6.

Because this prediction does not take into account the metabolic response to injury and illness, stress factors are added to adjust for activity, elevated body temperature, disease processes, surgery, burns, trauma, and sepsis (see Table 31–4). The following is an example of

---

> ### BOX 31–6 Harris–Benedict Equation
> **Adjusted Weight**
>
> Adjusted weight (kg) = Actual weight (kg) − Ideal weight (kg) × 0.25 + Ideal weight (kg)

Table 31–4 Estimation of Energy Expenditure in Commonly Encountered Conditions: The Harris–Benedict Equation and Stress Factors

Common Clinical Condition	Associated Stress Factor
Well nourished, unstressed	1
Maintenance	
• Mild stress	1–1.2
• Moderate stress	1.4
• Severe stress	1.6
Surgery	
• Minor	1.2
• Major	1.2–1.5
• Cancer	1–1.5
Fever	1.0 (for each °C above the normal body temperature)
Acute phase sepsis	
• Hypotensive	1.2–1.6
• Normotensive	1–1.4
Recovery phase of sepsis	1–1.2
Acute phase multiple trauma	
• Hypotensive	1.2–1.6
• Normotensive	1–1.5
Recovery phase of multiple trauma	1–1.2
Burn injury (before grafting)	
• 10% BSA*	1.25
• 20% BSA	1.5
• 30% BSA	1.5
• 40% BSA	1.75
• Greater than 40% BSA	2
Burn injury (after graft)	1–1.4

*BSA = Body surface area.
SOURCE: Data from Heimburger (2014).

use of the Harris–Benedict equation to estimate daily caloric need:

If a patient with multiple trauma was estimated by the Harris–Benedict equation to have an energy expenditure of 2,000, this figure would be multiplied by 1.1 to 1.5 to obtain an energy expenditure of 2,200 to 3,000. This patient would require 2,200 to 3,000 nonprotein kilocalories per day.

Simple Method of Calculating REE   If the stress factor coefficients to the Harris–Benedict equation are not readily accessible or indirect calorimetry is unavailable, the recommended way to calculate the resting energy expenditure (REE) is to use the simple equation in Box 31–7.

If the patient weighs more than 25% of ideal body weight (IBW), then the Harris–Benedict Equation for Adjusted Weight should be used. It is further recommended that a dry weight be used in this equation so that excess fluid volume is not accounted for in disease states such as acute heart failure or liver failure. Furthermore, the simple REE equation does not account for medications such as propofol that are lipid containing (the intake must be calculated) or patients with excess weight that may alter the energy requirements of the acutely ill adult (McClave et al., 2016).

BOX 31–7   Harris–Benedict Equation

Calculating Resting Energy Expenditure (REE)

REE (kcal/day) = 25 × actual body weight (kg)

Section Six Review

1. What is oxygen consumption used to measure?
   A. Oxygen delivery
   B. Resting energy expenditure
   C. Metabolic state
   D. Anaerobic metabolism

2. What does indirect calorimetry calculate?
   A. Caloric requirements
   B. Resting energy expenditure
   C. Resting energy demands
   D. Carbon dioxide production

3. What does the Harris–Benedict equation measure?
   A. REE
   B. IBW
   C. BMI
   D. PCM

4. The extraction of oxygen by the tissues to meet metabolic needs can be measured using which reading?
   A. Oxygen saturation of arterial blood (SaO_2)
   B. Oxygen saturation of venous blood (SvO_2)
   C. Partial pressure of arterial carbon dioxide ($PaCO_2$)
   D. Partial pressure of arterial oxygen (PaO_2)

Answers: 1. C, 2. B, 3. A, 4. B

Clinical Reasoning Checkpoint

JQ, a 42-year-old female, has a 25-year history of heavy smoking and now has advanced-stage chronic obstructive pulmonary disease (COPD). She has been admitted to the Pulmonary ICU for severe respiratory distress. In examining JQ, you find that she has a thoracic cage with a 1:1 diameter (barrel chest), typical of advanced COPD patients. Her limbs appear wasted with little muscle or fat present. An arterial blood gas is drawn showing hypoxemia as well as acute respiratory acidosis. A serum albumin is also drawn, and the result is an albumin level of 3.0.

1. Explain what information JQ's serum albumin level can give us that may be helpful in evaluating her status.
2. Further testing shows that JQ is in a negative nitrogen balance. What does this mean?
3. The pulmonary team orders indirect calorimetry to be done on JQ. Briefly explain what this test measures.
4. Evaluating respiratory quotient (RQ) may be especially valuable in JQ's situation since she has COPD. What does RQ measure, and why would it be helpful in nutritional treatment for COPD patients?

Chapter 31 Review

1. A client admitted to the intensive care unit 3 days ago with several fractures and multiple abrasions required splenectomy and is now spiking intermittent fevers. No nutritional support is occurring. How would the nurse explain this client's primary metabolic state?
   1. Catabolic
   2. Anabolic
   3. Anaerobic
   4. Glycolytic

2. A severely injured client is having difficulty maintaining oxygenation. To evaluate the client for excessive anaerobic metabolism, the nurse would expect which serum laboratory test to be drawn?
   1. Lactic acid
   2. Nicotinic acid dehydrogenase (NAD+)
   3. Pyruvate
   4. Glucose

3. The ability of a severely injured client to heal depends on nutritional state. Evaluation of the client's macro-nutrient status would include which nutrients? (Select all that apply.)
   1. Minerals
   2. Proteins
   3. Vitamins
   4. Fats
   5. Carbohydrates

4. The client who is severely injured is not eating enough protein. If this poor intake results in low protein levels, how will recovery be affected? (Select all that apply.)
   1. Impaired wound healing
   2. Decreased fluid shifts

3. Increased risk for gut bacterial translocation
4. Inhibited immune function
5. Reduced growth hormone

5. A client is admitted to the intensive care unit after sustaining a severe throat injury when falling from a tree. The nurse would evaluate imbalance of which electrolyte as indicating possible injury to the parathyroid glands?
   1. Calcium
   2. Sodium
   3. Potassium
   4. Magnesium

6. The nurse is assessing a client just admitted to the intensive care unit following severe injury in a building explosion. Which assessments are important in determining which nutritional approach is indicated? (Select all that apply.)
   1. Is the client conscious?
   2. Is the client alert?
   3. Can the client swallow?
   4. Does the client have a gag reflex?
   5. What is the client's weight?

7. A client who was admitted to the intensive care unit after serious trauma 10 days ago has been receiving parenteral nutrition and has since stabilized. To monitor the effects of this nutritional plan, the nurse will check which serum laboratory test result?
   1. Albumin
   2. Prealbumin
   3. Nitrogen
   4. Total lymphocyte count

8. Cellular immunity-delayed cutaneous hypersensitivity screening is planned for a client who has been hospitalized 2 weeks for treatment of serious trauma. Which nursing interventions are necessary? (Select all that apply.)

   1. Inject the test dose intradermally.

   2. Monitor the client for immediate itching after the dose is administered.

   3. Give a test dose of the antigen by mouth 2 hours before the test begins.

   4. Plan to assess for induration in 24 and 48 hours.

   5. Keep the client NPO for 8 hours after the test.

9. Which nursing interventions can directly decrease the metabolic oxygen demands of a critically ill client? (Select all that apply.)

   1. The nurse administers antipyretic medications to reduce fever.

   2. The nurse keeps the client covered with a blanket as much as possible during initial resuscitation.

   3. The nurse offers the client pain medication on a routine basis.

   4. The nurse maintains sterile technique when changing dressings.

   5. The nurse encourages visitors to talk to an unconscious client.

10. A client's respiratory quotient (RQ) is 1.3. What intervention does the nurse anticipate providing?

    1. Increasing the client's tidal volume on the mechanical ventilator

    2. Increasing the rate of the client's maintenance IV

    3. Decreasing the rate of the client's parenteral feeding

    4. Decreasing the amount of IV diuretic the client is receiving

---

Answers to questions found inside your textbook are available on the faculty resources site. Please consult with your instructor.

References

Aldebayan, S., Nooh, A., Aoude, A., Weber, M., & Harvey, E. (2016). Hypoalbuminaemia—a marker of malnutrition and predictor of postoperative complications and mortality after hip fractures. *Injury,* 1–5. doi:10.1016/j.injury.2016.12.016

Aldeguer, Y. R. T., Wilson, S., & Kohli-Seth, R. (2017). Chapter 29: Nutrition support. In J. M. Oropello, V. Kvetan, & S. M. Pastores (Eds.), *Lange critical care.* New York, NY: McGraw Hill Education.

Barrett, K. E., Barman, S. M., Boitano, S., & Brooks, H. L. (2016). Chapter 19: The thyroid gland. In K. E. Barrett, S. M. Barman, S. Boitano, & H. L. Brooks (Eds.), *Ganong's review of medical physiology* (25th ed.). New York, NY: McGraw-Hill. Retrieved March 14, 2017, from http://accessmedicine.mhmedical.com.ezproxy.uky.edu/content.aspx?bookid=1587&sectionid=97164051

Dwyer, J. (2014). Nutrient requirements and dietary assessment. In K. D. Kasper, A. Fauci, S. Hauser, D. Longo, J. Jameson, & J. Loscalzo (Eds.), *Harrison's principles of internal medicine* (19th ed.). New York, NY: McGraw-Hill. Retrieved March 14, 2017, from http://accessmedicine.mhmedical.com.ezproxy.uky.edu/content.aspx?bookid=1130&sectionid=79728843

Else, T., & Hammer, G. D. (2013) Disorders of the adrenal cortex. In G. D. Hammer & S. J. McPhee (Eds.), *Pathophysiology of disease: An introduction to clinical medicine* (7th ed.). New York, NY: McGraw-Hill. Retrieved March 14, 2017, from http://accessmedicine.mhmedical.com.ezproxy.uky.edu/content.aspx?bookid=961&sectionid=53555702

Forbes, H., & Watt, E. (2016). *Jarvis's physical examination and health assessment* (2nd ed.). New South Wales, Australia: Elsevier Australia.

Giacalone, M., Martinelli, R., Abramo, A., Rubino, A., Pavoni, V., Iacconi, P., . . . Forfori, F. (2015). Rapid reversal of severe lactic acidosis after thiamine administration in critically ill adults: A report of 3 cases. *Nutrition in Clinical Practice: Official Publication of the American Society for Parenteral and Enteral Nutrition, 30*(1), 104–110. doi:10.1177/0884533614561790

Hall, J. E. (2016). *Guyton and Hall textbook of medical physiology* (13th ed.). Philadelphia, PA: Elsevier.

Hamwi, G. J. (1964). Changing dietary concepts. In T. S. Danowsi (Ed.), *Diabetes mellitus: Diagnosis and treatment.* New York, NY: American Diabetes Association.

Harris, J. A., & Benedict, F. G. (1919). *A biometric study of basal metabolism in man.* Publication No. 279. Washington, DC: Carnegie Institute of Washington.

Heimburger, D. C. (2014). Chapter 97: Malnutrition and nutritional assessment. In K. D. Kasper, A. Fauci, S. Hauser, D. Longo, J. Jameson, & J. Loscalzo (Eds.), *Harrison's principles of internal medicine* (19th ed.). New York, NY: McGraw-Hill. Retrieved March 15, 2017, from http://accessmedicine.mhmedical.com.ezproxy.uky.edu/content.aspx?bookid=1130&sectionid=63653604

Hiesmayr, M. (2012). Nutrition risk assessment in the ICU. *Current Opinion in Clinical Nutrition and Metabolic Care, 15*(2), 174–180. doi:10.1097/MCO.0b013e328350767e

Janson, L. W., & Tischler, M. E. (2012). Chapter 7. Lipid Metabolism. In *The big picture: Medical biochemistry.* New York, NY: McGraw-Hill. Retrieved May 23, 2017, from http://accessmedicine.mhmedical.com.ezproxy .uky.edu/content.aspx?bookid=397&sectionid =39898613

Jellinge, M. E., Henriksen, D. P., Hallas, P., & Brabrand, M. (2014). Hypoalbuminemia is a strong predictor of 30-day all-cause mortality in acutely admitted medical patients: A prospective, observational, cohort study. *PLoS One, 9*(8), e105983. doi:10.1371/journal .pone.0105983

Jensen, G. L., Compher, C., Sullivan, D. H., & Mullins, G. E. (2013). Recognizing malnutrition in adults: Definitions and characteristics, screening, assessment, and team approach. *Journal of Parenteral and Enteral Nutrition, 37*(6), 802–807.

Jensen, G. L., Hsiao, P. Y., & Wheeler, D. (2012). Chapter 9: Screening and assessment. In C. M. Mueller (Ed.), *A.S.P.E.N. adult nutrition support core curriculum* (2nd ed., pp. 155–170). Silver Spring, MD: American Society for Parenteral and Enteral Nutrition.

Joosten, A., Alexander, B., & Connesson, M. (2015). Defining goals of resuscitation in the critically ill patient. *Critical Care Clinics, 31*(1), 113–132. doi:10.106/j .ccc.2014.08.006

Kee, J. L. (2014). *Laboratory and diagnostic tests with nursing implications* (9th ed.). Hoboken, NJ: Pearson.

Lyons, O., Whelan, B., Bennett, K., O'Riordan, D., & Silke, B. (2010). Serum albumin as an outcome predictor in hospital emergency medical admissions. *European Journal of Internal Medicine, 21*(1), 17–20. doi:10.1016/j .ejim.2009.10.010

Maday, K. R. (2017). The importance of nutrition in critically ill patients. *Journal of American Academy of Physician Assistants, 30*(1), 32–36. doi:10.1097/01 .JAA.0000502861.28599.c6

Marino, P. (2014). Nutritional requirements. In P. Marino (Ed.), *The ICU book* (4th ed.). Philadelphia, PA: Lippincott Williams & Wilkins.

McClave, S., Taylor, B., Martindale, R., Warren, M., Johnson, D., Braunschweig, C., . . . The Society of Critical Care Medicine and the American Society for Parenteral and Enteral Nutrition. (2016). Guidelines for the provision and assessment of nutrition support therapy in the adult critically ill patient: Society of Critical Care Medicine (SCCM) and American Society for Parenteral and Enteral Nutrition (A.S.P.E.N.). *Journal of Parenteral and Enteral Nutrition, 40*(2), 159–211. doi:10.1177/0148607115621863

Mogensen, K. M., Robinson, M. K., Casey, J. D., Gunasekera, N. S., Moromizato, T., Rawn, J. D., & Christopher, K. B. (2015). Nutritional status and mortality in the critically ill. *Critical Care Medicine, 43*(12), 2605–2615. doi:10.1097/CCM.0000000000001306

Molina, P. E. (2013a). Chapter 1: General principles of endocrine physiology. In P. E. Molina (Ed.), *Endocrine physiology* (4th ed.). New York, NY: McGraw Hill Medical. Retrieved March 14, 2017, from http:// accessmedicine.mhmedical.com.ezproxy.uky.edu /content.aspx?bookid=507&sectionid=42540504

Molina, P. E. (2013b). Chapter 4: Thyroid gland. In P. E. Molina (Ed.), *Endocrine physiology* (4th ed.). New York, NY: McGraw-Hill Medical. Retrieved March 14, 2017, from http://accessmedicine.mhmedical.com.ezproxy .uky.edu/content.aspx?bookid=507&sectionid =42540504

Mueller, C. (2012). *The A.S.P.E.N. adult nutrition support core curriculum* (2nd ed., pp. 155–169, 234–244, and 377–391). Silver Spring, MD: American Society for Parenteral and Enteral Nutrition.

National Heart, Lung, and Blood Institute. (2016). *Classification of overweight and obesity by BMI, waist circumference, and associated disease risks.* Retrieved May 31, 2017, from https://www.nhlbi.nih.gov /health/educational/lose_wt/BMI/bmi_dis.htm

Nicoll, D., Mark Lu, C., & McPhee, S. J. (2017). Lab tests. In D. Nicoll, C. Mark Lu, & S. J. McPhee (Eds.), *Guide to diagnostic tests* (7th ed.). New York, NY: McGraw-Hill. Retrieved March 14, 2017, from http://accessmedicine .mhmedical.com.ezproxy.uky.edu/content.aspx?bookid =2032&sectionid=152254910

Packer, M. (2016). Cobalt cardiomyopathy: A critical reappraisal in light of a recent resurgence. *Circulation Heart Failure, 9*(12), 1–10. doi:10.1161 /CIRCHEARTFAILURE.116.003604

Tao, K., Li, X., Yang, L., Yu, W., Lu, Z., Sun, Y., & Wu, F. (2014). Glutamine supplementation for critically ill adults. *The Cochrane Database of Systematic Reviews, 9,* CD010050. doi:10.1002/14651858.CD010050.pub2

Weitzel, L. R., & Wischmeyer, P. E. (2010). Glutamine in critical illness: The time has come, the time is now. *Critical Care Clinics, 26*(3), ix–x, 515–525.

White, J. V., Guenter, P., Jensen, G., Malone, A., Schofield, M., Academy Malnutrition Work Group, . . . A.S.P.E.N. Board of Directors. (2012). Consensus statement of the Academy of Nutrition and Dietetics/American Society for Parenteral and Enteral Nutrition: Characteristics recommended for the identification and documentation of adult malnutrition (undernutrition). *Journal of the Academy of Nutrition and Dietetics, 112*(5), 730–738.

Chapter 32
Metabolic Response to Stress

⌄ Learning Outcomes

32.1 Examine the neuro-endocrine response of the hypothalamic–pituitary–adrenal axis, the thyroid, the pancreas, and the liver to acute and prolonged stress from critical illness.

32.2 Demonstrate knowledge of the diagnosis and collaborative management of adrenal dysfunction in critical illness.

32.3 Demonstrate clinical judgment and critical thinking around the diagnosis and collaborative management of thyroid dysfunction in critical illness.

32.4 Examine the evidence base supporting the collaborative management of hyperglycemic syndromes during critical illness.

When the endocrine system is not functioning at its best, a variety of disorders may occur. Critical illness can result in stress-related neuro-endocrine responses that, if not anticipated or left untreated, may complicate recovery and contribute to poor outcomes. It is important to understand how stress from critical illness can affect endocrine response.

Section One: Introduction to Responses to Stress in Acute and Critical Illness

Neuro-endocrine and metabolic responses to stress can have serious implications. Often, severe and prolonged activation of the stress response can place increased demands on the adrenal and thyroid glands, altering their function. These responses are introduced here but are presented in more depth in later sections of this chapter.

Neuro-endocrine Stress Response

The acute phase response to physiologic stress of acute and critical illness involves rapid release of the catecholamines *epinephrine* and *norepinephrine* by the sympathetic nervous system into the circulation—the "fight-or-flight" response. Epinephrine, also known as adrenaline, is released by the adrenal medulla and causes an increase in

blood flow to the brain, heart, lung, and skeletal muscles. Comparatively, blood flow is decreased to other vital organs such as those in the abdomen, including the liver, pancreas, and intestines (both small and large). Severe stress that triggers the sympathetic nervous system simultaneously activates the hypothalamic–pituitary–adrenal axis (an essential homeostatic mechanism necessary for life); stress also affects thyroid and pancreatic organ systems. This response is particularly strong at the onset of physiological stress and diminishes with prolonged critical illness. Prolonged activation of this stress response decreases the ability of the body to respond to potential complications such as inflammation, infection, and trauma that may negatively affect outcomes for the patient being treated for a critical illness.

Hypothalamic–Pituitary–Adrenal Axis   The **hypothalamic–pituitary–adrenal (HPA) axis** is composed of the hypothalamus, anterior pituitary gland, and adrenal cortex; it is a major component of the stress response (Long & Cakmak, 2015; Schimmer & Funder, 2011) (see Figure 32–1). It is an integrated negative feedback loop that moderates hormones within the body. Three major hormones are involved in the HPA axis: corticotropin-releasing hormone (CRH), adrenocorticotropic hormone (ACTH), and cortisol. When stress occurs, the hypothalamus responds by secreting CRH. Available CRH stimulates the anterior pituitary gland to secrete ACTH, and then ACTH stimulates the adrenal cortex to secrete glucocorticoids, primarily cortisol (Hall, 2016). As cortisol levels rise, the hypothalamus eventually responds by reducing secretion of CRH, thereby

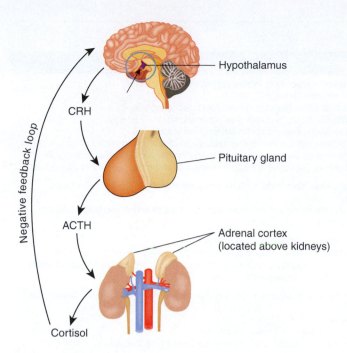

Figure 32–1 HPA axis response to physical or emotional stress. CRH, corticotropin hormone; ACTH, adrenocorticotropic hormone.

reducing cortisol secretion and establishing a negative feedback loop.

Cortisol release is protective during stress, and levels increase significantly with a normally functioning adrenal gland. Cortisol plays multiple roles in helping the body cope with stress, such as the following:

- Increases insulin resistance, resulting in increased serum glucose and increased consumption of fats for energy
- Triggers increased hepatic glycogenolysis to increase the amount of glucose released into the circulation by the liver
- Alters carbohydrate, fat, and protein metabolism so that energy is immediately available for use by vital organs such as the brain, heart, and skeletal muscles
- Works with growth hormone (GH) to increase protein catabolism for energy and tissue building
- Increases serum sodium by causing water retention and increased movement of extravascular water into the intravascular space to support circulating blood volume

The hypothalamus and pituitary glands also stimulate the stress response through other means. The hypothalamus controls the response to stress of both the anterior and posterior pituitary gland. When the posterior pituitary is stimulated, it releases antidiuretic hormone (ADH), also known as vasopressin (pitressin). The primary function of ADH is to conserve water; however, it is also a potent vasoconstrictor. Along with epinephrine and norepinephrine, these endogenous hormones increase the heart rate and raise the blood pressure quickly to restore cardiac output. The anterior pituitary gland also releases

the anabolic growth hormone (GH) into the circulation, which triggers the increased consumption of amino acids to build protein for tissue repair. Furthermore, the pituitary gland increases endogenous opioids, which provide some analgesia during the stress response. While HPA axis function is capable of providing a short-term compensatory response to stress, it is unable to maintain that response over a prolonged period of time, as seen in critical illness that lasts more than a week (Bosmann & Ward, 2013; Preiser, Ichai, Orban, & Groeneveld, 2014; Rosenthal & Moore, 2015). Eventually, chronic stress causes the HPA axis to become under- or nonresponsive, adrenal fatigue or exhaustion occurs, and the patient will begin to decompensate. When function decreases, cortisol levels remain elevated but corticotropin and growth hormone levels decrease. The nurse should suspect inadequate adrenal function if, despite resuscitation efforts, the patient remains unstable (e.g., hypotensive, vasopressor dependent, requiring prolonged mechanical ventilation). Older adults are particularly susceptible to adrenal dysfunction as they are more vulnerable to common causes of adrenal insufficiency such as head injury related to falls, cancer with metastasis, and infections (fungal and tuberculosis). Other common causes of adrenal dysfunction include tumors affecting the pituitary gland, adrenal hemorrhage, removal of the adrenal gland (adrenalectomy), and long-term glucocorticoid use (Puar, Stikkelbroeck, Smans, Zelissen, & Hermus, 2016).

In addition to the decreased HPA axis function, the liver, pancreas, and thyroid gland function can become impaired during prolonged stress response. Glucagon is a hormone that is produced in the liver to stimulate hepatic production of glucose to increase serum glucose levels during stress (gluconeogenesis). Insulin production by the pancreas remains relatively unchanged in the face of increased serum glucose levels. This imbalance in insulin production and increased serum glucose levels is believed to be responsible for the relative insulin resistance that develops in the peripheral tissues (Via & Mechanick, 2016). Insulin resistance means that the tissues are not able to use available insulin to transport glucose into the cells during times of severe stress. Therefore, hyperglycemia is common during physiological stress because of the combination of insulin resistance and increased serum glucose levels. It is important to manage glycemic levels with insulin administration to maintain glucose within normal limits as hyperglycemia can lead to poor wound healing, decreased immune function, increased susceptibility to infection, and longer hospitalizations (Marín-Peñalver, Martín-Timón, & del Cañizo-Gómez, 2016).

Stress-related imbalances in thyroid hormones also can occur during prolonged illness. Levels of circulating thyroid hormone (T3 and T4) decrease and thyroid-stimulating hormone (TSH) secretion is suppressed (Van den Berghe, 2017). Thyroid function follows a pattern similar to the HPA axis function in response to prolonged critical illness and should be assessed in patients with increased catabolism with symptoms of physical deconditioning. Restoration of circulating thyroid hormone has been found to have a positive relationship with the anabolism of skeletal muscle and

Table 32–1 Endocrine Stress Response

Hormone	Initiating Gland or Organ	Physiological Response During Stress
Cortisol (glucocorticoid)	Adrenal cortex	Inhibits glucose uptake and metabolism, increasing serum glucose levels Stimulates lipolysis for additional energy Increases liver release of glucose (gluconeogenesis) and glycogenolysis Decreases protein synthesis, increases breakdown of amino acids for energy Increases serum sodium levels, increasing circulating blood volume Suppresses immune system and wound healing through direct anti-inflammatory effects, including decreased histamine release; decreased circulating lymphocytes, monocytes, eosinophils, basophils; reduced connective-tissue fibroblasts; release of immature neutrophils (bandemia)
Mineralocorticoid	Adrenal cortex	Increases aldosterone release; decreases sodium and water excretion; results in increased intravascular volume Increases potassium and hydrogen ion excretion; can cause hypokalemia and helps to buffer against metabolic acidosis
Epinephrine and norepinephrine	Adrenal medulla	Increases endogenous endorphins/opioids and analgesia Increases heart rate, cardiac contractility and output, blood pressure, coronary artery dilation, insulin production, and glycogenolysis for increased glucose release; causes bronchodilation Decreases peristalsis, perfusion to peripheral organs
Corticotropin (ACTH) and growth hormone (GH)	Anterior pituitary	Increases aldosterone release; decreases sodium and water excretion, to increase intravascular blood volume Increases cortisol release Increases breakdown of protein amino acids for energy Increases thyroid-stimulating hormone (TSH) to increase production of thyroxine
Antidiuretic hormone (ADH)	Posterior pituitary	Increases vasoconstriction, water retention to restore circulating blood volume
Thyroxine	Thyroid	Increases heart rate and cardiac contractility Stimulates lipolysis for energy production Increases protein breakdown
Sex hormones	Gonads	Diverts energy and oxygen supply to brain, heart, skeletal muscles, and liver
Insulin and glucagon	Pancreas and liver	Increases insulin resistance of peripheral tissues, results in hyperglycemia Glucagon is a hormone that stimulates the liver to release glucose into the bloodstream and contributes to hyperglycemia

SOURCE: Data from Bauer & McPhee (2013); Else, Hammer, & McPhee (2014); Preiser et al. (2014).

bone. This is likely to promote rehabilitation and recovery after critical illness; therefore, it is important to monitor serum levels during the high-acuity phase of illness (Van den Berghe, 2017). Table 32–1 lists the hormones involved in the metabolic stress response, the initiating gland or organ, and the physiological response.

The Metabolic Stress Response

In addition to the powerful neuro-endocrine influences of stress on the body, there is a coupled metabolic response as well. Together, the combination of neuro-endocrine and metabolic stress responses can induce major adaptive and protective cellular mechanisms; however, prolonged stress in the form of critical illness may lead to organ dysfunction or failure.

The metabolic responses to physiologic stress such as infection, trauma, and surgery are fairly predictable. Two distinct phases of this response have been identified (Cuthbertson, 1979) and defined (Little & Girolami, 1999). The initial phase is called the ebb phase, which lasts about 24 hours after the occurrence of tissue injury. The ebb phase is followed by the flow phase. The duration of the flow phase is highly variable and is associated with the patient's clinical condition.

Ebb Phase The individual's metabolic rate is likely to be initially unchanged or slightly decreased during the first 24 hours after injury. Exceptions to this are patients with burns and patients with a severe head injury who have a Glasgow Coma Scale score of 8 or less and an increased metabolic rate. A slightly hypothermic body temperature may be observed in the body's attempt to decrease oxygen consumption and preserve energy. Increases in blood glucose and lactate levels are common.

Alterations in both carbohydrate and lipid metabolism are observed in the ebb phase, often with an increase in blood glucose and fatty acids. The body increases blood glucose production after an injury has occurred in an attempt to provide energy for wound healing. There is an increased release of stress hormones, such as epinephrine, glucagon, and cortisol, that stimulate the conversion of glycogen stores to glucose. Coupled with decreased production of insulin along with insulin resistance in peripheral tissues, this contributes to hyperglycemia following injury.

Recent literature has redefined nutrition as a therapy instead of a supportive intervention to prevent lean muscle mass depletion while a patient is hospitalized (McClave et al., 2016). Nutrition therapy is now a foundation for mediating the body's metabolic, immune, and inflammatory response to stress; it is now seen in ways similar to how medical therapies are viewed. The most recent guidelines from the Society of Critical Care Medicine (SCCM) and the American Society for Parenteral and Enteral Nutrition (A.S.P.E.N., 2016) recommend early enteral nutrition (EN) within 24 to 48 hours of intensive care admission. Initiation of EN during this essential ebb phase has been shown to reduce mortality, decrease the deaths associated with infections, decrease length of stay, and significantly reduce the incidence of pneumonia in multiple meta-analyses of data from randomized control trials (McClave et al., 2016). Specifically, early EN is beneficial to the critically ill patient as it maintains the integrity of the gut, which is at risk for decreased permeability from the time of injury due to systemic inflammatory and immune modulated responses (McClave et al., 2016). The influence of early EN has been reported to be positive. Data on multiple organ failure (MOF) is limited.

Although evidence supports early EN, controversy still exists regarding the utility of providing nutrition during the ebb phase. It is the current recommendation that EN be withheld if there is hemodynamic compromise (resulting in low cardiac output or instability) for complications such as ischemia of the microcirculation; the bowel is most at risk for this complication (McClave et al., 2016). Specifically, contraindications to early EN during the ebb phase include a mean arterial pressure (MAP) of less than 50 mmHg, requiring vasopressor support (such as epinephrine or norepinephrine), and patients whose requirements of vasopressors are steadily increasing due to circulatory collapse. Early EN may also be inappropriate for patients who are intolerant to EN and show signs of decreased absorption (resulting in watery diarrhea), decreased bowel motility, and increasing abdominal distension (McClave et al., 2016).

During the ebb phase, the fat stored in adipose tissue is susceptible to catabolism to contribute to energy needs. As fats are oxidized, fatty acids are produced and contribute to increases in lactic acid levels. Serum lactate, a by-product of anaerobic metabolism, will increase as anaerobic metabolism occurs in injured, ischemic tissues. Subsequently, the increasing quantity of lactate is converted to glucose by the liver, further contributing to hyperglycemia (Else et al., 2014; Funk, 2014).

Flow Phase   The onset of the flow phase begins 24 to 36 hours following the physiologic insult. The flow phase is characterized by increased oxygen consumption and calorie demands to provide for wound healing. Typical symptoms of the flow phase include the onset of tachycardia, tachypnea, increased cardiac output, and fever. **Hypercatabolism** (breakdown of body proteins) is prominent as stored protein is metabolized to help meet the sudden increase in oxygen consumption and energy expenditure. Increased oxygen consumption and energy expenditure along with hypercatabolism comprise the clinical condition known as **hypermetabolism**. Hyperglycemia is frequently observed after tissue injury, for the reasons presented with the HPA axis discussion earlier in this section. Administration of insulin may be ineffective in controlling elevated glucose levels during the metabolic stress response.

Patient prognosis worsens as hypermetabolism persists; this may occur in patients with severe tissue trauma, such as the burn injury patient or patients with septic shock. Hypermetabolism in combination with GI dysfunction, including decreased motility, absorption, and blood flow, may be especially harmful in patients with severe sepsis or septic shock; this places them at a high nutritional risk. There is little evidence to compare patients who receive early EN to patients who have late EN, but early EN is likely to be associated with favorable clinical outcomes (McClave et al., 2016). Particularly, patients with tissue trauma experience a reduced ability to use carbohydrates, proteins, and lipids, another factor that contributes to malnutrition in the high-acuity patient.

The peak of the hypermetabolic response usually occurs 3 to 4 days following the initiating event. In the patient without complications, the hypermetabolic stress response usually lasts 7 to 10 days; however, the hypermetabolic high-acuity patient is rarely without complications. Exacerbation of the hypermetabolic response occurs with repeated episodes of tissue ischemia, localized infections, or septicemia. The metabolic alterations occurring with hypermetabolism and hypercatabolism can become a vicious cycle leading to further clinical deterioration if the patient does not receive adequate metabolic support and nutritional therapies within the first few days of the precipitating event. Table 32–2 provides a synopsis of the metabolic stress response.

Table 32–2 Summary of the Stress Response

Characteristics	Ebb Phase	Flow Phase
Duration	First 24 hours after physiologic insult*	Variable but usually begins 24–36 hours after physiological insult and peaks in 3–4 days, lasting 7–10 days or longer for persistent insult
Goal	Prevent tissue injury	Repair injured tissue
Stress hormone release (epinephrine, glucagon, cortisol)	Increased ("flight" stress response)	Increased ("fight" and tissue repair)
Metabolism	Unchanged or slightly decreased	Increased (hypermetabolic and hypercatabolic)
Body temperature	Decreased	Increased
Oxygen consumption	Decreased	Increased
Blood glucose levels	Increased (decreased insulin production, increased insulin resistance)	Increased (same as ebb phase)
Blood lactate levels	Increased (increased fat metabolism for energy)	Increased (same as ebb phase)
Primary fuel sources for energy production	Glucose and fat	Glucose, fat, and branched chain amino acids from breakdown of lean muscle mass

*Physiologic insult can be due to trauma, ischemia, or infection.

Section One Review

1. Which hormone stimulates hepatic production of glucose?
   A. ACTH
   B. Insulin
   C. Thyroxine
   D. Glucagon

2. The ebb phase of the metabolic and neuro-endocrine stress response is characterized by which physiological responses? (Select all that apply.)
   A. Hypermetabolism
   B. Alteration in carbohydrate/lipid metabolism
   C. Increased release of glucagon and cortisol
   D. Hypercatabolism
   E. Increased production of insulin

3. The hypothalamic–pituitary–adrenal (HPA) axis is an important negative feedback hormone mechanism that involves which hormones? (Select all that apply.)
   A. Antidiuretic hormone (ADH)
   B. Corticotropin-releasing hormone (CRH)
   C. Adrenocorticotropic hormone (ACTH)
   D. Growth hormone (GH)
   E. Cortisol

4. High levels of prolonged physiologic stress cause which alteration in thyroid hormones?
   A. No associated changes
   B. Increased T3 and T4 levels
   C. Decreased T3 and increased T4 levels
   D. Suppression of thyroid-stimulating hormone

Answers: 1. D, 2. (B, C), 3. (B, C, E), 4. D

Section Two: Acute Adrenal Insufficiency During Critical Illness

The adrenal gland plays a major role in the adaptive response to stress. Acute adrenal insufficiency has been associated with critical illness. For example, a relatively new concept in the critical care literature is critical illness–related corticosteroid insufficiency (CIRCI), a type of insufficiency in which there is inadequate corticosteroid activity to meet the needs of the critically ill patient (Graves, Faraklas, & Cochran, 2012). CIRCI is often reversible and primarily focuses on dysfunction of the HPA axis and tissue corticosteroid resistance associated with a prolonged inflammatory response (Graves et al., 2012; Marino, 2014). This section provides an overview of acute adrenal insufficiency and its implications during critical illness.

Types of Adrenal Insufficiency

Adrenal insufficiency can be a primary disorder (inability of the gland to secrete cortisol or aldosterone) or a secondary disorder (inability of the HPA axis to release ACTH). Acute adrenal insufficiency may result from pre-existing or previously undiagnosed chronic disease of the adrenal glands or HPA axis, or acute conditions affecting these endocrine structures. The presence of chronic diseases is a risk factor for the development of acute adrenal insufficiency precipitated by infection or other stressors. Also, relative or absolute insufficiency of glucocorticoid (cortisol) or mineralocorticoid (aldosterone) production can cause functional impairments in the patient during critical illness; however, the insufficiency

usually reverses with recovery from the illness. Table 32–3 lists causes of adrenal insufficiency due to chronic and acute conditions.

Signs and Symptoms of Adrenal Insufficiency

No specific signs and symptoms are associated with adrenal insufficiency, making recognition of the disorder difficult. The hallmark characteristic of adrenal insufficiency is often refractory hypotension despite adequate fluid and/or blood volume resuscitation (Marino, 2014). Clinical manifestations that suggest adrenal insufficiency include

---

Table 32–3 Chronic and Acute Conditions That Cause Adrenal Insufficiency

Type	Conditions Causing Adrenal Insufficiency
Acute	**Critical illness** Hypotension, hypoperfusion Cytokine effects (altered cortisol metabolism)
	Acute adrenal hemorrhage Disseminated intravascular coagulation (DIC) Anticoagulation (heparin, warfarin, or other drugs) Severe sepsis and thrombocytopenia
Chronic	**Adrenal glands** Autoimmune disease HIV infection Tuberculosis Primary or metastatic malignancy Drug effects Other infections (fungal, viral, bacterial)
	Hypothalamic–pituitary–adrenal (HPA) axis Withdrawal from chronic glucocorticoid (steroid) therapy Hypopituitarism from tumors, infarction, radiation Head trauma Cerebrovascular disease and stroke

Table 32–4 Clinical Manifestations Suggesting Adrenal Insufficiency

Parameter	Manifestations
Vital signs	Fever Tachycardia Orthostatic hypotension Hypotension that is refractory to volume or vasopressor agent administration
Gastrointestinal	Nausea and vomiting Abdominal pain
Laboratory	Hyponatremia and hyperkalemia Acidosis Hypoglycemia Eosinophilia Increased serum creatinine and blood urea nitrogen (BUN)
Other	General weakness

alterations in vital signs, gastrointestinal symptoms, and abnormal laboratory values (see Table 32–4). The patient may develop increased serum creatinine and blood urea nitrogen (BUN) associated with a prerenal etiology for acute kidney injury (AKI) associated with circulating volume deficit or dehydration. Much like in Addison disease, a common form of adrenal insufficiency, the patient with CIRCI may have changes in serum electrolytes such as hyponatremia and hyperkalemia (Marino, 2014). In the event that adrenal insufficiency is due to acute adrenal hemorrhage, the patient may have acute pain in the back, flank, or abdomen. These clinical and laboratory manifestations are nonspecific and overlap significantly with those of other critical illnesses, such as sepsis. Adrenal insufficiency should be suspected in any patient who is seriously ill, develops hypotension of unclear etiology, has hypotension that fails to respond to fluid resuscitation and vasopressor agents, or has persistent fever without an apparent source.

Evaluation of Adrenal Insufficiency

The diagnostic test of choice for adrenal insufficiency in critically ill patients is the rapid ACTH stimulation test (or short cosyntropin test) along with baseline serum cortisol levels (Carroll, Aron, Findling, & Tyrrell, 2011; Kee, 2014; Nicoll, Mark Lu, & McPhee, 2017). The rapid ACTH stimulation test evaluates adrenal reserve by evaluating the ability of the adrenal cortex to respond to exogenous ACTH by increasing the level of cortisol. To perform this test, an arterial blood sample is obtained for plasma cortisol level, and synthetic ACTH (cosyntropin 250 mcg) is administered IV or IM. A blood sample for a second plasma cortisol level is obtained 60 to 90 minutes later. An abnormally low response indicates reduced adrenal reserve and helps to establish the diagnosis of adrenal insufficiency (Carroll et al., 2011). The rapid ACTH stimulation test can be performed at any time of the day or night because it is not influenced by diurnal variations in cortisol secretion; these are often absent in critically ill patients. If the rapid ACTH stimulation test

is abnormal, plasma ACTH levels are drawn to further differentiate whether it is primary or secondary adrenal insufficiency. If ACTH levels are elevated, primary adrenal insufficiency is present; however, if ACTH levels are normal or lower than normal, secondary insufficiency is suspected to be present (Carroll et al., 2011; Via & Mechanick, 2016).

Diagnostic Criteria for Adrenal Insufficiency

Glucocorticoid levels are normally elevated in response to stress, so a very low baseline plasma cortisol (less than 3 mcg/dL) in the setting of critical illness is diagnostic of adrenal insufficiency. Cortisol levels of 36 mcg/dL or greater indicate appropriate or adequate adrenal function (Marino, 2014). However, if a cortisol level less than 15 mcg/dL is present in the setting of hypotension and refractory shock despite adequate volume resuscitation and vasopressor agent administration, adrenal insufficiency should be considered. A baseline cortisol level greater than 23 mcg/dL is sufficient to rule out adrenal insufficiency. After cosyntropin (synthetic ACTH used for diagnosis of cortisol problems) administration, an increase in serum cortisol of less than 9 mcg/dL suggests adrenal insufficiency and helps identify patients who would likely benefit from glucocorticoid therapy such as intravenous hydrocortisone (Via & Mechanick, 2016). Ideally, cortisol and ACTH levels should be drawn before any empiric therapy is begun. Treatment decisions are based on clinical grounds and severity of symptoms. Improvement in hemodynamic function after administration of hydrocortisone may be an important physiologic indicator of true adrenal insufficiency.

Treatment

Emergent treatment is indicated in critically ill patients, even if the diagnosis is not firmly established. Hydrocortisone is the drug of choice as it provides both corticosteroid and mineralocorticoid effects. If the patient's status improves following glucocorticoid (hydrocortisone) administration, treatment should be continued until resolution of the critical illness or for 7 days. Tapering of steroid therapy may avoid rebound effects associated with abrupt discontinuation of the drug such as increased inflammatory mediators; tapering should occur over a few days (Marino, 2014). Patients with evidence or history of persistent adrenal insufficiency (chronic or newly diagnosed) should be converted to oral steroid therapy; this may include drugs such as prednisone. It is important to note that high-dose steroid therapy during critical illness has been de-emphasized, as supporting research evidence is lacking. Treatment with steroids is reserved for critically ill patients that show no improvement despite maximal medical therapies. Treatment steps for adrenal insufficiency associated with critical illness are outlined in the "Related Pharmacotherapy: Corticosteroid Treatment for Adrenal Insufficiency" feature.

Related Pharmacotherapy

Corticosteroid Treatment for Adrenal Insufficiency

Corticosteroid Therapy

Hydrocortisone
Fludrocortisone

Action and Uses

Corticosteroid replacement therapy to normalize cortisol levels. Steroid treatment reserved for critically ill patients with the following: (1) Vasopressor-dependent shock despite adequate volume resuscitation (vasopressor-dependent shock defined as needing a dosage of norepinephrine or equivalent 0.05–0.1 mcg/kg/min within 12 hours of onset); (2) failure to respond to appropriate fluid administration; (3) progressive acute respiratory distress syndrome after 48 hours of supportive care.

Dosages (Adult)

Hydrocortisone: Initial dosing: 50 mg IV every 6 hours or 100 mg bolus followed by 10 mg/hour continuous infusion for at least 7 days with option of treatment for 10–15 days. Taper dosing: 50 mg IV every 8 hours for 3–4 days, then 50 mg IV/PO every 12 hours for 3–4 days, then 50 mg IV/PO daily for 3–4 days. If there is recurrence of shock or worsening oxygenation, then reinstitution of full-dose hydrocortisone should be considered.

Fludrocortisone: 50 mcg PO once daily to replace mineralocorticoid insufficiency should be considered in patients with known primary adrenal insufficiency or if methylprednisolone is used in place of hydrocortisone. Hydrocortisone is known to have good mineralocorticoid activity, so the addition of fludrocortisone is considered adjunctive therapy (Marino, 2014).

Major Adverse Effects

Potentially serious multiple system effects including Cushingoid syndrome

Most severe: Anaphylactoid reactions, masking or aggravation of infection, thrombocytopenia

Nursing Implications

Hydrocortisone and methylprednisolone are considered interchangeable for their combined glucocorticoid and mineralocorticoid effectiveness; methylprednisone has better anti-inflammatory properties.

Vasopressor therapy indicating resolution of shock should not be required before beginning taper.

Patients who receive steroids are at increased risk of developing infections. Nurses should have a low threshold for initiating blood, urine, sputum, or other appropriate cultures if infection is suspected.

Patients are at increased risk of hyperglycemia; this has implications that delay wound healing. Nurses should monitor serum blood glucose and initiate insulin therapy as appropriate.

Patients are at increased risk of myopathy and should monitor muscular strength; initiate early activity and physical therapy in patients with prolonged immobility.

Neuromuscular blocking agents should be avoided in patients who receive steroids.

SOURCE: Data from Marino (2014); Via & Mechanick (2017); Wilson, Shannon, & Shields (2017).

Section Two Review

1. The inability of the adrenal gland to secrete cortisol suggests which condition?
   A. Primary adrenal dysfunction
   B. Primary hypothalamic–pituitary dysfunction
   C. Secondary adrenal dysfunction
   D. Secondary hypothalamic–pituitary dysfunction

2. Acute adrenal insufficiency may result from which conditions? (Select all that apply.)
   A. Undiagnosed disease of the HPA axis
   B. Infection
   C. Hypothyroidism
   D. Preexisting adrenal disease
   E. Prolonged critical illness

3. Which abnormal finding commonly occurs with adrenal insufficiency?
   A. Hypernatremia
   B. Hyperglycemia
   C. Hypertension
   D. Persistent shock

4. In a client who is critically ill, the serum cortisol level is 5 mcg/dL. The client is hypotensive and is receiving IV vasopressor agents and fluids. What medication should be considered for this client?
   A. Propranolol
   B. Levothyroxine
   C. Hydrocortisone
   D. Insulin

Answers: 1. A, 2. (A, B, D, E), 3. D, 4. C

Section Three: Thyroid Dysfunction During Critical Illness

Previously diagnosed thyroid disorders that have been treated in the outpatient setting do not generally result in crisis. However, in patients with undiagnosed thyroid disorders who become critically ill, serious life-threatening complications can occur. Abnormalities in thyroid function can develop either as a primary disorder of the thyroid gland itself (primary hyperthyroidism or hypothyroidism) or as a secondary disorder, a problem that occurs outside of the thyroid gland but affects its function. This section briefly reviews thyroid hormones and primary thyroid diseases but focuses on nonthyroid illness syndrome, a secondary hypothyroid condition seen in the critically ill patient.

Thyroid Hormones

Thyroid hormone regulates metabolic rate, increases myocardial contractility and heart rate, and regulates systemic vascular resistance (SVR) to optimize cardiac output. Thyroid-stimulating hormone (TSH) controls the production and release of thyroid hormone and is secreted by the anterior pituitary gland. The anterior pituitary gland, in turn, is regulated by thyrotropin-regulating hormone (TRH), which is secreted by the hypothalamus. TSH stimulates the breakdown of thyroglobulin (stored form of thyroid hormone) to release T3 (triiodothyronine) and T4 (levothyroxine) into the bloodstream. Both T3 and T4 are stored in the form of thyroglobulin and are highly protein bound. Thus, TSH and TRH secretions are under a negative regulation feedback loop: as the level of active thyroid hormone in the circulation rises, the release of TRH and TSH is inhibited, which decreases thyroid hormone synthesis.

TSH levels give the best indication of thyroid function in nonthyroid-related illness (Marino, 2014). They also distinguish between primary and secondary thyroid conditions. Therefore, if thyroid deficiency is suspected in critical illness, this test should be performed first. Serum TSH levels have diurnal variations, with the highest levels present during hours of rest or sleep; lab draws should be assessed based on this pattern. The normal serum TSH level is 0.3 to 4.5 mU/dL. It is important to note that TSH levels can be suppressed during critical illness from conditions such as sepsis or pharmacologic therapies such as corticosteroid administration (Marino, 2014).

Thus, it is recommended that the assessment of TSH levels should be combined with T4 levels during critical illness; free T3 levels are less available (Marino, 2014). This is because the thyroid gland itself is able to convert only a small amount of thyroglobulin directly into T3, with the majority of T3 being produced in the peripheral tissues from conversion of T4, a pro-hormone, to T3, an active hormone (Economidou, Douka, Tzanela, Nanas, & Kotanidou, 2011; Marino, 2014). Assessment of T4, which is highly protein bound, may give a better indication of thyroid function

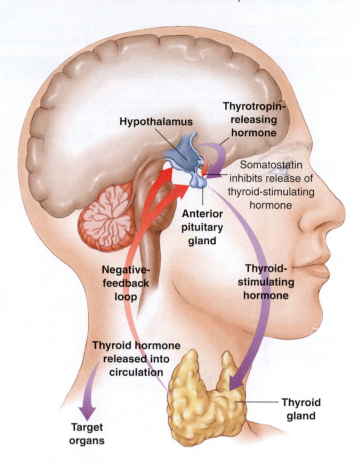

Figure 32–2 The thyroid feedback loop. The hypothalamus controls the anterior pituitary, which in turn controls the thyroid gland. Negative feedback loops prevent the oversecretion of hormones.

SOURCE: Martini, Frederick. H; Bartholomew, Edwin F.; Bledsoe, Bryan E.; *Anatomy and Physiology for Emergency Care*, 2nd Ed., © 2008, pp. 527, 373, 390. Reprinted by permission of Pearson Education, Inc., Upper Saddle River, New Jersey.

because of alterations in protein metabolism during critical illness (Marino, 2014). Figure 32–2 illustrates the thyroid feedback loop.

Primary Hyperthyroidism and Hypothyroidism

Severe derangements in thyroid function can precipitate a metabolic crisis. While thyroid crises are rare, they can be life-threatening, requiring rapid diagnosis and treatment.

Hyperthyroidism Hyperthyroidism, or thyrotoxicosis, is a condition in which there is an overproduction of thyroid hormones. The major causes are autoimmune disorders of the thyroid gland (e.g., Graves disease) that stimulate hormone production (Jameson, Mandel, & Weetman, 2015). Signs and symptoms reflect systemic increases in metabolic functions (see Table 32–5).

Hyperthyroid Crisis/Thyroid (Thyrotoxic) Storm. A severe exacerbation of hyperthyroid signs and symptoms known as *thyroid storm* can be precipitated by acute illness, infection, withdrawal of antithyroid medications, or surgery.

Table 32–5 Comparison of Characteristics of Hypothyroidism and Hyperthyroidism

System	Hyperthyroidism	Hypothyroidism
Cardiac	Tachycardia Systolic hypertension; widened pulse pressure (or hypotension if cardiovascular complications occur) Hyperdynamic heart failure and shock ECG: atrial fibrillation/flutter; myocardial ischemia Chest pain	Bradycardia Hypotension Heart failure in patients with underlying cardiac disease Angina ECG: low voltage Pericardial effusions
Pulmonary	Dyspnea Tachypnea	Shortness of breath Hypoventilation Pleural effusions Ventilatory failure and increased PCO_2 levels
Gastrointestinal	Hyperactive bowel; diarrhea Malabsorption	Hypoactive bowel; constipation (reduced intestinal motility) Paralytic ileus
Neurological	Agitation, tremors Anxiety Emotional lability Altered LOC Lethargy (in older adults)	Dull mentation Dementia Decreased deep tendon reflexes Altered LOC
Musculoskeletal	Weakness and fatigue	Weakness and fatigue
Other	Weight loss Heat sensitivity Hyperthermia Diaphoresis Anemia and leukocytosis	Weight gain Cold sensitivity Hypothermia Nonpitting edema Hyponatremia Increased serum creatinine More common in females and older adults

SOURCE: Data from Idrose (2016) and Jameson et al., 2015).

No definitive signs differentiate thyroid storm from severe hyperthyroidism. Hyperthyroid crisis is characterized by severe agitation, high fever, tachyarrhythmias, and heart failure (with high cardiac output), which may progress to shock, coma, and death if not recognized and treated. As seen in many other conditions in older adults, patients may exhibit signs of lethargy that are called *apathetic thyrotoxicosis* (Marino, 2014). These patients may have a goiter, heart failure, atrial fibrillation, and/or flutter, tremor, diaphoresis, diarrhea, elevated liver function tests, and psychosis. Both hyperthyroid crisis and thyroid storm will be accompanied by elevated T3 or T4 levels and a decreased TSH level, which may be so low that it is undetectable with laboratory diagnostics (Marino, 2014).

Management of thyroid storm is both therapeutic and supportive. Treatment is threefold: (1) decrease thyroid hormone production, (2) inhibit conversion of T4 to active T3, and (3) block the effects of metabolically active thyroid hormone. Methimazole and propylthiouracil (PTU) are most commonly used to decrease the production of thyroxine. Nursing considerations for these drugs include monitoring for liver dysfunction with physical assessment findings (jaundice) and diagnostics (liver function tests); agranulocytosis may also result from the use of PTU. Severe cases of thyroid storm may require iodine therapy, which blocks the conversion of T4 to T3 and is usually given in an oral form called Lugol's solution. Adrenal insufficiency may be an unanticipated consequence of thyroid storm; glucocorticoid treatment may be indicated if severe.

Symptom management of thyroid storm is mostly supportive with other pharmacotherapies that target the body systems affected by thyrotoxicosis and thyroid storm. The most frequently seen defining symptoms of thyroid storm—including agitation, tachycardia, and tremors—are usually treated with propranolol (Marino, 2014). This is a nonselective beta-receptor blocker and the drug of choice in thyroid storm. It is included in the management of most patients with thyroid storm and in large doses can block the conversion of T4 to T3. It can be given orally or intravenously and is not recommended for patients whose medical history includes asthma (it is a nonselective beta-receptor antagonist). Supportive care also includes treatment of fever with antipyretics, aggressive fluid resuscitation to replace excessive fluid losses (related to vomiting and diarrhea), and nutritional support (Fitzgerald, 2017; Marino, 2014; Via & Mechanick, 2016). Additional management information is provided in the "Nursing Care: The Patient with Hyperthyroidism" and "Related Pharmacotherapy: The Patient with Hyperthyroid Crisis/Thyroid Storm" features.

Hypothyroidism Hypothyroidism is a condition in which there is a deficiency of thyroid hormone. Characteristically, serum levels of T4 are decreased, but levels of TSH in primary hypothyroidism are elevated (Marino, 2014). In secondary hypothyroidism, the hypothalamic–pituitary axis is involved, and TSH levels may be reduced in cases of, for example, pituitary tumors. Hypothyroidism often affects adults, particularly older adults. Common causes are iodine deficiency, autoimmune diseases that destroy the thyroid (e.g., Hashimoto thyroiditis), pituitary tumors, and consequences of treatment of hyperthyroidism such as thyroidectomy or radioiodine therapy (Jameson et al., 2015; Marino, 2014). Hypothyroidism is associated with a slowing of metabolism characterized by a systemic reduction in body functions (see Table 32–5). Because thyroid hormone regulates free water in the circulation, hypothyroid patients are at increased risk of developing hyponatremia from increased free water accumulation in the blood, causing dilution. Cortisol clearance is enhanced when thyroid hormone is administered, so it is always important to remember that patients treated with thyroid hormone replacement are at increased risk of adrenal insufficiency.

Hypothyroid Crisis/Myxedema Coma. Myxedema coma is a severe form of hypothyroidism characterized by altered mental status ranging from lethargy to psychosis, hypothermia, bradycardia, hypotension, hypoventilation, hyponatremia, and hypoglycemia. Myxedema is rare and is differentiated from simple hypothyroidism by hypothermia, central nervous system dysfunction, and hypotension. Myxedema coma can occur acutely in patients with preexisting, untreated, or inadequately treated hypothyroidism who experience physiological stress from acute illness, exposure to cold temperatures, or sedative drugs; myxedema coma occurs most commonly in older adult women (Leung, 2016).

Advances in myxedema management have reduced overall mortality to 20% to 25%. Risk factors for poor prognosis include lower Glasgow Coma Scale score, prolonged bradycardia or hypothermia, multiple organ dysfunction, and older age (Jameson et al., 2017; Klubo-Gwiezdzinska & Wartofsky, 2012). Myxedema can be a cause of several common syndromes responsible for critical illness, including severe ileus associated with bowel obstruction, respiratory failure or failure to wean from a ventilator, heart failure, hypothermia, and coma. TSH levels are extremely elevated in myxedema coma due to primary thyroid disease. TSH may be low or normal if the hypothyroidism is due to central or pituitary dysfunction.

Treatment of myxedema with intravenous thyroid hormone should be initiated immediately. Supportive therapy may include passive warming to treat hypothermia, fluid resuscitation, and/or vasopressors for shock, positive pressure ventilator support for hypoventilation, IV glucose to treat and prevent hypoglycemia, and adrenal hormone replacement with glucocorticoids. When hypothyroidism is suspected, adrenal function should also be assessed because treatment for hypothyroidism can precipitate adrenal crisis and may warrant administration of doses of glucocorticoids while awaiting the results of the adrenal function studies (ACTH stimulation test and serum cortisol levels) (Fitzgerald, 2017). Refer to the "Nursing Care: The Patient with Hypothyroidism" feature for additional information.

In both hyperthyroidism and hypothyroidism, respiratory muscles are weakened, which can precipitate ventilatory failure, which is particularly pronounced in patients with underlying pulmonary diseases. Primary thyroid disorders (hyperthyroidism and hypothyroidism) are characterized by changes in both T3 and T4 levels. They are increased with hyperthyroidism and decreased with hypothyroidism, with reciprocal changes in the serum TSH levels (decreased in hyperthyroidism and increased in hypothyroidism). Table 32–5 compares characteristics of hyperthyroidism with hypothyroidism in critically ill patients.

Nonthyroid Illness Syndrome

Critically ill patients have stress-related changes in hormone balance. The most common thyroid disorder seen in the critically ill patient population is not due to dysfunction of the thyroid gland itself. In fact, severe illness (and stress) can cause abnormal thyroid findings in the absence of underlying thyroid disease from primary and secondary etiologies (Jameson et al., 2015; Van den Berghe, 2014). Nonthyroid-illness syndrome (NTIS), or *sick euthyroid syndrome*, is the most common form of thyroid dysfunction in the critically ill population and is a type of hypothyroidism. In NTIS, low serum concentrations of T3 or T4 coexist with normal TSH levels; this relationship is not reflected in either hypothyroidism or hyperthyroidism (Van den Berghe, 2014). A decline in T3 or T4 levels may be related to the inflammatory process, in which cytokines are released into the bloodstream, and to the consequences of hypoxemia that the high-acuity patient often experiences (Van den Berghe, 2014). The role of NTIS in the acute phase of critical illness can be attributed to fasting, resulting in a lack of macronutrients and subsequent poor nutrition; the body decreases T3 concentrations as a protective mechanism to prevent catabolism and reduce energy expenditure (Cuesta & Singer, 2012; Van den Berghe, 2014). However, after full nutritional support has been implemented and the patient remains critically ill past the acute phase of disease, thyroid function may be altered. In prolonged critical illness, elevated cortisol levels in the body can potentiate hypothyroidism in addition to a heightened response to low T3 levels by the peripheral tissues that increase the amount of thyroid hormone available. It remains controversial whether NTIS should be treated because of confounding factors, including drugs that suppress thyroid hormone production, the status of nutritional support, and the effects of critical illness on metabolism. High-quality evidence is limited; therefore, thyroid function should be assessed based on timing and duration of critical illness, as well as on baseline thyroid function (Van den Berghe, 2014).

The most common form of NTIS is characterized by a thyroid hormone pattern of decreased T3 levels with normal T4 and TSH levels; however, in severe critical illness, the T4 may drop significantly, which has been associated with a poor prognosis (Jameson et al., 2015). In critically ill patients, thyroid hormones may not bind well to receptors in the peripheral tissues, and the production of T3 in the peripheral tissues is suppressed by conditions common to the critical care setting (see Box 32–1). Furthermore, certain drug therapies are known to suppress thyroid hormone production. Critical illness can have numerous effects on thyroid tests, in some cases simulating thyroid disease when none is present and in other cases obscuring true thyroid disease (Economidou et al., 2011).

Nursing Care
The Patient with Hyperthyroidism

Expected Patient Outcomes and Related Interventions

Outcome 1: Early recognition of hyperthyroidism.

Assess and compare to established normal, patient baselines, and trends:
> Health history: other diseases, family history of thyroid disease, when manifestations began, severity of symptoms, intake of thyroid medications, menstrual history, changes in weight, bowel elimination patterns
> Physical assessment: muscle strength, tremors, vital signs, cardiovascular and peripheral vascular systems, integument, size of thyroid gland, presence of bruit over thyroid, eyes and vision

Outcome 2: Regain and maintain euthyroid state.

Administer related drug therapy and monitor for therapeutic and nontherapeutic effects.
> Antithyroid medications—methimazole (Tapazole), propylthiouracil (PTU), radioactive iodine therapy
> Beta-blocker medications—propranolol, atenolol, esmolol
> Glucocorticoid medications—hydrocortisone, dexamethasone, prednisone

Intervene to regain/maintain euthyroid state.
> Administer drugs at the same time each day.
> Monitor for signs and symptoms of hypothyroidism (fatigue, weight gain).

Outcome 3: Maintain normal cardiac output.

Assess and compare to established normal, patient baselines, and trends:
> Blood pressure, pulse rate and rhythm, respiratory rate, and breath sounds
> Monitor for peripheral edema, jugular vein distention, and increased activity intolerance.
> Monitor oxygenation status: hemoglobin and hematocrit, arterial blood gases, pulse oximetry, SvO_2 (mixed or central).

Implement interventions to optimize cardiac output and oxygenation.
> Keep ambient room temperature cool.
> Prevent stress by explaining interventions, relaxation to reduce stress, and oxygen demands.
> Assess for and manage pain.

Outcome 4: Maintain normal body temperature.

Assess and compare to established normal, patient baselines, and trends:
> Monitor temperature.

Implement interventions to normalize body temperature.
> Comfort measures as patient may be intolerant to heat.
> Offer fan to circulate the air.
> Reduce ambient room temperature.
> Utilize light bedclothes, coverings that are comfortable and nonrestrictive.
> Offer tepid sponge bath and cold-pack applications to groin and axilla.
> Use cooling blanket for fever greater than 102°F.

Administer antipyretic medications and monitor for therapeutic and nontherapeutic effects.
> Acetaminophen
> Ibuprofen

Outcome 4: Rehydrate and correct metabolic derangements.

Assess and compare to established normal, patient baselines, and trends:
> Temperature, heart rate, rhythm, diaphoresis, vomiting, and diarrhea
> Serum electrolyte levels (potassium, sodium, calcium, phosphorous)
> Kidney function—blood urea nitrogen (BUN), creatinine (Cr), potassium, hourly urine output

Implement interventions to optimize nutrition, fluids, and electrolyte balance.
> Replace fluids and electrolytes as indicated.
> Administer isotonic IV fluids as ordered.
> Monitor glucose.
> Provide nutrition support and early nutrition consult.
> Record daily weights.
> Monitor nutrient intake (calories, protein).
> Monitor serum protein nutrition indicators (e.g., serum albumin, prealbumin).

Administer medications as ordered to treat hyperglycemia.
> Insulin via continuous infusion or subcutaneous injection

Related Pharmacotherapy
The Patient with Hyperthyroid Crisis/Thyroid Storm

Beta-Adrenergic Blocking Agents
Propranolol (Inderal)

Action and Uses
Nonselective beta-adrenergic receptor antagonist. Blocks catecholamine receptor sites, reducing heart rate and cardiac contractility.

Dosages (Adult)
Initial Therapy: 1–3 mg/min initially; repeat every 2–5 min to desired HR or a total of 5 mg; after 5 mg is given, then additional drug should not be administered until 4 hours later to control tachycardia along with stress-dose glucocorticoids (see Corticosteroids below)

Adverse Effects
Most common: confusion, fatigue, drowsiness, bradycardia, shortness of breath or wheezing, paresthesia of hands, insomnia, nausea, vomiting, diarrhea, or constipation
Most severe: allergic reaction, Stevens-Johnson syndrome, exfoliative dermatitis, agranulocytosis

Nursing Implications

Monitor vital signs closely (especially blood pressure and heart rate).

Beta-adrenergic blocking agents contraindicated with respiratory diseases, such as asthma and COPD.

Assess BP and HR prior to each dose and contact provider if below established parameters.

Monitor for signs and symptoms of heart failure.

Corticosteroids

Hydrocortisone

Action and Uses

Reduces conversion of T4 to T3 and prevents adrenal insufficiency that commonly occurs because endogenous cortisol is rapidly metabolized during thyroid storm. See "Related Pharmacotherapy: Corticosteroid Treatment for Adrenal Insufficiency" feature for additional information.

Dosages (Adult)

100 mg hydrocortisone IV every 8 hours

Thyroid Hormone Suppressants

Propylthiouracil (PTU)

Methimazole (Tapazole)

SOURCE: Data from Fitzgerald (2017) and Wilson, Shannon, & Shields (2017).

Action and Uses

Suppression of thyroid hormone production

Dosages (Adult)

PTU: Initial dose of PTU is 200–300 mg PO every 4–6 hours, and then reduced gradually to a maintenance dose of 100–150 mg/day PO daily divided every 8–12 hours

Methimazole: 20–30 mg daily divided every 6–12 hours PO, and then reduced to a maintenance dose of 5–15 mg per day divided every 8–12 hours

Adverse Effects

Hypothyroid signs and symptoms (refer to Table 32–5)

Nursing Implications

PTU is generally preferred because it also blocks conversion of T4 to its biologically active form of T3 in the peripheral tissues.

Allergic reactions are more common with PTU compared with methimazole. PTU also can cause elevations in the WBC count.

Monitor closely for development of hypothyroid signs and symptoms.

BOX 32–1   Conditions That Suppress Production of T3 in the Peripheral Tissues

- Malnutrition
- Diabetes characterized by insulin resistance or relative insulin deficiency
- Release of circulating proinflammatory cytokines
- High levels of circulating free fatty acids from catabolism and muscle breakdown
- Chronic and prolonged illness
- Hepatic and renal failure
- Certain drugs, such as amiodarone, dopamine, dobutamine, beta blockers, corticosteroids
- Surgical procedures

SOURCE: Data from Economidou et al. (2011); Jameson et al., (2015).

Abnormal glucocorticoid levels seen in the critically ill can also impact thyroid hormone levels. Patients under severe physiological stress from trauma or infection have elevated cortisol levels because of endogenous elevations resulting from the stress response and due to glucocorticoid (steroid) therapy. Cortisol suppresses both TRH and TSH. It is common for these patients to have decreased levels of TSH, T3, and T4. In fact, during prolonged critical illness, stress-related alterations in the peripheral metabolism of thyroid hormones result in thyroid hormone imbalance associated with an early decrease in serum thyroid hormones consistent with NTIS.

Laboratory Assessment   Thyroid function tests can be difficult to interpret and therefore may not be diagnostic during critical illness. With NTIS, decreases in T3 levels occur within hours of the onset of illness. As illness severity increases, T4 levels decrease. With prolonged critical illness, the TSH levels also decline. Table 32–6 lists the variations seen with laboratory results in both primary thyroid disease (hyperthyroidism and hypothyroidism) and NTIS.

Treatment Considerations   Many healthcare professionals maintain that treatment to replace thyroid hormone in NTIS will only provide small benefits related to the patient's response to a pathological process without significant decrease in mortality (DeGroot, 2015). However, there are no randomized controlled trials available to contribute to the knowledge base for treatment recommendations for NTIS (Fliers, Bianco, Langouche, & Boelen, 2015; Van den Berghe, 2014). Treatment with thyroid hormone may vary from patient to patient as nutritional status, metabolic rate, and drug therapies are different with varying degrees of critical illness and disease processes (Fliers et al., 2015). Differences in opinion also exist because treatment in the form of thyroid hormone replacement in patients with NTIS is thought to be protective in that it reduces catabolism and metabolic energy requirements.

In summary, for patients without a prior diagnosis of thyroid disease in which there exists evidence of new or undiagnosed thyroid dysfunction, a full thyroid panel (TSH, free T3, T4) should be ordered to assess for primary thyroid dysfunction. Patients with known or preexisting hypothyroidism should continue to receive their usual dose of thyroid hormone and do not usually require dosage adjustment during serious illness. It is also appropriate to obtain an endocrine consultation to assist with treatment decisions and individualize the patient's plan of care.

Nursing Care

The Patient with Hypothyroidism

Expected Patient Outcomes and Related Interventions.

Outcome 1: Early diagnosis of hypothyroidism.

Assess and compare to established normal, patient baselines, and trends:

On all patients with known or suspected hypothyroid state, conduct:

Health history: pituitary or adrenal diseases, patient or family history of thyroid disease and treatment with medications or radioactive iodine, thyroid surgery, treatment of head or neck cancer with radiation, diet and intake of iodized salt, bowel elimination, depression, muscle or joint pain, cold intolerance, swelling, respiratory difficulties

Physical assessment: muscle strength, deep tendon reflexes, vital signs, cardiovascular and peripheral vascular systems, integument, thyroid gland, and weight

Outcome 2: Regain and maintain euthyroid state.

Assess and compare to established normal, patient baselines, and trends:

Serum thyroid-stimulating hormone (TSH) levels

Administer related drug therapy and monitor for therapeutic and nontherapeutic effects.

Levothyroxine (Synthroid)—thyroxine replacement medication

Outcome 3: Maintain stable hemodynamic and oxygenation parameters.

Assess and compare to established normal, patient baselines, and trends:

Blood pressure, pulse rate and rhythm, respiratory rate, and breath sounds. Monitor for widening pulse pressure.

Continuous ECG monitoring for signs of severe depression (flattened or inverted *T* waves, or prolonged *QT* or *PR* intervals) *or* ventricular arrhythmias

Monitor oxygenation status—hemoglobin and hematocrit, arterial blood gases, pulse oximetry, SvO₂ (mixed or central).

Monitor for respiratory failure.

Monitor for peripheral edema, jugular vein distention, and increased activity intolerance.

Echocardiogram may be needed to assess cardiac function and/or presence of pericardial effusion

Chest x-ray or ultrasound can be used to assess for pleural effusion

Implement interventions to optimize cardiac output and oxygenation.

Intervene to increase oxygen supply and decrease oxygen demand.

Administer sedatives and opiates with caution.

Administer intravenous fluids cautiously, observing for pleural effusion and heart failure.

Outcome 4: Maintain normal temperature.

Assess and compare to established normal, patient baselines, and trends:

Temperature

Intervene to normalize body temperature.

Keep room warm.

Warm patient passively, using blankets.

Assess body temperature continuously; avoid too rapid heating and vasodilation, which can cause hypotension.

Table 32–6   Laboratory Derangements in NTIS and Primary Thyroid Disease Compared

Type of Thyroid Condition	T3	T4	TSH
Nonthyroid-illness syndrome (NTIS)			
• Early critical illness	Decreased	Normal	Normal
• Prolonged critical illness greater than 72 hours	Decreased	Decreased	Decreased or normal
Primary thyroid disease (preexisting or not adequately treated)			
• Primary hyperthyroidism	Increased	Increased	Decreased
• Primary hypothyroidism	Decreased	Decreased	Increased

SOURCE: Data from Economidou et al. (2011) and Van den Berghe (2014).

Section Three Review

1. Where is TRH secreted, and what does it regulate?
   A. By the hypothalamus and regulates thyroid-stimulating hormone (TSH)
   B. By the pituitary and regulates growth hormone (GH)
   C. By the thyroid and regulates T₄ (thyroid hormone) level in the peripheral tissues
   D. By the adrenal gland and regulates cortisol secretion

2. Which description best fits the action of thyroid hormones?
   A. Suppresses cardiac contractility
   B. Inhibits anti-inflammatory process
   C. Regulates metabolic rate
   D. Enhances insulin resistance

3. Amiodarone is an anti-arrhythmic medication that can precipitate which response?
   A. Decreased proinflammatory cytokine release
   B. Increased T4 to T3 conversion in the thyroid gland
   C. Increased T3 to T4 conversion in the pituitary gland
   D. Decreased T4 to T3 conversion in the peripheral tissues

4. Hypothyroidism is characterized by which manifestation?
   A. Widened pulse pressure
   B. Bradycardia
   C. Atrial fibrillation
   D. Diarrhea

Answers: 1. A, 2. C, 3. D, 4. B

Section Four: Hyperglycemic Syndromes in the High-Acuity Patient

Hyperglycemia is common in diabetic and nondiabetic patients with critical illness. Approximately 75% of all patients have a blood glucose greater than 110 mg/dL at the time of admission, and up to 20% of patients have a blood glucose greater than 200 mg/dL (Hsu, 2012). Factors contributing to hyperglycemia are release of stress hormones (glucagon, epinephrine, cortisol, and TNF-α), medications (exogenous glucocorticoids, vasopressors, lithium, and beta blockers), overfeeding, intravenous dextrose and parenteral nutrition administration, immobility, increased insulin resistance (type 2 diabetes mellitus), deficient insulin secretion (type 1 diabetes mellitus) (Hsu, 2012).

Patients diagnosed with diabetes almost always need higher than usual levels of insulin to achieve glycemic control when they are sick. Even those without diabetes will experience a hypermetabolic state likely contributing to increased glucose production and insulin resistance (Hsu, 2012). Hyperglycemia in this setting is due to factors that can precipitate a cascade of physiological responses that place patients at risk for complications, particularly for infection (Ingels, Vanhorebeek, & Van den Berghe, 2017). It is important to maintain glycemic control in critically ill patients because sustained hyperglycemia has been linked to poor outcomes, especially increasing hospital mortality. This may be attributed to the impact of hyperglycemia on the immune response, which may be reduced, increasing the risk for the development of nosocomial infections while hospitalized (Ingels et al., 2017). This section provides a brief overview of hyperglycemic issues commonly associated with critical illness; however, Chapter 33 describes hyperglycemic syndromes in detail, including pathophysiology, collaborative management, and nursing care, as well as intensive insulin therapy.

Normal fasting blood glucose is between 80 and 110 mg/dL and does not increase to more than 200 mg/dL even with large amounts of glucose in the bloodstream when there is normal uptake of glucose at the tissue level and subsequent normal insulin production (Ingels et al., 2017). A known cause of hyperglycemia includes the release of circulating hormones and inflammatory mediators, which increases glucose production. Glycogenolysis, combined with increased insulin resistance in the periphery, creates a situation where the insulin-producing pancreatic beta cells cannot keep up with insulin demand, resulting in hyperglycemia. Figure 32–3 illustrates the effects of stress on glucose and potential sequelae.

Several factors contribute to hyperglycemia during critical illness. First, increased endogenous stress hormone (cortisol) is produced from an exaggerated and often prolonged stress response and glucocorticoid therapy. Second, proinflammatory mediators/cytokines are released by the endothelial system in response to stress, infection, trauma, and/or iatrogenic causes common to critically ill populations (mechanical ventilation, invasive devices). Third, overfeeding during critical illness along with the effects of immobility (inflammation, vasodilatation, decreased cardiac output) also contribute to hyperglycemia. Hyperglycemia places the patient at increased risk for poor wound healing, especially in patients with diagnosed diabetes or who are immunocompromised from chronic illness. Hyperglycemia also impairs immune response to infection, increases inflammation, and precipitates endothelial dysfunction, all leading to increased risk for illness and death. Contributing factors to hypoglycemia are severe sepsis, trauma/surgery, diabetes mellitus (DM), prior insulin or glucocorticoid treatment, heart failure, and intensive insulin therapy (Finfer et al., 2012).

Hyperglycemia, Hypoglycemia, Glycemic Variability, and Patient Outcomes: The Evidence

Severe hyperglycemia is a marker of illness severity, rather than a direct cause of poor outcome (Marik & Bellomo, 2013) and may subside after the acute or critical injury or illness has resolved (Dungan, Braithwaite & Preiser, 2009; Van den Berghe, 2014). In acute or critical injury or illness, hyperglycemia occurs as a result of insufficient insulin secretion to overcome the hyperglycemic effect of catecholamine release during stress (Harp, Yancopoulos, & Gromada, 2016). Insulin resistance may also contribute to hyperglycemia in patients with chronic disease–associated end-organ tissue injury (Dungan et al., 2009; Harp et al., 2016). For example, patients with preexisting DM often have persistent hyperglycemia that is due to insulin resistance (type 2 diabetes mellitus) or insulin absence (type 1 diabetes mellitus), and hyperglucagonemia because of the disease process itself, which results in stress-induced hyperglycemia that can be more severe in diabetic patients (type 1 or type 2) than in nondiabetic patients, and more likely to require control with insulin and strict glucose monitoring (Harp et al., 2016).

Hyperglycemia and glycemic variability have been noted to be independent predictors of mortality in critically ill patients (Finney, Zekveld, Elia, & Evans, 2003;

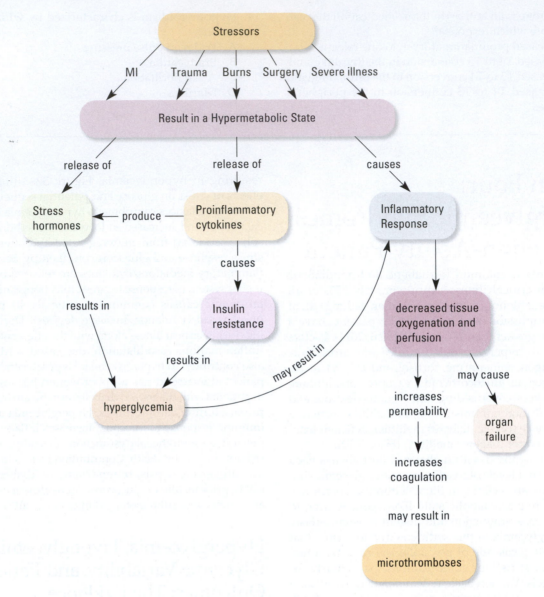

Figure 32–3 Hyperglycemia during critical illness.

Krinsley, 2008; Marik & Bellomo, 2013; Norhammar, Ryden, & Malinberg, 1999). The effect of hyperglycemia on the immune response includes decreased functioning and availability of neutrophils, altered macrophage phagocytosis, and reduced opsonization (targeting) of bacteria (Hsu, 2012; Ingels et al., 2017; Van den Berghe, 2014). Hyperglycemia can also potentiate the body's inflammatory response, which can lead to various complications of critical illness. It is not clear whether measures to control hyperglycemia improve patient outcomes, and which patient populations benefit from these measures. Early studies of "tight" intensive glucose control (serum glucose between 80 and 110 mg/dL) suggested a decreased risk for mortality but lead to higher rates of hypoglycemia. Tight glycemic control with a blood glucose level less than 140 mg/dL positively correlated with reduced hospital length of stay, decreased ventilator days, and a lower rate of intensive care–related mortality (Hsu, 2012). There also has been evidence to suggest that tight glycemic control has no influence on mechanical ventilation use, vasopressor use, renal replacement therapies, and the need for blood

transfusions (Hsu, 2012). The results of the Van den Berghe studies influenced the introduction of intensive insulin therapy based on algorithms and protocols as the standard of care for hyperglycemia management for the high-acuity patient. The goal was to improve one of the primary adverse events of tight blood glucose control: hypoglycemia.

The Normoglycemia in Intensive Care Evaluation–Survival Using Glucose Algorithm Regulation (NICE-SUGAR) trial was a large (6,014 critically ill patients) randomized prospective trial in which the intensive glucose protocol was compared directly with a less restrictive conventional protocol (serum glucose less than or equal to 180 mg/dL) (Finfer et al., 2009). The trial found a higher risk of death (increased mortality at 90 days of 2.6 %) with the intensive glucose control group and a higher incidence of hypoglycemia as well (Finfer et al., 2009). Hypoglycemia is an unintended consequence and can have negative effects on mental status and in severe cases lead to death. In diabetic patients, particularly those with persistent hyperglycemia, significantly lowering glucose levels and strict glycemic control may lead to symptomatic and life-threatening hypoglycemia and glycemic variability (Marik & Egi, 2014).

In patients with persistent hyperglycemia, aggressive lowering of serum glucose with strict glycemic control may cause symptomatic and life-threatening hypoglycemia and glycemic variability (Marik & Egi, 2014). Glycemic variability, defined as acute glycemic fluctuations between hyperglycemia and hypoglycemia, is associated with increased oxidative stress that can contribute to endothelial dysfunction and vascular damage (Marik & Egi, 2014; Monnier, Colette, & Owens, 2008). Glycemic variability is associated with an increased risk of mortality in critically ill patients (Krinsley, 2008; Krinsley, 2009), with an increased risk by 25.7% in critically ill nondiabetic patients. Monnier, Colette, and Owens (2008) propose a range of 40 mcg/dL as the acceptable glycemic variability range in critically ill patients; however, consensus on this range has not yet been fully established.

On the other hand, hypoglycemia is also very dangerous for both diabetic and nondiabetic critically ill patients. Evidence suggests that hypoglycemia is associated with an increased risk of cardiovascular mortality among both diabetic and nondiabetic patients in critical care (Kalfon et al., 2015; Robinson, Harris, Ireland, Macdonald, & Heller, 2004; Saisho, 2014; Svensson, McGuire, Abrahamsson, & Dellborg, 2005). Further studies are needed to determine the effects of glycemic variability on outcomes in the critically ill patient population.

Given the theoretical and research findings to date, critical care providers have a greater appreciation for intensive insulin protocols and a recognition that the risks associated with their use in patients with hypoglycemia outweigh the benefits of tight glucose control in critically ill patients. More liberal glucose control than originally thought is the current trend as evidenced by multiple clinical practice guidelines (American Diabetes Association [ADA], 2015; Society of Critical Care Medicine [SCCM], 2012). Therefore, evidence supports that in critically ill patients, insulin therapy should be initiated for persistent hyperglycemia, starting at a blood glucose level of no greater than 180 mg/dL. Maintaining a blood glucose range of 140 to 180 mg/dL is recommended (ADA, 2012; SCCM, 2012). Intravenous insulin continuous infusions are most effective at achieving and maintaining glycemic control. During the intravenous insulin therapy, frequent monitoring (hourly) of blood glucose and early interventions are necessary to minimize and treat hypoglycemia and, thus, achieve optimal glucose control. More research is needed to further explore glycemic variability in conjunction with the use of moderately intensive anti-hyperglycemia protocols and the specific benefits.

Prevention of Insulin-induced Hypoglycemia

Administration of insulin "drips" or continuous infusions requires astute nursing supervision and monitoring to achieve blood glucose targets and to minimize life-threatening hypoglycemia. Hourly blood glucose measurement is typically done using a handheld device that tests a drop of blood obtained by fingerstick. There should also be serial measurements of blood glucose obtained via venipuncture as results from different types of blood sampling and glucose measurement methods may yield slightly different results. At a minimum, a patient on an insulin drip should have serum glucose measurements via venipuncture every 12 hours (SCCM, 2012). The institutional protocol for blood sampling, insulin infusion, and glucose management targets should be followed to achieve consistency and minimize the risk of adverse events.

Interruption of nutrition due to occlusion or inadvertent removal of feeding tubes or invasive lines, prolonged NPO status, and less-than-adequate point-of-care blood glucose testing during insulin administration may precipitate hypoglycemia. It is important to administer a source of glucose (10% dextrose) in the event of an interruption of nutrition or glucose intake to prevent hypoglycemia.

To treat hyperglycemia and decrease the risk of hypoglycemia after initial stabilization, recent international guidelines from the SCCM (2012) and the Surviving Sepsis Campaign (Professional Practice Committee for the Standards of Medical Care in Diabetes, 2016; Rhodes et al., 2017) recommend the following:

1. Following initial stabilization, hyperglycemia should be treated with IV insulin.

2. A valid evidence-based protocol should be used to treat hyperglycemia, with a suggested target blood glucose range between 140 and 180 mg/dL.

3. All patients receiving IV insulin must receive a glucose calorie source and must have blood glucose monitoring every 1 to 2 hours until levels are stable, then every 4 hours (assuming that nutrition is not interrupted, in which case blood glucose testing should revert back to hourly).

4. Hypoglycemia from capillary blood (fingerstick) point-of-care testing should be confirmed with a full blood or plasma sample.

When transitioning patients from an insulin drip to subcutaneous insulin, the first dose of long-acting insulin (usually NPH insulin, twice daily) should be given at least 2 hours prior to discontinuation of the infusion. The total daily dose of long-acting NPH insulin (divided into two daily doses) should be half the total insulin dose administered intravenously over the preceding 24 hours. The remainder of the insulin requirement is provided using a sliding scale of regular or fast-acting insulin (Schnipper, 2017).

Hyperglycemic Syndromes: Collaborative Management

Life-threatening hyperglycemic syndromes include diabetic ketoacidosis (DKA) and hyperglycemic hyperosmolar state (HHS). Clinical manifestations result from hyperglycemia in both syndromes and from excess ketone production in DKA. Hyperglycemia causes hyperosmolality, osmotic diuresis, fluid and electrolyte loss/imbalance, and dehydration, resulting in intravascular volume depletion. DKA is characterized by metabolic acidosis with a high anion gap secondary to volume depletion. An elevated serum sodium concentration suggests severe dehydration

Emerging Evidence

- Thyrotoxicosis, or thyroid storm, has high morbidity and mortality; it is a life-threatening endocrine emergency. Treatment often involves pharmacotherapies such as methimazole, PTU, and radioactive iodine therapies to decrease circulating thyroid hormone. A euthyroid state is the goal prior to thyroidectomy. Thyroid arterial embolization may be considered for treatment of patients who are refractory to medical therapies and/or not a surgical candidate due to hemodynamic compromise or significant comorbidity. It is viewed as a bridge to thyroidectomy once the patient is more stable. Thyroid arterial embolization involves induction of atrophy of the thyroid gland without further potentiation of thyroid storm *(Rohr, Kovaleski, Hill, & Johnson, 2016)*.

- Stress-induced hyperglycemia is glucose intolerance that often presents during the acute phase of illness. The risk for the development of type II diabetes after survival from a critical illness is increased if a patient suffers from stress-induced hyperglycemia (without concomitant diabetes). In a study of 17,074 patients without diabetes admitted to the ICU, 821 or 4.8% went on to develop type II diabetes following critical illness; this was approximately double the risk of those patients who did not experience hyperglycemia during critical illness within the first 24 hours after admission *(Plummer et al., 2016)*.

- In recent years, research has found that cortisol metabolism is decreased during critical illness, which explains why serum cortisol levels are elevated in the high-acuity patient. In a randomized controlled trial of 4640 critically ill patients, those who received early parenteral nutrition (PN) were compared to those who received late parenteral nutrition. It was found that early PN did not impact serum ACTH levels any differently than it would affect those levels in healthy subjects. Thus, it is possible that fasting and reduced macronutrient caloric intake may not be responsible for activation of the hypothalamic–pituitary–adrenal (HPA) axis. In addition, early PN may be responsible for the increased number of patients with septic shock and may be harmful to patients in sepsis or severe sepsis; corticosteroid administration may increase the progression of their critical illness *(Meersseman et al., 2015)*.

in either condition. Both syndromes are associated with serum potassium deficit or excess, hypophosphatemia, and hypomagnesemia. After an initial assessment of the patient's mental and volume status, laboratory studies should be obtained to assess CBC, electrolytes, renal function, blood glucose, serum ketones, and arterial blood gas. Also, cultures should be obtained to determine source of infection that may have caused the hyperglycemic state.

The treatment goals for hyperglycemic syndromes are as follows (ADA, 2015; SCCM, 2012; Schnipper, 2017):

1. Restore fluid and electrolyte balance.
2. Provide IV insulin.
3. Replace glucose once blood levels are lower than 250 mg/dL.
4. Identify causative factors.

Section Four Review

1. Which finding suggests severe dehydration in a client with diabetic ketoacidosis (DKA)?
   A. Elevated serum glucose
   B. Decreased capillary sample glucose
   C. Elevated serum sodium
   D. Elevated serum magnesium

2. Hyperglycemia in critical illness results from which conditions? (Select all that apply.)
   A. Insulin resistance
   B. Increased cortisol production
   C. Inability to take oral nutrition
   D. Increase in inflammatory mediators
   E. Immobility

3. Insulin therapy should be initiated for which persistent blood glucose levels?
   A. No greater than 200 mg/dL
   B. Less than 200 mg/dL
   C. No greater than 180 mg/dL
   D. Less than 180 mg/dL

4. Which management strategy is appropriate in clients with hyperglycemic syndrome (DKA or HHS)?
   A. Restore electrolyte balance.
   B. Measure blood glucose levels every 12 hours.
   C. Restrict all fluids.
   D. Administer SQ insulin before consideration of IV insulin.

Answers: 1. C, 2. (A, B, D, E), 3. C, 4. A

Critical Reasoning Checkpoint

QP, a 74-year-old Caucasian female, presents to a local emergency department with a 2-day history of worsening shortness of breath, increasing weakness, and swelling of her lower extremities and face. She is drowsy, answering questions with short phrases. She denies pain but appears to be having difficulty breathing. She denies increased sputum production, cough, nausea, vomiting, or diarrhea but does admit to having a decreased appetite. Her husband reports that she has been increasingly bedridden for the past month, walking only between bed, couch, and bathroom, and has become unable to stand today. He also reports that her face and legs began to swell yesterday, becoming much worse today. He also says that she has become incontinent and confused. The husband states that she has been responsible for managing her own medications but seems to be forgetting to take them regularly.

Past Medical History: Hypertension, hyperlipidemia, coronary artery disease, type II diabetes, and hypothyroidism.

Home Medications: Synthroid, metformin, hydrochlorothiazide, Lipitor, and aspirin.

Current Assessment: BP 89/60, HR 50–60 with sinus bradycardia showing on the cardiac monitor, RR 20 breaths per minute, temp 96°F, SpO_2 ranges from 82%–94%. Patient is increasingly lethargic and more difficult to arouse. Pupils are equal and reactive to light, mucous membranes are pale and dry, significant peri-orbital edema makes it difficult for her to open her eyes, her skin is extremely dry, pale, and cool to touch; her hair is thin; neck is supple without stiffness; no jugular venous distention or thyroid enlargement is noted. Lung sounds are diminished at bases, and she has occasional expiratory wheezing, no crackles.

Laboratory and Diagnostic Study Results

Test	Results
ABG	ph 7.29, PCO_2 68, PaO_2 65, SaO_2 84% while wearing 100% FiO_2 non-rebreathing mask
Serum glucose	Normal
Serum electrolytes	Serum sodium 122 mg/dL; others are normal
Serum BUN and creatinine	Normal
CBC	WBC: 12,000; hemoglobin and hematocrit levels normal; platelets normal
Cardiac markers	Normal
Chest radiograph	Clear of infiltrates or evidence of pulmonary edema
Thyroid panel	Serum TSH is elevated at 66 mg/dL; serum thyroid hormone levels are decreased (Free T3 is 0.56 mg/dL, and T4 is 0.56 mg/dL.)

1. Based on QP's medical history, clinical presentation, and test results, what type of endocrine problem could she be experiencing? Based on which data?

2. Based on her history, what might have precipitated this acute event?

3. How will this acute crisis be immediately treated?

Chapter 32 Review

1. A client was severely injured 4 days ago. Which findings would the nurse interpret as meaning the compensatory response of the hypothalamic–pituitary–adrenal (HPA) axis is no longer adequate? (Select all that apply.)
   1. Corticotropin levels begin to elevate.
   2. Growth hormone levels decrease.
   3. Adrenal dysfunction occurs.
   4. Serum glucose is elevated.
   5. Serum sodium is elevated.

2. The nurse would evaluate that slight hypothermia, increased blood glucose, and increased lactate levels would be expected findings in which clients? (Select all that apply.)
   1. A 75-year-old man who had a massive myocardial infarction 16 hours ago
   2. A 24-year-old woman who sustained full thickness burns over 30% of her body 12 hours ago
   3. An 18-year-old man with a traumatic brain injury that occurred 5 hours ago and whose first Glasgow Coma Scale was 8
   4. A 30-year-old who was just admitted with a stab wound to the abdomen
   5. A 56-year-old woman admitted a week ago with gastrointestinal bleeding

3. A rapid ACTH stimulation test done on a client this morning reveals a low response, and a plasma ACTH level has been drawn. What response will the nurse evaluate as supporting a presumed diagnosis of primary adrenal insufficiency?
   1. Elevation of ACTH level
   2. Normal ACTH level
   3. ACTH level below that of the ACTH stimulation test result
   4. ACTH level equal to that of the ACTH stimulation test result

4. A client has been receiving hydrocortisone 50 mg IV every 6 hours for the last 12 days. An order to begin tapering the dose by administering the same dose every 8 hours for the next 3 days has been written. The nurse would question this order if which condition exists?
   1. The client has a documented infection.
   2. The client is receiving vasopressors.
   3. The client's blood glucose has been decreasing for the last 2 days.
   4. The client has weakness in the left arm and hand.

5. A severely ill client has developed hyperthyroidism. Which nursing interventions are indicated? (Select all that apply.)
   1. Keep the room temperature warm.
   2. Have visitors talk with the client to maintain stimulation.
   3. Untuck sheets from the foot of the bed.
   4. Monitor isotonic IV fluid administration.
   5. Offer frequent high-carbohydrate snacks.

6. A client with long-standing hypothyroidism has been admitted with a diagnosis of pneumonia. The nurse would immediately contact the primary health care provider if which condition occurs?

   1. The client's temperature elevates to 38.7°C (101.6°F).
   2. The client does not recognize a visiting grandchild.
   3. The client's blood pressure is 140/98 mmHg.
   4. The client refuses to eat lunch due to nausea.

7. A client with long-standing thyroid deficiency has been hospitalized following a motorcycle crash. How would the nurse anticipate providing thyroid support for this client?

   1. The oral dose of thyroid medication will be increased.
   2. Thyroid medication will be discontinued until traumatic brain injury is ruled out.
   3. The client's normal dose of thyroid medication will be maintained.
   4. Thyroid medication will be changed to a parenteral form.

8. A nurse discovers that the tube delivering a client's gastric feeding is disconnected and leaking on the bed. The client is receiving a continuous insulin infusion, and the last blood glucose, done 1 hour ago, was 150 mg/dL. What should be the nurse's priority intervention?

   1. Report the finding to the primary care provider.
   2. Check the gastric tube for occlusion.
   3. Do a fingerstick blood glucose.
   4. Provide hygiene care, a clean gown, and dry sheets.

9. A client who is receiving an insulin drip has a fingerstick blood glucose reading of 142 mg/dL. The client's skin is cool and moist, heart rate is 110 and irregular, and the client is restless. What is the nurse's priority intervention?

   1. Contact the primary health care provider.
   2. Administer 10% glucose IV.
   3. Call for a venipuncture blood glucose measurement.
   4. Increase the rate of the insulin drip.

10. A severely ill client is diagnosed with diabetic ketoacidosis (DKA) after being hospitalized for 3 days. Which laboratory results would the nurse evaluate as commonly occurring in clients with this diagnosis? (Select all that apply.)

    1. Hypernatremia
    2. Hypokalemia
    3. Hyperphosphatemia
    4. Hypermagnesemia
    5. Hyperosmolality

Answers to questions found inside your textbook are available on the faculty resources site. Please consult with your instructor.

References

American Diabetes Association (ADA). (2015). Standards of medical care in diabetes—2015. *Diabetes Care, 38*(Suppl 1), S4–S63.

Bauer, D., & McPhee, S. J. (2013). Thyroid disease. In G. D. Hammer & S. J. McPhee (Eds.), *Pathophysiology of disease: An introduction to clinical medicine* (7th ed., pp. 549–570). New York, NY: McGraw Hill Medical. Retrieved March 15, 2017, from http://accessmedicine.mhmedical.com.ezproxy.uky.edu/content.aspx?bookid=961&sectionid=53555701

Bosmann, M., & Ward, P. A. (2013). The inflammatory response in sepsis. *Trends in Immunology, 34*, 129–136.

Carroll, T. B., Aron, D. C., Findling, J. W., & Tyrrell, B. (2011). Glucocorticoids and adrenal androgens. In D. G. Gardner & D. Shoback (Eds.), *Greenspan's basic & clinical endocrinology* (9th ed.). Retrieved February 3, 2013, from http://www.accessmedicine.com/content.aspx?aID=8403322

Cuesta, J. M., & Singer, M. (2012). The stress response and critical illness: A review. *Critical Care Medicine, 40*, 3283–3289.

Cuthbertson, D. P. (1979). Second annual Jonathan E. Rhoads lecture. The metabolic response to injury and its nutritional implications: Retrospect and prospect. *Journal of Parenteral and Enteral Nutrition, 3*, 108–129.

DeGroot, L. (2015). The non-thyroidal illness syndrome. In L. J. De Groot, G. Chrousos, K. Dungan, K. R. Feingold, A. Grossman, J. Hershman, . . . A. Vinik (Eds.), *Endotext* [Internet]. South Dartmouth, MA. Retrieved June 3, 2017, from: https://www.ncbi.nlm.nih.gov/books/NBK285570

Dungan, K. M., Braithwaite, S. S., & Preiser, J. C. (2009). Stress hyperglycemia. *Lancet, 373*, 1798–1807. doi:10.1016/S0140-6736(09)60553-5

Economidou, F., Douka, E., Tzanela, M., Nanas, S., & Kotanidou, A. (2011). Thyroid function during critical illness. *Hormones, 10*(2), 117–124.

Else, T., Hammer, G. D., & McPhee, S. J. (2014). Chapter 21: Disorders of the adrenal cortex. In G. D. Hammer & S. J. McPhee (Eds.), *Pathophysiology of disease: An introduction to clinical medicine* (7th ed., pp. 571–583). New York, NY: McGraw Hill Medical. Retrieved March 15, 2017, from http://accessmedicine.mhmedical.com.ezproxy.uky.edu/content.aspx?bookid=961&sectionid=53555702

Finfer, S., Chittock, D. R., Su, S. Y., Blair, D., Foster, D., Dhingra, V., . . . Ronco, J. J. (2009). NICE-SUGAR study. *New England Journal of Medicine, 360*(13), 1283–1297.

Finney, S. J., Zekveld, G., Elia, A., & Evans, T. W. (2003). Glucose control and mortality in critically ill patients. *JAMA, 290*(15), 2041–2047.

Fitzgerald, P. A. (2017). Endocrine disorders. In M. A. Papadakis, S. J. McPhee, & M. W. Rabow (Eds.), *CURRENT medical diagnosis & treatment 2017.* New York, NY: McGraw-Hill. Retrieved March 15, 2017, from http://accessmedicine.mhmedical.com.ezproxy.uky.edu/content.aspx?bookid=1843&sectionid=135718249

Fliers, E., Bianco, A., Langouche, L., & Boelen, A. (2015). Thyroid function in critically ill patients. *The Lancet. Diabetes & Endocrinology, 3*(10), 816–825. doi:10.1016/S2213-8587(15)00225-9

Funk, J. L. (2014). Disorders of the endocrine pancreas. In G. D. Hammer & S. J. McPhee (Eds.), *Pathophysiology of disease: An introduction to clinical medicine* (7th ed., pp. 497–522). New York, NY: McGraw Hill Medical. Retrieved March 15, 2017, from http://accessmedicine.mhmedical.com.ezproxy.uky.edu/content.aspx?bookid=961&sectionid=53555699

Graves, K. K., Faraklas, I., & Cochran, A. (2012). Identification of risk factors associated with critical illness related corticosteroid insufficiency in burn patients. *Journal of Burn Care & Research, 33*(3), 330–335.

Hall, J. E. (2016). Chapter 61: The autonomic nervous system and the adrenal medulla. In J. E. Hall (Ed.), *Guyton and Hall textbook of medical physiology* (13th ed.), pp. 773-794. Philadelphia, PA: Elsevier.

Harp, J. B., Yancopoulos, G. D., & Gromada, J. (2016). Glucagon orchestrates stress induced hyperglycaemia. *Diabetes Obesity and Metabolism, 18*, 648–653. doi:10.1111/dom.12668

Hsu, C. (2012). Glycemic control in critically ill patients. *World Journal of Critical Care Medicine, 1*(1), 31–39. doi:10.5492/wjccm.v1.i1.31

Idrose, A. M. (2016). Chapter 229: Hypothyroidism and Chapter 230: Hyperthyroidism. In J. E. Tintinalli, J. Stapczynski, O. Ma, D. M. Yealy, G. D. Meckler, & D. M. Cline (Eds.), *Tintinalli's emergency medicine: A comprehensive study guide* (8th ed.). New York, NY: McGraw-Hill. Retrieved March 15, 2017, from http://accessmedicine.mhmedical.com.ezproxy.uky.edu/content.aspx?bookid=1658&sectionid=109444027

Ingels, C., Vanhorebeek, I., & Van den Berghe, G. (2017). Glucose homeostasis, nutrition and infections during critical illness. *Clinical Microbiology & Infection,* 1–6. doi:10.1016/j.cmi.2016.12.033

Jameson, J., Mandel, S. J., & Weetman, A. P. (2015). Disorders of the thyroid gland. In D. Kasper, A. Fauci, S. Hauser, D. Longo, J. Jameson, & J. Loscalzo (Eds.), *Harrison's principles of internal medicine* (19th ed.). New York, NY: McGraw-Hill. Retrieved March 15, 2017, from http://accessmedicine.mhmedical.com.ezproxy.uky.edu/content.aspx?bookid=1130&sectionid=79751787

Kalfon, P., Le Manach, Y., Ichai, C., Bréchot, N., Cinotti, R., Dequin, P. F., . . . Riou, B. (2015). Severe and multiple hypoglycemic episodes are associated with increased risk of death in ICU patients. *Critical Care, 19*, 153. doi:10.1186/s13054-015-0851-7

Kee, J. L. (2014). *Laboratory and diagnostic tests with nursing implications* (9th ed.). Upper Saddle River, NJ: Pearson Prentice Hall.

Klubo-Gwiezdzinska, J., & Wartofsky, L. (2012). Thyroid disorders and diseases: Thyroid emergencies. *Medical Clinics of North America, 96*(2), 385–403.

Krinsley, J. S. (2008). Glycemic variability is a strong predictor of mortality in critically ill patients. *Critical Care Medicine, 36*(11), 3008–3013. doi:10.1097/CCM.0b013e31818b38d2

Krinsley, J. S. (2009). Glycemic variability and mortality in critically ill patients: The impact of diabetes. *Journal of Diabetes Science and Technology, 3*(6), 1292–1301.

Leung, A. (2016). Thyroid emergencies. *The Art and Science of Infusion Nursing, 39*(5), 281–286. doi:10.1097/NAN.0000000000000186

Little, R. A., & Girolami, A. (1999). Trauma metabolism—ebb and flow revisited. *British Journal of Intensive Care, 9*, 142–146.

Long, R. K., & Cakmak, H. (2015). Hypothalamic & pituitary hormones. In B. G. Katzung & A. J. Trevor (Eds.), *Basic & clinical pharmacology* (13th ed.). New York, NY: McGraw-Hill. Retrieved March 15, 2017, from http://accessmedicine.mhmedical.com.ezproxy.uky.edu/content.aspx?bookid=1193&sectionid=69109543

Marik, P. E., & Bellomo, R. (2013). Stress hyperglycemia: An essential survival response! *Critical Care Medicine, 17*(2), 305.

Marik, P. E., & Egi, M. (2014). Treatment thresholds for hyperglycemia in critically ill patients. *Intensive Care Medicine, 40*(7), 1049–1051. doi:10.1007/s00134-014-3344-2

Marino, P. L. (2014). Chapter 50: Adrenal and thyroid dysfunction. In P. L. Marino (Ed.) *Marino's The ICU Book* (4th ed., pp. 887–897). Philadelphia, PA: Wolters Kluwer Health/ Lippincott Williams & Wilkins.

Marín-Peñalver, J. J., Martín-Timón, I., & del Cañizo-Gómez, F. J. (2016). Management of hospitalized type two diabetes mellitus patients. *Journal of Translational Internal Medicine, 4*(4), 155–161. doi:10.1515/jtim-2016-0027

McClave, S., Taylor, B., Martindale, R., Warren, M., Johnson, D., Braunschweig, C. . . . Society of Critical Care Medicine and the American Society for Parenteral and Enteral Nutrition. (2016). Guidelines for the provision and assessment of nutrition support therapy in the adult critically ill patient. *Journal of Parenteral and Enteral Nutrition, 40*(2), 159–211. doi:10.1177/0148607115621863

Meersseman, P., Boonen, E., Peeters, B., Vander Perre, S., Wouters, P., Langouche, L., & Van den Berghe, G. (2015): Effect of early parenteral nutrition on the HPA axis and on treatment with corticosteroids in intensive care patients. *The Journal of Clinical Endocrinology and Metabolism, 100*(7), 2613–2620. doi:10.1210/jc.2016-1846

Monnier, L., Colette, C., & Owens, D. R. (2008). Glycemic variability: The third component of the dysglycemia in diabetes. Is it important? How to measure it? *Journal of Diabetes Science and Technology, 2*(6), 1094–1100. doi:10.1177/193229680800200618

Nicoll, D., Mark Lu, C., & McPhee, S. J. (2017). Lab tests. In D. Nicoll, C. Mark Lu, & S. J. McPhee (Eds.), *Guide to diagnostic tests* (7th ed.). New York, NY: McGraw-Hill. Retrieved March 15, 2017, from http://accessmedicine.mhmedical.com.ezproxy.uky.edu/content.aspx?bookid=2032&sectionid=152254910

Norhammar, A. M., Ryden, L., & Malinberg, K. (1999). Admission plasma glucose: Independent risk factor for long-term prognosis after myocardial infarction even in non-diabetic patients. *Diabetes Care, 22*(11), 1827–1831.

Plummer, M., Finnis, M., Phillips, L., Kar, P., Bihari, S., Biradar, V., . . . Deane, A. (2016). Stress induced hyperglycemia and the subsequent risk of type 2 diabetes in survivors of critical illness. *Public Library of Science, 11*(11), e0165923. doi:10.1371/journal.pone.0165923

Preiser, J. C., Ichai, C., Orban J. C., & Groeneveld, A. B. J. (2014). Metabolic response to the stress of critical illness. *British Journal of Anaesthesia, 113*, 945–954.

Professional Practice Committee *for the Standards of Medical Care in Diabetes—2016*. (2016). *Diabetes Care, 39*(Suppl 1), S107–S108. doi:10.2337/dc16-S018

Puar, T., Stikkelbroeck, M., Smans, L., Zelissen, P., & Hermus, R. (2016). Adrenal crisis: Still a deadly event in the 21st century. *The American Journal of Medicine, 129*(3), 339.e1–339.e9. doi:10.1016/j.amjmed.2015.08.021

Rhodes, A., Evans, L. E., Alhazzani, W., Levy, M. M., Antonelli, M., Ferrer, R., . . . Dellinger, R. P. (2017). Surviving sepsis campaign: International guidelines for management of sepsis and septic shock: 2016. *Intensive Care Medicine, 43*(3), 304–377. doi:10.1007/s00134-017-4683-6

Robinson, R. T., Harris, N. D., Ireland, R. H., Macdonald, I. A., & Heller, S. R. (2004). Changes in cardiac repolarization during clinical episodes of nocturnal hypoglycaemia in adults with Type 1 diabetes. *Diabetologia, 47*(2), 312–315. doi:10.1007/s00125-003-1292-4

Rohr, A., Kovaleski, A., Hill, J., & Johnson, P. (2016). Thyroid embolization as an adjunctive therapy in a patient with thyroid storm. *Journal of Vascular and Interventional Radiology, 27*(3), 449–451. doi:10.1016/j.jvir.2015.11.037

Rosenthal, M. D., & Moore, F. A (2015). Persistent inflammatory, immunosuppressed, catabolic syndrome (PICS): A new phenotype of multiple organ failure. *Journal of Advanced Nutrition and Human Metabolism, 1*, e784.

Saisho, Y. (2014). Glycemic variability and oxidative stress: A link between diabetes and cardiovascular disease? *International Journal of Molecular Science, 15*, 18381–18406.doi:10.3390/ijms151018381

Schimmer, B. P., & Funder, J. W. (2011). ACTH, adrenal steroids, and pharmacology of the adrenal cortex. In L. L. Brunton, B. A. Chabner, & B. C. Knollmann (Eds.), *Goodman & Gilman's the pharmacological basis of therapeutics* (12th ed.). Retrieved February 1, 2013, from http://accessmedicine.mhmedical.com.ezproxy.uky.edu/content.aspx?bookid=1613&sectionid=102162158.

Schnipper, J. L. (2017). Inpatient management of diabetes and hyperglycemia. In S. C. McKean, J. J. Ross, D. D. Dressler, & D. B. Scheurer (Eds.), *Principles and practice of hospital medicine* (2nd ed.). New York, NY: McGraw-Hill. Retrieved March 15, 2017, from http://accessmedicine.mhmedical.com.ezproxy.uky.edu/content.aspx?bookid=1872&sectionid=146981442

Society of Critical Care Medicine (SCCM). (2012). SCCM guidelines for the use of an insulin infusion for the management of hyperglycemia in critically ill patients. *Critical Care Medicine, 40*(12), 3251–3276.

Svensson, A. M., McGuire, D. K., Abrahamsson, P., & Dellborg, M. (2005). Association between hyper- and hypoglycaemia and 2 year all-cause mortality risk in diabetic patients with acute coronary events. *European Heart Journal, 26*, 1255–1261. doi:10.1093/eurheartj/ehi230

Van den Berghe, G. (2014). Non-thyroidal illness in the ICU: A syndrome with different faces. *Thyroid, 24*(10), 1456–1465. doi:10.1089/thy.2014.0201

Van den Berghe, G. (2017). The 2016 ESPEN Sir David Cuthbertson lecture: Interfering with neuroendocrine and metabolic responses to critical illness: From acute to long-term consequences. *Clinical Nutrition, 36*(2), 348–354. doi:10.1016/j.clnu.2016.10.011

Van den Berghe, G., Wilmer, A., & Hermans, G. (2006). Intensive insulin therapy in the medical ICU. *New England Journal of Medicine, 354*(5), 449–461.

Van den Berghe, G., Wouters, P., & Weekers, F. (2001). Intensive insulin therapy in the critically ill patient. *New England Journal of Medicine, 345*(19), 1359–1367.

Via, M. A., & Mechanick, J. I. (2016). Endocrine dysfunction leading to critical illness. In J. M. Oropello, S. M. Pastores, & V. Kvetan (Eds.), *Critical care*. New York, NY: McGraw-Hill. Retrieved March 15, 2017, from http://accessmedicine.mhmedical.com.ezproxy.uky.edu/content.aspx?bookid=1944&sectionid=143518760

Wilson, B. A., Shannon, M. T., & Shields, K. M. (2017). *Pearson nurse's drug guide 2017*. Hoboken, NJ: Pearson.

Chapter 33
Diabetic Crises

Learning Outcomes

33.1 Differentiate the two major types of diabetes mellitus and the effects of insulin deficit on the body.

33.2 Discuss the precipitating factors, pathophysiology, clinical presentation, and collaborative management of a hypoglycemic crisis.

33.3 Describe the precipitating factors, pathophysiology, and clinical presentation of diabetic ketoacidosis.

33.4 Discuss the precipitating factors, pathophysiology, and clinical presentation of a hyperglycemic hyperosmolar state.

33.5 Apply knowledge of collaborative management to the patient experiencing a hyperglycemic crisis.

33.6 Explain the use of exogenous insulin therapy as a treatment strategy for management of the patient with a hyperglycemic crisis and the use of insulin for glycemic control in the critical care patient.

33.7 Demonstrate an understanding of the acute care nursing implications of caring for the diabetic patient with chronic diabetes complications.

Diabetes mellitus represents a complex set of metabolic disorders associated with insulin deficiency and insulin resistance. Three types of acute glucose-related crises may occur with diabetes, all of which are considered medical emergencies: hypoglycemic crisis, a crisis of low blood glucose; and two hyperglycemic crises, diabetic ketoacidosis (DKA) and hyperglycemic hyperosmolar state (HHS). Understanding the pathophysiological basis for each of these crises enhances the understanding of the clinical presentation of the patient. Early recognition and timely, aggressive management of a diabetic crisis is crucial for positive patient outcomes. Furthermore, many patients with diabetes are admitted to the hospital with diagnoses other than their chronic diabetic state; however, the physiologic stress created by the acute problem may precipitate a diabetic crisis, which further complicates the patient's prognosis. Insulin therapy is a key component of effective management of hyperglycemic crises and is also recognized as an important intervention in maintaining glycemic control in critically ill patients.

Section One: Review of Diabetes Mellitus and Insulin Deficit

Diabetes mellitus (diabetes) refers to several complex metabolic disorders characterized by hyperglycemia. The exact contributing factors to development of hyperglycemia vary with the etiology of the diabetes and include increased production of glucose, reduced glucose utilization, and decreased insulin production (Powers, 2014a). A person with diabetes mellitus has either an absolute or a relative insulin deficit with some degree of insulin resistance. According to the Centers for Disease Control and Prevention (CDC) (2016a), there are more than 29 million people in the United States with diabetes, with about 25% unaware of its presence, and another 86 million with prediabetes.

Types of Diabetes Mellitus

There are two predominant forms of diabetes mellitus (DM) in the general population, type 1 and type 2. While both are metabolic disorders associated with elevated serum glucose, they have some distinctly different characteristics. This section provides a brief review of type 1 and type 2 DM.

Type 1 Diabetes Mellitus Type 1 DM, previously called juvenile-onset diabetes or insulin-dependent DM (IDDM), occurs when there is an absolute (or near absolute) lack of endogenous insulin. It is caused by destruction of the pancreatic beta cells and is of autoimmune or idiopathic origin (Centers for Disease Control and Prevention [CDC], 2014; Powers, 2014a). It can develop at any age but most commonly develops before the age of 20 and accounts for only about 5% to 10% of all diabetes cases. There are only a few known risk factors for development of type 1 DM, including a positive family history and genetics (see "Genetic Considerations: Type 1 Diabetes" feature). A genetic predisposition seems to be insufficient to result in active disease development. It is believed that some trigger is required, such as a viral or chemical agent or an environmental trigger. Treatment of type 1 DM centers on replacement insulin therapy and dietary management.

Type 2 Diabetes Mellitus Type 2 DM, previously called adult-onset DM or non-insulin-dependent DM (NIDDM), refers to a set of disorders with characteristics that include varying degrees of insulin resistance, increased glucose production by the liver, impaired insulin secretion, and abnormal fat metabolism (Powers, 2014a). It accounts for most DM cases (90%–95%) in the United States (Centers for Disease Control and Prevention [CDC], 2014). Type 2 DM is usually diagnosed after the age of 45 but is becoming more prevalent in children and adolescents. Obesity (particularly central distribution type) in the presence of hereditary tendencies is a major risk factor for development. Other risk factors include a history of impaired metabolism, older age, race or ethnicity (e.g., African Americans, Hispanics, and Latinos), and physical inactivity (Centers for Disease Control and Prevention [CDC], 2014). Treatment of type 2 DM centers on weight loss, dietary management, and healthy lifestyle changes. Oral antidiabetic agents or insulin replacement therapy may eventually be required.

Effects of Insulin Deficit

Recall from normal physiology that insulin plays a crucial role in regulation of fats, carbohydrates, and protein metabolism. Carbohydrates are the major sources of glucose. Insulin is required by the insulin-dependent cells (most cells in the body) for uptake of glucose into the cells.

The pathophysiologic basis for the clinical findings associated with hyperglycemic diabetic crises is largely due to the effects of insulin deficiency, which results in disordered carbohydrate, protein, and fat metabolism. In the absence of insulin, the liver initiates conversion of glycogen to glucose. The principal metabolic alterations associated with insulin deficiency include (1) impaired cellular uptake and use of glucose, (2) increased extracellular (serum) glucose, (3) increased mobilization of fats, and (4) tissue depletion of protein (Figure 33–1). Movement of glucose into

Genetic Considerations
Type 1 Diabetes

Multiple genes have been identified that make a person susceptible to type 1 diabetes; however, chromosome 6 is the major "susceptibility gene." The chromosome 6 human leukocyte antigen haplotypes HLA DR-3, DR-4, or both, have been strongly associated with the occurrence of type 1 DM, accounting for 40% to 50% of type 1 diabetes cases. These haplotypes are responsible for presenting antigens to the immune system's T-helper cells, thereby activating the immune response (Powers, 2014a).

insulin-dependent cells occurs in direct proportion to the amount of insulin available. When insulin-dependent tissues are deprived of glucose as a result of either insulin deficiency or insulin resistance, their functional capacities become restricted. Table 33–1 summarizes the effects of insulin deficiency on insulin-dependent tissues.

Insulin Deficit and Carbohydrate Metabolism Insulin deficit dramatically alters carbohydrate metabolism. Carbohydrates are the major suppliers of simple and complex sugars, producing glucose as the primary energy source. An absolute insulin deficit causes cessation in glucose uptake by insulin-dependent cells and a decrease in glucose use by the cells. The combination of decreased glucose uptake and decreased glucose use causes a rapid increase of serum glucose, known as hyperglycemia. Moreover, insulin normally increases the synthesis and storage of glycogen by the liver and decreases **gluconeogenesis** (production of glucose from noncarbohydrate sources). However, when an insulin deficit exists, the liver converts glycogen to glucose (**glycogenolysis**) and increases gluconeogenesis, with both actions contributing to hyperglycemia.

In an insulin-poor environment, insulin-dependent cells are starving, and although abundant potential energy is available in the form of glucose, it is of no use to the cells because insulin is not present for glucose transfer into cells. Other sources of energy are used once fat reserves are depleted, including fatty acids (the primary backup energy source) and amino acids. Clinically, dysfunctional carbohydrate metabolism is evidenced as hyperglycemia. If not controlled, **ketosis** (elevated total ketone bodies) and **aminoacidemia** (elevated blood amino acids) may result, each with its own set of complications.

Insulin Deficit and Fat Metabolism Insulin deficit alters fat metabolism by increasing lipolysis (fat breakdown) and decreasing lipogenesis (fat formation). The decreased availability of intracellular glucose results in increased breakdown of stored triglycerides by hormone-sensitive lipase, causing lipolysis. Free fatty acids become the major energy source for the tissues, with the major exception of the brain. Clinically, this is evidenced as increased blood levels of free fatty acids and glycerol. The liver also converts some of the excess fatty acids into cholesterol and phospholipids. Excess fatty acid breakdown causes increased levels of acetylcoenzyme A (acetyl-CoA), used by the liver for energy. The excess is converted into acetoacetic acid. Some of the acetoacetic acid is further converted into β-hydroxybutyric acid and acetone (dimethyl

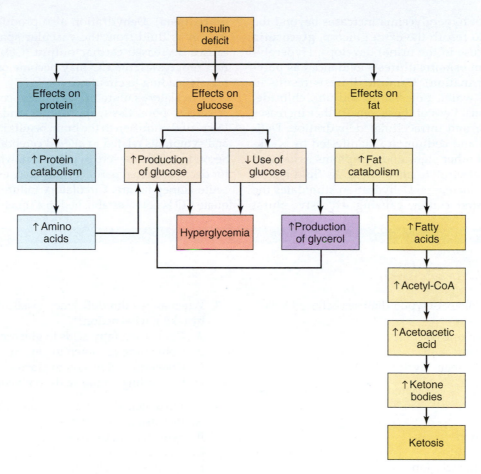

Figure 33–1 Consequences of insulin deficit.

ketone). These three substances (acetoacetic acid, β-hydroxybutyric acid, and acetone) move into the circulation as ketone bodies.

Clinically, this sequence of events has both acute and chronic consequences. Acutely, the increased levels of ketone bodies result in *ketosis* and *ketonuria*. When ketosis is extreme, severe **metabolic acidosis** and coma result

Table 33–1 Effects of Insulin Deficit on Insulin-dependent Tissues

Tissues and Cells	Effects
Glucose Transport Problems	
Skeletal muscle	Fatigue; decreased strength
Cardiac muscle	Weaker contractions; decreased cardiac output; decreased peripheral circulation
Smooth muscle	Poor bowel tone; decreased vascular tone
Leukocytes	Depressed leukocyte function; impaired inflammatory response
Crystalline lens of eye	Opacity or cataracts
Fibroblasts	Impaired healing
Pituitary gland	Retarded growth; impaired regeneration of tissue; other endocrine problems
Insulin Resistance Problem	
Adipose tissue	Lipolysis; lipidemia; elevated serum ketone levels

(e.g., diabetic ketoacidosis). The use of fat as energy is evident as a significant increase in plasma lipoproteins (as much as three times normal). In the long term, high levels of lipoproteins are associated with the rapid onset of atherosclerosis, especially when high cholesterol levels are present. Many of the complications of diabetes mellitus are secondary to atherosclerotic changes.

Insulin Deficit and Protein Metabolism Without insulin, the body is unable to store protein. There is an increase in protein catabolism and cessation of protein synthesis. Protein catabolism causes large quantities of amino acids to move into the circulation. The amino acids are then used either directly as an energy source or as part of the **gluconeogenesis** process.

Clinically, protein catabolism is evidenced by muscle wasting, multiple organ dysfunction, aminoacidemia, and increased urine nitrogen. If nitrogenous wastes accumulate in the body faster than they can be excreted in the urine, the patient will exhibit an altered level of consciousness and mentation. In addition, as gluconeogenesis is initiated, hyperglycemia is further aggravated.

Insulin Deficit and Fluid and Electrolyte Balance When an insulin deficit exists, the serum glucose level increases, creating increased plasma osmotic pressure. The resulting change in pressure produces a shifting of body fluids from the tissues into the intravascular compartment. This shifting of fluids leads to intracellular dehydration.

As the level of hyperglycemia increases beyond the kidney's ability to resorb the extra glucose, **glycosuria** (excretion of glucose in the urine) develops. Hyperglycemia produces an **osmotic diuresis** evidenced as **polyuria** (excessive urination). Osmotic diuresis results in excessive loss of water, potassium, sodium, chloride, and phosphate ions. Loss of these ions further increases both extracellular and intracellular dehydration. Deficits in potassium and sodium are manifested by weakness, fatigue, and other signs and symptoms associated with the specific electrolyte imbalances. As fluid is lost, serum osmolality increases. Dehydration stimulates the hypothalamic thirst center, causing excessive thirst

(**polydipsia**). Dehydration also produces hemoconcentration as fluid from the vascular space is lost, which causes decreased cardiac output (CO). If the dehydration progresses, the CO may become critically low, ultimately leading to circulatory failure.

Circulatory failure has two major consequences. First, it causes poor tissue perfusion and tissue hypoxia. Decreased perfusion to the brain results in cerebral hypoxia and symptoms related to altered cerebral tissue perfusion. Second, it causes severe hypotension, which is responsible for decreased renal perfusion and may eventually result in acute kidney failure. Circulatory failure is fatal if an adequate CO is not re-established in a timely manner.

Section One Review

1. What is the etiology of type 1 diabetes believed to be?
   A. Obesity
   B. An autoimmune reaction
   C. A bacterial infection
   D. General pancreatic dysfunction

2. Type 2 diabetes is associated with which major risk factor?
   A. Smoking
   B. Viral infection
   C. Obesity
   D. Autoimmune reaction

3. When an insulin deficiency exists, the liver responds by taking what action?
   A. Converting fatty acids to glucose
   B. Converting glycogen to glucose
   C. Converting glucagon to glucose
   D. Converting amino acids to glucose

4. Insulin deficit alters fat metabolism by doing what?
   A. Increasing lipogenesis
   B. Synthesizing triglycerides
   C. Increasing lipolysis
   D. Synthesizing glycerol

Answers: 1. B, 2. C, 3. B, 4. C

Section Two: Hypoglycemic Crisis

Hypoglycemia (abnormally low blood glucose level) is the most common diabetic complication and can occur with any type of diabetes. According to the American Diabetes Association, more than 280,000 visits to the emergency room in 2011 had hypoglycemia as a first diagnosis and diabetes as a secondary diagnosis (American Diabetes Association, 2016). A hypoglycemic episode is triggered by imbalances in exercise, diet, or medication. It most commonly is caused by medications, usually excessive administration of insulin or oral antidiabetes agents (Cryer & Davis, 2014). Patients receiving oral antidiabetic agents (e.g., sulfonylureas) are at highest risk for severe and prolonged symptoms of hypoglycemia because of the extended half-life of these agents. Additional precipitating factors for hypoglycemia are listed in Box 33–1. Intensive insulin therapy (IIT) is an important potential cause of severe hypoglycemia in the critical care unit and is discussed in Section Six of this chapter.

Clinical Diagnosis and Presentation

Hypoglycemia occurs from a relative excess of insulin in the blood and results in excessively low blood glucose

---

BOX 33–1   Common Precipitating Factors of Hypoglycemia

Drug Related (Most common)
- Excessive dose of insulin or oral antidiabetes agent
- Change in medication regimen
- Potentiating effects of medications or drugs (e.g., propranolol and alcohol)

Physiology Related
- Increase in insulin sensitivity (e.g., better glycemic control)
- Decrease in endogenous glucose production (e.g., post-alcohol intake)
- Decrease in insulin clearance (e.g., kidney failure)

Lifestyle Related
- Consumption of too little food
- High activity levels

Critical-illness Related
- Hormonal deficiencies (e.g., cortisol, glucagon, epinephrine)
- Kidney, liver, or heart failure
- Sepsis

SOURCE: Data from Cryer & Davis (2014).

Table 33–2 Hypoglycemia Levels of Severity

Level	Criteria
1 Mild	Serum glucose: 70 mg/dL (3.9 mmol/L) or less
2 Clinically significant	Serum glucose: less than 54 mg/dL (3.0 mmol/L); should be reported
3 Severe	Serum glucose: variable; major criterion = severe cognitive impairment that requires external treatment for recovery

SOURCE: Data from American Diabetes Association (ADA) (2016) and Goyal & Schlichting (2016).

levels. It is defined clinically by meeting three criteria: the presenting symptoms are those of hypoglycemia, the serum glucose is low (less than 70 mg/dL), and symptoms cease with administration of glucose (American Diabetes Association [ADA], 2015a). Hypoglycemia can be classified as mild, clinically significant, or severe; however, the point at which hypoglycemic symptoms occur varies. Some patients may develop symptoms with a serum glucose of greater than 70 mg/dL, whereas others may develop symptoms when serum glucose drops rapidly. Table 33–2 lists three levels of severity of hypoglycemia.

Onset of hypoglycemic symptoms is usually rapid; and the clinical presentation primarily reflects neuroglycopenic and autonomic nervous system (NS) effects. If hypoglycemia becomes severe, the patient can slip into a stuporous or comatose state, a condition referred to as *hypoglycemic coma*. Severe hypoglycemia can cause irreversible brain damage and death; thus, early recognition with rapid reversal through administration of glucose is needed for optimal patient outcomes.

Neuroglycopenic Effects   Neuroglycopenic (low CNS glucose) effects are a direct result of the inability of brain cells to function normally in the absence of an adequate glucose energy source, causing diminishing cognitive (mental) abilities and altered balance and coordination. Table 33–3 lists neuroglycopenic symptoms that develop as hypoglycemia worsens.

Autonomic Nervous System and Catecholamine Effects The lack of circulating glucose stimulates the autonomic nervous system (ANS; sympathetic nervous system branch) and increases secretion of the stress hormone

Table 33–3 Clinical Manifestations of Hypoglycemia

Neuroglycopenic Effects	Autonomic Effects
• Slowed thinking	• Tachycardia, palpitations
• Changing mental status	• Hunger
• Emotional lability	• Sweating
• Headache, dizziness	• Anxiety
• Thickened, slurred speech	• Tremors, nervousness
• Loss of coordination	• Cold, clammy skin
• Loss of proprioception	• Hyperventilation
• Numbness	• Tingling in extremities
• Drowsiness	• Nausea and vomiting
• Convulsions	
• Coma	

epinephrine, subsequently increasing glucose production from alternate body sources. The increased level of epinephrine triggers a sympathetic nervous system physiologic response. This stress response accounts for many of the fight-or-flight symptoms associated with hypoglycemia, such as listed in Table 33–3.

Hypoglycemia-associated Autonomic Failure Hypoglycemia-associated autonomic failure (HAAS) refers to a potentially severe, sometimes fatal hypoglycemic phenomenon that mostly develops following a recent iatrogenic (therapy-related) hypoglycemic episode. Other, less common triggering factors are exercise related and sleep related. HAAS is associated with individuals who have an absolute lack of endogenous insulin (i.e., type 1 or advanced type 2 diabetes). It is most common in patients with type 1 diabetes. The concept of HAAS involves two syndromes: (1) a defect in the counterregulation of glucose and (2) hypoglycemia unawareness (hypoglycemia that develops without warning symptoms) (Cryer, 2004; Cryer & Davis, 2014).

The pathophysiologic basis of HAAS is not fully understood. Usually, as serum glucose levels fall, the body increases the glucose level by suppressing insulin secretion while increasing glucagon and epinephrine secretion. However, in the complete absence of insulin production by pancreatic beta cells, the normal glucose counterregulatory responses to hypoglycemia become defective. In individuals who produce no insulin (type 1 and advanced type 2 DM), the normal glucose counterregulation mechanisms fail. As glucose levels fall, there is no corresponding decrease in circulating insulin or increase in glucagon and epinephrine levels (Cryer & Davis, 2014). Thus, the characteristic sympathetic nervous system neural responses and catecholamine clinical manifestations fail to appear, masking the presence of hypoglycemia. The lack of classic hypoglycemia signs and symptoms significantly increases the risk of the patient developing severe, possibly life-threatening hypoglycemia (Cryer, 2004; Cryer & Davis, 2014; Goyal & Schlichting, 2016).

Other Determinants of Hypoglycemic Symptoms

The rate of onset and the patient's age influence the type of symptoms that predominate.

Rate of Onset: Rapid   When the onset of hypoglycemia is rapid, ANS or catecholamine symptoms often predominate. A significant, rapid drop of blood glucose level stimulates the sympathetic nervous system, which initiates secretion of epinephrine. Epinephrine causes gluconeogenesis in the liver, thereby increasing the serum glucose level. Concurrently, growth hormone and cortisol are secreted to assist in increasing glucose levels by decreasing glucose use by the cells.

Rate of Onset: Slow   When the onset of hypoglycemia is slow, the ANS does not respond to the slow decline as it does with rapid-onset hypoglycemia. Given sufficient time, the body is able to adapt to a slow decline in blood glucose. Brain cells are not insulin dependent and take in

Table 33–4 Treatment of Hypoglycemia in the Conscious Hospitalized Adult Patient

Interventions	Description
Glucose replacement	Administer 15 to 20 g of glucose. Example glucose sources: 5–6 oz regular soda, 8 oz juice (glucose content varies), 2 tablespoons cake icing, 1 tube 40% glucose oral gel, or 4 glucose tablets
Assessments	• Assess for safety of administering oral therapies; if patient is unable to safely cooperate or swallow, move to treating as for hypoglycemia in the patient with altered mental status. • Repeat blood glucose levels every 15 minutes until glucose levels normalize, then continue to periodically measure as ordered by provider or agency protocol. • Following correction of blood glucose, monitor closely for relapse of symptoms of hypoglycemia, keeping in mind that relapse may reoccur.
Other	• When normal glucose levels are achieved, patient should eat a meal or snack. • Report hypoglycemic episode promptly to provider. • Document occurrence in detail, including assessments and all interventions taken.

SOURCE: Data from American Diabetes Association (ADA) (2016) and Goyal & Schlichting (2016).

glucose directly. Sympathetic nervous system (SNS) symptoms, therefore, are caused by lack of available glucose, rather than an insulin deficit. The brain is a high-energy tissue, requiring large amounts of glucose to maintain normal functioning. Without glucose, particularly over a prolonged period, the brain can sustain permanent damage that may be either minor or severe (irreversible coma).

The Influence of Age   The age of the patient has an impact on the clinical presentation of hypoglycemia. Older adult patients tend to have more severe symptoms and may become symptomatic at higher serum glucose levels. SNS (cognitive) symptoms, particularly those relating to altered levels of consciousness, may be misdiagnosed in chronically ill older adult if the onset is exceptionally slow as it may be taken for worsening dementia.

Collaborative Interventions

The major goal of hypoglycemia-related interventions is rapid restoration of intravascular fluid levels and normal serum glucose levels, which includes treating the underlying cause. The specific type of intervention is based partially on the patient's level of consciousness.

If a hospitalized adult patient with diabetes exhibits acute onset of mental alterations or hypoglycemia is diagnosed, the following interventions are recommended:

1. Evaluate airway, breathing, and circulation (ABCs); initiate intravenous access if not present.

2. If patient is unconscious or becomes unconscious, reposition to side-lying position to reduce risk of aspiration unless contraindicated.

3. Obtain a STAT blood glucose level prior to initiating therapy. In the absence of equipment to check capillary blood glucose, glucose administration should not be delayed until a blood sample is available. A delay in treating severe hypoglycemia may be detrimental to patient outcomes.

4. Based on level of consciousness and severity of hypoglycemia, implement appropriate hypoglycemic patient protocol per agency policy, provider order, or evidence-based practice if no policy or orders are available.

The Alert Hypoglycemic Patient   Reversal of hypoglycemia in the conscious patient is relatively simple to accomplish and usually centers on oral replacement of glucose. A variety of foods (e.g., graham crackers), beverages (regular sodas or juices), and commercial products (e.g., glucose oral gel or glucose tablets) can be used as a glucose source. Many high-carbohydrate foods can be used; however, they should have a high glucose content to be most effective. Table 33–4 provides information on management of the conscious hospitalized patient experiencing hypoglycemia.

The Unconscious Hypoglycemic Patient   The unconscious hypoglycemic patient requires rapid correction of serum glucose levels; therefore, the mainstay of emergency glucose therapy is intravenous dextrose. Glucagon can be substituted for dextrose if there is no IV access or dextrose is not available. Table 33–5 lists major management recommendations for treating severe hypoglycemia in an adult patient with altered mental status. The American Association of Clinical Endocrinologists (AACE, n.d.) also has a recommended hypoglycemic protocol (see Figure 33–2).

The Patient with Hypoglycemia-associated Autonomic Failure (HAAS)   Hypoglycemia-associated autonomic failure has important clinical implications, especially when the patient is in a critical care setting where tight glycemic control is emphasized to improve patient outcomes. Aggressive insulin therapy to control glucose levels significantly increases the risk for development of HAAS (Clain, Ramar, & Surani, 2015). While this syndrome is reversible, current recommendations emphasize the importance of preventing hypoglycemia in at-risk patients. Because HAAS is triggered by an event (usually a recent episode of hypoglycemia), maintaining glycemic

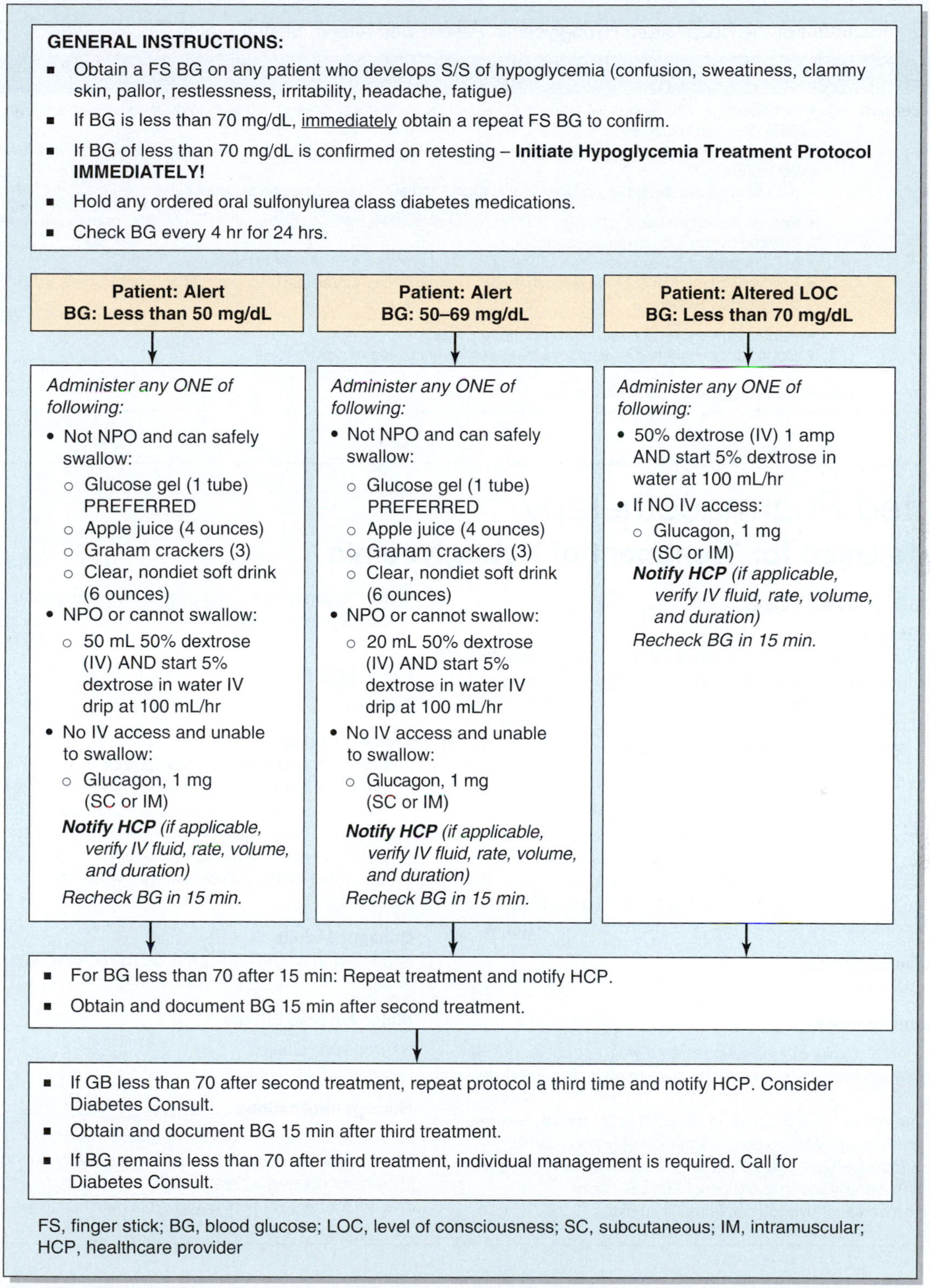

GENERAL INSTRUCTIONS:

- Obtain a FS BG on any patient who develops S/S of hypoglycemia (confusion, sweatiness, clammy skin, pallor, restlessness, irritability, headache, fatigue)
- If BG is less than 70 mg/dL, <u>immediately</u> obtain a repeat FS BG to confirm.
- If BG of less than 70 mg/dL is confirmed on retesting – **Initiate Hypoglycemia Treatment Protocol IMMEDIATELY!**
- Hold any ordered oral sulfonylurea class diabetes medications.
- Check BG every 4 hr for 24 hrs.

Patient: Alert BG: Less than 50 mg/dL	Patient: Alert BG: 50–69 mg/dL	Patient: Altered LOC BG: Less than 70 mg/dL

Administer any ONE of following:
 	
• Not NPO and can safely swallow:
  o Glucose gel (1 tube) PREFERRED
  o Apple juice (4 ounces)
  o Graham crackers (3)
  o Clear, nondiet soft drink (6 ounces)
• NPO or cannot swallow:
  o 50 mL 50% dextrose (IV) AND start 5% dextrose in water IV drip at 100 mL/hr
• No IV access and unable to swallow:
  o Glucagon, 1 mg (SC or IM)
Notify HCP *(if applicable, verify IV fluid, rate, volume, and duration)*
Recheck BG in 15 min.
	Administer any ONE of following:
	
	• Not NPO and can safely swallow:
	  o Glucose gel (1 tube) PREFERRED
	  o Apple juice (4 ounces)
	  o Graham crackers (3)
	  o Clear, nondiet soft drink (6 ounces)
	• NPO or cannot swallow:
	  o 20 mL 50% dextrose (IV) AND start 5% dextrose in water IV drip at 100 mL/hr
	• No IV access and unable to swallow:
	  o Glucagon, 1 mg (SC or IM)
	Notify HCP *(if applicable, verify IV fluid, rate, volume, and duration)*
	Recheck BG in 15 min.
		Administer any ONE of following:
		
		• 50% dextrose (IV) 1 amp AND start 5% dextrose in water at 100 mL/hr
		• If NO IV access:
		  o Glucagon, 1 mg (SC or IM)
		Notify HCP *(if applicable, verify IV fluid, rate, volume, and duration)*
		Recheck BG in 15 min.

- For BG less than 70 after 15 min: Repeat treatment and notify HCP.
- Obtain and document BG 15 min after second treatment.

- If GB less than 70 after second treatment, repeat protocol a third time and notify HCP. Consider Diabetes Consult.
- Obtain and document BG 15 min after third treatment.
- If BG remains less than 70 after third treatment, individual management is required. Call for Diabetes Consult.

FS, finger stick; BG, blood glucose; LOC, level of consciousness; SC, subcutaneous; IM, intramuscular; HCP, healthcare provider

Figure 33–2 Hypoglycemia treatment protocol.

SOURCE: Data from the American Association of Clinical Endocrinologists (AACE) (n.d.; rev. 2011).

control is critical (Cryer, 2015). Furthermore, if an episode of hypoglycemia has already occurred, steps should be taken to prevent a recurrent episode. The American Diabetes Association recommends that the target level for glycemic control be reset to a higher range in patients who have experienced repeated severe hypoglycemia or hypoglycemia unawareness (American Diabetes Association [ADA], 2017b).

A summary of glucose or dextrose and glucagon pharmacologic agents is available in the "Related Pharmacotherapy: Agents Used for Treatment of Hypoglycemia" feature.

Table 33–5   Treatment of the Hospitalized Hypoglycemic Patient with Altered Mental Status

Interventions	Descriptions
Glucose replacement	• Administer an intravenous (IV) bolus of 50% dextrose in water at dosage of 0.5–1 g/kg; or administer a 50 mL bolus of 50% dextrose solution. • Follow the glucose bolus with a continuous IV glucose infusion (10%) to maintain the plasma glucose at a level greater than 100 mg/dL. • If no IV access is available, administer glucagon 1 mg subcutaneous or intramuscular (IM).
Assessments	• Repeat blood glucose levels every 30 minutes until glucose levels normalize, then continue to periodically measure as ordered by provider or agency protocol. • Monitor level of consciousness and vital signs closely throughout interventional period. • Following correction of blood glucose levels, monitor closely for relapse of symptoms of hypoglycemia keeping in mind that relapse may reoccur.
Other	• Report hypoglycemic episode promptly to provider. • Document occurrence in detail, including assessments and all actions taken.

SOURCE: Data for glucose replacement therapy from Bosse (2015) and Kefer (2016).

Related Pharmacotherapy
Agents Used for Treatment of Hypoglycemia

Glucose or Dextrose

Action and Uses
When delivered orally, dextrose is rapidly absorbed in the intestine and is taken up and used by tissues. Delivered intravenously, it causes a rapid increase in serum glucose levels and provides relief of hypoglycemic states. Dextrose can be used for providing energy and is the primary therapy for treatment of hypoglycemia.

Dosages (Adult)
Mild hypoglycemia: administer 15 to 20 g of glucose.

Hypoglycemia with altered mental status: Administer an intravenous (IV) bolus of 50% dextrose in water at dosage of 0.5–1 g/kg or administer a 50 mL bolus of 50% dextrose solution. Follow the glucose bolus with a continuous IV glucose infusion (10%) to maintain the plasma glucose at a level greater than 100 mg/dL.

Major Adverse Effects
Hyperglycemia

Nursing Implications
Obtain an initial capillary blood glucose level when possible, but do not delay administration if blood glucose cannot be immediately drawn.

Acute treatment of hypoglycemia in an adult is 50 mL of dextrose 50% given as an IV bolus on confirmation of hypoglycemia.

Prolonged management in an adult is glucose 10% in water delivered via a central line to avoid peripheral vein injury.

Monitor for reversal of hypoglycemia manifestations.

Monitor capillary blood glucose via bedside glucometer if accuracy has been established.

Glucagon
Glucagen

Action and Uses
This naturally occurring hormone produced by the alpha cells of the pancreas increases production of glucose by the liver and relaxes the muscles of the GI tract. Glucagon has a longer action-onset time, and if glycogen stores have already been depleted, it will not be an effective therapy (Bosse, 2015). It is used as alternative treatment of hypoglycemia only when there is no available IV access.

Dosages (Adult)
Usual dose in an adult is 1–2 mg; can be administered subcutaneously or IM.

Major Adverse Effects
Nausea and vomiting
Hypersensitivity reaction

Nursing Implications
Assess for nausea and vomiting during therapy.

Monitor glucose levels via bedside glucometer during treatment and several hours posttreatment.

Monitor for reversal of hypoglycemia manifestations.

Section Two Review

1. Which statement is true regarding hypoglycemia?
   A. It is defined only in terms of blood glucose levels.
   B. It is defined only in terms of clinical presentation.
   C. It becomes symptomatic only when excessive insulin is present.
   D. It becomes symptomatic at different blood glucose levels.

2. Which conditions increase the risk of hypoglycemia?
   A. Too little exercise
   B. High-fat diet
   C. Dietary fasting
   D. Too little insulin

3. The clinical presentation of hypoglycemia partially reflects which condition?
   A. Lack of glucose within the cells
   B. Excessive glucose within the cells
   C. Stimulation of parasympathetic nervous system
   D. Excessive circulating insulin

4. A client experiencing rapid-onset hypoglycemia is most likely to have predominantly what symptom?
   A. Cell dysfunction
   B. Gastrointestinal
   C. Stimulated sympathetic nervous system
   D. Stimulated parasympathetic nervous system

Answers: 1. D, 2. C, 3. A, 4. C

Section Three: Hyperglycemic Crisis— Diabetic Ketoacidosis

Two major diabetic crises are associated with high serum glucose levels: diabetic ketoacidosis (DKA) and hyperglycemic hyperosmolar state (HHS), with DKA being much more common than HHS. Both of these potentially life-threatening complications of diabetes result from a relative or absolute deficiency in insulin and some degree of insulin resistance. The mortality rate associated with hyperglycemic crises has steadily decreased over the past three decades (Centers for Disease Control and Prevention [CDC], 2012; Hamdy, 2017). In adults, the mortality rate associated with DKA is less than 0.2% to 2%; however, in older adults and those with concurrent critical illnesses, it is higher (Hamdy, 2017). The mortality rate associated with HHS is significantly higher than that of DKA, at an estimated 5% to 10% (Avichal, 2017). Much of the pathophysiology, clinical findings, and treatment strategies are similar for both crises; however, for clarity, they will be discussed separately over two sections.

Diabetic ketoacidosis (DKA) results from an absolute or relative deficiency in insulin. It is a potentially severe, sometimes life-threatening complication characterized by elevated total ketones (ketosis), metabolic acidosis, and uncontrolled hyperglycemia.

Patient Profile and Precipitating Factors

There are known patient characteristics and precipitating factors for development of DKA.

Patient Profile Diabetic ketoacidosis is seen most commonly in individuals with type 1 diabetes; however, it can develop in patients with type 2 diabetes. Individuals who are at higher risk for developing DKA have type 1 diabetes and are of younger age (younger than 45), non-White, and female, although gender is almost equally distributed (Centers for Disease Control and Prevention [CDC], 2012; Nyce, Lubkin, & Chansky, 2016). In addition, it is estimated that up to 30% of DKA cases occur in individuals with newly diagnosed type 2 diabetes (Nyce et al., 2016).

Precipitating Factors Any condition or situation that increases insulin deficit can precipitate a hyperglycemic crisis such as DKA—for example, insufficient insulin therapy coverage, insufficient food intake, acute illness events

(e.g., infection, stroke, myocardial infarction, trauma), alcohol abuse, and certain drugs (e.g., thiazide diuretics, corticosteroids, pentamidine, and sympathomimetic agents) (American Diabetes Association [ADA], 2015b; Nyce et al., 2016). In about 20% of cases, no specific precipitating event is found, in which case the DKA is sometimes referred to as unprovoked DKA.

Infection and Stress. Infection is a major precipitating factor for DKA; however, increased physiologic stress is also an important factor that warrants consideration. Table 33–6 lists causes of increased risk for infection in diabetic patients. Illness and infection increase the production of glucocorticoids by the adrenal gland, stimulating the production of new glucose by the liver (gluconeogenesis). Epinephrine and norepinephrine levels are also increased, causing further breakdown of glycogen into glucose (glycogenolysis). An increased level of stress causes increased production of stress hormones (e.g., epinephrine, growth hormone, and cortisol). When secreted, these hormones increase blood glucose levels by either increasing conversion of glycogen to glucose or decreasing cellular use of glucose. When the stress is severe, as in a severe acute infection or illness, the increase in glucose can be substantial, precipitating an imbalance in the glucose–insulin relationship.

Table 33–6 Causes of Increased Risk for Infection in Diabetic Patients

Underlying Dysfunction	Description
Diminished early warning system	Impaired vision and peripheral neuropathy contribute to a decreased ability to perform self-monitoring. Breaks in skin integrity may not be seen or felt because of the underlying disease process.
Tissue hypoxia	Vascular disease causes tissue hypoxia. When skin integrity is broken, there is a decreased ability to heal, secondary to lack of oxygen. Glycosylated hemoglobin in RBCs decreases release of oxygen to the tissues, thus contributing to hypoxia.
Rapid proliferation of pathogens	Once inside the body, pathogens rapidly multiply because of increased glucose in body fluids, which acts as an energy source for the pathogens.
Impaired leukocytes	Diabetes is associated with the development of abnormal white blood cells, particularly phagocytes, and it also alters chemotaxis (movement of WBCs to the site of infection).
Impaired circulation	A diminished blood supply decreases the ability of WBCs to move into the infected area.

Significant infection is typically accompanied by hyperthermia (fever), which increases the metabolic rate, thus greatly increasing cellular need for insulin. Therefore, in the presence of infection, there is both an increased supply and an increased demand for glucose. In such a situation, ideally a balance in supply and demand of glucose would exist. However, this is not the case in the type 1 diabetic patient; a supply-and-demand glucose balance can be maintained or regained only when sufficient exogenous insulin is made available to meet the increased glucose needs of the cells. Diabetic ketoacidosis is precipitated by a relative exogenous insulin deficiency in this situation. If insulin dosage is not increased in response, there is insufficient insulin to meet the increased glucose supply in addition to the increased metabolic demand—and thus circulating glucose levels increase while the cells become starved.

A similar situation can occur in a patient with type 2 diabetes whose condition normally is controlled by diet, oral antidiabetes agents, or both. In situations of high stress (e.g., infection, trauma, surgery), the level of insulin secretion in the pancreas often is insufficient to meet the increased supply of and demand for glucose, creating a relative endogenous insulin deficiency. Thus, this type of patient clinically develops hyperglycemia, which often requires temporary exogenous insulin therapy. Temporary adjusted-dosing (e.g., sliding scale) insulin is often required until the level of physiologic stress is sufficiently reduced and balance is regained between the glucose level and the endogenous insulin supply.

Pathophysiologic Basis of DKA

The major characteristics of DKA include hyperglycemia, ketosis, high-anion-gap metabolic acidosis, and osmotic diuresis, which account for most signs and symptoms of DKA. The following provides an overview of the pathophysiologic findings.

Hyperglycemia   Recall that the origin of **hyperglycemia** is an absolute or relative deficit in insulin, which prevents the uptake of glucose into cells. Rather than being taken in and used by the cells, the glucose continues to circulate and accumulate, causing increased serum glucose levels. In response to insufficient glucose available to the cells, the body turns to fat to produce energy. Fat is converted into free fatty acids (FFAs) through an oxidation process, making FFA readily available as an energy source. The liver also causes glycogenolysis, which converts glycogen to glucose. All these factors contribute to worsening hyperglycemia.

A major diagnostic criterion of DKA is serum glucose of greater than 250 mg/dL. However, about 10% of patients presenting with DKA have ketoacidosis with serum glucose levels below the 250 mg/dL, a condition called *euglycemic ketoacidosis* (Nyce et al., 2016). This unusual presentation is usually seen in younger patients with vomiting, patients with liver failure or alcohol abuse, or patients with depression, pregnancy, or recent low dietary intake (Nyce et al., 2016). The severity of a DKA episode is largely based on the serum glucose level and may range from mild to severe.

Ketosis   While FFAs provide needed energy, they produce acidic ketone bodies which accumulate in the circulation causing ketosis. Acetone, which is contained in ketone bodies, is excreted through the lungs (ketone breath) and the kidneys (ketonuria).

Metabolic Acidosis (High Anion Gap Type)   As the level of circulating ketone bodies increases, there is a resulting decrease in pH; and as the pH falls below 7.20, the respiratory center is stimulated to excrete carbonic acid via the lungs in the form of carbon dioxide and water (Kussmaul breathing). In response, conservation and secretion of bicarbonate attempts to compensate for the worsening ketosis. Eventually, bicarbonate reserves become overwhelmed and then exhausted by the severity and prolonged state of acidosis, which is clinically noted as a drop in serum bicarbonate levels and further lowering of the pH.

Diabetic ketoacidosis is only one cause of metabolic acidosis. Measuring **anion gap** is one way to help differentiate DKA from some other acidotic conditions. Metabolic acidosis exists either as normal anion gap acidosis (from loss of bicarbonate ions) or as high anion gap acidosis (from an accumulation of fixed acids in the serum). Recall from basic chemistry that anions are negatively charged particles (e.g., CO_2^-, HCO_3^-, and Cl^-), whereas cations are positively charged particles (e.g., Na^+ and K^+). Normally, cations and anions exist in balance with each other. Anion gap represents the level of unmeasurable anion excess that exists in the body. Measurement of the anion gap is helpful in identifying the type of metabolic acidosis present. It is expressed as

$$\text{Anion gap} = (Na^+ + K^+) - (Cl^- + HCO_3^-)$$

Anion gap has a normal range of 8–16 mEq/L (Laposata, 2014). This normal range incorporates unmeasured serum anions such as phosphates, sulfates, ketones, and lactic acid. An anion gap of greater than 17 mEq/L indicates an accumulation of these unmeasured anions and warrants immediate attention. Abnormal states such as starvation, lactic acidosis, and DKA cause a high anion gap—an excess of unmeasured anions. A patient who is suspected of a hyperglycemic crisis such as DKA may have an anion gap calculation performed. Although anion gap alone is nonspecific for DKA, it is used as adjunctive data for differential diagnosis and monitoring purposes.

Osmotic Diuresis   Elevated serum glucose levels increase intravascular osmotic pressure, and the increased pressure draws extravascular fluids into the intravascular compartment. As the levels of glucose and intravascular volume increase, the kidneys respond by dramatically increasing excretion of glucose and urine—**osmotic diuresis**. This is associated with increased loss of electrolytes, hemoconcentration, increasing dehydration, and decreasing blood pressure.

As a compensatory response to the osmotic diuresis, the renin-angiotensin-aldosterone system (RAAS) is activated to increase sodium and water resorption. Antidiuretic hormone (ADH) is secreted by the posterior pituitary to cause retention of water and sodium. Urine output also is controlled by compensatory vasoconstriction, which limits renal blood flow. The autonomic nervous system is stimulated to secrete catecholamines and glucocorticoids, which results in vasoconstriction, thereby increasing the blood pressure and decreasing urine output. As a result, blood pressure, pulse, and respirations are all increased.

If an episode of DKA is prolonged or severe, the patient will eventually decompensate. Decompensation represents exhaustion of compensatory mechanisms, which rapidly leads to cardiovascular collapse and death. The level of consciousness deteriorates, and blood pressure and pulse can no longer maintain adequate organ perfusion. The supply of catecholamines becomes exhausted, causing the body to lose its ability to maintain peripheral vasoconstriction. Urine output decreases and ceases as hypoperfusion to the kidneys causes them to fail.

Table 33–7 provides a summary of the major characteristics and associated signs and symptoms of DKA.

Laboratory Parameters   Measurement of certain laboratory parameters is a crucial part of evaluating hyperglycemic crises. Some parameters can also help differentiate DKA from HHS or other metabolic crises. Standard parameters to be monitored include serum glucose, ketones (acetone and acetoacetate), arterial blood gases (pH and bicarbonate), and serum electrolytes (particularly potassium). Since infection is a major precipitating event for development of a hyperglycemic crisis, a complete blood cell count (CBC) is usually ordered. Some degree of leukocytosis ($10,000$–$15,000$ mm^3) is expected during hyperglycemic crises related to circulating proinflammatory factors that increase during the active crisis period; however, a significantly elevated WBC count (higher than $25,000$ mm^3) strongly suggests ongoing infection (Gosmanov, Gosmanova, & Kitabchi, 2015).

Other parameters that may be measured include serum osmolality, anion gap, blood urea nitrogen (BUN), free fatty acids, and serum β-hydroxybutyrate. β-hydroxybutyrate is the primary ketone body present in ketoacidosis; therefore, when measurement is available, it may provide useful diagnostic data. In addition, stress hormone levels (e.g., cortisol, human growth hormone, and catecholamines) may be ordered and evaluated since they increase during hyperglycemic crises, contributing to the glucose load.

Table 33–7   Major Characteristics and Associated Signs and Symptoms of DKA

Characteristics	Major Signs and Symptoms
Hyperglycemia	Elevated serum glucose (greater than 250 mg/dL [13.8 mmol/L]) Elevated urine glucose
Ketosis	Elevated serum and urine ketones (ketonuria); ketone breath (sweet fruity odor)
Metabolic acidosis (high anion gap)	ABG —pH less than 7.30; HCO_3 less than 15 mEq/L [15 mmol/L]; $PaCO_2$ less than 35 mmHg High anion gap (greater than 10 mEq/L [10 mmol/L]) Elevated respiratory rate and depth (Kussmaul breathing)
Osmotic diuresis	Hypotension Polyuria and polydipsia Dehydration: weight loss, poor skin turgor, dry mucous membranes and skin, weakness, elevated serum BUN and creatinine Electrolyte abnormalities Elevated serum osmolality (but less than 350 mg/dL) Vomiting

SOURCE: Data from Nyce et al. (2016).

Section Three Review

1. Which set of laboratory results best reflects diabetic ketoacidosis?
   A. pH 7.28, HCO_3 34 mEq/L, blood glucose 70 mg/dL
   B. pH 7.18, HCO_3 13 mEq/L, blood glucose 100 mg/dL
   C. pH 7.26, HCO_3 14 mEq/L, blood glucose 450 mg/dL
   D. pH 7.38, HCO_3 24 mEq/L, blood glucose 620 mg/dL

2. Ketosis results from the mobilization of which component?
   A. Amino acids
   B. Glucagon
   C. Glucose
   D. Fatty acids

3. A high anion gap acidosis is consistent with which problem?
   A. Diarrhea
   B. High intake of chloride
   C. Starvation
   D. High intake of sodium

4. What is a common precipitating factor for development of diabetic ketoacidosis?
   A. Infection
   B. Decreased exercise
   C. A stress-free lifestyle
   D. Food–insulin balance

Answers: 1. C, 2. D, 3. C, 4. A

Section Four: Hyperglycemic Crisis—Hyperglycemic Hyperosmolar State

Hyperglycemic hyperosmolar state (HHS) is a hyperglycemic complication of diabetes mellitus that results from insulin deficiency and insulin resistance. Historically, it has been known by many names, such as hyperglycemic hyperosmolar nonketotic coma (HHNC) and hyperglycemic hyperosmolar nonketotic syndrome (HHNKS), among others. It has a slower onset than DKA, with symptoms slowly increasing over several days to several weeks. HHS is less common than DKA and has a higher mortality rate because of the severity of metabolic derangements, extreme dehydration, older age, and often poorer health of the patient.

Patient Profile and Precipitating Factors

HHS is typically seen in older adults persons with new onset or previously diagnosed type 2 diabetes. The person usually has underlying diseases, frequently is residing in a long-term-care facility, and often is unable to readily access fluids without assistance. The precipitating factors for development of HHS are essentially those of DKA, with infection being the leading trigger. Because patients who develop HHS often are debilitated physically or mentally, the presenting signs and symptoms may be misinterpreted as worsening dementia, delaying diagnosis until the HHS becomes severe.

Pathophysiologic Basis of HHS

Recall from the previous section that DKA is characterized by hyperglycemia, ketosis, high anion gap metabolic acidosis, and osmotic diuresis. HHS has only two of the DKA characteristics: extreme hyperglycemia and severe osmotic diuresis. In addition, severe alterations in mental status are more common in HHS.

Extreme Hyperglycemia　The degree of hyperglycemia is usually significantly higher in HHS than in DKA. The patient with type 2 diabetes may produce moderate levels of insulin. In the presence of a precipitating event, such as infection, the relative lack of insulin in these patients can trigger hyperglycemia by way of acceleration of hepatic gluconeogenesis and decreased peripheral glucose utilization. The result of these events is extreme hyperglycemia (usually over 600 mg/dL but may be more than 2000 mg/dL).

Osmotic Diuresis　The degree of osmotic diuresis and dehydration is typically worse in the HHS patient than in the DKA patient because of the extreme levels of hyperglycemia associated with HHS. The patient experiences severe dehydration and hypotension. Excess glucose accumulates in the extracellular spaces because it cannot be transported into the cells or metabolized normally, resulting in a progressive increase in osmolality. As extracellular osmolality increases, water is pulled from the intracellular spaces into the extracellular spaces. When the level of hyperglycemia eventually exceeds the renal threshold, osmotic diuresis significantly increases, precipitating progressive dehydration of intracellular and extracellular spaces with substantial loss of electrolytes.

Neurological Alterations　While both DKA and HHS can cause mental status changes, the patient with DKA is often fully alert throughout the entire crisis unless the metabolic derangements are severe. HHS is associated with more severe neurologic signs (e.g., stupor, coma, or seizures), and mental status changes may progress insidiously over a period of days. There is a direct relationship between serum osmolality and level of consciousness; thus, as osmolality increases, the patient with HHS will develop increasing deterioration of LOC. If the serum osmolality increases to 320 mOsm/L or higher, the patient may develop hyperosmolar coma.

Absence of Ketoacidosis　Failure of the patient with type 2 diabetes to develop significant ketoacidosis is attributed to the ability of the pancreas to produce sufficient insulin to prevent or minimize lipolysis and formation of ketone bodies but not enough insulin to effectively prevent increasing serum glucose levels. Without significant increases in circulating ketone bodies, ketoacidosis usually does not develop; if present, it is usually minor.

Clinical Presentation

On admission, it is important to differentiate whether the patient is experiencing DKA or HHS. While these two hyperglycemic crises share many clinical features, others can help distinguish them. Table 33–8 presents a comparison of diagnostic criteria for DKA and HHS.

Quality and Safety
Differentiating HHS and DKA

Hyperosmolar hyperglycemic nonketotic syndrome (HHS) is often difficult to differentiate from diabetic ketoacidosis (DKA), which leads to misdiagnosis and inappropriate management. A nurse-based practice-improvement project was developed to (1) determine the frequency with which HHS is correctly diagnosed and (2) develop an evidence-based protocol to assist with making a differential diagnosis of HHS. A review of 991 patient records was conducted, using the ICD-9 codes for hyperglycemia, HHS, and DKA. Investigators found that HHS was correctly identified in only 5% of patients (n = 9) with type 2 diabetes. Of the patients who were misdiagnosed as having DKA, 39% (n = 74) exhibited the clinical features of HHS, and 36% (n = 24) required readmission within 2 weeks. The investigators concluded that development of an HHS-specific diagnostic algorithm is essential to decrease misdiagnosis, provide appropriate management, decrease mortality, and decrease length of stay and readmission occurrences. Based on their findings and a review of literature, the practice-improvement project group developed an algorithm for making a differential diagnosis of DKA versus HHS based on type of diabetes and serum laboratory tests (C-peptides, serum glucose, serum osmolality, pH, anion gap, bicarbonate, and ketones) (McCombs, Appel, & Ward, 2014).

Table 33–8 A Comparison of DKA and HHS

	DKA	HHS
Age of patient	Usually less than 45 years old	Usually less than 60 years old
Associated type of diabetes	Primarily type 1	Primarily type 2
Plasma glucose level	Greater than 250 mg/dL but less than 600 mg/dL	Greater than 600 mg/dL
Mental status	Varies with severity	Stuporous or comatose
Bicarbonate concentration	Low (10–18)	Normal (greater than 18)
Ketone bodies	Positive (++++)	Negative or low (+/−)
Arterial pH	6.8–7.3	Greater than 7.3
Serum osmolality	Variable but typically 300–320 mOsm/kg	Usually greater than 320 mOsm/kg
Mortality	Less than 1%*	5%–20% mortality
Subsequent course	Insulin therapy required in virtually all cases	Insulin therapy may not be required
Anion gap	High	Normal to slightly elevated

*Mortality is significantly higher in extremes of age.
SOURCE: Data from Powers (2014b).

Section Four Review

1. Which statement is correct regarding HHS?
   A. It has a high mortality rate.
   B. It is most common in type 1 diabetes.
   C. It causes severe fluid volume overload.
   D. Death occurs from severe metabolic acidosis.

2. Common precipitating events causing HHS include which conditions?
   A. Hemodialysis
   B. Infection
   C. Loop diuretic therapy
   D. High fat diet

3. HHS does not cause ketosis for what reason?
   A. Lipolysis does not occur.
   B. Protein catabolism is occurring.
   C. High glucagon levels prevent it.
   D. Hyperglycemia is not sufficiently severe.

4. Which statement regarding the differences between DKA and HHS is correct?
   A. The onset of HHS is faster.
   B. Dehydration is less severe in HHS.
   C. Hyperosmolality is more severe in HHS.
   D. Mental status changes more rapidly in HHS.

Answers: 1. A, 2. B, 3. A, 4. C

Section Five: Management of Hyperglycemic Crises

Many of the medical goals and treatment strategies for management of patients with DKA and HHS are the same. In fact, with its most recent update of the protocols for management of DKA and HHS, the ADA consensus statement combined the two separate protocols into one. A general summary of major aspects of this protocol is presented in Table 33–9.

Collaborative Interventions

The ADA protocol for management of adult patients with DKA or HHS includes recommendations regarding IV fluids, insulin therapy, and electrolyte replacement (e.g., sodium bicarbonate, potassium, sodium, and phosphate)

(Joint British Diabetes Societies Inpatient Care Group [JBDS ICG], 2013; Kitabchi, Umpierrez, Miles, & Fisher, 2009).

Treatment Goals for Hyperglycemic Crises

1. Restore intravascular fluid volume.
2. Correct electrolyte imbalances.
3. Clear ketones and correct acidosis.
4. Normalize serum glucose.
5. Closely monitor patient's status.
6. Identify precipitating cause.
7. Prevent further complications.

Restore Intravascular Fluid Volume. Fluid resuscitation is the highest priority when a person first presents with a hyperglycemic crisis. Osmotic diuresis precipitated by elevated glucose levels can severely deplete body fluids

Table 33–9 General Management of Diabetic Ketoacidosis and Hyperglycemic Hyperosmolar State*

Therapies	Determinants of Therapy	Management
IV fluids	Hydration status and corrected serum sodium level	**Mild dehydration:** Depending on corrected serum Na$^+$, administer 0.45% or 0.9% NaCl at rate of 250–500 mL/hr. **Severe hypovolemia:** Administer 0.9% NaCl at rate of 1 L/hr. **Cardiogenic shock:** Initiate hemodynamic monitoring and vasopressor drugs. **Endpoint therapy:** Switch to 5% dextrose in 0.45% NaCl when serum glucose reaches 200 mg/dL (DKA) or 300 mg/dL (HHS).
Bicarbonate	pH	**pH less than 6.9:** Administer IV sodium bicarbonate with potassium chloride (KCl), and repeat (and re-evaluate serum K$^+$) every 2 hrs until pH rises to 7.0 or higher or anion gap normalizes.
Insulin (Regular)	Serum glucose level	**Option 1:** Administer 0.1 unit/kg (IV bolus) then 0.1 unit/kg continuous infusion. **Option 2:** Administer 0.14 unit/kg/hr continuous infusion. **Both options:** After 1 hr, if serum glucose has not decreased by 10% or more, administer 0.14 unit/kg and return to previous (option 1 or 2) therapy. **Endpoint therapy (DKA):** Reduce dose of IV insulin therapy (or begin administering rapid-acting insulin subcutaneously) when serum glucose is 200 mg/dL. Maintain serum glucose between 150–200 mg/dL until DKA is resolved. **Endpoint therapy (HHS):** Reduce IV insulin dose when serum glucose is 300 mg/dL. Maintain serum glucose at 200–300 mg/dL until patient becomes alert.
Potassium	Serum potassium level	**K$^+$ greater than 5.2 mEq/L:** Check levels every 2 hrs. **K$^+$ less than 3.3 mEq/L:** Hold insulin; administer KCl 20–30 mEq/L per hour. **Endpoint therapy:** K$^+$ of greater than 3.3 mEq/L; maintain K$^+$ at 4–5 mEq/L; add 20–30 mEq of K$^+$ to each liter of IV fluid.
Other	Kidney and electrolyte status	Periodic monitoring of lab values: Check glucose, BUN and creatinine, and electrolytes every 2–4 hours while unstable.

*The detailed ADA Protocol for Management of Adult Patients with DKA and HHS is available in Kitabchi et al. (2009).
SOURCE: Data from Kitabchi et al. (2009).

sufficiently to cause hypovolemic shock. The patient's initial management requires rapid rehydration upon determination of the patient's current hydration status. The dehydration resulting from HHS is usually significantly more severe than seen in DKA due to the extreme hyperglycemia. Initial fluid replacement will be with one-half normal (0.45%) or normal (0.9%) saline. As soon as the serum glucose level is decreased to approximately 200 mg/dL, IV fluids containing glucose (e.g., 5% dextrose with 0.45% NaCl [D$_5$ ½ NS]) are started, replacing normal saline intravenous fluids. The patient will receive nothing by mouth until the crisis state is resolved.

The nurse is responsible for ensuring that the correct IV fluids are hung to run at the ordered rate. Hydration status is closely monitored throughout the fluid resuscitation period. Vital signs, intake and output balance, skin turgor, and heart and lung assessments are performed frequently to assess hydration progress and ensure that complications of fluid overload do not occur.

Correct Electrolyte Imbalances. Potassium, sodium, and phosphate are three of the major electrolytes requiring replacement during a DKA episode. Care is taken in managing potassium replacement because serum levels decrease when potassium shifts back into the cells as the acidotic state is corrected and normal urine output is regained. In cases of severe hypokalemia, insulin treatment should be delayed until potassium levels are greater than 3.3 mEq/L to decrease the risk for cardiac dysrhythmias or cardiac arrest. Sodium is replaced primarily during the initial rehydration phase of treatment using 0.9% and 0.45% normal saline IV solutions. Phosphate, a buffer, may become depleted during periods of acidosis, particularly if

the acidosis is prolonged. Adequate levels of phosphate are important in managing the acidosis. Phosphate replacement therapy is not routinely recommended; however, it may be considered in specific situations: serum phosphate less than 1 mg/dL, cardiac dysfunction, anemia, or respiratory depression (Kitabchi et al., 2009).

The nurse is responsible for ensuring that ordered labs are drawn and that abnormal electrolyte levels are immediately relayed to the provider. The nurse assesses the patient for signs and symptoms of electrolyte imbalances, closely monitors the cardiac rhythm, and is responsible for ensuring that electrolyte replacements are carried out as ordered. The nurse then assesses the patient's status for therapeutic and nontherapeutic effects of the replacement electrolytes.

Clear Ketones and Correct Acidosis. Diabetic ketoacidosis often corrects itself with the use of insulin, electrolyte therapy, and IV fluid replacement. Sodium bicarbonate (NaHCO$_3$) was once the drug of choice for rapid correction of most metabolic acidosis problems. However, with DKA, treatment with sodium bicarbonate is controversial and not recommended for routine management because as ketone levels decrease, bicarbonate levels increase. When ketoacidosis is corrected too rapidly, it can precipitate cerebrospinal fluid (CSF) acidosis, causing potentially severe neurologic complications. Cerebrospinal fluid acidosis is difficult to correct because sodium bicarbonate does not cross the blood–brain barrier.

Sodium bicarbonate may be recommended with severe cases of metabolic acidosis if the arterial pH is 6.9 or less. In such cases, it is recommended to infuse 100 mmol over a 2-hour period in a water solution with 20 mEq of potassium chloride, repeating as needed until the pH rises above 7.0.

The nurse is responsible for ensuring that the IV fluid, electrolyte, and insulin therapeutic strategy is carried out as ordered and closely monitoring the effects of the therapy, including ketone levels, bicarbonate, and pH. The nurse keeps the healthcare provider informed of changes in the patient's status and follows the agency's hyperglycemic crisis protocol or provider orders.

Normalize Serum Glucose. Correction of the hyperglycemic state depends on careful use of intravenous (IV) insulin. During the crisis state, only short-acting insulins are used because of their rapid onset and short half-life, which facilitate better titration control and rapid reduction of glucose levels. Insulin management generally is via continuous, low-dose IV infusion with regular insulin. An initial bolus of insulin is not necessary; however, the American Diabetes Association (ADA) protocol includes it as one option. The recommended insulin dose is 0.1 unit/kg/hr continuous IV drip with an increase to 0.14 unit/kg/hr if the patient's blood glucose does not reduce by 10% over the first hour of treatment. The patient's glucose levels should be monitored hourly while receiving insulin IV. The protocol provides recommendations for when and how the patient should be switched to subcutaneous insulin therapy.

The nurse is responsible for ensuring that the insulin therapy strategy is carried out as ordered and closely monitoring serum glucose. The nurse keeps the healthcare provider informed of changes in the patient's status and follows the agency's hyperglycemic crisis protocol or provider orders. As the patient's blood glucose approaches normal and ketosis is resolved, the nurse can anticipate a change in insulin and/or IV fluid orders. Also, as the glucose level normalizes, the nurse should monitor the patient closely for development of hypoglycemia as IV and subcutaneously administered insulin dosages change.

Closely Monitor Patient's Status. The patient's status will be closely monitored throughout the crisis period, and the patient is often admitted to an intensive care setting. Initially, frequent close monitoring of serum pH, glucose, ketone bodies (e.g., acetone and β-hydroxybutyrate), osmolality, anion gap, and electrolytes is necessary. An electrocardiogram (ECG) and cardiac monitoring will be ordered to monitor serum potassium effects on the heart. A culture and gram stain of potentially infected secretions or fluids confirm the type of organism so that appropriate IV antibiotic therapy can be administered.

The aggressive emergency treatment plan requires close monitoring of the patient during initial therapy, evaluating status changes for possible early signs of complications. Frequent drawing of blood samples is necessary to monitor the changing status of the patient's metabolic derangements. These blood samples may be drawn by the nurse for point-of-care serum analysis or may be drawn by laboratory personnel and sent to the laboratory for analysis. Either way, the nurse is responsible for ensuring that the blood tests are drawn and abnormal values are communicated to the healthcare provider with appropriate follow-up of orders.

Identify Precipitating Cause. A key to successful management of a hyperglycemic crisis is finding and aggressively treating the underlying cause. If an infection is the underlying problem, antibiotic therapy is initiated, and if a wound is present (such as an open ulcer), it may be surgically debrided of necrotic tissue to facilitate healing. The pathophysiologic effects of diabetes prevent the patient from healing well, which increases the patient's risk for developing a worsening infection or sepsis.

The nurse obtains a history and performs a physical assessment to investigate potential sources of the triggering event. Clinical findings that suggest a possible etiology of the precipitating cause are communicated to the healthcare provider. Once the underlying cause is identified, the nurse carries out orders and evaluates the patient for therapeutic and nontherapeutic effects of those orders.

Prevent Further Complications. The patient history should include questions regarding chronic medical conditions and current medication regimen that may impact the hyperglycemic crisis therapeutic plan. For example, if the patient has chronic cardiac disease, fluid resuscitation may require careful adjustment to reduce the risk of heart failure. Effective and rapid reversal of the hyperglycemic crisis reduces the risk of the complications that can arise as the severity of the hyperglycemic crisis worsens, such as kidney failure, cardiac arrest, or irreversible neurological damage.

For a summary of major nursing considerations of patients during the acute phase of DKA or HHS, refer to the "Nursing Care: The Patient in a Hyperglycemic Crisis" feature.

Nursing Care
The Patient in a Hyperglycemic Crisis

Expected Patient Outcomes and Related Interventions*

Outcome 1: Regains normovolemic state

Assess and compare to established norms, patient baselines, and trends.

Cardiovascular status: arterial blood pressure, heart rate, and rhythm

Hemodynamic status (as available)—cardiac output and cardiac index, CVP, PAP, PAWP

Urine output, intake-to-output ratio

Laboratory test results: BUN, creatinine, hemoglobin, hematocrit

Jugular vein status (flat or collapsed)

Report abnormal assessments and worsening trends

Interventions to replace fluids

Insert large-bore intravenous catheter; central line may be indicated.

Initiate fluid resuscitation with 0.9% NaCl based on degree of hypovolemia (see Table 33–9).

Monitor for therapeutic and nontherapeutic effects of fluid replacement therapy.

Maintain urine output at greater than 50 mL/hr.

Encourage intake of fluids if fluid volume deficit exists.

Administer related drug therapy and monitor for therapeutic and nontherapeutic effects.

Possible vasopressor therapy for severe hypovolemia if unresponsive to fluid replacement

Outcome 2: Normalization of glucose and ketones

Assess and compare to established norms, patient baselines, and trends.

Capillary glucose, serum and urine ketones

ABG (monitor pH), anion gap

Kussmaul respirations (elevated rate and depth of breathing)

Level of consciousness

Intervene to normalize glucose and ketones.

Monitor for hyperglycemia and ketonemia, ketonuria, and hypoglycemia.

Initiate insulin therapy (intravenous route).

Monitor for therapeutic and nontherapeutic effects of insulin replacement therapy.

Monitor and document dietary intake.

Encourage intake of prescribed diet.

Administer related drug therapy and monitor for therapeutic and nontherapeutic effects.

Insulin therapy (see Table 33–9)

Outcome 3: Normalization of electrolytes

Assess and compare to established norms, patient baselines, and trends.

Serum electrolytes (focus on potassium and bicarbonate trends)

ABG (monitor pH and bicarbonate)

Signs and symptoms of metabolic acidosis

Intervene to regain electrolyte stability.

Monitor laboratory (e.g., serum electrolytes) and other test results and report abnormal results or worsening trends.

Monitor for therapeutic and nontherapeutic effects of electrolyte and acidosis drug therapy; report abnormal effects.

Monitor ECG for changes consistent with electrolyte imbalance, such as dysrhythmias, *T* wave changes, *ST* segment changes.

Encourage intake of appropriate nutrients.

Restrict intake of undesirable nutrients based on electrolyte levels.

See "Bicarbonate" and "Potassium" in Table 33–9.

Administer related drug therapy and monitor for therapeutic and nontherapeutic effects.

Possible potassium, bicarbonate, or other electrolyte replacement

Outcome 4: Prevention of future hyperglycemic crisis episodes

Assess and compare to established norms, patient baselines, and trends.

Identify etiology of current hyperglycemic episode.

Identify learning needs of patient and family regarding diabetes, DKA or HHS, and prevention of future occurrences.

Interventions to prevent future hyperglycemic crisis episodes

Provide diabetes and DKA or HHS teaching, based on assessed knowledge deficits.

*Note: It is crucial to rapidly identify and treat the underlying cause of the hyperglycemic crisis to improve patient outcomes.

Section Five Review

1. Which intervention has priority in the management of the client with a hyperglycemic crisis?
   A. Correct acidosis
   B. Fluid resuscitation
   C. Initiating insulin therapy
   D. Normalization of serum glucose

2. Protocols typically recommend initial fluid replacement using which IV fluids? (Select all that apply.)
   A. 5% dextrose, 0.45% normal saline
   B. Lactated Ringer's solution
   C. 0.9% normal saline
   D. 0.45% normal saline
   E. 5% dextrose in water

3. Which serum electrolyte is the primary focus when managing hyperglycemic crises?
   A. Potassium
   B. Sodium
   C. Chloride
   D. Magnesium

4. During a hyperglycemic crisis, ADA recommended insulin therapy consists of which of the following?
   A. Slow-acting insulin
   B. Short-acting insulin
   C. Medium-acting insulin
   D. Long-acting insulin

Answers: 1. B, 2. (C, D), 3. A, 4. B

Section Six: Insulin Therapy During Crises

Individuals who experience a hyperglycemic crisis require insulin therapy as a key part of their emergency treatment strategy. This section addresses several insulin administration concepts that are important in high-acuity settings, including continuous low-dose IV insulin infusion, subcutaneous insulin, and adjusted or sliding-scale insulin. Intensive insulin therapy (IIT) is also presented here, not as therapy for hyperglycemic crises but, rather, as a therapy to control blood glucose in critically ill patients. IIT is also a major cause of severe hypoglycemia in critically ill patients.

Continuous Low-dose Intravenous Insulin Infusion

Historically, treatment of DKA and HHS in their early phases consisted of administering large doses of insulin (hundreds of units) (Fleckman, 1993). Over time, clinicians found that continuous low-dose IV insulin made regulation easier and provided better control of glucose levels. Other advantages of low-dose IV insulin infusions include fewer complications associated with hypokalemia and hypoglycemia, as well as rapid rate of insulin dissipation.

During a hyperglycemic crisis, a continuous infusion of regular insulin may be ordered to provide better control of serum insulin levels. When preparing to administer IV insulin, it is important to remember the following:

- Only regular insulin is administered intravenously.
- Insulin binds to polyvinylchloride in IV bags and tubing, lowering the insulin concentration in the fluid. One form of insulin, Velosulin, has been buffered with phosphate, which prevents the insulin from binding to plastic tubing.
- Blood glucose levels must be monitored frequently, at least hourly, to adequately monitor the effects of therapy and to avoid hypoglycemia.

Sliding-scale Insulin Administration

During periods of physiologic stress, glucose levels may be extremely unstable, requiring supplemental insulin in addition to the patient's usual insulin coverage. Treatment of hospitalized type 1 and type 2 diabetic patients requires an insulin regimen that is responsive to glycemic variation secondary to the admitting condition and its treatment, including surgery. During hospitalization for an acute illness, glucose control in type 2 diabetic patients often cannot be managed using their usual oral antidiabetic medications because of the risk of hypoglycemia from not eating and the slower response of these medications to correct hyperglycemia. Consequently, insulin dosage must reflect current blood glucose levels. Orders may be written to adjust (titrate) the insulin dose to specific glucose levels. This type of insulin regimen is called *adjusted* or *sliding-scale insulin* coverage. Table 33–10 provides an example of a sliding-scale insulin order.

Table 33–10 Example of Sliding-scale Insulin Regimen

Blood Glucose Level	Regular Insulin Dose (Subcutaneously)
200–250 mg/dL	5 units
251–300 mg/dL	10 units
301–350 mg/dL	12 units
351–400 mg/dL	15 units
> 400 mg/dL	Call provider

It is recommended that sliding-scale insulin administration be carried out based on blood glucose rather than urine glucose measurements. Urine glucose does not reflect hour-by-hour changes in serum glucose levels. Thus, its value for tight glucose control is diminished.

Intensive Insulin Therapy

Stress hyperglycemia refers to elevated blood glucose levels that develop because of the stress response. Most patients in critical care units develop some degree of hyperglycemia (Bassily-Marcus & Khachaturova, 2016). During times of crisis, the stress response triggers an outflow of stress hormones, particularly cortisol, which significantly increase blood glucose levels. Multiple studies (e.g., Capes, Hunt, Malmberg, & Gerstein, 2000; Kitabchi et al., 2009; Malmberg, Norhammar, Wedel, & Ryden, 1999; Van den Berghe et al., 2001) found that hyperglycemia in ICU patients increases mortality and the risk of complications.

Initial recommendations in the early 2000s called for extremely tight glycemic control with a target goal of 80 mg/dL to 110 mg/dL (Van den Berghe et al., 2001); however, it became evident that this degree of control actually increased patient mortality. Current recommendations from the American Association of Clinical Endocrinologists (AACE) and the American Diabetes Association (ADA) are to maintain glucose levels at 140 mg/dL to 180 mg/dL for critically ill patients with the understanding the patients might benefit most with glucose levels maintained at the lower end of that range (American Diabetes Association [ADA], 2009).

Section Six Review

1. Continuous low-dose IV insulin therapy is the treatment of choice for hyperglycemic crises for which reason?
   - A. It reduces acidosis.
   - B. It is easy to titrate.
   - C. It is long acting.
   - D. It stabilizes sodium levels.

2. The recommendation by AACE and ADA for intensive insulin therapy is to control glucose levels between which parameters?
   - A. 80–110 mg/dL
   - B. 100–140 mg/dL
   - C. 140–180 mg/dL
   - D. 180–200 mg/dL

3. The major complication of intensive insulin therapy is which of the following?
   A. Severe hypoglycemia
   B. Cerebral edema
   C. Thromboembolism
   D. Stroke

4. Adjusted or sliding-scale insulin therapy is primarily used for which purpose?
   A. As an alternative therapy during an HHS episode
   B. To control glucose levels in type 1 diabetics during surgical procedures
   C. As an alternative therapy during a DKA episode
   D. To temporarily treat stress hyperglycemia in type 2 diabetes

Answers: 1. B, 2. C, 3. A, 4. D

Section Seven: Acute Care Implications of Chronic Complications

Many factors, such as preexisting chronic diseases, influence patient outcomes in the acutely ill. Diabetes is a chronic disease that profoundly affects patient outcomes because of the many acute and chronic complications that can result from it. Patients with diabetes may be admitted to the hospital with a primary diagnosis directly related to their diabetes, or they may be admitted with a diagnosis completely unrelated to their chronic diabetic disorder. Regardless of the admitting diagnosis, the patient's diabetes has broad implications for nursing care. For this reason, when a patient with diabetes is admitted to a high-acuity hospital setting, the nursing history and assessment should include an evaluation of the diabetes, medication regimen, and presence of any chronic complications.

Major long-term complications of diabetes include heart disease and stroke, hypertension, blindness, kidney disease, nervous system disease, and peripheral vascular disease (that may result in the need for amputation) (Centers for Disease Control and Prevention [CDC], 2016b). These complications stem from three different underlying chronic pathologic processes, including peripheral neuropathies, microvascular disease, and macrovascular disease. This section presents an overview of major long-term complications associated with diabetes mellitus and acute-care nursing implications.

Diabetic Peripheral Neuropathies

Peripheral neuropathies are the most common complications of diabetes mellitus. They begin early in the course of the disease, affecting both type 1 and type 2 diabetics. Peripheral neuropathies primarily alter sensory perception. The underlying cause of neuropathies is poorly understood. They may result from thickening of vessel walls that supply peripheral nerves, thus impairing nutrition to the nerves. They also may result from a segmental demyelinization that results in slowed or disrupted conduction. There is also some evidence that sorbitol may accumulate in the nerve cells, impairing conduction. Whatever the cause, the result is an alteration in sensory perception.

Neuropathies initially may cause pain or abnormal sensations or both. As nerve degeneration progresses, the patient may experience loss of the ability to discriminate fine touch, a decrease in proprioception, and local anesthesia. The autonomic nervous system also may be affected. As the myelin sheath undergoes degenerative changes, functions governed by the autonomic nerves are affected adversely. The patient may experience an increase in gut motility and diarrhea, postural hypotension, or other autonomic nervous system–related complications. The neuropathies experienced by diabetics vary in type, severity, and clinical manifestations. Because of this diversity, it is not possible to predict which neuropathy any individual will develop.

Acute Care Implications Patients with diabetes should be assessed for the presence and degree of peripheral neuropathy. The presence of a diminished sense of touch and pain may mask injury or infection. The patient must be protected from injury at all times to prevent damage to affected tissues. The diabetic patient must also be protected from hyperthermic burns. Excessive heat may not be sensed, which increases the risk of burns by heating pads, hyperthermia blankets, and bathing. Some neuropathies are associated with progressive, permanent damage to the neurons. However, others are reversible when good glucose control is maintained.

Microvascular Disease

Microvascular disease is associated with capillary membrane thickening, which causes **microangiopathy** (small blood vessel disease). As the capillary membrane thickens, the tissues become increasingly hypoperfused, and organs become hypoxic and ischemic. Prolonged ischemia eventually causes **infarction** (death of tissue). The degree of microvascular disease may be influenced most by the duration of diabetes rather than the level of glucose control. Two organs at high risk for microvascular disease secondary to diabetes mellitus are the retina of the eyes (retinopathy) and the kidneys (nephropathy).

Retinopathy Diabetic retinopathy is responsible for a significant portion of newly diagnosed blindness in the United States. It is caused by an underlying microangiopathy of the retina, leading to retinal microvascular occlusion. Once occlusion exists, the retina undergoes development of increasing areas of ischemia and infarction,

Emerging Evidence

- A retrospective review of 244 adult patients who entered the ED in a large academic-based medical center focused on management of hypoglycemia and identification of characteristics related to refractory and recurrent hypoglycemia. Investigators found that 12% of patients with a serum glucose of 50 mg/dL or lower were not treated in the ED for hypoglycemia. Point-of-care glucose testing decreased the time required for receiving treatment when compared to serum glucose testing. Refractory or recurrent hypoglycemia was found in about one third of the patients, with infection being the only associated characteristic with refractory or recurrent hypoglycemia. Patients with recurrent hypoglycemia were less likely to receive dextrose-containing IV solutions when compared to those without recurrent hypoglycemia *(Bilhimer, Treu, & Acquisto, 2017)*.

- A retrospective records review was conducted of 12 adult patients in a large academic-based medical center who developed DKA within 90 days after undergoing bariatric surgery. Investigators found that 8 of 12 (67%) patients had a history of type 1 diabetes and 4 had type 2 diabetes. All patients had poor glycemic control prior to surgery, and 8 patients (67%), had a history of problems with medical noncompliance or inadequate insulin therapy. The median time for development of DKA was 12 days postsurgery. Three patients developed DKA prior to hospital discharge, with major precipitating factors being infection, inadequate insulin coverage, stress of surgery, and poor oral intake. Clinical presentation of DKA in the study cohort included nausea and vomiting, as well as abdominal pain, which may be erroneously identified as a surgical complication (e.g., abscess or leak) *(Aminian et al., 2016)*.

- A large population-based cohort study was conducted to investigate the association between specifically identified critical illnesses and frequency of newly diagnosed type 2 diabetes. The critical illnesses of interest were acute myocardial infarction (AMI), stroke, septicemia, and septic shock. Investigators found that patients with a diagnosis of septicemia or septic shock were at highest risk for developing newly diagnosed type 2 diabetes followed by acute myocardial infarction *(Hsu et al., 2016)*.

- A large observational cohort study of hospitalized patients admitted with acute illnesses was conducted to explore whether relative or absolute hyperglycemia was more strongly related to critical illness. Relative hyperglycemia was identified using the stress hyperglycemia ratio (SHR) (i.e., admission glucose ÷ estimated average glucose [from glycosylated hemoglobin]). Absolute hyperglycemia was identified using serum glucose measurements in mmol/L. Patients with a critical illness were identified based on admission to critical care or in-hospital death. Investigators concluded that SHR is a better biomarker of critical illness than absolute hyperglycemia and that SHR identifies patients at risk for development of critical illness *(Roberts et al., 2015)*.

eventually leading to blindness. Damage occurs in two complex stages. Stage I is associated with increased capillary permeability, aneurysm formation, and hemorrhage. Stage II is associated with increasing retinal ischemia and eventual infarction, causing blindness. Diabetic retinopathy is associated with both type 1 and type 2 diabetes.

Acute Care Implications. The acutely ill diabetic patient may have moderate to severe visual impairment. Early assessment of visual status is important, either by questioning the patient directly or by interviewing the family. Medical and nursing management and teaching must be altered to meet the needs of a visually impaired patient. In the high-acuity patient, blindness affects pupillary changes and must be taken into consideration when performing a neurologic assessment. A visually impaired patient in a critical care environment may have more difficulty making sense of distracting noises and equipment surrounding the bedside. Frequent explanation and reorientation may be necessary.

Nephropathy Diabetic nephropathy is a disease of the glomeruli. The glomerular basement membrane becomes thickened, resulting in intracapillary glomerulosclerosis (hardening and thickening of the glomeruli). Glomeruli become enlarged and eventually are destroyed, ultimately resulting in renal failure. As the degree of renal injury increases, the patient may require a decreased insulin dosage to prevent hypoglycemia. Reduced renal function decreases the ability of the kidneys to metabolize insulin. Insulin not metabolized remains available to facilitate glucose metabolism.

Acute Care Implications. The acutely ill patient with some degree of preexisting renal impairment is at risk for further impairment from hypotensive episodes, nephrotoxic drug therapy, or the multisystemic complications associated with many acute illnesses. Kidney function must be carefully monitored at regular intervals. Drug therapy may need to be altered based on kidney function. Kidney failure, as a disease entity, has its own set of actual and potential complications.

Macrovascular Disease

Macrovascular disease (**macroangiopathy**) refers to atherosclerosis. **Atherosclerosis** is a form of arteriosclerosis (thickening and hardening of arterial walls), characterized by plaque deposits of lipids, fibrous connective tissue, calcium, and other blood substances. Atherosclerosis affects only medium and large arteries (excluding arterioles). The cause of rapid development of atherosclerosis in the diabetic patient is related to altered fat metabolism.

Macrovascular disease is associated with the development of coronary artery disease, peripheral vascular disease, stroke, and increased risk of infection. Type 2 diabetes is more closely associated with macrovascular diseases than type 1 diabetes. Peripheral vascular disease and increased risk of infection have important implications in the care of the acutely ill patient.

Peripheral Vascular Disease Progressive atherosclerotic changes in peripheral arterial circulation lead to decreasing arterial blood flow to peripheral tissues. As the disease progresses, small arteries become occluded, precipitating a tissue ischemia or infarction sequence of events. In the type 2 diabetic, this is typically noted as small isolated patches of gangrene, particularly on the feet and toes. As circulation becomes increasingly compromised, areas of gangrene become larger and amputation may be required.

Acute Care Implications. The patient with peripheral vascular disease is at increased risk for complications secondary to poor tissue perfusion and loss of skin integrity. Of high concern in the acutely ill patient is the development of pressure ulcers and infection, each of which could lead to gangrene and possible amputation. Careful limb positioning, excellent skin hygiene, and close monitoring of skin integrity are extremely important.

Increased Risk of Infection

As discussed in Section Three, the diabetic patient is at increased risk for development of infection for a variety of reasons (refer to Table 33–6) related to the diabetes disease

process and chronic vascular complications. Infection may be the triggering event leading to admission to the hospital, or infection can occur as a complication of hospitalization.

Acute Care Implications   The acutely ill diabetic patient is at increased risk for the development of severe, difficult-to-treat infections. Any infection, no matter how minor, may become life-threatening in this population. Close monitoring for infection and rapid, aggressive interventions are needed. Remember that decreased kidney function may be a complicating factor in aggressive antibiotic therapy. Wound healing is impaired in the diabetic for several reasons. Impaired tissue perfusion, especially in the distal extremities, interferes with healing in those areas because of lack of circulation and tissue hypoxia. Hyperglycemic states adversely affect wound healing by interfering with collagen concentrations in a wound. Good control of blood glucose significantly facilitates wound healing.

Section Seven Review

1. Peripheral neuropathies primarily affect which functions?
   A. Motor functions
   B. Sensory functions
   C. Optic functions
   D. Vascular functions

2. Microvascular diseases are associated with which of the following?
   A. Deposits of lipoproteins
   B. Deposits of calcium products
   C. Large blood vessel disease
   D. Small blood vessel disease

3. Diabetic retinopathy causes blindness as a result of what condition?
   A. Glucose deposits on the retina
   B. Thickening of the retina
   C. Destruction of the optic nerve
   D. Infarction of retinal tissue

4. Diabetes increases a client's chance of infection as a result of which of the following?
   A. Abnormal white blood cells
   B. Abnormal platelet function
   C. Slow proliferation of pathogens
   D. Decreased body fluid glucose levels

Answers: 1. B, 2. D, 3. D, 4. A

Clinical Reasoning Checkpoint

Marcel M., 32 years old, is brought into the emergency department by his wife. She informs the nurse that her husband has been not been feeling well over the past few days with a gastrointestinal problem and that his mental state has slowly shifted from being anxious and "foggy headed" to drowsy. About 1 hour prior to arrival at the ED, Marcel reportedly experienced a seizure. His wife relates that her husband is a type 1 diabetic who has been on insulin most of his life. Over the past 3 days, he has been trying to eat but has been vomiting up his food. He has continued to administer his usual dosage of insulin until today. The nurse suspects that Mr. M. may be experiencing a hypoglycemic crisis.

1. Assuming that Mr. M. has developed a hypoglycemic crisis, what common symptoms would you anticipate finding during your assessment?

2. Briefly explain the pathophysiologic basis for the classic signs and symptoms of hypoglycemia.

3. Mr. M. is now unconscious. What interventions are appropriate at this time?

4. A STAT bedside glucometer reading cannot be obtained at this time. Should Mr. M.'s drug therapy of either glucose or glucagon be held until his blood sugar level is confirmed? Why or why not?

Chapter 33 Review

1. A client is admitted for treatment of diabetes mellitus. History reveals that the client's mother also has diabetes. The client was diagnosed at age 32 and has required daily insulin injections since the time of diagnosis. The client is 5 feet 5 inches (16.5 meters) tall and weighs 173 pounds (78.6 kg). Which data is most suggestive of type I diabetes?

   1. The client's mother also has diabetes.
   2. The client was diagnosed at age 32.
   3. The client is 5 feet 5 inches (16.5 meters) tall and weighs 173 pounds (78.6 kg).
   4. The client has required daily insulin injections since the time of diagnosis.

2. A client who has type 1 diabetes has been NPO since midnight for a test scheduled for 8:00 a.m. The usual morning insulin was administered. The test has been delayed, and it is now noon. The nurse would monitor for which signs of hypoglycemia? (Select all that apply.)

   1. Slowed thinking
   2. Headache
   3. Fever
   4. Bradycardia
   5. Tingling in extremities

3. A client has experienced and been successfully treated for a hypoglycemic episode while hospitalized. The client says, "What if this happens to me at home? What should I do?" What instruction should the nurse provide?

   1. "You should drink a can of diet cola."
   2. "You should carry a small package of peanuts and eat them if you feel hypoglycemic."
   3. "The best treatment is to avoid becoming hypoglycemic in the first place."
   4. "Eating hard candy or drinking juice is a good method of correcting hypoglycemia."

4. A client with type 1 diabetes is admitted for treatment of influenza. The client is hypotensive and very weak. Which serum glucose level would suggest that this client is in diabetic ketoacidosis?

   1. 85 mg/dL
   2. 100 mg/dL
   3. 145 mg/dL
   4. 260 mg/dL

5. A client who has type 2 diabetes is admitted to the emergency department after becoming unconscious at home. The client's plasma glucose is 910 mg/dL, arterial pH is 7.30, and serum osmolality is 310 mOsm/kg. Which information suggests that this client has hyperglycemic hyperosmolar state (HHS) rather than diabetic ketoacidosis (DKA)?

   1. The client is unconscious.
   2. The client's plasma glucose is 910 mg/dL.
   3. The client's arterial pH is 7.30.
   4. The client's serum osmolality is 310 mOsm/kg.

6. A client is diagnosed with hyperglycemic hyperosmolar state (HHS). Which initial collaborative management technique would the nurse expect to restore this client's intravascular fluid volume?

   1. Encourage the client to drink water by keeping ice water at the bedside.
   2. Offer the client milk or juice at least every hour.
   3. IV infusion of D_5 0.45% NS
   4. IV infusion of 0.45% NS

7. A nurse is providing care to a client receiving intensive insulin therapy (IIT). What is the priority nursing assessment?

   1. Monitor IV site for infiltration.
   2. Monitor availability of IV solution to reduce therapy interruption.
   3. Monitor for hypoglycemia.
   4. Monitor for decrease in urine output.

8. A client with type 2 diabetes reports numbness in the toes of one foot. Which nursing interventions are indicated? (Select all that apply.)

   1. Encourage the client to soak the foot in warm water each evening.
   2. Teach the client to visually assess the feet daily.
   3. Talk to the client about the importance of controlling blood glucose levels.
   4. Have the client sleep with the foot wrapped in an elastic bandage.
   5. Discuss the need for shoes that fit properly.

9. A client with diabetic retinopathy is admitted after suffering a traumatic brain injury. What nursing interventions are indicated? (Select all that apply.)

   1. Assess the client's level of vision.
   2. Frequently reorient the client to the environment.
   3. Defer the visual portions of neurological exams.
   4. Keep the room lights dimmed.
   5. Obtain teaching material written in braille.

10. A client with type 1 diabetes is admitted after developing an infection. Her temperature is 100°F (37.8°C) orally. She responds to verbal stimuli but then immediately closes her eyes and begins groaning. What laboratory result would support a diagnosis of diabetic ketoacidosis in this client?

    1. pH 7.34
    2. Anion gap 18 mEq/L
    3. HCO_3 17 mEq/L
    4. $PaCO_2$ 28 mmHg

Answers to questions found inside your textbook are available on the faculty resources site. Please consult with your instructor.

References

American Association of Clinical Endocrinologists (AACE). (n.d.). Documentation of hypoglycemia treatment protocol (2011 update). Retrieved March 31, 2017, from http://inpatient.aace.com/protocols-and-order-sets

American Diabetes Association (ADA). (2009, May 8). Press release. Diabetes experts issue new recommendations for inpatient glycemic control—call for systemic changes in hospitals nationwide. Retrieved April 1, 2017, from http://www.diabetes.org/newsroom/press-releases/2009/diabetes-experts-issue-new-2009.html

American Diabetes Association (ADA). (2015a). Hypoglycemia (low blood glucose). Retrieved March 29, 2017, from http://www.diabetes.org/living-with-diabetes/treatment-and-care/blood-glucose-control/hypoglycemia-low-blood.html

American Diabetes Association (ADA). (2015b). DKA (ketoacidosis) & ketones. Retrieved April 1, 2017, from http://www.diabetes.org/living-with-diabetes/complications/ketoacidosis-dka.html

American Diabetes Association (ADA). (2016). Position statement: Hypoglycemia. Press release November 22, 2016. Retrieved March 29, 2017, from http://www.diabetes.org/newsroom/press-releases/2016/ada-issues-hypoglycemia-position-statement.html

American Diabetes Association (ADA). (2017a). Glucose concentrations of less than 3.0 mmol/L (54 mg/dL) should be reported in clinical trials: A joint position statement of the American Diabetes Association and the European Association for the Study of Diabetes. *Diabetes Care, 40,* 155–157.

American Diabetes Association (ADA). (2017b). Sec. 14. Diabetes care in the hospital. In Standards of Medical Care in Diabetes—2017. *Diabetes Care, 40*(Suppl. 1), S120–S127.

Aminian, A., Kashyap, S. R., Burguera, B., Punchai, S., Sharma, G., Froylich, D., . . . Schauer, P. R. (2016). Incidence and clinical features of diabetic ketoacidosis after bariatric and metabolic surgery. Retrieved April 2, 2017, from http://care.diabetesjournals.org.ezproxy.uky.edu/content/39/4/e50

Avichal, D. (2017). Hyperosmolar hyperglycemic state: Epidemiology. Retrieved April 1, 2017, from http://emedicine.medscape.com/article/1914705-overview#a5

Bassily-Marcus, A., & Khachaturova, I. (2016). Chapter 74: Controversies—Is glucose control relevant? In J. M. Oropello, S. M. Pastores, V. Kvetan (Eds.), *Critical Care.* Retrieved April 1, 2017, from http://accessmedicine.mhmedical.com.ezproxy.uky.edu/content.aspx?bookid=1944&sectionid=143521451

Bilhimer, M. H., Treu, C. N., & Acquisto, N. M. (2017). Current practice of hypoglycemia management in the ED. *American Journal of Emergency Medicine, 35*(1), 87–91. Retrieved April 2, 2017, from http://ezproxy.uky.edu/login?url=http://search.ebscohost.com/login.aspx?direct=true&db=c8h&AN=120942089&site=ehost-live&scope=site

Bosse, G. M. (2015). Antidiabetics and hypoglycemics. In R. S. Hoffman, L. S. Nelson, L. R. Goldfrank, M. A. Howland, N. A. Lewin, & N. E. Flomenbaum (Eds.), *Goldfrank's toxicologic emergencies* (9th ed.). Retrieved March 31, 2017, from http://accessemergencymedicine.mhmedical.com.ezproxy.uky.edu/content.aspx?bookid=1163&sectionid=65095317

Capes, S. E., Hunt, D., Malmberg, K., & Gerstein, H. C. (2000). Stress hyperglycemia and increased risk of death after myocardial infarction in patients with and without diabetes: A systematic overview. *The Lancet, 355,* 773–778.

Centers for Disease Control and Prevention (CDC). (2012). Number of deaths for hyperglycemic crises as underlying cause, United States, 1980–2009. Retrieved June 1, 2017, from https://www.cdc.gov/diabetes/statistics/mortalitydka/fnumberofdka.htm

Centers for Disease Control and Prevention (CDC). (2014). Diabetes fact sheets: General information. Atlanta, GA: U.S. Department of Health and Human Services, Centers for Disease Control and Prevention. Retrieved June 9, 2017, from https://www.cdc.gov/diabetes/pdfs/data/2014-report-GeneralInformation.pdf

Centers for Disease Control and Prevention (CDC). (2016a). At a glance 2016—diabetes: Working to reverse the US epidemic. Retrieved June 9, 2017, from https://www.cdc.gov/diabetes/managing/problems.html

Centers for Disease Control and Prevention (CDC). (2016b). Managing diabetes: Prevent complications. Retrieved April 1, 2017, from https://www.cdc.gov/diabetes/managing/problems.html

Clain, J., Ramar, K., & Surani, S. R. (2015). Glucose control in critical care. *World Journal of Diabetes, 6*(9), 1082–1091.

Cryer, P. E. (2004). Diverse causes of hypoglycemia-associated autonomic failure in diabetes. *New England Journal of Medicine, 350*(22), 2272–2279.

Cryer, P. E. (2015). Minimizing hypoglycemia in diabetes. *Diabetes Care, 38,* 1583–1591.

Cryer, P. E., & Davis, S. N. (2014). Chapter 420: Hypoglycemia. In D. L. Kasper, A. S. Fauci, S. L. Hauser, D. L. Longo, J. L. Jameson, & J. Loscalzo (Eds.), *Harrison's principles of internal medicine* (19th ed.). Retrieved March 29, 2017, from http://accessmedicine.mhmedical.com.ezproxy.uky.edu/content.aspx?bookid=1130&sectionid=79753191

Fleckman, A. M. (1993). Diabetic ketoacidosis. *Endocrinology Metabolic Clinics of America, 22*(2), 181–206.

Gosmanov, A. R., Gosmanova, E. O., & Kitabchi, A. E. (2015). Hyperglycemic crises: Diabetic ketoacidosis (DKA), and hyperglycemic hyperosmolar state (HHS). In L. J. De Groot, G. Chrousos, K. Dungan et al. (Eds.), *Endotext* (Internet). Retrieved April 1, 2017, from https://www.ncbi.nlm.nih.gov/books/NBK279052

Goyal, N., & Schlichting, A. B. (2016). Chapter 223: Type 1 diabetes mellitus. In J. E. Tintinalli et al. (Eds.), *Tintinalli's emergency medicine: A comprehensive study guide* (10th ed.). Retrieved March 30, 2017, from http://accessemergencymedicine.mhmedical.com .ezproxy.uky.edu/content.aspx?bookid=1658&sectionid =109443541

Hamdy, O. (2017). Diabetic ketoacidosis: Prognosis. Retrieved April 1, 2017, from http://emedicine .medscape.com/article/118361-overview#a7

Hsu, C. W., Lin, C. S., Chen, S. J., Lin, S. H., Lin, C. L., & Kao, C. H. (2016). Risk of type 2 diabetes mellitus in patients with acute critical illness: A population-based cohort study. *Intensive Care Medicine, 42*(1), 38–45.

Joint British Diabetes Societies Inpatient Care Group (JBDS ICG). (2013). The management of diabetic ketoacidosis in adults. Retrieved April 1, 2017, from http://www.diabetologists-abcd.org.uk/JBDS /JBDS_IP_DKA_Adults_Revised.pdf

Kefer, M. P. (2016). Chapter 129. Diabetic emergencies. In R. K. Cydulka, D. M. Cline, O. Ma, M. T. Fitch, S. Joing, & V. J. Wang (Eds.), *Tintinalli's emergency medicine manual* (8th ed.). Retrieved March 31, 2017, from http:// accessemergencymedicine.mhmedical.com.ezproxy .uky.edu/content.aspx?bookid=1759&sectionid =154655608

Kitabchi, A. E., Umpierrez, G. E., Miles, J. M., & Fisher, J. N. (2009). Consensus statement: Hyperglycemic crises in adult patients with diabetes. *Diabetes Care, 32*(7), 1335–1343. Retrieved August 26, 2012, from http://care.diabetesjournals.org/content/32/7/1335 .full.pdf+html

Laposata, M. (Ed.). (2014). Clinical laboratory reference values. In M. Laposata (Ed.), *Laboratory medicine: The diagnosis of disease in the clinical laboratory*. Retrieved April 1, 2017, from http://accessmedicine.mhmedical .com.ezproxy.uky.edu/content.aspx?bookid =1069&sectionid=60775149

Malmberg, K., Norhammar, A., Wedel, H., & Ryden, L. (1999). Glycometabolic state at admission: Important risk marker of mortality in conventionally treated patients with diabetes mellitus and acute myocardial infarction. *Circulation, 99*, 2626–2632.

McCombs, D. G., Appel, S. J., & Ward, M. E. (2014). Quality improvement report: Expedited diagnosis and management of inpatient hyperosmolar hyperglycemic nonketotic syndrome. *Journal of the American Association of Nurse Practitioners, 27*(8), 426–432.

Nyce, A. L., Lubkin, C. L., & Chansky, M. E. (2016). Chapter 225: Diabetic ketoacidosis. In J. E. Tintinalli, J. Stapczynski, O. Ma, D. M. Yealy, G. D. Meckler, & D. M. Cline (Eds.), *Tintinalli's emergency medicine: A comprehensive study guide* (8th ed.). Retrieved April 1, 2017, from http://accessemergencymedicine .mhmedical.com.ezproxy.uky.edu/content.aspx?bookid =1658&sectionid=109443771

Powers, A. C. (2014a). Chapter 417: Diabetes mellitus: Diagnosis, classification, and pathophysiology. In D. Kasper, A. Fauci, S. Hauser, D. Longo, J. Jameson, & J. Loscalzo (Eds.), *Harrison's Principles of Internal Medicine* (19th ed.). Retrieved March 29, 2017, from http://accessmedicine.mhmedical.com.ezproxy.uky .edu/content.aspx?bookid=1130&sectionid=79752868

Powers, A. C. (2014b). Chapter 418: Diabetes mellitus: Management and therapies. In D. Kasper, A. Fauci, S. Hauser, D. Longo, J. Jameson, & J. Loscalzo (Eds.), *Harrison's principles of internal medicine* (19th ed.). Retrieved April 1, 2017, from http://accessmedicine .mhmedical.com.ezproxy.uky.edu/content.aspx?bookid =1130&sectionid=79752952

Roberts, G. W., Quinn, S. J., Valentine, N., Alhawassi, T., O'Dea, H., Stranks, S. N., . . . Doogue, M. P. (2015). Relative hyperglycemia, a marker of critical illness: Introducing the stress hyperglycemic ratio. *The Journal of Clinical Endocrinology and Metabolism, 100*(12), 4490–4497. doi:10.1210/jc.2015-2660

Van den Berghe, G., Wouters, P., Weekers, F., Verwaest, C., Bruyninckx, F., Shetz, M., . . . Bouillon, R. (2001). Intensive insulin therapy in critically ill patients. *New England Journal of Medicine, 345*(19), 1359–1367.

Chapter 34
Determinants and Assessment of Oxygenation

Learning Outcomes

34.1 Explain the concept of oxygenation.

34.2 Differentiate the components of gas exchange.

34.3 Explain how cardiac output alters oxygen delivery and consumption.

34.4 Describe oxygen consumption in terms of aerobic and anaerobic metabolism.

 xygenation problems may develop as a complication of many diagnoses, particularly in the high-acuity patient population. All tissues are subject to hypoxia if any of the three oxygenation components (pulmonary gas exchange, oxygen delivery, or oxygen consumption) breaks down. If hypoxia is not relieved quickly in the affected tissues, ischemia and cell death result. When hypoxia is isolated to a small area (e.g., ischemic stroke or acute myocardial infarction), ischemic damage is localized; however, if hypoxia is systemic (e.g., acute respiratory failure or shock states), ischemia ultimately affects all tissues. In problems of oxygenation, the nurse assesses and intervenes primarily with two major oxygenation issues: decreased oxygen supply and increased oxygen demand.

This chapter is an introduction to the complex physiologic processes involved in oxygenation. It provides the basis for a better understanding of multisystem disease processes that can profoundly impair oxygenation, such as shock states, severe burns, multiple trauma, systemic inflammatory response syndrome (SIRS), and multiple organ dysfunction syndrome (MODS). The information provided here focuses on the global concept of oxygenation and does not go into depth reviewing material covered elsewhere in the book—in particular, pulmonary gas exchange (Chapter 11: Determinants and Assessment of Pulmonary Function) and cardiac output (Chapter 13: Determinants and Assessment of Cardiac Function). It is recommended that those two chapters be reviewed prior to beginning this one.

Section One: Introduction to Oxygenation

Oxygenation cannot be understood solely by understanding the respiratory or the cardiovascular system. It is a concept of multisystem integration and coordination in the intake, delivery, and use of oxygen for energy metabolism, involving cardiovascular, respiratory, neurologic, hematologic, and metabolic processes.

The term *oxygenation* refers to the use of oxygen for energy through aerobic metabolism. All cells require a continuous energy supply via adenosine triphosphate (ATP) and prefer to use the metabolic process of *oxidative phosphorylation* to obtain the energy (Kibble & Halsey, 2014). Cellular oxidative phosphorylation occurs in the cell mitochondria. Mitochondria are organelles located within cells that act as powerhouses, producing energy for cells to carry out their activities. Through the Krebs (or citric acid) cycle, respiratory enzymes convert adenosine diphosphate (ADP) to ATP, the energy source. Mitochondria require oxygen to produce the energy (aerobic metabolism); therefore, when insufficient oxygen is available to meet cellular demands, cell functions rapidly deteriorate. The Krebs cycle and aerobic metabolism are discussed in more detail later in this chapter.

To provide a continuous supply of oxygen to the cells, the body must take in oxygen from the atmosphere and deliver it to the cells. It does this through a complex set of physiologic processes primarily involving three organ systems: the lungs, heart, and blood (Kibble & Halsey, 2014). Unlike the heart, which has intrinsic rhythmic properties to work independently, the respiratory system requires continuous input from the nervous system. Depending on various internal and external stimuli, the nervous system regulates the respiratory system to meet identified body needs for oxygen.

Oxygen is brought into the internal environment via the respiratory system during the process of ventilation. Oxygen crosses alveolar–capillary membranes by diffusion, combines with hemoglobin, and is transported via the pulmonary vein to the left side of the heart. The heart pumps oxygenated blood into the vascular system, where it is transported to cells. Oxygenated blood then leaves the capillaries by diffusion and enters the cells. Each cell extracts the amount of oxygen it needs to fulfill its metabolic requirements. Cells use oxygen to convert nutrients into energy. Carbon dioxide and "unused" oxygen are carried to the right side of the heart and back to the lungs for elimination or reuse.

The process of oxygenation involves three physiologic components for the intake, delivery, and use of oxygen for energy: pulmonary gas exchange, oxygen delivery, and oxygen consumption, as illustrated in Figure 34–1. The adequacy of oxygenation depends on the integration of these physiologic components. **Pulmonary gas exchange** involves the intake (inhalation) of oxygen from the external environment into the internal environment and is carried out by the processes of ventilation, diffusion, and pulmonary perfusion. **Oxygen delivery (DO$_2$)** is the process of transporting oxygen to the cells and has four components: cardiac output, the oxygen content of arterial blood, autoregulation, and autonomic nervous system innervation. **Oxygen consumption (VO$_2$)** involves the use of oxygen at the cellular level to generate energy for cells to perform their specific functions.

Impaired oxygenation can result from impaired pulmonary gas exchange, decreased oxygen delivery, or impaired oxygen consumption. Any condition or disease that affects one or more of these components (e.g., acute respiratory distress syndrome, anemia, and hyperventilation)

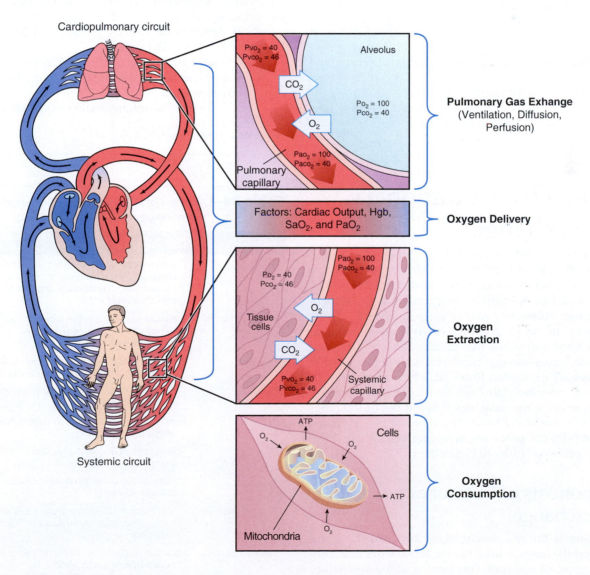

Figure 34–1 Components of oxygenation.

will result in impaired oxygenation. These conditions represent a continuum of oxygen disturbances. Life-threatening oxygenation impairments usually involve deficiencies in all three oxygenation components.

Monitoring oxygenation is an important component of a nursing assessment, particularly in the high-acuity patient. Accurate assessment and treatment of oxygenation disturbances may determine whether or not a patient survives. Identification of impaired oxygenation requires an understanding of the three components of oxygenation. Each component may respond independently to pathophysiologic conditions and therapeutic interventions; therefore, it is necessary to accurately assess all three components when assessing oxygenation status. There are two goals in the assessment of oxygenation: (1) to determine the overall adequacy of oxygenation and (2) to determine which component of oxygenation dysfunction should be manipulated.

Section One Review

1. Which statement best describes oxygenation?
   A. It occurs in the cardiovascular system.
   B. It involves only pulmonary ventilation, diffusion, and perfusion.
   C. It specifically refers to transportation of oxygen to cells.
   D. It involves the intake, delivery, and use of oxygen for energy metabolism.

2. What are the major physiologic components of oxygenation?
   A. Pulmonary gas exchange, oxygen delivery, and consumption
   B. Diffusion, ventilation, perfusion
   C. Cardiac output, hemoglobin saturation with oxygen
   D. Pulmonary and cardiovascular systems

3. How is pulmonary gas exchange carried out?
   A. Inspiration of oxygen by the process of ventilation
   B. Expiration of carbon dioxide by the process of diffusion
   C. Ventilation, diffusion, perfusion
   D. Ventilation, oxygen consumption, perfusion

4. Which statement correctly describes oxygen consumption?
   A. It depends on cardiac output and hemoglobin saturation with oxygen.
   B. It refers to the use of oxygen to generate energy.
   C. It involves the intake of oxygen from the external environment.
   D. It is the process of transporting oxygen to cells.

Answers: 1. D, 2. A, 3. C, 4. B

Section Two: Pulmonary Gas Exchange

An understanding of basic gas exchange terminology is necessary to fully comprehend the discussion in this section. A brief review of important terms is provided in Table 34–1.

The initial component of oxygenation is pulmonary gas exchange. Pulmonary gas exchange involves the intake and delivery of oxygen from the external environment to the alveoli and diffusion across the alveolar–capillary (a–c) membrane, where oxygen combines with hemoglobin in the pulmonary capillaries. Pulmonary blood flow must be adequate to move blood through the lungs for gas exchange and then to carry the oxygenated blood out of the lungs into the left side of the heart. These functions are carried out by physiologic processes involving ventilation, diffusion, and perfusion (refer to Figure 34–1).

Components of Pulmonary Gas Exchange

Ventilation is the movement of air between the atmosphere and the lungs. It involves the actual work of breathing and requires adequate functioning of the ventilatory muscles, thorax, lungs, conducting airways, and nervous

Table 34–1 Review of Pulmonary Gas Exchange Terminology

Term	Definition
FiO_2	Fraction of inspired oxygen (O_2 concentration) being delivered to the patient, expressed as a decimal. For example, if the patient is receiving 40% oxygen, the FiO_2 would be 0.4.
Minute ventilation ($\dot{V}_E$ or M)	Total volume of air expired in 1 minute; calculated as tidal volume (V_T) × respiratory rate (f) [$\dot{V}_E = V_T \times f$].
P/F ratio	Estimate of intrapulmonary shunt; calculated as $PaO_2 \div FiO_2$. Normal values: 350–450.
$PaCO_2$	Partial pressure of carbon dioxide in arterial blood. Normal range: 35–45 mmHg
P_AO_2	Partial pressure of oxygen in the alveoli. Normal range: 100–105 mmHg
PaO_2	Partial pressure of oxygen dissolved in arterial blood. Normal range: 75–100 mmHg
PvO_2	Partial pressure of oxygen in venous blood. Normal average: 40 mmHg
Tidal volume (V_T)	Amount of air that moves in and out of the lungs with each normal breath. Normal range: 7–9 mL/kg (ideal body weight)
Vital capacity (VC)	Maximum amount of air expired (exhaled) after a maximal inspiration (inhalation). Normal range: 4.8 L (adult male) and 3.2 L (adult female)

system. Decreased functioning of any one of these ventilatory components affects ventilation and can ultimately impair oxygenation.

Diffusion is the movement of gas across a pressure gradient from an area of high concentration to one of low concentration. Diffusion is the mechanism by which oxygen moves across the alveoli and into the pulmonary capillaries. Three factors affect diffusion across the a–c membrane: pressure gradient, surface area, and thickness. The greater the difference between alveolar oxygen (P_AO_2) and pulmonary capillary oxygen (PaO_2) pressures, the greater the diffusion of oxygen from the alveoli to the pulmonary capillaries. The greater the available a–c membrane surface area, the greater the amount of oxygen that can diffuse across it. Many conditions can cause a significant reduction in functional surface area. The thickness of the a–c membrane affects diffusion of oxygen from the alveoli to the pulmonary capillary. Conditions that increase the thickness of the a–c membrane can decrease diffusion.

The third component of gas exchange is **perfusion**. When discussing components of pulmonary gas exchange, perfusion refers to pulmonary perfusion of the pulmonary capillaries. Pulmonary perfusion does not refer to perfusion of the body, which is part of the oxygen delivery discussed in the next section. Three factors affect pulmonary perfusion: hemoglobin (Hgb) concentration, affinity of oxygen to Hgb, and blood flow. When oxygen diffuses across the a–c membrane into the blood, it binds to iron atoms in the Hgb in red blood cells and is carried to the left side of the heart. Certain factors affect the affinity of oxygen to Hgb, such as body temperature, acid–base balance, 2,3 diphosphoglycerate (2,3 DPG), and $PaCO_2$ (Glass, 2016; Kibble & Halsey, 2014). The amount of blood flowing past the alveoli also has an effect on oxygenation. A decrease in blood flow through the pulmonary vasculature results in an imbalance between ventilation and perfusion. Any disease or condition that impairs pulmonary perfusion impairs pulmonary gas exchange.

Factors That Impair Pulmonary Gas Exchange The matching of ventilation to perfusion is essential for gas exchange; otherwise, impaired oxygenation occurs. Conditions such as pulmonary embolus, which decreases perfusion, or pneumothorax, which decreases ventilation, can produce ventilation–perfusion mismatching. This mismatching is a common cause of hypoxemia, a condition characterized by an inadequate amount of oxygen in the blood as a result of impaired gas exchange. Hypoxemia is frequently quantified as a PaO_2 of less than 60 mmHg. If allowed to progress, hypoxemia can result in hypoxia. Some conditions and diseases that affect oxygenation as a result of impaired gas exchange are summarized in Table 34–2.

Assessment of Pulmonary Gas Exchange

Assessment of gas exchange must include techniques to assess ventilation, diffusion, and perfusion. Techniques to assess for pulmonary gas exchange are summarized in Box 34–1.

Table 34–2 Conditions That Impair Pulmonary Gas Exchange

Impairment	Associated Conditions
Ventilation	Inspiratory muscle weakness or trauma (Guillain-Barré, spinal cord injury) Decreased level of consciousness Obstruction or trauma to airways, lung, thorax (flail chest, mucous plug) Restrictive pulmonary disorders
Diffusion	Decrease in a–c membrane surface area (atelectasis, lung tumors, pneumonia) Increase in a–c membrane thickness (acute respiratory distress syndrome, pulmonary edema, pneumonia) Decreased pressure gradient between alveolar P_AO_2 and pulmonary capillary PaO_2.
Perfusion	Increased affinity of oxygen to Hgb (alkalosis) Decreased availability of Hgb (anemia, carbon monoxide poisoning) Decreased perfusion to the lungs ($\downarrow$ CO, hemorrhage) Pulmonary vasoconstriction (pulmonary hypertension, hypoxemia)

Auscultation of the Lungs Auscultation of the lungs is a technique for assessing ventilation. The key physiologic disturbance that auscultation detects is a change in airflow. Often there are no adventitious breath sounds or changes in chest radiographs during the early stages of alteration in pulmonary gas exchange. However, when changes do occur, it is important for the nurse to document the change and convey the assessment to the healthcare provider. Adventitious sounds can result from airway edema, bronchoconstriction, bronchospasm, airway obstruction, and airway fluid or secretions. Furthermore, no lung sounds will be auscultated if the airway becomes sufficiently obstructed by any of these conditions, such that there is little or no airflow distal to the obstruction or over the area of a pneumothorax.

Measurement of Carbon Dioxide Ventilation is the body's only internal mechanism for eliminating carbon dioxide (CO_2); therefore, assessment of $PaCO_2$ provides valuable information about the adequacy of ventilation. Ventilatory failure is commonly defined as a $PaCO_2$ greater than 50 mmHg with a pH of less than 7.30. Carbon dioxide can also be assessed using end-tidal CO_2 measurements, whereby a sensor is placed at the end of the endotracheal tube to measure the amount of exhaled CO_2. Hypercapnia results from alveolar hypoventilation—that is, an abnormally elevated $PaCO_2$ level secondary to inadequate elimination of CO_2 from the alveoli.

BOX 34–1 Assessment of Pulmonary Gas Exchange

- ABG (PaO_2, $PaCO_2$)
- Auscultation
- End-tidal CO_2
- Assessment of respiratory muscle efficiency via pulmonary function testing (e.g., tidal volume)
- PaO_2/ FiO_2 ratio

Pulmonary Function Tests Pulmonary function testing (PFT) measures ventilation by evaluating respiratory muscle strength, endurance, and efficiency. It is an essential tool for diagnosing pulmonary diseases, identifying and quantifying changing pulmonary status, and monitoring the effects of therapies (Kibble & Halsey, 2014). Many PFTs can be performed at the bedside, such as tidal volume (V_T), minute ventilation $\dot{V}_E$ vital capacity (VC), and maximum inspiratory pressure (MIP). Other tests require that the patient go to a special procedure area for more sophisticated measurements. PFTs provide valuable information on changes in ventilation, suggesting worsening or improving respiratory muscle strength and effort. They are generally indicated when determining the need for initiation or termination of mechanical ventilation.

Estimation of Intrapulmonary Shunt Intrapulmonary shunt is the proportion of blood that flows past alveoli without participating in gas exchange and is a major contributor to hypoxemia (Petersson & Glenny, 2014; Schumann, 2013). Normally, only a small percentage of blood does not take part in gas exchange; however, in high-acuity patients, pulmonary disorders such as pulmonary edema (common to heart failure or acute respiratory distress syndrome), atelectasis, or pneumonia can significantly increase the amount of shunt.

Multiple measures can be used to estimate shunt, with the most accurate measures requiring complex formulae. Rougher estimates of intrapulmonary shunt are simpler to measure and are sufficiently accurate for bedside assessment of shunt trends. The most common estimate of shunt used by nurses is the PaO_2/FiO_2 (P/F) ratio. It is a simple calculation that consists of the patient's PaO_2 divided by the concurrent FiO_2. The normal range is 350 to 450. The P/F ratio is used as part of the acute respiratory distress syndrome (ARDS) definition (ARDS = P/F ratio less than

Table 34–3 Nasal Cannula Oxygen: Liters/Minute – FiO_2 Equivalents

O_2 Flow Rate	Approximate FiO_2
0 (room air)	21%
1 LPM	24%
2 LPM	27%
3 LPM	30%
4 LPM	33%
5 LPM	35%
6 LPM	38%

LPM = liters per minute.

200) (Glass, 2016; Kibble & Halsey, 2014). For example, if a patient has PaO_2 of 80 mmHg while receiving oxygen at a concentration of 40% (0.40 FiO_2), the P/F ratio is 200 (80/0.40), which meets the ARDS criterion.

The P/F ratio can also be obtained if the patient has a nasal cannula in place; however, the oxygen flow rate in liters/minute (LPM) must be converted to FiO_2 before it will fit the formula. The following conversion formula can be used: $FiO_2 = (O_2$ flow rate $\times 4) + 21\%$, in which flow rate is in LPM, 4 represents 4% FiO_2 for each liter of oxygen being used, and 21% is the FiO_2 of room air. For example, a patient is receiving 4 LPM of oxygen via a nasal cannula. Using the conversion formula, the FiO_2 would be calculated as follows: (4 [LPM] $\times 4) + 21\% = 38\%$ (0.38) FiO_2. It is important to note that calculating FiO_2 when a patient has a nasal cannula in place yields only a rough estimate because the actual quantity of oxygen entering the lungs is unpredictable with this method of oxygen delivery. Table 34–3 lists the approximate FiO_2 and liters/minute equivalent for oxygen delivered by nasal cannula using the conversion formula.

Section Two Review

1. Which condition has an effect on perfusion?
   A. Low hemoglobin levels
   B. Upper airway obstruction
   C. Pulmonary embolism
   D. Hypovolemic shock

2. A P_AO_2 of 100 mmHg and a PaO_2 of 40 mmHg would have which effect on the respiratory process?
   A. Facilitate diffusion
   B. Decrease diffusion
   C. Decrease ventilation
   D. Facilitate perfusion

3. Atelectasis decreases the functional alveolar–capillary membrane surface area, altering gas exchange in which way?
   A. Increased alveolar–capillary pressure gradient
   B. Decreased alveolar–capillary pressure gradient
   C. Decrease in oxygen diffusion across alveolar–capillary membranes
   D. Increase in oxygen diffusion across alveolar–capillary membranes

4. Anemia affects which component of the gas exchange process?
   A. Ventilation
   B. Diffusion
   C. P_AO_2
   D. Perfusion

Answers: 1. A, 2. A, 3. C, 4. D

Section Three: Oxygen Delivery

The second component of oxygenation is oxygen delivery (DO_2), which is the primary function of the heart and lungs (Alarcon & Fink, 2015). Oxygen delivery involves the process of transporting oxygen to the cells.

Components of Oxygen Delivery

Factors that affect DO_2 include cardiac output (CO), autoregulation, oxygen content of arterial blood (CaO_2), and autonomic nervous system innervation. Table 34–4 provides a quick review of terms critical to understanding this section.

Cardiac Output **Cardiac output (CO)** is the amount of blood pumped by the heart each minute and is determined by two factors: heart rate and stroke volume (which consists of preload, afterload, and contractility). Recall that the equation to calculate cardiac output is $CO = SV \times HR$, where CO is cardiac output, SV is stroke volume, and HR is heart rate. The greater the cardiac output, the greater the amount of oxygen delivered to the tissues per minute; and, conversely, conditions that cause a decrease in cardiac output result in a decrease in the amount of oxygen delivered to the tissues per minute.

Autoregulation Under normal circumstances, the volume of oxygenated blood pumped by the heart is proportional to the body's demands. When tissues require more oxygen, the heart rate increases in an attempt to augment cardiac output and deliver more oxygenated blood. Tissues regulate their own blood supply by dilating or constricting local blood vessels through the mechanism of **autoregulation**. Tissues have varying energy requirements and use autoregulation to meet their metabolic demands. When the body is at rest, not all tissue capillaries are open at the same time. An increased metabolic rate (e.g., during exercise) and arterial hypoxemia (decreased PaO_2) open more tissue capillaries, allowing more oxygen to be extracted by tissue beds. Autoregulation serves to protect tissues locally by controlling blood flow and oxygen delivery in response to individual local tissue needs.

Oxygen Content of Arterial Blood Oxygen is carried in arterial blood in two forms: combined with hemoglobin or dissolved in the plasma. The content of oxygen in arterial blood (CaO_2) largely depends on the concentration of Hgb available to carry oxygen, the amount of oxygen carried in the blood in a dissolved form (PaO_2), and the saturation of Hgb with oxygen (SaO_2) (called oxyhemoglobin [$HgbO_2$]). Almost 97% of all oxygen delivered to cells is in the form of $HgbO_2$, and the remaining 3% is delivered dissolved in plasma (PaO_2) (Levitizky, 2013). Total oxygen content in the blood can be manipulated by only two interventions: administering red blood cells to increase hemoglobin or supplementing oxygen to increase SaO_2 and PaO_2 (Glass, 2016; Kibble & Halsey, 2014).

Oxyhemoglobin Each molecule of Hgb carries four oxygen molecules (O_2) that are attached to four atoms of iron. When Hgb is fully saturated with oxygen, oxyhemoglobin ($HgbO_2$) is formed. The measurement of SaO_2 by arterial blood gas (ABG) analysis (or SpO_2 when measured using pulse oximetry) is a measurement of the percentage of available sites on hemoglobin that are bound with oxygen. For example, if the SaO_2 or SpO_2 is 95%, it can be interpreted that 95% of all the available binding sites are occupied by oxygen. Because the majority of oxygen is carried to the tissues by Hgb, any condition or disease that decreases Hgb content severely decreases the amount of oxygen carried to the tissues. Furthermore, any condition that reduces the amount of available iron (e.g., iron-deficiency anemia) reduces oxygen-carrying capacity.

Autonomic Nervous System Innervation The autonomic nervous system exerts partial control of oxygen delivery through excitatory or inhibitory effects on the heart, lungs, and blood vessels. The stimulation of specific cell receptors

Table 34–4 Review of Oxygen Delivery (DO_2) Terminology

Term	Definition
Afterload	Resistance against which the ventricle pumps blood. Normal range: 800–1200 dynes · sec · cm^{-5}
Cardiac output (CO)	Amount of blood pumped by the heart each minute. Normal range: 4–8 LMN
Content of arterial blood (CaO_2)	Total amount of oxygen carried in arterial blood; represents the combination of oxyhemoglobin (SaO_2) and dissolved oxygen (PaO_2)
Contractility	Force of myocardial contraction
Oxygen delivery (DO_2)	Process by which oxygen is transported to the cells, comprising four components: cardiac output (CO), oxygen content of arterial blood (CaO_2), autoregulation, and autonomic nervous system innervation. Calculated as [product of CO and CaO_2]: $$DO_2 = (CO \times [Hgb \times 1.34 \times SaO_2] + [PaO_2 \times 0.003]) \times 10^*$$
Oxyhemoglobin ($HgbO_2$)	Hemoglobin that is fully saturated with oxygen
Preload	Amount of stretch in the myocardial fibers at the end of diastole
Saturation of arterial blood (SaO_2 and SpO_2)	Ratio of $HgbO_2$ to total hemoglobin (Hgb). The abbreviation SpO_2 is used when the measurement is obtained through pulse oximetry.
Stroke volume	Volume of blood pumped with each heartbeat. Normal range: 50–100 mL/beat

* 10 is a conversion factor.

in the cardiovascular and respiratory systems results in a target cell response based on local tissue needs. Two major types of cell receptors are alpha$_1$ (α_1) receptors, whose therapeutic effects are vasoconstriction of the vascular, visceral, and integumentary tissues to increase the blood pressure; and beta$_1$ (β_1) receptors, whose therapeutic effects are inotropic and include increased heart rate and force of contraction to increase cardiac output. Drugs can stimulate or inhibit these receptors through their mechanisms of action. For example, adrenergic agonist drugs activate the adrenergic receptor sites, thereby stimulating the sympathetic nervous system and causing vasoconstriction; whereas adrenergic antagonist (blocking) agents block the receptor sites, usually causing vasodilation.

Factors That Impair Oxygen Delivery Many conditions impair oxygen delivery (DO$_2$). High-acuity patients are particularly at risk for impaired DO$_2$ as a result of a decrease in heart function, such as that occurring with dysrhythmias or heart failure. An uncompensated decrease in cardiac output, Hgb, or SaO$_2$ can significantly reduce DO$_2$. Patients who have what may appear to be clinically insignificant decreases in all three factors can have a significant decrease in DO$_2$ when these factors are considered together. Furthermore, it is important for the nurse to be aware of any drugs being given to a patient that cause vasoconstriction (e.g., norepinephrine or vasopressin) or vasodilation (e.g., nitroglycerin), as these will impact DO$_2$.

Assessment of Oxygen Delivery

Assessment of DO$_2$ requires assessing parameters that reflect each of its components: cardiac output (CO), Hgb, SaO$_2$, and PaO$_2$. CO can be assessed directly or indirectly.

Indirect assessment is performed during a focused cardiovascular assessment, whereas more direct measurements require additional invasive or noninvasive technology devices.

Assessing Cardiac Output An indirect assessment of cardiac output includes evaluation of heart rate and two components of stroke volume (preload and afterload). However, there are no indirect assessments that specifically focus on contractility. Decreased contractility is most commonly caused by myocardial ischemia and infarction (MI) (Alarcon & Fink, 2015); therefore, it is important to determine whether the patient is experiencing cardiac ischemia or acute MI or has a history of either of these disorders. Table 34–5 lists bedside assessments that reflect the components of cardiac output. The patient's basic neurologic status is also important, particularly the level of consciousness (LOC), as an inadequate cardiac output reduces cerebral blood flow, resulting in a reduction in LOC (e.g., restlessness, confusion).

Direct measurement of cardiac output requires invasive catheterization of the pulmonary artery. Thermodilution methods employ a special pulmonary artery catheter that measures cardiac output intermittently or continuously. Direct measurement techniques provide the most accurate data and are of most value when the patient has a severely unstable hemodynamic status, as in shock states. Hemodynamic monitoring is usually reserved for patients

Table 34–5 Indirect Bedside Assessments of Cardiac Output

CO Parameter	Assessments
Heart rate (with cardiac assessment)	Palpation of peripheral pulses Heart auscultation: assess for rate, regularity, strength; note any extra heart sounds Cardiac monitor: rate and rhythm, wave configuration; note any dysrhythmias, including type and frequency
Stroke volume • Preload	Fluid balance status: • Fluid deficit (e.g., poor skin turgor, dry mucous membranes, decreased urine output, hypotension, fever) • Fluid overload (e.g., weight gain, lung crackles, dependent edema, + jugular vein distention [JVD], hepatic tenderness and enlargement, frothy sputum, shortness of breath, orthopnea, fatigue) • Intake and output balance • Central venous pressure (CVP) Heart sounds: noting abnormal presence of S$_3$ or S$_4$ Oxygenation status: SpO$_2$ or SaO$_2$
• Afterload	No indirect assessments that specifically target afterload Assessments that may be meaningful include blood pressure, pulse pressure Assess for patient factors that alter afterload, such as shock, vasopressor drugs, mechanical ventilation, positive end–expiratory pressure (PEEP), spinal cord injury
• Contractility	No specific bedside measures for evaluating; reflected in preload assessments History of previous myocardial infarction Acute myocardial ischemia or infarction

in critical care units. Using the data provided by pulmonary artery catheters, the nurse can monitor the patient's hemodynamic status on an ongoing basis. Measurements that can be obtained include heart pressures (e.g., pulmonary artery pressure and pulmonary artery wedge pressure, central venous pressure, cardiac output or cardiac index, and systemic vascular resistance [SVR]).

Newer hemodynamic monitoring technologies have gained in popularity for measuring CO and its components using noninvasive or minimally invasive methods. Two examples are impedance cardiography and Doppler echocardiography. Impedance cardiography measures CO and other hemodynamic parameters (e.g., stroke volume) using small high-frequency electrical current through the aorta to measure beat-by-beat blood flow (Neligan & Fuchs, 2015; Nguyen, Huang, & Pinsky, 2016). Doppler echocardiography uses ultrasound technology to measure blood flow velocity, determining CO, preload, afterload, and contractility (Neligan & Fuchs, 2015; Nguyen et al., 2016). Although hemodynamic measurements using noninvasive methods are not as accurate as pulmonary artery catheter measurements, the results are considered acceptable and involve fewer risks for complications. A more in-depth discussion of these CO measuring technologies is provided in Chapter 8.

Assessing Hemoglobin, PaO$_2$, and SaO$_2$ Direct measurement of PaO$_2$ and SaO$_2$ is made with an arterial blood gas (ABG), and Hgb is obtained as part of a complete blood cell count or separately, in a venous or capillary blood specimen. Of the three parameters, Hgb and SaO_2 are the most important to monitor, as they quantify the available oxygen carriers and how well they are saturated with oxygen. Although PaO_2 contributes to a smaller extent to oxygen delivery (less than 3% of all oxygen delivered to tissues), it is still important in the evaluation and calculation of oxygen delivery and also plays a significant role in oxygenation as one of two components of the oxyhemoglobin dissociation curve.

The primary indirect measure of oxygen saturation is obtained through pulse oximetry. Pulse oximetry is used for continuous (or intermittent) noninvasive measurement of arterial oxygenation saturation and is referred to as SpO_2 to differentiate it from the direct measure, SaO_2. SpO_2 monitoring is recommended for any patient at risk for hypoxemia. Certain factors alter the interpretation and accuracy of SpO_2, such as cardiac output, anemia (low Hgb), HgbCO (hemoglobin saturated with carbon monoxide), shock, vasoconstriction at the location of the sensor, and hypothermia.

Calculating Oxygen Delivery Oxygen delivery (DO_2) can also be calculated; however, it is not usually the responsibility of the nurse to obtain or monitor this value. This calculation requires a CO measurement, serum Hgb analysis, and ABG analysis for SaO_2 and PaO_2 (see Table 34–4).

Section Three Review

1. How is oxygen delivery defined?
   A. Amount of oxygen in arterial blood
   B. Process of transporting oxygen to cells
   C. Process of using oxygen for energy
   D. Amount of blood pumped by the heart per minute

2. Which set of factors affects oxygen delivery?
   A. Ventilation, diffusion, perfusion
   B. Cardiac output, hemoglobin concentration, ventilation
   C. Cardiac output, autoregulation, oxygen content of venous blood
   D. Cardiac output, autoregulation, oxygen content of arterial blood, autonomic nervous system innervation

3. A client who has suffered a myocardial infarction is at risk for impaired oxygenation primarily related to which condition?
   A. Overactive autoregulation
   B. Impaired autonomic nervous system innervation
   C. Decreased cardiac output
   D. Decreased oxygen content of arterial blood

4. The client's latest SaO_2 value is 97%. The nurse is aware that SaO_2 represents which aspect of oxygenation?
   A. Oxyhemoglobin
   B. Partial pressure of oxygen
   C. Dissolved oxygen
   D. Oxygen bound to proteins

Answers: 1. B, 2. D, 3. C, 4. A

Section Four: Oxygen Consumption

The third component of oxygenation is **oxygen consumption (VO$_2$)** which is the rate at which oxygen is used by the cells to generate energy (see Figure 34–1). Once oxygen is delivered to the tissue-level circulation, it must be taken into the cells (a process called **oxygen extraction**). The cells take in only the amount of oxygen required to meet their energy needs, a tightly regulated supply-and-demand situation. In this way, oxygen does not go to waste, making unused oxygen available for use by active tissues through a process of autoregulation.

Aerobic Metabolism

The majority of the body's energy needs are met through aerobic metabolism, which requires oxygen; however, as a backup energy source in the absence of oxygen, the body produces smaller amounts of energy through anaerobic metabolism. The primary value of oxygen is its ability to develop adenosine triphosphate (ATP). In the presence of oxygen, ingested carbohydrates, fats, and proteins are broken down into substrates that are converted in the Krebs cycle into energy in the form of ATP, a process called **aerobic metabolism** (Figure 34–2). The purpose of forming ATP is to create intracellular energy stores; and when energy is required, ATP is broken down and energy is released. Aerobic metabolism results in the creation of 36 molecules of ATP, which the cells use as their energy source to perform all necessary functions. Without the ATP energy stores, cellular processes break down, and the cells cannot function. The by-products of aerobic metabolism are water and carbon dioxide, which are readily eliminated from the body.

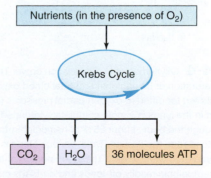

Figure 34–2 Aerobic metabolism.

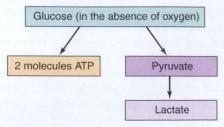

Figure 34–3 Anaerobic metabolism.

Anaerobic Metabolism

As a "backup" mechanism, cells can generate energy in the absence of oxygen by the process of **anaerobic metabolism** (Figure 34–3). Carbohydrates are the only food substrate that can be broken down to generate ATP without the use of oxygen; therefore, when anaerobic metabolism is required, carbohydrates become the source of ATP. Anaerobic metabolism is not an efficient energy source, producing only two ATP molecules and two potentially harmful by-products, pyruvate and lactate. When local tissues rely on anaerobic metabolism, lactate (an acid) accumulates in the tissue and results in local tissue lactic acidosis (e.g., ischemic stroke). However, if a patient becomes globally hypoxic (e.g., cardiopulmonary arrest), a large proportion of tissue shifts to anaerobic metabolism, and, if prolonged, the patient develops lactic acidosis (increased serum lactate, acidic pH, low bicarbonate, and base deficit). The acidic environment alters cellular structure and greatly impairs cellular function.

Oxygen Extraction

Recall that oxygen extraction is the process by which cells take oxygen from the blood. Normal oxygen consumption

is approximately 1000 mL/min, and approximately 250 mL of this oxygen is required by tissue metabolic processes; therefore, the usual oxygen extraction is 25%. In other words, about 25% of the oxygen is taken up by the cells, and about 75% returns to the right side of the heart in the venous circulation (measurable as SvO_2).

Oxyhemoglobin Dissociation Curve and Oxygen Extraction Under normal circumstances, oxygen is loosely attached to hemoglobin so that it is readily released from the hemoglobin when it arrives at the tissues. The degree to which hemoglobin and oxygen are attracted is called **affinity**. The affinity of oxygen to hemoglobin is demonstrated by the oxyhemoglobin dissociation curve (Figures 34–4 and 34–5), which depicts the relationship between oxyhemoglobin (represented on the curve as SaO_2) and PaO_2. This relationship changes when conditions alter certain physiologic factors (e.g., pH, temperature, $PaCO_2$, and 2,3 DPG), causing a shift in the curve to the left or right. The organic phosphate in RBCs known as 2,3 DPG affects the affinity of hemoglobin for oxygen and is an important component of respiratory compensation to hypoxemia (Kibble & Halsey, 2014). Table 34–6 summarizes information about left and right shifts of the curve.

Left Shift. A shift to the left increases the affinity of hemoglobin for oxygen and decreases the unloading of oxygen to the tissues. Major physiologic factors that cause a left shift include alkalosis, hypothermia, hypocapnia (decreased $PaCO_2$), and decreased 2,3 DPG. Oxygen dissociates from hemoglobin in response to local tissue oxygen demands, and tissues' demands are lower with a left shift. For example, if a person develops hypothermia, metabolic processes decrease, reducing tissue demands for oxygen, and the curve shifts to the left.

Right Shift. A shift of the curve to the right results in decreased affinity of hemoglobin for oxygen, and oxygen is readily released from hemoglobin at the tissue level. Major

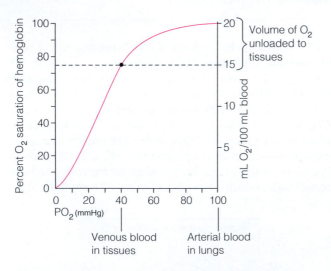

Figure 34–4 Oxyhemoglobin dissociation curve. The percent O_2 saturation of hemoglobin and total blood oxygen volume are shown for different oxygen partial pressures (PO_2). Arterial blood in the lungs is almost completely saturated. During one pass through the body, about 25% of hemoglobin-bound oxygen is unloaded to the tissues. Thus, venous blood is still about 75% saturated with oxygen. The steep portion of the curve shows that hemoglobin readily off-loads and on-loads oxygen at PO_2 levels below 50 mmHg.

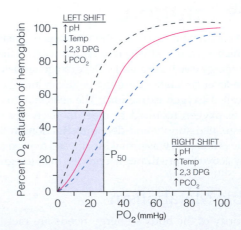

Figure 34–5 Oxyhemoglobin dissociation curve right and left shifts. Normally, when hemoglobin is 50% saturated with oxygen (P_{50}), the PaO_2 will be 27 mmHg. The P_{50} changes when physiologic factors are altered, shifting the curve. A shift to the left increases the affinity of oxygen to hemoglobin, inhibiting its release to tissues. A shift to the right decreases the affinity of oxygen to hemoglobin, making it release to tissues more readily.

Table 34–6 Alterations of the Oxyhemoglobin Dissociation Curve

	Left Shift	Right Shift
Physiologic factors	Alkalosis ($\uparrow$ pH), hypocapnia ($\downarrow$ PaCO$_2$), or hypothermia ($\downarrow$ temp) (Alkalosis and hypocapnia often occur together.)	Acidosis ($\downarrow$ pH), hypercapnia ($\uparrow$ PaCO$_2$), or hyperthermia ($\uparrow$ temp) (Acidosis and hypercapnia often occur together.)
Effects on tissue oxygenation	Increases affinity of hemoglobin for oxygen In lungs: Hemoglobin readily binds with oxygen (high HgbO$_2$/SaO$_2$). At tissues: Hemoglobin does not readily release oxygen; therefore, less oxygen is extracted and cells can become hypoxic. More oxygen remains in the blood as it flows back to the heart through the venous system.	Decreases affinity of hemoglobin for oxygen In lungs: Hemoglobin does not bind as readily with oxygen (low HgbO$_2$/SaO$_2$). At tissues: Hemoglobin readily releases oxygen; therefore, oxygen is extracted rapidly, possibly leaving insufficient oxygen for all tissues. Less oxygen remains in blood as it flows back to the heart through the venous system.
Associated assessments	ABG: $\uparrow$ SaO$_2$ Pulse oximetry: $\uparrow$ SpO$_2$ SvO$_2$: $\uparrow$	ABG: $\downarrow$ SaO$_2$ Pulse oximetry: $\downarrow$ SpO$_2$ SvO$_2$: $\downarrow$
Examples of precipitating conditions	Environmental exposure (cold-water near-drowning, cold-weather exposure), induced hypothermia (e.g., surgery) Hyperventilation GI-associated loss of acid or gain of alkaline (e.g., vomiting, nasogastric [NG] drainage) Administration of sodium bicarbonate	Respiratory failure High fever Metabolic acidosis

physiologic factors that cause a right shift include acidosis, hyperthermia (fever), hypercapnia (elevated PaCO$_2$), and increased 2,3 DPG. When the cells demand more energy, they extract more oxygen from the blood. For example, during exercise, muscle cells extract more oxygen than they do at rest to meet their increased oxygen needs. Another example is what occurs when a person develops a fever; metabolic processes and oxygen needs both increase, and the curve shifts to the right.

Clinical Implications. The curve shifts become clinically significant if they are prolonged or severe due to factors that alter acid–base balance, body temperature, PaCO$_2$, or 2,3 DPG because they can significantly alter oxygen extraction. In high-acuity patients, a right shift is more common than a left shift because of the increased likelihood of development of the physiologic factors underlying the shift (e.g., acidosis, fever, or hypercapnia). Body temperature is sometimes clinically controlled to reduce oxygen consumption. For example, in a randomized controlled trial, Schortgen et al. (2012) investigated the use of external cooling to maintain normothermia in 200 febrile patients with septic shock and requiring vasopressors, mechanical ventilation, and sedation. Body temperature was significantly lower in the cooling group after 2 hours, vasopressor dose significantly decreased from 12 hours of treatment, and mortality was significantly lower. In this study, fever control using external cooling was safe and decreased vasopressor requirements and early mortality in septic shock. Zobel et al. (2012) studied the effectiveness of mild therapeutic hypothermia (MTH) in 20 patients with cardiogenic shock. After successful resuscitation from out-of-hospital cardiac arrest, patients were cooled to 33°C (91.4°F) for 24 hours. They found that patients' metabolic rate decreased by about 8% for every degree of Celsius temperature reduction, which reduced oxygen consumption as well as CO$_2$ production. There was a significant decrease in HR, increase in MAP, and lower cumulative doses of vasopressors and inotropes. The use of MTH resulted in decreased use of catecholamine drug therapy and increased patient survival compared to patients with cardiogenic shock who did not undergo MTH.

Factors That Alter Oxygen Consumption

Numerous conditions alter the oxygen consumption of high-acuity patients (Table 34–7), and coexisting conditions can have an additive effect. For example, the oxygen consumption of a patient with a fever, infection, and increased work of breathing may be two times the resting oxygen consumption. Nursing care also affects oxygen consumption. In a classic study, Swinamer, Phang, Jones, Grace, and King (1987) found that routine nursing care increases energy expenditure and oxygen consumption in critically ill mechanically ventilated patients. In a prospective observational study, Jakob et al. (2009) investigated the impact of nursing care (e.g., ventilator-related procedures, hygiene, and changing the patient's position) on splanchnic oxygen extraction in 36 mechanically ventilated ICU patients. Activities, such as weighing a patient on a sling-type bed scale, repositioning, and chest physiotherapy resulted in increased energy expenditure above resting levels (36%, 31%, and 20%, respectively); the actual contribution of these activities to total energy expenditure was small (1.1%, 2.1%, and 3.6%, respectively). Most decreases

Table 34–7 Conditions That Alter Oxygen Consumption

Alteration	Associated Conditions
Increased consumption	Hyperventilation, hyperthermia, trauma, sepsis, anxiety, stress, hyperthyroidism, increased muscle activity
Decreased consumption	Hypoventilation, hypothermia, sedation, neuromuscular blocking agents, anesthesia, hypothyroidism, inactivity

Table 34–8 Activities That Increase Oxygen Consumption

Activity	Approximate Increase Above Resting Oxygen Consumption
Nursing assessment	10%
Repositioning patient	30%
Dressing change	10%
Bed bath	20%
Weighing patient on sling bed scale	40%
Visitors	18%
Restlessness or agitation	18%

SOURCE: Data from Jakob et al. (2009) and Swinamer et al. (1987).

in splanchnic oxygen saturation were caused by airway suctioning, assessing level of sedation, turning the patient, and combinations of procedures. Table 34–8 lists some routine activities that increase oxygen consumption.

Assessment of Oxygen Consumption

Ideally, assessment of oxygen consumption would include techniques that directly assess the availability and use of oxygen at the cellular level. However, in the clinical setting, this type of assessment is not currently possible. There are no physical assessment parameters that can be used to evaluate oxygen consumption, and traditional means of assessing oxygenation (e.g., ABGs, cardiac output) do not reflect oxygen availability at the cellular level. Current methods of assessing oxygen consumption are limited to indirect measurement techniques, including measurement of serum lactate levels, base deficit, and venous oxygen saturation monitoring.

Serum Lactate Levels Under conditions of inadequate oxygen delivery, cells convert from aerobic metabolism to anaerobic metabolism. The by-product of anaerobic metabolism is lactate, which can lead to lactic acidosis. Normal serum lactate levels are less than 2 mmoL (Kee, 2014). Serum lactate levels, evaluated using serial measurements (e.g., every 4 to 8 hours), can be used as an indicator of improving or worsening oxygen delivery in relation to oxygen consumption. Serum lactate levels must be interpreted with caution in patients with certain disorders, such as cancer, liver failure, renal disease, and alcoholism because levels may also increase for reasons not directly related to worsening oxygen delivery. For example, in patients with cancer, aerobic (rather than anaerobic) glycolysis is often the preferred metabolic process by which tumor cells meet their energy needs, resulting in increased glucose uptake and release of lactic acid (Dhup, Dadhich, Porporato, & Sonveaux, 2012). Lactate is also produced in the breakdown of certain amino acids, such as glutamine (glutaminolysis), associated with tumor cell metabolism. Furthermore, patients with liver failure cannot clear serum lactate adequately, maintaining elevated lactate levels that

may not accurately reflect tissue hypoxia (Illuzzi & Gillespie, 2017; Neligan & Fuchs, 2015).

Base Deficit Base deficit is defined as the amount of base (mmoL) required to titrate 1 liter of arterial blood to a normal pH. It is calculated from an ABG and is used as an approximation of metabolic acidosis. A base deficit results from an imbalance between oxygen delivery and oxygen consumption, which results in lactic acidosis secondary to anaerobic metabolism. Normal base deficit is +2 mmoL to –2 mmoL. Positive values reflect metabolic alkalosis, and negative values reflect metabolic acidosis. Base deficit can be classified in three categories: mild (–3 to –5 mmoL), moderate (–6 to –14 mmoL), and severe (greater than –15 mmoL). A deficit of greater than 15 mmoL is associated with a 70% mortality rate (Zuckerbraun, Peitzman, & Billiar, 2015).

Venous Oxygen Saturation and Central Venous Oxygen Saturation (SvO$_2$ and ScvO$_2$) Venous oxygen saturation (SvO$_2$) reflects oxygen extraction by the tissues and the balance between oxygen supply and oxygen demand (Neligan & Fuchs, 2015; Nguyen et al., 2016). Measuring SaO$_2$ or SpO$_2$ provides information about the oxygen saturation of *arterial* blood. Measuring SvO$_2$ provides information about the oxygen saturation of *venous* blood. Monitoring both parameters allows clinicians to assess the amount of oxygen delivered to and returned from tissues. Abnormally low values indicate either excessive oxygen consumption or inadequate oxygen delivery (Nguyen et al., 2016; Zuckerbraun et al., 2015).

The Physiologic Basis of SvO$_2$. When the supply of oxygen to the tissues is sufficient, the tissues extract the amount needed for their metabolic processes. Each organ system requires a different amount of oxygen, and each organ extracts a certain percentage of the oxygen according to its metabolic rate. The kidneys have a relatively low demand for oxygen because much of their function uses passive transport, and the oxygen saturation of the venous blood leaving the kidneys averages 74%. Conversely, the heart requires a large amount of oxygen for its work, and the oxygen saturation of blood leaving the coronary circulation averages only 30% (Nguyen et al., 2016).

The Clinical Significance of SvO$_2$. If the oxygen delivery to tissues is adequate for tissue demands, oxygen saturation of the blood in the pulmonary artery will be about 70% because the body normally uses 20% to 40% of the oxygen delivered (Nguyen et al., 2016; Siegal, 2017). When evaluating SvO$_2$, the nurse should also be aware of the four factors that influence it: SaO$_2$, Hgb, CO, and oxygen consumption; abnormal levels of any of these factors will influence SvO$_2$. A low SvO$_2$ means that less oxygen is returning to the right heart; the cells are not getting enough oxygen to meet their needs. Treatment to increase the SvO$_2$ may include blood transfusion (if low Hgb) or inotropic drug therapy (if low CO) (Siegal, 2017). The nurse should also look for ways to decrease oxygen demand. A normal SvO$_2$ indicates that oxygen delivery is adequate for tissue

Table 34–9 Causes of Decreased and Increased SvO$_2$

Causes of Decreased SvO$_2$	Causes of Increased SvO$_2$*
Decreased oxygen supply	*Increased oxygen supply*
Decreased cardiac output	Increased cardiac output
Heart failure	Inotropic drugs
Hypovolemia	Intra-aortic balloon pump
Dysrhythmias	Afterload reduction
Cardiac depressants (e.g., beta blockers)	Increased oxygen saturation
	Increased FiO$_2$ (inspired oxygen)
Decreased oxygen saturation	Improvement in lung problem
Respiratory failure	Increased hemoglobin
Pulmonary infiltrates	Blood transfusion
Suctioning	
Ventilator disconnection	
Decreased hemoglobin	
Anemia	
Hemorrhage	
Increased oxygen consumption	*Decreased oxygen demand*
Hyperthermia	Hypothermia
Seizures	Fever reduction
Shivering	Sepsis (late stages)
Pain	Paralysis
Increased work of breathing	Pain relief
Increased metabolic rate	Anesthesia
Exercise	
Agitation	

* A wedged pulmonary artery catheter may result in a falsely elevated SvO$_2$.

oxygen demands. Causes of decreased and increased SvO$_2$ are summarized in Table 34–9.

Measuring SvO$_2$. SvO$_2$ is measured in two ways: as a mixed sample or as a central value.

Mixed Venous Oxygen Saturation (Mixed SvO$_2$). The venous blood transported to the pulmonary artery is actually a "mixture" of blood from all organ systems and is referred to as "mixed" by the time it reaches the pulmonary artery. The saturation of this mixed venous blood represents an average of the venous saturation of blood from all parts of the body and is called mixed SvO$_2$ (or SmvO$_2$, to differentiate it from ScvO$_2$, central venous O$_2$ saturation [Nguyen et al., 2016]). Mixed SvO$_2$ can be measured intermittently by blood gas analysis of a mixed venous blood sample drawn from the distal port of a pulmonary artery catheter. Intermittent sampling methods, however, may cause a delay in the discovery of an oxygenation problem because they capture only one moment in time. Mixed SvO$_2$ can also be measured continuously through the use of a special fiber optic pulmonary artery catheter. A fiber optic filament in the catheter emits a constant beam of light on the red blood cells flowing past it in the pulmonary artery. The amount of emitted light reflected back to the computer depends on the oxygen saturation of the red blood cells. The computer uses this information to determine the oxygen saturation of mixed venous blood. A digital readout of the SvO$_2$ is updated several times each minute. Normal mixed venous oxygen saturation is 60% to 80%. Trends in SvO$_2$ can be used to assess patient tolerance and response to resuscitation interventions.

Central Venous Oxygen Saturation (ScvO$_2$). This method measures venous oxygen saturation only from the upper body rather than, as mixed SvO$_2$ does, from the whole body. It is considered a minimally invasive procedure because it requires placement of a central line catheter into the jugular or subclavian vein rather than a pulmonary artery catheter. Normal values are slightly lower (2%–3%) than mixed SvO$_2$; in shock states, values are usually 5% to 10% higher than mixed SvO$_2$ (Nguyen et al., 2016). It can be measured intermittently, by obtaining a venous blood gas, or continuously, with a special monitoring system. The values obtained using this method are considered to run parallel and closely reflect values obtained using mixed SvO$_2$ pulmonary artery sampling. This makes ScvO$_2$ a viable alternative for use in patients in whom minimally invasive monitoring procedures are preferred.

Emerging Evidence

- In a randomized, controlled trial, 105 patients with a PaO$_2$/FiO$_2$, ratio less than or equal to 300 immediately before extubation were placed on a Venturi mask (n = 52) or nasal high-flow (n = 53) for 48 hours postextubation. Nasal high-flow resulted in better oxygenation and was associated with increased comfort, fewer desaturations and lower reintubation rate compared to the Venturi mask group (*Maggiore et al., 2014*).
- A prospective, multicenter, observational study of 363 patients with severe sepsis or septic shock with an initial ScvO$_2$ below 70% was conducted to determine if there was an association with mortality. ScvO$_2$ was measured at inclusion and 6 hours later by blood sampling. Results showed a low ScvO$_2$ in the first hour of admission to the ICU for severe sepsis, and septic shock was common even when clinical resuscitation end points were achieved and arterial lactate normalized. A low ScvO$_2$ below 70% in the first hours of admission and 6 hours later was associated with day-28 mortality (*Boulain et al., 2014*).
- A prospective, randomized, cross-over trial was conducted on 34 intubated and ventilated patients to compare the effect of positioning on gas exchange, respiratory mechanics, and hemodynamics. Subjects were passively mobilized out of bed into a seated position (from a supine to a semi-recumbent position greater than 450 degrees elevation in bed). Measurement of arterial blood gas (PaO$_2$/FiO$_2$ and A-a O$_2$ gradient) respiratory mechanics, heart rate, and mean arterial blood pressure were collected in supine position, 5 minutes and 30 minutes after repositioning. There were no clinically significant changes in arterial blood gas or in respiratory mechanic or hemodynamic values due to either position. Patients being weaned from the ventilator can safely tolerate position changes during weaning (*Thomas, Paratz, & Lipman, 2014*).

Section Four Review

1. Which statement is correct concerning a continuous supply of oxygen?
   A. It is not necessary because oxygen is stored in cells.
   B. It is required for adequate ATP synthesis.
   C. It depends on the amount of blood ejected from the left ventricle.
   D. It depends on adequate supplies of hemoglobin.

2. A blood sample for a newly admitted trauma client reveals a high level of lactate. What does this indicate?
   A. Adequate oxygen delivery
   B. Anaerobic metabolism
   C. Adequate oxygen consumption
   D. Aerobic metabolism

3. Which condition increases oxygen consumption?
   A. Hypoventilation
   B. Sedation
   C. Bed rest
   D. Temperature of 38.9°C (102°F)

4. Which statement about direct measurement of oxygen consumption is correct?
   A. It is not clinically possible to measure it.
   B. It is made using transcutaneous oxygen measurements.
   C. It can be measured using SvO_2 monitoring.
   D. It can be calculated as the product of cardiac output and oxygen content of arterial blood.

Answers: 1. B, 2. B, 3. D, 4. A

Clinical Reasoning Checkpoint

Mr. T. is a 69-year-old male admitted to the high-acuity unit with right lower-lobe pneumonia. He has a history of chronic renal failure, anemia, and a myocardial infarction. He is currently receiving 4 liters O_2 by nasal cannula and IV antibiotics. His vital signs are BP 90/60 mmHg, HR 108/min, RR 34/min, temperature 38.5°C (101.5°F).

1. Identify conditions present in Mr. T. that impair pulmonary gas exchange.

2. Identify conditions present in Mr. T. that impair oxygen delivery.

3. Identify conditions present in Mr. T. that alter oxygen consumption.

4. What parameters could the nurse use to assess Mr. T.'s pulmonary gas exchange?

5. What parameters could the nurse use to assess Mr. T.'s oxygen delivery?

6. What parameters could the nurse use to assess Mr. T.'s oxygen consumption?

Chapter 34 Review

1. A client's cardiac output is low. The nurse must take into consideration that the client has a disorder of which physiologic component of oxygenation?
   1. Pulmonary gas exchange
   2. Oxygen delivery
   3. Oxygen consumption
   4. Capillary membrane porosity

2. What are the nurse's goals when assessing a client's oxygenation? (Select all that apply.)
   1. To reverse the effects of poor oxygenation
   2. To determine if the client is adequately oxygenated
   3. To determine which medications should be administered
   4. To identify which part of oxygenation needs manipulation
   5. To identify how to reduce the need for oxygen

3. The nurse is caring for a client who is tetraplegic. The nurse plans care based on a disorder of which component of pulmonary gas exchange?
   1. Ventilation
   2. Diffusion
   3. Perfusion
   4. Dilution

4. The client who is receiving oxygen at 60% concentration and is breathing 14 breaths/min has a PaO_2 of 84 mmHg. The client's heart rate is 114 bpm. The nurse calculates the client's P/F ratio as _____.

5. A client's SaO_2 is measured at 80%. How should the nurse interpret this information?
   1. The client's hemoglobin is 80% saturated with oxygen.
   2. The client's hemoglobin is 80%.
   3. The client's plasma is 80% saturated with oxygen.
   4. The client's cardiac output has dropped to 80%.

6. Because a client is hemorrhaging, the nurse realizes that stroke volume is diminished. What effect would the nurse expect as the client's body attempts to compensate for this change? (Select all that apply.)
   1. Respirations will increase.
   2. Temperature will increase.
   3. Heart rate will increase.
   4. Blood pressure will increase.
   5. The skin will flush.

7. A client who is in respiratory failure has a decreased SaO_2, decreased SpO_2, and decreased SvO_2. Because of these values, the nurse identifies which change in the client's oxyhemoglobin dissociation curve?
   1. There is no change.
   2. There is a right shift.
   3. There is a left shift.
   4. There is an upward shift.

8. A client's mixed SvO_2 is measured at 78%. How does the nurse interpret this information?
   1. The client's cardiac cells are not extracting normal amounts of oxygen.
   2. Not enough oxygen is being delivered in arterial blood.
   3. The client's cells are likely adequately oxygenated.
   4. Too much oxygen is being delivered to tissues.

9. A client's oxygenation is impaired due to problems with oxygen delivery. The nurse anticipates interventions directed at which processes to improve oxygen delivery? (Select all that apply.)
   1. Improving cardiac output
   2. Enhancing oxygen content of arterial blood
   3. Restricting autoregulation
   4. Augmenting ventilation
   5. Supporting action of mitochondria

10. A client's poor oxygenation is thought to be related to decreased contractility. Which assessment findings would the nurse evaluate as supporting that decrease? (Select all that apply.)
   1. The client has a history of two myocardial infarctions.
   2. There is ECG evidence of current myocardial ischemia.
   3. Troponin levels indicate an acute myocardial infarction.
   4. The nurse auscultated an S3 heart sound.
   5. Crackles are present in lung bases bilaterally.

Answers to questions found inside your textbook are available on the faculty resources site. Please consult with your instructor.

References

Alarcon, L. H., & Fink, M. P. (2015). Chapter 12: Physiologic monitoring of the surgical patient. In F. C. Brunicardi, D. K. Andersen, T. R. Billiar, D. L. Dunn, J. G. Hunter, J. B. Matthews, & R. E. Pollock (Eds.), *Schwartz's principles of surgery* (10th ed.). New York, NY: McGraw-Hill. Retrieved March 20, 2017, from http://accessmedicine.mhmedical.com.ezproxy.uky.edu/content.aspx?bookid=980&sectionid=59610854

Boulain, T., Garto, D., Vignon, P., Lascarrou, J., Desachy, A., Botoc, V., . . . Dequin, P. (2014). Prevalence of low central venous oxygen saturation in the first hours of intensive care unit admission and associated mortality in septic shock patients: A prospective multicenter study. *Critical Care, 18*(609), 1–12.

Dhup, S., Dadhich, R. K., Porporato, P. E., & Sonveaux, P. (2012). Multiple biological activities of lactic acid in cancer: Influences on tumor growth, angiogenesis and metastasis. *Current Pharmaceutical Design, 18*(10), 1319–1330.

Glass, C. (2016). Blood gases. In J. E. Tintinalli, J. Stapczynski, O. Ma, D. M. Yealy. G. D. Meckler, & D. M. Cline (Eds.), *Tintinalli's emergency medicine: A comprehensive study guide* (8th ed.). New York, NY: McGraw-Hill. Retrieved March 25, 2017, from http://accessmedicine.mhmedical.com.ezproxy.uky.edu/content.aspx?bookid=1658&sectionid=109385181

Illuzzi, E., & Gillespie, M. (2017). Physical examination in the ICU. In J. M. Oropello, S. M. Pastores, & V. Kvetan (Eds.), *Critical care*. New York, NY: McGraw-Hill. Retrieved March 25, 2017, from http://accessmedicine.mhmedical.com.ezproxy.uky.edu/content.aspx?bookid=1944&sectionid=143515966

Jakob, S. M., Parviainen, I., Ruokonen, E., Hinder, R., Uusaro, A., & Takala, J. (2009). Increased splanchnic oxygen extraction because of routine nursing procedures. *Critical Care Medicine, 37*(2), 483–489.

Kee, J. L. (2014). *Laboratory and diagnostic tests with nursing implications* (10th ed.). Hoboken, NJ: Pearson.

Kibble, J. D., & Halsey, C. R. (2014). Pulmonary physiology. In J. D. Kibble & C. R. Halsey (Eds.), *Medical physiology: The big picture*. New York, NY: McGraw-Hill. Retrieved March 25, 2017, from http://accessmedicine.mhmedical.com.ezproxy.uky.edu/content.aspx?bookid=1291&sectionid=75576764

Levitizky, M. G. (2013). Chapter 7. Transport of oxygen and carbon dioxide in the blood. In M. G. Levitzky (Ed.), *Pulmonary physiology* (8th ed.). New York, NY: McGraw-Hill. Retrieved March 21, 2017, from http://accessmedicine.mhmedical.com.ezproxy.uky.edu/content.aspx?bookid=575&sectionid=42512985

Maggiore, S., Idone, F., Vaschetto, R., Cataldo, A., Antonicelli, F., Montini, L., . . . Antonelli, M. (2014). Nasal high-flow versus Venturi mask oxygen therapy after extubation. *American Journal of Respiratory and Critical Care Medicine, 190*(3), 282–288.

Neligan, P. J., & Fuchs, B. D. (2015). Hemodynamic and respiratory monitoring in acute respiratory failure. In M. A. Grippi, J. A. Elias, J. A. Fishman, R. M. Kotloff, A. I. Pack, R. M. Senior, & M. D., Siegel (Eds.), *Fishman's pulmonary diseases and disorders* (5th ed.). New York, NY: McGraw-Hill. Retrieved March 25, 2017, from http://accessmedicine.mhmedical.com.ezproxy.uky.edu/content.aspx?bookid=1344&sectionid=81211113

Nguyen, H. B., Huang, D. T., & Pinsky, M. R. (2016). Hemodynamic monitoring. In J. E. Tintinalli, J. S. Stapczynski, O. J. Ma, D. M. Yealy, G. D. Meckler, & D. M. Cline (Eds.), *Tintinalli's emergency medicine: A comprehensive study guide* (8th ed.). New York, NY: McGraw-Hill. Retrieved March 25, 2017, from http://accessmedicine.mhmedical.com.ezproxy.uky.edu/content.aspx?bookid=1658&sectionid=109427770

Petersson, J., & Glenny, R. W. (2014). Gas exchange and ventilation-perfusion relationships in the lung. *European Respiratory Journal, 44*(4), 1023–1041. doi:10.1183/09031936.00037014.

Schortgen, F., Clabault, K., Katsahian, S., Devaquet, J., Mercat, A., Deye, N., . . . Brochard, L. (2012). Fever control using external cooling in septic shock: A randomized controlled trial. *American Journal of Respiratory and Critical Care Medicine, 185*(10), 1088–1095.

Schumann, L. L. (2013). Respiratory function and alterations in gas exchange. In L. Copstead & J. Banasik (Eds.), *Pathophysiology* (5th ed., pp. 449–474). St. Louis, MO: Elsevier.

Siegal, E. M. (2017). Acute respiratory failure. In S. C. McKean, J. J. Ross, D. D. Dressler, & D. B. Scheurer (Eds.), *Principles and practice of hospital medicine* (2nd ed.). New York, NY: McGraw-Hill. Retrieved March 25, 2017, from http://accessmedicine.mhmedical.com.ezproxy.uky.edu/content.aspx?bookid=1872&sectionid=146980188

Swinamer, D. L., Phang, P. T., Jones, R. L., Grace, M., & King, E. G. (1987). Twenty-four-hour energy expenditure in critically ill patients. *Critical Care Medicine, 15*(7), 637–643.

Thomas, P., Paratz, J., & Lipman, J. (2014). Seated and semi-recumbent positioning of the ventilated intensive care patient—effect on gas exchange, respiratory mechanics and hemodynamics. *Heart & Lung: The Journal of Acute and Critical Care, 43*, 105–111.

Zobel, C., Adler, C., Kranz, A., Seck, C., Pfister, R., Hellmich, M., . . . Reuter, H. (2012). Mild therapeutic hypothermia in cardiogenic shock syndrome. *Critical Care Medicine, 40*(6), 1715–1723.

Zuckerbraun, B. S., Peitzman, A. B., & Billiar, T. R. (2015). Shock. In F. C. Brunicardi, D. K. Andersen, T. R. Billiar, D. L. Dunn, J. G. Hunter, J. B. Matthews, & R. E. Pollock (Eds.), *Schwartz's principles of surgery* (10th ed.). New York, NY: McGraw-Hill. Retrieved March 25, 2017, from http://accessmedicine.mhmedical.com.ezproxy.uky.edu/content.aspx?bookid=980&sectionid=59610846

Chapter 35
Multiple Trauma

Learning Outcomes

35.1 Discuss traumatic injury, including categories of injury and risk factors that influence injury patterns.

35.2 Describe blunt trauma, including its associated forces and the clinical assessment of a patient with blunt trauma.

35.3 Discuss penetrating trauma, including its associated forces and the clinical assessment of a patient with penetrating trauma.

35.4 Demonstrate an understanding of the mechanisms of injury and mediators of the response to injury when caring for a patient with traumatic injury.

35.5 Apply the clinical assessment format used to identify life-threatening injuries during the primary and secondary surveys of an injured patient.

35.6 Describe trauma resuscitation and nursing responsibilities based on the trimodal distribution of trauma-related mortalities.

35.7 Discuss the management of selected traumatic injuries, including chest, pulmonary, cardiac, abdominal, and pelvic.

35.8 Link posttrauma complications and interventions with the physiology of a traumatic injury and preexisting risk factors.

Injuries are the cause of significant morbidity and mortality in the United States (Figure 35–1). In 2012, the three leading trauma-injury–related reasons for seeking medical assistance were falls, being struck by a person or object, and transportation-related injury (Centers for Disease Control and Prevention [CDC], 2014). In a final report on causes of death in the United States in 2014, unintentional injury, the fifth-leading cause of death in 2012, became the fourth-leading cause in 2014, and intentional self-harm (suicide) ranked tenth (Centers for Disease Control and Prevention [CDC], 2016a). While assault (including homicide) dropped below the top 15 in 2010, it remained a significant cause of death in 2014 (CDC, 2016a). Adjusting for age, homicide remains among the 15 leading causes of death (CDC, 2016a).

This chapter provides an overview of traumatic injury. Particular focus is given to the mechanism of injury in both blunt and penetrating trauma as an assessment factor that should raise the index of suspicion for certain injuries.

Many important complications are associated with severe multiple trauma injury. This chapter briefly profiles the major complications; however, the reader is referred to specific textbook chapters for more detailed information, as follows: acute respiratory distress syndrome (Chapter 12); abdominal compartment syndrome (Chapter 22); acute kidney injury (Chapter 27); disseminated intravascular coagulation (Chapter 29); shock, including septic shock (Chapter 37); and multiple organ dysfunction syndrome (Chapter 38).

Section One: Overview of the Injured Patient

Understanding injury enables the nurse to approach a patient in crisis with a level-headed, systematic plan based on a solid body of nursing knowledge. Historically, injuries or accidents were viewed as the result of random chance beyond human control. Now, injury is viewed as an event with an identifiable cause: the interaction of energy and force with a recipient. The recipient may be an inanimate object, such as a motor vehicle, or an animate object, such as a person.

Injury results from acute exposure to energy, such as kinetic energy (e.g., a motor vehicle crash [MVC], fall, or bullet); from chemical, thermal, electrical, or ionizing radiation;

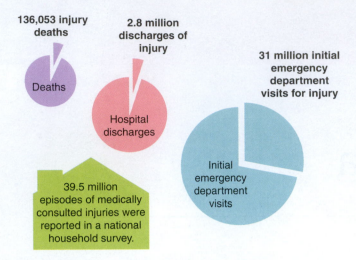

Figure 35–1 Injuries in the United States.

SOURCE: Centers for Disease Control and Prevention (2014); Centers for Disease Control and Prevention (2016b); National Hospital Discharge Survey (2016b); National Vital Statistics System (2016b).

or from a lack of essential agents (e.g., oxygen [drowning] or heat [frostbite]). The injury occurs because of the body's inability to tolerate excessive exposure to the energy source. The term **traumatic injury**, the focus of this chapter, is specific to injuries caused by kinetic injury. The CDC (2016a) published the National Vital Statistics for 2014, including the number of injury deaths by mechanism, as well as the percentages of the top three trauma-related causes of death: motor vehicle traffic (17%), firearms (17%), and falls (16%) (CDC, 2016a) (Figure 35–2).

Categories of Kinetic Injury

Although usually unintentional, traumatic injuries may be intentional (e.g., assault or murder) or self-inflicted (suicide). Although intent varies, the categories of traumatic injury remain the same: either blunt or penetrating, depending on the injuring agent.

Blunt trauma is any traumatic injury in which there is tissue deformation without interruption of skin integrity. Blunt trauma may be life-threatening because the extent of

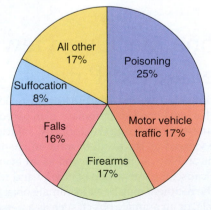

Figure 35–2 Injury death by mechanism: United States, 2014.

SOURCE: From National Vital Statistics Reports—Deaths (2014).

the injury may be covert, making diagnosis difficult. The nature of the injury is related to both the transfer of energy and the anatomic structure involved.

Penetrating trauma refers to injury sustained by the transmission of energy to body tissues from a moving object that interrupts skin and tissue integrity. Penetrating trauma may also cause surrounding tissue deformation based on the energy transferred by the penetrating object.

Deformation and displacement of body tissue and organs occur in both forms of injury because of the transfer of energy. Injury takes place as the structural limits of a particular tissue or organ are exceeded. Injury may be localized, as in hematoma formation, or systemic, as in shock states. The local response varies according to the tissue or organ involved, such as bone fractures and bleeding vessels.

Risk Factors for Traumatic Injury

Traumatic injuries, like other diseases, do not occur at random. Identifiable risk factors are associated with specific injury patterns. These risk factors include age, gender, and alcohol use, as well as race, income, and geography.

Age Unintentional injury continues to be the leading cause of death in all Americans ages 1 through 45 (Centers for Disease Control and Prevention [CDC], 2016b). The death rate from injury is highest for persons over 65 years old. The highest injury rate is for persons between the ages of 15 through 24 because of their participation in high-risk activities (including poor judgment with the use of alcohol, drugs, and driving practices). The highest homicide rate occurs among persons between 18 and 24 years of age.

Older adults are predisposed to trauma because of age-related changes in reaction time, balance and coordination, and sensory motor function; falls are the leading mechanism of injury in people 65 years and older (CDC, 2016b). Trauma in older adults is associated with higher mortality and morbidity with less severe injury. For example, a 79-year-old with multiple rib fractures will have a very different clinical course than an 18-year-old with the same injuries. This is attributed to preexisting medical conditions and the older person's diminished ability to compensate for severe injury (known as *limited physiological reserve*) (Adams & Holcomb, 2015; Joseph et al., 2017). Limited physiological reserve is the concept of limited organ function in the face of a physiologic challenge. Organ dysfunction may not appear in the resting state, but in a physiological stress situation (such as traumatic injury), the ability of the organs to augment function is compromised (Adams & Holcomb, 2015; Joseph et al., 2017). Moreover, the reduced physiological response to traumatic injury may mask the seriousness of the older patient's condition, causing delayed diagnosis and treatment.

Gender Injury rates are highest for 15- to 24-year-old males. The risk for men is 2.5 times that for women, possibly because of male involvement in hazardous activities. Women are at higher risk for fall injury than are men (CDC, 2014).

Alcohol Motor vehicle crashes (MVCs) involving alcohol-impaired drivers were responsible for about one third of all traffic-related deaths in 2014 (CDC, 2016a). Alcohol use and abuse increase the likelihood of virtually all types of injury, even among young teenagers. An alcohol-related MVC kills someone every 53 minutes, at an associated annual cost of over $44 billion (Centers for Disease Control [CDC], 2016c). Alcohol-related trauma is a major public health problem. Communities have enacted programs to reduce alcohol-related MVCs, including lowering the legal blood alcohol level to 0.08% and initiating sobriety checkpoints.

Severity of Injury, Mortality, and Payer Source

According to the 2016 American College of Surgeons National Trauma Data Bank Annual Report (NTDB), of 861,888 trauma patients, almost half (45.29%) sustained minor injuries, and just less than one third (32.69%) had moderate injuries based on the Injury Severity Score (ISS), a system for stratifying injury severity (Chang, 2016). The ISS ranges from 1 to 75, and the risk of mortality increases with a higher score. An ISS between 1 and 8 is minor trauma, between 9 and 15 is moderate trauma, between 16 and 24 is severe trauma, and greater than 24 is very severe. The case fatality rate increases as injury severity increases to as high as 30%. Mortality rates for all severity levels is higher for patients ages 75 and older. Length of stay in acute care hospitals increases as injury severity increases. Private or commercial insurance has now overtaken Medicare as the single largest payment source at 35.10%, with Medicare coming in second at 27%. Medicaid is the third largest payer source at 16.28% (Chang, 2016).

The overall mortality rate for all causes of trauma is 4.39% with the largest number of deaths being due to fall-related injuries, followed by MVCs and firearm-related injuries. Fatality rates are higher in patients 75 years or older, with firearm injuries having the highest fatality rates in all age groups (Chang, 2016).

Age, Gender, Mechanism of Injury, and Geography

Trauma injuries initially peak in ages 14 to 29 from MVC injuries, then peak again between the ages of 40 to 50 due to an increase in fall-related trauma injuries. Falls peak in children at ages 5 to 9 years of age and in adults over the age of 65. Men account for 70% of all trauma-related injuries up to age 70; after age 71, women account for most trauma-related injuries. Falls accounted for 44.18% of cases in the NTDB, with these injuries peaking in children under age 7 and adults over age 75. MVC injuries accounted for 25.97% of cases in the NTDB, with peaks between ages 16 and 26 years. Suffocation, drowning or submersion, and firearm injuries have the highest case fatality rates (suffocation 27.12%, firearm 15.30%, and drowning or submersion 19.20%). At 12 years of age, firearm injuries double and steadily increase until age 22, then they are followed by a decrease (Chang, 2016).

Rural areas account for a higher unintentional injury rate, and a higher intentional injury rate is seen in urban areas (Chang, 2016). Behaviors associated with unintentional injuries in rural areas may include greater use of recreational vehicles and employment in high-risk occupations such as farming. Intentional injuries in urban areas are usually related to homicide attempts (Chang, 2016).

Section One Review

1. The death rate from injury is highest for which age group?
   - A. 24 to 42 years old
   - B. 15 to 24 years old
   - C. 5 to 14 years old
   - D. Over 65 years old

2. Why do older adults with traumatic injury have higher mortality and morbidity rates?
   - A. They have limited physiological reserve.
   - B. They are exposed to high-risk activities.
   - C. They drink more alcohol.
   - D. They have poor judgment.

3. How does the risk for injury among men compare to the risk among women?
   - A. It is 2.5 times lower.
   - B. It is 2.5 times higher.
   - C. It is 5 times higher.
   - D. The risks are equal.

4. Reducing legal blood alcohol to what level has been shown to decrease alcohol-related MVCs?
   - A. 0.10%
   - B. 0.05%
   - C. 0.08%
   - D. 0.04%

Answers: 1. D, 2. A, 3. B, 4. C

Section Two: Mechanism of Injury: Blunt Trauma

Blunt trauma is most commonly associated with MVCs, motor vehicles striking pedestrians, and falls from significant heights. One of the most basic principles of physics can be used to explain trauma: the law of conservation of energy. Energy can be neither created nor destroyed; it is only changed from one form to another. Blunt trauma is the translation of energy from one form to another, through force.

Forces Associated with Blunt Trauma

Force is a physical factor: the push or pull that changes the state of an object that is either at rest or already in motion. Injury resulting from force is related to the velocity of energy transmission, the surface area to which the energy is applied, and the elasticity of the tissues affected. The more slowly the force is applied, the more slowly energy is released, with less subsequent tissue deformation. The forces most often applied are shearing, acceleration, deceleration, and compression (Ali, 2014; Cameron & Knapp, 2016).

Shearing Force   **Shearing** refers to a tearing injury that results when two structures, or two parts of the same structure, slide in opposite directions or at different speeds. For example, shearing forces are frequently the cause of spinal injury at the C7–T1 juncture because the mobile cervical spine attaches at that point to the relatively immobile thoracic spine. Shearing forces are often the cause of aortic tears, splenic and renal injuries, and liver, brain, or heart injuries. These structures have a relatively immobile section connected to a relatively mobile section and are therefore subject to shearing forces (Roccaforte, 2017).

Acceleration and Deceleration Forces   **Acceleration** is an increase in the rate of velocity of a moving body or body structure. Velocity is the most significant determinant of the amount of injury sustained. As velocity increases, so does tissue damage, because a greater amount of energy is involved. The concept of acceleration is illustrated by the following example: Upon impact with a solid object (e.g., another car, a brick wall, or a telephone pole), the driver of a car is suddenly propelled forward. He experiences a sudden acceleration of body mass determined by the rate of speed at which he was traveling and his body mass.

Body weight × mph = pounds per square inch of impact

A person weighing 100 pounds, traveling at 35 miles per hour (mph), will impact at 3500 pounds per square inch. This is equivalent to jumping head-first from a three-story building.

Deceleration is a decrease in the rate of velocity of a moving object. The same driver in the preceding example who is moving forward after hitting a solid object will experience a sudden deceleration after he comes into contact with the mass that impedes his forward (or backward) progression (e.g., the steering wheel, a tree, the road, or another passenger).

Acceleration and deceleration injuries are most common with blunt trauma and are closely associated with shearing-force injuries—for example, injuries involving the thoracic aorta. MVCs and falls from 20 feet or higher precipitate stretching, bowing, and shearing in major vessels. Any or all layers of the vessel wall may be damaged. The vessel wall can tear, dissect, rupture, or form an aneurysm immediately or at any time post-injury. Shearing damage occurs in the vessels when deceleration occurs at a different rate than that occurring in other internal structures. For example, the relatively mobile ascending aorta continues to move after the relatively stationary descending aorta has stopped moving, resulting in a shearing injury.

Compression Force   **Compression** is the process of being pressed or squeezed together with a resulting reduction in volume or size. For example, sudden acceleration or deceleration during an MVC can cause compression of the heart and lung parenchyma between the posterior and anterior chest walls. The small bowel may be compressed between the vertebral column and the lower part of the steering wheel or an improperly placed seat belt. The bowel may rupture. The same mechanism can cause compression of the liver, causing it to burst.

Injuries Associated with Blunt Trauma

Injuries associated with blunt traumatic forces include head injuries (the movement of the brain inside the skull with acceleration, deceleration, and shearing coup injury), spinal cord injuries (the instability and poor support of the cervical spine predispose it to shearing and acceleration or deceleration injury), fractures (from shearing and compression), and abdominal injuries, especially to the spleen and liver (from shearing and compression).

Each type of tissue has its own characteristic tensile strength—that is, the tissue's ability to withstand injury from the applied forces of shearing, acceleration, deceleration, and compression. Tissue deformation is generally the result of **tensile forces** (those that stretch and extend tissue) or shear forces. The tensile strength of a specific tissue is the greatest longitudinal stretch or stress it can withstand without tearing apart. Joint dislocations, muscle sprains, and strains are frequently the result of tensile forces (Roccaforte, 2017).

Section Two Review

1. What is the term for a decrease in the velocity of a moving object?
   A. Acceleration
   B. Deceleration
   C. Compression
   D. Shearing

2. What is the force that causes two structures to slide in opposite directions or at different speeds?
   A. Acceleration
   B. Deceleration
   C. Compression
   D. Shearing

3. The process of being pressed or squeezed is known by what term?
   A. Acceleration
   B. Deceleration
   C. Compression
   D. Shearing

4. Which forces cause tissues to stretch?
   A. Tensile
   B. Shearing
   C. Mass
   D. Compression

Answers: 1. B, 2. D, 3. C, 4. A

Section Three: Mechanism of Injury: Penetrating Trauma

Penetrating trauma is often quickly discovered because, unlike blunt trauma, the skin has been broken, providing an obvious clue to the injury. However, although it is easier to discover, the severity of internal injury is more difficult to ascertain. Understanding the forces involved in penetrating trauma will facilitate rapid assessment and management of patients with penetrating injuries.

Forces Associated with Penetrating Trauma

Penetrating trauma is the result of the transmission of energy from a moving object (referred to as a missile) into body tissues as the object disrupts the integrity of the skin and the underlying structures. The amount of kinetic energy transmitted by the object has a direct bearing on the degree of tissue damage. With tissue or organ penetration, the severity of the injury depends on the organs and tissues damaged by the transmission of the energy. A penetrating object can be almost anything—for example, a knife, a bullet, shrapnel, an arrow, a stick, a metal rod, a fork, or a gear shift.

The amount of kinetic energy available to be transmitted to tissues depends on the surface area of the point of impact, the density of the tissue, and the velocity of the projectile at the time of impact. Weapons are usually classified by the amount of energy they are capable of producing: low-energy weapons include knives, arrows, or any type of hand missile; medium-energy weapons include handguns and some rifles; and high-energy weapons include hunting rifles and shotguns (Ali, 2014; Cameron & Knapp, 2016).

Low- to Medium-energy Missiles

Low- to medium-energy missiles travel less than 2000 feet per second. The injury sustained usually results from the missile contacting the tissue. Typically, damage is localized to those structures directly in the missile's path (Figure 35–3). However, special consideration must be given when injury occurs where body cavities lie in close proximity to one another. This principle is of critical importance when considering the close proximity of the thoracic and abdominal cavities, especially with injuries occurring near the diaphragm, which offers very little resistance to the penetrating

object. Penetrating injuries to the chest below the nipple line, the sixth rib, or the scapula may involve both thoracic and abdominal structures.

If the offending missile (e.g., knife, stick, or metal rod) is impaled in the body, it is critical that it be left in place and protected from further movement until definitive surgical intervention is available. For example, if a knife is impaled in the abdomen, protective padding such as gauze rolls or abdominal pads can be placed around the externally exposed blade and handle. A protective device, such as a plastic cup, may be used to secure the protruding part of the missile. Impaled missiles may actually control hemorrhage from damaged structures, and removal may precipitate exsanguination.

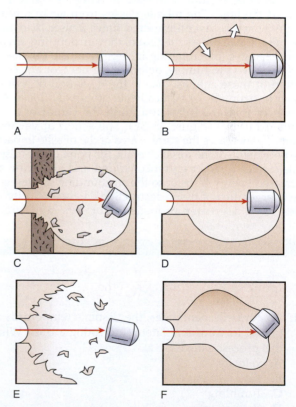

Figure 35–3 Patterns of tissue injury secondary to gunshot wounds. A, Low velocity, small entrance, and exit wounds. B, Higher velocity, cavitation present with energy dispersion outward from missile path (blast effect). C, Same velocity as in B but with penetration of bone and greater blast effect because of projections of bone being spread through tissue. D, Higher velocity than in B or C with greater cavitation effect, small entrance and exit wounds. E, Same velocity as in D, but person or extremity hit is thinner, resulting in large exit wound. F, Asymmetrical cavitation as bullet begins to yaw and tumble.

High-energy Missiles

High-energy missiles are those traveling more than 2000 feet per second. Also referred to as high-velocity missiles, they transmit more kinetic energy than low-energy missiles. As the missile penetrates the tissue, the transmission of kinetic energy displaces tissues forward and laterally to form a temporary cavity, a process known as **cavitation** (see Figure 35–3). The degree of cavitation is directly related to the amount of kinetic energy transmitted to the tissues, which in turn is determined by the velocity of the missile. The size of the cavity may be up to 30 times the diameter of the missile. Tissue surrounding the missile tract is exposed to tensile (stretching), compressing, and shearing forces, which produce damage outside the direct path of the missile. Vessels, nerves, and other structures that are not directly damaged by the missile may be affected. The phenomenon of injury to structures outside the direct missile path is referred to as blast effect. Higher-velocity missiles produce more serious injury because of the destructive process of cavitation and blast effect on surrounding tissue and organs.

Missile Trajectory   In addition to the amount of kinetic energy (low, medium, or high) associated with the missile, its trajectory (path of the missile) is also an important consideration. Consider a missile moving in stable flight toward the host. The missile passes from air into human tissue, which is several hundred times denser than air. As the missile penetrates the tissue, the surrounding environment changes, precipitating instability in the missile. The missile may yaw, tumble, deform, fragment, or any combination of these actions. *Yaw* is the deviation of a missile either horizontally or vertically about its axis. *Tumble* is the action of forward rotation around the center of a mass (somersaulting) (Figure 35–3F). The action of yawing or tumbling increases the surface area of the missile impacting the body (side of the missile versus the point of the missile). This creates a larger entrance wound and also allows for increased energy transfer to the surrounding tissues, creating a larger area of tissue destruction. Higher-velocity missiles have a greater propensity for yaw and tumble.

Moreover, the missile can *fragment*, or break into multiple pieces, which increases internal deformation and damage.

Secondary Missiles

Another injury mechanism to consider when analyzing the effects of penetrating injury is the creation of secondary missiles by the penetrating object. A missile or its fragments may impart sufficient kinetic injury to dense tissue, such as bone or teeth, to create highly destructive secondary missiles. Furthermore, the primary missile can fragment into multiple secondary missiles. These secondary missiles may take erratic, unpredictable courses, resulting in additional injury.

Injuries Associated with Penetrating Trauma

Wounds caused by the missile must be evaluated, noting their location, size, and shape. It is also important to determine whether there is any foreign substance on the surrounding tissue, such as gunpowder, and whether the wound is actively bleeding.

If there are two wounds, noting the location of each gives the clinician information regarding the trajectory the missile may have taken if the same missile caused both wounds. Missiles usually take the path of least resistance, so the path may not be a straight line between the two wounds. Entrance wounds are usually smaller than exit wounds. However, the characteristics of a wound depend on the forces causing the injury, such as velocity, cavitation, and blast effect. Identifying the entrance and exit wounds is not necessary and should be left to experienced personnel. Simply identifying the wounds as wound 1 and wound 2 will suffice. The presence of two wounds does not necessarily mean one is an entrance wound and one is an exit wound, as there may be two entrance wounds from two separate missiles. Not all medium- and high-energy penetrating injuries have a resulting exit wound because the missile may remain inside the body (Roccaforte, 2017).

Section Three Review

1. As a missile penetrates, the tissue is temporarily displaced forward and laterally, creating a tract. What is this process called?
   A. Velocity
   B. Yaw
   C. Tumbling
   D. Cavitation

2. What is the term for structure injury outside the direct missile path?
   A. Cavitation
   B. Blast effect
   C. Yaw
   D. Tumbling

3. How do yaw and tumble affect the area of tissue destruction caused by a missile?
   A. Decrease it
   B. Increase it
   C. Minimize it
   D. Do not affect it

4. A client has an impaled knife in the upper abdomen. What should the nurse do?
   A. Remove the knife and apply pressure.
   B. Manipulate the knife to facilitate assessment of injured organs.
   C. Stabilize the knife without removal and with minimal manipulation.
   D. Leave the knife alone.

Answers: 1. D, 2. B, 3. B, 4. C

Section Four: Mechanism of Injury: Patterns and Mediators of Injury Response

The mechanism of injury is associated with certain possible injury patterns. This fact makes it possible to associate the type and extent of injuries based on the mechanism involved. In addition, when a multiple-trauma patient is admitted, the nurse should be aware of mediators that may influence the seriousness and extent of injury.

Mechanisms of Injury and Injury Patterns

Certain mechanisms of injury result in predictable injury patterns (Table 35–1). Thus, the events surrounding the injury, such as pedestrian–motor vehicle injuries, motor vehicle driver and passenger injuries, fall injuries, and missile injuries, should increase suspicion for certain patterns of injured structures.

The following example demonstrates the importance of understanding the mechanism of injury. A 21-year-old unrestrained male driver crashes into another vehicle head-on (Figure 35–4). Traveling speed was in excess of 95 mph. Both the steering wheel and windshield were broken. A high index of suspicion must be maintained for the following potential injuries:

1. Intracranial injury because of the high rate of speed and shattered windshield

2. Cervical vertebrae injury because of acceleration or deceleration at a high rate of speed and the broken windshield

3. Intrathoracic injuries because of the broken steering wheel—suspect rib fractures, myocardial and pulmonary contusions, and great vessel injury

4. Intra-abdominal injuries because of the broken steering wheel and acceleration or deceleration mechanism; could include splenic or liver lacerations, small bowel injuries, and great vessel injuries

5. Long-bone fractures, especially femur fractures or posterior hip fracture–dislocation, because of the impact of the knees on the dashboard

6. Multiple skin lacerations, avulsions, punctures from impact with various parts of the vehicle interior

Factors Affecting the Response to Injury

Many clinical conditions affect a patient's response to injury, including underlying medical disorders, substance use, and physiological alterations such as pregnancy and advancing age.

Comorbidities It is extremely important to identify comorbidities or underlying medical conditions when considering the patient's physiological and hemodynamic response to trauma. Chronic conditions such as heart disease, kidney disease, or diabetes and the medications used to control their manifestations may alter the physiological response to trauma. The patient with COPD who sustains a minor pulmonary contusion related to blunt trauma may require prompt, life-saving intubation because of the alteration in

Table 35–1 Commonly Seen Injuries

Mechanism of Injury	Predictable Injury Pattern
Pedestrian hit by automobile	
Adult	Fractures of femur, tibia, and fibula on side of impact; ligamental damage to impacted knee; mild contralateral brain injury
Child	Fractures of femur, chest injury, contralateral brain injury
Unrestrained driver	Head and/or facial injury, rib fractures, sternum with underlying myocardial or pulmonary contusion, cervical spine fractures, laryngotracheal injuries, spleen injuries, liver injuries, small bowel injuries, posterior fracture–dislocation of hip, femur fractures
Unrestrained front seat passenger	Head and/or facial injuries, laryngotracheal injuries, posterior fracture–dislocation of femoral head, femur or patellar fractures
Restrained driver (lap and shoulder harness)	Contusions of structures underlying harness (e.g., pulmonary contusion, contusion of small bowel)
Restrained passenger (lap belt only)	Flexion-distraction fractures, especially lumbar vertebrae (L1–L4), duodenal injuries, cervical spine injuries
Fall injuries	Compression fractures of lumbosacral spine and calcaneous fractures; fractures of radius or ulna, patella if victim falls forward
Vehicular ejection	Multiple injuries, especially head and cervical spine injuries; injury risk increases by 300% when ejection occurs
Low-velocity impalement	Local tissue or organ disruption, little or no cavitation
High-velocity missile, short missile path	Entrance wound larger than missile caliber; large ragged exit wound with cavitation
High-velocity missile, long missile path	Entrance wound larger than missile caliber; exit wound slightly larger than or equal to missile caliber; extensive cavitation (blast effect to deep structures absorbing lost kinetic energy)
High-velocity missile hitting bone or teeth	Entry wound larger than missile caliber; possibly no exit wound with missile fragmentation; secondary missile injury in unpredictable, erratic pattern

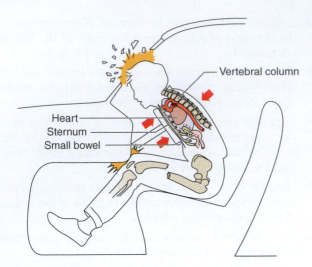

Figure 35–4 Typical injuries of an unrestrained driver.

the ventilation–perfusion ratio, inability to compensate, and lack of pulmonary reserve. Beta blockade used for coronary artery disease to minimize oxygen demands by the heart could prevent a normal response to hypovolemia (i.e., tachycardia). The patient with a brain injury who has a history of stroke may experience an altered level of consciousness, difficulty in communication, or sensory or motor dysfunction from the prior stroke and not the acute brain injury. Eliciting a complete medical history, including comorbidity information, is crucial during the initial assessment. This is especially important in older adults who are most likely to be admitted with at least one comorbid illness; it is estimated that 80% of people 65 years of age or older have comorbid illnesses (Adams & Holcomb, 2015).

Substance Use Disorders

Substance use disorders (as it is now called, changed from the previous classification: substance abuse and substance dependence) are characterized by recurrent and clinically significant adverse consequences related to the repeated use of substances. The DSM-V definition for substance use includes meeting two or three (mild substance use diagnosis), four or five (moderate), and six or seven (severe) of the following criteria: (1) taking the substance in larger amounts or for longer than intended, (2) wanting to cut down or stop, but not managing to, (3) spending a lot of time getting, using, or recovering from use, (4) having cravings and urges to use, (5) knowing work, home, or school obligations are affected, (6) continuing to use, even with relationship problems, (7) giving up social, occupational, or recreational activities, (8) using substances again and again, despite dangers, (9) continuing to use, even knowing a physical or psychological problem is made worse by the substance, (10) needing an increasing amount of the substance to have desired effect, and (11) developing withdrawal symptoms (American Psychiatric Association, 2013).

The high incidence of alcohol as a contributing factor to injury has been demonstrated (National Highway Traffic Safety Administration [NHTSA], 2016). The effects of alcohol on the level of consciousness make it extremely difficult to obtain an accurate baseline assessment of the patient. Alcohol is a central nervous system (CNS) depressant, and

its effects on the brain are concentration dependent. The most sensitive tool for evaluating brain injury is level of consciousness. Therefore, alcohol or other CNS-depressant intake is a critical consideration because it can delay accurate evaluation for potential brain injury.

Blood alcohol concentration (BAC) is a measurement of intoxication, given in either milligrams per deciliter (mg/dL) or grams per deciliter (g/dL). Legal intoxication in all states, as well as the District of Columbia and Puerto Rico, is a BAC of 80 mg/dL (0.08 g/dL); however, the effects of alcohol on the brain are apparent at a level of 20 mg/dL (0.02 g/dL) (NHTSA, 2016; Kee, 2014). A history of alcohol use should be obtained because a degree of tolerance develops with frequent alcohol ingestion. As plasma levels increase, sedation, lack of motor coordination, ataxia, and impaired psychomotor performance become apparent. The concomitant use of alcohol and other CNS depressants (e.g., barbiturates, opiates, sedative–hypnotics) potentiates each drug's effects, creating a synergistic effect. CNS stimulants such as cocaine can also alter the level of consciousness in an injured patient. Neurologically, changes in mental status range from anxiety to acute paranoid psychosis. For the high-acuity nurse, it is very difficult to obtain a baseline level of consciousness when the patient is intoxicated with alcohol or other drugs that cloud his or her sensorium.

Pregnancy The pregnant trauma patient presents with anatomical and physiological changes that must be carefully considered. Major trauma affects 8% of pregnant patients (Jain et al., 2015). Familiarity with trauma assessment and management during pregnancy is important for the nurse in the high-acuity setting. Pregnancy testing may be done on any woman of childbearing age who presents with multiple trauma (Roccaforte, 2017).

Anatomic Changes. Anatomic rearrangement occurs in the pregnant woman as the uterus progressively enlarges in the anterior abdomen and presses many of the abdominal organs to a more posterior abdominal location. During early pregnancy, the uterus and fetus are well protected within the pelvis and lower abdomen; in later pregnancy, however, the prominent anatomic location of the uterus places both the uterus and fetus at higher risk of injury (Jain et al., 2015; Limmer et al., 2016). Therefore, different patterns of injury may occur to the mother, as well as to the fetus, depending on the stage of pregnancy. Blunt abdominal trauma in the pregnant patient is associated with different injuries from those in the nonpregnant patient.

Hemodynamic Changes. After the tenth week of pregnancy, cardiac output increases by up to 50%. A high-output, low-resistance hemodynamic state is characteristic in pregnancy. Maternal heart rate increases by 10 to 15 beats per minute throughout pregnancy, with a slight increase in stroke volume. Blood pressure decreases by 5 mmHg to 15 mmHg (Jain et al., 2015). It is important to remember that some women experience profound hypotension when placed in the supine position (especially during the third trimester). This is known as the *vena cava syndrome* and is caused by the enlarged uterus compressing the inferior vena cava against the spinal column, which decreases venous return and preload. The hypotension can be relieved by turning the patient to the left lateral decubitus position.

Blood Volume and Composition. During pregnancy, maternal blood volume increases by 50% by the end of the third trimester, with maximal volume expansion by 28 to 32 weeks gestation (Jain et al., 2015). Therefore, mild blood loss as a result of traumatic injury is usually well tolerated. Because of the hypervolemic state associated with pregnancy, a 30% to 40% (up to 2000 mL) blood loss may occur in a pregnant patient before signs and symptoms of hypovolemia occur; however, the patient may deteriorate rapidly once a 2500 mL blood loss has occurred.

During pregnancy, a physiological anemia results as plasma volume increases by 50% and red blood cell volume increases by only 30%. Late in pregnancy, the hemoglobin may fall to 10.5 to 11 g/dL and the hematocrit to 31% to 35%. The white blood cell count increases during pregnancy (15,000 to 18,000/mm^3) and during labor may be as high as 25,000/mm^3 (Jain et al., 2015).

Advancing Age Physiological changes associated with aging (65 years and older), such as delayed reaction times, disturbances of gait and balance, diminished visual acuity, and hearing loss, predispose older adults to traumatic injury. Also, age-related deterioration in body systems alters the older adult trauma victim's response to injury and increases the risk for complications. The most common mechanism of injury in this age group is falls, followed by motor vehicle crashes, pedestrian-versus-automobile crashes, and penetrating trauma.

Chronic Disease States. Chronic disease states exacerbate or compound the patient's response to traumatic injury. The most commonly encountered chronic conditions in older Americans include hypertension, heart disease, stroke, cancer, diabetes, chronic obstructive pulmonary disease (COPD), arthritis, and asthma (Federal Interagency Forum on Aging-Related Statistics, 2016). The patient not only may have a chronic medical condition but also may be following with a polypharmaceutical regimen that could affect the response to a traumatic injury.

Limited Physiologic Reserve. Recall from Section One that the higher morbidity and mortality rates associated with trauma and advancing age can be attributed to limited physiological reserve, most often in the cardiorespiratory, neurological, and musculoskeletal systems.

Cardiorespiratory Changes Cardiorespiratory changes include decreased distensibility of blood vessels, increased systolic blood pressure and systemic vascular resistance, increased vascular resistance, decreased coronary blood flow, decreased cardiac output, decreased respiratory muscle strength, limited chest expansion, and decreased number of functioning alveoli. These alterations combine to reduce greatly the ability to sustain adequate tissue perfusion and oxygenation. Mild anemia is also common in this age group and potentiates alterations in oxygenation by limiting oxygen transport capabilities.

Neurologic Changes Neurologic changes associated with advancing age include short-term memory loss and reduced cerebral blood flow. Preexisting neurologic conditions, such as senility, dementia, and Alzheimer disease, may significantly affect evaluation of the patient's neurologic status. Head injuries are common in older adults. A high index of suspicion for a potential head injury, awareness of the patient's preexisting neurologic status, and frequent, thorough neurologic assessments are necessary to avoid detrimental delays in diagnosis and intervention.

Musculoskeletal Changes Osteoporosis and decreasing muscle mass contribute to the high incidence of fractures. The incidence of rib fractures with blunt chest trauma is 10% to 76% (Dehghan, de Mestral, McKee, Schemitsch, & Nathens, 2014). Patients of advancing age have twice the mortality and morbidity rates of younger patients. Mortality increases with the number of rib fractures. Normal aging processes diminish blood supply to the skin and result in delayed healing of soft-tissue injuries and the development of pressure ulcers.

Shock During the initial assessment, difficulties related to normal aging may be noted by the clinician. Shock is difficult to diagnose secondary to age-related changes that affect the patient's response to trauma, including decreased cardiac output, decreased maximal heart rate, and increased peripheral vascular resistance (Adams & Holcomb, 2015; Calland et al., 2012). Because of the decline in gag and cough reflexes, airway patency may be difficult to maintain. Shock may be difficult to detect because of older adults' propensity toward hypertension. Thus, normal blood pressures may actually indicate low perfusion states. Aggressive care and resuscitation significantly improve patient outcomes; therefore, older adults require a more aggressive approach during their initial emergency management than do younger patients with similar injuries (Calland et al., 2012).

Section Four Review

1. A restrained driver (lap and shoulder harness) involved in an MVC can receive what type of injuries from the restraints?
   A. Pulmonary contusions
   B. Lumbar fractures
   C. Femur fractures
   D. Facial injuries

2. Which statement about vehicular ejection is true?
   A. It increases the risk for injury.
   B. It decreases the risk for injury.
   C. It is not related to the risk for injury.
   D. It is associated with seat belt use.

3. A broken steering wheel should induce a high suspicion of injury to which part of the body?
   A. Head
   B. Neck
   C. Abdomen
   D. Long bones of the legs

4. Why is eliciting a medical history crucial during the initial assessment? (Select all that apply.)
   A. Comorbidities alter the physiologic response to trauma.
   B. It is essential to determining mechanism of injury.
   C. A medical history helps to identify the cause of injury.
   D. The client may be comatose later.

Answers: 1. A, 2. A, 3. C, 4. A

Section Five: Primary and Secondary Surveys

Trauma should always be approached as a multisystem disease. The nurse must develop a rapid, systematic approach to assessing each trauma patient to identify injuries. Trauma presents myriad potentially life-threatening injuries that must be evaluated quickly, with immediate interventions. Trauma care based on Advanced Trauma Life Support (ATLS) principles is divided into three phases: primary survey, resuscitation, and secondary survey, with the primary survey and resuscitation phases occurring simultaneously (Cameron & Knapp, 2016; Roccaforte, 2017). This section provides an overview of the ATLS survey process.

The Primary Survey

The purpose of the primary survey is to identify life-threatening injuries and intervene appropriately. The primary survey is done using the ABCDE approach:

- **A—Airway (with cervical spine immobilization):** The nurse assesses the patient for airflow from nose and mouth, normal chest movements, the presence of foreign bodies in the mouth, and abnormal breathing sounds that suggest airway obstruction.
- **B—Breathing:** The nurse assesses breathing rate, rhythm and depth and pattern, abnormal breathing sounds, use of accessory respiratory muscles, and oxygen saturation.
- **C—Circulation:** The nurse assesses blood pressure; heart rate, rhythm, and quality; bleeding; and signs of shock.
- **D—Disability:** The nurse assesses the patient's level of consciousness and motor function.
- **E—Exposure and evacuation:** The nurse completely undresses the patient to allow visualization of external causes of injury. If the severity of the patient's injury exceeds the capability of the hospital, the patient should be transported to a hospital with the appropriate level of trauma care.

Each step of the primary survey is explored in more detail here, providing information needed to assess the patient with multiple injuries using critical thinking and problem-solving strategies.

A–Airway   The first step in the primary survey is assessment of the patency of the patient's airway. The goal of airway management is to maintain an open airway while protecting the cervical spine. An injury to the cervical spine should always be assumed in the patient with multisystem trauma, especially in the patient with an injury above the clavicle. Excessive manipulation of the head, face, or neck, such as hyperextension or hyperflexion of the cervical spine, while performing airway management may convert a fracture without neurologic deficits into a fracture–dislocation with spinal cord contusion, laceration, compression, or transection. Therefore, cervical immobilization is imperative during airway assessment.

Airway Obstruction.   Potential causes of partial or complete airway obstruction include the tongue falling back into the oropharynx; blood, vomitus, secretions, or foreign objects in the airway; and fractures of the facial bony structures or crushing injuries of the laryngotracheal tree. Signs and symptoms of an inadequate airway are listed in Box 35–1.

Airway Management Techniques.   Airway management techniques range from simple positional maneuvers to complex surgical procedures. During all maneuvers, it is critical that the cervical spine be maintained by in-line immobilization, applied either by a caregiver or with a hard cervical collar, with the patient's head in the neutral position (Figure 35–5). Disposable head blocks or towel rolls may be placed on both sides of the patient's head with tape across the forehead to immobilize the cervical spine. These actions prevent forward flexion, hyperextension, and lateral rotation of the cervical spine. Sandbags are no longer an acceptable means of lateral cervical immobilization because of the increased lateral pressure to the cervical spine that occurs with turning or tilting of the backboard (Sundstrom, Asbjornsen, Habiba, Sunde, & Wester, 2014).

Simple Airways.   The first and simplest maneuver used to open the airway is a chin lift or modified jaw thrust (Figure 35–6). The airway can be suctioned for debris, secretions, blood, or vomitus. An oropharyngeal or nasopharyngeal airway may be used to facilitate airway maintenance. The oropharyngeal airway should be used only in patients who are unconscious and have no gag reflex. Using this airway in a conscious patient may precipitate gagging, vomiting, and potential aspiration. Improper placement of the

BOX 35–1 Inadequate Airway, Breathing, and Circulation in the Trauma Patient: Manifestations and Immediate Interventions

Airway

- *Signs and symptoms:*
  o No signs of breathing; no air heard or felt at nose and mouth
  o Presence of foreign bodies in airway
  o Abnormal chest movements or breathing effort limited to abdominal breathing
  o Partial obstruction: nasal flaring; abnormal sounds, such as stridor, hoarseness, snoring, gurgling
  o Conscious patient: difficulty or inability to speak, or raspy or hoarse voice quality

- *Potential immediate interventions:*
  o Open airway (e.g., jaw-thrust maneuver); oro- or nasopharyngeal airway
  o Suction airway
  o Assess for or to remove foreign bodies

Breathing

- *Signs and symptoms:*
  o Rate, rhythm, or depth outside of normal parameters
  o Absent or diminished breath sounds
  o Abnormal breathing sounds, such as gurgling, crowing, gasping

  o Cyanosis
  o Use of accessory respiratory muscles
  o Hypoxemia, hypercapnia

- *Potential immediate interventions:*
  o Apply oxygen at high-flow (usually 100%)
  o Inspect for signs of chest trauma
  o Position on side after neck is stabilized
  o Positive pressure ventilation (e.g., bag-valve-mask with manual ventilation; intubation, mechanical ventilation)
  o Rescue breathing if respiratory arrest

Circulation

- *Signs and symptoms:*
  o Pulse, blood pressure outside of normal parameters; weak or absent peripheral pulses; poor capillary refill
  o Bleeding
  o Skin: pale coloring, cool temperature

- *Potential immediate interventions:*
  o Control bleeding
  o Treat for shock
  o Perform CPR if cardiac arrest develops

SOURCE: Data from Limmer et al. (2016), Section 5: Trauma Emergencies.

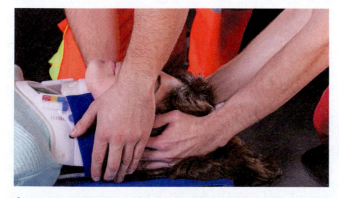

Figure 35–5 Neutral neck positioning and placement of cervical collar for neck stabilization.

SOURCE: Katarzyna Bialasiewicz/123RF.com

oropharyngeal airway may cause airway obstruction (Figure 35–7). The nasopharyngeal airway can be used in the conscious victim with an intact gag reflex. However, it should be avoided if a basal skull fracture is suspected.

Endotracheal Intubation. If the aforementioned procedures are inadequate in establishing an airway, more aggressive measures must be taken. Endotracheal intubation is achieved either orally or nasally. Nasotracheal intubation may be performed in the injured patient because hyperextension of the neck is minimized. With the nasotracheal method, the tube is advanced during the inspiratory effort

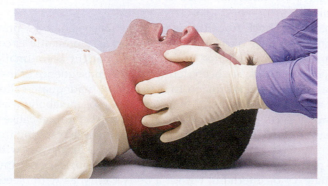
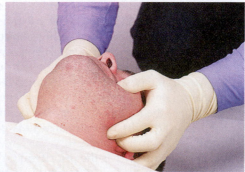

Figure 35–6 Jaw-thrust maneuver. Note that the fingers are positioned at the angle of the lower jaw directly below the ears. Lift lower jaw by gently pushing the angle of the lower jaw forward.

SOURCE: Michal Heron/Pearson Education, Inc.

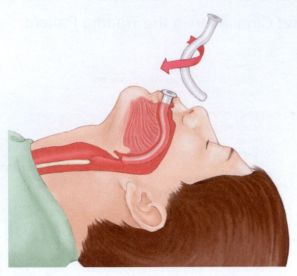

Figure 35–7 Proper placement of oropharyngeal airway. The airway is inserted with curved end up, advanced over the tongue, then turned 180 degrees to point down.

when the epiglottis is open. Orotracheal intubation is necessary when the patient is apneic or a cribriform plate fracture is suspected, as with basilar skull fractures. With fractures of the cribriform plate, the nasally inserted endotracheal tube could pass into the cranial vault, injuring brain tissue. If orotracheal intubation is necessary, vigilant care must be taken to avoid hyperextension of the cervical spine. The most important determinant when choosing the method of intubation is the experience of the provider. The clinician should first auscultate over the epigastrium for gurgling sounds to rule out an esophageal intubation. After intubation is achieved, breath sounds are auscultated to confirm tracheal intubation. Repeated assessment of breath sounds in any intubated patient is a critical nursing action.

Surgical Airway.   The indication for a surgical airway is the inability to intubate the trachea, which may result from edema of the glottis, laryngeal fracture, severe oropharyngeal hemorrhage, or gross instability of the midface. A surgical airway can be achieved by a needle cricothyroidotomy, surgical cricothyroidotomy, or tracheostomy. Surgical cricothyroidotomy is performed by making an incision through the cricothyroid membrane and passing an endotracheal or tracheostomy tube into the trachea. Tracheostomy must be considered in the patient with suspected laryngeal trauma. Symptoms of laryngeal injury include tenderness, hoarseness, subcutaneous emphysema, and intolerance of the supine position. The supine position is poorly tolerated by these patients because, on assuming the position, the airway will collapse where the laryngeal injury has occurred. With the patient sitting upright, an open airway is maintained even though the larynx is injured.

Assurance of airway integrity is the priority in the primary survey. Airway integrity does not ensure adequate ventilation, but the airway must be opened and secured before ventilation is assessed. After a definitive airway has been secured, placement of a gastric tube decompresses the stomach.

B–Breathing   The next step in the primary survey is to assess adequacy of ventilation. The primary goal of ventilation is to achieve maximum cellular oxygenation by providing an oxygen-rich environment. All trauma patients should receive high-flow oxygen during the initial evaluation.

Breathing is evaluated by the *look*, *listen*, and *feel* parameters. Look to detect the presence of respiratory excursion, listen for breath sounds, and feel for breathing. Positive pressure ventilation (PPV) may be required in some patients and is provided in a number of ways: mouth-to-mask, bag-valve-mask, or mechanical ventilator. A frequent complication of ventilation with PPV is gastric distention. Increased risks secondary to distention include vomiting, aspiration, and diaphragmatic impingement. Gastric distention can be minimized by not using too large a volume or too many breaths.

The adequacy of ventilation and oxygenation is confirmed by evaluating the PaO_2 and $PaCO_2$ obtained from an arterial blood gas (ABG) or by continuous monitoring of end-tidal carbon dioxide and arterial oxygen saturation using noninvasive measures. Other signs and symptoms of inadequate breathing and immediate interventions are listed in Box 35–1. If arterial blood gases are inadequate, the airway patency is re-evaluated and the patient is assessed for the presence of pneumothorax, hemothorax, hemopneumothorax, or tension pneumothorax (discussed in Section Seven). Tube thoracostomy is indicated for all of these conditions because they are life-threatening injuries.

C–Circulation   The third step in the primary survey is assessment of circulation. The trauma patient is at very high risk of hypovolemic shock from acute blood loss and the shifting of fluid from inside the blood vessels to the interstitial space. The trauma team must identify hypovolemia quickly and search for the etiology. Inadequate circulation is manifested as shock, a clinical state characterized by inadequate organ perfusion and tissue oxygenation. Assessment for adequate circulation includes palpating for strength, rate, rhythm, and symmetry of carotid, radial, femoral, and pedal pulses. Skin temperature is evaluated, as is capillary refill. Adequacy of tissue perfusion is reflected in the patient's level of consciousness. Signs and symptoms of inadequate circulation and immediate interventions are listed in Box 35–1.

Shock from Trauma.   Shock is considered a preventable cause of death. One of the most frequently encountered clinical states in the injured patient is traumatic shock. Shock has been defined as the consequence of insufficient tissue perfusion that results in inadequate cellular oxygenation and the accumulation of metabolic wastes (Ali, 2014; Roccaforte, 2017). The most common cause of shock in the injured patient is hypovolemia resulting from acute blood loss. Blood loss can occur externally, as with lacerations, open fractures, avulsion injuries, or amputations, or internally within a body cavity, as with bleeding into the chest cavity, abdominal cavity, retroperitoneum, or soft tissue.

Exsanguination is the most extreme form of hemorrhage. There is an initial loss of 40% of the patient's blood volume, with a rate of blood loss, or hemorrhage, exceeding 250 mL per minute. If uncontrolled, the patient may lose 50% of the entire blood volume within a very few minutes. Loss of up to 15% of circulating volume (700 to 750 mL for a patient weighing 70 kg) may produce little in terms of obvious symptoms, whereas loss of up to 30% of circulating volume (1.5 L) may result in mild tachycardia, tachypnea, and anxiety. Hypotension, marked tachycardia (pulse 110 to 120 beats per minute), and confusion may not be evident until more than 30% of blood volume has been lost. Loss of 40% of circulating volume (2 L) is immediately life-threatening. Most injuries precipitating exsanguination are from penetrating trauma. Regardless of the mechanism of injury, exsanguination leads to hypovolemic shock (Cameron & Knapp, 2016; Roccaforte, 2017).

D–Disability   After airway, breathing, and circulation are assessed and adequately managed, the fourth step in the primary survey is quick initial assessment of neurologic disability. The purpose of the neurologic examination in the primary survey is to quickly establish the patient's level of consciousness, and to assess pupil size and reactivity. Level of consciousness is determined using the AVPU scale.

- **A**—Alert
- **V**—Responds to verbal stimulation
- **P**—Responds to painful stimulation
- **U**—Unresponsive

A more detailed neurologic examination is included in the secondary survey.

E–Exposure   At this point in the primary survey, the patient is completely disrobed in preparation for the secondary survey. Exposure to the cold ambient temperatures of resuscitation areas, infusion of large volumes of room temperature IV fluids and/or cold blood products, and wet clothing all predispose the trauma patient to hypothermia. The need for careful attention to the maintenance of body temperature cannot be overemphasized.

The Secondary Survey

The secondary survey begins after the primary survey is completed and all immediately life-threatening injuries have been addressed. A head-to-toe approach is used, with a thorough examination of each body system. A critical point to remember is that if the patient becomes hemodynamically unstable at any point during the secondary survey, immediately return to the primary survey format (ABCDE) to troubleshoot the problem. During the secondary survey, the trauma patient requires repeated re-evaluation so that any new signs or symptoms are not overlooked. Other life-threatening problems may appear, or exacerbation of previously treated injuries may occur (such as tension pneumothorax, pericardial tamponade, or intracranial bleeding). Continuous monitoring of vital signs is critical. Key points in the secondary survey are presented in Table 35–2.

Table 35–2 Key Points in the Secondary Survey

Surveyed System	Evaluated Criteria
Head	Complete neurologic examination using a tool such as the Glasgow Coma Scale (GCS); re-evaluation of pupil size and reactivity; inspection and palpation of cranium for lacerations, fractures, contusions, hemotympanum, cerebrospinal fluid leakage, and edema
Maxillofacial	Assessment for facial fractures via inspection; palpation for open fractures, lacerations, and mobility or instability of facial structures
Cervical spine or neck	Inspection and palpation of neck anteriorly (maintaining cervical spine immobilization); palpation anteriorly and posteriorly for pain, crepitus, bony step-offs indicating fracture–dislocation, neck vein distention, and tracheal deviation
Chest	Inspection for paradoxical movement, flail segments, open chest wounds, and ecchymosis; palpation for rib fractures, subcutaneous emphysema, respiratory excursion, and sternal fractures; auscultation for quality, equality of breath sounds, and presence of adventitious sounds; auscultation of heart sounds for quality, extra heart sounds, murmurs, or pericardial friction rubs possibly indicating pericardial effusion
Abdomen	Inspection and auscultation before palpation to prevent precipitation of misleading bowel sounds by manual manipulation; inspection for abrasions, contusions, lacerations, and distention; auscultation for bowel sounds in four quadrants, bruits, and breath sounds; light and deep palpation precipitating a painful response may indicate intraperitoneal bleeding and should be quickly attended
Pelvis, perineum, genitalia	Inspection of pelvis for deformation; palpation for stability; inspection of perineum and genitalia for bleeding at the meatus, hematoma, vaginal bleeding, and lacerations; rectal examination to evaluate rectal wall integrity, presence of blood, position of prostate, presence of palpable pelvic fractures, and quality of sphincter tone
Musculoskeletal	Visual evaluation of extremities for contusions or deformities; palpation of all extremities for tenderness, crepitation, or abnormal range of motion, which may raise index of suspicion for fracture; all peripheral pulses should be evaluated, and capillary refill, skin color, temperature rechecked
Back	All patients should be log-rolled with careful attention to spinal immobilization to afford clinician a full view of patient's posterior surfaces, including neck, back, buttocks, and lower extremities, which should be carefully inspected and palpated to detect any area of injury
Complete neurologic examination	Motor and sensory evaluation of the extremities; re-evaluation of the patient's GCS score and pupils; any evidence of paralysis or paresis should prompt immediate immobilization of the entire patient if not already done

SOURCE: Data from Ali (2014); Cameron & Knapp (2016); Roccaforte (2017).

Section Five Review

1. When are life-threatening injuries detected?
   - A. Primary survey
   - B. Resuscitation
   - C. Secondary survey
   - D. Tertiary survey

2. During the secondary survey, a client becomes hemodynamically unstable. What should the nurse do?
   - A. Stop the secondary survey and reinstitute the primary survey.
   - B. Finish the secondary survey, looking for potential etiologies of instability.
   - C. Start again at the beginning of the secondary survey.
   - D. Re-evaluate patency and flow rates of IVs.

3. What is the purpose of the secondary survey?
   - A. To identify and intervene with life-threatening injuries
   - B. To identify all injuries
   - C. To facilitate treatment of airway and breathing
   - D. To assess response to resuscitative interventions

4. The presence of abdominal pain on light or deep palpation in the injured client usually indicates which condition?
   - A. Gastritis
   - B. Presence of intraperitoneal blood
   - C. Pelvic fracture
   - D. Intracerebral pathology

Answers: 1. A, 2. A, 3. B, 4. B

Section Six: Trauma Resuscitation

During the primary survey and resuscitation phases, which occur simultaneously, other therapies are also initiated. For example, a Foley catheter is inserted (unless contraindicated) and a nasogastric tube is placed to prevent aspiration. This section discusses management of the trauma patient based on changing priorities through the crisis period.

Trimodal Distribution of Trauma Deaths

In 1975, Cowley (1976) introduced the concept of the "golden hour" for resuscitation of the severely injured patient. The first hour following the trauma was the most opportune time to increase the chances of survival through primary assessment, diagnostic testing, and initiating definitive therapy (resuscitation, stop bleeding, hemodynamic stabilization, and surgical care). In a seminal paper published in 1983, Trunkey described trauma mortality as having a trimodal distribution based upon the time interval from injury to death—that is, death from trauma has three peak periods of occurrence (Figure 35–8) (Cameron & Knapp, 2016; Trunkey, 1983). The first peak occurs within minutes of the injury, before the patient arrives at the hospital. These deaths usually result from devastating injuries to the brain, upper spinal cord, heart, aorta, or other major blood vessel. The second peak occurs minutes to hours after arrival in the emergency department, and death usually is related to subdural or epidural hematoma(s), hemopneumothorax, ruptured spleen, lacerated liver, fractured femur(s), or other injuries resulting in significant blood loss. The third peak occurs days to weeks after the injury, usually in the intensive care unit, and death results from complications of systemic inflammatory response syndrome (SIRS), multiple organ dysfunction syndrome (MODS), or sepsis (Cameron & Knapp, 2016).

Comprehensive trauma healthcare systems targeting all three peak times for trauma deaths have developed over the past 25 years to improve the outcomes of trauma patients (West, Trunkey, & Limm, 1979). Evidence-based programs to reduce trauma mortality include injury prevention, use of prehospital and emergency department advanced life support interventions, rapid transport, designated trauma centers with personnel and resources to care for the injured trauma patient, evidence-based protocols for acute care, advances in critical care medicine, multidisciplinary care approaches, and an emphasis on rehabilitation and reintegration back into the community (West et al., 1979). More recent studies have shown that trauma-related deaths now have a largely bimodal, rather than a trimodal distribution with diminished late peak in deaths that could reflect improvements in access to better trauma, resuscitation, and critical care (Abdelrahman et al., 2014; Evans et al., 2010; Gunst et al., 2010). The golden hour is still important as the majority of deaths occur rapidly following a severe injury.

How does an understanding of this distribution enhance clinical practice? It can empower the nurse to anticipate the needs of the patient based on time from injury and physiological manifestations. If a patient is received within minutes of injury, what are the life-threatening injuries that may cause death in this time frame? Has the patient experienced brainstem compression or laceration resulting in respiratory center dysfunction? What assessments and interventions must be performed to identify and treat these injuries?

If an unstable patient arrives within 30 minutes of injury, the injuries that pose a risk for trauma-related death during this time frame must be assessed and monitored to

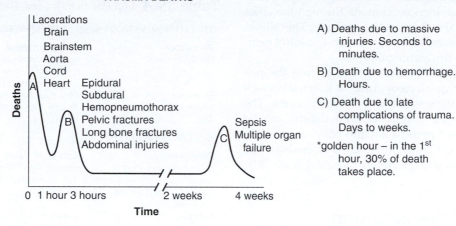

Figure 35–8 Trimodal distribution of trauma deaths.

anticipate a life-threatening situation. These injuries might include hemopneumothorax (assess respiratory effort, lung sounds, possible need for a chest tube), ruptured spleen or lacerated liver (assess for a tense and painful abdomen, hypotension with no signs of obvious blood loss), and fractured femur (assess for a painful leg with obvious fracture).

The high-acuity nurse caring for a patient 3 days post-injury anticipates quite different causes for trauma-related death during this time frame. The nurse identifies precipitating or contributing factors in a patient experiencing sepsis or MODS, such as overhydration during the first 24 to 48 hours, with development of acute respiratory distress syndrome (ARDS) or a missed intra-abdominal injury that predisposes the patient to sepsis.

Trauma Resuscitation

Of the causes of early post-injury deaths in the hospital that are amenable to effective treatment, hemorrhage is predominant. The most common cause of shock in the injured patient is hypovolemia resulting from acute blood loss. Successful treatment of shock depends on early recognition, controlling obvious hemorrhage, and fluid resuscitation, with fluid resuscitation being the fundamental treatment for hypovolemic shock until definitive surgical intervention is available to treat the site (or sites) of injury.

Recognition of the source of blood loss is critical. Blood volume loss in quantities large enough to produce a shock state can occur in any of five areas: chest, abdomen, pelvis and retroperitoneum, femur fractures, and external hemorrhage. See Table 35–3 for more details. Because of the potential for large-volume hemorrhage from abdominal and pelvic trauma, rapid evaluation of these two areas is critical (Cameron & Knapp, 2016; Roccaforte, 2017).

Resuscitation of the patient who is exsanguinating is based on the aggressive application of basic principles of circulation management. Intravenous access is established quickly with large-bore (e.g., 14- or 16-gauge) catheters. Because the underlying source of the hypotension is hypovolemic shock, administering fluids (usually normal

Table 35–3 Estimating Potential Blood Volume Loss

Location	Volume Loss
Chest	In the adult, 2.5 L of blood can be lost in each hemothorax. Thus, a total of 5 L can be lost inside the chest, which would be the total blood volume of a person weighing 70 kg.
Abdomen	As much as 6 L of blood can be lost via intraperitoneal bleeding from damaged organs or vessels.
Pelvis and retroperitoneum	Unstable pelvic fractures, especially those involving the posterior elements of the pelvis, can precipitate liters of blood loss. A patient may actually exsanguinate from an unstable pelvic fracture involving posterior bony elements.
Femur fractures	For each femur fracture, 500 to 1000 mL of blood can be lost.
External hemorrhage	Bleeding wounds are a consideration. A scalp laceration, in particular, requires proper hemostasis because a significant amount of blood can be lost with this injury.

saline) is crucial. Vasopressors are not given to treat hypotension until fluid volume has been restored. Blood and blood products may be given in addition to IV fluids. Type-specific blood should be given, but in an emergency situation low-titer O-positive blood may be given to men and O-negative to women of childbearing age.

Other infusion devices are available in the acute phase of resuscitation of the patient with exsanguination. Rapid infusion devices are available that can deliver large amounts of crystalloid and colloid quickly (up to 1400 mL/minute). The use of autotransfusion devices facilitates resuscitative efforts in patients with chest tubes by transfusing the patient's own blood during massive bleeding from trauma. Major advantages of autotransfusion are that it reduces the usual risks of banked-blood transfusions (e.g., transfusion reactions and transmission of disease [McGinty, 2017]). Emergency department open resuscitative thoracotomy also may be performed to manage the exsanguinating patient, especially if exsanguination is suspected to be related to injury to the great vessels (e.g., aorta) or the heart.

Open resuscitative thoracotomy is an emergency last-resort procedure in which an incision is made through the chest wall to gain access to the chest and its contents. This allows direct viewing of the heart and great vessels to control hemorrhage and treat life-threatening injuries.

Critical analysis of assessment data during the primary assessment and quick recognition of traumatic shock are essential skills in the resuscitative phase of trauma. The number of preventable trauma-related deaths can be reduced with improved prehospital and hospital care provided by highly skilled clinicians trained to evaluate the injured patient rapidly and effectively (Sanddal et al., 2011; Vioque et al., 2014).

End Points of Resuscitation

How is it determined that a patient has been adequately resuscitated? The goal of the resuscitation is to treat shock so it does not progress to an irreversible state. Determining when tissue perfusion has been restored is a challenge. Traditional signs of sufficient tissue perfusion alone (normal blood pressure, heart rate, and urine output) cannot be used in shock states because seemingly "normal" vital signs and urine output may be the result of compensatory mechanisms (renin-angiotensin-aldosterone system, or RAAS) and the sympathetic nervous system. Currently, the best indicators of adequate tissue perfusion in shock include traditional hemodynamic parameters, global parameters, and organ-specific parameters (Table 35–4).

The nurse should not be lulled into a false sense of security when vital signs and basic hemodynamic parameters

Table 35–4 End Points in Trauma Resuscitation

TRADITIONAL HEMODYNAMIC PARAMETERS	
Parameter	End-point Value
Blood pressure	Systolic blood pressure greater than 90 mmHg; mean arterial pressure (MAP) greater than 70 mmHg
Heart rate	Less than 100 beats per minute
Urine output	Greater than 30 mL per hour
Skin	Warm, dry
GLOBAL PARAMETERS	
Parameter	End-point Value
Oxygen delivery index	Greater than 500 mL/min/m^2
Oxygen consumption index	125 mL/min/m^2
Systemic mixed venous oxygen saturation	65% to 80%
Lactate	Less than 2.2 mmol/L
Base deficit	± 3 mmol/L
Tissue arteriovenous carbon dioxide gradient	Less than 11 mmHg
Sublingual capnography	Less than 70
Gastric pH$_i$	pH$_i$ greater than 7.35

have been restored to normal values. During resuscitation from traumatic hemorrhagic shock, normalization of blood pressure, heart rate, and urine output are not adequate, as occult hypoperfusion, oxygen debt, and ongoing tissue acidosis (compensated shock) may be present, which may lead to organ dysfunction and death. Optimizing hemodynamic variables to improve cardiac output or index, oxygen delivery, and oxygen consumption may be beneficial.

Emerging Evidence

- Goldsmith, Curtis, and McCloughen (2017) explored immediate post-hospitalization incidence, intensity, and impact of pain in recently discharged adult trauma patients at 2 weeks post-discharge from a level one trauma center. Ninety-eight percent experienced a blunt injury. Eighty-two patients completed a pain inventory questionnaire assessing their injury-related pain experience (pain severity, impact of pain) 2 weeks postdischarge from the hospital. The questionnaire assessed injury severity and impact of pain through a score from 0 to 10. Eighty patients (98%) reported experiencing pain since discharge, with 65 patients still experiencing the pain 2 weeks after discharge. These trauma patients reported that their normal work patterns were most affected by their pain, with an average score of 6.6 out of 10 on the Brief Pain Inventory, followed by effect on general activity (6.1/10) and enjoyment of life (5.7/10). The highest pain severity was reported by those with injuries from road trauma, with low injury severity scores reported by those who were female and did not speak English at home. The authors concluded that pain was common in this sample of trauma patients; it was intense, enduring, and interfered with quality of life. This study has implications in the importance for nurses and physicians to identify barriers to effective pain management while implementing interventions to address the barriers in order to manage pain and optimize functional outcomes of trauma patients (*Goldsmith et al., 2017*).

- Leske, McAndrew, Brasel, and Feetham (2017) examined the effects of family presence during resuscitation (FPDR) in patients who survived trauma from motor vehicle crashes (MVCs) and gunshot wounds (GSWs). Family members of 140 trauma patients

(MVC = 110, 79%; GSW = 30, 21%) participated in the study within 3 days of admission to the critical care unit. Results indicate that participation in the FPDR may help family members to be better able to assist the patient during the initial critical care period. Participation in FPDR significantly reduced family reports of anxiety ($p = .04$) and stress ($p = .005$) and fostered family reports of well-being ($p = .001$). There was no statistically significant difference in satisfaction with critical care ($p = .78$) between the FPDR group and the no-FPDR group. Family resources moderated the stress in the FPDR group participants ($p = .01$) (*Leske et al., 2017*).

- Harada et al. (2017) conducted a retrospective review of medical records of 1571 trauma patients who sustained moderate to severe injury and who received crystalloid resuscitation in the ED at an urban level one trauma center (1) to characterize how the center has responded to changes in crystalloid resuscitation practice trauma practices and (2) to describe associated patient outcomes over time. They compared clinical characteristics and outcomes between high- and low-volume resuscitation patients. Of these patients, 82% (n = 1282) received low-volume resuscitation and 18% (n = 289) received high-volume resuscitation. The patients in the low-volume group presented to the ED with a higher mean arterial pressure ($p < 0.001$). Low-volume patients had lower injury severity compared to high-volume patients ($p < 0.001$); mortality was lower in the low-volume group ($p < 0.001$). Decreased high-volume resuscitation with crystalloids was associated with a reduced mortality over the 10-year study period, and mortality was higher in those patients who received high-volume resuscitation (*Harada et al., 2017*)

Section Six Review

1. Trauma-related mortalities exhibit which distribution?
   A. Modal
   B. Bimodal
   C. Trimodal
   D. Bell shaped

2. Which shock state is most common in injured clients?
   A. Hypovolemic
   B. Cardiogenic
   C. Neurogenic
   D. Septic

3. Which parameter is the BEST indication that resuscitation efforts have improved the shock state?
   A. MAP greater than 80 mmHg
   B. Heart rate 110 beats per minute
   C. Urine output 20 mL per hour
   D. Lactate less than 2.2 mmol

4. Why are traditional signs of tissue perfusion such as heart rate and urine output unreliable indicators of sufficient tissue perfusion?
   A. The effects of base deficit
   B. The effects of RAAS
   C. Effects of parasympathetic response to injury
   D. Effects of fluid administration on hemodynamics

Answers: 1. B, 2. A, 3. D, 4. B

Section Seven: Management of Selected Injuries

The focus of this section is to provide a profile of the management of chest, abdominal, and pelvic injuries, which are commonly seen in trauma patients in high-acuity units. Some of these injuries require interventions during the primary survey.

Chest Injuries

Injuries to the chest are usually a result of an MVC or a violent crime and are a major cause of death in North America. Chest injuries involve trauma to the chest wall, lungs, and heart.

Rib Fractures   Rib fractures are typically caused by blunt trauma. Multiple ribs can be fractured. Rib fractures are very painful; the pain is aggravated by any movement of the chest wall, even breathing. Therefore, the patient with rib fractures often takes shallow breaths. Atelectasis can develop, and the patient is at risk for developing pneumonia. Nonsteroidal anti-inflammatory agents, intercostal nerve block, thoracic epidural analgesia, and narcotics may be used to optimize pain management. There is no treatment for nondisplaced rib fractures other than to let the fractures heal naturally over time. Incentive spirometry reduces atelectasis and risk for pneumonia (Kaafarani et al., 2016). Trauma patients with blunt trauma to the torso should be evaluated for rib fractures that could result in pleural or diaphragmatic injury.

Flail Chest   Flail chest results when two or more rib fractures occur in two or more places, causing the flail segment to separate from the rib cage (Figure 35–9). The flail portion

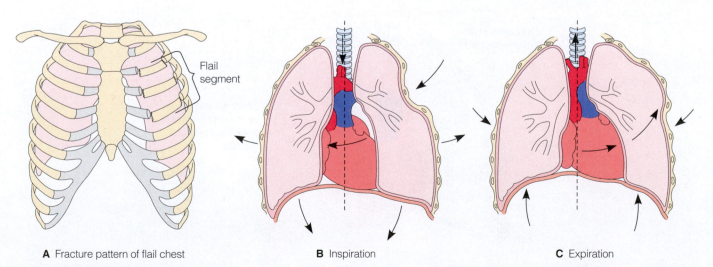

A Fracture pattern of flail chest   **B** Inspiration   **C** Expiration

Figure 35–9 Flail chest. Physiologic function of the chest wall is (A) impaired as the flail segment (B) is sucked inward during inspiration and (C) moves outward with expiration.

of the chest wall does not have bony support and moves independently of the normal chest wall movement. Complications develop as a result of extreme pain with inspiration and expiration, and hypoxemia often results from inadequate respiratory effort. Signs of a flail chest include uncoordinated, paradoxical movement of the flail portion of the chest wall, crepitus, and hypoxemia on blood gas. Flail chest requires immediate treatment during the primary survey to stabilize breathing. Treatment goals are directed at preventing and treating hypoxemia. Positive-pressure mechanical ventilation may be required.

Pulmonary Injuries

Traumatic injury to the lungs can be readily assessed in some instances—for example, a penetrating gunshot wound to the chest—or it can be initially hidden, particularly when it is associated with blunt chest trauma. Pulmonary injuries are potentially life-threatening because the lungs are necessary for gas exchange and tissue oxygenation. (See Table 35–5.)

Table 35–5 Traumatic Injuries and Associated Sequelae

Condition	Pathophysiology	Complication
Thoracic Trauma		
Great vessel tears	Hemorrhage	DIC, AKI
Hemothorax	Decreased gas exchange	ARDS
Tension pneumothorax	Decreased gas exchange	ARDS
Open pneumothorax	Disruption in skin integrity	Sepsis
Abdominal Trauma		
Perforation of intestine	Extravasation of GI contents into peritoneum	Sepsis
Liver or splenic laceration	Hemorrhage	DIC, ACS, AKI
Orthopedic Trauma		
Femur or pelvis fracture	Hemorrhage	DIC, AKI
Long-bone fractures	Disruption of fat-containing tissue, increased flow of fat globules in microcirculation	ARDS, AKI

DIC = disseminated intravascular coagulation; AKI = acute kidney injury; ARDS = acute respiratory distress syndrome; ACS = abdominal compartment syndrome

Pulmonary Contusions Blunt trauma to lung parenchyma can result in a unilateral or bilateral pulmonary contusion, or bruising. These injuries can be quite serious because the bruising can lead to alveolar hemorrhage, edema, and inflammation within the lung. A large pulmonary contusion can result in respiratory failure. Clinical manifestations of pulmonary contusion may not appear for several days. A chest x-ray may reveal pulmonary infiltrates. Crackles may be auscultated. Because the patient is at risk for impaired gas exchange, nursing care must focus on improving gas exchange through deep breathing exercises, ambulation, and removal of secretions. The patient is monitored for worsening respiratory status. Intubation and mechanical ventilation may be required if signs of respiratory failure are present. As with rib fractures, pain management is paramount.

Tension Pneumothorax A tension pneumothorax occurs when air leaks from the lung or through the chest wall. Air trapped in the thoracic cavity without means of escape collapses the affected lung (Figure 35–10). As intrathoracic pressure continues to increase, it is transmitted to the heart, causing decreased venous return and cardiac output. Tension pneumothorax is characterized by chest pain, air hunger, respiratory distress, tachycardia, neck vein distention, trachea displaced from midline, and absent breath sounds on the affected side. It is treated during the primary survey to stabilize breathing. In an emergent situation, the increased intrathoracic pressure is relieved by needle thoracotomy using a large-bore (14-gauge) needle or immediate placement of a chest tube.

The nurse can distinguish hypotension resulting from hypovolemia from that associated with increased pericardial pressure by assessing for the presence of a paradoxical pulse (**pulsus paradoxus**), a decrease of 10 mmHg or more in the systolic blood pressure on inspiration that occurs in the presence of tension pneumothorax. In these conditions, the increased thoracic pressure from inspiration further decreases left ventricle filling and results in blood backing up into the right heart, compromising CO. If a right atrial pressure (RAP) catheter or pulmonary arterial catheter is

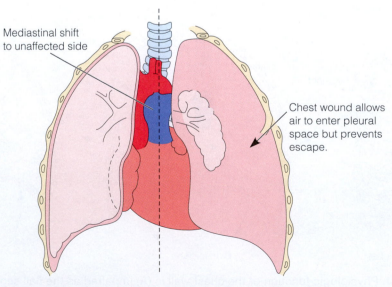

Mediastinal shift to unaffected side

Chest wound allows air to enter pleural space but prevents escape.

Figure 35–10 Tension pneumothorax.

in place, the RAP reading is elevated because of increased right atrial filling with decreased emptying. A RAP reading greater than 15 cm H_2O is significant. Jugular venous distention will be present. Hypotension resulting from hypovolemia is associated with flat neck veins. Decreased pedal pulses and pale or mottled skin also may be present.

Open Pneumothorax   An open pneumothorax is a penetrating chest wall injury that sucks air, causing intrathoracic pressure and atmospheric pressure to equilibrate (Figure 35–11). The clinical manifestations are the same as for a tension pneumothorax. Initial treatment includes covering the wound with a sterile occlusive dressing taped on three sides, which creates an occlusion with inspiration (the dressing is sucked into the wound as the patient breathes in), with an outlet through the lower edge for expiration. Open pneumothorax is treated during the primary assessment to stabilize breathing with placement of a chest tube. Surgery may also be required.

Massive Hemothorax   Massive hemothorax is defined as the accumulation of more than 1500 mL of blood in the chest cavity (Roccaforte, 2017). Usually, the cause is a penetrating wound that disrupts the great vessels. Assessment findings may include decreased breath sounds or dullness to percussion on the affected side and hypotension. Management would be aimed at restoring blood volume and decompressing the chest cavity with a chest tube and would occur during the primary survey to stabilize breathing. An autotransfusion device may be attached to the chest tube collection chamber. Surgery may be required for patients who have continued bleeding requiring persistent transfusions and changes in physiologic status (McGinty, 2017).

Cardiac Injuries

Cardiac injuries are potentially life-threatening and should always be suspected when a patient is admitted with potential chest trauma.

Cardiac Tamponade   Whether from penetrating or blunt trauma, cardiac tamponade causes the pericardium (the sac around the heart) to fill with blood. This restricts the heart's ability to pump and impedes venous return. Signs and symptoms include Beck's triad (elevated right atrial pressure with neck vein distention, hypotension, and muffled heart sounds), pulsus paradoxus, and pulseless electrical activity (PEA). Cardiac tamponade would be treated during the primary survey to stabilize circulation. Treatment is initially directed at volume resuscitation until pericardiocentesis can be performed (Figure 35–12).

Blunt Cardiac Injury   Blunt cardiac injury, formerly called cardiac contusion, is bruising of the myocardium. Chest discomfort, sinus tachycardia, and hypotension are suggestive of this injury, but many patients are asymptomatic. Electrocardiogram (ECG) changes may also be present and may include *ST* changes, dysrhythmias, or heart block. If the ECG is abnormal on admission, the patient is admitted to the high-acuity unit for continuous ECG monitoring for 24 to 48 hours (Clancy et al., 2012). An echocardiogram may be done to evaluate cardiac function, as well as troponin lab values.

Abdominal Injuries

Blunt trauma creates potentially life-threatening abdominal injuries. In a motor vehicle crash, a compression and possibly shearing injury from a steering wheel or seat belt may rupture solid organs such as the liver or spleen. Deceleration may cause lacerations to the spleen and liver because these organs are movable from the fixed structures surrounding them. The incidence of injury to the spleen is the highest (40%–55%), followed by injury to the liver (35%–45%) (Cameron & Knapp, 2016). Penetrating trauma from stab wounds most commonly involves the liver, small bowel, diaphragm, or colon. Gunshot wounds have a greater kinetic energy and more often involve the small bowel, colon, liver, and abdominal vascular structures.

Spleen Injuries   The spleen is located in the left upper quadrant of the abdomen and is the organ most commonly

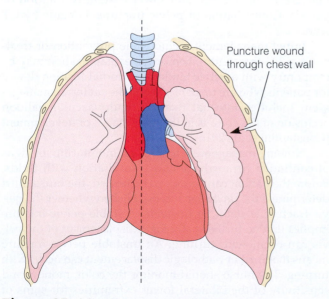

Figure 35–11 Open pneumothorax.

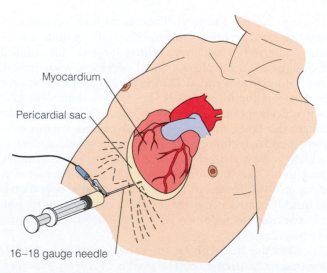

Figure 35–12 Pericardiocentesis.

injured in blunt trauma to the abdomen. The spleen has important immunologic functions; therefore, steps are taken to let the spleen wound heal after injury instead of removing it. Diagnosis of injury to the spleen is made by focused assessment with sonography in trauma (FAST) and CT scan. Patients are admitted to a high-acuity unit for serial monitoring of vital signs, abdominal exam, and hematocrit. It is crucial to monitor vital signs for evidence of continued bleeding in or around the spleen. Continued hemodynamic instability may indicate the need for angiography for embolization or surgical intervention (Hildebrand et al., 2014). Patients who do have a splenectomy are at risk for infections and require vaccinations prior to discharge from the hospital.

Liver Injuries Although anterior and lateral portions of the liver are protected by the lower rib cage, the liver remains vulnerable to injury in blunt or penetrating trauma. The majority of liver injuries are minor and do not require surgery. However, mortality may be greater than 50% with a complex liver injury, and death is usually the result of hemorrhage. Diagnosis of liver injury is made by CT scan. Liver injuries are graded on a scale of 1 to 6, with 6 being a complete hepatic avulsion and the worst injury possible. Bleeding is the most common complication, and patients must be monitored for changes in vital signs and continued decline in hematocrit values.

Patients with liver injuries are usually admitted to a high-acuity unit for serial monitoring of vital signs and hematocrit. Medical management may include hepatic arteriography to embolize any bleeding in the liver, or surgery may be required to stop the bleeding. In the event the patient becomes hemodynamically unstable from continued bleeding and develops hypovolemic shock, the high-acuity nurse must be prepared to implement volume resuscitation as ordered. This may include crystalloids and blood or blood products. Coagulopathies may be corrected with fresh-frozen plasma, platelets, or cryoprecipitate. It is crucial that the nurse monitor the patient's response to these interventions. Continued hemodynamic instability may require surgical interventions to find and control the source of hemorrhage within the liver.

Damage Control Surgery Patients with abdominal injuries that need an operative procedure may require a technique referred to as *damage control surgery*. This surgical technique has three phases: initial operation, resuscitation, and definitive restoration. During the initial operation, time in the operating room (OR) is kept to a minimum. The goal is to quickly locate and control sources of hemorrhage. The longer this takes, the greater the risk of three conditions—hypothermia, continued bleeding, and systemic acidosis—which create a self-propagating cycle that can eventually lead to an irreversible physiological insult (Cameron & Knapp, 2016). Therefore, the goal of this initial operation is to quickly control hemorrhage, which may be done by simply packing the abdomen with sterile dressing to control the bleeding.

After this initial phase, the patient is taken to the ICU for trauma resuscitation. The goal is to correct hypothermia, acidosis, and coagulopathies. Serial measurements of lactate and base deficit are assessed for signs of improving metabolic acidosis. Coagulopathies are corrected with blood and blood products. During this time, the patient is assessed for abdominal compartment syndrome.

Abdominal Compartment Syndrome. Abdominal compartment syndrome (ACS) is essentially intra-abdominal hypertension, or too much pressure within the abdominal cavity. It is caused by continued bleeding or visceral edema. Signs and symptoms include a taut distended abdomen, decreased cardiac output, elevated central venous pressure and pulmonary capillary wedge pressure, increased peak pulmonary pressures, and decreased urine output (Kirkpatrick et al., 2013). ACS is discussed in Chapter 22.

Intra-abdominal pressures may be indirectly measured via a Foley catheter. Fluid is instilled to create a fluid-filled column that transmits pressure from the bladder to the transducer. The transducer should be leveled and zeroed to the midaxillary line with the patient in the supine position. The measurement is obtained at end expiration (Kirkpatrick et al., 2013). These pressures can be monitored intermittently or continuously, as ordered. Abdominal pressures greater than 15 to 25 mmHg are considered high and may indicate that the abdomen needs to be opened to relieve the pressure (Kirkpatrick et al., 2013).

Once the hypothermia, acidosis, and coagulopathies are corrected (usually within 72 hours of the initial operation), the patient is returned to the OR for definitive repair of injuries.

Pelvic Injuries

Pelvic fractures can be life-threatening injuries. They are associated with blunt trauma—an MVC or a crushing injury to the pelvic region. Because the pelvis protects major blood vessels, patients with pelvic fractures are at high risk for hemorrhage. Signs of a pelvic fracture include perianal ecchymosis, pain on palpation or "rocking" of the iliac crests, hematuria, and lower extremity rotation or paresis. Confirmation of pelvic fractures is made by CT scan.

Initial management includes the prevention or treatment of life-threatening hemorrhage. Stabilization may be temporary with a pelvic binder or external fixation device for patients who are unstable. While the preferred management includes internal fixation, endovascular balloon occlusion of the aorta is in the early stages of development (Constantini et al., 2016).

Nursing management focuses on monitoring for signs of continued hemorrhage and resuscitation with fluids. Before the patient can be moved or turned, the nurse must determine if the physician has established whether the pelvic fracture is stable or unstable. A stable pelvic fracture implies that no further pathologic displacement of the pelvis can occur with turning. An unstable pelvic fracture means that further pathologic displacement can occur with turning. The nurse should monitor the color, motion, and sensitivity of the bilateral lower extremities for signs of neurologic or vascular compromise.

Section Seven Review

1. What is an important intervention for the client with multiple rib fractures?
   A. Chest tube placement
   B. Needle aspiration
   C. Pain management and pulmonary hygiene
   D. Placing a gauze dressing over the wound

2. Clients with injuries to the spleen or liver may require operative repair under which condition?
   A. Their abdominal girth increases.
   B. They have a change in level of consciousness.
   C. The hematocrit increases.
   D. They become hemodynamically unstable.

3. During damage control surgery, the initial operation time is restricted to prevent which conditions?
   A. Cardiac dysrhythmias
   B. Coagulopathy
   C. Metabolic alkalosis
   D. Hyperthermia

4. Before turning a client with a pelvic fracture, what must the nurse do first?
   A. Medicate the client.
   B. Determine if the fracture is stable or unstable.
   C. Remove the fixation device.
   D. Assess the color, motion, and sensitivity of the legs.

Answers: 1. C, 2. D, 3. B, 4. C

Section Eight: Complications of Traumatic Injury

As discussed in Section Six, trauma deaths occur in three peaks. The third (final) peak occurs days to weeks after the injury event; death is usually attributable to complications of critical illness. This section focuses on common complications during this phase.

The primary responsibilities of the nurse caring for a trauma patient in the final phase are prevention and surveillance. Treatment of trauma sequelae is controversial because research in this area, compared to trauma resuscitation research, is still in its infancy. Therefore, the goal of nursing care is to prevent complications.

Patients with traumatic injuries are at increased risk for multiple complications, such as venous thromboembolism (VTE), undernutrition, acute respiratory distress syndrome (ARDS), disseminated intravascular coagulation (DIC), acute kidney injury (AKI), and multiple organ dysfunction syndrome (MODS). All of these complications are discussed in detail in other chapters of this text, but they are reviewed here briefly, as they relate to the patient with traumatic injuries.

Risks for Complications

Several types of injuries predispose the trauma patient to complications. Table 35–5 summarizes traumatic injuries and their associated sequelae. Thoracic trauma may produce massive hemorrhage in addition to disruption in the lung parenchyma. Thus, the thoracic trauma patient is at high risk for DIC and ARDS. Abdominal trauma increases the likelihood of hemorrhage, abdominal compartment syndrome, and infection. Orthopedic trauma predisposes the patient to VTE and prolonged immobility, which may negatively impact gas exchange should pulmonary complications occur, such as pulmonary embolus or severe atelectasis. The physiological complications of trauma are interrelated, as it is common for a patient to have a combination of complications. Although the etiologies of these complications may differ slightly, the result is the same: inadequate oxygen delivery to the tissues. For this reason, it is important to keep in mind that the patient may be at higher risk for one complication because of the initial injury, but in reality, any one—or more than one—complication may develop.

Metabolic Response to Injury: Risk for Undernutrition

The metabolic response to stress after injury occurs in two phases: ebb phase and flow phase. The ebb phase occurs in the first 3 days during acute resuscitation. Characteristics of the ebb phase are summarized in Table 35–6. The body

Table 35–6 Metabolic Response to Trauma

Ebb Phase (first 72 hours after injury)	Flow Phase (begins 72 hours after injury)
• Hypometabolism	• Hypermetabolism
• Decreased energy expenditure	• Increased energy expenditure
• Normal glucose production with insulin resistance	• Increased glucose production
• Decreased oxygen consumption	• Increased oxygen consumption
• Mild protein catabolism	• Profound protein catabolism
• Increased glucocorticoids	• Increased glucocorticoids
• Increased catecholamines	• Increased catecholamines
• Decreased cardiac output	• Increased potassium and sodium losses
• Decreased body temperature	• Loss of serum proteins through wounds, exudates, drains, and hemorrhage
• Vasoconstriction	

requires a large amount of glucose during this time, which is supplied by the breakdown of glycogen stores through glycogenolysis. Prolonged glycogenolysis depletes skeletal muscle protein and can lead to wasting. This phase typically ends after the resuscitative phase, about 72 hours after injury. The second phase is the flow phase, which is characterized by a hypermetabolic response. This phase results in catabolism of lean body mass, negative nitrogen balance, and altered glucose metabolism (Ali, 2014).

Nutritional support is required to supply amino acids and adequate energy for protein synthesis as new tissues are synthesized and wounds are repaired. Starting nutritional support as early as possible is essential in the trauma patient as malnutrition is associated with increased morbidity and mortality, whereas those patients whose nutritional requirements are adequately met experience reduced time on a ventilator, fewer complications, and shorter time in rehabilitation (Kaafarani et al., 2016). Following nutritional guidelines helps ensure patients receive adequate nutritional support. The use of algorithms encourages early initiation and rapid achievement of therapeutic nutritional support goals to ensure optimal delivery of nutrition to patients (Simmons & Adam, 2014).

Venous Thromboembolism

Venous thromboembolism (VTE) encompasses deep vein thrombosis (DVT) and pulmonary embolism (PE), both of which constitute a major health problem with significant morbidity and mortality. Trauma patients have one of the highest incidences of VTE among hospitalized patients for myriad reasons, including stasis from immobility and increased coagulability from the inflammatory process of injury (Van & Schreiber, 2016). Prophylaxis in the trauma patient may be difficult because injuries with a high risk of bleeding preclude anticoagulant use, and lower-extremity injuries hinder the use of pneumatic sequential compression devices, or SCDs (Toker, Hak, & Morgan, 2011). The high-acuity nurse must be ever vigilant in ensuring the use of SCDs when indicated and in monitoring for complications of VTE.

Sepsis

Sepsis is the SIRS phenomenon in the presence of blood-borne infection, and septic shock is the severe physiologic response to an infection that results in hemodynamic instability. Gram-negative and gram-positive bacteria, viruses, and fungi can produce sepsis. The offending pathogens may be part of the patient's normal flora or may be present in the external environment. The patient with traumatic injuries is at particular risk for infection and sepsis because of so many potential ports of entry, including urinary catheters, endotracheal tubes, surgical wounds, invasive hemodynamic monitoring catheters, and IV catheters. Foreign devices in the nose, such as a nasotracheal tube, represent a major risk factor for the development of healthcare-associated sinusitis, which itself is a risk factor

---

BOX 35–2   Risk Factors for Infection in the Patient with Traumatic Injury

- High injury severity
- Shock on admission
- Prolonged ICU length of stay
- Age greater than 60 years
- Size of ICU (more than 10 beds)
- Parenteral nutrition
- Days with arterial catheter
- Days with mechanical ventilation
- Days with central venous catheters
- Tracheostomy
- Neurologic failure at day 3
- ICP monitor

---

for the development of pneumonia. Additional risk factors for infection are summarized in Box 35–2.

Acute Respiratory Distress Syndrome

The trauma patient is at risk for acute respiratory distress syndrome (ARDS) as a result of direct and indirect lung injury. Primary lung injury includes direct blunt or penetrating injury to the lungs, aspiration, and inhalation. Indirect injuries include sepsis, fat embolism, ischemia or reperfusion, and missed injuries. ARDS is characterized by acute dyspnea and hypoxemia within hours to days of the inciting event. In 2011, with agreement among the European Society of Intensive Care Medicine, the American Thoracic Society, and the Society of Critical Care Medicine, a new definition was developed to better describe ARDS (Fanelli et al., 2013). ARDS is defined as the presence of early (within 1 week) onset, bilateral pulmonary infiltrated, and respiratory failure (not explained by cardiac failure or fluid overload). Oxygenation status is characterized as mild (PaO_2/FiO_2 ratio < 300), moderate (PaO_2/FiO_2 < 200), and severe (PaO_2/FiO_2 < 100), all with PEEP requirements of 5 cm H_2O (Fanelli et al., 2013).

Disseminated Intravascular Coagulation

Acute disseminated intravascular coagulation (DIC) is an exaggerated response to a condition such as sepsis or multiple trauma that causes excessive clotting. Excessive systemic clotting leads to depletion of clotting factors and platelets and results in serious bleeding (MacLeod, Winkler, McCoy, Hillyer, & Shaz, 2014). Normal clotting is a localized reaction to injury, whereas DIC is a systemic response. The healthy individual maintains a balance between clot formation and lysis. In trauma, both the extrinsic and intrinsic pathways of coagulation may be stimulated. Brain injury can precipitate the release of tissue thromboplastin (extrinsic pathway). Hypoxia and acidosis also stimulate the extrinsic pathway. Crush injuries, burns, and sepsis result in blood cell injury as well as platelet aggregation (intrinsic pathway).

Acute Kidney Injury (AKI)

In the trauma patient, kidney failure rarely occurs as a result of direct trauma to the kidneys. Often AKI is the result of acute tubular necrosis from renal hypoperfusion or toxin-mediated damage to the tubules. Toxin-mediated kidney injury may be caused by many of the drugs trauma patients frequently receive, including aminoglycosides, nonsteroidal anti-inflammatory agents, and radiologic contrast dyes used for CT scanning. Myoglobin from crushed skeletal muscle can accumulate in the tubules and cause obstruction and renal failure.

Systemic Inflammatory Response Syndrome and Multiple Organ Dysfunction Syndrome

Underlying the high mortality associated with severe trauma injury is systemic inflammatory response syndrome (SIRS) and multiple organ dysfunction syndrome (MODS). The pathophysiologic basis of SIRS provides an explanation for the injury and failure of one or more organs, leading to MODS. When SIRS is severe and MODS involves multiple organs, the probability of death is high. Specific risk factors for development of MODS in trauma patients include severe injury; massive volumes of fluid resuscitation, including blood products, crystalloids, and fresh-frozen plasma; multiple preexisting comorbidities, particularly liver disease; and development of significant shock (with prolonged abnormal base deficit and lactate levels) (Frohlich et al., 2014; Minei et al., 2012). For an explanation of the SIRS and MODS phenomena, see Chapter 38: Multiple Organ Dysfunction Syndrome.

Nursing Assessment and Diagnosis

Complications may develop at any time in the post-injury phase. Baseline laboratory and diagnostic data are important in the trauma patient. With these data, the nurse can monitor for subtle changes which indicate that a complication is developing. The following assessment data would indicate the presence of a posttrauma complication:

- Elevation of white blood cell count
- Fever
- Change in characteristics of wound drainage (foul odor, thick, and colored)
- Decreasing oxygenation (e.g., decreasing SpO_2, PaO_2)
- Decreasing level of responsiveness (related to decreased oxygenation or increased serum ammonia levels)
- Decreased urine output

- Diaphoresis
- Cool, mottled skin
- Presence of bleeding (melena, hemoptysis, hematemesis, petechiae, or hematuria)
- Changing trends in vital signs or hemodynamic readings (e.g., elevated CO, decreased systemic vascular resistance, SVR)

Nursing diagnoses that pertain to the trauma patient can be clustered into the two broad areas of pulmonary gas exchange and perfusion.

Pulmonary Gas Exchange   Without adequate pulmonary gas exchange, the tissues do not receive the oxygen they require. Therefore, meticulously managing the airway and optimizing oxygenation are major priorities in the care of the trauma patient. Alterations in pulmonary gas exchange can occur due to increased capillary permeability, decreased alveolar surface area for gas exchange, or obstruction in pulmonary capillary perfusion. Ventilation impairments result from abnormal breathing patterns from respiratory muscle fatigue or brain injury. Fatigue, decreased level of consciousness, and inability to clear secretions can interfere with the ability to adequately ventilate.

Perfusion   Optimizing perfusion is often a challenge, particularly during the initial phases of trauma care related to hemorrhage with significant loss of circulating blood volume. Hypovolemia can impair tissue perfusion and results from bleeding and interstitial fluid shift from leaky vessels that occur due to systemic inflammatory response and shock. Tissue perfusion can also be affected by capillary obstruction from vasoconstriction that occurs with bleeding. Decreased vascular volume and systemic vascular resistance can impair cardiac output.

In addition, trauma patients may experience acute kidney failure from obstruction (microemboli and myoglobin) of renal blood flow. In the period following a traumatic injury, patients have an acute catecholamine release with activation of inflammatory response resulting in a hypermetabolic state with decreased or absent oral intake leading to nutritional compromise. There is also an increased risk for infection because of open wounds, invasive procedures, surgical incisions, debilitated state, and altered nutrition.

Psychosocial Nursing Considerations

The emphasis here has been on physical manifestations of posttrauma complications; however, psychosocial aspects must not be ignored. These patients may remain in high-acuity environments for prolonged periods and are susceptible to sensory disturbances. Extensive rehabilitation may be necessary to regain skeletal muscle mass and neurologic function. Quality-of-life issues should be considered by the patient and the family. The family's standard of living may decline because of financial factors related to healthcare costs and changes in the patient's role.

Section Eight Review

1. What risk is associated with the delay in treatment of open fractures?
   A. The client will not be able to produce the same number of immunoglobulins.
   B. The client will have a higher microorganism count because of the delay in wound debridement.
   C. The client is at higher risk for antibiotic resistance.
   D. The client will be unable to mount a local inflammatory response.

2. When crush injuries occur, DIC may develop because of which factor?
   A. Activation of the intrinsic pathway via platelet aggregation
   B. Activation of the extrinsic pathway via platelet release
   C. High microorganism count
   D. Long-bone injury

3. Which statement best describes the relationship between ARDS and MODS?
   A. Decreased pulmonary gas exchange leads to decreased tissue oxygenation and cellular death.
   B. Pulmonary edema produces a fluid volume deficit and hypoperfusion of tissues.
   C. Organ death releases endotoxins that kill pulmonary epithelial cells.
   D. Increased carbon dioxide retention stimulates peripheral vasodilation and hypoperfusion of tissue.

4. Which statements best describe nutritional support for the trauma client?
   A. It should be instituted when the client has bowel function.
   B. It is difficult to use protocols because every case is different.
   C. It should be instituted as early as possible.
   D. It should be instituted as soon as the client is removed from mechanical ventilation.

Answers: 1. B, 2. A, 3. A, 4. C

Clinical Reasoning Checkpoint

An 82-year-old male unrestrained driver hit another vehicle head-on while driving at 45 miles per hour. He was brought to the ED via helicopter. On arrival, his vital signs were BP 125/85 mmHg, HR 110/min, RR 34/min, and temperature 37°C (98.6°F). His past medical history includes myocardial infarction and hypertension.

1. Given the patient's mechanism of injury, for what injuries is he at risk?

2. On arrival at the ED, how would you begin to assess this patient?

Clinical update: During your secondary survey, the patient becomes hypotensive. You note his blood pressure is lower on expiration than inspiration. His heart sounds are now muffled.

3. Based on the clinical update, what should you do, and what is your interpretation of his condition?

Chapter 35 Review

1. A nurse is advised that a client with multiple blunt trauma is expected to arrive in the emergency department. What preparations should the nurse make?
   1. Stock the receiving room with suture kits.
   2. Alert radiology staff that x-rays will be required.
   3. Check the available supply of dressings and bandages.
   4. Prepare a chest tube drainage tray.

2. A client has experienced blunt trauma in a motor vehicle crash. The ED nurse would consider which forces while discussing mechanism of injury with the paramedic team? (Select all that apply.)
   1. Acceleration
   2. Axial loading
   3. Deceleration
   4. Mass
   5. Shearing

3. A client is admitted to the emergency department with two gunshot wounds. What can the nurse determine from the presence of these wounds? (Select all that apply.)

   1. One is an entrance wound and one is an exit wound.
   2. The location of the wounds provides a hint of the trajectory the missile might have taken if the same missile caused both wounds.
   3. The client was shot twice.
   4. The internal injuries will lie on a straight line between these two wounds.
   5. It will be necessary to inspect both wounds closely for the presence of gunpowder.

4. A client admitted after a motor vehicle crash is 36 weeks pregnant. After spinal injury has been ruled out, how should the nurse position the client?

   1. Supine with head of bed flat
   2. Prone
   3. Supine with head of bed raised 30 degrees
   4. Left lateral decubitus

5. A client, admitted after falling, is unconscious and has open fractures to both femurs. Initial assessment reveals diminished breath sounds bilaterally despite chest wall movements of breathing. What is the nurse's priority intervention?

   1. Roll the client to the left side.
   2. Tilt the client's head back to open the airway.
   3. Do a blind finger sweep of the oral pharynx.
   4. Perform a modified jaw thrust maneuver.

6. Paramedics report that a client was the restrained driver of a vehicle that struck a bridge abutment. Time of injury was approximately 30 minutes ago. Which assessment findings would alert the nurse to the possibility of a ruptured spleen? (Select all that apply.)

   1. Decreased lung sounds on the right side
   2. Hypotension with no obvious hemorrhage
   3. Presence of seat belt abrasions
   4. Distention of the abdomen
   5. Client is unconscious

7. A client who was admitted to the emergency department after a gunshot wound to the chest is hemorrhaging. What interventions should the nurse anticipate? (Select all that apply.)

   1. Initiation of IV access with two large-bore catheters
   2. Administration of IV vasopressors
   3. Administration of packed red blood cells
   4. Rapid administration of IV fluid
   5. Open resuscitative thoracotomy

8. Which assessment would alert the nurse to the presence of flail chest?

   1. Paradoxical chest wall movement
   2. Tachycardia
   3. Tachypnea
   4. Splinting

9. A client has been admitted with multiple trauma injury. What assessments should make the nurse suspect that a posttrauma complication has occurred? (Select all that apply.)

   1. Warm, dry skin
   2. Decreased urine output
   3. Decreased white blood cell count
   4. Decreased level of consciousness
   5. Changing wound drainage characteristics

10. A client required a colostomy following a gunshot wound to the abdomen. The nurse would evaluate which assessment finding as indicating development of a common complication of this type of injury?

    1. Excessive bleeding from puncture sites for laboratory testing
    2. Decreased urine output
    3. Fever
    4. Bradycardia

Answers to questions found inside your textbook are available on the faculty resources site. Please consult with your instructor.

References

Abdelrahman, H., El-Menyar, A., Al-Thani, H., Consunji, R., Zarour, A., Peralta, R., . . . Latifi, K. (2014). Time-based trauma-related mortality patterns in a newly created trauma system. *World Journal of Surgery, 38*(11), 2804–2812. doi:10.1007/s00268-014-2705-x

Adams, S. D., & Holcomb, J. B. (2015). Geriatric trauma. *Current Opinion in Critical Care, 21,* 520–526.

Ali, J. (2014). Priorities in multisystem trauma. In J. B. Hall, G. A. Schmidt, & J. P. Kress (Eds.), *Principles of critical care* (4th ed.). New York, NY: McGraw-Hill. Retrieved March 26, 2017, from http://accessmedicine.mhmedical.com.ezproxy.uky.edu/content.aspx?bookid=1340&sectionid=80026930

American Psychiatric Association. (2013). *Diagnostic and statistical manual of mental disorders: DSM-V*. Washington, DC: American Psychiatric Association.

Calland, J. E., Ingraham, A. M., Martin, N., Marshall, G. T., Schulman, C. L., Stapleton, T., . . . Eastern Association for the Surgery of Trauma. (2012). Evaluation and management of geriatric trauma: An Eastern Association for the Surgery of Trauma practice management guideline. *Journal of Trauma Acute Care Surgery, 73*(5, suppl. 4), S345–S350.

Cameron, P., & Knapp, B. J. (2016). Trauma in adults. In J. E. Tintinalli, J. Stapczynski, O. Ma, D. M. Yealy, G. D. Meckler, & D. M. Cline (Eds.), *Tintinalli's emergency medicine: A comprehensive study guide* (8th ed.). New York, NY: McGraw-Hill. Retrieved March 26, 2017, from http://accessemergencymedicine.mhmedical.com.ezproxy.uky.edu/content.aspx?bookid=1658&sectionid=109387355

Centers for Disease Control and Prevention (CDC). (2014). *Summary health statistics for the U.S. population: National health interview survey, 2012*. Retrieved December 13, 2016, from http://www.cdc.gov/nchsdata/series/sr_10/sr10_260.pdf

Centers for Disease Control and Prevention (CDC). (2016a). *National vital statistics reports—Deaths: Final data for 2014*. Retrieved December 13, 2016, from http://www.cdc.gov/nchs/nvsr65/nvsr65_04.pdf

Centers for Disease Control and Prevention (CDC). (2016b). *NCHS data on accidents or unintentional injuries*. Retrieved December 14, 2016, from www.cdc.gov/nchs/fastats/accidntal-injury.html

Centers for Disease Control and Prevention (CDC). (2016c). *Impaired driving; Get the facts*. Retrieved December 13, 2016, from http://www.cdc.gov/motorvehiclesafety/impaired_driving/impaired-drv_factsheet.html

Chang, M. C. (Ed.). (2016). *Committee on Trauma, American College of Surgeons: National trauma data bank annual report 2016*. Chicago, IL: American College of Surgeons. Retrieved March 26, 2017, from https://www.facs.org/~/media/files/quality%20programs/trauma/ntdb/ntdb%20annual%20report%202016.ashx

Clancy, K., Velopulos, C., Bilaniuk, J., Collier, B., Crowley, W., Kurek, S., . . . Haut, E. (2012). Screening for blunt cardiac injury: An Eastern Association for the Surgery of Trauma practice management guideline. *Journal of Trauma and Acute Care Surgery, 73*(5), 301–305.

Constantini, T., Coimbra, R., Holcomb, J., Podbielski, J., Catalano, R. Blackburn, A., . . . Moore, F. (2016). Current management of hemorrhage from severe pelvic fractures: Results of an American Association for the Surgery of Trauma multi-institutional trial. *Journal of Trauma and Acute Care Surgery, 80*, 717–725.

Cowley, R. A. (1976). The resuscitation and stabilization of major multiple trauma patients in a trauma center environment. *Clinical Medicine, 83*, 16–22.

Dehghan, N., de Mestral, C., McKee, M., Schemitsch, E., & Nathens, A. (2014). Flail chest injuries: A review of outcomes and treatment practices from the National Trauma Data Bank. *Journal of Trauma and Acute Care Surgery, 76*(2), 462–468.

Evans, J. A., van Wessem, K. S., McDougall, D., Lee, K. A., Lyons, T., & Balogh, Z. (2010). Epidemiology of traumatic deaths: Comprehensive population-based assessment. *World Journal of Surgery, 34*(1), 158–163.

Fanelli, V., Vlachou, A., Ghannadian, S., Simonetti, U., Slutsky, A., & Zhang, H. (2013). Acute respiratory distress syndrome: New definition, current and future therapeutic options. *Journal of Thoracic Disease, 5*(3), 326–334.

Federal Interagency Forum on Aging-Related Statistics. (2016). *Older Americans 2016: Key indicators of well-being*. Retrieved July 6, 2017, from https://agingstats.gov/docs/LatestReport/Older-Americans-2016-Key-Indicators-of-WellBeing.pdf

Frohlich, M., Lefering, R., Probst, C., Paffrath, T., Schneider, M. M., Maegele, M., . . . Committee on Emergency Medicine Intensive Care and Trauma Management of the German Trauma Society. (2014). Epidemiology and risk factors of multiple organ failure after multiple trauma: An analysis of 31,154 patients from the Trauma Register DGU. *Journal of Trauma Acute Care Surgery, 76*(4), 921–927.

Goldsmith, H., Curtis, K., & McCloughen, A. (2017). Incidence, intensity, and impact of pain in recently discharged adult trauma patients: An exploratory study. *Journal of Trauma Nursing, 24*(2), 102–109.

Gunst, M., Ghaenmaghami, V., Gruszecki, A., Urban, J., Frankel, H., & Shafi, S. (2010). Changing epidemiology of trauma deaths leads to a bimodal distribution. *Proceedings (Baylor University Medical Center), 23*(4), 349–354.

Harada, M. Y., Ko, A., Barmparas, G., Smith, E. J., Patel, B. K., Dhillon, N. K., . . . Ley, E. J. (2017). Ten-year trend in crystalloid resuscitation: Reduced volume and lower mortality. *International Journal of Surgery, 38*, 78–82. doi:10.1016/j.ijsu.2016.12.073

Hildebrand, D., Ben-Sassi, A., Ross, N., Macvicar, R., Frizelle, F., & Watson, A. (2014). Modern management of splenic trauma. *The British Medical Journal, 348*, 1864–1866.

Jain, V., Chari, R., Maslovitz, S., Farine, D., Bujold, E., Gagnon, R., . . . Sanderson, F. (2015). Guidelines for the management of a pregnant trauma patient. *Journal of Obstetrics and Gynaecology Canada, 37*(6), 553–571.

Joseph, B., Jokar, T. O., Hassan, A., Azim, A., Mohler, M. J., Kulvatunyou, N., . . . Rhee, P. (2017). Redefining the association between old age and poor outcomes after trauma: The impact of frailty syndrome. *Journal of Trauma and Acute Care Surgery, 82*(3), 575–581.

Kaafarani, H., Lee, J., King, D., DeMoya, N., Fagenholz, P., & Butler, K. (2016). Adequate nutrition may get you home: Effect of caloric/protein deficits on the discharge distribution of critically ill surgical patients. *Journal of Parenteral and Enteral Nutrition, 40*(1), 37–44.

Kee, J. K. (2014). *Laboratory and diagnostic tests with nursing implications* (10th ed.). Hoboken, NJ: Pearson.

Kirkpatrick, A., Roberts, D., De Waele, J., Jaeschke, R., Malbrain, M., De Keulenaer, B., . . . Olvera, C. (2013). Intraabdominal hypertension and the abdominal compartment syndrome: Updated consensus definitions and clinical practice guidelines from the World Society of the Abdominal Compartment Syndrome. *Intensive Care Medicine, 39*, 2187–2190.

Leske, J. S., McAndrew, N. S., Brasel, K. J., & Feetham, S. (2017). Family presence during resuscitation after trauma. *Journal of Trauma Nursing, 24*(2) 85–96.

Limmer, D., O'Keefe, M. F., Grant, H., Murray, B., Bergeson, J. D., & Dickinson, E. T. (Eds.) (2016). Section 5: Trauma emergencies. In *Emergency care* (13th ed.). Boston, MA: Prentice Hall/Brady.

MacLeod, J. B., Winkler, A. M., McCoy, C. C., Hillyer, C. D., & Shaz, B. H. (2014). Early trauma induced coagulopathy: Prevalence across the injury spectrum. *Injury, 45*(5): 910–915.

McGinty, K. (2017). Autotransfusion. In D. L. Wiegand (Ed.), *AACN procedure manual for critical care* (7th ed., pp. 164–168). St. Louis, MO: Elsevier.

Minei, J. P., Cuschieri, J., Sperry, J., Moore, E. E., West, M. A., Harbrecht, B. G., . . . Maier, R. V. (2012). The changing pattern and implications of multiple organ failure after blunt injury with hemorrhagic shock. *Critical Care Medicine, 40*(4), 1129–1135.

National Highway Traffic Safety Administration (NHTSA). (2016). *The ABCs of BAC: A guide to understanding blood alcohol concentration and alcohol impairment.* Washington, DC: NHTSA. Retrieved December 13, 2016, from http://www.nhtsa.gov /Driving-Safety/Impaired-Driving

Roccaforte, J. (2017). Posttrauma care. In J. M. Oropello, S. M. Pastores, & V. Kvetan (Eds.), *Critical care.* New York, NY: McGraw-Hill. Retrieved March 26, 2017, http://accessmedicine.mhmedical.com.ezproxy.uky. edu/content.aspx?bookid=1944&sectionid=143519714

Sanddal, T. A. L., Esposito, T. J., Whitney, J. R., Hartford, D., Taillac, P. P., Mann, N. C., & Sanddal, N. D. (2011). Analysis of preventable trauma deaths and opportunities for trauma care improvement in Utah. *Journal of Trauma, 70*(4), 970–977.

Simmons, J., & Adam, L. (2014). Principles of postoperative critical care. In J. B. Hall, G. A. Schmidt, & J. P. Kress (Eds.), *Principles of critical care* (4th ed.). New York, NY: McGraw-Hill. Retrieved March 27, 2017, from http://accessmedicine.mhmedical.com .ezproxy.uky.edu/content.aspx?bookid=1340&sectionid =80026410

Sundstrom, T., Asbjornsen, H., Habiba, S., Sunde, G., & Wester, K. (2014). Prehospital use of cervical collars in trauma patients: A critical review. *Journal of Neurotrauma, 31*(6), 531–540.

Toker, S., Hak, D. J., & Morgan, S. J. (2011). *Deep vein thrombosis prophylaxis in trauma patients. Thrombosis.* Retrieved September 7, 2012, from http://www.ncbi. nlm.nih.gov/pmc/articles/PMC3195354/. doi:10.1155/ 2011/505373

Trunkey, D. D. (1983). Trauma. *Scientific American, 249*(2), 28–35.

Van, P. Y., & Schreiber, M. A. (2016). Contemporary thromboprohylaxis of trauma patients. *Current Opinion in Critical Care, 22*(6), 607–612.

Vioque, S., Kim, P., McMaster, J., Gallagher, J., Allen, S., Holena, D., . . . Pascual, J. (2014). Classifying errors in preventable and potentially preventable trauma deaths: A 9-year review using the Joint Commission's standardized methodology. *American Journal of Surgery, 208*(2), 187–194.

West, J. G., Trunkey, D. D., & Limm, R. C. (1979). Systems of trauma care. A case of two counties. *Archives of Surgery, 114*(4), 455–460.

Chapter 36
Acute Burn Injury

Learning Outcomes

36.1 Explain the mechanisms of burn injury.

36.2 Differentiate burn wound descriptors based on the level of dermis and tissue involved, including criteria for transferring a burn patient to a burn center.

36.3 Discuss the cardiovascular and pulmonary effects of burn injury during the resuscitative phase.

36.4 Describe the neurologic and psychologic effects of burn injury during the resuscitative phase.

36.5 Discuss the metabolic and renal effects of burn injury during the resuscitative phase.

36.6 Explain burn wound healing, wound care, and closure.

36.7 Describe the psychosocial and physical mobility needs of the patient with burn injury during the acute rehabilitative phase.

36.8 Discuss nursing interventions related to physical conditioning, protection of new skin, scar management, and psychosocial adjustment during the long-term rehabilitative phase of burn care.

Nearly 500,000 people are burned each year in the United States, resulting in more than 3200 deaths (American Burn Association [ABA], 2016). Burn injuries account for approximately 40,000 admissions to acute-care hospitals every year (ABA, 2016). The economic costs of treatment and recovery from burn injury rise into the billions of dollars per year, as do the costs of days lost from work and of physical and vocational rehabilitation (Centers for Disease Control and Prevention [CDC], 2014; U.S. Fire Administration [USFA], 2016).

Most burn injuries occur in the home (ABA, 2016). Children and older adults are most prone to burn injuries. Older adults have impaired senses and slower reaction times and tend to assess risk inaccurately. They also have thinner skin, diminished microcirculation, and an increased susceptibility to infection (Wysocki, 2016). All of these factors not only put older adults at greater risk for burn injuries but also lead to heightened morbidity and mortality. Furthermore, diabetes increases the risk for burn injury, particularly of the feet, because of diminished ability to sense temperature extremes secondary to distal sensorimotor polyneuropathy.

This chapter focuses primarily on the management of the first two phases of severe burn injury—the resuscitative and acute rehabilitative phases—but a brief overview of the third phase (long-term rehabilitative) is also provided. During the first two phases, every system in the body can be adversely affected, making acute burn care a challenge. Management is complex and requires a multidisciplinary team approach for the best patient outcomes.

Section One: Mechanisms of Burn Injury

Burn injury may be caused by exposure to heat (flames, steam, hot objects and liquids), chemicals (household or industrial), electricity (current or lightning), radiation (sun exposure, tanning or radiography), or extreme cold. The severity of the injury depends on factors that may be specific to the type of burn, such as length of exposure, temperature of the offending substance, tissue conductance, and substance concentration.

Thermal Burns

Thermal burns are caused by exposure to dry sources (fire or flame) or wet sources (scalds) and account for 80% of all burns (Rowan et al., 2015). They produce microvascular and inflammatory responses within minutes of the injury (Figure 36–1). The effects of these two responses can last 2 to 3 days. Inflammatory mediators (e.g., histamine and serotonin) released by damaged cells increase vascular permeability, causing fluid, electrolytes, and proteins to leak into the interstitial space. These mediators also contribute to cell wall changes that permit intravascular fluid and proteins to leak into the interstitial spaces. Both of these responses contribute to burn edema formation. Burn edema is usually limited to the injured tissues in smaller burns. Severe thermal injuries over a large surface area (roughly 20% of body surface) also produce edema in uninjured tissues. However, the fluid shift from intravascular to interstitial spaces may cause a hypovolemic shock state. Fluid loss by evaporation from the burn wound also contributes to the volume deficit. This hypovolemic shock state is frequently referred to as **burn shock** (Rowan et al., 2015).

Chemical Burns

Chemical burns are the result of exposure to acid, alkali, or organic substances and result in 2% to 6% of admissions to burn units (Cox, 2015). The extent of injury depends on the amount and concentration of the substance, the length of exposure, and the mechanism of chemical action. An acid substance (e.g., hydrochloric or sulfuric acid) causes an **eschar** (dead sloughing tissue) type of wound, resulting from coagulation necrosis. The eschar formation from coagulation necrosis is not limited to chemical burns; eschar can also occur with burns over large body surface areas and burns from other causes. The eschar prevents continued tissue damage beneath the

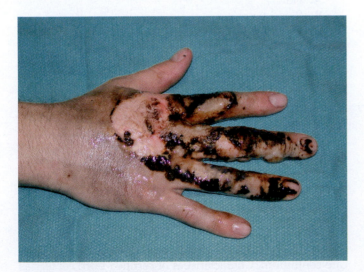

Figure 36–1 Thermal burn.
SOURCE: Pearson Education/PH College.

layer of eschar. An alkaline substance (e.g., sodium hydroxide [lye] or ammonium hydroxide [ammonia]) usually causes more tissue damage than an acid substance (given the same volume) because alkalis cause protein liquefaction, producing a soupy wound that allows continued tissue damage into deeper structures. Damage occurs rapidly and continues until the pH returns to a normal physiologic level.

Organic substances (e.g., cresols, phenols) produce a thermal component and may be absorbed systemically, producing renal and hepatic toxicity. Inhalation of chemical substances can cause direct parenchymal lung injury, as can inhalation of noxious smoke from a fire. Absorption of a chemical either through the pulmonary system or through direct skin contact can cause systemic effects involving the pulmonary, cardiovascular, renal, or hepatic systems.

Electrical Burns

Electrical burns result from the conversion of electrical energy into heat. Electrical burns account for 3% to 5% of admissions to burn units and cause 2% to 3% of pediatric emergency department burn visits (Cushing, 2016). The extent of dermal injury depends on the type of current, the pathway of current flow, local tissue resistance, and the duration of contact. All tissues are conductive to some extent, but there are differences in resistance to current flow. Externally, the skin is the primary resistor to electrical current. Its ability to resist electrical current depends on its thickness and amount of moisture. Internally, nerves and blood vessels are the best electrical conductors. Because of the internal damage that can be caused by electrical injuries, the severity of an electrical burn is difficult to determine on initial exam.

Electrical contact injuries can be caused by low-voltage lines. These lines, most commonly found in homes and offices, usually conduct alternating current (AC). Typically, household current carries 110 volts up to 240 volts. Because AC flows back and forth in a cyclical manner, the former terminology describing an entrance and exit wound is incorrect. Alternating current causes a more severe injury than does direct current (DC) because it produces tetanic muscle contractions that do not allow disengagement from the current source. Direct current hurls the person away from the current source. These differences between AC and DC are significant only with low voltages.

High-voltage burn injuries are caused by a current that moves from the electrical source in an arc, either into or over the person. The arc can generate temperatures up to 5000°C (9032°F), causing thermal injuries. High voltage may be categorized as low as 500 to 1000 volts, and industrial high-tension power lines carry as much as 100,000 volts of electricity (Cushing, 2016).

Another type of electrical burn is the electrical flash burn, which involves no electrical contact and is a true thermal injury caused by electrical arcs that pass over the skin. Differentiating the types of electrical burns helps the healthcare provider determine depth of injury, as well as possible associated injuries.

Radiation and Extreme Cold Burns

Radiation burns result from the transfer of radiant energy to the body and the production of cellular toxins. The effect is most evident in cells that reproduce rapidly, such as those of the skin, blood vessels, intestinal lining, and bone marrow. Greater exposure to radiation causes more significant damage to varying cell types than does less exposure. A radiation victim's injury usually results from radiation therapy or from an industrial or laboratory incident.

Exposure to severe cold temperatures can cause frostbite injuries (Figure 36–2). They result from microvascular stasis and occlusion, direct damage to cells from cold and the formation of ice crystals, and reperfusion injury (Mechem, 2017). While frostbite injuries may not seem to be burn injuries, frostbite is a thermal injury to the skin. Therefore, the treatment of severe frostbite can be very similar to the treatment of burn injuries. Conditions that increase susceptibility to this type of injury include decreased muscle and fat, which reduces insulation from cold; poor nutrition; the inability to generate sufficient body heat through physical activity; alcohol and drug abuse, which affects judgment and can lead to prolonged cold exposure; and a diminished ability to shiver. Older adults are at greater risk for this type of injury because of vasoconstriction and their

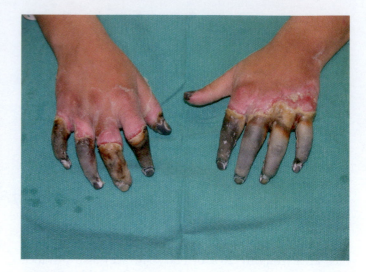

Figure 36–2 Frostbite injury.

SOURCE: Pearson Education/PH College.

reduced ability to generate heat. Frostbite injuries are treated conservatively because it may be weeks before there is a clear demarcation between viable and nonviable tissue.

Section One Review

1. Which groups are at greatest risk for burn injuries? (Select all that apply.)
   A. Middle adults
   B. Older adults
   C. Children
   D. Teenagers
   E. Young adults

2. Which type of burn is characterized by deep penetration of tissues and necrosis continuing for several hours after injury?
   A. Acidic burn
   B. Alkaline burn
   C. Electrical burn
   D. Flash burn

3. Severe electrical contact injuries are often caused by low-voltage lines in which form?
   A. Alternating current
   B. Direct current
   C. Current source
   D. Reflex arc

4. Which areas are most prone to injury as a result of radiation exposure? (Select all that apply.)
   A. Skin
   B. Blood vessels
   C. Intestinal lining
   D. Bone marrow
   E. Heart

Answers: 1. (B, C), 2. B, 3. A, 4. (A, B, C, D)

Section Two: Burn Wound Classification and Burn Center Transfer

The primary goal in the initial emergency management of the burned patient is to stop the burning, whether that means putting out the fire, removing the chemical substance in an appropriate manner, or otherwise stopping the burn process. Once the burning is stopped, the next priority is to protect the airway, as oral–pharyngeal edema can quickly occlude the airway and compromise the patient, and to stabilize

breathing and circulation. Once the patient is stabilized, the goal is then to assess the extent of the injuries and take appropriate measures to treat them. On assessment, if the patient meets established burn-related criteria, it is recommended that the patient be transferred to a burn center. Burn centers provide comprehensive, highly skilled care to patients with critical burns. Patient care processes are evidence based, and continuous quality assessments are a part of the delivery of care continuum. Characteristics of certified burn centers as mandated by the American Burn Association (ABA) Verification Committee and the American College of Surgeons Committee on Trauma (ACS-COT) are listed in the "Quality and Safety: Selected Qualities of Certified Burn Centers" feature.

Burn wound assessment is a high-priority skill for nurses who care for patients with severe burn injuries. After the patient is stabilized, the nurse assists in assessing and classifying the burn wound based on the level of dermis and tissue involved and calculating the extent of total body surface area affected.

Burn Classification

Burns are classified according to depth of injury and extent of body surface area involved. Most burns are not uniform in depth, and often the edges of the wound are more shallow than the center; a burn injury is classified by the deepest tissue destruction. Early burn classification is crucial because it heavily influences the early resuscitative plan.

Burn Depth   Burn depth was traditionally described as first, second, or third degree (Figure 36–3). Currently, burn wounds are more specifically differentiated by the level of dermis and subcutaneous tissue involved (Table 36–1), which is more descriptive of damage. However, it is important to understand that many agencies still utilize the degree classification. **Superficial burns** involve only epidermis tissues—for example, a sunburn. **Superficial partial-thickness burns** involve the epidermis and the superficial layer of the dermis. These burns may occur after brief contact with hot objects. **Deep partial-thickness burns** involve the epidermis and deep layer of the dermis—for example, a hot tar burn (thermal burn). **Full-thickness burns** involve the epidermis, dermis, and subcutaneous layers of skin and tissue. Prolonged

exposure to flames, electricity, or chemicals can cause these very severe burns. **Subdermal burns**, also referred to as **deep full-thickness burns**, usually involve all layers of the skin and may include injury to muscle, tendons, or bone as a result of prolonged contact with flames, hot objects, or electricity. This more accurate and specific classification of burns is often the lexicon for specialized burn units.

Wound Conversion.   The depth of the burn is often difficult to assess initially. Calculation of the extent of injury should be re-evaluated after the initial wound debridement (dead tissue removal) and over the course of the ensuing 72 hours. With extensive and deep wounds, surgical debridement may be postponed for up to 72 hours to allow the wound to fully evolve.

Wound conversion (or wound progression) is the spontaneous progression of a burn wound into deeper tissue after the initial burn insult (e.g., a partial-thickness burn progressing to a full-thickness burn). Wound conversion sometimes occurs whereby viable tissue becomes nonviable, increasing the depth of the wound. Risk factors for wound conversion include impaired oxygenation of tissues, infection, mechanical trauma, and malnutrition (Evans, 2016).

Zones of Injury.   Each thermal burn consists of three zones of injury from the most severe inner area to the least severe outer area of the burn (Evans, 2016). The area of greatest damage is called the **zone of coagulation**. The zone of coagulation is typically closest to the heat source, and all tissue in this zone is damaged. Surrounding this central zone is the **zone of stasis**, which can easily convert to nonviable tissue (wound conversion) if blood flow is not adequately restored. Only some of the tissue in this zone is damaged. The outermost area is termed the **zone of hyperemia**; it blanches with pressure and heals in 7 to 10 days as long as the tissue is perfused. It is red in color because of a prolonged inflammatory response (Evans, 2016). In instances of prolonged hypoperfusion, this area can also undergo wound conversion, progressing to a zone stasis injury, or, in severe cases of hypoperfusion, an ischemic area. Appropriate fluid resuscitation and possible release of constriction by escharotomy is essential in ensuring adequate tissue perfusion and oxygenation.

Total Body Surface Area   The extent of injury is expressed by the percentage of total body surface area (TBSA) burned. Mild superficial burns are not included in this calculation. The most accurate guide in determining the extent of injury is the Lund and Browder Chart, which adjusts TBSA for age (Figure 36–4). This is important because a child's body is proportioned differently from an adult's. For example, a child's head is allowed a greater TBSA percentage than the head of an adult.

To use the guide, one assesses all partial- and full-thickness burns and shades the figure accordingly. The percentage of each anatomic area involved is determined, and then the percentages are totaled. For example, if an adult were to sustain a scald injury to the right lower arm and hand, the TBSA burned would be 5.5%.

Another guide used to calculate TBSA is the rule of nines (Figure 36–5). This method divides the body into areas of 9% or multiples of 9%. The head is 9%, each upper extremity is 9%, each lower extremity is 18%, the back is 18%, the trunk (front) is 18%, and the perineum is 1%, for a total of

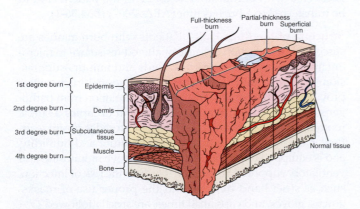

Figure 36–3 Burn injury classification according to the depth of burn.

Table 36–1 Descriptions of Burn Depth

Depth of Burn	Description
Superficial burn	Involves epidermis only May be caused by the sun or brief exposure to hot liquids Erythema, pain, minimal edema No blisters, dry skin Heals in 3 to 7 days via sloughing of the epidermal layer, no scarring
Superficial partial-thickness burn	Involves the epidermis and the papillary layer of the dermis (superficial layer) May be caused by hot liquids, brief contact with hot objects, or flash flame Erythema, brisk capillary refill, blisters, moistness Moderate edema, very painful Heals in 10 to 14 days via re-epithelialization No scarring; potential for hypo- or hyperpigmentation
Deep partial-thickness burn	Involves the epidermis and the reticular layer of the dermis (deep layer) May be caused by flame, hot liquids, radiation, tar, or other hot objects and materials Erythematous or pale, sluggish or absent capillary refill Moist or dry, no blisters Significant edema and altered sensation Heals in 21 days or longer Potential for scarring and hypo- or hyperpigmentation May require skin grafting for optimal function or appearance
Full-thickness burn	Involves the epidermis, dermis, and subcutaneous layer May be caused by flame, electricity, or chemicals Dry, leathery, white Absent capillary refill Generally requires skin grafting Heals via contraction and granulation tissue formation Autografting is required for healing Scarring and hypo or hyperpigmentation
Subdermal burn	Involves the epidermis, dermis, subcutaneous layer, and muscle, tendon, or bone May be caused by electricity, prolonged contact with flame, or a hot object or material Charred, dry appearance Requires skin grafting, flap, or amputation

SOURCE: Data from Evans (2016).

100%. This method is quick and easy but less accurate than the Lund and Browder method—particularly for children, whose proportions are different from those of adults.

Another method of evaluating burn injuries, especially those that are irregularly shaped or occur in patches, is to use the palmar surface (accounts for 0.5% of TBSA) of the patient's hand (accounts for approximately 1% of TBSA). For example, if a patchy burn to the torso comprises four burned areas, each approximately the size of the patient's palm, the TBSA involved would be 2%.

Burn Center Transfer

Patients with complex and/or critical burn injuries are ideally treated in highly specialized burn centers. Criteria are available to guide the decision of when an acutely burned patient should be transferred.

Burn Center Referral Criteria   While the extent and depth of the burn injury are classified as part of the assessment process, the severity of the injury is also evaluated. The more complex the burn injuries, the more complex the physiological and psychosocial needs of the patient. A **burn center** is a specific area in the hospital with specialized equipment, resources, and staff designated for the treatment of patients who have experienced burn injuries. The interdisciplinary staff working in these areas receive special training and continuing education to maintain and enhance their expertise. The American Burn Association has established criteria that indicate the need to transfer a patient to a burn center. As a general rule, if more than 10% of the TBSA is covered with partial-thickness burns, the patient should be transferred to a burn center (ABA, 2007) (Box 36-1).

Structure of the Burn Unit   Patients with burn injuries are susceptible to infection because of altered resistance to microorganisms as a result of open wounds and immunosuppression. The burn unit in an accredited regional burn center provides an environment that promotes isolation from pathogens and prevents infection. Each patient occupies a single room that is access restricted. The room provides positive airflow, has individual controls for temperature and humidity, and is equipped to provide standard invasive monitoring and ventilatory support. Protocols that reduce the risk of infection, such as strict hand hygiene and the proper use of masks, gowns, gloves, and caps at all times, are strictly followed.

Hydrotherapy or whirlpool facilities are often located in burn units because patients may require hydrotherapy to

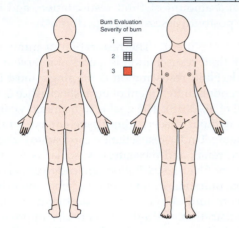

Area	Age (years)					% 1	% 2	% 3	% Total
	0–1	1–4	5–9	10–15	Adult				
Head	19	17	13	10	7				
Neck	2	2	2	2	2				
Ant. trunk	13	13	13	13	13				
Post. trunk	13	13	13	13	13				
R. buttock	2½	2½	2½	2½	2½				
L. buttock	2½	2½	2½	2½	2½				
Genitalia	1	1	1	1	1				
R.U. arm	4	4	4	4	4				
L.U. arm	4	4	4	4	4				
R.L. arm	3	3	3	3	3				
L.L. arm	3	3	3	3	3				
R. hand	2½	2½	2½	2½	2½				
L. hand	2½	2½	2½	2½	2½				
R. thigh	5½	6½	8½	8½	9½				
L. thigh	5½	6½	8½	8½	9½				
R. leg	5	5	5½	6	7				
L. leg	5	5	5½	6	7				
R. foot	3½	3½	3½	3½	3½				
L. foot	3½	3½	3½	3½	3½				
					Total				

Burn Evaluation
Severity of burn

1
2
3

Figure 36–4 The Lund and Browder chart.

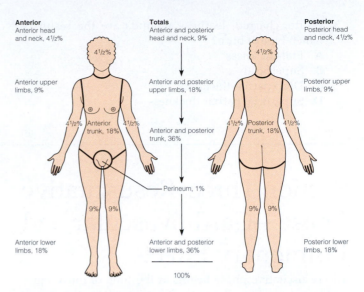

Figure 36–5 The rule of nines.

Anterior
Anterior head
and neck, 4½%

Anterior upper
limbs, 9%

4½% Anterior 4½%
trunk, 18%

Anterior lower
limbs, 18%

Totals
Anterior and posterior
head and neck, 9%

Anterior and posterior
upper limbs, 18%

Anterior and posterior
trunk, 36%

Perineum, 1%

Anterior and posterior
lower limbs, 36%

100%

Posterior
Posterior head
and neck, 4½%

Posterior upper
limbs, 9%

4½% Posterior 4½%
trunk, 18%

Posterior lower
limbs, 18%

debride tissue and promote wound healing. Operating room suites may also be located within or near the burn unit.

Burn Team Members Care of the critically injured burn patient is complex and requires an interdisciplinary team approach. Burn team members include, but are not limited to, nurses, physicians (plastic and general surgeons), advanced practice nurses, physical therapists (PTs), occupational therapists (OTs), pharmacists, dietitians, discharge planners, social workers, chaplains, and psychologists (ABA, 2007). Additional team members and services may also be necessary. Nurses who work in burn centers participate in an orientation program that documents nursing competencies specific to the age-appropriate care and treatment of burn patients, including critical care, wound care, and rehabilitation. They must also attend burn-related continuing education courses annually (ABA, 2007). Personnel working in a regionally accredited burn center should be

trained in the principles of Advanced Burn Life Support (ABLS) (ABA, 2007). ABLS is a certification program sponsored by the ABA that provides advanced training in burn care to best ensure competent, best-practice care.

BOX 36–1 Specialized Burn Center Referral Criteria

1. Partial thickness burns greater than 10% total body surface area (TBSA)
2. Burns that involve the face, hands, feet, genitalia, perineum, or major joints
3. Third-degree burns in any age group
4. Electrical burns, including lightning injury
5. Chemical burns
6. Inhalation injury
7. Burn injury in patients with preexisting medical disorders that could complicate management, prolong recovery, or affect mortality
8. Any patient with burns and concomitant trauma (such as fractures) in which the burn injury poses the greatest risk of morbidity or mortality
9. Burned children in hospitals without qualified personnel or equipment for the care of children
10. Burn injury in patients who will require special social, emotional, or rehabilitative intervention

SOURCE: Data from American Burn Association (ABA) (2007).

Section Two Review

1. An adult client received partial-thickness flash burns to the anterior neck, chest, and both upper arms above the elbow. Estimate the extent of the injury according to the Lund and Browder Chart.
   A. 21%
   B. 18%
   C. 14%
   D. 7%

2. Using the rule of nines, calculate the extent of burn for a client with burns to the posterior head and posterior trunk.
   A. 22.5%
   B. 18%
   C. 20%
   D. 13%

3. White, charred, leathery wounds are the result of which type of burn?
   A. Full-thickness
   B. Superficial
   C. Deep partial-thickness
   D. Superficial partial-thickness

4. Which thermal burn zone is an area of immediately nonviable tissue?
   A. Zone of hyperemia
   B. Zone of ischemia
   C. Zone of coagulation
   D. Zone of stasis

Answers: 1. B, 2. A, 3. A, 4. C

Section Three: Resuscitative Phase—Cardiovascular and Pulmonary Effects

The resuscitative phase begins at the time of burn injury and lasts from 48 to 72 hours after injury. Activities during this phase focus on fluid resuscitation and a thorough evaluation of any additional injuries and comorbid conditions (Stoddard, Ryan, & Schneider, 2014). For example, traumatic injuries such as brain trauma, internal injuries, and fractures that may occur concurrently with burn injuries are identified and treated early in this phase. Stabilization of the cardiovascular and pulmonary systems is an early priority.

Cardiovascular Effects of Burn Injury

Burns covering more than 40% of the total body surface area produce significant myocardial dysfunction, with myocardial contractility and cardiac output decreasing within the first few minutes of injury.

Related Pathophysiology Within a few hours postburn, intravascular volume drops as fluid shifts from the intravascular space into the interstitium in both burned and unburned tissues, and large volumes of plasma leak out from the burn wound surfaces. The combination of fluid shifts and plasma loss results in hemodynamic instability, decreased cardiac output (CO), and a combination of distributive and hypovolemic shock called *burn shock*, which can rapidly lead to cardiovascular collapse. The pathophysiology of these cascading events are multifactorial and are largely unclear, but they are critical (Snell, Loh, Mahambrey, & Shokrollahi, 2013). Stabilization of cardiac output can take 24 to 48 hours after injury (Snell et al., 2013).

Chemical and vasoactive mediators produced as a result of burn injury cause arterial vasoconstriction initially; this is followed by vasodilation and increased capillary permeability, referred to as a loss of capillary seal. The loss of capillary seal leads to massive fluid and electrolyte shifts from intravascular spaces to the interstitium. Hypovolemic shock is a complication of loss of capillary seal and other factors. Although the exact mechanisms for vascular and fluid changes are not well understood, the capillary seal is usually restored within 36 hours after injury (Kasten, Makley, & Kagan, 2011; Latenser, 2009).

Related Assessment Findings Adults with large burns are frequently tachycardic (heart rate between 110 and 125 beats per minute) due to the pain and compensatory mechanism response to hypovolemia and hypoperfusion. Generalized edema develops within the first 24 hours following a severe burn and is influenced by the burn size, the type and amount of fluid resuscitation, and timing (when the postburn assessment is performed).

Related Management The restoration of intravascular volume by fluid resuscitation is a critical intervention for burn shock. Fluid resuscitation is the single most important intervention in treatment of burn shock (Rice & Orgill, 2015; Snell et al., 2013). The goal is to maintain vital organ perfusion without exacerbating tissue edema, which can be challenging. Under-resuscitation can lead to ischemia of pulmonary, renal, and mesenteric vascular beds and can worsen injury. Over-resuscitation can lead to upper-airway obstruction, pulmonary and cerebral edema, and extremity compartment and abdominal compartment syndromes. The administration of fluids dramatically improves outcomes for the burn patient. Fluid resuscitation is usually initiated in adult patients with greater than 15% to 20% TBSA involvement and in the older adult with greater than 5% to 15% TBSA involvement (Rice & Orgill, 2015; Snell et al., 2013). Because the older adult is less able to tolerate the stress of injury and is sensitive to fluid overload, volume replacement must be implemented very carefully.

Fluid resuscitation is guided by urine production and measures of hypoperfusion. The routine use of invasive hemodynamic monitoring to guide fluid resuscitation in patients with burn injury is not recommended because of the risk of infections. The patient's physiologic responses, such as urine output, vital signs, mentation, capillary refill, and peripheral pulses guide fluid administration efforts, and, of these, urine output is the most important parameter (Rice & Orgill, 2015; Snell et al., 2013). Volume resuscitation should be titrated to a urine output of at least 0.5 mL/kg/hr in adults. If these goals are not met, the fluid administration rate should be increased gradually each hour until the urine output is adequate (Rice & Orgill, 2015). Laboratory values, such as serum sodium concentration and serum and urine glucose concentrations, as well as body weight changes, clinical examination, and intake and output records, are monitored to assist in the process of fluid replacement. Fluids are infused at a steady rate through two large-bore (14- to 16-gauge) intravenous (IV) catheters placed through unburned skin if possible. If an IV catheter must be inserted into a burned area, the cannula is threaded into a long vein so that edema does not push the hub out of the vessel and cause infiltration.

A number of formulas are used to guide crystalloid fluid administration during the first 24 hours. Each formula must be modified according to the patient's response.

One of the most frequent formulas used is the Parkland formula (with TBSA expressed as a whole number):

4 mL Ringer's lactate × TBSA % burned × patient weight (kg)

With the Parkland formula, half of the amount is infused during the first 8 hours after injury. This is followed by the second half over the next 16 hours. For example, a patient weighing 68 kilograms has a 50% TBSA burn. This patient's fluid needs would be calculated as 4 (mL of Ringer's lactate) × 50 (TBSA) × 68 (kg) = 13,600 mL total fluids. This patient would require 6800 mL of IV fluids during the first 8 hours after injury and a subsequent infusion of 6800 mL during the next 16 hours. It is important to note that the Parkland formula (or other formulas such as the Brooke formula) should be regarded as a starting point for calculating fluid needs following critical burn injury (Sheridan, 2014). These formulas cannot account for clinical changes; therefore, burn team members with experience and expertise are the best care providers to assess, administer, and evaluate fluid resuscitation (Rice & Orgill, 2015; Snell et al., 2013).

Fluid administration requirements are altered under certain circumstances. Patients with inhalation injuries in conjunction with thermal burns require increased amounts of fluid initially (40% to 50% more). Normally, the lungs are only a minor source of insensible water loss; however, with inhalation injury, there is a significant increase in water loss through the lungs secondary to hyperventilation (especially if the patient is intubated) and hypermetabolism (Nicol & Huether, 2012). Patients with electrical burns and associated trauma, extensive deep thermal burns, or alcohol intoxication; those receiving delayed resuscitation (more than 2 hours after the time of injury); and those with preexisting medical conditions (e.g., patients receiving diuretic therapy) may require increased amounts of fluid according to their physiological responses.

Isotonic crystalloid fluids are used for patients with less than 40% TBSA involvement and no pulmonary injury. Dextrose solutions are not given because as the body uses the glucose from the 5% dextrose in water (D_5W), the solution becomes hypotonic and the fluid shifts out of the vascular space into the interstitial spaces. All resuscitation formulas should be viewed as guidelines that require individualization according to patient assessments. Burn resuscitation fluids should be used until the volume infused is maintaining adequate urine output (at least 0.5 mL/kg/hr in adults) and is equal to the IV fluid maintenance rate (normal maintenance volume plus estimated evaporative water loss) (Rice & Orgill, 2015).

Electrical Burns. Patients who have been exposed to electrical currents may have necrosis of the myocardium and may be predisposed to cardiac dysrhythmias, including sinus tachycardia, nonspecific *ST* or *T* wave changes, *QT* segment prolongation, ventricular ectopy, atrial fibrillation, bundle branch block, ventricular fibrillation, varying degrees of atrioventricular heart blocks, supraventricular tachycardia, and asystole. Patients who experience lethal dysrhythmias (ventricular fibrillation or asystole) from contact with electricity or lightning receive aggressive resuscitation, which has a high rate of success. Cardiac monitoring continues for at least 24 hours after injury even for patients who had electrical contact but do not appear to have any obvious cardiovascular injury. Because the potential for cardiac demise is high, close monitoring, especially in the first 24 to 48 hours following electrical injury is crucial (Marques et al., 2014).

Peripheral Vascular Effects of Burn Injury

A peripheral vascular assessment of each extremity is part of the initial assessment and is repeated every hour thereafter throughout the resuscitative phase. Each extremity is evaluated for color, temperature, pulses, capillary refill, sensation, pain, and motor movement. Signs and symptoms of limb tissue ischemia include pain on passive stretching of the muscle, reduced sensation, weakness, swelling, and pain beyond that expected for the injury sustained. A Doppler ultrasound device may be required to better assess peripheral pulses because edema can interfere with palpation. Increased pressure within the limb from edema can cause tissue ischemia. It is important to remember that the presence of Doppler pulses does not confirm adequate perfusion of the underlying structures and that further evaluations may be necessary if compartment syndrome is suspected. Elevating burned extremities above the level of the heart reduces edema, and jewelry and constricting clothing are removed as soon as possible.

Peripheral blood flow in the limbs can be compromised by eschar or compartment syndrome, either of which can cause limb ischemia. It is crucial that nurses who work with patients with acute burns become proficient at recognizing the need to relieve pressure or tension and prevent further tissue damage.

Eschar   Eschar is stiff (nonelastic), tough, dead tissue covering a full-thickness burn that is unable to expand in response to increasing edema, which can compromise limb circulation, particularly in circumferential burns. If limb blood flow becomes compromised, an emergency **escharotomy** is performed, in which an incision is made through the eschar to expose the fatty tissue below, thereby relieving the pressure and returning blood flow. Escharotomies are performed in a longitudinal fashion midlateral or midmedial in the supinated extremity through the entire involved area, as shown in Figure 36–6. Escharotomy is also used to relieve pulmonary compromise from circumferential burns of the chest. Continued close monitoring is necessary to ensure that the area was adequately released and that elevated pressures have not returned.

Burn-induced Compartment Syndrome   Compartment syndrome occurs when the tissue pressure within a muscle compartment exceeds microvascular pressure and causes an interruption in perfusion at the cellular level. In burn injury, it results from excess fluid in the extravascular space, which increases compartment pressures. To treat burn-induced compartment syndrome, a fasciotomy may be needed, in which a surgical incision is made into the fascia to relieve pressure or tension.

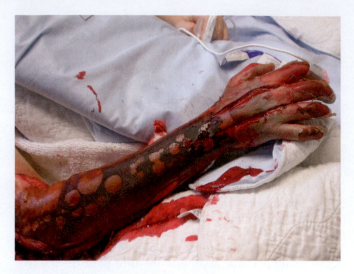

Figure 36–6 Escharotomy of the hand.

SOURCE: Pearson Education/PH College.

Pulmonary Effects of Burn Injury

Alterations in pulmonary function can occur as part of the systemic response to burn injury or from direct inhalation injury. The systemic response results in increased systemic vascular resistance, with a corresponding increase in pulmonary vascular resistance from generalized vasoconstriction of microcirculation. This results in increased pulmonary artery pressure and pulmonary artery wedge pressure. Pulmonary edema is common during the resuscitative phase related to hypoproteinemia (from plasma loss), which decreases vascular oncotic pressure, and it is related to fluid resuscitation efforts. A decrease in pulmonary perfusion from vasoconstriction results in decreased diffusion of oxygen at the capillary level. Respiratory insufficiency can occur at two points after injury: immediately during the resuscitative phase and 10 days to 2 weeks after injury during the acute rehabilitation phase. Respiratory failure during the resuscitative phase is usually a result of inhalation injury; in the acute rehabilitation phase it is usually a result of infection.

Circumferential (or near circumferential) full-thickness burns on the chest can also cause alterations in pulmonary function because stiff eschar does not allow for adequate expansion of the chest. If these eschar chest wounds are circumferential, the patient cannot adequately expand the chest to ventilate effectively, and respiratory distress will develop. Escharotomy incisions may be performed at the bedside to allow movement of the chest wall and restore adequate ventilation.

Upper-airway Injury Upper-airway injuries are supraglottic, resulting from either heat or chemicals dissolved in water. Heat causes immediate injury to the mucosa. Thermal burns from hot air are usually isolated to the supraglottic area because of the ability of the nasopharynx to absorb the heat and a reflex closure of the glottic opening when exposed to heat. Evaluation of patients with upper-airway burns may reveal facial burns, singed nasal hairs, facial erythema and edema, tachypnea, dyspnea, hoarseness, a brassy cough or stridor, and ulceration, especially of the nasopharynx.

Initial treatment for upper-airway injury is humidified 100% oxygen via a snugly fitting nonrebreather mask. Careful observation is necessary to identify impending airway obstruction. When airway edema develops, patients can rapidly experience an airway occlusion. Patients with hoarseness, stridor, or pharyngeal burns are intubated and stabilized and then transferred to a burn center. Upper-airway edema peaks within 48 hours after injury. If not contraindicated, the head of the bed is elevated to reduce edema. Circumferential burns to the neck can cause airway obstruction as a result of edema, and compression, escharotomy, and endotracheal intubation are required to maintain an open airway.

An **inhalation injury** is suspected in the patient who presents with an altered level of consciousness or was retrieved from a confined space in a burning environment. Inhalation injury is a leading cause of death in adult burn patients (Rice & Orgill, 2015; Walker et al., 2015). The diagnosis is made if there is a history of exposure to products of combustion and if bronchoscopy reveals evidence of carbonaceous material or signs of edema or ulceration below the glottis. Bronchoscopy often cannot reach distal lung structures, so there may be limitations with ascertaining the extent of injury in the more distal lung areas (Walker et al., 2015). Clinical indicators of inhalation injury are listed in Box 36–2. The composition and amount of inhaled substance correlates with the severity of the injury.

Lower-airway Injury Lower-airway injury (infraglottic) is usually caused by the gaseous and chemical by-products of combustion contained in inhaled smoke. When these products come into contact with the pulmonary mucosa, complications develop, such as ulceration of mucous membranes, edema, excessive secretions, decreased ciliary action, reactive bronchospasms, inactivation of surfactant, and atelectasis. The end result is an airflow obstruction causing hypoxemia and deteriorating pulmonary function. These patients develop respiratory failure, acute respiratory distress syndrome (ARDS), and pulmonary infections.

BOX 36–2 Clinical Indicators of Inhalation Injury

- Facial burns with charred lips and tongue
- Carbonaceous sputum
- Wheezing or rhonchi on auscultation
- Stridor
- Cough
- Tachypnea
- Singed nasal hair
- Altered level of consciousness
- Injury in enclosed space
- History of flash burn
- Elevated carboxyhemoglobin levels
- Abnormal arterial blood gases

The onset of symptoms of lower-airway injury is unpredictable. Patients may present without symptoms to the emergency department. However, they also may present with the signs and symptoms of upper-airway injury, in addition to cough, carbonaceous (sooty) sputum, signs of hypoxemia (agitation, anxiety, cyanosis, and impaired mental status), chest tightness, flaring nostrils, grunting, crackles, rhonchi, or wheezing. If the potential for inhalation injury exists, the patient is monitored closely for at least 24 hours after injury. Parenchymal lung injuries may take longer to evolve. Diagnostic tests for determining the effects and extent of inhalation injury include physical examination, arterial blood gases (partial pressure of oxygen may be normal initially), chest computerized tomography (CT), fiber-optic bronchoscopy (to visualize tracheobronchial injuries), radionuclide imaging with Xenon, and pulmonary function testing (Rice & Orgill, 2015; Walker et al., 2015). It can be difficult to ascertain the severity of inhalation injuries (Walker et al., 2015).

Treatment for lower-airway injury is supportive, involving aggressive pulmonary toileting and often mechanical ventilation (Walker et al., 2015). Any patient with the potential for inhalation injury must receive high-flow humidified oxygen (100% by nonrebreather mask) while immediate preparations are made for intubation (Walker et al., 2015). Once the patient is intubated, mechanical ventilation is initiated to provide positive pressure ventilation. In the early stages of mechanical ventilator support, the patient should be sedated and, if necessary, paralyzed to provide the optimal ventilation support. In situations where traditional positive pressure mechanical ventilation is unsuccessful due to high airway pressures, high-frequency percussive ventilation may be initiated. Patients who do not require intubation and who can spontaneously breathe may receive intrapulmonary percussive ventilation administered through a face mask, which can result in significant improvement of hypoxia and persistent atelectasis (Walker et al., 2015).

One of the major aspects of nursing care for the critically burned patient is to provide aggressive pulmonary support. Ensuring that the patient engages in coughing and deep breathing exercises, as well as turning the patient, suctioning the airway, providing early ambulation, administering chest physiotherapy, carrying out therapeutic bronchoscopy, and performing pharmacologic interventions, are actions that promote optimal pulmonary functioning (Walker et al., 2015). Repeated assessment and

documentation of respiratory status are necessary for effective interdisciplinary communication and collaboration.

Ventilatory support is tailored to each patient's needs with the ultimate goal of improvement to the point that support is no longer required and the patient can be extubated. Ensuring that the endotracheal tube is secured is very important. Accidental displacement of an endotracheal tube in a patient with airway edema can have catastrophic results; securing the airway and preventing pressure ulcers from the ties can be challenging in the presence of facial burns and associated edema.

Carbon Monoxide Poisoning Carbon monoxide (CO) poisoning is a chemical inhalation injury that has an action different from that of other inhaled chemicals. CO is a colorless, odorless gas that is a by-product of the combustion of organic material. It is more than 200 times more likely to bind to hemoglobin than oxygen. In the presence of CO, hemoglobin becomes saturated with CO rather than oxygen. This results in hypoxemia. The diagnosis of CO poisoning is made by obtaining a history of exposure to by-products of combustion, especially in an enclosed space, and by drawing a serum **carboxyhemoglobin** level (percentage of CO bound to hemoglobin).

CO poisoning is the result of exposure to either low levels of CO for prolonged periods or higher levels for a shorter duration. The severity of poisoning depends on several factors, such as underlying patient health, length of exposure, and concentration of CO inhaled. Symptoms are the result of the CO replacing O_2 on the hemoglobin. The most common symptoms are headache, malaise, nausea, difficulty with memory, personality changes, and gross neurologic dysfunction. An elevated carboxyhemoglobin (COHgb) level confirms CO poisoning. Although carboxyhemoglobin levels may be greater than 70%, the carboxyhemoglobin level is not indicative of the level of neurologic injury.

The treatment for CO poisoning consists of the administration of high fractional concentrations of supplemental oxygen. Early, aggressive hyperbaric oxygen therapy (HBOT) may reduce the negative sequelae of CO poisoning. HBOT refers to giving the patient 100% oxygen while in a chamber that is pressurized to a higher-than-normal atmospheric pressure. Serial carboxyhemoglobin levels are monitored to evaluate patient response to treatment. Pulse oximetry does not differentiate between hemoglobin saturated with oxygen and hemoglobin saturated with CO, so readings may be falsely high.

Section Three Review

1. The resuscitative phase of burn injury lasts how long after the time of injury?
   A. 24 to 48 hours
   B. 36 to 60 hours
   C. 48 to 72 hours
   D. 60 to 84 hours

2. Critically burned clients are at high risk for which complication during the resuscitative phase?
   A. Burn shock
   B. Neurogenic shock
   C. Contractures
   D. Myocardial infarction

3. An adult client has a 55% TBSA burn and weighs 75 kilograms. Using the Parkland formula, calculate fluid resuscitation requirements for the first 8 hours.
   A. 8250 mL
   B. 16,500 mL
   C. 4125 mL
   D. 12,375 mL

4. What is a primary component of treatment for carbon monoxide poisoning?
   A. Hyperbaric oxygen therapy
   B. Hypertonic saline
   C. Keeping peak inspiratory pressure less than 40 cm H_2O
   D. Pulmonary hygiene

Answers: 1. C, 2. A, 3. A, 4. A

Section Four: Resuscitative Phase—Neurologic and Psychologic Effects

The effects of burn injury on nerves depend on a number of variables, such as the depth of the burn (e.g., partial thickness or full thickness) and its location, extent, and type. Furthermore, burn patients often experience psychologic issues such as anxiety, stress, and delirium.

Neurologic Effects

Neurologic effects are most common with electrical and lightning injuries. Nerve tissue offers low resistance to electrical current and is easily damaged. Electric current enters the body at the point of contact in electrical injuries and can enter from any site in lightning strikes. Although it is usually transient, respiratory paralysis can occur, and loss of consciousness is frequent, especially with high-voltage injury. Patients may experience confusion, exhibit a flat affect, lose the ability to concentrate, or have short-term memory problems. Seizures, headaches, peripheral nerve damage, and loss of muscle strength may be observed. Long-term or permanent numbness, prickling, tingling, heightened sensitivity, or paralysis may also occur. The spinal cord can be damaged by high-voltage burns, and although the injury mechanisms are complex and not well understood, they may include direct nerve injury (e.g., demyelinization) or injury to the vessels supplying blood to the cord. The onset of clinical manifestations may be acute or delayed; however, they are more commonly delayed.

Pain and Itching   All burns are painful initially. Burn pain is very unpredictable, and this variation is due to the complex physiology connected to the burn injury and the treatment of the burn injury. Pain presence and expression are also linked to psychosocial coping, as well as any preburn existing behavior issues (Wiechman, Jeschke, & Collins, 2015). Despite advances in burn care, effective pain control remains a challenge and is difficult to achieve consistently in many patients. There are no foolproof methodologies or guidelines as this type of pain is highly variable. Burn pain is a major cause of distress in patients and pain may continue for years after discharge from a burn unit (Wiechman, Sharar, Jeschke, & Collins, 2017). Superficial partial-thickness burns are the most painful. In some instances, air movement across the damaged skin can be quite painful. Moderate superficial burns result in moderate to severe pain as the pain receptors are damaged at this level of injury. Full-thickness and deep burns are typically characterized as absent of pain. However, in patients with deeper burns, there may be an aching sensation likely related to the inflammatory response that is difficult to relieve (Wiechman, Jeschke, & Collins, 2015).

Pain in burn patients is often classified as either procedural or nonprocedural pain. *Procedural pain* is related to wound care or stretching of the patient's scar tissue. *Nonprocedural* (or now frequently called "background") *pain* is the discomfort experienced at rest. Breakthrough pain is an unexpected spike in pain and can be related to anxiety, inadequate pain treatment, or other factors. Postoperative pain is a temporary and expected increase in pain after burn excision or grafting; the duration of this pain is generally 2 to 5 days. Chronic pain is the sensation of discomfort that lasts more than 6 months and is present long after burns are healed. This pain is often classified as neuropathic pain because of damage to nerve endings secondary to the burn (Wiechman, Sharar, Jeschke, & Collins, 2017).

Pain assessment in burns is ascertained in the very same way as other pain. There is no evidenced-based pain assessment that is better than another to assess burn pain. The most important principle in pain assessment in the burn patient is the consistent use of the same pain assessment techniques. This provides predictability for the patient and the nurse and promotes better and more consistent pain management (Wiechman, Jeschke, & Collins, 2015).

Optimum pain management of burn patients is a central component of care in all phases of burn injury. During initial critical care, intravenous (IV) administration of medication is preferred, because of the impaired pharmacokinetics with severe burns. Opioid analgesics are most commonly used (morphine, fentanyl), and intramuscular administration of medications is not recommended due to fluid shifts, the pain of injections, and potentially poor medication absorption (Wiechman, Jeschke, & Collins, 2015). It is recommended that the opioid analgesic be combined with an anxiolytic because anxiety can escalate the feeling of acute pain. Benzodiazepines are frequently used, and lorazepam, specifically, has been demonstrated to reduce acute pain scores (Wiechman, Jeschke, & Collins, 2015). Also beneficial to patients with burns is the use of nonopioid analgesics such as ketamine for short-term pain relief during procedures such as dressing changes. Background pain is best managed with patient-controlled analgesia after the resuscitative phase. Mild opioid analgesics, acetaminophen, or nonsteroidal anti-inflammatory drugs may be given for pain control. Analgesics are most effective when they are given on a regularly scheduled basis rather than intermittently or as needed.

Nonpharmacologic therapies play an important role in addressing the psychological factors that exacerbate pain, as well as directly affecting the pain itself. These therapies include classical conditioning, relaxation therapy, cognitive interventions, distraction (music therapy), hypnosis, and massage therapy.

Pruritus is one of the most common subjective symptoms after burn injury, occurring in 90% of burn patients and continuing for years postburn in 40% of burn patients (Kim, 2015). The mechanism is not well understood, but predictors of pruritus include deep dermal injury, the extent of the burn, and early posttraumatic stress syndromes (Stoddard, Ryan, & Schneider, 2014). Scratching can further injure the skin, leading to graft loss and skin breakdown, and it can impede exercise or sleeping. A recently proposed postburn pruritus protocol suggests pharmaceutical and nonpharmaceutical treatments for this phenomenon based on the status of the burn: prehealing, healing, or healed. This protocol includes oral medications (including gabapentin, pregalbin, cetirizine, pheniramine, cyproheptadine, and naltrexone), as well as topical medications, massage therapy, laser therapy, muscle relaxation therapy, and moisturizing body shampoos (Kim, 2015). Postburn pruritus, like pain, is subjective and labile, and it requires an individualized treatment plan, as often a combination of interventions is needed to control this symptom (Stoddard et al., 2014).

Anxiety and Psychiatric Issues

Patients with critical burns experience increased levels of anxiety, especially related to the treatment and outcome of their injuries. Anticipatory anxiety related to treatment can lead to perceptions of increased pain, which in turn further increases anxiety. Relaxation techniques have been useful in reducing anxiety in the burn patient population (Park, Oh, & Kim, 2013).

Common psychiatric symptoms during the emergency and acute-care phases may include delirium, acute stress and posttraumatic stress disorder symptoms, sleep disturbances, and depression. The causes of these symptoms are often multifactorial and include preburn illnesses (physical and mental), the presence of preburn alcoholism or substance abuse, and current physiological processes (Stoddard et al., 2014). Delirium may be caused by disturbances in fluids and electrolytes or glucose, altered cerebral perfusion, and history of substance abuse. During the acute phase, a significant number of burn survivors experience posttraumatic stress disorder (PTSD) symptoms, including intrusive memories of injury, hypervigilance, and disturbed sleep patterns. Antipsychotic phenothiazines are commonly used in the acute-burn phase to address delirium and/or combative, uncooperative behavior such as pulling off dressings, attempting to get out of bed, or striking out at caregivers. Antidepressants may be administered to treat depression (Stoddard et al., 2014).

Section Four Review

1. In general, how are full-thickness burns best described?
   A. Not painful
   B. Mildly painful
   C. Moderately painful
   D. Extremely painful

2. Neurological effects such as seizure or respiratory paralysis is most common with which type of burn injury?
   A. Thermal
   B. Acid
   C. Electrical
   D. Alkali

3. Which burn injury is associated with pain that is exceptionally sensitive and painful even to an air current passing over it?
   A. Full-thickness
   B. Partial-thickness
   C. Third-degree
   D. Electrical

4. The nurse anticipates administering a medication from which class to address acute-burn phase delirium?
   A. Opioid
   B. NSAID
   C. Antipsychotic phenothiazine
   D. Anabolic steroid

Answers: 1. A, 2. C, 3. B, 4. C

Section Five: Resuscitative Phase—Metabolic and Renal Effects

During the resuscitative phase, the metabolic response to stress causes the patient's metabolism to change dramatically, making it a challenge to meet metabolic needs. The kidneys are also challenged due to the altered metabolic state and decreased perfusion, placing the patient at risk for acute kidney injury during this phase.

Metabolic Effects

The metabolic changes that occur in the burn patient, although similar to what happens for other high-acuity patients, are related to the extent of the injury and, in severe burn injury, have been found to persist for more than 3 years postburn (Gauglitz, 2014). The changes in metabolic rate increase proportionally to the size of the burn. Patients with severe burns covering more than 25% of TBSA can experience hypermetabolic rates of up to 120%. Patients with burns over 40% of the body experience a period of physiologic stress, hypermetabolism, and inflammation; these mechanisms result in glycolysis, proteolysis, lipolysis, and hypermetabolism that is in excess of 180% or more of baseline (Gauglitz, 2014).

Patients with severe burn injury experience the metabolic stress response, which consists of two phases: ebb and flow. The *ebb phase* begins at the time of injury and lasts up to 48 hours after injury (Gauglitz, 2014). It is characterized by a state of hypometabolism, with a decrease in both oxygen consumption and metabolic rate. The ebb phase is followed by the *flow phase*, a hyperdynamic state that stems from massive heat loss from the burn wounds. The flow phase is characterized by an extreme state of hypermetabolism and catabolism, with persistent elevation of cortisol, cytokines, catecholamines, and glucose, which generally plateaus approximately 5 days after injury (Gauglitz, 2014). Patients experience an increase in cardiac output, oxygen consumption, carbon dioxide production, caloric requirements, energy consumption, heart rate, respiratory rate, and body temperature. This hypermetabolic response impacts both acute recovery and rehabilitation. Stress-induced hyperglycemia occurs in patients with burn injury as it does in patients with other critical illnesses or injuries. Administration of insulin in severely burned patients has been shown to improve muscle protein synthesis, accelerate healing time, attenuate the loss of lean body mass, and reduce the acute phase response. Insulin administration is beneficial in both diabetic and nondiabetic burn patients (Gaugliz, 2014). The ebb and flow phases of the metabolic stress response are presented in more detail in Chapter 32.

Meeting Nutritional Needs Nutritional requirements are strongly influenced by the metabolic response to stress; severe burn injury results in an extreme catabolic state. Skeletal muscle protein becomes the major fuel source, which leads to significant wasting of lean body mass

within days of burn injury; visceral proteins are also consumed. Large amounts of protein are also lost from the body as protein-rich plasma shifts to the burn wound surface. Adequate nutritional intake is essential to meet the patient's considerable caloric needs for wound healing and maintaining the immune system. Trace elements and vitamins are also supplemented to facilitate healing and recovery. Unfortunately, there are no current optimal dosing guidelines for proteins or amino acids (Weijs et al., 2014). However, there are multiple formulas for estimating the caloric, energy, and protein needs of burn patients.

Enteral nutrition is initiated early—ideally within 24 hours after injury (Cochran, 2015). Early nutritional support reduces cumulative caloric deficits, stimulates insulin secretion, and conserves lean body mass. A formula that provides at least 50% of calories as carbohydrates, 35 percent as protein, and no more than 15 percent as fat, supplemented with micronutrients and macronutrients and glutamine, is recommended for the severely burned patient (Cochran, 2015). Enteral nutrition is preferred over parenteral nutrition because it maintains gastrointestinal motility and reduces the translocation of bacteria. Parenteral nutrition is reserved for patients with prolonged ileus or intolerance to enteral feedings. Nutritional status is closely monitored via clinical examination of wound healing, serial weights, prealbumin levels, and indirect calorimetry.

Renal Effects

Acute renal failure is a major complication of burn injury and is associated with a high mortality rate. It occurs in up to 30% of burn patients (Emara & Alzaylai, 2013). Most renal failure occurs either immediately following burn injury or later when sepsis ensues and the failure is associated with multiple organ failure (Emara & Alzaylai, 2013). Etiologic factors include fluid shifts, stress-related hormones, myocardial depression, inflammatory mediators, denatured proteins, and nephrotoxic substances (Emara & Alzaylai, 2013). Renal replacement therapy may be used for supportive treatment of acute renal failure.

Emerging Evidence

- A systemic review and meta-analysis of 15 randomized controlled trials were performed to evaluate the efficacy of the use of the anabolic steroid oxandrolone in patients with severe burns. The review found that oxandrolone did not affect mortality, liver failure, or infection in this population. In the catabolic phase of burn injury, the use of the drug led to shortened length of stay, increased the time interval between surgical procedures, increased donor site healing time, and significantly reduced weight loss and nitrogen balance issues. In the rehabilitative phase of burn healing, weight loss was decreased, as was the loss of lean body mass, even after 12 months. This may be an important medication in the treatment of burned patients to enhance the quality outcomes, both short and long term (Li, Guo, Yang, Roy, & Guo, 2016).

- Ventilator-associated pneumonia (VAP) is a common cause of mortality in burn patients. VAP bundles that are implemented during the hospital care of burn patients may have an effect on mortality

rates. A 2-year retrospective chart review revealed that patients with an inhalation injury and a large burn injury were at increased risk for developing VAP. In this sample of patients, the risk for and incidence of VAP were significantly reduced with the use of VAP prevention bundles (Sen, Johnston, Greenhalgh, & Pamieri, 2016).

- Characterizing burn sizes that are associated with an increase in mortality can be helpful in the determination of optimal treatment, including innovative, experimental, or novel treatments. In six major burn centers in North America, the data for 573 burn patients with more than 20% TBSA burns and within 96 hours of injury (including 226 children) were reviewed for mortality, infection or sepsis, pneumonia, acute respiratory distress syndrome, and multi-organ failure. Findings included that children with TBSA burns of 60% or more and adults with 40% TBSA burns or more were at high risk for morbidity and mortality even in specialized burn units. These findings provide information to assist with the benchmarking of modern burn care (Jeschke et al., 2015).

If a patient has experienced muscle damage from exposure to an electrical current, direct thermal injury, or compartment syndrome, then release of **myoglobin** and free hemoglobin may occur (Ibrahim, Sarhane, Fagan, & Goverman, 2013). Myoglobin in the urine may change the urine color to red or reddish-brown. Myoglobin is released from damaged muscle tissue and can precipitate in and obstruct the renal tubules, causing intrinsic renal failure, especially in the face of inadequate fluid resuscitation, shock, or acidosis. If myoglobin is present in the urine (**myoglobinuria**), adequate urine output (0.8–1 mL/kg/hour) that reflects adequate perfusion pressure must be maintained through IV fluid administration to prevent myoglobinuric renal failure (Emara & Azaylai, 2013). This rate of urine output is maintained as long as there is pigment in the urine. In addition to increasing the amount of fluids administered, alkalizing the urine also prevents myoglobin from crystallizing in the tubules and causing an obstruction. The solubility of myoglobin increases in an alkaline environment, so maintaining alkaline urine will increase the rate of myoglobin clearance. An osmotic diuretic, such as mannitol, may be used to increase diuresis and promote the clearance of myoglobin.

In addition to myoglobin, hemoglobin released from damaged red blood cells can also turn the urine red to reddish-brown. It is difficult to distinguish myoglobin from hemoglobin by looking at the urine, so until laboratory tests confirm the presence of one or both of these substances, all red to reddish-brown discoloration should be treated as if it were myoglobin. Both myoglobin and hemoglobin are excreted more readily if the urine pH is alkaline.

Section Five Review

1. Which statement reflects current recommendations for meeting the hypermetabolic needs of a burn client?
   A. Total parenteral nutrition should be started within 24 hours after injury.
   B. Enteral nutrition should be started within 24 hours after injury.
   C. The client should not be fed until bowel sounds are present.
   D. Enteral nutrition should be started after 48 hours of admission.

2. What occurs metabolically during the ebb phase of severe burn injury?
   A. Hypometabolism
   B. Hyperdynamics
   C. Extreme catabolism
   D. Elevation of catecholamines

3. Which injury places the burn client at the highest risk for developing renal failure?
   A. Full-thickness burn to the perineum
   B. Full-thickness burn to the flank
   C. Electrical or crush-type injury
   D. Traumatic brain injury

4. What is the effect of alkalizing the urine of a client with a serious burn injury?
   A. Promotes renal clearance of myoglobin
   B. Promotes hepatic clearance of myoglobin
   C. Increases urine output
   D. Concentrates myoglobin so it can be removed more easily

Answers: 1. A, 2. A, 3. C, 4. A

Section Six: Burn Wound Healing

The cellular and biochemical events that occur during the healing of burn injuries are similar to those that occur in the healing of other wounds. The major difference is that the phases of wound healing in the burn occur more slowly and last longer. Patients with larger burns enter a more prolonged period of hypermetabolism, chronic inflammation, and lean body mass wasting, all of which may impair wound healing (Rowan et al., 2015). Wound healing begins immediately after the injury occurs with the inflammatory response. The *inflammatory phase* lasts approximately 2 weeks, extending into the acute rehabilitative phase; thus, overall wound repair is delayed. At the end of the inflammatory phase, the *proliferative phase* begins. This phase lasts up to 1 month, during which time collagen synthesis, revascularization, and reepithelialization occur. Collagen layers are not as organized as they are in other wounds, which contributes to excessive scar tissue (Figure 36–7).

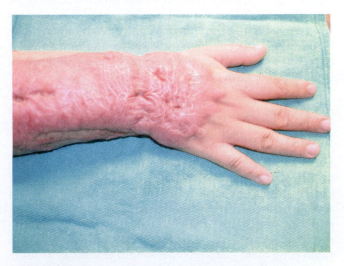

Figure 36–7 Disorganized collagen layers lead to excessive scar tissue.

SOURCE: Pearson Education/PH College.

The *maturation phase* of wound healing follows the proliferative phase and can last 6 to 18 months or longer, depending on the wound. New collagen layers are formed, strengthening the wound, and old collagen layers are broken down. Excessive deposits of collagen during this time produce hypertrophic scars that are characteristic of deep partial- and full-thickness burns. Hypertrophic scars contract while maturing, which can lead to contractures. Wound contraction can produce both cosmetic and functional deformities.

Initial Wound Care

The first step in caring for the burn wound during the resuscitative phase is to ensure the burning process has stopped. The longer the patient's skin is in contact with the burning agent and the higher the temperature, the deeper the cellular damage. Clothing, jewelry, belts, or anything containing heat is removed from the patient (adhered clothing or tar is left in place and cooled with water because removing it will cause further damage to the skin). Dry chemicals are brushed from the patient (taking care not to contaminate the caregiver), and continuous water lavage is initiated.

The initial assessment of the burn wound takes place in the secondary assessment after the head-to-toe evaluation has been completed. Burned extremities are elevated above the level of the heart to reduce edema formation. The head of the bed is also elevated to reduce upper-body and head edema if not contraindicated by trauma or hemodynamic instability. Tetanus prophylaxis is administered.

Initial care of the burn wound depends on the severity of the burn. If the patient meets criteria for transfer to a burn center, the patient is covered with a clean, dry sheet. Care is taken to avoid hypothermia. If time permits, the wound is gently cleansed with sterile saline or a mild soap. Creams or ointments are not applied as they must be removed on arrival at the burn center to allow evaluation of the wound. Removal of topical medications and dressings is a painful procedure, so unless directed to do so by the receiving physician, the nurse leaves the wound clean and covers the patient with a sheet. An escharotomy may be required for a circumferential burn. Definitive care of the wound begins once the patient has been admitted to the hospital or burn center.

Acute Rehabilitative Phase Wound Management

The *acute rehabilitative phase* of burn care occurs after the resuscitative phase, beginning 2 to 3 days after injury and lasting until wound closure. The goals of burn wound management include prevention and control of infection, preservation of viable tissue, and promotion of wound closure with minimal complications. Interventions aimed at supporting these goals include wound cleansing, debridement, topical antimicrobial therapy, and wound closure. Early excision and closure of burn wounds in patients with thermal burn injuries have become the gold standard and have led to a substantial reduction in resting energy requirements and subsequent improvement in mortality rates (Rowan et al., 2015).

Inpatient burn wound care begins with cleansing with water and a mild soap to remove exudate and devitalized tissue. This can be accomplished by showering if the patient is able, or by placing the patient on a table where the wounds are washed and rinsed with running water from spray hoses. If these methods are contraindicated, the wounds can be cleansed while the patient is in the hospital bed. Once the wound has been cleaned, it must be debrided.

Wound Debridement Wound **debridement** is the removal of debris and nonviable tissue from a wound. Burn blisters are usually left intact initially; however, after the patient arrives at a burn center, larger blisters may be debrided. Wound debridement can be achieved mechanically, biologically, chemically, or surgically.

Mechanical Debridement. In burn injury management, mechanical debridement includes *hydrotherapy* and *wound irrigation*. Hydrotherapy uses water to soften and remove dead tissue to improve healing. The two major forms of hydrotherapy are whirlpool and pulsatile lavage. Whirlpool therapy involves immersing the patient (or affected body part) in a bath of warm flowing water in a large metal tank. Pulsatile lavage is a local therapy that applies pulsating water to debride the wound. Wound irrigation applies water (or other solution) to a local wound area in a steady positive pressure flow.

With all methods of mechanical debridement, care is taken to avoid disrupting newly formed granulation tissue or epithelial buds in the healing wound. Wound irrigation and pulsatile lavage are easier to control than hydrotherapy, but all can cause disruption of newly formed tissue. The use of wet-to-dry dressings is no longer recommended because this is a nonselective form of debridement that causes harm to newly formed tissue and is also very painful.

Biodebridement. The biodebridement approach, also known as *biosurgical* or *maggot debridement therapy* (MDT), uses sterilized living fly larvae (maggots) to ingest dead tissue and wound debris while sparing healthy tissues. For many years it has been successfully used to treat acute and chronic wounds, including burn wounds, though it is often used as a last resort (National Pressure Ulcer Advisory Panel [NPUAP], European Pressure Ulcer Advisory Panel [EPUAP], & Pan Pacific Pressure Injury Alliance [PPPIA], 2014). It is theorized that maggots excrete or secrete proteolytic enzymes such as collagenase, allantoin, and other substances that rapidly break down necrotic tissue (NPUAP et al., 2014).

Chemical Debridement. The chemical approach to debridement involves the application of an enzymatic or fibrinolytic preparation to the burn eschar to digest necrotic tissue and hasten eschar separation. Removal of eschar prevents bacterial colonization of dead tissue.

Surgical Debridement. The surgical approach is accomplished under anesthesia in the operating room and usually takes place during the resuscitative phase or within the first week postburn. The two methods of burn wound excision are tangential and fascial. The method used depends on the depth and extent of the burn. *Tangential excision* involves shaving away thin layers of eschar until viable tissue is exposed (Figure 36–8). This method gives a better cosmetic result than fascial excision; however, significant blood loss may occur, causing hypovolemia. *Fascial excision* involves removing nonviable tissue down to the fascial or subcutaneous planes. This method is often used for patients with a large component of full-thickness burns because it is less stressful. The cosmetic result is less satisfactory than with tangential excision; however, if the injury is such that the patient will not survive the stress of tangential excision, fascial excision is performed.

Infection   Bacteria are present in all burn wounds; however, the presence of bacteria alone does not indicate an infection. The nurse must perform diligent surveillance of burn wounds to identify any changes in appearance. Local signs of burn wound infection include conversion of a partial-thickness injury to a full-thickness wound, worsening cellulitis of surrounding normal tissue, eschar separation, and tissue necrosis (Fonseca, 2016). However, an **invasive infection**—defined as the presence of pathogens in a burn wound at sufficient concentrations (in conjunction with depth, surface area involved, and age of the patient) to cause supportive separation of eschar or graft loss, invasion of adjacent unburned tissue, or the systemic response of sepsis syndrome—should be recognized early as invasive infection is highly lethal in the burned patient (Rowan et al., 2015). Early suppurative separation of the eschar, graft loss with involvement of unburned tissue, the presence of a systemic response consistent with sepsis, change in wound color (focal areas of red, brown, or black), or green discoloration of subcutaneous fat indicate a dangerous invasive infection (Fonseca, 2016; Rowan et al., 2015).

Topical Antimicrobial Therapy.   Initially, the burn wound surface is colonized by gram-positive bacteria. After the first week, the surface becomes colonized by gram-negative bacteria. Burn wounds are typically treated with a topical antimicrobial to control bacterial proliferation. Systemic antibiotics are not used prophylactically but, rather, are initiated when there is clinical evidence of an infection and culture confirmation. To prevent the formation of antibiotic-resistant strains of bacteria, the healthcare provider chooses an antibiotic based on sensitivity results. Additional information can be found in the "Related Pharmacotherapy: Topical Antimicrobials" feature.

The topical agent is applied using aseptic technique once or twice daily. Dressing the wound in a silver hydrofiber or 1% silver sulfadiazine dressing covered by a layer of gauze provides a clean, protective environment. The silver ions act as an antimicrobial agent. Silver hydrofiber dressings can reduce the amount of pain and time to wound closure in patients experiencing partial-thickness burns. This type of dressing is effective for up to 7 or more days without reapplication of a topical agent. This allows optimal healing as the wound base is undisturbed for a period of time.

Once the antimicrobial has been applied, an open- or closed-dressing technique is used. The open method leaves the antimicrobial-covered wound open to air. This method

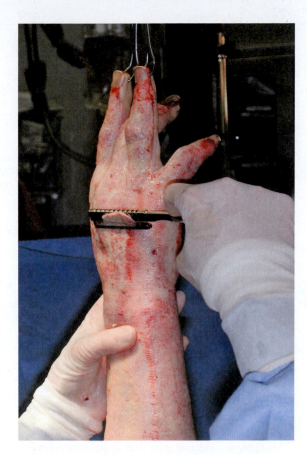

Figure 36–8 Tangential excision.
SOURCE: Pearson Education/PH College.

is primarily used for burns to the face and ears. The closed method involves the application of gauze dressings over the antimicrobial agent. Proponents of this method argue its superiority because it assists with debridement and protects granulation tissue and fragile epithelial buds while also decreasing the evaporative fluid loss from the wounds. Disadvantages to the closed method include fewer opportunities to evaluate the wound. It is crucial that the dressings are applied with function in mind. The dressings should be tight enough to stay in place with motion but not so tight as to restrict motion.

Temporary Burn Coverings   Biological, synthetic, and biosynthetic materials act as skin substitutes and are used to temporarily cover a burn. The type used depends on the depth of the wound and the goal of therapy. The functions of temporary wound coverings are listed in Box 36–3.

BOX 36–3   Functions of Temporary Wound Coverings

- Decrease bacterial proliferation
- Prevent desiccation
- Control heat loss
- Decrease protein loss in wound exudate
- Increase patient comfort
- Protect underlying structures
- Stimulate healing
- Prepare and test wound bed for autografting

Related Pharmacotherapy
Topical Antimicrobials

Sulfonamide

Silver sulfadiazine (Silvadene)

Action and Uses

Silver salt is slowly released and exerts its bactericidal effect only on the bacterial cell membrane and wall; has broad antimicrobial activity, including many gram-negative and gram-positive bacteria and yeast.

Dosages (Adult)

Apply a thickness of approximately $\frac{1}{16}$ inch (1.5 mm) to skin 1–2 times/day

Major Side Effects

Potential for toxicity if applied to extensive areas of the body surface

Nursing Implications

Apply with sterile, gloved hands to cleansed, debrided burned areas. Reapply cream to areas where it has been removed by patient activity; cover burn wounds with medication at all times.

Reapply after bathing.

Dressings are not required but may be used if necessary. Drug does not stain clothing.

Store at room temperature, away from heat.

Pain may be experienced upon application; intensity and duration depend on depth of burn.

Pseudo-eschar (nonviable tissue) may form on wound if it is not *completely* cleansed from burned areas with each dressing change.

Sulfonamide Derivative

Mafenide acetate (Sulfamylon)

Action and Uses

Produces marked reduction of bacterial growth in vascular tissue; active in presence of purulent matter; bacteriostatic against many gram-positive and gram-negative organisms.

Dosages (Adult)

Apply a thickness of approximately $\frac{1}{16}$ inch (1.5 mm) to skin 1–2 times/day

Major Side Effects

Intense pain, burning, or stinging at application sites

Nursing Implications

Apply to cleansed, debrided burn areas with sterile, gloved hands 1–2 times daily. Reapply cream to areas where it has been removed by patient activity; cover burn wounds with medication at all times.

Reapply after bathing.

Dressings are not required but may be used if necessary. Drug does not stain clothing.

Store in a light-resistant container; avoid extremes of heat.

Pain may be experienced upon application; intensity and duration depend on depth of burn.

- Biological dressings obtained from animals (frequently pigs) are referred to as **xenografts or heterografts**. Biological dressings obtained from humans are called **allografts** or **homografts**. These grafts are used to cover clean, superficial partial-thickness burns maintain a moist wound environment; protect the ungrafted wound; and test the receptivity of the wound to autografting. **Autografting** is the process of transplanting skin from one part of the body to fill in another part that has been injured. It is a method of permanent burn wound closure and uses either full-thickness or split-thickness skin grafts. If an infection or necrotic tissue is present, the biological dressing will not adhere to the wound, and it is considered a failure. Failure of a biological dressing is preferable to failure of a valuable donor site autograft. Biological dressings are occlusive, so they also help to reduce pain.

- Synthetic materials such as thin film dressings are used to cover donor sites and to protect small, clean, superficial wounds. These dressings are waterproof and transparent, reduce pain, and maintain moisture in the wound to promote healing. Examples include OpSite and Tegaderm.

- Biosynthetic dressings may be used to cover clean, superficial partial-thickness burns, meshed autografts, donor sites, and exudative wounds. An example is Biobrane. TransCyte is a human-fibroblast–derived temporary skin that can be used on middermal (partially damaged dermis) to indeterminate-depth partial-thickness burns, as well as middermal burns after debridement.

Nonbiologic dressings can be used on superficial and superficial partial-thickness burns to provide a moist wound-healing environment. Examples of nonbiologic dressings include Mepitel and Xeroform.

Negative pressure wound therapy, such as vacuum-assisted closure (VAC), provides negative-pressure wound therapy to promote wound healing. The VAC promotes the formation of granulation tissue, decreases wound size, removes exudate, and provides an environment for moist wound healing. This treatment device is typically used postdebridement; the goals are to reduce the wound size prior to grafting or to promote graft success by placing it on top of skin grafts. These dressings easily conform to the wound beds, facilitate removal of exudate, and expedite granulation.

Growth factor is another type of topical wound covering that can be used on burn injuries to stimulate healing. This is an area of great interest currently, but few studies have been conducted to determine its efficacy.

Nursing care related to temporary wound coverings includes the periodic application and removal of the dressing material. It is imperative that dressings and the surrounding tissues be inspected for dislodgment, suppuration, fluid accumulation, and cellulitis. Most of these complications can be prevented by stabilizing the temporary covering with gauze, keeping it dry, and preventing contamination and wound shearing. It is important to note that wounds are dynamic, and wound-management choices should be based on the state of the wound at a particular time. Wounds are evaluated at regular intervals and dressings changed accordingly.

Wound Closure   Superficial partial-thickness burns heal by spontaneous re-epithelialization within 7 to 10 days. Small full-thickness burns may be allowed to heal on their own by granulation tissue formation and contraction. Full-thickness burns are typically grafted for several reasons, including better cosmetic appearance, improved function, decreased risk of infection, and a faster return to a pre-injury lifestyle. A large TBSA or a deep partial-thickness burn is also grafted because healing usually takes more than 14 days, and without grafting, significant scarring usually occurs.

The early excision and closure of burn wounds have several advantages, including improved survival rates, reduction in incidences of infection, reduced in-hospital stays, decrease in amount of grafting required, improved cosmetic results, and better functional outcomes. Once the wound has been excised, steps are taken to close it. Small wounds are closed via primary wound closure. Larger wounds are closed via skin grafts, flaps, or skin substitutes.

When the skin is removed down to the subcutaneous layer for autografting, it is termed a *full-thickness skin graft* (Figure 36–9). Full-thickness skin grafts (0.64–0.76 mm thick) are used to cover areas that need the extra thickness and durability they provide, such as the palm of the hand, or to cover a point that will be exposed to pressure, such as the elbow or the scapula. When skin is removed for a full-thickness graft, the donor site becomes a full-thickness skin defect. This defect is closed by either suturing or using a split-thickness skin graft. Full-thickness grafting is used for small areas only.

Split-thickness skin grafts (0.2–0.3 mm thick) are not as thick as full-thickness grafts. The donor site is a partial-thickness skin defect that will heal within 10 to 14 days. A split-thickness skin graft can be used as a sheet graft or a meshed graft. Skin is harvested from a donor site using an instrument called a dermatome. The sheet graft is taken from the donor site and placed on the recipient wound (Figure 36–10). To make a meshed graft, the skin is taken

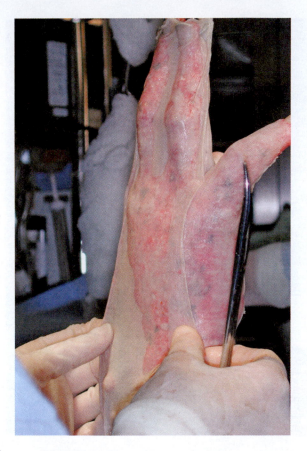

Figure 36–10 Sheet graft taken from donor site and placed on recipient's wound.

SOURCE: Pearson Education/PH College.

from the donor site and then expanded with a mesh dermatome (Figure 36–11). The mesh dermatome makes multiple small slits in the skin, giving it the appearance of netting. A meshed graft is expanded to cover a larger area; however, the wider the mesh is spread, the longer it takes the wound to close, increasing scar formation (Figure 36–12). Sheet grafts usually provide a better cosmetic appearance than meshed grafts. They are typically used on conspicuous sites such as the face and hands and provide the most optimal coverage for burns less than 40% TBSA.

Skin grafts are adhered to the recipient site with serum applied between the two layers. Soon a fibrin matrix forms, which better secures the donor graft to the recipient site. Within 48 hours, the wound takes on a pink or red color, indicating that graft vascularization has taken place.

Flaps are another choice for burn wound coverage. Flaps are typically chosen for full-thickness burns over tendons and subdermal burns where the wound either will not support skin graft coverage or would benefit from a thicker and more stable covering.

One product, Integra Dermal Regeneration Template, is a dermal replacement layer consisting of cross-linked bovine tendon collagen and chondroitin-6-sulfate covered with a silicone layer. Typically, Integra is applied to an excised full-thickness burn wound and provides a structure for a more organized neodermis to form (Figure 36–13). Approximately 2 to 3 weeks after placement, the silicone layer is removed and a thin epidermal autograft is placed.

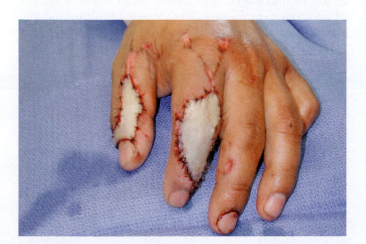

Figure 36–9 Full-thickness skin grafts on fingers.

SOURCE: Pearson Education/PH College.

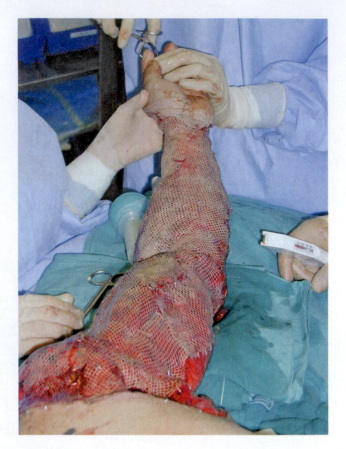

Figure 36–11 Placement of mesh graft on arm.

SOURCE: Pearson Education/PH College.

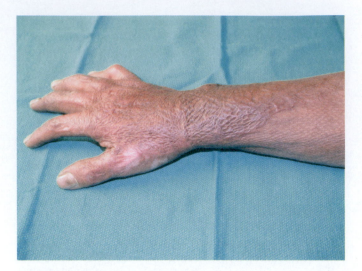

Figure 36–12 Mature mesh graft on hand.

SOURCE: Pearson Education/PH College.

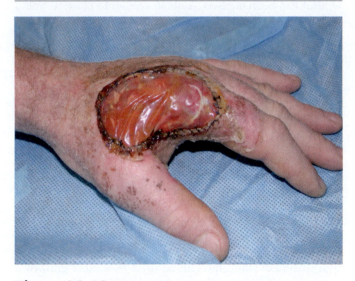

Figure 36–13 Integra artificial skin.

SOURCE: Pearson Education/PH College.

This product allows for early coverage of extensive full-thickness burns. Integra also has been used in conjunction with cultured skin substitutes. Further applications include burn wound reconstruction.

Nursing Considerations Nursing care of the burn wound includes monitoring for infection. Signs of noninvasive wound infection include reddened wound edges, generalized wound discoloration, change in the color of the wound exudate, foul-smelling exudate, loss of a healed skin graft, and an increase in wound pain. Signs of more severe invasive infection include conversion of a partial-thickness injury to a full-thickness injury, early separation of eschar, small necrotic subcutaneous vessels, tenderness

at the wound edges, and edema. Burn wounds are not always easy to evaluate, so surface wound culture and sensitivity tests are frequently performed. A burn wound biopsy is performed if an infection is suspected.

Section Six Review

1. When does the initial evaluation of burn wounds take place?
   A. Immediately on arrival
   B. At the end of the primary assessment
   C. At the end of the head-to-toe evaluation during the secondary assessment
   D. On admission to the burn center

2. The nurse is caring for a client with 60% TBSA burns in the emergency department. The client is to be transferred to a regional burn center within 20 minutes. What is the appropriate initial wound care management while awaiting transfer?
   A. Cleanse the wounds and cover the client with a dry sheet.
   B. Place Neosporin ointment on all open burn wounds.
   C. Put antibiotic cream on all wounds.
   D. Cleanse the wounds and leave them open to the air to dry out.

3. Which method of dead tissue removal harms newly formed tissue?

- **A.** Mechanical debridement
- **B.** Biodebridement
- **C.** Chemical debridement
- **D.** Wet-to-dry dressing debridement

4. Nursing care related to temporary wound coverings includes inspection for which primary factor?

- **A.** Dislodgement
- **B.** Permanent adherence
- **C.** Autograft integrity
- **D.** Scar formation

Answers: 1. C, 2. A, 3. D, 4. A

Section Seven: Acute Rehabilitative Phase— Psychosocial Needs and Physical Mobility

In addition to physical recovery, emotional recovery must also continue during the rehabilitative phase of burn injury. Furthermore, while the pain experienced in the acute rehabilitative phase may be different from pain experienced in the resuscitative phase, it remains an important care priority. Moreover, severe burn injury can cause severe physical mobility complications that must be attended to during the acute rehabilitative phase.

Psychosocial Needs

The ramifications of the injury eventually become apparent to the patient, and patient response is varied. The ability to cope with the injury depends in part on coping mechanisms the patient has learned in the past. These mechanisms may be healthy, or they may be dysfunctional. Problems most frequently experienced by burn patients include anxiety, fear, grief, depression, sleep problems, acute stress disorder, and aggressive or regressive behavior.

Personally meaningful rehabilitation and recovery from burn injuries can be greatly facilitated through the use of behavioral and image-enhancement strategies. Psychological and emotional problems can be minimized by involving the patient in self-care activities soon after the injury is sustained. To improve their self-concept, patients should participate in wound care, feeding, exercising, and administering medications as soon as they are physically and emotionally able. Fear and anxiety can be reduced with repeated and consistent explanations in understandable terms. Nurses play an important role in facilitating the involvement of family and friends in the recovery and rehabilitation of burn survivors. Visits by recovered burn patients allow patients to discuss their concerns with nonmedical personnel who can offer practical advice on coping with burns. Recovery can be facilitated by a long-term therapeutic relationship (Sheridan, 2014). This can be arranged by contacting a peer support group such as the national office of the Phoenix Society, a support group for burn survivors. Moderate depression can be expected in many patients and may be magnified if optimal recovery potential has not been reached because of inadequate therapy (Sheridan, 2014). Formal counseling and even medication may be needed in assisting treatment of depression.

Pain   During the acute rehabilitative phase, patients generally experience decreasing levels of pain. However, pain continues to occur as chronic or background pain and as procedural pain. Procedures, surgery, or infection delay the easement of pain. Interventions vary depending on the duration and severity of the pain.

Patients achieve better pain control when they are given opportunities to choose interventions that work best for them. As the patient stabilizes and pain levels decline, oral analgesics are used with greater frequency. Nonpharmacologic interventions for pain control include, but are not limited to, biofeedback, hypnosis, relaxation therapy, and guided imagery. Thorough pain assessments are conducted on a regular basis throughout the patient's recovery, and the plan of care is adjusted accordingly.

Physical Mobility

Physical mobility problems during the acute rehabilitative phase of burn care are directly related to the healing wound itself and to the therapeutic interventions necessary to maintain life and close the wound. During the resuscitative phase, excessive edema develops in the extremities and mobility is restricted by edema and pain. Later, this problem is compounded by the limitations placed on mobility to protect healing grafts from shearing. As the wound heals, mobility is restricted by burn scar formation and contraction and the patient's desire to assume a position of comfort, which is typically flexed. Therefore, the treatment goals related to physical mobility during the acute rehabilitative phase include the following:

- Returning to the pre-injury level of functioning
- Maintaining musculoskeletal, cardiopulmonary, and respiratory function
- Promoting wound healing
- Protecting healing skin grafts
- Preventing contractures and soft tissue deformity
- Preserving and strengthening extremity function
- Scar management
- Achieving maximum functional recovery
- Patient and family education

The physical therapist (PT), occupational therapist (OT), and nursing staff all have important roles in managing the patient's physical mobility issues. The OT and PT develop a treatment plan, fashion appliances, and perform daily treatments. The role of the nursing staff is to integrate the treatment plan into their delivery of care and to provide assessment feedback to the OT and PT. In addition, nurses play a pivotal role in gaining patient adherence because they have continuous contact with the patient and many opportunities to support the patient toward these rehabilitation goals.

Interventions Interventions to promote physical mobility during the acute phase of burn care employ many techniques and devices. Antideformity positioning begins at the time of admission unless contraindicated by a complicating condition. Its use is imperative during the acute phase because it reduces scar contracture across flexor surfaces that often compromises joint mobility and functional capacity.

Joint function is also preserved by active and passive range-of-motion exercises. The administration of analgesics prior to therapy may improve mobility outcomes and is discussed with the patient.

Early total body mobilization is important because of the beneficial impact of upright positioning on cardiopulmonary functioning. Patients are assisted out of bed and ambulated early in the acute phase after hemodynamic stabilization. To prevent venous stasis, it is important to apply compression wraps on the lower extremities before getting the patient out of bed. If extremities are not wrapped, the patient is at risk for capillary bed bleeding, which could cause autograft failure or delay donor-site healing. Venous pooling coupled with prolonged immobility also predisposes the patient to deep-vein thromboses. Wrapping the extremities continues until all wounds are healed and pressure garments are applied.

Section Seven Review

1. Which statement about pain associated with burn injury is true?
   A. Burn wounds are ischemic, so burn clients do not experience pain.
   B. Pain generally increases during the acute rehabilitative phase.
   C. Clients achieve better pain control when they can choose the interventions that work best for them.
   D. Nonpharmacologic interventions have been tried in burn clients, but without success.

2. Which treatment goals are related to physical mobility during the acute rehabilitative phase? (Select all that apply.)
   A. Return to pre-injury functioning
   B. Promotion of wound healing
   C. Scar management
   D. Walking independently
   E. Acknowledging that life will not be the same postburn

3. When should antideformity positioning begin?
   A. After skin grafting
   B. After the client can walk again
   C. At the time of admission
   D. On discharge from the high-acuity area

4. Which statements are correct regarding mobility after a burn injury? (Select all that apply.)
   A. During the acute resuscitative phase, clients have decreased mobility due to treatments to maintain life.
   B. During the resuscitative phase, edema is no longer an issue.
   C. Clients may be allowed limited mobility to protect healing grafts from shearing.
   D. As wounds heal, mobility may be restricted by scar formation.
   E. Clients often identify extension as their position of comfort.

Answers: 1. C, 2. (A, B, C), 3. C, 4. (A, C, D)

Section Eight: Overview of Long-term Rehabilitative Phase

Traditionally, the rehabilitative phase was thought to begin when all wounds were healed and continued throughout the patient's life span. From this paradigm it would seem that the rehabilitative phase would not fall into the realm of high-acuity nursing. However, it is important to recognize that preventive rehabilitative interventions actually begin during the resuscitative phase and directly involve high-acuity nurses.

Interventions related to physical conditioning, protection of new skin, scar management, and psychosocial adjustment during the long-term rehabilitative phase are crucial to the successful treatment of a critically burned patient.

Physical Conditioning Patients recovering from a severe burn injury are likely to have experienced prolonged bed rest and restricted physical activity for weeks or possibly months, which results in muscle atrophy, weakness, and activity intolerance. As the burn patient moves into the long-term rehabilitative phase, the body requires reconditioning to regain lost strength and mobility. A physical conditioning plan is developed, usually by a physical therapist, based on the individual needs of the patient. It may include activities to increase range of motion, muscle strength, functional mobility, and aerobic endurance. Physical conditioning begins in the burn unit but is mainly accomplished after discharge. Physical conditioning programs have no set parameters as a standard and are individualized. However, the benefits of such a program include a documented reduced number of surgeries needed for scar release, improved muscle strength, and muscle mass growth. The ultimate goal of burn rehabilitation is to assist in restoring functional capacity and independence among patients experiencing serious burn injuries (Diego et al., 2013).

Care of Healing Skin   Interventions related to the care of healing skin include protection of newly formed epithelium, scar management, and prevention of burn scar contractures. The epithelium over healing burn wounds is extremely fragile. Daily skin care includes cleansing with a mild soap and the generous application of a high-quality emollient. Patients are instructed to apply this emollient several times a day because their sebaceous glands have been destroyed in the burning and grafting process. The skin is also protected from mechanical traumas such as shearing and pressure. Finally, patients are instructed to protect their scar from sun exposure for 1 year or until the scar turns silvery white. The application of a sunscreen product with a sun protection factor of at least 15 (greater is better) is recommended for scars prior to sun or UV light exposure (Stoddard et al., 2014). Otherwise the scar will "tan" and remain permanently pigmented, leaving the patient with a less satisfactory cosmetic result.

Scar Management   Scar management is achieved by wearing compression garments (Figure 36–14). These garments are custom made and costly. The constant pressure from the garment assists in remodeling irregular collagen

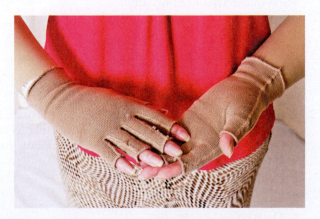

Figure 36–14 Hand compression garment. The patient may wear it for 6 months to 1 year postgraft.

SOURCE: Alistair Heap/Alamy Stock Photo

into a more parallel pattern to improve both function and appearance. Because hypertrophic scars are also hypervascular, pressure therapy may also help to reduce local blood supply, thereby improving the scar's appearance. Patient compliance is difficult to obtain because the garments are hot, difficult to put on, and require continuous wearing (except when bathing). Compression garments are worn until scars are mature, as evidenced by a flat, white, and avascular appearance, which is usually achieved in 12 to 18 months. Patients with burn wounds over a joint are at risk for future limited functional mobility. Preventive measures include compression garments, night splinting, silicone gel sheets to reduce scarring, serial splinting or casting, and range-of-motion exercises. Should a burn scar contracture and functional deficit occur, surgical intervention may be necessary to provide full mobility.

Psychosocial Adjustment   For the vast majority of burn survivors, social and psychological rehabilitation is profoundly more important than the recovery of physical functioning. Psychosocial adjustment is a major task of the rehabilitative phase. The physical and emotional consequences postburn differ widely and are dependent upon the individual's resilience, genetic and genomic risk, and time of life when the burns occur. Consequently, the younger the person is at the time of the burn, the longer the psychosocial impact of the burn as contrasted with the life cycle of an older patient (Stoddard et al., 2014). During this postburn recovery time, patients begin to renew their interests in the outside world, invest in their rehabilitation, and reintegrate their identities. Burn-unit nurses may witness some of these behaviors, but the majority of the behaviors occur after discharge. The burn team is challenged to find appropriate community resources for discharged patients as they adapt to postburn alterations in appearance, level of physical functioning, and role concept. For example, patients with facial burns may struggle with their altered body image and have difficulty resuming their preburn lifestyle. It may be helpful to refer these patients to a licensed esthetician familiar with scar therapy and camouflage makeup techniques. The Phoenix Society maintains a registry of these professionals and can assist with appropriate referrals.

A growing body of evidence suggests a high prevalence of psychological distress syndromes following burn injury, including posttraumatic stress disorder (PTSD) in burn patients of all ages (Bakker, Maertens, Van Son, & Van Loey, 2013; Sareen, 2014) and in their family members (Bronson, 2014). PTSD can occur after someone experiences a serious accident or a life-threatening event, and a critical burn injury can manifest as either of these descriptors (Anxiety and Depression Association of America, 2016). In children with burns, parental guilt is a pervasive factor in the parent–child relationship (Stoddard et al., 2014). Grief over loss is much different from a traumatic response to burn injury, and grief may require ongoing treatment and attention. It cannot be stressed enough that burn patients and significant others who are experiencing psychological distress symptoms should be referred to a mental health professional for treatment.

Section Eight Review

1. Rehabilitative interventions begin during which phase of burn care?
   A. Resuscitative
   B. Acute rehabilitative
   C. Long-term rehabilitative
   D. Transitional

2. Interventions during the rehabilitation phase are focused on which factor? (Select all that apply.)
   A. Physical conditioning
   B. Care of healing skin
   C. Support of psychosocial adjustment
   D. Transfer to rehabilitation centers
   E. Scar management

3. How do pressure garments improve immature scars?
   A. By thinning hypertrophic epithelium
   B. By remodeling irregular collagen
   C. By reducing skin friction
   D. By increasing arterial blood flow

4. Most burn survivors indicate which outcome as being their primary goal?
   A. Social rehabilitation
   B. Returning to their preburn physical condition
   C. Adaptation to severe pain
   D. Avoiding scarring from the burn

Answers: 1. A, 2. (A, B, C, E), 3. B, 4. A.

Clinical Reasoning Checkpoint

Sally P, a 65-year-old retired nurse, is found unresponsive in her apartment after a major fire in the building and is transported to the nearest hospital. Upon her arrival at the emergency department, the healthcare team assesses and documents burns to her anterior trunk, anterior lower limbs bilaterally, and left anterior arm.

1. The nurse determines the percentage of TBSA burn injury by using the rule of nines. Describe the appropriate calculation for Ms. P's injuries.

2. Using the Parkland formula, calculate Ms. P's fluid requirements for the first 24 hours based on her weight of 100 kg.

Clinical update: Further physical examination reveals new data. Ms. P's left arm is erythematous and has brisk capillary refill and blisters. Her anterior chest is dry, leathery, and white. Her lower extremities are pale and dry; there are no blisters, and capillary refill is absent.

3. Based on this description, identify the depth of burn of each of the following areas:
   • Left arm
   • Anterior chest
   • Lower extremities

4. Burn injuries to Ms. P's chest place her at risk for at least three postburn complications. What are they? What assessment findings would confirm the development of these complications?

5. Describe the wound care Ms. P should receive before she is transferred to a burn unit.

Chapter 36 Review

1. A nurse is developing educational materials on burn prevention. The nurse would discuss which reasons that older adults are prone to burn injury? (Select all that apply.)
   1. Older adults often have impaired senses.
   2. Older adults spend the majority of their time alone.
   3. As people age, their reaction times slow.
   4. Aging increases people's tendency toward risk-taking behaviors.
   5. Risk assessment skills decline with aging.

2. A client's burned arm is erythematous and blistered. Capillary refill is brisk, and the client complains of severe pain. How should the nurse document this burn?
   1. Full-thickness
   2. Superficial partial-thickness
   3. Deep partial-thickness
   4. First-degree

3. An emergency department uses the American Burn Association's criteria for transfer to a burn center. The nurse would anticipate that which client would require transfer?

   1. A client with superficial partial-thickness burns on 5% of TBSA
   2. A client with superficial burns on 50% of TBSA
   3. A client with deep partial-thickness burns over the entire face
   4. A client with deep partial-thickness burns on less than 5% of TBSA

4. A client has an inhalation injury. The nurse would prepare to assist with which tests specific to this injury?

   1. Electrocardiogram, thallium scan
   2. Arterial blood gases, bronchoscopy
   3. Serum potassium, serum sodium levels
   4. Pulmonary angiograms, hemoglobin level

5. Which assessment finding is most important for the nurse to monitor during initial fluid resuscitation of a seriously burned client?

   1. Hemoglobin
   2. Pain level
   3. Thirst
   4. Urine output

6. A client had an immediate hypermetabolic response to a severe burn and is now experiencing a hypermetabolic hyperdynamic state. Which assessment findings would the nurse anticipate? (Select all that apply.)

   1. Increased heart rate
   2. Decreased cardiac output
   3. Decreased temperature
   4. Increased respiratory rate
   5. Decreased serum glucose

7. The surgeon has planned tangential excision of eschar on a severely burned client. How would the nurse explain this procedure to the client's family? (Select all that apply.)

   1. "Your loved one is too unstable for the other option, which is fascial excision."

2. "This procedure can result in blood loss, so we may need to transfuse."
   3. "The cosmetic results of this procedure are better than those of the alternatives."
   4. "This procedure will be done under anesthesia in the operating room."
   5. "This is a form of biological debridement."

8. A severely burned client is in the resuscitative phase of burn care. How can the nurse help to minimize psychological and emotional problems in this client?

   1. Involve the client in self-care activities as soon as medically feasible.
   2. Keep the client sedated as long as possible while healing continues.
   3. Shelter the client from any negative interactions about the future.
   4. Do not allow mirrors on the burn unit.

9. The nurse is working with a physical therapist and an occupational therapist to promote antideformity positioning in a burned client. What criterion should the positions meet?

   1. The position should be comfortable for the client.
   2. The position should maintain joint extension.
   3. The position should allow for maximum joint flexion.
   4. The position should be easily altered by the client.

10. The nurse teaches a client to apply an emollient to healing burn wounds several times a day. Which rationale should the nurse offer for this instruction? (Select all that apply.)

    1. "This will help keep your skin moist."
    2. "You do not have as many sebaceous glands as you did before the injury."
    3. "If you use this lotion, you will not need soap, which can be drying."
    4. "Emollients will protect your skin from shearing pressures while you are in bed."
    5. "This lotion will protect your skin from the sun."

Answers to questions found inside your textbook are available on the faculty resources site. Please consult with your instructor.

References

American Burn Association (ABA). (2007). Guidelines for the operation of burn centers. *Journal of Burn Care & Research, 28*(1), 134–141.

American Burn Association (ABA). (2016). *Burn incidence and treatment in the United States: 2016 fact sheet.* Retrieved June 23, 2016, from http://www.ameriburn .org/resources_factsheet.php

American Burn Association. (2017). *Burn Center Verification Review Program.* Retrieved February 16, 2017, from http://www.ameriburn.org/Verification /CriterionDeficiencies.pdf

Anxiety and Depression Association of America. (2016). *Posttraumatic stress disorder (PTSD).* Retrieved July 1, 2016, from http://www.adaa.org/understanding -anxiety/posttraumatic-stress-disorder-ptsd

Bakker, A., Maertens, K. J. P., Van Son, M. J. M., & Van Loey, N. E. E. (2013). Psychological consequences of pediatric burns from a child and family perspective: A review of the empirical literature. *Clinical Psychology Review, 33*(3), 361–371.

Bronson, M. (2014). *Psychological and emotional impact of a burn injury.* Phoenix Society. Retrieved June 12, 2017, from https://www.phoenix-society.org /resources/entry/psychological-and-emotional-impact

Centers for Disease Control and Prevention (CDC). (2014). *Web–based Injury Statistics Query and Reporting System (WISQARS)* [online]. Retrieved June 17, 2016, from http://www.cdc.gov/injury/wisqars

Cochran, A. (2015). Nutritional demands and enteral formulas for moderate to severe burn patients. *UpToDate.* Retrieved June 30, 2016, from https://www .uptodate.com/contents/nutritional-demands-and -enteral-formulas-for-moderate-to-severe-burn -patients?source=see_link

Cox, R. D. (2015). Chemical burns. *Medscape.* Retrieved June 20, 2016, from http://emedicine.medscape.com /article/769336-overview#a6

Cushing, T. A. (2016). Electrical injuries in emergency medicine. *Medscape.* Retrieved April 20, 2017, from http://emedicine.medscape.com/article/770179 -overview#a6

Diego, A. M., Serghiou, M., Padmanabha, A., Porro, L. J., Herndon, D. N., & Suman, O. E. (2013). Exercise training following burn injury: A survey of practice. *Journal of Burn Care and Research, 34*(6). doi:10.1097 /BCR.0b013e3182839ae9

Emara, S. S., & Alzaylai, A. A. (2013). Renal failure in burn patients: A review. *Annals of Burns and Fire Disasters.* Retrieved June 30, 2016, from http://www.medbc .com/meditline/articles/vol_38/num_1/text /vol38n1p821.pdf

Evans, J. (2016). Burns. In R. A. Bryant & D. P. Nix, *Acute & chronic wounds: Current management concepts* (5th ed., pp. 446–460). St. Louis, MO: Elsevier.

Fonseca, J. A. (2016). Burn wound infections clinical presentation. *Medscape.* Retrieved July 1, 2016, from http://emedicine.medscape.com/article/213595-clinical

Gauglitz, G. G. (2014). Hypermetabolic response to severe burn injury: Recognition and treatment. *UpToDate.* Retrieved June 28, 2016, from https://www.uptodate .com/contents/hypermetabolic-response-to -severe-burn-injury-recognition-and-treatment

Ibrahim, A. E., Sarhane, K. A., Fagan, S. P., & Goverman, J. (2013). Renal dysfunction in burns: A review. *Annals of Burns and Fire Disasters, 26*(1), 16–25. PMCID: PMC3741002

Jeschke, M. G., Pinto, R., Kraft, R., Nathens, A. B., Finerty, C. C., Gamelli, R. L., . . . Herndon, D. N. (2015). Morbidity and survival probability in burn patients in modern burn care. *Critical Care Medicine, 43*(4), 808–815. doi:10.1097/CCM.0000000000000790

Kasten, K. R., Makley, A. T., & Kagan, R. J. (2011). Update on the critical care management of severe burns. *Journal of Intensive Care Medicine, 26*(4), 223–236.

Kim, Y. S. (2015). *Post-burn pruritis relief protocol.* (Unpublished doctoral thesis). California State University, Fullerton, California. Retrieved July 1, 2016, from http://nursing.fullerton.edu/programs/pdf /dnp/finalprojects/2015/Kim_YeonSook_DNP_Final _Project_2015.pdf

Latenser, B. A. (2009). Critical care of the burn patient: The first 48 hours. *Critical Care Medicine, 37*(10), 2819–2826.

Li, H., Guo, Y., Yang, Z., Roy, M., & Guo, Q. (2016). The efficacy and safety of oxandrolone treatment for patients with severe burns: A systematic review and meta-analysis. *Burns, 42*(4), 717–727. http://dx.doi .org/10.1016/j.burns.2015.08.023

Marques, E., Pereira, G. A., Neto, B. F. M., Freitas, R. A., Yaegashi, L. B., Almeida, C. E. F., & Farina, J. A. (2014). Visceral injury in electrical shock trauma: Proposed guideline for the management of abdominal electrocution and literature review. *International Journal of Burns and Trauma, 4*(1), 1–6. PMCID: PMC3945822

Mechem, C. C. (2017). Frostbite. *Medscape.* Accessed April 26, 2017 from http://emedicine.medscape.com /article/926249-overview#a0104

Nicol, N. H., & Huether, S. E. (2012). Structure, function, and disorders of the integument. In K. L. McCance & S. E. Huether, *Understanding pathophysiology* (5th ed., pp. 1038–1069). St. Louis, MO: Elsevier.

National Pressure Ulcer Advisory Panel (NPUAP), European Pressure Ulcer Advisory Panel (EPUAP), & Pan Pacific Pressure Injury Alliance (PPPIA). (2014). *Prevention and treatment of pressure ulcers: Quick reference guide.* E. Haesler (Ed.), Cambridge Media: Osborne Park, Western Australia. Retrieved June 10, 2017, from http://www.npuap.org/wp-content/uploads/2014 /08/Updated-10-16-14-Quick-Reference-Guide -DIGITAL-NPUAP-EPUAP-PPPIA-16Oct2014.pdf

Park, E., Oh, H., & Kim, T. (2013). The effects of relaxation breathing on procedural pain and anxiety during burn care. *Burns, 39*(6), 1101–1106.

Rice, P. L., & Orgill, D. P. (2015). Emergency care of moderate and severe thermal burns in adults. *UpToDate.* Retrieved June 30, 2016, from http://www .uptodate.com/contents/emergency-care-of-moderate -and-severe-thermal-burns-in-adults

Rowan, M. P., Leopoldo, C. C., Elster, E. A., Burmeister, D. M., Rose, L. F., Shanmugasundaram, N., . . . Chung, K. K. (2015). Burn wound healing and treatment: Review and advancements. *Critical Care, 19*(243). doi:10.1186/s13054-015-0961-2

Sareen, J. (2014). Posttraumatic stress disorder in adults: Impact, comorbidity, risk factors, and treatment. *Canadian Journal of Psychiatry, 59*(9), 460–467.

Sen, S., Johnston, C., Greenhalgh, D., & Palmieri, T. (2016). Ventilator-associated pneumonia prevention bundle significantly reduces the risk of ventilator-associated pneumonia in critically ill burn patients. *Journal of Burn Care & Research, 37*(3), 143–195.

Sheridan, R. L. (2014). Burn rehabilitation. *Medscape.* Retrieved June 29, 2016, from http://emedicine .medscape.com/article/318436-overview

Snell, J. A., Loh, N., Mahambrey, T., & Shokrollahi, K. (2013). Clinical review: The critical care management of the burn patient. *Critical Care, 17*(241). doi:10.1186/ cc12706

Stoddard, F. J., Ryan, C. M., & Schneider, J. C. (2014). Physical and psychiatric recovery from burns. *Surgical Clinics of North America, 94,* 863–878. http://dx.doi .org/10.1016/j.suc.2014.05.007

U.S. Fire Administration (USFA). (2016). *U.S. fire statistics.* Retrieved June 17, 2016, from https://www.usfa.fema .gov/data/statistics

Walker, P. F., Buehner, M. F., Wood, L. A., Boyer, N. L., Driscoll, I. A., Lundy, J. B . . . Chung, K. K. (2015). Diagnosis and management of inhalation injury: An updated review. *Critical Care, 19*(351). doi:10.1186 /s13054-015-1077-4

Weijs, P. J. M., Cynober, L., DeLegge, M., Kreymann, G., Wernerman, J., & Wolfe, R. R. (2014). Proteins and amino acids are fundamental to optimal nutrition support in critically ill patients. *Critical Care, 18,* 591. doi:10.1186/s13054-014-0591-0

Wiechman, S., Jeschke, M. G., & Collins, K. A. (2015). Burn pain: Principles of pharmacologic and nonpharmacologic management. *UpToDate.* Retrieved June 22, 2017, from https://www.uptodate.com/contents/burn-pain- principles-of-pharmacologic-and-nonpharmacologic- management?source=search_result&search =burn%20pain%20principles&selectedTitle=1~150

Wiechman, S., Sharar, S., Jeschke, M. G., & Collins, K. A. (2017). Paradigm-based treatment approaches for burn pain control. *UpToDate.* Retrieved June 22, 2017, from https://www.uptodate.com/contents/paradigm -based-treatment-approaches-for-burn-pain -control?source=search_result&search=burn%20pain &selectedTitle=2~150

Wysocki, A. (2016). Anatomy & physiology of skin and soft tissue. In R. A. Bryant & D. P. Nix, *Acute & chronic wounds: Current management concepts* (5th ed., 45–62). St. Louis, MO: Elsevier.

Chapter 37
Shock States

Learning Outcomes

37.1 Discuss the general concepts associated with shock states, including physiologic response to shock and shock progression.

37.2 Assess a patient who may be experiencing signs of shock.

37.3 Demonstrate competency in collaborative management of the patient experiencing shock based on interventions that optimize oxygen delivery and reduce oxygen consumption.

37.4 Discuss the use of pharmacotherapy in the management of shock states.

37.5 Describe cardiogenic shock, including pathophysiology, clinical manifestations, diagnosis, and management.

37.6 Discuss hypovolemic shock, including pathophysiology, clinical manifestations, diagnosis, and management.

37.7 Explain the septic type of distributive shock, including pathophysiology, clinical manifestations, diagnosis, and management.

37.8 Discuss the neurologic and anaphylactic types of distributive shock, including the pathophysiology, clinical manifestations, diagnosis, and management of each type.

37.9 Describe the major causes of obstructive shock, including the pathophysiology, clinical manifestations, diagnosis, and management of each cause.

To understand shock states, it is important to first have a basic understanding of oxygen delivery and oxygen consumption. It is therefore recommended that Chapter 34: Determinants and Assessment of Oxygenation be read prior to beginning this one.

The major function of the cardiovascular system is to deliver blood, oxygen, and nutrients to the cells, tissues, and organs of the body and to remove metabolic wastes. When this fails to occur, a state of shock develops. However, defining shock is more complex than defining other disease entities. It is difficult to agree on one concise definition because **shock** is a syndrome, a complex presentation of signs and symptoms that describe a sequence of changes that occur when tissue oxygen supply does not meet oxygen demand. In this chapter, the relationship between oxygen supply and oxygen demand (consumption) serves as the conceptual framework for shock. The chapter first presents global concepts common to all forms of shock and then provides an overview of each of the four shock states, including unique clinical findings and management.

Section One: Introduction to Shock States

A characteristic of shock states is circulatory insufficiency (failure) that causes an imbalance between tissue oxygen supply (availability for delivery) and demand (consumption). An imbalance between oxygen supply and demand results in inadequate oxygen delivery to meet cellular oxygen demands, which can cause end-organ injury. Shock is circulatory failure whereby oxygen transport to and uptake by tissues is impaired. This type of circulatory collapse can result from four conditions:

- Reduced intravascular volume
- Failure of the cardiac pump
- Obstruction in the circulatory system
- Maldistribution of the peripheral circulation (Edul, Ince & Dubin, 2016)

Table 37–1 Types of Shock

Type	Underlying Dysfunction	Associated Disorders
Cardiogenic	Heart fails to function as a pump	Acute myocardial infarction, severe heart failure
Hypovolemic	Inadequate circulating volume	Hemorrhage, severe dehydration
Distributive (subtypes: septic, neurogenic, anaphylactic)	Relative hypovolemia; impaired blood flow distribution and excessive vasodilation (low peripheral vascular resistance)	Sepsis (most common cause), systemic inflammatory response syndrome (SIRS), toxic shock syndrome (TSS), systemic anaphylaxis, spinal cord injury
Obstructive	Mechanical obstruction to blood flow into or out of the heart	Pulmonary embolism, tension pneumothorax, cardiac tamponade, mitral or aortic stenosis

Regardless of the underlying cause, all forms of shock are characterized by decreased tissue perfusion and microvascular dysfunction (De Backer, Orbegozo, Donadello, & Vincent, 2014; Tachon et al., 2014; Zuckerbraun, Peitzman, & Billiar, 2015). Shock states can be conceptualized by etiology, underlying pathophysiologic mechanisms, or functional alterations. For the purposes of this chapter, shock is classified into four categories: cardiogenic, hypovolemic, distributive, and obstructive (Table 37–1).

Physiologic Response to Shock

Shock occurs when oxygen delivery does not support tissue oxygen demands. In an attempt to stabilize this life-threatening imbalance, a pattern of responses, or compensatory mechanisms, is set in motion.

Compensation in Shock   In response to the development of shock, the body triggers a series of complex neuro-endocrine responses to overcome ineffective circulating blood volume. Low-pressure stretch receptors in the right atrium sense a decrease in circulating blood volume when there is a decrease in venous return to the right atrium. Baroreceptors in the aorta and carotid arteries sense a decrease in blood volume and cardiac output (CO). Carotid body chemoreceptors sense alterations in pH and partial pressure of arterial carbon dioxide ($PaCO_2$). The baroreceptors and chemoreceptors alert the hypothalamus to activate the sympathetic nervous system's fight-or-flight response. This system releases a massive amount of norepinephrine, epinephrine, and cortisol, which initiates several compensatory mechanisms (Table 37–2). The beneficial effects of these mechanisms are an increase in venous return, an increase in CO, and an increase in O_2 delivery.

In response to the shock state, the endocrine system is activated in ways to increase oxygen delivery by increasing blood volume during stress (Figure 37–1). The hypothalamus releases corticotropin-releasing hormone (CRH). The anterior hypothalamus releases adrenocorticotropic hormone (ACTH) in response to CRH. ACTH stimulates secretion of glucocorticoids such as cortisol from the adrenal cortex. Cortisol release is protective during stress. Increased cortisol levels cause insulin resistance, thus triggering

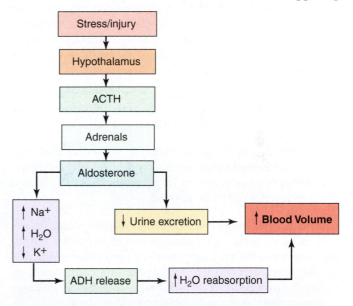

Figure 37–1 ACTH, aldosterone, and ADH release.

Table 37–2 Sympathetic Nervous System's Fight-or-Flight-Response

Physiologic Response	Physiologic Rationale
Increased heart rate	To deliver needed oxygen rapidly
Increased respiratory rate	To increase tidal volume, thereby increasing available oxygen
Increased glycolysis, gluconeogenesis, mobilization of free fatty acids	To increase availability of glucose for energy
Decreased urine output	To conserve fluid volume; to return more blood volume to cardiovascular system to increase volume and blood pressure
Decreased blood flow to internal organs (e.g., kidneys, gastrointestinal tract, liver)	To allow more blood flow to more vital organs (e.g., heart and lungs)
Decreased intestinal peristalsis	To shunt blood to vital organs; no need for digestion as body energy is redirected to lifesaving measures
Cool skin	To produce (by alpha receptors) peripheral vasoconstriction to shunt blood to more vital organs
Diaphoresis	To release heat as a by-product of metabolism

hepatic glycogenolysis, resulting in increased serum glucose availability for energy. Cortisol works with growth hormone (GH) to increase protein catabolism for energy and tissue building and alters carbohydrate, fat, and protein metabolism so that energy is immediately available for use by vital organs during shock states. Along with aldosterone and antidiuretic hormone (ADH), cortisol release increases serum sodium by causing water retention and increased movement of extravascular water into the intravascular space to support circulating blood volume during shock states.

Cardiac output (CO) must be augmented in shock to ensure adequate tissue perfusion. CO increases in response to increased venous return; therefore, to increase venous return, sodium and water are retained by aldosterone and ADH. In addition, another mechanism, the renin–angiotensin–aldosterone system (RAAS), is activated to increase blood volume and venous return (Figure 37–2). As a result of reduced blood flow to the kidneys, the juxtaglomerular (JG) cells in the kidneys excrete renin. Renin catalyzes angiotensinogen in the liver, which then converts to angiotensin I in the circulation. Once in the lungs, angiotensin I converts to angiotensin II, which is a potent vasoconstrictor. The vasoconstriction produced by angiotensin II increases blood pressure by increasing afterload. Angiotensin II stimulates the release of aldosterone. The net effects of these hormonal mechanisms are increased blood pressure through vasoconstriction, increased venous return through retention of sodium and water, and decreased urine output.

Progression of Shock There are four stages of shock: initial, compensatory, progressive, and refractory. These stages are common to all classifications of shock.

Initial Stage. In the initial stage, decreased cardiac output and decreased tissue perfusion occur. Decreased oxygen delivery to cells results in anaerobic metabolism and the development of lactic acidosis.

Compensatory Stage. In the compensatory stage, neuroendocrine responses are activated to restore cardiac output and oxygen delivery. Compensatory mechanisms function to restore oxygen delivery by augmenting cardiac output, redistributing blood flow, and restoring blood volume. Compensatory signs and symptoms are evident.

Progressive Stage. When compensatory mechanisms cannot restore homeostasis and if prompt and proper treatment has not been instituted, shock enters the third stage. Progressive shock results in the major dysfunction of many organs. The continued low blood flow, poor tissue perfusion, inadequate oxygen delivery, and buildup of metabolic wastes over time lead to multiple organ dysfunction syndrome (MODS).

Refractory Stage. The final stage of shock is the refractory stage, in which the shock state is so profound and cell destruction is so severe that death is inevitable. The organs of the body become refractory, or resistant, to conventional therapy. Profound hypotension develops despite the administration of potent vasoactive drugs. The patient remains hypoxemic despite high levels of oxygen therapy. A state of intractable circulatory failure leads to total body failure and death.

Not every patient progresses through all four stages, and often the progression from one stage to the next is not obvious. If the shock state is assessed early and appropriate treatment is instituted, the progression is reversed, the O_2 supply-and-demand balance is restored, and the patient recovers.

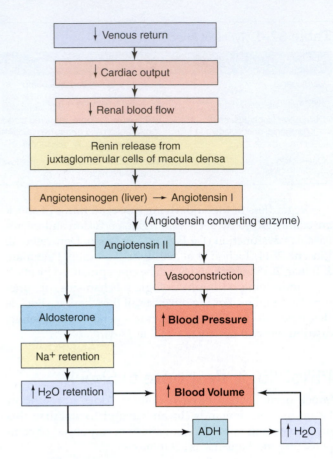

Figure 37–2 Renin–angiotensin–aldosterone system.

Section One Review

1. All forms of shock have which characteristic in common?
   A. Inadequate circulating fluid levels
   B. Loss of sympathetic nervous system innervation
   C. Tissue oxygen supply in excess of oxygen demand
   D. Imbalance between tissue oxygen supply and oxygen demand

2. When shock develops, the body attempts to meet the crisis through which mechanism?
   A. Releasing cortisol, norepinephrine, and epinephrine
   B. Activating the parasympathetic nervous system
   C. Decreasing venous return to the right heart
   D. Inhibiting the release of aldosterone

3. Angiotensin II plays an important role in increasing blood pressure through which action?
   A. Decreasing afterload
   B. Blocking aldosterone release
   C. Vasoconstriction
   D. Stimulating secretion of renin

4. How is the compensatory stage of shock best characterized?
   A. Anaerobic metabolism and lactic acidosis begin.
   B. Neuroendocrine responses are activated.
   C. Organ function becomes compromised.
   D. The client becomes resistant to treatment.

Answers: 1. D, 2. A, 3. C, 4. B

Section Two: Assessment of Shock States

Clinical manifestations of all shock states are the result of inadequate oxygen delivery and the activation of compensatory mechanisms. Shock affects essentially all body systems. Objective data such as pH, serum lactate level, and base excess more accurately reflect tissue oxygenation than do more traditional but less sensitive parameters such as blood pressure and level of consciousness. Thus they are important to obtain and evaluate when a shock state is suspected. It is important for the nurse and other providers to monitor the trends of these values to assess whether the shock state is improving or worsening.

Traditional Parameters

Traditional assessment parameters such as appearance (e.g., cold, clammy skin and cyanosis), vital signs (e.g., low blood pressure; rapid, weak pulse; and rapid breathing), level of consciousness (e.g., confusion or unconsciousness), and low urine output provide supportive data. However, they are inadequate to accurately assess shock states. The absence of the traditional presentation does not exclude the presence of shock, as different types of shock are characterized by varying clinical presentations. The traditional parameters often underestimate the degree of oxygen debt or imbalance between oxygen supply and demand at the cellular or tissue level.

For example, the significance of a patient's blood pressure is hard to evaluate because it is so individualized. A blood pressure of 90/60 mmHg may be normotensive for one patient but hypotensive for another patient. There are many factors that precipitate tachycardia, including anxiety, pain, dysrhythmia, and fever. Mentation may be hard to assess because of the presence of brain injury, alcohol, drugs, or chronic diseases (e.g., Alzheimer). Adequacy of urine output (UO) can be difficult to determine because UO is influenced by many factors, such as the neuro-endocrine response to shock, hyperglycemia, or diabetes insipidus.

Objective Parameters of Shock

Each type of shock has certain unique physiologic characteristics that help the practitioner differentiate one type from the other. There are a growing number of direct and indirect measures of tissue perfusion and oxygenation that more accurately reflect the patient's physiologic status in all types of shock. This section provides a brief overview of some of the major parameters that are monitored to assess the status of the patient experiencing shock.

Arterial pH The pH is a measure of hydrogen ions that determines the acid or alkaline state of the arterial blood. It is one of the standard values provided by the arterial blood gas (ABG). Analysis of the ABG indicates whether the acidosis is respiratory or metabolic or both. In adults, the normal pH range is 7.35 to 7.45; a value of less than 7.35 is acidosis, and a value greater than 7.45 is alkalosis (Kee, 2014). While pH is important to establish, it does not provide sufficient information to determine the underlying cause because the acidosis can develop as a respiratory problem or a metabolic problem. Therefore, it is important to consider other supportive data when investigating the etiology of an acidotic pH. When a shock state is suspected, two other important parameters to be evaluated in addition to the pH are the serum lactate and base excess or base deficit measures. Chapter 11 contains an in-depth discussion of pH.

Serum Lactate Normal serum lactate levels are less than 2 mmol/L (Kee, 2014). A diagnosis known as lactic acidosis is confirmed with a plasma lactate of 5 mmol/L or higher with an arterial pH of less than 7.35 (Kee, 2014). Lactate, or lactic acid, is the metabolic by-product of pyruvate, which is formed as a result of anaerobic metabolism. Lactic acidosis can be divided into two types based on etiology. Type A lactic acidosis arises from impaired tissue oxygenation (e.g., shock states, respiratory failure, or ischemic bowel); type B occurs with normal tissue oxygenation but in the presence of elevated metabolic acids (e.g., diabetic ketoacidosis [DKA], severe alcoholism, salicylate toxicity, or metformin toxicity) (Sabatine, 2014).

Serum lactate levels can be used as an indirect measure of impaired oxygenation and shock (type A lactic acidosis). In the presence of shock, oxygen delivery is insufficient to meet cellular oxygen demand, which results in anaerobic metabolism when compensatory mechanisms fail. The level of lactate increase reflects the degree of hypoperfusion; a level greater than 5 mEq/L is considered critical (panic level) (Kee, 2014). Because lactic acidosis can develop in the presence of normal tissue oxygenation, elevated lactate levels should be evaluated within the broader context of the patient's clinical presentation.

Base Excess and Base Deficit Base excess or base deficit is the amount of base required to titrate 1 liter of arterial blood to a normal pH of 7.40 (Zuckerbraun et al., 2015). It reflects metabolic acid–base status based on the amount of buffer present, particularly bicarbonate (HCO_3). The base excess or base deficit value is obtained from an arterial blood gas, where it is usually identified as *base excess* or *BE*. Base excess or base deficit exists as a continuum that normally ranges from a base excess of +2 mmol to a base deficit of −2 mmol/L (Kee, 2014). In shock states, a base deficit develops from the buildup of lactic acidosis resulting from impaired tissue oxygenation. Base deficit is classified as mild (−3 to −5 mmol/L), moderate (−6 to −9 mmol/L), or severe (−10 mmol/L or greater) (Zuckerbraun et al., 2015). Ongoing or worsening base deficit may indicate the need for further evaluation for an ongoing shock state.

Venous Oxygen Saturation

Venous oxygen saturation (SvO_2) indirectly measures the amount of oxygen uploaded into the tissues before the venous blood returns to the lungs for reoxygenation. It provides information on the balance between oxygen supply and demand. Normally, when oxygen supply and demand are in balance, hemoglobin is about 60% to 80% saturated (average is 70%) after leaving the tissues. An abnormally low SvO_2 suggests a problem with O_2 delivery or increased demand (i.e., supply is not meeting demand).

The two major measurements of SvO_2 are mixed venous oxygen saturation ($SmvO_2$) and central venous oxygen saturation ($ScvO_2$). Measuring $SmvO_2$ requires an invasive pulmonary artery (PA) catheter, while $ScvO_2$, a newer, less invasive technology, requires only a centrally located venous access rather than a PA catheter. Detailed information on SvO_2 can be found in Chapter 34.

Emerging Technologies

During a shock episode, circulation becomes compromised, causing end organ hypoperfusion. There can be regional microcirculation hypoperfusion even after systemic hemodynamic parameters have returned to normal (De Backer et al., 2014; Edul et al., 2016; Tachon et al., 2014). A successful surveillance of the microcirculation in the individual patient may guide diagnostic and treatment strategies in order to optimize organ perfusion and oxygenation, subsequently leading to an individualized therapy (De Backer & Durand, 2014; Jung & Kelm, 2015). Noninvasive technologies to assess shock include gastric tonometry, near-infrared spectroscopy, Doppler ultrasonography, pulse contour analysis, and impedance cardiography (Ince, 2014).

Gastric Tonometry

Gastric tonometry is a minimally invasive technology that is used to estimate gastric tissue perfusion. A special nasogastric tube is inserted into the stomach that samples the gastric mucosa carbon dioxide (CO_2) level and provides a tissue partial pressure of CO_2 ($PtCO_2$) reading. Using $PtCO_2$ values, intestinal mucosal pH (called pHi) is calculated (normal pHi = greater than 7.3). The use of gastric tonometry as a prognostic indicator of regional tissue perfusion is based on the assumption that pHi values will drop below 7.3 as gastric tissue perfusion worsens, causing gastric CO_2 to accumulate. Moreover, the $PtCO_2$ (gastric CO_2) and $PaCO_2$ (partial pressure of dissolved carbon dioxide in the plasma of arterial blood) can be compared because there is a normal gap between the two values; a gap greater than 15 mmHg is associated with increased mortality. Gastric tonometry has been critiqued as being partially based on assumptions of questionable

validity, and the use of pHi as an endpoint in resuscitation remains controversial (Zuckerbraun et al., 2015).

Near-infrared Spectroscopy

Near-infrared spectroscopy (NIRS) is a noninvasive technology that measures regional tissue microoxygenation, through the use of multiple light wavelengths through tissue (Orbegozo, Puflea, De Backer, Creteur, & Vincent, 2015). The technology is similar to that of pulse oximetry; however, pulse oximetry reads pulsatile blood flow to measure arterial oxyhemoglobin, whereas NIRS measures the differences between oxyhemoglobin (oxygen-saturated hemoglobin) and deoxyhemoglobin (oxygen-poor hemoglobin) to measure the uptake of oxygen in the tissue beds, providing a measurement of regional tissue oxygen saturation, referred to as rSO_2 or StO_2 (tissue oxygen saturation) (Orbegozo et al., 2015). NIRS measurements in the assessment of tissue status in critically ill neonates has been shown to provide useful information regarding peripheral circulation and microoxygenation and is thus a promising tool (Holler et al., 2015). Currently, the accuracy and effectiveness of NIRS in the assessment of regional tissue perfusion status in adult patients during shock continues to be examined. Further studies are needed to help ascertain if there is clinical significance in the use of StO_2 in the setting of shock.

Doppler Ultrasonography

Doppler ultrasound is a technique used at the bedside for a goal-directed rapid assessment and continuous monitoring of the high-acuity patient. This is a test that bounces high-frequency ultrasonic sound waves off moving erythrocytes in the bloodstream (Alarcon & Fink, 2014). This method is used on high-acuity patients to study diagnostic indicators of shock, such as cardiac function, via the examination of right and left ventricle diameter and inferior vena cava diameter and collapsibility. Two different approaches can be used in Doppler ultrasound. The first method is transthoracic and is therefore noninvasive and uses an ultrasound transducer that is placed on the suprasternal notch in order to examine the aortic root. This approach requires a highly skilled clinician in order to obtain relevant results (Alarcon & Fink, 2014). Conversely, the second approach with the Doppler ultrasound is transesophageal, thus more invasive; however, it seems to be more promising. With the transesophageal approach, a continuous-wave Doppler is placed into the esophagus. The probe is connected to a monitor that displays continuous blood flow velocities in the aorta (Alarcon & Fink, 2014). Nevertheless, research suggests that rapid goal-directed transthoracic ultrasonography may be an excellent noninvasive diagnostic method to evaluate the etiology of shock status at the bedside when conducted by a well-trained clinician (Volpicelli et al., 2013).

Pulse Contour Analysis

Pulse contour analysis is an approach for determining cardiac output with an estimation of stroke volume on a beat-to-beat basis (Hollenberg, 2013). This method uses an arterial waveform as a model of the systemic circulation in order to determine the flow of the circulatory system throughout the cardiac cycle. Pulse contour monitoring is much less invasive and is comparable to the pulmonary artery catheter thermodilution techniques (Alarcon & Fink, 2014). Despite its current and more widespread use in the high-acuity setting, further studies supporting the clinical accuracy of pulse contour monitoring need to be conducted (Pinsky, 2014).

Impedance Cardiography Bioimpedance cardiography is a noninvasive technology that measures the flow of transthoracic electrical conductivity and its changes in time. This technique estimates cardiac output (CO) using conversions to stroke volume via mathematical algorithms (Hollenberg, 2013). Despite its attractive noninvasive quality and minimal need for training, the measurements obtained from bioimpedance are not completely reliable and, in fact, may have weak correlation with thermodilution (Alarcon & Fink, 2014).

Section Two Review

1. Which two underlying shock-related factors cause the majority of clinical manifestations associated with shock?
   A. Fluid deficiencies and electrolyte imbalances
   B. Activation of compensatory mechanisms and inadequate oxygen delivery
   C. Impaired alveolar oxygenation and increased cardiac output
   D. Loss of organ function and decreased oxygen carrying capacity of the blood

2. Which statement best describes the use of traditional parameters (e.g., blood pressure, heart rate, and appearance) to assess a client for the presence of shock?
   A. They accurately reflect a shock state.
   B. They are of little use in the assessment of shock states.
   C. They provide supportive data but cannot be relied on.
   D. They can be used for diagnosis of some shock states but not others.

3. In the assessment of shock, arterial pH can be measured in conjunction with which two parameters to evaluate the client's acid–base status?
   A. Serum lactate and base excess/deficit
   B. Pulse oximetry and blood pressure
   C. Gastric tonometry and gastric pH
   D. Venous oxygen saturation and pulmonary artery wedge pressure

4. A client's lactate level is 5.3 mmol/L. What would this value indicate to the nurse?
   A. The client's arterial pH is likely to be alkalotic.
   B. The client is receiving oxygen therapy at too high a concentration.
   C. The client is likely to be experiencing tissue hyperperfusion.
   D. The client is experiencing significant anaerobic metabolism.

Answers: 1. B, 2. C, 3. A, 4. D

Section Three: General Management of Shock States

Each type of shock has certain specific treatment strategies, and interventions to optimize oxygen delivery and minimize oxygen consumption are implemented for all patients in shock. This section provides a brief overview of general shock management based on two major therapeutic goals: optimizing oxygen delivery and reducing oxygen consumption. Interventions that are specific to each type of shock are presented in their respective sections later in this chapter. Vasoactive drugs used in the treatment of shock are presented in Section Four.

Interventions to Optimize Oxygen Delivery

Shock of any type involves an imbalance between tissue oxygen supply and oxygen demand (consumption). To optimize oxygen delivery, the patient may require supplemental oxygen and/or fluid resuscitation.

Oxygen Therapy Supplemental oxygen is administered to improve oxygen delivery to hypoxic tissues. For patients who are conscious, are spontaneously breathing, and have adequate arterial blood gas levels, oxygen delivered by nasal cannula or mask may be all that is necessary. If the patient who is experiencing moderate-to-severe shock is unconscious or is demonstrating respiratory distress, intubation and mechanical ventilation are usually required. Intubation and mechanical ventilation serve multiple functions, including protecting the airway, optimizing gas exchange, and reducing the work of breathing. Oxygen therapy support is crucial, and careful attention to the oxygen concentration delivered is important because oxygen is a drug that can have toxic effects on cells. Hyperoxia, caused by the delivery of oxygen at too high a concentration, may impair an innate immune response and increase the susceptibility to infectious complications and cause tissue damage (Helmerhorst, Schultz, van der Voort, de Jonge, & van Westerloo, 2015).

Fluid Resuscitation Administration of IV fluids assists in restoring optimal tissue perfusion by restoring preload and increasing the cardiac output (CO) component of oxygen delivery. The question of which fluid is best suited for shock states remains controversial; however, a combination of crystalloids and colloids is usually administered. Crystalloid solutions (e.g., normal saline or lactated Ringer's solution) restore interstitial and intravascular fluid volumes, increase preload and CO, and are the initial fluid of choice in the resuscitation of septic shock (Dellinger et al., 2013).

Colloids, which include albumin (a natural plasma protein) and artificial plasma expanders (e.g., starches or dextrans), have oncotic capabilities not inherent in crystalloids. The administration of colloids rapidly expands the circulating volume, and colloids remain in circulation significantly longer than crystalloids. Blood or blood products (e.g., packed red blood cells) are given when necessary to provide adequate hemoglobin concentration and to increase oxygen-carrying capacity or maintain adequate circulatory volume. Vasopressor medications are considered only when volume resuscitation has not been sufficient to adequately improve oxygenation (Nicks & Gaillard, 2016).

The patient's response to treatment must be assessed frequently for signs of improved oxygen delivery, including improving trends in cardiac output/cardiac index, arterial blood gases (especially PaO_2 and SaO_2), hemoglobin, urine output, and mean arterial pressure (MAP).

Interventions to Decrease Oxygen Consumption

In addition to optimizing oxygen delivery, interventions should include measures to decrease oxygen consumption. Such interventions are directed toward decreasing total body work, reducing pain and anxiety, and maintaining normothermia.

Decreasing Total Body Work Decreasing total body work during shock reduces the oxygen demands of all tissues. This can be accomplished through interventions that reduce the work of breathing and the activity of the voluntary muscles.

In the lungs, compensatory hyperventilation occurs in an effort to increase oxygenation and gas exchange to meet the high O_2 demands associated with the shock state and as a compensatory response to metabolic acidosis (e.g., lactic acidosis). However, increasing ventilation requires a great deal of respiratory muscle effort, and the patient can rapidly develop respiratory distress. Mechanical ventilation plays an important role in decreasing oxygen consumption by minimizing respiratory muscle oxygen demands by taking over the work of breathing.

Muscle work can be reduced through sedation, analgesia, controlling body temperature, and, when necessary, neuromuscular blocking agents (NMBAs).

Neuromuscular Blocking Agents (NMBA). Oxygen consumption by voluntary muscles can be reduced through the use of NMBAs such as pancuronium (Pavulon) or vecuronium (Norcuron), which paralyze the muscles. These drugs eliminate voluntary muscle activity, thereby allowing oxygen to be redirected for use in involuntary muscles, such as the heart. The use of NMBAs requires intubation and mechanical ventilation of the patient prior to initiation of the drug because NMBAs paralyze the respiratory muscles. Furthermore, NMBAs have no sedation or analgesia properties; therefore, adjunct sedation/anesthetic (e.g., propofol) and analgesia (morphine or fentanyl) are used. The level of paralysis is measured using a train of four (TOF) series of electrical impulses to the ulnar nerve at the forearm and observing for adduction of the thumb. NMBAs are presented in more detail in the Chapter 17 feature, "Related Pharmacotherapy: Neuromuscular Blocking and Reversal Agents."

The use of NMBAs for a patient in shock with acute respiratory distress syndrome (ARDS) has been controversial. Historically, research has suggested that a neuromuscular blockade is not ideal for long-term management of mechanically ventilated patients. NMBAs increase the time to extubation and time in ICU, contribute to muscle wasting in high-acuity patients and are associated with increased incidence of intensive care unit acquired weakness (ICU-AW) (Arroliga et al., 2005; Puthucheary et al., 2012). However, more recent studies have suggested that the short-term use of NMBAs reduces hospital mortality, reduces barotrauma, and is not associated with an increase in ICU-acquired weakness (Alhazzani et al., 2013; Hraiech, Dizier, & Papazian, 2014).

Although, NMBAs are considered high-alert drugs, current evidence suggests that the use of nonsteroidal NMBAs has no association with a risk of ICU-AW when they are used for a short duration. That said, it is recommended that their use be reserved for cases of acute phase ARDS in which more conservative therapies—such as benzodiazepines, opioids, and propofol—fail to meet therapeutic goals (Hraiech et al., 2014; Papazian et al., 2010).

Sedation. The use of propofol (Diprivan), an IV anesthetic agent, is often the preferred initial therapy for reducing oxygen consumption because it quickly induces deep sedation and has a short half-life, which makes it very titratable (Kress & Hall, 2013). When propofol is administered, mental status can be evaluated daily because the patient is arousable within minutes upon discontinuing the drug, and deep sedation returns rapidly on its resumption. In addition, research has shown that ICU patients who were treated with propofol had a statistically lower risk for ICU mortality, an overall decrease in ICU and hospital length of stay, and fewer ventilator days (Lonardo et al., 2014). Benzodiazepines (e.g., diazepam and lorazepam) have been used for sedation, to control anxiety, and as hypnotics for many years in critical care units. These drugs have a longer half-life than propofol and, when used for heavy sedation, can take a prolonged period of time to reverse, particularly if the patient has kidney or liver dysfunction. In addition, benzodiazepines have been associated with an increase in mortality, duration of ICU stay, time of mechanical ventilator support, ICU delirium, and other related ICU complications when compared to propofol (Lonardo et al., 2014). ICU delirium alone has been shown to have a strong dose-dependent association with long-term cognitive impairment (Pandharipande et al., 2013). Propofol is discussed in more detail in the Chapter 17 feature, "Related Pharmacotherapy: Adjunct Sedation and Analgesia Agents."

Reducing Pain and Anxiety Pain and anxiety stimulate the sympathetic nervous system to release catecholamines (e.g., epinephrine and norepinephrine), which increase the metabolic rate and, therefore, oxygen consumption. Appropriate analgesics and anxiolytics are administered to minimize pain and anxiety.

Maintaining Normothermia Hyperthermia increases metabolic demands and oxygen requirements. This is controlled with antipyretic drugs, such as acetaminophen, or physical cooling measures, such as a fan or cooling blanket. Some interventions to cool the body, such as cooling blankets or fans, can cause shivering. Shivering must be noted and managed because it increases metabolism and oxygen consumption.

Maintaining Normal Serum Glucose Level Stress-induced hyperglycemia in critically ill patients is associated with a longer hospital stay, an increased risk of complications, and an increased mortality (Bodawi, Waite, Fuhrman, & Zuckerman, 2012; Gomez & Umpierrez, 2014). It is recommended that IV insulin therapy be initiated if the patient's blood glucose rises above 180 mg/dL on two consecutive occasions; this approach should have a target of less than 180 mg/dL (Dellinger et al., 2013). However, stringent intensive insulin therapy to maintain normal glucose levels (80–110 mg/dL) is no longer recommended because of the risk for severe hypoglycemic episodes (Dellinger et al., 2013). Intensive insulin therapy is described in detail in Chapter 33.

Nursing Considerations

Fluid resuscitation requires frequent, accurate monitoring of the patient's hemodynamic and oxygenation status as the primary indicators of the patient's progress during the resuscitation phase. In addition, the nurse should monitor the patient closely for signs of continued or renewed bleeding. If massive fluid resuscitation is required, fluids, including blood or blood products, are warmed to prevent complications associated with hypothermia. The nurse can expect to rapidly change out bags of IV fluids, which requires close attention to hanging the correct fluids, documenting intake and output, and monitoring for signs of overhydration. Intravenous catheter insertion sites should be monitored closely for signs of extravasation and inflammation and/or infection.

Maintaining patient comfort is largely in the nurse's purview. Pain is regularly assessed and comfort measures provided as needed. Controlling pain and anxiety not only addresses the patient's comfort needs but also reduces oxygen consumption. Special attention is given to providing care that increases oxygen supply while reducing oxygen demand. A sedation protocol should be in place for patients requiring mechanical ventilation.

Protocols should be in place to reduce the risk of complications associated with critical illness such as deep vein thrombosis and stress ulcers. Deep vein thrombosis is prevented by administering either low-dose unfractionated heparin or low-molecular-weight heparin. Administering H_2 receptor inhibitors or proton pump inhibitors prevents the formation of stress ulcers.

Communication with the patient and family must include realistic treatment goals and likely outcomes. Decisions to limit or withdraw support may be in the patient's best interest, so the information must be clearly presented and carefully considered.

Emerging Evidence

- The Transfusion Requirements in Septic Shock (TRISS) trial examined transfusion thresholds in 998 patients diagnosed with sepsis. This randomized multicenter study assigned patients to two hemoglobin transfusion threshold groups. When comparing the two groups, the one with the transfusion threshold of 7.0 g/dL had fewer transfusions received, similar mortality at 90 days, similar use of life support, and a similar number of days alive out of the hospital when compared to the group with the hemoglobin threshold of 9.0 g/dL. This study suggests that a transfusion threshold of 7.0 g/dL is safe for the majority of patients with septic shock (*Holst et al., 2014*).

- A meta-analysis examining the use of procalcitonin (PCT) as a prognosticator in septic patients was designed to explore diagnostic accuracy of a single PCT concentration and PCT nonclearance in predicting all-cause mortality in septic patients. The study determined that elevated procalcitonin concentrations were strongly associated with all-cause mortality in septic patients. The authors found that elevated procalcitonin levels were associated with a higher risk of death in patients who were diagnosed with sepsis. However, it was also determined that procalcitonin levels may not be a completely useful indicator for assessing prognosis due to its moderate diagnostic accuracy. Despite its moderate diagnostic accuracy, the evidence from this meta-analysis may contribute additional information for the clinical utility of procalcitonin and may further help guide therapeutic interventions (e.g., antibiotic therapy) (*Liu, Su, Han, Yan, & Xie, 2015*).

- In a large multicenter retrospective observational analysis of 2,849 patients diagnosed with septic shock, investigators found that mortality was the lowest when vasopressor therapy was delayed by 1 hour and then initiated from 1 to 6 hours after the onset of shock. Investigators concluded that the first hour of therapy should consist of aggressive fluid administration. Delaying the start of vasopressor therapy in the first hour may allow for aggressive fluid resuscitation (*Waecher et al., 2014*).

- The current consensus definition of septic shock requires sepsis-induced hypotension that continues despite adequate fluid resuscitation or vasopressor therapy. Within the shock patient population, some patients present with hypotension and an elevated serum lactate (tissue dysoxic shock), and others present with hypotension alone and a normal serum lactate (vasoplegic shock). This study compared the outcomes of patients with tissue dysoxic versus vasoplegic septic shock. In a secondary analysis of a large randomized controlled trial, the investigators found that the group with vasoplegic shock had a lower Sequential Organ Failure Assessment (SOFA) than did the group with tissue dysoxic shock (5.5 vs. 7.0 points; $p = 0.0002$). The investigators concluded that there was a significant difference in in-hospital mortality between dysoxic and vasoplegic septic shock, which suggests a need to consider these differences when examining future shock therapies (*Sterling et al., 2013*).

- In a small study of 52 patients who were diagnosed with shock in the emergency department, early bedside sonographic exams were conducted for diagnostic accuracy and consistency in predicting shock type in critically ill patients. Multiorgan sonography was performed on the participants based on the Rapid Ultrasound for Shock and Hypotension (RUSH) protocol that was designed to help clinicians better recognize the etiology of shock in an expeditious time frame. The investigators found that patients who presented in a shock state and within the care of an emergency physician with ultrasonography expertise had an initial clinical diagnosis that was congruent with the patient's final diagnosis (Kappa index = 0.70). Thus, appropriate initial treatment and goal-directed therapies could be administered with greater confidence with the performance of an ultrasonography examination performed by a provider with expertise (*Ghane et al., 2015*).

Section Three Review

1. Which therapy would most effectively increase the cardiac output component of a client's oxygen delivery?
   A. O_2 therapy by nasal cannula
   B. Normal saline at 200 mL/hr
   C. Low-dose dopamine
   D. Acetaminophen

2. Why is it important to closely monitor the oxygen concentration being delivered to a client in shock?
   A. High oxygen concentrations can impair the immune system.
   B. High oxygen concentrations can reduce venous return to the heart.
   C. High oxygen concentration decreases creatinine clearance by the kidney.
   D. High oxygen concentration can result in tissue hypoxia.

3. Why would the nurse be alert for shivering in a client who is receiving physical cooling measures?
   A. Shivering indicates cooling has reached its maximum effectiveness.
   B. Once shivering begins, cooling measures should be discontinued.
   C. Shivering increases metabolism and oxygen consumption.
   D. The onset of shivering indicates hypothermia is reversing.

4. A client in septic shock has an NMBA initiated. Which other drug is most likely to be administered in conjunction with the NMBA?
   A. Propofol
   B. Lorazepam
   C. Diazepam
   D. Norepinephrine

Answers: 1. B, 2. A, 3. C, 4. A

Section Four: Vasoactive Pharmacotherapy in Shock Treatment

Vasoactive drugs alter blood vessel diameter through vasodilation or vasoconstriction and are an important part of the treatment strategy for shock. All of the shock states described in this chapter either have altered vascular tone as part of their pathophysiologic progression or would potentially benefit from manipulation of vascular tone.

As a general rule in the treatment of shock, vasoactive drug therapy is initiated when fluid resuscitation efforts have failed to adequately improve the patient's perfusion status and should be used early (Zhou et al., 2015). In most circumstances, a combination of drugs may be advantageous. Combining a positive inotropic drug (which affects the force of contraction) with a vasopressor or a vasodilating drug can manipulate different aspects of the patient's hemodynamic status, lending better hemodynamic support than if the drugs are given alone. Vasoactive drugs are temporary supportive agents because they do not treat the underlying cause of shock; it is crucial that the cause of the shock be identified rapidly and resolved to improve patient outcomes. This section describes three different types of drugs: vasopressors, inotropes, and vasodilators.

Vasopressors

Vasopressors are vasoactive drugs whose action causes peripheral vasoconstriction. Recommended vasopressor agents in the treatment of shock include norepinephrine, dopamine, and vasopressin (Dellinger et al., 2013); however, phenylephrine and epinephrine can also be used (Hollenberg, 2011). Vasopressors are used to increase systemic blood pressure through constriction of the peripheral vasculature.

General Actions With the exception of vasopressin, vasopressor agents are classified as adrenergic agonists (sympathomimetics)—that is, they directly bind to and activate adrenergic receptors, mimicking sympathetic nervous system stimulation (Adams, Holland, & Urban, 2014). Vasopressors are subclassified into catecholamines or noncatecholamines based on specific chemical structure differences. Catecholamine agents cannot be administered orally, have a brief duration of action, and do not cross the blood–brain barrier; noncatecholamines can be administered orally, have a longer duration of action, and are able to cross the blood–brain barrier (Burchum & Rosenthal, 2015). With the exception of phenylephrine (Neo-Synephrine), the vasopressor agents commonly used in shock are all catecholamines.

As can be seen in Table 37–3, it is the $alpha_1$ and $beta_1$-adrenergic actions that provide the desired effects in the treatment of shock: vasoconstriction to increase blood pressure and positive inotropic effects to improve heart function. Vasopressor agents are called *nonselective* if they stimulate more than one type of receptor and selective if they stimulate only one type.

Adverse Effects of Vasopressor Therapy The vasopressor agents used to treat shock are delivered intravenously, and the onset of actions is almost immediate. Moreover, because they bind directly to receptor sites, their effects are strong. For these reasons, initial dosages are usually low and titrated in small dosage increments (often micrograms/kilogram) until the desired therapeutic effects are achieved.

As noted in Table 37–4, two of the listed vasopressors are nonselective, and this lack of selectivity increases the

Table 37–3 Effects of Alpha$_1$- and Beta$_1$-Adrenergic Receptor Stimulation

Receptor	Therapeutic Effects	Adverse Effects
alpha$_1$ (α_1)	Vasoconstriction (vascular, visceral, integumentary); increases blood pressure	Hypertension, tachycardia, or bradycardia Tissue ischemia and necrosis
beta$_1$ (β_1)	Heart: positive inotropic effect (increased heart rate and force of contraction, which increases CO)	Tachycardia and dysrhythmias Angina (increased oxygen demand in heart)

SOURCE: Data from Burchum & Rosenthal (2015).

risk of undesired effects of the drug as well as desired effects. For example, norepinephrine may be ordered to increase the patient's BP by its vasoconstriction effect. However, norepinephrine stimulates all four adrenergic receptor sites, and therefore—in addition to vasoconstriction (alpha$_1$)—it also exerts positive inotropic (beta$_1$) effects. The beta$_1$ effects increase heart rate and cardiac oxygen demand, which can precipitate cardiac complications in patients with marginal cardiac function.

The vasoconstrictive effects of alpha$_1$ vasopressors can also cause visceral and peripheral tissue ischemia and possibly necrosis, which when severe can result in limb ischemia with necrosis, and organ perfusion can become significantly reduced (Hollenberg, 2011).

Vasopressin Vasopressin, or antidiuretic hormone (ADH), has a different classification from the other vasoactive agents. As a naturally occurring hormone, vasopressin is secreted by the posterior pituitary gland in response to increased serum osmolality, reduced blood volume, or low blood pressure (Han, Cribbs, & Martin, 2015; Wilson, Shannon, & Shields, 2016). When secreted, vasopressin causes water conservation, decreasing urine output and increasing intravascular water. In addition, at higher blood concentrations, vasopressin causes systemic vasoconstriction of the arterioles and may also inhibit production of nitric oxide (NO), a powerful naturally occurring vasodilator (Hall, 2015; Hollenberg, 2011). Although current data do not recommend vasopressin as a single-line agent for the treatment and management of shock (Dellinger et al., 2013), potential benefits have been shown when used to help wean patients off catecholamines, and it is associated with a decreased mortality (Serpa Neto et al., 2012). Emerging research suggests that vasopressin is a reasonable second-line agent for use in those patients who need an

Table 37–4 Common Vasopressor Agents Used in Shock States

Classification	Receptors Activated
Catecholamines (nonselective) • Norepinephrine (Levophed, Levarterenol) • Dopamine	All alpha and beta receptors Alpha$_1$ (α_1), beta$_1$ (β_1), dopamine
Noncatecholamine (selective) • Phenylephrine (Neo-Synephrine)	Alpha$_1$ (α_1)

Table 37–5 Positive Inotropic Agents

Classification	Mechanism of Action
Dobutamine (Dobutrex)	Primary activity is as a beta$_1$-adrenergic (β_1-adrenergic) agonist
Milrinone (Primacor)	Intracellular cyclic-AMP phosphodiesterase inhibitor

increase in mean arterial pressure (MAP) and for those who are nonresponsive to norepinephrine (Dellinger et al., 2013; Pollard, Edwin, & Alaniz, 2015).

A profile of major vasopressor agents can be found in the "Related Pharmacotherapy: Vasopressor Agents" feature.

Inotropes

Inotropic agents manipulate heart contractility and, therefore, cardiac output. Inotropes are classified as negative (decrease contractility) or positive (increase contractility). Positive inotropic agents may be ordered as part of shock treatment strategy. Three major drug groups qualify as positive inotropic agents: cardiac glycosides (e.g., digoxin), sympathomimetics (e.g., dopamine and dobutamine), and phosphodiesterase inhibitors (e.g., milrinone) (Table 37–5). Cardiac glycoside therapy is used primarily for long-term heart failure therapy and will not be discussed further here.

Sympathomimetics generally have both vasopressor and inotropic actions, although these two actions are not necessarily balanced in strength. These drugs exert their vasopressive activities through their alpha$_1$ receptor influence. The positive inotropic actions are exerted through their beta$_1$ receptor influence, which increases the force of contraction and heart rate. Dopamine is a good example of a drug that has relatively strong vasopressor and positive inotropic capabilities. Dobutamine (Dobutrex) is the major sympathomimetic positive inotropic agent used to treat shock. It is a selective agent—that is, it is beta$_1$ specific, which significantly reduces undesirable alpha$_1$ effects.

Phosphodiesterase (PDE3) inhibitors influence intracellular cyclic AMP (cAMP) rather than beta$_1$-adrenergic receptors to produce positive inotropic effects. They inhibit the PDE3 enzyme that breaks down cAMP, allowing cAMP to accumulate inside the cell (Burchum & Rosenthal, 2015). The increased cAMP levels result in increased force of contraction. A disadvantage of PDE3 inhibitors, however, is that they also increase levels of cAMP in vascular smooth muscle, which results in vasodilation that can worsen hypotension in shock (Hollenberg, 2011). The effectiveness of PDE3 inhibitors (e.g., milrinone) for treatment in shock states remains uncertain; thus, they are not considered a first-line therapy but may be considered after more conventional therapies have been proven inadequate (Hollenberg, 2011).

A profile of dobutamine and milrinone can be found in the "Related Pharmacotherapy: Positive Inotropic Agents" feature.

Vasodilators

Afterload-reducing (vasodilating) drugs improve cardiac output and oxygen delivery. Peripheral arterial vasodilators

Related Pharmacotherapy
Vasopressor Agents

Nonselective Adrenergic Agent 1

Norepinephrine (Levarterenol, Levophed)

Action and Uses

Sympathomimetic agents that act directly on alpha-adrenergic receptors to cause peripheral vasoconstriction to increase blood pressure. Norepinephrine has moderate $beta_1$ positive inotropic activity.

Dosages (Adult)

Hypotension: Initial 0.5–1 mcg/min; titrate to response; usual range 8–30 mcg/min

Major Adverse Effects

Ventricular dysrhythmias, hepatic or renal necrosis, cerebral hemorrhage

Nursing Implications

Monitor BP closely for patient response. Titrate dose to target BP as ordered by provider. Give at lowest dose possible to maintain BP. Administer via infusion pump.

If administering drug via peripheral IV site, monitor site closely for infiltration. If infiltration does occur, stop infusion and call healthcare provider (HCP) immediately (infiltration can cause ischemia and necrosis of tissue).

Avoid abrupt withdrawal; when drug is discontinued, infusion rate is slowed gradually.

Nonselective Alpha-Adrenergic Agent 2

Dopamine hydrochloride

Action and Uses

Precursor of norepinephrine/epinephrine with dose-dependent adrenergic effects (less than 5 mcg/kg/min: dopaminergic receptors stimulated; 5–10 mcg/kg/min: $beta_1$ receptors predominate; doses greater than 10 mcg/kg/min: $alpha_1$ effects predominate) (Gahart, Nazareno, & Ortega, 2016). Dopamine also qualifies as a positive inotropic agent.

Dosages (Adult)

Shock: 2–5 mcg/kg/min increased gradually up to 20–50 mcg/kg/min if necessary

Major Adverse Effects

Tachycardia (particularly at higher doses), hypotension, aberrant cardiac conduction, tissue ischemia

Nursing Implications

Notify HCP of decreased urine output in absence of hypotension, increasing tachycardia, dysrhythmias, or signs of peripheral ischemia (pallor, cyanosis, mottling, coldness).

Monitor lung sounds in patients with pulmonary congestion or edema because of its vasoconstrictive properties; it can increase venous return to right side of the heart and can worsen pulmonary edema.

SOURCE: Data from Gahart et al. (2016).

Administration, infiltration, and drug withdrawal: refer to norepinephrine.

Selective Adrenergic Agents

Phenylephrine (Neo-Synephrine)

Action and Uses

Sympathomimetic agent that acts directly on $alpha_1$-adrenergic receptors to cause peripheral vasoconstriction and increase blood pressure. Has some $beta_1$ activity at high doses. No longer recommended for routine use for vasodilatory shock (Gahart et al., 2016).

Dosages (Adult)

Do not administer bolus. Severe hypotension/shock: 0.5–6 mcg/kg/min until BP stabilizes, then titrate for blood pressure goal (Gahart et al., 2016).

Major Adverse Effects

Tissue ischemia and necrosis, local tissue necrosis with extravasation, bradycardia or tachycardia

Nursing Implications

Monitor BP closely. Titrate dose to target BP as ordered by provider. Give at lowest dose possible to maintain BP.

Administration, infiltration, and drug withdrawal: refer to norepinephrine.

Antidiuretic Hormone

Vasopressin (Pitressin)

Action and Uses

Antidiuretic hormone (ADH) agent that causes increased intravascular volume and widespread arteriolar vasoconstriction. It may be used as adjunct therapy with IV catecholamines (e.g., norepinephrine) to increase arterial blood pressure in shock states associated with vasodilation.

Dosages (Adult)

No recommended standard dosages available for use in shock (off-label use). American Heart Association (AHA) recommends low dosages of 0.02 to 0.04 units/min with no added benefits of a dose greater than 0.08 units/min (Gahart et al., 2016).

Major Adverse Effects

Tissue ischemia and necrosis, local tissue necrosis with extravasation, bradycardia or tachycardia

Nursing Implications

Monitor BP closely. Titrate dose to target BP as ordered by provider. Give at lowest dose possible to maintain BP.

Administration, infiltration, and withdrawal: refer to norepinephrine.

(e.g., nitroglycerine) decrease systemic vascular resistance (SVR). When afterload is decreased, stroke volume is improved. The ventricles have less resistance to overcome and eject blood with less force. Vasodilators decrease preload, as well as afterload, and, therefore, should be used with caution when treating shock. Vasodilator therapy should be initiated only in patients who have adequate fluid volume. Intravenous nitroglycerine is the primary vasodilator agent used to reduce afterload and should be initiated only after the patient's blood pressure has been stabilized, usually to a systolic of greater than 100 mmHg (Hochman & Ingbar, 2015). While receiving a vasodilating

Related Pharmacotherapy
Positive Inotropic Agents

Selective Beta-Adrenergic Agonist
Dobutamine

Action and Uses
Acts on beta$_1$ receptors in the heart to increase inotropic activity (increase contractility) and increase conduction through the AV node (increase heart rate)

Dosages (Adult)
Cardiac decompensation: 0.5–1 mcg/kg/min, then titrate up to 2.5–15 mcg/kg/min (max: 40 mcg/kg/min)

Major Adverse Effects
Angina, increased myocardial workload, tachycardia

Nursing Implications
Monitor ECG and BP closely.
Administer via infusion pump.
Marked hypertension and tachycardia and appearance of dysrhythmias are usually reversed by promptly decreasing the dose.

SOURCE: Data from Gahart et al. (2016).

Phosphodiesterase (PDE3) Inhibitor
Milrinone

Action and Uses
Inhibits cyclic AMP phosphodiesterase in cardiac and smooth muscle, thereby increasing myocardial contractility (increased CO) and causing vasodilation (decreased pulmonary artery wedge pressure [PAWP], decreased systemic vascular resistance [SVR]). Little chronotropic activity, therefore does not significantly increase myocardial oxygen demand or increase HR.

Dosages (Adult)
Heart failure: **loading dose**, 50 mcg/kg IV over 10 minutes; **maintenance dose**, 0.375–0.75 mcg/kg/min

Major Adverse Effects
Ventricular dysrhythmias, hypotension

Nursing Implications
Monitor ECG and BP closely.
Administer via infusion pump.
In presence of significant hypotension, stop infusion, notify HCP.

agent, the patient must be monitored carefully so that the blood pressure does not become so low that reflex tachycardia occurs and coronary perfusion suffers.

A profile of IV nitroglycerine can be found in the "Related Pharmacotherapy: Vasodilator Agents" feature.

Vasoactive Agents: Nursing Implications

In treating shock, more than one vasoactive drug may be ordered to run concurrently, increasing the risk of nontherapeutic effects and drug toxicity. It is critical that the nurse have a strong understanding of the actions and adverse effects of each specific drug being delivered. As a group, IV vasoactive agents are incompatible with many other drugs, making it imperative that specific incompatibilities be checked prior to drug initiation. The nurse should closely

monitor the patient for therapeutic and nontherapeutic effects of each agent, keeping in mind that these agents in combination can either enhance or counteract each other's actions. Furthermore, when weaning the patient from vasoactive drug therapy, dosage is reduced in small increments to avoid destabilizing the patient's hemodynamic status, and the patient's response to the dosage changes is closely monitored.

Patients receiving IV vasoactive agents frequently have hemodynamic monitoring (e.g., arterial line, pulmonary artery catheter, or central venous catheter) to facilitate safe, effective drug dosage titration. When IV inotropic agents are used to increase contractility, direct measurement of cardiac output (CO) may still be advisable as CO is the primary method by which contractility can be evaluated (Hollenberg, 2011). During initial titration, parameters such as heart rate and blood pressure (and mean arterial pressure) may require documentation every 5 minutes until

Related Pharmacotherapy
Vasodilating Agents

Nitrate Vasodilator
Nitroglycerine

Action and Uses
Relaxes smooth muscles of vessels by converting to nitric oxide (NO), a natural vasodilator. Used for treatment of significant hypertension or refractory angina. In cardiogenic shock, it reduces cardiac preload and afterload, which increases cardiac tissue oxygenation.

SOURCE: Data from Hochman & Ingbar (2015).

Dosages (Adult)
Cardiogenic shock: 10–20 mcg/min IV if BP is greater than 100 mmHg

Major Adverse Effects
Hypotension, headache, circulatory collapse

Nursing Implications
Monitor ECG and BP closely.
Monitor for cardiac dysrhythmias.
Administer via infusion pump.

therapeutic effects are achieved and then frequently thereafter. Peripheral oxygenation is closely monitored through frequent evaluation of limb perfusion (pulses, coloring, temperature), and indirect measures of tissue oxygenation are monitored (e.g., arterial blood gas [ABG], serum lactate, base excess/base deficit, venous oxygen saturation [SvO_2], and laboratory measures of organ function).

The strong vasoconstrictive effects of vasopressors can result in local tissue ischemia and necrosis should the IV infiltrate into the subcutaneous tissue; therefore, infusing vasopressors through a central venous catheter (CVC) line is preferred. When a peripheral line must be used, if infiltration occurs the drug is stopped and the healthcare provider is contacted immediately to determine the best course of action. Interventions to reverse or minimize the tissue damage caused by extravasation vary with the specific agent and may include injecting the local area with an antidote such as phentolamine. In addition to causing local tissue destruction, the sudden cessation of the vasopressor may result in a rapid drop in BP and worsening of shock; therefore, it is critical that the nurse act quickly when extravasation occurs.

Section Four Review

1. In the treatment of shock, it is recommended that vasoactive drug therapy be considered at what point relative to fluid resuscitation?
   A. At the same time as fluid resuscitation
   B. As soon as fluid resuscitation has been completed
   C. Immediately, before starting fluid resuscitation initiatives
   D. If fluid resuscitation fails to sufficiently improve perfusion

2. All vasopressor drugs have which action in common?
   A. Vasodilation
   B. Increase heart contractility
   C. Vasoconstriction
   D. Increase stroke volume

3. The nurse is titrating norepinephrine on a client for treatment of shock. The healthcare provider has just ordered that the drug be discontinued. How should the nurse comply with this order?
   A. Stop the drip immediately.
   B. Gradually decrease the rate of flow over time.
   C. Increase the maintenance IV fluid rate prior to discontinuing.
   D. Decrease the rate over a 1-hour period and discontinue.

4. The provider has just ordered dobutamine for a client in shock. The nurse is aware that this type of drug has which physiologic effect?
   A. Vasodilation
   B. Vasoconstriction
   C. Increases contractility
   D. Decreases pulmonary vascular resistance

Answers: 1. D, 2. C, 3. D, 4. B

Section Five: Cardiogenic Shock

Cardiogenic shock, sometimes referred to as "pump" failure, occurs when the heart fails to function as a pump to deliver oxygenated blood to the tissues. Failure can occur when the right ventricle fails to pump the volume of blood it receives into the pulmonic circulation or when the left ventricle fails to pump oxygenated blood into the systemic circulation. The most common cause of cardiogenic shock is extensive left ventricular myocardial infarction (MI), particularly *ST*-segment elevation MI (STEMI) (Hochman & Ingbar, 2015; Khan, Corbett, & Hollenberg, 2014; Zuckerbraun et al., 2015). Other causes of cardiogenic shock include mechanical complications such as papillary muscle rupture, mitral or aortic stenosis, and ventricular septal rupture, as well as other pathologic heart conditions such as end-stage cardiomyopathy, myocarditis, and severe heart contusion. Mortality rates for cardiogenic shock are significant: an estimated 50% to 80% (Zuckerbraun et al., 2015). This section focuses on the left-ventricular-failure etiology of cardiogenic shock, as it is by far the most common cause.

Pathophysiology

A myocardial infarction produces necrotic myocardial tissue that can no longer contribute to heart muscle contraction; thus, it impairs cardiac contractility and cardiac output. The damaged ventricle is unable to propel oxygenated blood forward into the systemic circulation for delivery to tissues or the myocardium, resulting in progressive ischemia (Hochman & Ingbar, 2015). As stroke volume decreases, so do CO and systemic blood pressure. Decreased blood pressure results in decreased aortic diastolic pressure, which further compromises perfusion to the coronary arteries that are located in the aorta adjacent to the aortic valve. As coronary artery perfusion declines, oxygen delivery to the myocardium decreases, resulting in worsening myocardial ischemia. Blood begins to back up into the pulmonary system because the damaged left ventricle cannot pump all of its contents forward out of the heart, causing pulmonary congestion. Increased pulmonary congestion leads to increased capillary hydrostatic pressure, which in turn leads to pulmonary edema and increased afterload for the right ventricle.

The events that trigger cardiogenic shock can also trigger additional aggravating pathophysiologic events. For example, in the presence of an extensive myocardial infarction, systemic inflammatory response syndrome (SIRS) can develop, which causes the release of chemical mediators, some of which release nitric oxide (NO), causing widespread vasodilation that worsens oxygen delivery problems (Hochman & Ingbar, 2015). Moreover, progressive ischemia results in lactic acidosis, which further impairs the already decreased cardiac contractility (Hochman & Ingbar, 2015). These pathologic changes can occur rapidly or can progress over several days; however, about 75% of cardiogenic shock cases develop signs of shock within 24 hours of acute MI onset, and about 25% develop shock within 6 hours (Hochman & Ingbar, 2015; Zuckerbraun et al., 2015).

Clinical Manifestations and Diagnosis

The hemodynamic criteria for diagnosis of cardiogenic shock include sustained hypotension (systolic blood pressure [SBP] of less than 90 mmHg for 30 minutes or longer), an elevated pulmonary artery wedge pressure (PAWP) greater than 15 mmHg, and a low cardiac index (less than 2.2 L/min/m^2) (Zuckerbraun et al., 2015). Common clinical findings include continuing chest pain and manifestations of pulmonary congestion, including dyspnea, bilateral crackles, and hypoxemia. Other general signs of shock are usually present, such as reduced mentation, mottled and cool skin, diaphoresis, weak peripheral pulses, and tachycardia.

Confirmation of cardiogenic shock may require a variety of heart-specific diagnostic tests, such as electrocardiogram (ECG), cardiac echocardiogram, and serial cardiac enzymes, as well as more general tests, such as chest x-ray, arterial blood gases, and electrolytes (Zuckerbraun et al., 2015). It is critical that the specific etiology of the shock be rapidly identified to improve patient outcomes.

Management

Nursing and medical interventions for patients in cardiogenic shock are directed toward decreasing myocardial oxygen demand and improving myocardial oxygen supply. Emergency interventions should be initiated as soon as cardiogenic shock is suspected, with interventions and diagnostic testing performed simultaneously (Hochman & Ingbar, 2015). Initial management is centered on reducing pulmonary edema, increasing systemic blood pressure and cardiac output, and preventing or controlling cardiac dysrhythmias. The patient is usually intubated and placed on mechanical ventilation to optimize oxygen supply, decrease oxygen demand by taking over the patient's work of breathing, and protect the patient's airway. Other treatment options may include thrombolytic therapy, an intra-aortic balloon pump, percutaneous left ventricular assist devices, veno-arterial extra-corporeal membrane oxygenation, and revascularization (angioplasty or coronary artery bypass surgery).

Supporting Circulation   Because of the loss of a functioning heart pump associated with cardiogenic shock, supporting circulation is critical. Management that supports circulation includes IV drug therapies such as vasopressors, inotropic agents, and diuretics; invasive or noninvasive hemodynamic monitoring; aortic counterpulsation; percutaneous left ventricular assist devices; and possibly veno-arterial extra-corporeal membrane oxygenation.

Drug Therapy.   Treatment of cardiogenic shock may include the use of vasopressors and positive inotropes to improve myocardial oxygenation, contractility, and cardiac output, as described in Section Four. Vasopressors are used to increase the systemic blood pressure sufficiently to provide a coronary perfusion pressure above 50 mmHg to perfuse and oxygenate the myocardium (Hollenberg, 2011). Other drugs that may be ordered include a vasodilator, such as nitroglycerine, to reduce cardiac workload, and diuretics, such as furosemide (Lasix), to treat pulmonary congestion.

Hemodynamic Monitoring.   Continuous monitoring of the patient's cardiac rhythm status and oxygen saturation (e.g., pulse oximetry [SpO$_2$] or via arterial line [SaO$_2$]) helps evaluate the patient's shock status and response to therapy. In addition, research recommends the measurement of end-tidal CO$_2$ (ETCO$_2$), monitoring of serum lactate, kidney and liver function markers to assess the improvement or persistence of cardiogenic shock, and the monitoring of central venous oxygen saturation (ScvO$_2$) (Dellinger et al., 2013; Levy et al., 2015). Although increasingly controversial, the insertion of a pulmonary artery catheter may be considered to accurately measure cardiac output and filling pressures and optimize intravenous fluid use (Hochman & Ingbar, 2015). There is weak expert agreement for the use of a pulmonary artery catheter for hemodynamic monitoring (Levy et al., 2015). Conversely, the use of pulse contour analysis is less invasive than the pulmonary artery catheter and permits serial measurements of cardiac output, stroke volume, and ejection fraction (Hollenberg, 2013), and it can allow the titration of inotropic and vasopressor drugs to the minimum dose required to achieve optimal cardiac output. In addition, emerging data have shown stroke volume variance (SVV) to be a better predictor of fluid responsiveness in a study of 45 mechanically ventilated patients with acute circulatory failure who have been diagnosed with sepsis when compared to central venous pressure (CVP) (Angappan, Parida, Vasudevan, & Badhe, 2015).

Aortic Counterpulsation   An intra-aortic balloon pump (IABP) is an invasive technology that reduces afterload and augments coronary perfusion, which increases cardiac output and improves coronary blood flow. The IABP has a 40 mL balloon mounted on a catheter that is inserted into the femoral artery and until it is in the descending thoracic aorta. The IABP is synchronized with the patient's cardiac cycle. During ventricular diastole, the balloon inflates (Figure 37–3). With the balloon inflated, the blood distal to the balloon is forced back toward the aortic valve, where the coronary arteries are located. This supplies the coronary arteries with additional oxygenated blood to meet myocardial oxygen needs. Before ventricular systole, the balloon deflates, which decreases pressure in the aorta. This makes it easier for the left ventricle to contract and eject its stroke volume. Stabilization with the IABP is a temporary measure, as it does not reestablish coronary blood flow, but it does allow stabilization until definitive therapy can be

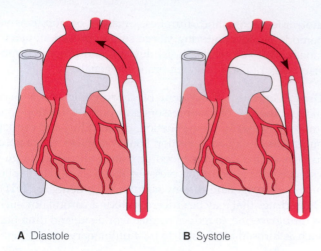

A Diastole   **B** Systole

Figure 37–3 Intra-aortic balloon pump. **A,** When inflated during diastole, the balloon supports cerebral, renal, and coronary artery perfusion. **B,** The balloon deflates during systole, so cardiac output is unimpeded.

instituted. The IABP has not demonstrated success in reversing hypotension and hypoperfusion problems in severe cardiogenic shock, and multiple randomized, controlled trials (RCTs) have failed to show clear evidence of IABP benefit (Curtis et al., 2012; Thiele et al., 2012). However, despite the evidence presented by these RCTs, the IABP still has a significant role in the stabilization of patients in cardiogenic shock (Khan et al., 2014).

Percutaneous Left Ventricular Assist Devices   Percutaneous left ventricular assist devices (pLVADs) are mechanical circulatory assist devices, inserted percutaneously, that are created to imitate or assist a functioning heart and relieve the workload on the failing left ventricle (Khan et al., 2014). Two types of pLVADs are left atrial to aorta-assist devices and left ventricle to aorta-assist devices (Khan et al., 2014). The left atrial to aorta-assist device is a transseptally placed left atrial cannula that pumps blood extracorporeally from the left atrium to the iliofemoral arterial system and in turn bypasses the left ventricle (Basra, Loyalka, & Kar, 2011). Conversely, the left ventricle to aorta-assist device has an axial flow pump and is inserted through the femoral artery and subsequently across the aortic valve. The pump then pulls blood from the left ventricle and pushes it into the ascending aorta (Khan et al., 2014). Data suggest that in the setting of severe cardiogenic shock, continuous pump devices such as pLVADs are likely to provide more benefit than the IABP (Khan et al., 2014).

Veno-arterial Extra-corporeal Membrane Oxygenation   Veno-arterial extra-corporeal membrane oxygenation (VA ECMO) is a mechanical circulatory support device that involves draining blood from the venous system, oxygenating it through a membrane oxygenator, and then returning the oxygenated blood into the systemic circulation through the use of a centrifugal pump (Hollenberg, 2013; Khan et al., 2014; Rihal et al., 2015). Specifically, VA ECMO cannulation involves central cannulation of the right atrium and aorta or peripheral cannulation of the femoral artery and vein (Khan et al., 2014). VA ECMO circulatory support is the preferred method of mechanical circulatory support with patients who present in cardiogenic shock and have impaired tissue oxygenation due to its ability to provide complete cardiopulmonary support (Rihal et al., 2015). However, VA ECMO presents many potential complications, including an increased risk of bleeding, clotting abnormalities, and a high risk of stroke. In addition, there are no RCTs or meta-analyses that examine prognosis post–VA ECMO in the cardiogenic shock patient, and, therefore, more research needs to be conducted.

Revascularization (Angioplasty or Coronary Artery Bypass Grafting)   Revascularization for patients with myocardial infarction (MI)–related cardiogenic shock can be performed through a percutaneous coronary intervention (PCI) procedure (i.e., coronary angioplasty) or through surgical methods (i.e., coronary artery bypass grafting [CABG]). The purpose of a PCI is to improve wall motion in the infarct area and increase perfusion of the infarct zone; it remains the gold standard in the treatment of acute MI. In addition, CABG may be considered in patients with cardiogenic shock who have multiple-vessel coronary artery disease, particularly if PCI cannot be performed (Mehta et al., 2010).

Acute myocardial infarction is responsible for over 70% of cardiogenic shock cases. In the case of patients who present with advanced cardiogenic shock refractory to IABP and PCI or coronary bypass surgery, the use of surgically placed pLVADs or VA ECMOs may be the only option for the improvement of hemodynamic compromise in the setting of cardiogenic shock. However, further studies are warranted in order to appropriately assess the need for the different types of emerging mechanical circulatory support devices and their utility in the treatment and management of cardiogenic shock.

A profile of care for the patient in cardiogenic shock can be found in the "Nursing Care: The Patient with Cardiogenic Shock" feature.

Nursing Care

The Patient with Cardiogenic Shock

Expected Patient Outcomes and Related Interventions

Outcome: Optimize cardiac output

Assess and compare to established norms, patient baselines, and trends.

Clinical manifestations of left ventricular failure: dyspnea, bilateral crackles, distant heart sounds, third or fourth sounds, elevated PAWP, low cardiac index (CI), sustained systolic hypotension

Clinical manifestations of right ventricular failure: peripheral edema, split S_2 heart sounds, elevated RAP in the presence of normal or low PAWP

Implement interventions to optimize oxygen delivery.

Administer supplemental oxygen as ordered.

Administer IV fluids as ordered.

Administer inotropic agents as ordered (dobutamine [Dobutrex]).
Administer afterload-reducing (vasodilating) drugs as ordered.
Implement IABP as ordered.

Implement interventions to decrease oxygen consumption.
Initiate mechanical ventilation as ordered.
Administer sedatives, analgesics, anxiolytics as ordered.
Implement nonpharmacologic interventions to reduce pain and anxiety.
Position the patient to maximize comfort.
Provide a calm, quiet environment.

Administer related drug therapy and monitor for therapeutic and nontherapeutic effects.
Diuretics (e.g., furosemide [Lasix])
Vasodilators (e.g., nitroglycerine)
Inotropic agents (e.g., PDE3 inhibitors [milrinone])
Thrombolytic therapy

Related nursing diagnoses
Risk for complications from acute myocardial ischemia or infarction, altered myocardial contractility and heart rate

Section Five Review

1. Which condition characterizes cardiogenic shock?
   A. Impaired cardiac contractility and cardiac output
   B. Increasing stroke volume in the face of decreasing cardiac output
   C. Increasing stroke volume in the face of increasing cardiac output
   D. Hypovolemic shock as the result of a massive myocardial infarction

2. Which combination of assessments should alert the nurse that the client may be developing cardiogenic shock? (Select all that apply.)
   A. Sustained systolic blood pressure (SBP) of less than 90 mmHg
   B. Cardiac index (CI) of less than 2.2 L/min/m^2
   C. Pulmonary artery wedge pressure (PAWP) of less than 4 mmHg
   D. Client report of continuing chest pain and dyspnea
   E. Reduced mentation

3. Initial management of cardiogenic shock focuses on which goals? (Select all that apply.)
   A. Reduce pulmonary edema.
   B. Provide fluid resuscitation.
   C. Control cardiac dysrhythmias.
   D. Increase BP.
   E. Increase cardiac output.

4. A client in cardiogenic shock is undergoing placement of a left ventricular assist device (LVAD). What is a major purpose of this procedure?
   A. To control cardiac dysrhythmias
   B. To decrease afterload
   C. To increase oxygen demand
   D. To rest the injured myocardium

Answers: 1. A, 2. (A, B, D, E), 3. (A, C, D, E), 4. D

Section Six: Hypovolemic Shock

Hypovolemic shock is the most common type of shock that occurs in trauma and surgical high-acuity patients (Zuckerbraun et al., 2015). It develops when inadequate circulating volume results in inadequate cardiac output to meet tissue oxygenation. Hypovolemic shock can result from an absolute fluid volume deficit (e.g., hemorrhage, severe dehydration, or skin loss via burns) or from a relative fluid volume deficit in which there may be adequate fluids in the body but they are located outside of the vascular space, as in third-spacing (e.g., severe ascites) or severe generalized edema (e.g., severe burns, severe hypoalbuminemia). Hemorrhage is by far the most common form of hypovolemic shock (often referred to as hemorrhagic shock) and is the primary focus of this section.

Pathophysiology

Diminished fluid volume leads to decreased cardiac output, resulting in impaired oxygen delivery to the tissues. Acute loss or displacement of a significant volume of intravascular fluid results in the inhibition of baroreceptors in the large arteries, which then triggers compensatory peripheral vasoconstriction and stimulation of the sympathetic nervous system (SNS) with the subsequent release of catecholamines (Zuckerbraun et al., 2015). The severity of shock depends on the percentage of circulating volume lost; a loss of 25% or greater is sufficient to precipitate clinical manifestations of hypovolemic shock (Zuckerbraun et al., 2015). Table 37–6 lists the levels of severity of hypovolemia by circulating volume loss in an adult who weighs 70 kilograms.

Clinical Manifestations

The severity of clinical manifestations associated with hypovolemic shock depends on the degree of volume depletion

Table 37–6 Severity of Hypovolemia by Circulating Volume Loss (70 kg patient)

Severity (% volume loss)	Volume Loss	Associated Manifestations
Mild (up to 15% loss)	0.7 to 0.75 L	Few, if any, overt manifestations
Moderate (up to 30% loss)	1.5 L	Anxiety, tachypnea, mild tachycardia
Severe (30%–40%)	1.5 to 2 L	Marked tachycardia (HR greater than 110), hypotension, confusion
Massive (40% or greater)	2 L or greater	Life-threatening

SOURCE: Data from Zuckerbraun et al. (2015).

Table 37–7 Clinical Manifestations of Hypovolemic Shock

Parameter	Related Manifestations
Hemodynamics	Hypotension: BP decreases as volume loss increases; systolic BP of less than 100 is considered significant Low: central venous pressure (CVP) and right atrial pressure (RAP), pulmonary artery wedge pressure (PAWP), pulmonary artery pressure (PAP), cardiac output (CO), venous capacitance Elevated: heart rate, systemic vascular resistance (SVR), stroke volume variation (SVV)
Urine output	Low
Skin and peripheral pulses	Cool, clammy, poor capillary refill Peripheral pulses faint or absent

SOURCE: Data from Zuckerbraun et al. (2015).

and the general age and health of the patient. Young, healthy adults are significantly more tolerant of hypovolemia than are older adults, who have diminished physiologic reserves and a reduced ability to muster sufficient compensatory activities (Zuckerbraun et al., 2015). Clinical manifestations are due primarily to decreased circulating volume and SNS stimulation (Table 37–7). The systemic vascular resistance (SVR) is elevated as vasoconstriction occurs in an effort to increase venous return and CO.

Treatment

Time is a critical factor in the successful treatment of hemorrhagic-type hypovolemic shock. The treatment priorities are to secure the patient's airway, support breathing, and concurrently control bleeding and restore fluid volume (Zuckerbraun et al., 2015). The source of the fluid loss must be rapidly identified and controlled. If large-vessel hemorrhage is present, immediate surgical intervention is required. The nurse should monitor the patient closely for signs of continued or renewed bleeding.

Fluid Resuscitation Refer to Section Three for general fluid resuscitation information. If hemorrhage is the underlying problem, blood products will likely be ordered to achieve a hemoglobin level of 7 to 9 g/dL (Zuckerbraun et al., 2015). Interestingly, overaggressive volume resuscitation that is initiated before controlling hemorrhage has been associated with negative patient outcomes. If the patient's blood pressure is driven too high, it reopens injured vessels that have already clotted, causing resumption of bleeding. Therefore, initial volume resuscitation prior to controlling hemorrhage may be limited to achieving a systolic blood pressure of about 90 mmHg—which is sufficient for tissue perfusion but not high enough to cause renewed bleeding (Zuckerbraun et al., 2015).

Section Six Review

1. Which clinical situation could result in a *relative* fluid volume deficit?
   - A. Ascites
   - B. Hemorrhage
   - C. Dehydration
   - D. Severe burns

2. Clinical manifestations of hypovolemic shock develop when the client has lost which percentage of fluid volume?
   - A. 10%
   - B. 15%
   - C. 20%
   - D. 25%

3. In clients experiencing hemorrhagic shock, blood or blood products are usually ordered to achieve a hemoglobin of which level?
   - A. 6 to 8 g/dL
   - B. 7 to 9 g/dL
   - C. 8 to 10 g/dL
   - D. 9 to 11 g/dL

4. For a client with ongoing severe hemorrhage, the fluid resuscitation goal is to achieve what systolic blood pressure?
   - A. 80 mmHg
   - B. 90 mmHg
   - C. 100 mmHg
   - D. 110 mmHg

Answers: 1. A, 2. D, 3. B, 4. B

Section Seven: Distributive Shock—Septic

The three types of distributive shock are septic, anaphylactic, and neurogenic. This section introduces the concept of distributive shock and then focuses on septic shock. The two other forms of distributive shock are discussed in the next section.

Introduction to Distributive Shock

Distributive shock states involve impaired oxygenation because of altered blood flow distribution. The vascular smooth muscle becomes incapable of constricting for one of two reasons: endothelial insult (septic and anaphylactic shock) or loss of sympathetic nervous system response (neurogenic shock). Regardless of the underlying cause, massive vasodilation is the primary characteristic of all forms of distributive shock. It causes significant expansion of the size of the intravascular compartment without increasing the volume of circulating blood, which results in a relative hypovolemia (decreased venous return and reduced ventricular filling pressure, stroke volume, and cardiac output). Hypotension results from the loss of vascular smooth muscle's ability to vasoconstrict (Zuckerbraun et al., 2015).

Pathophysiologic Basis of Septic Shock

The three forms of sepsis are uncomplicated sepsis, severe sepsis, and septic shock. Of approximately 750,000 cases of severe sepsis per year in North America, one fourth are fatal (Dellinger et al., 2013). Sepsis is associated with a significant mortality rate of about 20%; however, septic shock carries a high mortality burden of 40% to 60% (Felner & Smith, 2012).

The pathophysiology of sepsis and septic shock is complex and beyond the scope of this chapter; however, a basic overview is provided here. Septic shock is characterized by altered fluid volume related to vasodilation, increased capillary permeability, and maldistribution of circulating volume, in which some organs receive more blood than required as a result of vasodilation while other organs (skin, lungs, kidneys) do not receive the blood they require. The systemic response to infection triggers a complex series of cellular and humoral events (Figure 37–4). As pathogens (and bacterial endotoxins, if present) invade the bloodstream, they stimulate the release of inflammatory mediators such as innate humoral, cytokine, and host complement responses that impair the microvasculature and cause cellular dysfunction, resulting in increased capillary permeability and vasodilation (Han et al., 2015).

A multitude of metabolic, hematologic, and hemodynamic abnormalities occur as a systemic response to the invasion of microorganisms in the bloodstream. These abnormalities are part of a complex syndrome that may ultimately culminate in septic shock. The American College of Chest Physicians and Society of Critical Care Medicine (ACCP/SCCM) have clinically defined sepsis (Bone et al., 1992; Dellinger et al., 2013). Such clinical definitions aim to assist in the early recognition and treatment of these disorders, with the ultimate goal of improving patient outcomes. Key to the ACCP/SCCM definitions is the assumption that sepsis is the SIRS phenomenon in the presence of an actual or suspected infection. To date, the ACCP/SCCM sepsis definitions continue to dominate the scientific literature (Table 37–8). The Surviving Sepsis Campaign on the SCCM website (Rhodes et al., 2017) provides up-to-date information regarding sepsis.

The ACCP/SCCM definitions have been hailed as a major advancement in the understanding of the spectrum

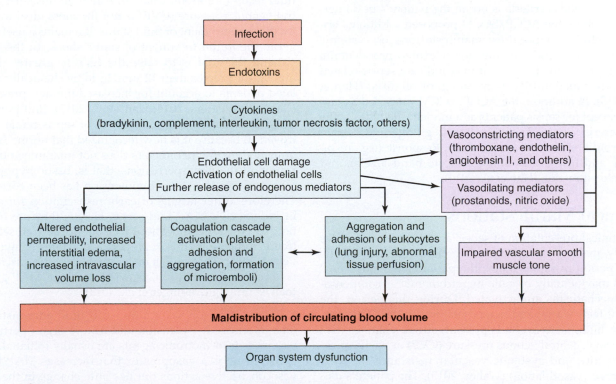

Figure 37–4 Pathophysiology of septic shock.

Table 37–8 ACCP/SCCM Definitions of Sepsis, Severe Sepsis, and Septic Shock

Term	Definition
Sepsis	Infection (confirmed or suspected) *and* systemic inflammatory response syndrome (SIRS) criteria: the presence of two or more of the following conditions: 1. Temperature greater than 38.3°C (100.9°F) or less than 36°C (96.8°F) 2. Heart rate greater than 90 bpm 3. Respiratory rate greater than 20 breaths/min 4. Plasma C-reactive protein 2 or more standard deviations greater than normal value 5. Procalcitonin 2 or more standard deviations greater than normal value 6. White blood cell count greater than 12,000/mL or less than 4,000/mL, or greater than 10% immature (band) forms
Severe sepsis	Sepsis associated with organ dysfunction, hypoperfusion, or hypotension Hypoperfusion and perfusion abnormalities that may include, but are not limited to, lactic acidosis, oliguria, or an acute alteration in mental status
Septic shock	Sepsis associated with hypotension despite adequate fluid resuscitation, along with the presence of perfusion abnormalities that may include, but are not limited to, lactic acidosis, oliguria, or an acute alteration in mental status

SOURCE: Data from Bone et al. (1992) and Dellinger et al. (2013).

of sepsis, and a fundamental principle of that definition is that clinical sepsis essentially represents an immune response to infection (Han et al., 2015). The foundational principle for the current definition of sepsis is having two of the SIRS criteria in conjunction with an infection or probable infection (Han et al., 2015). However, not every patient who presents with severe sepsis or septic shock will have SIRS criteria, and delaying care to wait on the presence of those criteria is not in the patient's best interest. Therefore, the ACCP/SCCM proposed additional criteria including laboratory manifestations of systemic illness that may indicate infection (elevated procalcitonin or C-reactive protein), or that may indicate sepsis-related organ dysfunction (ScvO$_2$, mottling, or oliguria) (Han et al., 2015). In addition, the ACCP/SCCM proposed a staging concept for sepsis patients as a model called PIRO. The characteristics are **P**redisposition (e.g., age and certain comorbidities), **I**nfection (or insult), **R**esponse (e.g., respiratory and heart rates and leukocyte band levels), and **O**rgan dysfunction (Han et al., 2014).

Clinical Manifestations

The clinical presentation of sepsis and septic shock varies widely, making early diagnosis a challenge. During the early period of septic shock, the patient's hemodynamic status may actually become hyperdynamic as compensatory mechanisms are activated. During this period, the patient feels warm, and hemodynamically the CO is normal or high, tachycardia is present, stroke volumes (SV) are normal, central venous pressure (CVP) or wedge pressure is low, and systemic vascular resistance (SVR) is decreased (vasodilation) (Walley, 2015). The patient's diastolic blood pressure decreases, causing a widening pulse

pressure (Walley, 2015). As the septic shock continues, compensatory mechanisms fail, myocardial depressant and hypoxemic effects predominate, and tissue hypoperfusion develops. This later stage of septic shock is sometimes referred to as the hypodynamic or cold phase. The patient's extremities are now cold and mottling may be present, serum lactate levels increase, and ScvO$_2$ decreases as tissue perfusion becomes increasingly compromised (Walley, 2015).

Treatment

The "Surviving Sepsis Campaign: International Guidelines for Management of Severe Sepsis and Septic Shock" are multidisciplinary guidelines that provide evidence-based recommendations for the care of patients with severe sepsis and septic shock (Dellinger et al., 2013). A summary of the major points of the guidelines is presented in the following paragraphs; however, the reader is encouraged to visit the Surviving Sepsis Campaign website to view the entire bundle (Rhodes et al., 2017).

A nursing priority is to administer antibiotics within 1 hour after a healthcare provider initiates the order; however, blood cultures should be obtained prior to initiating the antibiotics. A serum lactate level should be obtained immediately to evaluate end-organ hypoperfusion. A lactate level greater than 4 mmol/L is highly suspicious of significant tissue hypoperfusion and requires immediate fluid resuscitation and other interventions to relieve tissue hypoxia (e.g., decrease O$_2$ demand or increase O$_2$ supply). The patient's venous oxygen saturation (SvO$_2$), either mixed (SmvO$_2$) or central (ScvO$_2$), should be monitored with a goal level of 70% or greater.

Fluid Resuscitation Refer to Section Three for general fluid resuscitation information. Although measuring central venous pressure (CVP) is not the most ideal method for the measurement of fluid status, it remains a useful target in the initial treatment of septic shock. In the septic patient, the goal is to raise the CVP to greater than 8 mmHg (or greater than 12 mmHg in mechanically ventilated patients to account for increased thoracic pressures) (Cawcutt & Peters, 2014; Han et al., 2015). End points of fluid resuscitation in the treatment of sepsis remain controversial because it is now recognized that normalization of hemodynamic parameters does not guarantee normalization of the microperfusion—that is, tissue hypoperfusion may continue after hypotension has been corrected. Therefore, other targets of early resuscitation for sepsis include ScvO$_2$, MAP, and serum lactate; they are important to consider and should be monitored closely for trends indicating end-organ perfusion states (Cawcutt & Peters, 2014). That said, a major goal of fluid resuscitation is to relieve hypotension, as evidenced by a MAP greater than 65 mmHg (Dellinger et al., 2013).

Pharmacotherapy Interventions If fluid administration fails to relieve hypotension and restore organ perfusion, vasopressor or inotropic agents are usually initiated. Norepinephrine is a vasopressor that increases MAP by its vasoconstrictive actions but has little change in the heart rate and stroke volume. It is the first-choice vasopressor in the treatment of septic shock that is unresponsive to fluid resuscitation (Dellinger et al., 2013). Dobutamine, a sympathomimetic inotropic agent, is a second-line agent that is sometimes used in the treatment of septic shock to improve CO and splanchnic perfusion. Vasopressor and inotropic drug groups are presented in detail in Section Four.

Corticosteroid Therapy. Corticosteroids may be considered for patients with septic shock who have not responded adequately to fluid resuscitation and vasopressor therapy. The use of low-dose hydrocortisone for rapid reversal of shock can reduce the amount of time the patient requires vasopressors. The effectiveness of corticosteroids in sepsis to reduce long-term mortality remains controversial. In a substudy conducted by Povoa et al. (2015), the authors concluded that the use of systemic steroids for treating sepsis should not be used systematically. Moreover, there was no noticeable positive impact found from the intravenous use of steroids.

Activated Protein C. Research into the pathophysiologic processes involved in sepsis and septic shock has highlighted the role of the coagulation cascade. A key feature of this pathophysiology is microscopic clots that occlude blood flow to organs. Under normal circumstances, these clots are degraded by the body's fibrinolytic system. However, during septic shock, activated protein C (APC), a key component of fibrinolysis, is consumed at such a rate that clot dissolution is impeded. APC not only plays a role in the coagulation cascade but also has anti-inflammatory properties. Repletion of the stores of APC showed promise in the treatment of septic shock; for a number of years APC was available as drotrecogin alfa (Xigris) and was widely recommended for use with severe sepsis and septic shock. In 2011, it was withdrawn from the market because it failed to show any benefit to patient survival (Han et al., 2015; U.S. Food and Drug Administration, 2011).

Other Supportive Interventions The complex care inherent in managing the patient in septic shock is distinctly an interprofessional team effort. The nurse plays a pivotal role in minute-to-minute management at the bedside, seeing to the patient's physical and psychosocial needs and efficiently and accurately carrying out orders based on best-practice guidelines. The nurse monitors the many physiologic and laboratory parameters and their trends, interpreting the results and consulting with other team members as needed. The nurse also monitors the patient for therapeutic and nontherapeutic effects of interventions and closely monitors for the physiologic effects of the drug therapies.

Section Seven Review

1. The various forms of distributive shock have which characteristic in common?
   A. Endothelial injury
   B. Massive vasodilation
   C. Constriction of vascular smooth muscle
   D. Loss of sympathetic nervous system response

2. Which pathophysiologic events are characteristics of septic shock? (Select all that apply.)
   A. Altered fluid volume
   B. Increased capillary permeability
   C. Inhibition of inflammatory mediators
   D. Maldistribution of circulating volume
   E. Vasoconstriction

3. Which factor separates sepsis from septic shock?
   A. Bands greater than 10%
   B. Fever greater than 39.4°C (103°F)
   C. Sepsis interventions no longer effective
   D. WBC count greater than 12,000/mL or less than 4,000/mL

4. A client with septic shock has a high CO and tachycardia. The nurse recognizes that this combination of clinical signs suggests which type of shock?
   A. Hyperdynamic shock
   B. Hypodynamic shock
   C. Mild septic shock
   D. Severe septic shock

Answers: 1. B, 2. (A, B, D), 3. C, 4. A

Section Eight: Distributive Shock—Neurogenic and Anaphylactic

While both neurogenic and anaphylactic shock develop secondary to widespread vasodilation, the mechanisms by which vasodilation occurs are different, and the management of each form has unique features.

Neurogenic Shock

Neurogenic shock is associated with acute spinal cord injury (SCI), which most commonly results from blunt trauma injury to the cord. However, nontraumatic causes are also possible, such as tumors, disk degeneration, and inflammation/infection. Acute SCI is presented in detail in Chapter 20 and will not be discussed here.

Related Pathophysiology Two types of shock result from spinal cord injury: spinal shock and neurogenic shock. It is important to be able to differentiate them.

Spinal Shock. Spinal shock is the temporary loss of spinal reflex activity that develops below the level of cord injury. It is characterized by sensorimotor function loss, hypertension followed by hypotension, and flaccid paralysis that includes the bladder and bowel (Oropello, Mistry, & Ullman, 2015). Spinal shock, while temporary, can end within hours or last for weeks, resolving when the spinal reflex arc function returns.

Neurogenic Shock. When the spinal cord is injured above the midthoracic region (usually above T6), impulses from the sympathetic nervous system cannot reach the arterioles, resulting in unopposed vagal stimulation and loss of vasomotor tone (Oropello et al., 2015; Zuckerbraun et al., 2015). The loss of sympathetic innervation prohibits vasoconstriction of blood vessels, but blood vessels continue to receive parasympathetic innervation, allowing vasodilation. Blood then pools in the dilated peripheral venous system, creating a relative hypovolemia. The right heart receives an inadequate venous return, and cardiac output (CO) decreases. The hypovolemic state results in hypoperfusion to the spinal cord, further damaging the cord.

Clinical Manifestations In neurogenic shock, signs and symptoms are related to lost sympathetic innervation and unopposed parasympathetic innervation. There is a triad of expected signs: hypotension, bradycardia, and hypothermia. Persistent vasodilation leads to decreased systemic vascular resistance (SVR). The pooling of blood in dilated vessels results in diminished venous return, producing a low CVP and BP. The unopposed parasympathetic innervation to the heart causes bradycardia and also prevents compensatory reflex tachycardia as a response to the relative hypovolemia, and cardiac dysrhythmias may occur (Zuckerbraun et al., 2015). If the patient has a pulmonary artery catheter in place, the hemodynamic parameters would show a low SVR, RAP, PAP, PAWP, and CO. Peripheral vasodilation produces warm skin; however, sweating is absent below the level of the spinal cord injury.

Treatment The treatment goals for neurogenic shock are to maintain stability of the spine, optimize oxygen delivery, and restore intravascular volume. Continuous cardiac monitoring is required; if marked bradycardia occurs, medications to increase heart rate may be given. The patient's airway and mechanical ventilation support may

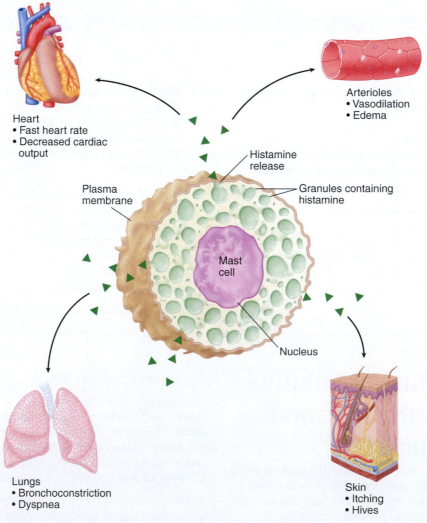

Heart
• Fast heart rate
• Decreased cardiac output

Arterioles
• Vasodilation
• Edema

Histamine release

Plasma membrane

Granules containing histamine

Mast cell

Nucleus

Lungs
• Bronchoconstriction
• Dyspnea

Skin
• Itching
• Hives

Figure 37–5 Pathophysiologic response to anaphylaxis.

Table 37–9 Example of a Drug Regimen for an Adult in Anaphylactic Shock

Drugs	Suggested Dosages	Purposes
Epinephrine (adrenergic agonist)	0.3–0.5 mg (0.3 to 0.5 mL 1:1000), IM in thigh IV route if IM injections not effective; suggested dose 100 mcg of 1:100,000 dilution; dilute 0.1 mL of 1:1000 in 10 mL NS; deliver over 5–10 min.	First-line therapy. Given immediately to restore vascular tone and blood pressure. Repeat every 5 minutes PRN.
Methylprednisolone (corticosteroid)	125 mg IV	Severe allergic reaction. Given to reverse allergic response; inhibits release of allergic substances.
Prednisone (corticosteroid)	60 mg PO	Mild allergic reaction. Given to reverse allergic response; inhibits release of allergic substances.
Diphenhydramine (H_1 histamine antagonist)	50 mg IV	Given to reverse allergic response by blocking histamine release at H_1 receptor sites.
Ranitidine (H_2 histamine antagonist)	50 mg IV	Given to reverse allergic response by blocking histamine release at H_2 receptor sites.
Albuterol (β-agonist)	2.5 mg inhaled	Bronchodilation
Ipratropium bromide (anticholinergic) and magnesium (electrolyte)	Ipratropium: 250 mcg inhaled Magnesium: 2 g IV (over 20–30 min)	Bronchodilation; used when bronchospasm is refractory to B-agonist therapy.

SOURCE: Data from Stern et al. (2014) and Wilson et al. (2016).

require protection, depending on the location of the spinal cord injury and the patient's general condition.

Anaphylactic Shock

Anaphylactic shock is a severe systemic allergic reaction to allergens such as foods (e.g., peanuts, fish, eggs, and milk), drugs (e.g., nonsteroidal anti-inflammatory drugs, antibiotics, and anesthetic agents), blood products, insect venom, and latex.

Related Pathophysiology Anaphylactic shock is predominantly a severe type I (anaphylactic) hypersensitivity response involving immunoglobulin IgE and mast cells. Massive amounts of vasoactive substances (e.g., histamine and kinins) are released from mast cells (Figure 37–5), flooding the circulation with mediators and leading to systemic vasodilation and increased capillary permeability. Vasodilation increases the size of the intravascular compartment, while increased capillary permeability allows fluid to shift from the blood vessels into the interstitium, resulting in potentially life-threatening edema. As fluid is lost from the vascular compartment, a relative hypovolemia develops. The net consequences of combined massive vasodilation and increased capillary permeability are a decrease in venous return, decrease in CO, and decrease in oxygen delivery.

Clinical Manifestations Severe anaphylactic shock frequently involves multiple organ systems, but the most life-threatening are those involving the cardiovascular and pulmonary systems. Anaphylactic shock can develop rapidly (5–30 min) or slowly (6–12 hours); however, rapid onset is often the most life-threatening because it makes seeking emergency medical attention difficult, if not impossible. Typical manifestations include hypotension, upper-airway obstruction (from angioedema, tongue or laryngeal edema, and laryngospasm), flushing, urticaria and pruritus, abdominal cramping, and diarrhea (Boyce & Austen, 2015; Stern, Cifu, & Altkorn, 2014). Severe upper-airway obstruction is the greatest threat as it can lead to rapid asphyxiation and death (Stern et al., 2014).

Treatment The immediate goals for treatment of anaphylactic shock are to maintain an airway and support blood pressure. Oxygen is administered as needed based on pulse oximetry readings. Early intubation is recommended if the patient develops respiratory distress, as waiting until upper-airway edema becomes severe makes intubation more difficult (Boyce & Austen, 2015). If the patient is hypotensive, aggressive fluid resuscitation is required to restore vascular volume. Drug therapies are the mainstay of stopping the hypersensitivity response and reversing manifestations. Table 37–9 lists drugs commonly used in the treatment of anaphylactic shock. Additional supportive therapies are initiated as needed to support the patient and treat specific clinical problems.

Section Eight Review

1. A client with a T5 spinal cord injury is in neurogenic shock. The nurse is aware that this type of shock results from which mechanism?
   A. Unopposed parasympathetic nervous system stimulation
   B. Loss of spinal reflex activity
   C. Overstimulation of the sympathetic nervous system
   D. Loss of vagal stimulation activity

2. The nurse is preparing to assess a client experiencing neurogenic shock. Which vital signs should the nurse anticipate?
   A. BP 132/74
   B. HR 53 bpm
   C. RR 14/min
   D. Temp 37.9°C (100.2°F)

3. Anaphylactic shock involves the interplay of what factors? (Select all that apply.)
   A. Immunoglobulin IgA
   B. Mast cells
   C. Immunoglobulin IgE
   D. Lymphocytes
   E. Immunoglobulin IgM

4. Anaphylactic shock is associated with increased capillary permeability. Based on this particular pathophysiologic problem, which assessment should the nurse focus on immediately?
   A. Severe diarrhea
   B. Respiratory distress
   C. Cardiac dysrhythmias
   D. Urticaria and pruritus

Answers: 1. A, 2. B, 3. (B, C), 4. B

Section Nine: Obstructive Shock States

Obstructive shock states occur as a result of a mechanical barrier to blood flow that blocks oxygen delivery to tissues. The major causes of obstructive shock states are pulmonary embolism, tension pneumothorax, and cardiac tamponade. All three are profiled here and discussed in detail in their respective chapters: pulmonary embolism, Chapter 11; tension pneumothorax, Chapter 34; and cardiac tamponade, Chapter 14.

Pulmonary Embolism

Pulmonary embolism refers to a clot, air, or tissue that obstructs blood flow through any part of the lungs. Pulmonary embolism can range from clinically unimportant thromboembolism to massive embolism with sudden death.

Related Pathophysiology   Hypercoagulability leads to the formation of thrombi in the deep veins of the legs, pelvis, or arms. The thrombi dislodge and embolize (cause an embolism), flowing with venous blood returning to the right heart and into the pulmonary artery blood flow via the vena cava. The affected pulmonary arteries become obstructed, which results in impaired gas exchange due to an increase in alveolar dead space and a ventilation–perfusion mismatch. Obstruction of the pulmonary arteries also causes right ventricular dysfunction. As blood flow becomes obstructed, hypoxia and pulmonary vasoconstriction result in increased pulmonary vascular resistance (PVR). Increased PVR forces the right heart to work harder to push blood into the lungs, leading to right heart strain. As right ventricular afterload increases, right ventricular dysfunction can occur. Shock states can develop because of impaired gas exchange and cardiac dysfunction, which compromise oxygen delivery. A massive pulmonary embolism rapidly leads to cardiovascular collapse and death.

Clinical Manifestations   The presenting signs and symptoms of pulmonary embolism are variable, making rapid diagnosis difficult. Dyspnea is the most frequent symptom, tachypnea the most frequent sign. Other common signs and symptoms include pleuritic pain, cough, wheezing, crackles, and tachycardia, and the patient may have evidence of a deep vein thrombosis (DVT) (unilateral leg pain and swelling); however, a DVT is present in less than one third of patients who present with a PE (Saha & Rao, 2014). Arterial blood gases (ABGs) may be normal or may indicate hypoxemia or hypercapnia. In patients with right ventricular failure caused by a large pulmonary embolism, echocardiography will show right ventricular enlargement and pulmonary hypertension. Perfusion lung scans, pulmonary angiography, spiral CT of the chest with contrast, or transthoracic echocardiography may be used in the diagnostic workup.

Treatment   The cornerstone of management for pulmonary embolism is early initiation of anticoagulant therapy (usually heparin) because it prevents additional thrombi from forming and permits fibrinolysis to dissolve some of the clot (Saha & Rao, 2014). Inferior vena cava filters may be used in the presence of active hemorrhage, contraindications to anticoagulation, or recurrent pulmonary embolism despite intensive prolonged anticoagulation (Saha & Rao, 2014). In the presence of hemodynamic instability and obstructive shock, the use of thrombolytic therapy or emergency surgical embolectomy may be necessary.

Tension Pneumothorax

Tension pneumothorax is the collapse of an area of the lung caused by increased pressure within the thoracic cavity. It usually results from a penetrating chest wound; however, it can also result from an internal lung problem, such as a burst bleb in a patient with chronic obstructive pulmonary disease (COPD).

Related Pathophysiology   A tension pneumothorax occurs when air enters the pleural space during inspiration but cannot leave during expiration (like a one-way valve). The progressive accumulation of air within the thoracic cavity leads to a shift of the mediastinal structures and compression of the opposite lung and soft tissues on the affected side (e.g., great vessels and heart). The increased pleural pressure impedes venous return and serves as a barrier to O_2 delivery.

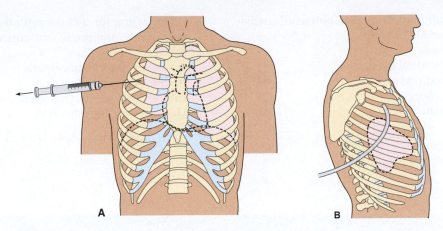

Figure 37–6 Needle thoracostomy. May be used in the emergency treatment of a tension pneumothorax. **A,** A large-gauge needle is introduced, and air and fluid are aspirated. **B,** Alternatively, a chest tube may be inserted and connected to a chest drainage system.

Clinical Manifestations   Increased pleural pressure as a result of a tension pneumothorax puts direct pressure on the heart, vena cava, and contralateral lung, which decreases venous return and CO. The patient typically experiences chest pain and air hunger and develops respiratory distress. Lung sounds will be absent on the affected side. As intrathoracic pressure increases, tracheal deviation may develop.

Treatment   For a tension pneumothorax, a healthcare provider decompresses trapped air with the insertion of a 14-gauge needle or a chest tube (Figure 37–6). The procedure is called a needle thoracostomy.

Cardiac Tamponade

Cardiac tamponade refers to pressure exerted on the heart that compresses the heart wall and restricts heart actions. It is a medical emergency.

Related Pathophysiology   Cardiac tamponade usually develops secondary to an accumulation of fluid, such as blood, in the pericardial sac. Chest trauma, blunt or penetrating, is the most common cause. As fluid in the sac accumulates, the heart chambers become compressed and cannot adequately fill, causing a significant decrease in CO. If CO becomes too compromised, cardiovascular collapse and death follow.

Clinical Manifestations   **Pulsus paradoxus** is one of the classic signs of cardiac tamponade. It is an exaggerated decrease (greater than 10 mmHg) of the systolic blood pressure during inspiration. Increased pericardial fluid may produce distant heart sounds. In tamponade, right arterial pressure (RAP) is usually elevated and is equaled by the pulmonary artery wedge pressure (PAWP). Beck's triad—elevated RAP, decreased blood pressure, and muffled heart sounds—may be present.

Treatment   Volume resuscitation may be initiated as preparations are made for the emergency removal of the pericardial fluid (pericardiocentesis). Needle pericardiocentesis is performed to rapidly decompress the pericardium; a long needle is inserted between the ribs into the pericardial sac, and the fluid is drawn off. The decompression should improve the heart's pumping ability at least temporarily; however, in severe cases, particularly if bleeding into the pericardial sac continues, a thoracotomy may be required to surgically control and decompress the tamponade.

Section Nine Review

1. In early management of pulmonary embolism, which drug is the highest priority to initiate?
   A. Dobutamine
   B. Morphine
   C. Aspirin
   D. Heparin

2. Which pathophysiologic mechanism is involved in tension pneumothorax?
   A. Air enters the thoracic cavity but cannot escape.
   B. Fluid accumulates in the pleural sac, compressing lung tissue.
   C. Increased pulmonary vascular resistance exerts pressure on lung tissue.
   D. Blood enters the thoracic cavity and compresses soft intrathoracic structures.

3. What are the major clinical manifestations of cardiac tamponade? (Select all that apply.)
   A. Pulsus paradoxus
   B. Decreased right atrial pressure
   C. Decreased blood pressure
   D. Muffled heart sounds
   E. Severe chest pain

4. When caring for a client who has developed cardiac tamponade, the nurse can anticipate which priority emergency action?
   A. Needle pericardiocentesis
   B. Surgical decompression
   C. Cardiopulmonary resuscitation
   D. IV vasopressor therapy

Answers: 1. A, 2. A, 3. (A, C, D), 4. A

Clinical Reasoning Checkpoint

Mr. H is an 82-year-old man admitted to the hospital from a nursing home with a diagnosis of urosepsis. Urine cultures revealed gram-negative bacteria, and he was started on Bactrim. He continued to be febrile despite antibiotic therapy. After 72 hours he was transferred to the ICU because of his declining mental status. He was intubated and placed on mechanical ventilation. Despite multiple fluid boluses and a norepinephrine infusion (5μg/min), his mean arterial pressure remains less than 60 mmHg.

1. Identify the functional classification of shock pertinent to Mr. H.

2. Describe the mechanism of impaired oxygenation for this shock state in this patient.

3. Describe the compensatory mechanisms that occurred in response to this shock state.

4. What stage of compensatory shock is Mr. H in?

5. What are the nursing implications for the patient receiving norepinephrine?

6. What other collaborative interventions may be initiated upon Mr. H's admission to the ICU?

Chapter 37 Review

1. A client is in refractory shock. What information should the nurse provide to the family?
   1. "You should prepare yourself for your loved one's death."
   2. "Recovery will be rapid once we complete fluid resuscitation."
   3. "Your loved one will be hospitalized for at least a week during this recovery."
   4. "Treatment will be prolonged and may not be successful."

2. A client who had abdominal surgery yesterday is cold, clammy, and confused. Which additional assessment findings would support concern that this client is in shock? (Select all that apply.)
   1. Pulse rapid and weak
   2. Arterial pH 7.49
   3. Serum lactate level 5.8 mmol/L
   4. Base excess 1 mmol/L
   5. BP 88/50 mmHg

3. A client having chest pain is being monitored for myocardial infarction. Which finding would the nurse evaluate as indicating the client is at risk for developing cardiogenic shock?
   1. The client did not take aspirin prior to presenting at the emergency department.
   2. The client has started having increased premature ventricular contractions.
   3. The client's temperature has risen to 37.7°C (99.8°F).
   4. The client is nauseated.

4. A client who had a myocardial infarction yesterday was pain free until 15 minutes ago. The client now says the pain is like it was when he originally came to the emergency department. Which assessments should the nurse conduct? (Select all that apply.)
   1. Auscultate bowel sounds.
   2. Palpate for cardiac lifts or heaves.
   3. Auscultate breath sounds.
   4. Evaluate cardiac rhythm.
   5. Review urinary output measurements.

5. A client has hypovolemic shock as a result of massive gastrointestinal bleeding. The client is given fluids and vasopressors. Which outcome indicates to the nurse that these treatments are having the desired effect?

   1. Base deficit is –6 mmol.

   2. Lactate levels are decreasing from admission levels.

   3. Urine output is normal.

   4. Blood pressure is now 90/60 mmHg.

6. A client in septic shock has been prescribed a vasopressor medication. Which assessment finding would the nurse evaluate as indicating the need to question this order?

   1. The client's mentation has not improved.

   2. The client's heart rate is 50 bpm.

   3. The client's urine output for the last hour was 10 mL.

   4. The client's breath sounds include crackles.

7. A client in septic shock is given IV insulin therapy. The nurse would increase this infusion if which blood glucose level was measured? (Select all that apply.)

   1. 110 mg/dL

   2. 136 mg/dL

   3. 156 mg/dL

   4. 184 mg/dL

   5. 200 mg/dL

8. A client is received in the emergency department from emergency medical services after sustaining a brain injury in a fall. She is on a spineboard and has a cervical collar in place. She is not moving her lower extremities. What would alert the nurse to the possible development of neurogenic shock?

   1. The client reports that she feels a tingling sensation in her lower extremities.

   2. The client's heart rate drops from 82 bpm to 68 bpm.

   3. The client's blood glucose is 134 mg/dL.

   4. The client's friend reports that the client was unconscious for a "few seconds" after the fall.

9. A client with a long history of chronic obstructive pulmonary disease (COPD) presents to the emergency department in respiratory distress. After assessing absence of lung sounds on the right and tracheal deviation, the nurse notifies the ED physician. What emergency intervention should the nurse anticipate?

   1. Intubation and mechanical ventilation

   2. Needle thoracostomy

   3. Administration of furosemide

   4. Pericardiocentesis

10. A client is receiving intravenous dobutamine, which the nurse is titrating to effect. Which assessment findings would indicate the need to reduce the rate of infusion? (Select all that apply.)

    1. The client complains of chest pain.

    2. The client's heart rate is 110 bpm.

    3. The client begins having ventricular dysrhythmias.

    4. The client's blood pressure is 160/110 mmHg.

    5. The client complains of headache.

Answers to questions found inside your textbook are available on the faculty resources site. Please consult with your instructor.

References

Adams, M. P., Holland, L. N., & Urban, C. Q. (2014). *Pharmacology for nurses: A pathophysiologic approach* (4th ed.). Hoboken, NJ: Pearson.

Alhazzani, W., Alshahrani, M., Jaeschke, R., Forel, J. M., Papazian, L., Sevransky, J., & Meade, M. O. (2013). Neuromuscular blocking agents in acute respiratory distress syndrome: A systematic review and meta-analysis of randomized controlled trials. *Critical Care, 17*(2), R43. doi:10.1186/cc12557

Alarcon, L. H., & Fink, M. P. (2014). Physiologic monitoring of the surgical patient. In F. Brunicardi, D. K. Andersen, T. R. Billiar, D. L. Dunn, J. G. Hunter, J. B. Matthews, & R. E. Pollock (Eds.), *Schwartz's principles of surgery* (10th ed.). New York, NY: McGraw-Hill.

Angappan, S., Parida, S., Vasudevan, A., & Badhe, A. S. (2015). The comparison of stroke volume variation with central venous pressure in predicting fluid responsiveness in septic patients with acute circulatory failure. *Indian Journal of Critical Care Medicine: Peer-Reviewed, Official Publication of Indian Society of Critical Care Medicine, 19*(7), 394–400. http://doi.org/10.4103/0972-5229.160278

Arroliga, A., Frutos-Vivar, F., Hall, J., Esteban, A., Apezteguía, C., Soto, L., & Anzueto, A. (2005). Use of sedatives and neuromuscular blockers in a cohort of patients receiving mechanical ventilation. *Chest, 128*(2), 496–506.

Badawi, O., Waite, M. D., Fuhrman, S. A., & Zuckerman, I. H. (2012). Association between intensive care unit-acquired dysglycemia and in-hospital mortality. *Critical Care Medicine 40*, 3180–88.

Basra, S. S., Loyalka, K., & Kar, B. (2011). Current status of percutaneous ventricular assist devices for cardiogenic shock. *Current Opinion in Cardiology, 26*(6), 548–554. doi:10.1097/HCO.0b013e32834b803c

Bone, R. C., Balk, R. A., Cerra, F. B., Dellinger, R. P., Fein, A. M., Knaus, W. A., . . . Sibbald, W. J. (1992). Definitions for sepsis and organ failure and guidelines for the use of innovative therapies in sepsis. The ACCP/SCCM Consensus Conference Committee. American College of Chest Physicians/Society of Critical Care Medicine. *Chest, 101*(6), 864–874.

Boyce, A., & Austen, K. (2015). Allergies, anaphylaxis, and systemic mastocytosis. In D. Kasper, A. Fauci, S. Hauser, D. Longo, J. Jameson, & Loscalzo, J. (Eds.), *Harrison's principles of internal medicine* (19th ed.). Retrieved September 24, 2015, from http://accessmedicine.mhmedical.com.ezproxy.uky.edu/content.aspx?bookid=1130&Sectionid=79749806

Burchum, J., & Rosenthal, L. (2015). *Lehne's pharmacology for nursing care* (9th ed.). St. Louis, MO: Saunders/Elsevier.

Cawcutt, K. A., & Peters, S. G. (2014). Severe sepsis and septic shock clinical overview and update on management. *Mayo Clinic Proceedings, 89*(11), 1572–1578.

Curtis, J. P., Rathore, S. S., Wang, Y., Chen, J., Nallamothu, B. K., & Krumholz, H. M. (2012). Use and effectiveness of intra-aortic balloon pumps among patients undergoing high risk percutaneous coronary intervention: Insights from the National Cardiovascular Data Registry. *Circulation Cardiovascular Qualitative Outcomes, 5*, 21–30.

De Backer, D., & Durand, A. (2014). Monitoring the microcirculation in critically ill patients. *Best Practice and Research: Clinical Anaesthesiology, 28*(4), 441–451.

De Backer, D., Orbegozo, C. D., Donadello, K., & Vincent, J. L. (2014). Pathophysiology of microcirculatory dysfunction and the pathogenesis of septic shock. *Virulence, 5*, 73–79.

Dellinger, R. P., Levy, M. M., Rhodes, A., Annane, D., Gerlach, H., Opal, S. M., . . . Moreno, R. (2013). Surviving Sepsis Campaign: International guidelines for management of severe sepsis and septic shock—2012. *Critical Care Medicine, 41*(2), 580–637.

Edul, V. S., Ince, C., & Dubin, A. (2016). What is circulatory shock? *Current Opinion in Critical Care, 21*, 245–252.

Felner, K., & Smith, R. L. (2012). Chapter 138. Sepsis. In S. C. McKean, J. J. Ross, D. D. Dressler, D. J. Brotman, & J. S. Ginsberg (Eds.), *Principles and practice of hospital medicine.* Retrieved September 22, 2015, from http://accessmedicine.mhmedical.com.ezproxy.uky.edu/content.aspx?bookid=496&Sectionid=41304118

Gahart, B. L., Nazareno, A. R., & Ortega, M. Q. (2016). *Gahart's 2016 intravenous medications: A handbook for nurses and health professionals* (32nd ed.) St. Louis, MO: Elsevier.

Ghane, M. R., Gharib, M., Ebrahimi, A., Saeedi, M., Akbari-Kamrani, M., Rezaee, M., & Rasouli, H. (2015). Accuracy of early rapid ultrasound in shock (RUSH) examination performed by emergency physician for diagnosis of shock etiology in critically ill patients. *Journal of Emergency Trauma Shock, 8*(1), 5–10. doi:10.5812/traumamon.20095

Gomez, A. M., & Umpierrez, G. E. (2014). Continuous glucose monitoring in insulin-treated patients in non-ICU settings. *Journal of Diabetes Science Technology, 8*(5), 930–936.

Hall, J. E. (2015). Pituitary hormones and their control by the hypothalamus. In J. E. Hall, *Guyton and Hall textbook of medical physiology* (13th ed.). St. Louis, MO: Elsevier/Saunders.

Han, J., Cribbs, S. K., & Martin, G. S. (2015). Sepsis, severe sepsis, and septic shock. In J. B. Hall, G. A. Schmidt, & J. P. Kress (Eds.), *Principles of critical care* (4th ed.). Retrieved September 22, 2015, from http://accessmedicine.mhmedical.com.ezproxy.uky.edu/content.aspx?bookid=1340&Sectionid=80033910

Helmerhorst, H. J., Schultz, M. J., van der Voort, P. H. J., de Jonge, E., & van Westerloo, D. J. (2015). Bench-to-bedside review: The effects of hyperoxia during critical illness. *Critical Care, 19*(1), 284. doi:10.1186/s13054-015-0996-4

Hochman, J. S., & Ingbar, D. H. (2015). Cardiogenic shock and pulmonary edema. In D. Kasper, A. Fauci, S. Hauser, D. Longo, J. Jameson, & J. Loscalzo (Eds.), *Harrison's principles of internal medicine* (19th ed.). Retrieved September 17, 2015, from http://accessmedicine.mhmedical/content.aspx?bookid=1130&Sectionid=79745930

Hollenberg, S. M. (2011). Vasoactive drugs in circulatory shock. *American Journal of Respiratory & Critical Care Medicine, 183*, 847–855.

Hollenberg, S. M. (2013). Hemodynamic monitoring. *Chest, 143*(5), 1480–1488.

Holler, H., Urlesberger, B., Mileder, L., Baik, N., Schwaberger, B., & Pichler, G. (2015). Peripheral muscle near-infrared spectroscopy in neonates: Ready for clinical use? A systematic qualitative review of the literature. *Neonatology, 108*, 233–245. doi:10.1159/000433515

Holst, L. B., Haase, N., Wettersley, J., Wernerman, J., Guttormsen, A. B., Karlsson, S., . . . for the TRISS Trial Group and the Scandinavian Critical Care Trials Group. (2014). Lower versus higher hemoglobin threshold for transfusion in septic shock. *The New England Journal of Medicine, 371*(15), 1383–1391.

Hraiech, S., Dizier, S., & Papazian, L. (2014). The use of paralytics in patients with acute respiratory distress syndrome. *Clinical Chest Medicine, 35*, 753–763.

Ince, C. (2014). The rationale for microcirculatory guided fluid therapy. *Current Opinion in Critical Care, 20*, 301–308.

Jung, C., & Kelm, M. (2015). Evaluation of the microcirculation in critically ill patients. *Clinical Hemorheology Microcirculation, 61*(2), 213–224.

Kee, J. L. (2014). *Laboratory and diagnostic tests with nursing implications* (9th ed.). Hoboken, NJ: Pearson.

Khan, M. H., Corbett, B. J., & Hollenberg, S. M. (2014). Mechanical circulatory support in acute cardiogenic shock. *F1000Prime Reports, 6*, 91. http://doi.org/10.12703/P6-91

Kress J. P., & Hall, J. B. (2013). Chapter 50: Pain control, sedation, and neuromuscular blockade. In M. J. Tobin (Ed.), *Principles and practice of mechanical ventilation* (3rd ed.). Retrieved September 11, 2015, from http://accessmedicine.mhmedical.com.ezproxy.uky.edu/content.aspx?bookid=520&Sectionid=41692297

Levy, B., Bastien, O., Benjelid, K., Cariou, A., Chouihed, T., Combes, A., . . . Kuteifan, K. (2015). Experts' recommendations for the management of adult patients with cardiogenic shock. *Annals of Intensive Care, 5*(17). doi:10.1186/s13613-015-0052-1

Liu, D., Su, L., Han, G., Yan, P., & Xie, L. (2015). Prognostic value of procalcitonin in adult patients with sepsis: A systematic review and meta-analysis. *PLoS ONE, 10*(6). doi:10.137.1371/journal.pone.0129450

Lonardo, N. W., Mone, M. C., Nirula, R., Kimball, E. J., Ludwig, K., Zhou, X., . . . Barton, R. G. (2014). Propofol is associated with favorable outcomes compared with benzodiazepines in ventilated intensive care unit patients. *American Journal of Respiratory and Critical Care Medicine. 189*(11), 1383–1394.

Mehta, R. H., Lopes, R. D., Ballotta, A., Frigiola, A., Sketch Jr., M. H., Bossone, E., & Bates, E. R. (2010). Percutaneous coronary intervention or coronary artery bypass surgery for cardiogenic shock and multivessel coronary artery disease? *American Heart Journal, 159*(1), 141–147.

Nicks, B. A., & Gaillard, J. (2016). Approach to shock. In J. E. Tintinalli, J. Stapczynski, O. Ma, D. M. Yealy, G. D. Meckler, & D. M. Cline (Eds.), *Tintinalli's emergency medicine: A comprehensive study guide,* (8th ed.). New York, NY: McGraw-Hill. Retrieved July 5, 2017, from http://accessemergencymedicine.mhmedical.com .ezproxy.uky.edu/content.aspx?bookid=1658&sectionid =109384946

Orbegozo, C. D., Puflea, F., De Backer, D., Creteur, J., & Vincent, J. L. (2015) Near infrared spectroscopy (NIRS) to assess the effects of local ischemic preconditioning in the muscle of healthy volunteers and critically ill patients. *Microvascular Research, 102,* 25–32. doi:10.1016/j.mvr.2015.08.002

Oropello, J. M., Mistry, N., & Ullman, J. S. (2015). Spinal injuries. In J. B. Hall, G. A. Schmidt, & J. P. Kress (Eds.), *Principles of critical care* (4th ed.). Retrieved September 24, 2015, from http://accessmedicine.mhmedical.com .ezproxy.uky.edu/content.aspx?bookid=1340&Sectio nid=80027179

Pandharipande, P. P., Girard, T. D., Jackson, J. C., Morandi. A., Thompson, J. L., Pun, B. T., . . . Ely, E. W. (2013). Long-term cognitive impairment after critical illness. *New England Journal of Medicine, 369*(14), 1306–1316. doi:10.1056/NEJMoa1301372

Papazian, L., Forel, J. M., Gacouin, A., Penot-Ragon, C., Perrin, G., Loundou, A., . . . Roch, A. (2010). Neuromuscular blockers in early acute respiratory distress syndrome. *New England Journal of Medicine, 363*(12), 1107–1116.

Pinsky, M. R. (2014) Assessing the circulation: Oximetry, indicator dilution, and pulse contour analysis. In J. B. Hall, G. A. Schmidt, & J. P. Kress (Eds.), *Principles of critical care (4th ed.).* New York, NY: McGraw-Hill. Retrieved April 04, 2017, from http://accessmedicine .mhmedical.com.ezproxy.uky.edu/content.aspx?bookid =1340&Sectionid=80030766

Pollard, S., Edwin, S. B., & Alaniz, C. (2015). Vasopressor and inotropic management of patients with septic shock. *Pharmacy and Therapeutics, 40*(7), 438–450.

Povoa, P., Salluh, J. I., Martinez, M L., Guillamat-Prats, R., Gallup, D., Al-Khalidi, H. R., . . . Artigas, A. (2015). Clinical impact of stress dose steroids in patients with septic shock: Insights from the PROWESS-Shock trial. *Critical Care, 19*(1), 193–203.

Puthucheary, Z., Rawal, J., Ratnayake, G., Harridge, S., Montgomery, H., & Hart, N. (2012). Neuromuscular blockade and skeletal muscle weakness in critically ill patients. *American Journal of Respiratory and Critical Care Medicine, 185*(9), 911–917.

Rhodes, A., Evans, L., Alhazzani, W., Levy, M. M., Antonelli, M., Ferrer, R., . . . Dellinger, R. P. (2017). Surviving Sepsis Campaign: International Guidelines for Management of Severe Sepsis and Septic Shock: 2016. *Intensive Care Medicine, 43*(3), 304–377.

Rihal, C. S., Naidu, S. S., Givertz, M., M., Szeto, W. Y., Burke, J. A., Kapur, N. K., . . . Tu, T. (2015). 2015 SCAI/ACC/HFSA/STS clinical expert consensus statement on the use of percutaneous mechanical circulatory support devices in cardiovascular care. *Journal of the American College of Cardiology, 65*(19), e7–e26.

Sabatine, M. S. (2014). *Pocket medicine: The Massachusetts General Hospital handbook of internal medicine* (5th ed.). Philadelphia, PA: Wolters Kluwer/Lippincott Williams & Wilkins.

Saha, S. A., & Rao, R. K. (2014). Chapter 29: Pulmonary embolic disease. In M. H. Crawford (Ed.), *Current diagnosis & treatment: Cardiology* (4th ed.). Retrieved September 25, 2015, from http://accessmedicine .mhmedical.com.ezproxy.uky.edu/content.aspx?bookid =715&Sectionid=48214563

Serpa Neto, A., Nassar, A. P., Cardoso, S. O., Manetta, J. A., Pereira, V. G., Espósito, D. C., . . . Russell, J. A. (2012). Vasopressin and terlipressin in adult vasodilatory shock: A systematic review and meta-analysis of nine randomized controlled trials. *Critical Care, 16*(4), R154. http://doi.org/10.1186/cc11469

Sterling, S. A., Puskarich, M. A., Shapiro, N. I., Trzeciak, S., Kline, J. A., Summers, R. L., & Jones, A. E. (2013). Characteristics and outcomes of patients with vasoplegic versus tissue dysoxic septic shock. *Shock, 40*(1), 11–14. doi:10.1097/SHK.0b013e318298836d

Stern, S. C., Cifu, A. S., & Altkorn, D. (2014). Hypotension. In S. C. Stern, A. S. Cifu, & D. Altkorn (Eds.), *Symptom to diagnosis: An evidence-based guide* (3rd ed.). Retrieved September 24, 2015, from http://accessmedicine .mhmedical.com.ezproxy.uky.edu/content.aspx?bookid =1088&Sectionid=61699701

Tachon, G., Harrois, A., Tanaka, S., Kato, H., Huet, O., Pottecher, J., . . . Duranteau, J. (2014). Microcirculatory alterations in traumatic hemorrhagic shock. *Critical Care Medicine, 42,* 1433–1441.

Thiele, H., Zeymer, U., Neumann, F. J., Ferenc, M., Olbrich, H. G., Hausleiter, J., . . . IABP-SHOCK II Trial Investigators. (2012). Intraaortic balloon support for myocardial infarction with cardiogenic shock. *New England Journal of Medicine, 367*(14), 1287–1296.

U.S. Food and Drug Administration (FDA). (2011). Xigris [drotrecogin alfa (activated)]: Market withdrawal—Failure to show survival benefit. Retrieved June 20, 2017, from https://www.fda.gov/Drugs/DrugSafety/ucm277114.htm

Volpicelli, G., Lamorte, A., Tullio, M., Cardinale, L., Giruado, M., Stefanone, V., . . . Frascisco, M. F. (2013). Point-of-care multiorgan ultrasonography for the evaluation of undifferentiated hypotension in the emergency department. *Intensive Care Medicine, 39*(7), 1290–1298.

Waecher, J., Kumar, A., Lapinsky, S. F., Marshall, J., Dodek, P., Arabi, Y., . . . Garland, A. (2014). Interaction between fluids and vasoactive agents on mortality in septic shock: A multicenter, observational study. *Critical Care Medicine, 42*(10), 2158–2168.

Walley, K. R. (2015). Shock. In J. B. Hall, G. A. Schmidt, & J. P. Kress (Eds.), *Principles of critical care* (4th ed.). Retrieved September 28, 2015, from http://accessmedicine.mhmedical.com.ezproxy.uky.edu/content.aspx?bookid=1340&Sectionid=80030826

Wilson, B. A., Shannon, M. T., & Shields, K. M. (2016). *Pearson nurse's drug guide 2016*. Hoboken, NJ: Pearson.

Zhou, F., Mao, Z., Zeng, X., Kang, H., Liu, H., Pan, L., & Hou, P. C. (2015). Vasopressors in septic shock: A systematic review and network meta-analysis. *Therapeutics and Clinical Risk Management, 11*, 1047–1059.

Zuckerbraun, B. S., Peitzman, A. B., & Billiar, T. R. (2015). Shock. In F. Brunicardi, D. K. Andersen, T. R. Billiar, D. L. Dunn, J. G. Hunter, J. B. Matthews, & R. E. Pollock (Eds.), *Schwartz's principles of surgery* (10th ed.). New York, NY: McGraw-Hill. Retrieved April 04, 2017, from http://accessmedicine.mhmedical.com.ezproxy.uky.edu/content.aspx?bookid=980&Sectionid=59610846

Chapter 38
Multiple Organ Dysfunction Syndrome

∨ Learning Outcomes

38.1 Explain the inflammatory process and the role of endothelium in that process.

38.2 Differentiate the major physiologic changes that occur with the systemic inflammatory response syndrome (SIRS).

38.3 Explain four pathophysiologic changes that occur with multiple organ dysfunction syndrome.

38.4 Apply knowledge of the seven most common organ systems that fail as a result of the SIRS process.

38.5 Demonstrate the collaborative management of the patient with multiple organ dysfunction syndrome.

ultiple organ dysfunction syndrome (MODS) is characterized by the progressive dysfunction of two or more organ systems. In critically ill patients it is usually the ominous consequence of a cascade of complex pathophysiologic events involving widespread endothelial injury and systemic inflammation. The clinical course of MODS typically results in prolonged hospital stays. Despite the expenditure of significant time, resources, and technology, the mortality rate from MODS remains high. Through identification of risk factors and early interventions, nurses play a crucial role in detecting and preventing this highly lethal cascade of events.

Section One: Inflammatory Response and Endothelium

To understand the complexity of systemic inflammatory response syndrome (SIRS) and multiple organ dysfunction syndrome (MODS), it is important to first have a basic understanding of the inflammatory response and the role of endothelium in that response. For a more detailed discussion of cells of immunity and inflammation, refer to Chapter 28.

Review of the Inflammatory Response

Inflammation is a localized immunologic response to tissue injury (e.g., foreign materials, trauma, allergens, and excessive heat or cold) or infection. It is important to point out that inflammation does not require infection—only tissue injury or irritation. Inflammation is a critical defense mechanism for protecting the body, restoring homeostasis, and paving the way for tissue repair.

Sequence of Events   On exposure to cell injury, **mast cells** located in the tissues near capillary beds, initiate the inflammatory process by releasing powerful **chemical mediators**, such as histamine, bradykinin, and prostaglandins (Table 38–1). The release of mediators results in a sequence of vascular events that trigger local vasodilation and increased vascular permeability. In addition, the immune system is activated, triggering events such as chemotaxis and the migration of immune cells to the site of injury to destroy the offending agent and clean the site in preparation for healing and reestablishing homeostasis. Figure 38–1 illustrates the chain of events of the inflammatory response.

Clinical Manifestations   The clinical manifestations of inflammation result from the activation of the chemical

Table 38–1 Major Chemical Mediators of the Inflammatory Response

Mediator	Major Sources	Functions
Histamine	Mast cells in tissues, basophils in circulation	Powerful vasodilation, increased vascular permeability
Bradykinin	Mast cells	Vasodilation, increased vascular permeability, constricts smooth muscle, stimulates pain receptors
Serotonin	Platelets	Vasoconstriction, increased vascular permeability
Prostaglandins	Mast cells	Increased vascular permeability, smooth muscle contraction, vasodilation; activate local nerve endings, causing pain
Proteolytic enzymes	Phagocytes	Break down proteins, including those of microbes or foreign material
Leukotrienes	Mast cells	Increased vascular permeability, platelet activation, stimulation of leukocyte adherence to endothelium, smooth muscle contraction, chemotaxis
Interleukins (IL)	As a group, produced by WBCs, primarily T cells	Attract neutrophils, lymphocyte activation, growth and differentiation, chemotaxis

mediators of inflammation and can be divided into two types: localized and systemic. Localized manifestations include redness (rubor), heat (calor), swelling (tumor), pain (dolor), and loss of function (functio laesa). Systemic manifestations include elevated leukocyte count, fever, malaise, and anorexia. The signs and symptoms depend on the severity and extent of the tissue insult. Table 38–2 provides additional information about the source and purposes of the various local and systemic manifestations.

Endothelium

The **endothelium** provides major barrier and chemical support to the vascular system and to the inflammatory response. Insults to the endothelium, if extensive, can significantly alter homeostasis and are a major contributor to the development of systemic inflammatory response syndrome (SIRS) and subsequent organ dysfunction.

Review of Anatomy and Physiology The endothelium is the thin, single-cell layer of cells that comprise the inner lining of all veins and arteries (tunica intima). Capillaries are composed only of endothelium surrounded on the outside by basement membrane (Figure 38–2). The endothelium is the only layer of blood vessels that directly interfaces with blood flowing by and acts as a selectively permeable barrier.

The endothelium is often referred to as an organ system because it has many important local homeostatic functions (Box 38–1). Endothelial cells are highly active and are constantly sensing and responding to alterations in the local cell environment. Endothelial cells cross-talk to other cells, including the blood cells and vascular smooth muscle

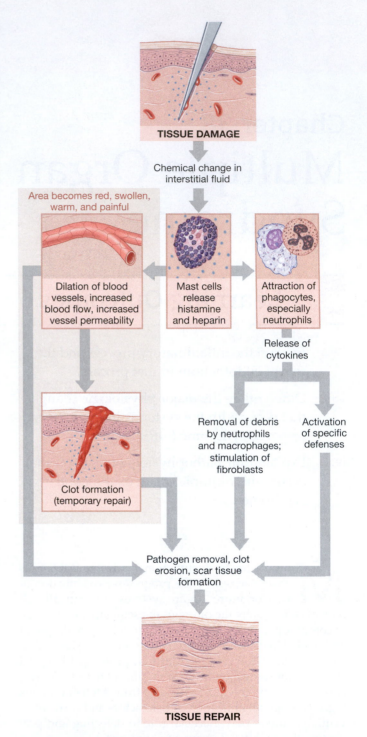

Figure 38–1 Events in inflammation.

cells. They respond to a variety of factors, including inflammatory mediators, stretch, changes in flow, and many circulating substances (Hajjar, Marcus, & Muller, 2015). Endothelial cells are activated by alterations in the local environment, such as minor trauma to blood vessels, transient bacteria, and stress. Their regulatory functions differ from one location in the body to another based on the function of local tissues.

Endothelial cell activation is a normal adaptive response under physiologic conditions, but it also occurs in response to pathophysiologic conditions. When bacteria invade local tissues or tissue is exposed to some other type

Table 38–2 Clinical Manifestations of Inflammation

Location	Manifestation	Source	Purpose
Local	Redness, heat, and swelling	Local vasodilation and increased capillary permeability	Facilitates entry of immune cells into area of injury
	Pain	Bradykinin Pressure on sensitive tissues or nerves Altered pH	Alerts host to presence of inflammation
	Loss of function	Local swelling and pain	Protects injury site
Systemic	Elevated leukocyte count	Increased production and release of leukocytes	Destroys infection or foreign material
	Fever	Release of pyrogens by IL-1, TNF-α, and prostaglandins	Destroys temperature-sensitive pathogens Increases important immune functions
	Increased heart rate and respirations	Increased metabolic processes secondary to fever	Compensatory mechanism Increases oxygen supply and CO_2 elimination

of irritant, endothelial cells are activated and release chemical mediators. These mediators stimulate the inflammatory response, recruit white blood cells to the area, and promote localized clotting to contain the infection. Table 38–3 lists major substances secreted by the endothelium, many of which have similar or counterbalancing functions. During inflammation, endothelial cells undergo necrosis and **apoptosis**, or programmed cell death, as tissues are repaired. The endothelium orchestrates this local physiologic response by promoting the adhesion and migration of white blood cells, altering local vasomotor tone, increasing permeability, inducing thrombin generation and fibrin formation, and triggering apoptosis. These activities are instrumental in containing the inflammatory activity

> **BOX 38–1** Major Functions of Endothelial Cells
>
> - Mediate vasomotor tone
> - Maintain vessel wall integrity
> - Control cellular and nutrient "traffic"
> - Regulate inflammatory and anti-inflammatory mediators
> - Participate in generating new blood vessels
> - Undergo apoptosis

locally, confining it to the site of infection. The goal of a local inflammatory response is to limit the extent of injury and promote healing. Normally, the inflammatory process

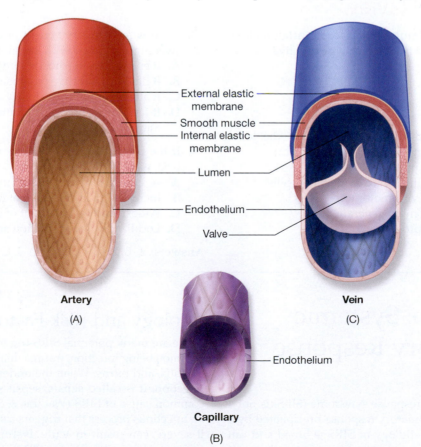

External elastic membrane
Smooth muscle
Internal elastic membrane
Lumen
Endothelium
Valve

Artery
(A)

Vein
(C)

Endothelium

Capillary
(B)

Figure 38–2 Comparative structures of arteries, capillaries, and veins.

Table 38–3 Critical Substances Secreted by the Endothelium

Substance	Function	Significance
Prostacyclin (PGI$_2$)	Anticoagulation Vasodilation	Prevents circulating platelets from activating (aggregating) prematurely Counterbalances thromboxane A$_2$, which is produced by platelets, causing vasoconstriction
Nitric oxide (NO)	Vasodilation	Diffuses to the smooth muscle cells, where it ultimately mediates vascular smooth muscle relaxation Decreases blood pressure
Endothelin-1 (ET-1)	Potent vasoconstriction Cardiac stimulation	Vasoconstricts vascular smooth muscle; increases blood pressure Increases cardiac contractility and heart rate (positive inotrope)
P-selectin	Proinflammatory	Mediates interaction of activated endothelial cells (or platelets) with leukocytes Facilitates movement of leukocytes from circulation to inflammatory site in tissues
Interleukins	Anti-inflammatory Help maintain endothelium barrier integrity	Specific interleukins counterbalance proinflammatory activities Maintain or reestablish barrier integrity

SOURCE: Data from Barrett et al. (2016), Kress & Hall (2015), and Rote (2017).

is contained within a local environment by a complex system of checks and balances, confining it to the site of infection through negative feedback mechanisms. The response of endothelial cells to alterations in the environment differs according to the host's genetics, age, and gender; the nature of the pathogen; and the location of the vascular bed.

It is essential to any discussion of SIRS and MODS to be aware that successful containment of the local inflammatory response limits damage to the host and preserves the integrity of uninvolved endothelial cells. If, for any reason, the host inflammatory response becomes uncontrolled and generalized, it escapes the well-developed local checks and balances, resulting in an unregulated inflammatory response with widespread involvement of endothelial cells and a more generalized activation of inflammation and coagulation. This type of generalized response can lead to SIRS and MODS, which are discussed in the next sections.

Section One Review

1. Mediators that stimulate the local inflammatory response are released from which type of activated cell?
   A. Platelets
   B. Endothelial cells
   C. Leukocytes
   D. Bacteria

2. How does the endothelium orchestrate the local inflammatory response? (Select all that apply.)
   A. By decreasing capillary permeability
   B. By promoting adhesion of white blood cells
   C. By altering local vasomotor tone
   D. By inducing thrombin generation
   E. By blocking apoptosis

3. What is the primary benefit of the redness, heat, and swelling associated with local inflammation?
   A. It encourages the host to protect the injury site.
   B. It destroys infective organisms.
   C. It alters the pH of the injury area.
   D. It facilitates entry of immune cells into the area of injury.

4. If the host inflammatory response becomes generalized, what is the result?
   A. A reduction in secretion of mediators
   B. Increased pain at the site of injury
   C. Widespread involvement of endothelial cells
   D. Localized vasoconstriction and coagulation

Answers: 1. B, 2. (B, C, D), 3. D, 4. C

Section Two: Systemic Inflammatory Response Syndrome

Systemic inflammatory response syndrome (SIRS) is not a disease; it is a proinflammatory response precipitated by a nonspecific insult. The etiology of SIRS is broad and can arise from both infectious and noninfectious stimuli, and it denotes systemic inflammation regardless of its cause.

Etiology and Risk Factors

There are many potential SIRS-triggering insults, the most common being infection, trauma, major surgery, acute pancreatitis, and burns. When the underlying cause of SIRS is infection, it is called **sepsis**; sepsis syndrome is the most common cause of SIRS (Watkins & Salata, 2016). Sepsis is an infectious process that triggers a systemic response that, if severe, can result in acute dysfunction of one or more organs (Kleinpell & Burns, 2014). Sepsis is discussed in detail in Chapter 37.

A number of patient-related risk factors for SIRS have been proposed, such as older age, baseline organ dysfunction, and malnutrition (Caserta et al., 2016); immunosuppression (Caserta et al., 2016); compromised gut integrity (Klingensmith & Coopersmith, 2016); and obesity (Andruszkow et al., 2013). Therapies have also been suggested as risk factors, including intraperative blood transfusion (Ferraris, Ballert, & Mahan, 2013) and cardiopulmonary bypass (Landis et al., 2014).

Clinical Manifestations

Systemic inflammatory response syndrome (SIRS) is said to be present when a patient meets any two of four clinical criteria first established by the American College of Chest Physicians/Society of Critical Care Medicine Consensus Conference (1992). The criteria include vital signs (temperature, heart rate, and respiratory rate) and leukocyte count. Box 38–2 lists the definitional criteria of SIRS for adults. The number of SIRS criteria reflects mortality rates: Meeting two criteria carries a 5% mortality risk; three criteria, 10%; and four criteria, 15% to 20% (Chen, Shapiro, Angood, & Makary, 2014).

Other common manifestations include decreased urine output and altered level of consciousness (Kleinpell & Burns, 2014). Manifestations reflect the underlying etiology of SIRS (e.g., infection, pancreatitis) and any organ dysfunctions that may develop as a complication (e.g., acute respiratory distress syndrome [ARDS], acute kidney injury [AKI], disseminated intravascular coagulation [DIC])—for example, if kidney function decreases, blood urea nitrogen and serum creatinine levels will elevate.

SIRS manifests on a continuum of mild to severe, depending on the etiology and comorbidities of the patient. Some patients develop only mild SIRS, with minor organ dysfunction that resolves rapidly; other patients exhibit a massive inflammatory reaction with multiple organ involvement and die from profound shock.

The SIRS–MODS Connection

Severe SIRS can progress to multiple organ dysfunction syndrome (MODS) when it overwhelms the body's ability to physiologically compensate and manage the widespread inflammation, thereby compromising organ function. The connection between SIRS and MODS is evident in the significant number of patients with severe sepsis who die with failure of multiple organs (mortality is estimated at 20%–50%) (Kleinpell & Burns, 2014). In fact, organ dysfunction is a pivotal criterion for defining severe sepsis and septic shock.

Section Two Review

1. The client is assessed with the following: temperature 39.5°C (103°F), heart rate 110 beats/min, respiratory rate 12/min, WBC 15,000 cells/mm^3 with greater than 10% bands. How many of the criteria for SIRS does this client exhibit?
   A. 1
   B. 2
   C. 3
   D. 4

2. Which statement about the pathogenesis of SIRS is accurate?
   A. It is not associated with MODS.
   B. It is an abnormal generalized proinflammatory response.
   C. It is an attempt to limit inflammation.
   D. It is associated with an excessive anti-inflammatory response.

3. What are risk factors for SIRS? (Select all that apply.)
   A. Older age
   B. Immunosuppression
   C. Gut hypoperfusion
   D. Low body mass index (BMI)
   E. Malnutrition

4. What are the most common underlying causes of SIRS? (Select all that apply.)
   A. Trauma
   B. Autoimmune disorders
   C. Acute pancreatitis
   D. Major surgery
   E. Infection

Answers: 1. C, 2. B, 3. (A, B, C, E), 4. (A, C, D, E)

Section Three: Multiple Organ Dysfunction Syndrome

Multiple organ dysfunction syndrome (MODS), also referred to as multiple system failure or multiple organ failure, is characterized by progressive dysfunction of two or more organ systems that persists beyond 24 hours (Kress & Hall, 2015). The prognosis worsens with each additional organ that fails; when five or more organs fail, mortality is about 90% (Casserly & Rounds, 2016).

Pathophysiologic Considerations

The physiologic derangements of MODS occur as the result of a severe insult that initiates the inflammatory response. Although sepsis (infection) is the most common insult, numerous other stimuli have been implicated. The pathophysiology of MODS is complex and not completely understood; hundreds of biochemical and cellular abnormalities have been described. Widespread endothelial injury with subsequent release of cytokines and other active molecules from the endothelial cells has been proposed as the likely major mechanism for MODS (Munford, 2015).

MODS Pathways   MODS appears to follow one of two distinct pathways, termed primary and secondary (Figure 38–3).

Primary MODS Pathway.   Primary MODS develops early (within the first 72 hours of admission) as the direct consequence of a well-defined initiating event, such as injury, hemorrhage, or hypoxemia (Nicks & Gaillard, 2016). Primary MODS is thought to be the result of inadequate oxygen delivery to cells and a failure of the microcirculation to remove metabolic end-products. As progressively more cells die, organ dysfunction and failure occur.

Secondary MODS Pathway.   The secondary MODS pathway involves the host response to toxins that occurs within the context of SIRS rather than as a direct response to the initiating insult (Nicks & Gaillard, 2016). The onset of secondary MODS is later in the patient's course, often weeks after the initial acute insult. The initial insult is thought to prime the inflammatory response, and a second insult reactivates it at an exaggerated level.

Pathologic Changes   The pathologic changes associated with MODS have four prominent explanations: uncontrolled systemic inflammation, tissue hypoxia, unregulated apoptosis, and microvascular coagulopathy.

Uncontrolled Systemic Inflammation.   Clinical evidence of systemic inflammation (SIRS) is evident in almost all patients with MODS. A large number of proinflammatory mediators (refer back to Table 38–1) have been implicated in initiating and potentiating a systemic inflammatory response, but the mechanisms through which these mediators induce organ injury are not clear. In sepsis, early activation of immune cells (monocytes, macrophages, lymphocytes, and neutrophils) is followed by downregulation of their activity that leads to a state of immune deficiency and an increased risk of superinfection. Proinflammatory mediators increase capillary permeability, resulting in edema in organs such as the lungs (ARDS) or brain (cerebral edema). Proinflammatory mediators cause the release of nitric oxide from endothelial cells, which results in vasodilation. Neutrophils induce the release of oxygen radicals and proteolytic enzymes and also potentiate increased vascular permeability.

Tissue Hypoxia.   The common pathway to organ dysfunction is global tissue hypoxia (Otero, Nguyen, & Rivers, 2016). Decreased oxygen delivery or reduced cellular use of oxygen inhibits normal cell function. Although the patient may appear clinically to have adequate oxygenation, regional tissue hypoxia may occur, particularly in the intestinal tract and brain.

Tissue hypoxia may result from derangements in the cellular use of oxygen in the presence of adequate oxygen delivery; as a result, a state of metabolic shutdown occurs because of an inadequate supply of energy to power the various cellular processes (i.e., a shift to anaerobic metabolism). As cells receive less oxygen for adenosine triphosphate (ATP) production, they cannot perform protein synthesis or maintain function of sodium–potassium pumps. When this derangement is widespread and severe, organ function becomes compromised.

Unregulated Apoptosis.   Derangements in the normal expression of apoptosis appear to be an important factor in the development of MODS. There appears to be an increase in apoptosis in some cell types (e.g., lymphocytes and GI epithelial cells) and delayed apoptosis in others (neutrophils). In addition, excessive apoptosis occurs in certain organ systems, such as the liver, kidney, and heart. The implications of unregulated apoptosis are reduced levels

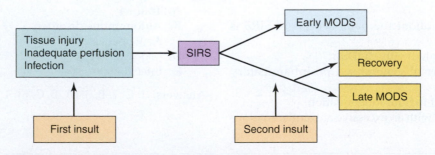

Figure 38–3 Primary and secondary MODS pathways.

of certain immune cells (increasing susceptibility to or worsening of infection) and an overabundance of other immune cells that increase tissue damage.

Microvascular Coagulopathy. Microvascular coagulopathy is abnormal clotting in the small blood vessels (microcirculation) that results in microthrombosis that obstructs blood flow. It is an important factor in the development of MODS. The mechanisms that regulate inflammation are linked with those that control coagulation. Coagulation is initiated through tissue factor (factor III) on the endothelial cell membrane, and tissue factor is released in response to the presence of endotoxin or inflammatory cytokines. Furthermore, tissue factor activates factor VII of the extrinsic pathway of the coagulation cascade, which ends in the formation of fibrin clots. Normally, fibrin clots play a critical role in restoring hemostasis and localizing microorganisms during the inflammatory response. However, under abnormal circumstances associated with widespread activation of tissue factor, microvascular clots can form in multiple tissues and organs, impeding blood flow and oxygen delivery to cells, which leads to the release of additional inflammatory mediators.

Risk Factors

Risk factors for primary MODS include increased severity of injury, shock, and SIRS. Risk factors for secondary MODS include infection, transfusion, and multiple surgical operations. Multiple host factors increase the risk for MODS, including age older than 45 years, because of reduced organ function associated with aging, decreased functional reserve, impaired stress response, and a higher number of preexisting conditions (e.g., cirrhosis, ischemic heart disease, chronic lung diseases, and diabetes).

Section Three Review

1. MODS is characterized by the dysfunction of how many organ systems?
   - **A.** One
   - **B.** Two or more
   - **C.** Three or more
   - **D.** Four or more

2. Primary MODS can develop in response to which factor?
   - **A.** The insult itself
   - **B.** Secondary complications
   - **C.** An exaggerated SIRS
   - **D.** Septic shock

3. Why is advancing age a risk factor for developing MODS?
   - **A.** Older adults do not have the money to pay for services.
   - **B.** Older adults do not take antibiotics as prescribed.
   - **C.** Older adults have decreased functional reserve.
   - **D.** Older adults have enhanced stress response.

4. Which pathophysiologic condition occurs as a result of anaerobic metabolism?
   - **A.** Metabolic shutdown
   - **B.** Apoptosis
   - **C.** Uncontrolled systemic inflammation
   - **D.** Microvascular coagulopathy

Answers: 1. B, 2. A, 3. C, 4. A

Section Four: Sequential Organ Involvement and Failure

As the pathophysiologic changes associated with MODS persist, organ dysfunction progresses and additional organ systems fail. Organ dysfunction can develop far from the initial injury site as a result of SIRS. There appears to be cross talk between organs through the activities of the chemical mediators, which is believed to facilitate the spread of injury from one organ to the next. The lungs and kidneys are particularly vulnerable to distant organ injury. This may be due to the leakage of mediators from an injury site into the systemic circulation. Examples include the translocation of endotoxin from the intestines into the portal circulation and the leakage of proinflammatory mediators from the lung into the circulation (Klingensmith & Coopersmith, 2016). Organ ischemia and cellular damage perpetuate SIRS, which perpetuates MODS. A vicious cycle develops; as each additional organ system fails, the risk of mortality escalates.

Assessing the Severity of Organ Dysfunction

Several different scoring systems and assessment tools have been proposed to quantify the extent of organ system dysfunction in MODS, but to date there has not been universal acceptance of any one tool. Most tools assess six major organ systems: respiratory, cardiovascular, neurologic, renal, hepatic, and hematologic. An evaluation of MODS severity involves assessment of several major organ systems for indicators of organ dysfunction.

One of the most commonly used tools is the Sequential Organ Failure Assessment (SOFA). The main purposes of the SOFA score are to determine the extent of organ function and to predict patient outcome. The scores for six organ systems (neurologic, cardiovascular, respiratory, hematologic, hepatic, and renal) can be calculated daily to provide an assessment of the patient's status during his or her ICU stay. The scores also provide general information on the effectiveness of the therapeutic interventions, as reflected in improved organ scores (McLymont & Glover, 2016) The SOFA scoring system is available for viewing at multiple public internet sites.

Sequential Organ Injury

A diagnosis of MODS requires dysfunction in two or more organs that persists for more than 24 hours. The organs tend to develop dysfunction in a fairly sequential order; however, other factors such as the patient's primary illness and comorbidities also impact the order in which the organs begin to fail. The clinical manifestations of MODS reflect the degree of organ injury; thus it is important for the nurse to have a strong understanding of which organs are most commonly affected, the associated risk factors, and major manifestations of individual organ dysfunction. This section provides an overview of the most common organ failures associated with MODS; details of each of the organs highlighted here are presented in other chapters.

Pulmonary Dysfunction   The lungs are usually the first organ system to fail and manifests as ARDS, which can progress rapidly from mild to severe. Many conditions have been associated with ARDS either as a direct result of injury to the lung or as a result of an indirect pulmonary response to a systemic insult. The most common direct predisposing factors are pneumonia and gastric aspiration; the most common indirect factors are sepsis and traumatic injury with shock that requires massive blood transfusions (Fahr, Jones, O'Neal, Duchesne, & Tatus, 2017).

The tissue damage specific to ARDS is injury to the alveolar–capillary membrane, with damage to both the capillary endothelium and alveolar epithelium. The damaged endothelium loses its barrier capabilities, allowing protein and water to leak out from the capillaries. This results in a noncardiogenic form of pulmonary edema. The damaged alveolar epithelium likewise loses its intactness, and fluid that has leaked out of the capillaries shifts into the alveoli. Ultimately, the injury to the alveolar–capillary membrane results in pulmonary shunt that is refractory (unresponsive) to oxygen therapy, causing profound hypoxia. Furthermore, injury to the alveolar epithelium includes injury to the surfactant-producing cells, with subsequent loss of surfactant necessary to keep the alveoli open. This results in widespread alveolar collapse and atelectasis. Two commonly monitored indicators of lung status in ARDS are arterial blood gases (ABG) and the PaO_2/FiO_2 (P/F) ratio (an estimate of pulmonary shunt).

Cardiovascular Dysfunction   The cardiovascular dysfunction associated with MODS includes dysrhythmias and hypotension that is unresponsive to fluid administration. In addition, peripheral vascular dysfunction occurs, including increased capillary permeability, edema, and alterations in regional blood flow. Cardiovascular failure is calculated as the product of heart rate (HR) times the central venous pressure (CVP) divided by the mean arterial pressure (MAP) (HR × CVP/MAP). This formula, called the pressure-adjusted heart rate (PAR), is analogous to the P/F ratio with ARDS and is used as a measure of cardiovascular dysfunction in MODS. Increasing values of the PAR reflect worsening cardiovascular function.

Acute Kidney Dysfunction   The development of acute kidney injury (AKI) is multifactorial and can occur as the result of ischemic or toxic insults to renal tubular cells.

Kidney dysfunction is frequently found in the intensive care setting (incidence of 20%–60%) and most frequently accompanies respiratory failure (Gaudry et al., 2016). Loss of renal function is characterized by a rise in serum levels of substances normally excreted by the kidneys, including creatinine, nitrogen, potassium, and drug metabolites. Regardless of the serum creatinine level, mortality appears to be lower when urine output is greater than 400 mL/day in an average-size adult. The mortality rate associated with AKI during critical illness correlates with the severity of the kidney injury and which specific organ system failures accompany it (e.g., AKI in the presence of neurologic or hepatic system failure carries the worst prognosis [Gaudry et al., 2016]).

Neurologic Dysfunction   Neurologic dysfunction is manifested in MODS as alterations in level of consciousness and peripheral neuropathy. Potential causes are many, and the pathogenesis of these neurologic changes is controversial. They may occur as a result of hypoperfusion, microvascular coagulopathy, or cerebral ischemia. Central nervous system dysfunction presents as altered level of consciousness (LOC) or delirium. Peripheral nervous system dysfunction presents as peripheral neuropathy and includes debility, muscle weakness, and atrophy. Risk factors include prolonged sedation or therapeutic paralysis and bed rest, aminoglycoside therapy, malnutrition, electrolyte abnormalities, and muscle deconditioning from disuse and lack of exercise. Despite its limitations in the sedated and mechanically ventilated patient, the Glasgow Coma Scale is the most widely used measure of neurologic function.

Liver Dysfunction   Hepatic injury involves progressive dysfunction. Abnormalities of its protein synthesis functions include low serum albumin, fibrinogen, and other clotting factors. Liver injury is believed to contribute to the development of sepsis as the liver loses its ability to destroy and clear pathogens and their toxins, thereby allowing them to migrate into the systemic circulation (Sun et al., 2017). Liver dysfunction typically manifests as high levels of serum bilirubin.

GI Dysfunction   It has been suggested that injury to the GI system is a driving force in the development of critical illness and SIRS (Klingensmith & Coopersmith, 2016). Intestinal hypoperfusion with subsequent GI injury or failure is associated with shock states, when critical blood flow is shunted away from the GI system to perfuse other organs. GI injury results in damage to the intestinal epithelial lining with release of proinflammatory mediators, leading to SIRS; furthermore, evidence suggests that it contributes to the development of sepsis (Klingensmith & Coopersmith, 2016). There are no reliable measures of GI function in MODS. The development of ileus or diarrhea may indicate GI dysfunction.

Hematologic Dysfunction   The most common hematologic dysfunction in MODS is thrombocytopenia secondary to increased platelet consumption, sequestration of platelets in the vasculature, and impaired thrombopoiesis as a result of bone marrow suppression. In its most severe form, the hematologic dysfunction of MODS is disseminated intravascular coagulation (DIC), which is characterized by widespread intravascular clotting with bleeding secondary to consumption of coagulation factors.

Section Four Review

1. What are the results of the respiratory dysfunction associated with MODS?
   A. A high P_ACO_2 with a high P_AO_2
   B. Increased diffusion across the alveolar membrane
   C. Refractory hypoxia
   D. Profound hemoptysis

2. Which finding reflects worsening cardiovascular function?
   A. High cardiac output
   B. Increasing PAR values
   C. Increasing P_AO_2/FiO_2
   D. Tachycardia

3. Mortality in MODS-related AKI is lower in which case?
   A. Urine output is greater than 400 mL/day.
   B. Serum creatinine is greater than 4.0 mg/dL.
   C. Neurologic function is maintained.
   D. Hemodialysis is delayed until absolutely necessary.

4. What is the most severe manifestation of hematologic dysfunction?
   A. Anemia
   B. Thrombocytopenia
   C. DIC
   D. Jaundice

Answers: 1. C, 2. B, 3. A, 4. C

Section Five: Management of MODS

The management of the patient with MODS is a tremendous medical challenge. There is currently no treatment that reverses the pathophysiologic processes involved in SIRS or MODS. This section provides an overview of major aspects of collaborative patient care management. Sepsis, the major contributor to the development of MODS, is discussed in detail in Chapter 37; an overview of sepsis-related MODS management is provided here.

Prevent SIRS and Sepsis

The management of MODS is complex, with unpredictable patient outcomes and high mortality rates. Prevention of complications such as SIRS and sepsis can offset the development and progression of MODS. Unfortunately, it is not always possible to prevent SIRS because underlying predisposing factors may be present on admission to the hospital, such as multiple trauma, cardiopulmonary arrest, or hemorrhage. Furthermore, treatments, such as cardiopulmonary bypass or massive transfusions, may increase the risk of SIRS.

A major focus of nursing care is to prevent infection through meticulous adherence to hand hygiene and universal precautions. If the patient is mechanically ventilated, an evidence-based ventilator bundle should be implemented to minimize the risk of ventilator-associated pneumonia (VAP) (Munaco, Dumas, & Edlund, 2014). Other significant potential sources of infection include urinary catheters, central venous catheters, and pressure ulcers; great care must be taken to follow hospital policies regarding assessment and management of invasive catheters and maintenance of skin integrity.

Detect Early SIRS, Sepsis, and MODS

Organ dysfunction, if treated in time, can potentially be reversed before the organ fails; however, the longer MODS persists, the worse the prognosis (Kress & Hall, 2015). SIRS and sepsis are often triggered by infection—for example, a urinary-catheter–related infection or postsurgical wound abscess (Kleinpell & Burns, 2014).

Nurses are in a prime position to assess and monitor patients who are at risk for MODS. Continuous monitoring of physiologic parameters, early recognition of changes, and early interventions are key to improving patient outcomes. Key parameters include monitoring of vital signs (with particular focus on temperature and mean arterial pressure [MAP]), electrocardiograms, oxygen saturation (arterial [SaO_2], central venous [$ScvO_2$], or mixed venous [$SmvO_2$]), central venous pressure, serum lactate, and cardiac output. Nursing assessments are crucial to early identification of patients who may be progressing from SIRS to MODS.

The nurse monitors for infection by considering potential sources for infection in the individual patient (e.g., invasive lines or tubes, skin breakdown). Temperature changes, either fever or hypothermia, should be carefully evaluated as a potential sign of sepsis. Fever may be the earliest manifestation of SIRS or sepsis and, in the intensive care environment, deserves further investigation. Serum white blood cell (WBC) with differential counts should be obtained regularly and trends closely monitored. When infection is suspected, blood cultures should be obtained prior to initiation of antibiotic therapy.

Parameters specific to organ function should be regularly evaluated. Focused assessments of the pulmonary, cardiovascular, renal, hepatic, neurologic, gastrointestinal, and hematopoietic systems are critical.

Implement a Treatment Plan

Current management of patients with MODS is focused on correcting the underlying problem while supporting organ function. There is no definitive treatment for MODS, and recommended treatments continue to evolve as new evidence becomes available. Identification and treatment of infection; glycemic control; and correction of hypoxia, hypotension, and impaired tissue oxygenation are priority goals. To meet these goals, management should focus on the following:

- Early recognition of sepsis or organ dysfunction
- Early hemodynamic resuscitation and continuous support
- Early and adequate antibiotic therapy for infection
- Tight glycemic control
- Mechanical ventilation

Glycemic Control Since 2001, considerable attention has been paid to the role of hyperglycemia in the pathogenesis of MODS based on a clinical study performed by Van den Berghe et al. (2001) who found that in a group of surgical ICU patients intensive insulin therapy with tight (aggressive) glycemic control (blood glucose 110 mg/dL or less) resulted in decreased mortality and morbidity. More recent clinical investigations, however, have not supported the findings of Van den Berghe and colleagues. Current evidence suggests that hypoglycemia is a common problem associated with aggressive glycemic control that results in increased morbidity and mortality (Clain, Ramar, & Surani, 2015; Finfer, 2014). New, more moderate glycemic control recommendations for patients with severe sepsis are that insulin therapy should be used to maintain blood glucose below 180 mg/dL (10 mmol/L), with the goal being a glucose level of approximately 150 mg/dL (Clain et al., 2015; Finfer, 2014; Society of Critical Care Medicine, 2009). Critically ill patients with stress hyperglycemia (blood glucose greater than 180 mg/dL [10 mmol/L]) may also require treatment to maintain blood glucose levels between 144 and 180 mg/dL (8–10 mmol/L (Finfer, 2014).

Nursing Considerations Even with the best of care, the patient with MODS may not survive. The nurse must be responsive to and supportive of the patient's family members, who may have limited understanding of the patient's crisis state or may feel lost in the environment of technical equipment, sounds, and high-intensity activities surrounding their loved one. Answering questions promptly and honestly, explaining equipment and procedures, and providing regular updates on the patient's condition may help the family cope with the situation. Should the management goals change from those focusing on lifesaving to those focusing on end-of-life and palliative care, the nurse continues to play a major role in supporting the family.

General nursing assessments and interventions that support the patient with MODS are presented in the "Nursing Care: The Patient with MODS" feature. Supporting oxygenation by performing interventions to increase oxygen supply and decrease oxygen demand is a major focus of care of the patient with MODS.

Nursing Care
The Patient with MODS

Expected Patient Outcomes and Related Interventions

Outcome: Optimize pulmonary gas exchange

Assess and compare to established norms, patient baselines, and trends.

Parameters and SOFA score

Respiratory rate, breath sounds, tidal volumes, peak and plateau pressures, assess for dyspnea or increased work of breathing (use of accessory muscles)

Temperature

Pulse oximetry and end-tidal CO_2 as ordered

Arterial blood gases

Sputum cultures as ordered

Timely and accurate serum antibiotic peak and trough levels as ordered

Implement interventions to optimize pulmonary gas exchange.

Implement mechanical ventilation settings and parameters as ordered.

Elevate head of bed at least 30 degrees.

Decrease patient oxygen needs by promoting rest, comfort, and relief of pain and anxiety.

Position patient to improve diaphragm excursion.

Provide tracheal suctioning as needed.

Administer related drug therapy and monitor for therapeutic and nontherapeutic effects.

IV antibiotics

Beta-adrenergic agents that promote bronchodilation

Outcome: Optimize tissue perfusion

Assess and compare to established norms, patient baselines, and trends.

Peripheral perfusion, capillary refill, skin temperature and color, peripheral pulses

Mean arterial pressure, pressure-adjusted heart rate, hemodynamic parameters (CVP, PAWP, CO), serum lactate, oxygen saturation (arterial and central or mixed venous)

Monitor ECG

Implement interventions to optimize tissue perfusion.

Supplemental oxygen as ordered

IV fluids as ordered

Implement interventions to decrease oxygen consumption.

Mechanical ventilation as ordered

Sedative, analgesics, anxiolytics as ordered

Nonpharmacologic interventions to decrease pain and anxiety

Position patient to maximize comfort

Calm, quiet environment

Offer support to decrease anxiety

Administer related drug therapy and monitor for therapeutic and nontherapeutic effects.

Administer inotropic agents as ordered (e.g., dobutamine [Dobutrex]).

Administer vasoconstricting agents as ordered (e.g., norepinephrine [Levophed]).

Emerging Evidence

- New criteria of sepsis were defined by The Society of Critical Care Medicine and the European Society of Intensive Care Medicine at a third international consensus conference in 2016 based on cohort studies, surveys, and systematic reviews. Updated criteria include: (1) vasopressors are required to maintain the patient's MAP at 65 mmHg or higher; and (2) serum lactate levels of greater than 2 mmol/L after the patient has received adequate fluid resuscitation. *(Shankar-Hari et al., 2016)*.

- In a retrospective 4.2-year study of 9,120 mixed-population critically ill adult patients in an ICU setting, the SOFA score was used to explore whether specific organ systems were more highly predictive of 30-day mortality than others. Investigators concluded that neurologic dysfunction, as measured by the CNS component of the SOFA score using the Glasgow Coma Scale, was most associated with 30-day mortality. Investigators recommended additional research to investigate whether the SOFA scoring system should be weighted differently, with special attention to neurologic function, for more accurate evaluation of MODS outcomes *(Knox et al., 2014)*.

- Pulmonary aspiration of gastric or oropharyngeal fluid is a serious complication of general anesthesia that can lead to the development of acute respiratory distress syndrome (ARDS) in up to 30% of patients, as well as the need for extracorporeal membrane oxygenation (ECMO), and a high risk of mortality. Patients often develop a SIRS response that can lead to hemodynamic instability and MODS, further complicating treatment. A recently introduced extracorporeal cytokine hemoadsorption device called CytoSorb (CytoSorbents Corporation, USA) has gained interest in the field of critical care and cardiac surgery as a strategy to help control severe SIRS. It works with standard hemodialysis or continuous renal replacement therapy (CRRT) machines to purify blood extracorporeally. An increasing number of case studies report use of this new technology in the setting of an extreme SIRS response, cytokine storm, ARDS, and severe hemodynamic impairment. This particular case study report was on a single 45-year-old patient with a small bowel obstruction who aspirated during anesthesia induction *(Träger et al., 2016)*.

Section Five Review

1. Which strategy is essential to reducing the mortality associated with MODS?
   - **A.** Early recognition and management of MODS
   - **B.** Administration of acetaminophen for febrile episodes
   - **C.** Prompt administration of aminoglycosides as ordered
   - **D.** Knowing how to operate a dialysis machine

2. What is the best way to prevent MODS?
   - **A.** Place the client on mechanical ventilation.
   - **B.** Initiate antibiotics with the onset of fever.
   - **C.** Ensure optimal oxygenation.
   - **D.** Prevent SIRS and sepsis.

3. Which nursing interventions decrease the incidence of infection? (Select all that apply.)
   - **A.** Monitoring vital signs every 2 hours
   - **B.** Strict adherence to hand hygiene
   - **C.** Use of a ventilator bundle
   - **D.** Meticulous catheter care
   - **E.** Maintenance of client skin integrity

4. The nurse has orders to obtain blood cultures and begin IV antibiotic therapy. Which statement is correct regarding these orders?
   - **A.** IV antibiotic should be started before obtaining blood cultures.
   - **B.** Blood cultures should be obtained before starting antibiotics.
   - **C.** The sequence in which the orders are carried out does not matter.
   - **D.** The prescribing provider should be consulted to clarify the orders.

Answers: 1. A, 2. D, 3. (B, C, D, E), 4. B

Clinical Reasoning Checkpoint

Mr. F, a 75-year-old male, was admitted to the high-acuity unit with a diagnosis of pneumonia. He was placed on IV hydration and antibiotics. Twenty-four hours later, he complains of shortness of breath and difficulty breathing. His blood pressure is 80/60 mmHg, pulse 125 bpm, respirations 30 bpm, temperature 39°C (102.4°F). A chest x-ray reveals diffuse bilateral infiltrates. Arterial blood gas results on 2 liters nasal cannula are pH 7.45, PaCO$_2$ 45,

PaO_2 44, SaO_2 82%. He is intubated and transferred to the ICU. His urine output for the past 24 hours is 400 mL, and his morning serum laboratory results are as follows:

Lab Parameter	Patient Value
Lactate	5.2 mmol/L
Glucose	320 mg/dL
Creatinine	2.8 mg/dL
WBC	25,000
Hgb/Hct	7.5/22.4%
Platelets	86,000

1. What are Mr. F's risk factors for developing SIRS?
2. What conditions does Mr. F have that meet the criteria for SIRS?
3. Based on the data given, what organ systems appear to be injured? Give data to support your answer.
4. Do you believe Mr. F, now in the ICU, has MODS? Explain your answer.
5. What is the pathophysiologic basis for MODS in this patient? How can a pulmonary infection on admission progress to MODS 48 hours later?
6. Should the nurse be concerned about Mr. F's hyperglycemia? Explain your answer.

Chapter 38 Review

1. The nurse explains that a client has multiple organ dysfunction syndrome that likely was caused by widespread inflammation. The client's spouse says, "But the doctor said he didn't have an infection." How should the nurse respond?
   1. "His infection was subclinical, so we did not know he had it."
   2. "Inflammation can occur even when there's no infection."
   3. "There must have been a lab error that caused us to miss the presence of the infection."
   4. "You must have misunderstood what the doctor said."

2. It is suspected that a client has a systemic inflammation. Which findings would the nurse interpret as supporting this suspicion? (Select all that apply.)
   1. WBC of $14,400/mm^3$
   2. Temperature of 38.0°C (100.4°F)
   3. Inability to sleep
   4. Decreased urine output
   5. General malaise and confusion

3. The spouse of a client asks why his wife has developed SIRS. The nurse reviews the client's history and discovers the client is 43 years old, is 5 feet 5 inches tall, weighs 200 pounds, has three children who were all born by cesarean section, has never smoked, and drinks wine with dinner three times a week. Which assessment finding would the nurse interpret as a risk factor for the development of SIRS?
   1. Female gender
   2. Age
   3. Increased body mass index
   4. History of multiple surgeries

4. It is suspected that a client is developing SIRS. Which assessment findings would the nurse interpret as supporting this suspicion? (Select all that apply.)
   1. Temperature 35.8°C (96.4°F)
   2. Heart rate 108/min
   3. $PaCO_2$ 28 mmHg
   4. WBC $10,000/mm^3$
   5. Respiratory rate 22/min

5. A client was admitted after being severely injured in an explosion. How long would the nurse monitor this client for the development of primary MODS?
   1. 12 hours
   2. 24 hours
   3. 48 hours
   4. 72 hours

6. The nurse is reviewing the serial SOFA scores of a client with MODS. What is the benefit of understanding this trend?
   1. The trend predicts whether the client will die.
   2. The trend can provide information about the efficacy of interventions.
   3. The trend predicts which organ system will fail next.
   4. The trend identifies when a client will require mechanical ventilation.

7. A client's pressure-adjusted heart rate (PAR) has increased since yesterday's measurement. Which information should the nurse provide to the client's family?
   1. "Her cardiovascular status has worsened."
   2. "She is having more cardiac arrhythmias."
   3. "Her heart rate is better."
   4. "Her blood pressure is improving."

8. The medical team is concerned that a client's gut may be injured. Which assessment findings would the nurse interpret as supporting that concern? (Select all that apply.)
   1. The client's bowel sounds are greatly diminished.
   2. The client has diarrhea.
   3. Tube feeding residuals are increasing.
   4. The client's creatinine is elevated.
   5. The client is jaundiced.

9. A hospital has seen an increase in the number of its clients who develop SIRS and MODS. Which statement by the nurse in charge of quality reflects correct initial management of this increase?

   1. "This increase shows we are not providing good care."
   2. "I will review the admission status of these clients."
   3. "We should review all our policies to see where we must make changes."
   4. "I will develop education modules on SIRS and MODS for all staff to review."

10. A client who has developed MODS has had an average blood glucose of 165 mg/dL over the last three days. How would the nurse interpret this finding?

    1. The client needs a higher insulin dosage.
    2. The client needs additional IV glucose.
    3. The client's glycemic control is adequate.
    4. The client needs additional potassium.

Answers to questions found inside your textbook are available on the faculty resources site. Please consult with your instructor.

References

American College of Chest Physicians & Society of Critical Care Medicine. (1992). The AACP–SCCM consensus conference on sepsis and organ failure. *Chest, 101,* 1481–1483.

Andruszkow, H., Veh, J., Mommsen, P., Zeckey, C., Hildebrand, F., & Frink, M. (2013). Impact of the body mass on complications and outcome in multiple trauma patients: What does the weight weigh? *Mediators of Inflammation.* Article ID 345702. http://dx.doi.org/10.1155/2013/345702

Barrett, K. M., Barman, S. M., Boitano, S., & Brooks, H. (2016). *Ganong's review of medical physiology* (25th ed.). New York, NY: McGraw-Hill.

Caserta, S., Kern, F., Cohen, J., Drage, S., Newbury, S. F., & Llewelyn, M. J. (2016). Circulating plasma microRNAs can differentiate human sepsis and systemic inflammatory response syndrome (SIRS). *Scientific Reports, 6,* 28006.

Casserly, B., & Rounds, S. (2016). Essentials in critical care medicine. In T. E. Andreoli, I. J. Benjamin, R. C. Griggs, & E. J. Wing (Eds.), *Cecil Essentials of Medicine* (9th ed., pp. 259–265). St. Louis, MO: Elsevier Saunders.

Chen, C. L., Shapiro, M. L., Angood, P. B., & Makary, M. A. (2014). Patient safety. In F. C. Brunicardi, D. K. Andersen, T. R. Billiar, D. L. Dunn, J. G. Hunter, J. B. Matthews, & R. E. Pollock (Eds.), *Schwartz's principles of surgery* (10th ed.). Retrieved December 12, 2016, from http://accessmedicine.mhmedical.com.ezproxy.uky.edu/content.aspx?bookid=980&Sectionid=59610853

Clain, J., Ramar, K., & Surani, S. R. (2015). Glucose control in critical care. *World Journal of Diabetes, 6*(9), 1082–1091.

Fahr, M., Jones, G., O'Neal, H., Duchesne, J., & Tatus, D. (2017). Acute respiratory distress syndrome incidence, but not mortality, has decreased nationwide: A national trauma data bank study. *The American Surgeon, 83*(4), 323–331.

Ferraris, V. A., Ballert, E. Q., & Mahan, A. (2013). The relationship between intraoperative blood transfusion and postoperative systemic inflammatory response syndrome. *The American Journal of Surgery, 205*(4), 457–465.

Finfer, S. (2014). Clinical controversies in the management of critically ill patients with severe sepsis: Resuscitation fluids and glucose control. *Virulence, 5*(1), 200–205.

Gaudry, S., Hajage, D., Schortgen, F., Martin-Lefevre, L., Pons, B., Boulet, E., . . . Markowicz. (2016). Initiation strategies for renal-replacement therapy in the intensive care unit. *The New England Journal of Medicine, 375*(2), 122–133.

Hajjar, K. A., Marcus, A. J., & Muller, W. A. (2015). Vascular function in hemostasis. In J. T. Prchal, K. Kaushansky, M. A. Lichtman, T. J. Kipps, & U. Seligsohn (Eds.), *Williams hematology* (9th ed.). Retrieved January 14, 2017, from http://accessmedicine.mhmedical.com.ezproxy.uky.edu/content.aspx?bookid=1581&Sectionid=101236970

Kleinpell, R. M., & Burns, S. M. (2014). Multisystem problems. In M. Chulay & S. M. Burns (Eds.), *AACN essentials of critical care nursing* (3rd ed., pp. 293–310). Philadelphia, PA: McGraw Hill.

Klingensmith, N. J., & Coopersmith, C. M. (2016). The gut as the motor of multiple organ dysfunction in critical illness. *Critical Care Clinics, 32*(2), 203–212.

Knox, D. B., Lanspa, M. J., Pratt, C. M., Kuttler, K. G., Jones, J. P. & Brown, S. M. (2014). Glasgow Coma Scale score dominates the association between admission Sequential Organ Failure Assessment score and 30-day mortality in a mixed intensive care unit population. *Journal of Critical Care, 29*(5), 780–785.

Kress, J. P., & Hall, J. B. (2015). Approach to the patient with critical illness. In D. L. Longo, A. S. Fauci, D. L. Kasper, S. L. Hauser, J. L. Jameson, & J. Loscalzo (Eds.), *Harrison's principles of internal medicine* (19th ed.). Retrieved January 25, 2017, from http://accessmedicine.mhmedical.com.ezproxy.uky.edu/content.aspx?bookid=1130&Sectionid=63651436

Landis, R. C., Brown, J. R., Fitzgerald, D., Likosky, D. S., Shore-Lesserson, L., Baker, R. A., & Hammon, J. W. (2014). Attenuating the systemic inflammatory response to adult cardiopulmonary bypass: A critical review of the evidence base. *The Journal of Extra-Corporeal Technology, 46*(3), 197–211.

Levy, M. M., Fink, M. P., Marshall, J. C., Abraham, E., Angus, D., Cook, D., . . . Ramsay, G. (2001). SCCM/ESICM/ACCP/ATS/SIS International Sepsis Definitions Conference. *Critical Care Medicine, 31*(4), 1250–1256.

McLymont, N., & Glover, G. W. (2016). Scoring systems for the characterization of sepsis and associated outcomes. *Annals of Translational Medicine, 4*(24), 527.

Munaco, S., Dumas, B., & Edlund, B. J. (2014). Preventing ventilator-associated events: Complying with evidence-based practice. *Critical Care Nursing Quarterly, 37*(4), 384–392.

Munford, R. S. (2015). Severe sepsis and septic shock. In D. L. Longo, A. S. Fauci, D. L. Kasper, S. L. Hauser, J. L. Jameson, & J. Loscalzo (Eds.), *Harrison's principles of internal medicine* (19th ed.). Retrieved January 25, 2017, from http://accessmedicine.mhmedical.com.ezproxy.uky.edu/content.aspx?bookid=1130&Sectionid=63651436

Nicks, B. A., & Gaillard, J. (2016). Approach to shock. In J. E. Tintinalli, J. S. Stapczynski, D. M. Cline, O. J. Ma, R. K. Cydulka, & G. D. Meckler (Eds.), *Tintinalli's emergency medicine: A comprehensive study guide* (8th ed.). Retrieved November 29, 2016, from http://accessmedicine.mhmedical.com.ezproxy.uky.edu/content.aspx?bookid=1658&Sectionid=109384946

Otero, R. M., Nguyen, H. B., & Rivers, E. P. (2016). Approach to the patient in shock. In J. E. Tintinalli, J. S. Stapczynski, D. M. Cline, O. J. Ma, R. K. Cydulka, & G. D. Meckler (Eds.), *Tintinalli's emergency medicine: A comprehensive study guide* (8th ed.). Retrieved January 9, 2017, from http://accessmedicine.mhmedical.com.ezproxy.uky.edu/content.aspx?bookid=1658&Sectionid=109384946

Rote, N. S. (2017). Innate immunity: Inflammation and wound healing. In S. Huether & K. McCance (Eds.), *Understanding pathophysiology* (6th ed., pp. 134–157). St. Louis, MO: Elsevier.

Shankar-Hari, M., Phillips, G. S., Levy, M., Seymour, C. W., Liu, V. X., Deutschman, C. S., . . . Singer, M. (2016). Developing a new definition and assessing new clinical criteria for septic shock. *Journal of the American Medical Association, 315*(8), 775–787.

Society of Critical Care Medicine. (2009). *Severe sepsis bundles, element 2: Maintain adequate glycemic control.* Retrieved May 9, 2012, from http://www.survivingsepsis.org/Bundles/Pages/SepsisManagementBundle.aspx

Society of Critical Care Medicine. (2016). *Critical care statistics.* Retrieved March 16, 2017, from http://www.sccm.org/Communications/Pages/CriticalCareStats.aspx

Sun, D.-Q., Zheng, C.-F., Liu, W.-Y., Van Poucke, S., Mao, Z., Shi, K.-Q., . . . Zheng, M.-H. (2017). AKI-CLIF-SOFA: A novel prognostic score for critically ill cirrhotic patients with acute kidney injury. *Aging (Albany NY), 9*(1), 286–296.

Träger, K., Schütz, C., Fischer, G., Schröder, J., Skrabal, C., Liebold, A., & Reinelt, H. (2016). Cytokine reduction in the setting of an ARDS-associated inflammatory response with multiple organ failure. *Case Reports in Critical Care,* 9852073.

Van den Berghe, G., Wouters, P., Weekers, F., Verwaest, C., Bruyninckx, F., Schetz, M., . . . Bouillon, R. (2001). Intensive insulin therapy in critically ill patients. *New England Journal of Medicine, 345*(19), 1359–1367.

Watkins, R. R., & Salata, R. A. (2016). Bacteremia and sepsis syndrome. In T. E. Andreoli, I. J. Benjamin, R. C. Griggs, & E. J. Wing (Eds.), *Cecil essentials of medicine* (9th ed., pp. 846–852). St. Louis, MO: Elsevier Saunders.

Chapter 39

Solid Organ and Hematopoietic Stem Cell Transplantation

⌄ Learning Outcomes

39.1 Discuss the history of organ transplantation.

39.2 Describe types of donors and transplant-related legal considerations.

39.3 Define brain and cardiac death and explain how death is determined.

39.4 Discuss organ donor management.

39.5 Explain the general organ procurement process and organ preservation.

39.6 Discuss the immunologic considerations of organ transplantation.

39.7 Describe how the need for organ transplantation is determined.

39.8 Discuss the major complications associated with organ transplantation.

39.9 Describe immunosuppressant therapy for prevention of graft rejection.

39.10 Explain hematopoietic stem cell transplantation.

39.11 Discuss the general concepts related to kidney transplantation, including implications for postprocedure management.

This chapter provides a broad picture of solid-organ transplantation and hematopoietic stem cell transplantation. The chapter is organized into two parts: The first part focuses on transplantation from the donor's perspective and includes a discussion of donor types, selection, and management. The second part focuses on transplantation from the recipient's (transplant candidate's) perspective, including eligibility for transplantation, complications, and management. To exemplify the general preoperative, perioperative, and immediate postoperative transplantation process, a profile of kidney transplantation is also provided.

Section One: Brief History of Organ Transplantation

For centuries, surgeons have attempted to **graft** body tissue—that is, to transfer it from one part of the body to a different part, or to transfer it from another donor source.

However, it was not until the dawn of the twentieth century that surgical skills and knowledge of immunology and immunosuppression were sufficiently advanced to facilitate tissue survival following transplantation. This section highlights strategic events in the development of modern organ transplantation as described by Dr. Joseph Murray, a pioneer in transplantation (Murray, 1991).

1910 to 1930: The Beginnings

The kidney was the early focal point of interest in organ transplantation. Surgeons had struggled with otherwise healthy young patients who were dying of end-stage renal failure. Prior to 1912, although there was interest in performing such transplants, surgeons had not yet developed a successful method of reconnecting the organ vasculature to make transplantation a feasible option. In 1912, the Nobel Prize winner Dr. Alexis Carrel developed a landmark method of successfully suturing and transplanting blood vessels and organs. During this period, animal researchers also began examining tissue survival following transplantation.

1930 to 1950: In Search of Long-term Success

In the early 1930s, experimentation in skin grafting as a treatment for burns contributed greatly to the advancement of transplantation knowledge. It was noted that skin grafts from family member donors survived longer than those provided by nonfamily members, although no skin grafts survived for long. In 1936 the first kidney transplant was performed, using a kidney from a person who had recently died; however, the patient died after the donor kidney was rejected. The reasons for tissue acceptance or *rejection*—the activation of the immune response against the transplanted tissue—were still unknown.

In the late 1940s, renal transplantation programs began to be developed in earnest. Following World War II, research focused on allograft (the transplantation of tissues between members of the same species) rejection. A common antigen was discovered between kidney and skin allografts that caused sensitization of a recipient for subsequent grafting. Scientists knew that for renal transplantation to be a feasible option they needed to get around the immunologic problems experienced thus far. By the end of the 1940s, transplanted kidneys were surviving for up to 6 months, but long-term organ transplant survival remained out of reach.

1950 to 1960: The Isograft and Immunosuppressant Discovery Years

In 1954, the first isograft—a transplant between identical human twins—took place. Tissue matching was performed by crossgrafting skin between twin brothers. The success of this isograft, a renal transplant, demonstrated that identical twins provided a method of bypassing the tissue incompatibility problem.

Research on the problem of tissue incompatibility continued. A total body x-ray was performed experimentally as a means to depress the immune system. After the x-ray treatments, bone marrow infusions were performed and the renal allograft transplant was completed. This method, however, yielded only marginal success in the short term and little success in the long term.

During this decade, research also focused on developing **immunosuppressants**—drugs that curb the body's immune response. In 1959, animal experimentation focused on 6-mercaptopurine (Purinethol), an antimetabolite, with encouraging success. Azathioprine (Imuran) was introduced the following year. Early use of azathioprine was associated with patient death from high-dose–related complications; after the correct dose was established, azathioprine was very successful in human clinical trials and continues to be a major component of immunosuppression therapy today. Not long after initiating the use of azathioprine, corticosteroids were introduced as adjunctive therapy.

In 1957, Dr. E. Donnall Thomas documented the first allogeneic hematopoietic marrow transplantations, which he performed on several patients with cancer (Applebaum, 2007). His initial attempts were not successful, primarily due to the lack of scientific knowledge at that time about cell antigenic markers and their impact on tissue compatibility (**histocompatibility**). The similarities in histocompatibility antigens between individuals determines the degree to which donated tissues will be accepted or rejected. However, after years of research, in 1969 Dr. Thomas finally realized success by using well-matched sibling marrow in patients with leukemia.

1961 to 1979: The Expansion Years

The 1960s saw a rapid increase in transplant knowledge. Renal transplant survival rates rose dramatically. New forms of immunosuppressive therapy were discovered. Organ procurement programs were initiated, both regionally and nationally. There was great enthusiasm to take what was learned from the renal transplantation programs and expand it to transplantation of other organs.

An important expansion in organ transplantation occurred during the mid-to-late 1960s; it was during this period that pancreas and kidney, and isolated pancreas, liver, and heart transplantation were first successful. Early attempts at heart transplantation did not have a high success rate. Cardiac transplantation is highly successful today, in part because of tissue typing and improved immunosuppressant therapy.

1980 to the Present

In 1977, cyclosporine, a drug with powerful immunomodulating properties, was discovered, and in 1983 it was approved for use in the United States (Linden, 2009). Cyclosporine opened the door to successful transplantation because it effectively suppressed rejection. Its discovery heralded a new age of immunosuppressant drug discovery and the expansion of transplant programs.

Following on the heels of success in the area of cardiac transplantation, surgeons turned to perfecting heart–lung, single-lung, and double-lung transplants in the early 1980s. In 1989, a transplantation milestone was achieved with the first successful living-donor liver transplantation; in 1990, the first successful living-donor lung transplant was performed.

Section One Review

1. What was the early focal point of interest in organ transplantation?
   A. Kidney
   B. Lungs
   C. Heart
   D. Liver

2. Skin grafts were first used experimentally as a treatment for which condition?
   A. Leg ulcers
   B. Traumatic injury
   C. Burn injury
   D. Skin cancer

3. What was one of the earliest immunosuppressants to be successfully used on transplant clients?
   A. Cyclosporine
   B. Azathioprine
   C. Corticosteroids
   D. 6-mercaptopurine

4. Early attempts at organ and hematopoietic cell transplantation failed for which underlying reason?
   A. Use of nonhuman donors
   B. Postoperative infections
   C. Primitive surgical techniques
   D. Lack of knowledge about histocompatibility

Answers: 1. A, 2. C, 3. B, 4. D

The Organ Donor

Section Two: Graft, Immunologic, and Legal Considerations

The transplantation of tissues and organs is known as grafting. The term *graft* refers to the transfer of tissue from one part of the body to a different part, or the transfer of tissue from one person (or animal), called the *donor*, to another person, the *recipient*. The donor source is a particularly important consideration because it dictates how the recipient's immune system will react to the new tissue or organ.

In the United States, organ donation is tightly regulated by law at the state and national levels. While there is a rising demand for organs, the number of willing donors remains relatively low, and organizations such as United Network for Organ Sharing (UNOS) and Donate Life America aim to educate the American public to encourage tissue and organ donation.

Types of Grafts

The three major types of grafts are autograft, heterograft, and allograft. Each type has its advantages and disadvantages.

Autograft   An **autograft** is the transplantation of tissue from one part of a person's body to another part of the body. It is the ideal situation for tissue compatibility and graft survival. A common example of autografting is the skin autograft. For example, when a person suffers severe burns, healthy tissue can be removed from an undamaged body area and transplanted over the burned area to promote healing and recovery. Autografting is not used for organ transplantation and thus will not be discussed further in this section.

Heterograft   A **heterograft**, also called a **xenograft**, is the transplantation of tissue between two different species. Examples of heterografts are porcine skin grafts and experimental baboon heart transplants. At this time, heterografts are used primarily as temporary transplantations until a permanent allograft becomes available. Tissue rejection occurs rapidly because of the dissimilarities of tissues between species.

Allograft   An **allograft** (also known as a *homograft)* is the transplantation of tissue between members of the same species. One form of allograft, the **isograft** or **syngraft**, is transplantation between identical twins. The allograft is the most common type of organ transplantation. With the exception of isografts, allografts trigger an immune reaction that causes rejection of the graft. Allografts are obtained from either live or deceased donors.

Types of Donors

Grafts can come from two sources, either a living donor or a deceased donor. The majority of grafts come from deceased donors.

Living Donor   A **living donor** is a person who volunteers to have an organ, part of an organ, or hematopoietic stem cells removed for transplantation into another person. Ideally, the living donor is related to the recipient as part of the immediate family (e.g., parents, siblings). Related donors are preferred because of increased histocompatibility and, therefore, longer graft life. When a related donor is not available, a nonrelated living donor may donate. In the case of an isograft (between identical twins), no rejection is expected because the two tissues are completely histocompatible.

The kidney is the solid organ most frequently recovered in its entirety from a living donor. Segmental (partial) organ donation, such as that involving one lobe of a liver or lung or part of the pancreas, is also performed using a living donor. Initially, segmental organ donation was performed primarily in pediatric patients, often parent–donor to child–recipient. A trend is growing toward adult-to-adult living donors due to the scarcity of whole-organ resources; the size of the organ waiting list continues to increase, while the number of available donors has not matched the need. For example, the waiting list for all organ transplants as of April 8, 2017, was 118,121. In January and February 2017, available donors numbered 2,555 (1,659 deceased and 896 living) (Organ Procurement and Transplantation Network [OPTN], 2017a).

Becoming a living donor is not without risk. For example, with the exception of hematopoietic stem cell donation, a living donor must undergo a major surgical procedure and is therefore at risk for developing postoperative complications such as infection and thromboembolism. The living donor may lose work days due to the surgery, which may have financial ramifications, and his or her life insurance rates may change. Furthermore, a live kidney donor may eventually develop disease in the remaining kidney, requiring a kidney transplant. Another concern relative to the live donor initiative in general is the potential for coercion or fear of rejection by family members if the donor refuses. It is important that the potential live donor and the recipient are both well informed of the risks and benefits associated with live organ transplantation.

Deceased Donor   The deceased (or cadaver) donor is one whose organs or tissues are recovered after death. Deceased donors are usually healthy individuals who die as the result of a traumatic event or sudden death. They comprise the majority of solid organ donors and must be initially evaluated for suitability. Strict laws and formal procurement protocols have been established to protect the potential donor's rights. The two types of deceased donors are those who die of cardiac death and those who die of brain death.

Donors Who Die of Cardiac Death.   *Cardiac death* refers to death by cessation of cardiac and respiratory function. Transplantable tissues may be limited to heart valves, corneas, eyes, saphenous veins, skin, and bones. These tissues must be recovered within 12 to 24 hours postdeclaration of death. On occasion, organs (e.g., kidneys and liver) may be recovered following cardiac death. This must be initiated within minutes of cardiac arrest with the appropriate personnel available to complete the organ recovery.

Donors Who Die of Brain Death.   *Brain death* refers to the cessation of function of the entire brain and brainstem. Loss of brainstem function destroys the vital centers for blood pressure, temperature, and respiratory control, making cardiopulmonary death imminent. Organ donations following brain death comprise the majority of deceased-donor organ transplants. Transplantable tissues from this group of donors include tissues, as well as solid organs such as the kidneys, lungs, heart, liver, pancreas, and small bowel.

Legal Aspects of Donation and Transplantation

Many laws are in place at both the national and state levels to protect the potential organ donor and to organize and facilitate organ procurement and distribution. The following are examples of some of this legislation in the United States.

Uniform Anatomical Gift Act   The Uniform Anatomical Gift Act (UAGA) was originally passed in 1968 to promote uniformity of donation throughout the United States. This act authorizes the donation of all parts of the human body for use in transplantation, research, and education (Uniform Law Commission, 2017a). Originally, the UAGA provided a way for individuals to make their wishes for donation known; but often the consent for donation was given by the legal next of kin. In 2006, most states in the United States began using electronic donor registries in which people legally document their wish to be donors.

In the absence of an individual's registered wish to donate, the act describes who can authorize donation and

the order of priority in giving consent. Many states have revised their UAGA to include "first person consent," which prevents a person other than the adult donor from altering or revoking the donor's expressed wishes to donate organs or tissues. The UAGA also seeks to limit the liability of healthcare providers who act on good-faith representations that a deceased patient meant to make an anatomical gift. The act also prohibits trafficking in human organs for profit.

Required-request Legislation   A section of the UAGA entitled "Routine Inquiry and Required Request: Search and Notification" stipulates hospitals' responsibilities for identifying potential donors and providing information to families to make them aware of opportunities to donate. Hospitals that do not comply with the required-request stipulations may be open to penalties or administrative actions.

National Organ Transplant Act   The National Organ Transplant Act of 1984 set up the national Organ Procurement and Transplantation Network (OPTN). The OPTN establishes national registries to track potential recipients and posttransplantation organ recipients. It also provides for a national system to match organs and potential recipients. In addition, the act prohibits the selling of human organs and tissues. This act has been adopted in all 50 states.

Uniform Determination of Death Act   The Uniform Determination of Death Act has been enacted as a guideline for states to establish a legal definition of death. Most states have adopted some form of this act. For example, in Kentucky, KRS 446.400 (Determination of Death—Minimal Conditions to Be Met) states:

> For all legal purposes, the occurrence of human death shall be determined in accordance with the usual and customary standards of medical practice, provided that death shall not be determined to have occurred unless the following minimal conditions have been met: (1) When respiration and circulation are not artificially maintained, and there is a total and irreversible cessation of spontaneous respiration and circulation; or (2) When respiration and circulation are artificially maintained, and there is a total and irreversible cessation of all brain function, including the brain stem, and that such determination is made by two licensed physicians.

42 CFR 482.45 Conditions of Participation: Organ, Tissue, and Eye Procurement   Federal guidelines enacted in 1998 specifically address the responsibilities of hospitals for notifying and working with their organ procurement organization (OPO) (U.S. Government Printing Office [GPO], 2016). Specifically, hospitals must report all deaths and imminent deaths to the OPO in a timely manner. If the OPO finds that a patient meets criteria for organ donation, the hospital must ensure that the family is offered the donation option. Those who communicate with the family about donation must be employed by the OPO or must have received training from the OPO on best practices for donation communication. If the patient becomes a potential organ donor, care of the patient is directed by the OPO. Death records are reviewed collaboratively by the OPO and the hospital, and the OPO provides education to the hospital as needed. The Standards for Privacy of Individually

Identifiable Health Information (164.512 of the Health Insurance Portability and Accountability Act [HIPAA] of 1996) allows the hospital to share information with the OPO concerning the patient without requiring that legal consent or authorization be obtained first.

Section Two Review

1. The transplantation of tissue between members of the same species is which type of graft?
   A. Autograft
   B. Heterograft
   C. Xenograft
   D. Allograft

2. Which term refers specifically to transplantation between identical twins?
   A. Isograft
   B. Autograft
   C. Heterograft
   D. Allograft

3. Initially segmental (partial) live-organ donations were usually between which two parties?
   A. Identical twins
   B. Husband and wife
   C. Parent and child
   D. Human and ape

4. Which major legislation authorizes the donation of all or part of the human body following death?
   A. National Organ Transplant Act
   B. Uniform Anatomical Gift Act
   C. Uniform Determination of Death Act
   D. Omnibus Reconciliation Act

Answers: 1. D, 2. A, 3. C, 4. B

Section Three: Determination of Death

Confirmation of brain death is more complex than confirmation of cardiac death. With brain death, the patient appears to be alive, although comatose; there is blood pressure and a pulse rate, and breathing is controlled through mechanical ventilation. This section focuses on the determination of brain death.

Definition of Death

The Uniform Determination of Death Act (UDDA) defines death in two ways: (1) total irreversible failure of the cardiorespiratory system or (2) irreversible loss of all brain functions, including the brainstem and neocortex. Death must be determined according to accepted medical standards (Uniform Law Commission, 2017b). Most states have adopted the UDDA definitions and have developed their own statutes that define criteria to determine death. Some states have also added amendments regarding physician qualifications, confirmation by a second physician, and religious exemptions.

Determination of Death

Brain death can be determined by a clinical exam, cerebral blood perfusion study, or electroencephalography (EEG). The type of testing used is determined by the physician, with consideration of the patient's injuries and hemodynamic stability and the presence or absence of toxic or

metabolic CNS depression. Determination of brain death requires measures that accurately reflect cessation of brain and brainstem function to ensure that the patient meets the legal definition.

Prerequisite Diagnostic Criteria   Four diagnostic criteria must be met before a clinical diagnosis of brain death can be made:

1. Clinical or neuroimaging evidence of an acute CNS catastrophe that is compatible with the clinical diagnosis of brain death

2. Exclusion of complicating medical conditions that may confound clinical assessment (no severe electrolyte, acid–base, or endocrine disturbance)

3. No drug intoxication or poisoning

4. Core temperature greater than or equal to 32°C (90°F) (American Academy of Neurology [AAN], 2010; Wijdicks, Varelas, Gronseth, & Greer, 2010).

To meet the four criteria, the UDDA requires the use of "accepted medical standards":

- To determine "cessation of all functions of the entire brain, including the brain stem," physicians must determine the presence of unresponsive coma, the absence of brainstem reflexes, and the absence of respiratory drive after a CO_2 challenge.

- To ensure that the cessation of brain function is "irreversible," physicians must determine the cause of coma, exclude mimicking medical conditions, and observe the patient for a period of time to exclude the possibility of recovery (AAN, 2010; Wijdicks et al., 2010).

Clinical Diagnosis of Brain Death

Clinical examination is probably the most cost-effective test to determine brain death and can be performed at the bedside. It cannot be performed if the patient has toxic or metabolic CNS depression or cannot initiate respiration as a result of other injuries or pathology. Each hospital should have policies in place outlining how many clinical tests are required and how often to test (e.g., two clinical exams 12 hours apart, with continued observation between the two exams).

The clinical diagnosis of brain death focuses on three cardinal signs: coma or unresponsiveness, absence of brainstem reflexes, and apnea (AAN, 2010; Wijdicks et al., 2010). Assessments and tests are conducted to evaluate the patient for each of these signs.

Coma or Unresponsiveness   Reversible causes of coma or unresponsiveness must be ruled out. Evaluating the patient for possible CNS depression requires investigating drug or chemical sources for CNS depression. Toxicology screening may be performed to confirm the absence of CNS depressant drugs or substances in the blood (AAN, 2010; Wijdicks et al., 2010). No neuromuscular blockades or residual paralytics can be present. The patient's body temperature must be sufficiently warm to rule out hypothermia as an etiology of unresponsiveness.

Absence of Brainstem Reflexes   The following conditions are evaluated to confirm absence of all brainstem reflexes:

- Glasgow Coma Score of 3
- No response to painful or verbal stimuli
- Absent reflexes, including pupillary light, oculomotor (no eye movement with head rotation), oculocephalic (no eye movement in response to cold-water ear irrigations), corneal, cough, and gag

Apnea   Apnea testing is performed at the time of the final clinical exam. The purpose of apnea testing is to determine whether a patient's respiratory drive is stimulated by an elevated $PaCO_2$. Prior to initiating the test, the patient is preoxygenated with 100% oxygen concentration. The patient is disconnected from the ventilator, and passive oxygenation is maintained via supplemental oxygen through an endotracheal or tracheostomy tube. During the test, the patient is observed for any respiratory movement as the $PaCO_2$ is allowed to rise. If any respiratory effort is seen, the patient is reconnected to the ventilator and care is continued, as this indicates continued brain function in the medulla. If no respiratory effort is seen, after 10 minutes an arterial blood gas (ABG) is drawn, and the patient is reconnected to the mechanical ventilator. If the ABG results show that the $PaCO_2$ is above 60 mmHg (or there is a 20 mmHg increase over the baseline $PaCO_2$) and no respiratory movement is noted during the test, the patient is considered apneic.

During the test, if the patient develops cardiac dysrhythmias or hypotension or oxygen saturation falls below 70%, an ABG is immediately drawn, and the patient is reconnected to the ventilator. If the patient requires reconnection to the ventilator before apnea testing is complete and the $PaCO_2$ is less than 60 mmHg at the time of ventilator reconnection, another type of testing may be considered or the apnea test is repeated after the patient is stabilized.

Confirmatory Tests   Although not required, confirmatory tests can be used with patients for whom specific components of clinical testing cannot be reliably performed or evaluated. They may also be used when the apnea test cannot be performed. Three cerebral blood flow studies can be used to confirm loss of blood flow to the brain: cerebral angiography, cerebral scintigraphy (HMPAO SPECT), and transcranial Doppler (TCD) ultrasonography. Other confirmatory testing includes CT angiography (CTA), magnetic resonance imaging (MRI) or magnetic resonance angiography (MRA), and somatosensory evoked potentials. Electroencephalography (EEG) can also be obtained to evaluate the presence or absence of brain electrical activity; findings of electrocerebral silence are consistent with the diagnosis of brain death.

Documenting Time of Death   The official time of death is determined upon completion and interpretation of the apnea test (or of confirmatory tests if they are used). The official time of death should be documented in the patient's medical record, and the family should be informed.

Section Three Review

1. According to the Uniform Determination of Death Act (UDDA), which aspects are included in the definition of brain death? (Select all that apply.)
   A. Irreversible
   B. Failure of cardiac function
   C. Loss of brainstem function
   D. Loss of all brain function
   E. Glasgow Coma Scale score of 3

2. Which diagnostic criterion must be met before a client can be clinically diagnosed with brain death?
   A. Core temperature of 32°C (90°F) or higher
   B. Arterial pH between 7.35 and 7.45
   C. Serum K between 3 and 5 mEq/L
   D. Serum glucose between 70 and 100 mg/dL

3. In apnea testing, the client is considered apneic if there is no respiratory effort and the $PaCO_2$ is above which level after 10 minutes off the ventilator?
   A. 40
   B. 45
   C. 50
   D. 60

4. Which confirmatory test for brain death evaluates blood flow to the brain?
   A. Electroencephalography
   B. Cerebral angiography
   C. Somatosensory evoked potentials
   D. Arterial blood gas

Answers: 1. (A, C, D), 2. A, 3. D, 4. B

Section Four: Donor Management

Donor management focuses on maintaining organ function after brain death occurs. Close monitoring and evaluation of the patient's body system functions are crucial for maintaining organ viability for eventual transplantation.

Donor Management

When brain death occurs, organ and gland function begin to fail over time. To preserve healthy organs for recovery, it is essential to meet their oxygenation and perfusion needs through interventions that restabilize the body systems as their functions deteriorate. It has been shown that by achieving a set of nine donor management goals (DMGs), more organs can be successfully recovered from a single donor (Patel et al., 2014) (Table 39–1).

Hemodynamic Instability   Hemodynamic instability develops related to sequelae of physiologic events that occur with brain death. These include diabetes insipidus, initial hypertension followed by hypotension, inability to regulate body temperature, and neurogenic pulmonary edema. When brain death occurs, the body responds by releasing massive amounts of catecholamines, which increase heart rate and blood pressure in an attempt to increase cerebral blood supply. Catecholamine-induced tachycardia and hypertension continue until the catecholamine supply is depleted, resulting in the onset of hypotension (Kumar, 2016). The hypotensive state persists unless catecholamine stores are replaced intravenously.

The goals of management are to maintain the potential donor within normal hemodynamic parameters (refer to Table 39–1). However, failing to meet those criteria does not mean donation cannot take place. The OPO reviews the hemodynamics and determines whether the instability is significant. Hemodynamic dysfunction—when recognized and treated early through aggressive fluid resuscitation, thyroid hormone therapy (to improve cardiac muscle function), and vasopressor therapy—can usually be controlled and hemodynamic stability restored and maintained. Intropin (dopamine) is the most common catecholamine used and generally corrects the hypotension; however, if dopamine therapy is not successful in achieving an acceptable arterial blood pressure, initiation of norepinephrine or epinephrine may be necessary. If the hypotension is not successfully treated, cardiac standstill is imminent, which compromises organ donation.

Loss of Thermoregulation   After brain death occurs, the hypothalamus loses thermoregulatory control and the patient can no longer regulate body temperature. Hypothermia is seen most often, and warming must be initiated as hypothermia significantly reduces cardiac output and organ perfusion. Left untreated, the body eventually assumes ambient temperature, which can cause cardiac dysrhythmias and cardiac standstill. Occasionally, hyperthermia develops and cooling blankets must be employed. Hyperthermia results in vasodilatation and worsening hypotension if untreated. The temperature should be maintained at 35.6°C to 37.8°C (96°F to 100°F).

Fluid and Electrolyte Instability   As the pituitary gland ceases functioning after brain death, antidiuretic hormone (ADH) is no longer secreted. The absence of ADH results in diabetes insipidus (DI). Symptoms of DI include urine output greater than 4 mL/kg/hr, urine-specific gravity of less than 1.005, and urine osmolality of less than 300 mOsm/kg. Placing a central line to monitor central venous pressure (CVP) is helpful in the measurement of fluid status. Replacement of ADH may be necessary to manage fluid balance. Desmopressin acetate (DDAVP) or

Table 39–1 Donor Management Goals (DMG)

Benchmarks	Parameter
Mean arterial pressure (MAP)	60–110 mmHg
Central venous pressure (CVP)	4–12 mmHg
Ejection fraction	50% or greater
Arterial blood gas (ABG)	pH 7.3–7.5
PaO_2/FiO_2 (P/F) ratio	300 or greater
Sodium (serum)	155 mEq/L or less
Glucose (serum)	150 mg/dL or less
Urine output	0.5 mL/kg/hr or greater over 4 hours
Numbers of vasopressors	1 or less used Plus: Dopamine of 10 mcg/kg/min or less, or Norepinephrine of 10 mcg/min or less, or Neosynephrine of 60 mcg/min or less

SOURCE: Data from Patel et al. (2014).

vasopressin is the usual drug of choice in treating diabetes insipidus (DI). Urine output should be maintained at 0.5 to 3 mL/kg/hr.

When DI is present, choosing the correct IV fluid can be challenging. IV fluids should be salt poor. If large amounts of dextrose-containing IV fluids are used, hyperosmolar diuresis can develop; therefore, serum glucose levels must be closely monitored and treated appropriately. The rapid loss of urine in DI can result in significant electrolyte and acid–base imbalances. Potassium, calcium, phosphorus, and magnesium are lost, whereas sodium is retained. Unresolved hypernatremia eventually causes liver dysfunction, which may result in primary nonfunction if the liver is transplanted. Serum electrolytes must be closely monitored and replaced as necessary to maintain optimal cell and organ function.

Pulmonary Dysfunction   Occasionally, brain death may precipitate neurogenic pulmonary edema. This is characterized by crackles, pink frothy secretions, and a decreasing PaO_2 and SpO_2. The chest x-ray shows "whited-out" lungs. Judicious treatment with ventilator support is required, maximizing the FiO_2 and positive end–expiratory pressure (PEEP) to maintain the PaO_2 above 100 mmHg, and low tidal volumes are used to minimize alveolar damage.

Hematopoietic Dysfunction   Coagulopathies are common in the patient with traumatic brain death. As brain death occurs, large amounts of tissue plasminogen activator (tPA), a thrombolytic enzyme, are released. Long-term hypothermia increases the likelihood of coagulopathy. Hemograms, prothrombin time (PT), partial thromboplastin time (PTT), and international normalized ratio (INR)

should be monitored. Blood or blood component therapy (e.g., fresh frozen plasma, cryoprecipitate) is administered as needed.

Loss of Endocrine Function   Brain death results in a loss of thyroid hormone production. In addition, cortisol production ceases and insulin production declines. The combination of these processes causes a shift from aerobic to anaerobic metabolism. The myocardial cells become oxygen depleted, and cellular death begins. Organ procurement organizations now use a thyroid protocol to reverse this process. A levothyroxine drip is started after an initial bolus and is continued throughout the organ recovery process to decrease vasopressor requirements and prevent cardiovascular collapse.

Table 39–2 provides a summary of some of the management of the functional instabilities that accompany brain death.

Nursing Considerations   The unit nurse assigned to the donor patient (or the organ procurement coordinator [OPC]) is responsible for maintaining the organ donor's status within a set of hemodynamic and physiologic parameters until the patient is taken to the surgical suite for organ recovery. After brain death, organ and gland functions fail; therefore, the nurse monitors the patient's status closely and intervenes as necessary to restabilize the patient. For example, close monitoring and aggressive management of the patient's hemodynamic status are imperative to maintain optimal organ health. Suboptimal care of the donor patient during this vulnerable period will result in recovery of suboptimal organs that will likely negatively impact the long-term success of the graft in the recipient.

Table 39–2 Summary of Organ Donor Management of Functional Instabilities

Functional Instability or Problem	Goals	Management Options
Hemodynamic (hypotension)	MAP 60–100 mmHg; ejection fraction greater than 50%; minimal use of vasopressors	Aggressive fluid resuscitation Levothyroxine (T4) IV catecholamine therapy—dopamine most common choice; norepinephrine or epinephrine drip may be considered if dopamine therapy is ineffective for maintenance of blood pressure
Thermoregulatory (hypothermia, occasionally hyperthermia)	Maintain body temperature at 35.6°C–37.8°C (96°F–100°F)	Warming blanket (hypothermia); cooling blanket (hyperthermia)
Renal or fluid and electrolytes (dehydration and electrolyte imbalances from diabetes insipidus [DI]; decreased renal perfusion resulting in organ deterioration)	Maintain UO at 0.5–3 mL/kg/hr and serum creatinine less than 1.5–2 mg/dL; maintain adequate electrolyte balance CVP 4–10 mmHg; serum sodium 135–155 mEq/L	Supportive measures to maintain cardiac output and tissue perfusion (e.g., fluid resuscitation); replace ADH if necessary (DDAVP [preferred] or vasopressin); IV fluids: salt-poor IV fluids and avoid hypo-osmotic fluids; placement of central line; close monitoring of urine output and replacement of fluid and electrolytes
Pulmonary (neurogenic pulmonary edema)	Maintain PaO_2 above 100 mmHg; PaO_2/FiO_2 ratio above 300	Mechanical ventilation; positive end–expiratory pressure (PEEP); high-frequency percussive ventilation
Hematopoietic (coagulopathy)	Maintain adequate hematopoietic status	Monitor Hgb/Hct; PT, PTT, and INR; replace blood as necessary; fresh frozen plasma, cryoprecipitate; factor VII
Endocrine (loss of thyroid hormone and cortisol production; decreased insulin production)	Maintain adequate hormone levels Serum glucose: less than 150 mg/dL	Replace hormones as necessary—thyroid protocol: IV bolus of levothyroxine followed by continuous intravenous infusion; given in conjunction with methylprednisolone, regular insulin, and dextrose

MAP = mean arterial pressure; UO = urine output; Hgb = hemoglobin; Hct = hematocrit; PT = prothrombin time; PTT = partial thromboplastin time; INR = international normalized ratio.

SOURCE: Data from Kumar (2016), Shapiro & DeVita (2016), and UpToDate (2017).

Section Four Review

1. What are major management goals in caring for the donor client? (Select all that apply.)
   A. Maintaining a stable hemodynamic status
   B. Maintaining infections at a minimum level
   C. Maintaining fluid balance
   D. Maintaining optimal oxygenation status
   E. Maintaining electrolyte balance

2. What is the most common underlying cause of hypotension in the donor?
   A. Depletion of catecholamine stores
   B. Cardiac failure
   C. Fluid overload
   D. Increased systemic vascular resistance

3. A client diagnosed with brain death who develops a coagulopathy may receive which therapy to counteract this problem?
   A. Dopamine
   B. Fresh frozen plasma
   C. Levothyroxine
   D. Solu-Medrol

4. Which medication is given to a potential organ donor to delay shift from aerobic to anaerobic metabolism?
   A. Glucose
   B. Epinephrine
   C. Insulin
   D. Levothyroxine

Answers: 1. (A, C, D, E), 2. A, 3. B, 4. D

Section Five: Organ Procurement

The specific procedures used to procure and distribute organs differ among transplant programs and organizations. This section describes the procurement process in general.

Referral to the Organ Procurement Organization

The Medicare conditions of participation state that all imminent deaths should be referred to the OPO. *Imminent death* refers to the potentially brain-dead patient, although the Department of Health and Human Services (DHHS) defines imminent death as that of a severely brain-injured patient with a Glasgow Coma Score of 5 or less. After the referral, the OPO makes a determination of suitability for organ donation and develops a plan of care with the medical staff regarding patient and family care. Should the patient become brain-dead, the early notification and evaluation facilitate timely communication between the OPO and the family.

It is often the emergency department or critical care nurse who first identifies a patient as a potential organ donor. To facilitate the referral process, the nurse can have specific data available to help the OPO begin the evaluation (Box 39–1).

Determination of Patient's Suitability for Organ Donation

Multiple factors must be considered in determining if a patient is a candidate for donation: type of death (as presented in Section Two), general health status, age, and

> **BOX 39–1**   Important Initial Information for Potential Donor Referral
>
> - Patient's name
> - Age, sex, race
> - Cause of brain injury
> - Height and weight
> - Current Glasgow Coma Score (GCS)
> - Past medical and social history
> - Laboratory data (if available): serum electrolytes, BUN, creatinine, AST, ALT, alk phos, WBC, Hgb, Hct
> - Hemodynamic status: blood pressure, mean arterial pressure, heart rate, O_2 saturation
> - Urine output (mL/hr)
> - Current inotropic support (drug name and dose)
> - Plan of care: brain death testing scheduled, DNR status

weight. Other significant factors that may impact donor suitability include the patient's medical and social history and compliance with medical treatments. In addition, the patient's current hemodynamic stability is important, as discussed in Section Four: Donor Management.

Medical and Social History   Past medical and social history considers the patient's illnesses and behaviors that affect function and the transmission of diseases. This information is helpful in determining the risks posed to a potential organ recipient. Certain other factors, although not necessarily precluding donation, are important to consider, including sepsis and any high-risk behaviors for disease transmission (e.g., IV drug abuse, male-to-male sex, extended time in jail, hemophilia, or blood contact with a person who has HIV/AIDS or hepatitis B). Having cancer does not necessarily eliminate a person as a potential donor, particularly if the cancer is in remission, localized, and not bloodborne.

Obtaining Consent

The Uniform Anatomical Gift Act defines the order of priority of those who give consent for donation. Individuals can indicate their wish to donate by registering on their state's donor registry or having it designated in a legal document. If the patient has not indicated a wish for donation in a legal document, the responsibility of consent lies with the legal next of kin. When the legal next of kin is to be approached, the order of priority is spouse, adult children, parent, adult sibling(s), and guardian.

Who Obtains Consent? Only persons who are employed by the OPO or have received training from the OPO in best practices in the consent process should discuss donation (Department of Health and Human Services, 2006). The OPO staff provides support to the family after receiving the patient referral. Their initial interactions focus heavily on facilitating the family's understanding of the patient's brain injury, poor prognosis, and imminent death. A significant amount of time may need to be devoted to helping the family understand the concept of brain death—that death has occurred although the patient will sustain a heartbeat for a period of time.

Donor Testing

After consent is obtained, care of the donor is transferred to the OPO, and an OPO coordinator initiates orders. Each organ is evaluated to ensure suitability for transplant. Serologic testing is performed to determine the absence or presence of transmittable diseases. Blood type and human leukocyte antigen (HLA) typing are determined. In addition to blood and tissue typing, the patient's health history is carefully examined for possible organ problems (e.g., history of heart failure or chronic renal insufficiency), and a battery of laboratory and other tests (e.g., CBC, BUN and creatinine, ECG, echocardiogram) will be obtained to evaluate organ function for possible recovery. Each organ requires its own battery of tests. After all tests are completed, the information is entered into the United Network for Organ Sharing (UNOS) system to identify matching recipients.

A specific algorithm matches each organ to a recipient. The UNOS Organ Center provides a centralized repository of data on the organ and on recipients on the waiting list. Critical information includes tissue and blood types, organ size, the potential recipient's medical urgency, time on the waiting list, and the geographic distance between the donor and the potential recipient (Organ Procurement & Transplantation Network [OPTN], 2017b). In general, priority is given to recipients within the donor's local area. A significant factor for the initial function and long-term survival of a transplanted organ is a decreased cold ischemic time, the period when circulation to the organ is stopped in the donor and restored in the recipient. If a matching recipient is not found within the local area, the search expands regionally, then nationally.

The Organ Recovery Process

The OPO plays an important role in the donor process: identifying potential donors, working with donor families and ensuring that the donation is truly based on informed consent, managing clinical care of the donor prior to organ recovery, entering donor data into the UNOS computer for matching purposes, and coordinating the organ recovery process (Organ Procurement and Transplantation Network [OPTN], 2017c). Once the recipients are located, the donor organ recovery is scheduled.

Organ Recovery At a prearranged time agreed to by all the transplant teams involved, the donor is taken to the operating room and prepared for surgery. When the donor is brought to the OR, the chart must contain the required documentation: date and time of the death declaration and the signed or recorded consent form. In addition, the hospital may require a signed death certificate or other documentation.

Each transplant team receiving an organ may be present for the organ recovery or may ask a transplant recovery team from the donor's location to recover the organ. In accordance with federal law, the donor's attending physician cannot be part of the recovery teams (OPTN, 2017c). Each recovery team must be present in the operating room to perform the recovery together. The donor is taken to the operating room, prepped, and draped as for any surgical procedure. The patient is kept on mechanical ventilation with anesthesia to maintain hemodynamic stability. Usually an abdominal surgical team begins the recovery process with an incision from the suprasternal notch to the symphysis pubis. The surgeon inspects the body for the presence of any unexpected disease, such as an undiagnosed cancer, and then begins the process of dissecting each organ from its surrounding anatomical structures. The organs are prepared for removal by each recovery team.

Organ Preservation When all the organs are ready to be removed, cannulas are placed in the thoracic aorta, pulmonary artery, portal vein, and abdominal aorta. A clamp is placed on the aorta, and perfusion of the organs begins with a cold preservation solution. The solution runs through each organ, removing the blood. This procedure slows the organ's metabolic rate and preserves it until the organ is transplanted. Once removed from the donor, the organ is packed in the preservative solution and sterile triple bagged. It is then placed on ice and transported to the recipient's hospital. Each organ has a certain window of time in which it can safely remain outside of the body, called *cold ischemic time* (see Table 39–3).

Table 39–3 Organ Preservation and Transplantation Ischemic Times

Organ	Transplantation Time Frame (hrs)
Heart	4–6
Lungs	4–6
Liver	12–24
Kidneys	48–72

Section Five Review

1. A client is declared brain dead after a serious head injury. His care has involved services of a trauma surgeon, a cardiology team, and an intensivist. Consent for donor status has been obtained. Who is in charge of the care of the donor?
   A. The trauma surgeon
   B. The cardiologist
   C. The organ procurement organization (OPO) coordinator
   D. The intensivist

2. Which statement best describes procedures related to organ recovery in the operating room?
   A. An anesthesiologist is not necessary.
   B. The donor's physician is not part of the recovery team.
   C. Only one organ recovery team can be present in the operating room.
   D. The recipient's physician must be part of the recovery team.

3. When the donor is brought to the OR for organ recovery, the chart must contain which required documentation? (Select all that apply)
   A. Signed OPO release form
   B. Signed or recorded consent form
   C. Time-of-death declaration
   D. Specification of which organs are to be recovered
   E. Date-of-death declaration

4. Which descriptors best represent how recovered organs are preserved for transport? (Select all that apply.)
   A. Preservation solution
   B. Shipped frozen
   C. Cold packing
   D. Electrolyte solution
   E. Warm packing

Answers: 1. C, 2. B, 3. (B, C, E), 4. (A, C)

The Organ Recipient

Section Six: Immunologic Considerations

Before the scientific discovery of human leukocyte antigens (HLAs), organ transplants were for the most part unsuccessful in the long term because a mismatch of HLA between the organ donor and the recipient (transplant candidate) resulted in organ rejection. An individual's HLA fingerprint consists of antigens on the surface of most cells in the body that allows the immune system to discriminate between self and nonself. The immune system ignores "self" cells and musters an immune response against "nonself" cells. Compatibility testing of donor and transplant candidate is crucial because, ultimately, the long-term success or failure of the graft is greatly dependent on the compatibility of the donor tissue with that of the recipient.

Donor–Recipient Compatibility Testing

The three tests used to evaluate the compatibility of the donor's tissues with the tissues of the transplant candidate are tissue typing, crossmatching, and ABO typing.

Tissue Typing   In humans, histocompatibility is identified through special cell surface antigens called human leukocyte antigens (HLAs). Tests of histocompatibility on the donor and recipient are crucial for optimizing success in organ transplantation. A perfect HLA match is only possible between identical twins; however, the HLA match between first-degree relations (parents and siblings) is generally much better than between nonrelations.

Tissue typing is the identification of the histocompatibility antigens of both the donor and the transplant candidate. It evaluates the degree to which the two sets of tissues are HLA matched. The closer the HLA match, the better the chances for long-term transplant success. The opposite is true as well.

Crossmatching   Crossmatching tests the potential recipient for antidonor (preformed) antibodies. When preformed antibodies are present, the transplant candidate has been presensitized to the donor. Histocompatibility can be tested by evaluating the degree of reactivity of the immune response to crossmatch testing of donor and recipient cells and serum. In serum crossmatching, a sample of the recipient's serum is exposed to the serum from a sample of the prospective donor's blood. The serum is analyzed for the formation of preformed antibodies (PRAs). The normal value is 0%. A prospective crossmatch is performed immediately prior to the transplant on patients with a PRA of 10% or higher. In order to suppress the preformed antibodies, the transplant candidate may undergo one or more treatment modalities, such as plasmapheresis, intravenous immunoglobulin (IVIg), or immunosuppressant therapy. A candidate can become sensitized to foreign HLA antigens through prior organ transplantation, blood transfusions, and pregnancy. In such cases, the reintroduction of a new organ containing the sensitized HLA antigens can cause rapid organ rejection and possibly organ or recipient death.

ABO Typing ABO typing identifies the blood group of the donor and the transplant candidate. ABO compatibility is an initial criterion for transplantation. The rules for blood type matching are the same as for transfusions: Unmatched protein types cause a rapid immune reaction.

The type O allograft is considered the universal transplant donor type because it can be transplanted safely into a recipient with any blood type. Type AB is considered the universal recipient because it can receive an allograft from all blood types. Types A and B can receive an allograft only from the same blood type or type O donors.

Section Six Review

1. Where on (in) the cell are HLA antigens located?
   A. Surface
   B. Nucleus
   C. Cytoplasm
   D. Mitochondria

2. The best histocompatibility matching is found between which relatives?
   A. Siblings
   B. Identical twins
   C. Parent and child
   D. Fraternal twins

3. What is the term for the identification of the histocompatibility antigens of both donor and recipient?
   A. Crossmatching
   B. ABO typing
   C. Antigen classifying
   D. Tissue typing

4. A recipient can become sensitized to foreign HLA antigens in which ways? (Select all that apply.)
   A. Pregnancy
   B. Donating blood
   C. Prior organ transplantation
   D. Receiving blood transfusions
   E. Some medications

Answers: 1. A, 2. B, 3. D, 4. (A, C, D)

Section Seven: Determination of Transplant Need

The scarcity of organs, along with the physical and financial costs involved, make determination of transplant need a major issue. Determining who will receive an organ is not a simple decision and is based on multiple factors. The criteria used to determine who is eligible for organ transplantation are multifaceted and vary among transplant programs.

Evaluation of the Transplant Recipient

The primary eligibility criterion for organ transplantation is end-stage organ disease, which is determined by thoroughly evaluating organ function. The patient is considered a transplant candidate only after maximum medical therapy has proven ineffective, leaving transplantation as the final option. Evaluation of the potential recipient is an extensive process and can vary based on the type of transplant required by the patient. Many factors are taken into consideration, such as comorbid illnesses, obesity, and older age—all factors that increase the risks of posttransplant complications and adverse patient outcomes (Brammer, Andersson, & Hosing, 2016; Gruessner et al., 2015).

Clinical Status Organ-specific diagnostic studies and laboratory testing are conducted. Preexisting or concurrent medical problems are closely scrutinized and discussed with the transplant candidate and family.

Nutritional Status Malnourished transplant candidates awaiting an organ transplant are at high risk for perioperative complications such as wound infection, graft failure, cytomegalovirus (CMV) infection, and bacterial infection. Nutritional intervention is crucial in the pretransplant stage and may even require enteral or parenteral feedings. Assessments should include regular physical assessments, weights, anthropometric measurements, and laboratory tests.

Psychosocial Status Certain psychosocial factors increase the risk of adverse recipient outcomes, including an active diagnosed psychiatric problem (especially mood disorders), history of poor adherence to treatment plan, inability to comprehend complex transplant management, and problems of financial support (Gruessner et al., 2015). Chronic illness and its treatment are known to have profound long-term psychological effects on the transplant candidate and family. Furthermore, it is known that certain psychological factors play a role in determining long-term adherence to the recommended drug regimen, which may have an impact on the long-term success of the transplant. In addition, the stresses associated with organ transplantation can further strain the recipient's coping abilities. While there are stressors associated with the receipt of a transplanted organ, some psychological relief may occur when the seriously ill patient moves from transplant candidate to recipient. An

Quality and Safety
Quality of Life for Transplant Patients

Quality of life (QOL) differences were examined in a survey of patients who were in the process of planning and receiving organ transplantation. Using a crisis theory framework, transplant candidates were considered to be in-crisis patients and transplant recipients were postcrisis patients in a study of 226 research participants. Stress, coping, and QOL were examined in transplant candidates and recipients and in healthy individuals who did not need transplantation. In this study sample, transplant candidates experienced lower QOL than organ recipients and those who did not require transplantation. Differences in stress or coping styles between groups were not noted, but stress did impact the patients' quality of life. These findings emphasize the importance of providing psychological support throughout the transplant process, especially during the organ candidacy phase (Denny, Kienhuir, & Gavidia-Payne, 2015).

exploration of psychological variables, including quality of life, during organ transplant candidacy and receipt is provided in the "Quality and Safety: Quality of Life for Transplant Patients" feature.

Financial Status   The total cost of organ transplantation varies with the organ being grafted. Costs include 30 days of pretransplant care, organ procurement, hospital admission, physician costs during transplant, and 180 days of posttransplant admission and immunosuppressant costs (United Network for Organ Sharing [UNOS], 2017). Solid-organ transplantation is expensive—the estimated average charges per transplant in 2014 ranged from $334,300 (kidney transplant) to more than $1,547,000 (intestine transplant) (Bentley, 2014). Nonmedical costs, such as transportation to and from the transplant center, food and lodging, child care, and lost wages, are also substantial. In addition, the patient may be required to relocate close to the transplant center for a designated period both pre- and posttransplant. Coverage varies widely among Medicare, state medical programs, and private health insurance and is often differentiated by the type of organ being transplanted. If financial resources are questionable, financial options are explored. Many transplant programs offer financial and social services to the public that provide information and other forms of support for transplant recipients.

Placement on UNOS Waiting List   Once the decision is made to accept a patient as a transplant candidate, the patient's name and vital information are entered into the computer bank at the United Network for Organ Sharing (UNOS). This organization is charged with distributing organs in an equitable and nondiscriminatory manner. The transplant candidate remains on the UNOS waiting list until an organ becomes available, the candidate is removed from the list, or the candidate dies. Periodic reevaluation of the transplant candidate's health status is recommended.

In anticipation of being placed on the UNOS waiting list, it is crucial that the transplant candidate and the family go into the transplant process with a thorough and realistic understanding of the entire process, including its risks and benefits, waiting time, costs, expectations, tests, and procedures. The nurse plays a major role in obtaining this essential information, helping the transplant candidate and family understand the process and access support resources. Table 39–4 lists major educational topics for organ transplant patients, which change as the patient moves through the transplant process.

Waiting Time   In April 2017, 118,088 patients were on the waiting list for transplants (Organ Procurement and Transplantation Network [OPTN], 2017d). Hundreds, possibly thousands, of transplant candidates are on the national waiting list for the same organ at any one time. Many will succumb to their disease before a donor organ becomes available. It is essential that the transplant candidate and family have a realistic expectation of waiting time, which is the length of time from placement on the UNOS waiting list to organ availability. Waiting times for deceased organ donors vary widely, depending on the patient's tissue and blood type and the organ to be transplanted. An organ may become available in as few as 30 days of being placed on the waiting list or as long as 5 years or more.

Providing basic information on how organs are allocated may help the transplant candidate and family understand the variability of the waiting time. Organs are allocated based on a point system established by the United Network for Organ Sharing (UNOS). The allocation policy for kidney transplants (United Network for Organ Sharing [UNOS], 2016) includes the following factors:

- Length of time spent on waiting list
- Whether the organ candidate is a child
- Body size of both donor and candidate

Table 39–4   Transplant Patient Education

Timing	Focus of Teaching
Preparing for UNOS waiting list	Waiting times Tests: tissue typing, ABO typing General organ evaluation to establish overall health status Preparations: costs and financial, medical, educational, spiritual, practical
Preparing for surgery	Proper cough and deep breathing methods Correct use of incentive spirometer Rating and control of pain postoperatively ICU environment (monitors, special devices) Overview of surgery and acute postop activities and expectations Possible postoperative complications (delayed graft functioning, graft thrombosis, rejection) and treatment Drug regimen
Preparing for discharging	Individual drugs in drug regimen and importance of adherence (should be able to identify each drug, its purpose, and common side effects) Symptoms of infection and rejection When to contact transplant professionals (e.g., symptoms of infection, rejection, adverse drug effects) Self-care at home (e.g., good hand hygiene, exercise, diet, self-monitoring, sexual adjustments, travel) Contacting donor family Important resources (e.g., transplant professionals, social services, rehabilitation, support)

- Tissue match between donor and candidate
- Blood type
- Antibody levels

Transplant Resources and Support In addition to resources provided by transplant professionals, multiple online resources can answer many common questions that the transplant candidate and family may have. Many national organizations, such as the National Kidney Foundation and the American Diabetes Association, offer transplantation information specific to their particular disorder. Box 39–2 lists three of the major national transplant-oriented resources.

> **BOX 39–2** National Transplant-Oriented Resources
>
> - Transplant Living (a service of UNOS): patient-oriented site that provides information and support. PO Box 2484, Richmond, VA 23218, www.transplantliving.org
> - National Foundation for Transplants (NFT): patient-oriented site that provides information and support. 5350 Poplar Ave., Suite 430, Memphis, TN 38119, www.transplants.org
> - United Network for Organ Sharing (UNOS): national clearinghouse of information and data. PO Box 2484, Richmond, VA 23218, www.transplantliving.org

Section Seven Review

1. What is true regarding financial implication of receiving an organ transplant?
   A. All costs are covered by Medicare.
   B. Costs are waived by the hospitals involved.
   C. There are substantial nonmedical costs.
   D. No private insurance plans cover transplant costs.

2. The decision to place a person on the organ transplant waiting list is usually made by whom?
   A. The client and family
   B. A multidisciplinary committee
   C. The organ procurement team
   D. The potential recipient's physician

3. Which factors are considered when allocating a kidney for transplant? (Select all that apply.)
   A. Length of time on the transplant list
   B. Age of the candidate
   C. Candidate body size
   D. Amount of insurance reimbursement
   E. Blood type

4. A transplant candidate undergoes basic psychological testing for which reason?
   A. There is a risk of posttransplant psychosis.
   B. A depressed state is a major contraindication for transplantation.
   C. A higher mortality is associated with pretransplant psychological distress.
   D. Certain psychological profiles increase the risk of posttransplant nonadherence to the drug regimen.

Answers: 1. C, 2. B, 3. (A, B, C, E), 4. D

Section Eight: Posttransplantation Complications

Each type of organ transplant has its own unique features and commonalities. This is true also of organ transplant complications. Three major types of complications are associated with transplantation:

- Technical complications
- Graft rejection
- Immunosuppressant-related problems

Technical Complications

The technical procedures involved in performing transplantation are not without risks. Three major groups of technical complications are associated with the surgical procedure: vascular thrombosis, bleeding, and anastomosis leakage.

Vascular Thrombosis **Vascular thrombosis** is a fairly rare complication that usually develops during the early postoperative period. As a complication of organ transplantation, it refers to a blood clot in the vasculature of the graft, often the major artery. The thrombosis may not be detected initially because the patient is frequently asymptomatic. Diagnostic tests may be performed soon after surgery (e.g., duplex ultrasonography) to ensure arterial patency. Early detection and immediate thrombectomy are essential if the graft is to survive. Even then, the graft is at high risk for failure. Any delay in detection of thrombosis frequently leads to loss of the graft.

Bleeding Postoperative transplantation bleeding is managed in a fashion similar to bleeding in other postsurgery patients, with the exception of liver transplants. In the liver transplant patient, it is often difficult to differentiate bleeding that is secondary to coagulopathy associated with a dysfunctional liver from bleeding that has resulted from a surgical (technical) problem. Postoperatively, a transplanted liver may have some degree of coagulopathy, which makes control of otherwise normal postoperative bleeding extremely difficult. The decision must be made whether to allow bleeding to continue until the coagulopathy resolves as liver function returns or to take the patient for exploratory surgery under the assumption that the cause is technical.

Anastomosis Leakage   The term **anastomosis** refers to the site at which the graft is sutured into the recipient. Problems at the anastomosis site usually occur 1 to 3 weeks following transplantation. The problem may be failure of the anastomosis to seal completely, usually at the epithelial layer, which results in leakage of fluids (e.g., urine following a postrenal graft, or air as in bronchial dehiscence). An anastomosis leak usually results from inadequate healing, possibly as a result of a deficient blood supply or steroid therapy. Anastomosis leaks usually require surgical exploration and repair.

Graft Rejection

Graft rejection is the activation of the immune response against a transplanted tissue or organ. The body recognizes the new tissue as nonself, triggering an autoimmune system attack to eliminate the invader. Graft rejection is primarily the result of T lymphocyte and B lymphocyte activities. The three types of graft rejection are based on the time and speed of onset and are called hyperacute, acute, and chronic.

Hyperacute Rejection   **Hyperacute rejection** is a type III (Arthus) hypersensitivity response—that is, a humoral response in which the B lymphocytes are activated to produce antibodies. It occurs within minutes to hours following transplantation and results from the presence of preformed graft-specific cytotoxic antibodies. Because the antibodies are already formed, as soon as the graft is placed the immune system recognizes the foreign tissue and increases graft-specific antibody production. In turn, the antibodies accumulate rapidly and trigger the agglutination of platelets, activation of the complement system, and phagocytic activities. Fortunately, hyperacute rejection is now rare in countries such as the United States, where donor–recipient screening and matching procedures have been greatly improved.

Acute Rejection   **Acute rejection** is characterized by its sudden onset and usually occurs within days or months following the transplant. Acute rejection begins as a type IV hypersensitivity response—that is, a cell-mediated immune response in which the T lymphocytes and macrophages of the host (recipient) attack and destroy the graft (donor) tissue. The graft's HLA antigens are recognized as foreign (nonself), thereby triggering T lymphocyte proliferation and attack. As the acute rejection continues, graft-specific cytotoxic antibodies are produced, further aggravating the rejection process. If this condition is recognized and treated promptly, organ function can be preserved.

Chronic Rejection   **Chronic rejection** is a humoral immune response in which antibodies slowly attack the graft. Chronic rejection may begin at any time following transplantation and may take years to render the graft nonfunctional. The antibodies trigger the same immune response seen in hyperacute rejection but at a very low level. In time, the organ becomes ischemic and dies.

Immunosuppressant-related Complications

Immunosuppressants are the cornerstone to successful long-term transplantation. However, this group of drugs is associated with adverse effects that can cause serious problems, such as infection, organ dysfunction, malignancy, and steroid-induced problems such as hyperglycemia.

Infection   Infection is a leading cause of morbidity and mortality in posttransplantation patients. Jani (2017) proposes the CREDIT framework for a risk assessment of infection. The CREDIT framework suggests that there are six pathways by which the organ recipient can develop infection: C for community acquired; R for reactivated pathogens; E for epidemiologic exposures; D for donor organ source; I for iatrogenic infections; and T for travel-associated infections. Table 39–5 summarizes the six components of the CREDIT framework.

Long-term immunosuppressant therapy and the frequent use of antibiotics to treat infections are not without risk, as they may precipitate an invasive fungal infection (e.g., *Clostridium difficile*, *Candida*, or *Aspergillus*). Furthermore, repeated runs of antibiotics increase the risk of development of resistant strains of pathogens such as ganciclovir-resistant cytomegalovirus (CMV), methicillin-resistant *S. aureus* (MRSA), and vancomycin-resistant *Enterococcus* (VRE), which complicates treatment significantly (Gruessner et al., 2015).

CMV is a major pathogen that can significantly impact outcomes in the posttransplant patient. The CMV may have already been present in the recipient, or it may have been introduced through the donor organ (Gruessner et al., 2015). CMV-seropositive patients may develop reactivation of the virus as a result of their immunosuppressed state. CMV infections may be mild or severe; a severe infection can potentially cause dysfunction of multiple organs. This is especially a problem in seronegative recipients who received a seropositive organ or CMV-positive blood products.

Infection is a major posttransplantation problem because immunosuppressant therapy compromises the immune system. The immunosuppressed patient is unable to muster the same response to acute infection as a person who is immunocompetent; therefore, infection presents itself in more subtle ways. The primary symptom of infection in this population is fever that is often low grade (about 38°C [100.5°F]). Other assessments may include tachypnea, fatigue, tachycardia, and pain. Development of a fever requires a rapid but thorough search for the source of the infection and aggressive treatment. The lungs and urinary tract are the most common sources of nosocomial infection.

Organ Dysfunction   Almost all solid-organ transplant patients receive a similar regimen of immunosuppressant therapy. Immunosuppressants are associated with multiple

Table 39–5   CREDIT Posttransplant Infections

Infection Sources	Description
C - Community acquired	Infections from exposure within the recipient's community living Includes many common pathogens such as cold viruses, respiratory viruses or bacteria, GI pathogens; can also include newer resistant strains (e.g., methicillin-resistant *S. aureus* [MRSA]), influenza and other specific viruses), and atypical organisms such as *Mycoplasma* and *Chlamydia*
R - Reactivation of previous infection	Infections that reactivate from a dormant state; pathogens may come from the donor organ Includes cytomegalovirus (CMV), *M. tuberculosis*, Epstein-Barr virus (EBV), parasites, herpes viruses, HIV, hepatitis viruses, and others
E - Epidemiologic exposure	Exposure to pathogens secondary to specific factors such as environments in which the recipient lives, works, or plays; comorbid conditions (e.g., diabetes), recreational habits (e.g., drugs, smoking) Thorough patient history: workplace conditions, hobbies (e.g., gardening), history of transfusions, sexual history, pets, medications, food and water, recreational habits, and many others
D - Donor-derived infections	Donor organs contaminated with active or dormant pathogens Includes viruses (e.g., CMV, herpes, HTLV, HIV), mycobacteria, *Meningococcus*, donor-derived drug-resistant bacteria, and others
I - Iatrogenic	Infection acquired in the hospital following transplantation Requires vigilance by healthcare workers in performing hand hygiene and maintaining sterile technique during procedures
T - Travel	Travel, both recent and past, increases risk of exposure to novel forms of pathogens (e.g., *E. coli*, *Plasmodium* species, *Mycobacterium leprae*) Patient history should include past travel destinations.

SOURCE: Data from Jain, A. A. (2017).

side effects, many of which target specific organs. Some degree of graft dysfunction is common immediately following organ transplantation. Development of nephrotoxicity and hepatotoxicity can occur with any organ transplant but are considered especially serious in kidney and liver transplants, respectively. The combination of postgraft dysfunction and the adverse effects of the immunosuppressant may precipitate a severe graft crisis. Immunosuppressant therapy is discussed in Section Nine.

Malignancy   In the United States, patients undergoing organ transplantation run a twofold risk of developing cancer. The increased cancer risk has been attributed to two major underlying factors: long-term immunosuppressant therapy and persistent viral infection. The immune system plays a major role in surveillance and destruction of neoplastic cells. Long-term immunosuppression significantly hinders the protection against cancer, thus increasing the risk for development of malignancy. Persistent viral infection with certain viruses has been associated with development of cancer (Mesri, Feitelson, & Munger, 2014). For example, persistent *H. pylori* infection has been attributed to gastric cancer (Zhang, Zhang, & Aboul-Soud, 2017). In posttransplant patients, Epstein-Barr virus (EBV) infection has been identified as a risk factor for development of non-Hodgkin lymphoma and other cancers (Souza et al., 2010; Wang & Kieff, 2014).

Posttransplant cancers may develop within 6 months to a year or as distantly as 10 to 15 years after transplantation. Engels and colleagues (2011) conducted a large study on the incidence of cancer in transplant patients. They found that the most common malignancies associated with kidney, liver, heart, and lung transplantation in the United States include non-Hodgkin lymphoma and cancers of the lung, liver, and kidney, with the highest incidence of cancers developing in the transplanted organ (e.g., lung cancer in transplanted lung). However, the incidence of cancer developing in the lung, liver, or kidney is increased regardless of which organ was transplanted. The incidence of non-Hodgkin lymphoma in lung transplant patients is highest in the first posttransplant year and peaks again 4 to 5 years posttransplant. The vast majority of liver cancer is diagnosed within the first 6 months following liver transplantation.

Other relatively common malignancies that have an increased incidence in posttransplant patients include nonmelanoma skin cancers (usually squamous or basal cell), Kaposi sarcoma, and Merkel cell carcinoma (Mesri et al., 2014), as well as melanoma and lung cancer (Hersh, 2016).

New-onset Diabetes After Transplant   Development of new-onset diabetes after transplant (NODAT) contributes significantly to patient morbidity and mortality and is a significant predictor of graft failure and cardiovascular complications (Tobin, Klein, & Brennan, 2017). According to this article, in renal transplant recipients NODAT is a relatively common complication, affecting up to 40% of the transplant population (Rohan, Kishi, McGillicuddy, & Nadig, 2017). Interestingly, in cardiac transplant patients, it is estimated that about 20% develop diabetes within the first year, but the percentage drops to about 15% by the end of 5 years, a statistic attributable to decreased steroid dosages (Yamani & Taylor, 2010). Risk factors may include older age, higher BMI following transplantation, positive family history for diabetes, use of steroid therapy or the immunosuppressant tacrolimus (Prograf, FK-506), infection, rejection, and low magnesium levels (Hayes, Boyle, Carroll, Bockenhauer & Marks, 2017; Shary, Chapman, & Herrmann, 2015).

Steroid-induced Problems   Long-term steroid therapy carries with it multiple potentially serious side effects. Steroid-induced hyperglycemia, significant weight gain, and metabolic bone disease are common problems, especially in the first year. Steroid therapy is discussed further in Section Nine.

Section Eight Review

1. What is the term used to describe organ rejection that takes place minutes to hours following transplantation and results from the presence of preformed graft-specific cytotoxic antibodies?
   A. Subacute
   B. Acute
   C. Hyperacute
   D. Chronic

2. Posttransplant clients are at particular risk for developing which infection, either from being seropositive prior to the transplant or after receiving a seropositive organ or blood transfusion?
   A. Cytomegalovirus
   B. Pneumonia
   C. Hepatitis A
   D. Wound

3. Posttransplant clients are at increased risk for malignancies secondary to which condition? (Select all that apply)
   A. Organ toxicity
   B. Persistent viral infections
   C. Underlying tissue incompatibility
   D. Prolonged immunosuppressant therapy
   E. Drug toxicities

4. What are some risk factors for posttransplant new-onset diabetes mellitus? (Select all that apply.)
   A. Older age
   B. Low BMI
   C. Steroid therapy
   D. Female gender
   E. Low magnesium levels

Answers: 1. C, 2. A, 3. (B, D), 4. (A, C, E)

Section Nine: Immunosuppressant Therapy

The long-term success of organ transplantation has been made possible by use of immunosuppressant therapy. Prior to the discovery and refinement of immunosuppressant therapy, tissue transplantation was considered only a short-term therapy, with the exception of identical-twin grafts. This section presents an overview of some of the major drug groups and drugs administered for their ability to alter immune function. Figure 39–1 shows the sites of action of immunosuppressive agents.

Calcineurin Inhibitors

Calcineurin inhibitors are a class of immunosuppressant drugs that inhibit interleukin-2 (IL-2) production in T cells, which leads to suppression of cytotoxic T cells (Azzi, Milford, Sayegh, & Chandraker, 2015). They are considered the most effective of the immunosuppressant agents. These agents do not, however, suppress bone marrow function.

Depending on the type of organ transplant (e.g., heart, kidney) calcineurin inhibitors are usually used in conjunction with other immunosuppressant drug groups. There are three major drugs in this group: cyclosporine (Gengraf, Sandimmune, Neoral), tacrolimus (Prograf, FK-506), and sirolimus (Rapamune, Rapamycin). In addition to infection—the major adverse effect of all immunosuppressants—the adverse effects of this drug group include renal toxicity and cancer (lymphoma). A summary of this drug group is presented in the "Related Pharmacotherapy: Calcineurin Inhibitors" feature.

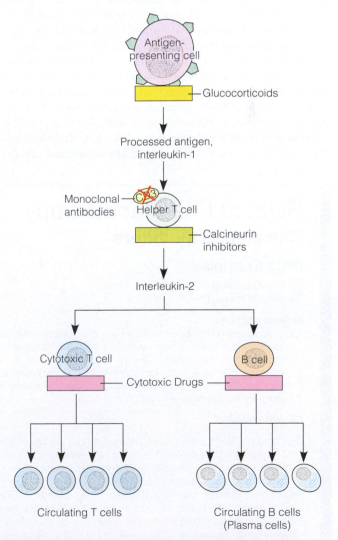

Figure 39–1 Sites of action of immunosuppressive agents.

Cyclosporine (Gengraf, Sandimmune, Neoral) is an immunosuppressant agent for the prevention of allograft rejection (Adams & Urban, 2016). Cyclosporine is notable for being highly incompatible with other drugs, and great care should be taken to avoid incompatibilities, which can be life-threatening.

Tacrolimus (Prograf, FK-506) is a powerful and commonly used immunosuppressant. Following transplantation, tacrolimus is administered through oral, sublingual, or intravenous routes with a goal of 8 to 12 ng/mL trough levels during the first 3 months, then tapering down to 6 to 10 ng/mL thereafter (Gruessner et al., 2015).

Sirolimus (Rapamune, Rapamycin) is currently approved for use only in kidney transplant rejection and is recommended for use in conjunction with cyclosporine and prednisone (Adams & Urban, 2016). Hyperlipidemia is the most notable additional side effect; however, concomitant use with cyclosporine potentiates the nephrotoxicity, leading the manufacturer to recommend that sirolimus be given 4 hours after cyclosporine.

Glucocorticoids

Glucocorticoids are steroid hormones produced by the adrenal glands. They are used for a wide variety of disorders because of their anti-inflammatory and immunosuppressive capabilities. Prednisone is a synthetic corticosteroid that is commonly used as adjunct immunosuppressant therapy following organ transplantation and is also used in the treatment of acute rejection. In the posttransplant patient, glucocorticoids are administered in large doses to achieve the desired immunosuppressant effects, increasing adverse effects such as severe bone disorders, diabetes mellitus, and cataracts. A summary of glucocorticoid use for immunosuppression is presented in the "Related Pharmacotherapy: Glucocorticoids" feature.

Cytotoxic Agents

Cytotoxic agents have the capability of destroying target cells. Certain drugs target immunocompetent cells and therefore are of use as immunosuppressants. Two cytotoxic agents are azathioprine (Imuran, Azasan) and mycophenolate mofetil (MMF; CellCept). Before the introduction of cyclosporine, azathioprine was the drug of choice in the prevention of graft rejection; however, with the advent of newer cell-cycle-specific drugs such as MMF, azathioprine is no longer a drug of choice because of the number of severe adverse effects associated with it. MMF is approved for organ rejection prophylaxis and is used in conjunction with glucocorticoids and cyclosporine (Adams & Urban, 2016). Its action primarily targets B and T lymphocytes by inhibiting proliferation. Additional information on this drug group is provided in the "Related Pharmacotherapy: Cytotoxic Agents" feature.

Antibodies (Monoclonal and Polyclonal)

Antibodies are a newer form of immunosuppressive therapy than are many of the other immunosuppressants. The two major antibody preparations are monoclonal and polyclonal. Both are formed from foreign proteins, derived from animals that may cause the formation of recipient antibodies and resulting in the patient's sensitization and the possible development of serum sickness or anaphylactic reactions. Antibodies direct their attack narrowly by targeting the lymphocyte subsets responsible for the immune

---

Related Pharmacotherapy
Calcineurin Inhibitors

Drug Examples

Cyclosporine (Gengraf, Sandimmune, Neoral)
Tacrolimus (Prograf, FK-506)

Actions and Uses

The powerful immunosuppressant activities of calcineurin inhibitors are directed primarily against cytotoxic T cells without suppressing bone marrow function. Although they may be used alone, recommended use is in combination therapy with corticosteroids to prevent rejection. They are also effective agents in preventing graft-versus-host disease (GVHD).

Dosages (Adult)

Cyclosporine: Initial preoperative dosing—14–18 mg/kg (PO) [or 5–6 mg/kg IV] administered 4–12 hours before transplantation and continued for 1–2 weeks postsurgery; taper dose 5%/week to 10 mg/kg/day. Maintenance—(PO) 5–10 mg/kg/day.

Tacrolimus (dosage based on organ transplanted): 0.075–0.2 mg/kg/day PO in divided dosage administered every 12 hours (or 0.01–0.05 mg/kg/day continuous IV) to begin 6 or more hours posttransplant. To be switched to PO for maintenance.

Major Adverse Effects

Most common: nephrotoxicity and infection
Other: hepatotoxicity, neurotoxicity, hyperglycemia, hirsutism, gingival hyperplasia

Nursing Implications

Monitoring for hypersensitivity reaction, infection, kidney and liver function

Regular monitoring of plasma drug levels

Cautious concurrent use with other immunosuppressants except glucocorticoids

Patient education: important cyclosporin interaction—grapefruit juice (increases drug concentration). Provider and pharmacist should be aware of all prescription and nonprescription drugs, including nutritional supplements, to avoid untoward interactions or adverse effects.

SOURCE: Data from Adams & Urban (2016), Gruessner (2015), and Wilson, Shannon, & Shields (2016).

Related Pharmacotherapy
Glucocorticoids

Drug Examples

Prednisone (Deltasone)
Methylprednisolone (Solu-Medrol)

Action and Uses

Corticosteroids significantly reduce the number of lymphocytes, particularly T lymphocytes, by interfering with the production and secretion of interleukin-2. In addition, large doses of corticosteroids suppress immune globulin production, particularly IgG and IgA, and significantly impair monocyte–macrophage function. Steroid therapy is useful in preventing rejection and is used in rescue therapy for organ rejection; however, long-term use is associated with severe bone disorders, diabetes mellitus, and cataracts.

Dosages (Adult)

Prednisone: rejection prevention dosing 0.5–2 mg/kg
Methylprednisolone: acute rejection dosing 500–1500 mg (IV)

Major Adverse Effects

When used postoperatively to prevent rejection, steroids can cause decreased wound healing, increased risk of dehiscence, or tearing of the anastomosis.

Long term: Cushing syndrome (hyperglycemia, bruising, redistribution of fat, bone weakening, and multisystem problems), gastric ulcers

Nursing Implications

Patient teaching:
    Take with milk or food.
    Do not stop taking drug abruptly.
    Take at the same time every day.
Monitor:
    Serum glucose
    Blood pressure
    Weight
    Serum electrolytes

SOURCE: Data from Adams & Urban (2016) and Wilson et al. (2016).

---

rejection reaction, which allows the other immune cell components to continue providing protection.

Basiliximab (Simulect) is the only approved monoclonal antibody (mAB) used for immunosuppression in transplant patients (Adams & Urban, 2016). It binds to the IL-2 receptors on T lymphocytes, preventing T-cell activation. Side effects are typically mild; however, anaphylaxis can occur on rare occasions. It is approved for prevention of kidney transplant rejection during the acute period following surgery and is used in conjunction with cyclosporine and glucocorticoid therapy.

Lymphocyte immune globulin (antithymocyte globulin; Atgam, Thymoglobulin), a polyclonal antibody, is produced from horse- or rabbit-derived antibodies that have been injected with human T lymphocytes (Adams & Urban, 2016). It is administered directly following the transplantation to reduce the function of T lymphocytes and is approved for prevention of renal transplant rejection. It is also used off label to treat myelodysplastic syndrome and graft-versus-host disease (Adams & Urban, 2016). Because this product comes from animal sera, mild to moderate reactions can occur, and, while rare, anaphylactic reactions are possible. Additional information on this drug group can be found in the "Related Pharmacotherapy: Monoclonal and Polyclonal Antibodies" feature.

Related Pharmacotherapy
Cytotoxic Agents

Drug Example

Mycophenolate mofetil (MMF; CellCept)

Action and Uses

Interferes with cell proliferation by inhibiting DNA and RNA synthesis. B- and T-cell lymphocytes are targeted. MMF has been shown to be more effective than azathioprine in preventing acute rejection and is effective in rejection rescue therapy.

Dosages (Adult)

Within 24 hours of transplant; administer 720 mg twice per day PO or IV, given in combination with cyclosporine and corticosteroids

Major Adverse Effects

Bone marrow suppression: neutropenia, infection (including sepsis)
Gastrointestinal: nausea, vomiting, and diarrhea
Infection

Nursing Implications

Monitor: CBC, liver enzymes; GI hypersensitivity (severe nausea and vomiting)

SOURCE: Data from Adams & Urban (2016).

Related Pharmacotherapy
Monoclonal and Polyclonal Antibodies

Drug Examples

Basiliximab (Simulect)

Lymphocyte immune globulin (antithymocyte globulin [ATG] [Atgam])

Action and Uses

Basiliximab binds to and blocks the interleukin-2 receptor alpha subunit on the surface of activated T-cell lymphocytes. Lymphocyte immune globulin targets T lymphocytes and is used primarily to treat renal graft rejection, but it can be used prophylactically in the immediate posttransplant period.

Dosages (Adult)

Basiliximab: 2 hours before surgery, 20 mg is given IV; the second dose is given 4 days after transplantation

Lymphocyte immune globulin (Atgam): prevention of rejection 10–30 mg/kg IV daily

Major Adverse Effects

Anaphylaxis (uncommon)

Infection

Hypertension

Gastrointestinal symptoms

Nursing Implications

Have epinephrine and cardiopulmonary resuscitation equipment available

Monitor for hypersensitivity reactions, gastrointestinal disturbances

SOURCE: Data from Adams & Urban (2016).

Nursing Considerations

Patients who have an allograft organ transplant face a rigid, lifelong medication regimen to ensure the long-term health of the graft. Adherence to the recommended drug regimen is often a challenge for the patient and family; however, nonadherence can end in loss of the graft. Despite the high stakes associated with nonadherence, a significant number of transplant patients do not fully adhere to the recommended immunosuppressive therapeutic regimen (Berben, Dobbels, Kugler, Russell, & De Geest 2011).

Risk factors for nonadherence to the medication regimen center around psychosocial, educational, age, medication, and provider factors (Table 39–6) (National Kidney Foundation/Kidney Disease Improving Global Outcomes [NKF/KDIGO], 2009). The NKF/KDIGO recommends early identification of high-risk posttransplant patients followed by increased intensity of adherence monitoring. Patient and family education may not be sufficient to ensure adherence, and it is recommended that a combination approach include educational, counseling, and psychological interventions to improve outcomes. In addition,

Table 39–6 NKF/KDIGO Risk Factors for Nonadherence to Medication Regimen

Factor	Risk Factors
Psychosocial	Pattern of nonadherence behaviors before surgery Personality disorders or psychiatric illness Poor social support History of substance abuse or other high-risk behavior
Educational	High education level Inadequate pretransplant education
Age	Adolescence
Medications	Drug adverse effects Complexity of drug regimen
Provider	Inadequate follow-up by transplant professionals

SOURCE: Based on National Kidney Foundation/Kidney Disease Improving Global Outcomes (KDIGO) (2009).

it is recommended that adherence be evaluated at every follow-up visit to the provider. These interventions should begin early in the transplantation preparation process, then continue perioperatively, postoperatively, and on a regular basis postdischarge.

Section Nine Review

1. Which drugs are considered the most effective of the immunosuppressant agents?
   A. Glucocorticoids
   B. Cytotoxic agents
   C. Calcineurin inhibitors
   D. Antibodies

2. Long-term posttransplantation steroid therapy is particularly associated with potentially severe disorders of which structure?
   A. Heart
   B. Bone
   C. Liver
   D. Blood

3. What is a major adverse effect of most cytotoxic agents?
   A. Nausea
   B. Rash
   C. Metallic taste in the mouth
   D. Constipation

4. What is a major concern associated with the administration of cyclosporine?
   A. It can only be given orally.
   B. It is highly incompatible with other drugs.
   C. It is often implicated in causing graft-versus-host disease (GVHD).
   D. It must be administered with an antihistamine.

Answers: 1. C, 2. B, 3. A, 4. B

Section Ten: Hematopoietic Stem Cell Transplantation

Hematopoietic stem cell transplantation (HSCT), formerly referred to as bone marrow transplantation, is a therapy in which healthy stem cells are infused into a recipient for the purpose of restoring normal bone marrow function in patients who have a hematologic malignancy or bone marrow failure. HSCT can be used to treat a variety of disorders, such as leukemia, multiple myeloma, lymphomas, autoimmune disorders, and aplastic anemia. In some disorders, such as relapsed acute myelogenous leukemia (AML), it is the only curative therapeutic option.

HSCT allows patients with cancer to receive higher doses of chemotherapy than the bone marrow can usually tolerate. High-dose chemotherapy, while more effectively destroying the malignancy, also destroys bone marrow function. With HSCT, high-dose therapy can be administered, after which healthy stem cells are reintroduced to restore bone marrow function and speed up hematologic recovery time. HSCT has also been used to correct certain genetic disorders such as severe combined immunodeficiency (SCID) (Aster & Antin, 2017).

Types of HSCT

There are two major types of HSCT: autologous and allogeneic. Each is useful under certain circumstances.

Autologous Transplantation Autologous stem cells come from the recipient's own blood or bone marrow, providing the perfect HLA match, no graft-rejection complications, and significantly reduced morbidity and mortality. To qualify for autologous stem cell transplantation, the patient's blood and bone marrow must be free of malignant cells. The stem cells are not harvested until all tests are negative for malignant cells during a full disease remission period. The primary disadvantage of autologous transplantation is the increased potential for malignancy relapse due to the possible reintroduction of essentially undetectable numbers of the patient's own malignant cells when the autologous cells are reintroduced. However, hematopoietic stem cell (HSC) transfer between identical twins, a syngeneic transplant, can avert this complication (Aster & Antin, 2017).

Allogeneic Transplantation Allogeneic stem cells come from a carefully selected donor other than the patient. Close HLA matching is essential, and when possible, the patient's siblings are tested first, as they are likely to provide the best HLA match. If a related donor cannot be found, an unrelated donor may be found through a registry or HLA testing of the blood of potential donors. Because the donor's stem cells and immune cells cannot be separated, grafting allogeneic stem cells can precipitate two complications: either host-versus-graft (HVG) effect or graft-versus-host disease (GVHD) (Leukemia & Lymphoma Society [LLS], 2013). HVG effect is a type of graft rejection in which the recipient's immune system attacks the donor stem cells; with GVHD, the donor cells attack the tissues of the recipient. GVHD is discussed in further detail later in this section.

Sources of Hematopoietic Stem Cells

The two major sources of hematopoietic stem cells are the bone marrow and the peripheral blood. Umbilical cord blood is a recent addition to potential sources; however, it is not a common source at this time.

Bone Marrow Bone marrow was the original source for hematopoietic stem cells. Harvesting is performed under general anesthesia in the operating room and requires about two hours to complete. The volume removed varies with the recipient's size; up to a liter of bone marrow may be aspirated. A large-bore needle is inserted multiple times into easily accessible bone marrow locations, usually the iliac crests. Complications of this procedure are rare and include bleeding and infection. The patient may report localized discomfort at the site of the harvesting.

Peripheral Blood The peripheral blood is now the major source of stem cells for transplantation. Stem cells can be identified and measured through their CD marker, the CD34 antigen; thus they are referred to as CD34+ cells. These cells normally exist in the peripheral circulation but only in small numbers; however, CD34+ cell concentration can be increased significantly using growth factors, such as granulocyte colony-stimulating factor (G-CSF) (Filgrastim). In preparation for donation, the donor receives daily injections of Filgrastim for about 5 days. Daily blood samples are taken to measure the number of CD34+ cells. When a sufficient number of cells are present, they are harvested by **apheresis**, which can be performed in an ambulatory setting such as a blood bank facility. The procedure takes 3 to 4 hours and requires no anesthesia. The cells can then be frozen for extended periods.

Transplanting Procedure

HSCT is a multistep process that includes preparing the patient for the engraftment, delivering the stem cells, and then waiting for the stem cells to produce new blood cells. The entire process can take a month or more to complete.

Preparing for HSCT Preparation for stem cell engraftment (called "conditioning") involves eradication of the disease for which the person is to receive the HSCT and immunosuppressant therapy to prevent rejection of the graft. In general, disease eradication procedures include a regimen of high-dose chemotherapy and possibly radiation therapy (Aster & Scadden, 2017). The preparatory regimen can follow many different protocols, but the overriding goal is to essentially clear the patient's dysfunctional bone marrow of as much disease as possible—and optimize the engraftment potential of the donor's hematopoietic stem cells.

Stem Cell Delivery and Engraftment The donor stem cells are delivered to the patient through a simple transfusion process through a central line in a large blood vessel, much like a blood transfusion. By mechanisms that are poorly understood, the donor's stem cells migrate to the patient's bone marrow. After transplantation, there is a period of waiting for **engraftment**—for the donor's stem cells to take hold in the patient's marrow and start producing normal hematopoietic cells. Engraftment can take as long as 5 weeks, during which time the transplant patient is maintained in a protective environment, described later in this section.

Post-HSCT Complications

The major negative outcomes and complications of HSCT are graft failure (the donor marrow does not successfully take hold or engraft) and graft-versus-host disease (the donor marrow sees the patient as foreign and attacks the patient's tissues). Despite the significant progress that has been made in the area of HSCT, graft failure can occur. The outcomes of allogeneic HSCT depend on multiple factors, such as the patient's overall clinical status, age, disease process, and compatibility with the donor.

Graft-versus-host disease (GVHD) is a complication that develops in allogeneic HSCT patients. It occurs when donor T cells, along with the hematopoietic stem cells, are infused into the host (the recipient). The donor T cells see the recipient's tissues as nonself (foreign) and muster an attack. The incidence of GVHD is highest when a matched but unrelated donor is used. GVHD can be acute or chronic and is difficult to treat successfully; thus, prophylactic drug therapy is generally initiated 1 or 2 days before stem cell infusion and may be continued for a prolonged period after engraftment to prevent development of GVHD (Leukemia & Lymphoma Society [LLS], 2013).

Table 39–7 Clinical Manifestations and Management of Major Complications of HSCT

Complication	Clinical Manifestations	Management
Mucositis (oral or intestinal)	Oropharyngeal pain Nausea, abdominal cramping, diarrhea	Pain control: • Topical analgesics • Systemic opioids Prophylactic: • Growth factors (e.g., palifermin [Kepivance], amifostine [Ethiofos])
Severe pancytopenia	Leukopenia: • < 500 cells/mcL (often < 100) • Prolonged neutropenia (2–4 weeks) Thrombocytopenia: • < 50,000 (often < 10,000) Erythrocytopenia (anemia)	Prophylaxis: • Recombinant hematopoietic growth factors (e.g., filgrastim [Zarxio, Granix, Neupogen]) • Recombinant erythropoietin • Antibiotic, antifungal, and/or antiviral therapy Infection: • Empiric broad-spectrum antibiotics, antifungals, antivirals Thrombocytopenia: • Platelet transfusions Anemia: • RBC transfusions Other infection prophylaxis: • Positive-air-pressure sealed rooms with HEPA filter • Strict hand hygiene
Graft-versus-host disease (GVHD) (mild, moderate, or severe)	Acute: • Skin rash and blisters (similar to burns) • Abdominal pain (severe) • Severe diarrhea • Hyperbilirubinemia, jaundice (liver injury) Chronic: • Onset: after third month posttransplant • Skin rash and itching; possible loss of patches of skin • Skin texture and color changes • Skin scarring • Dry oral mucous membranes and eyes • Hyperbilirubinemia (liver injury)	Prophylaxis to reduce occurrence: • T-cell depletion of graft • Immunosuppressant therapy (e.g., cyclosporine, tacrolimus, methotrexate) Treatment: • Corticosteroids • Cyclosporine (Successful treatment is often disappointing, making prophylaxis a better option.)
Graft failure (poor function or complete failure)	Severe pancytopenia Clinical manifestations of: • Infection • Anemia • Thrombocytopenia	Prevention: • Well–HLA-matched donor • Improving marrow function • Growth factors (e.g., G-CSF) • Erythropoietin • Second stem cell infusion

SOURCE: Data from Aster & Antin (2017) and LLS (2013).

Table 39–7 summarizes the common complications of HSCT, including clinical manifestations and treatments.

Management of the Immediate Post-allogeneic HSCT Patient

Within 2 to 3 days after an allogeneic HSCT transplant, the patient's bone marrow function drops to its lowest level (nadir) from the conditioning treatment regimen (LLS, 2013). Until engraftment occurs and bone marrow function adequately recovers, the patient is at extreme risk of contracting fatal infections, particularly lethal fungal or viral infections; thus, a protective environment must be provided. For this reason, many transplant centers have specific units that house only transplant patients; alternatively, the patient may be placed in an intensive care unit. Both settings can provide the specialized protective and supportive care required for these patients.

Nursing Considerations Prevention of complications is the major focus of nursing care following HSCT. When bone marrow function is low, the patient is at high risk for blood-cell–related complications such as anemia (erythrocytopenia), infection (leukopenia), and bleeding (thrombocytopenia). Laboratory values of the complete blood cell count (CBC) are closely monitored as an indicator of bone marrow status, degree of risk of complications, and the need for specific interventions. The patient is placed in a protective environment that includes a positive-air-pressure sealed room with special HEPA filters and protective protocols to guard against potential contamination from people and the hospital environment.

Meticulous hand hygiene must be maintained and protective clothing must be worn to reduce the risk of contaminating the patient with pathogens from the outside environment. Because the patient may develop feelings of isolation during this period, it is important to encourage the family to visit and to provide psychosocial support. Prior to allowing family into the room, the nurse must ensure that family members understand and adhere to the protective regimen—for example, showing them where (and how) to properly wash their hands and how to wear protective clothing. The family also needs a clear understanding of what can be brought into the room, as gifts and flowers or plants may contaminate the environment.

Emerging Evidence

- Postreperfusion syndrome can occur during orthotopic liver transplant (OLT)—that is, a donor liver replaces the recipient's liver in the same anatomical location. Low mean arterial pressure and cardiac output can result in cardiac arrest and poor graft function when postreperfusion is evident. Several etiologies for the syndrome are suspected, and the presence of oxygen-free radicals that interfere with tissue oxygenation is a known contributor to this complication. Researchers examined the effect of mannitol, a free-radical scavenger, on oxygenation parameters before and after the declamping of the portal vein during liver transplant surgery. Liver transplant patients ($n = 53$) were randomized into two groups; one received 1 g/kg mannitol, and one received normal saline intravenously during surgical clamping procedures. No significant changes occurred in mean arterial pressure, cardiac output, or central venous oxygen saturation before and after portal vein declamping in the mannitol group; the saline group experienced significantly lower values of these measures after declamping ($p = .003$, $p = .001$, and $p < .001$, respectively). Consequently, the infusion of mannitol during liver transplantation may improve perfusion outcomes in patients receiving this surgical intervention (*Sahmeddini et al., 2014*).

- Patient and family education and advanced care planning are essential components of critical care nursing. In a qualitative study of advanced care planning perceptions, six patients receiving HSCT, five family members, and eight clinicians described perceived barriers and facilitators with advanced care planning. Perceived barriers included lack of a planning process, time, or resources; a desire to focus on the positives of the treatment; and unpredictability of the disease and outcomes. Facilitators included integrating advanced care planning as part of routine HSCT care, using a multidisciplinary team approach, and starting the education and planning process early and reinforcing frequently (*Booker, Simon, & Bouchal, 2016*).

Section Ten Review

1. Allogeneic hematopoietic stem cell transplantation to treat cancer has which major advantage?
   A. It can cure all types of leukemia.
   B. It has fewer complications than other treatments for cancer.
   C. Remaining cancer cells can be filtered out during apheresis.
   D. A high-dose chemotherapy regimen can be used to eradicate the cancer.

2. What is the major drawback of using autologous stem cells for transplantation?
   A. It has a higher risk for graft rejection than that associated with allogeneic grafts.
   B. It has a higher risk of reintroducing malignant cells into the blood.
   C. It requires high doses of immunosuppressant drug therapy.
   D. It is not as effective as allogeneic stem cell transplant in restoring marrow function.

3. When a donor's peripheral blood is to be used as the source of hematopoietic stem cells for grafting purposes, what step must be taken before cells are harvested?
   A. The final round of cancer chemotherapy is completed.
   B. Growth factors are administered to maximize stem cells.
   C. Total body irradiation therapy has been administered.
   D. Immunosuppressants are administered to decrease the numbers of immune cells.

4. Which statement regarding graft-versus-host disease (GVHD) is correct?
   A. It usually targets the heart and lungs.
   B. It is treated using apheresis.
   C. It requires aggressive antibiotic therapy.
   D. It is difficult to successfully treat.

Answers: 1. D, 2. B, 3. B, 4. D

Section Eleven: Kidney Transplantation: An Overview

Transplantation of the kidney represents almost 80% of all organ transplantations. Kidney transplants have been in the literature since the early 1930s, when a kidney was transplanted into the thigh of a young woman in Russia. Today, kidney transplants are a highly successful mode of therapy.

Major Indications for Renal Transplantation

End-stage renal disease (ESRD) is the primary indicator for kidney transplant. However, a diagnosis of ESRD does not necessitate kidney transplantation because dialysis can be used as an alternative therapy. ESRD can result from many causes, the most common being hypertension, diabetes mellitus, and glomerulonephritis, which account for more than half of all cases. A patient who is being considered for transplantation is carefully screened to determine whether the probability of a successful transplant is sufficient to warrant transplantation rather than continuing use of dialysis. When a renal transplant is successful, it is significantly less costly than long-term dialysis therapy. Transplant success by way of graft survival rates are influenced by the genetic characteristics of the donor and are described in the "Genetic Considerations: Survival Rates for Kidney Transplants" feature.

Genetic Considerations
Survival Rates for Kidney Transplants

With renal transplantation, the kidney can be obtained from cadaver sources or voluntary living donors. Graft survival rates after 1 year are 5% to 7% higher when first-degree relatives donate a kidney compared to deceased donors. Five-year survival rates are better with at least a partially human leukocyte antigen (HLA)–matched family donor when compared to a randomly selected deceased donor. In all donors, 5-year outcomes are poor when there is a complete mismatch (Azzi et al., 2015).

Preparation of the Recipient

When a kidney becomes available, the recipient is admitted to the hospital and pretransplant orders are initiated. Admission may take place the day before a scheduled surgery if there is a living donor. If a deceased donor kidney is made available, the preparatory time is much shorter. On notification, the patient is admitted to the transplant center, with surgery rapidly following admission. Preoperative hemodialysis is often performed to normalize fluid and electrolyte balance. Before the patient goes to surgery, crossmatching is performed. If the results are negative, an initial dose of an immunosuppressant and prophylactic antibiotics are administered either before or after the patient is transferred to the operating room. Figure 39–2 illustrates a renal transplant.

Postoperative Management

Following transplantation, the patient is monitored closely for the first 24 hours, often in an intensive care setting. Medical and nursing priorities depend on the level of graft

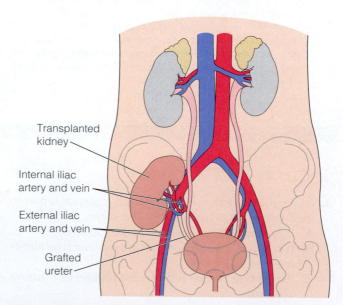

Figure 39–2 Placement of a transplanted kidney in the iliac fossa with anastomosis to the hypogastric artery, iliac vein, and bladder.

Transplanted kidney

Internal iliac artery and vein

External iliac artery and vein

Grafted ureter

function and the development of any complications. Risks for complications are particularly high when the graft has undergone a prolonged cold ischemic time. Graft dysfunction and failure are more commonly noted in deceased donor grafts than in live ones. In the deceased donor transplant, organ ischemia is more likely a result of the increased length of time the organ was preserved. Renal ischemia may lead to acute tubular necrosis, which causes oliguria or anuria. If the dysfunction lasts more than 48 hours, hemodialysis may be necessary until the graft begins functioning sufficiently. It takes several weeks posttransplantation for the grafted kidney to become fully functional.

Hypertension is a common problem in the kidney transplant patient. This condition can be exacerbated during the postoperative recovery period because of fluid volume imbalances precipitated by the high volume of IV fluids used to maintain a high urine flow. Antihypertensive agents may be ordered preoperatively and postoperatively to maintain the blood pressure within an acceptable range for the patient.

The patient's nutrition must also be taken into consideration because end-stage renal disease is often associated with decreased appetite and poor nutrition status. Malnutrition impairs healing and must be addressed early in admission. Typical postoperative management considerations are included in the "Nursing Care: The Postoperative Kidney Transplant Patient" feature.

Evaluation of Kidney Function In addition to laboratory tests, several procedures can be performed to evaluate function of the kidney graft. A needle biopsy using ultrasound is performed to examine renal tissue. This is considered the most valuable indicator of renal function. Ultrasound of the kidney may be ordered to look for hydronephrosis, obstruction, or collections of fluid. A renal scan using radioactive isotopes also evaluates renal function.

Postrenal Transplant Complications General complications associated with organ transplantation are presented in Section Seven. The 1-year graft survival rate for deceased-donor renal transplants is about 96%, and for living-donor transplants about 99% (Organ Procurement & Transplant Network [OPTN], 2017e). The most common long-term complication of renal transplantation is graft rejection.

Nursing Care
The Postoperative Kidney Transplant Patient

Expected Patient Outcomes and Related Interventions

Outcome 1: Fluid and electrolyte balance

Assess and compare to established normal, patient baselines, and trends.
Fluid—intake and output balance with hourly urine outputs, weight, breath sounds, jugular veins, extremities, hemodynamic monitoring values (BP, CVP, MAP)
Electrolytes—particularly potassium, sodium, bicarbonate, calcium, and phosphorous
Acid–base balance—arterial blood gases

Administer related drug therapy and monitor for therapeutic and nontherapeutic effects.
Diuretics (e.g., furosemide [Lasix])

Outcome 2: Maintain or regain kidney function

Assess and compare to established normal, patient baselines, and trends.
Kidney function: blood urea nitrogen (BUN), creatinine (Cr), potassium, hourly urine output
Monitor for blood clots in urinary catheter, which can obstruct the catheter
Monitor oxygenation status: hemoglobin and hematocrit, arterial blood gases, pulse oximetry, SvO_2 (mixed or central)

Implement interventions to optimize kidney graft function.
IV fluids at a rate sufficient to keep urine output greater than 100 mL/hr; rate may also be titrated based on hourly urine outputs
Oxygen therapy, as ordered

Outcome 3: Prevent patient complications

Assess and compare to established normal, patient baselines, and trends.
Signs and symptoms of acute infection (temperature, WBC)
Signs and symptoms of acute rejection
Signs of hemodynamic instability: either fluid volume excess or deficit
Monitor blood levels of immunosuppressant drugs (e.g., cyclosporine, tacrolimus, and sirolimus)
Monitor for signs of technical complications: vascular thrombosis, bleeding, anastomosis leakage (see Section Seven)

Administer related drug therapy and monitor for therapeutic and nontherapeutic effects.
Antibiotics as ordered

Outcome 4: Patient will have improved nutrition status

Assess and compare to established normal, patient baselines, and trends.
Daily weights
Monitor nutrient intake (calories, protein)
Monitor serum protein nutrition indicators (e.g., serum albumin, prealbumin)

Implement interventions to optimize kidney graft function.
Early nutrition consult
Enteric feedings or total parenteral nutrition as ordered

SOURCE: Data from Chandraker & Yeung (2016) and Kapadia & Oropello (2017).

Section Eleven Review

1. The major indication for kidney transplantation is end-stage renal disease, which most commonly results from which problems? (Select all that apply.)
   A. Diabetes mellitus
   B. Hypertension
   C. Glomerulonephritis
   D. Heart disease
   E. Spinal cord dysfunction

2. Dysfunction of a kidney graft is most commonly associated with which factor?
   A. Preoperative condition of the donor
   B. Preoperative condition of the recipient
   C. Length of time the organ was preserved
   D. Length of time required to perform the transplant

3. What is the most common long-term complication of renal transplantation?
   A. Rejection
   B. Hypoperfusion
   C. Development of hypertension
   D. Posttransplant new-onset diabetes mellitus

4. Directly following transplant surgery, the nurse can anticipate initiating interventions to maintain urine output at which level?
   A. 30 mL/hr
   B. 50 mL/hr
   C. 75 mL/hr
   D. 100 mL/hr

Answers: 1. (A, B, C), 2. C, 3. A, 4. D

Clinical Reasoning Checkpoint

Marty Q, a 36-year-old middle school teacher, has been diagnosed with acute myelogenous leukemia (AML). After hearing his treatment options and conferring with his family, he decides to undergo aggressive high-dose chemotherapy, total body irradiation (TBI), and hematopoietic stem cell transplantation (HSCT).

1. The oncologist explains to Marty two HSCT options: autologous and allogeneic. How would you respond if Marty asked you to clarify the pros and cons of these two options?

2. Marty opts to have an allogeneic transplant. His younger sister volunteers to donate. It is decided to use the peripheral blood method rather than a bone marrow aspiration to obtain the stem cells. Marty asks you what his sister will experience. Explain what you can about this procedure.

Clinical update: Marty has gone through the preparation, or conditioning, for stem-cell engraftment.

3. What is the purpose of conditioning?

4. How will total body irradiation be performed?

Clinical update: Marty has had his hematopoietic stem-cell transplant and is now awaiting engraftment.

5. While Marty waits for engraftment, how will his environment be controlled?

6. List at least three common complications of hematopoietic stem-cell transplant that the nurse will need to monitor for posttransplant.

Chapter 39 Review

1. What improvements have made cardiac transplantation a highly successful option for today's client and surgeon? (Select all that apply.)
   1. Improved immunosuppressive therapy
   2. Routine use of syngraft donors
   3. Improved tissue typing
   4. Wide use of xenografting techniques
   5. Less focus on histocompatibility

2. A client is determined to be near death, and the organ procurement organization (OPO) has been notified. Which persons should discuss the possibility of organ donation with the client's family? (Select all that apply.)
   1. An employee of the OPO
   2. The client's primary nurse
   3. The client's primary provider
   4. The unit's chaplain
   5. A specially trained employee

3. Brain-death testing is being conducted at the bedside of a client critically injured in an explosion. Which results would the nurse interpret as indicating that brain death has occurred? (Select all that apply.)
   1. Glasgow Coma Scale (GSC) score of 5
   2. No doll's-eye reflex to head rotation
   3. No eye movement to cold-water ear irrigations
   4. Weak cough response to deep suctioning
   5. No pupillary response to light

4. An adult client has been declared brain dead and is being managed until organ donation can occur. The nurse works to maintain at least which mean arterial pressure (MAP) level in this client?
   1. 110 mmHg
   2. 100 mmHg
   3. 80 mmHg
   4. 60 mmHg

5. The sister of a client who needs a kidney transplant says, "I would donate my kidney, but I have type O blood and his blood is type A." How should the nurse respond?
   1. "If you were type A and he was type O, a transplant would be possible."
   2. "You would have to be type A to donate to your brother."
   3. "Blood type is no longer used as a criterion for donation."
   4. "The transplant may still be possible."

6. A client who has developed chronic renal failure says, "I really don't want to wait until I need to go on dialysis. Let's just go ahead and do a transplant now." How should the nurse respond?
   1. "If your insurance and your personal finances will cover the surgery and aftercare, you can go on the transplant list."
   2. "It often takes months to find a suitable organ for transplant."
   3. "The primary criterion for transplant is end-stage renal disease, which you have not reached."
   4. "If this is your desire, we need to get you started on a nutritional support plan."

7. A client who received a kidney transplant 2 years ago has been diagnosed with chronic rejection of the graft. If this rejection is not effectively managed, what will happen?
   1. The client will have to take additional immunosuppressant drugs for up to 4 years.

2. The kidney will become ischemic and die.
3. Because it has taken 2 years for the rejection to occur, there will be little effect on the client's health.
4. The client will develop acute renal failure and will likely die.

8. A client is scheduled for an allogenic hematopoietic stem cell transplant. What education should the nurse provide to the client and family? (Select all that apply.)
   1. The policy of no visitors for the first 2 to 3 days until the client passes nadir
   2. A demonstration of how to don protective clothing before visiting
   3. The need to supplement the client's diet with fresh fruits and vegetables after the transplant
   4. Hand hygiene protocol and demonstration
   5. The need to avoid bringing flowers in the room

9. A client is being prepared for a heart–lung transplant. The nurse is assessing the client and family for risks for nonadherence to the posttransplant drug regimen. Which statements would the nurse interpret as indicating an increased risk? (Select all that apply.)
   1. "My heart medicines sure make me nauseated."
   2. "I hope I can remember how to take all these medicines."
   3. "When I'm nervous, I still want a cigarette."
   4. "Thanks so much for spending so much time teaching us how to do all this."
   5. "I can expect to discuss my medicines at every doctor visit."

10. A client says, "I just had a kidney transplant two days ago. Now the doctor says I have to go on dialysis for two weeks. I don't understand all of this." How should the nurse respond?
    1. "Your transplant was not successful, so dialysis is necessary."
    2. "Because your transplant was not from a living donor, it may take a while for the kidney to recover."
    3. "We told you about this before surgery. Don't you remember?"
    4. "I'm afraid your kidney was not a good match. We have to support you with dialysis while we look for another kidney to transplant."

Answers to questions found inside your textbook are available on the faculty resources site. Please consult with your instructor.

References

Adams, M. P., & Urban, C. Q. (2016). Immunostimulants and immunosuppressants. In M. P. Adams & C. Q. Urban (Eds.), *Pharmacology: Connections to nursing practice* (3rd ed.). Retrieved April 15, 2017, from https://bookshelf.vitalsource.com/#/books/9780133896848

American Academy of Neurology (AAN). (2010). *Brain injury and brain death (reaffirmed 2014)*. Retrieved April 9, 2017, from https://www.aan.com/Guidelines/Home/ByTopic?topicId=13

Applebaum, F. R. (2007). Hematopoietic-cell transplantation at 50. *New England Journal of Medicine, 357*(15), 1472–1475.

Aster, J. C., & Antin, J. H. (2017). Hematopoietic stem cell transplantation. In J. C. Aster & H. Bunn (Eds.), *Pathophysiology of blood disorders* (2nd ed.). Retrieved April 15, 2017, from http://accessmedicine.mhmedical.com.ezproxy.uky.edu/Content.aspx?bookid=1900&sectionid=137395909

Aster, J. C., & Scadden, D. (2017). Hematopoiesis. In J. C. Aster & H. Bunn (Eds.), *Pathophysiology of blood disorders* (2nd ed.). Retrieved April 15, 2017, from http://accessmedicine.mhmedical.com.ezproxy.uky.edu/Content.aspx?bookid=1900&sectionid=137394642

Azzi, J., Milford, E. L., Sayegh, M. H., & Chandraker, A. (2015). Transplantation in the treatment of renal failure. In D. Kasper, A. Fauci, S. Hauser, D. Longo, J. Jameson, & J. Loscalzo (Eds.), *Harrison's principles of internal medicine* (19th ed.). Retrieved April 14, 2017, from http://accessmedicine.mhmedical.com.ezproxy.uky.edu/content.aspx?bookid=1130&sectionid=79746670

Bentley, T. S. (2014). 2014 U.S. organ and tissue transplant cost estimates and discussion. *Milliman Research Report*, 1–20, Retrieved April 13, 2017, from http://www.milliman.com/uploadedFiles/insight/Research/health-rr/1938HDP_20141230.pdf

Berben, L., Dobbels, F., Kugler, C., Russell, C., & De Geest, S. (2011). Interventions used by health professionals to enhance medication adherence in transplant patients: A survey of current clinical practice. *Progress in Transplantation, 21*(4), 322–331.

Booker, R., Simon, J., & Bouchal, S. R. (2016). Patient, family member, and clinician perspectives on advance care planning (ACP) in hematology and hematopoietic stem cell transplantation (HSCT). *Journal of Clinical Oncology, 34*(suppl 26S; abstract 7). Retrieved April 16, 2017, from http://meetinglibrary.asco.org/content/172875-180

Brammer, J. E., Andersson, B. S., & Hosing, C. (2016). Allogeneic transplantation. In H. M. Kantarjian & R. A. Wolff (Eds.), *The MD Anderson manual of medical oncology* (3rd ed.). Retrieved April 13, 2017, from http://accessmedicine.mhmedical.com.ezproxy.uky.edu/content.aspx?bookid=1772&sectionid=121897922

Chandraker, A., & Yeung, M. Y. (2016). Overview of care of the adult kidney transplant recipient. *UpToDate.* Retrieved April 17, 2017, from https://www.uptodate.com/contents/overview-of-care-of-the-adult-kidney-transplant-recipient?source=machineLearning&search=nursing%20care%20renal%20transplant&selectedTitle=1~150&sectionRank=2&anchor=H25671032#H25671032

Denny, B., Kienhuir, M., & Gavidia-Payne, S. (2015). Explaining the quality of life of organ transplant patients by using crisis theory. *Progress in Transplantation, 25*(4), 324–331.

Department of Health and Human Services. (2006). *42CFR Parts 413, 441, et al. Medicare and Medicaid programs; conditions for coverage for organ procurement organizations (OPOs); final rule.* Retrieved April 13, 2017, from https://www.cms.gov/Regulations-and-Guidance/Regulations-and-Policies/QuarterlyProviderUpdates/Downloads/cms3064f.pdf

Engels, E., Pfeiffer, R., Fraumeni, J., Kasiske, B., Israni, A., Snyder, J., . . . Lin, M. (2011). Spectrum of cancer risk among U. S. solid organ transplant recipients: The transplant cancer match study. *Journal of the American Medical Association, 306*(17), 1891–1901.

Gruessner, A. C., Jie, T., Papas, K., Porubsky, M., Rana, A., Smith, M., . . . Gruessner, R G. (2015). Transplantation. In F. Brunicardi, D. K. Andersen, T. R. Billiar, D. L. Dunn, J. G. Hunter, J. B. Matthews, & R. E. Pollock (Eds.), *Schwartz's principles of surgery* (10th ed.). Retrieved April 13, 2017, from http://accessmedicine.mhmedical.com.ezproxy.uky.edu/content.aspx?bookid=980&sectionid=59610852

Hayes, W., Boyle, S., Carroll, A., Bockenhauer, D., & Marks, S. D. (2017). Hypomagnesemia and increased risk of new-onset diabetes mellitus after transplantation in pediatric renal transplant recipients. *Pediatric Nephrology, 32*, 879–884.

Hersh, C. A. (2016). Advances in the study of cancer risk among organ transplant patients: Clues to the role of the immune system in cancer etiology. *National Cancer Institute.* Retrieved April 13, 2017, from https://dceg.cancer.gov/news-events/linkage-newsletter/2016-11/research-publications/cancer-organ-transplants

Jani, A. A. (2017). *Infections after solid organ transplantation.* Retrieved April 15, 2017, from http://emedicine.medscape.com/article/430550-overview#aw2aab6b7

Kapadia, P., & Oropello, J. M. (2017) Posttransplantation care. In J. M. Oropello, S. M. Pastores, & V. Kvetan (Eds.). *Critical care.* Retrieved April 15, 2017, from http://accessmedicine.mhmedical.com.ezproxy.uky.edu/content.aspx?bookid=1944&sectionid=143519625

Kumar, L. (2016). Brain death and care of the organ donor. *Journal of Anesthesiology Clinical Pharmacology, 32*(2), 146–152.

Leukemia & Lymphoma Society (LLS). (2013). *Blood and marrow stem cell transplantation.* Retrieved April 15, 2017, from http://www.lls.org/sites/default/files/file_assets/PS40_BloodMarrow_booklet_6_16reprint.pdf

Linden, P. K. (2009). History of solid organ transplantation and organ donation. *Critical Care Clinics, 25*(1), 165–184.

Mesri, E. A., Feitelson, M., & Munger, K. (2014). Human viral oncogenesis: A cancer hallmarks analysis. *Cell Host & Microbe, 15*(3), 266–282.

Murray, J. E. (1991). Nobel Prize lecture: The first successful organ transplants in man. In P. I. Terasaki (Ed.), *History of transplantation: Thirty-five recollections* (pp. 123–138). Los Angeles, CA: UCLA Tissue Typing Laboratory.

National Kidney Foundation/Kidney Disease Improving Global Outcomes (NKF/KDIGO). (2009). Managing your adult patients who have a kidney transplant. Retrieved April 15, 2017, from http://www.kdigo.org/pdf/KDIGO_TX_PCP_Tool.pdf

Organ Procurement and Transplantation Network (OPTN). (2017a). *Data*. Retrieved April 8, 2017, from https://optn.transplant.hrsa.gov/data

Organ Procurement & Transplantation Network (OPTN). (2017b). *How organ allocation works*. Retrieved April 13, 2017, from https://optn.transplant.hrsa.gov/learn/about-transplantation/how-organ-allocation-works

Organ Procurement & Transplantation Network (OPTN). (2017c). *Donor matching system*. Retrieved April 13, 2017 from https://optn.transplant.hrsa.gov/learn/about-transplantation/donor-matching-system

Organ Procurement & Transplantation Network (OPTN). (2017d). *At a glance*. Retrieved April 13, 2017, from https://optn.transplant.hrsa.gov

Organ Procurement & Transplant Network (OPTN). (2017e). *National data*. Retrieved April 15, 2017, from https://optn.transplant.hrsa.gov/data/view-data-reports/national-data

Patel, M. S., Zatarain, J., Cruz, S. D. L., Sally, M. B., Ewing, T., Crutchfield, M., . . . Malinoski, D. J. (2014). The impact of meeting donor management goals on the number of organs transplanted per expanded criteria donor: A prospective study from the UNOS Region 5 Donor Management Goals Workgroup. *JAMA Surgery, 149* (9), 969–975.

Rohan,V. S., Kishi, E., McGillicuddy, J. W., & Nadig, S. N. (2017). Transplant surgery. In S. C. McKean, J. J. Ross, D. D. Dressler, & D. B. Scheurer (Eds.), *Principles and practice of hospital medicine* (2nd ed.). Retrieved April 14, 2017, from http://accessmedicine.mhmedical.com.ezproxy.uky.edu/content.aspx?bookid=1872&sectionid=146975062

Sahmeddini, M. A., Zahiri, S., Khosravi, M. B., Ghaffaripour, S., Eghbal, M. H., & Shokrizadeh, S. (2014). Effect of mannitol on postreperfusion cardiac output and central venous oxygen saturation during orthotopic liver transplant: A double-blind randomized clinical trial. *Progress in Transplantation, 24*(2), 121–125.

Shapiro, R., & DeVita, M. A. (2016). Management of the potential deceased donor. *UpToDate*. Retrieved April 11, 2017, from https://www.uptodate.com/contents/management-of-the-potential-deceased-donor#H5

Shary, T. M., Chapman, E. A., & Herrmann, V. M. (2015). Surgical metabolism & nutrition. In G. M. Doherty (Ed.), *CURRENT diagnosis and treatment: Surgery* (14th ed.). Retrieved April 13, 2017, from http://

accessmedicine.mhmedical.com.ezproxy.uky.edu/content.aspx?bookid=1202&sectionid=71516511

Souza, E. M., Baiocchi, O. C., Zanichelli, M. A., Alves, A. C., Assis, M. G., Eiras, D. P., . . . Oliveira, J. S. (2010). Impact of Epstein-Barr virus in the clinical evolution of patients with classical Hodgkin's lymphoma in Brazil. *Hematological Oncology, 28*(3), 137–141.

Tobin, G. S., Klein, C. L., & Brennan, D. C. (2017). New-onset diabetes after transplant (NODAT) in renal transplant recipients. *UpToDate*. Accessed April 27, 2017, from https://www.uptodate.com/contents/new-onset-diabetes-after-transplant-nodat-in-renal-transplant-recipients

Uniform Law Commission (2017a). *Anatomical Gift Act (2006) Summary*. Retrieved April 16, 2017, from http://www.uniformlaws.org/ActSummary.aspx?title=Anatomical%20Gift%20Act%20%282006%29

Uniform Law Commission. (2017b). *Determination of death act summary. The National Conference of Commissioners on Uniform State Laws*. Retrieved April 16, 2017, from http://uniformlaws.org/ActSummary.aspx?title=Determination%20of%20Death%20Act

United Network for Organ Sharing (UNOS). (2016). *Questions & answers for transplant candidates about kidney allocation policy*. Retrieved April 15, 2017, from http://www.unos.org/wp-content/uploads/unos/Kidney_Brochure.pdf

United Network for Organ Sharing (UNOS). (2017). *Transplant living: Costs*. Retrieved April 13, 2017, from https://transplantliving.org/before-the-transplant/financing-a-transplant/the-costs

UpToDate. (2017). *Levothyroxine: Drug information*. Retrieved April 11, 2017, from https://www.uptodate.com/contents/levothyroxine-drug-information?source=see_link

U.S. Government Printing Office (GPO). (2016). *42 CFR 482.45 Condition of participation: Organ, tissue, and eye procurement*. Retrieved April 9, 2017, from https://www.gpo.gov/fdsys/pkg/CFR-2016-title42-vol5/pdf/CFR-2016-title42-vol5-sec482-45.pdf

Wang, F., & Kieff, E. (2014). Medical virology. In D. Kasper, A. Fauci, S. Hauser, D. Longo, J. Jameson, & J. Loscalzo (Eds.), *Harrison's principles of internal medicine* (19th ed.). Retrieved April 13, 2014, from http://accessmedicine.mhmedical.com.ezproxy.uky.edu/content.aspx?bookid=1130&sectionid=79737992

Wijdicks, E., Varelas, P., Gronseth, G., & Greer, D. (2010). Evidence-based guidelines update: Determining brain death in adults. *Neurology, 74*, 1911–1918.

Wilson, B. A., Shannon, M. T., & Shields, K. M. (2016). *Pearson nurse's drug guide 2016*. Retrieved April 15, 2017, from https://bookshelf.vitalsource.com/#/books/9780134070728/cfi/6/2!/4/2@0:0

Yamani, M. H., & Taylor, D. O. (2010). Heart transplantation. Section 2: Cardiology. In *Cleveland Clinic: Current Clinical Medicine* (2nd ed., pp. 180–186). St. Louis, MO: Elsevier Saunders.

Zhang, X., Zhang, P., & Aboul-Soud, M. A. M. (2017). From inflammation to gastric cancer: Role of *Helicobacter pylori*. *Oncology Letters, 13*(2), 543–548.

Glossary

abdominal compartment syndrome (ACS)   Occurs when the intra-abdominal pressure increases to a point where vascular tissue is compromised with subsequent loss of tissue viability and function.

abrasion   Partial-thickness denudation of skin caused by friction or scraping. Top layer of the skin has been removed, revealing the top layer of the dermis.

absolute refractory period   The period after an action potential when a stimulus cannot produce a second action potential no matter how strong the stimulus.

absolute shunt   The sum of anatomic shunt and capillary shunt; refractory to oxygen therapy.

acceleration   An increase in the rate of velocity or speed of a moving body.

accessory muscles   Muscles not normally used during quiet breathing that are available for assisting either inspiration or expiration during times of increased work of breathing.

acids   Substances that dissociate or lose ions.

acinus   The exocrine functional unit of the pancreas; composed of acinar cells that produce, store, and secrete digestive enzymes and ductal cells that secrete bicarbonate and water (plural: acini).

action potential   A change in cell polarity. Signal produced from rapid change in membrane permeability that is transmitted from one part of the nerve or muscle cell to another.

active acquired immunity   A type of immunity that results from exposure to a specific antigen and subsequent formation and programming of antibodies.

acute coronary syndrome (ACS)   Coronary artery insufficiency typically resulting from disruption of intracoronary plaque, and further resulting in partial or total occlusion of the artery with subsequent ECG changes and cardiac biomarker release.

acute disseminated intravascular coagulation (DIC)   A type of coagulopathy associated with systemic activation of the coagulation cascade.

acute GI bleeding   A potentially life-threatening abdominal emergency that remains a common cause of hospitalization.

acute kidney injury   Abruptly diminished renal function with many possible causes and typically having the presenting characteristics of oliguria, as well as elevations of serum BUN and creatinine.

acute liver failure   Clinically defined by coagulation abnormalities, with an international normalized ratio (INR) greater than 1.5; the onset of encephalopathy in someone who has no previously known hepatic cirrhosis; and a duration of less than 26 weeks.

acute lung injury (ALI)/acute respiratory distress syndrome (ARDS)   ALI and ARDS are syndromes with a range of increasing severity of lung injury with damage to cells and structures of the alveolar capillary membrane.

acute lymphocytic leukemia (ALL)   A type of acute leukemia characterized by the proliferation of immature lymphoblasts that cannot carry on normal immune functions.

acute myelogenous leukemia (AML)   A type of acute leukemia characterized by the proliferation of malignant blast cells from myeloid stem cells.

acute rejection   A cell-mediated immune response in which the T lymphocytes and macrophages of the host suddenly attack and destroy the graft tissue; it occurs within days, months, or even years following the transplant.

acute respiratory distress syndrome (ARDS)   A type of respiratory failure caused by diffuse injury to the alveolar–capillary membrane, resulting in noncardiogenic pulmonary edema.

acute respiratory failure (ARF)   A life-threatening state caused by an imbalance in supply and demand; develops when the cardiopulmonary system is unable to maintain adequate gas exchange.

acute tubular necrosis   A kidney disorder involving damage to the tubule cells of the kidneys.

acute ventilatory failure (AVF)   A state of respiratory decompensation in which the lungs are unable to maintain adequate alveolar ventilation, losing the ability to eliminate carbon dioxide.

addiction (psychological dependence)   A chronic neurologic and biologic disease characterized by behaviors that include one or more of the following: impaired control of drug use, compulsive use despite harm to self or others, craving, and use of drug for purposes other than pain relief.

adenosine triphosphate (ATP)   A nucleotide that contains large amounts of chemical energy stored in high-energy phosphate bonds; when it is broken down by a process called hydrolysis, energy is released and utilized for metabolic processes.

aerobic metabolism   The mechanism used by the body for energy generation in the presence of oxygen.

affinity   The degree to which hemoglobin releases oxygen.

afterload   The resistance against which the ventricle pumps blood.

agnosia   A perceptual impairment resulting in the failure to recognize familiar objects by the senses even though sensation is intact; types include tactile, visual, or auditory.

agranulocytosis   An absolute neutrophil count (ANC) of less than 100 cells/mcL; a potentially life-threatening degree of neutropenia.

air trapping   The abnormal retention of air in the lungs on exhalation.

akinesis   Lack of myocardial wall movement.

albumin   The major protein produced in the liver.

allograft   Tissue that is transplanted between members of the same species; also referred to as a *xenograft*.

aminoacidemia   Amino acids in the blood.

amylase   A pancreatic enzyme that breaks down starch; when found in the blood may be indicative of acute pancreatitis.

anabolism   A constructive metabolic process whereby simple molecules are converted into more complex molecules.

anaerobic metabolism   The mechanism used by the body for energy generation in the absence of oxygen.

anaphylactic shock   A form of hypovolemic shock; the extreme result of type I hypersensitivity response with mediator-induced generalized vasodilatation and increased vascular permeability causing rapid loss of plasma into interstitial spaces.

anaphylaxis   A severe type I hypersensitivity response caused by the massive release of chemical mediators and other substances from mast cells.

anastomosis Site at which a graft is sutured into a recipient.

anatomic shunt Movement of blood from the right heart and back into the left heart without coming into contact with alveoli.

anemia A condition marked by decreased numbers of RBCs, decreased hemoglobin, or decreased hematocrit.

anergy Lack of immune response.

aneurysm An abnormal localized dilation of an artery that results from a weakened arterial wall.

angina pectoris Chest pain that is usually precipitated by exercise and relieved by rest.

anginal equivalents Symptoms suggestive of coronary artery disease but that do not include angina (e.g., dyspnea, fatigue, dizziness).

angiogenesis Formation of new blood vessels in order to reestablish perfusion to the wound bed.

anion gap A measurement of excessive unmeasurable anions.

anions Negatively charged ions.

anosognosia A severe form of neglect in which the patient fails to recognize his or her illness or paralysis.

antigen A substance capable of triggering an immune response.

antigen-presenting cells (APCs) Special cells that process antigen and present a fragment for recognition by the T and B lymphocytes.

antrum The terminal portion of the stomach, located between the gastric body and the pyloric sphincter.

anuria No urine, as defined as less than 100 mL/day.

aortic valve regurgitation (AR) Aortic valve insufficiency that allows blood to flow back into the left ventricle from the aorta during diastole.

aortic valve stenosis (AS) A narrowing of the aortic valve orifice so that blood flow is obstructed from the left ventricle into the aorta during systole.

aphasia The inability to understand language, use language, or both.

apheresis A therapeutic procedure in which blood is removed from the body and run through a special cell-separating apparatus to remove specific blood components, such as platelets, plasma, or hematopoietic stem cells.

apical–radial pulse deficit The difference between the apical and radial pulse rates, which reflects the number of heartbeats too weak to be transmitted to the periphery.

aplastic anemia A clinical syndrome characterized by a significant reduction in the formation of all blood cells in the bone marrow, resulting in pancytopenia (abnormally low numbers of all blood cell types) and hypocellular bone marrow.

apoptosis Programmed cell death.

APP Assume pain present.

apraxia A perceptual and cognitive impairment resulting in an inability to perform movements voluntarily in the presence of intact motor power, sensation, or coordination; may move automatically but not purposefully; types of apraxia include dressing, ideational, ideomotor, motor, and constructional.

aromatherapy Use of oils to reduce stress and anxiety.

arousal The component of consciousness concerned with the ability of an individual simply to respond to environmental stimuli, such as opening the eyes to speech or turning the head toward a noise; degree of alertness or responsiveness to stimuli.

ascites An abnormal accumulation of fluid in the peritoneal cavity; often occurs with renal or liver failure.

assist-control (AC) mode A mechanical ventilation mode that combines two single modes: assist, a patient-sensitive mode; and control, a time-triggered mode.

asterixis Bilateral flapping tremor most often seen in the wrist with dorsiflexion.

asystole No heartbeat.

ataxia Impaired gait characterized by unsteadiness, poor balance, and lack of coordination (lesion site: cerebellum).

atheroma Complicated atherosclerotic lesion that is calcified and contains hemorrhage, ulceration, and scar tissue deposits.

atherosclerosis A form of arteriosclerosis characterized by plaque deposits in the intimal lining of medium and large arteries.

atrial gallop Abnormal S4 heart sound caused by atrial contraction.

Auer rods Abnormal, large, granule-containing, needlelike rods in the cytoplasm; most commonly found in blast cells of the bone marrow and blood in patients with AML (acute myelogenous [myelocytic] leukemia).

autodigestion Breakdown of pancreatic tissues by its own enzymes.

autograft Transplantation of tissue from one part of a person's body to another part.

autografting Transplanting tissue from one part of the patient's body to another part of the patient's body.

autoimmunity A destructive response in which the immune system recognizes self as foreign and begins to destroy the body's own cells and tissues.

autolytic debridement Use of dressing materials that allow endogenous enzymes to liquefy necrotic tissue.

automaticity Ability to initiate an impulse.

autonomic dysreflexia Potentially life-threatening complication following spinal cord injury; caused by excessive sympathetic nervous system stimulation that produces extreme vasoconstriction and hypertension.

auto-PEEP The unintentional buildup of positive end-expiratory pressure caused by air trapping.

autoregulation Mechanism used by tissues to regulate their own blood supply by dilating or constricting local blood vessels; the localized matching of cerebral blood flow with cerebral metabolism.

autosplenectomy Destruction of the spleen.

awareness Having or showing realization, perception, or knowledge of surroundings, situation, circumstances.

axon A long slender projection of a nerve cell or neuron, that conducts electrical or chemical signals away from the neuron to effect a change in distant cells.

azotemia Accumulation of abnormally large amounts of nitrogenous waste products in the blood.

bacteremia The presence of bacteria in the blood.

BALT See *bronchial- and tracheal-associated lymphoid tissue.*

band (stab) An immature neutrophil.

bariatric surgery is a treatment option for obesity when attempts at losing weight using diet, exercise, and/or medication strategies are unsuccessful.

baroreceptors Pressure receptors located in the arch of the aorta and carotid sinus that detect arterial pressure changes.

barotrauma Injury to pulmonary tissues as a result of excessive pressures.

base deficit (BD) The amount of base required to titrate 1 liter of arterial blood to a normal pH. It is calculated from an arterial blood gas. A person can develop a base excess (metabolic alkalosis) or a base deficit (metabolic acidosis).

base excess (BE)   A measure of the amount of buffer required to return the blood to a normal pH state; used in reference to metabolic acid–base states. A person can develop a base excess (metabolic alkalosis) or a base deficit (metabolic acidosis).

bases   Substances capable of accepting ions.

Beck's triad   Classic signs of cardiac tamponade that include elevated right atrial pressure, hypotension, and muffled heart sounds.

bigeminy   A cardiac dysrhythmia of one SA node–generated beat followed by one premature ventricular contraction.

bile   A substance produced by the hepatocytes that is essential to normal digestion, particularly for fats.

bilirubin   The end product of hemoglobin degradation.

bioburden   The degree of foreign material and debris resulting from bacteria and tissue injury that cause a delay in the wound healing process.

biofilm   A group of mixed microorganisms embedded in a matrix that is permanently attached to the wound.

biosurgical (maggot) debridement   Form of debridement that uses sterile larvae that are introduced into the wound bed.

bleb   A type of cyst (or blister) of gas that develops in the visceral pleura of the lung.

blood–brain barrier   A network of cells and membranes that control brain volume and contents by controlling permeability.

blunt trauma   Injury without interruption of skin integrity.

body (gastric)   The largest portion of the stomach located between the fundus and the antrum.

body mass index (BMI)   The reference standard for normal body weight.

bradycardia   Heart rate less than 60 bpm.

brain death   Irreversible cessation of all brain function, including brainstem function.

brainstem   Contains the midbrain, pons, and medulla oblongata.

Broca's (expressive) aphasia   Inability to express language through speech or writing.

bronchial- and tracheal-associated lymphoid tissue (BALT)   Specialized cells that support immune function in the respiratory tract; cellular clusters of these lymphoid tissues engage in surveillance and early detection of foreign substances.

B-type natriuretic peptide (BNP)   Hormone released from the ventricles in response to increased preload; causes urinary excretion of sodium and diuresis. Its action results in reduced preload.

buffer   A substance that reacts with acids and bases to maintain a neutral environment of stable pH.

burn center   A specific area in the hospital with resources and staff designated for treating patients who have experienced burn injuries.

burn shock   Hypovolemic shock that develops secondary to fluid shifts occurring with burn injury.

burnout   A syndrome of emotional exhaustion, depersonalization, and reduced personal accomplishments that occurs among individuals who work with people on a daily basis.

cachetic   Relating to having cachexia.

cachexia   Observable wasting of body mass caused by malnutrition.

canaliculi   Small channels or canals that branch out and connect to lacunae.

capillary shunt   Normal flow of pulmonary blood past completely unventilated alveoli.

capnogram   Graphic representation of carbon dioxide levels during respiration.

capnography   The noninvasive graphic display of CO_2 concentration that is exhaled by the patient during breathing.

capnometry   Measurement of carbon dioxide in expired gas.

carbohydrates   Nutritional substances composed of complex and simple sugars.

carboxyhemoglobin   A compound formed by carbon monoxide and hemoglobin.

cardiac cycle   The heart muscle activities associated with one complete heartbeat.

cardiac index (CI)   Cardiac output divided by body surface area.

cardiac markers   Proteins released by necrotic myocytes into the blood; when present in the serum, they signal myocardial damage.

cardiac output (CO)   The amount of blood pumped by the heart each minute.

cardiac tamponade   A life-threatening postoperative complication of coronary artery bypass surgery caused by bleeding into the pericardial sac.

cardiogenic shock   Impaired oxygenation because the heart fails to function as a pump to deliver oxygenated blood.

cardioplegic   Intentional and temporary cessation of cardiac activity.

carina   The junction of the Y formed by the right and left mainstem bronchi in the lungs.

catabolism   Process by which complex nutrients are converted into more basic elements, such as glucose, fatty acids, and amino acids; breakdown of a substance.

central line-associated blood stream infection (CLABSI)   Infection due to lack of sterility during placement of central lines and inadequate precautions taken during maintenance of the central line and insertion site (e.g., changing tubing, dressings, bags).

catheter-related sepsis (CRS)   A potentially lethal complication of total parenteral nutrition (TPN); microorganisms are introduced through the TPN catheter, eventually causing a systemic infection (sepsis).

cations   Positively charged ions.

cavitation   Creation of a temporary cavity as tissues are stretched, compressed, and displaced forward and laterally, creating a tract from a penetrating missile.

CD markers   Refers to "clusters of differentiation" cell surface antigens markings on lymphocytes.

cell differentiation   Development of specific cell functions through a maturation process.

cell-mediated immunity   A type of protection against invading antigens characterized by surveillance and direct attack of foreign material; the primary effector cell is the T lymphocyte.

central stimulation   Involves the trunk or central portion of the body and produces an overall body response; should be used for initial introduction of pain; refers to stimulation of the cerebral hemispheres rather than spinal cord.

central sensitization   The increased excitability of neurons in the CNS that is a complex abnormal response to a barrage of prolonged nociceptive activation.

cerebral blood flow (CBF)   Blood flow to the brain is maintained at a constant rate by vasodilation of the vessels to increase the flow or vasoconstriction to decrease the flow.

cerebral hematomas   A group of focal cerebral injuries associated with the accumulation of blood in the cranial vault.

cerebral perfusion pressure (CPP)   An estimate of the adequacy of cerebral circulation; perfusion pressure to the brain that is the difference between the mean systemic arterial pressure and the mean intracranial pressure. It is calculated as follows: CPP = MAP − ICP.

cerebral salt wasting (CSW)   A state of fluid overload with the end result being the loss of sodium into the urine causing water to follow.

chemical debridement   Use of topical enzymes applied to a wound to remove necrotic tissue; also known as *enzymatic debridement*.

chemical mediators   Chemicals (such as histamine, bradykinin, and prostaglandins) that initiate the inflammatory process.

chemotaxis   The movement of leukocytes along an increasing concentration of chemical stimulus (chemotactic factors) toward an area of inflammation.

chief cells   The particular cells of gastric glands that secrete pepsinogen, a precursor of pepsin for protein digestion.

cholecystokinin (CCK)   Hormone that stimulates pancreatic enzymes, increases contractility of the gallbladder, and inhibits gastric motility.

chronic kidney failure (CKF)   The gradual loss of renal function.

chronic obstructive pulmonary disease (COPD)   Chronic airflow limitation disease; a group of pulmonary diseases that cause obstruction to expiratory airflow.

chronic rejection   A humoral immune response in which antibodies slowly attack and destroy a graft.

Chvostek sign   The facial nerve is tapped directly in front of the ear; a positive sign is present when the facial muscles contract on the same side of the face as the tapping.

chyme   The mixture of partially digested food and secretions of digestion found in the stomach and small bowel.

circle of Willis   An area in the brain where carotid arteries and vertebral arteries unite to provide collateral blood flow to either side of the brain.

CO₂ narcosis   A state of hypercapnic encephalopathy caused by toxic levels of $PaCO_2$ that produces drowsiness, stupor, or coma.

cognition   Thinking skills that include language use, calculation, perception, memory, awareness, reasoning, judgment, learning, intellect, social skills, and imagination.

collagen   Major component of new connective tissue that gives tensile strength to the wound.

colonization   The replication of microflora that do not adversely affect wound healing.

coma   A state of unconsciousness from which one cannot be aroused and is the most severe of the alterations of consciousness.

committed stem cell   A pluripotential stem cell that has committed its development to either the myeloid or lymphoid cell line.

compartment syndrome   Pressure within a muscle compartment rises and exceeds microvascular pressure, thereby interfering with cellular perfusion.

compassion fatigue   Results when the compassionate energy that has been expended by the nurse exceeds the ability to personally reenergize.

compensated   A state in which the pH is within normal limits with the acid–base imbalance being neutralized but not corrected.

complement system   A progressive, sequential cascade of events produced by substances found naturally in the circulating sera; components of the system must be triggered individually and cause cellular lysis of antigens.

complementary and alternative therapies (CAT)   Therapies used in lieu of, or along with, standard medical treatment.

complete spinal cord injury   A traumatic injury that results in the loss of motor and sensory function below the level of injury, extending to the lowest sacral segment.

compliance   (C_L) Measurement of the relative ease with which an organ can expand; reflects relative stiffness of the organ; in the lungs, it is the amount of force required to expand the lungs; measured in mL/cm H_2O; normal is 50 to 100 mL/cm H_2O.

compression   The process of being pressed or squeezed together, resulting in reduction in size or volume.

compromised wound   Wound that contains devitalized tissue.

concussion   Mild traumatic brain injury caused by blunt trauma to the head.

conductivity   The ability of the cardiac stimulus to transmit throughout the myocardium.

conjugated bilirubin   Bilirubin that has been joined with glucuronic acid to make it water soluble.

consciousness   State of general awareness of oneself and the environment; made up of the components of arousal and content.

conservative sharp debridement   The removal of necrotic tissue with a clean method and does not generally result in blood loss.

contamination   The presence of nonreplicating microbes.

content   The component of consciousness concerned with interpreting environmental stimuli; includes thinking, memory, problem solving, orientation, and speech.

continuous positive airway pressure (CPAP)   The application of positive pressure to the airway of a spontaneously breathing person. See *positive end-expiratory pressure* [*PEEP*]).

contractility   The ability of a muscle to shorten when stimulated; in particular, the force of myocardial contraction.

contraction (wound)   Wound margins begin to pull toward the center of the wound to decrease the wound surface area.

controlled mandatory ventilation (CMV)   See *assist-control mode* (*AC*).

contusion   Injury to superficial tissues, with disruption of blood vessels (bruising) with extravasation into the skin; in brain injury it is a moderate-to-severe injury with bruising of brain tissue.

cor pulmonale   Right ventricular hypertrophy and dilation secondary to pulmonary disease, resulting in pulmonary hypertension.

corrected   A state in which all acid–base parameters have returned to normal ranges after a state of acid–base imbalance.

crackles   Adventitious breath sounds associated with fluid or secretions or both in small airways or alveoli.

C-reactive protein (CRP)   Peptide released by the liver in response to inflammation, infection, and tissue damage; downstream marker for inflammation now considered a major risk factor for heart disease.

critical colonization   A level of microorganism burden that affects skin cell proliferation and tissue repair, altering wound healing but not invading the wound tissue.

CT angiography   A contrast-enhanced, spiral computed tomographic angiogram.

Cullen's sign   A bluish discoloration around the umbilicus seen in hemorrhagic pancreatitis.

cultural competence   An awareness of one's own thoughts and feelings without letting them influence caring for patients with different backgrounds.

Cushing's triad   Vital sign changes that occur where the pulse pressure widens until ICP equals MAP and includes (1) increased systolic blood pressure, (2) decreased diastolic blood pressure, and (3) bradycardia.

cytokines Special secreted cellular proteins that serve as messengers for activation of components of the immune system and other hematopoietic functions.

cytotoxic agents Drugs that have the capability of destroying target cells.

D-dimer A protein that is released into the circulation during the breakdown of fibrin blood clots.

debridement Removal of necrotic tissue, devitalized tissue, or debris from the wound bed.

deceleration A decrease in the rate of velocity or speed of a moving body.

decerebrate posturing Abnormal extension; neck is extended with jaw clenched; arms pronate and extend straight out; feet are plantar flexed.

decorticate posturing Abnormal flexion; upper arms move upward to the chest; elbows, wrists, and fingers flex; legs extend with internal rotation; feet flex.

decreased or absent breath sounds Caused by diminished or absent air flow to an area of the lungs.

deep full-thickness burn (subdermal burn) Burn that destroys all layers of the skin and may include injury to muscle, tendons, or bone.

deep partial-thickness burn Burn that involves the epidermis and deep layers of the dermis.

defibrillation An unsynchronized direct-current electrical countershock that depolarizes all the cells simultaneously, allowing the SA node to resume the pacemaker role.

delirium Acute onset of fluctuating awareness, impaired ability to attend to environmental stimuli, and disorganized thinking. May include hallucinations or delusions; difficulty in focusing attention and sleeping; and emotional, physical and autonomic overactivity.

dementia A progressive, often irreversible decline in mental functioning that involves increasing deficits of reasoning, judgment, abstract thought, comprehension, learning, task execution, and speech.

depolarization A wave of electrical current that causes cardiac cells to become positively charged; should result in cardiac muscle contraction.

dermatome A cutaneous section of the body innervated by a spinal or cranial nerve.

dermis Middle layer of skin, referred to as true skin.

dexmedetomidine A sedative agent typically used to provide moderate sedation in the mechanically ventilated patient especially when performing a procedure.

diabetes insipidus (DI) A condition associated with improper water balance and characterized by the decrease or absence of antidiuretic hormone (ADH) secreted by the posterior pituitary gland; this loss of ADH secretion results in diuresis.

diabetes mellitus (diabetes) A complex metabolic disorder in which the person has either an absolute or a relative insulin deficiency; this insulin deficiency results in impaired carbohydrate, protein, and fat metabolism.

diabetic ketoacidosis (DKA) A potentially devastating form of metabolic acidosis, characterized by a clinical syndrome of symptoms associated with elevated blood glucose, blood ketone levels and metabolic acidosis.

dialysate Fluid used to remove or add solute to the plasma water.

diapedesis The movement of WBCs through an intact vessel wall using ameboid movement.

diastole The relaxation of a heart chamber, when blood fills the chamber in preparation for the next cardiac cycle and the coronary arteries fill with blood.

diastolic dysfunction Heart failure characterized by impairment of ventricular relaxation.

diencephalon Located deep within the cerebrum and superior to the brainstem, consists of the thalamus, hypothalamus, pituitary gland, and the epithalamus.

diffuse axonal injury (DAI) Injury that occurs when shearing forces disrupt the structure of neurons and their nearby blood vessels.

diffuse injuries Occur in several areas of the brain and may occur with concussion and diffuse axonal injury.

diffusion Movement of gases across a pressure gradient from an area of high concentration to one of low concentration.

dilated cardiomyopathy Condition associated with left ventricular dilation and decreased ejection fraction.

direct calorimetry Measurement of the body's heat production while the individual is isolated in a chamber or room specifically equipped for this purpose.

distributive shock Involves impaired oxygenation because of altered blood flow distribution.

doll's eye movements Oculocephalic reflex; reflexive movements of the eyes in the opposite direction of head rotation.

dysarthria Impairment of the muscles that control speech.

dyskinesis Myocardial wall movement in the opposite direction.

dysphagia Dysfunction of one or more parts of the swallowing process.

dysphasia Impaired capacity to interpret, formulate, or express meaningful language by speaking, writing, or gesturing (expressive or Broca's dysphasia); the inability to understand the written or spoken language (receptive or Wernicke's dysphasia).

dyspnea Subjective sensation of difficulty breathing.

dysrhythmias Abnormal heart rhythms.

echocardiography Imaging technique used to assess functional structures of the heart using ultrasound waves.

edema Excess accumulation of fluid in interstitial spaces.

ejection fraction (EF) The amount of blood ejected from the left ventricle per each heartbeat; normal is above 50 percent.

elastase A proteolytic pancreatic enzyme; its proenzyme, proelastase, requires trypsin to become activated; responsible for erosion of blood vessels contributing to hemorrhage in severe acute pancreatitis.

electrocardiogram (ECG) Graphic representation of the electrical, not mechanical, activity of the heart.

electrodes Small adhesive patches with conducting gel placed on the skin to pick up (sense) electrical impulses and send them through attached lead wires to a cable on the ECG machine or cardiac monitor where the ECG rhythm can be viewed or printed out on special paper.

electrolytes Electrically charged microsolutes found in body fluids.

empyema Abnormal accumulation of purulent fluid in the intrapleural space as a result of inflammation or infection.

endocardium The innermost layer of the heart.

endogenous Internal to the body.

endoscopic retrograde cholangiopancreatography (ERCP) An invasive endoscopic test that allows cannulation and direct viewing of the ampulla of Vater, as well as the pancreatic and bile ducts.

endothelium Thin inner layer of blood vessels composed of endothelial cells.

energy The ability to do work; synonymous with calories; most common sources are carbohydrates and fats.

engulfment   The swallowing up of antigens by the phagocyte, for purposes of destruction or neutralization.

engraftment   The donor's stem cells take hold in the patient's marrow and start producing normal hematopoietic cells.

enteral nutrition   Nutrition delivered into the gastrointestinal tract through a feeding tube; it is a lactose-free, nutritionally complete formula composed of protein, carbohydrates, fats, electrolytes, vitamins, and minerals.

enterocutaneous fistula (ECF)   A passageway that develops between a segment of the gastrointestinal tract and the skin.

enzymes   Catalyst substances found in cells that assist in cellular activities.

epicardium   A tough fibrous covering surrounding the outside of the heart that helps maintain the heart in position and contributes to its structure; also called pericardium.

epidermis   Outermost layer of skin.

epidural hematoma (EDH)   Bleeding in the space between the dura mater and the skull.

epithelialization   Migration of epithelial cells along the wound surface.

erythrocytes   Red blood cells; part of the hematopoietic stem cell line; produced in the bone marrow.

erythropoiesis   Refers to production of erythrocytes.

erythropoietin   A circulating hormone, produced by the kidneys, that regulates production of erythrocytes.

eschar   A tough, dry, inelastic wound indicative of a full-thickness burn.

escharotomy   Surgical incision of the eschar and superficial fascia of a circumferentially burned limb or trunk in order to restore blood flow distal to the affected area.

esophageal varices   Dilated and tortuous vessels found in the distal esophagus and stomach.

ethnicity   A set of social, cultural, and political beliefs held by a group of individuals.

exogenous   External to the body.

expressive aphasia   The inability to write or use language appropriately.

exsanguination   The most extreme form of hemorrhage, with an initial loss of blood volume of 40% and a rate of hemorrhage exceeding 250 mL per minute.

external respiration   Movement of gases across the alveolar–capillary membrane.

extracellular   Fluid compartment within the body composed of plasma and interstitial fluid.

extrinsic pathway   A coagulation cascade of events triggered by blood being exposed to extravascular tissue that results in clot formation.

extubation   Removal of an endotracheal or tracheostomy tube from the patient's airway.

exudate   Fluid produced by wounds.

failure to capture   The situation in which the pacemaker initiates an impulse but the stimulus is not strong enough to produce depolarization.

failure to fire   Situation in which a pacemaker fails to send out an electrical impulse at the appointed time.

failure to sense   Situation in which the pacemaker competes with the patient's own impulse generation.

fatty streaks   Type II atherosclerotic skin lesions characterized by macrophage migration across the endothelium and smooth muscle cells that contain lipid droplets.

fibrinolytic   A group of drugs capable of breaking down the protein fibrin, which is the main constituent of blood clots.

fibrous atheromatous plaque   Basic lesion associated with atherosclerosis; lesion filled with lipids, collagen, scar tissue, and vascular smooth muscle cells.

fistula   Tubelike passages that form connections between different sites of the gastrointestinal tract.

flaccid paralysis   Damage to lower motor neurons, producing loss of both voluntary and involuntary movement.

focal injuries   Two types of traumatic brain injury; typically occur in a well-defined area of the brain and may be the result of a hematoma.

forced expiratory volume (FEV)   Measure of how rapidly a person can forcefully exhale air after a maximal inhalation; a measurement of dynamic lung function.

fraction of inspired oxygen (FIO$_2$)   That portion of the total gas being inspired that is composed of oxygen; expressed in decimals from 0.21 to 1.0.

full-thickness burn   A burn that destroys epidermis, dermis, and portions of subcutaneous tissues (formerly known as third- and fourth-degree burns).

full-thickness wound   Injury to the epidermis and dermis with exposure of subcutaneous tissue.

fundus   The anatomic area of the stomach located above the lower esophageal sphincter, appearing as a bulge at the top of the stomach.

GALT   See *gut-associated lymphoid tissue.*

gastric inhibitory peptide (GIP)   Hormone that helps digest carbohydrates and fats.

gastric tonometry   A technique to assess gut perfusion by using a gastric balloon to measure the mucosal CO_2 level.

gastrin   A hormonal regulator produced by cells located in the pyloric region of the stomach; stimulates gastric glands to produce hydrochloric acid and pepsinogen.

gastrocolic reflex   A mass movement of the contents of the colon, frequently preceded by a similar movement in the small intestine, which sometimes occurs immediately following the entrance of food into the stomach.

G-cells   Gastrin secreting cells located in the mucosa of the pyloric area of the stomach and duodenum.

Glasgow Coma Scale (GCS)   An objective neurological assessment tool that was originally developed to standardize measurement of the ability of the patient with a traumatic brain injury (TBI) to interact with the environment.

global aphasia   The inability to use or understand language.

gluconeogenesis   Formation of glucose from protein and fat stores in the body; seen in the ebb phase and flow phase; formation of glycogen in the liver from a noncarbohydrate substance.

glycogenesis   Process by which excess glucose that is not needed for cellular activities is stored as glycogen in the liver and muscle cells.

glycogenolysis   Conversion of glycogen to glucose in the liver and muscles; seen in the ebb phase of the metabolic stress response.

glycosuria   Excretion of glucose in the urine.

graft   The transfer of tissue or organ from one part of the body to a different part, or from another donor source.

graft-versus-host disease (GVHD)   A complication of hematopoeitic stem cell transplantation in which donor T cells, after being implanted in the recipient, recognize the recipient's tissues as being foreign and muster an attack.

granulation tissue   Tissue in a wound with a characteristic pink-red color.

granulocyte A type of blood cell with granules located in the cytoplasm.

granulocyte-monocyte colony-stimulating factors (GM-CSF) A group of cytokines involved in the division and differentiation of neutrophils and monocytes and other chemical mediator activities.

Grey Turner's sign A bluish discoloration of the flank region seen in hemorrhagic pancreatitis.

guided imagery A complementary alternative therapy that uses patients' past experiences to promote a vision or fantasy that encourages relaxation.

gut Refers to the bowel or intestine.

gut-associated lymphoid tissue (GALT) All lymphoid tissue associated with the gastrointestinal tract, including the tonsils, appendix, and Peyer's patches.

hard palate Bony surface against which the tongue forces food during chewing.

Harris–Benedict equation Estimates caloric requirements of a resting, fasting, unstressed individual based on the individual's height, weight, age, and sex; expressed in kilocalories.

haustral churning Movement of the large intestine.

health literacy The degree to which patients and families have the ability to obtain, process, and understand basic health information to make informed decisions about their healthcare.

healthy practice environment A practice environment that supports quality client care and high levels of nurse satisfaction.

healthy work environment A work environment that supports quality patient care and high levels of nurse satisfaction.

heart failure (HF) Clinical syndrome that can result from structural or functional cardiac disorders that decrease the ability of the ventricle to fill or eject.

hematemesis Vomiting of bright red blood or blood that resembles "coffee grounds."

hematochezia Bright red blood or maroon-colored stool secondary to bleeding.

hemiplegia Paralysis or loss of voluntary movement of one side of the body.

hemodynamics A physiologic term that refers to the forces involved in the flow of blood as it circulates through the cardiovascular system.

hemoglobin (Hgb) The oxygen-carrying protein found on erythrocytes.

hemolytic anemia Breakdown (pathologic destruction) of red blood cells.

hemopneumothorax Abnormal accumulation of air and blood in the intrapleural space.

hemoptysis Expectoration of bloody sputum.

hemorrhagic cystitis Severe bladder irritation resulting in gross bleeding.

hemostasis Stoppage of bleeding; stagnation of blood flow.

hemothorax Abnormal accumulation of blood in the intrapleural space.

hepcidin The major iron-regulating hormone produced in the liver.

herniation A catastrophic shifting or displacement of brain tissue, which causes pressure and traction on cerebral structures and produces clinical symptoms.

heterograft Transplantation of tissue between two different species (e.g., animals and humans); can be used as a temporary biological dressing; also referred to as *xenograft*.

high-density lipoprotein (HDL) Lipoprotein molecule that has a high density (amount) of protein and a small amount of cholesterol; commonly known as the "good" cholesterol.

histocompatibility The ability of cells and tissues to live without interference from the immune system.

homocysteine A naturally occurring amino acid.

homograft Tissue transplanted from another individual to be used as a biological dressing.

homonymous hemianopsia Hemineglect syndrome.

humoral immunity The type of protection against foreign antigens provided by antibody formation from B lymphocytes.

hydrocephalus A clinical syndrome caused by an increased production of cerebrospinal fluid that exceeds the absorption rate.

hydrochloric acid Secreted by the parietal cells to lower gastrointestinal pH and to regulate bacterial growth.

hyperalgesia Characterized by increasing pain despite repeated upward titration of opioids.

hyperacute rejection A humoral immune response in which the B lymphocytes are activated to produce antibodies against the donor organ; it occurs within minutes to hours following transplantation.

hypercapnia Abnormally high level of carbon dioxide in the blood.

hypercatabolism Breakdown of total body protein; skeletal muscle protein is used initially for conversion to glucose through gluconeogenesis; visceral (organ) protein is used after skeletal muscle protein; occurs in the flow phase of the metabolic stress response.

hypercholesterolemia High levels of serum cholesterol.

hyperemia A state in which cerebral blood flow is higher than cerebral metabolic needs; also known as *luxury perfusion*.

hyperglycemia Abnormally high level of glucose in the blood.

hyperglycemic hyperosmolar state (HHS) A hyperglycemic complication of diabetes mellitus that results from insulin deficiency or insulin resistance; previously referred to as hyperglycemic hyperosmolar nonketotic syndrome (HHNS).

hyperlipidemia A condition manifested by high levels of lipids in the blood.

hypermetabolism An increased metabolic rate in response to a major bodily insult requiring increased quantities of oxygen and nutrients to meet the increased metabolic needs; occurs in the flow phase of the metabolic stress response.

hypersensitivity An exaggerated response of the immune system to an antigen or antigens otherwise considered nonpathogenic; an allergy to a certain substance is an example of a hypersensitivity reaction.

hypertonic A high-osmolarity state in which the concentration of particles is greater on one side of a membrane than on the other side; in the body, the solution has a higher osmolarity than exists inside of the cells.

hypertrophic cardiomyopathy Condition associated with left ventricular hypertrophy that decreases the ability of the chamber to relax (diastolic dysfunction).

hypervolemia Excess volume of circulating fluids.

hypoalbuminemia Low serum albumin levels.

hypochromic The abnormal pale coloring of RBCs, indicating reduced hemoglobin content.

hypodermis A subcutaneous layer below the dermis that consists of adipose tissue and blood vessels.

hypoglycemia Abnormally low level of glucose in the blood.

hypokinesis Decreased myocardial wall movement resulting from myocardial ischemia or injury.

hypothalamic–pituitary–adrenal (HPA) axis An integrated negative feedback hormone mechanism composed of the hypothalamus, anterior pituitary gland, and adrenal cortex.

hypotonic A low-osmolarity state in which the concentration of particles in a solution is greater on one side of a membrane than on the other side; in the body, the solution has a lower osmolarity than exists inside of the cells.

hypovolemia Decreased volume of circulating fluids.

hypovolemic shock Impaired oxygenation because of inadequate cardiac output as a result of decreased intravascular volume.

ideal body weight (IBW) The expected weight of an individual based on age, sex, and height.

immunity A normal adaptive response to the external environment; it functions to protect the body from disease by means of both resistance to offending organisms and attack on offending organisms.

immunodeficiency A deficiency of T cells or B cells or both resulting from illnesses, chemotherapy, radiation therapy, or a direct pathogenic attack on the immune system.

immunodeficiency state A general term referring to a state of deficient immune activity.

immunoglobulin (Ig) The product of plasma cells in the humoral immune response following exposure to a specific antigen; the five classes of immunoglobulins are IgA, IgD, IgE, IgG, and IgM; antibodies.

immunosuppressants Drugs that suppress the immune response.

incomplete spinal cord injury Trauma to the spinal cord that leads to partial loss of sensory or motor function below the neurological level of injury; includes the lower sacral segment.

indirect calorimetry A technique of estimating an individual's metabolic or energy expenditure through the measurement of oxygen consumed (VO_2) and carbon dioxide produced (VCO_2); can also calculate respiratory quotient (RQ).

infarction Death of tissue.

infective endocarditis (IE) A disease caused by microbial infection of the endothelial lining of the heart, usually presenting with microorganisms called vegetations on a heart valve.

injectate A 10-mL bolus of IV normal saline that is injected through the proximal injectate port of the PA catheter into the right atrium.

inhalation injury Burn-associated injury caused by inhaling products of combustion.

innate (natural) immunity Species-specific protection composed of natural resistance and the activities of certain leukocytes.

inotropes Factors that influence contractility.

inotropic Factor that influences myocardial contractility; a positive inotrope increases myocardial contractility; a negative inotrope decreased myocardial contractility.

interferon (INF) A cytokine involved in the signaling between cells of the immune system and in protection against viral infections. See *cytokines*.

interleukin (IL) A cytokine involved in signaling between cells of the immune system. See *cytokines*.

intermediate care unit (IMC) High-acuity nursing unit that provides an efficient distribution of resources for the patient whose acute illness requires less use of monitoring equipment and staffing than an intensive care unit.

internal respiration Movement of gases across the systemic capillary–cell membrane in the tissues.

intestinal strangulation Intestine twists to such an extent that circulation to the twisted area is impaired.

intra-abdominal hypertension (IAH) Abnormally high pressure within the abdominal cavity.

intracellular Fluid compartment within the body's cells; composes approximately two thirds of the total body water.

intracerebral hematoma (ICH) Accumulation of blood in the parenchyma of brain tissue.

intracranial hypertension Increased intracranial pressure.

intracranial pressure Pressure exerted by the cerebrospinal fluid within the ventricles of the brain; normal pressure is 0 to 15 mmHg.

intraparenchymal hematoma (IPH) Accumulation of blood in the parenchyma or tissue of the brain rather than between the meningeal layers.

intrathecal Within a sheath (e.g., cerebrospinal fluid that is contained within the dura mater).

intravenous (IV) Into a vein.

intravascular Fluid compartment in the blood vessels; fluid is available for exchange of nutrients and oxygen.

intrinsic factor (IF) Secreted by the parietal cells; necessary for vitamin B_{12} absorption.

intrinsic pathway A coagulation cascade of events triggered by direct exposure of blood to subendothelial vascular tissue that results in clot formation.

intrinsic kidney injury Caused by problems that target the kidney parenchyma (renal tissue) where the injury occurs.

invasive infection The presence of pathogens in a burn wound at sufficient concentrations (in conjunction with depth, surface area involved, and age of the patient) to cause supportive separation of eschar or graft loss, invasion of adjacent unburned tissue, or the systemic response of sepsis syndrome.

isoenzymes A subgrouping of parent enzymes that are more specific to a particular cell type.

isograft Transplantation of tissues between identical twins; also referred to as a *syngraft*.

isotonic The concentration of particles in a solution on one side of a membrane is the same as it is on the other side of the membrane; in the body, it closely approximates normal serum plasma osmolality.

jaundice A yellow cast of the skin, sclera, and mucous membranes caused by elevated bilirubin, a yellow pigment.

kallikrein An enzyme found in plasma, body tissues, and urine that forms kinin; it normally circulates in the plasma in its inactive state, as the proenzyme kallikreinogen; when activated by trypsin, it is an extremely potent vasodilator.

ketamine Provides analgesia by blocking specific receptors within the neurons.

ketosis The presence of ketones in the blood.

Kupffer cells Fixed tissue macrophages found in the liver.

kwashiorkor A state of malnutrition in which there is a prolonged deficiency for absence of protein in the presence of adequate carbohydrate intake.

LaPlace's law States that wall tension (T) is equal to the pressure (P) being exerted against the wall, multiplied by the wall radius (R), or $T = P \times R$; therefore, as an artery dilates, it increases the force on the arterial wall, which then causes more dilation.

leukocytes White blood cells or WBCs.

lipase A lipolytic pancreatic enzyme; its action contributes to necrosis of fatty tissue surrounding the pancreas in the presence of pancreatitis.

lipogenesis The liver's production of lipids from glucose or amino acid.

lipolysis Breakdown or splitting of fat.

lipolytic Facilitating the breakdown of fats.

lipoprotein Cholesterol bound to protein and carried in the blood.

living donor A person who volunteers to have an organ, part of an organ, or hematopoietic stem cells removed for transplantation into another person while still alive.

loading dose A dosage of medication administered at the beginning of a treatment regimen; it is usually a large dose to achieve the most therapeutic effects from.

lobectomy Surgical procedure that removes one or more lobes of the lung.

lobule The functional unit of the liver.

low-density lipoprotein (LDL) Lipoprotein molecule that has a low density (amount) of protein and a large amount of cholesterol; commonly known as the "bad" cholesterol.

lower esophageal sphincter (LES) Structure with high resting muscle tone at the distal end of the esophagus to prevent gastroesophageal reflux.

low tidal volume ventilation (LTVV) Reduces the damaging effects (volutrauma) of excessive stretching of lung tissue and alveoli that occurs with higher tidal volumes; is the standard of care for people with ARDS requiring mechanical ventilation.

lysosomes Sacs inside the cell containing digestive enzymes.

macrocytic Abnormally large RBCs.

macroangiopathy Macrovascular disease; refers to atherosclerosis.

macronutrients Carbohydrates, lipids (fats), and proteins.

macrophages Activated, mature monocytes that ingest and digest antigens, then carry the antigen to the T cells and B cells; the link between the immune response and the inflammatory response.

magnetic resonance cholangiopancreatography (MRCP) A test using magnetic resonance imaging to produce images of the hepatobiliary tree.

maintenance dose The dosage of medication required to maintain the desired steady state of a drug in the body.

major histocompatibility complex (MHC) A group of genes located on the sixth chromosome responsible for coding histocompatibility antigens for discrimination of self from nonself.

malnutrition A state of poor nutrition that arises from a lack of meeting the body's minimum nutritional requirements of carbohydrates, proteins, lipids, and other essential nutrients; may be caused by anorexia, poor diet, or malabsorption of nutrients in the gastrointestinal tract.

MALT See *mucosa-associated lymphoid tissue.*

marasmus A state of malnutrition in which there is inadequate intake of protein and calories and generalized wasting is evident.

margination The movement and adhering of circulating WBCs to the capillary wall in preparation for shifting out of the vessel to move to the site of injury.

mast cells Large granule-containing tissue cells that are located in connective tissue throughout the body.

mean arterial pressure Common measurement used clinically to reflect adequacy of perfusion.

mean corpuscular volume (MCV) A measurement of the size (volume) of RBCs.

mechanical debridement Use of moist dressings, irrigation, or whirlpool to remove foreign material from a wound.

medical futility A situation in which the continuation or initiation of medical treatment might have the expected medical effect, yet there is no benefit to the client.

megakaryocytes Cells that produce thrombocytes.

melena Black, tarry, foul-smelling stools containing blood.

meninges The protective connective tissue that covers the brain and spinal cord, forms the divisions that separate the lobes and structures of the brain, and contains venous sinuses.

mentation Refers to mental activity.

microangiopathy Small blood vessel disease.

microcytic Abnormally small RBC.

micronutrients Electrolytes, vitamins, minerals, and trace elements.

microvascular disease Disease of the capillaries.

microvilli Fingerlike projections covering the villi.

migration The movement of leukocytes to the site of injury via the chemotaxis process after they have escaped through the capillary wall.

minute ventilation ($\dot{V}_E$) The total volume of expired air in 1 minute.

mitral valve regurgitation (MR) Incompetent mitral valve allows blood to flow back into the left atrium during systole because the mitral valve does not fully close.

mitral valve stenosis (MS) A narrowing of the mitral valve orifice so that blood flow is obstructed from the left atrium into the left ventricle during diastole.

mitral valve prolapse A type of mitral valve insufficiency that occurs when one or both of the mitral valve cusps flow into the atria during ventricular systole.

Magnet designation Accreditation awarded to hospitals that create working environments which are successful in recruiting and retaining professional nurses.

moderate sedation Sedation ("level two") primarily used to induce relaxation while minimally disturbing the vital signs when cooperation is needed for a procedure.

modifiable risk factors Risk factors that can be altered through either lifestyle modification or medications (e.g., obesity and smoking).

modulation The body's attempt to modulate (alter) pain transmission in response to specific physiologic events, such as pain and stress.

monocytes Large, single-nucleus cells that provide the second line of defense.

mucosa Innermost layer of the GI wall.

mucosa-associated lymphoid tissue (MALT) Provides immunologic defense; includes the bronchial- and tracheal-associated and gut-associated lymphoid tissues.

mucositis Inflammation of any or all of the oral mucous membranes (i.e., tongue, gums, pharynx, lips, and cheeks).

multifocal Premature contractions originating from more than one ectopic pacemaker.

multimodal analgesia A balanced approach to pain treatment that targets several pain-signaling pathways and matches the treatment to the type of pain.

multiple organ dysfunction syndrome (MODS) The presence of altered organ function in an acutely ill patient such that homeostasis cannot be maintained without intervention.

muscularis Muscular layer of the GI wall.

myocardium The thick middle layer of the heart.

myoglobin An oxygen-binding protein similar to hemoglobin and primarily found in muscle; substance released from damaged muscle tissue.

myoglobinuria The presence of myoglobin in the urine.

myopathy Any muscle disease that is marked by focal or diffuse muscular weakness.

myxedema coma An extreme form of hypothyroidism characterized by altered mental status ranging from lethargy to psychosis, hypothermia, bradycardia, hypotension, hypoventilation, hyponatremia, and hypoglycemia.

neointimal hyperplasia The overgrowth of cells in the internal stent wall.

neurogenic shock Condition that occurs with an injury above T6; manifested by hypotension, bradycardia, decreased cardiac output, and inability to sweat below the level of the injury.

neuroplasticity Changes in the structure and function of the spinal segment of the nervous system.

neuropathic pain Occurs when there is a direct injury to a peripheral nerve, spinal cord, or the brain.

neutropenia Abnormally low number of neutrophils.

neutropenic enterocolitis (necrotizing enteritis or ileocecal syndrome) A necrotizing infectious process that affects the bowel.

neutrophil Segmented granulocyte of the myeloid cell line.

nitrogen A basic unit of protein (amino acid) breakdown; excreted primarily in urine in the form of urea; a 24-hour urinary urea nitrogen (UUN) measures nitrogen losses for a 24-hour period.

nitrogen balance The difference between nitrogen output and nitrogen intake.

nociception The activation of pain receptors and the pain pathway by a noxious stimulus of sufficient strength to threaten tissue integrity.

nociceptors Refers to pain receptors; sensory receptors that, when stimulated, cause the sensation of pain.

noninvasive intermittent positive pressure ventilation (NIPPV or NPPV) The application of positive pressure ventilation using a mechanical ventilator and a mask in place of an artificial airway.

noninvasive positive pressure ventilation (NPPV) A noninvasive alternative to conventional mechanical ventilatory support that does not require intubation.

nonmodifiable risk factors Risk factors that, regardless of therapy, cannot be altered (e.g., genetics and age).

nonspecific The general, nonadaptive natural protection.

nonvolatile (metabolic) acids Metabolic acids that cannot be converted to a gas, requiring excretion through the kidneys.

normochromic The normal coloring of RBCs, indicating normal hemoglobin content.

normocytic Normal-size cells.

nuchal rigidity Neck pain or stiffness.

nutrients Elements and compounds required for growth and maintenance of life; consist of macro- and micronutrients.

nutrition A complex process by which an organism takes in and uses food substrates for the purpose of providing energy for growth, maintenance, and repair; nutrition involves ingestion, digestion, absorption, and metabolism.

nystagmus Lateral tonic deviation of the eyes toward a stimulus.

obstruction Common surgical complication, often the result of adhesions that develop following abdominal surgery.

occult blood Blood present in the GI tract but not really visible.

oculovestibular reflex (cold caloric test) May be performed when determining brainstem function. Instilling cold water into the ear canal causes **nystagmus** (lateral tonic deviation of the eyes) toward the stimulus.

oligoanalgesia Treating pain with minimal drug use.

oliguria Production of an abnormally small amount (less than 400 mL) of urine per 24 hours; can be a symptom of kidney disease or obstruction of the urinary tract.

opiates Naturally occurring alkaloids such as morphine or codeine.

opioid pseudoaddiction Term applied to patients who develop behaviors that mimic those associated with addiction.

opioids Broadly describes all compounds that work at the opioid receptor sites.

opiophobia The fear of prescribing or consuming adequate amounts of opiates for therapeutic results.

opsonization A process by which an antigen is modified, making it more susceptible to phagocytosis.

orthopnea Difficulty breathing while laying down, relieved in the upright position.

orthostatic (postural) hypotension A drop in blood pressure greater than 20 mmHg or an increase in heart rate greater than 20 bpm when going from sitting to standing or lying to sitting position.

osmolality The solute concentration per volume of a solution (refers to body fluids).

osmolarity The solute concentration per volume of a solution (refers to outside of body).

osmoreceptors Neurons that detect changes in osmotic pressure.

osmosis The net diffusion of water from an area of greater concentration to an area of lesser concentration across the cell membrane; occurs as the result of osmotic pressure.

osmotic diuresis Excessive urinary excretion caused by osmotic shifting of fluids.

otorrhea The drainage of cerebral spinal fluid through the ear; indicates possible tear in the meninges.

oxygen consumption (VO_2) The amount of oxygen used by the body; described as a product of cardiac output and the difference between arterial oxygen content and venous oxygen content.

oxygen delivery (DO_2) The process of transportation of oxygen to cells, dependent on cardiac output, hemoglobin saturation with oxygen, and the partial pressure of oxygen in arterial blood.

oxygen extraction The process by which cells take oxygen from the blood.

oxygenation failure A respiratory crisis in which the primary problem is one of hypoxemia; clinically, it is defined as a PaO_2 of less than 60 mmHg.

oxyhemoglobin dissociation curve A graphic representation of the relationship between oxygen saturation of hemoglobin (SaO_2) and the partial pressure of oxygen (PaO_2) in the plasma.

pacemaker cells Specialized cardiac nervous tissue that is able to initiate an electrical impulse, resulting in contraction of the heart; an artificial pulse generator used to provide electrical stimulus to the heart when the heart fails to conduct or generate impulses on its own at a rate that maintains cardiac output.

pain An unpleasant sensory and emotional experience typically associated with actual or impending tissue damage.

pain behavior A person's physical reaction to the conscious perception of pain.

palliative care An interdisciplinary approach to patient care to relieve suffering and improve quality of life.

palpitations Subjective feeling of heart rhythm abnormalities; perceived as a "skipping" or "thumping"; related to premature cardiac beats.

pancreatitis Inflammation of the pancreas; it may occur as an acute or chronic condition.

pancytopenia   Deficiency of all three cell lines of the blood: white blood cells, red blood cells, and platelets.

PaO$_2$ Partial pressure of oxygen in the arterial blood.

paraplegia   Injury to the thoracolumbar region of the spine, causing loss of motor function in the lower extremities.

paresthesias   Abnormal sensations, such as burning or tingling of the skin, often occurring during stroke recovery.

parietal cells   A fundic gland that secretes hydrochloric acid for pH regulation and intrinsic factor for vitamin B$_{12}$ absorption.

parietal pleura   The moist membrane that adheres to the thoracic walls, diaphragm, and mediastinum.

paroxysmal nocturnal dyspnea (PND)   A symptom usually associated with transient pulmonary edema secondary to heart failure; patient awakens from sleep with severe orthopnea.

partial pressure   Pressure each gas exerts in a total volume of gases.

partial-thickness wound   Injury to the epidermis and part of the dermis.

partially compensated   A state in which the pH is abnormal but the body buffers and regulatory mechanisms have started to respond to the imbalance.

passive acquired immunity   A temporary immunity acquired through transfer of antibodies from one individual to another or from some other source to an individual. Examples include breast feeding (antibodies transferred to baby through milk) and gamma globulin (antibodies transferred through injection).

pathogens   Disease-producing microorganisms.

peak inspiratory pressure (PIP)   Amount of pressure required to deliver a volume of gas.

penetrating trauma   The result of the transmission of energy from a moving object into the body tissue as the object disrupts the integrity of the skin and the underlying structures.

penumbra   An ischemic zone of viable, threatened tissue surrounding the brain infarct.

pepsinogen   An enzyme secreted by chief cells; converts to its active form of pepsin for protein digestion.

percutaneous coronary intervention (PCI)   The use of angioplasty balloons and coronary stents to alleviate stenoses of arteries and reestablish blood flow to ischemic myocardium.

perfusion   The pumping or flow of blood into tissues and organs.

perfusionist   A specially trained technician who controls the cardiopulmonary bypass machine during coronary artery bypass surgery.

pericardiocentesis   Pericardial drainage in the operating room.

pericardium   Tough fibrous covering surrounding the outside of the heart that helps maintain the heart in position and contributes to its structure; also called epicardium.

peripheral nerve block (PNB)   A pain management procedure that involves injecting a local anesthetic at the origin of the pain.

peripheral sensitization   Maintenance of pain intensity or persistent noxious stimulation, causing cell damage and release of additional chemical mediators; results in expansion of the number of involved nociceptors, with pain developing over a larger area.

peripheral stimulation   Pain stimulus that is delivered more distally in extremities and is important in the differentiation between hemispheric conditions and spinal cord injury.

peritoneum   Serous membrane that lines the abdominal cavity and abdominal organs.

persistent vegetative state (PVS)   A specific type of coma in which the patient continues to maintain the arousal component of consciousness but not awareness.

Peyer's patches   Lymph tissue on the outer wall of the intestine.

pH   Represents free hydrogen ion concentration.

phagocytosis   An important innate immune response whereby invading foreign materials or injured cells are ingested and destroyed by phagocytic cells, such as neutrophils, macrophages, or NK cells.

pharmacologic multimodal analgesia   Addition of nonopioid and adjuvant therapies to further enhance the effects of opioid therapy and reduce side effects by decreasing the amount of opioids needed to achieve analgesia.

phlebostatic axis   An imaginary point determined by the intersection of two lines; 4th intercostal space midpoint between the anterior and posterior diameter; this is the correct level for positioning transducers used for hemodynamic monitoring.

phospholipase A   A lipolytic pancreatic enzyme, activated by either bile salts or trypsin; contributes to the development of pulmonary complications (acute respiratory distress syndrome [ARDS]) by decreasing surfactant in the lungs.

physical dependence   A physical adaptation of the body to the presence of opioids, existing when rapid drug withdrawal produces signs and symptoms.

plateau phase   Part of the repolarization when the calcium channels open to allow movement of calcium into the cell to help maintain the cell in a depolarized state.

platelet activating factor (PAF)   A potent proinflammatory phospholipid mediator whose inappropriate activation results in inflammatory disease states.

platelet factor 4   A protein located in the platelet alpha granules.

platelet plug   A rapid-onset hemostatic function of platelets in which the platelets aggregate and adhere to each other at the site of a vessel injury to form a temporary seal and facilitate clot formation.

pleural effusion   Abnormal accumulation of fluid in the intrapleural space.

pleural infusion   A pain management route in which a catheter is inserted between the parietal and visceral pleura; often used when the patient has fractured ribs.

pleural rub   Adventitious breath sound caused by inflammation of the pleural membrane.

pleurisy   Pain caused by inflammation of the parietal pleura.

pleuritis   See *pleurisy.*

pluripotential hematopoietic stem cells (PHSC)   Stem cells produced in the bone marrow that have the potential to become erythrocytes, leukocytes, or thrombocytes.

pneumonectomy   Surgical procedure that removes one entire lung.

pneumothorax   Abnormal presence of air in the intrapleural space.

poikilothermia   Loss of internal temperature control whereby the patient assumes the temperature of the environment.

polarized   Negatively charged.

polycythemia   Abnormally elevated red blood cell mass.

polycythemia vera (PV)   An acquired form of primary polycythemia: a rare clonal myeloproliferative disease involving the pluripotential hematopoietic stem cells.

polydipsia   Excessive thirst.

polymorphonuclear   The presence of multiple nuclei in a cell (e.g., segmented neutrophils).

polypharmacy   The use of multiple medications, increasing the potential for drug interactions, metabolic changes, and cognitive changes that could lead to the misinterpretation of new disease onset.

polyuria   Excessive urination.

positive end-expiratory pressure (PEEP) Provides pressure at the end of expiration, to prevent alveolar collapse.

prealbumin A transport protein that binds retinol-binding protein and thyroxin, a thyroid hormone.

prerenal kidney injury resulting from an absolute decrease in effective blood volume (e.g., hemorrhage, severe dehydration), relative decrease in blood volume (e.g., relative hypovolemia from vasodilation and peripheral pooling that causes an ineffective blood volume), or arterial occlusion.

preload The degree of stretch in myocardial fibers at the end of diastole.

pressure gradient Difference between the partial pressures of a gas; influences rate of diffusion.

pressure support ventilation (PSV) A type of mechanical ventilatory support in which a preset level of positive pressure augments the inspiratory effort required to attain a tidal volume, thereby decreasing the work of breathing.

pressure-regulated volume-controlled (PRVC) A dual mode of mechanical ventilation where the pressure support is adjusted breath to breath to deliver a set tidal volume.

priapism Persistent penile erection produced by reflex activity.

primary injury Occurs when neurons sustain direct injury at the moment of impact.

primary intention Method of wound closure using sutures or tape.

primary response The initial humoral response to antigen exposure.

Prinzmetal's angina See *variant angina*.

progressive care unit (PCU) Also referred to as an intermediate care unit (IMC).

proliferative phase Phase of wound healing that lasts for several weeks after injury; wound is restored with a functional barrier.

propofol Primarily used as an anesthetic to decrease level of consciousness and to produce amnesia during procedures.

proprioception The ability to determine spatial position; knowing where the body or a body part is positioned in space.

protein-calorie malnutrition An undernutrition problem involving insufficient protein and calories.

proteolytic Facilitating the breakdown of proteins.

pseudocyst A combination of pancreatic enzymes, necrotic tissue, and possible blood that is enclosed by pancreatic or adjacent tissues.

pulmonary artery diastolic (PAD) pressure Reflects diastolic filling pressure in the left ventricle.

pulmonary artery pressure (PAP) normally reflects both right and left heart pressures and is read as a systolic and diastolic pressure.

pulmonary artery systolic (PAS) pressure Pressure generated by the right ventricle during systole.

pulmonary artery wedge pressure (PAWP) Pressure obtained when the inflated balloon wedges in a small branch of the pulmonary artery, reflecting pressures from the left heart.

pulmonary embolism Blockage of a pulmonary vessel caused by lodging of a thromboembolism or other bloodborne material.

pulmonary gas exchange The process that involves the intake of oxygen from the external environment into the internal environment and is carried out by ventilation, diffusion, and perfusion.

pulmonary shunt (true shunt or physiologic shunt) The percentage of cardiac output that flows from the right heart and back into the left heart without undergoing pulmonary gas exchange or without achieving normal levels of PaO_2 because of abnormal alveolar functioning.

pulmonary vascular resistance (PVR) Afterload of the right ventricle; the resistance the right ventricle must overcome to open the pulmonic valve and eject the stroke volume into the pulmonary artery.

pulse oximetry Noninvasive technique for monitoring arterial capillary hemoglobin saturation.

pulse pressure Difference between diastolic and systolic pulse pressure.

pulsus alternans Alternating weak and strong pulses.

pulsus paradoxus Exaggerated decrease (greater than 10 mmHg) in systolic blood pressure during inspiration.

Purkinje fibers Special conductive fibers that carry electrical impulses directly to ventricular muscle cells.

pus A thin liquid residue that is an important indicator of inflammation.

quadriplegia Injury to cervical or thoracic regions of the spinal cord that may result in impaired function of the arms, trunk, legs, and pelvic organs; also known as tetraplegia.

race Human biological variation.

receptive aphasia The inability to understand written or spoken words.

refeeding syndrome (RFS) A nutritional complication associated with reinitiating nutritional support in a significantly malnourished person, characterized by electrolyte imbalances.

reflexes Rapid, involuntary, predictable motor responses to a stimulus.

refractory hypoxemia Hypoxemia that is not significantly affected by administration of increasing levels of oxygen.

regurgitation Backward blood flow through the chambers of the heart.

relative refractory period The period after an action potential when a stimulus can produce a second action potential if the stimulus is greater than the threshold level.

remodeling/maturation phase Final wound repair process; lasts up to 2 years; final product is the scar.

repolarization Return of the cellular membrane to its resting membrane potential; should result in cardiac muscle relaxation.

respiration The process by which the body's cells are supplied with oxygen and carbon dioxide is eliminated from the body; also refers to breathing, the movement of air in and out of the lungs.

respiratory insufficiency A state of pulmonary compensation in which a normal blood pH is maintained only at the expense of the cardiopulmonary system.

respiratory quotient (RQ) A ratio of carbon dioxide ($\dot{V}CO_2$) to oxygen consumed ($\dot{V}O_2$) provides information about fuel composition used by the body; $\dot{V}CO_2$ and $\dot{V}O_2$ are obtained from an indirect calorimetry study.

resting membrane potential Point at the end of repolarization when the membrane is relatively permeable to potassium but is almost impermeable to sodium; thus, intracellular concentration of potassium is greater than extracellular concentration.

restrictive cardiomyopathy Condition associated with a stiff noncompliant left ventricle that fills inadequately during diastole.

restrictive disorders Pulmonary disorders associated with a decrease in lung volume.

reticular activating system (RAS) A pathway of neurons and neuronal connections for transmission of sensory stimuli from the lower brainstem to the cerebral cortex; the anatomic basis of the arousal component of consciousness.

reticulocytes   Immature RBCs.

reticuloendothelial system   A group of cells found throughout the body that are capable of ingesting particles; cells include macrophages, reticular cells, and other tissue macrophages.

retroperitoneal bleeding   Bleeding from the abdominal cavity below the peritoneum.

rhinorrhea   The drainage of cerebral spinal fluid through the nose; indicates possible tear in the meninges.

rhonchi   Adventitious breath sounds associated with an accumulation of fluid or secretions in the larger airways.

right atrial pressure (RAP)   A measure of the pressure in the right ventricle at end diastole; represents right ventricular preload.

R **on** *T* **phenomenon**   A potentially life-threatening dysrhythmia.

right ventricular (RV) pressure (or RVP)   Measured as a systolic and diastolic pressure; systolic pressure represents the pressure necessary to exceed the pressure in the pulmonary artery (RV afterload), open the pulmonary valve, and eject blood into the pulmonary circulation; right end-diastolic pressure directly reflects the preload status of the right ventricle and should approximate the RAP.

SaO₂   A direct measure of arterial blood oxygen saturation.

schistocytes   RBC fragmentation.

secondary injury   Injury that occurs in response to a primary (direct) injury; involves complex biochemical processes that occur within minutes of a primary injury and can last for days to weeks.

secondary intention   Method of wound closure in which the wound is allowed to heal gradually, using the biological phases of wound healing to fill in a cavity or defect.

secondary response   The humoral response to subsequent exposures to the same antigen; immune response is heightened, and antibody formation is triggered more quickly than in the primary response.

secretin   A hormone present in the small bowel mucosa that stimulates sodium bicarbonate secretion by the pancreas and bile secretion by the liver; decreases gastrointestinal peristalsis and motility.

sedation   A state of drowsiness and clouding of mental activity that may be accompanied by impaired reasoning ability.

segmentectomy   Surgical procedure that removes a portion of a lobe of the lung.

segmented cells (segs)   Mature neutrophils.

seizure activity   A complication of traumatic brain injury.

sensory perceptual alterations   The amount, character, or intensity of stimuli that exceeds the person's minimum or maximum threshold of tolerance for sensory input; accompanied by a diminished, exaggerated, distorted, or impaired response.

sepsis   A pathologic state in which microorganisms, or their toxins, are present in the bloodstream; syndrome of systemic inflammation in response to infection; a subcategory of systemic inflammatory response syndrome (SIRS).

septic encephalopathy   Generalized brain dysfunction marked by varying degrees of impairment of speech, cognition, orientation, and arousal that is associated with systemic inflammatory response syndrome or septicemia.

seroconversion   Stage in which sufficient antibodies develop against a virus to be measurable in the blood.

serosa   Outermost layer of the GI wall.

severe acute respiratory syndrome (SARS)   An atypical pneumonia caused by a novel form of coronavirus called SARS-CoV.

sharp debridement   Removal of necrotic areas in wounds using scissors or a scalpel.

shearing   Structures sliding in opposite directions causing a tearing or degloving type of injury.

shock   A syndrome; a complex of signs and symptoms that describe a sequence of changes that occur when tissue oxygen supply does not meet oxygen demand.

shunting   The state in which pulmonary capillary perfusion is normal but alveolar ventilation is lacking.

shuntlike effect   Effect created by an excess of perfusion in relation to alveolar ventilation.

sigh   Intermittent hyperinflation of the lungs.

sinusoids   A type of blood vessel that serves as a location and conduit for oxygen-rich blood from the hepatic artery and the nutrient-rich blood from the portal vein.

slough   Moist, stringy, thick, yellow tissue that is dying.

sodium–potassium pump (Na⁺/K⁺ pump)   An active transport ion gradient mechanism that maintains intracellular sodium and potassium homeostasis.

soft palate   Includes the uvula and rises as a reflex to close off the oropharynx.

somatic pain   Occurs when nerves from skin, subcutaneous tissue, bones, muscle, and blood vessels are activated.

spastic paralysis   Damage to upper motor neurons resulting in the inability to carry out a skilled movement.

spinal shock   The absence of all reflex activity, flaccidity, and loss of sensation below the level of the injury.

spiral CT scan   A specialized computerized axial tomography scan (CT scan) that continuously moves the patient through the scan quickly; provides greater visualization of blood vessels.

spirituality   A sense of faith and transcendence.

splanchnic circulation   The combination of the portal venous and arterial circulatory systems of the viscera; blood flow through the gut, spleen, pancreas, and liver.

SpO₂   The saturation of oxygen when measured using pulse oximetry.

spontaneous breaths   Breaths that use the patient's own respiratory effort and mechanics.

stable angina   Chest pain that is predictable and relieved with rest or nitrates.

stabs (bands)   A commonly used alternative name for immature neutrophils.

status asthmaticus   A life-threatening emergency of acute airway obstruction that does not respond to usual therapy.

status epilepticus   Continuous seizure activity without a pause— that is, without an intervening period of normal brain function; a life-threatening emergency.

stenosis   Valve leaflets fuse together and cannot fully open or close.

stridor   A type of wheeze heard loudest over the neck, suggesting obstruction of the trachea or larynx.

stroke   A brain attack; an acute neurologic deficit that occurs when impaired blood flow to a localized area of the brain results in injury to brain tissue.

stroke volume (SV)   The volume of blood pumped with each heartbeat.

subarachnoid hemorrhage (SAH)   Accumulation of blood between the arachnoid layer of the meninges and the brain.

subdermal burn (deep full-thickness burn)   Burn that destroys all layers of the skin and may include injury to muscle, tendons, or bone.

sublingual capnometry A simple, noninvasive technology that provides immediate measures of partial pressure of sublingual carbon dioxide (PslCO$_2$).

subdural hematoma (SDH) Accumulation of blood between the dura and arachnoid layers of the meninges.

submucosa Layer of the GI wall that contains blood and lymphatic vessels.

summation gallop S3 and S4 heart sounds are present; indicative of severe heart failure.

superficial burn Burn that destroys the epidermis only.

superficial partial-thickness burn Burn that destroys the epidermis and superficial layer of the dermis.

supranormal period The period after an action potential during which a stimulus that is slightly less than normal can precipitate another action potential.

surfactant A lipoprotein produced by type II alveolar cells that reduces the surface tension of the alveolar fluid lining.

susceptible host A patient who has some degree of local or systemic impairment of resistance to bacterial invasion.

synapse The space or junction between nerve fibers that contains neurotransmitters (presynaptic end) and receptors (postsynaptic end) and permits a nerve fiber (axon) to pass an impulse or signal to another neuron.

synchronous intermittent mandatory ventilation (SIMV) A mechanical ventilator mode that allows the patient to breathe spontaneously through ventilator circuitry while interspersing mandatory mechanical breaths at even intervals via a preset rate. The mandatory breaths are synchronized to the patient's own breathing cycle.

syncope Temporary loss of consciousness followed by complete, spontaneous recovery.

syndrome of inappropriate antidiuretic hormone (SIADH) The retention of water due to the excessive secretion of antidiuretic hormone (ADH); characterized by the production of small amounts of concentrated urine with an associated decrease in serum sodium.

syngraft See *isograft*.

systemic vascular resistance (SVR) Afterload of left ventricle; the resistance the left ventricle must overcome to open the aortic valve and eject the stroke volume into the aorta.

systole The contraction of a heart chamber, whereby blood is ejected into either an adjacent ventricle (atrial systole) or the pulmonary artery or aorta (ventricular systole).

systolic dysfunction Heart failure characterized by ejection fraction less than 40 percent.

T lymphocytes (T cells) Lymphocytes primarily responsible for direct attack and destruction of invading antigens and for primary cell-mediated immunity.

tachycardia Heart rate greater than 100 bpm.

target organ damage Dysfunction that occurs in organs affected by high blood pressure.

tensile forces Forces that cause tissues to stretch or extend.

tentorium cerebelli An extension of the dura mater.

terminal weaning The intentional removal of the mechanical ventilator when the patient is expected to die without it.

tertiary intention Method of wound closure in which a combination of primary and secondary intention is used.

tetraplegia Injury to cervical or thoracic regions of the spinal cord that may result in impaired function of the arms, trunk, legs, and pelvic organs; also known as quadriplegia.

third-spacing Shift of fluid from the intravascular compartment to a third-space (transcellular space), usually a serous cavity.

thirst The awareness of the desire to drink.

thrombocytes Platelets.

thrombocytopenia An abnormally low platelet count.

thymus Organ in the mediastinum primarily responsible for differentiating lymphocytes into various types of T cells for cell-mediated immunity.

tidal volume (TV or VT) The volume of air moved into and out of the lungs during one normal breath. It is also an important setting on a mechanical ventilator; if set too high the patient is hyperventilated, and if set too low the patient is hypoventilated.

tissue typing Identification of the HLA antigens of both the donor and the recipient.

tolerance A decrease in effectiveness or diminishing side effects for the same dose that had previously been effective or caused the side effects.

tongue The muscle responsible for mixing the food with saliva during chewing, forming the food into a bolus (mass); assists with licking and swallowing.

tonicity Osmolarity of an intravenous fluid.

total lymphocyte count (TLC) An easily obtained indicator of overall immune status and adequacy of protein.

total parenteral nutrition (TPN) A nutritionally complete, IV-delivered solution composed of protein, carbohydrate, fat, electrolytes, vitamins, and trace elements; TPN with a glucose concentration of greater than 10 percent is administered through a central vein.

tracheomalacia Weakening or erosion of the tracheal cartilage.

transfer anxiety Anxiety experienced by the individual who is moved from a familiar, somewhat secure environment to an environment that is unfamiliar.

transferrin A plasma protein that binds with and transports iron to cells.

transient ischemic attacks (TIAs) Episodes of focal neurologic deficits that usually resolve in a few minutes or hours.

traumatic brain injury (TBI) Injury that results from any mechanical disruption of brain tissue from an impact or injury to the head.

traumatic injury Injury caused by kinetic injury.

trigeminy A cardiac dysrhythmia of two normal *QRS* complexes followed by one premature ventricular contraction.

troponin A protein found in cardiac muscle; when present in the blood, it is used as a marker of myocardial cell death.

Trousseau sign A blood pressure cuff is inflated on the upper arm to a level directly above the patient's systolic blood pressure for 2 minutes; a positive sign is present when the hand flexes (carpopedal spasm) in response to the test.

true shunt Flow of blood from the right heart, through the lungs, and on into the left heart without taking part in alveolar–capillary diffusion or oxygen exchange.

tumor necrosis factor (TNF) A cytokine involved programmed cell death.

tunneling Narrow passageway created by the separation of, or destruction to, fascial planes.

type I (allergic) hypersensitivity response A hypersensitivity immune response that involves an interaction between IgE and mast cells; its systemic form is anaphylaxis.

type II (cytotoxic) hypersensitivity response A hypersensitivity immune response; IgM and IgG react directly with cell-surface antigens, injuring or destroying targeted cells.

type III (immune complex-mediated) hypersensitivity response   A hypersensitivity immune response involving antigen–antibody complexes with IgG and IgM; complexes are deposited vessel walls or tissues causing an inflammatory response.

type IV (cell-mediated) hypersensitivity response   A delayed hypersensitivity immune response involving tissue injury by direct T-cell attack in the absence of antibody activity.

uncompensated   An acid–base state in which the pH is abnormal because other buffer and regulatory mechanisms have not begun to correct the imbalance.

unconjugated bilirubin   Fat-soluble bilirubin that has not yet joined with glucuronic acid.

undermining   Can be likened to a cliff without tissue underneath it. The undermined space is usually broader than a tunnel.

undernutrition   A state of malnutrition that arises when the body's minimum nutritional requirements of carbohydrates, proteins, lipids, and other essential nutrients are not met.

unifocal   Premature contractions originating from one ectopic pacemaker.

unstable angina   Chest pain that is not predictable and that occurs with rest or with minimal activity.

unstable spinal injury   An injury to two or more of the spinal columns; vertebral and ligamentous structures are unable to support and protect the injured area.

urea   A nitrogen substance produced by the liver from ammonia.

urobilinogen   Bilirubin in the urine.

valvular prolapse   An abnormal condition in which a heart valve (almost always the mitral) cusps balloon (bulge) up into the atrium during ventricular systole.

variant angina   Chest pain that is not predictable, may occur at night, and is caused by coronary artery spasm; also known as Prinzmetal's angina.

vascular thrombosis   A blood clot in the vasculature of the graft.

venous admixture   The effect that a physiologic shunt has on the oxygen content of the blood as it drains into the left heart.

ventilation   The gross movement of air into and out of the lungs; airflow between the atmosphere and alveoli.

ventilatory failure   A condition caused by alveolar hypoventilation; clinically, it is called acute respiratory acidosis.

ventricles   Chambers that contain cerebral spinal fluid (CSF).

ventricular gallop   S3 heart sound caused by decreased ventricular compliance.

ventricular response   Impulses that pass through the AV node triggering ventricular depolarization and contraction.

ventricular stroke work index (VSWI)   Amount of work involved in moving blood in the ventricle with each heartbeat.

villi   Fingerlike projections covering intestinal folds.

visceral pain   Involves the internal organs or body cavity linings such as chest (lungs or heart) and abdomen, bladder or intestinal distention, or organ metastasis.

visceral pleura   The moist membrane that adheres to the lung parenchyma and is adjacent to the parietal pleura.

vital capacity (VC)   The volume of air that can be exhaled after maximum inhalation; an indication of respiratory muscle strength; normal is 65 to 75 mL/kg.

volatile acids   Acids that can convert to a gas form for excretion.

$\dot{V}/\dot{Q}$ ratio   A ratio expressing the relationship of ventilation to perfusion.

wedge resection   Surgical procedure that removes a wedge-shaped section of the peripheral portion of the lung.

Wernicke's (receptive) aphasia   Inability to understand written or spoken words.

wheeze   Adventitious breath sound caused by air passing through constricted airways.

wound conversion (wound progression)   The spontaneous progression of a burn wound into deeper tissue after the initial burn insult.

wound infection   The multiplication of microorganisms that invade body tissues.

xanthomas   Cholesterol-filled lesions commonly seen around the eyes.

xenograft   Biological dressings or grafts obtained from animals; also referred to as heterografts.

zone of coagulation   The innermost zone of a thermal burn, an area of immediately nonviable tissue.

zone of hyperemia   The zone of a thermal burn surrounding the central zone; can easily convert to nonviable tissue (wound conversion) if blood flow is not adequately restored.

zone of stasis   The outermost zone of a thermal burn; blanches with pressure and heals in 7 to 10 days as long as the tissue is perfused.

Abbreviations

2,3-DPG	2,3-diphosphoglycerate
5-FU	5-Fluorouracil
5′-N	5′-nucleotidase
α_1	Alpha$_1$
A	Alveolar ventilation
AA	Abdominal aorta
AAA	Abdominal aortic aneurysm
AAA	Aromatic amino acid
AACN	American Association of Critical Care Nurses
AAPHN	American Academy of Hospice and Palliative Medicine
ABCDE	Awakening and Breathing Coordination, Delirium monitoring/management, and Early exercise/mobility
ABCs	Airway, breathing, and circulation
ABG	Arterial blood gas
ABLS	Advanced Burn Life Support
ABO	Refers to the A, B, and O blood types
a–c	Alveolar–capillary
AC	Alternating current
AC	Assist-control
ACC	American College of Cardiology
ACCM	American College of Critical Care Medicine
ACE	Angiotensin-converting enzyme
ACh	Acetylcholine
ACLS	Advanced cardiac life support
ACS	Abdominal compartment syndrome
ACS	Acute coronary syndromes
ACTH	Adrenocorticotropic hormone
AD	Autonomic dysreflexia
ADD	Acute Aortic Dissection Diagnostic (Risk Score)
ADH	Antidiuretic hormone
ADL	Activities of daily living
ADP	Adenosine diphosphate
ADR	Adverse drug reaction
AED	Automatic external defibrillator
AFib	Atrial fibrillation
AFL	Atrial flutter
AFP	Alpha-fetoprotein
AHA	American Heart Association
AHCPR	Agency for Health Care Policy and Research
AHF	Acute hepatic failure
AI	Anemia of inflammation
AI	Aortic insufficiency
AICD	Automatic implantable cardioverter-defibrillator
AIDS	Acquired immune deficiency syndrome
AIHA	Autoimmune-induced hemolytic anemia
AIS	Acute ischemic stroke
AIS	ASIA Impairment Scale
AKI	Acute kidney injury
ALF	Acute liver failure
ALG	Antilymphocyte globulin
ALI	Acute lung injury syndrome
Alk phos	(ALP) Alkaline phosphatase; previously SGOT
ALL	Acute lymphocytic leukemia
ALP	Alk phos; alkaline phosphatase
ALT	Amino alanine aminotransferase (SGPT)
ALTRA	All-trans-retinoic acid
AMI	Acute myocardial infarction
AML	Acute myelogenous (myelocytic) leukemia
AMSN	Academy of Medical-Surgical Nurses
ANA	American Nurses Association
ANA	Antinuclear antibody
ANC	Absolute neutrophil count
AND	Allow natural death
ANF	Atrial natriuretic factor
ANP	Atrial natriuretic peptide
ANS	Autonomic nervous system
AP	Anteroposterior
AP	Acute pancreatitis
APC	Activated protein C
APC	Antigen-presenting cell
APP	Abdominal perfusion pressure
APRV	Airway pressure release ventilation
APS	American Pain Society
aPTT	Activated partial thromboplastin time
APWCA	American Professional Wound Care Association
AR	Aortic regurgitation
ARB	Angiotensin receptor blocker; angiotensin II receptor blocker
ARDS	Acute respiratory distress syndrome
ARF	Acute respiratory failure
ARS	Adjective Rating Scale
ART	Antiretroviral therapy
AS	Aortic stenosis
ASA	Acetylsalicylic acid (aspirin)
ASA	American Society of Anesthesiologists
ASCVD	Atherosclerotic cardiovascular disease

ASIA	American Spinal Injury Association		**CAD**	Coronary artery disease
ASPEN	American Society for Parenteral and Enteral Nutrition		**CAM**	Confusion Assessment Method
ASPM	American Society for Pain Management Nursing		**CAM-ICU**	Confusion Assessment Method for the ICU
AST	Aspartate aminotransferase (*or* SGOT)		**cAMP**	Cyclic AMP
ATC	Around the clock		**CaO$_2$**	Oxygen content of arterial blood
ATG	Antithymocyte globulin		**CAP**	Community-acquired pneumonia
ATLS	Advanced Trauma Life Support		**CAPC**	Center to Advance Palliative Care
ATN	Acute tubular necrosis		**CAPM**	Continuous airway pressure monitoring
ATP	Adenosine triphosphate		**CARS**	Compensatory anti-inflammatory response syndrome
AV	Atrioventricular		**CAT**	Complementary and alternative therapies
AV block	Atrioventricular block		**CAUTI**	Catheter-associated urinary tract infection
AVAPS	Average volume-assured pressure support		**CAVH**	Continuous arterial venous hemofiltration
AVF	Acute ventilatory failure		**CBC**	Complete blood count
AVM	Arteriovenous malformation		**CBF**	Cerebral blood flow
AVP	Arginine vasopressin		**CBT**	Cognitive behavioral therapy
AVPU	Alert–AZT Azidothymidine		**CBV**	Cerebral blood volume
β$_1$	beta$_1$		**CCB**	Calcium channel blocker
B cells	Bursa cells		**CCK**	Cholecystokinin
BAC	Blood alcohol concentration		**CCO**	Continuous cardiac output
BAL	Bronchoalveolar lavage		**CCSC**	Canadian Cardiology Society Classification
BB	Beta blocker		**CD**	Clusters of differentiation
BBB	Blood–brain barrier		**CDC**	Centers for Disease Control & Prevention
BBB	Bundle branch block		**CEA**	Carcinoembryonic antigen
BCAA	Branched-chain amino acid		**CEO$_2$**	Cerebral oxygen extraction
BCMA	Barcode medication administration		**CFU**	Colony-forming units
BCR	Bulbocavernosus reflex		**CHD**	Coronary heart disease
BCR-ABL	Breakpoint cluster region-Abelson (oncogene)		**CHI**	Closed-head injury
BD	Base deficit		**CI**	Cardiac index
BDNF	Brain-derived neurotrophic factor		**CI**	Confidence interval
BE	Base excess		**CIC**	Clean intermittent catheterization
BG	Blood glucose		**CIM**	Critical illness myopathy
BISAP	Bedside Index of Severity in Acute Pancreatitis		**CIP**	Critical illness polyneuropathy
BMI	Body mass index		**CIRCI**	Critical illness–related corticosteroid insufficiency
BMS	Bare-metal stents		**CISD**	Critical incident stress debriefing
BMZ	Basement membrane zone		**CK**	Creatine kinase
BNP	Brain natriuretic peptide		**CKD**	Chronic kidney disease
BNP	B-type natriuretic peptide		**CKF**	Chronic kidney failure
BPM	Beats per minute		**CK-MB**	Creatine kinase–myocardial bands
BPM	Breaths per minute		**Cl**	Chloride
BPOC	Barcode point-of-care		**CL**	Lung compliance, expressed in cm H_2O/mL
BPS	Behavioral Pain Scale		**CLABSI**	Central line–associated bloodstream infection
BSA	Body surface area		**CLL**	Chronic lymphocytic leukemia
BUN	Blood urea nitrogen		**CLRT**	Continuous lateral rotation therapy
BVM	Bag-valve-mask		**cm H_2O**	Centimeters of water pressure
C	Celsius		**CML**	Chronic myelogenous (myelocytic) leukemia
C	Cervical vertebrae (C1–C7)		**CMO**	Comfort measures only
Ca	Calcium		**CMS**	Centers for Medicare & Medicaid Services
CABG	Coronary artery bypass graft		**CMV**	Controlled mandatory ventilation
CAC	Coronary artery calcium		**CMV**	Cytomegalovirus
			CN	Cranial nerve

CNPI	Checklist of Nonverbal Pain Indicators	**DC**	Direct current
CNS	Central nervous system	**DCD**	Donation after cardiac death
CO	Carbon monoxide	**DDAVP**	Desmopressin acetate
CO	Cardiac output	**DES**	Drug-eluting stents
CO$_2$	Carbon dioxide	**DI**	Diabetes insipidus
COPD	Chronic obstructive pulmonary disease	**DIC**	Disseminated intravascular coagulation
CoV	Coronavirus	**DKA**	Diabetic ketoacidosis
CP	Chronic pancreatitis	**DM**	Diabetes mellitus
CPAP	Continuous positive airway pressure	**DMG**	Donor management goal
CPB	Cardiopulmonary bypass	**DNA**	Deoxyribonucleic acid
CPK	Creatine phosphokinase	**DNI**	Do not intubate
CPOE	Computerized provider order entry	**DNR**	Do not resuscitate
CPOT	Critical Care Pain Observation Tool	**DO$_2$**	Oxygen delivery
CPP	Cerebral perfusion pressure	**DPPHR**	Duodenum-preserving pancreatic head resection
CPP	Coronary perfusion pressure	**DVT**	Deep vein thrombosis
CPR	Cardiopulmonary resuscitation	**EBL**	Estimated blood loss
Cr	Creatinine	**EBP**	Evidence-based practice
CrCl	Creatinine clearance	**EBV**	Epstein-Barr virus
CRF	Chronic renal failure	**ECF**	Enterocutaneous fistula
CRH	Corticotropin-releasing hormone	**ECF**	Extracellular fluid
CRNA	Certified registered nurse	**ECF-A**	Eosinophil chemotactic factor of anaphylaxis
CRP	C-reactive protein	**ECG**	Electrocardiogram
CRRT	Continuous renal replacement therapy	**ECMO**	Extracorporeal membrane oxygenation
CRS	Catheter-related sepsis, cytokine-release syndrome	**EDH**	Epidural hematoma
CRT	Cardiac resynchronization therapy	**EEG**	Electroencephalogram
CSF	Cerebrospinal fluid	**EEG**	Electroencephalography
CSI	Cervical spine injury	**EF**	Ejection fraction
CSICU	Cardiac surgical ICU	**EGD**	Esophagogastroduodenoscopy
CSW	Cerebral salt wasting	**EGDT**	Early goal-directed therapy
CT	Computed tomography	**ELISA**	Enzyme-linked immunosorbent assay
CTA	CT angiogram; CT angiography	**EMS**	Emergency medical services
CTD	Cognitive Test for Delirium	**EN**	Enteral nutrition
CTH	CT of the head	**EPAP**	Expiratory positive airway pressure
cTn	Cardiac troponin	**EPO**	Erythropoietin
cTnI	Cardiac troponin-I	**EPS**	Electrophysiology study
cTnT	Cardiac troponin-T	**ERCP**	Endoscopic retrograde cholangiopancreatography
CTSI	Computed tomography severity index	**ERV**	Expiratory reserve volume of lungs
CVA	Cerebrovascular accident	**ESR**	Erythrocyte sedimentation rate
CVC	Central venous catheter	**ESRD**	End-stage renal disease
CVD	Cardiovascular disease	**EST**	Endoscopic sphincterotomy
CvO$_2$	Oxygen content of venous blood	**EST**	Exercise stress test
CVP	Central venous pressure	**ET**	Endotracheal
CVVH	Continuous venovenous hemofiltration	**ET-1**	Endothelin-1
CVVH-D	Continuous venovenous hemofiltration dialysis	**EtCO$_2$**	End tidal carbon dioxide
CVVHDF	Continuous venovenous hemodiafiltration	**ETOH**	Ethanol (alcohol)
CyA	Cyclosporine (or CsA)	**EUS**	Endoscopic ultrasound
DAI	Diffuse axonal injury	**EVAR**	Endovascular aneurysm repair
DASH	Dietary approaches to stop hypertension	**EVD**	External ventricular drain
dBA	Decibel	**f**	Frequency, rate of breathing
DBP	Diastolic blood pressure	**f**	Respiratory force

f	Respiratory rate expressed in breaths per minute
FAST	Focused assessment with sonography in trauma
FDP	Fibrin degradation product
FeNa	Fractional excretion of sodium
FEV	Forced expiratory volume
FEV_1	Forced expiratory volume in 1 second
FFA	Free fatty acid
FFP	Fresh-frozen plasma
FG	Fournier gangrene
FH	Familial hypercholesterolemia
FHF	Fulminant hepatic failure
FiO_2	Fraction of inspired oxygen
FLIE	Functional Living Index Emesis
FPDR	Family presence during resuscitation
FPS-R	FACES Pain Scale Revised
FRC	Functional residual capacity
FSP	Fibrin split products
ft	Foot (measurement)
FTc	Corrected flow time
FVC	Forced vital capacity
FVD	Fluid volume deficit
FVE	Fluid volume excess
GALT	Gut-associated lymphoid tissue
GAS	Group A beta-hemolytic streptococci
GCS	Glasgow Coma Scale
GCS	Graduated compression stocking
G-CSF	Granulocyte-colony stimulating factor
g/dL	Grams per deciliter
GDS	Geriatric Depression Scale
GERD	Gastroesophageal reflux disease
GFR	Glomerular filtration rate
GGT	Gamma glutamyl transferase
GGT	Γ-glutamyltranspeptidase
GH	Growth hormone
GI	Gastrointestinal
GIP	Gastric inhibitory peptide
g/kg	Gram per kilogram
GLN	Glutamine
GM-CSF	Granulocyte- macrophage colony-stimulating factor
GP	Glycoprotein
GRV	Gastric residual volume
GSW	Gunshot wound
GU	Genitourinary
H^+	Hydrogen ion
H_2	Histamine
H_2CO_3	Carbonic acid
H_2O	Water
H_2RA	Histamine-2 receptor antagonist
HAAS	Hypoglycemia-associated autonomic failure
HAP	Hospital-acquired (nosocomial) pneumonia
HAPU	Hospital-acquired pressure ulcer
HAV	Hepatitis A virus
Hb (Hgb)	Hemoglobin
Hb A	Hemoglobin A; adult hemoglobin
Hb A_{1c}	Glycosylated hemoglobin
Hb F	Hemoglobin F; fetal hemoglobin
HbO_2	Oxyhemoglobin
HBOT	Hyperbaric oxygen therapy
Hb S	Hemoglobin S; sickle hemoglobin
HBsAg	Hepatitis B surface antigen
HBV	Hepatitis B virus
HCAP	Healthcare-associated pneumonia
HCO_3	Bicarbonate
HCP	Healthcare provider
Hct	Hematocrit
HCV	Hepatitis C virus
HDL	High-density lipoprotein
HDL-C	High-density lipoprotein cholesterol
HDV	Hepatitis D virus
HE	Hepatic encephalopathy
HEV	Hepatitis E virus
HF	Heart failure
HFNC	High-flow nasal cannula
HFV	High-frequency ventilation
HFOV	High-frequency oscillating ventilation
HFPV	High-frequency percussive ventilator
Hgb (Hb)	Hemoglobin
HgbCO	Hemoglobin saturated with carbon monoxide
$HgbO_2$	Oxyhemoglobin
HHNC	Hyperglycemic hyperosmolar nonketotic coma
HHNKS	Hyperglycemic hyperosmolar nonketotic syndrome; now known as HHS
HHS	Hyperglycemic hyperosmolar state
HIPAA	Health Insurance Portability and Accountability Act
HIT	Heparin-induced thrombocytopenia
HIV	Human immunodeficiency virus
HIV/AIDS	Human immunodeficiency virus/acquired immunodeficiency disease syndrome
HLA	Human leukocyte antigen
HLA DR	Human leukocyte antigen DR
HO	Heterotopic ossification
HOB	Head of bed
HPNA	Hospice and Palliative Nurses Association
HR	Heart rate
HRS	Hepatorenal syndrome
HSCT	Hematopoietic stem-cell transplantation
HSV	Herpes simplex virus
HTLV	Human T cell lymphotropic virus
HTLV-1	Human T cell leukemia virus type I
IABP	Intra-aortic balloon pump

IAH	Intra-abdominal hypertension		K	Potassium
IAP	Increased abdominal pressure		kcal	Kilocalorie
IBD	Inflammatory bowel disease		kg	Kilogram
IBW	Ideal body weight		KIM-1	Kidney injury molecule-1
ICD	Implantable cardioverter-defibrillator		KODA	Kentucky Organ Donor Affiliates
ICDSC	Intensive Care Delirium Screening Checklist		L	Lumbar vertebrae (L1–L5)
ICF	Intracellular fluid		LA	Left atrium
ICG	Impedance cardiography		LAD	Left anterior descending artery
ICH	Intracerebral hematoma		LCX	Left circumflex artery
ICH	Intracranial hemorrhage		LDH	Lactic dehydrogenase
ICP	Intracranial pressure		LDL	Low-density lipoprotein
ICU	Intensive care unit		LDL-C	Low-density lipoprotein cholesterol
ICUAW	Intensive care unit acquired weakness		LES	Lower esophageal sphincter
ICU-LOS	Intensive care unit length of stay		LFT	Liver function test
IDDM	Insulin-dependent diabetes mellitus		LGIB	Lower GI bleed
IE	Infective endocarditis		LGL	Large granulated lymphocytes (NK cells)
I:E	inspiratory-to-expiratory (ratio)		LIMA	Left internal mammary artery
IF, IFN	Intrinsic factor		LMCA	Left main coronary artery
Ig	Immunoglobulin		L/min	Liters per minute
IgG	Immunoglobulin G		LMN	Lower motor neuron
IgM	Immunoglobulin M		LMWH	Low molecular weight heparin
IHD	Intermittent hemodialysis		LOC	Level of consciousness
IHI	Institute of Health Improvement		LOS	Length of stay
IIT	Intensive insulin therapy		LP	Lumbar puncture
IK-18	Interleukin-18		LPM	Liters per minute
IL	Interleukin		LR	Lactated Ringer's
IL-6	Interleukin-6		LRINEC	Laboratory risk indicator for necrotizing fasciitis
IM	Intramuscular		LST	Life-sustaining therapy
IMC	Intermediate-care unit		LTVV	Low tidal volume ventilation
INF	Interferon		LV	Left ventricle
iNO	Nitric oxide		LVAD	Left ventricular assist device
INR	International normalized ratio		LVD	Left ventricular dysfunction
INV-2	Rhodes Index of Nausea and Vomiting		LVEDP	Left ventricular end diastolic pressure
IOM	Institute of Medicine		LVSWI	Left ventricular stroke work index
IPAP	Inspiratory positive airway pressure		$M_{\dot{V}}$	Minute ventilation; also $\dot{V}_E$
IPPB	Intermittent positive pressure breathing		mAb	Monoclonal antibody
IR	Immediate release		MABP	Mean arterial blood pressure (or MAP)
IRI	Ischemia reperfusion injury		MAC	*Mycobacterium avium-intracellulare* complex
IRV	Inspiratory reserve volume		MALT	Mucosa associated lymphoid tissue
ISNCSCI	International Standards for Neurological Classification of Spinal Cord x Injury		MANE	Morrow Assessment of Nausea and Emesis
ISP	Intraspinal pressure		MAP	Mean arterial pressure
ISS	Injury Severity Score		MAPS	Multidimensional Affect and Pain Survey
ITP	Immunologic thrombocytopenic purpura		MARS	Mixed antagonistic response syndrome
IV	Intravenous		MARS	Molecular adsorbent recirculating system
IVC	Intraventricular catheter		MB	Myocardial band
IVIG	Intravenous immunoglobulin		MCAs	Middle cerebral arteries
J	Joules		mcg	Micrograms
JG	Juxtaglomerular		MCH	Mean corpuscular hemoglobin
JVD	Jugular venous distention, jugular vein distention		MCHC	Mean corpuscular hemoglobin concentration
			mcL	Microliter

mcm	Micrometer
MCV	Mean corpuscular volume
MDF	Myocardial depressant factor
MDI	Metered-dose inhaler
MDMA	Ecstasy (3,4-methylenedioxymethamphetamine)
MDT	Maggot debridement therapy
mEq/L	Milliequivalents per liter
MERS	Middle East Respiratory Syndrome
Mg	Magnesium
mg/dL	Milligram/deciliter
MHC	Major histocompatibility complex
MHD	Maintenance hemodialysis
MI	Myocardial infarction
MIDCAB	Minimally invasive direct coronary artery bypass
MIND	Modifying the Incidence of Delirium
MIP	Maximum inspiratory pressure
mL	Milliliter
MMF	Mycophenolate mofetil
mmHg	Millimeters of mercury
mmoL	Millimoles per liter
MMR	Measles, mumps, and rubella
MMV	Mandatory minute ventilation
MODS	Multiple organ dysfunction syndrome
MOF	Multiple organ failure
MOLST	Medical Orders for Life-Sustaining Treatment
mOsm	Milliosmole
MOsm/L	Milliosmoles per liter
MPI	Myocardial perfusion imaging
MPQ	McGill Pain Questionnaire
MPV	Microprocessor ventilator
MR	Mitral valve regurgitation
MRA	Magnetic resonance angiography
MRCP	Magnetic resonance cholangiopancreatography
MRI	Magnetic resonance imaging
MRSA	Methicillin-resistant *Staphylococcus aureus*
MS	Mitral stenosis
MSB	Maximal sterile barrier
MSSA	Methicillin-susceptible *S. aureus*
mTBI	Mild traumatic brain injury
MTH	Mild therapeutic hypothermia
mU/dL	Milliliter/deciliter
MUGA	Multigated angiographic scan
MVC	Motor vehicle crash
N_2O	Nitrous oxide
Na	Sodium
Na^+/K^+	Sodium/potassium ions
NAC	N-acetylcysteine
NAD^+	Nicotinic acid dehydrogenase
$NaHCO_3$	Sodium bicarbonate
NANDA	North American Nursing Diagnosis Association

NASW	National Association of Social Workers
N-BNP	N-terminal pro-BNP
NCF	Neutrophil chemotactic factor
NCP	National Consensus Project for Quality Palliative Care
NF	Necrotizing fasciitis
NG	Nasogastric
NGAL	Neutrophil gelatinase-associate lipocalin
NGT	Nasogastric tube
NHPCO	National Hospice and Palliative Care Organization
NICHE	Nurses Improving Care for Healthsystem Elders
NIDDM	Non-insulin-dependent diabetes mellitus
NIF	Negative inspiratory force
NIPPV	Noninvasive intermittent positive pressure ventilation
NIRS	Near-infrared spectroscopy
NK	Natural killer
NKF	National Kidney Foundation
NMB	Neuromuscular blockade
NMBA	Neuromuscular blocking agent
NNRTI	Non-nucleoside reverse transcriptase inhibitors
NO	Nitrous oxide
NODAT	New-onset diabetes after transplant
NP	Nurse practitioner
NPCRC	National Palliative Care Research Center
NPO	Nothing by mouth
NPPV	Noninvasive positive pressure ventilation
NPUAP	National Pressure Ulcer Advisory Panel
NPWT	Negative pressure wound therapy
NQF/AHRC	National Quality Forum/Agency for Healthcare Research and Quality
NRS	Numeric Rating Scale
NRTI	Nucleoside and nucleotide reverse transcriptase inhibitors
NS	Nervous system
NS	Normal saline
NSAID	Nonsteroidal anti-inflammatory drug
NSR	Normal sinus rhythm
NSTEMI	Non-ST elevation myocardial infarction
NSTI	Necrotizing soft-tissue infection
NTIS	Nonthyroid-illness syndrome
NYHA	New York Heart Association
O_2	Oxygen
OCT	Ornithine carbamoyl transferase
O_2ER	Oxygen extraction ratio
OLT	Orthotopic liver transplant
OPC	Organ procurement coordinator
OPCAB	Off-pump coronary artery bypassing
OPO	Organ procurement organization
OPTN	Organ Procurement and Transplantation Network

OR	Operating room
ORT	Opioid Risk Tool
OSA	Obstructive sleep apnea
OSR	Open surgical repair
OT	Occupational therapist
OTC	Over-the-counter (nonprescription)
P	Pancreaticoduodenectomy
$P_{0.1}$	Airway Occlusion Pressure
PA	Pulmonary artery
PA	Mean airway pressure
PAC	Premature atrial contraction
PAC	Pulmonary artery catheter
P_ACO_2	Partial pressure of alveolar carbon dioxide in the alveoli
$PaCO_2$	Partial pressure of dissolved carbon dioxide in the plasma of arterial blood
PAD	Peripheral artery disease
PAD	Pulmonary artery diastolic
PAF	Platelet activating factor
PAG	Periaqueductal gray
PAIN-AD	Pain Assessment in Advanced Dementia Scale
PaO_2	Partial pressure of oxygen in the arterial blood
P_AO_2	Partial pressure of oxygen in the alveoli
PAOP	Pulmonary artery occlusion pressure
PAP	Peak airway pressure; proximal airway pressure
PAP	Pulmonary artery pressure
PAR	Pressure-adjusted heart rate
PAS	Pulmonary artery systolic
PAV+	Proportional assist ventilation plus
PAWP	Pulmonary artery wedge pressure
$PbtO_2$	Brain tissue oxygen partial pressure
PC	Potential complication
PCA	Patient-controlled analgesia
PCAs	Posterior cerebral arteries
PCD	Pneumatic compression device
PDE3	Phosphodiesterase
PCEA	Patient-controlled epidural analgesia
PCI	Percutaneous coronary intervention
PCO_2	Partial pressure of carbon dioxide
PCP	*Pneumocystis carinii* pneumonia
PCR	Polymerase chain reaction
PCS	Postconcussion syndrome
PCU	Progressive care unit
PCWP	Pulmonary capillary wedge pressure
PD	Peritoneal dialysis
PDA	Personal digital assistant
PDA	Posterior descending artery
P_{dias}	Diastolic BP
PE	Pulmonary embolism
PEA	Pulseless electrical activity

PEEP	Positive end–expiratory pressure
PEP	Postexposure prophylactic
PET	Positron emission tomography
$PETCO_2$	Partial pressure of end-tidal carbon dioxide
P/F	PaO_2/FiO_2 ratio
PF	PaO_2/FiO_2
PF4	Platelet activating factor 4
PFT	Pulmonary function test/testing
pH	Free hydrogen ion concentration
Ph1	Philadelphia chromosome
pHi	Intestinal mucosal pH
PHSC	Pluripotential hematopoietic stem cell
PI	Protease inhibitor
PICC	Peripherally inserted central catheter
PICS	Post intensive care syndrome
PIM	Potentially inappropriate medication
P_{Imax}	Maximum inspiratory pressure
PIP	Peak inspiratory pressure
PIP	Performance improvement and patient safety
PJP	*Pneumocystis jiroveci* pneumonia
PLISSIT	Permission, Limited Information, Specific Suggestions, and Intensive Therapy
pLVAD	Percutaneous left ventricular assist device
PMBV	Percutaneous mitral balloon valvuloplasty
PMI	Point of maximal impulse
PMN	Polymorphonuclear neutrophil
PMV	Prolonged mechanical ventilation
PN	Parenteral nutrition
PND	Paroxysmal nocturnal dyspnea
PNS	Parasympathetic nervous system
PNS	Peripheral nervous system
PO	Oral route
PO_2	Partial pressure of oxygen or oxygen tension, expressed in mmHg
PO_4	Phosphate
POD	Postoperative days
POLST	Provider/Physician Orders for Life Sustaining Treatment
POSS	Pasero Opioid-Induced Sedation Scale
P_{Peak}	Peak airway pressure
PPI	Proton pump inhibitor
PPV	Positive pressure ventilation
PR	Peripheral resistance
PRA	Preformed antibody
PRN	As needed
PRVC	Pressure-regulated volume-controlled
PS	Pressure support
PSA	Prostate-specific antigen
PSI	Pneumonia Severity Index
psi	Pounds per square inch
$pslCO_2$	Sublingual carbon dioxide

PSV	Pressure support ventilation	RR	Respiratory rate
P_{sys}	Systolic BP	RRT	Rapid response team
PT	Physical therapist	RRT	Renal replacement therapy
PT	Prothrombin time	rSO_2	Regional tissue oxygen saturation
PTA	Plasma thromboplastin antecedent	r-tPA	Recombinant tissue plasminogen activator
PTC	Plasma thromboplastin component	RUQ	Right upper quadrant
PTCA	Percutaneous transluminal coronary angioplasty	RUSH	Rapid Ultrasound for Shock and Hypotension
$PtCO_2$	Partial pressure of CO_2	RV	Residual volume of lungs
PTFE	Polytetrafluoroethylene	RV	Right ventricle
PTH	Parathyroid hormone	RVEDP	Right ventricular end diastolic pressure
PTSD	Post-traumatic stress disorder	RVEDV	Right ventricular end diastolic volume
PTT	Partial thromboplastin time	RVEF	Right ventricular ejection fraction
PTU	Propylthiouracil	RVP	Right ventricular pressure
PUD	Peptic ulcer disease	RVSWI	Right ventricular stroke work index
PUSH	Pressure Ulcer Scale for Healing	RYB	red-yellow-black (RYB) system
PVC	Premature ventricular contraction	SA node	Sinoatrial node
$PvCO_2$	Partial pressure of carbon dioxide in the venous blood	SAH	Subarachnoid hemorrhage
PVD	Peripheral vascular disease	SaO_2	Oxygen saturation of arterial blood
PvO_2	Partial pressure of oxygen in the venous blood	SARS	Severe acute respiratory syndrome
PVR	Pulmonary vascular resistance	SAS	Sedation-Agitation Scale
PVRI	Pulmonary vascular resistance index	SAT	Spontaneous Awakening Trials
PVS	Persistent vegetative state	SB	Sinus bradycardia
Q	Perfusion	SBP	Systolic blood pressure
$\dot{Q}$	Perfusion	SBT	Spontaneous Breathing Trials
QOL	Quality of life	SCAP	Severe Community Acquired Pneumonia (score)
Qs/Qt	Intrapulmonary shunt	SCC	Spinal cord compression
RA	Right atrium	SCCM	Society of Critical Care Medicine
RAAS	Renin-angiotensin-aldosterone system	SCD	Sequential compression devices
RAP	Right atrial pressure	SCI	Spinal cord injury
RASS	Richmond Agitation-Sedation Scale	SCID	Severe combined immune deficiencies
R_{aw}	Airway resistance	SCI-IDS	Spinal Cord Injury-Induced Immune Depression Syndrome
RBC	Red blood cell	SCPP	Spinal cord perfusion pressure
RCA	Right coronary artery	SCUF	Slow continuous ultrafiltration
RCT	Randomized controlled trial	$ScvO_2$	Central venous oxygen saturation
RDOS	Respiratory Distress Observation Scale	SDH	Subdural hematoma
RDW	Red blood cell distribution width	sDTI	Suspected deep-tissue injury
REALM	Rapid Estimate of Adult Literacy in Medicine	SE	Side effect
REE	Resting energy expenditure	SEPs	Somatosensory-evoked potentials
REM	Rapid eye movement	SF-MPQ	Short-form McGill Pain Questionnaire
RFS	Refeeding syndrome	SG	Specific gravity
rhTM	Recombinant human soluble thrombomodulin	SGA	Subjective Global Assessment of Nutritional Status
RIFLE	Risk, Injury, Failure, Loss, End-stage kidney disease	SGOT	Serum glutamic oxaloacetic transaminase (*or* AST)
RIMA	Right internal mammary artery	SGPT	Serum glutamic pyruvic transaminase (ALT)
RLE	Right lower extremity	SHR	Stress hyperglycemia ratio
RN	Registered nurse	SIADH	Syndrome of inappropriate antidiuretic hormone
RNA	Ribonucleic acid	SICU	Surgical intensive care unit
ROM	Range of motion	SIMI	Stress-induced mucosal injury
RQ	Respiratory quotient	SIMV	Synchronous intermittent mandatory ventilation
RR	Relative risk	SIRS	Systemic inflammatory response syndrome

SjO$_2$	Jugular venous oximetry		TJC	The Joint Commission
SLE	Systemic lupus erythematosus		TLC	Total lung capacity
SLP	Speech and language pathologist		TLC	Total lymphocyte count
SmvO$_2$	Mixed venous oxygen saturation (Mixed SvO$_2$)		TLS	Tumor lysis syndrome
SNS	Sympathetic nervous system		TMP-SMX	Trimethoprim-sulfamethoxazole
SOAPP	Screener and Opioid Assessment for Patients with Pain		TNF	Tumor necrosis factor
			TNFα	Tumor-necrosis factor alpha
SOFA	Sequential Organ Failure Assessment		TOF	Train of four
SPA	Sensory perceptual alteration		tPA	Tissue plasminogen activator
SPECT	Single photon emission computed tomography		TPN	Total parenteral nutrition
SpO$_2$	Saturation of arterial capillary hemoglobin determined by pulse oximetry		TRA	Thrombopoietin receptor agonist
			TRALI	Transfusion-related acute lung injury
SQ	Subcutaneous		TRH	Thyrotropin-regulating hormone
SRMD	Stress-related mucosal disease		T$_S$ cell	T suppressor cell
ST	Sinus tachycardia		TSH	Thyroid-stimulating hormone
S/T	Spontaneous-timed		TTE	Transthoracic echocardiography
STD	Sexually transmitted disease		TTP/HUS	Thrombotic thrombocytopenic purpura/hemolytic uremic syndrome
STEMI	*ST* segment elevation myocardial infarction			
StO$_2$	Tissue oxygen saturation		TV	Tidal volume
STSG	Split-thickness skin graft		UA	Unstable angina
SV	Spontaneous ventilation		UAGA	Uniform Anatomical Gift Act
SV	Stroke volume		UAP	Unlicensed assistive personnel
SVC	Superior vena cava		UDDA	Uniform Determination of Death Act
SVG	Saphenous vein graft		UGIB	Upper GI bleed
SVI	Stroke volume index		UH	Unfractionated heparin
SvO$_2$	Mixed venous oxygen saturation		UMN	Upper motor neuron
SVR	Systemic vascular resistance		UNOS	United Network for Organ Sharing
SVRI	Systemic vascular resistance index		UO	Urine output
SVT	Supraventricular tachycardia		US	Ultrasound
SVV	Stroke volume variance		UTI	Urinary tract infection
T	Thoracic vertebrae (T1–T12)		UUN	Urine urea nitrogen
TBGH	Traumatic basal ganglia hemorrhage		V	Ventilation
TBI	Total body irradiation		V̇	Ventilation
TBI	Traumatic brain injury		V̇$_A$	Alveolar ventilation
TBSA	Total body surface area		VA ECMO	Veno-arterial extra-corporeal membrane oxygenation
T$_C$	T cytotoxic		VAC	Vacuum-assisted closure
TCA	Tricyclic antidepressant		VAD	Ventricular assist device
TCD	Transcranial Doppler		VAE	Venous air embolism
TCOM	Transcutaneous oxygen measurement		VAE	Ventilator-associated event
TE	Tracheoesophagealx		VAI	Vertebral artery injury
TECAB	Total endoscopic coronary artery bypass		VAP	Ventilator-associated pneumonia
TEE	Transesophageal echocardiogram		VAS	Visual Analog Scale
TEE	Transesophageal echocardiography		VATS	Video-assisted thoracoscopic surgery
TENS	Transcutaneous electrical nerve stimulation		VC	Vital capacity
TF	Tissue factor		V̇CO$_2$	Carbon dioxide produced
T$_H$ cells	Helper T cells		VDS	Verbal Descriptor Scale
TH	Induced or therapeutic hypothermia		V̇$_E$	Minute ventilation; also M$_{V̇}$
TIA	Transient ischemic attack		VFib	Ventricular fibrillation
TICU	Trauma intensive care unit		VILI	Ventilator-induced lung injury
TIPS	Transjugular intrahepatic portosystemic shunt		V̇O$_2$	Oxygen consumption

$\dot{V}/\dot{Q}$ **ratio**	Ventilation to perfusion ratio	**VT**	Ventricular tachycardia
VRE	Vancomycin-resistant *Enterococci*; vancomycin-resistant *Enterococcus*	**VTE**	Venous thromboembolism
		WBC	White blood cell
VSW	Ventricular stroke work	**WHO**	World Health Organization
VSWI	Ventricular stroke work index	**WOCN**	Wound Ostomy Continence Nurses (Society)
V_T	Tidal volume		

Index

Note: Page numbers with *f* indicate figures; those with *t* indicate tables.